Clinical Magnetic Resonance Imaging

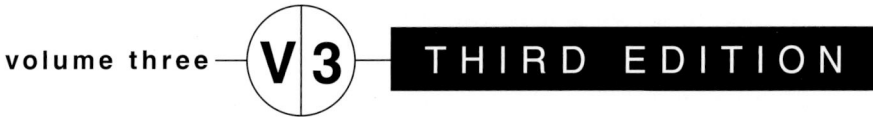

volume three — V3 — THIRD EDITION

EDITED BY

ROBERT R EDELMAN, MD
Professor of Radiology, Feinberg School of Medicine, Northwestern University;
William B and Catherine Graham Chairman of Radiology, Department of
Radiology, Evanston Northwestern Healthcare, Evanston, Illinois, USA

JOHN R HESSELINK, MD FACR
Professor of Radiology and Neurosciences, University of California, San Diego
School of Medicine; Chief of Neuroradiology, Vice Chair of Clinical and Academic
Affairs, Department of Radiology, San Diego Medical Center, San Diego,
California, USA

MICHAEL B ZLATKIN, MD FRCP(C)
President, National Musculoskeletal Imaging Inc., Weston, Florida; Voluntary Professor
of Radiology, University of Miami School of Medicine, Miami, Florida, USA

JOHN V CRUES III, MD
Medical Director, RadNet Management, Inc. (Primedex Health Systems, Inc.);
MRI Fellowship Director, Beverly Radiology Medical Group, Los Angeles;
Volunteer Clinical Professor of Radiology, University of California San Diego,
San Diego, California, USA

SAUNDERS

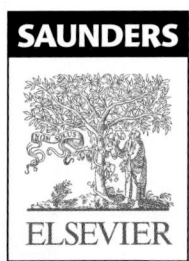

ELSEVIER

SAUNDERS
ELSEVIER

1600 John F. Kennedy Blvd.
Ste 1800
Philadelphia, PA 19103-2899

CLINICAL MAGNETIC RESONANCE IMAGING

Vol I: 9-9960-1949-7
Vol II: 9-9960-1955-1
Vol III: 9-9960-1961-6
ISBN-13: 978-0-7216-0306-3
ISBN: 0-7216-0306-8
e-dition: 1-4160-3081-6

Copyright © 2006, Elsevier Inc.

Notice

Knowledge and best practice in this field are constantly changing. As new research and experience broaden our knowledge, changes in practice, treatment and drug therapy may become necessary or appropriate. Readers are advised to check the most current information provided (i) on procedures featured or (ii) by the manufacturer of each product to be administered, to verify the recommended dose or formula, the method and duration of administration, and contraindications. It is the responsibility of the practitioner, relying on their own experience and knowledge of the patient, to make diagnoses, to determine dosages and the best treatment for each individual patient, and to take all appropriate safety precautions. To the fullest extent of the law, neither the Publisher nor the Editors assumes any liability for any injury and/or damage to persons or property arising out or related to any use of the material contained in this book.

First Edition 1990. Second Edition 1996

Library of Congress Cataloging-in-Publication Data

Clinical magnetic resonance imaging/ [edited by] Robert R. Edelman… [et al.].—3rd ed.
   p. ; cm.
     Includes bibliographical references and index.
     ISBN 0-7216-0306-8
1. Magnetic resonance imaging.   I. Edelman, Robert R.
     [DNLM: 1. Magnetic Resonance Imaging –methods. WN 185 C641 2006]
     RC78.7.N83C56 2006
616.07'548—dc22   2005047246

Acquisitions Editor: Allan Ross
Developmental Editor: Ann Ruzycka Anderson
Book Designer: Ellen Zanolle

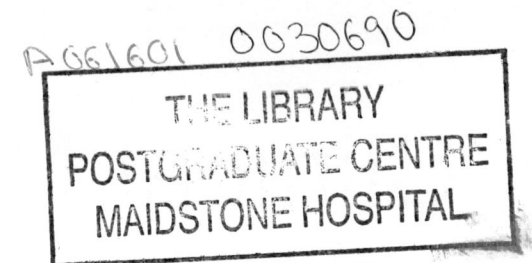
Printed in China

Last digit is the print number : 9 8 7 6 5 4 3 2 1

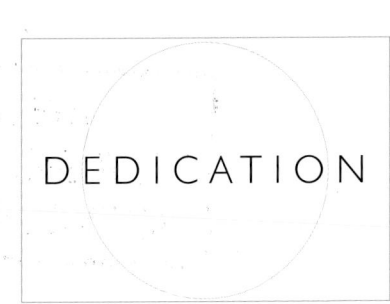

DEDICATION

To my wife, Melissa, and children Daniel, Laura, Amanda, and Alexis, for their love and bemused tolerance of my many foibles, and to Dr Sven Paulin, for his guidance and unwavering support during the formative stages of my career.

RRE

To my wife, Kay, my son, André, and his wife, Sara.

JRH

To my wife, Marilyn, and my children, Nancy, Robert, Alyssa, and Chad. Thank you for your support, patience, and understanding while I toiled on this book.

MBZ

To my wife, Maribeth, without whose support and patience my involvement in this book would have been impossible.

JVC

LIST OF CONTRIBUTORS

Essam Abou-Bieh MSc
Department of Radiology, Urology and Nephrology
Center, Mansoura University, Mansoura, Egypt

David Alsop PhD
Associate Professor, Department of Radiology,
Beth Israel Deaconess Medical Center, and Harvard
Medical School, Boston, Massachusetts, USA

Charles M Anderson MD PhD
Associate Professor of Radiology, University of
California, San Francisco; Chief of MRI, San Francisco
Veterans Administration Medical Center, San Francisco,
California, USA

Evan Appelbaum MD
Department of Medicine, Cardiovascular Division,
Beth Israel Deaconess Medical Center and Harvard
Medical School, Boston, Massachusetts, USA

Vincent J Argiro PhD
Founder and Chief Technology Officer, Vital Images Inc.,
Minnetonka, Minnesota, USA

Manohar Aribandi MD
Academic Chief of Neuroradiology; Associate,
Department of Radiology, Geisinger Medical Center,
Danville, Pennsylvania, USA

Susan M Ascher MD
Director, Division of Abdominal Imaging, Professor,
Department of Radiology, Georgetown University
Medical Center, Washington DC, USA

Laila Ashkar MD FRCPC
Fellow, Magnetic Resonance Imaging, McGill University
Health Center, Montreal, Quebec, Canada

Mark H Awh MD
President, Radsource, Brentwood, Tennessee, USA

Till R Bader MD
Associate Professor of Radiology, Department of
Radiology, Medical University Vienna, Vienna, Austria

Behnam Badie MD
Associate Professor, Department of Neurosurgery,
University of Wisconsin Hospital and Clinics, Madison,
Wisconsin, USA

William S Ball MD
Professor of Biomedical Engineering, Radiology and
Pediatrics; Attending Neuroradiologist,Department of
Radiology and Medical Imaging, Children's Hospital
Medical Center, University of Cincinnati, Cincinnati,
Ohio, USA

Roland Bammer PhD
Assistant Professor of Radiology, Lucas MRS/I Center,
Stanford University, Stanford, California, USA

Jelle O Barentsz MD PhD
Professor, Department of Radiology, Universitair
Medisch Centrum, St Radboud, Nijmegen,
The Netherlands

James A Barkovich MD
Professor of Radiology, Neurology, Pediatrics and
Neurological Surgery, University of California
San Francisco School of Medicine, San Francisco,
California, USA

Ahmed Ba-Ssalamah MD
Associate Professor of Radiology, Department of
Radiology, University of Vienna, Vienna, Austria

Peter J Basser PhD
Senior Investigator, National Institutes of Health,
Bethesda, Maryland, USA

Carlos Bazan III MD
Clinical Professor of Radiology, Director of
Neuroradiology, Department of Radiology, University
of Texas Health Science Center at San Antonio,
San Antonio, Texas, USA

Ricardo J Becerra
MR Chief Engineer, Diagnostic Imaging, GE Healthcare,
Waukesha, Wisconsin, USA

Roland Bejm RT(R)(MR)
Assistant Manager, Department of Radiology, Evanston
Northwestern Healthcare, Evanston, Illinois, USA

Javier Beltran MD FACR
Chairman, Department of Radiology, Maimonides
Medical Center; Clinical Professor of Radiology,
Mount Sinai School of Medicine; Director of Medical
Education, Franklin and Seidelmann, Inc., Virtual
Subspecialty Radiologists, New York, New York, USA

Rita G Bhatia MBBS MD
Assistant Professor of Clinical Radiology, Department of Radiology, University of Miami School of Medicine, Miami, Florida, USA

George S Bisset III MD
Vice-Chairman, Department of Radiology, Duke University Medical Center, Durham, North Carolina, USA

Chris Boesch MD PhD
Professor, Department of Clinical Research (MR Spectroscopy and Methodology), University of Bern, Bern, Switzerland

Eddy B Boskamp PhD
Applied Science Lab, GE Healthcare, Waukesha, Wisconsin, USA

René M Botnar PhD
Department of Medicine, Cardiovascular Division, Beth Israel Deaconess Medical Center and Harvard Medical School, Boston, Massachusetts, USA

Robert D Boutin MD
Vice President, Musculoskeletal Radiology, Med-Tel International, Davis, California, USA

Bryan C Bowen MD PhD
Professor, Departments of Radiology, Neurology and Neurological Surgery, University of Miami, Miami, Florida, USA

Barton F Branstetter IV MD
Assistant Professor of Radiology and Otolaryngology, Director of Head and Neck Imaging, Associate Director of Radiology Informatics, Departments of Radiology and Otolaryngology, University of Pittsburgh School of Medicine, Pittsburgh, Pennsylvania, USA

Richard A Bronen MD
Professor of Diagnostic Radiology and Neurosurgery, Department of Diagnostic Radiology, Yale University School of Medicine, New Haven, Connecticut, USA

Gregory G Brown PhD
Chief Psychology Service, SDVAHS; Professor of Psychiatry and Cognitive Science, University of California, San Diego; Co-Director Laboratory of Cognitive Imaging, La Jolla, California, USA

Jeffrey J Brown MD FACR
Professor of Radiology, Mallinckrodt Institute of Radiology, Washington University School of Medicine, St. Louis, Missouri, USA

Michele Brown MD
Assistant Professor of Radiology, Department of Radiology, University of California San Diego Medical Center, San Diego, California, USA

James A Brunberg MD MHSA
Professor and Chair, Department of Radiology, University of California Davis Medical Center, Sacramento, California, USA

Deborah Burstein PhD
Associate Professor of Radiology at Harvard Medical School, Beth Israel Deaconess Medical Center, Boston, Massachusetts, USA

Richard B Buxton PhD
Professor of Radiology, Director, Center for Functional MRI, Department of Radiology, University of California San Diego, La Jolla, California, USA

Julie Bykowski MD
Stroke Diagnostics and Therapeutics Section, Stroke Branch, NINDS, NIH, Bethesda, Maryland, USA

Peter Caravan PhD
Principal Scientist, EPIX Pharmaceuticals, Cambridge, Massachusetts, USA

John A Carrino MD MPH
Assistant Professor of Radiology, Harvard Medical School; Clinical Director, Magnetic Resonance Therapy Program, Co-Director, Spine Intervention Service, Brigham and Women's Hospital, Department of Radiology, Boston, Massachusetts, USA

Timothy J Carroll PhD
Biomedical Engineering and Radiology, Northwestern University, Chicago, Illinois, USA

M Allison Cato PhD
MIRECC Fellow, Psychology Service, VASDHS; Laboratory of Cognitive Imaging, La Jolla, California, USA

Kim M Cecil PhD
Research Associate Professor of Radiology, Pediatrics and Neuroscience; Senior MR Spectroscopist, Imaging Research Center, Department of Radiology and Medical Imaging, Children's Hospital Medical Center, University of Cincinnati, Cincinnati, Ohio, USA

Sridhar R Charagundla MD PhD
Assistant Professor, Department of Radiology, University of Pennsylvania Medical Center, Philadelphia, Pennsylvania, USA

Oliver S Chen MD
Clinical Assistant Professor, Department of Radiology, New York University Medical Center, New York, New York, USA

Neeraj B Chepuri MD
Neuroradiology Section, Consulting Radiologists Ltd., Abbott Northwestern Hospital, Minneapolis, Minnesota, USA

Daisy Chien PhD
Director, Cardiac MR Research and Development, Cedars-Sinai Medical Center, Los Angeles, California, USA

Brian W Chong MD FRCP(C)
Professor of Radiology, Mayo Clinic Scottsdale, Scottsdale, Arizona, USA

Christine B Chung MD
Associate Professor of Radiology, Department of
Radiology, University of California, San Diego; Director,
Radiology Research, VA Healthcare System, La Jolla,
San Diego, California, USA

Alessandro Cianfoni MD
Clinical MRI Fellow, Department of Radiology, University
of California San Diego, San Diego, California, USA

Paul D Clifford MD
Chief, Musculoskeletal Section, Department of
Radiology, University of Miami School of Medicine,
Miami, Florida, USA

Fergus V Coakley MD
Associate Professor and Chief, Abdominal Imaging,
Department of Radiology, University of California
San Francisco, San Francisco, California, USA

Steven M Cohen MD
RadNet Management, Inc., (Primedex Health Systems,
Inc.); Beverly Radiology Medical Group, Los Angeles,
California, USA

Patrick M Colletti MD
Professor of Radiology, University of Southern California,
Keck School of Medicine, Los Angeles; Chief of MRI,
LAC-USC Imaging Science Center, Los Angeles,
California, USA

John V Crues III MD
Medical Director, RadNet Management, Inc. (Primedex
Health Systems, Inc.); MRI Fellowship Director, Beverly
Radiology Medical Group, Los Angeles; Volunteer
Clinical Professor of Radiology, University of California
San Diego, San Diego, California, USA

Terry Cunningham BS RT(MR)
Northwestern Memorial Hospital, Chicago, Illinois, USA

Oliver A Cvitanic MD
Medical Director, Southwest Oklahoma MRI,
Oklahoma City, Oklahoma, USA

Jevan Damadian BSEE
Fonar Corporation, Melville, New York, USA

Raymond V Damadian MD
Fonar Corporation, Melville, New York, USA

Peter G Danias MD PhD
Cardiac MR Center, Hygeia Hospital, Athens, Greece; Tufts
University Medical School, Boston, Massachusetts, USA

Jörg F Debatin MD MBA
Professor and Medical Director, Chief Executive
Director, University Medical Center Hamburg-
Eppendorf, Hamburg, Germany

Mony J de Leon EdD
Professor and Director, Center for Brain Health,
Department of Psychiatry, New York University Medical
Center, New York, USA

Vibhas S Deshpande PhD
Siemens Medical Solutions USA, Inc., Los Angeles,
California, USA

Rosalind B Dietrich MB ChB
Professor of Radiology, Chief of MRI, Department of
Radiology, University of California San Diego Medical
Center, San Diego, California, USA

Tomas Duby PhD
GE Magnet Engineering, GE Healthcare, Florence,
South Carolina, USA

David J Dubowitz MD PhD
Associate Professor, Center for Functional MRI,
Department of Radiology, University of California
San Diego, La Jolla, California, USA

Eugene E Dunkle RT(R)(MR)
Evanston Northwestern Healthcare Center for
Advanced Imaging, Evanston, Illinois, USA

Jay S Dworkin PhD
Fonar Corporation, Melville, New York, USA

James P Earls MD
Vice President and Medical Director, Fairfax
Radiological Consultants PC, Fairfax, Virginia;
Department of Radiology, Inova Fairfax Hospital,
Falls Church, Virginia, USA

Gregory Eckel MD MA
Assistant Clinical Professor of Radiological Sciences,
University of California, David Geffen School of
Medicine, Los Angeles; Faculty Radiologist, Department
of Radiology, Harbor-UCLA Medical Center, Torrance,
California, USA

Robert R Edelman MD
Professor of Radiology, Feinberg School of Medicine,
Northwestern University; William B and Catherine
Graham Chairman of Radiology, Department of
Radiology, Evanston Northwestern Healthcare,
Evanston, Illinois, USA

John C Egelhoff DO
Professor of Radiology and Pediatrics; Attending
Neuroradiologist, Department of Radiology and Medical
Imaging, Children's Hospital Medical Center, University
of Cincinnati, Cincinnati, Ohio, USA

Tarek A El-Diasty MD
Department of Radiology, Urology and Nephrology
Center, Mansoura University, Mansoura, Egypt

Steven Falcone MD
Assistant Professor of Clinical Radiology, Neurological
Surgery and Ophthalmology, Assistant Professor of
Clinical Radiology, Department of Radiology,
University of Miami School of Medicine, Miami, Florida,
USA

Charles Facanati BS RT(MR)
Northwestern Memorial Hospital, Chicago, Illinois, USA

Julia R Fielding MD
Associate Professor of Radiology; Chief, Abdominal Radiology, Department of Radiology, University of North Carolina at Chapel Hill, North Carolina, USA

J Paul Finn MD
Professor of Radiological Sciences; Chief, Diagnostic Cardiovascular Imaging; Director, Magnetic Resonance Research, Department of Radiology, David Geffen School of Medicine at UCLA, Los Angeles, California, USA

David N Firmin BSc PhD
Professor of Biomedical Imaging, CMR Unit, Royal Brompton Hospital/Imperial College London, London, UK

Michael Fogli MD
Fellow, Department of Internal Medicine, University of Texas Southwestern Medical Center at Dallas, Dallas, Texas, USA

Richard J Friedland MD
DRA Imaging and Vassar Brothers Medical Center, Poughkeepsie, New York, USA

Russell C Fritz MD
National Orthopedic Imaging Associates, Greenbrae, California, USA

Peter D Gatehouse BSc PhD
Research Assistant, CMR Unit, Royal Brompton Hospital, Imperial College of Science, Technology and Medicine, London, UK

Mark Gelbien MD
Fonar Corporation, Melville, New York, USA

Lindell R Gentry MD
Professor of Radiology, Neurology and Neurosurgery, Department of Radiology (E3/311), University of Wisconsin Hospital and Clinics, Madison, Wisconsin, USA

Ajax E George MD
Professor of Radiology, New York University Medical Center, New York, New York, USA

Bassem Georgy MD
Assistant Clinical Professor of Radiology, University of California San Diego Medical Center, San Diego, California, USA

Tal Geva MD
Senior Associate, Department of Cardiology; Director, Cardiac MRI Program; Children's Hospital Boston; Associate Professor of Pediatrics (Radiology), Harvard Medical School, Boston, Massachusetts, USA

Mary Gianni RT (R)(MR)
Fonar Corporation, Melville, New York, USA

James Golomb MD
Clinical Instructor, Department of Neurology, New York University Medical Center, New York, New York, USA

R Gilberto González MD PhD
Director of Neuroradiology, Massachusetts General Hospital, Professor of Radiology, Harvard Medical School, Boston, Massachusetts, USA

Charles A Green
Fonar Corporation, Melville, New York, USA

John F Greenhalgh PhD
Fonar Corporation, Melville, New York, USA

Ceylan C Guclu PhD
Diagnostic Imaging, GE Healthcare, Waukesha, Wisconsin, USA

John K Hald MD PhD
Chief, Section of Neuroradiology, Department of Radiology, Rikshospitalet, Oslo, Norway

Michael J Harsh
Engineering Manager, GE Medical Systems Global MR Engineering, Niskayuna, New York, USA

Hiroto Hatabu MD PhD
Director, Residency Program and Pulmonary Functional Imaging; Associate Professor of Radiology, Harvard Medical School; Department of Radiology, Beth Israel Deaconess Medical Center, Boston, Massachusetts, USA

Victor M Haughton MD
Professor of Radiology, Department of Radiology (E3/311), University of Wisconsin Hospital and Clinics, Madison, Wisconsin, USA

Thomas H Hauser MD
Instructor, Department of Medicine, Cardiovascular Division, Beth Israel Deaconess Medical Center and Harvard Medical School, Boston, Massachusetts, USA

Timothy J Havens PhD
GE Magnet Engineering, GE Healthcare, Florence, South Carolina, USA

John F Healy MD FACR
Professor of Radiology, Department of Neuroradiology, University of California San Diego, San Diego, California, USA

Thomas Helmberger MD PhD
Institute for Radiology, University of Lübeck, Lübeck, Germany

Roland G Henry PhD
Associate Professor of Radiology, Center for Molecular and Functional Imaging, University of California San Francisco, San Francisco, California, USA

John R Hesselink MD FACR
Professor of Radiology and Neurosciences, University of California San Diego School of Medicine; Chief of Neuroradiology, Vice Chair of Clinical and Academic Affairs, Department of Radiology, San Diego Medical Center, San Diego, California, USA

Richard J Hicks MD
Assistant Professor, Diagnostic Radiology, Tufts University School of Medicine, Boston Massachusetts; Director of MRI, Department of Radiology, Baystate Medical Center, Springfield, Massachusetts, USA

R Scott Hinks PhD
Applied Science Lab, GE Healthcare, Waukesha, Wisconsin, USA

Fredric A Hoffer MD FAAP FSIR
Pediatric and Interventional Radiologist, Division of Diagnostic Imaging, Department of Radiological Sciences, Member and Chair of the Clinical Staff, St Jude Children's Research Hospital, Memphis, Tennessee, USA

Caroline L Hollingsworth MD
Assistant Professor, Department of Radiology, Duke University Medical Center, Durham, North Carolina, USA

Andrei I Holodny MD
Associate Attending Neuroradiologist, Director of the Functional MRI Laboratory, Memorial Sloan-Kettering Cancer Center, New York; Associate Professor of Radiology, Weill Medical College of Cornell University, New York, New York, USA

Shahid M Hussain MD PhD
Chief, Section of Abdominal Imaging, Department of Radiology, Erasmus Medisch Centrum, Rotterdam, The Netherlands

Roy Irwan MSc PhD
Department of Radiology, University Medical Center Groningen, Groningen, The Netherlands

Katsuyoshi Ito MD
Department of Radiology, Yamaguchi University School of Medicine, Yamaguchi, Japan

Terry L Jernigan PhD
Clinical Research Psychologist, SDVAHS; Professor of Psychiatry and Radiology, University of California San Diego, San Diego; Co-Director, Laboratory of Cognitive Imaging, La Jolla, California, USA

Michael Jerosch-Herold PhD
Associate Professor, Departments of Cardiology and Radiology, Oregon Health and Science University, Portland, Oregon, USA

J Randy Jinkins MD FACR FEC
Senior Research Fellow, Fonar Corporation, Melville, New York, USA

Ferenc A Jolesz MD
B Leonard Holman Professor of Radiology, Vice Chairman for Research, Director, Division of MRI and Image Guided Therapy Program, Department of Radiology, Harvard Medical School at Brigham and Women's Hospital, Boston, Massachusetts, USA

Blaise V Jones MD
Associate Professor of Radiology and Pediatrics, Chief, Section of Pediatric Neuroradiology, Department of Radiology and Medical Imaging, Cincinnati Children's Hospital Medical Center, University of Cincinnati, Cincinnati, USA

Robert M Judd PhD
Co-Director, Duke Cardiovascular Magnetic Resonance Center, Associate Professor of Medicine and Radiology, Duke University Medical Center, Durham, North Carolina, USA

Sanjeeva P Kalva MD
Fellow, Division of Cardiovascular Imaging and Intervention, Massachusetts General Hospital, Boston, Massachusetts, USA

Spyros K Karampekios MD
Assistant Professor of Radiology, Department of Radiology, School of Medicine, University of Crete, Heraklion, Crete; Chief of Neuroradiology, Department of Radiology, University Hospital of Heraklion, Crete, Greece

Sasan Karimi MD
Assistant Professor of Radiology, Cornell University Weill Medical College, New York; Staff Neuroradiologist, Department of Radiology, Memorial Sloan-Kettering Cancer Center, New York, New York, USA

Charles W Kerber MD
Clinical Professor, Department of Radiology, University of California San Diego Medical Center, San Diego, California, USA

Claus Kiefer
Physicist (claus.kiefer@insel.ch), Department of Diagnostic and Interventional Neuroradiology, University of Bern, Bern, Switzerland

Raymond J Kim MD
Co-Director, Duke Cardiovascular Magnetic Resonance Center, Associate Professor of Medicine and Radiology, Duke University Medical Center, Durham, North Carolina, USA

Karen Kinkel MD PD
Fondation de Grangettes, Geneva, Switzerland

Kraig V Kissinger BS RT(R)(MR)
Senior MR Technologist, Cardiac MR Center, Beth Israel Deaconess Medical Center, Boston, Massachusetts, USA

Michael V Klein MD
Staff Neuroradiologist, Department of Radiology, Huntington Memorial Hospital, Pasadena, California; Former Clinical Instructor, Department of Radiology, University of California San Diego Medical Center, San Diego, California, USA

Michel Kliot MD
Associate Professor and Chief, Department of Neurosurgery, University of Washington and Puget Sound VA Health Care Center, Seattle, Washington DC, USA

Michael V Knopp MD PhD
Professor, Department of Radiology, The Ohio State University Hospitals, Columbus, Ohio, USA

Kimberly Knox
Research Associate, Department of Radiology, University of California San Diego Medical Center, San Diego, California, USA

Frank Korosec PhD
Professor of Medical Physics and Radiology, University of Wisconsin Medical School, Madison, Wisconsin, USA

Jonathan B Kruskal MD PhD
Director, Body Imaging, Beth Israel Deaconess Medical Center; Associate Professor of Radiology, Harvard Medical School, Boston, Massachusetts, USA

John Kurhanewicz PhD
Associate Professor of Radiology, Pharmaceutical Chemistry and Bioengineering, University of California San Francisco, San Francisco, California, USA

Susanne C Ladd MD
Assistant Professor of Radiology, Department of Diagnostic and Interventional Radiology and Neuroradiology, University Hospital Essen, Essen, Germany

Charles F Lanzieri MD
Professor and Chairman, Department of Radiology, Case Western Reserve University, Cleveland, Ohio, USA

Andrew C Larson PhD
Assistant Professor, Department of Radiology, Feinberg School of Medicine, Northwestern University, Chicago, Illinois, USA

Randall B Lauffer PhD
Founder, EPIX Pharmaceuticals, Cambridge, Massachusetts, USA

Meng Law MD FRACR
Assistant Professor of Radiology and Neurosurgery, Department of Radiology and Neurosurgery, New York University School of Medicine, New York, New York, USA

Martin L Lazarus MD
Associate Professor of Clinical Radiology, Feinberg School of Medicine, Northwestern University; Director, Sports Medicine Imaging; Section Chief, Musculoskeletal Radiology, Department of Radiology, Evanston Hospital, Evanston, Illinois, USA

Ralph E Lee RT(R)(MR) EdD
Manager of Clinical Marketing: MRI, Toshiba America Medical Systems, Tustin, California, USA

Robert E Lenkinski PhD
Professor of Radiology, Harvard Medical School, Head of MR Research, Department of Radiology, Beth Israel Deaconess Medical Center-East, Boston, Massachusetts, USA

Deborah Levine MD
Associate Professor of Radiology, Co-chief of Ultrasound, Beth Israel Deaconess Medical Center, Boston, Massachusetts, USA

Frank J Lexa MD
Professor, Department of Marketing; Project Faculty and Country Manager, Global Consulting Practicum, Wharton School-Graduate Division, University of Pennsylvania; Clinical Associate Professor of Radiology, University of Pennsylvania Medical Center, Philadelphia, Pennsylvania, USA

John R Leyendecker MD
Associate Professor of Radiology, Clinical Director, MRI, Department of Radiology, Wake Forest University School of Medicine, Winston-Salem, North Carolina, USA

Debiao Li PhD
Professor of Radiology and Biomedical Engineering, Director, Cardiovascular MR Research, Northwestern University, Chicago, Illinois, USA

Wei Li MD
Research Associate Professor of Radiology, Northwestern University Feinberg School of Medicine, Evanston, Illnois, USA

Alexander Lin BS
Senior Scientist, Rudi Schulte Research Institute; Director of Clinical Services, Huntington Medical Research Institutes, Pasadena, California, USA

Chunlei Liu PhD
Lucas MRS/I Center, Department of Radiology and Department of Electrical Engineering, Stanford University, Stanford, California, USA

Russell N Low MD
Department of Radiology, Sharp Memorial Hospital; Medical Director, Sharp and Children's MRI Center, San Diego, California, USA

Mahmood F Mafee MD FACR
Professor of Radiology, Chief of Head and Neck
Radiology, Department of Radiology, University of
Illinois, Chicago, Illinois, USA

Sharad Maheshwari MD MBBS
Fellow, Abdominal Imaging, McGill University Health
Center, Montreal, Quebec, Canada

Jeffrey H Maki MD PhD
Diagnostic Radiology Specialist, University of
Washington Medical Center, Veteran's Administration
Medical Center, Seattle, Washington, USA

Warren J Manning MD
Professor of Medicine, Cardiovascular Division,
Beth Israel Deaconess Medical Center, Harvard Medical
School, Boston, Massachusetts, USA

Kenneth R Maravilla MD
Professor, Director of MRI Research, Departments of
Radiology and Neurological Surgery, University of
Washington, Seattle, Washington, USA

Maria da Graca M Martin MD
Neuroradiology Research Fellow, Neuroradiologist at
the Clinics Hospital in the University of Sao Paulo,
Sao Paulo, Brazil

Thomas J Masaryk MD
Head, Section of Neuroradiology, Department of
Radiology, Cleveland Clinic Foundation, Cleveland,
Ohio, USA

Heinrich P Mattle MD
Professor, Department of Neurology, Inselspital,
University of Bern, Bern, Switzerland

Robert F Mattrey MD
Professor, Department of Radiology, University of
California San Diego School of Medicine, MRI Institute,
San Diego, California, USA

Michael P McNamara Jr MD
Associate Professor of Radiology; Chief, Breast Imaging
and Intervention, Case School of Medicine, MetroHealth
Medical Center, Cleveland, Ohio, USA

Tushar Mehta MPPM PhD
www.tushar-mehta.com, Consultants in Technology
and Workflow Productivity Integration, Rochester,
New York, USA

Michael S Middleton MD PhD
Assistant Professor of Radiology (Voluntary),
Department of Radiology, University of California,
San Diego, California, USA

Scott A Mirowitz MD
Professor and Director, MR Services, Department of
Radiology, Thomas Jefferson University Hospital,
Philadelphia, Pennsylvania, USA

Donald G Mitchell MD
Professor, Department of Radiology, Thomas Jefferson
Medical College, Philadelphia, Pennsylvania, USA

Raad H Mohiaddin MD PhD FRCR FRCP FESC
Consultant and Reader in Cardiovascular Imaging,
Royal Brompton Hospital and Imperial College of
Science, Technology and Medicine, London, UK

Chad H Moritz MD
Department of Radiology, University of Wisconsin
Hospital and Clinics, Madison, Wisconsin, USA

Elizabeth A Morris MD
Director, Breast MRI, Department of Radiology,
Memorial Sloan-Kettering Cancer Center, New York,
New York, USA

Michael E Moseley PhD
Professor of Radiology, Lucas MRS/I Center,
Department of Radiology, Stanford University Medical
Center, Stanford, California, USA

John P Mugler III PhD
Professor of Radiology and Biomedical Engineering,
Departments of Radiology, University of Virginia School
of Medicine, Charlottesville, Virginia, USA

Pratik Mukherjee MD PhD
Assistant Professor of Radiology and Bioengineering,
Attending Neuroradiologist, Diagnostic Neuroradiology,
Department of Radiology, University of California
San Francisco, San Francisco, California, USA

Asako Nakai MD
Research Fellow, Magnetic Resonance Imaging, McGill
University Health Center, Montreal, Quebec, Canada

Marvin D Nelson Jr MD MBA
Radiologist in Chief, Department of Radiology,
Children's Hospital, Los Angeles; Professor of Radiology,
University of Southern California, Keck School of
Medicine, Los Angeles, California, USA

Mizuki Nishino MD
Research Fellow, Department of Radiology, Beth Israel
Deaconess Medical Center, Harvard Medical School,
Boston, Massachusetts, USA

Jeffrey P Noonan
Diagnostic Imaging, GE Healthcare, Waukesha,
Wisconsin, USA

Alexander M Norbash MD MHCM
Professor and Chairman, Department of Radiology,
Boston University School of Medicine, Boston,
Massachusetts, USA

Niels Oesingmann PhD
MR Research and Development, Siemens Medical
Solutions USA, Inc., Malvern, Pennsylvania; Center for
Biomedical Imaging, New York University School of
Medicine, New York, New York, USA

Reed A Omary MD MS
Director of Research, Associate Professor of Radiology
and Biomedical Engineering, Department of Radiology,
Northwestern University, Chicago, Illinois, USA

Matthijs Oudkerk MD PhD
Professor and Chairman, Department of Radiology,
University Medical Center Groningen, Groningen,
The Netherlands

Neeraj J Panchal
Resident, Department of Radiology, University of
California San Diego, San Diego, California, USA

Mini N Pathria MD
Professor, Department of Radiology, University of
California San Diego Medical Center, San Diego,
California, USA

Wallace W Peck MD
Assistant Clinical Professor in Radiology, University of
California San Diego, San Diego; Director of MRI and
Chief of Neuroimaging and Head and Neck Radiology,
St Joseph Hospital and Children's Hospital of Orange
County, Orange, California, USA

Ivan Pedrosa MD
Assistant Professor of Radiology, Harvard Medical
School, Department of Radiology, Beth Israel Deaconess
Medical Center, Boston, Massachusetts, USA

F Scott Pereles MD
Associate Professor of Radiology, Director of MRI,
Body MRI, Northwestern University SMaRT; Associate
Professor of Cardiac MRI, Northwestern University
Feinberg School of Medicine, Chicago, Illinois, USA

John Perl II MD
Neuroradiology Section, Consulting Radiologists, Ltd.,
Abbott Northwestern Hospital, Minneapolis, USA

Ronald M Peshock MD
Professor, Departments of Radiology and Internal
Medicine, University of Texas Southwestern Medical
School at Dallas, Dallas, Texas, USA

William T Peterson
Diagnostic Imaging, GE Healthcare, Waukesha,
Wisconsin, USA

Stanley J Piepenburg
Diagnostic Imaging, GE Healthcare, Waukesha,
Wisconsin, USA

Julia Po MD
Research Assistant, Lucas MRS/I Center, Department of
Radiology, Stanford University, Stanford, California, USA

Hollis G Potter MD
Chief, Magnetic Resonance Imaging, Hospital for Special
Surgery; Professor of Radiology, Cornell University Weill
Medical College, New York, New York, USA

Andrew J Powell MD
Associate, Department of Cardiology; Children's
Hospital Boston; Assistant Professor of Pediatrics,
Harvard Medical School, Boston, Massachusetts, USA

Pottumarthi V Prasad PhD
Director of Physiological Imaging Laboratory,
Department of Radiology, Evanston Northwestern
Healthcare, Evanston, Illinois, USA

Gary A Press MD
Chief of Neuroradiology and Director of Magnetic
Resonance, Kaiser-Permanente Medical Center,
San Diego, California, USA

Josephine Pressacco MD PhD
Fellow, Magnetic Resonance Imaging, McGill University
Health Center, Montreal, Quebec, Canada

Martin R Prince MD PhD
Professor of Radiology, Cornell University Weill Medical
College, New York; Professor of Radiology, Chief of MRI,
New York Hospital, Columbia College of Physicians
and Surgeons, New York, New York, USA

Aliya Qayyum MBBS FRCR
Assistant Professor, Department of Radiology, University
of California San Francisco, San Francisco, California, USA

Vikram A Rao MD
Instructor, Department of Radiology, Feinberg School
of Medicine, Northwestern University, Chicago, Illinois,
USA

John D Reeder MD FACR
Chief, Musculoskeletal Imaging Division, Proscan
Imaging, Columbia, Maryland, USA

Peter Reimer MD PhD
Department of Radiology, Klinikum Karlsruhe,
Academic Teaching Hospital of the University of
Freiberg, Moltkestrasse, Karlsruhe, Germany

Sharon Reimold MD
Associate Professor, Department of Internal Medicine,
University of Texas Southwestern Medical Center at
Dallas, Dallas, Texas, USA

Caroline Reinhold MD MSc
Professor, Departments of Radiology, Gynecology and
Gastroenterology, Director, MR Imaging; Director of
Research, McGill University Health Center, Montreal,
Quebec, Canada

Kent B Remley MD
Center for Diagnostic Imaging, Indianapolis, Indiana,
USA

Luca Roccatagliata MD
Department of Radiology, Massachusetts General
Hospital, Harvard Medical School, Boston,
Massachusetts, USA

Neil M Rofsky MD
Associate Professor of Radiology, Harvard Medical
School; Chief of MRI, Beth Israel Deaconess Medical
Center, Boston, Massachusetts, USA

Brian D Ross MD FRCS FRCPath DPhil(Oxen)
Director, Magnetic Resonance Spectroscopy Unit;
Visiting Associate, Chemistry and Chemical Engineering,
California Institute of Technology, Pasadena, California;
Professor of Clinical Medicine, University of Southern
California, Keck School of Medicine, Los Angeles,
California, USA

Marc Rothenberg SM CMPE CHE CHFP
Cary, North Carolina, USA

Armando Ruiz MD
Voluntary Faculty, Department of Radiology,
University of Miami School of Medicine,
Miami, Florida, USA

Dushyant V Sahani MD
Director of CT, Department of Radiology, Division
of Abdominal Imaging and Intervention,
Massachusetts General Hospital, Boston; Instructor
in Radiology, Harvard Medical School, Boston,
Massachusetts, USA

Ken E Sakaie PhD
Departments of Biomedical Engineering and
Radiology, Northwestern University, Chicago, Illinois,
USA

John C Salanitri MD
Fellow, Department of Radiology, Northwestern
University Feinberg School of Medicine, Chicago,
Illinois, USA

David Saloner PhD
Professor of Radiology; Director, Vascular Imaging
Research Center, University of California San Francisco,
San Francisco, California, USA

Pamela W Schaefer MD
Associate Director of Neuroradiology, Neuroradiology
Fellowship Director, Clinical Director of MRI,
Massachusetts General Hospital; Associate Professor
of Radiology, Harvard Medical School, Boston,
Massachusetts, USA

Peter D Schellinger MD PhD
Department of Neurology, University of Heidelberg,
Heidelberg, Germany

Wolfgang Schima MD PhD
Department of Radiology, University of Vienna,
Währinger Gürtel, Vienna, Austria

Gerhard Schroth MD
Professor, Department of Diagnostic and Interventional
Neuroradiology, University of Bern, Bern, Switzerland

Abraham Seidmann PhD
Xerox Chair Professor of Computers and Information
Systems, Electronic Commerce, and Operations
Management, W E Simon Graduate School of Business
Administration, University of Rochester, New York, USA

Richard C Semelka MD
Director of MR Services, Professor and Vice Chair of
Research, Department of Radiology, University of
North Carolina, Chapel Hill, North Carolina, USA

Farid F Shafaie MD
Director of Neuroradiology, Department of Radiology,
MacNeal Hospital, Berwyn, Illinois, USA

Dipan J Shah MD
Director, Nashville Cardiovascular Magnetic Resonance
Institute, The Heart Group, PLLC, Brentwood, Tennessee;
Assistant Consulting Professor of Medicine, Duke
University Medical School, Durham, North Carolina, USA

Frank G Shellock PhD FACC FACSM
Adjunct Clinical Professor of Radiology and Medicine,
Keck School of Medicine, University of Southern
California; Institute for Magnetic Resonance Safety,
Education, and Research, Los Angeles, California, USA

Marilyn J Siegel MD
Professor of Radiology and Pediatrics, Mallinckrodt
Institute of Radiology, Washington University School of
Medicine, St. Louis, Missouri, USA

Evan S Siegelman MD
Associate Professor, Section Chief, MRI, Department of
Radiology, University of Pennsylvania Medical Center,
Philadelphia, Pennsylvania, USA

Bettina Siewert MD
Assistant Professor of Radiology, Beth Israel Deaconess
Medical Center, Harvard Medical School, Boston,
Massachusetts, USA

Orlando P Simonetti PhD
Associate Professor of Internal Medicine and Radiology;
Director, Cardiovascular MR and CT Research, Davis
Heart and Lung Research Institute, The Ohio State
University, Columbus, Ohio, USA

Claude B Sirlin MD
Assistant Professor of Radiology, Body Imaging Division,
University of California San Diego, San Diego, California,
USA

Evelyn M L Sklar MD
Professor of Clinical Radiology and Neurological
Surgery, Department of Radiology, University of Miami
School of Medicine, Miami, Florida, USA

Daniel K Sodickson MD PhD
Assistant Professor of Radiology and Medicine,
Harvard Medical School; Director, Laboratory for
Biomedical Imaging Research, Beth Israel Deaconess
Medical Center, Boston, Massachusetts, USA

Carolyn M Sofka MD
Assistant Attending in Radiology, Hospital for
Special Surgery; Assistant Professor of Radiology,
Cornell University Weill Medical College,
New York, New York, USA

Michael E Stadnick MD
Medical Director, Radsource, Brentwood, Tennessee,
USA

Arthur E Stillman MD PhD
Head, Division of Cardiovascular MRI, Department of
Radiology, Cleveland Clinic Foundation, Cleveland,
Ohio, USA

Robert S Stormont
Diagnostic Imaging, GE Healthcare, Waukesha,
Wisconsin, USA

Pippa Storey PhD
Research Scientist, Department of Radiology, Evanston
Hospital, Evanston, Illinois, USA

Clare M C Tempany MD
Professor of Radiology and Director of Clinical MRI,
Brigham and Women's Hospital, Boston, Massachusetts,
USA

H Thomas Temple MD
Professor, Orthopedics and Pathology; Chief,
Orthopedic Oncology Division, University of Miami
School of Medicine, Florida, USA

Kathleen Thangaraj RT(MR)
Chief Technologist, MRI Department, McLean Hospital,
Belmont, Massachusetts, USA

Keith R Thulborn MD PhD
Professor of Radiology, Physiology and Biophysics,
Director of Center for Magnetic Resonance
Research, University of Illinois at Chicago, Chicago,
Illinois, USA

Robert Troiano MD
Associate Professor of Radiology, Obstetrics and
Gynecology, Weill Medical College of Cornell University,
New York; Attending Physician, New York Presbyterian
Hospital, New York Weill Cornell Medical Center,
New York, New York, USA

Patrick A Turski MD FACR
Professor, Departments of Radiology, Neurology and
Neurosurgery, University of Wisconsin Medical School,
Madison, Wisconsin, USA

Kâmil Uludağ
Research Scientist, Center for Functional MRI,
Department of Radiology, University of California
San Diego, La Jolla, California, USA

Raul N Uppot MD
Instructor in Radiology, Harvard Medical School,
Department of Radiology, Division of Abdominal
Imaging and Intervention, Massachusetts General
Hospital, Boston, Massachusetts, USA

Robert M Vavrek MSEE
Diagnostic Imaging, GE Healthcare, Waukesha,
Wisconsin, USA

Louis-Gilbert Vézina MD
Director, Program in Neuroradiology, Children's
National Medical Center; Associate Professor of
Radiology and Pediatrics, The George Washington
University School of Medicine and Health Sciences,
Washington DC, USA

Steven Warach MD PhD
Chief, Stroke Diagnostics and Therapeutics Section,
Stroke Branch, NINDS, NIH, Bethesda, Maryland, USA

Oliver M Weber PhD
Assistant Professor of Radiology, University of California
San Francisco, San Francisco, California, USA

Jane L Weissman MD FACR
Professor of Radiology, Ophthalmology and
Otolaryngology, Department of Radiology, Oregon
Health Sciences University, Portland, Oregon, USA

Gary J Wendt MD MBA
Vice Chair of Informatics, Associate Professor of
Radiology, Enterprise Director of Medical Imaging,
Department of Radiology, University of Wisconsin
Hospital and Clinics, Madison, Wisconsin, USA

Piotr A Wielopolski PhD
Department of Radiology, Erasmus Medisch Centrum,
Rotterdam, The Netherlands

Richard D White MD FACC FAHA
Division of Radiology, Cleveland Clinic Foundation,
Cleveland, Ohio, USA

Norbert Wilke MD
Associate Professor of Radiology and Cardiology,
Chief, Cardiovascular MR and CT Imaging, University
of Florida, Jacksonville, Florida, USA

Robert B Wolf BS
Fonar Corporation, Melville, New York, USA

Wade Wong DO FACR
Professor of Radiology, Interventional Neuroradiology
Section, University of California San Diego Medical
Center, San Diego, California, USA

Gongyu Yang MD
Clinical Assistant Professor of Radiology, University
of Illinois, Chicago, Illinois, USA

Susan B Yeon MD JD
Department of Medicine, Cardiovascular Division,
Beth Israel Deaconess Medical Center and Harvard
Medical School, Boston, Massachusetts, USA

Honglei Zhang
Fellow, Department of Radiology, Cornell University
Weill Medical College, New York, New York, USA

Michael B Zlatkin MD FRCP(C)
President, National Musculoskeletal Imaging Inc.,
Weston, Florida; Voluntary Professor of Radiology,
University of Miami School of Medicine, Miami,
Florida, USA

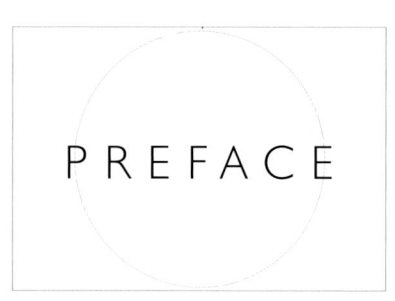

PREFACE

TO THE THIRD EDITION OF *CLINICAL MAGNETIC RESONANCE IMAGING*

This is the third edition of *Clinical Magnetic Resonance Imaging*. It has been almost a decade and a half since the publication of the first edition, which came into existence at a time when the field of MRI was still very much in its infancy. Back in the era defined by the first edition, MRI was a fledgling modality. Although well accepted as a helpful tool in the field of brain imaging, MRI had little clinical utility in other areas. Scans often took 15 minutes or longer and the MR images were routinely plagued with artifacts. MRI of the knee was just coming into its own, and other musculoskeletal applications were in their infancy. The only contrast agents available were nonspecific and used much like iodine-based agents for computed tomography (CT).

The second edition was published at a time when MRI was on firmer footing as a diagnostic tool in the fields of brain, spine, and joint imaging. Abdominal and pelvic applications appeared promising, whereas cardiovascular applications suffered from severe technological limitations and were seldom successful or useful. Fast imaging techniques were entirely hardware based and available only to a handful of academic investigators.

Nine long years have passed since the second edition. Over that period, we have all experienced the physical passage of time, perhaps hair a bit grayer, joint aches a bit more frequent, maybe even a tad less spry in our step. Yet over the same period, MRI has grown and prospered to a degree that would have been difficult to imagine in years past. There has been exponential growth in the number of MRI systems across the globe. New whole-body scanner installations include systems at field strengths of 3 T to 9.4 T, which at the time of the first edition would have been considered impossible by many top investigators in the field. Nowadays, echo planar imaging is routinely used for diagnosis of stroke and other disorders of the brain. MRI can easily depict brain function based on changes in blood oxygenation or flow, and is considered superior in many ways to positron emission tomography. Contrast-enhanced angiograms that rival digital subtraction angiography in quality are the routine, with new contrast agents and imaging techniques in development that might allow MR angiography to surpass even that long-recognized gold standard.

Advances in molecular imaging permit imaging of stem cells in vivo, tracking of cell migration, and identification of specific receptors in cancer. Novel therapies such as MR-guided focused ultrasound are used to noninvasively annihilate uterine fibroids, breast tumors, and even brain tumors without the morbidity expected from an invasive surgical procedure. Advances in the technology for cardiac imaging have made this a routine test that is beginning to compete with established nuclear and echocardiographic tests for the diagnosis of heart disease. Abdominal images can be acquired within a comfortable breath-hold with quality that rivals multi-detector CT. High-field imaging has reinforced the diagnostic value of musculoskeletal imaging, which is now one of the most common applications of MRI, whereas open-architecture low-field systems offer greater patient convenience and eliminate problems with claustrophobia.

The progress seems unstoppable. New developments in other areas such as hyperpolarized contrast agents, parallel imaging, spectroscopy, and scanner hardware promise to propel the field to ever-greater clinical utility, while offering the scientist endless possibilities for clinical investigation.

The third edition of *Clinical Magnetic Resonance Imaging* is greatly expanded in size and scope compared with the previous editions. We have endeavored to explore all significant aspects of the field, including the basic principles, techniques, and clinical applications. The chapters are written by internationally recognized experts in their respective fields. Moreover, we have endeavored to maintain some of the more appreciated qualities of the previous editions: clarity in writing, practicality, and utility for day-to-day practice. New features include extensive use of color illustrations and an accompanying website (*http://www.clinicalmri.com*) that will keep the reader up to date with the latest developments and interesting cases, and provide continuing medical education credits.

The preparation of this textbook was a huge task, but it was also an endeavor of love that provided the editors with great satisfaction. We hope that it provides you with a useful guide to one of the most exciting fields in medicine today.

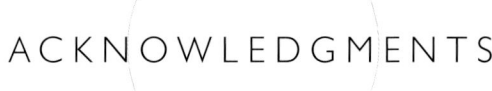

ACKNOWLEDGMENTS

I thank my assistant, Sally Gartman, who diligently and patiently handled the many tasks concerning all aspects of this textbook that were assigned to her; my assistant Angela Love-Bradford, for helping to keep my Radiology department—and me—sane throughout the lengthy editorial and publication process; Nora Naughton, Sarah Abel, Samantha Gear, Kathy Syplywczak, and Amanda Sancto, who did such a fine job in copyediting and other key aspects of the publication process; our Production Manager, Joan Sinclair, our Developmental Editor, Ann Ruzycka Anderson, and our Executive Editor, Allan Ross, for hanging in there through "thick and thin" and investing the necessary resources for this ambitious project. Most of all I would like to thank the numerous contributors, all experts in their respective fields, who gave so freely of their time and effort to ensure the highest scientific standards and greatest educational benefit to the reader.

RRE

I thank Julie Wise, my assistant, who helped coordinate all phone calls, mailings and the many inquiries about this project. I also thank the fellows and residents who helped me collect all the case material for the textbook.

JRH

I thank Elaine Pieroni for her assistance with preparing material for this book.

MBZ

I thank Angela, my assistant, who faithfully coordinated manuscript transfers and communication for several years as the book was being forged. I appreciate the assistance of my radiology partners and our MRI fellows, especially Timothy Chen and Muhammad Ali, for help and advice. I also thank Radnet Management, especially Howard Berger, for encouragement and support.

JVC

TABLE OF CONTENTS

Volume 3

VI. BODY

VII. MUSCULOSKELETAL SYSTEM

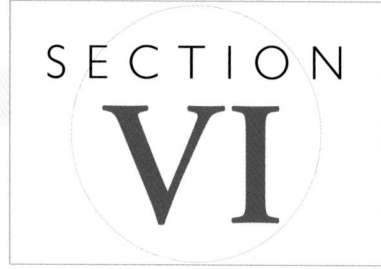

SECTION VI

BODY

CHAPTER 76

THORAX

Mizuki Nishino ● Hiroto Hatabu

INTRODUCTION

Although radiologic science including magnetic resonance imaging (MRI) has changed medicine dramatically in the past decades, MRI is probably underutilized in chest imaging. Currently, the chest radiograph and computed tomography (CT) are modalities of choice for clinical practice in medicine. The chest radiograph provides instant and inexpensive imaging of the cardiopulmonary system, and plays a primary role in outpatient, emergency medicine, and intensive care units. CT provides exquisite three-dimensional (3D) data of the thorax. The CT scan is an essential part of oncologic imaging including screening and staging of lung cancer. High-resolution CT yields detailed images of lung parenchyma. MRI is a valuable problem-solving tool for specific clinical problems, which include evaluation of the aorta and great vessels, mediastinal masses, superior sulcus tumor, chest wall, and diaphragm. The advantages of MRI include multiplanar capability, high tissue contrast, flow sensitivity, and use of less nephrotoxic contrast agents such as gadolinium.[1]

This chapter presents: 1. magnetic resonance (MR) application for imaging the great vessels; 2. summary of current applications in the thorax, including lung cancer, mediastinum, pleura, diaphragm, and chest wall; and 3. newer applications in the thorax, i.e., MR imaging of pulmonary function.

GREAT VESSELS

MRI is an excellent modality for noninvasive morphologic and functional evaluation of the thoracic aorta. The advantages of MRI include its inherent multiplanar imaging capability, intrinsic contrast between blood flow and vascular structures, and absence of radiation exposure. Multiplanar imaging is helpful in visualizing the extent of abnormalities of the thoracic aorta, including the aortic valve and annulus and the origin of the arch vessels. MRI can be performed with or without contrast enhancement, and is suitable for follow-up of patients requiring sequential imaging examinations.[1-3]

Assessment of the thoracic aorta requires visualization of the lumen, aortic wall, and periaortic region to define intraluminal, mural, and extramural pathology.[1] As MRI combines attributes of echocardiography, angiography, and CT, it is sometimes considered suitable for nonemergent evaluation of the thoracic aorta.[4]

Clinical Indications

The combination of MR images and MR angiography is an effective noninvasive technique applicable to most aortic pathology. Some of the specific indications for MRI in assessing thoracic aortic disease are listed in Box 76-1.[1,5] Of these, the major pathology of the thoracic aorta diagnosed with MRI includes aortic dissection, penetrating aortic ulcers, aortic aneurysms, and congenital abnormalities of the aorta such as coarctation.[6]

Technical Considerations

Conventional SE Imaging

The most common pulse sequence used for thoracic imaging is a conventional spin-echo (SE) sequence gated to the cardiac cycle in a multislice mode. T1-weighted SE axial and left anterior oblique (LAO) images with

Box 76-I	Clinical Indications for MRI in Assessing Thoracic Aortic Disease

Evaluation of abnormal aortic contour or size
Distinguishing a mediastinal mass from vascular abnormality
Diagnosis and follow-up of aortic dissection in hemodynamically stable patients, including postsurgical evaluation
Diagnosis of aortic arch anomalies
Diagnosis and assessment of the dimensions of aortic aneurysms as well as evaluation for possible leakage
Diagnosis and assessment of the extent of aortitis
Monitoring the aorta in Marfan syndrome and annuloaortic ectasia
Establishing the source of peripheral embolization
Diagnosis and assessment of the severity of coarctation, including postangioplasty evaluation
Diagnosis of periaortic abscess or infectious pseudoaneurysm in bacterial endocarditis of the aortic valve
Assessment of the origin and proximal extent of great vessels for possible causes of cerebrovascular disease

electrocardiographic (ECG) gating can show the thoracic aorta dimensions without significant blurring from adjacent cardiac motion.

Fast Spin-echo Imaging

Fast SE T2-weighted images provide shorter imaging times and better image resolution than conventional SE images. It also has the advantage of decreasing respiratory motion artifacts. Chemical shift-fat suppression may be used due to the high signal intensity of fat on fast SE images. Dark-blood half-Fourier single-shot turbo SE (HASTE) imaging can be performed instead of ECG-triggered T1-weighted SE images.[7]

Cine Gradient-echo Imaging

Cine imaging for cardiac MR imaging consists of a motion picture loop of various phases of the cardiac cycle. The cine gradient-echo technique uses the ECG signal retrospectively to "freeze" cardiac motion and provide useful data regarding cardiac dimensions and valvular flow.[8] Fast time-of-flight techniques have been performed with breath-hold imaging to minimize respiratory motion.[9]

MR Angiography

Gadolinium-enhanced 3D MR angiography has been shown to be capable of depicting the aortic arch and upper descending thoracic aorta. This technique has fewer limitations compared with other sequences.[10] Compared with 2D techniques, 3D pulse sequences provide: 1. stronger signal enhancement of vessels compared with the background; 2. greater spatial resolution; and 3. less artifactual signal loss from dephasing within a voxel. Maximum intensity projections and multiplanar reformations provide images that appear comparable to conventional angiographic images. The advent of phased-array coils and head-and-neck coils allows for increased

signal-to-noise ratio while maintaining higher resolution as well as a decrease in contrast dose.[7] Early gadolinium-enhanced 3D imaging was performed with a continuous infusion of contrast over a 2- to 5-minute acquisition. While these images were an improvement over prior techniques, they were limited by respiratory-induced motion artifacts and artifacts from enhancing veins.[11] As technology improved, it became possible to perform breath-hold studies of the thoracic aorta, but appropriate timing of the contrast bolus became critical to avoid overlap of brachiocephalic arterial enhancement with jugular venous enhancement.[12] A timing injection method was used to precisely match peak arterial enhancement to the acquisition of the central lines of k-space.[13]

Imaging Plane

MR can image the heart and great vessels in any plane regardless of the availability of acoustic windows. In routine imaging, transverse, sagittal, and coronal planes are generally sufficient to solve most of the common clinical problems encountered. Sagittal, LAO sagittal, and coronal T1-weighted SE images are helpful in evaluating aortic dissection, coarctation, and vascular rings.

Aortic Dissection

Thoracic aortic dissection is the most frequent cause of aortic emergency, and is a life-threatening condition that requires immediate diagnosis and treatment.[14] It occurs more commonly in elderly male patients.[15] The clinical symptoms include acute onset of sharp pain radiating to the chest, back, or neck, which is seen in 95% of patients. More than one third of patients with aortic dissection show signs and symptoms indicating systemic involvement.[14]

Hypertension is the most common risk factor of aortic dissection, and is found in approximately 75% of patients. Other predisposing factors include: Marfan syndrome, Ehlers-Danlos syndrome and other connective tissue diseases, Turner syndrome, aortic valvular disease, aortic coarctation, aortic aneurysm, aortitis, and pregnancy.[16,17] Cocaine use has been reported to predispose aortic dissection in healthy, normotensive patients.[18]

Dissection is classified as acute if symptoms last less than 2 weeks and chronic if longer than 2 weeks.[19] Three quarters of deaths from this entity occur within 2 weeks after the initial manifestation.[20] Aortic dissection is also classified based on the site and extent of aortic involvement. Stanford type A (or DeBakey type 1 or II) aortic dissection involves the ascending aorta proximal to the origin of the left subclavian artery. Urgent surgical repair is required because of the risk of intrapericardial rupture and subsequent cardiac tamponade. Stanford type B (or DeBakey type III) denotes dissections involving only the descending aorta, and is usually more stable and may be managed medically (Fig. 76-1) .

The indications for surgery include: 1. acute ascending thoracic aortic dissections; 2. acute descending thoracic aortic dissections with hemodynamic instability; and

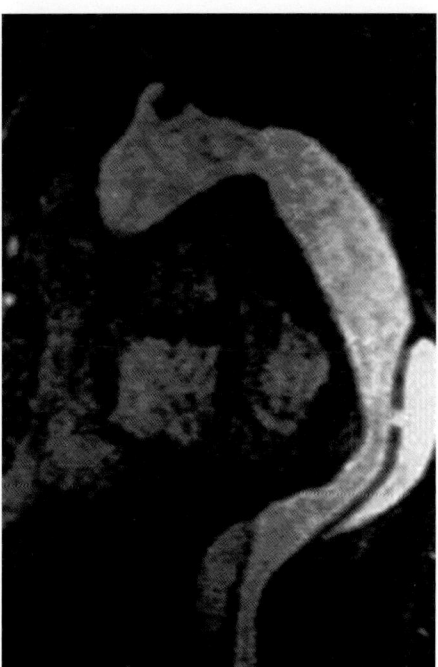

FIGURE 76-1

3D MRA after administration of Gd-DTPA showing dissection of the descending thoracic aorta extending into the upper abdominal aorta. The entry site and dissection flap are well demonstrated.

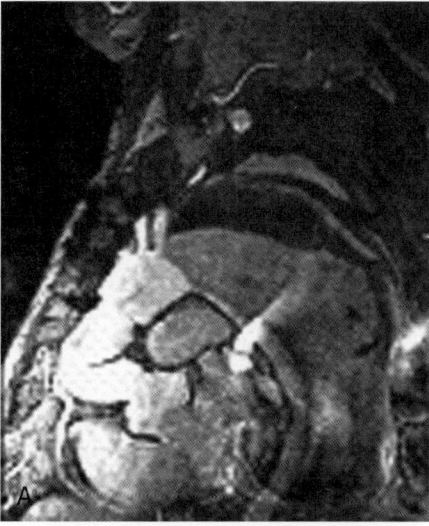

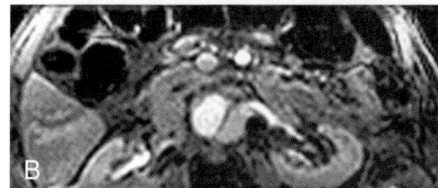

FIGURE 76-2

A, Contrast-enhanced saggital MIP image of a 72-year-old man with chest pain shows dissecting aneurysm beginning at the level of the left subclavian artery and extending into the descending aorta, with contrast-filled compressed true lumen and expanded false lumen posterior to it. The right brachiocephalic and left carotid arteries are proximal to the origin of the dissection. **B,** Axial images at the level of renal arteries show left renal artery arising from the false lumen.

3. chronic dissections that are symptomatic, growing more than 1 cm in diameter per year, or exceeding 5 cm in diameter.[21]

Potential life-threatening complications of aortic dissection include acute aortic regurgitation, pericardial tamponade, aortic rupture, and major branch-vessel obstruction causing ischemia to the myocardium, brain, or abdominal viscera. Recognition of the complications that often accompany aortic dissection is important for achieving accurate diagnosis and effective treatment.[14] These three forms of aortic dissection: typical dissection, intramural hematoma, and penetrating aortic ulcer, which are clinically indistinguishable, can be differentiated based on imaging findings.[14]

Typical Aortic Dissection

Typical aortic dissection occurs when an intimal tear allows blood to enter the medial layer of the aortic wall, separating into two lumina: true lumen and false lumen.[14] With its multiplanar capability, MRI provides complete assessment of the aortic valves, sinotubular complex, ascending and descending segments of the aorta, and branch vessels.[22] In patients suspicious of systemic involvement, the entire aorta should be evaluated in order to determine the distal extent of the dissection and to detect ischemic disease (Fig. 76-2).

It has been reported that MRI using only axial T1-weighted SE sequences had a greater sensitivity and specificity for the diagnosis of aortic dissection compared to transthoracic echocardiography, transesophageal echocardiography, and nonhelical contrast-enhanced CT.[23] T1- and T2-weighted sequences have been shown to be useful for accurate detection of thrombus in the false lumen created by aortic dissection.[24]

Cine MRI and 3D gadolinium-enhanced MR angiography are useful in evaluating false lumen patency and identifying the origin of branch vessels. Cine MRI sequences can be used to detect an intimal flap, and help to distinguish a dissection with chronic thrombosis from aneurysm with mural thrombosis.

General rules for distinguishing between a thrombus-filled false lumen in dissection and a thoracic aortic aneurysm with mural thrombosis are as follows:

1. The patent lumen is noncircular and compressed in a dissection.
2. A change in the location of the thrombosis, usually right-sided in the ascending aorta and left-sided in the descending aorta, is a sign of a false lumen of a dissection.
3. The extension of the thrombus over more than 7 cm, which is seen typically in a dissection.[25]

3D gadolinium-enhanced MR angiography is suitable for demonstrating the entry and exit sites. Delayed sequences of 3D MR angiography can show the false lumen with slower flow and increased signal or hetero-geneous signal intensity relative to the true lumen. 3D gadolinium-enhanced MR angiography also helps to assess the distal intra-abdominal extent of the dissection by providing a large field of view.[26] It helps to determine whether aortic branches including the great vessels, celiac, superior mesenteric, and renal arteries arise from the true or false lumen. Patency of these arteries can also be assessed by the presence of a flow void in the visceral vessels.[27]

Intramural Hematoma

Intramural hematoma (IMH) is caused by a spontaneous localized hemorrhage of the vasa vasorum of the medial layer, which weakens the media in the absence of an intimal tear.[28] The clinical manifestations and risk factors in intramural hematoma are similar to those in typical aortic dissection. Approximately 13% of acute aortic dissection is caused by intramural hematoma.[29]

As in typical aortic dissection, classification of intra-mural hematoma uses the Stanford system, which recom-mends surgical treatment in cases of IMH of Stanford type A.[30,31] Because of the high mortality and morbidity associated with aortic surgery, it has been suggested that supportive medical treatment with frequent follow-up imaging may be a rational management option.[32,33] It is also reported that noninvasive imaging study including CT, MRI and transesophageal echocardiography provides important prognostic information in the medical treatment of acute type A intramural hematoma, with the initial hematoma thickness being the best index for predicting an adverse clinical outcome.[34]

On MRI, T1-weighted SE and cine gradient-echo sequences may demonstrate a crescent-shaped high signal in the aortic wall, as well as focal thickening, indicative of intramural hematoma. In this aortic pathology, focal aortic wall thickening may be the only finding. Thoracic aortic wall thickening can be associated with dissection of the abdominal aorta, which evokes the need for careful evaluation of the complete aorta, including the level of the bifurcation. Routine follow-up approximately every 3 months is also recommended to monitor pro-gression of the intramural hematoma.[30] Resolution of intramural hematomas during follow-up suggests a favorable prognosis and is unlikely to be associated with dissection[35] (Fig. 76-3).

Penetrating Aortic Ulcer

Penetrating atherosclerotic ulcer is a distinct radiologic and pathologic entity in which an ulceration of atheromatous plaque erodes the inner, elastic layer of the aortic wall, reaches the medial layer, and produces a hematoma in the media.[36] It is usually associated with intramural hematoma and, potentially, aortic rupture.[37] Penetrating atherosclerotic ulcers are most often seen in elderly patients with severe atherosclerosis. The most accepted treatment for penetrating atherosclerotic

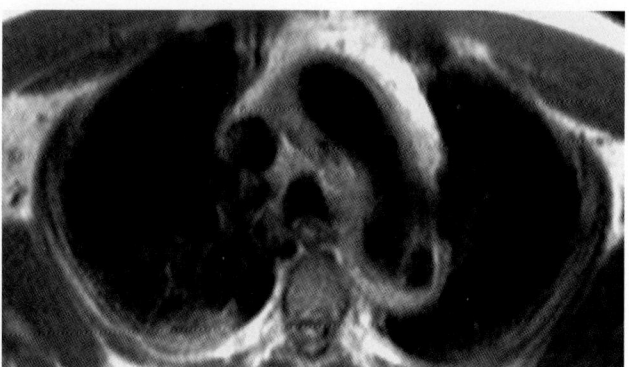

FIGURE 76-3

Axial HASTE image in a 55-year-old man shows wall thickening of the aortic arch, suggesting intramural hematoma.

ulcers is medical therapy. Surgery is reserved for patients with hemodynamic instability, persistent pain, aortic rupture, distal embolization, or rapid enlargement of the aortic diameter.[14]

3D MR angiography may demonstrate the penetrating atherosclerotic ulcers with intramural hematoma, which require surgical repair.[38] T1- and T2-weighted SE images depict the ulcer as an area of high signal within the aortic wall. The ulcer is typically located in the middle to distal portions of the descending thoracic aorta, from which subsequent subintimal dissection occurs. With the penetrating atherosclerotic ulcer, the aorta usually progressively enlarges, and eventually develops saccu-lar aneurysms, which sometimes rupture.[39] In some cases when atherosclerotic disease and medial fibrosis are present, the dissection may be of focal limited pro-gression (Fig. 76-4).

Aortic Aneurysm

An aorta with a diameter greater than 4 cm is considered dilated, and a diameter greater than 5 cm is aneurismal (Fig. 76-5). Aneurysms greater than 6 cm in diameter carry a risk of rupture, which exceeds 30% over the short term.[40] Surgical mortality is approximately 10% for elective repairs and more than 20% for emergent repairs.[41]

Aortic aneurysms vary in size and shape. Saccular aneurysms involve less than the entire circumference of the aorta and are usually localized, whereas fusiform aneurysms involve the entire circumference of the aorta and may extend over the thoracic or thoracoabdominal aorta. True aneurysms denote those composed of all layers of the aortic wall, whereas false aneurysms result from a focal disruption of the aortic wall surrounded by the adventitial layer or fibrous tissue. True aneurysms tend to be fusiform with more extensive involvement. False aneurysms are often saccular and have a shorter length than true aneurysms. The most frequent cause of a true aneurysm is atherosclerosis, which usually

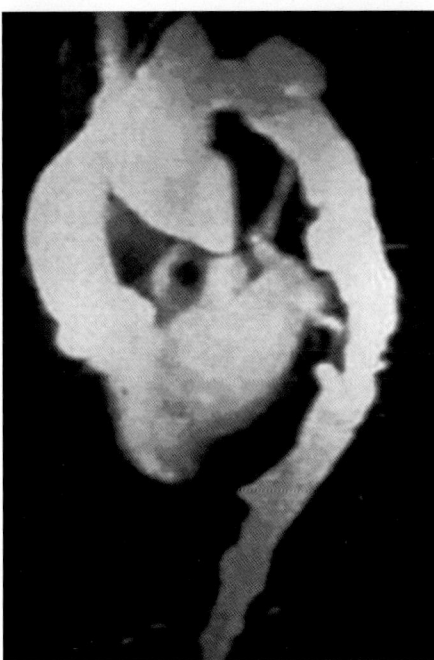

FIGURE 76-4

3D MRA in a patient with diabetes mellitus shows a diffusely athero-sclerotic thoracic and upper abdominal aorta with multiple penetrating ulcers in the descending thoracic aorta. Also noted is a large pseudo-aneurysm extending off the aortic arch and around the region of the ligamentum arteriosum.

involves both the ascending and descending aorta. Other causes include trauma, syphilis, Marfan syndrome, Takayasu's arteritis and other connective tissue diseases, and infection with resultant mycotic aneurysms. Trauma and infection can frequently cause false aneurysms. Up to 30% of patients with thoracic aneurysms have concomitant infrarenal abdominal aortic aneurysms, requiring imaging of the abdominal aorta[42] (Figs 76-6, 76-7).

The role of imaging studies in evaluating aneurysms is to: 1. measure the diameter of the aneurysm; 2. assess the longitudinal extent of the aneurysm; 3. determine involvement of arch branches; 4. detect periaortic hematoma or other signs of leakage; and 5. identify additional aneurysms at other sites.[1] In addition, MRI is a practical method for monitoring the progression of thoracic aortic aneurysms.[3]

Axial T1-weighted spin-echo images with ECG gating demonstrate the concentric enlargement of the ascending or descending aorta in patients with thoracic aortic aneurysm, visualizing the outer diameter of the aneurysm and size of the residual lumen. This technique is useful for accurate measurement of the diameter of the aneurysm when there is wall thickening or mural thrombus. Sagittal or oblique sagittal images can help determine the longitudinal extent of the aneurysm.

Effacement of the sinotubular junction with aortic root aneurysm may be caused by Marfan syndrome, syphilitis aortitis, annuloaortic ectasia, and, possibly, severe aortic valve insufficiency. This effacement is not seen in aortic stenosis, in which the poststenotic dilatation occurs distal to the sinotubular region.

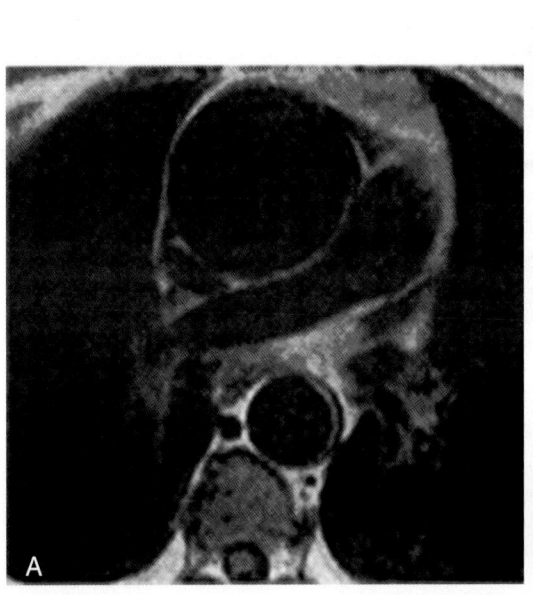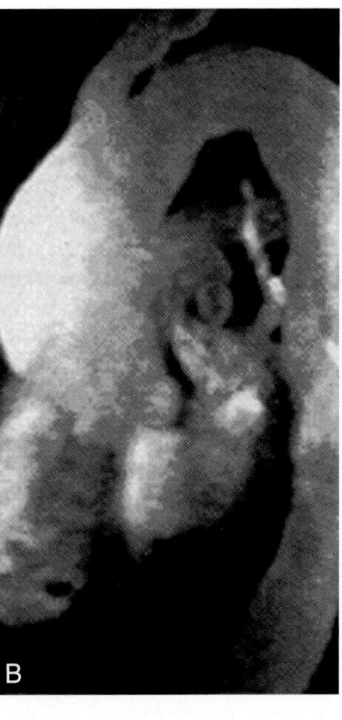

FIGURE 76-5

A, T1-weighted MR image demonstrates a remarkably enlarged ascending thoracic aorta with a normal caliber descending thoracic aorta. **B,** 3D MRA confirms a contrast-filled aneurysmal ascending aorta and normal caliber descending thoracic aorta. No evidence of dissection was found.

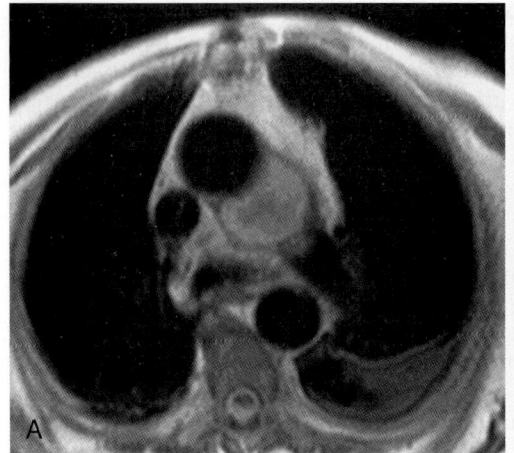

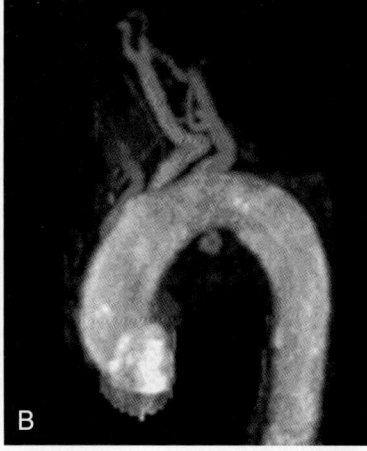

FIGURE 76-6

A, Axial HASTE image of an 81-year-old man shows a pseudoaneurysm with contained hematoma of high signal intensity. **B,** Contrast-enhanced 3D MRA shows the contrast-filled lumen of the pseudoaneurysm.

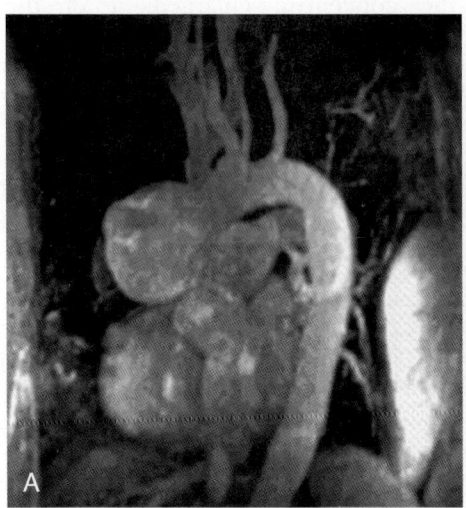

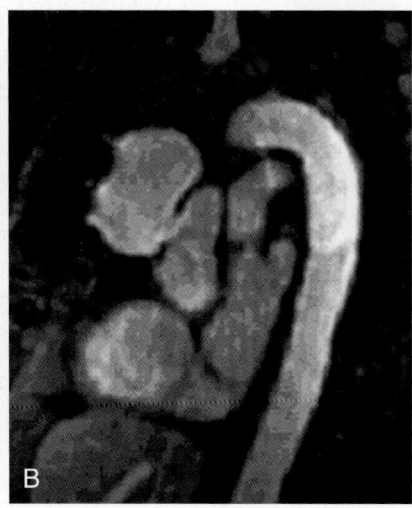

FIGURE 76-7

A, Contrast-enhanced 3D angiogram of a 54-year-old woman with history of ascending aortic dissection and surgical repair shows a new large pseudoaneurysm originating from the anterior wall of the ascending aorta. **B,** Contrast-enhanced sagittal image shows the neck of the pseudoaneurysm continuing from the ascending aorta

Areas of periaortic or mediastinal bleeding can be detected as high signal intensity on T1-weighted images produced by hematoma. It can be difficult to distinguish between periaortic hematoma due to a leaking aneurysm and chronic thrombosis in an aortic dissection. Periaortic hematoma tends to be more diffuse compared to the thrombus within a false lumen. Acute hemorrhage usually demonstrates low signal intensity on T1-weighted images, although there are cases of acute aortic rupture with blood in the mediastinum demonstrating high T1 signal.[43]

Aortitis

As MR imaging resolution improves, its role in diagnosing aortitis increases. ECG-gated T1-weighted LAO and coronal SE images demonstrate moderate wall thickening and high T1 signal consistent with chronic inflammatory vascular disease.[1] Takayasu's arteritis, one of the major causes of aortitis, usually affects young women of Asian descent. The early stage of this disease presents with mural thickening of the aorta, which can be best seen on T1-weighted SE images supplemented with breath-hold T2-weighted images (i.e., HASTE) or short tau inversion recovery.[44] The contrast-enhanced T1-weighted SE images may demonstrate dilated inflammatory vessels in the thickened aortic wall and markedly enhanced periaortic tissue in acute or chronic active patients.[45] The chronic occlusive phase results in aorta or branch vessel narrowing or occlusion. Aneurysms and aortic insufficiency may be identified. Cine MRI is helpful in evaluation of aortic insufficiency.[45] Typically, there are regions of normal-appearing aortic wall between the affected sites.[46] Contrast-enhanced MR angiography can also delineate the classic "skip lesions" in the great vessels and their branches[4] (Fig. 76-8).

Coarctation

Coarctation, the most common congenital anomaly of the thoracic aorta, refers to focal narrowing of the aortic lumen in the proximal descending thoracic aorta. It arises from a defect in the aortic media.[47,48] Coarctation usually occurs in the aortic isthmus, between the left

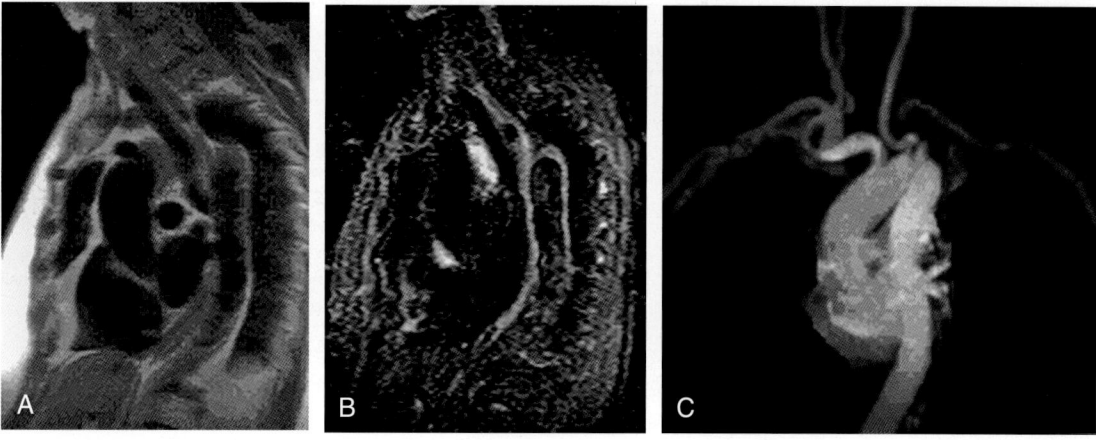

FIGURE 76-8

A and **B,** Sagittal HASTE images in a 72-year-old woman with aortitis show diffuse wall thickening of the descending aorta with prominent enhancement, suggesting active inflammation. **C,** Contrast-enhanced 3D angiogram shows occlusion of the proximal left subclavian artery, suggesting subclavian steal.

subclavian artery and the ductus.[48] It is often associated with tubular hypoplasia of the transverse portion of the aortic arch with dilated supraaortic vessels, causing upper extremity hypertension. Coarctation has been classified as postductal (adult) or preductal (infantile) depending on the site of narrowing, relative to the ductus or ligamentum arteriosum. Coarctation can be effectively treated by surgical correction or by percutaneous balloon dilatation. However, restenosis at the repair site is a frequent complication that has been reported in up to 42% of patients.[49]

Preoperative imaging study is used for evaluation of the extent and severity of the coarctation as well as visualization of collateral vessels.[1] Coarctation is best seen on the LAO ECG-gated T1-weighted SE sequence. Cine gradient-echo images obtained in the LAO projection are able to detect a hemodynamically significant flow jet through the coarctation; however, this flow jet is not always present and not 100% specific for hemodynamically significant coarctation.[50] 3D gadolinium-enhanced MR angiography can help determine the severity of coarctation by demonstrating collateral vessels. 3D gadolinium-enhanced MR angiography is useful in distinguishing high-grade coarctation from an interrupted aortic arch, because it can demonstrate whether the aortic arch and descending aorta are continuous or not. It has also been reported that direct visualization of collateral vessels by MRA and percent increase in flow from proximal to distal descending thoracic aorta as measured by velocity-encoded cine MRI are reliable indicators of hemodynamic significance.[49]

Mediastinal Veins

MRI is considered the primary modality in evaluating suspected mediastinal venous obstruction, providing more comprehensive information than catheter venog-raphy on central venous anatomy and blood flow.[51] MRI can detect and localize the extent of venous obstruction including the jugular, subclavian, and brachiocephalic veins, and the superior vena cava. It is also reported that MRI is useful in distinguishing intraluminal clot or tumor from extrinsic compression by adjacent mediastinal masses.

MR venography (MRV) is increasing its usefulness in clinical settings because placement and complications of central venous access devices are becoming more common. MRV is used to determine the presence of collaterals, the presence of thrombus, and venous patency. Although contrast venography is the gold standard, it can evaluate only a single draining system with each venipuncture. In contrast, MRV is a comprehensive, well-tolerated and highly accurate examination for visualizing all veins to help guide successful placement of central venous catheters and may be predictive of unsuccessful outcomes.[52] MRV is obtained utilizing 2D time-of-flight gradient-echo scans in the transverse plane for the internal jugular veins and the sagittal plane for the subclavian veins. Maximal intensity projections demonstrate the site of occlusion and visualize collaterals. It has been reported that 3D gadolinium-enhanced MRV is 100% sensitive, specific, and accurate in the diagnosis of abnormalities affecting the large central veins of the body.[53] It has also been reported that, in the evaluation of central venous thrombo-occlusive disease in the chest, gadolinium-enhanced MRV did not miss any findings seen on sonography, conventional venography, or CT. In addition, the complete extent of disease, regarding involvement of superior vena cava, subclavian, brachiocephalic, internal jugular, or axillary veins, was successfully characterized in 94% of patients.[54] However, interpretation of MR venography may be difficult in patients with extensive occlusion because of complex collateral drainage patterns[55-58] (Figs 76-9, 76-10).

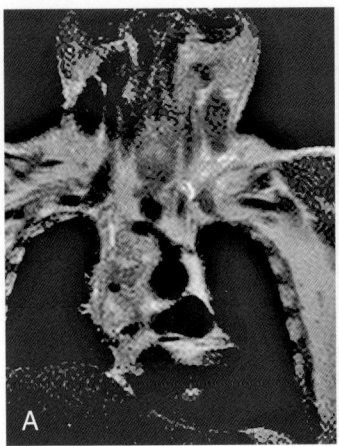 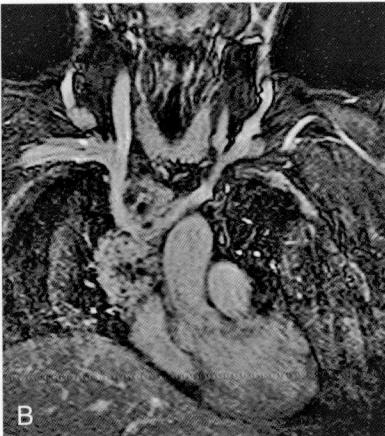

FIGURE 76-9

Coronal HASTE image (**A**) and contrast enhanced angiography (**B**) of a 48-year-old man with lung cancer and SVC syndrome demonstrate an irregular mass in the right upper lobe causing marked compression on the left brachiocephalic vein and obliteration of the SVC.

Pulmonary Vasculature

Pulmonary Hypertension

Pulmonary hypertension occurs when the pulmonary vascular flow increases to such an extent that the available extra channels are saturated, or because of vasoconstriction or structural change in the small pulmonary vessels, resulting in increased pulmonary arterial pressure and pulmonary vascular resistance. Pulmonary hypertension can be idiopathic or due to a variety of causes, including congenital and valvular heart diseases, obstructive or interstitial lung diseases, primary myocardial disease, pulmonary thromboembolic disease, arterial hypoxemia with hypercapnia, collagen vascular disease, parasitic disease, sickle-cell anemia, intravenous drug abuse, granulomatous lung disease, and chronic liver disease.[59]

Von Schulthess et al[60] first reported the use of MRI for noninvasive assessment of pulmonary hypertension and showed the ability of MR images to provide information on blood flow, suggesting a role for MR in assessing the severity of pulmonary hypertension. Cine gradient-echo sequences with high flow sensitivity and high temporal resolution can provide combined anatomic and dynamic flow-related information.[61] Cine MRI demonstrates dilatation of the central pulmonary arteries with attenuation of peripheral branches and loss of normal systolic distention and diastolic collapse in the proximal right pulmonary artery, indicating decreased pulmonary arterial compliance.[1] Velocity mapping with cine MRI shows inhomogeneity of flow in the main pulmonary arteries. It is also reported that velocity-encoded MRI can provide accurate pulmonary arterial blood flow measurements, with high correlation with the estimates of right-sided heart catheterization, making it possible to distinguish patients with high pulmonary vascular resistance from subjects with normal pulmonary vascular resistance.[62]

Vasculitis Involving the Pulmonary Arteries

MRI may be informative in depicting various vascular lesions associated with vasculitis, involving the pul-

monary arteries. Takayasu arteritis is a chronic inflammatory disease of unknown etiology affecting the aorta, its branches, as well as the pulmonary arteries. In a series of 77 patients, pulmonary arterial abnormalities were observed in 70% of patients and included dilatation (17%), thrombi (3%), and an abnormal tree-like appearance of the peripheral pulmonary vascular branches, indicating occlusive disease (66%).[44] Behçet disease is a multisystem, chronic relapsing vasculitis with a classic clinical triad of recurrent oral and genital ulcers, and a relapsing uveitis. Pleuropulmonary involvement occurs in about 5% of patients, predominantly males. Pulmonary vasculitis and thrombosis of pulmonary vessels may result in infarction, hemorrhage, or atelectasis. Hemoptysis is often a dominant and life-threatening complication, commonly caused by infarction and rupture of pulmonary artery aneurysms. Behçet's disease is the leading cause of pulmonary artery aneurysm.[63]

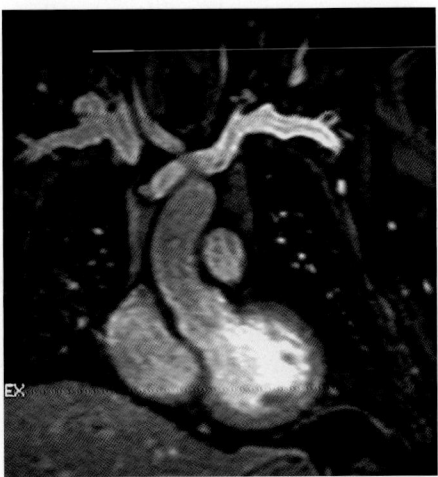

FIGURE 76-10

Contrast-enhanced coronal image of a 52-year-old man demonstrates a structure contiguous with the right central venous system at the confluence of the right subclavian vein and brachiocephalic vein with contrast enhancement, suggesting venous diverticulum.

Pulmonary artery aneurysms can be true or false, are often multiple, and can be either unilateral or bilateral. MRI is the modality of choice for detecting pulmonary artery aneurysms because these aneurysms may not be seen by conventional angiography if completely thrombosed. Subacute or chronic thrombus in pulmonary artery aneurysms may demonstrate high signal intensity on both T1- and T2-weighted images.[64] The aneurysms may become smaller or disappear with medical treatment. MRI is suitable for the follow-up as a noninvasive technique.

Pulmonary Artery Dissection

Pulmonary artery dissection is a rare but usually fatal complication of chronic pulmonary arterial hypertension. In a case reported by Stern et al,[65] SE MRI failed to show either the intimal flap or any intraluminal signal defects, but cine MRI outlined the intimal flap by demonstrating different signal intensities within the true and false lumens of the dissection.

Primary Pulmonary Artery Sarcoma

Primary pulmonary artery sarcoma is an uncommon cause of pulmonary arterial mass or occlusion. Growing within the pulmonary arterial lumen, the mass may initially be mistaken for chronic thrombi.[66-68] MRI is also useful in evaluating the extent of the tumors. Sarcomas demonstrate high signal intensity on T2-weighted images and show considerably greater degree of contrast enhancement than thrombi, which helps to differentiate sarcomas from thrombi (Fig. 76-11).[66-69]

Total and Partial Anomalous Pulmonary Venous Connection

MRI is useful in demonstrating partial anomalous pulmonary venous connection (PAPVC), as well as total anomalous pulmonary venous connection (TAPVC).[70,71] It has been reported in a retrospective review of 11 patients with PAPVC that MRI successfully identified all anomalous pulmonary venous connections.[71] In 13 patients with TAPVC, the combination of axial and coronal MRI visualized 96% of the individual anomalous pulmonary veins and 100% of the common pulmonary veins. Stenosis of a common pulmonary vein or the superior vena cava was detected by MRI in all cases[70] (Fig. 76-12).

Pulmonary Arteriovenous Malformations

MRI can be a rapid, noninvasive method to evaluate pulmonary arteriovenous malformations (AVMs), depicting the vascular nature of an atypical pulmonary nodule.[72,73] Breath-hold cine gradient-echo images clearly visualize AVMs, although pulsatile signal intensity changes during the cardiac cycle are seen.[73] It has been reported that 3D MR angiography is a promising technique in detecting pulmonary AVM, and in demonstrating the size and number of feeding arteries prior to treatment, although small (< 5 mm) AVMs may be more difficult to identify with this technique[74] (Fig. 76-13).

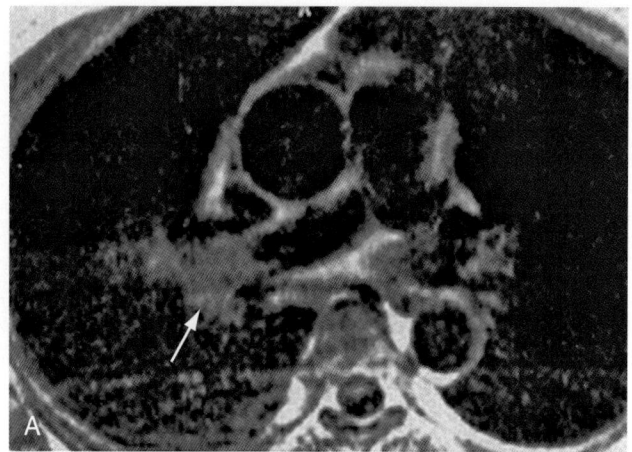
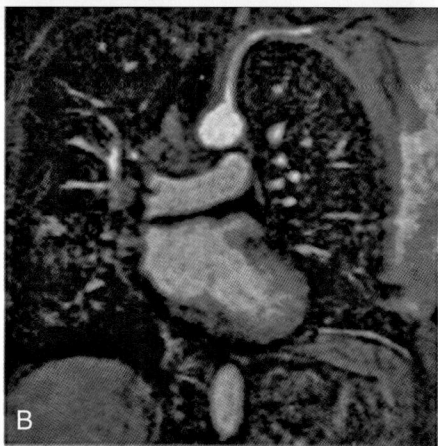

FIGURE 76-11

A, Axial T1-weighted spin-echo sequence demonstrates an irregular mass in the distal right main pulmonary artery *(arrow)* in a patient with pulmonary artery leiomyosarcoma. **B,** Coronal 3D MRA showed abrupt cutoff of right main pulmonary artery in the right pulmonary hilar region.

Pulmonary Embolism

Pulmonary embolism (PE) is one of the most frequently encountered clinical emergencies, and is a leading cause of morbidity and mortality accounting for 50,000 deaths per year in the USA.[75] Pulmonary embolism can be considered to be a complication of deep venous thrombosis (DVT), and 70% to 90% of patients with PE also have demonstrable deep leg vein thrombosis. Both pulmonary embolism and DVT are components of more general thromboembolic disorders.

Several diagnostic strategies have been employed for the diagnosis of PE, usually combining several modalities.[76] Conventional pulmonary angiography is regarded as the "gold standard" for the diagnosis of PE, and can be performed relatively safely with appropriate monitoring of the patients. However, it is invasive and can be accompanied by complications, especially for patients with severe pulmonary hypertension. Morbidity and mortality rates between 0.2% and 4% have been reported.[77-80]

Until recently, radionuclide ventilation-perfusion (V-P) scintigraphy has been the main imaging method used in the diagnosis of PE. It is noninvasive and serves as an

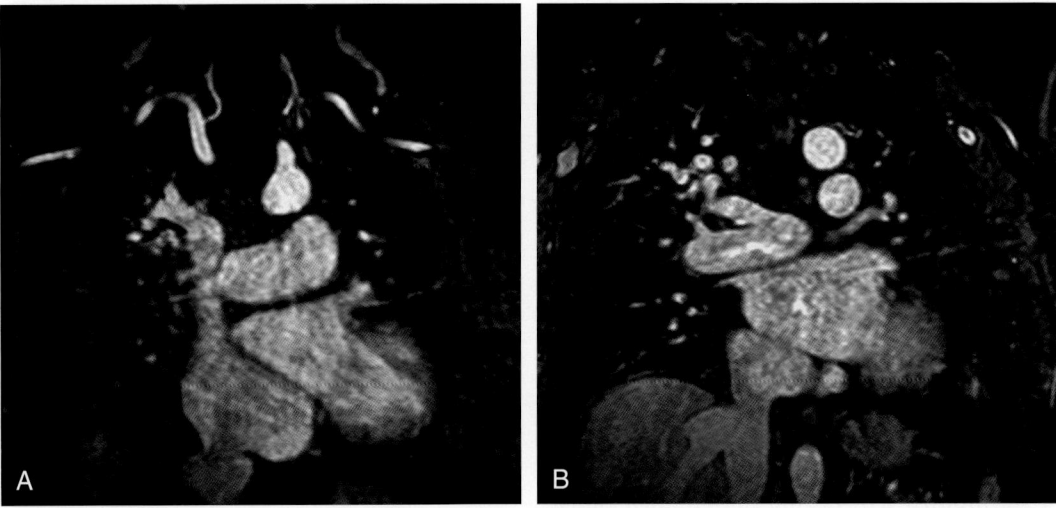

FIGURE 76-12

MR venogram of a 77-year-old woman shows the right upper lobe pulmonary vein draining into the posterior aspect of the SVC, compatible with partial anomalous pulmonary venous return.

excellent screening modality. However, a major limitation of V-P scintigraphy is the high percentage of nondiagnostic intermediate probability scans. It has been reported that even expert interpretation of V-P scans results in uncertain diagnosis in up to 73% of cases. In addition, only 41% of patients with documented pulmonary embolism had high-probability scans.[81-83]

Other methods employed relatively recently include plasma D-dimer (a breakdown product of fibrin) with high negative predictive value, ultrasonography of the leg veins to help prove the disease,[84,85] and, most prominently, the development of helical CT with CT-pulmonary angiography.[86,87] CT is accurate, rapid, and noninvasive. With contrast enhancement, it directly demonstrates intraluminal clot as a filling defect. In addition, in patients without PE, CT is often able to provide alternative diagnoses.[88-92] With the recent advent of multi-detector row CT, it is now possible to evaluate subsegmental pulmonary arteries.[93]

MRI has the potential to be a promising modality in visualizing intravascular filling defects and in providing information about the regional distribution of ventilation and perfusion.[94] Early studies using electrocardiography (ECG)-gated SE MRI showed that the embolus is demonstrated as an intraluminal lesion with intermediate to moderately high signal intensity.[95-97] On MRI, it may often be difficult to differentiate emboli and a low–flow-related signal, which is frequently seen in patients with pulmonary hypertension.

Because of the inherent limitations due to respiratory and cardiac motion artifacts, gradient-recalled echo imaging techniques during suspended respiration have been applied, including cine gradient-recalled acquisition in the steady state (GRASS), which is sensitive to blood flow and typically demonstrates the clot as a low-signal intensity area.[10,98] The spatial modulation of magnetization (SPAMM) technique produces tagging stripes

on MR images, and helps to distinguish slow–flow-related signal from embolism.[99]

With the advancements in MR techniques, MR pulmonary angiography has become an important imaging method.[69,100-102] It has been reported that MR angiography is as accurate as CT angiography in demonstrating lobar and segmental emboli.[103] In a study by Erdman et al,[95] MRI had a sensitivity of 90% and a specificity of 77%, whereas in a study by Gupta et al,[103] MR had a sensitivity of 85% and a specificity of 96%. MR demonstrates perfusion and ventilation of the lung parenchyma, which will be discussed in detail later. With a combination of IV bolus administration of gadolinium-diethylene-triamine penta-acetic acid (Gd-DTPA), 3D MR pulmonary angiography with breath-hold is able to provide detailed pulmonary vascular anatomy including subsegmental branches (Fig. 76-14).[104-106]

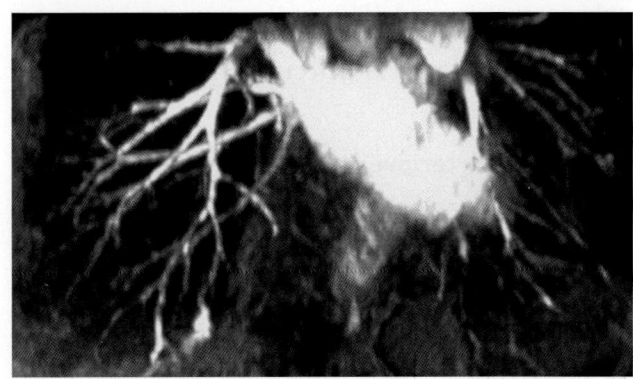

FIGURE 76-13

Contrast-enhanced 3D MRA of a 63-year-old woman with arteriovenous malformation demonstrate serpiginously enhancing lesion at the right posterior lung base with a pair of feeding pulmonary arteries and a draining vein.

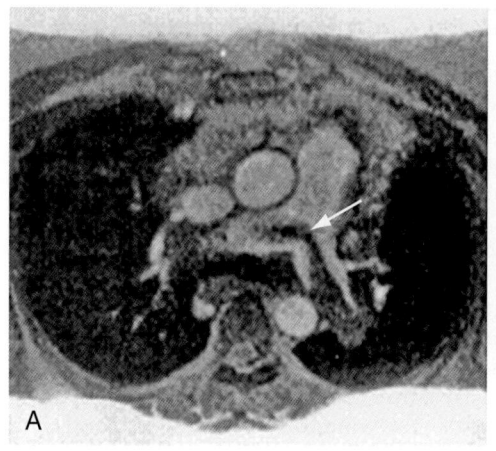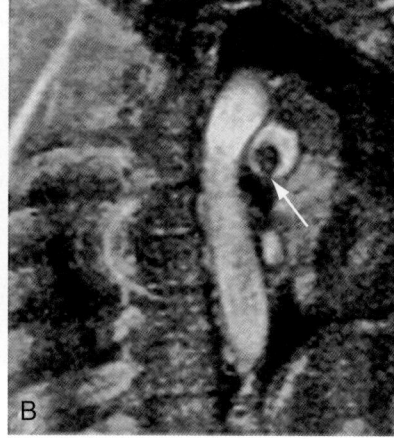

FIGURE 76-14

A, Axial gradient-echo image demonstrates a saddle embolus extending into both right and left main pulmonary arteries from the main pulmonary artery *(arrow).* **B,** Oblique sagittal 3D MRA shows an embolus in the left main pulmonary artery *(arrow).*

Although currently playing a limited role, MRI is considered able to remain a competitive modality for diagnosis of pulmonary embolism, because it:

1. does not require radiation or administration of iodinated contrast media
2. can evaluate the pulmonary vasculature and deep veins in one study
3. can evaluate pulmonary perfusion and ventilation as well as the pulmonary vasculature.[1]

LUNG CANCER AND OTHER NEOPLASMS OF THE LUNG

Lung Cancer

Currently, CT is the first modality of choice for evaluation of patients with lung cancer. Compared to MRI, CT is less costly and offers better spatial resolution with a shorter examination time. In addition, CT is more sensitive in detecting calcification. On the other hand, MRI has some advantages due to its superiority in tissue contrast, multiplanar capability, and demonstration of thoracic vessels. MRI has been utilized in lung cancer assessment in selected cases, including superior sulcus (Pancoast) tumors, tumors invading the vessels, medi-

astinum, pericardium, chest wall or spine.[1,107] It has been reported that in selected patients, MRI is more accurate in separating stage IIIa (generally resectable) and stage IIIb (generally unresectable) tumors.[1,108] In lung cancer patients with iodinated contrast material intolerance, MRI should be considered in addition to CT for assessing hilar and mediastinal involvement and nodal metastases. Recently, there have been attempts to characterize solitary pulmonary nodules using contrast-enhanced dynamic MRI, correlating the findings with the necessity for further evaluation and treatment,[109] or with tumor vascularity and prognosis.[110]

This section describes the role of MRI in evaluation of: 1. superior sulcus tumors; 2. mediastinal lymphadenopathy; 3. secondary changes due to atelectasis, penumonitis, surgery and radiation; 4. mediastinal and chest wall invasion; 5. distant metastasis; and 6. solitary pulmonary nodules with recent advancement.

Superior Sulcus (Pancoast) Tumors

Superior sulcus or Pancoast tumor refers to lung cancers that invade the lower cord of brachial plexus and sympathetic chain, resulting in arm and shoulder pain and Horner syndrome. MRI is superior to CT in evaluating the extent of this type of tumor due to its multiplanar imaging capabilities and better tissue contrast (Fig. 76-15).[111]

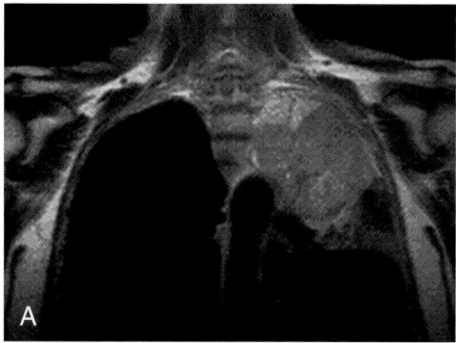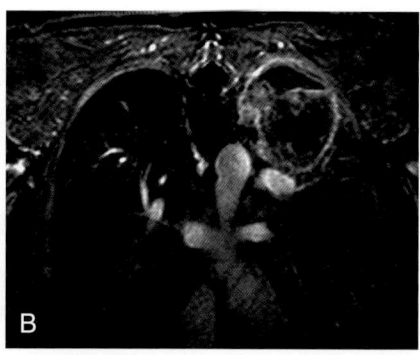

FIGURE 76-15

A, Coronal HASTE image in a 70-year-old woman with lung cancer and left shoulder pain shows a heterogeneous mass invading the mediastinum and abutting the aortic arch and the paraspinal soft-tissues. The mass also abuts the chest wall superiorly and laterally. **B,** Subtraction image shows slight asymmetric enhancement of left apical chest wall, suggesting invasion.

Mediastinal Lymphadenopathy

Accurate nodal staging is directly related to surgical indication and thus, extremely important in evaluating and managing lung cancer patients. MRI and CT have been reported to have similar accuracy in detecting mediastinal lymph node metastasis, with a sensitivity of approximately 65% and a specificity of approximately 72%, but lesser values have also been reported.[112] For both modalities, diagnosis is based on the short-axis diameter of the lymph nodes, with a threshold of 10 mm. The limitations of this diagnostic method include the fact that: 1. some reactive lymph nodes can be greater than 10 mm without tumor involvement and some lymph nodes with small metastases can be smaller than 10 mm; and 2. residual mediastinal masses may persist during or after therapy, without any viable tumor. It has been reported that 17% of lymph nodes smaller than 1.5 cm contained metastases and more than 33% of nodes measuring 2 to 4 cm were reactive nodes without tumor. Thus, there indeed is a limitation in size-based evaluation of lymph nodes. Fluorodeoxyglucose-positron emission tomography (FDG-PET) imaging is one solution to this problem, although false positives can occur due to active infection or inflammation.

There have been attempts to utilize MRI for better identification of metastatic lymph nodes. In one study with nine patients by Laissy et al,[113] metastatic mediastinal lymph nodes demonstrated peak enhancement at 60 to 80 s, whereas granulomatous and anthracotic lymph nodes displayed no peak within 6 minutes.

Recently, use of short time inversion recovery (STIR) MRI has been discussed to differentiate between metastatic and nonmetastatic lymph nodes.[107,114-117] Takenaka et al reported that using the ratios of signal intensity of lymph nodes to 0.9% saline phantoms, sensitivity, specificity, and accuracy for differentiating metastatic lymph node from nonmetastatic lymph node per patient were 100%, 75%, and 88%, respectively.[118]

Secondary Changes Due to Atelectasis, Pneumonitis, Surgery and Radiation

MRI can be used to distinguish between central tumor and adjacent atelectasis.[1,107] On contrast-enhanced T1-weighted images, atelectasis normally shows higher and earlier peak signal intensity compared to tumor due to a better blood supply. However, this relationship changes if the tumor obstructs the pulmonary artery. On T2-weighted images, postobstructive atelectasis or pneumonitis show higher signal intensity than tumor.[107] MRI is also capable of demonstrating tumor necrosis after radiation therapy. Gadolinum-enhanced imaging improves the detection of viable tumor and necrosis. Some studies suggest T2-weighted MRI may be helpful in differentiating recurrent tumor from fibrosis, with mature fibrosis being hypointense and tumor tissue being hyperintense. Although CT is the modality of choice for routine follow-up, MRI may add some useful information when CT is nondiagnostic or equivocal.[119]

Mediastinal and Chest Wall Invasion

The sensitivity and specificity of CT in evaluating mediastinal invasion of lung cancer has been reported to range from 40% to 84%, and 57% to 94%, respectively.[120-130] On the other hand, MRI was reported to be significantly more accurate than CT in the diagnosis of mediastinal invasion.[131,132] Recently, multiphase 3D contrast-enhanced MRA with cardiac synchronization was reported to increase the diagnostic accuracy of hilar or mediastinal invasion of lung cancer, with sensitivity and specificity of 89% to 90% and 83% to 87%, respectively.[120]

Chest wall invasion by lung cancer can also be demonstrated by MRI, with a sensitivity of 90% and a specificity of 86%.[133] Owing to its better spatial and time resolutions and multiplanar capability, MRI is superior to CT in showing the extent of chest wall invasion, especially for superior sulcus tumors. Signs of invasion include demonstration of soft-tissue extension into the chest wall, the loss of the subpleural fat stripe between pleura and cancer, and bone destruction. Cine MRI may be used to depict chest wall involvement that is difficult to diagnose by routine examinations. Cine MR images were obtained at an orthogonal section to the chest wall during slow, deep breathing every 1.2 s with fast spoiled GRASS sequence, and were analyzed with cine-loop display. In a study of 11 patients, eight cases were correctly diagnosed by this technique.[134]

Distant Metastasis

Distant metastasis is frequently associated with lung cancer, and can involve many organs. The adrenal glands are one of the frequent sites of metastatic spread in patients with lung cancer. Adrenal masses are detected in up to 21% of routine CT studies for lung cancer staging.[1] In patients with non-small cell lung cancer, isolated adrenal mass is more likely to be benign than metastatic.[135,136] MR study with chemical shift imaging is useful in differentiating adrenal adenomas by demonstrating fat (or lipid) within the adrenal mass.[137] The adenomas demonstrate lower signal intensity on out-of-phase images than on in-phase images, whereas adrenal masses without lipid, such as metastasis, do not show signal loss. With the chemical shift technique, the reported sensitivity and specificity in differentiating adenomas from metastases ranges from 81% to 100% and 94% to 100%, respectively.[138-144]

Recently, whole-body MRI techniques with a moving table platform have been applied in patients with breast cancer to detect distant metastasis,[115] in patients with metastatic cancer with unknown primary,[116] and in patients with bone metastasis.[145] Whole-body MRI can be a single cost-effective imaging test, but its role in the evaluation of lung cancer patients remains to be determined.

Other Neoplasms of the Lung

Bronchial carcinoid is an uncommon tumor of the lung, comprising only 1% to 2% of all lung tumors. Most

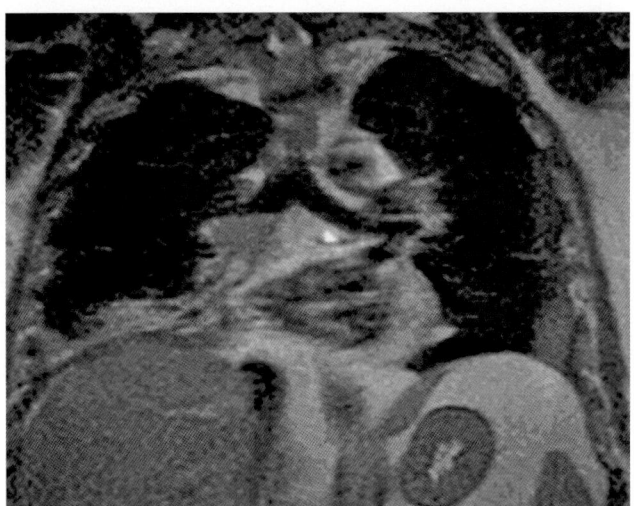

FIGURE 76-16

Coronal HASTE image of a 54-year-old man with bronchial carcinoid tumor demonstrates a well-circumscribed soft-tissue mass, involving the right main stem bronchus and bronchus intermedius.

carcinoids primarily present as endobronchial lesions. Chest radiograph and CT are the preferred imaging modalities. MRI may be useful in differentiating mucoid-filled bronchi from centrally located tumors based on the signal intensities on T2-weighted images[146] (Fig. 76-16).

Mucinous cystadenocarcinoma, an extremely rare tumor of the lung, demonstrates a cystic mass with thin septum. MRI helps to demonstrate mucinous material in the cyst as a high signal on T2-weighted imaging and the septum within the cyst as a low-signal intensity structure[147] (Fig. 76-17).

MEDIASTINUM

Anterior Mediastinal Compartment

Thyroid

On MRI, the normal thyroid gland reveals low signal intensity on T1-weighted images and intermediate signal intensity on T2-weighted images.[148] MRI is indicated for evaluating large thyroid masses, especially mediastinal extension of large goiters.[149,150] Axial, coronal, and sagittal images 3 mm thick using T1- and T2-weighted images with or without gadolinium are used.[151]

A multinodular goiter is an aggregate of multiple discrete nodules of either colloid or true adenomas. Up to 75% to 80% of the mediastinal goiters extend from the neck into the superoanterior mediastinum, with up to 25% extending posteriorly and superiorly.[152] On MR, multinodular goiters exhibit heterogeneous signal intensity on T1- and T2-weighted imaging. MRI is particularly useful in showing the extent of the goiter and displacement of neighboring structures, providing useful information for surgical planning. However, differentiation of benign and malignant thyroid masses is not possible based on MRI.[153] The frequency of a carcinoma evolving in the multinodular goiter is approximately 7.5%.[154]

Parathyroid

Most patients with primary hyperparathyroidism can be treated successfully with surgery without prior imaging evaluation.[1] MRI is useful in assessing patients who remain hypercalcemic even after the initial surgery.[155-157] MRI and isotope scintigraphy are used for presurgical localization of ectopic parathyroid glands, which can

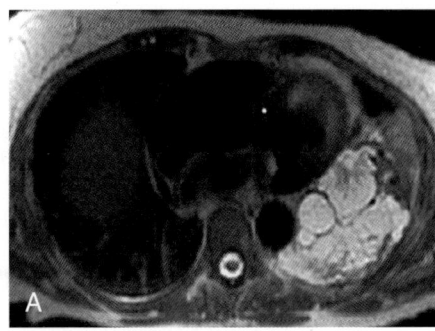

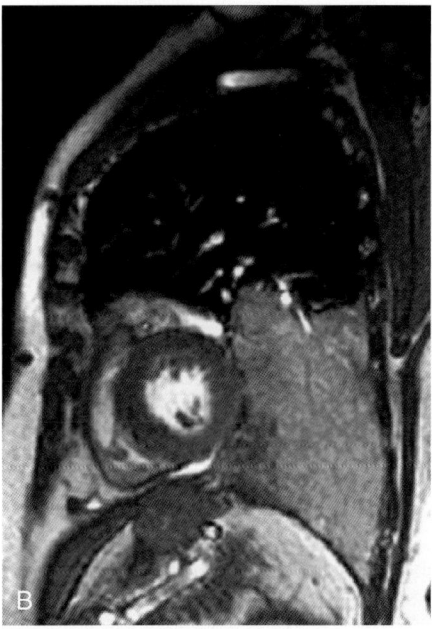

FIGURE 76-17

A, Axial HASTE image of an 80-year-old woman shows a mass in the left lower lobe which demonstrates high signal intensity with septation, suggesting a fluid/mucinous filled air-space disease. **B,** Sagittal TrueFISP image shows the mass infiltrating the left lower lobe. Surgical resection was performed, and the pathology showed mucinous adenocarcinoma of the lung.

be located anywhere in the mediastinum.[158-160] The parathyroid tissue is typically hypo- to isointense relative to muscle on T1-weighted images, and hyperintense on T2-weighted MR images. Fat-suppressed MR images and gadolinium-based contrast agent injections may be useful for better visualization of parathyroid tissue. MRI with gadolinium and fat suppression is also indicated to evaluate parathyroid carcinoma, which comprises less than 1% of parathyroid tumors, in presurgical assessment and follow-up for recurrence.

Teratoma and Other Germ Cell Neoplasms

Teratoma and other germ cell neoplasms may contain fat, calcifications, and cystic components, which help to narrow differential diagnosis. These components are characterized by signal intensities on MRI (Fig. 76-18).[161]

Thymic Tumors

The thymus is a triangular- or bilobar-shaped organ located in the anterior mediastinum. It reaches its maximum weight in puberty and subsequently undergoes fatty involution. The entities that can cause mass lesions in the thymus include thymoma (invasive or noninvasive), thymic cyst, thymic hyperplasia, thymolipoma, thymic cancer, and thymic carcinoid. Thymic tissue represents nonspecific MR signal intensities, but most

commonly demonstrates low to intermediate signal on T1-weighted images and high signal on T2-weighted images.[162] MRI is used to demonstrate the extent of the tumor, the relationship to vascular structures, and soft-tissue invasion. Thymic masses containing fat suggest the diagnosis of thymolipoma[163,164] (Fig. 76-19).

Lymphoma and Other Diseases

MRI is used along with CT to stage and monitor mediastinal lymphoma.[165] Lymphoma is represented by homogeneous, relatively low signal intensity on T2-weighted MRI. MRI is adequate for demonstrating the relationship between the mass and vessels, which is useful for radiation planning.[166,167] MR signal intensity changes after therapy can also play a role in the follow-up:

- Low signal intensity on T2-weighted images precludes relapse in most cases[168]
- High signal intensity on T2-weighted images within the first 6 months of therapy is a nonspecific finding but after 6 months it suggests recurrent lymphoma.

MR can provide an overall accuracy similar to that of gadolinium-67 scintigraphy.[165,169-171]

Castleman's disease is a rare entity that manifests with nodal enlargement, and can involve the mediastinum.[172] The nodal masses may contain calcifications and enhance after IV contrast administration.

Fibrosing mediastinitis is a rare, benign disorder caused by proliferation of fibrous tissue within the mediastinum, which can show a localized pattern of calcified lymph nodes or a diffuse pattern.[173,174] Because the mass can encase and constrict the mediastinal vessels, MRI is helpful in assessing vascular patency.

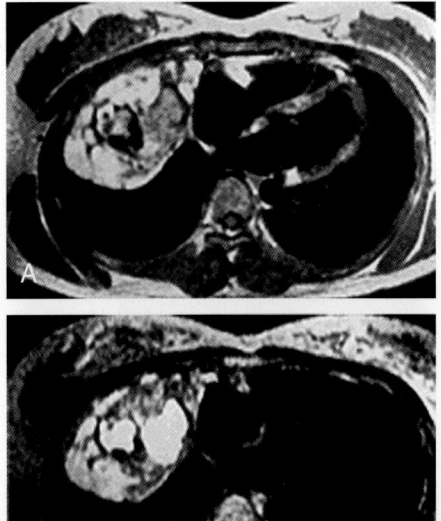

FIGURE 76-18

A, Axial spin-echo T1-weighted image demonstrates a well-delineated mass lesion in the anterior mediastinum, which contains fat and dark signal, indicating teeth. **B,** Axial T2-weighted spin-echo image demonstrates a well-delineated anterior mediastinal mass. Note the teeth as a dark signal area and cystic component. The diagnosis of teratoma is possible from these MR images.

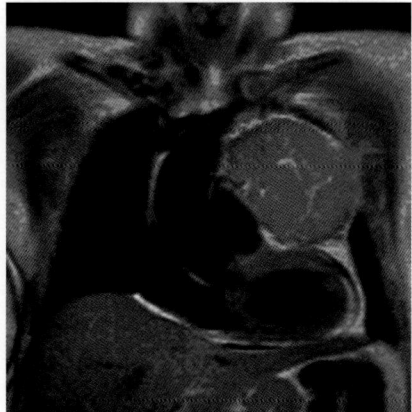

FIGURE 76-19

A coronal HASTE image in a 66-year-old woman with thymoma demonstrates a large, smoothly marginated anterior mediastinal mass with slightly higher signal intensity than muscle. Note a lobulated internal architecture separated by linear areas of low signal intensity. A well-delineated fat plane separating the mass from the transverse aorta and the pulmonary artery suggests absence of vascular invasion.

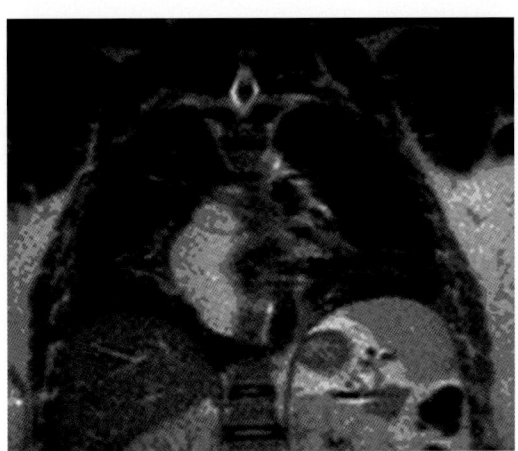

FIGURE 76-20

A coronal HASTE image of a 45-year-old woman with bronchogenic cyst shows a cystic mass with bright signal intensity with longitudinal extension.

Middle Mediastinal Compartment and Paracardiac Space

While infectious and neoplastic lymphadenopathies are the most common space-occupying lesions in the middle mediastinum, these lesions have been discussed previously with mediastinal lymphadenopathy and lymphomas.

Benign congenital cystic lesions are commonly encountered in the middle mediastinal compartment, including bronchogenic cysts (frequently near the carina), esophageal duplication cysts (near the esophagus), and pericardial cysts.[175] Mediastinal cystic masses are well-marginated, round, epithelium-lined lesions with fluid, which exhibit various signal intensities depending on content.[176] Pure serous fluid has a low signal intensity on T1-weighted images and high signal intensity on T2-weighted images, just like water. Cysts with protein-rich content demonstrate higher signal intensities on T1- and lower intensities on T2-weighted images. When hemorrhagic, the mass may exhibit complex signal intensities depending on the age of hemorrhage. In the protein-rich or hemorrhagic cyst, CT images may demonstrate high attenuation, making it difficult to determine if the lesion is solid or cystic. In these situations, MRI may be helpful for definite characterization of the mass and its content. With multiplanar capability, MRI is superior in demonstrating the lesion in relation to neighboring organs and vessels, and can assist in surgical planning[177] (Figs 76-20, 76-21).

Other benign masses in the middle mediastinum include thymolipomas, hemangiomas, Morgagni hernias, and those associated with the pericardium. Hemangiomas demonstrate bright signal intensity on T2-weighted images and show extensive growth between the normal structures in the mediastinum (Fig. 76-22). Pericardial lesions include pericardial fat pad; pericardial cyst; pericardial metastasis; and primary tumors of the pericardium, including fibroma, lipoma, lymphangiomas, hemangiomas, mesothelioma, and liposarcoma.[178]

Posterior Mediastinal Compartment

Various entities can involve this compartment, including primary and metastatic neoplasms, congenital lesions and infection. These lesions are mainly located in paraspinal or periaortic areas.

Neurogenic tumors are commonly encountered in the paraspinal area. Schwannomas and neurofibromas can manifest as a dumbell-shaped paraspinal mass, with one component within the spinal canal and the other component expanding the neural foramen. The MR signal intensities of schwannomas depend on the types of tissue they contain; myxoid tissue is hyperintense on T2-weighted images, cellular tissue is hypointense on both T1- and T2-weighted images, and solid fibrous tissue enhances on contrast-enhanced images.[179] Neurofibromas tend to demonstrate high signal intensity on T2-weighted MR images and can be multiple and associated with neurofibromatosis. Ganglioneuroma and neuroblastomas should be considered in younger patients.

Another cause of paraspinal mass is osteomyelitis, which may result in a paraspinal pyogenic or tuberculous abscess. Further differential diagnosis includes extramedullary hematopoiesis. MRI is useful in demonstrating the extent of these lesions in relation to the spinal structures.

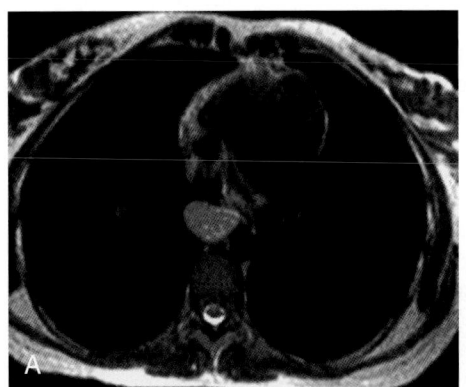 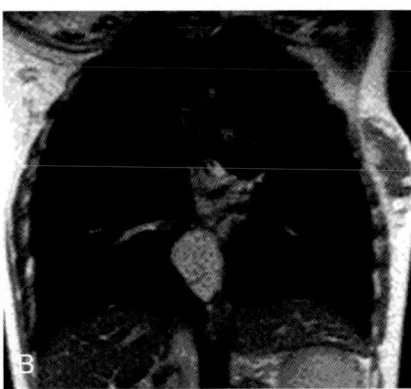

FIGURE 76-21

A, Axial HASTE image of a 21-year-old woman with an esophageal duplication cyst shows a well-circumscribed distal para-esophageal mass with high signal intensity both on T1- (not shown) and T2-weighted images, reflecting the proteinaceous content of the cyst. **B,** Coronal HASTE image shows a thin septation within this lesion.

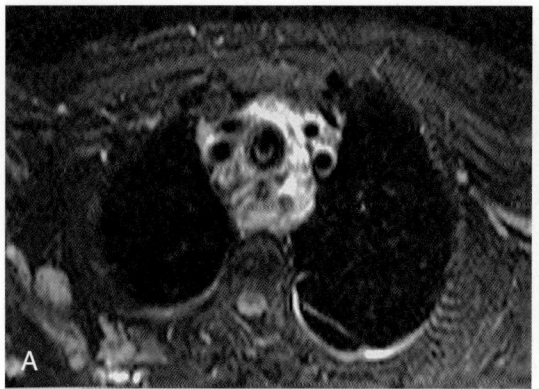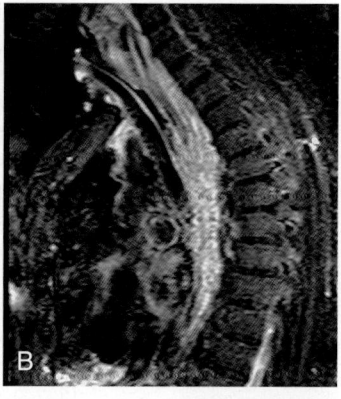

FIGURE 76-22

A, Axial STIR image of a 74-year-old woman with hemangiomatosis demonstrates an extensive lesion with a vascular-like structure presenting a bright signal in the anterior and superior mediastinum as well as in the right chest wall. **B,** Sagittal STIR images demonstrate the mediastinal lesion extending posteriorly and inferiorly, along with aorta and esophagus.

Periaortic masses include lymphoma, metastatic lymph nodes, lung cancer with direct extension, and rarely, paraganglioma. In these lesions MRI is superior to CT in localizing the tumor and defining its relationship to neighboring structures.

PLEURA

For evaluation of pleural diseases, chest radiography, CT scans, and ultrasonography remain the primary imaging modalities,[180,181] but MRI may provide useful information in selected patients.[1]

The characterization of the pleural fluid collections, either transudates or exudates, can be determined by MRI to some extent. Exudative pleural effusions show a higher degree of enhancement after IV gadolinium-based contrast administration than transudative pleural effusions.[182] Diffusion-weighted imaging with an echo-planar imaging sequence may differentiate exudates from transudates based on the apparent diffusion coefficient (ADC) value.[183] High signal intensity on T1-weighted images identifies a chylothorax.[184] Subacute and chronic hematoma can be recognized in the pleural space based on its signal characteristics.[184] These noninvasive techniques can be used to characterize pleural fluid collection and may obviate the need for thoracentesis, especially in high-risk patients.

MRI is also useful in detection and evaluation of patients with malignancy. It has been reported that MRI can differentiate benign (low signal intensity) from malignant (high signal intensity) pleural nodules with T2-weighted and proton density-weighted images with a specificity of 87%.[185-187] The most common pleural tumor is metastasis. In patients with pleural mesothelioma, MRI is helpful in distinguishing tumor tissue from adjacent effusions and showing extension of the tumor into the mediastinum, chest wall, opposite pleural space, and into the abdomen.[188]

DIAPHRAGM

MR imaging is able to display diaphragmatic anatomy and pathology in sagittal and coronal planes, which helps to demonstrate the lesions.[189] MR can demonstrate tumor invasion into the diaphragm or diaphragmatic hernias or rupture.[190] MRI has not been suitable for acute traumatic patients, but with the development of faster imaging sequences, improved MR-compatible physiologic monitoring, and improved life-support equipment, MRI can now be applied to most hemodynamically stable trauma patients.[191] MRI is also able to assess diaphragm motion and may provide some physiologic information.

CHEST WALL AND THORACIC OUTLET

As described previously, MRI is the primary modality for demonstrating chest wall invasion by primary lung cancer or by infectious diseases such as actinomycosis.

A variety of benign and malignant neoplasms of vascular, neurogenic, osseous or mesenchymal origin can occur in the chest wall. The most common mesenchymal tumor is lipoma, in which MRI, as well as CT scans, can make a specific diagnosis.[192] Other common benign tumors include hemangioma and neurogenic tumors. Malignant tumors include liposarcoma, leiomyosarcoma, rhabdomyosarcoma, angiosarcoma, and chondro/osteosarcoma. MRI shows tumor extension and is helpful in planning biopsy or surgery.

Primitive neuroectodermal (or Askin) tumor of the chest wall is a rare malignancy that occurs in young adults.[193,194] It typically shows a heterogeneous signal intensity on T1- and T2-weighted MR images, and can invade the adjacent lung. Another rare malignancy seen in young adults is dermatofibrosarcoma, which is located in the skin and has a high propensity for local invasion and recurrence. MRI findings are nonspecific and may include heterogeneous foci of hemorrhage, myxoid change, or necrosis.[195]

The thoracic outlet includes the interscalene triangle, the costoclavicular space, and the retropectoralis minor space (subcoracoid tunnel). Narrowing of these spaces with neurovascular compression causes thoracic outlet syndrome. It has been reported that sagittal and coronal MRI with the postural maneuver may be helpful in demonstrating the location and cause of arterial or nervous compressions.[196,197]

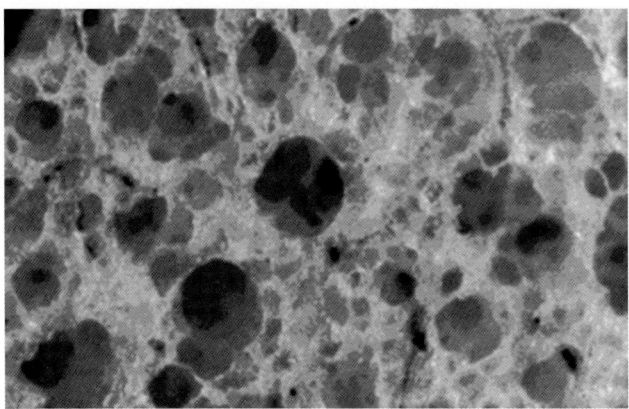

FIGURE 76-23

3D geometric structure of alveoli and alveolar walls, which have different magnetic susceptibilities, thus dephasing the signal from the lung parenchyma. The human lung contains approximately 300 million anatomic alveoli measuring 200-300 μm in diameter, with a total surface area of 50 to 70 m². *(Reprinted from European Journal of Radiology, Vol. 29, Hatabu H, Chen Q, Stock KW, et al, Fast MR imaging of the lung, pages 114-132, Copyright 1999, with permission from the Association of University Radiologists.)*

PULMONARY FUNCTIONAL IMAGING

Recent development of fast MRI techniques has opened a new window for functional assessment of the lung.[198] The lung is an organ of gas exchange, which acquired its unique morphology through the evolution of animals and humans[199] (Fig. 76-23). For this specific function of incorporating oxygen into blood from the atmosphere

and excreting carbon dioxide, blood flow (perfusion), air flow (ventilation), lung motion, diaphragm, and chest wall (biomechanics) must be exquisitely coordinated. MRI provides a noninvasive technique to observe, record, and quantify these pulmonary functions without the use of ionizing radiation.

The difficulties in MRI of the lung have been posed by lung morphology and physiological motion. The lung has a proton density of only 10% to 20%, which is much lower than that of other organs. The lung moves according to respiratory and cardiac motions. Moreover, multiple air-soft-tissue interfaces generated by its unique 3D structure of alveoli result in heterogeneous magnetic susceptibility, which produce large local magnetic field gradients.[200-202] The local gradients act to dephase the MR signal from the lung.[203,204] Therefore, initial preliminary studies focused on pulmonary vasculature rather than lung parenchyma.[69,205] Fast MR imaging techniques with a very short TE are overcoming the problem of inhomogeneous magnetic susceptibility.[206-208] In addition, the single-shot fast SE sequence can now depict the lung parenchyma, providing a platform for functional imaging of the lung.[209,210]

Pulmonary perfusion can be assessed using T1-weighted ultra-short TE sequence and contrast agents[104,211,212] (Fig. 76-24). By fitting a portion of the time-intensity curve to a gamma variate function, flow parameters such as peak time, apparent mean transient time, and blood volume are calculated.[213] Such parametric analysis of pulmonary perfusion can be performed pixel by pixel, which generates a map of regional perfusion parameters throughout the lung.[214] The natural extension of the 2D technique is breath-hold contrast-enhanced 3D MR

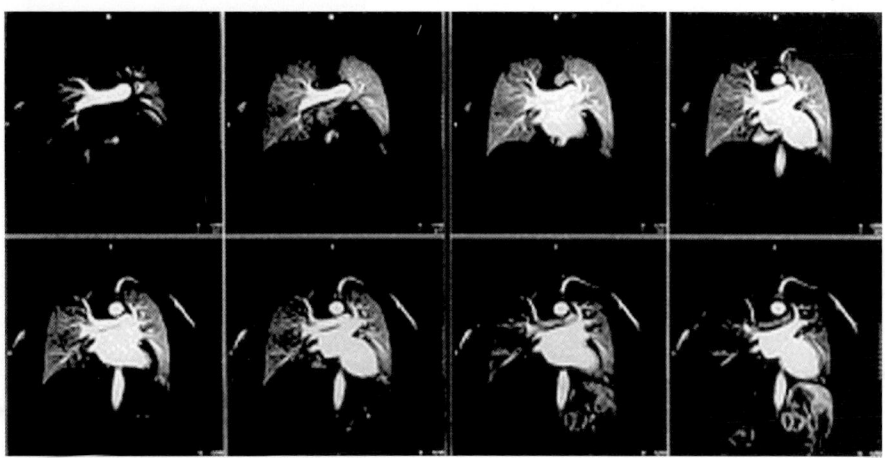

FIGURE 76-24

Dynamic contrast-enhanced MR imaging of pulmonary perfusion in a normal volunteer using an ultra-short TE inversion recovery (IR)-turbo Fast Low Angle Shot (FLASH) sequence (TR/TE/TI/flip angle = 3.5 ms/1.4 ms/400 ms/8 degrees, 10 mm section thickness, 128 × 128 matrix, 42 cm field of view). 5 ml of Gd DTPA was administered over 1 s. Eight consecutive coronal images are shown from the total of 45 coronal images obtained every 1 s in the plane of the pulmonary hila. For the purpose of image subtraction, a mask image was used (acquired prior to vascular enhancement). The pulmonary arterial tree was visualized beyond the segmental branches followed by a faint diffuse blush of lung parenchyma. Diffuse gradual increase in signal intensity of the lung parenchyma was observed. *(From Hatabu H, Tadamura E, Levin DL, et al: Quantitative assessment of pulmonary perfusion with dynamic contrast-enhanced MRI. Magn Reson Med 42:1033-1038, 1999, with permission.)*

with short TR and TE, which enables simultaneous evaluation of pulmonary perfusion and vasculature.[215] With the advancement of parallel imaging techniques, 3D pulmonary perfusion mapping is now feasible[216-218] (Fig. 76-25). Preliminary reports have shown the feasibility of the MR perfusion technique in the evaluation of patients with pulmonary embolism,[219] unilateral lung transplantation,[220] solitary pulmonary nodule, and arteriovenous malformation.[109,221,222]

Another approach to the evaluation of pulmonary perfusion is utilization of arterial spin labeling (ASL) techniques, which use blood water as an endogenous, freely diffusible tracer. The pulsed ASL method called signal targeting alternating radiofrequency (STAR) uses pulsed magnetic labeling of arterial blood flowing into the organ of target.[223] For image acquisition, a modified fast gradient-echo or single-shot turbo SE pulse sequence is used instead of echo-planar imaging, which is more prone to magnetic susceptibility artifacts in the lung. Within each breath-holding period, two sets of images are acquired. In only one set of images, an RF pulse is applied to the right ventricle and main pulmonary artery in order to invert the magnetization of blood within those structures. After an inflow period (TI), which is on the order of a few hundred milliseconds to seconds, data are acquired using fast gradient-echo or single-shot, half-Fourier, turbo SE (HASTE) pulse sequences. The subtraction of the two images results in the perfusion image.[224-226] The merits of this technique lie in its potential to provide a noninvasive method for the absolute measurement of pulmonary perfusion by the application of a mathematical model[226] (Fig. 76-26). Mai et al have reported on the application of flow-sensitive alternating inversion recovery (FAIR) with an extra radiofrequency pulse (FAIRER).[227-230] Pulmonary perfusion imaging using a steady-state ASL method has also been reported.[231-233] Subtraction of diastolic and systolic HASTE images has also been utilized to show pulmonary perfusion.[234,235]

Oxygen modulates MR signals of blood and fluid through two different mechanisms: 1. the paramagnetic property of deoxyhemoglobin; and 2. the paramagnetic property of molecular oxygen itself.[236,237] Molecular oxygen is weakly paramagnetic with a magnetic moment of 2.8 Bohr magnetrons.[238,239] Young et al demonstrated reduction in T1 relaxation time of blood at 0.15 T after inhalation of oxygen.[237,239] After inhalation of 100% oxygen, the concentration of dissolved oxygen in arterial blood increases by approximately five times. They demonstrated the feasibility of oxygen inhalation to evaluate regional pulmonary ventilation and examined the effect of oxygen inhalation on relaxation times in various tissues.[240,241] Signal changes from the right upper quarter of the right lung following alternate administration of 10 L/minute air (21% oxygen) and 100% oxygen via a mask were demonstrated. Calculated T1 values of the lung with various TIs before and after administration of oxygen were 1336 ± 46 ms and 1162 ± 33 ms, respectively. The observed change in T1 value confirms that molecular oxygen can be used as an effective T1 shortening agent in the assessment of ventilation in humans. Ventilation demonstrated by

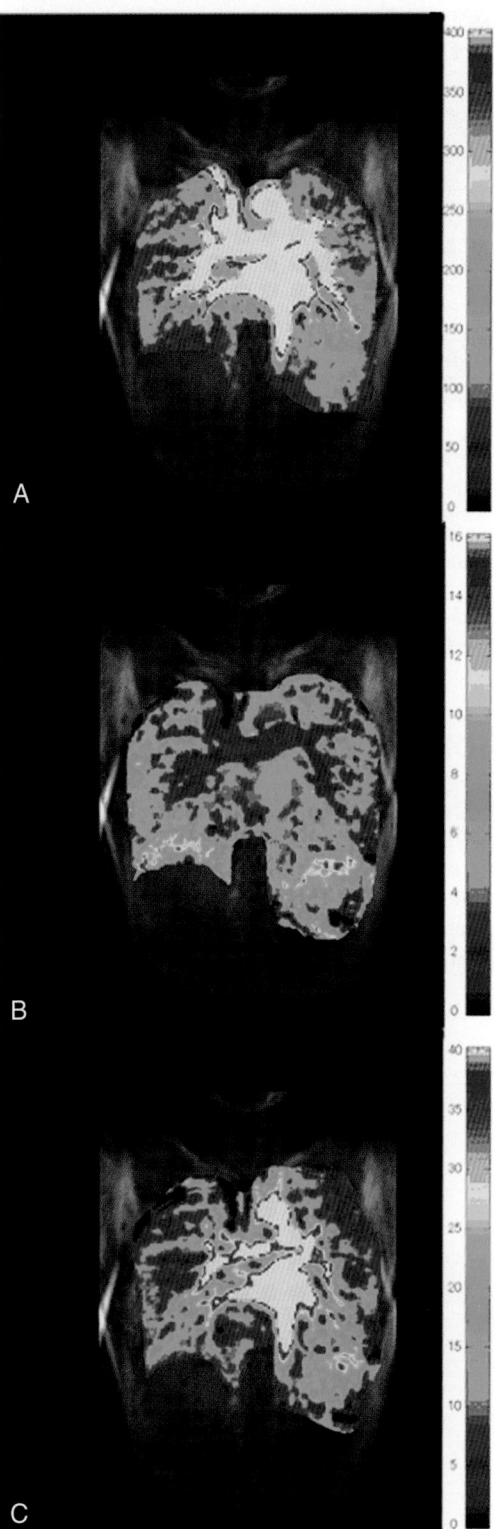

FIGURE 76-25

31-year-old healthy male volunteer. **A,** Image maps (L to R = ventral to dorsal) of pulmonary blood flow (PBF) demonstrated regional changes of PBF in the gravitational and isogravitational directions. **B,** Image maps (L to R = ventral to dorsal) of mean transit time (MTT) demonstrated regional changes of MTT in the gravitational and isogravitational directions. **C,** Image maps (L to R = ventral to dorsal) of pulmonary blood volume (PBV) demonstrated regional changes of PBV in the gravitational and isogravitational directions. *(Courtesy of Dr Ohno, Kobe University, Japan.)*

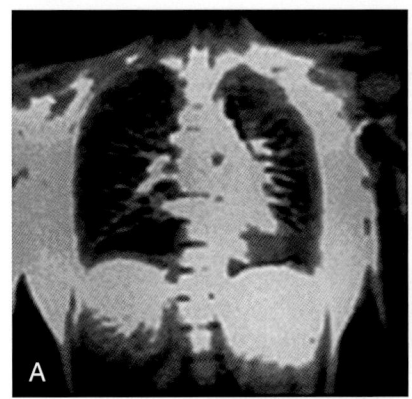

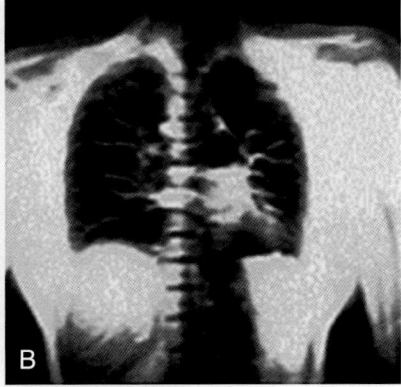

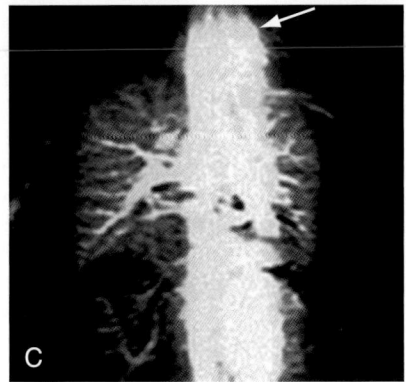

FIGURE 76-26

Coronal HASTE images of the chest in a healthy volunteer without (**A**) and with (**B**) an RF inversion pulse applied to the right ventricle and pulmonary artery with a TI time of 600 ms, as well as a subtraction image between (**A**) and (**B**) for pulmonary perfusion (**C**). Note the adiabatic RF inversion pulse to tag the proton spins (*arrow*). (*From Hatabu H, Tadamura E, Prasad PV, et al: Noninvasive pulmonary perfusion imaging by STAR-HASTE sequence. Magn Reson Med 44: 808-812, 2000, with permission.*)

oxygen-enhanced MRI is a dynamic process.[242] When correlated with pulmonary function tests, oxygen-enhancement has high correlation with diffusion capacity[243,244] (Figs 76-27, 76-28). Preliminary reports showed successful clinical applications.[245-247] The oxygen-enhanced MR ventilation technique utilizes conventional proton-based MRI. Oxygen is available in most MR units for patients and its administration is safe and inexpensive. Thus the oxygen-enhanced MRI

technique for assessing pulmonary ventilation has the potential to provide a noninvasive means of assessing regional pulmonary ventilation at high resolution. Combined with MRI perfusion studies, this technique has the potential to have a major impact on the diagnosis and assessment of a variety of pulmonary disorders.[101]

Laser-polarized ^{129}Xe and ^{3}He have been proposed for ventilation MRI.[248-251] These noble gases can be hyperpolarized using an optical pumping technique.

FIGURE 76-27

A 67-year-old male with pulmonary emphysema. **A,** CT image at the lower lung area shows severe pulmonary emphysema bilaterally, and bulla in left lower lobe. Note the decreased lung volume of the left lower lobe with scar. **B,** HASTE image (TE = 16 ms, ES = 4 ms, TI = 720 ms) obtained at baseline demonstrates a bulla (*arrow*) in the left lower lobe. **C,** Relative enhancement map obtained after oxygen inhalation shows inhomogeneous and decreased enhancement (light blue) of both lungs. Maximum mean relative enhancement ratio by oxygen inhalation was 18.0%SI. **D,** Mean relative enhancement time course curve of the dynamic oxygen-enhanced MR imaging. Maximum mean relative enhancement ratio was 18.0%SI. (*From Ohno Y, Hatabu H, Takenaka D, et al. Dynamic oxygen-enhanced MRI reflects diffusing capacity of the lung. Magn Reson Med. 47:1139-1144, 2002, with permission.*)

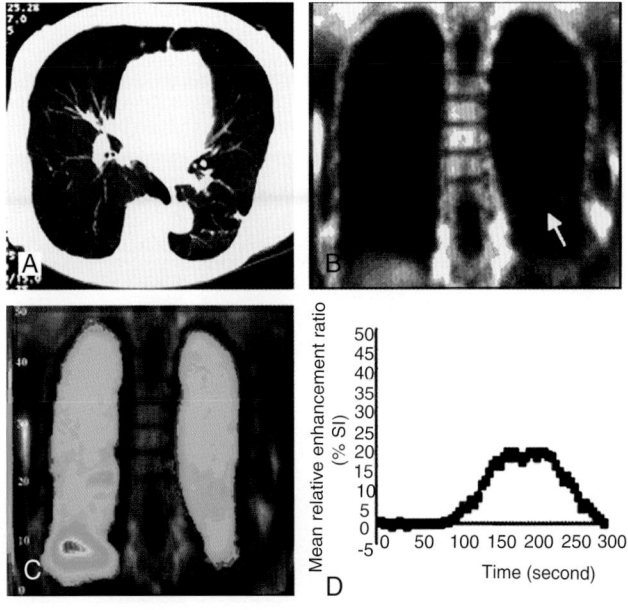

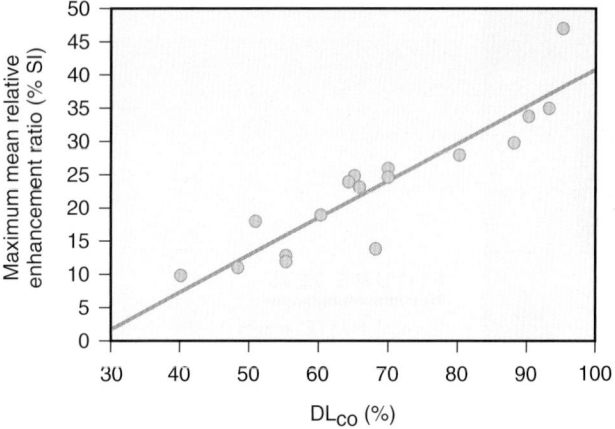

FIGURE 76-28

Correlation between maximum mean relative enhancement and diffusion lung capacity (percentage predicted). Graph shows excellent correlation between maximum mean relative enhancement and % DL_{CO} ($y = 0.56x - 15.0$, $r^2 = 0.83$, $P < 0.0001$). *(From Ohno Y, Hatabu H, Takenaka D, et al. Dynamic oxygen-enhanced MRI reflects diffusing capacity of the lung. Magn Reson Med. 47:1139-1144, 2002, with permission.)*

MR signal from these noble gases may be increased by 100,000 times compared with the MR signal in a thermal equilibrium state. The strong signal from the noble gases enables the acquisition of the data from gas itself. Using ^{3}He MRI: 1. gas density MRI with high spatial resolution display of gas distribution; 2. dynamic imaging with high temporal resolution; 3. diffusion-weighted imaging; and 4. oxygen-sensitive imaging are possible.[252] Gas density ^{3}He MRI provides whole-lung imaging with a pixel size of $3 \times 3 \times 10$ mm, which is higher than that available with nuclear medicine. The images are acquired during a 10-second breath-hold. In human subjects without lung disease, homogenous distribution of signal intensity with only a few small and transient ventilation defects was observed. Ventilation defects are frequently observed in patients with a history of smoking, chronic obstructive lung disease with and without emphysema, bronchiectasis, asthma, bronchiolitis obliterans following lung transplantation, pulmonary fibrosis and neoplasms[253-261] (Fig. 76-29). Compared with other modalities, ^{3}He MRI has a very high sensitivity for detecting ventilation defects.[261] Dynamic ^{3}He MRI requires sequences that will provide a high temporal resolution of 30 to 130 ms.[252] Ultrafast FLASH sequence, echo-planar imaging or spiral imaging have been utilized.[262-265] In normal subjects, homogenous and fast distribution of ^{3}He-3 gas through the trachea with a peak time of 260 ms as well as alveoli with a peak time of 910 ms have been observed.[262] In patients with emphysema, irregular and delayed distribution patterns have been observed. The quantification will be the key to further define and characterize dynamic ventilation abnormality.[266] Diffusion-weighted ^{3}He MRI measures random molecular movement of gases. During a breath-hold with hyperpolarlized ^{3}He gas inhalation, bipolar diffusion gradients are applied before data acquisition.[267] Spins with random molecular diffusion result in signal decrease. The random movement of gas is restricted by the normal 3D alveolar structure. When the normal alveolar structure is destroyed, the random motion of gas will be freed from the alveolar walls. In normal subjects, ADC ranges between 0.17 and 0.28 cm^2/s.[268-271] In patients with emphysema, increases in ADC values ranging 0.4 to 0.9 cm^2/s have been observed.[265,271] Moreover, ADC values show an inhomogenous distribution with broadening in histogram distribution.[268,272] Anisotropy of diffusive gas motion indicating nonspherical geometric change was also observed in the diseased lung.[273,274] Oxygen-sensitive ^{3}He MRI provides regional analysis of alveolar partial pressure of oxygen, which reflects regional pulmonary perfusion, ventilation-perfusion ratio, and oxygen uptake.[252] Because molecular oxygen has paramagnetic properties, it destroys magnetization of ^{3}He gas when oxygen and hyperpolarized ^{3}He are mixed together. Saam et al demonstrated the linear relationship between the partial pressure of oxygen and the loss of magnetization of ^{3}He.[275] Using this principle, regional partial pressure of oxygen can be estimated from ^{3}He MRI.[276-278] Application

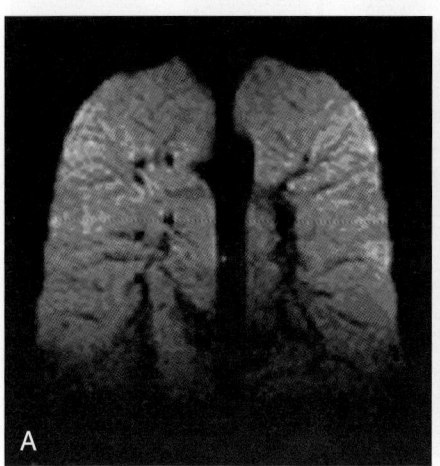

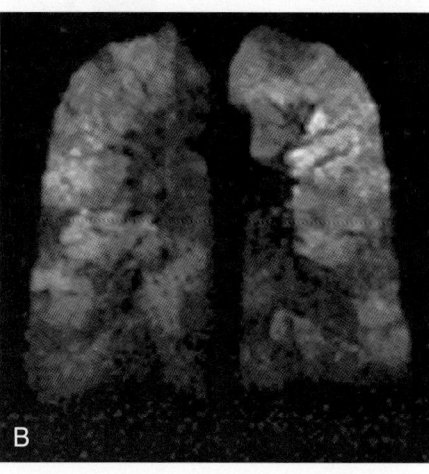

FIGURE 76-29

Coronal hyperpolarized ^{3}He MR ventilation images from an asymptomatic asthmatic (**A**) immediately before (FEV1 80% predicted), and (**B**) 5 minutes after treatment with inhaled methacholine (FEV1 40% predicted). Numerous ventilation defects appear following methacholine challenge. *(From Altes TA, de Lange EE: Applications of hyperpolarized helium-3 gas magnetic resonance imaging in pediatric lung disease. Top Magn Reson Imaging 14:231-236, 2003, with permission.)*

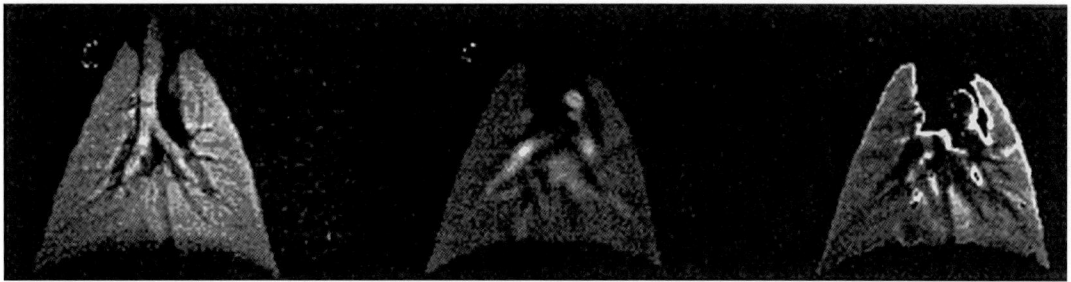

FIGURE 76-30

Registered 3He ventilation image (*left*), blood flow map (*center*), and V/Q ratio map (*right*) of a swine. Normal V/Q patterns are observed. The V/Q ratio map shows heterogeneous distribution in the lung. Low V/Q values are demonstrated for the pulmonary artery. *(Reprinted from Academic Radiology, Vol. 10, Hasegawa I, Uematsu H, Gee JC, et al, Voxelwise mapping of magnetic resonance ventilation-perfusion ratio in a porcine model by multimodality registration: technical note, pages 1091-1096, Copyright 2003, with permission from the Association of University Radiologists.)*

of the hyperpolarized noble gas technique is particularly attractive for pediatric patients with asthma and cystic fibrosis due to its minimum radiation exposure.[279]

Hyperpolarized ^{129}Xe has a high solubility in lipid as well as water, and demonstrates a large chemical shift (200 ppm) upon dissolution.[280] These properties have been exploited for imaging dissolved-phase compartments throughout bodies.[281-285] Spectroscopic studies have also been performed to characterize ^{129}Xe spectral properties in animal lungs.[286-294] T1 of ^{129}Xe depends on the blood oxygenation level, which demonstrated the feasibility of ^{129}Xe as intravascular contrast agent.[295-301] Recently, the difference in chemical shift between gas-phase and dissolved-phase xenon was utilized for depicting regional xenon gas exchange.[302,303]

Imaging of ventilation can be performed using the hyperpolarized noble gas technique or oxygen-enhanced MRI. Both methods are relatively new and novel. The hyperpolarized noble gas technique demonstrates the flow of gas itself, while oxygen-enhanced MRI shows transfer of molecular oxygen indirectly through enhancement of protons in lungs by the paramagnetic effect of molecular oxygen.

MR assessment of pulmonary ventilation-perfusion is possible when combined with the recent first-pass contrast-enhanced MR perfusion technique using Gd-DTPA.[100,101,104,215] The combination of ventilation-perfusion techniques is particularly interesting when airway obstruction and pulmonary embolism, two classic disease models of the lung with contrasting radiographic manifestations, are studied. Airway obstruction causes regional hypoxemia, which elicits hypoxic vasoconstriction, resulting in an accompanying decreased regional perfusion. Therefore, matched regional ventilation-perfusion deficit is expected when a combined ventilation-perfusion imaging study is performed.

In contrast, pulmonary embolism does not cause airway obstruction. Therefore, regional perfusion deficit without ventilation deficit (mismatched ventilation-perfusion) is expected on the combined ventilation-perfusion imaging study.[101,304]

Various combinations of methods for MR ventilation-perfusion imaging have been reported.[305-307] The registration of quantified ventilation and perfusion images is crucial to generate accurate ventilation-perfusion maps. However, the fact that ventilation requires lung motion poses a fundamental challenge for registration of ventilation-perfusion images. Ventilation images obtained during respiration must be matched to perfusion images obtained with a breath-hold. The multimodality registration technique has been utilized for this purpose[305] (Figs 76-30, 76-31). At the same time, a physics-based approach to registration of lung imaging provides a unique mathematical description of lung mechanics.[308-310] Using serial MR images during respiration, the motion of

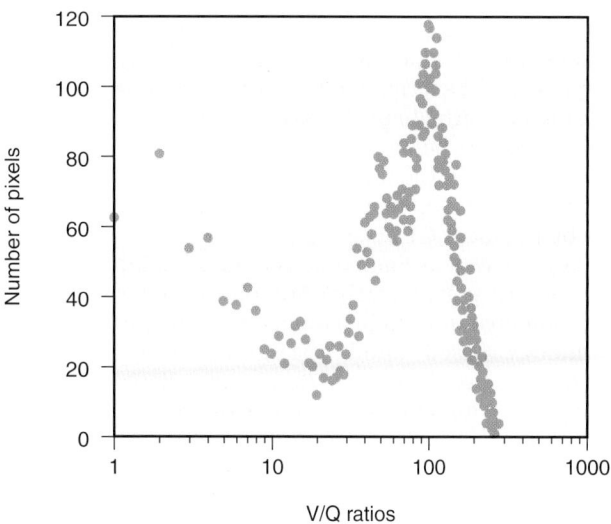

FIGURE 76-31

Semi-logarithmic scatter plots of V/Q ratios against the number of voxels. Note that the scale of the Y axis (number of voxels) is linear. Low V/Q values are indicated for the pulmonary artery. Plots of the V/Q ratios are similar to the logarithmic normal distribution. *(From Hasegawa I, Uematsu H, Gee JC, et al: Voxelwise mapping of magnetic resonance ventilation-perfusion ratio in a porcine model by multimodality registration: technical note. Acad Radiol 10:1091-1096, 2003, with permission.)*

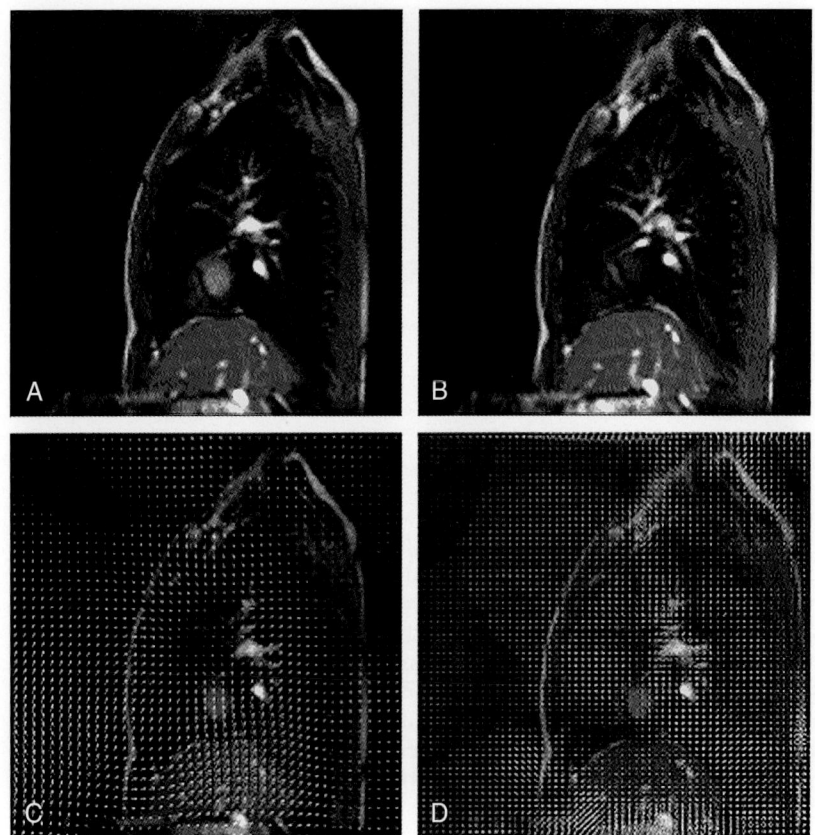

FIGURE 76-32

Illustration of the estimated lung motion between two consecutive frames (**A, B**) in a sequence of MRIs. The registration transformation between the images, represented as a field of displacement vectors, is shown superimposed on the first image (**C**), where the vectors indicate the corresponding locations in the second image and thus provide a direct, quantitative measure of the lung motion between the images. The strain induced by the motion is also shown (**D**), where each strain tensor is depicted using an ellipse with major and minor axes directed along its eigenvectors, respectively, and scaled by the corresponding principal strain values. *(Reprinted from Academic Radiology, Vol. 10, Gee J, Sundaram T, Hasegawa I, et al, Characterization of regional pulmonary mechanics from serial magnetic resonance imaging data, pages 1147-1152, Copyright 2003, with permisison from the Association of University Radiologists.)*

individual portions of the lung is demonstrated as a vector field. The strain tensor can also be calculated and projected over the images of the lung[311] (Fig. 76-32). Such computational tools produced using image processing provide new insight for analyzing lung parenchyma. Determination of regional biomechanical parameters in the lung holds the potential to assist early or localized pathological processes.

Finally, with the availability of high-resolution CT, should the development of lung parenchymal imaging by MR be pursued? CT diagnosis is based on morphological findings as well as limited density information (calcium, fat, contrast enhancement). MR, on the other hand, has the potential for multi-parametric characterization of pathology based upon relaxation times, perfusion, ventilation, proton density (lung water determination), diffusion, biomechanics, and susceptibility-induced T2* changes as reflections of alveolar architecture. Fast MR imaging is opening a new, exciting window into multifunctional MR imaging of the lung.[198] Ventilation, perfusion, and biomechanics are three major components of lung function. MRI provides a powerful tool for 21st-century functional imaging of the lung.

Acknowledgment

The authors would like to thank Donna Wolfe, MFA, for assistance in manuscript preparation.

REFERENCES

1. Hatabu H, Stock KW, Sher S, et al: Magnetic resonance imaging of the thorax. Past, present, and future. Clin Chest Med 20:775-803, viii-ix, 1999.
2. Reddy GP, Higgins CB: MR imaging of the thoracic aorta. Magn Reson Imaging Clin N Am 8:1-15, vii, 2000.
3. Matsunaga N, Hayashi K, Okada M, et al: Magnetic resonance imaging features of aortic diseases. Top Magn Reson Imaging 14:253-266, 2003.
4. Link KM, Lesko NM: The role of MR imaging in the evaluation of acquired diseases of the thoracic aorta. Am J Roentgenol 158:1115, 1992.
5. Higgins CB: The thoracic aorta. In Higgins CB, Hricak H, Helms CA (eds): Magnetic Resonance Imaging of the Body, 3rd ed. New York: Lippincott-Raven Press, 519, 1997.
6. Hartnell GG, Finn JP, Zenni M, et al: MR imaging of the thoracic aorta: Comparison of spin-echo, angiographic, and breath-hold techniques. Radiology 191:697, 1994.
7. Krinsky G, Reuss PM: MR angiography of the thoracic aorta. Magn Reson Imaging Clin N Am 6:293, 1998.
8. Pflugfelder PW, Landzberg JS, Cassidy MM, et al: Comparison of cine MR imaging with Doppler echocardiography for the evaluation of aortic regurgitation. Am J Roentgenol 152:729, 1989.
9. Pearlman JD, Edelman RR: Ultrafast magnetic resonance imaging. Segmented turboflash, echo-planar, and real-time nuclear magnetic resonance. Radiol Clin North Am 32:593, 1994.
10. Posteraro RH, Sostman HD, Spritzer CE, et al: Cine-gradient-refocused MR imaging of central pulmonary emboli. Am J Roentgenol 152:465, 1989.
11. Krinsky G, Rofsky NM, DeCorato DR, et al: Thoracic aorta: Comparison of gadolinium-enhanced three-dimensional MR angiography with conventional MR imaging [abstract]. Radiology 202:183, 1997.
12. Krinsky G, Rofsky N, Flyer M, et al: Gadolinium-enhanced three-dimensional MR angiography of acquired arch vessel disease. Am J Roentgenol 167:981, 1996.
13. Earls JP, Rofsky NM, DeCorato DR, et al: Breath-hold single-dose gadolinium-enhanced MR aortography: Usefulness of a timing examination and MR power injector. Radiology 201:705, 1996.
14. Castaner E, Andreu M, Gallardo X, et al: Radiographics. CT in nontraumatic acute thoracic aortic disease: typical and atypical features and complications, 23:S93-110, 2003.
15. Crawford ES: The diagnosis and management of aortic dissection. JAMA 264:2537, 1990.

16. De Sanctis RW, Doroghazi RM, Austen WG, et al: Aortic dissection. N Engl J Med 317:1060-1067, 1987
17. Larson EW, Edwards WD: Risk factors for aortic dissection: a necropsy study of 161 cases. Am J Cardiol 53:849-855, 1984.
18. Fisher A, Holroyd BR: Cocaine-associated dissection of thoracic aorta. J Emerg Med 10:723-727, 1992.
19. Prete R, Von Segesser LK: Aortic dissection. Lancet 349:1461-1464, 1997.
20. Hirst AE, Johns VR, Klime SW: Dissecting aneurysm of the aorta: a review of 505 cases. Medicine 37:217-279, 1958.
21. Ergin MA, Griepp RB: Dissections of the aorta. In Baue AE (ed): Glenn's Thoracic and Cardiovascular Surgery. New York, Appleton & Lange, 2273, 1996.
22. Link KM, Loehr SP, Baker DM, et al: Magnetic resonance imaging of the thoracic aorta. Semin Ultrasound CT MR 14:91, 1993.
23. Nienaber CA, von Kodolitsch Y, Nicolas V, et al: The diagnosis of thoracic aortic dissection by noninvasive imaging procedures. N Engl J Med 328:1, 1993.
24. Kaminaga T, Yamada N, Takamiya M, et al: Sequential MR signal change of the thrombus in the false lumen of thrombosed aortic dissection. Magn Reson Imaging 13:773, 1995.
25. Ambos MA, Rothberg M, Lefleur RS, et al: Unsuspected aortic dissection: The chronic "healed" dissection. Am J Roentgenol 132:221, 1979.
26. Ho VB, Prince MR: Thoracic MR aortography: Imaging techniques and strategies. Radiographics 18:287, 1998.
27. Amparo EG, Higgins CB, Hricak H, et al: Aortic dissection: Magnetic resonance imaging. Radiology 155:399, 1985.
28. Yamada T, Tada S, Harada J: Aortic dissection without intimal rupture: diagnosis with MR imaging and CT. Radiology 1988; 168:347-352.
29. Nienaber CA, von Kodolitsch Y, Peterson B, et al: Intramural hemorrhage of the thoracic aorta: diagnostic and therapeutic implications. Circulation 92:1465-1472, 1995.
30. Murray JG, Manisalli M, Flamm SD, et al: Intramural hematoma of the thoracic aorta: MR imaging findings and their prognostic implication. Radiology 204:349-355, 1997.
31. Rerkpattanapipat P, Jacobs LE, Makornwattana P, et al: Meta-analysis of 143 reported cases of aortic intramural hematoma. Am J Cardiol 86:664-668, 2000.
32. Song JK, Kim HS, Kang DH, et al: Different clinical features of aortic intramural hematoma versus dissection involving the ascending aorta. J Am Coll Cardiol 37:1604-1610, 2001.
33. Sueyoshi E, Matsuoka Y, Sakamoto I, et al: Fate of intramural hematoma of the aorta: CT evaluation. J Comput Assist Tomogr 21:931-938, 1997.
34. Song JM, Kim HS, Song JK, et al: Usefulness of the initial noninvasive imaging study to predict the adverse outcomes in the medical treatment of acute Type A aortic intramural hematoma. Circulation 108:II-324, 2003.
35. Oliver TB, Murchison JT, Reid JH: Serial MRI in the management of intramural haemorrhage of the thoracic aorta. Br J Radiol 70:1288, 1997.
36. Stanson AW, Kazmier FJ, Hollier LH, et al: Penetrating atherosclerotic ulcers of the thoracic aorta: natural history and clinicopathologic correlations. Ann Vasc Surg 1:15-23, 1986.
37. Troxler M, Mavor AI, Homer-Vanniasinkam S: Penetrating atherosclerotic ulcers of the aorta. Br J Surg 88:1169-1177, 2001.
38. Yucel EK, Steinberg FL, Egglin TK, et al: Penetrating aortic ulcers: Diagnosis with MR imaging. Radiology 177:779, 1990.
39. Kazerooni EA, Bree RL, Williams DM: Penetrating atherosclerotic ulcers of the descending thoracic aorta: Evaluation with CT and distinction from aortic dissection. Radiology 183:759, 1992.
40. Joyce JW, Fairbairn JF, Kincaid OW, et al: Aneurysms of the thoracic aorta: A clinical study with special reference to prognosis. Circulation 29:176, 1964.
41. Coady MA, Rizzo JA, Hammond GL, et al: What is the appropriate size criterion for resection of thoracic aortic aneurysms? J Thorac Cardiovasc Surg 113:476, 1997.
42. Prince MR, Narasimham DL, Jacoby WT, et al: Three-dimensional gadolinium-enhanced MR angiography of the thoracic aorta. Am J Roentgenol 166:1387, 1996.
43. Gomori JM, Grossman RI, Goldberg HI, et al: Intracranial hematomas: Imaging by high-field MR. Radiology 157:87, 1985.
44. Yamada I, Numano F, Suzuki S: Takayasu arteritis: Evaluation with MR imaging. Radiology 188:89, 1993.
45. Choe YH, Kim DK, Koh EM: Takayasu arteritis: diagnosis with MR imaging and MR angiography in acute and chronic active stages. J Magn Reson Imaging 10:751-757, 1999.
46. White RD, Dooms GC, Higgins CB: Advances in imaging thoracic aortic disease. Invest Radiol 21:761, 1986.
47. von Schulthess GK, Higashino SM, Higgins SS, et al: Coarctation of the aorta: MR imaging. Radiology 158:469, 1986.
48. Sebastia C, Quiroga S, Boye R: Aortic stenosis: spectrum of diseases depicted at multisection CT. Radiographics 23:S79-91, 2003.
49. Araoz PA, Reddy GP, Tarnoff H: MR findings of collateral circulation are more accurate measures of hemodynamic significance than arm-leg blood pressure gradient after repair of coarctation of the aorta. J Magn Reson Imaging 17:177-183, 2003.
50. Simpson IA, Chung KJ, Glass RF, et al: Cine magnetic resonance imaging for evaluation of anatomy and flow relations in infants and children with coarctation of the aorta. Circulation 78:142, 1988.
51. Finn JP, Zisk JH, Edelman RR, et al: Central venous occlusion: MR angiography. Radiology 187:245, 1993.
52. Shinde TS, Lee VS, Rofsky NM, et al: Three-dimensional gadolinium-enhanced MR venographic evaluation of patency of central veins in the thorax: initial experience. Radiology 213:555-560, 1999.
53. Thornton MJ, Ryan R, Varghese JC, et al: A three-dimensional gadolinium-enhanced MR venography technique for imaging central veins. Am J Radiol 173:999-1003, 1999.
54. Kroencke TJ, Taupitz M, Arnold R, et al: Three-dimensional gadolinium-enhanced magnetic resonance venography in suspected thrombo-occlusive disease of the central chest veins. Chest 120:1570-1576, 2001.
55. Rose SC, Gomes AS, Yoon HC: MR angiography for mapping potential central venous access sites in patients with advanced venous occlusive disease. Am J Roentgenol 166:1181, 1996.
56. Hansen ME, Spritzer CE, Sostman HD: Assessing the patency of mediastinal and thoracic inlet veins: Value of MR imaging. Am J Roentgenol 155:1177, 1990.
57. Li W, David V, Kaplan R, et al: Three-dimensional low dose gadolinium-enhanced peripheral MR venography. J Magn Reson Imaging 8:630, 1998.
58. Earls JP, Shaves SC: MR angiography of the thoracic, abdominal, and extremity venous system. Magn Reson Imaging Clin N Am 6:417, 1998.
59. Rich S: Primary pulmonary hypertension. In Isselbacher KJ, Braunwald E, Wilson JD, et al (eds): Harrison's Principles of Internal Medicine, 13th ed., vol 2. New York: McGraw-Hill, 1211, 1994.
60. von Schulthess GK, Fisher MR, Higgins CB: Pathologic blood flow in pulmonary vascular disease as shown by gated magnetic resonance imaging. Ann Intern Med 103:317, 1985.
61. Gefter WB, Hatabu H, Dinsmore BJ, et al: Pulmonary vascular cine MR imaging: A noninvasive approach to dynamic imaging of the pulmonary circulation. Radiology 176:761, 1990.
62. Mousseaux E, Tasu JP, Jolivet O, et al: Pulmonary arterial resistance: non-invasive measurement with indexes of pulmonary flow estimated at velocity-encoded MR imaging—preliminary experience. Radiology 212(3):896-902, 1999.
63. Tunaci A, Berkman YM, Gokmen E: Thoracic involvement in Behçet disease: Pathologic, clinical, and imaging features. Am J Roentgenol 164:51, 1995.
64. Numan F, Islak C, Berkmen T, et al: Behçet disease: Pulmonary arterial involvement in 15 cases. Radiology 192:465, 1994.
65. Stern EJ, Graham C, Gamsu G, et al: Pulmonary artery dissection: MR findings. J Comput Assist Tomogr 16:481, 1992.
66. Bressler EL, Nelson JM: Primary pulmonary artery sarcoma: Diagnosis with CT, MR imaging, and transthoracic needle biopsy. Am J Roentgenol 159:702, 1992.
67. Smith WS, Lesar MS, Travis WD, et al: MR and CT findings in pulmonary artery sarcoma. J Comput Assist Tomogr 13:906, 1989.
68. Weinreb JC, Davis SD, Berkmen YM, et al: Pulmonary artery sarcoma: Evaluation using Gd-DTPA. J Comput Assist Tomogr 14:647, 1990.
69. Hatabu H, Gefter WB, Kressel HY, et al: Pulmonary vasculature: High-resolution MR imaging. Work in progress. Radiology 171:391, 1989.
70. Choe YH, Lee HJ, Kim HS, et al: MRI of total anomalous pulmonary venous connections. J Comput Assist Tomogr 18:243, 1994.
71. Verdant A, Cossette R, Page A, et al: Aneurysms of the descending thoracic aorta: Three hundred and sixty-six consecutive cases resected without paraplegia. J Vasc Surg 21:385, 1995.
72. Brown JJ, Gilbert T, Gamsu G, et al: MR imaging of low signal intensity pulmonary lesions using flow-sensitive techniques. J Comput Assist Tomogr 12:560, 1988.
73. Dinsmore BJ, Gefter WB, Hatabu H, et al: Pulmonary arteriovenous malformations: Diagnosis by gradient-refocused MR imaging. J Comput Assist Tomogr 14:918, 1990.
74. Maki DD, Siegelman ES, Roberts DA, et al: Pulmonary arteriovenous malformations: three-dimensional gadolinium-enhanced MR angiography-initial experience. Radiology 219:243-246, 2001.
75. Moser KM: Pulmonary thromboembolism. In Isselbacher KJ, Braunwald E, Wilson JD, et al (eds): Harrison's Principles of Internal Medicine. New York: McGraw-Hill, 1214, 1994.
76. van Beek EJ, Wild JM, Fink C, et al: MRI for the diagnosis of pulmonary embolism. J Magn Reson Imaging 18(6):27-40, 2003.
77. Mills SR, Jackson DC, Older RA, et al: The incidence, etiologies, and avoidance of complications of pulmonary angiography in a large series. Radiology 136:295, 1980.
78. Mills SR, Jackson DC, Sullivan DC, et al: Angiographic evaluation of chronic pulmonary embolism. Radiology 136:301, 1980.
79. Nicod P, Peterson K, Levine M, et al: Pulmonary angiography in severe chronic pulmonary hypertension. Ann Intern Med 107:565, 1987.
80. Rich S, Levitsky S, Brundage BH: Pulmonary hypertension from chronic pulmonary thromboembolism. Ann Intern Med 108:425, 1988.
81. Value of the ventilation/perfusion scan in acute pulmonary embolism: results of the prospective investigation of pulmonary embolism diagnosis (PIOPED)-the PIOPED investigators. JAMA 263:2753-2759, 1990.
82. Bell WR, Simon TL: A comparative analysis of pulmonary perfusion scans with pulmonary angiograms. From a national cooperative study. Am Heart J 92:700, 1976.
83. Biello DR, Mattar AG, McKnight RC, et al: Ventilation-perfusion studies in suspected pulmonary embolism. Am J Roentgenol 133:1033, 1979.

84. Perrier A, Bounameaux H, Morabia A, et al: Diagnosis of pulmonary embolism by a decision analysis-based strategy including clinical probability, D-dimer levels, and ultrasonography: a management study. Arch Intern Med 156:531-536, 1996.

85. Turkstra F, Kuijer PMM, van Beek EJR, et al: Value of compression ultrasonography for the detection of deep venous thrombosis in patients suspected of having pulmonary embolism. Ann Intern Med 126:775-781, 1997.

86. Ghaye B, Remy J, Remy-Jardin M: Non-traumatic thoracic emergencies: CT diagnosis of acute pulmonary embolism: the first 10 years. Eur Radiol 12:1886-1905, 2002.

87. Ghaye B, Dondelinger RF: Non-traumatic thoracic emergencies: CT venography in an integrated diagnostic strategy of acute pulmonary embolism and venous thrombosis. Eur Radiol 12:1906-1921, 2002.

88. Han D, Lee KS, Franquet T, et al: Thrombotic and nonthrombotic pulmonary arterial embolism: spectrum of imaging findings. Radiographics 23(6):521-539, 2003.

89. Fishman EK, Horton KM: CT of suspected pulmonary embolism: study design optimization. Am J Roentgenol 175:1002-1003, 2000.

90. Mayo JR, Remy-Jardin M, Müller NL, et al: Pulmonary embolism: prospective comparison of spiral CT with ventilation-perfusion scintigraphy. Radiology 205:447-452, 1997.

91. Lomis NNT, Yoon HC, Moran AG, et al: Clinical outcomes of patients after a negative spiral CT pulmonary arteriogram in the evaluation of acute pulmonary embolism. J Vasc Intervent Radiol 10:707-712, 1999.

92. Goodman LR, Lipchik RJ, Kuzo RS, et al: Subsequent pulmonary embolism: risk after a negative helical CT pulmonary angiogram-prospective comparison with scintigraphy. Radiology 215:535-542, 2000.

93. Ghaye B, Szapiro D, Mastora I, et al: Peripheral pulmonary arteries: how far in the lung does multi-detector row spiral CT allow analysis? Radiology 219:629-636, 2001.

94. Hatabu H, Uematsu H, Nguyen B, et al: CT and MR in pulmonary embolism: a changing role for nuclear medicine in diagnostic strategy. Semin Nucl Med 32:183-192, 2002.

95. Erdman WA, Peshock RM, Redman HC, et al: Pulmonary embolism: Comparison of MR images with radionuclide and angiographic studies. Radiology 190:499, 1994.

96. Fisher MR, Higgins CB: Central thrombi in pulmonary arterial hypertension detected by MR imaging. Radiology 158:223, 1986.

97. White RD, Winkler ML, Higgins CB: MR imaging of pulmonary arterial hypertension and pulmonary emboli. Am J Roentgenol 149:15, 1987.

98. Gefter WB, Palevsky HI, Axel L, et al: MR evaluation of chronic central pulmonary artery thromboemboli in patients with pulmonary hypertension. In Book of Abstracts. New York: Society of Magnetic Resonance in Medicine, 293, 1990.

99. Hatabu H, Gefter WB, Axel L, et al: MR imaging with spatial modulation of magnetization in the evaluation of chronic central pulmonary thromboemboli. Radiology 190:791, 1994.

100. Hatabu H: MR pulmonary angiography and perfusion imaging: Recent advances. Semin Ultrasound CT MR 18:349, 1997.

101. Hatabu H, Chen Q, Levin DL, et al: Ventilation-perfusion MR imaging of the lung. Magn Reson Imaging Clin N Am 7:379, 1999.

102. Wielopolski PA, Haacke EM, Adler LP: Three-dimensional MR imaging of the pulmonary vasculature: Preliminary experience. Radiology 183:465, 1992.

103. Gupta A, Frazer CK, Ferguson JM, et al: Acute pulmonary embolism: diagnosis with MR angiography. Radiology 210:353-359, 1999.

104. Hatabu H, Gaa J, Kim D, et al: Pulmonary perfusion: qualitative assessment with dynamic contrast-enhanced MRI using ultra-short TE and inversion recovery turbo FLASH. Magn Reson Med 36:503-508, 1996.

105. Hatabu H, Tadamura E, Chen Q, et al: Pulmonary ventilation: dynamic MRI with inhalation of molecular oxygen. Eur J Radiol 37:172-178, 2001.

106. Meaney JF, Weg JG, Chenevert TL, et al: Diagnosis of pulmonary embolism with magnetic resonance angiography. N Engl J Med 336:1422, 1997.

107. Ohno Y, Sugimura K, Hatabu H: MR imaging of lung cancer. Eur J Radiol 44:172-181, 2002.

108. Gefter WB: Magnetic resonance imaging in the evaluation of lung cancer. Semin Roentgenol 25:73, 1990.

109. Ohno Y, Hatabu H, Takenaka D, et al: Solitary pulmonary nodules: potential role of dynamic MR imaging in management initial experience. Radiology 224(2):503-511, 2002.

110. Fujimoto K, Abe T, Müller NL, et al: Small peripheral pulmonary carcinomas evaluated with dynamic MR imaging: correlation with tumor vascularity and prognosis. Radiology 227:786-793, 2003.

111. Manfredi R, Pirronti T, Bonomo L, et al: Accuracy of computed tomography and magnetic resonance imaging in staging bronchogenic carcinoma. MAGMA 4:257, 1996.

112. Gdeedo A, Van Schil P, Corthouts B, et al: Comparison of imaging TNM ((i)TNM) and pathological TNM (pTNM) in staging of bronchogenic carcinoma. Eur J Cardiothorac Surg 12:224, 1997.

113. Laissy JP, Gay-Depassier P, Soyer P, et al: Enlarged mediastinal lymph nodes in bronchogenic carcinoma: assessment with dynamic contrast-enhanced MR imaging. Work in progress. Radiology 191:263, 1994.

114. Fujimoto K, Edamitsu O, Meno S, et al: MR diagnosis for metastasis or non-metastasis of mediastinal and hilar lymph nodes in cases of primary lung cancer: detectability, signal intensity, and MR-pathologic correlation. Nippon Acta Radiol 55:162-171, 1995.

115. Walker R, Kessar P, Blanchard R, et al: Turbo STIR magnetic resonance imaging as a whole-body screening tool for metastases in patients with breast carcinoma: preliminary clinical experience. J Magn Resonance Imaging 11:343-350, 2000.

116. Eustace S, Tello R, DeCarvalho V, et al: Whole body turbo STIR MRI in unknown primary tumor detection. J Magn Resonance Imaging 8:751-753,1998.

117. Takenaka D, Ohno Y, Hatabu H, et al: Respiratory-triggered STIR turbo spin-echo imaging: potential role for management of mediatinal lymph nodes. Radiology 221:536, 2001.

118. Takenaka D, Ohno Y, Hatabu H, et al: Differentiation of metastatic versus non-metastatic mediastinal lymph nodes in patients with non-small cell lung cancer using respiratory-triggered short inversion time inversion recovery (STIR) turbo spin-echo MR imaging. Eur J Radiol 44:216-224, 2002.

119. Heelan RT, Panicek DM, Burt ME, et al: Magnetic resonance imaging of the postpneumonectomy chest: Normal and abnormal findings. J Thorac Imaging 12:200,1997.

120. Ohno Y, Adachi S, Motoyama A, et al: Multiphase ECG-triggered 3D contrast-enhanced MR angiography: utility for evaluation of hilar and mediastinal invasion of bronchogenic carcinoma. J Magn Reson Imaging 13:215-224, 2001.

121. Baron RL, Levitt RG, Sagel SS, et al: Computed tomography in the preoperative evaluation of bronchogenic carcinoma. Radiology 145:727-732, 1982.

122. Martini N, Heelan R, Westcott J, et al: Comparative merits of conventional, computed tomographic, and magnetic resonance imaging in assessing mediastinal involvement in surgically confirmed lung carcinoma. J Thorac Cardiovasc Surg 90:639-648, 1985.

123. Rendina EA, Bognolo DA, Mineo TC, et al: Computed tomography for evaluation of intrathorascic invasion by lung cancer. J Thorac Cardiovasc Surg 94:57-63, 1987.

124. Herman SJ, Winton TL, Weisbrod GL, et al: Mediastinal invasion by bronchogenic carcinoma: CT sign. Radiology 190:841-846, 1994.

125. Quint LE, Glazer GM, Orringer MB: Central lung mass: prediction with CT of need for pneumonectomy versus lobectomy. Radiology 165:735-738, 1987.

126. Quint LE, Francis IR, Wahl R, et al: Preoperative staging of non-small cell carcinoma of the lung: imaging methods. Am J Roentgenol 164:309-312, 1995.

127. Glazer HS, Kaiser LR, Anderson DJ, et al: Tumor invasion of chest wall and mediastinum in bronchogenic carcinoma: CT evaluation. Radiology 173:37-42, 1989.

128. Venuta E, Rendina EA, Ciriaco P, et al: Computed tomography for preoperative assessment of T3 and T4 bronchogenic carcinoma. Eur J Cardiothorac Surg 6:238-241, 1992.

129. White PG, Adams H, Crane MD, et al: Preoperative staging of carcinoma of the bronchus: can computed tomographic scanning reliably identify stage III tumors? Thorax 49:951-957, 1994.

130. Takahashi M, Shimoyama K, Murata K, et al: Hilar and mediastinal invasion of bronchogenic carcinoma: evaluation by thin-section electron-beam computed tomography. J Thorac Imaging 12:195-199, 1997.

131. Webb WR, Gastonis C, Zerhouni EA, et al: CT and MR imaging in staging non-small cell bronchogenic carcinoma: Report of Radiologic Diagnostic Oncology Group. Radiology 178:705-713, 1991.

132. Webb WR: The role of magnetic resonance imaging in the assessment of patients with lung cancer: a comparison with computed tomography. J Thorac Imaging 4:65-75, 1989.

133. Padovani B, Mouroux J, Seksik L, et al: Chest wall invasion by bronchogenic carcinoma: Evaluation with MR imaging. Radiology 187:33, 1993.

134. Yokozaki M, Nawano S, Nagai K, et al: Cine magnetic resonance imaging, computed tomography and ultrasonography in the evaluation of chest wall invasion of lung cancer. Hiroshima J Med Sci 46:61, 1997.

135. Burt M, Heelan RT, Coit D, et al: Prospective evaluation of unilateral adrenal masses in patients with operable non-small-cell lung cancer. Impact of magnetic resonance imaging. J Thorac Cardiovasc Surg 107:584, 1994.

136. Oliver TW Jr, Bernardino ME, Miller JI, et al: Isolated adrenal masses in nonsmall-cell bronchogenic carcinoma. Radiology 153:217, 1984.

137. Boraschi P, Braccini G, Grassi L, et al: Incidentally discovered adrenal masses: Evaluation with gadolinium enhancement and fat-suppressed MR imaging at 0.5 T. Eur J Radiol 24:245, 1997.

138. Mayo-Smith WW, Boland GW, Noto RB, et al: State-of-the-art adrenal imaging. Radiographics. 21(4):995-1012, 2001.

139. Mayo-Smith WW, Lee MJ, McNicholas MM, et al: Characterization of adrenal masses (<5 cm) by use of chemical shift MR imaging: observer performance versus quantitative measures. Am J Roentgenol 165:91-95, 1995.

140. Bilbey JH, McLoughlin RF, Kurkjian PS, et al: MR imaging of adrenal masses: volume of chemical-shift imaging for distinguishing adenomas from other tumors. Am J Roentgenol 164:637-642, 1995.

141. Outwater EK, Siegelman ES, Radecki PD, et al: Distinction between benign and malignant adrenal masses: value of T1-weighted chemical-shift MR imaging. Am J Roentgenol 165:579-583, 1995.

142. Korobkin M, Lombardi TJ, Aisen AM, et al: Characterization of adrenal masses with chemical-shift and gadolinium-enhanced MR imaging. Radiology 197:411-418, 1995.

143. Tsushima Y, Ishizaka H, Matsumoto M: Adrenal masses: differentiation with chemical-shift, fast low-angle shot MR imaging. Radiology 186:705-709, 1993.

144. Heinz-Peer G, Honigschnabl S, Schneider B, et al: Characterization of adrenal masses using MR imaging with histopathologic correlation. Am J Roentgenol 173:15-22, 1999.

145. Lauenstein TC, Freudenberg LS, Goehde SC, et al: Whole-body MRI using a rolling table platform for the detection of bone metastases. Eur Radiol 12:2091-2099, 2002.

146. Jeung MY, Gasser B, Gangi A, et al: Bronchial carcinoid tumors of the thorax: spectrum of radiologic findings. Radiographics 22:351-365, 2002.

147. Gaeta M, Blandino A, Scribano E, et al: Mucinous cystadenocarcinoma of the lung: CT-pathologic correlation in three cases. J Comput Assist Tomogr 23:641-643, 1999.

148. Mancuso AA, Dillon WP: The neck. Radiol Clin North Am 27:407-434, 1989.

149. Noma S, Kanaoka M, Minami S: Thyroid masses. MR imaging and pathologic correlation Radiology 168:759-764, 1988.

150. Sandler MP, Patton JA, Sacks GA, et al: Evaluation of intrathoracic goiter with I-123 scintigraphy and nuclear magnetic resonance imaging. J Nucl Med 12:673, 1984.

151. Weber AL, Randolph G, Aksoy FG: The thyroid and parathyroid glands. CT and MR imaging and correlation with pathology and clinical findings. Radiol Clin North Am 38:1105-1129, 2000.

152. Brown LR, Aughenbaugh LG: Masses of the anterior mediastinum: CT and MR imaging. Am J Roentgenol 157:1171-1180, 1991.

153. Nakahara H, Noguchi S, Murakami N, et al: Gadolinium-enhanced MR imaging of thyroid and parathyroid masses. Radiology 202:765, 1997.

154. Koh KB, Chang KW: Carcinoma in multinodular goiter. Br J Surg 79:266-267, 1992.

155. Kang YS, Rosen K, Clark OH, et al: Localization of abnormal parathyroid glands of the mediastinum with MR imaging. Radiology 189:137, 1993.

156. Lee VS, Spritzer CE, Coleman RE, et al: The complementary roles of fast spin-echo MR imaging and double-phase 99m Tc-sestamibi scintigraphy for localization of hyperfunctioning parathyroid glands. Am J Roentgenol 167:1555, 1996.

157. McDermott VG, Fernandez RJM, Meakem TJ 3rd, et al: Preoperative MR imaging in hyperparathyroidism: Results and factors affecting parathyroid detection. Am J Roentgenol 166:705, 1996.

158. Ishibashi M, Nishida H, Hiromatsu Y, et al: Localization of ectopic parathyroid glands using technetium-99m sestamibi imaging: Comparison with magnetic resonance and computed tomographic imaging. Eur J Nucl Med 24:197, 1997.

159. Ishibashi M, Nishida H, Hiromatsu Y, et al: Comparison of technetium-99m-MIBI, technetium-99m-tetrofosmin, ultrasound and MRI for localization of abnormal parathyroid glands. J Nucl Med 39:320, 1998.

160. Moka D, Voth E, Larena-Avellaneda A, et al: Location of a small mediastinal parathyroid adenoma using Tc-99m MIBI SPECT. Clin Nucl Med 23:186, 1998.

161. Rosado-de-Christenson ML, Templeton PA, Moran CA: From the archives of the AFIP: Mediastinal germ cell tumors: Radiologic and pathologic correlation. Radiographics 12:1013, 1992.

162. Kushihashi T, Fujisawa H, Munechika H: Magnetic resonance imaging of thymic epithelial tumors. Crit Rev Diagn Imaging 37:191, 1996.

163. Gregory AK, Connery CP, Resta-Flarer F, et al: A case of massive thymolipoma. J Pediatr Surg 32:1780, 1997.

164. Rosado-de-Christenson ML, Pugatch RD, Moran CA: Thymolipoma: Analysis of 27 cases. Radiology 193:121, 1994.

165. Bendini M, Zuiani C, Bazzocchi M, et al: Magnetic resonance imaging and ^{67}Ga scan versus computed tomography in the staging and in the monitoring of mediastinal malignant lymphoma: A prospective pilot study. MAGMA 4:213, 1996.

166. Carlsen SE, Bergin CJ, Hoppe RT: MR imaging to detect chest wall and pleural involvement in patients with lymphoma: Effect on radiation therapy planning. Am J Roentgenol 160:1191, 1993.

167. Flentje M, Zierhut D, Schraube P, et al: Integration of coronal magnetic resonance imaging (MRI) into radiation treatment planning of mediastinal tumors. Strahlenther Onkol 169:351, 1993.

168. Rahmouni A, Tempany C, Jones R, et al: Lymphoma: Monitoring tumor size and signal intensity with MR imaging. Radiology 188:445, 1993.

169. Devizzi L, Maffioli L, Bonfante V, et al: Comparison of gallium scan, computed tomography, and magnetic resonance in patients with mediastinal Hodgkin's disease. Ann Oncol 8(Suppl 1):53, 1997.

170. Hill M, Cunningham D, MacVicar D, et al: Role of magnetic resonance imaging in predicting relapse in residual masses after treatment of lymphoma. J Clin Oncol 11:2273, 1993.

171. Setoain FJ, Pons F, Herranz R, et al: ^{67}Ga scintigraphy for the evaluation of recurrences and residual masses in patients with lymphoma. Nucl Med Commun 18:405, 1997.

172. McAdams HP, Rosado-de-Christenson M, Fishback NF, et al: Castleman disease of the thorax: Radiologic features with clinical and histopathologic correlation. Radiology 209:221, 1998.

173. Rholl KS, Levitt RG, Glazer HS: Magnetic resonance imaging of fibrosing mediastinitis. Am J Roentgenol 145:255, 1985.

174. Sherrick AD, Brown LR, Harms GF, et al: The radiographic findings of fibrosing mediastinitis. Chest 106:484, 1994.

175. LeBlanc J, Guttentag AR, Shepard JA, et al: Imaging of mediastinal foregut cysts. Can Assoc Radiol J 45:381, 1994.

176. Jeung MY, Gasser B, Gangi A, et al: Imaging of cystic masses of the mediastinum. Radiographics 22:S79-S93, 2002.

177. Suen HC, Mathisen DJ, Grillo HC, et al: Surgical management and radiological characteristics of bronchogenic cysts. Ann Thorac Surg 55:476, 1993.

178. Wang ZJ, Reddy GP, Gotway MB, et al: CT and MR imaging of pericardial disease. Radiographics 23:S167-S180, 2003.

179. Glazen HS, Semenkovich JW, Gutierrez FR: Mediastinum. In Lee JKT, Sagel SS, Stanley RJ, Heiken JP (eds): Computed body tomography with MRI correlation, 3rd ed. Philadelphia: Lippincott-Raven, 261-350, 1996.

180. Heelan RT: CT and MR imaging in the evaluation of pleural masses. Chest Surg Clin N Am 4:431, 1994.

181. McLoud TC: CT and MR in pleural disease. Clin Chest Med 19:261, 1998.

182. Fiola C, Cantoni S, Turtulici I, et al: Transudative vs exudative pleural effusions: Differentiation using Gd-DTPA-enhanced MRI. Eur Radiol 7:860, 1997.

183. Baysal T, Bulut T, Gokirmak M, et al: Diffusion-weighted MR imaging of pleural fluid: differentiation of transudative vs exudative pleural effusions. Eur Radiol Aug 1 (Epub ahead of print), 2003.

184. McLoud TC, Flower CD: Imaging the pleura: Sonography, CT, and MR imaging. Am J Roentgenol 156:1145, 1991.

185. Falaschi F, Battolla L, Mascalchi M, et al: Usefulness of MR signal intensity in distinguishing benign from malignant pleural disease. Am J Roentgenol 166:963, 1996.

186. Ferretti GR, Chiles C, Cox JE, et al: Localized benign fibrous tumors of the pleura: MR appearance. J Comput Assist Tomogr 21:115, 1997.

187. Padovani B, Mouroux J, Raffaelli C, et al: Benign fibrous mesothelioma of the pleura: MR study and pathologic correlation. Eur Radiol 6:425, 1996.

188. Lorigan JG, Libshitz HI: MR imaging of malignant pleural mesothelioma. J Comput Assist Tomogr 13:617, 1989.

189. Gierada DS, Slone RM, Fleishman MJ: Imaging evaluation of the diaphragm. Chest Surg Clin N Am 8:237, 1998.

190. Shanmuganathan K, Mirvis SE, White CS, et al: MR imaging evaluation of hemidiaphragms in acute blunt trauma: Experience with 16 patients. Am J Roentgenol 167:397, 1996.

191. Iochum S, Ludig T, Walter F, et al: Imaging of diaphragmatic injury: a diagnostic challenge? Radiographics 22:S103-S116; discussion S116-S118, 2002.

192. Fortier M, Mayo JR, Swensen SJ, et al: MR imaging of chest wall lesions. Radiographics 14:597, 1994.

193. Sabate JM, Franquet T, Parellada JA, et al: Malignant neuroectodermal tumour of the chest wall (Askin tumour): CT and MR findings in eight patients. Clin Radiol 49:634, 1994.

194. Winer-Muram HT, Kauffman WM, Gronemeyer SA, et al: Primitive neuro-ectodermal tumors of the chest wall (Askin tumors): CT and MR findings. Am J Roentgenol 161:265, 1993.

195. Kransdorf MJ, Meis-Kindblom JM: Dermatofibrosarcoma protuberans: radiologic appearance. Am J Roentgenol 163:391-394, 1994.

196. Demondion X, Bacqueville E, Paul C, et al: Thoracic outlet: assessment with MR imaging in asymptomatic and symptomatic populations. Radiology 227:461-468, 2003.

197. Demondion X, Boutry N, Drizenko A, et al: Thoracic outlet: anatomic correlation with MR imaging. Am J Roentgenol 175:417-422, 2000.

198. Hatabu H, Chen Q, Stock KW, et al: Fast MR imaging of the lung. Eur J Radiol 29:114-132, 1999.

199. Itoh H, Nakatsu M, Yoxtheimer LM, et al: Structural basis for pulmonary functional imaging. Eur J Radiol 37:143-154, 2001.

200. Cutillo AG, Ganesan K, Ailion DC, et al: Alveolar air-tissue interface and nuclear magnetic resonance behavior of lung. J Appl Physiol 70:2145-2154, 1991.

201. Ailion DC, Case TA, Blatter DD, et al: Application of NMR spin imaging to the study of lungs. Bull Magn Reson 6:130-139, 1984.

202. Case TA, Durney CH, Ailion DC, et al: A mathematical model of diamagnetic line broadening in lung tissue and similar heterogenous systems: calculations and measurements. J Magn Reson 73:304-314, 1987.

203. Bergin CJ, Pauly JM, Macovski A: Lung parenchyma: projection reconstruction MR imaging. Radiology 179:777-781, 1991.

204. Bergin CJ, Glover GH, Pauly JM: Lung parenchyma: magnetic susceptibility in MR imaging. Radiology 180:845-848, 1991.

205. Hatabu H, Gefter WB, Konishi J, et al: Magnetic resonance approaches to the evaluation of pulmonary vascular anatomy and physiology. Magn Reson Q 7:208-225, 1991.

206. Hatabu H, Alsop DC, Listerud J, et al: T2* and proton density measurement of normal human lung parenchyma using submillisecond TE gradient echo MR imaging. Eur J Radiol 29:245-252, 1999.

207. Hatabu H, Alsop D, Bonnet M, et al: Approaches to MR imaging of lung parenchyma utilizing ultrashort TE gradient echo and fast SE sequences. Proceedings, Society of Magnetic Resonance, Second Meeting, August 6-12, 1994, San Francisco, 1474.

208. Alsop DC, Hatabu H, Bonnet M, et al: Multi-slice, breathhold imaging of the lung with submillisecond echo times. Magn Reson Med 33:678-692, 1995.

209. Hatabu H, Gaa J, Tadamura E, et al: Lung parenchyma: MRI with a half-Fourier single-shot turbo SE (HASTE) sequence. Proceedings, Society of Magnetic Resonance, Fourth Meeting, 1996, New York, 771.

210. Hatabu H, Gaa J, Tadamura E, et al: MR imaging of pulmonary parenchyma with a Half-Fourier Single-Shot TurboSE (HASTE) Sequence. Eur J Radiol 29:152-159, 1999.

211. Uematsu H, Levin DL, Hatabu H: Quantification of pulmonary perfusion with MR imaging: recent advances. Eur J Radiol 37: 155-163, 2001.
212. Uematsu H, Ohno Y, Hatabu H: Recent advances in magnetic resonance perfusion imaging of the lung. Top Magn Reson Imaging 14:245-251, 2003.
213. Hatabu H, Tadamura E, Levin DL, et al: Quantitative assessment of pulmonary perfusion with dynamic contrast-enhanced MRI. Magn Reson Med 42:1033-1038, 1999.
214. Levin DL, Chen Q, Zhang M, et al: Evaluation of regional pulmonary perfusion using ultrafast magnetic resonance imaging. Magn Reson Med 46:166-171, 2001.
215. Hatabu H, Gaa J, Kim D, et al: Pulmonary perfusion and angiography: evaluation with breath-hold enhanced three-dimensional fast imaging steady-state precession MR imaging with short TR and TE. Am J Roentgenol 167:653-655, 1996.
216. Fink C, Bock M, Puderbach M, et al: Partially parallel three-dimensional magnetic resonance imaging for the assessment of lung perfusion—initial results. Invest Radiol 38:482-488, 2003.
217. Ohno Y, Higashino T, Takenaka D, et al: MR angiography with sensitivity encoding (SENSE) for suspected pulmonary embolism: Comparison with MDCT and ventilation-perfusion scintigraphy. Am J Roentgenol 183:91-98, 2004.
218. Fink C, Puderbach M, Bock M, et al: Regional lung perfusion: assessment with partially parallel three-dimensional MR imaging. Radiology 231:175-184, 2004.
219. Amundsen T, Kvaerness J, Jones RA, et al: Pulmonary embolism: detection with MR perfusion imaging of lung—a feasibility study. Radiology 203:181-185, 1997.
220. Berthezene Y, Croisille P, Bertocchi M, et al: Lung perfusion demonstrated by contrast-enhanced dynamic magnetic resonance imaging. Application to unilateral lung transplantation. Invest Radiol 32:351-356, 1997.
221. Guckel C, Schnabel K, Deimling M, et al: Solitary pulmonary nodules: MR evaluation of enhancement patterns with contrast-enhanced dynamic snapshot gradient-echo imaging. Radiology 200:681-686, 1996.
222. Ohno Y, Hatabu H, Takenaka D, et al: Contrast-enhanced MR perfusion imaging and MR angiography: utility for management of pulmonary arteriovenous malformations for embolotherapy. Eur J Radiol 41:136-146, 2002.
223. Edelman RR, Siewert B, Adamis M, et al: Signal targeting with alternating radiofrequency (STAR) sequences: application to MR angiography. Magn Reson Med 31:233-238, 1994.
224. Hatabu H, Wielopolski PA, Edelman RR: Pulmonary perfusion MR imaging with ultrashort TR/TE GRE sequence and signal targeting with alternating RF. Radiology 197(P):231, 1995.
225. Hatabu H, Wielopolski P, Tadamura E: An attempt of pulmonary perfusion imaging utilizing ultrashort TE turbo FLASH sequence with signal targeting and alternating radio-frequency. Eur J Radiol 29:160-163, 1999.
226. Hatabu H, Tadamura E, Prasad PV, et al: Noninvasive pulmonary perfusion imaging by STAR-HASTE sequence. Magn Reson Med 44:808-812, 2000.
227. Mai VM, Hagspiel KD, Christopher JM, et al: Perfusion imaging of the human lung using flow-sensitive alternating inversion recovery with an extra radiofrequency pulse (FAIRER). Magn Reson Imaging 17: 355-361, 1999.
228. Mai VM, Berr SS: MR perfusion imaging of pulmonary parenchyma using pulsed arterial spin labeling techniques: FAIRER and FAIR. J Magn Reson Imaging 9:483-487, 1999.
229. Kwong KK, Belliveau JW, Chesler DA, et al: Dynamic magnetic resonance imaging of human brain activity during primary sensory stimulation. Proc Natl Acad Sci USA 89: 5675-5679, 1992.
230. Kim SG: Quantification of relative cerebral blood flow change by flow-sensitive alternating inversion recovery (FAIR) technique: application to functional mapping. Magn Reson Med 34:293-301, 1995.
231. Detre JA, Leigh JS, Williams DS, et al: Perfusion imaging. Magn Reson Med 23:37-45, 1992.
232. Roberts DA, Gefter WB, Hirsch JA, et al: Pulmonary perfusion: respiratory-triggered three-dimensional MR imaging with arterial spin tagging—preliminary results in healthy volunteers. Radiology 212:890-895, 1999.
233. Roberts DA, Rizi RR, Lipson DA, et al: Dynamic observation of pulmonary perfusion using continuous arterial spin-labeling in a pig model. J Magn Reson Imaging 14:175-180, 2001.
234. Tadamura E, Hatabu H: Assessment of pulmonary perfusion using a subtracted HASTE image between diastole and systole. Eur J Radiol 37:179-183, 2001.
235. Suga K, Ogasawara N, Okada M, et al: Lung perfusion impairments in pulmonary embolic and airway obstruction with noncontrast MR imaging. J Appl Physiol 92:2439-2451, 2002.
236. Pauling L, Coryell C: The magnetic properties and structure of the hemochromogens and related substances. Proc Natl Acad Sci USA 22:159-163, 1936.
237. Young IR, Clarke GJ, Bailes DR, et al: Enhancement of relaxation rate with paramagnetic contrast agents in NMR imaging. J Comput Tomogr 5:543-546, 1981.
238. Gore JC, Doyle FH, Pennock JM: Relaxation rate enhancement observed in vivo by NMR imaging. In Partain CL, James AE, Rollo FD, et al (eds): Nuclear Magnetic Resonance (NMR) Imaging. Philadelphia: WB Saunders, 94-106, 1983.
239. Tripathi A, Bydder GM, Hughes JMB, et al: Effect of oxygen tension on NMR spin-lattice relaxation rate of blood in vivo. Invest Radiol 19:174-178, 1984.
240. Edelman RR, Hatabu H, Tadamura E, et al: Noninvasive assessment of regional ventilation in the human lung using oxygen-enhanced magnetic resonance imaging. Nature Med 2:1236-1239, 1996.
241. Tadamura E, Hatabu H, Li W, et al: Effect of oxygen inhalation on relaxation times in various tissues. J MRI 7:220-225, 1997.
242. Hatabu H, Tadamura E, Chen Q, et al: Pulmonary ventilation: dynamic MRI with inhalation of molecular oxygen. Eur J Radiol 37:172-178, 2001.
243. Ohno Y, Hatabu H, Takenaka D, et al: Dynamic oxygen-enhanced MRI reflects diffusing capacity of the lung. Magn Reson Med 47:1139-1144, 2002.
244. Muller CJ, Schwaiblmair M, Scheidler J, et al: Pulmonary diffusing capacity: assessment with oxygen-enhanced lung MR imaging preliminary findings. Radiology 222: 499-506, 2002.
245. Ohno Y, Hatabu H, Takenaka D, et al: Oxygen-enhanced MR ventilation imaging of the lung: preliminary clinical experience in 25 subjects. Am J Roentgenol 177:185-194, 2001.
246. Nakagawa T, Sakuma H, Murashima S, et al: Pulmonary ventilation-perfusion MR imaging in clinical patients. J Magn Reson Imaging 14:419-424, 2001.
247. Ohno Y, Sugimura K, Hatabu H: Clinical oxygen-enhanced magnetic resonance imaging of the lung. Top Magn Reson Imaging 14:237-243, 2003.
248. Albert MS, Cates GD, Driehuys B, et al: Biological magnetic resonance imaging using laser-polarized [129]Xe. Nature 370:199-201, 1994.
249. Middleton H, Black RD, Saam B, et al: MR imaging with hyperpolarized [3]He gas. Magn Reson Med 33:271-275, 1995.
250. MacFall JR, Charles HC, Black H, et al: Human lung air spaces: potential for MR imaging with hyperpolarized He-3. Radiology 200:553-558, 1996.
251. Ebert M, Grossmann T, Heil W, et al: Nuclear magnetic resonance imaging with hyperpolarised helium 3. Lancet 1996; 347:1297-1299.
252. Kauczor HU: Hyperpolarized helium-3 gas magnetic resonance imaging of the lung. Top Magn Reson Imaging 14:223-230, 2003.
253. Kauczor HU, Hofmann D, Kreitner KF, et al: Normal and abnormal pulmonary ventilation: visualization at hyperpolarized He-3 MR imaging. Radiology 201(2):564-568, 1996.
254. Kauczor HU, Ebert M, Kreitner KF, et al: Imaging of the lungs using [3]He MRI: preliminary clinical experience in 18 patients with and without lung disease. J Magn Reson Imaging 7:538-543, 1997.
255. Kauczor H-U, Surkau R, Roberts T: MRI using hyperpolarized noble gases. Eur Radiol 8:820-827, 1998.
256. Guenther D, Eberle B, Hast J, et al: [3]He MRI in healthy volunteers: Preliminary correlation with smoking history and lung volumes. NMR Biomed 13:182-189, 2000.
257. deLange E, Mugler J, Brookeman J, et al: Lung air spaces: MR imaging evaluation with hyperpolarized He gas. Radiology 210:851-857, 1999.
258. Donnelly LF, MacFall JR, McAdams HP, et al: Cystic fibrosis: Combined hyperpolarized [3]He-enhanced and conventional proton MR imaging in the lung—preliminary observations. Radiology 212:885-889, 1999.
259. Altes T, Powers P, Knight-Scott J, et al: Hyperpolarized [3]He MR lung ventilation imaging in asthmatics: Preliminary findings. J Magn Reson Imag 13:378-384, 2001.
260. McAdams H, Palmer SM, Donnelly L, et al: Hyperpolarized [3]He-enhanced MR imaging of lung transplant recipients: preliminary results. Am J Roentgenol 173:955-959, 1999.
261. Gast K, Viallon M, Eberle B, et al: MR imaging in lung transplant recipients using hyperpolarized [3]He: comparison with CT. J Magn Reson Imag 15: 268-274, 2002.
262. Schreiber W, Weiler N, Kauczor H-U, et al: Ultraschnelle MRT der Lungenventilation mittels hochpolarisiertem Helium-3. Fortschr Röntgenstr 172:129-133, 2000.
263. Saam B, Yablonskiy DA, Gierada DS: Rapid imaging of hyperpolarized gas using EPI. Magn Reson Med 42:507-514, 1999.
264. Salerno M, Altes T, Brookeman J, et al: Dynamic spiral MRI of pulmonary gas flow using hyperpolarized [3]He: Preliminary studies in healthy and diseased lungs. Magn Reson Med 46: 667-677, 2001.
265. Gierada D, Saam B, Yablonskiy D, et al: Dynamic echo planar MR imaging of lung ventilation with hyperpolarized He-3 in normal subjects and patients with severe emphysema. NMR Biomed 13:176-181, 2000.
266. Gast K, Puderbach M, Rodriguez I, et al: Dynamic ventilation [3]He MRI with lung motion correction: gas flow distribution analysis. Invest Radiol 37:126-134, 2002.
267. Moeller H, Chen X, Saam B, et al: MRI of the lungs using hyperpolarized noble gases. Magn Reson Med 47:1029-1051, 2002.
268. Mugler J, Brookeman J, Knight-Scott J, et al: Regional measurement of the [3]He diffusion coefficient in the human lung. ISMRM 6th Scientific Meeting, Sydney, 1998.
269. Hanisch G, Schreiber W, Diergarten T, et al: Investigation of intrapulmonary diffusion by [3]He MRI. Eur Radiol 10:S345, 2000.
270. Salerno M, Brookeman J, deLange E, et al: Detection of regional microstructural changes of the lung in emphysema using hyperpolarized [3]He diffusion MRI. Proc Intl Soc Mag Reson Med 9, 2000.
271. Saam B, Yablonskiy D, Kodibagkar V, et al: MR imaging of diffusion of [3]He gas in healthy and diseased lungs. Magn Reson Med 44:174-179, 2000.
272. Salerno M, deLange E, Altes T, et al: Emphysema: hyperpolarized Helium3 diffusion MR imaging of the lungs compared with spirometric indexes—initial experience. Radiology 222:252-260, 2002.
273. Hanisch G, Schreiber W, Kauczor H-U, et al: Determination of diffusion anisotropy in the lung by Helium-3 MRI. Eur Radiol 10: G3, 2000.

274. Yablonskiy D, Sukstanskii A, Leawoods J, et al: Quantitative in vivo assessment of lung microstructure at the alveolar level with hyperpolarized ^{3}He diffusion MRI. Proc Natl Acad Sci USA 99:3111-3116, 2002.

275. Saam B, Happer W, Middleton H: Nuclear relaxation of ^{3}He in the presence of O2.Phys Rev A 52: 862-865, 1995.

276. Markstaller K, Eberle B, Deninger A, et al: Flip angle considerations in quantification of intrapulmonary oxygen concentration by Helium-MRI. NMR Biomed 13:190-193, 2000.

277. Deninger A, Eberle B, Ebert M, et al: Quantitation of regional intrapulmonary oxygen partial pressure evaluation during apnoe by ^{3}He-MRI. J MRI 141:207-216, 1999.

278. Deninger A, Eberle B, Bermuth J, et al: Assessment of a single-acquisition imaging sequence for oxygen-sensitive ^{3}He MRI. Magn Reson Med 47:105-114, 2002.

279. Altes TA, de Lange EE: Applications of hyperpolarized helium-3 gas magnetic resonance imaging in pediatric lung disease. Top Magn Reson Imaging 14:231-236, 2003.

280. Miller KW, Reo NV, Schoot Uiterkamp AJM, et al: Xenon NMR: chemical shifts of a general anesthetic in common solvents, proteins, and membranes. Proc Natl Acad Sci U S A 78:4946-4949, 1981.

281. Mugler JP 3rd, Driehuys B, Brookeman JR, et al: MR imaging and spectroscopy using hyperpolarized ^{129}Xe gas: preliminary human results. Magn Reson Med 37:809-815, 1997.

282. Albert MS, Tseng CH, Williamson D, et al: Hyperpolarized ^{129}Xe MR imaging of the oral cavity. J Magn Reson 111:204-207, 1996.

283. Swanson SD, Rosen MS, Agranoff BW, et al: Brain MRI with laser-polarized ^{129}Xe. Magn Reson Med 38:695-698, 1997.

284. Swanson SD, Rosen MS, Coulter KP, et al: Distribution and dynamics of laser-polarized ^{129}Xe magnetization in vivo. Magn Reson Med 42:1137-1145, 1999.

285. Kilian W, Seifert F, Rinnerberg H: Chemical shift imaging of human brain after inhaling hyperpolarized ^{129}Xe gas. In: Proceedings of the 10th Annual Meeting of ISMRM, 2002, Honolulu, 758.

286. Wagshul ME, Button TM, Li HF, et al: In vivo MR imaging and spectroscopy using hyperpolarized ^{129}Xe. Magn Reson Med 36:183-191, 1996.

287. Bifone A, Song YQ, Seydoux R, et al: NMR of laser-polarized xenon in human blood. Proc Natl Acad Sci U S A 93:12932-12936, 1996.

288. Maier T, Driehuys B, Hinton DP, et al: In: Proceedings of the 6th Annual Meeting of ISMRM, 1998, Sydney, Australia, 1907.

289. Wolber J, Doran SJ, Leach MO, et al: Measuring diffusion of xenon in solution with hyperpolarized ^{129}Xe NMR. Chem Phys Lett 296:391-396, 1998.

290. Wolber J, Santoro D, Leach MO, et al: Diffusion of hyperpolarized ^{129}Xe in biological systems: effects of chemical exchange. In: Proceedings of the 8th Annual Meeting of ISMRM, 2000, Denver, 754.

291. Wolber J, McIntyre DJ, Rodrigues LM, et al: In vivo hyperpolarized ^{129}Xe NMR spectroscopy in tumors. Magn Reson Med 46:586-591, 2001.

292. Sakai K, Bilek AM, Oteiza E, et al: Temporal dynamics of hyperpolarized ^{129}Xe resonance in living rats. J Magn Reson 111:300-304, 1996.

293. Ruppert K, Brookeman JR, Hagspiel KD, et al: NMR of hyperpolarized ^{129}Xe in the canine chest: spectral dynamics during a breath-hold. NMR Biomed 13:220-228, 2000.

294. Venkatesh AK, Hong KS, Kubatina L, et al: Direct observation of the transport of ^{129}Xe from the lung-gas to the tissue and the blood. In: Proceedings of the 9th Annual Meeting of ISMRM, 2001, Glasgow, Scotland, 954.

295. Wolber J, Cherubini A, Leach MO, et al: On the oxygenation–^{129}Xe T1 in blood. NMR Biomed 13: 234-237, 2000.

296. Cross A, McPhee D, Santyr GE, et al: Effects of dilution and oxygenation on T_1 of ^{129}Xe in perfluorocarbon emulsions. In: Proceedings of the 9th Annual Meeting of ISMRM, 2001, Glasgow, Scotland, 953.

297. Lavini C, Payne GS, Leach MO, et al: Intravenous delivery of hyperpolarized ^{129}Xe: a compartmental model. NMR Biomed 13:238-244, 2000.

298. Venkatesh AK, Zhao L, Balamore D, et al: Evaluation of carrier agents for hyperpolarized xenon MRI. NMR Biomed 13:245-252, 2000.

299. Duhamel G, Choquet P, Grillon E, et al: Xenon-129 MR imaging and spectroscopy of rat brain using arterial delivery of hyperpolarized xenon in a lipid emulsion. Magn Reson Med 46:208-212, 2001.

300. Wallace JC, Cross AR, Santyr GE, et al: Pharmacokinetics of hyperpolarized ^{129}Xe in a perfluorocarbon emulsion injected in a hollow-fibre capillary model of a breast tumor. In: Proceedings of the 10th Annual Meeting of ISMRM, 2002, Honolulu, 2002.

301. Goodson BM, Song Y, Taylor RE, et al: An In vivo NMR and MRI using injection delivery of laser-polarized xenon. Proc Natl Acad Sci USA 23(94):14725-14729, 1997.

302. Ruppert K, Brookeman JR, Hagspiel KD, et al: Probing lung physiology with xenon polarization transfer contrast (XTC). Magn Reson Med 44:349-357, 2000.

303. Ruppert K, Mata JF, Brookeman JR, et al: Exploring lung function with (hyperpolarized ^{129}Xe) nuclear magnetic resonance. Magn Reson Med 5:676-687, 2004.

304. Chen Q, Levin DL, Kim D, et al: Pulmonary disorders: ventilation-perfusion MR imaging with animal models. Radiology 213:871-879, 1999.

305. Hasegawa I, Uematsu H, Gee JC, et al: Voxelwise mapping of magnetic resonance ventilation-perfusion ratio in a porcine model by multimodality registration: technical note. Acad Radiol 10:1091-1096, 2003.

306. Berthezene Y, Vexler V, Clement O, et al: Contrast-enhanced MR imaging of the lung: assessments of ventilation and perfusion. Radiology 183:667-672, 1992.

307. Mai VM, Liu B, Polzin JA, et al: Ventilation-perfusion ratio of signal intensity in human lung using oxygen-enhanced and arterial spin labeling techniques. Magn Reson Med 48:341-350, 2002.

308. Napadow VJ, Mai V, Bankier A, et al: Determination of regional pulmonary parenchymal strain during normal respiration using spin inversion tagged magnetization MRI. J Magn Reson Imaging 13(3):67-74, 2001.

309. Chen Q, Mai VM, Bankier AA, et al: Ultrafast MR grid-tagging sequence for assessment of local mechanical properties of the lungs. Magn Reson Med 45(1):4-8, 2001.

310. Hatabu H, Ohno Y, Uematsu H, et al: Lung biomechanics via non-rigid registration of serial MR images. Radiology 221(P):630, 2001.

311. Gee J, Sundaram T, Hasegawa I, et al: Characterization of regional pulmonary mechanics from serial magnetic resonance imaging data. Acad Radiol 10:1147-1152, 2003.

CHAPTER 77

BREAST CANCER

Elizabeth A. Morris

INTRODUCTION

MRI has become an important and powerful tool in breast imaging. The performance and clinical uses of breast MRI are more standardized and defined than they were several decades ago. In recent years, great strides have been made in the realm of breast intervention with new coils and needles now available. More sequences are available from manufacturers with an increase in image quality and speed of acquisition. Breast MRI is no longer just a research tool in an academic setting. It is now available in many community practices. In fact, by using breast MRI, many current algorithms in the detection and treatment of breast cancer may change.

The strength of breast MRI lies in the detection of cancer that is occult on conventional imaging, such as mammography and sonography.[1,2] Many studies have shown that breast MRI is used best in situations where there is a known cancer, suspected cancer, or a high probability of finding cancer. For example, in the preoperative evaluation of the patient with a known cancer, the ability of MRI to detect multifocal (within the same quadrant of the breast) and multicentric (within different quadrants) disease that was previously unsuspected (Fig. 77-1) facilitates accurate staging.[3-10] Incidental synchronous contralateral carcinomas have also been detected when screening the contralateral breast in patients with known cancer (Fig. 77-2).[4,11,12] In the patient with positive margins following an initial attempt at breast conservation, MRI can detect residual disease (Fig. 77-3),[13-15] and in the patient with inoperable locally advanced breast cancer, MRI can assess response to neoadjuvant chemotherapy (Fig. 77-4).[16-20] Suspected recurrence can be confirmed with MRI in the previously treated breast (Fig. 77-5)[21-23] and breast MRI is absolutely indicated in the patient with axillary node metastases with unknown primary (Fig. 77-6).[24-28] Another indication that may be promising, though not yet validated by randomized trials, is the use of MRI for high-risk screening (Fig. 77-7).[29-35]

In recent decades, as breast MRI has been incorporated into the clinical evaluation of the breast, it has become apparent that standardization of image acquisition and terminology is important. The American College of Radiology Committee on Standards and Guidelines has drafted a document for the performance of breast MRI, which was published in 2004 and the recent publication of the Breast Imaging Reporting and Data System (BI-RADS®) lexicon (see later)[36] includes a section on breast MRI so that standardized terminology can be used when describing findings on breast MRI. The existence of standardized guidelines in image acquisition and interpretation will possibly help further disseminate this technology from academic centers into the community.

PREOPERATIVE STAGING

Traditional preoperative planning for breast cancer involves clinical examination and a mammogram. It has been shown from a study of 282 mastectomy specimens (performed for unifocal breast cancer, assessed clinically and mammographically) that the majority of breasts (63%) have additional sites of cancer that were undetected by clinical examination or mammography.[37] Additional foci of cancer were found pathologically in 20% of cases within 2 cm of the index cancer and in 43% more than 2 cm away from the index cancer; 7% had additional foci of carcinoma more than 4 cm away from

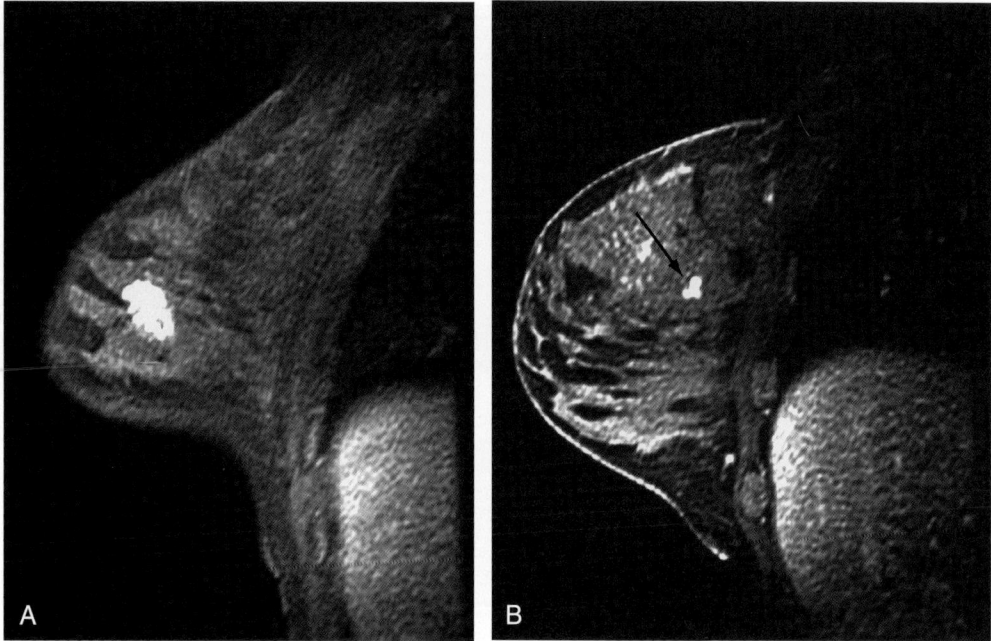

FIGURE 77-1

Multicentric carcinoma. This and all subsequent images are contrast-enhanced fat-suppressed 3D fast-spoiled gradient-echo (FSPGR) (TR/TE 17.1/2.4). **A,** 31-year-old woman presents with a palpable mass seen on ultrasound but not on a mammogram. Biopsy showed invasive ductal carcinoma. MRI performed for staging prior to surgery due to the patient's age and extreme breast density. MRI demonstrates the palpable mass. **B,** In a separate quadrant a 4-mm irregular mass (*arrow*) is identified that was subsequently biopsied, yielding invasive ductal carcinoma compatible with multicentric disease. The patient underwent mastectomy.

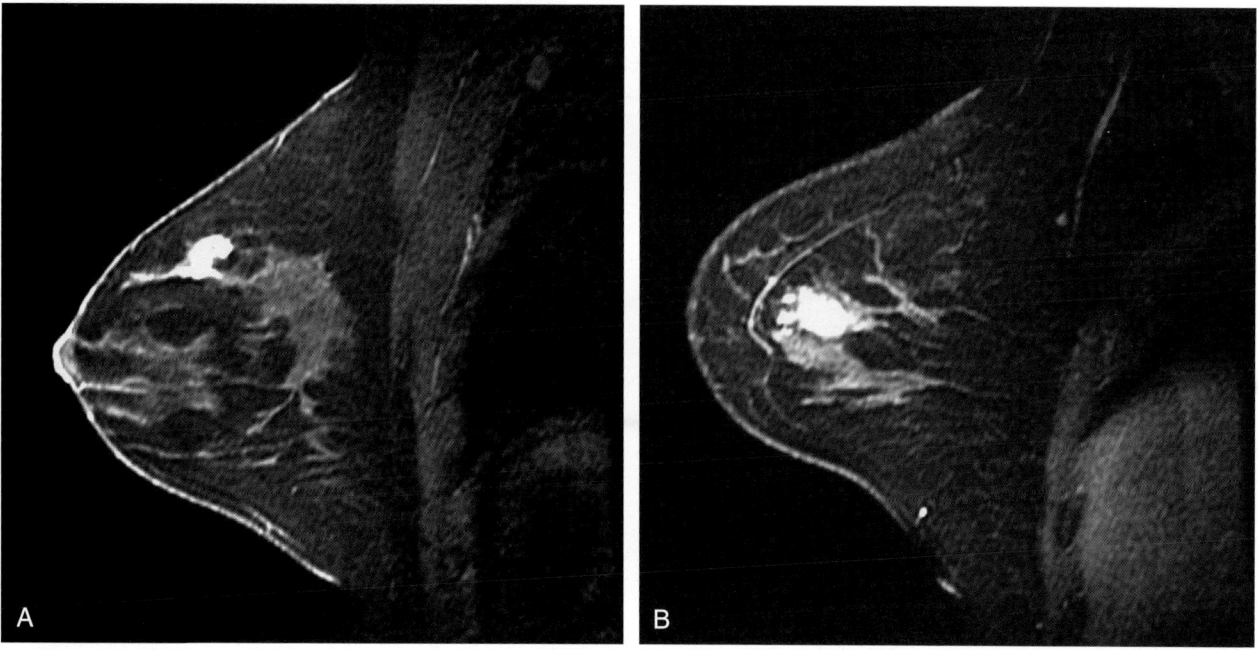

FIGURE 77-2

Contralateral carcinoma. **A,** 35-year-old woman palpated a mass in the left breast. Biopsy proved malignant. MRI demonstrates the index invasive ductal carcinoma with no additional suspicious findings in the left breast. **B,** Screening of the contralateral right breast demonstrates an irregular heterogeneously enhancing oval mass that represented a synchronous poorly differentiated invasive carcinoma with lobular features occult to physical examination and mammography.

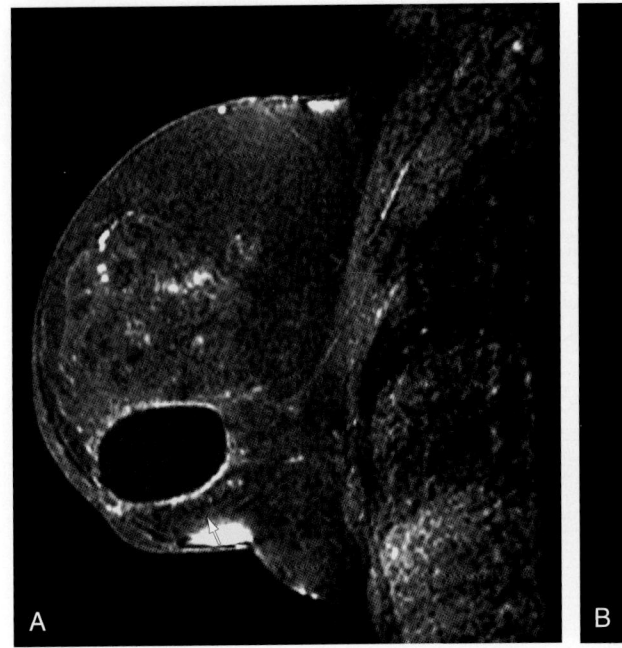

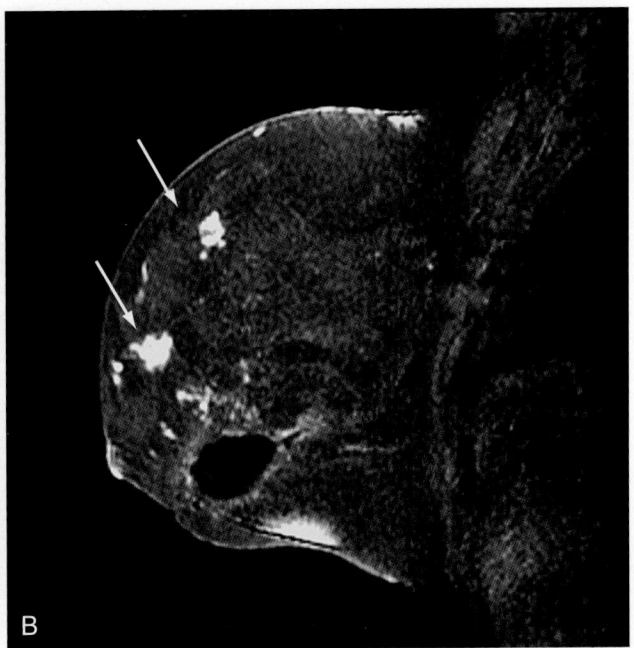

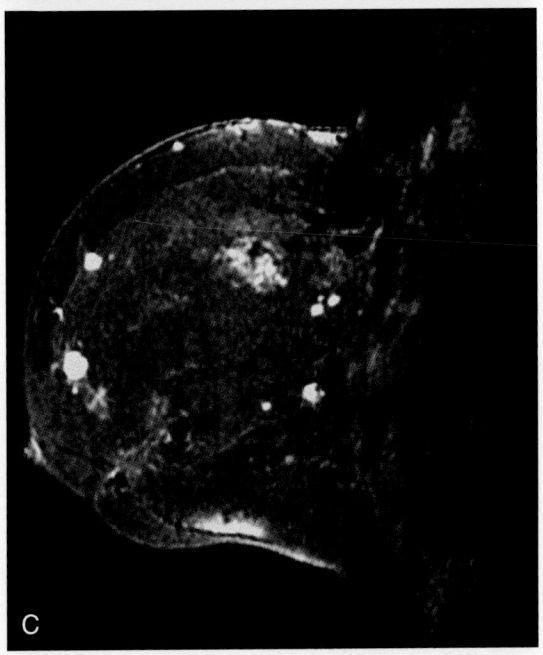

FIGURE 77-3

Residual disease. **A,** 30-year-old woman underwent removal of a palpable mass yielding invasive ductal carcinoma with positive margins. The postoperative seroma cavity is identified (*arrow*) with thin rim enhancement that is compatible with the postoperative state. No bulky residual disease is noted at the lumpectomy site. **B,** In a separate quadrant from the lumpectomy site there are two suspicious masses (*arrows*) which were subsequently biopsied yielding multicentric carcinoma for which the patient underwent mastectomy. **C,** Laterally multiple additional suspicious masses are identified that represented additional sites of carcinoma.

the index cancer, likely representing cancer within a separate breast quadrant. The presence of undetected residual disease that is not removed entirely at surgery is the rational for performing postoperative radiation therapy in patients who are treated with breast conservation therapy.

It has been known that disease may or may not be left behind in the breast; however, it has not been possible without the addition of MRI to reliably identify which patients have additional multifocal or multicentric cancer. Many studies have shown that MRI is able to detect additional foci of cancer in the breast that have been overlooked by conventional techniques. Several

investigators have shown that MRI is able to detect additional foci of disease (Fig. 77-8) in up to one third of patients,[3,4] possibly resulting in a treatment change.[8,9] MRI can potentially provide valuable information for preoperative planning in the single-stage resection of breast cancer.[10,11] By using breast MRI as a complementary test to conventional imaging techniques, more precise information can be obtained about the extent of breast cancer, improving patient care.

Patient selection for preoperative breast MRI may include the young patient, the patient with dense or moderately dense breasts, and the patient with difficult tumor histology, such as infiltrating lobular carcinoma

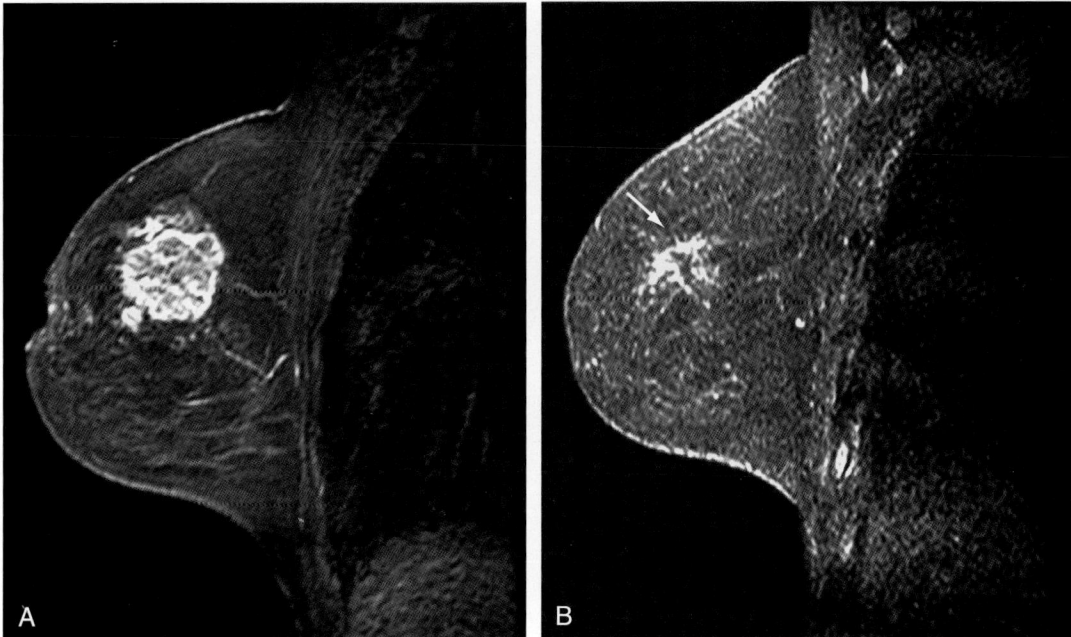

FIGURE 77-4

Neoadjuvent chemotherapy response. **A,** 39-year-old woman with locally advanced invasive ductal carcinoma. Pretreatment MRI demonstrates a large irregular mass with heterogeneous enhancement. **B,** Post-treatment MRI demonstrates very faint residual enhancement (*arrow*). At mastectomy prominent inflammatory changes were identified with no evidence of residual tumor.

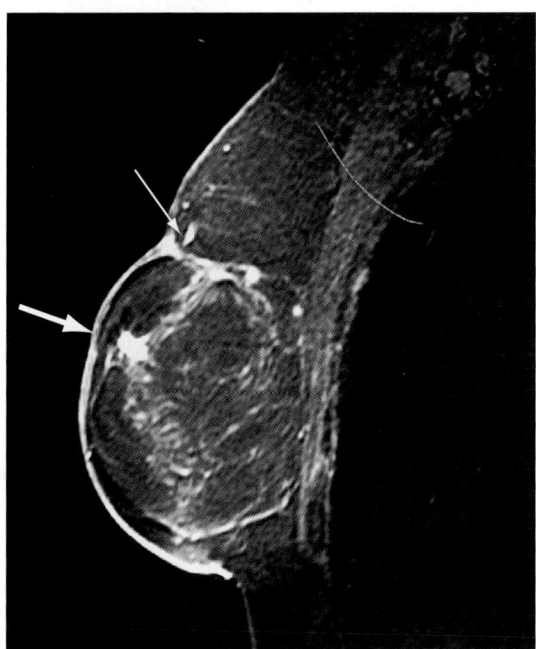

FIGURE 77-5

Recurrence. 53-year-old woman treated with conservation therapy for invasive ductal carcinoma 5 years previously. Screening MRI examination was performed. Recent mammography was negative. The lumpectomy site is identified in the superior breast with distortion and scarring extending to the skin (*thin arrow*). In the inferior breast an irregular mass is identified (*thick arrow*) that was subsequently identified on targeted ultrasound. Biopsy was performed yielding poorly differentiated invasive ductal carcinoma. The patient then underwent mastectomy.

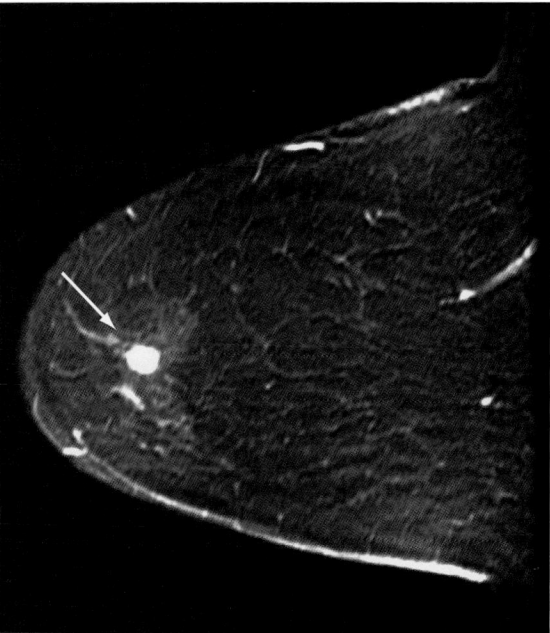

FIGURE 77-6

Unknown primary. 52-year-old woman with a palpable enlarged right axillary lymph node, biopsy positive for adenocarcinoma. Mammogram and physical examination were negative. MRI demonstrates an enhancing mass in the anterior breast which represents the patient's primary tumor (*arrow*). Biopsy showed invasive ductal carcinoma. The patient was then able to undergo breast conservation therapy in lieu of mastectomy.

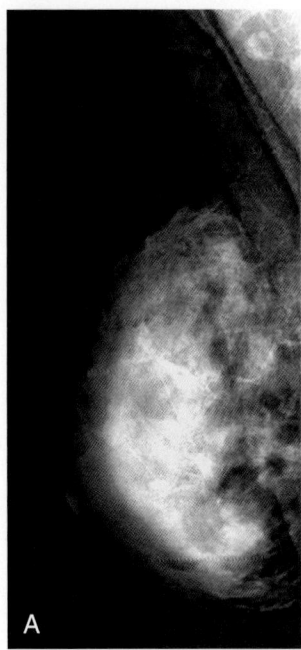
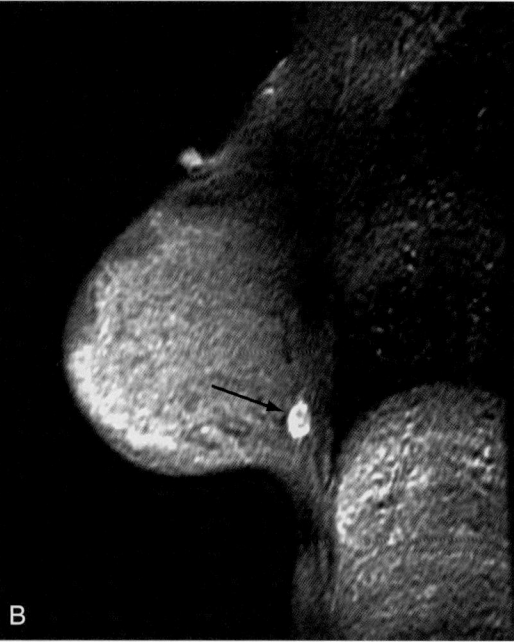

FIGURE 77-7

High-risk screening. **A,** 41-year-old, BRCA 2-positive woman underwent screening mammography, demonstrating a dense breast with no suspicious findings. **B,** Screening MRI obtained on the same day demonstrates an irregular rim-enhancing mass in the posterior breast (*arrow*). Targeted ultrasound was able to identify this area and biopsy was performed yielding invasive ductal carcinoma. The patient elected to undergo bilateral mastectomy. Sentinel lymph nodes were negative.

and tumors with extensive intraductal component, where assessment of tumor size is difficult.[10] Infiltrating lobular carcinoma is known to be difficult to detect on mammography and MRI has been shown to assess the correct extent of disease with infiltrating lobular carcinoma (Fig. 77-9) better than mammography.[38,39] MRI has also been shown to demonstrate unsuspected (DCIS) (Fig. 77-10), which can be helpful when assessing extent of disease in preoperative testing.[40-42] Extensive intraductal component (EIC) is associated with a known invasive carcinoma when greater than 25% of the tumor is DCIS. EIC is associated with residual carcinoma and positive margins after lumpectomy and there is some evidence that the presence of EIC may indicate an increased risk of local recurrence.

Breast MRI can give helpful information for staging, on tumor size, and presence or absence of multifocal or multicentric disease, as well as whether the chest wall or pectoralis muscle is invaded.[43] MR defines the anatomic extent of disease more accurately than mammography, particularly in tumors with difficult histologies, as discussed earlier. Chest wall involvement is an important consideration for the surgeon prior to surgical planning. Mammography does not image the ribs, intercostal muscles and serratus anterior muscle that comprise the chest wall. Tumor involvement of the chest wall changes the patient's stage to IIIB (Fig. 77-11), indicating that the patient may benefit from neoadjuvant chemotherapy prior to surgery (Fig. 77-12). Tumor involvement of the pectoralis muscle does not alter staging and surgery can usually proceed (Fig. 77-13); however, knowledge that the muscle is involved may alter the surgeon's plan. For example, if the full thickness of the pectoralis major muscle is involved with tumor, the surgeon may be more inclined to perform a radical instead of a modified radical mastectomy.

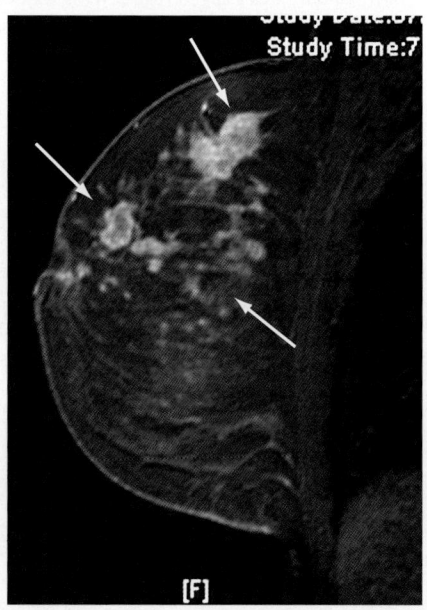

FIGURE 77-8

Extent of disease evaluation. 42-year-old woman with palpable masses in the upper outer quadrant of the right breast. MRI demonstrates multiple spiculated and irregular masses (*arrows*), some with rim enhancement corresponding to the palpable findings. Although only one quadrant was involved, negative margins could not be obtained with good cosmetic result and therefore the patient underwent mastectomy.

Controversy exists regarding the use of MRI to stage breast cancer. It is argued that MRI may identify cancer that is currently adequately treated with adjuvant chemotherapy and radiation therapy, especially DCIS, thus resulting in over treatment of the patient's breast cancer. For example, many women who may be

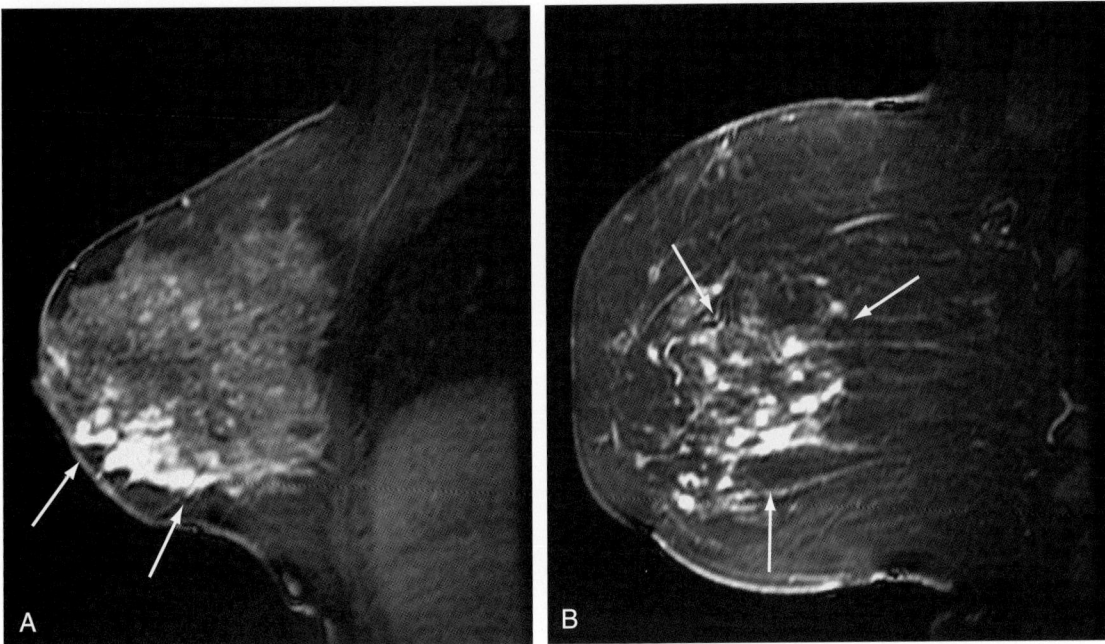

FIGURE 77-9

Infiltrating lobular carcinoma. **A,** 37-year-old woman with a palpable mass in the inferior breast. Mammogram and ultrasound were negative. MRI demonstrates a regional area of enhancement in the inferior breast that corresponded to a large 6-cm invasive lobular carcinoma (*arrows*). The patient underwent mastectomy. **B,** 39-year-old patient with a suspicious mass noted on mammography. Based on the mammogram the patient was considered to be a candidate for conservation therapy. MRI demonstrated multiquadrant involvement with clumped and masslike enhancement throughout the central breast (*arrows*). MRI evaluation better delineated the extent of disease.

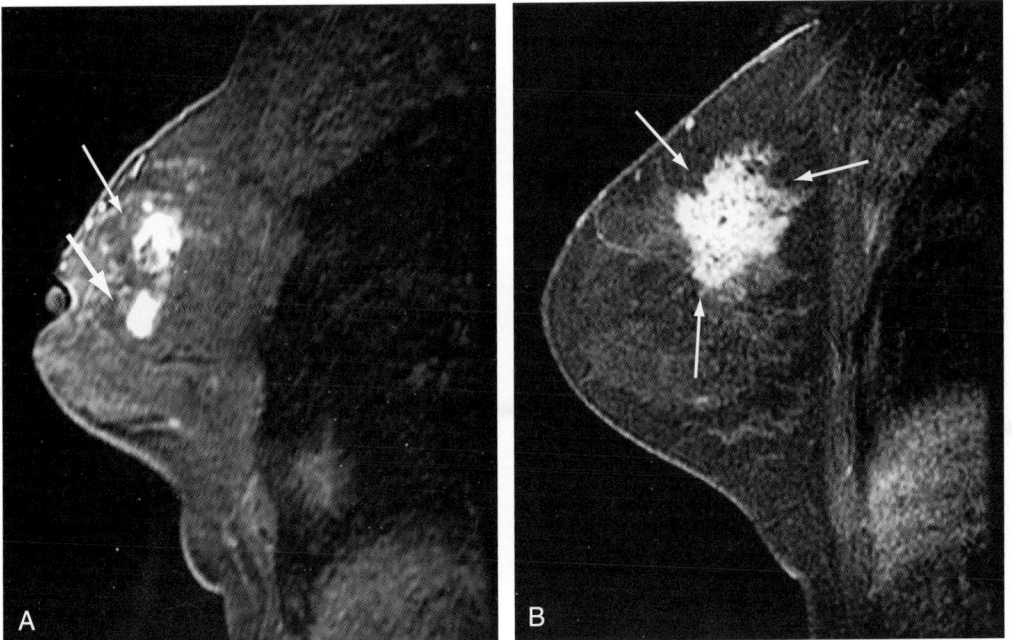

FIGURE 77-10

Unsuspected ductal carcinoma in situ (DCIS). **A,** 45-year-old woman with dense breasts presents with a palpable lump. Fine needle aspiration of the palpable lump (*thick arrow*) yielded adenocarcinoma. MRI was performed to evaluate disease extent. Extensive clumped enhancement is seen in the upper breast (*thin arrow*), corresponding to DCIS that comprised more than 40% of the tumor compatible with extensive intraductal component. **B,** 32-year-old woman presents with palpable mass that corresponds to a regional area of clumped enhancement on MRI (*arrows*) that yielded DCIS on biopsy. Mammography in both cases was negative without suspicious calcifications.

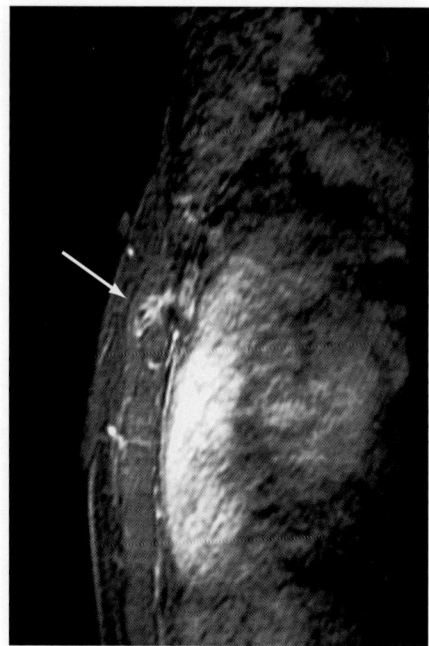

FIGURE 77-11

Chest wall involvement. 35-year-old high-risk woman presents with a palpable lump. Percutaneous core biopsy demonstrated poorly differentiated invasive ductal carcinoma. MRI was performed for staging. Abnormal enhancement is seen medially along the chest wall and extending into the intercostal muscles (*arrow*), which is compatible with chest wall involvement, indicating this patient is no longer a surgical candidate.

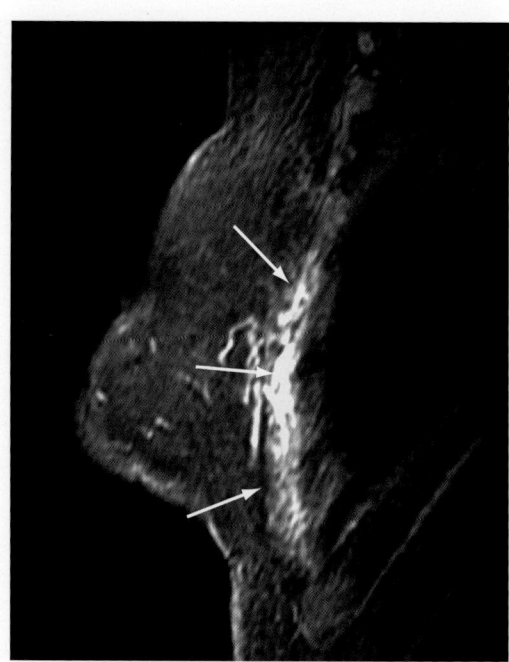

FIGURE 77-12

Chest wall invasion. 43-year-old woman with prior history of breast cancer presents with chest wall pain. MRI demonstrates enhancement of the serratus muscles (*arrows*). Biopsy yielded recurrent invasive ductal carcinoma with chest wall involvement.

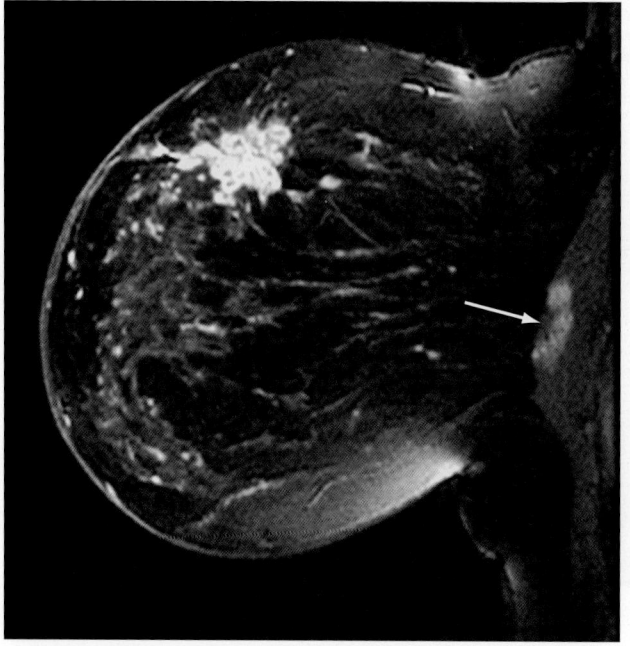

FIGURE 77-13

Pectoralis major invasion. 41-year-old with locally advanced breast cancer. MRI demonstrates a spiculated mass in the upper breast and pectoralis major muscle invasion (*arrow*). Invasion of the pectoralis major muscle does not preclude surgery.

candidates for breast conservation therapy may be over treated with mastectomy based on MRI results where additional disease is found elsewhere. These issues raise many questions, such as what size lesion can be safely ignored on MRI as perhaps MRI is too sensitive in detecting cancer in general. For current treatment algorithms, MRI may be detecting subclinical disease that may not be clinically relevant. On the other hand, MRI may detect additional disease that would not be treated with adjuvant therapy. The challenge is in knowing what is and what is not clinically significant disease. At this time, identification of significant disease that will not be treated with radiation therapy is not possible and all additional disease is treated surgically. Performing breast MRI to possibly prevent recurrence may be of benefit to the minority of breast conservation patients, namely those who will recur. Further complicating matters is that the ability to decrease the recurrence rate may have no overall effect on patient mortality. Trials that involve radiologists as well as radiation oncologists and surgeons are needed to answer these perplexing questions.

NEOADJUVANT CHEMOTHERAPY RESPONSE

Response to neoadjuvant chemotherapy for locally advanced breast cancer can be assessed with MRI. A complete pathologic response (elimination of tumor) following neoadjuvant therapy is strongly predictive

of excellent long-term survival (Fig. 77-14). Minimal response (Fig. 77-15) suggests a poor long-term survival regardless of postoperative therapy. MRI may find a role in being able to predict at an earlier time point, perhaps after a single cycle of chemotherapy, which patients are responding to neoadjuvant chemotherapy. Early knowledge of suboptimal response may allow substitution of alternative treatment regimens earlier rather than later. Unless the response is dramatic, it currently takes longer to predict response, as the mammogram and physical examination may be compromised due to fibrosis. Investigators have demonstrated that residual tumor measurements on MRI correlate with the pathologic residual disease following neoadjuvant chemotherapy.[44] Patterns of response are being evaluated in the hope that these findings may predict recurrence and survival. These patterns may hold more information because the mere presence or absence of enhancement may be misleading, as fibrosis, a consequence of treatment, may enhance or residual tiny islands of tumor may exist after treatment which are below the detection level of MRI.

ASSESSMENT OF RESIDUAL DISEASE

For patients who have undergone lumpectomy with positive margins, MRI can be helpful in the assessment of residual tumor load (Fig. 77-16). Postoperative mammography is able to detect residual calcifications, though

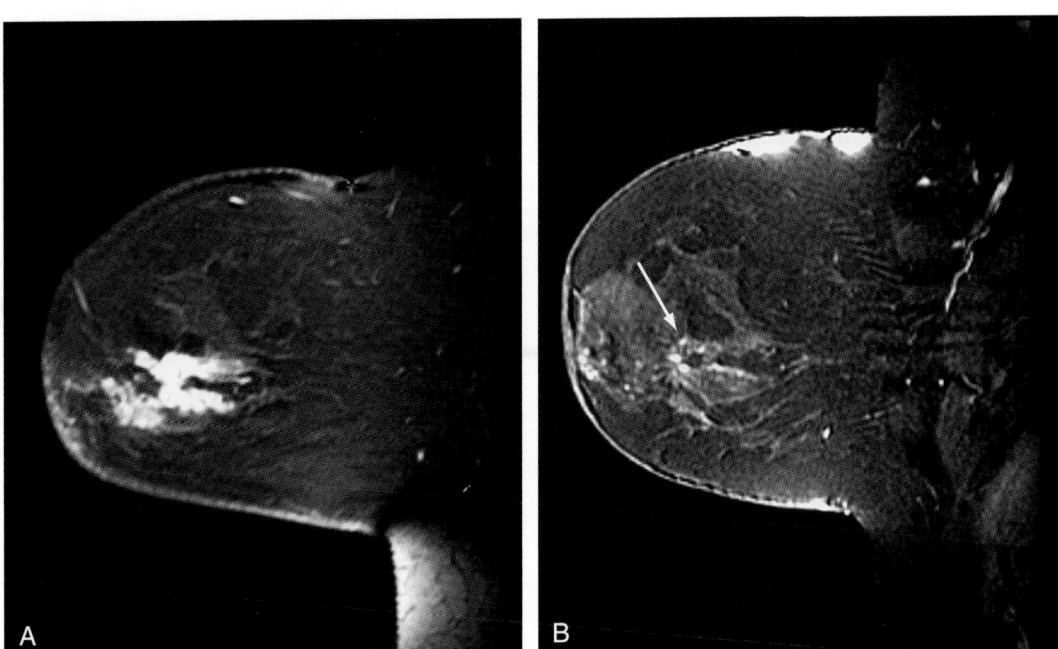

FIGURE 77-14

Complete clinical response. **A,** 57-year-old woman with inflammatory breast carcinoma involving the skin (not shown). Pretreatment MRI demonstrates a large irregular heterogeneously enhancing mass in the anterior breast. **B,** Post-treatment MRI following several cycles of chemotherapy demonstrates a tiny amount of residual enhancement (*arrow*). At mastectomy a few scattered foci of high-grade ductal carcinoma in situ were identified with no areas of invasion.

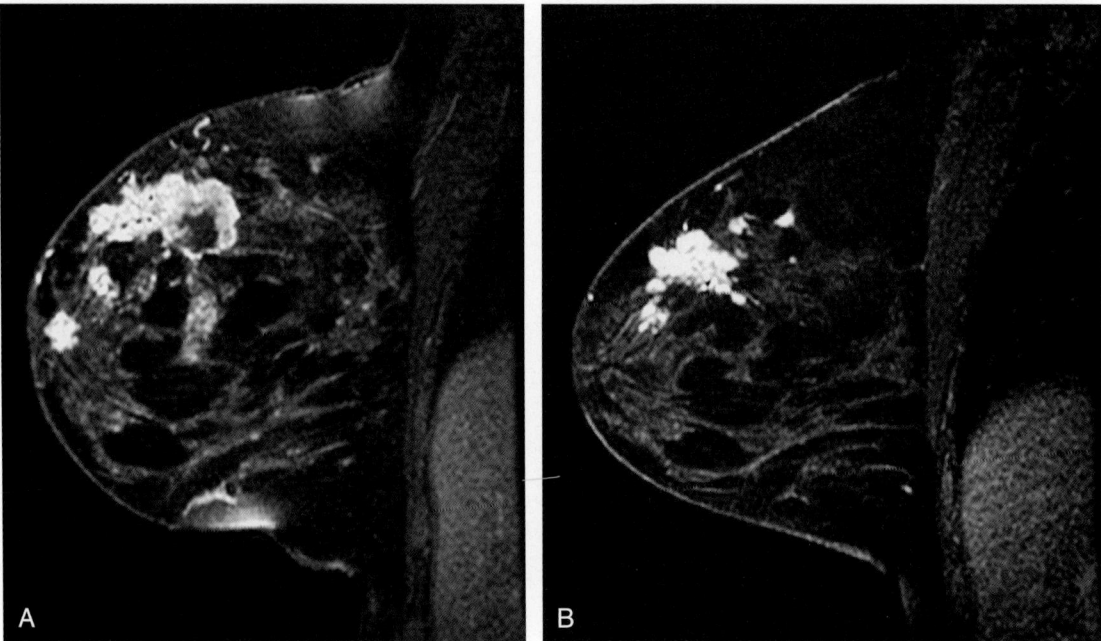

FIGURE 77-15

Partial clinical response. **A,** 52-year-old woman with locally advanced breast carcinoma. In the superior breast a large mass is identified on the pretreatment MRI. **B,** Post-treatment MRI following several cycles of chemotherapy demonstrates some response but persistence of the mass. The mastectomy specimen demonstrated several foci of residual invasive ductal carcinoma measuring up to 3 cm.

it is limited in the evaluation of residual uncalcified DCIS or residual mass. MRI is able to detect bulky residual disease at the lumpectomy site (Fig. 77-17) as well as residual disease in the same (multifocal) (Fig. 77-18) or different quadrant (multicentric) (Fig. 77-19). Determination of whether the patient would be best served with directed re-excision (residual disease at the lumpectomy site or multifocal disease) or whether she warrants mastectomy (multicentric disease) is where MRI can be helpful. Evaluation for microscopic residual disease directly at the lumpectomy site is not the role of MRI as the surgeon will perform re-excision based on pathologic margins and not MRI results. If multicentric disease is identified on MRI prior to mastectomy, it is important to sample and verify this impression. A study has shown that MRI is able to detect residual disease in 23 of 33 (70%) patients and alone identified multifocal or multicentric disease in 9 of 33 (27%) patients.[14] We looked at 100 women who underwent MRI for positive margins: 58 had residual disease at surgery (20 multicentric, 15 multifocal, and 23 unifocal). MR identified 18 of 20 (90%) cases of multicentric, 14 of 15 (93%) cases of multifocal, and 18 of 23 (78%) cases of unifocal residual disease. Eight false-negative findings included two cases of multicentric DCIS occult to MR imaging and six cases of residual disease (four subcentimeter invasive and two microscopic DCIS) directly at the lumpectomy site. Overall sensitivity for detection of residual cancer was 86% (50 of 58 cases) and specificity was 68% (28 of 41).

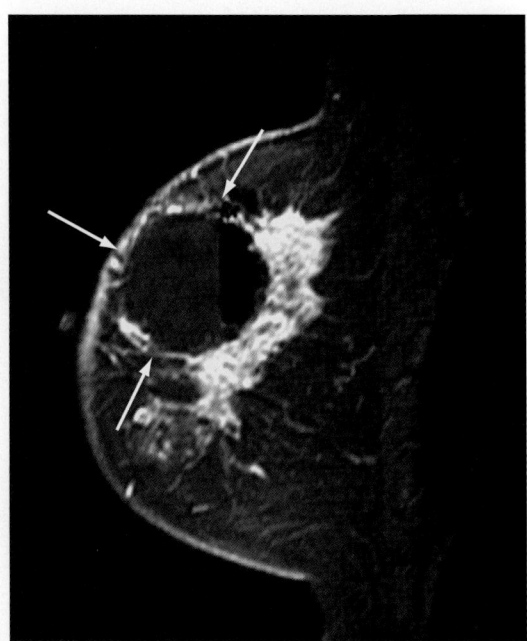

FIGURE 77-16

Residual tumor. 42-year-old woman who presented for breast reduction surgery and was found to have a mass. Excisional biopsy yielded invasive lobular carcinoma with the tumor extending to the cauterized margins. Postexcision MRI demonstrates the seroma cavity (*arrows*) with air-fluid level and extensive enhancement surrounding the posterior aspect of the seroma. Biopsy confirmed the presence of residual disease at the lumpectomy site.

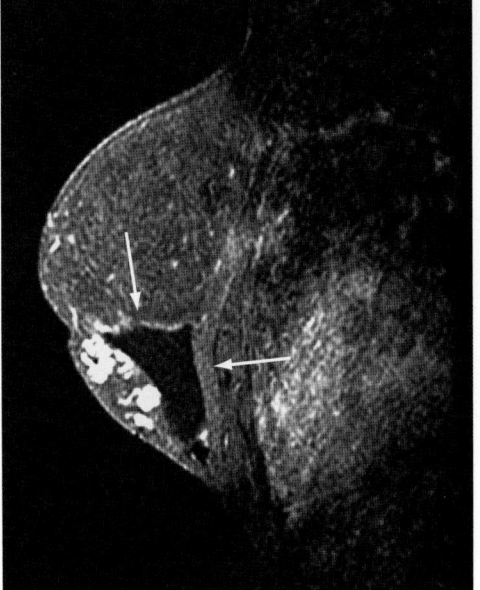

FIGURE 77-17

Residual disease at the lumpectomy site. 45-year-old woman with dense breasts presents with a palpable abnormality that was biopsied surgically yielding ductal carcinoma in situ (DCIS) with positive margins. Postexcision MRI demonstrates a seroma cavity (*arrows*) with residual clumped enhancement surrounding the anterior aspect of the cavity. Biopsy yielded residual DICS.

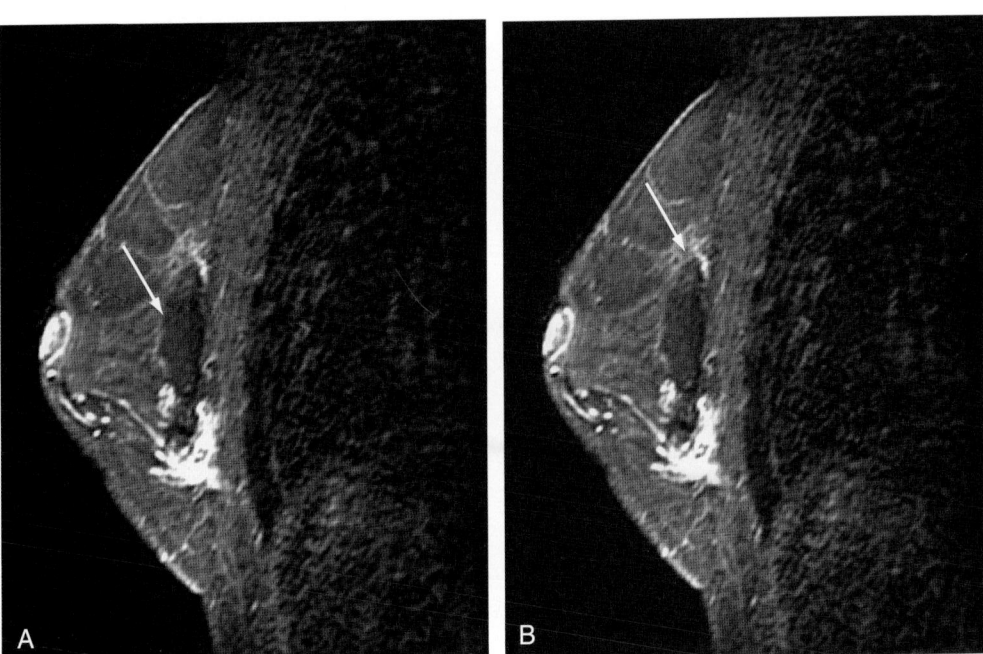

FIGURE 77-18

Residual multifocal disease. **A,** 37-year-old BRCA 1-positive patient presents with a palpable mass and suspicious findings on mammography and ultrasound. Biopsy yielded mixed ductal and lobular invasive carcinoma with positive margins. Postexcision MRI demonstrates the seroma cavity (*arrow*) and residual disease along the inferior aspect of the cavity. **B,** 36-year-old woman presented with a palpable mass. Surgery was performed yielding a 3-cm invasive ductal carcinoma with positive margins. Postexcision MRI demonstrates seroma (*arrow*) with residual enhancement anterior to the cavity compatible with residual cancer. The patient ultimately underwent a mastectomy as the disease proved to be too extensive for conservation.

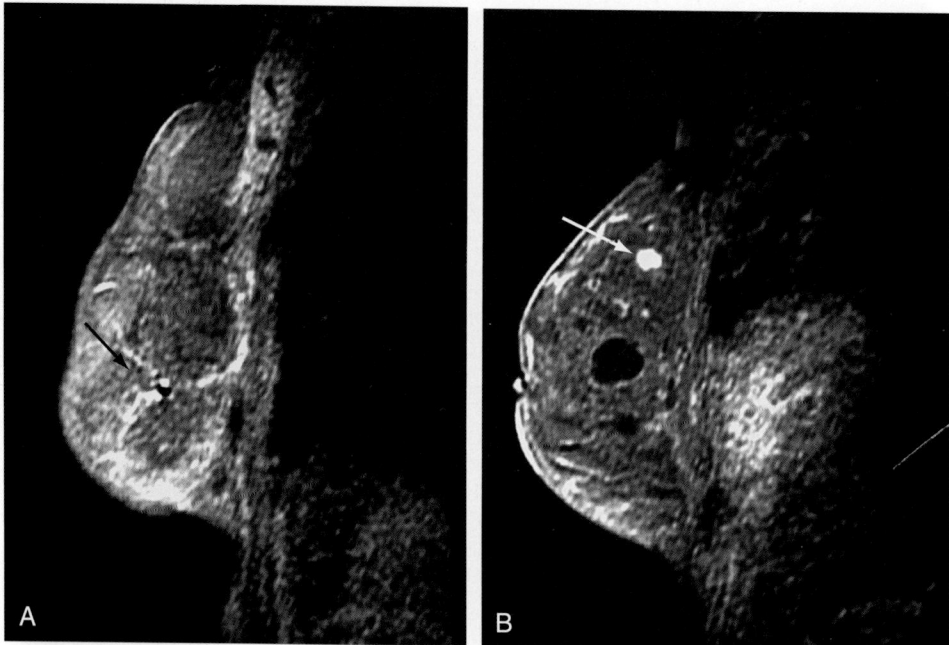

FIGURE 77-19

Residual multicentric disease. **A,** 59-year-old woman who underwent breast conservation 1 year previously at an outside institution. Pathologic margins were questionable at the time of surgery; however, she went on to receive a full course of chemotherapy and radiation therapy. MRI was performed to ensure the absence of any suspicious findings due to the questionable pathology margins. MRI demonstrates the lumpectomy site (*arrow*) with distortion and clip artifact. No suspicious findings are present at the site of surgery. **B,** In a separate quadrant, however, there is an irregular heterogeneously enhancing mass (*arrow*) that was subsequently seen with targeted ultrasound and biopsied yielding invasive ductal carcinoma.

TUMOR RECURRENCE AT THE LUMPECTOMY SITE

Tumor recurrence after breast conservation occurs at an overall rate of 1% to 2% per year. Recurrence directly at the lumpectomy site occurs earlier than elsewhere in the breast and usually peaks several years following conservation therapy (Fig. 77-20). Evaluation of the lumpectomy site by mammography is extremely limited due to postoperative scarring, and physical examination may have greater sensitivity in the detection of recurrence. Mammography is able to detect 25% to 45% of recurrences and is more likely to detect recurrent tumors associated with calcifications than recurrences without calcifications. All recurrences in one study[21] enhanced with nodular enhancement in all cases of invasive carcinoma (Fig. 77-21) and linear enhancement was observed in cases of DCIS recurrence. The majority of scars showed no enhancement.

When to image for potential recurrence is problematic as scar tissue can enhance for years following surgery. As recurrence peaks in the first few years following surgery and the most likely site of recurrence is the lumpectomy site, the usefulness of the information obtained from a costly MRI study needs to be weighed against that obtained from a potentially less expensive needle biopsy of the area.

OCCULT PRIMARY BREAST CANCER

Patients presenting with axillary metastases suspicious for breast primary cancer but a negative physical examination and negative mammogram should undergo breast MRI.[26,27] In patients with this rare clinical presentation, MRI has been able to detect cancer in 90% to 100% of cases, if a tumor is indeed present. The tumors are generally small in size, under 2 cm, thus they may evade detection by conventional imaging and physical examination (Fig. 77-22).

The identification of the site of malignancy is important therapeutically. Patients traditionally undergo mastectomy as the site of malignancy is unknown. Whole breast radiation can be given though this is generally not recommended as survival is the same but the recurrence rate is higher, up to 23%. Thus, if a site of malignancy can be identified, the patient can be spared mastectomy and offered breast conservation therapy, thereby having a significant impact on patient management. In one study, the results of the MR examination changed therapy in approximately one half of cases, usually allowing conservation in lieu of mastectomy.[28] In our practice, if a site of malignancy is not identified on MRI, the patient receives full breast radiation with careful follow-up with MRI examination.

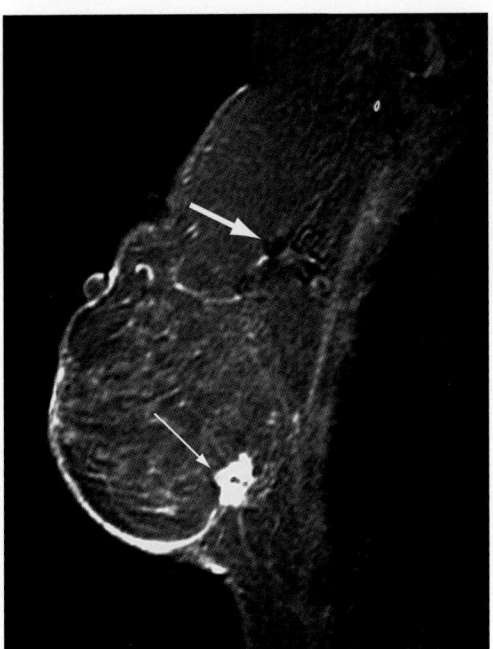

FIGURE 77-20

Recurrence. 53-year-old woman with a history of breast cancer was treated with lumpectomy (*thick arrow*) 3 years previously. Bilateral reduction mammoplasty had been performed 10 years previously. She complained of thickening of her lumpectomy scar. Mammogram and ultrasound were negative. MRI demonstrates an irregular mass associated with her post-reduction mammoplasty scar (*thin arrow*). Biopsy yielded poorly differentiated invasive ductal carcinoma. The patient subsequently received mastectomy.

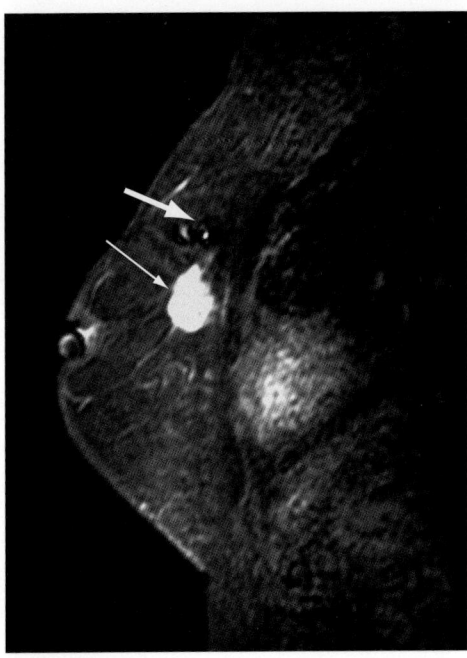

FIGURE 77-21

Recurrence. 76-year-old woman with a history of lumpectomy (*thick arrow*) for invasive ductal carcinoma 7 years previously. Patient presents with peri-incisional fullness. Mammogram was negative. MRI demonstrates an irregular heterogeneously enhancing mass compatible with recurrence (*thin arrow*). Pathology yielded invasive ductal carcinoma and ductal carcinoma in situ and the patient then underwent mastectomy.

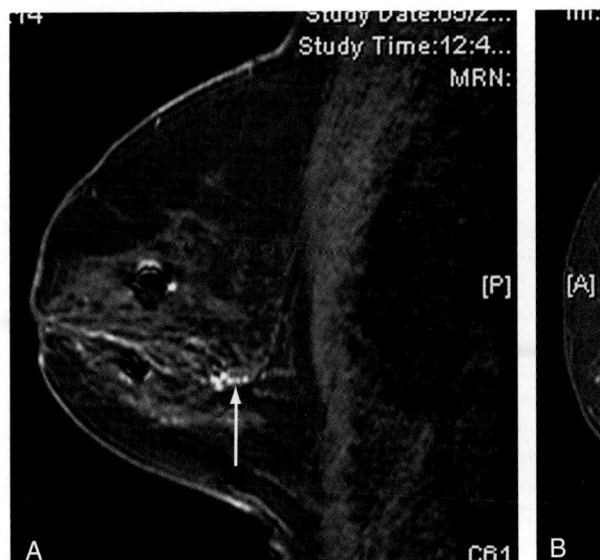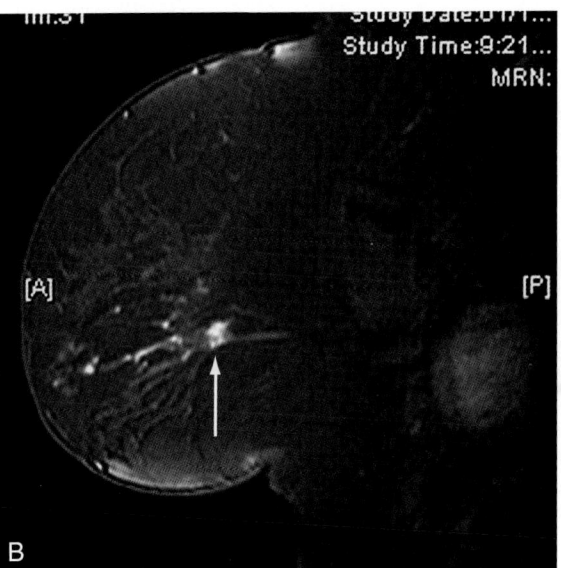

FIGURE 77-22

Unknown primary carcinoma. **A,** 64-year-old woman with an enlarged left axillary lymph node, biopsy positive for adenocarcinoma, and suspicious for breast primary. Mammogram and physical examinations were negative. Screening ultrasound resulted in two benign biopsies (clips seen). MRI demonstrates linear enhancement in the lower outer quadrant of the breast (*arrow*). MR biopsy yielded extensive lobular carcinoma in situ and invasive lobular carcinoma compatible with the patient's primary tumor. **B,** 64-year-old woman with a palpable 3-cm left axillary lymph node and negative mammogram and physical examination. MRI demonstrates an irregular mass (*arrow*) with surrounding clumped enhancement. Biopsy yielded invasive carcinoma compatible with the patient's primary tumor.

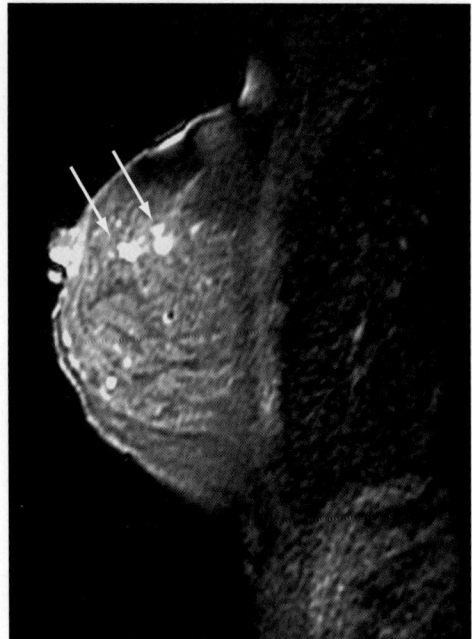

FIGURE 77-23

High-risk screening. 51-year-old with a history of benign biopsy yielding lobular carcinoma in situ, a high-risk lesion. MRI screening identifies two suspicious irregular masses in the superior breast (*arrows*). Biopsy yielded multiple foci of invasive ductal carcinoma. Sentinel lymph node biopsy was negative.

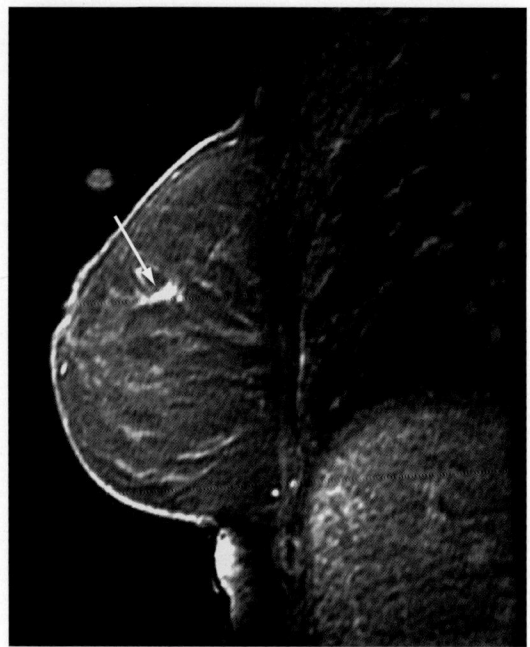

FIGURE 77-24

Screening detection of ductal carcinoma in situ (DCIS). 66-year-old woman with a history of right mastectomy. Screening MRI demonstrates irregular linear enhancement in the upper breast (*arrow*). Biopsy under MR guidance yielded high-grade DCIS. Patient elected for mastectomy.

HIGH-RISK SCREENING

A probable future use of breast MRI is screening for patients who are at high risk for developing breast cancer (Fig. 77-23). As mammography has an overall false-negative rate of up to 20% in the general population, it is evident that all cancers are not detected by conventional means. The rate of false-negative examinations may be even higher in premenopausal women with dense breasts and therefore alternative screening methods such as full breast ultrasound and MRI have been explored. Of the available methods, MRI holds perhaps the most promise, mostly due to its high-resolution capabilities, full documentation of the examination, and the potential to detect preinvasive DCIS (Fig. 77-24). The use of breast MRI in the high-risk population is still experimental, but the data to determine the appropriateness of MR for screening high-risk patients are accumulating in several ongoing studies in the United States and elsewhere.[34] Furthermore, no information exists for screening "dense, difficult to examine" breasts in patients who are not high risk. Screening by MRI in this population where the incidence of breast cancer is low would very likely result in too many false-positive biopsies to justify its use, though no data exist to support this view.

What exactly constitutes high risk can be variable. In general, high risk includes BRCA 1 or 2 heterozygotes, a personal history of breast cancer, a family history of breast cancer in a first-degree relative, prior benign biopsy yielding a high-risk lesion [lobular carcinoma in situ (LCIS), atypical ductal hyperplasia (ADH), atypical lobular hyperplasia (ALH), radial scar], history of thoracic radiation, or a known syndrome (Li-Fraumeni or Cowden's).

BRCA 1 and 2 carriers have an up to 85% risk of developing breast cancer over their lifetime. The onset of inherited breast cancer is earlier than sporadic cases and the prevalence of bilaterality is higher (Fig. 77-25). A study showed that MRI was able to detect mammographically and sonographically occult breast cancers in a group of patients who were known or suspected carriers of either the BRCA 1 or 2 genes.[29] Nine cancers were detected in a group of 192 patients and three (2%) of these cancers were detected on MRI only. All were pT1 and node negative. Preliminary results from another study of 105 BRCA patients,[45] of whom 38% had a prior history of breast cancer, have shown that MRI detected occult breast cancers in 7%. These cancers were both DCIS and invasive cancer and were identified in pre- and post-menopausal patients. Although these results are encouraging, applying this technology to the population at large is not advocated at this time.

Larger studies need to be performed to validate these data. If validated, a definition of what constitutes "high risk" is needed. Studies that have included patients at a lower risk than the heterozygote patients[30,34,35] have demonstrated that MRI still finds occult breast cancer though at lower rates. It appears that the lower the patient's risk, the lower the prevalence of MRI-detected

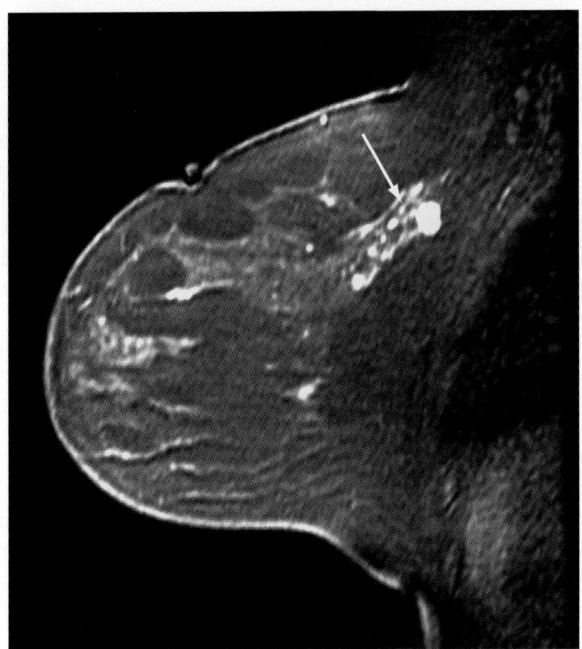

FIGURE 77-25

High-risk screening. 42-year-old, BRCA 1-positive woman underwent screening MRI. An irregular rim-enhancing mass (*arrow*) is seen with surrounding clumped enhancement. Pathology yielded invasive ductal carcinoma and ductal carcinoma in situ. Patient received conservation therapy.

Fibroadenomas
Recent scars
Inflammatory processes
Proliferative and nonproliferative changes
Atypical duct hyperplasia
Atypical lobular hyperplasia
Sclerosing adenosis
Radial scar
Lobular carcinoma in situ

cancer. Studies that include patients with an overall cumulative lifetime risk of developing breast cancer of approximately 30% show that MRI is able to detect cancer in approximately 1% to 3% of patients. Ultimately, MRI needs to be shown to not only detect a high prevalence of breast cancer on the initial screen, but also a high incidence (cancer found on subsequent screens) of breast cancer. Screening with MRI will also need to show a reduction of breast cancer mortality in the screened high-risk population and not result in too many false-positive biopsies.

SENSITIVITY AND SPECIFICITY

Breast MRI for cancer detection relies almost exclusively on the neovascularity associated with invasive carcinomas. The administration of an intravenous contrast agent such as gadolinium-diethylenetriamine penta-acetic acid (Gd-DTPA) allows these lesions to be well visualized, particularly if subtraction imaging or chemical fat-suppression sequences are used. Leaky capillaries and arteriovenous shunts allow contrast agents to leave the lesion rapidly over time resulting in the characteristic washout time intensity curves that can be seen with most but not all malignancies.[46-50] Detection of invasive breast carcinoma is extremely reliable on MR imaging as the sensitivity approaches 100%. As the sensitivity for cancer detection is high, the negative predictive value of breast MRI is high. If no enhancement is present in the

breast, and any possible technical mishap such as intravenous contrast extravasation has been excluded, there is an extremely high likelihood that no invasive carcinoma is present. Specificity is lower than sensitivity and therefore false positives can pose a problem in interpretation. Several causes of false-positive findings are listed in Box 77-1. It should be noted that false negatives have been reported with some well-differentiated invasive ductal carcinomas as well as invasive lobular carcinoma.[51]

Although the sensitivity is high for invasive carcinoma, the same may not be true for DCIS. The sensitivity has been reported to be low,[52,53] possibly secondary to more variable angiogenesis associated with these lesions. More recent evidence suggests that the sensitivity for DCIS detection may actually be higher than previously reported now that high-resolution scanning techniques are more available and widely used.[42] Also, it is recognized that morphology may be more important than kinetics in the evaluation of DCIS. Although more work needs to be performed in the MR assessment of in situ disease, MRI does not have as high a negative predictive value for DCIS as with invasive cancer; therefore, MRI is not able to exclude DCIS with current technology.

A negative MRI examination should not deter biopsy of a suspicious lesion (BIRADS 4 or 5) on mammography or ultrasound. Mammographically suspicious findings, such as suspicious calcifications, spiculated masses or areas of distortion, warrant appropriate biopsy, regardless of a negative MR examination. The MRI should ideally be interpreted in conjunction with all other pertinent imaging studies, such as mammograms and ultrasounds, to arrive at the best treatment option for the patient. With these limitations, breast MRI is best used as an adjunct test to conventional imaging, complementing but not replacing mammography and sonography.

BREAST MRI ANALYSIS

BI-RADS™ MRI Lexicon

Enhancement alone is not sufficient for determination of malignancy as any area of increased vascularity will be evident on the post-contrast images. By analyzing both the morphology and kinetic behavior of a lesion, the specificity of breast MRI is improved.[54-57] Breast MRI analysis incorporates the morphology and kinetics of the lesion. The American College of Radiology recently published a lexicon that standardizes terminology and reporting. The ACR MRI lexicon is modeled on the BI-RADS™ lexicon[36] for mammography using morphology as well as incorporating the dynamic enhancement properties of the lesions.

When reporting findings, it is recommended that the report includes a clinical statement as well as the technique used. The report should also include a final assessment BI-RADS™ category 0-6, which is used to direct the next step in management. The referring clinician is thus able to understand the next appropriate step in the work-up of the lesion. The report should use standardized terminology from the breast MRI lexicon. In addition to providing descriptions of the morphologic and kinetic findings, the MRI report should give a final recommendation to convey the level of suspicion to the referring physician. If a recommendation for biopsy is made, it should be clearly reported in the final impression and a final assessment category should be specified, as in mammography.

Morphology

When analyzing an enhancing lesion on MRI, the first distinction is to decide if the lesion is a focus, mass, or nonmass lesion. Further description of the lesion will depend on this distinction. It is often difficult to differentiate a focus from a mass. A focus is defined as a tiny spot of enhancement, i.e., a dot that does not occupy space (Fig. 77-26). Most tiny foci of enhancement are

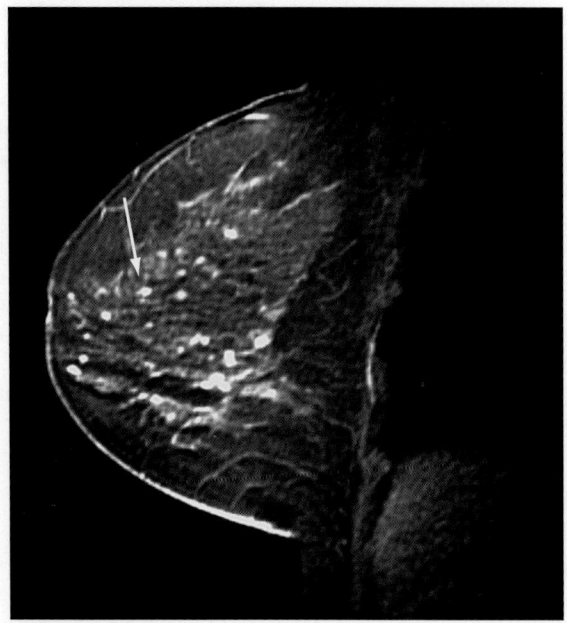

FIGURE 77-26

Focus. 59-year-old woman with a history of successfully treated invasive lobular carcinoma, underwent screening MRI. Numerous small foci of enhancement are seen (*arrow*) compatible with benign findings.

a few millimeters in size and appear round and smooth. When innumerable foci are present the breast has a characteristically benign "stippled" appearance (Fig. 77-27).

How should foci of enhancement be managed? If the lesion meets the criteria of a focus and is not a space-occupying mass then the decision may be made to do nothing, though long-term follow-up studies have not documented this approach. If at all concerned when interpreting an examination, short-term follow-up (usually 6 months) may be warranted, though again this has yet to be proven as cost-effective and efficacious.[58] Shorter-term follow-up of weeks or months may be an option in a premenopausal patient or a postmenopausal patient on hormones in whom there is suspicion that the foci are hormone related.[59,60] If hormone-related enhancement is suspected then follow-up in the premenopausal patient's next cycle (days 7-14) may be warranted, or cessation of hormone replacement therapy (HRT) for several weeks in the post-menopausal patient may be needed to document that the findings are indeed benign (see "Hormone-Related Enhancement"). Hormonal enhancement would be expected to decrease or diminish on the follow-up examination.

In patients with known cancer the presence of foci may be more ominous. Studies have shown that small areas of enhancement, when present in patients with a known primary breast carcinoma,[61] are more likely to represent malignancy, though long-term follow-up of these findings is also needed.

Investigators have analyzed architectural features of MR-detected masses and nonmass lesions, resulting in the development of interpretation models.[62-64] These studies have shown that smooth or lobulated borders have a high negative predictive value for carcinoma (95% and 90%, respectively). Other studies, however, have shown that due to the lower resolution of the MR image compared to mammography, many cancers may exhibit benign characteristics such as smooth margins and homogeneous enhancement.[65,66] Spiculated and irregular margins had high positive predictive value for malignancy (91% and 81%, respectively). Rim enhancement is a feature that has an 86% predictive value for malignancy. If several morphologic findings coexist, the most suspicious feature becomes the most pertinent finding and directs further work-up.

Nonmass enhancement such as ductal enhancement has a positive predictive value of malignancy of 85%. Clumped enhancement can be arranged within a single ductal system generating a segmental enhancement pattern on MRI. When seen, this is suspicious for DCIS.[67] Regional enhancement can be seen with both benign and malignant disease and has a negative predictive value of 53%.[64] A unique descriptor that is used in the case of inflammatory carcinoma with diffuse enhancement is reticular/dendritic where there is no underlying mass and the enhancement pattern appears lacelike.

Classic morphologic signs can be seen, such as non-enhancing bands in a fibroadenoma (Fig. 77-28) or the reniform shape of a lymph node (Fig. 77-29) so that the interpreter of the breast MRI can be confident that the lesion is likely benign. T2-weighted images can aid in

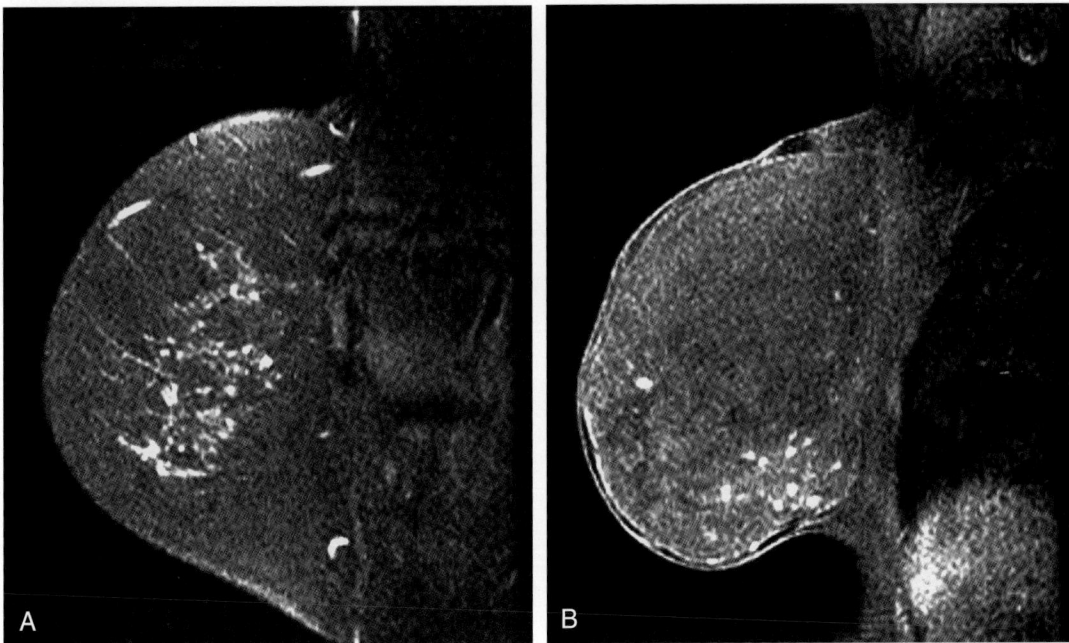

FIGURE 77-27

Stippled. **A,** 61-year-old woman with a strong family history of breast carcinoma. Routine MRI study demonstrates numerous foci of enhancement compatible with a benign stippled pattern. **B,** 47-year-old woman with prior history of breast carcinoma undergoes screening MRI. Regional scattered stippled enhancement is seen. Note that the foci are uniform in appearance, a few millimeters in size, and do not exhibit mass characteristics.

interpretation as benign lymph nodes and fibroadenomata can mimic breast cancer dynamically.[68] Lymph nodes and myxoid fibroadenomas are solid cellular breast masses that demonstrate high signal on T2-weighted images. It is not common for cancers to be very high in signal on T2-weighted imaging unless necrotic or of the mucinous or colloid type of invasive ductal carcinoma.

A spiculated mass (Fig. 77-30) or area of linear clumped enhancement (Fig. 77-31) is very likely to represent malignancy and therefore these lesions should be biopsied regardless of additional findings. Other findings that are suspicious are masses that demonstrate central enhancement (Fig. 77-32), rim enhancement (Fig. 77-33), and enhancing bands (Fig. 77-34). Two benign lesions that demonstrate rim enhancement and can be easily distinguished from invasive carcinoma: inflammatory cysts (Fig. 77-35) and fat necrosis (Fig. 77-36). Cysts can be confirmed on T2-weighted images and fat necrosis usually has central fat associated with it and a history of prior surgery or trauma.

If classic malignant or benign lesion morphology is not seen, time intensity curves can be extremely helpful in deciding whether to biopsy a lesion (Fig. 77-37).[69,70] If the time intensity curve does not exhibit washout or plateau kinetics (characteristic of malignant lesions), careful watchful waiting may be an option over biopsy, though this approach has yet to be validated clinically. A proposed algorithm for image analysis is presented in Figure 77-38.

Kinetics

Enhancement kinetics evaluates what happens to the intravenous contrast within a lesion over a period of time; therefore, repeat imaging of the lesion is necessary. Signal intensity increase following contrast administration (SI_{post}) is measured relative to the precontrast level (SI_{pre}):

$$\left[(SI_{post} - SI_{pre})\right] \times 100\% \qquad \text{(Eq. 77-1)}$$

When plotted, time-signal intensity curves are generated that can be analyzed to provide further information about the vascular properties of a lesion. They generally require at least several time points, with the first being at time zero when there is no contrast within the lesion. To generate these time points, the breast must be scanned and rescanned many times following intravenous contrast bolus injection. The more time points desired in a certain time frame, the faster the acquisition. Just what constitutes an adequate time-signal intensity curve is a matter of debate. Most imagers agree that each dynamic scan should be less than 2 minutes; however, the faster the dynamic scan, the less the spatial resolution and therefore a compromise must be reached.

In general, three types of time-signal intensity curves have been described.[69,70] Type I is continuous progressive enhancement over time indicating that contrast accumulates within the lesion, typically seen with benign

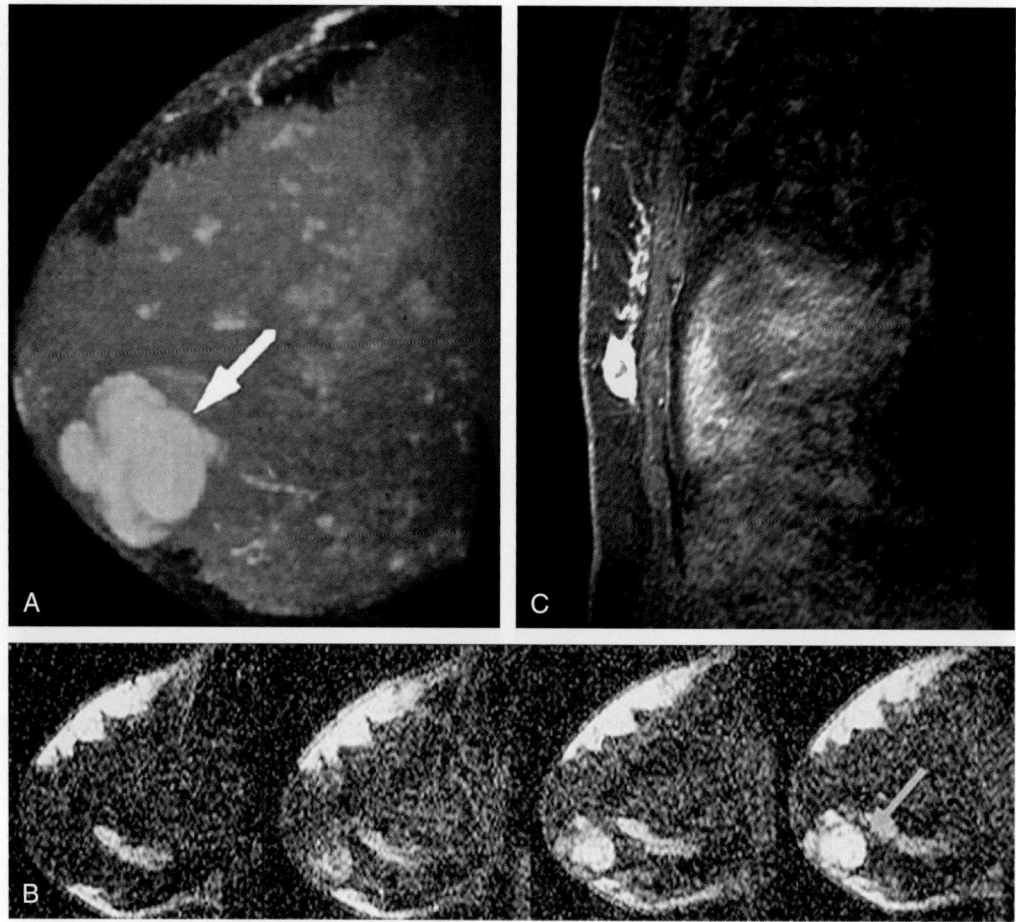

FIGURE 77-28

Fibroadenoma. **A,** Classic fibroadenoma. Maximum intensity projection of delayed contrast-enhanced MRI with fat suppression shows the lesion has smooth, lobulated margins (*arrow*). **B,** On serial dynamic MR images acquired over several minutes, there is gradual enhancement of the fibroadenoma (*arrow*) without washout. **C,** Atypical fibroadenoma. Morphologic characteristics are suspicious with rim enhancement and irregular margins. Biopsy under ultrasound guidance yielded fibroadenoma. (**A** and **B** *courtesy of Robert Edelman, MD.*)

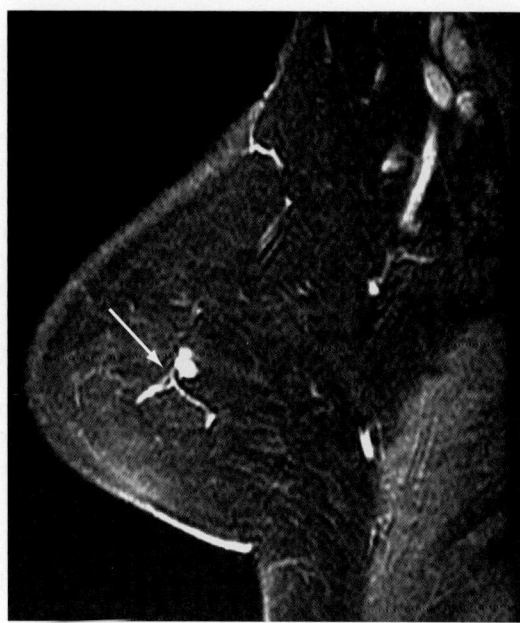

FIGURE 77-29

Lymph node. 57-year-old woman with a strong family history of breast carcinoma underwent screening MRI examination. An enhancing reniform mass is identified in the upper outer quadrant (*arrow*) compatible with lymph node. Lymph nodes are usually high in signal on T2-weighted images which can confirm impression.

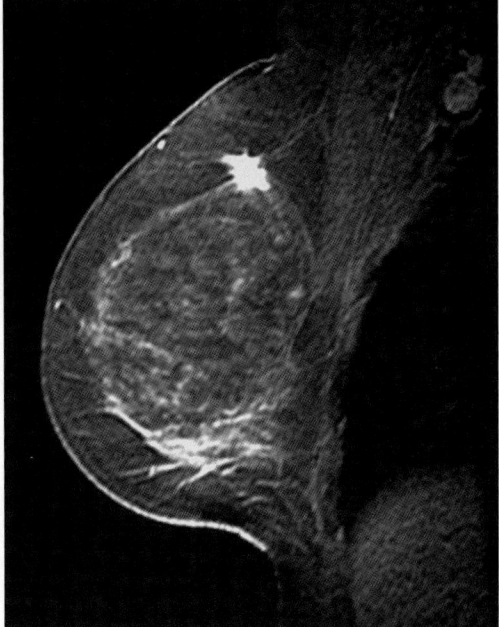

FIGURE 77-30

Spiculated mass. 48-year-old woman with invasive lobular carcinoma.

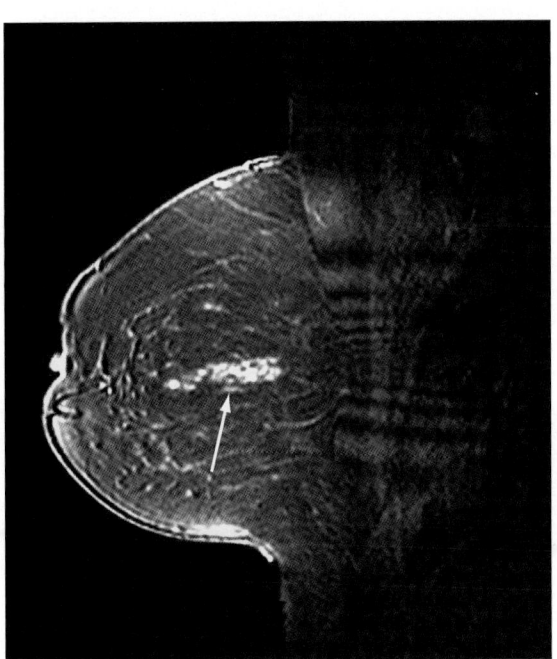

FIGURE 77-31

Clumped enhancement. 49-year-old woman with ductal carcinoma in situ (DCIS). Clumped linear enhancement (*arrow*) represented DCIS.

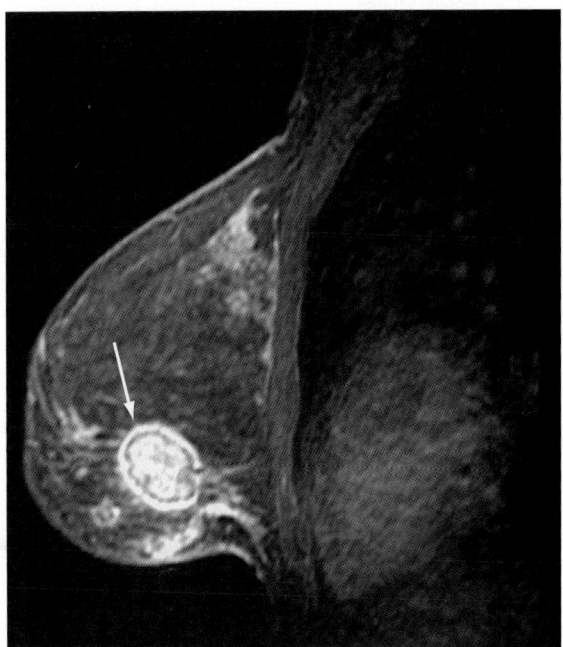

FIGURE 77-32

Central enhancement. 28-year-old woman with poorly differentiated invasive ductal carcinoma. MRI demonstrates an oval smooth mass with rim and central enhancement (*arrow*), compatible with carcinoma. Note the scattered areas of parenchymal enhancement.

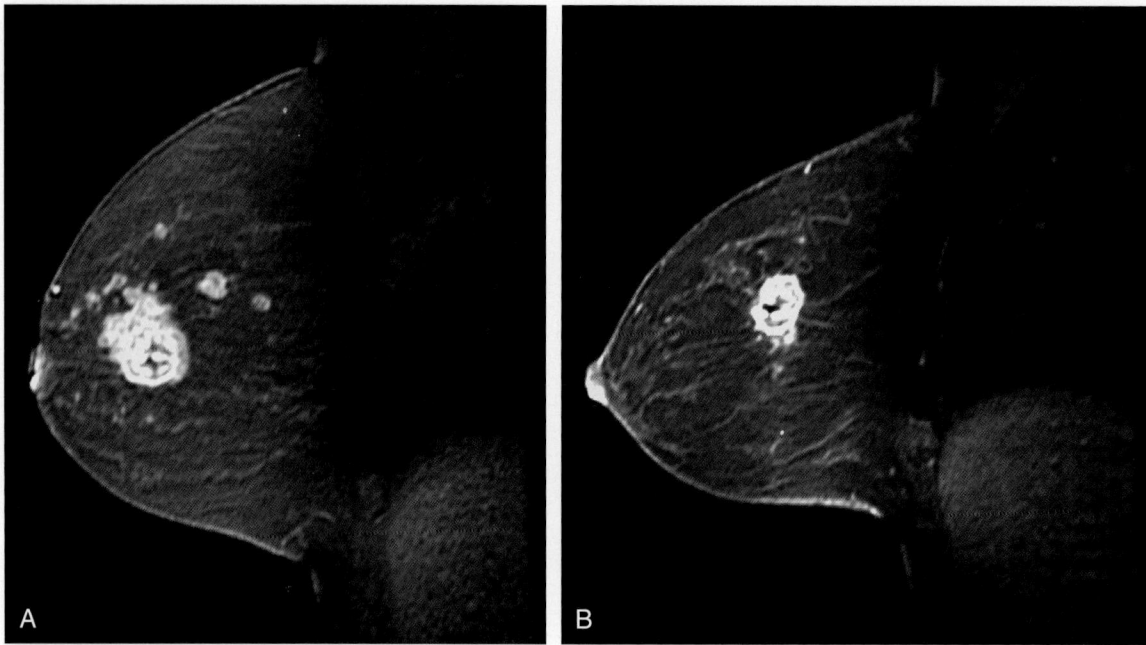

FIGURE 77-33

Rim enhancement. **A,** 44-year-old woman with a strong family history of breast carcinoma (sister died at age 36) presents with a palpable mass. MRI demonstrates a dominant mass with rim enhancement and enhancing bands compatible with a diagnosis of invasive ductal carcinoma. Note the satellite lesions. **B,** 47-year-old woman with a new mass on mammogram. Biopsy under ultrasound yielded invasive ductal carcinoma. MRI demonstrates a unifocal mass with rim enhancement. Note artifact centrally for clip placed following ultrasound biopsy.

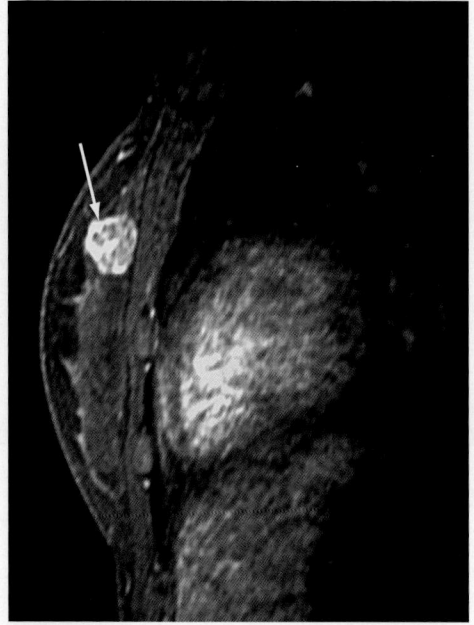

FIGURE 77-34

Enhancing band. 33-year-old woman with biopsy-proven invasive ductal carcinoma. MRI demonstrates rim enhancement with a central enhancing band (*arrow*).

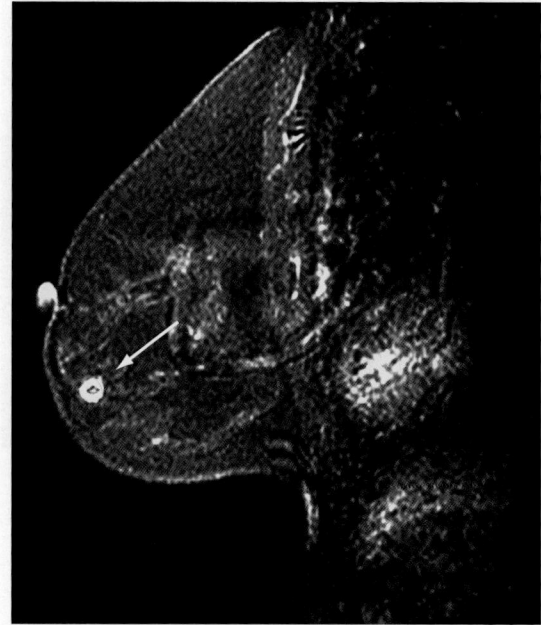

FIGURE 77-35

Inflammatory cyst. 56-year-old woman with a history of contralateral mastectomy undergoes screening MRI. A round, smooth, rim-enhancing mass is seen (*arrow*). T2-weighted images (*not shown*) confirmed the presence of an inflammatory cyst.

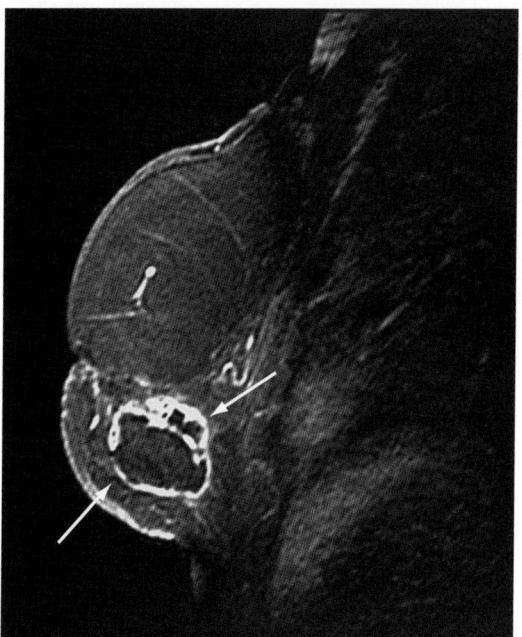

FIGURE 77-36

Fat necrosis. 49-year-old woman with mastectomy and transrectus abdominus flap (TRAM) reconstruction. MRI was performed to evaluate a mass suspicious for recurrence. MRI demonstrates a large inferior rim-enhancing mass (*arrows*) with central low signal compatible with fat necrosis. Non–fat-suppressed images (*not shown*) confirmed the presence of fat centrally.

findings. Type III is a washout curve indicating that after the lesion takes up contrast, the contrast promptly washes out, presumably from leaky capillaries and shunts found in malignant lesions. Type II is a plateau curve that is a combination of the type I and III curves and can be seen with both benign and malignant lesions.

Algorithm

An approach to breast MRI interpretation is outlined. Initial evaluation of T2-weighted images is performed to determine if high signal masses, such as cysts (Fig. 77-39), lymph nodes, or myxoid fibroadenomas are present. Evaluation of the nonenhanced T1-weighted images documents the presence of high-signal hemorrhagic or proteinaceous cysts as well as high signal within dilated ducts (Fig. 77-40). The post-contrast T1-weighted images will demonstrate the presence of any enhancing masses or non-masslike areas of enhancement. Morphologic analysis of the architectural features of a mass would then determine if the margins are irregular or spiculated, findings that would be highly suggestive of malignancy. At this point, biopsy would be recommended. A search for the mass by ultrasound may be helpful to allow percutaneous biopsy.

If the mass demonstrates smooth margins and rim enhancement biopsy would be recommended (once the false-positive causes of rim enhancement, such as inflamed cyst and fat necrosis, have been excluded) as rim enhancement is the only predictive of malignancy. Similarly, ductal enhancement that is irregular or clumped will be suspicious for DCIS and biopsy will generally result from this finding (Fig. 77-41).

If however the mass is smoothly marginated and enhances homogeneously, kinetic analysis can be extremely helpful (Fig. 77-42). Kinetics can determine whether this is indeed likely benign (type I curve) or possibly malignant (type II or III curve), prompting biopsy. Because a homogeneously enhancing smooth mass with a type I or II curve has been reported in some malignant lesions, short-term follow-up in 6 months may be advisable if this combination of findings is found to document benignity. There are no published reports to validate 6-month follow-up; however, there is some evidence to suggest that unlike mammography where the rate of malignancy for 6-month follow-up is less than 2%, the rate of malignancy on MRI for lesions that are followed at 6 months is much higher, approaching 10% possibly depending on patient population.[58]

For areas of non-masslike enhancement, kinetic analysis may be very helpful as findings such as regional enhancement can be found in both benign and malignant breast pathology, such as proliferative changes and DCIS. There is evidence, however, that kinetic curves are unreliable in DCIS and that "typical" type III curves may not be present. Therefore, morphologic analysis may play a more important role in lesions that are suspicious for DCIS.

HORMONE-RELATED ENHANCEMENT

Breast parenchyma in the pre- and post-menopausal patient can demonstrate enhancement that can be problematic.[59,60] These areas of enhancement can appear and disappear in different phases of the menstrual cycle and are different from the stippled appearance of the fibrocystic breast (Fig. 77-43). Hormone-related enhancement occurs primarily in the premenopausal patient as well as the post-menopausal patient on HRT who has parenchymal enhancement similar to that seen in

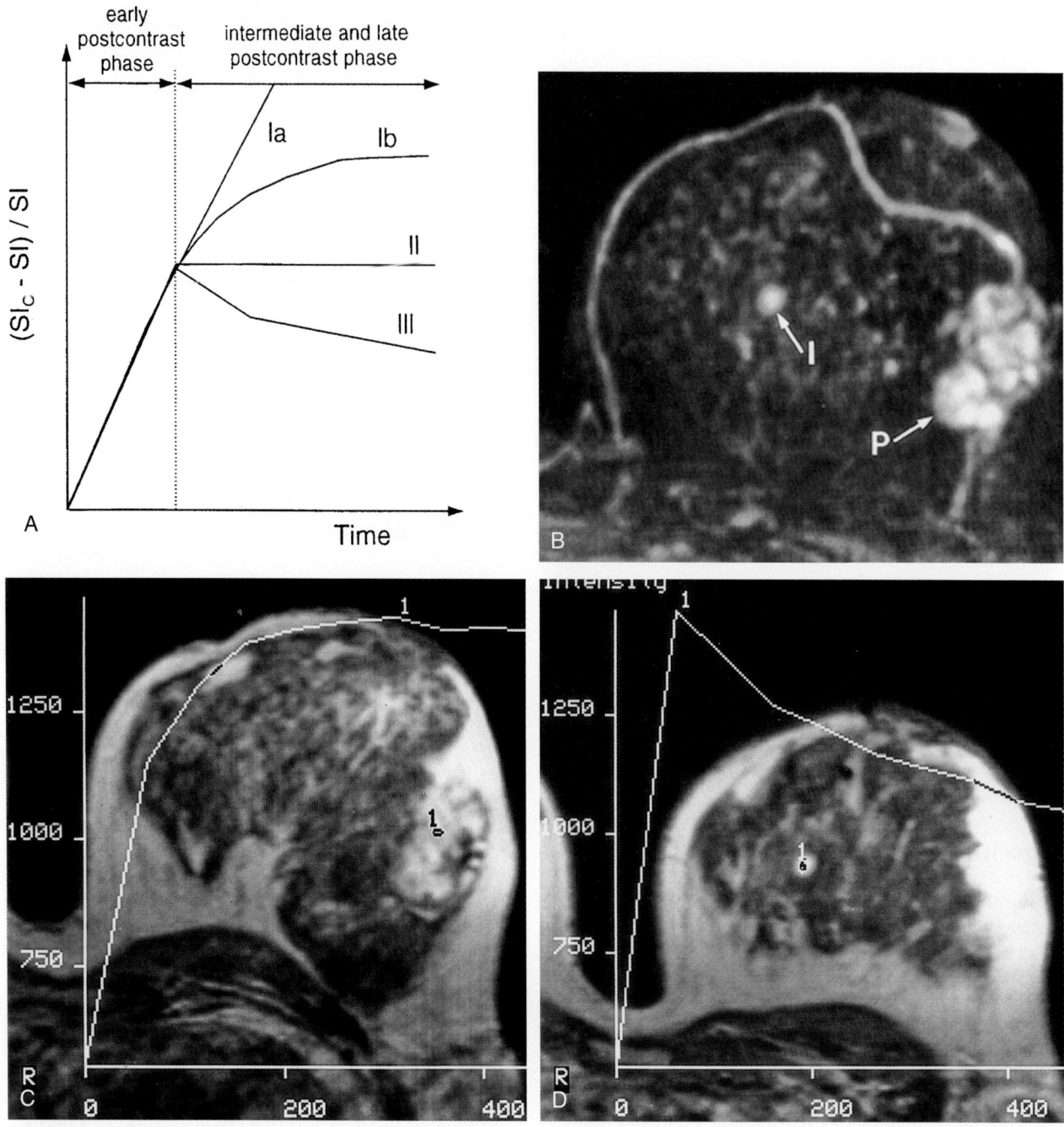

FIGURE 77-37

Time-signal intensity curves. **A,** Schematic drawing of time–signal intensity curve types for dynamic contrast-enhanced breast MRI, classified as steady (type I), plateau (type II), or washout (type III). A type III time course is a strong indicator of malignancy independent of other criteria. In breast cancers, plateau or washout time courses (type II or III) prevail. Benign lesions more commonly exhibit steadily progressive signal intensity time courses (type I); both benign tumors and fibrocystic changes share these enhancement kinetics. The distribution of curve types for breast cancers was type I, 8.9%; type II, 33.6%; and type III, 57.4%. The distribution of curve types for benign lesions was type I, 83.0%; type II, 11.5%; and type III, 5.5%. **B-D,** Breast MRI acquired in a 55-year-old patient with a palpable mass in the left upper outer quadrant. The mass had been rated as probably benign on the basis of mammographic and US findings. **B,** Axial maximum intensity projection MR image from an early postcontrast subtracted data set depicts two lesions (*arrows*): the expected palpable mass (*P*) and a nonpalpable, incidental lesion (*I*) in the left breast. **C,** Time–signal intensity curve of the palpable mass shows a type I time course. The x axis shows the time following contrast administration in seconds, and the y axis shows the signal intensity in arbitrary units. The palpable mass exhibits a suggestively strong early-phase enhancement, but it is well circumscribed, has a lobulated appearance, and reveals internal septations, which are all findings consistent with fibroadenoma. The signal intensity time course corresponds to a type Ib curve. **D,** Time–signal intensity curve of the incidental lesion shows a type III time course, which prompted the prospective diagnosis of an occult breast cancer, together with a fibroadenoma, in the same breast. Histologic confirmation of a 6 mm invasive ductal breast cancer pT1bN0M0 was obtained for the small incidental lesion and myxoid fibroadenoma was confirmed for the larger palpable lesion. (*Adapted from Kuhl CK, Mielcareck P, Klaschik S, et al. Dynamic Breast MR Imaging: Are Signal Intensity Time Course Data Useful for Differential Diagnosis of Enhancing Lesions? Radiology 1999; 211:101-110, with permission.*)

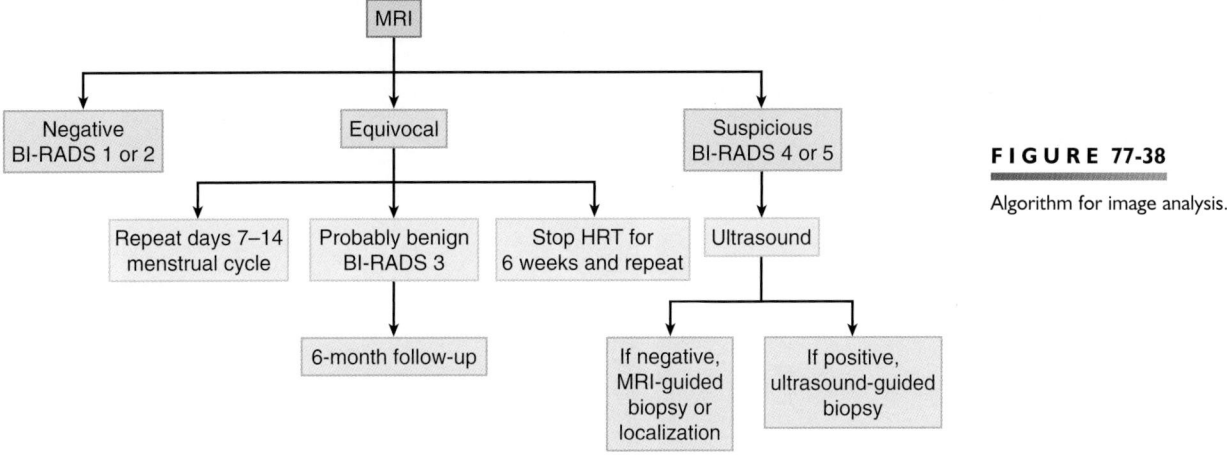

FIGURE 77-38

Algorithm for image analysis.

the premenopausal state. Exogenous and endogenous hormones can cause increased blood flow due to a histamine type of effect. In most cases, there is no mass effect associated with the enhancement and the kinetics of the enhancement is generally progressive or continual over time. Sometimes, these areas of normal parenchyma can enhance intensely and appear masslike, causing concern.

In general, premenopausal patients should be scheduled in the second week of their menstrual cycle (days 7-14), when proliferative changes are at their lowest, in order to minimize this potential enhancement. If this is not possible and parenchymal enhancement is suspected, we bring the patient back in week two of a subsequent menstrual cycle for short-term follow-up. In the case of post-menopausal patients on HRT, the hormones can be stopped if necessary and a short-term follow-up in 6 to 8 weeks can be performed (Fig. 77-44).

BREAST MRI PROGRAM

Image Acquisition

There is no gold standard technique for performing breast MR imaging. Many techniques are available and widely used depending on hardware and software capabilities and personal preferences. There are however a few minimal technical requirements that should be adhered to.[54] The basic sequence for breast MRI involves a T1-weighted sequence that is obtained as rapidly and with as high resolution as possible before and after gadolinium-DTPA administration. High-resolution techniques favor lesion morphologic analysis and rapid acquisition is used for assessing enhancement profiles. T2-weighted sequences are useful for identifying breast cysts that can be simple or hemorrhagic in addition to myxoid fibroadenomas and lymph nodes that can be high in signal intensity on this sequence.

Certain minimal technical requirements have been proposed by the International Working Group[54] with the aim of detecting small lesions by assessing lesion morphology and enhancement kinetics. A dedicated breast coil must be used, preferably one with localization or biopsy capability for MRI-only detected lesions. So far in the literature, 1.5-T systems have been validated, as these provide a high signal-to-noise ratio and allow fat suppression to be performed. To detect lesions and

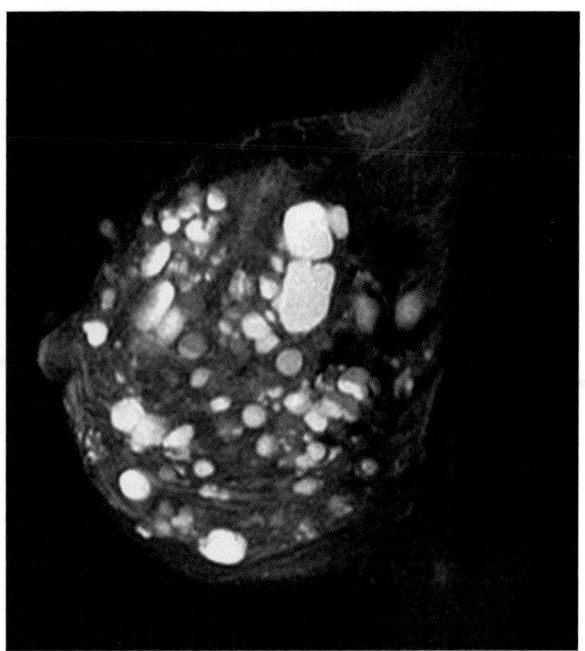

FIGURE 77-39

Cysts. 46-year-old woman with a history of lumpectomy has innumerable high signal cysts on T2-weighted imaging. A marker has been placed over the nipple and a palpable abnormality in the superior breast.

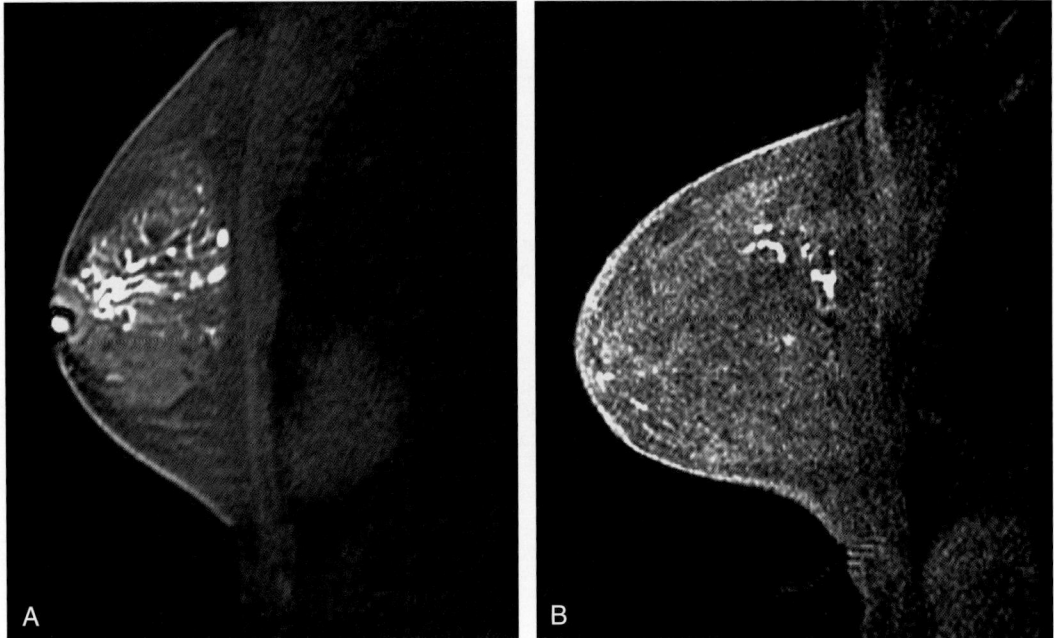

FIGURE 77-40

Dilated ducts. **A,** 46-year-old woman with a history of benign biopsy yielding a high-risk lesion of atypia. Precontrast MRI demonstrates a linear-branching high signal in a segmental distribution involving an entire ductal system compatible with duct ectasia. High signal in ducts is thought to represent proteinaceous debris or hemorrhage. **B,** 48-year-old woman with a history of lobular carcinoma in situ, a high-risk lesion. Precontrast MRI demonstrates high signal in several ducts in the superior breast compatible with duct ectasia. No enhancement of this area was noted on the post-contrast images.

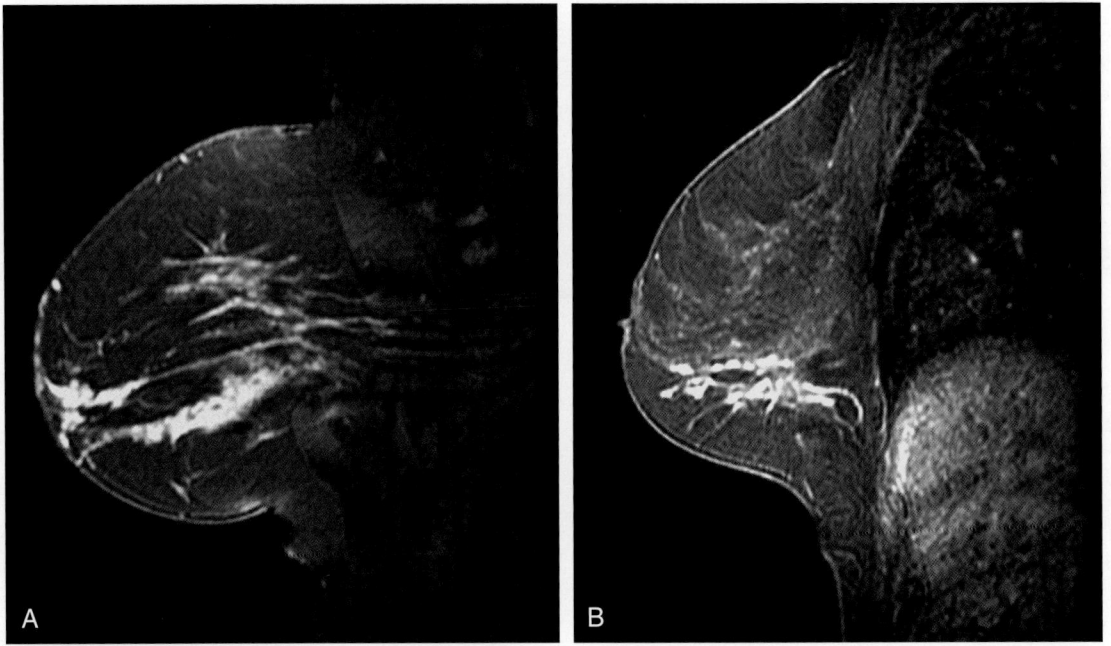

FIGURE 77-41

Ductal enhancement. **A,** 45-year-old woman presents with Paget's disease of the nipple. Mammogram and physical examination are negative. MRI demonstrates extensive clumped enhancement representing extensive ductal carcinoma in situ. The patient underwent mastectomy. **B,** 67-year-old woman with contralateral invasive lobular carcinoma diagnosed 1 year previously. MRI demonstrates clumped linear enhancement in the inferior breast. Biopsy yielded extensive ductal carcinoma in situ.

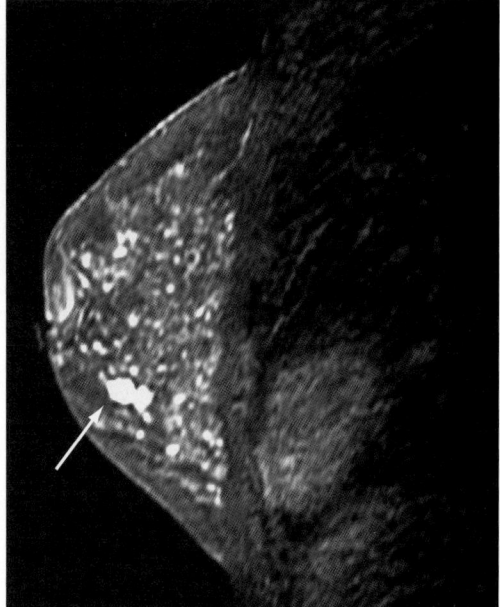

FIGURE 77-42

Smooth homogeneously enhancing mass. 43-year-old woman with extremely dense breasts has known carcinoma of the contralateral breast. Screening MRI demonstrates a bilobed smooth homogeneously enhancing mass (*arrow*). Kinetic analysis demonstrated washout (*not shown*). Biopsy showed simultaneous bilateral breast carcinoma. Note the background stippled enhancement.

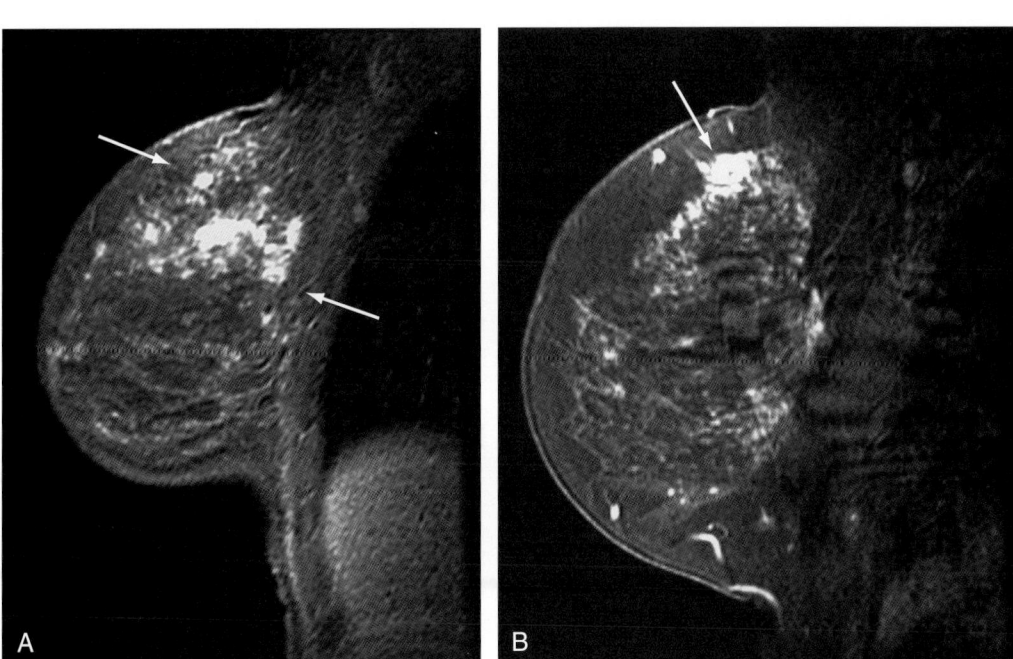

FIGURE 77-43

Hormonal enhancement (premenopausal). **A,** 32-year-old high-risk woman undergoes screening MRI. Patchy regional enhancement is identified in the upper outer quadrant (*arrows*). Kinetic analysis demonstrated a type I or continuous curve. A 6-month follow-up MRI (*not shown*) was performed to document the transient nature of this finding. The follow-up MRI demonstrated no enhancement. Both MRI examinations were performed in the second week of the patient's cycle (days 7-14). **B,** 44-year-old woman with patchy enhancement in the upper breast (*arrow*) that disappeared on follow-up examination.

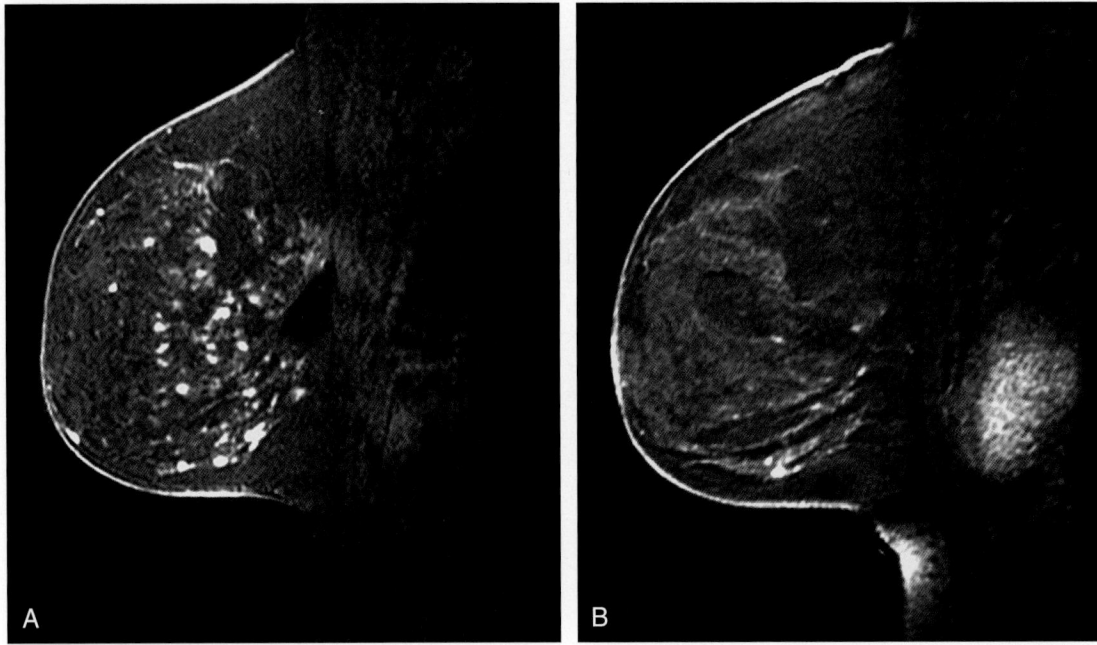

FIGURE 77-44

Hormone replacement therapy (HRT). **A,** 53-year-old woman on HRT demonstrates enhancement throughout the breast. Although most of these areas appear as foci, others border on clumped enhancement. **B,** On a follow-up MRI after discontinuing hormones for several weeks these findings regressed or disappeared.

analyze morphology, high spatial resolution is recommended (1-1.5 mm in all planes). To detect small lesions and to decrease volume averaging, slice thickness should be approximately 2-3 mm with no gap. High temporal resolution is recommended to facilitate enhancement kinetic data gathering; each post-contrast sequence should be performed in under 2 minutes.

New imaging sequences that are based on parallel imaging allow both high spatial and temporal resolution so that neither one needs to be sacrificed.[71] Additionally, these sequences allow simultaneous high-resolution sagittal imaging of both breasts without increasing imaging time. The increased efficiency that parallel imaging affords can be invested in decreasing examination time, improving image quality, and improving spatial and temporal resolution. Parallel imaging is advantageous in that resolution is increased with a concomitant decrease in scan time, artifacts, and acoustic noise. Parallel imaging is a major advantage to those who prefer sagittal small field of view imaging of the breast to axial large field of view imaging. Even for those who prefer axial bilateral imaging, parallel imaging techniques offer advantages and these techniques will likely become standard in the future.

The suppression of signal from fat is important for increasing conspicuity of breast lesions relative to the breast background tissue which can contain variable amounts of fat. Signal from fat can be suppressed by performing a fat-suppression technique or subtracting the post- from the pre-contrast image. For diagnostic purposes, if subtraction is the only method used,

misregistration from patient movement between the pre- and post-contrast images may result, possibly rendering the examination uninterpretable.

Newer post-processing techniques offered by several manufacturers have correction algorithms so that misregistration is not an issue. Nevertheless, chemical selective fat suppression is often preferred and can be performed without excessively lengthening the imaging time.

MSKCC Protocol

At our institution, an MRI Devices immobilization/biopsy coil is used to perform breast MR imaging on a 1.5-T GE Signa magnet. This system allows for compression for diagnostic imaging as well as interventional procedures. Sagittal fat-suppressed T2-weighted images are obtained to assess for cystic changes in the breast, and detection of high signal solid masses such as lymph nodes and myxomatous fibroadenomata. The entire breast is imaged using a three-dimensional fat-suppressed T1-weighted fast-spoiled gradient-echo (FSPGR) sequence. After gadolinium-DTPA administration (0.1 mmol/kg) the same sequence is then repeated a total of three times immediately following one another. Slice thickness is 2 to 3 mm without a gap, depending on breast thickness in compression; TR 17.1; TE 2.4; flip angle 35 degrees; bandwidth 31.25; matrix 256 × 192; 1 NEX; frequency in the anteroposterior direction. Image acquisition takes approximately 2 minutes. Subtraction imaging is performed in addition to fat suppression in

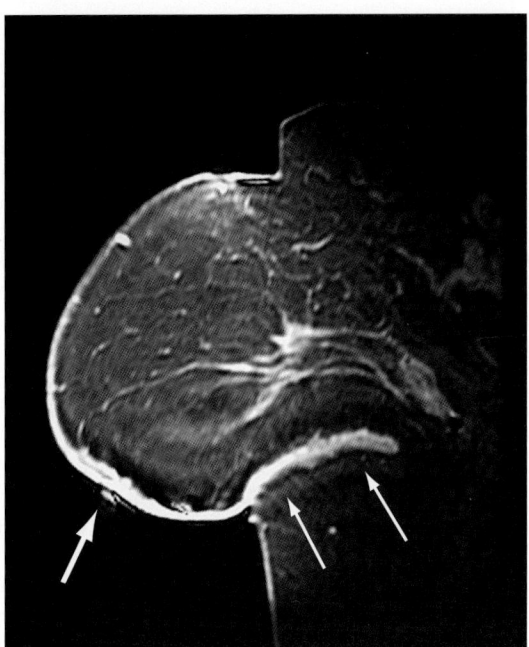

FIGURE 77-45

Positioning of breast. 45-year-old woman with a prior history of breast carcinoma. Note the poor positioning of the breast. The nipple (*thick arrow*) is directed towards the feet instead of towards the table. There is a redundant skinfold (*thin arrows*) that limits evaluation of the surrounding tissue. Note that the posterior breast tissue is incompletely visualized as it has not been pulled into the coil.

order to evaluate possible enhancement of high signal areas on the T1-weighted images and maximum intensity projection (MIP) images are generated in each case. Images are read out on a GE picture archiving and communication system (PACS), which is ideal for comparing prior studies and for windowing appropriately. Prior mammograms and breast ultrasounds are available, if needed. If a time-signal intensity curve needs to be generated, a workstation is available. We are currently evaluating several post-processing parametric imaging techniques and perform spectroscopy in a research setting.

Technologist Training

For performing diagnostic breast MRI, an MRI technologist, who can be trained in positioning of the breast within the breast coil, is essential (see Fig. 77-45). As with mammography, image quality depends on optimal positioning. The breast should be pulled away from the chest wall by the MRI technologist as much as possible and placed in the center of the coil in order to image the entire breast and reduce artifacts. If a compression plate is used for immobilization, this can be adjusted so that the medial breast tissue and axillary tail are not excluded. It is helpful for the MRI technologist to have a calm and reassuring manner, in order to facilitate patient cooperation and decrease movement. For interventional

procedures we have found it helpful to include the mammography technologist who is trained in interventional breast procedures, in addition to the MRI technologist who is trained in image acquisition.

Image Interpretation

To facilitate image interpretation, at our institution detailed clinical and physical examination information is required on the MRI requisition. A breast imager protocols the examination in advance. When the patient arrives, a nurse performs an intake questionnaire that gathers information important for interpretation on surgical history, family history, last menstrual period, HRT, and date and place of last mammogram and ultrasound, if not brought with the patient or not performed at our institution. The nurse draws on a preprinted diagram any scars, areas of discoloration or lumps, and then marks on the breast with vitamin E capsules any areas of palpable abnormality and prior sites of surgery. The patient's prior films are available at the time of interpretation so that correlation with the mammogram and sonogram can be made.

MR Intervention

Interventional procedures are essential to any breast MRI program. Many different types of interventional coils are currently available and can be easily used to perform needle localizations and biopsies. In our practice if a suspicious mass (usually >5 mm) or nonmass area of enhancement is identified on MRI and we think the lesion may be able to be identified on ultrasound, a targeted ultrasound will be performed. If we can reliably find a corresponding ultrasound finding, we will biopsy that lesion under ultrasound guidance.[72] However, solely relying on targeted ultrasound following breast MRI examination to identify suspicious lesions is not sufficient. Breast MRI intervention is still essential as cancers exist that are identified on MRI but not on ultrasound (Fig. 77-46).

For the purposes of MR intervention, imaging parameters should be the same as the diagnostic examination to ensure lesion conspicuity.[73] Lesions can disappear on the day of the examination and if this occurs it is necessary to ensure no mishap in contrast administration or imaging. In our experience this occurs less than 5% of the time, though other investigators have reported a much higher figure. In general, these areas are likely related to hormone effects. It is our practice to routinely have these patients return in 6 months to ensure that the lesion is not evident.

MR intervention is fairly straightforward for the radiologist who is familiar with routine breast interventional procedures.[74] Procedures under MR guidance, however, have unique considerations. First and foremost, there is currently no equivalent to the specimen radiograph so that lesion retrieval can be confirmed following a needle localization procedure. Therefore, accuracy of needle placement is paramount so that the

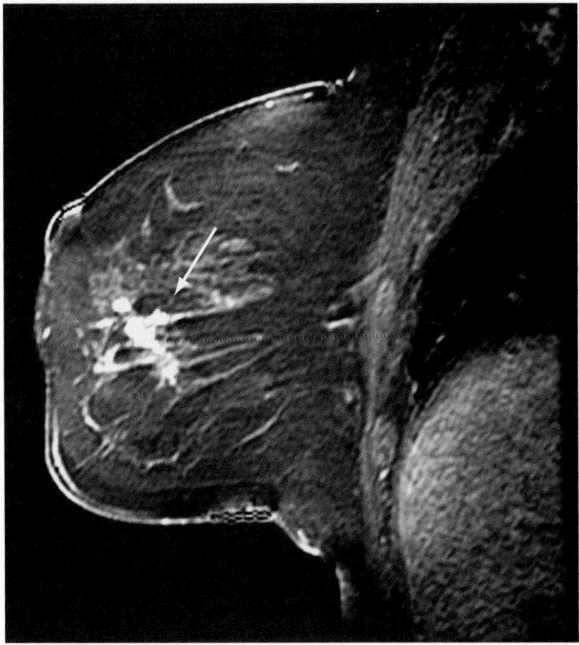

FIGURE 77-46

MR only detected infiltrating lobular carcinoma. 58-year-old woman with a history of contralateral breast cancer 15 years previously and treated with mastectomy. Screening MRI of the remaining breast demonstrates an area of clumped enhancement centrally (*arrow*) that was not seen on mammography or targeted ultrasound. MR biopsy yielded invasive lobular carcinoma. Sentinel node analysis was negative. The patient elected to undergo a mastectomy.

surgeon can have the best chance at lesion removal. The lack of a specimen that can be confirmed also means that the radiologist performing the procedure must perform careful correlation between the pathologic and MRI findings to ensure that the lesion that was localized was removed. If there is any discordance, a postoperative MRI examination can be performed. A second consideration is the fact that the contrast does not stay within the lesion forever; there is washout particularly in malignant lesions. Therefore, it is important that the radiologist is quick and accurate when performing the procedure and that the imaging parameters optimize speed. If for some reason the contrast washes out of the lesion before the needle has been placed, a repeat injection of contrast will often reidentify the lesion.

The basic design of breast MR localization/biopsy systems incorporates many of the same techniques as mammographic localization or stereotactic biopsy. To accomplish this, ideally, the breast is immobilized and all parts of the breast are accessible. Intervention of the breast under MR guidance is generally performed with the patient in a prone position. Prone positioning is generally preferred as the breast is pendant and away from the chest wall and needle direction is generally parallel to the chest wall. Some investigators have found that placing the patient in the prone oblique position facilitates access to the axillary tail and posterior breast tissue.[75]

Fixing the breast in the prone position has many advantages, including decreased movement of the breast when placing a needle. Immobilization of the breast tissue for most systems is performed in the mediolateral plane between compression plates that allow access to the breast from whatever direction compression is obtained. A variety of compression plates are available: perforated holes to accommodate needles as well as flexible moveable horizontal bands. Several coils allow needle placement from both the lateral and medial aspects of the breast, so that the minimum amount of breast tissue is traversed. We use a breast coil and grid biopsy device manufactured by MRI Devices (Waukesha, WI). The compression plates consist of a grid into which a needle guide is inserted in order to direct the needle in a horizontal fashion. These compression plates provide immobilization of the breast as well as a guide that acts as a coordinate system to enable accurate targeting of the lesion.

A potential problem with MR image-guided localizations relates to the fact that the wire is deployed with the breast in compression parallel to the direction of needle placement. This allows for an "accordion effect": during compression, structures that were far apart are brought close together, and when compression is released, structures that were close together move further apart. Any error in the depth direction (parallel to the axis of needle placement) can therefore be exaggerated when compression is released. Keeping compression to the minimum necessary to achieve immobilization can minimize the accordion effect. Following needle deployment it may be helpful to release the breast from the compression plates, massage it, and then reimage in the orthogonal plane (axial if the localization was performed in the sagittal plane) so that the depth of the needle can be seen with respect to the lesion.

To place a needle at the desired location in the breast, the position of the lesion must be related to the overlying grid system. One way to accomplish this is to place a fiducial marker on the grid system somewhere (usually close to the suspected location of the underlying lesion). The fiducial marker can be a vial filled with gadolinium-DTPA or a vitamin E capsule taped to the grid and skin. The fiducial marker is visualized as high signal on the initial post-contrast image and the exact insertion site over the lesion can be determined by measuring the lesion location relative to it. The depth of the lesion from the level of the grid and skin surface can be calculated by multiplying the number of sagittal slices by the slice thickness.

To introduce the needle into the breast in a grid system a needle guide can be inserted into the desired grid hole to facilitate needle placement. The guides are advantageous in that they allow the needle to remain relatively straight and horizontal to the chest wall. For biopsy procedures these guides support and fix the coaxial guides in the breast. Several MR-compatible needles are commercially available (Tumor Localizer, 18 or 20 gauge, Daum Medical Systems, Schwerin, Germany; MRI Breast Lesion Marking System, 20 gauge, E-Z-EM, Westbury, NY; and MReye Modified Kopans Spring Hook Localization Needle, 20 gauge, Cook,

Bloomington, IN). Although artifact can be a nuisance on MR images, visualization of artifact can be used to recognize the presence and position of the wire or needle. Some of these wires have reinforced portions that may be desirable.

When performing biopsy, the optimal probe is a directional vacuum-assisted device. Several are available on the market at this time and use a coaxial guide for probe placement. Available probes are 9 and 11 gauge (ATEC™ System, Suros Surgical Systems, Indianapolis; VACORA™, Bard Biopsy Systems, Tempe, Arizona). As with stereotactic biopsy, there has been a trend with MR biopsy to obtain more tissue,[76,77] thus decreasing underestimation of the sampled lesion, as well as ensuring lesion removal. Because many of the pathologic diagnoses of the breast rely on architectural analysis, the more tissue removed the more accurate the diagnosis. Other advantages of some of the probes are that once the probe is inserted into the breast it does not need to be removed and small movements in the coaxial guide with subsequent erroneous positioning do not occur. These biopsy systems also allow localizing clip placement which can be advantageous for patients who require surgery after MR biopsy, as the clip can be localized under mammographic guidance.

CONCLUSION

The availability of breast MRI has improved knowledge of breast cancer and breast disease. It can provide important information in a number of clinical scenarios and may have significant impact in the future in breast cancer screening. Many of the improvements in the past few years can be attributed to improved coil design, improved biopsy systems, and availability of MR-compatible interventional needles and probes. Having the ability to biopsy MR-visible lesions has allowed this technology to disseminate from academic centers into the community. A breast MRI program not only involves image acquisition and interpretation but also MRI intervention. This way MRI can be ideally incorporated into the performance of high-quality breast imaging.

REFERENCES

1. Heywang SH, Wolf A, Pruss E, et al: MR imaging of the breast with Gd-DTPA: use and limitations. Radiology 171:95-103, 1989.
2. Kaiser WA, Zeitler E: MR imaging of the breast: fast imaging sequences with and without Gd-DTPA. Radiology 170:681-686, 1989.
3. Orel SG, Schnall MD, Powell CM, et al: Staging of suspected breast cancer: effect of MR imaging and MR-guided biopsy. Radiology 196:115-122, 1995.
4. Fischer U, Kopka L, Grabbe E: Breast carcinoma: Effect of preoperative contrast-enhanced MR imaging on the therapeutic approach. Radiology 213:881-888, 1999.
5. Liberman L, Morris EA, Dershaw DD, et al: MR imaging of the ipsilateral breast in women with percutaneously proven breast cancer. Am J Roentgenol 180:901-910, 2003.
6. Mumtaz H, Hall-Craggs MA, Davidson T, et al: Staging of symptomatic primary breast cancer with MR imaging. Am J Roentgenol 169:417-424, 1997.
7. Schelfout K, Van Goethem M, Kersschot E, et al: Contrast-enhanced MR imaging of breast lesions and effect on treatment. Eur J Surg Oncol 30:501-507, 2004.
8. Bedrosian I, Mick R, Orel SG, et al: Changes in the surgical management of patients with breast carcinoma based on preoperative magnetic resonance imaging. Cancer 98: 468-473, 2003.
9. Esserman L, Hylton N, Yassa L, et al: Utility of magnetic resonance imaging in the management of breast cancer: evidence for improved preoperative staging. J Clin Oncol 17:110-119, 1999.
10. Berg WA: Imaging the local extent of disease. Semin Breast Dis 4:153-173, 2001.
11. Liberman L, Morris EA, Kim CM, et al: MR imaging findings in the contralateral breast of women with recently diagnosed breast cancer. Am J Roentgenol 180:333-341, 2003.
12. Lee SG, Orel SG, Woo IJ, et al: MR imaging screening of the contralateral breast in patients with newly diagnosed breast cancer: preliminary results. Radiology 226:773-778, 2003.
13. Frei K, Kinkel K, Bonel HM, et al: MR imaging of the breast in patients with positive margins after lumpectomy: Influence of the time interval between lumpectomy and MR imaging. Am J Roentgenol 175:1577-1584, 2000.
14. Orel SG, Reynolds C, Schnall MD, et al: Breast carcinoma: MR imaging before re-excisional biopsy. Radiology 205:429-436, 1997.
15. Faverly DR, Hendriks JH, Holland R: Breast carcinomas of limited extent: frequency, radiologic-pathologic characteristics, and surgical margin requirements. Cancer 91:647-659, 2001.
16. Esserman L, Kaplan E, Partridge S, et al: MRI phenotype is associated with response to doxorubicin and cyclophosphamide neoadjuvant chemotherapy in stage III breast cancer. Ann Surg Oncol 8:549-559, 2001.
17. Wasser K, Klein SK, Fink C, et al: Evaluation of neoadjuvant chemotherapeutic response of breast cancer using dynamic MRI with high temporal resolution. Eur Radiol 13:80-87, 2003.
18. Delille JP, Slanetz PJ, Yeh ED, et al: Invasive ductal breast carcinoma response to neoadjuvant chemotherapy: noninvasive monitoring with functional MR imaging pilot study. Radiology 228:63-69, 2003.
19. Knopp MV, Brix G, Junkermann HJ, et al: MR mammography with pharmacokinetic mapping for monitoring of breast cancer treatment during neoadjuvant therapy. MRI Clin North Am 2:633-658, 1997.
20. Hylton NM, Esserman LJ, Partridge SC, et al: Contrast MRI for characterization of tumor response to neoadjuvant chemotherapy and prediction of recurrence in stage III breast cancer [abstract]. Eur Radiol 10:F10-11, 2000.
21. Gilles R, Guinebretiere JM, Shapeero LG, et al: Assessment of breast cancer recurrence with contrast-enhanced subtraction MR imaging: preliminary results in 26 patients. Radiology 188: 473-478, 1993.
22. Dao TH, Rahmouni A, Campana F, et al: Tumour recurrence versus fibrosis in the irradiated breast: differentiation with dynamic gadolinium-enhanced MR imaging. Radiology 187:751-755, 1993.
23. Lewis-Jones HG, Whitehouse GH, Leinster SJ, et al: The role of magnetic resonance imaging in the assessment of local recurrent breast carcinoma. Clin Radiol 43:197-294, 1992.
24. Schorn C, Fischer U, Luftner N, et al: MRI of the breast in patients with metastatic disease of unknown primary. Eur Radiol 9:470-473, 1999.
25. Campana F, Fourquet A, Ashby MA, et al: Presentation of axillary lymphadenopathy without detectable breast primary (T0N1b breast cancer): experience at Institut Curie. Radiother Oncol 15:321-325, 1989.
26. Morris EA, Schwartz LH, Dershaw DD, et al: MR imaging of the breast in patients with occult primary breast cancer. Radiology 205:437-440, 1997.
27. Orel SG, Weinstein SP, Schnall MD, et al: Breast imaging in patients with axillary node metastases and unknown primary malignancy. Radiology 212:543-549, 1999.
28. Olson JA, Morris EA, Van Zee KJ, et al: Magnetic resonance imaging facilitates breast conservation for occult breast cancer. Ann Surg Oncol 7:411-415, 2000.
29. Kuhl CK, Schmutzler RK, Leutner CC, et al: Breast MR imaging screening in 192 women proved or suspected to be carriers of a breast cancer susceptibility gene: preliminary results. Radiology 215:267-279, 2000.
30. Lo LD, Rosen MA, Schnall MD, et al: Pilot study of breast MR screening of a high-risk cohort. Radiology 221:432(P), 2001.
31. Warner E, Plewes DB, Shumak RS, et al: Comparison of breast magnetic resonance imaging, mammography, and ultrasound for surveillance of women at high risk for hereditary breast cancer. J Clin Oncol 19:3524-3531, 2001.
32. Stoutjesdijk MJ, Boetes C, Jager GJ, et al: Magnetic resonance imaging and mammography in women with a hereditary risk of breast cancer. J Natl Cancer Inst 93:1095-1102, 2001.
33. Tilanus-Linthorst MMA, Obdeijn IMM, Bartels KCM, et al: First experiences in screening women at high risk for breast cancer with MR imaging. Breast Cancer Res Treat 63:53-60, 2000.
34. Leach MO, Eeles RA, Turnbull LW, et al: The UK national study of magnetic resonance imaging as a method of screening for breast cancer (MARIBS). J Exp Clin Cancer Res 21:107-14, 2002.
35. Morris EA, Liberman L, Ballon DJ, et al: MRI of occult breast carcinoma in a high-risk population. Am J Roentgenol 181:619-626, 2003.
36. American College of Radiology: Breast Imaging Reporting and Data System (BI-RADS). Reston, VA, American College of Radiology, 2003.
37. Holland R, Veling SH, Mravunac M, et al: Histologic multifocality of Tis, T1-2 breast carcinomas. Implications for clinical trials of breast-conserving surgery. Cancer 56:979-990, 1985.
38. Quan ML, Sclafani L, Heerdt AS, et al: Magnetic resonance imaging detects unsuspected disease in patients with invasive lobular cancer. Ann Surg Oncol 10:1048-1053, 2003.
39. Weinstein SP, Orel SG, Heller R, et al: MR imaging of the breast in patients with invasive lobular breast cancer. Am J Roentgenol 176:399-406, 2001.

40. Hwang ES, Kinkel K, Esserman LJ, et al: Magnetic resonance imaging in patients diagnosed with ductal carcinoma-in-situ: Value in the diagnosis of residual disease, occult invasion and multicentricity. Ann Surg Oncol 10:381-388, 2003.

41. Viehweg P, Lampe D, Buchmann J, et al: In situ and minimally invasive breast cancer: morphologic and kinetic features on contrast enhanced MR imaging. MAGMA 11:129-137, 2000.

42. Menell JH, Morris EA, Dershaw DD, et al. Determination of presence and extent of pure ductal carcinoma in situ by mammography and MR [abstract]. Am J Roentgenol 182:60, 2004.

43. Morris EA, Schwartz LH, Drotman MB, et al: Evaluation of pectoralis major muscle in patients with posterior breast tumors on breast MR imaging: Preliminary experience. Radiology 214:67-72, 2000.

44. Partridge SC, Gibbs JE, Lu Y, et al: Accuracy of MR imaging for revealing residual breast cancer in patients who have undergone neoadjuvant chemotherapy. Am J Roentgenol 179:1193 1199, 2002.

45. Podo F, Sardanelli F, Canese R, et al: The Italian multi-centre project on evaluation of MRI and other imaging modalities in early detection of breast cancer in subjects at high genetic risk. J Exp Clin Cancer Res 21:115-124, 2002.

46. Hayes C, Padhani AR, Leach MO: Assessing changes in tumour vascular function using dynamic contrast-enhanced magnetic resonance imaging. NMR Biomed 15:154-163, 2002.

47. Knopp MV, Weiss E, Sinn HP, et al: Pathophysiologic basis of contrast enhancement in breast tumors. J Magn Reson Imaging 10:260-266, 1999.

48. Esserman L, Hylton N, George T, Weidner N: Contrast-enhanced magnetic resonance imaging to assess tumor histopathology and angiogenesis in breast carcinoma. Breast J 5:13-21, 1999.

49. Mussurakis S, Buckley DL, Bowsley SJ, et al: Dynamic contrast-enhanced magnetic resonance imaging of the breast combined with pharmacokinetic analysis of gadolinium-DTPA uptake in the diagnosis of local recurrence of early stage breast carcinoma. Invest Radiol 30:650-662, 1995.

50. Hylton NM: Vascularity assessment of breast lesions with gadolinium-enhanced MR imaging. Magn Reson Imaging Clin N Am 7:411-420, 1999.

51. Boetes C, Strijk SP, Holland R, et al: False-negative MR imaging of malignant breast tumors. Eur Radiol 7:1231-1234, 1997.

52. Fischer U, Westerhof JP, Brinck U, et al: Ductal carcinoma in situ by dynamic MR-mammography at 1.5T. Rofo Forschr Geb Rontgenstr Neuen Bildgeb Verfahr 164:290-294, 1996.

53. Sittek H, Kessler M, Heuck AF, et al: Morphology and contrast enhancement of ductal carcinoma in situ in dynamic 1.0T MR mammography. Rofo Fortschr Geb Rontgenstr Neuen Bildgeb Verfahr 167:247-251, 1997.

54. Harms SE (ed): Technical report of the International Working Group on Breast MRI. J Magn Reson Imaging 10:978-1015, 1999.

55. Schnall MD, Ikeda DM: Lesion diagnosis working group report. J Magn Reson Imaging 10:982-990, 1999.

56. Ikeda DM, Baker DR, Daniel BL: Magnetic resonance imaging of breast cancer: clinical indications and breast MRI reporting system. J Magn Reson Imaging 12:975-983, 2000.

57. Morris EA: Illustrated breast MR lexicon. Semin Roentgenol 36:238-249, 2001.

58. Liberman L, Morris EA, Benton CL, et al: Probably benign lesions at breast magnetic resonance imaging: preliminary experience in high-risk women. Cancer 98:377-388, 2003.

59. Kuhl CK, Bieling HB, Gieseke J, et al: Healthy premenopausal breast parenchyma in dynamic contrast-enhanced MR imaging of the breast: normal contrast medium enhancement and cyclical phase dependency. Radiology 203:137-144, 1997.

60. Muller-Schimpfle M, Ohmenhauser MD, Stoli P, et al: Menstrual cycle and age: influence on parenchymal contrast medium enhancement in MR imaging of the breast. Radiology 203:145-149, 1997.

61. Lee CH, Smith RC, Levine JA, et al: Clinical usefulness of MR imaging of the breast in the evaluation of the problematic mammogram. Am J Roentgenol 173:1323-1329, 1999.

62. Nunes LW, Schnall MD, Siegelman ES, et al: Diagnostic performance characteristics of architectural features revealed by high spatial-resolution MR imaging of the breast. Am J Roentgenol 169:409-415, 1997.

63. Nunes LW, Schnall MD, Orel SG, et al: Breast MR imaging: Interpretation model. Radiology 202.833-841, 1997.

64. Nunes LW, Schnall MD, Orel SG, et al: Correlation of lesion appearance and histologic findings for the nodes of a breast MR imaging interpretation model. Radiographics 19:79-92, 1999.

65. Kim SJ, Morris EA, Liberman L, et al: Observer variability and applicability of BI-RADS terminology for breast MR imaging: invasive carcinomas as focal masses. Am J Roentgenol 177:551-557, 2001.

66. Liberman L, Morris EA, Lee MJ, et al: Breast lesions detected on MR imaging: features and positive predictive value. Am J Roentgenol 179:171-178, 2002.

67. Liberman L, Morris EA, Dershaw DD, Tan LK: Ductal enhancement on MR imaging of the breast. Am J Roentgenol 181:519-525, 2003.

68. Gallardo X, Sentis M, Castaner E, et al: Enhancement of intramammary lymph nodes with lymphoid hyperplasia: a potential pitfall in breast MRI. Eur Radiol 8:1662-1665, 1998.

69. Kuhl CK, Schild HH: Dynamic image interpretation of MRI of the breast. J Magn Reson Imaging 12:965-974, 2000.

70. Kuhl CK, Mielcareck P, Klaschik S, et al: Dynamic breast MR imaging: Are signal intensity time course data useful for differential diagnosis of enhancing lesions? Radiology 211:101-110, 1999.

71. Sodickson DK, Griswold MA, Jakob PM: SMASH imaging. Magn Reson Imaging Clin N Am 7:237-254, 1999.

72. LaTrenta LR, Menell JH, Morris EA, et al: Breast lesions detected with MR imaging: utility and histopathologic importance of identification with US. Radiology 227:856-861, 2003.

73. Morris EA, Liberman L, Dershaw DD, et al: Preoperative MR imaging-guided needle localization of breast lesions. Am J Roentgenol 178:1211-1220, 2002.

74. Liberman L, Morris EA, Dershaw DD, et al: Fast MRI-guided vacuum-assisted breast biopsy: initial experience. Am J Roentgenol 181:1283-1293, 2003.

75. Kuhl CK, Morakkabati N, Leutner CC, et al: MR imaging—guided large-core (14-gauge) needle biopsy of small lesions visible at breast MR imaging alone. Radiology 220:31-39, 2001.

76. Heywang-Kobrunner SH, Heinig A, Pickuth D, et al: Interventional MRI of the breast: lesion localisation and biopsy. Eur Radiol 10:36-45, 2000.

77. Perlet C, Heinig A, Prat X, et al: Multicenter study for the evaluation of a dedicated biopsy device for MR-guided vacuum biopsy of the breast. Eur Radiol 12:1463-1470, 2002.

CHAPTER 78

BREAST IMPLANTS

Michael S. Middleton ● Michael P. McNamara Jr

INTRODUCTION

Magnetic resonance (MR) imaging is capable of providing essential information that can assist physician and patient decisions when breast implant rupture or soft tissue silicone is known or suspected.[1] Understanding breast implant-related findings also is important when interpreting MR imaging of patients being evaluated for breast cancer.[2]

Modern breast augmentation began in the late 1940s with silicone fluid injections (in Japan[3]) and sponge implants.[4] The first silicone gel-filled breast implants were placed in March 1962,[5] and saline-filled implants were introduced circa 1965.[6] Although 14 types of breast implant have been described[2,7-10] (see Table 78-1) the majority encountered in clinical practice are either single-lumen silicone gel-filled, saline-filled, standard double-lumen (inner-lumen silicone gel, outer-lumen saline), or reverse double-lumen (inner-lumen saline, outer-lumen silicone gel) implants. Saline-filled implants often can be evaluated by physical examination alone since deflation, when it occurs, is usually rapid and complete. This chapter will focus mostly on the other three types*.

Using the Eklund ("push-back") technique, adequate mammography usually is possible for breast cancer screening, albeit with diminished sensitivity.[11,12] However, aside from special circumstances‡ mammography should not be relied upon to evaluate breast implant-related problems. An implant that appears intact mammographically may or may not be intact. Soft-tissue silicone from current or prior implant rupture often is poorly or incompletely seen mammographically, or not seen at all.

It is now known that implant rupture is common, but most often is *mammographically* silent. In the FDA Breast Implant Study, MR imaging showed that 77% of the 344 women studied had clear MR findings, or strong suspicion of rupture of one or both implants, and 21% of the women studied had strong MR imaging evidence of extracapsular soft-tissue silicone.[13] However, in a study of 350 women, on the basis of mammography alone Destouet et al only detected rupture in 5%.[14]

---

*An illustrated listing of implant types, styles and sizes, including less commonly seen types, are included in the book and CDROM from Middleton and McNamara.[2]

‡There are three circumstances where mammography can provide valuable information about breast implants: 1) Saline-filled implants easily can be recognized as such, and can be seen to be inflated (or deflated); 2) standard double-lumen implants with saline still present in the outer lumen easily can be recognized as such, and in those cases the presence of saline in the outer lumen is a reliable indication of implant integrity; and 3) the textured outer surface of some implants (Dow Corning SILASTIC MSI and McGhan Biocell) may be appreciated on mammography. The absence of that appearance may suggest rupture because escaped silicone gel may "fill in" the outer textured implant surface.[2]

TABLE 78-1 Types of Breast Implants

Type	Configuration
1. Single-lumen, silicone gel-filled	Silicone gel-filled
2. Single-lumen, adjustable	Prefilled with silicone gel, optional saline addable through a valve
3. Saline-, dextran-, or PVP-filled	Prefilled, or fillable through a valve
4. Standard double-lumen	Inner silicone gel-filled lumen, outer lumen fillable through a valve with saline
5. Reverse double-lumen	Outer silicone gel-filled lumen, inner lumen fillable through a valve with saline
6. Reverse adjustable double-lumen	Outer lumen silicone gel-filled, inner lumen silicone gel-filled, optional saline added to inner lumen through a valve
7. Gel-gel double-lumen	Inner high profile lumen silicone gel-filled, outer moderate profile lumen silicone gel-filled (all prefilled, no valve)
8. Triple-lumen	Inner high profile lumen silicone gel-filled, middle moderate profile lumen silicone gel-filled, outer lumen fillable with saline through a valve
9. Cavon	Silicone gel only, no shell
10. Custom	Created upon prescription to individualized specifications for a particular patient
11. Pectus	Solid pectus muscle replacement implant
12. Sponge	Sponge made of Ivalon, Etheron, or another material, simple or complex
13. Sponge adjustable	Sponge inside a silicone elastomer shell, inflatable with dextran or saline
14. Other	Soy bean oil-filled, etc.

Adapted from Middleton and McNamara: Breast Implant Imaging. Philadelphia: Williams & Wilkins, 2003.

Most rupture also is *clinically* silent. In the FDA study, only 8% of the women studied had pre-test suspicion or concern for rupture,[13] and in the study by Gabriel et al[15] (in which MR imaging was not used), only 5% of 749 patients had rupture at time of implant removal. Hence physical examination alone to detect implant rupture is notoriously inadequate.

Most rupture can be detected with MR imaging. Middleton reported 87% accuracy in the determination of rupture (75% sensitivity, 99% specificity) for 853 surgically removed single-lumen silicone gel-filled implants.[7] Some early references understate the accuracy of breast implant MR imaging because breast surface coils were not available, and some early rupture was classified only as "gel bleed".*

At this time, MR imaging is used to evaluate breast implants when the findings could affect patient care significantly, and is the noninvasive gold standard for evaluating silicone gel-filled breast implants in the current FDA breast implant approval process. MR imaging is also used to evaluate breast implants and soft-tissue silicone in patients for whom there is a concern for, or a diagnosis of, breast cancer.

Ultrasound can be very useful, and the reader is referred to other references since that is outside the scope of this work.[2,16]

---

*All "intact" silicone gel-filled breast implants "bleed" small amounts of silicone fluid by diffusion through the implant shell. This is not rupture. The diffusing silicone *fluid* consists of un-crosslinked silicone molecules. Diffused silicone fluid can be evident when an implant is examined directly, even before it is placed in the patient, but rarely is evident on MR imaging. At time of removal, however, implants in a state of uncollapsed or even minimally collapsed rupture, with clearly evident shell defects and abundant escaped silicone gel, may be misleadingly described as showing "gel bleed". Hence rupture prevalence in some early studies was understated, and clinically is likely underreported.

CLINICAL CONSIDERATIONS

Implant History and Prior Studies

Obtaining breast implant-related history and reviewing prior imaging studies and medical records is important for optimal breast MR imaging and interpretation:

- patient symptoms
- reason for implant placement
- reason for current requested evaluation
- current implant type, style, and size
- date of placement
- anatomic plane of placement (subglandular, submuscular, etc.)
- history of prior implants
- history of prior implant rupture
- history of breast trauma or capsulotomy (open or closed)
- history of TRAM or latissimus flap reconstruction.

Medical records and prior imaging studies can reveal implant type, as well as the state of the implants. If a patient has saline-filled implants, or standard double-lumen implants known still to have saline in their outer lumen (by mammography or ultrasound), MR imaging probably is not necessary. These findings can be evident on prior mammography, ultrasound, and MR imaging.[2]

Some women with breast implants avoid mammography because of concern that it may cause implant rupture.[2,17,18] Relating those concerns in the MR report may help the referring physician reinforce ACR/ACS mammography screening guidelines with the patient.

Plane of Placement

Implants usually are placed in the submuscular or the subglandular plane (Fig. 78-1). If there has been latissimus flap reconstruction, an implant may be placed

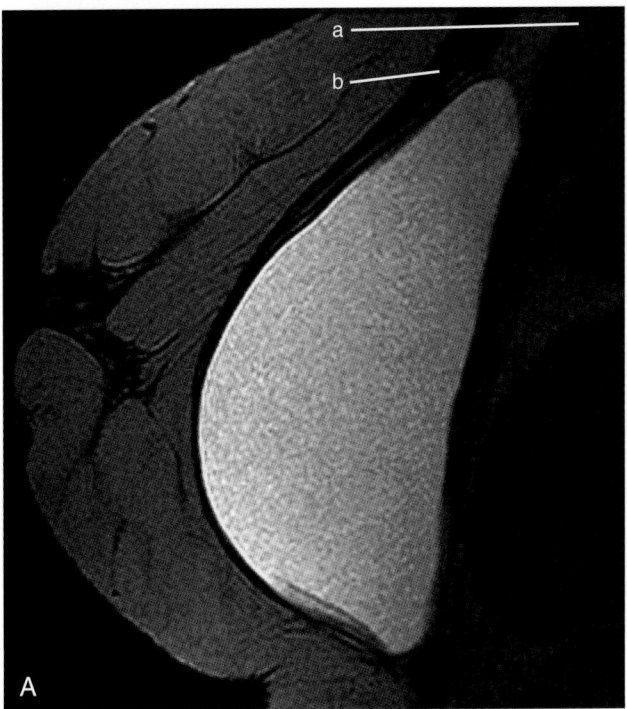 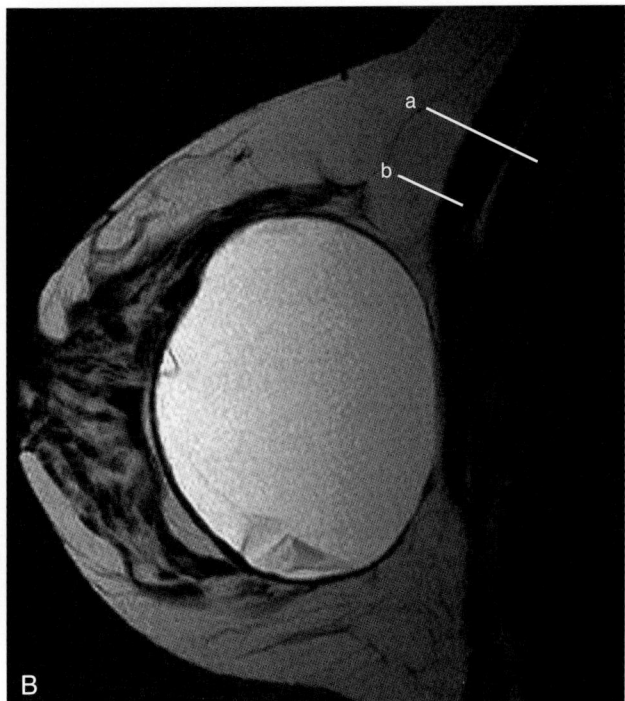

FIGURE 78-1

Planes of implant placement, pectoralis minor marked 'a', pectoralis major marked '**b**' (single-lumen silicone gel-filled, T2-weighted fast spin-echo, water suppression). **A,** Submuscular (intact, placed 1977, implant age 23.7 years). **B,** Subglandular (uncollapsed rupture, placed 1987, implant age 6.9 years).[2]

under it (Fig. 78-2). Brown et al[13] reported a 6 to15-fold increase in prevalence of rupture for submuscular implants compared to subglandular implants.[‡]

An implant in one plane can be replaced with one in another plane. Rarely, sizeable seroma/hematoma develops after replacement of a prior implant, which can be mistaken for a "2nd implant" on a current imaging study (Fig. 78-3). Two, or even three implants can be placed in a given breast, usually in a reconstructive setting (Fig. 78-4).

Fibrous Capsule Formation

A fibrous capsule starts to form around all breast implants very soon after placement. In animals it has been shown to begin forming within 2 days.[19,20] The Baker scale is used to describe capsular contracture:[21]

Grade I Prosthesis cannot be seen or felt
Grade II Prosthesis cannot be seen, but can be felt
Grade III Prosthesis can be seen and felt
Grade IV Breast is hard and tender or painful, with marked distortion and possibly cold.

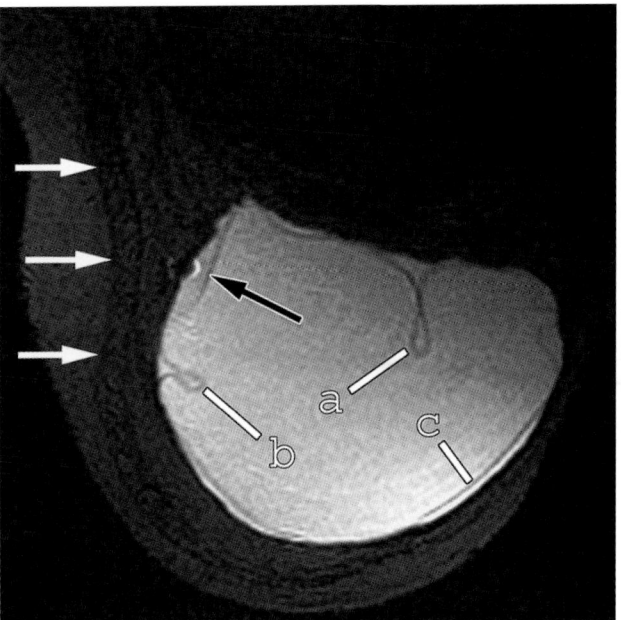

FIGURE 78-2

Placement under latissimus flap. White *arrows* mark lateral edge of latissimus flap, black *arrow* marks susceptibility from probable gas bubble within implant. **a,** keyhole sign; **b,** pull-away sign; **c,** subcapsular line sign (single-lumen silicone gel-filled, minimally collapsed rupture, T2-weighted fast spin-echo, water suppression, placed 1991, implant age 3.0 years).[2]

[‡]At study site 1, the odds ratio (OR) was 6.02, with a 95% confidence interval (CI) of 2.35 to 15.45; at study site 2, the OR was 15.87, with a 95% CI of 4.19 to 60.05.

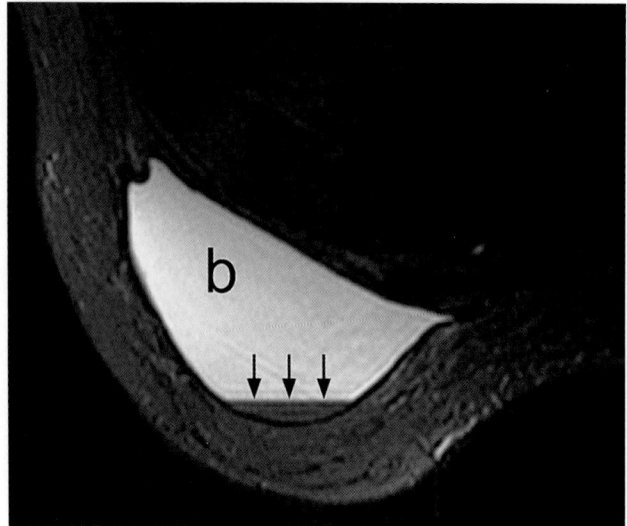

FIGURE 78-3

Sizeable seroma/hematoma mistaken for an implant showing a fluid-fluid level; capsular residual silicone from prior ruptured implant isointense to tissue and so not evident on this image (bright fluid of seroma marked **b**; *arrows* mark fluid-fluid level; T2-weighted fast spin-echo, silicone suppression).[2]

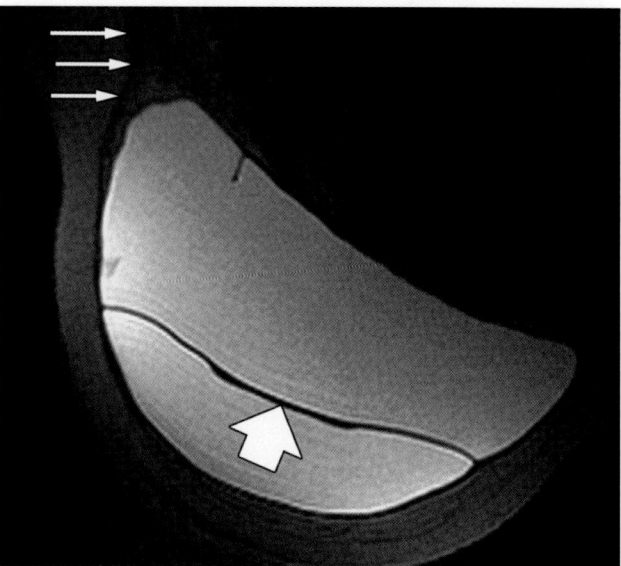

FIGURE 78-4

Stacked implants. *Thin arrows* mark lateral edge of latissimus flap, which split around lateral edge of implant. *Wide arrow* marks posterior shell patch of anterior implant (both intact, silicone gel-filled single-lumen, T2-weighted fast spin-echo, water suppression. Anterior one placed 1990, implant age 2.7 years; posterior one placed 1989, implant age 3.8 years).[2]

Capsular contracture is well evaluated by physical examination alone, and so although evidence of it may be seen on imaging studies, imaging is not needed to evaluate it. On T2-weighted imaging of extracapsular rupture the fibrous capsule can be evident as a thin irregular layer of dark signal between the extracapsular silicone and silicone gel that remains confined by the fibrous capsule. It also may be seen as an incisure or indentation in the contour of the implant (Fig. 78-5).

Implant Folds

Breast implants are composed of a silicone elastomer shell (or shells), intentionally underfilled with silicone gel, saline, or both. Because they are underfilled, infoldings of the shell occur as implants accommodate to the space allotted to them within the body (Fig. 78-6). The presence of folds by itself is not a sign of rupture. Folds will be evident on almost all breast implant MR imaging; they are theoretically less common in overfilled, thick-shelled, and very large implants, but in practice almost all implants exhibit folds while in the body.

Folds can have normal and abnormal appearances, and distinguishing intact from ruptured implants is based upon recognizing the differences. Appreciating the normal appearances of implant folds is the most important single aspect of breast implant MR image interpretation. After reviewing this chapter the interested reader is referred to Chapter 4 in Middleton and McNamara,[2] which contains 67 figure parts showing the various appearances of normal implant shell folds.

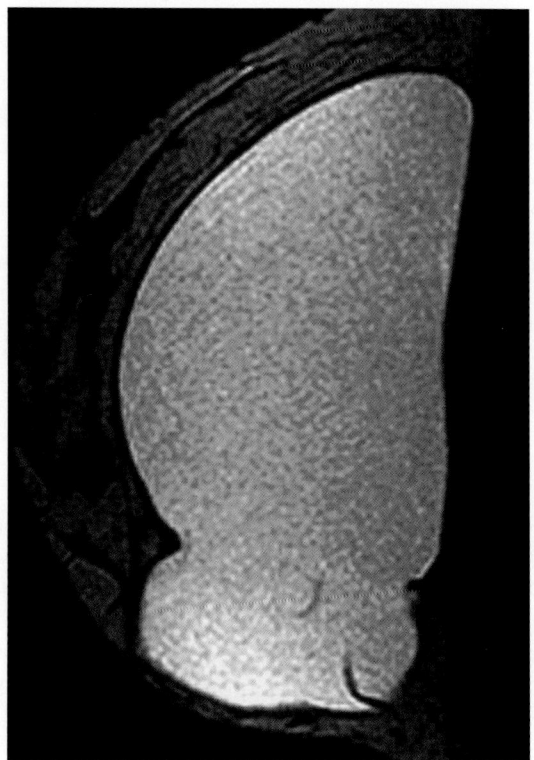

FIGURE 78-5

Herniation through fibrous capsule; incisures indicate boundaries of original fibrous capsule. This implant was in a state of uncollapsed rupture, which was not evident on MR imaging (subglandular, single-lumen silicone gel-filled, T2-weighted fast spin-echo, water suppression, placed 1984, implant age 9.1 years).[2]

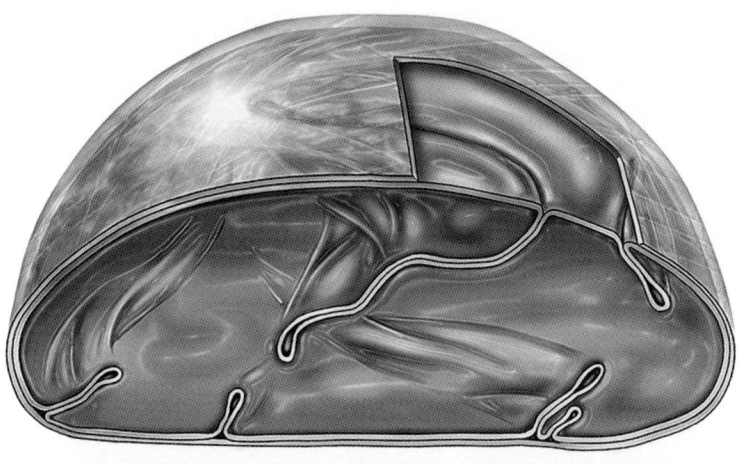
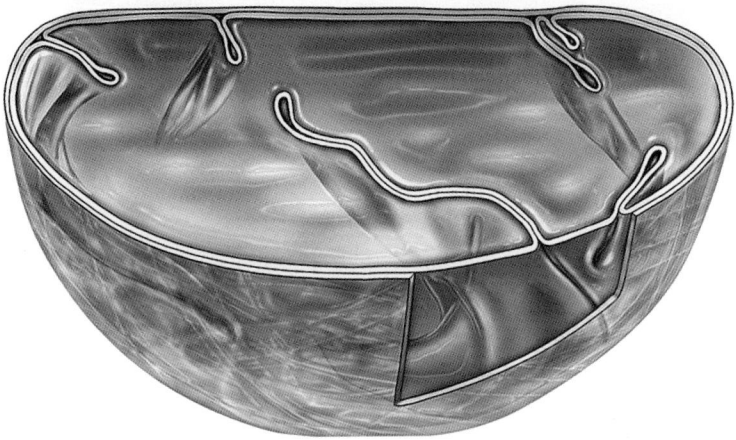

FIGURE 78-6

Schematic showing cutaway of implant folds of an intact single-lumen silicone gel-filled implant. The fibrous capsule is shown containing the implant.[2]

Rupture

Rupture prevalence has been shown to be correlated with implant age,[13,22,23] and certain types of implants may be more likely than others to rupture.[24,25] Rupture can be *intracapsular* (silicone gel constrained by the fibrous capsule) or *extracapsular* (silicone gel present outside the fibrous capsule) (Fig. 78-7). It can be helpful to categorize MR-detected rupture as follows (Fig. 78-8):

1. Uncollapsed rupture—silicone gel seen only within folds
2. Minimally collapsed rupture—silicone gel seen not only within folds, but also between implant shell and fibrous capsule
3. Partially collapsed rupture—implant shell partially submerged into the silicone gel
4. Fully collapsed rupture (also called "frank rupture" by others)—implant shell collapsed, surrounded by the silicone gel that was once within the implant.

Of fully collapsed rupture it has been said "the gel should be in the shell, not the shell in the gel".[7] The term "frank rupture" corresponds most closely to collapsed rupture, and also implies that it is in some sense clinically evident or unmistakable. However, as noted earlier, most rupture is clinically silent, and so only considering implants ruptured if they are "frankly" ruptured would grossly underestimate the prevalence of rupture.

Although the term "rupture" is used to describe implant failure, it should be understood that implants rarely burst. Most implant failure probably is a slow oozing of silicone gel through a rent in the shell that develops as a result of mechanical stress at the tip, or apex of a fold (so called "fold-flaw failure"). This may be more common in patients with capsular contracture. Shell defects also can occur at other sites of mechanical stress such as the junction of shell with a shell or fixation patch. Shell defects can be small, and so sometimes are described as "microhole rupture". If that is not appreciated when implants are removed, often they are described incorrectly as being "essentially intact" or as showing "only gel bleed" when in fact they are in a failed, or ruptured state. Even when shell defects are large they are only very rarely directly observable on MR imaging; the signs of implant rupture are all indirect and depend on observation of silicone outside the implant shell (see later in this chapter).

The term "leakage" is discouraged because it can mislead both physicians and patients. This term has been used to describe everything from the expected and universal "bleed" of silicone fluid from intact silicone gel-filled implants, to fully collapsed rupture with gross and extensive extracapsular silicone. Patients can be falsely reassured that their implants are "only leaking, not ruptured". Recognition of rupture can be delayed, which may have clinical consequences.

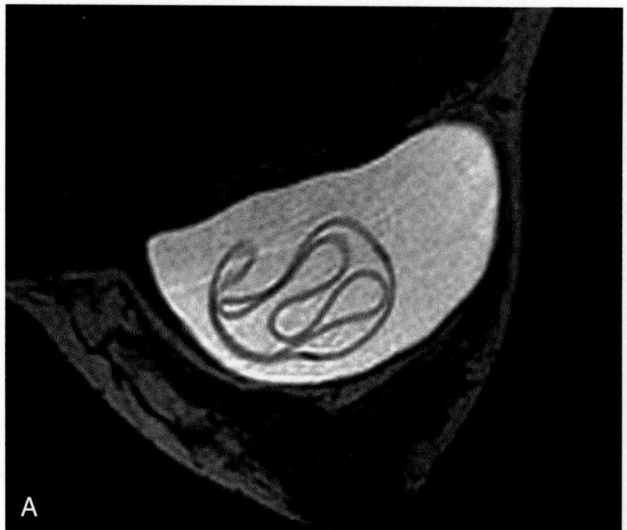
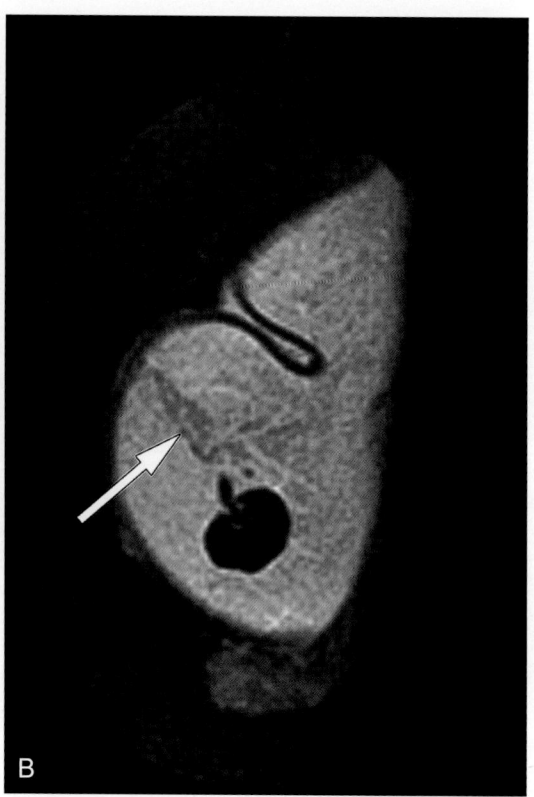

FIGURE 78-7

Implant rupture (T2-weighted fast spin-echo, water suppression). **A,** Fully collapsed intracapsular rupture, showing classic wavy-line sign (submuscular, single-lumen silicone gel-filled, placed 1987, implant age 5.7 years).[47] **B,** Minimally collapsed extracapsular rupture, showing inferior silicone granuloma, and internal baffle marked by *white arrow.* Area of dark signal within implant is a collection of water-like fluid (subglandular, single-lumen silicone gel-filled, Ashley polyurethane-coated, placed 1969, implant age 24.2 years).[8]

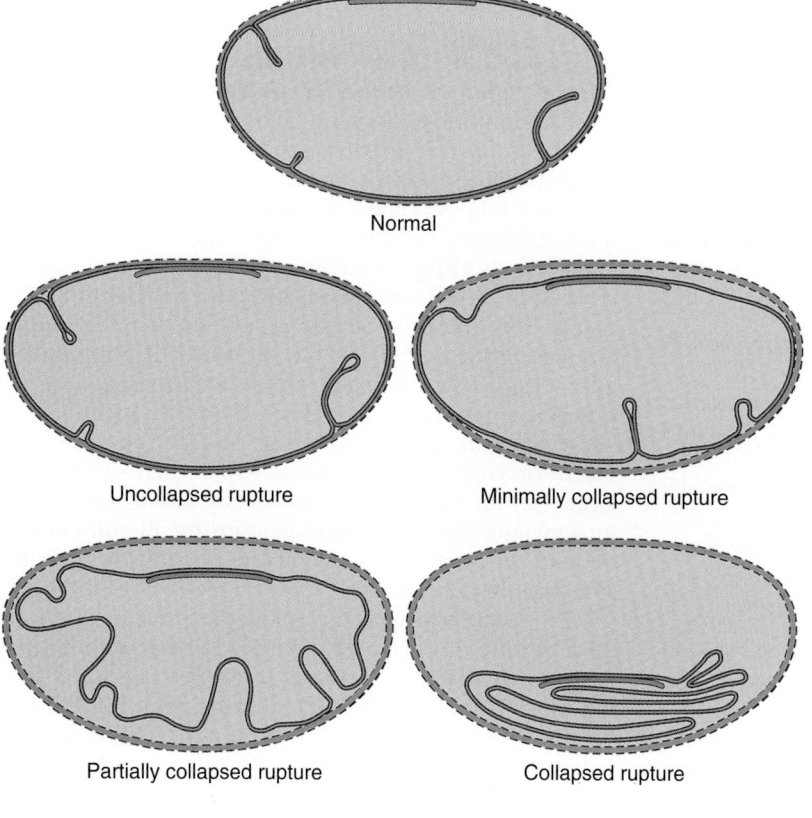

Normal

Uncollapsed rupture

Minimally collapsed rupture

Partially collapsed rupture

Collapsed rupture

Fibrous (i.e., biological) capsule   Implant shell   Silicone gel

FIGURE 78-8

Schematic showing progression from an intact shell fold pattern through fully collapsed rupture.[2]

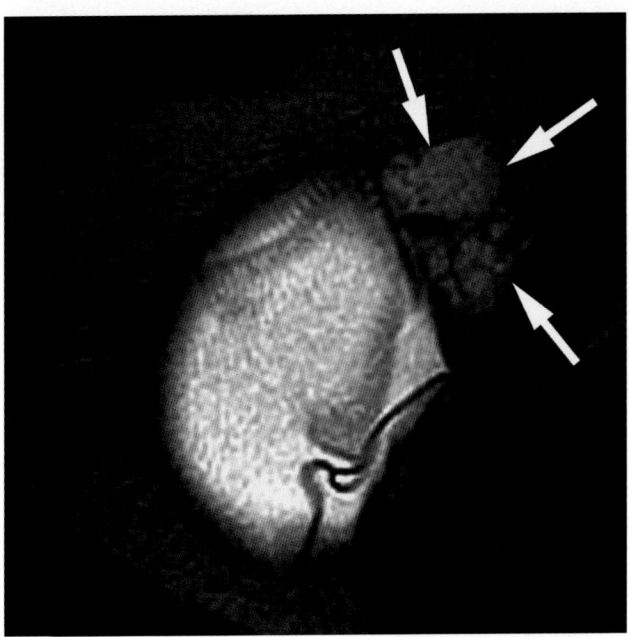

FIGURE 78-9

Silicone granuloma (outlined by *arrows*) from prior implant rupture (intact current subglandular implant, single-lumen silicone gel-filled, T2-weighted fast spin-echo, water suppression, placed 1986, implant age 6.9 years).[2]

Soft-tissue Silicone

Silicone from current or prior ruptured implants (or from silicone fluid injections) can migrate into surrounding soft tissues for varying distances.[26,27] The MR imaging appearance of extracapsular rupture in the FDA Breast Implant Study was reported by Berg et al.[28]

Soft-tissue migration of silicone usually is superior to the implant, with medial and lateral migration also being common. Occasionally migration across the midline is seen. The least likely direction is inferior. Silicone also can migrate anteriorly along Cooper's ligaments, or along an incision. Migration from subglandular implants can extend to the submuscular space, and migration from any plane of placement to the brachial plexus area can occur.

The three main appearances of soft-tissue silicone are *granuloma, gel extrusion,* and *gel cyst.* Often more than one appearance is seen in any given case. Silicone granuloma and gel extrusion are more common endpoints for soft-tissue silicone than gel cyst formation. Less common appearances are infiltration, capsular silicone and silicone adenopathy.

Silicone granuloma, also called siliconoma, is a foreign-body response to silicone fluid* or gel.[29] Silicone granulomas are typically rubbery, firm, off-yellow in color, and

"greasy" to the touch, and can be thought of as silicone-soaked scar tissue. On T2-weighted water-suppression MR imaging, increased inhomogeneous signal is seen (Fig. 78-9). If the concentration of silicone is too low, silicone granuloma may not be evident on MR imaging (but still may be evident on ultrasound).[2] Water suppression is necessary so that signal from bright unsuppressed water does not interfere with interpretation (Fig. 78-10).

Silicone gel from ruptured implants can persist indefinitely in soft tissues in its "gel state"—an appearance that can be noted as an extrusion (Fig. 78-11) or as a gel cyst (Fig. 78-12). The MR signal of silicone gel in an extrusion or cyst is indistinguishable from that of silicone gel still contained within the implant. In extrusion the gel is continuous with silicone gel still contained by the fibrous capsule, and develops its own fibrous capsule, where it comes into contact with breast tissue. Gel cysts are completely separated from gel within the fibrous capsule, and are completely surrounded by their own fibrous capsule. Gel extrusions can be small or large, but gel cysts typically are small, usually no more than 1 to 2 cc.

Silicone granuloma also can be entirely incorporated within a fibrous capsule, in which case it can be thought of as being *capsular* soft-tissue silicone. This can be difficult or impossible to distinguish from extracapsular silicone granuloma immediately adjacent to and outside the fibrous capsule.

Detectable silicone adenopathy can occur for patients with intact as well as ruptured implants, and should not, as an isolated finding be considered as evidence of rupture.[2] One suggested possible mechanism is that silicone gel or fluid may be engulfed by macrophages which migrate to node(s).[30]

Silicone Fluid Breast Injections

Silicone fluid breast injections began in Japan in about 1946. They were first performed in the USA c. 1961 to 1962, with the majority occurring before 1972. Several deaths were reported from silicone fluid embolism. The authors have seen one patient who was injected in the USA (Georgia) in the year 2000 by a non-physician (illegally). Silicone fluid injections are still given in other countries into the breast and other parts of the body. Silicone fluid injections are still used in the USA to correct facial wrinkling.[31]

Silicone fluid injections have a characteristic appearance on MR imaging. Silicone granuloma formation is common, as is silicone fluid cyst formation. An infiltrative appearance invariably is seen, usually with skin involvement. Migration of silicone fluid can be extensive: down the abdominal wall, into the axillae, or even around the back.[2] Infiltration of the pectoralis muscles and the presternal area is very common. On T2-weighted, water-suppression, dark-fat MR imaging, infiltrated silicone fluid will appear bright with a characteristic wispy lacey appearance (Fig. 78-13). It is important to recognize this infiltrative appearance so that soft-tissue silicone from injection of silicone fluid is not misinterpreted as evidence of extracapsular rupture (Fig. 78-14).

---

*It has been argued that the observed foreign-body response to some injected silicone fluid is actually a response to adulterants that may have been added before injection.

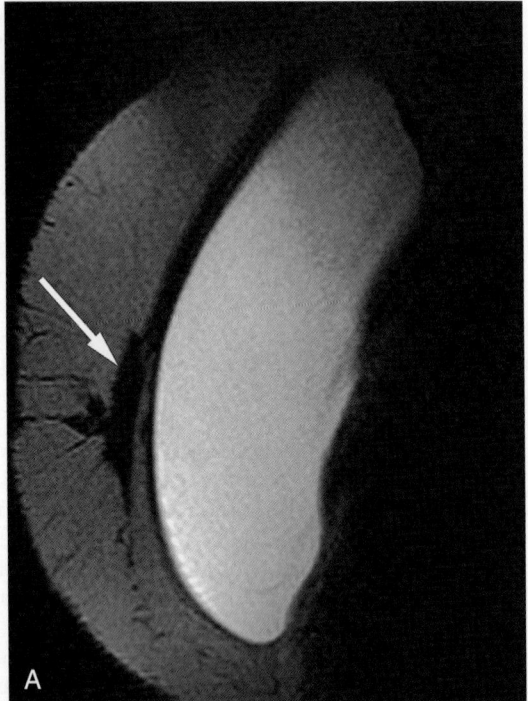

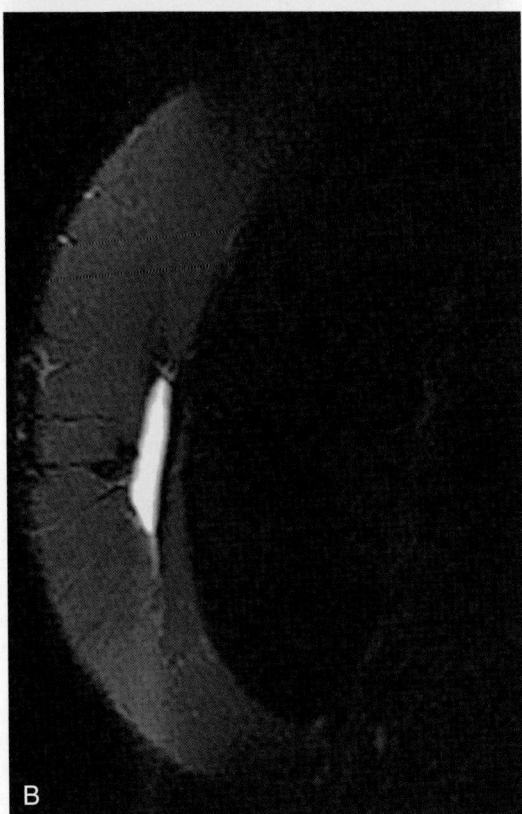

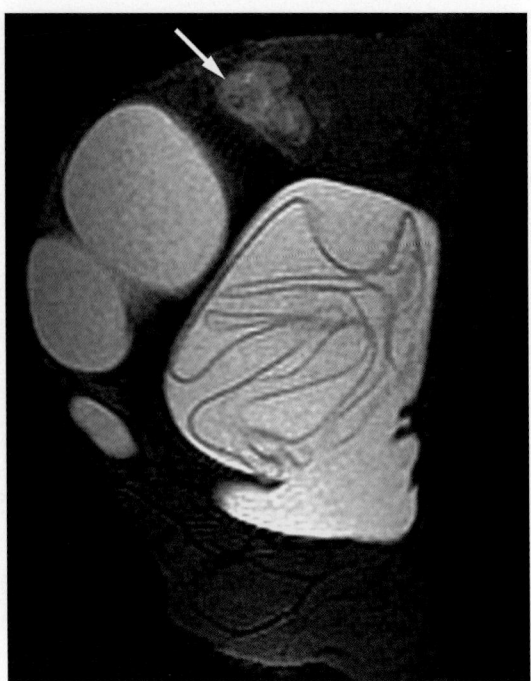

FIGURE 78-11

Massive gel extrusion. Collapsed implant shell remains within the original fibrous capsule, and massive amounts of silicone gel extrude into the breast soft tissues. When all images are viewed, it can be seen that all of the anterior gel was part of a single extruded gel collection that had continuity with gel still remaining within the original fibrous capsule. Silicone granuloma was also evident on this (*arrow*) and other images (subglandular, single-lumen silicone gel-filled, T2-weighted fast spin-echo, placed 1980, implant age 13.4 years).[2]

FIGURE 78-10

Water suppression necessary to interpret study. The current submuscular implant is intact. At the site of the prior subglandular implant there is a small seroma with no evidence of residual soft-tissue silicone (single-lumen silicone gel-filled, T2-weighted fast spin-echo, placed 1983, implant age 9.6 years). **A,** Water suppression image showing decreased signal at site of seroma (*arrow*). **B,** Silicone suppression image at same location, confirming that the subglandular area of increased signal in Part '**A**' does not represent residual soft-tissue silicone.[2]

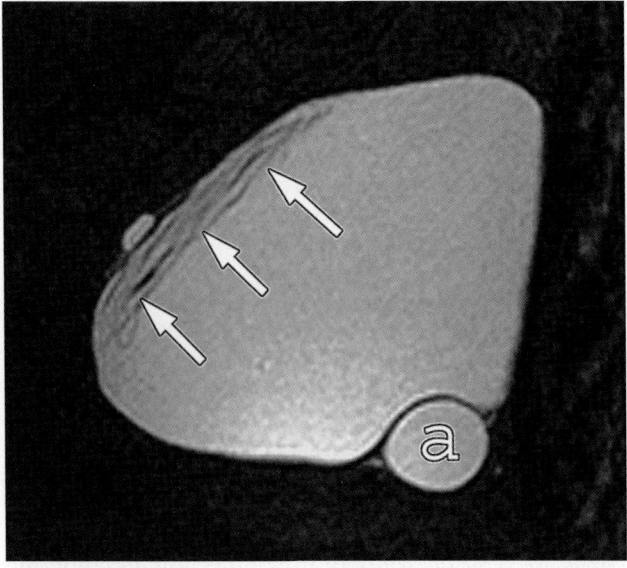

FIGURE 78-12

Gel cyst (**a**), completely surrounded by its own fibrous capsule. White arrows indicate collapsed implant shell within the fibrous capsule (subglandular, fully collapsed rupture, single-lumen silicone gel-filled, T2-weighted fast spin-echo inversion recovery, water suppression, placed 1978, implant age 16.3 years).[2]

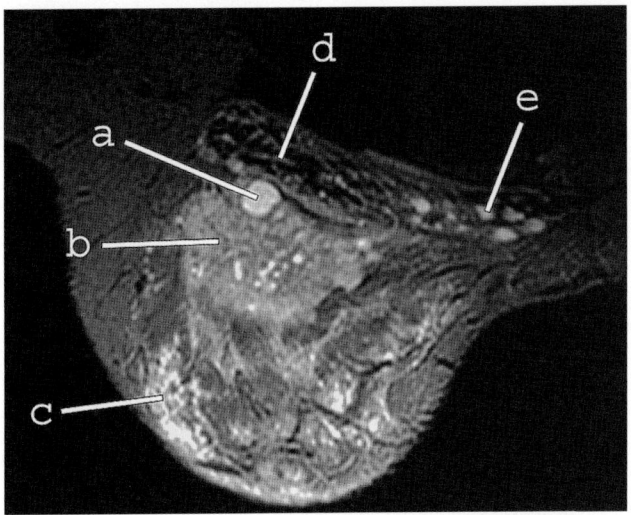

FIGURE 78-13

Silicone fluid injections. **a**, silicone fluid cyst; **b**, silicone granuloma; **c**, wispy-lacey infiltrative appearance that often extends all the way to the skin; **d**, infiltration of pectoralis major; and **e**, globules of silicone fluid with the substance of pectoralis major (T2-weighted fast spin-echo, water suppression, 1965 injections).[10]

SILICONE CHEMISTRY AND IMPLANT CONSTRUCTION

The Silicon (no final 'e') atom has atomic number 14, a chemical weight of 28.086, and is located in the periodic table just below carbon. In occurs naturally as a combination of ^{28}Si (92.2%), ^{29}Si (4.7%), and ^{30}Si (3.1%).[32] Silicon, like carbon, is tetravalent allowing for long-chain molecule formation, with two sites available for bonding to other atoms or molecules.

Silicones (with a final 'e') are a class of variable-length molecules which were described in the late 19th century as "uninviting glues".[33] They consist of a siloxane (– Si – O –) backbone, for medical applications mostly with attached methyl (CH_3) groups. A schematic of a typical subunit of silicone and its MR spectrum are shown in Fig. 78-15.

Silicone gel in breast implants can be thought of as a combination of long strands of silicone gel cross-linked to each other (the *matrix*) immersed in a bath of (*un-crosslinked*) silicone *fluid*. Silicone fluid alone (as a component of the gel used in breast implants) is a viscous liquid. Silicone gel (matrix and fluid combined) in breast implants can be extremely cohesive and tenacious, invariably is sticky to the touch, and exhibits stranding when observed between examining (gloved) fingers. In contrast, silicone fluid bleed can be appreciated as a slight oiliness of the implant shell surface, palpable and observable even before implantation.

The silicone elastomer sheeting making up the implant shell of (most) breast implants consists of silicone with a higher percentage of cross-linking than silicone gel.

The basic breast implant consists of a silicone elastomer shell filled with silicone gel. The term

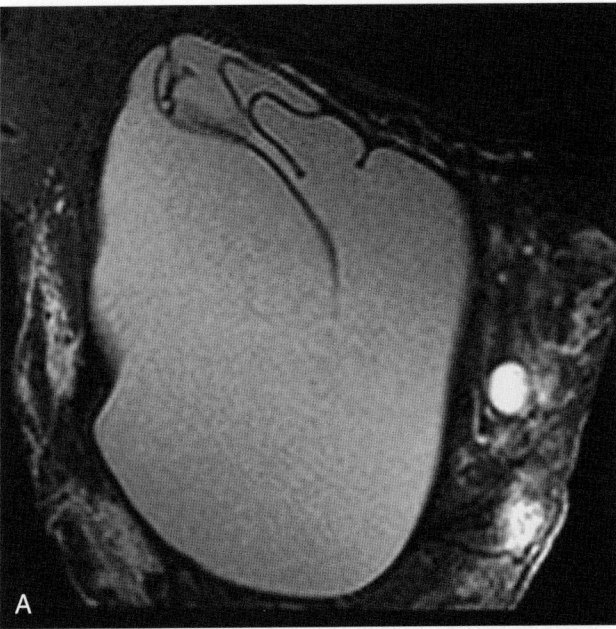

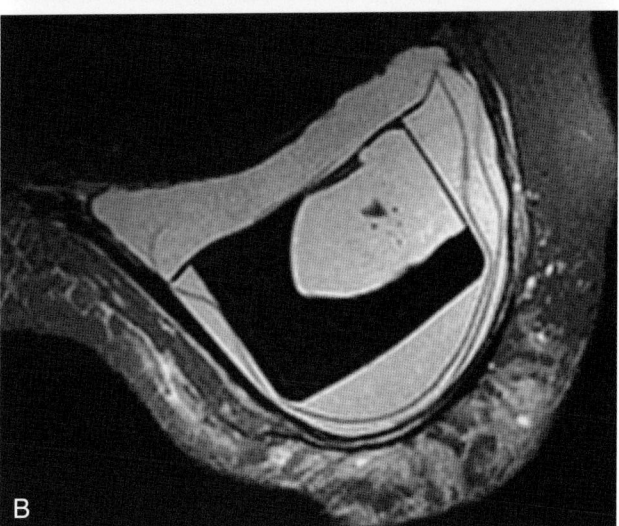

FIGURE 78-14

Implants and silicone fluid injections (T2-weighted fast spin-echo, water suppression). **A,** Intact implant, complex folds (subglandular, single-lumen silicone gel-filled, placed 1988, implant age 2.3 years, 1971 injections). **B,** Ruptured implant (submuscular, reverse double-lumen adjustable, placed 1985, implant age 12.4 years, 1965 injections).[2]

"capsule" should be reserved for the biological fibrous tissue capsule that surrounds implants, and should not be confused with the silicone elastomer shell.

Most breast implants from the 1960s and many from the 1970s had fixation patches attached to their posterior surface which were intended to induce tissue ingrowth to prevent movement after placement. Some can be seen on MR imaging. When they are seen, they appear as thickened areas of implant shell, sometimes with a zebra-stripe appearance (Fig. 78-16).

Most early and many later implants have a "smooth" outer shell surface. From about the mid-1980s, the outer

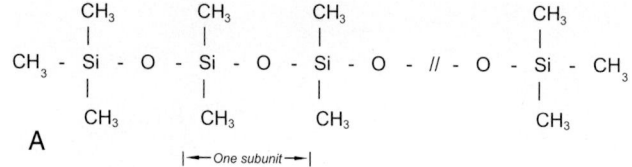

A

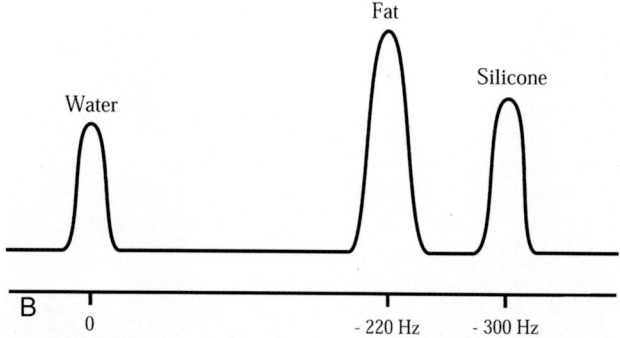

B

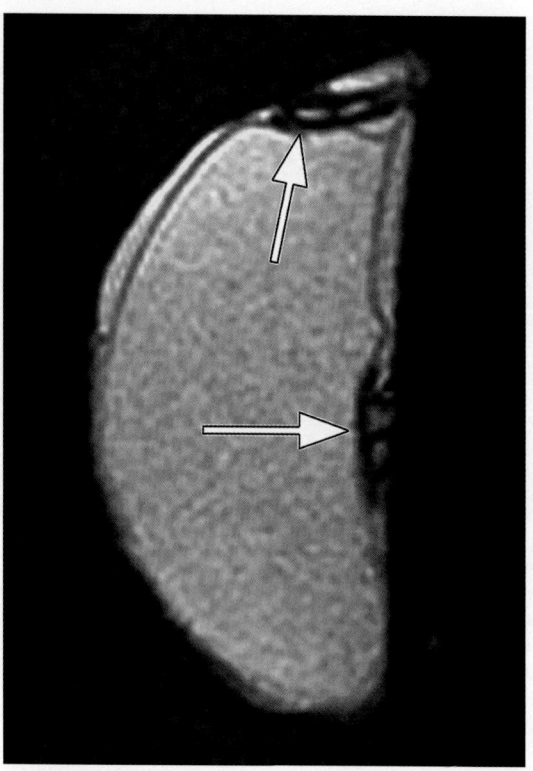

FIGURE 78-15

Structure and spectrum of silicone. **A,** Structure of silicone showing a typical subunit. The hydrogen atoms on the methyl (-CH$_3$) subunits are the source of the MR imaging signal from silicone.[2] **B,** Schematic spectrum of silicone at 1.5 T. Some scanner manufacturers show the spectrum as shown here (water on the left), and others show it with water on the right.[16]

FIGURE 78-16

Zebra-stripe appearance of fixation patches. Cross sections through two of the Dacron mesh-reinforced circular posterior fixation patches are shown here (*arrows*). The zebra-stripe appearance comes from infiltration of the fixation patches with silicone from the ruptured implant (subglandular, minimally collapsed rupture, single-lumen silicone gel-filled, T2-weighted fast spin-echo, water suppression, placed 1972, implant age 22.2 years).[2]

surface of the shell of some implants was textured in an attempt to inhibit capsular contracture (i.e., Bioplasty MISTI, Cox-Uphoff Microcell, Dow Corning SILASTIC MSI, McGhan Biocell, and Mentor Siltex).[2,7,34] Most breast implants currently being used are textured (see section on this later in this chapter).

Some breast implants are coated with a layer of polyurethane foam, also an attempt to reduce capsular contracture.* The earliest polyurethane-coated implants were called Natural-Y, or Ashley implants, produced from the late 1960s until the early 1980s. When examined with MR imaging most are ruptured by this time, but shell collapse usually does not progress further than minimal to partial collapse because their shells are thick and stiff (Fig. 78-7B). Later polyurethane-coated implants included the Même ME, Même MP, Vogue, Optimam, and Replicon. The Même ME implants have been reported to be much more likely to fail than other implants, and the Replicon implants to be less likely.[24] Polyurethane-coated implants commonly induce the presence of intracapsular water-like fluid, just like textured-surface silicone elastomer shell implants. If the implant is intact, the fluid can be seen as a layer outside the shell, within the fibrous capsule (Figs 78-18C, 78-23B, 78-38).

---

*Polyurethane-coated implants are just ordinary implants, usually single-lumen silicone gel filled, that have been coated with a layer of silicone adhesive, over which has been placed a thin layer of polyurethane foam.

PRINCIPLES OF BREAST IMPLANT MR IMAGING

The most useful MR images to evaluate the integrity of silicone gel-filled breast implants have bright silicone signal, dark fat signal, and dark signal from water-like fluids (Fig. 78-17). This allows the implant shell and its infoldings, which are dark on all sequences, to be visualized well against a background of bright silicone gel. In practice, when enough silicone gel is present outside an implant to be detected on MR imaging, either between the implant and the fibrous capsule, or within infoldings of shell, the implant is ruptured.[7]

Moderate resolution axial and sagittal imaging using a breast surface coil (20 cm FOV, 256 × 256 matrix, 4 mm slice thickness without skips) of each breast separately is sufficient to detect almost all advanced rupture, and most early rupture. For thin shell implants (manufactured between 1973 and the mid 1980s), it can be necessary to use higher resolution imaging (15 cm FOV, 256 × 256 matrix, 3 mm slice thickness without skips).

T2-weighted imaging is used because silicone has a relatively long T2 (~ 100 ms), and so it will be brighter than muscle and fat. However, the T2 of water is longer

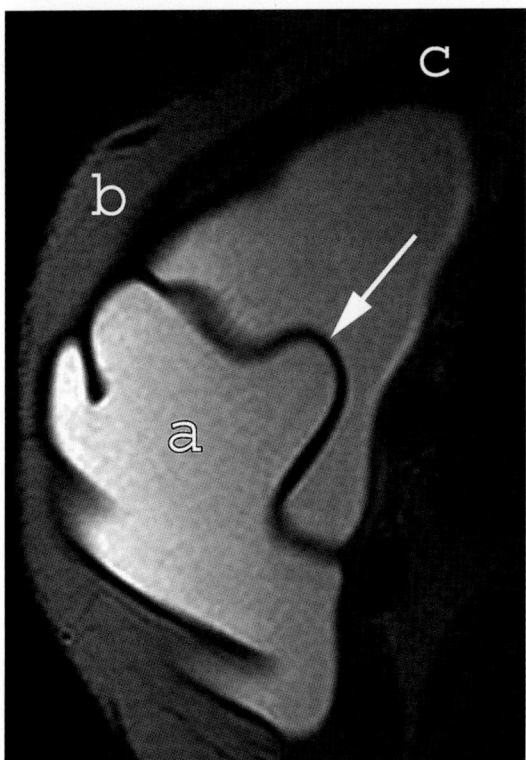

FIGURE 78-17

T2-weighted MR image. **a**, bright silicone signal; **b**, gray fat signal; **c**, dark muscle signal (submuscular, intact, single-lumen silicone gel-filled, textured surface. Surface texturing consists of an even layer of short 'micropillars' covering implant surface. T2-weighted fast spin-echo, water suppression, placed 1991, implant age 1.9 years).[2] *White arrow* indicates a normal shell fold, apparently thickened because of intracapsular water-like fluid surrounding the implant which is dark because of water-suppression.

than that of silicone, and so water will be brighter than silicone. Hence water suppression is used to reduce signal from water. Finally, to detect silicone reliably when fat is present, signal from fat should be reduced. This can be achieved using a long TE (so that signal from fat is low), but is accomplished better by nulling fat signal using inversion recovery.

T1-weighted imaging rarely is useful for breast implant-related evaluation because dark silicone gel cannot be distinguished as easily from dark implant shell, fibrous capsule, or breast tissue (Fig. 78-18). Silicone-suppression T2-weighted imaging can be helpful to show the relationship of findings to breast anatomy, to confirm the presence of extracapsular soft-tissue silicone, and to exclude failure of water suppression (Fig. 78-19).

The sequences described earlier are, with some variation, available from all major manufacturers of 1.5 T MR imaging scanners. Most breast implant-related imaging requires strong signal, and so performance on scanners with field strengths of <1.5 T predictably is worse. Breast implant imaging at 1.0 T will produce good and usually adequate results if findings are obvious, and the implant shell is not of the early, thin type. Imaging at and below 0.5 T is likely to be inadequate.

NORMAL AND ABNORMAL MR IMAGING APPEARANCES OF BREAST IMPLANTS

Single-lumen Silicone Gel-filled Implants

Breast implant contour can range from undulating to spherical with increasing capsular contracture (Fig. 78-20). Bulges are nonspecific. An (intact or ruptured) implant is *herniated* through the fibrous capsule when the shell is bulging through a defect in the fibrous capsule (Fig. 78-21). The term "extrusion" is used to describe movement of silicone gel (without accompanying implant shell) of a ruptured implant through the fibrous capsule, where that extruded gel remains continuous with gel still inside the fibrous capsule (Fig. 78-11).

Normal folds can have a variety of appearances. On T2-weighted imaging, folds of the implant shell appear as dark lines "surrounded" by bright silicone. Typical normal folds are twice as thick as the shell, often have a slight rounded thickening at their tip, and extend all the way to the implant perimeter. They can be simple or complex, straight or curved, floppy or crook-necked, and may "bisect" or "trisect" any given image (Fig. 78-22). The mere presence of folds, therefore, without any additional findings, does not indicate rupture or suspicion of rupture. Recognizing the normal appearance of implant folds is the key to not overcalling rupture.

Textured-surface and polyurethane-coated implants commonly develop a thin layer of water-like fluid between the implant and the inner surface of the fibrous capsule that can be seen on MR imaging (Figs 78-18C, 78-23, 78-38). This usually is not of any clinical significance. This appearance should be distinguished from the normal appearance of a standard double-lumen implant (Fig. 78-33).

Small water-like bubbles can be seen within single-lumen silicone gel-filled implants when an antibiotic or steroid has been intentionally added directly to the implant at the time of placement (Fig. 78-24). Since very thin needles were used and placement typically was through thickened locations on the implant shell patch, often these implants remain (otherwise) intact. This can have a similar appearance to single-lumen adjustable implants,[2,7] in which saline is meant to be added directly to the silicone gel in the implant through a valve which is part of the implant (Fig. 78-25).

The various signs of breast implant rupture are all based upon recognizing that silicone gel is present outside the implant as a whole (Fig. 78-8). False-positive interpretation can result when: a) a normal (intact) implant shell fold pattern is misinterpreted as showing silicone gel outside the implant, b) water suppression is inadequate; or c) an intact implant of an unusual type is not recognized as such. False-negative interpretation can occur when characteristic findings of rupture are not recognized, or when the amount of silicone gel outside a ruptured implant is too small to be detected. Hence false positives are largely avoidable, and some false negatives are to be expected.

The main MR imaging sign of partially and fully collapsed rupture is the continuous wavy line sign,[7] also

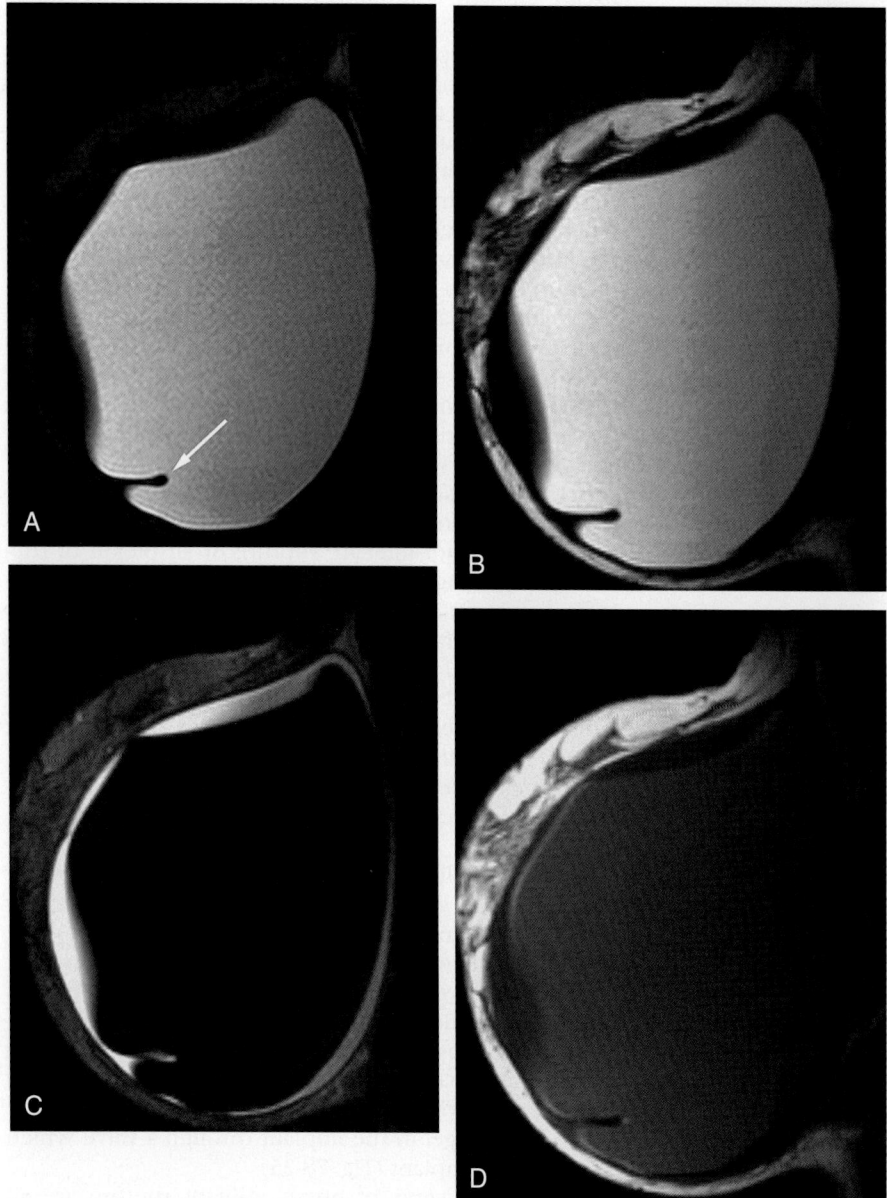

FIGURE 78-18

MR imaging appearance of breast implants on commonly used pulse sequences is shown. See Figure 78-38 for the appearance of this implant on a T2-weighted sequence with no suppression (intact, single-lumen silicone gel-filled, textured implant surface, placed 1999, implant age 15.0 years). **A,** T2-weighted fast spin-echo, inversion recovery fat-nulled, water suppression. This sequence is useful to evaluate the soft tissues outside the fibrous capsule. Note that suppressed (dark) water-like fluid within folds gives the appearance of the folds being widened (*arrow*). **B,** T2-weighted fast spin-echo, water suppression. This sequence is useful to evaluate implant shell fold patterns, especially at higher resolutions. **C,** T2-weighted fast spin-echo, silicone suppression. This sequence is useful to confirm that extracapsular silicone is or is not present. **D,** T1-weighted spin-echo, no suppression. Silicone is darker on this sequence, and folds are not as well seen as they are on T2-weighted imaging. Hence T1-weighted imaging should not be used to evaluate breast implants. Note the marked chemical shift artifact at the interface between intracapsular water-like fluid and the silicone gel of the implant, giving a dark stripe posteriorly and a bright stripe anteriorly. Compare to Figure 78-38, which shows the unsuppressed T2-weighted appearance of this same implant at this slice position.

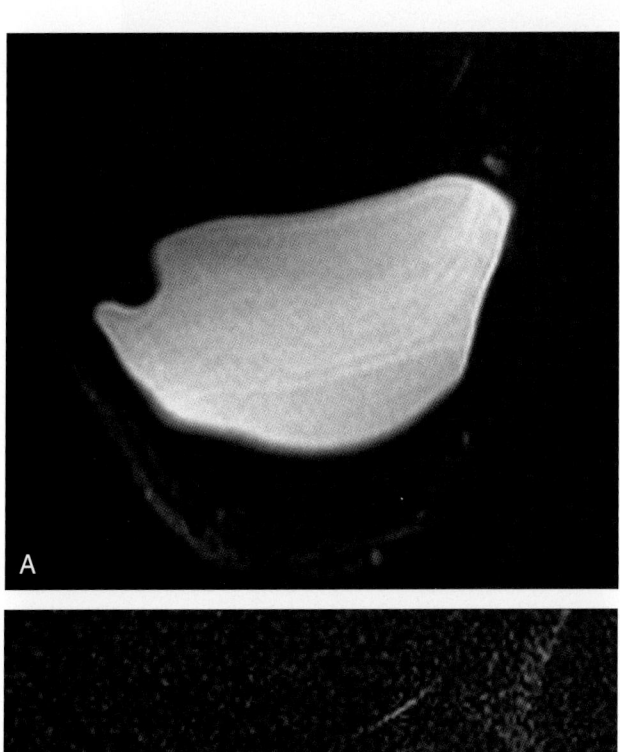

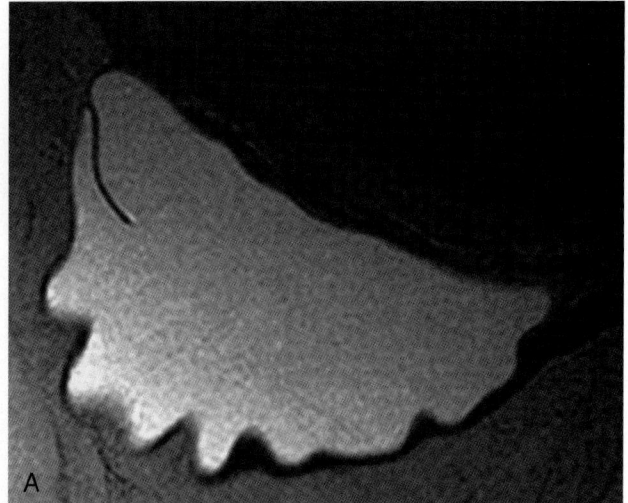

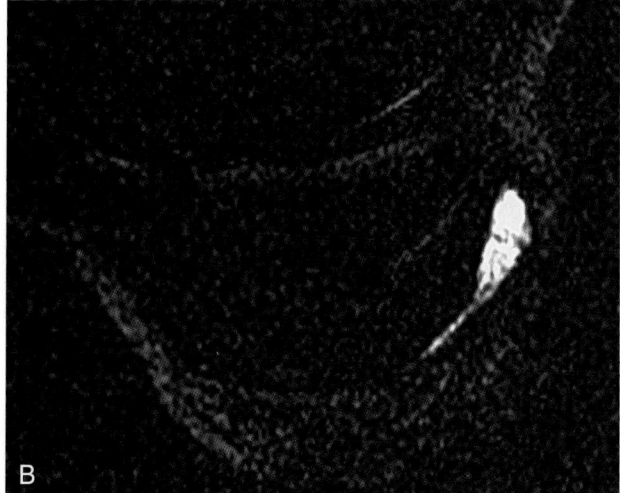

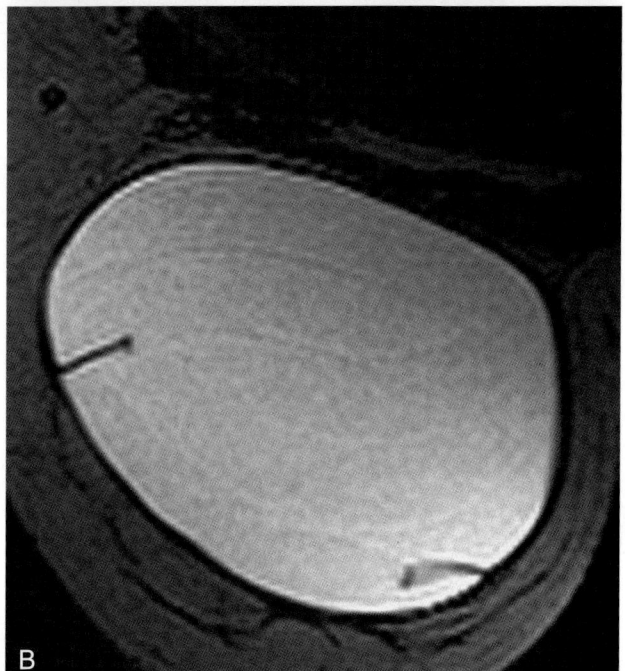

FIGURE 78-19

Silicone granuloma from a prior rupture adjacent to an inflated submuscular saline-filled implant (T2-weighted fast spin-echo). **A,** Silicone suppression image showing inflated saline-filled implant, and dark signal at site of silicone granuloma lateral to implant. **B,** Fat nulled (inversion recovery), water suppression image showing exactly the converse—dark saline implant signal, and bright inhomogeneous signal lateral to the implant from the silicone granuloma.[2]

FIGURE 78-20

Undulating and spherical implant contours (both intact, single-lumen silicone gel-filled, T2-weighted fast spin-echo, water suppression). **A,** Anterior contour of submuscular implant is softly undulating, and implant is soft, Baker Grade I (placed 1987, implant age 5.7 years). **B,** Implant contour of subglandular implant is essentially spherical, and implant is hard, Baker Grade IV (placed 1987, implant age 5.9 years).[2]

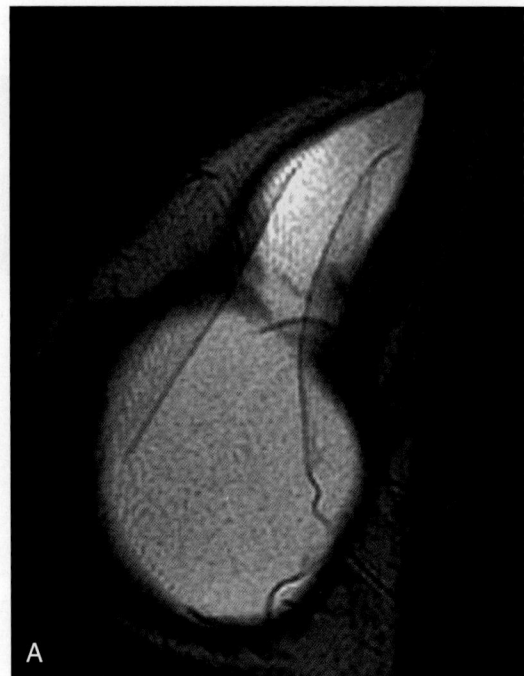
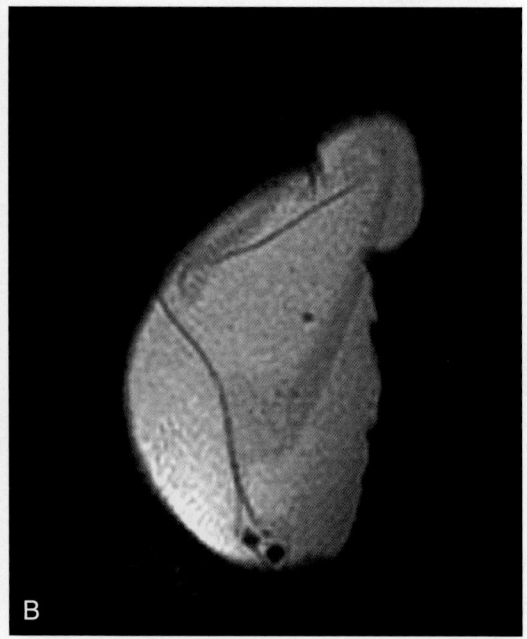

FIGURE 78-21

Intact and ruptured herniation (T2-weighted, water suppression). **A,** Superior herniation through the fibrous capsule is clearly demonstrated in this subglandular *intact* implant, with the characteristic appearance of folds bending inwards towards the center of the herniation (fast spin-echo, placed 1982, implant age 11.6 years).[8] **B,** Superior herniation through the fibrous capsule is clearly demonstrated for this submuscular *ruptured* implant, also with folds seen going into and through area of herniation (fat-nulled inversion recovery, placed 1987, implant age 7.0 years).[2]

described by Gorczyca et al as the linguini sign[35,36] (Fig. 78-26). This sign can be difficult to recognize if the imaging resolution is too low to visualize the implant shell.

The MR imaging signs of minimally collapsed rupture involve visualizing silicone gel between the implant shell and the fibrous capsule.[2,7,37] These signs are:

- *Anterior spiculation sign.* Silicone gel between the implant shell and clumpy irregular internal fibrous capsule calcification indicates rupture (Fig. 78-27).
- *Back patch sign.* Silicone gel outside the posterior shell patch (hence the term "back" patch) of a single-lumen silicone gel-filled implant indicates rupture (Fig. 78-28).
- *Subcapsular line sign.* Silicone gel between the implant shell and fibrous capsule was described by Soo et al as the subcapsular line sign.[37] Caution should be exercised because in some cases the normal implant shell folds can mimic this sign (Fig. 78-29). By the time this sign is present, usually there are other corroborating signs of rupture.

The MR imaging signs of uncollapsed rupture involve visualizing silicone gel only "within" folds, but not between implant shell and fibrous capsule. The two main signs of uncollapsed rupture are:[2,7,38-41]

- *Keyhole sign.* By the time silicone can be visualized within folds on MR imaging, uncollapsed rupture (at

least) is extremely likely. The keyhole appearance results when the sides of the fold are touching, and (bright) silicone gel is seen at the tip and the base of the fold (Fig. 78-30). This sign has also been called the *noose sign, teardrop sign,* and *inverted teardrop sign.* Silicone fluid from an intact implant will very rarely accumulate in an amount sufficient to be mistaken for this appearance on MR imaging. Of the 262 University of California, San Diego, cases of uncollapsed rupture as per MR imaging, two were false positives. In both cases no evidence of rupture was found upon examination at the time of removal.

- *Pull-away sign.* This sign is similar to the keyhole sign, but the sides of the fold are separated by silicone gel (Fig. 78-31). This sign has also been called the *open loop* sign.

If the MR imaging appearance is suspicious but not certain for uncollapsed rupture, the findings are 'indeterminate', in that most, but not all implants with this appearance will be ruptured.[2,8]

Standard Double-lumen Implants

Standard double-lumen breast implants are of two types: those with a shared posterior shell patch for the inner- and outer-lumen shells, and those with a separate posterior patch for each shell (Fig. 78-32). A summary of

Text continues on page 2473

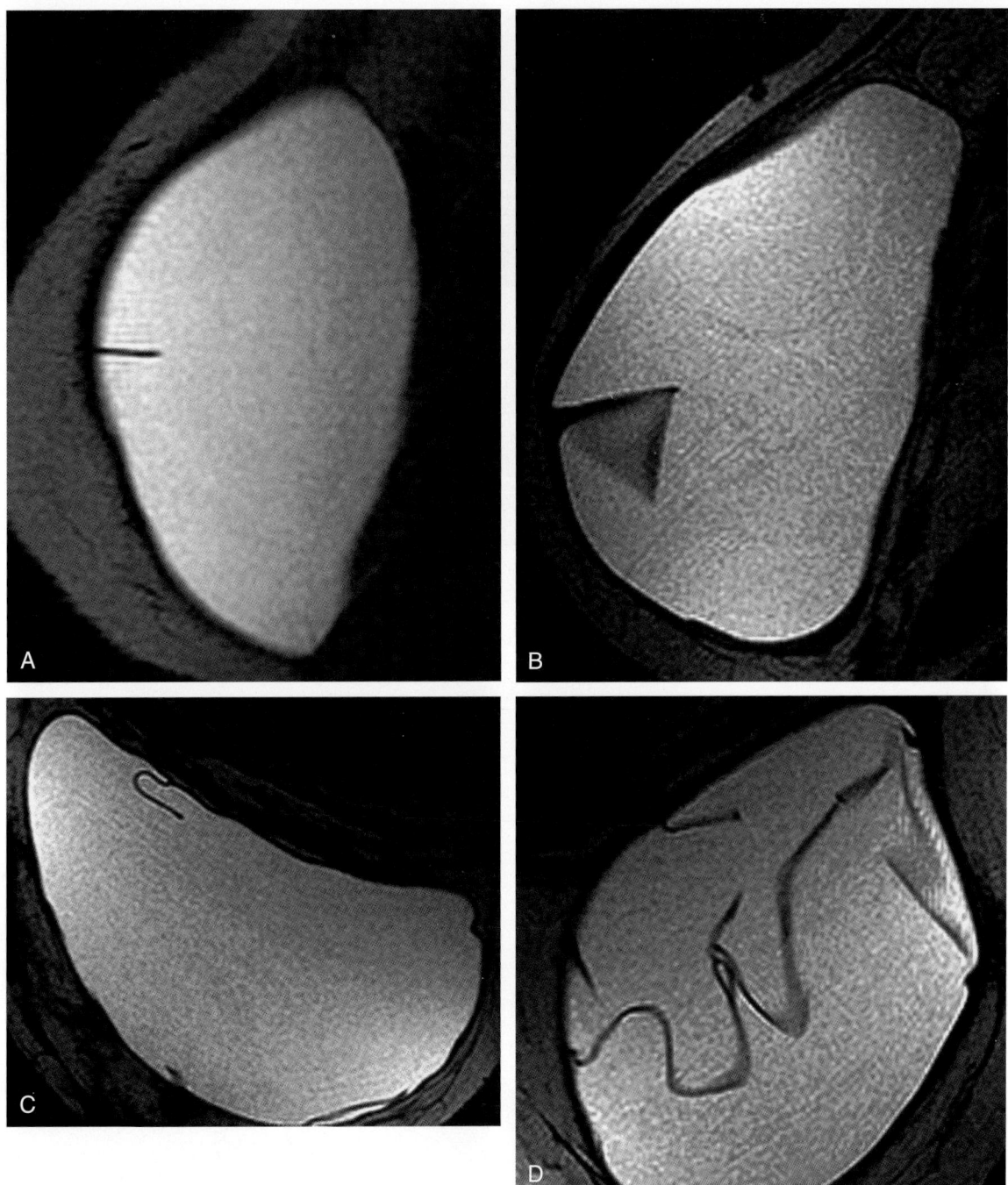

FIGURE 78-22

Normal fold examples of intact implants, verified as intact at and after removal (single-lumen silicone gel-filled, T2-weighted fast spin-echo, water suppression). **A,** Simple straight fold (submuscular, placed 1986, implant age 5.9 years). **B,** Traveling fold (volume averaging; submuscular, textured surface, placed 1992, implant age 5.2 years). **C,** Curved fold (subglandular, placed 1988, implant age 5.7 years). **D,** Complex folds (subglandular, placed 1987, implant age 6.2 years).[2]

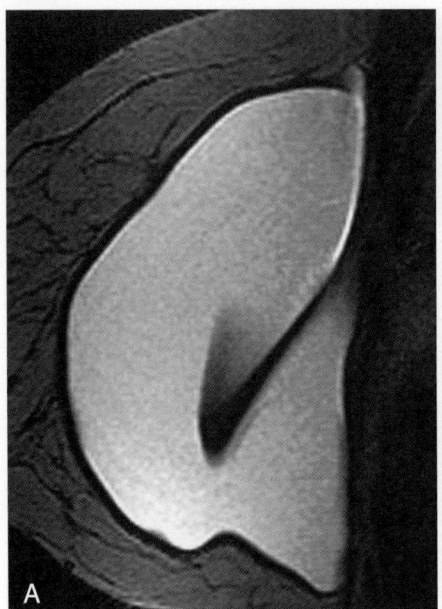
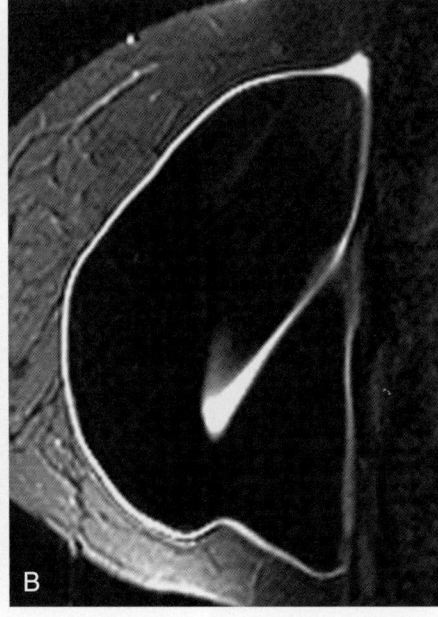

FIGURE 78-23

Textured-surface subglandular implant showing an intracapsular layer of water-like fluid surrounding the implant. This is the normal appearance for implants of this type. If an implant acquires more fluid on one side than the other, or there are signs of infection, this finding may be abnormal (intact, single-lumen silicone gel-filled, T2-weighted fast spin-echo, placed 1991, implant age 4.0 years). **A,** Water suppression image, showing incomplete suppression of water-like fluid within folds and surrounding the implant. **B,** Silicone suppression image, showing the intracapsular water-like fluid with bright signal.[2]

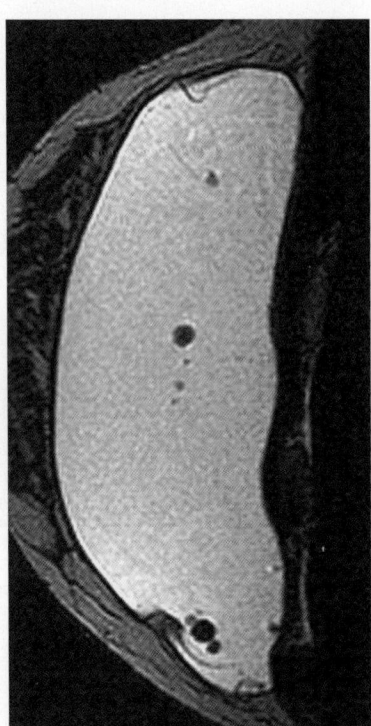

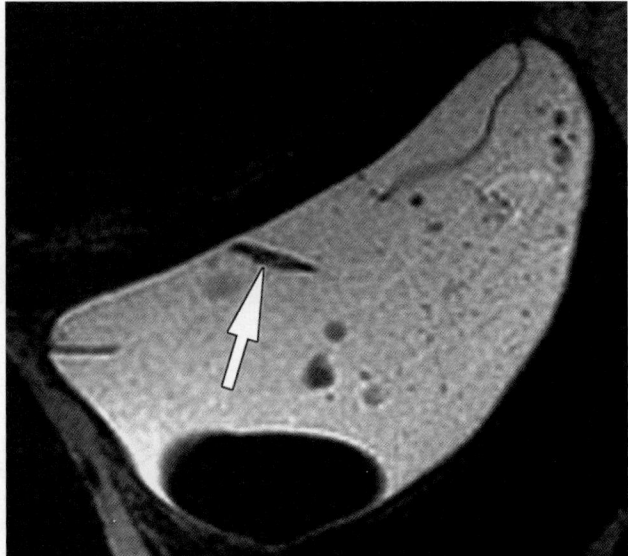

FIGURE 78-24

Intact subglandular single-lumen silicone gel-filled implant, to which small amounts of saline have been added using a small needle placed directly through the implant shell patch at time of placement (T2-weighted fast spin-echo, water suppression, placed 1983, implant age 10.0 years).[16]

FIGURE 78-25

Intact subglandular single-lumen adjustable implant, to which moderate amounts of saline have been added through a fill valve at time of placement. The fill valve (in cross-section) is indicated by the *arrow*. Note that the water bubbles can be quite large (T2-weighted fast spin-echo, water suppression, placed 1982, implant age 11.0 years).[2]

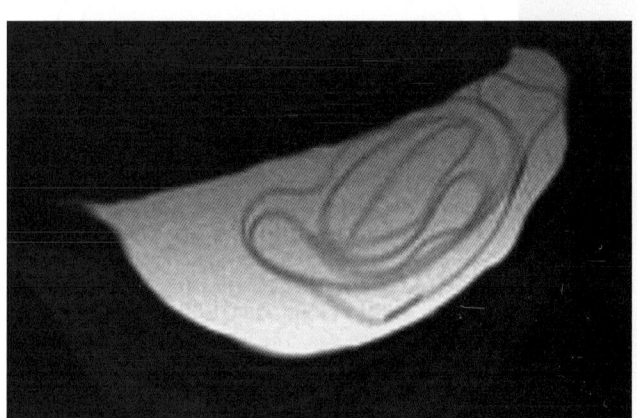

FIGURE 78-26

Fully collapsed rupture, showing classic wavy-line sign (submuscular, single-lumen silicone gel-filled, T2-weighted fast spin-echo, water suppression, fat-nulled inversion recovery, placed 1986, implant age 17.2 years).

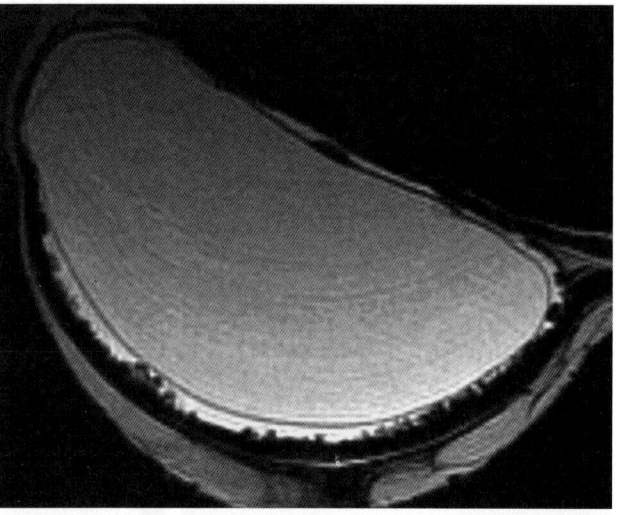

FIGURE 78-27

Minimally collapsed rupture, showing classic anterior spiculation sign. This appearance results from silicone gel from the ruptured implant filling the interstices between clumps of calcified tissue along the inner surface of the fibrous capsule (submuscular, single-lumen silicone gel-filled, T2-weighted fast spin-echo, water suppression, placed 1990, implant age 13.7 years).

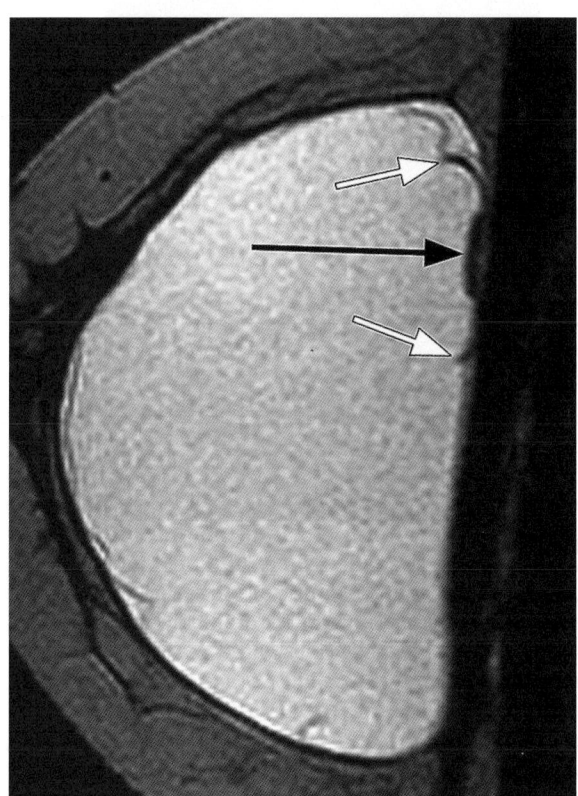

FIGURE 78-28

Minimally collapsed rupture, showing the back-patch sign, so named because silicone gel posterior to the shell patch of a single-lumen silicone gel-filled implant is necessarily outside the implant as a whole, indicating rupture. The black arrow indicates an approximate 12 mm reinforcement disc placed internal to the shell patch that was used on some breast implants through the 1970s. The edges of the shell patch, behind which silicone gel is clearly seen (indicating rupture), are marked with *white arrows* (subglandular, single-lumen silicone gel-filled, T2-weighted fast spin-echo, water suppression, placed 1978, implant age 16.4 years).[2]

15. Gabriel SE, Woods JE, O'Fallon M, et al: Complications leading to surgery after breast implantation. N Engl J Med 336:677-682, 1997.

16. Middleton MS, McNamara MP Jr: MR and ultrasound imaging of breast implants and soft-tissue silicone. Imaging 9:201-226, 1997.

17. Brown SL, Todd JF, Luu H-MD: Breast implant adverse events during mammography: Reports to the Food and Drug Administration. J Womens Health 13:370-378, 2004.

18. Middleton MS. Editorial on Brown et al: (reference 17 above). J Womens Health 13:379-380, 2004.

19. Vistnes LM, Ksander GA, Kosek J: Study of encapsulation of silicone rubber implants in animals. A foreign body reaction. Plast Reconstr Surg 62:580-588, 1978.

20. Vistnes LM, Ksander GA: Tissue response to soft tissue silicone prostheses: capsule formation and other sequelae. In Rubin LR (ed): Biomaterials in Reconstructive Surgery. St Louis: Mosby, 1983, pp 516-528.

21. Baker JL, Bartels RJ, Douglas WM: Closed compression technique for rupturing a contracted capsule around a breast implant. Plast Reconstr Surg 58:137-141, 1976.

22. Malata CM, Feldberg L, Coleman DJ, et al: Textured or smooth implants for breast augmentation? Three-year follow-up of a prospective randomized controlled trial. Br J Plast Surg 50:99-105, 1997.

23. Feng LJ, Amini SB: Analysis of risk factors associated with rupture of silicone gel breast implants. Plast Reconstr Surg 104:955-963, 1999.

24. Cross JL: Factors associated with the failure of silicone gel-filled breast implants. UCSD/SDSU doctoral dissertation, 1997.

25. Middleton MS, Soo MS, Berg WA, et al: Rupture prevalence and MR imaging appearance of the Hartley double-lumen breast implant. 86th Scientific Assembly and Annual Meeting of the RSNA, Chicago, November 2000.

26. Capozzi A, Du Bou R, Pennisi VR: Distant migration of silicone gel from a ruptured breast implant. Plast Reconstr Surg 62:302-303, 1978.

27. Argenta LC: Migration of silicone gel into breast parenchyma following mammary prosthesis rupture. Aesthetic Plast Surg 7:253-254, 1983.

28. Berg WA, Nguyen TK, Middleton MS, et al: MR imaging evaluation of extracapsular silicone from breast implants: diagnostic pitfalls. Am J Roentgenol 178(2):465-472, 2002.

29. Winer LH, Sternberg TH, Lehman R, et al: Tissue reactions to injected silicone liquids. Arch Dermatol 90:588-593, 1964.

30. Hardt NS, Emery JA, Steinbach BG, et al: Cellular transport of silicone from breast prostheses. Int J Occup Med Tox 4:127-134, 1995.

31. Jones DH, Carruthers A, Orentreich D, et al: Highly purified 1000-cSt silicone oil for treatment of human immunodeficiency virus-associated facial lipoatrophy: an open pilot trial. Dermatol Surg 30:1279-1286, 2004.

32. Waser J, Trueblood KN, Knobler CM: Chem One. New York: McGraw Hill, 1976.

33. McGregor RR: Silicones and their Uses. New York: McGraw-Hill, 1954.

34. Lesesne CB: Textured surface silicone breast implants: histology in the human. Aesthetic Plast Surg 21:93-95, 1997.

35. Gorczyca DP, Sinha S, Ahn CY, et al: Silicone breast implants in vivo: MR imaging. Radiology 185:407-410, 1992.

36. Gorczyca DP, DeBruhl ND, Mund DF, et al: Linguine sign at MR imaging: does it represent the collapsed silicone implant shell? Radiology 191:576-577, 1994.

37. Soo MS, Kornguth PJ, Walsh R, et al: Intracapsular implant rupture: MR findings of incomplete shell collapse. JMRI 7:724-730, 1997.

38. Berg WA, Caskey CI, Hamper UM, et al: Single and double-lumen silicone breast implant integrity: Prospective evaluation of MR and US criteria. Radiology 197:45-52, 1995.

39. Gorczyca DP, Schneider E, DeBruhl ND, et al: Silicone breast implant rupture: comparison between three-point Dixon and fast spin echo MR imaging. Am J Roentgenol 162:305-310, 1994.

40. Soo MS, Kornguth PJ, Georgiade GS, Sullivan DC: Seromas in residual fibrous capsules after explantation: mammographic and sonographic appearances. Radiology 194:863-866, 1995.

41. Everson LI, Parantainen H, Detlie T, et al: Diagnosis of breast implant rupture: imaging findings and relative efficacies of imaging techniques. Am J Roentgenol 163:57-60, 1994.

42. Camilleri IG, Malata CM, McLean NR: A review of 120 Becker permanent tissue expanders in reconstruction of the breast. Br J Plast Surg 49:346-351, 1996.

43. Brinton LA, Lubin JH, Burich MC, et al: Breast cancer following augmentation mammoplasty (United States). Cancer Causes Control, 11:819-827, 2000.

44. Brinton LA, Lubin JH, Burich MC, et al: Cancer risk at sites other than the breast following augmentation mammoplasty. Ann Epidemiol 11:248-256, 2001.

45. Brinton LA, Lubin JH, Burich MC, et al: Mortality among augmentation mammoplasty patients. Epidemiology 12:321-326, 2001.

46. Cheung YC, Lee KF, Ng SH, et al: Sonographic features with histologic correlation in two cases of palpable breast cancer after breast augmentation by liquid silicone injection. J Clin Ultrasound 30:548-551, 2002.

47. Brown JJ, Wippold FJ II: Practical MRI: a teaching file. Philadelphia: Lippincott-Raven, 1996, p 311.

..

CHAPTER 79

MR CHOLANGIOPANCREATOGRAPHY

Laila Ashkar ● Sharad Maheshwari ● Josephine Pressacco
● Asako Nakai ● Robert R. Edelman ● Caroline Reinhold

INTRODUCTION

Magnetic resonance cholangiopancreatography (MRCP) uses heavily T2-weighted sequences to noninvasively image the biliary tree and pancreatic duct. Compared with endoscopic retrograde cholangiopancreatography (ERCP), MRCP is noninvasive, faster, and provides comparable diagnostic information. ERCP may be complicated by pancreatitis, bleeding, sepsis, and duodenal perforation. In addition, ERCP is unsuccessful in as many as 5% to 10% of procedures, and often cannot define the anatomy proximal to a severe obstruction or after certain operative procedures (Fig. 79-1). Conversely, drawbacks of MRCP include an inferior spatial resolution relative to ERCP, limited evaluation of the ampulla, nondistension of the biliary system, and no biopsy or treatment capability.

In this chapter, technical issues for anatomic and functional MRCP will be reviewed. The advantages and disad-

vantages, along with cost-benefit considerations, will be discussed. Normal anatomy and anatomical variants of the biliary system will be covered, followed by in-depth considerations of the various clinical indications.

Advantages and Disadvantages of MRCP

Although the impact of MRCP in the management of patients with suspected bile duct obstruction needs to be further defined, MRCP has gained widespread clinical acceptance. This is largely because MRCP is a non-invasive procedure without risks, provided patients are adequately screened for contraindications. The rate of complications secondary to ERCP, however, range from 5% to 8%, with an overall mortality rate of up to 1.5%.[1-5] MRCP examinations cannot be performed or are technically incomplete in less than 5% of cases, while the rate of failed ERCP is reported to range from 5% to 20%.[3-5]

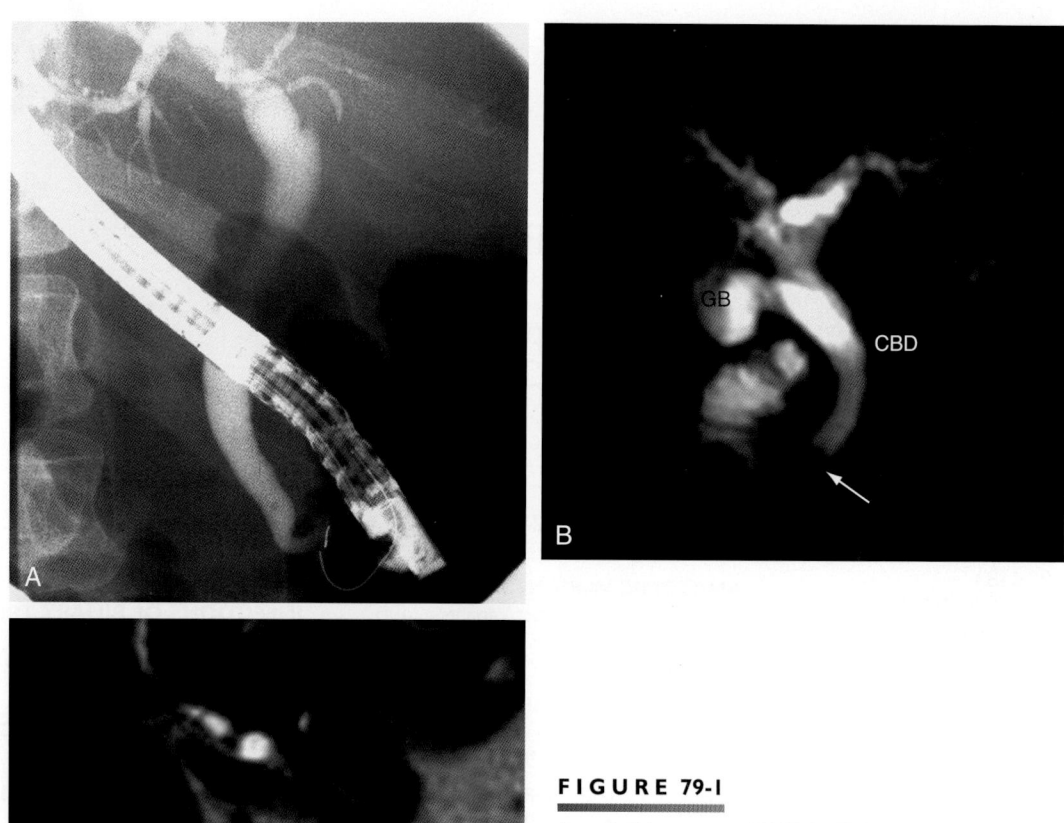

FIGURE 79-1

A to **C,** False-negative ERCP. **A,** ERCP demonstrates dilated intra- and extrahepatic bile ducts. It was interpreted as negative for stone. **B,** 40 mm coronal SSFSE rapid acquisition with relaxation enhancement (RARE) SLAB MRCP (TE 969) and **C,** 5 mm coronal SSFSE T2 MRCP (TE 180) demonstrate a distal common bile duct (CBD) stone (*arrow*). GB, gallbladder.

In addition, MRCP does not require radiation exposure, intravenous contrast agents, or a highly skilled operator.[6] MRCP is less expensive, can be performed on an outpatient basis and has excellent interobserver agreement.[7]

MRCP frequently demonstrates the anatomy of the biliary tree to a better advantage than ERCP as overlapping structures can be avoided by viewing the biliary tree in different projections and imaging planes. When compared to direct cholangiography, MRCP is superior in visualizing the bile ducts proximal to a site of obstruction as it can demonstrate the biliary tree above and below a high-grade stenosis.[8] When performed with simultaneously acquired T1-weighted postgadolinium MR images, MRCP can provide additional information on extraductal parenchymal abnormalities, vascular structures, lymph nodes and distant metastases.[9,10]

Major disadvantages of MRCP compared with ERCP include: 1. lack of an immediate therapeutic solution and inability to obtain tissue for diagnosis; 2. inability to provide information about the rate of biliary drainage or cystic duct patency; and 3. a lower spatial resolution and lack of distension by contrast limits visualization of non-dilated peripheral bile ducts and assessment of stricture morphology.[11] Unit availability, claustrophobia and the inability to evaluate patients with pacemakers or ferromagnetic implants are other drawbacks.

Clinical Indications for MRCP

A number of clinical indications for MRCP have evolved over the past decade and include situations where ERCP is technically unsuccessful, or deemed difficult such as in patients with Billroth II gastrectomy or Roux-en-Y diversions.[12-17] Other indications include patients in whom the indication for ERCP is not judged strong enough to justify its risks (e.g., jaundice/elevated liver enzymes with a low clinical probability of obstruction; acute pancreatitis; follow-up of benign asymptomatic biliary strictures including sclerosing cholangitis, postliver transplant, preoperative cholecystectomy with a moderate risk of choledocholithiasis, nonspecific abdominal pain, children, and pregnancy). MRCP may give more information than ERCP in hilar strictures, and lesions associated with complete biliary obstruction, for example, a transected aberrant right posterior hepatic duct.[18]

Cost-benefit Considerations

MRCP is a technique that has matured sufficiently to be in widespread clinical use. However, its role in the management of patients with suspected biliary disease remains in evolution. Although a large body of literature focusing on its diagnostic performance relative to ERCP has been published during the past decade, only a few articles have addressed the impact of MRCP in the management of patients with suspected bile duct obstruction.[19-22] Therefore, the precise role of MRCP in the evaluation of patients with bile duct obstruction remains somewhat unclear, as does its impact on health economics.

True-to-life situations frequently differ from what is predicted based on decision modeling or test performance. For example, at the Hospital Erasme in Brussels, concurrent with a marked increase in the number of MRCPs performed from 1995 to 1997, there was only a slight decrease in the total number of ERCPs (approximately one diagnostic or therapeutic ERCP less for every four additional MRCPs performed).[23] Preliminary results from a prospective randomized trial ($n = 162$) comparing ERCP with MRCP performed at the current authors' institution demonstrated a 51% rate of subsequent ERCPs in the MRCP arm, with no differences between the groups in the rate of subsequent complications based on an intention-to-treat analysis.[24] Similarly, a study by Sahai et al[25] assessed the ability of MRCP to change the differential diagnosis and to avoid diagnostic and/or therapeutic ERCPs. It was shown that the mean number of differential diagnoses did not change significantly when adding MRCP information to diagnostic ERCP information and prevented no therapeutic ERCP. Furthermore, adding MRCP to clinical information (without performing ERCP) reduced the differential diagnosis significantly only for the surgeon and radiologist, and would have prevented 3% of diagnostic and therapeutic ERCP examinations for all physicians. The authors concluded that the added value of MRCP may be limited in the face of inappropriate patient selection and may differ according to physician specialties.

It is clear that further studies are needed to better define the clinical context in which performing MRCP may obviate the need for diagnostic ERCP, thereby reducing complications and costs. More outcome trials are needed to better assess the influence of MRCP on clinical decision making and patient outcome.

Ultimately, these data should allow us to propose cost-effective imaging algorithms for the evaluation of patients with suspected biliary disease. For example, patients with a high pre-test probability of common bile duct (CBD) stones using risk-stratification have little to gain by undergoing MRCP since more than 90% will have CBD stones requiring therapeutic ERCP.[26] The principle of risk-stratification was also prospectively applied by Liu et al[27] to classify patients undergoing laparoscopic cholecystectomy (LC) according to their risk of harboring CBD stones into one of four groups: 1. an extremely high-risk group of patients who underwent preoperative ERCP; 2. a high-risk group who underwent MRCP; 3. a moderate risk group who underwent LC with intra-operative cholangiogram (IOC); and 4. a low-risk group who underwent LC without IOC. Overall, ERCP was performed in 8.9% of patients and MRCP was performed in 9.4%. This stratification resulted in the diagnosis of CBD stones during preoperative ERCP in 92.3% of the patients, while unsuspected CBD stones were found in only 1.4% of patients. Farrell et al[28] studied the potential impact of MRCP on patient outcome and overall ERCP workload if MRCP were the primary investigation in patients referred for ERCP because of abdominal pain. In this study it was shown that if MRCP had been used as the primary imaging investigation in patients referred for abdominal pain, 44% of patients would potentially have avoided ERCP, and the overall ERCP workload would have been reduced by 22%. Furthermore, 3.5% of major ERCP-related complications and 0.35% of ERCP-related deaths would also potentially have been prevented. The patient population in this study was unusual in that more than 50% of patients had probable sphincter of Oddi dysfunction, which benefited from endoscopic intervention and/or biliary manometry. This explains the relatively small decrease in ERCP workload among these patients despite a normal MRCP. Typically, most patients presenting with abdominal pain do not require subsequent therapeutic ERCP since a high proportion of them have normal ducts without biliary pathology.

These examples serve to illustrate that in the appropriate clinical setting, MRCP can indeed reduce the need for ERCP, thereby diminishing the complication rate and cost associated with ERCP. Sahai et al[29] proposed a number of tests and patient characteristics that need to be met if a new imaging test is to be cost effective in the work-up of patients with suspected biliary disease. These characteristics include the following: 1. the cost of the new imaging test must be 60% or less of the cost of ERCP; 2. the new test must have a diagnostic accuracy greater than 90%; and 3. the probability of the etiology requiring a therapeutic ERCP must be less than 40%. If these conditions cannot be met, then ERCP should remain the dominant strategy. The relative cost of MRCP and ERCP will vary according to regional differences. The diagnostic accuracy of MRCP for diagnosing bile duct obstruction and common biliary pathology in most efficacy studies exceeded 90%.[30] Therefore, the appropriateness of using MRCP in a particular clinical setting will depend largely on the probability of the etiology requiring a therapeutic ERCP.

MRCP TECHNIQUES AND IMAGING PROTOCOLS

Patient Preparation

The patient needs to be fasting for a minimum of 3 to 4 hours prior to the examination to allow gallbladder filling, gastric emptying, and to reduce unwanted secretions and fluid signal from the intestine. The high-signal intensity fluid may otherwise be volume averaged with bile duct fluid, thereby obscuring underlying pathology, which would interfere with the single section acquisitions. An oral contrast agent that shortens the T2 relaxation time of bile, such as dilute geritol, blueberry juice, or iron oxide agent, may be ingested to suppress the signal from fluid within the gastrointestinal tract. In addition, an antispasmodic agent (glucagon 1 mg IV or IM, or hyoscine butyl bromide 40 mg IM) may be administered at the onset of the examination.

Pulse Sequences

Most anatomic imaging methods for MRCP rely on the principle that only stationary fluids (such as bile) will be visible on strongly T2-weighted images.[18,31-33] Such images can be obtained using fast spin-echo pulse sequences with echo times (TE) in the order of 1 s, or by use of balanced steady-state free precession (SSFP) techniques such as true Fast Imaging with Steady-State Precession (FISP) or Fast Imaging Employing Steady-State Acquisition (FIESTA). Whereas only fluids appear bright on strongly T2-weighted fast spin-echo images, fluids, blood, and fat appear bright on SSFP images. Both fast spin-echo and SSFP are amenable to single-shot approaches wherein each image is taken within a fraction of a second.[31,34-37] This short acquisition time avoids misregistration and motion artifacts, and leads to images with reduced signal-to-noise ratio and increased contrast.

A single-shot, partial Fourier, fast spin-echo sequence such as Half-fourier Acquisition Single-Shot Turbo Spin-Echo (HASTE), Single-Shot Fast Spin-Echo (SSFSE), using a short inter-echo spacing, minimizes susceptibility artifacts from metallic surgical clips, vascular stents and surgical drainage catheters.[38] This sequence benefits image interpretation in patients who are post cholecystectomy or have undergone biliary enteric anastomosis or liver transplantation.

If a thick (e.g., 25 mm to 100 mm) slice is acquired, then a large portion of the biliary system is displayed in a single image. A thick slice can only be used with a very long TE fast spin-echo sequence (e.g., SSFSE). Background tissues have substantial signal intensity on HASTE images acquired with short-to-moderate TE (e.g. < 200 ms), so that thin slices should be acquired. Fat suppression is optional, but increases sensitivity to magnetic field inhomogeneity (which can be a problem near air-containing bowel loops or surgical clips). Alternatively, a respiratory-gated 2D fast spin-echo, or a breath-hold or respiratory-gated 3D sequence, enables the acquisition of thinner slices, thereby permitting a

maximum intensity projection that can be rotated. It is important to acquire thin-slice images in the axial and coronal planes, in addition to the thick-slice SSFSE acquisition, in order to improve the confidence for detecting small stones, strictures and disease outside of the biliary system.

Although large portions of the biliary tree can be evaluated with thick-slice MRCP images, each slice only provides a single view so that key structures may overlap and limit interpretation. Some institutions include a series of maximum-intensity projections (MIPs) in multiple orientations. Like thick-slice images, MIP images appear similar to conventional cholangiograms and allow complete visualization of the pancreatico-biliary ducts. However, in neither case is information on depth available.[39] In addition, partial volume averaging of tissue edema or ascites may obscure the biliary structures on these images. Consequently, thin-slice source images need to be carefully assessed for each patient.[40] Volume-rendering methods widely used for MR angiography may have benefits for the diagnosis of choledocholithiasis compared with MIP or thick-slice MRCP.[39]

Conventional MR imaging with nonenhanced T1- and less heavily T2-weighted images provide added value for the diagnostic accuracy in differentiating benign from malignant causes of biliary dilatation. Routine MRCP sequences used at present at the current authors' institution include a combination of breath-hold coronal and transverse thin-section SSFSE, as well as oblique thick-slab SSFSE sequences. For clarification of indeterminate or subtle findings they find the addition of a high-resolution, fat-suppressed, 3D fast recovery fast spin-echo (FRFSE) or 2D fast spin-echo (FSE) sequence with respiratory triggering to be helpful.[41,42] However, others may choose to use only breath-hold techniques. Spatial resolution is not as high as with respiratory-gated methods but study duration is significantly reduced.

Typical pulse sequences and imaging parameters for MRCP are provided in Table 79-1.

Contrast Enhancement

Administration of a gadolinium chelate (0.1 mmol/kg given IV at 2 cc/s) is helpful for evaluation of suspected neoplasm and infection. Images are acquired pre-contrast, as well as in the arterial (~20 s), portal (~50 s), and systemic (~2 minutes) postcontrast phases using either a fat-suppressed 2D gradient-echo sequence or a fat-suppressed 3D sequence such as Volumetric Interpolated Breath-hold Examination (VIBE), Fast Acquisition with Multiphase Eggre 3D (FAME), or Liver Acquisition with Volume Acceleration (LAVA). T1-weighted sequences with fat suppression before and after contrast administration are essential to evaluate duct walls, periductal tissue, parenchymal lesions and tumor infiltration.[43]

Functional MR Cholangiography (fMRC)

Functional MR cholangiography (fMRC) involves the administration of a hepatobiliary contrast agent (see

TABLE 79-1 Typical Imaging Parameters for Various MRCP Acquisitions

	Localizer	SSFSE (HASTE)	SSFSE (HASTE)	MRCP (Thick Slice)	FRFSE 3D	2D FSE	3D T1 (pre-/post-gad)
Plane	3 Plane	Coronal	Transverse	Oblique, multiple orientations	Coronal	Transverse	Transverse
Mode		2D	2D	2D	3D	2D	3D
Pulse Seq.		SSFSE	SSFSE	SSFSE	FRFSE	FSE	SPGR
Imaging Opt.		Fast	Fast	Fast	Fast		ZIP×2, ZIP512
No. of Echoes					1	31	1
TE		180	180	1 s	500-600	150-250	In-phase
TR		3000	3000	3000	~4000	~4000	Min
Optional		(resp.trig./ ASSET)	(resp.trig./ ASSET)		(resp. trig.)	(resp. trig.)	
Flip Angle		—	—	—	—	—	12
BW		62	62	50	31	31	62
Saturation					Fat	Fat	Fat, special
FOV	40	32-40	32-40	28-38	32-40	32-40	32-40
Slice Thickness (mm)	8	4-5 mm	4-5 mm	40 mm	1.6 mm	3 mm	3-4 mm
Spacing (mm)	2	0	0	—	(zip2 & zip512)	0.3	0
Matrix	256×128	384×224	384×224	320×320	256×256	384×256	256×192
NEX	1	0.5	0.5	1	1	2	0.75

Gad, gadolinium; Opt, option; Seq, sequence; resp trig, respiratory triggering; TE, time to echo; TR, time to repetition; BW, band width; FOV, field of view; NEX, number of excitations; ASSET, Array Spatial Sensitivity Encoding Technique.

Chapter 14) and image acquisition using a 3D gradient-echo sequence with high spatial resolution. Hepatobiliary contrast agents include manganese dipyridoxal diphosphate (Mn)-DPDP, iron HBED [bis (2-hydroxybenzyl) ethylenediamine diacetic acid], iron-EHPG [ethylenebis-(2-hydroxyphenylglycine)], and gadolinium-EOB [(ethoxybenzyl)-DTPA (diethylene-triamine pentaacetic acid)].[44-53] These agents are lipophylic, and are taken up by hepatocytes and excreted into the biliary ductal system. They lead to bright signal of contrast-enhanced bile on T1-weighted images, using 2D or 3D T1-weighted gradient-echo techniques.

If needed, standard MRCP images should be acquired before hepatobiliary contrast administration, since the contrast agent shortens T2 in addition to T1 and will impair visualization of the bile ducts on the long TE SSFSE images. The authors' current technique involves the acquisition of images in coronal and transverse planes approximately 10 to 20 minutes following injection of mangafodipir trisodium (dose = 5 μmol/kg or 0.5 mL/kg administered at 2 to 3 mL/min). Biliary excretion of mangafodipir trisodium usually occurs within 10 minutes of injection in nondilated biliary systems.[54,55] However, excretion is delayed in the setting of obstruction or impaired hepatocyte function. At a minimum of 2-hour intervals, and up to 24 hours after injection, additional delayed imaging is performed until there is visualization of contrast in the gallbladder and duodenum.[56]

Although SSFSE sequences are accurate for diagnosing bile duct obstruction, the sensitivity and specificity of MR was increased significantly in one study when fMRC was added.[56] Imaging with fMRC is particularly advantageous in early obstructions, since in these cases the

bile ducts may be of normal caliber and obstruction can therefore be missed with conventional MRCP. In addition, conventional MRCP may misdiagnose resolved prior obstruction in which the biliary tree remains dilated. Further indications for fMRC include patients in whom conventional MRCP is rendered nondiagnostic by overlying fluid-containing structures or ascites. Finally, Lee et al[55] found that fMRC is able to depict anatomical relationships between the ducts with increased confidence compared with conventional MRCP, and thus is a useful adjunct in preoperative planning to conventional MRCP.

However, for most clinical indications including the detection of strictures, filling defects, and ductal dilation, the addition of fMRC to conventional MRC resulted in a diagnostic performance similar to that of MRCP imaging alone.[56]

Another potential tool for the functional evaluation of the biliary tree is fMRC with IV secretin.[57] Secretin stimulation is clearly helpful for depicting the pancreatic duct on MRCP. However, the method may not be as useful in depicting the bile ducts.[58-60]

Kinematic MRCP

Kinematic, or dynamic MRCP, is performed by acquiring a series of thick-slice SSFSE images in a single plane and then displaying them as a cine loop. No contrast media or antispasmodic medication is given. Initially, the biliary tract and pancreatic duct are localized in the coronal and transverse planes. Thick-slice MRCP images are then obtained in the coronal and sagittal planes as well as in the 15-degree, 30-degree, and 45-degree left and right oblique planes. An optimal plane for the visualization of the sphincteric segment is determined from these images. Usually the 15-degree or 30-degree left anterior oblique coronal plane is chosen. Finally, 20 consecutive single thick-slice SSFSE images are obtained in the predetermined optimal plane.[59]

Kinematic MRCP can be used to assess the sphincteric segment of the ampulla of Vater.[57] By using this technique to evaluate the distal portion of the common bile duct, researchers have found that pathologic stenosis may be distinguished from nonvisualization of the sphincteric segment caused by physiologic contraction of the sphincter of Vater. The lack of visualization of the sphincteric segment was found to indicate ampullary or periampullary lesions.[36,61-65] Kinematic MRCP after the ingestion of a fatty meal or cholecystokinin may be useful in reducing the number of false negatives and false positives by inducing transient biliary dilatation.[59] It may also be helpful in patients with biliary dilatation to determine the necessity of therapeutic intervention.

DIAGNOSTIC PITFALLS OF MRCP INTERPRETATION

Various pitfalls may be encountered during interpretation of MRCP examinations that can simulate or mask disease processes of the biliary tree. This section will review the more frequently encountered pitfalls, and suggest strategies for their avoidance and recognition. Familiarity with the existence and prevalence of these diagnostic pitfalls should prevent misinterpretation of MRCP examinations. These can be broadly divided into four categories: 1. technical; 2. extraductal; 3. intraductal; and 4. normal variants.[66]

Technical Factors

Thick-slab MRCP examinations resemble conventional cholangiograms and are familiar to many clinicians. Nonetheless, spatial resolution is degraded because of volume-averaging effects, and can result in small luminal filling defects and strictures being overlooked. The multislice sequence (source images) provides greater spatial resolution, and should be carefully scrutinized in every case (Fig. 79-2).[67] MIP reconstructed images completely obscure small filling defects when surrounded by hyperintense bile (Fig. 79-3). In addition, the limited spatial resolution of MIP reconstructions may also overestimate ductal narrowing, giving a pseudostricture appearance.[68]

Misregistration artifacts from breathing during the acquisition result in respiratory motion artifacts. The biliary ducts may appear blurred, duplicated or disconnected (Fig. 79-4). This may be resolved by using single-section MRCP, which has a short imaging time, and careful interpretation of coronal source images.[66,68]

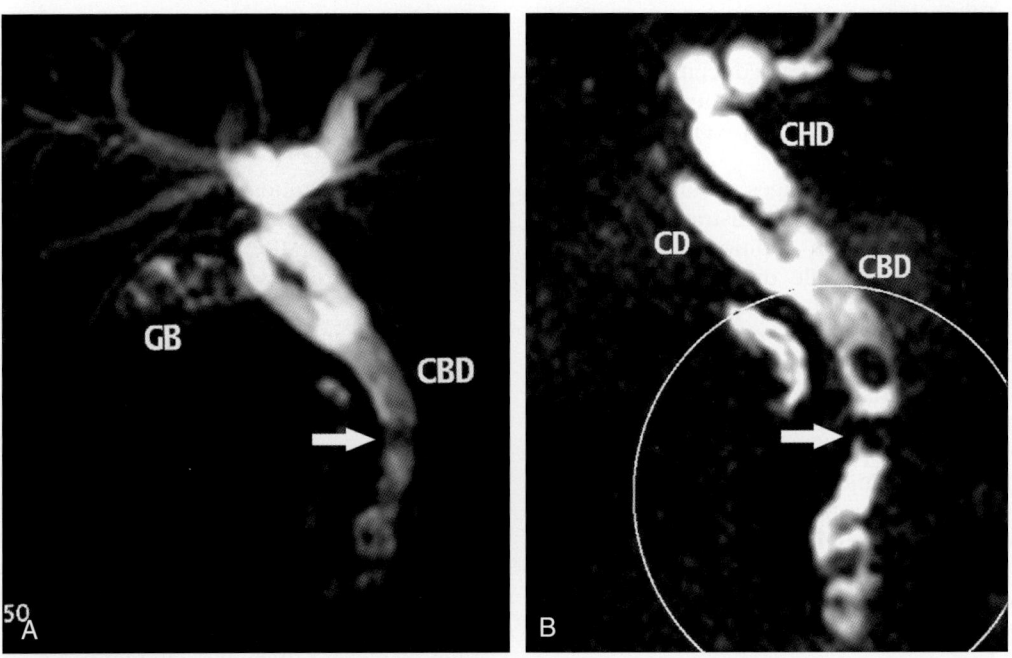

FIGURE 79-2

A and **B,** Thick SLAB vs. MULTISLICE. **A,** 70 mm coronal SSFSE RARE SLAB MRCP (TE 969) and **B,** 4 mm coronal fat-suppressed SSFSE MULTISLICE T2 MRCP (TE 180). Bile duct calculi, seen as multiple hypointense defects (*white arrow*), are better visualized in **B** due to higher spatial resolution. There is intra- and extrahepatic bile duct dilatation. CD, cystic duct; CHD, common hepatic duct; CBD, common bile duct; GB, gallbladder.

Extraductal Factors

Various extraductal factors can influence the anatomic visualization of the biliary tree. Common extraductal factors include: 1. pulsation artifacts from adjacent vessels; 2. susceptibility artifacts from metallic clips and gas in the bowel; and 3. overlapping of other stationary fluids such as adjacent bowel, ascites and cystic lesions in the upper abdomen.

Pulsatile vascular compression may cause non-pathologic bile duct narrowing and pseudo-obstruction of the bile duct. In order of decreasing frequency pulsatile vascular compression is most commonly noted in the region of the common hepatic duct, followed by the left hepatic duct and the mid portion of the common bile duct. This artifact is mostly caused by the hepatic and gastroduodenal arteries, which are anatomically closely related to the bile ducts. The extrinsic impression, caused by a right hepatic artery passing posterior to the proximal portion of the common hepatic duct, may create the appearance of an intraluminal filling defect or a signal void focus (Fig. 79-5).[69,70] This can usually be resolved with a transverse or coronal T2-weighted sequence, which will visualize the hepatic duct crossing over the right hepatic artery. Alternatively, a flow-sensitive sequence can be used to identify the right hepatic artery passing anterior to the portal vein and identify its characteristic location. The gastroduodenal artery may compress the mid portion of the common bile duct at its right anterolateral aspect, which may result in pseudo-obstruction. This artifact can also occur in the intrapancreatic portion of the common bile duct where branches of the pancreaticoduodenal artery run alongside the common bile duct.[70] The distinction between an extrinsic vascular impression and a bile duct stone can be achieved by viewing several contiguous images dynamically.

Surgical clips create susceptibility artifacts, which may obscure the region of interest by producing areas of signal void (Fig. 79-6). The artifact can also mimic a stone. Single-shot sequences with short echo spacing will minimize this artifact. Nowadays, surgical clips used for laparoscopic cholecystectomy do not cause much signal loss since they are made of nonmagnetic titanium.

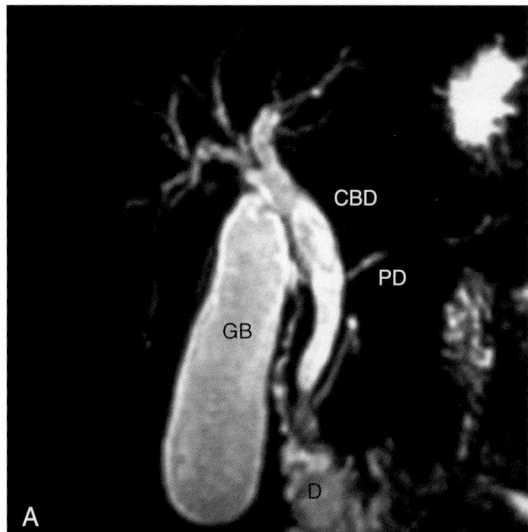

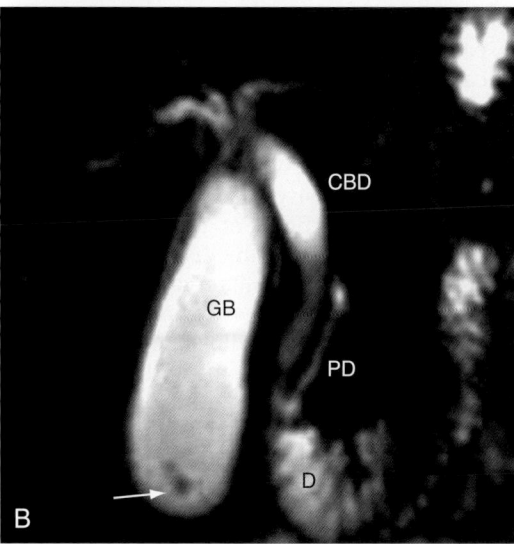

FIGURE 79-3

A and **B,** MIP reconstruction artifact. **A,** Coronal MIP and **B,** 40 mm coronal SSFSE RARE SLAB MRCP (TE 969). Coronal MIP image obscures small gallbladder calculi (*white arrow*), visualized on corresponding coronal RARE SLAB. GB, gallbladder; CBD, common bile duct; PD, pancreatic duct; D, duodenum.

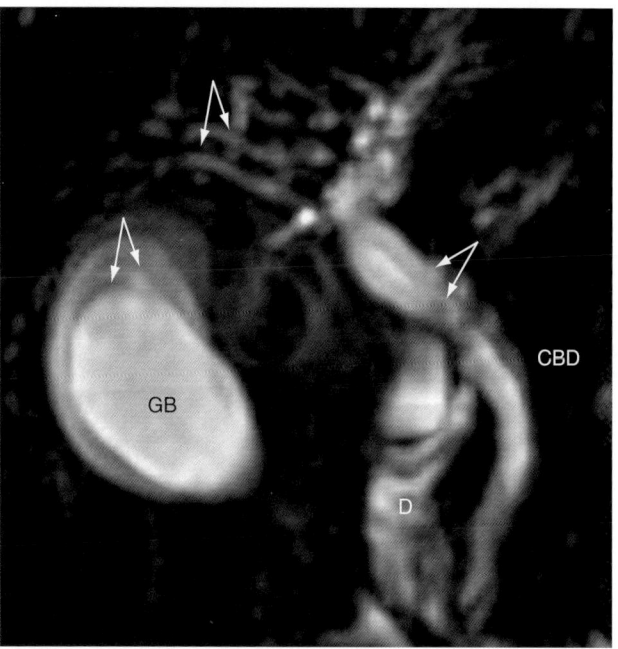

FIGURE 79-4

MIP reconstruction artifact: respiratory motion. Coronal MIP image from a study performed during quiet respiration, demonstrates duplication of the biliary tree (*arrows*) and gallbladder (GB). CBD, common bile duct; D, duodenum.

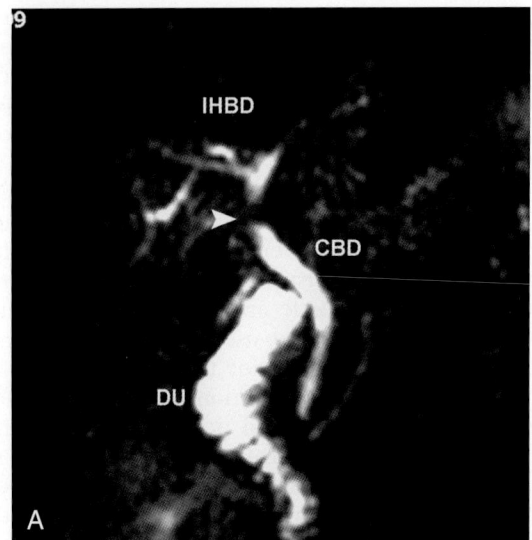

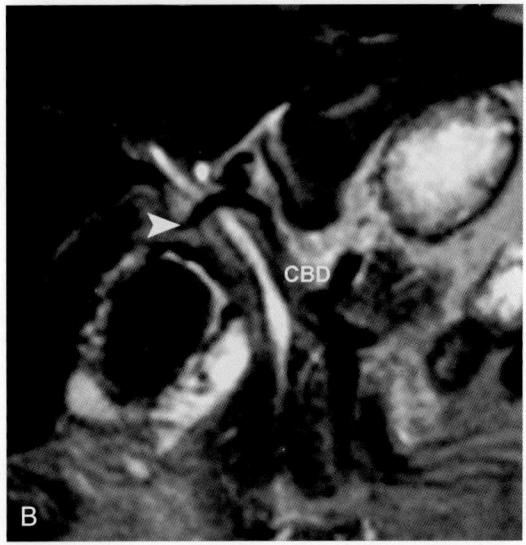

FIGURE 79-5

A and **B,** Artifact: vascular impression. **A,** 40 mm coronal SSFSE RARE SLAB MRCP (TE 969) and **B,** 6 mm coronal SSFSE T2 MRCP (TE 180). Focal hypointensity (*arrowhead*) at the level of the common hepatic duct (CHD) represents a vascular impression from the hepatic artery (*small arrow*) as it traverses the CHD. CBD, common bile duct; DU, duodenum; IHDB, intrahepatic bile duct.

However, other metallic foreign bodies, older surgical clips, or endovascular coils may produce adjacent signal loss or cause pseudo-obstruction.[70] The stomach and duodenum when filled with gas may also produce a susceptibility artifact which is most pronounced with fat-suppressed images.

Obscuration of the biliary tract, or a pseudostricture appearance, may be caused by overlapping intestinal or other stationary fluids. All these artifacts may be overcome by using different section thickness and performing MRCP from different angles. Alternatively, this may be resolved by using a negative oral contrast agent such as high concentrate ferric ammonium citrate (Fig. 79-7).[71]

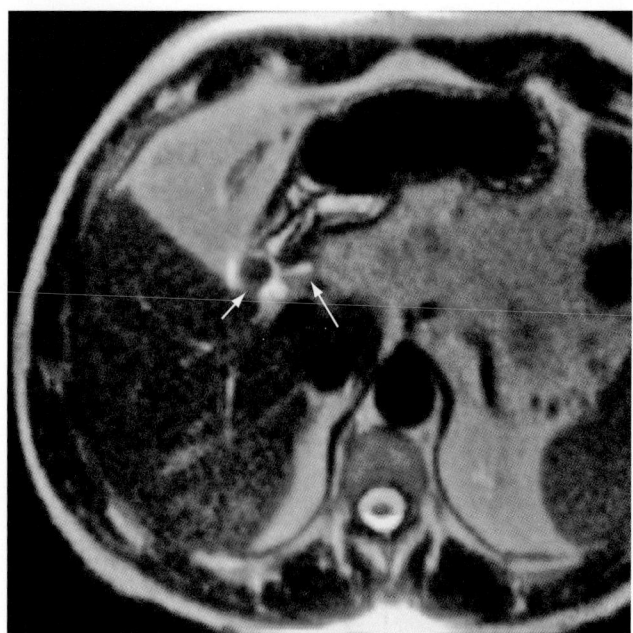

FIGURE 79-6

Clip artifact: 5 mm transverse SSFSE T2 MRCP (TE 90) image demonstrates a hypointense clip artifact (*small arrow*) from a cholecystectomy clip. *Long arrow* indicates cystic duct remnant.

Intraductal Factors

The signal intensity of bile may be reduced by several intraductal factors, such as gas, debris, hemorrhage, tumor, flow phenomenon and iodinated contrast material, all of which can produce an appearance of pseudo-obstruction, false filling defects or nonvisualization of the bile ducts.[66]

Pneumobilia may be misinterpreted as bile duct stones, particularly on coronal MRCP images. Diagnostic pitfalls caused by pneumobilia can be avoided by scanning in the transverse plane by which air bubbles rise to a nondependent position anteriorly, while stones typically layer in a dependent position posteriorly (Fig. 79-8).[66,72,73] Extensive biliary air may cause failure of visualization of portions of the biliary tree. MRCP should not be performed immediately after ERCP since dense iodinated contrast material injected into the biliary tree may result in nonvisualization of the extrahepatic bile ducts and gallbladder.

A flow artifact may result from swirling flow in dilated ducts and at the point of insertion of the cystic duct. Flow of bile may result in signal void, which may be mistaken for a stone. However, this signal void is usually seen in the nondependent, central portion of the bile duct over several sections, whereas stones are usually situated in the dependent portion of the bile ducts (Fig. 79-9). Sugita et al concluded on phantom studies, that flow artifact could be seen on images in which the ratio between the inlet and the outlet diameters in the phantom was equal to or greater than 1:4.[69] Careful interpretation of coronal source MR images and transverse T2-weighted MR images is necessary to differentiate

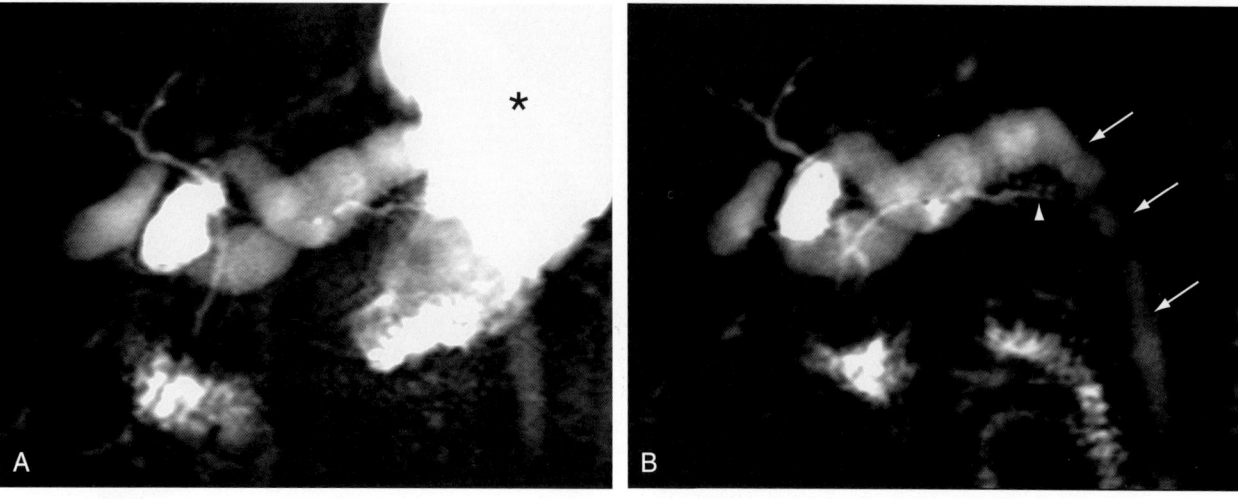

FIGURE 79-7

A and **B,** Overlapping of intestinal fluid: 70 mm coronal SSFSE RARE SLAB MRCP (TE 969) sequence. **A,** Portions of the pancreatic duct are obscured by a fluid-filled stomach (*asterisk*). **B,** On repeat MRC in the same imaging plane after administration of an oral negative contrast agent (ferric ammonium citrate), the obscured parts of the pancreatic duct (*arrowhead*) are visualized. (*Arrows* = fluid-filled small bowel).

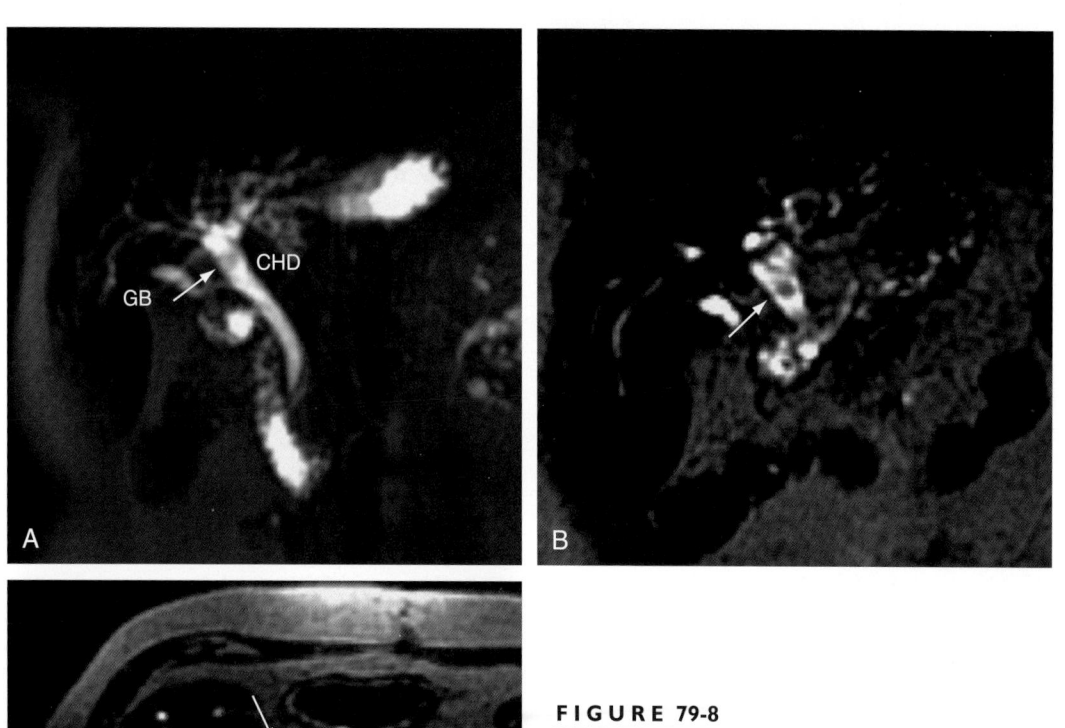

FIGURE 79-8

A, B and **C,** Pitfall related to choledocholithiasis: pneumobilia. **A,** 40 mm coronal SSFSE RARE SLAB MRCP (TE 969) demonstrates an area of hypointensity (*arrow*) in the common hepatic duct (CHD). **B,** 10 mm coronal SSFSE RARE SLAB MRCP (TE 969) confirms the hypointensity (*arrow*), which is better appreciated because of increased spatial resolution. **C,** 5 mm transverse SSFSE T2 MRCP (TE 90) demonstrates the hypointensity to be nondependent (*arrow*) within the CHD, consistent with pneumobilia. GB, gallbladder.

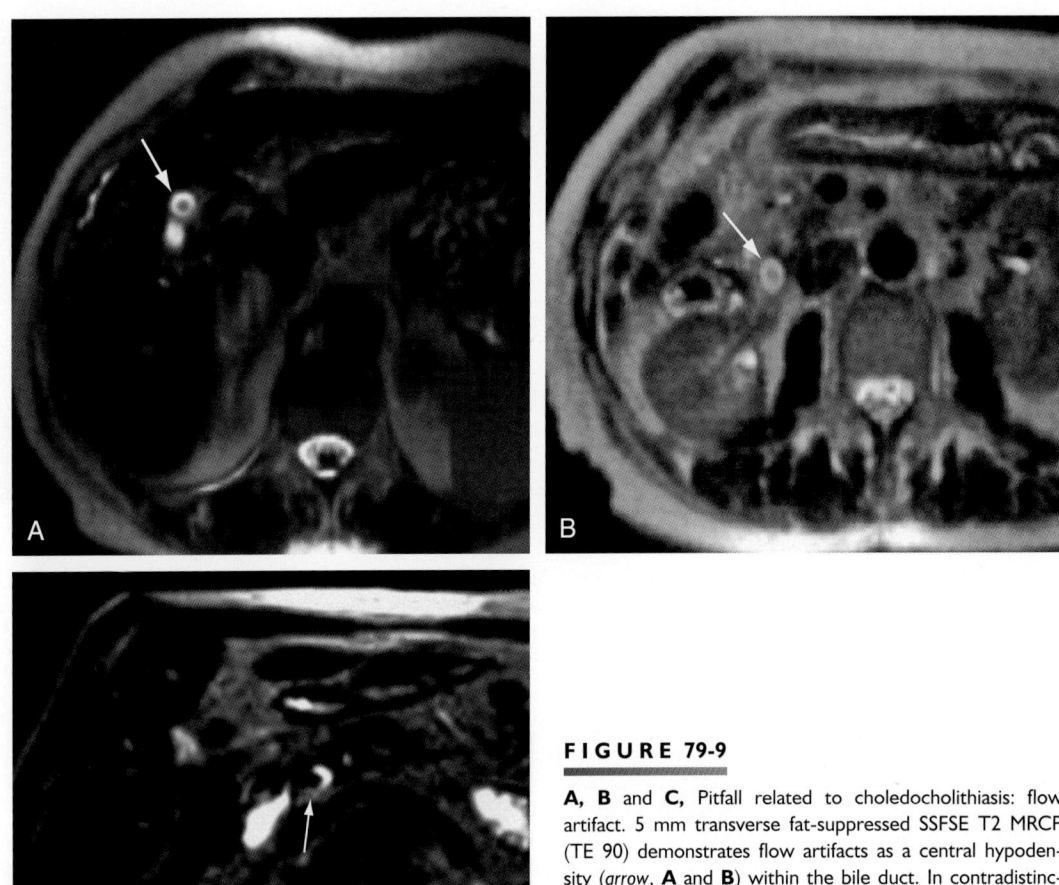

FIGURE 79-9

A, B and **C,** Pitfall related to choledocholithiasis: flow artifact. 5 mm transverse fat-suppressed SSFSE T2 MRCP (TE 90) demonstrates flow artifacts as a central hypodensity (*arrow,* **A** and **B**) within the bile duct. In contradistinction, stones are typically located in a dependent position (*arrow,* **C**).

pseudofilling defects related to flow artifacts from true filling defects (e.g., choledocholithiasis). All MRCP images and other transverse MR images should not show the exact same pseudofilling defects since bile juice flows only intermittently. If necessary this could also be resolved by using flow-sensitive MR imaging, such as time-of-flight MR angiography.[70,74]

Normal Variants

Several normal variants may simulate the presence of pathology. The en face insertion of the cystic duct into the bile duct can be mistaken for an intraductal filling defect such as a stone.[64,68,75] A long cystic duct running parallel to the common bile duct may simulate a dilated common bile duct (Fig. 79-10). These pitfalls can be avoided by using multiple imaging planes. On MRCP, the duodenal papilla can have a bulging appearance

and this may be mistaken for an impacted stone. Transverse T2-weighted images with short echo times, and 3 to 4 mm-thin sections, may clarify this pitfall (Fig. 79-11).[64,68] Contraction of the choledochal sphincter may also be confused with an impacted stone or stricture in the distal bile duct. However, this defect is transient and is called a pseudocalculus sign. In this instance only the superior margin of the defect is outlined by high-signal intensity bile. To overcome this pitfall, kinematic or repeat MRCP imaging should be performed (Fig. 79-12).[70]

NORMAL BILIARY ANATOMY

The major anatomical components of the biliary tree are the gallbladder and the intra- and extrahepatic bile ducts (Fig. 79-13).

FIGURE 79-10

Normal anatomic variant: low insertion of cystic duct. 40 mm coronal SSFSE RARE SLAB MRCP (TE 969) demonstrates a medial and low insertion of the cystic duct (*arrows*), giving an apparent widening of the lower common bile duct. Incidentally note the presence of a liver cyst (C). CHD, common hepatic duct; PD, pancreatic duct.

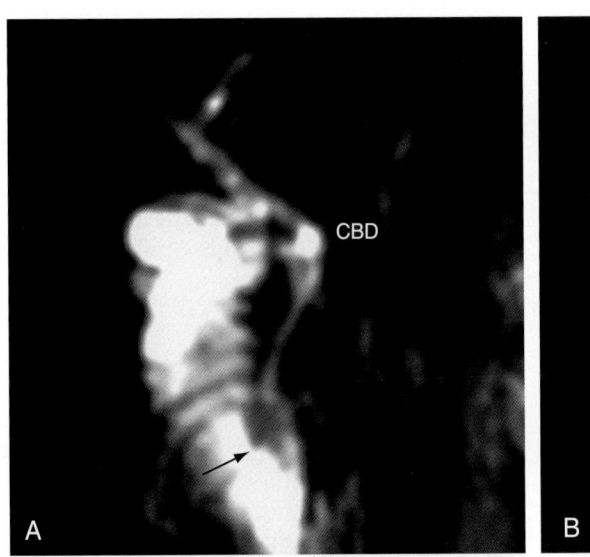

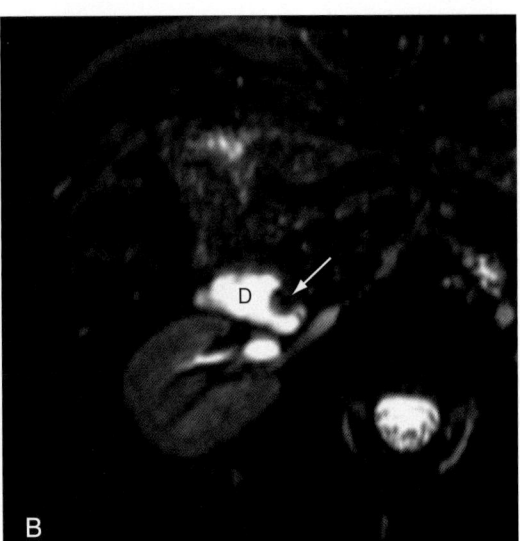

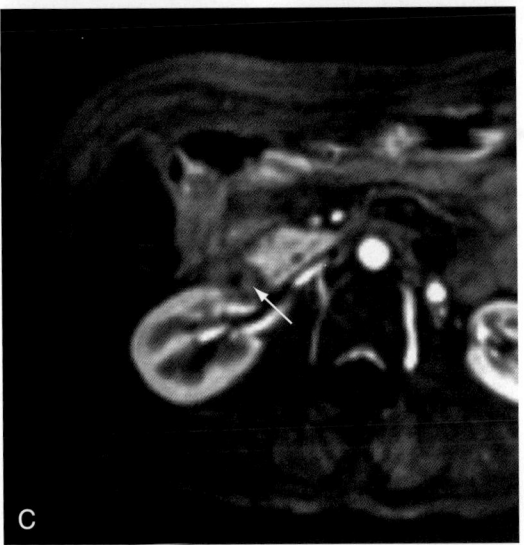

FIGURE 79-11

A, B and **C,** Pitfall: normal ampulla. **A,** 40 mm coronal SSFSE RARE SLAB MRCP (TE 969) demonstrates a focal hypointensity (*black arrow*) in the expected region of the ampulla. The common bile duct (CBD) is not dilated. **B,** 3 mm transverse fat-suppressed FSE T2 MRCP (TE 140) and **C,** 5 mm transverse fat-suppressed postgadolinium T1-weighted image demonstrates the prominent hypointensity, but normal ampulla (*arrow*, **B** and **C**).

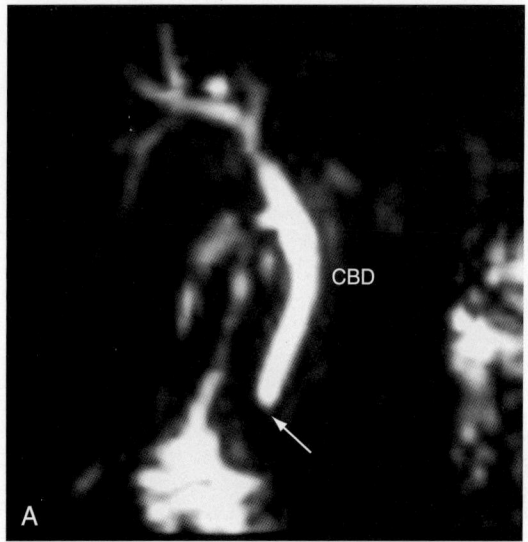

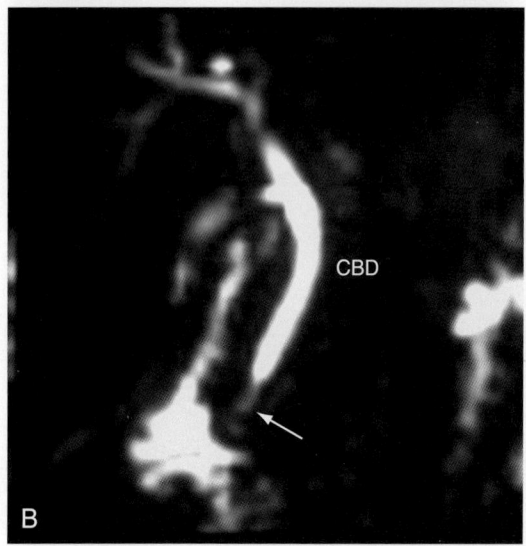

FIGURE 79-12

A and **B,** Choledochal sphincter spasm: kinematic MRC. Sequential: 20 mm coronal SSFSE RARE SLAB MRCP (TE 969). The narrowing (*arrow*) demonstrated in distal common bile duct (CBD) in image **A** was due to spasm of the choledochal sphincter.

Intrahepatic Bile Ducts

The intrahepatic bile ducts typically follow the portal veins along their anterior aspect.[76,77] The common hepatic duct divides into the right and left hepatic biliary ducts, which branch into segmental branches and then into subsegmental branches. The right hepatic duct is composed of an anterior branch, which drains Couinaud's segments 5 and 8 of the liver, and a posterior branch, which drains segments 6 and 7. The right anterior duct is vertically oriented whereas the right posterior duct is more horizontally oriented. The left hepatic duct drains segments 2, 3 and 4 of the liver.[78] The bile duct from the caudate lobe usually joins the origin of the left and right hepatic ducts.[79] At the level of

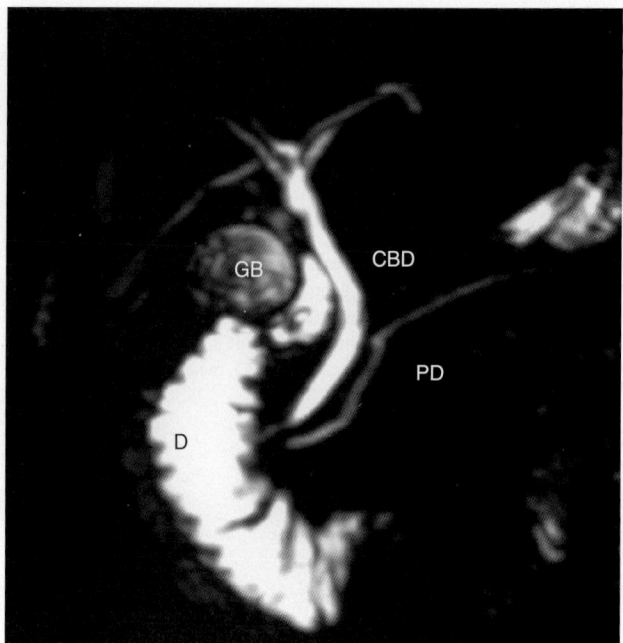

FIGURE 79-13

Normal MRCP: normal biliary anatomy on a coronal MIP reconstruction of 3D Fast Recovery Fast-Spin-Echo (FRFSE)/TE 560) sequence. CBD, common bile duct; D, duodenum; GB, gallbladder.

the porta hepatis, both hepatic ducts join and form a confluence, but at times this confluence may be situated more inferiorly.

Gallbladder

The gallbladder usually lies in the gallbladder fossa caudal to the right and left lobes of the liver at the junction of Couinaud's segments 4 and 5. A normal gallbladder usually measures 7 to 10 × 2 to 3.4 cm with a normal wall thickness that should not exceed 3 mm. However, it varies in size and shape depending on the dietary status. The cystic duct connects the gallbladder to the extrahepatic bile duct.

Extrahepatic Bile Ducts

The point of insertion of the cystic duct into the extrahepatic bile duct marks the division between the common bile duct and the common hepatic duct. The cystic duct contains several spiral valves, which are oriented concentrically and are called the valves of Heister. The diameter of the cystic duct is variable, ranging from 1 to 5 mm and follows a tortuous course. Its length varies from 1.5 to 9.5 cm, typically joining the extrahepatic bile duct halfway between the ampulla of Vater and the porta hepatis.[80] The point of insertion into the extrahepatic bile duct is variable, but in 49% it enters the extrahepatic bile duct from the right lateral aspect.[80]

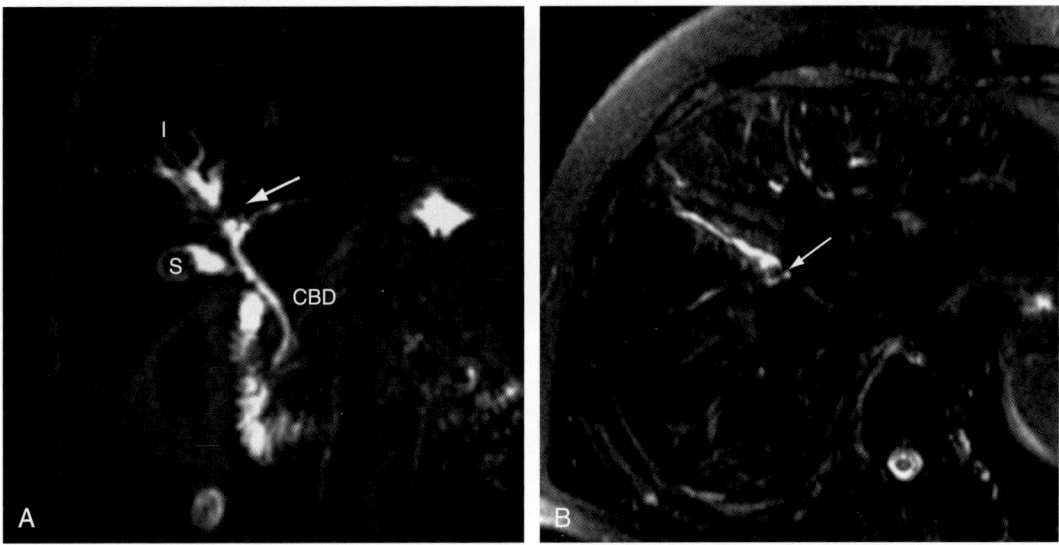

FIGURE 79-18

A, and **B,** Intrahepatic bile duct stricture and stone. **A,** 40 mm coronal SSFSE RARE SLAB MRCP (TE 969) demonstrates dilated intrahepatic ducts (I) in segment VIII of the liver. Indraductal hypointensity (*arrow*) may represent a stricture or stone. Incidentally a stone (S) is present in the gallbladder. **B,** 5 mm transverse fat-suppressed FSE T2 MRCP (TE 140) demonstrates a stone (*small arrow*) within the dilated duct proximal to the stricture. CBD, common bile duct.

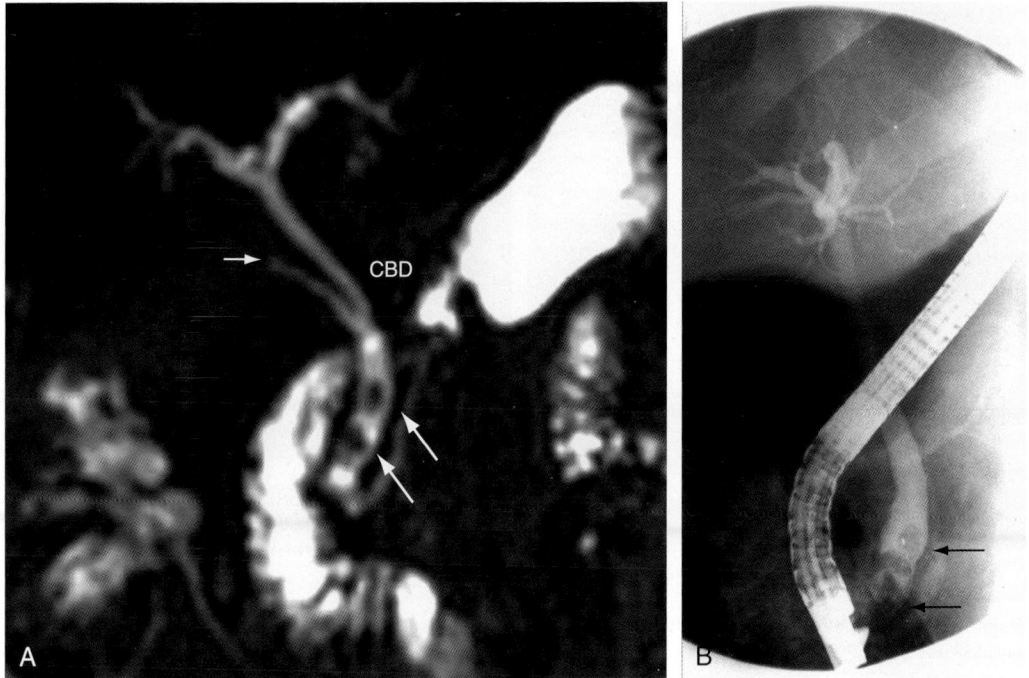

FIGURE 79-19

A, and **B,** Bile duct stones. **A,** 40 mm coronal SSFSE RARE SLAB MRCP (TE 969) and **B,** ERCP demonstrate multiple calculi (*large arrows*) in distal common bile duct (CBD). There is a low insertion of the cystic duct (*small arrow*, **A**).

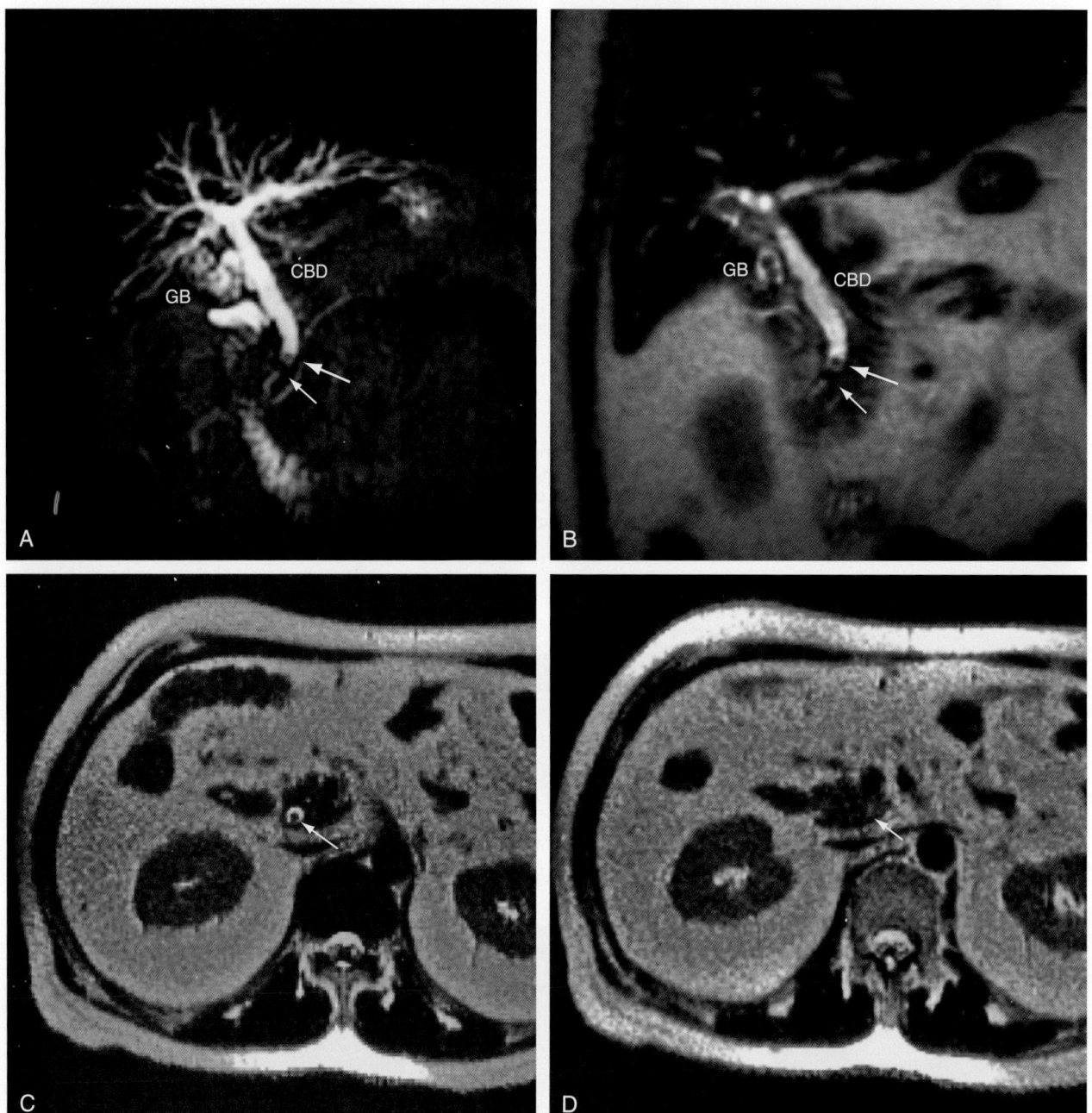

FIGURE 79-20

A, B, C and **D,** Pitfall related to choledocholithiasis: poor visualization of impacted stone. **A,** 40 mm coronal SSFSE RARE SLAB MRCP (TE 969) and **B,** 5 mm coronal SSFSE T2 MRCP (TE 180) demonstrate dilated intra- and extrahepatic bile ducts. There are two stones (*large and small arrow*) in the distal common bile duct (CBD). The caudal stone (*small arrow*) is impacted and is poorly visualized on the SLAB MRCP in **A** but is easily depicted in **B**. Multiple stones are present in the gallbladder (GB). **C** and **D,** 5 mm transverse SSFSE T2 MRCP (TE 180) demonstrate the more cranial stone as a dependent hypointensity (*large arrow*, **C**); while the distal impacted stone (*small arrow*, **D**) is not visualized, since it is not surrounded by hyperintense bile.

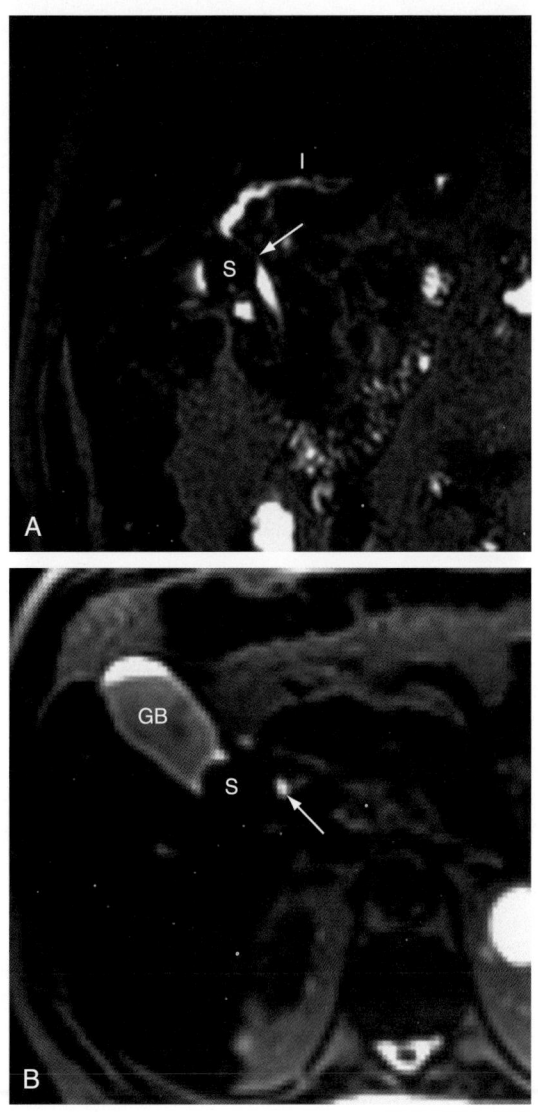

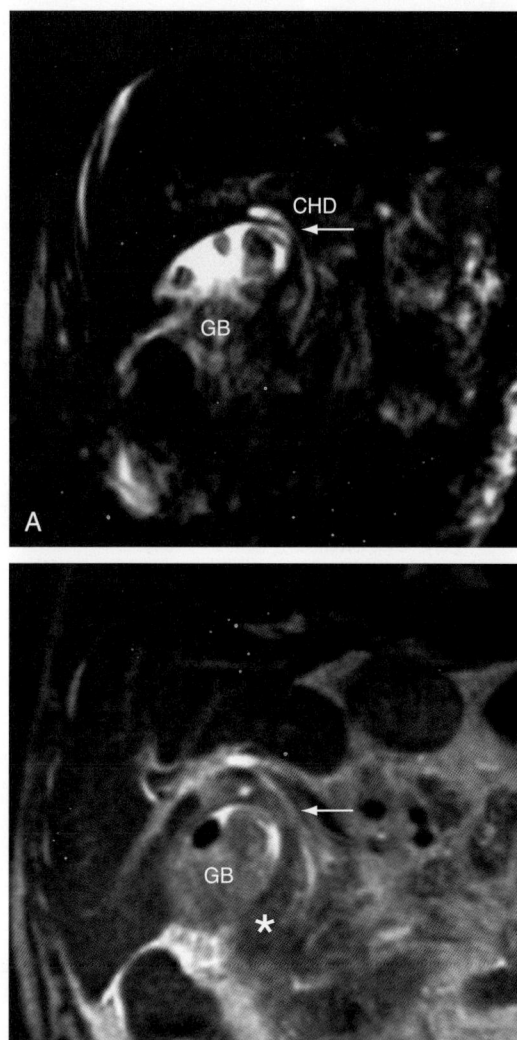

FIGURE 79-21

A and **B,** Mirizzi syndrome. **A,** 10 mm coronal SSFSE RARE SLAB MRCP (TE 969) and **B,** 5 mm transverse SSFSE T2 MRCP (TE 180) demonstrate an impacted stone (S) in the neck of the gallbladder (GB) compressing the common hepatic duct (*arrow*). There is intrahepatic bile duct dilatation (I). I, intrahepatic bile ducts.

FIGURE 79-22

A and **B,** Extramural compression: inflammatory changes secondary to acute cholecystitis. **A,** 10 mm coronal SSFSE RARE SLAB MRCP (TE 969) and **B,** 5 mm coronal SSFSE T2 MRCP (TE 180) demonstrate multiple stones within the gallbladder (GB) and pericholecystic inflammatory changes (*, **B**). There is mass effect (*arrow*) on the common hepatic bile duct (CHD) and early proximal bile duct dilatation.

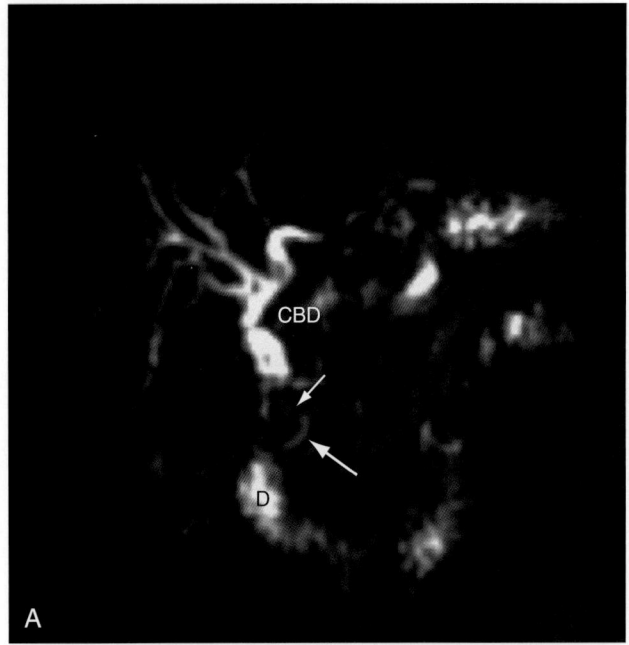

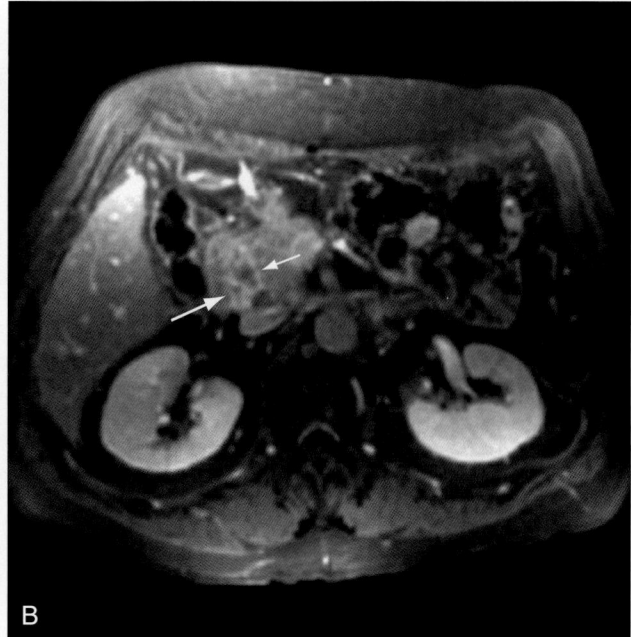

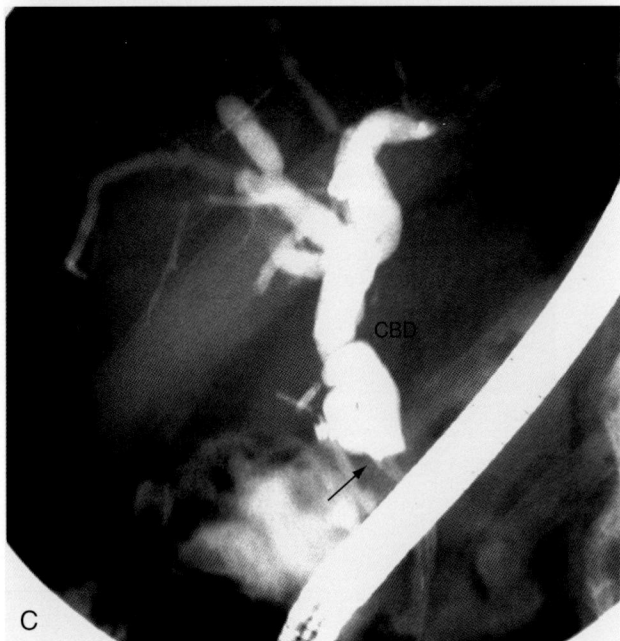

FIGURE 79-23

A, B and **C,** Extramural compression from lymphadenopathy in a patient with colorectal malignancy. **A,** 40 mm coronal SSFSE RARE SLAB MRCP (TE 969) demonstrates abrupt narrowing of the mid portion (*small arrow*) of the common bile duct (CBD). The proximal CBD and intrahepatic bile ducts are dilated. The intrapancreatic portion of the CBD, distal to the obstruction (*large arrow*) is not dilated. **B,** 5 mm transverse fat-suppressed postgadolinium SPGR T1-weighted image demonstrates necrotic lymph nodes (*small arrow*) compressing the CBD (*large arrow*). **C,** ERCP confirms obstruction of the mid CBD (*black arrow*). Biopsy of the lymph nodes revealed poorly differentiated adenocarcinoma. D, duodenum.

Ampullary Stenosis/Ampullary Fibrosis

Ampullary stenosis and ampullary fibrosis are commonly caused by surrounding inflammatory changes secondary to the passage of stones in the context of choledo-cholithiasis. Clinical presentation consists of recurrent, intermittent abdominal pain, abnormal liver function tests and CBD dilatation. MR imaging findings in the acute phase (Fig. 79-25), when the ampulla is swollen and edematous include: 1. bile duct obstruction; 2. enlargement of the ampulla; and 3. increased signal intensity of the ampulla on T2-weighted images. Once these changes become chronic, the ampulla returns to its normal size and appears to be of low-signal intensity on T2-weighted images due to progressive fibrosis (Fig. 79-26). Uncommonly, the ampulla may be enlarged secondary to proliferative fibrotic changes, and therefore mimic the appearance of an obstructing tumor. T1-weighted images with gadolinium are useful to show normal enhancement of the ampullary region versus the poorly enhanced tissue of a periampullary tumor.[61] However, in this setting a biopsy with ERCP is often necessary to exclude a small periampullary carcinoma.[41,82]

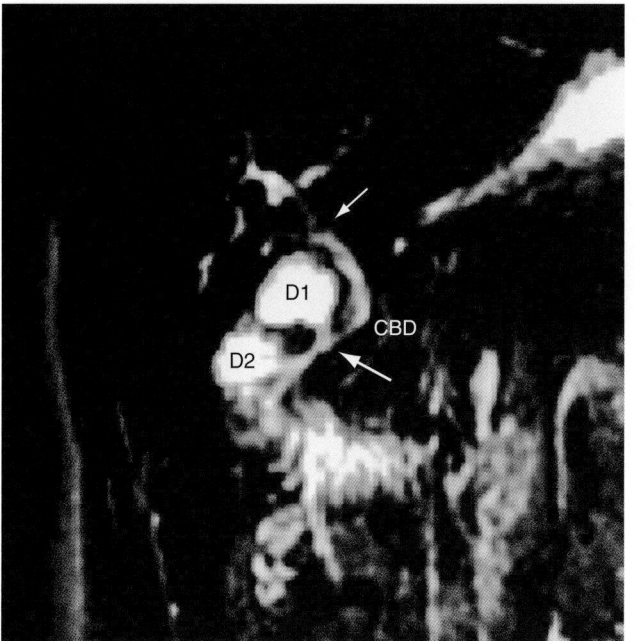

FIGURE 79-24

Choledochoduodenal fistula: 10 mm coronal SSFSE RARE SLAB MRCP (TE 969) demonstrates a fistulous communication (*large arrow*) between the common bile duct (CBD) and the first stage of the duodenum (D1). There is pneumobilia (*small arrow*) in the common hepatic duct. D2, second stage of duodenum.

Sphincter of Oddi Dysfunction

Sphincter of Oddi dysfunction includes spasm of the sphincter of Oddi and abnormalities of the rate of sphincteric contraction, causing functional stenosis.[126] Sphincter of Oddi dysfunction results in obstruction of the biliary tree at the level of the papilla, with delayed drainage of the common bile duct. The Sphincter of Oddi is approximately 1 cm long and is composed of smooth muscle from the choledochopancreatic and ampullary sphincters. It normally contracts phasically and these pressure changes produce either flow resistance or eject small volumes of bile or pancreatic juice into the duodenum.[82]

ERCP has several advantages in the evaluation of patients with suspected sphincter of Oddi dysfunction since the dynamics of biliary flow can be assessed fluoroscopically and manometry can be performed. Routine MRCP is a passive examination that is only able to assess bile ducts in the resting state. Nonvisualization of the sphincteric segment on routine MRCP can be a normal finding and can be caused by contractility of the sphincter of Oddi or by its small diameter. Sphincteric motility on MRCP is typically visualized in 97% of healthy patients.[65] MRCP is useful to establish the diagnosis of sphincter of Oddi dysfunction by excluding other causes of distal bile duct obstruction. The morphology and contractility of the sphincter of Oddi may be examined by the acquisition of kinematic MRCP images.[59]

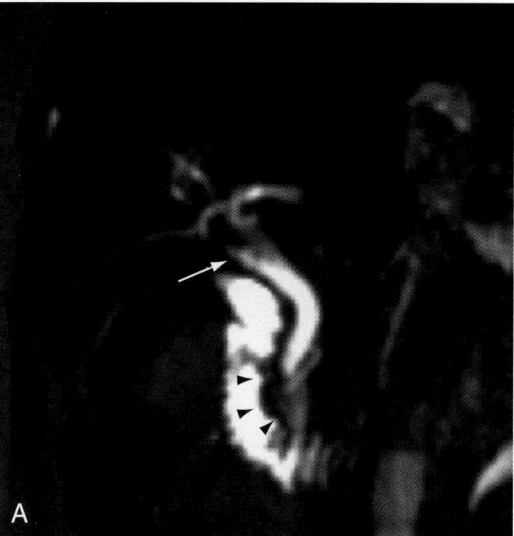

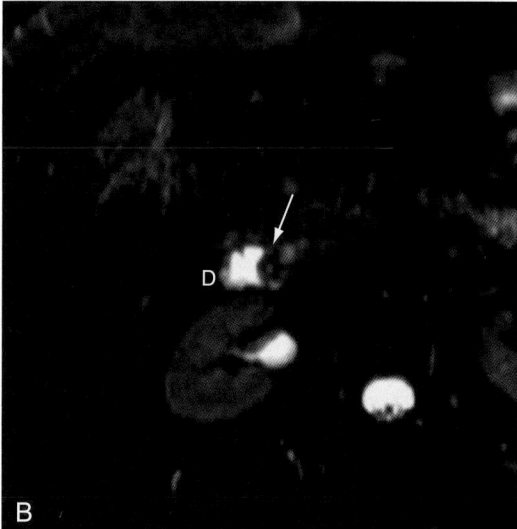

FIGURE 79-25

A and **B,** Edematous ampulla following passage of stone. **A,** 40 mm coronal SSFSE RARE SLAB MRCP (TE 969) demonstrates mild intra- and extrahepatic ductal dilatation. There is prominence of the ampulla (*arrowheads*). The cystic duct remnant is well visualized (*arrow*) in this patient with remote cholecystectomy. **B,** 5 mm transverse fat-suppressed FSE T2 MRCP (TE 140) demonstrates to better advantage the bulging and swollen papilla (*arrow*). Endoscopy confirmed the presence of a swollen papilla. Biopsy was negative for tumor. D, duodenum.

Sphincteric relaxation is usually visualized in all patients without periampullary disease on kinematic MRCP. Conversely, nonvisualization of sphincteric relaxation on kinematic MRCP implies the presence of an ampullary or periampullary lesion, which indicates the need for biliary intervention. In one study, kinematic MRCP achieved a sensitivity of 88% and a specificity of 100% in diagnosing obstruction at the level of the ampulla.[59] The accuracy of kinematic MRCP may be further improved by inducing transient biliary dilatation with the ingestion of a fatty meal or cholecystokinin administration. In patients with

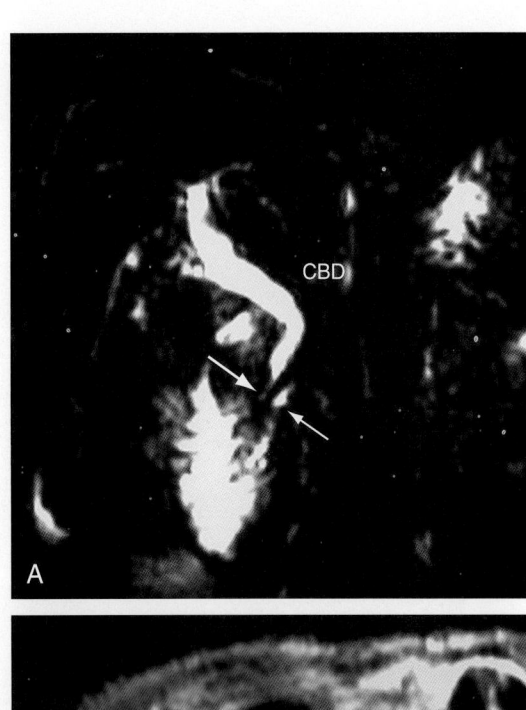

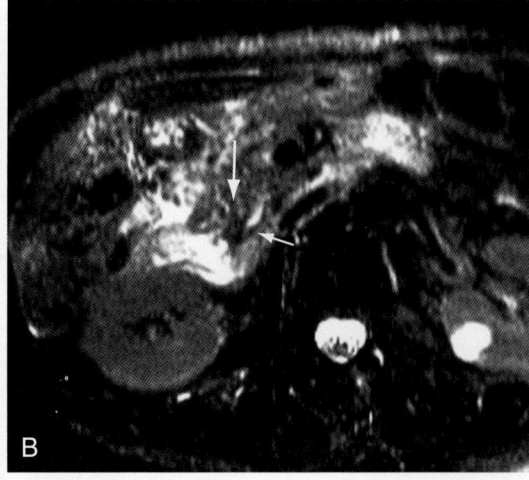

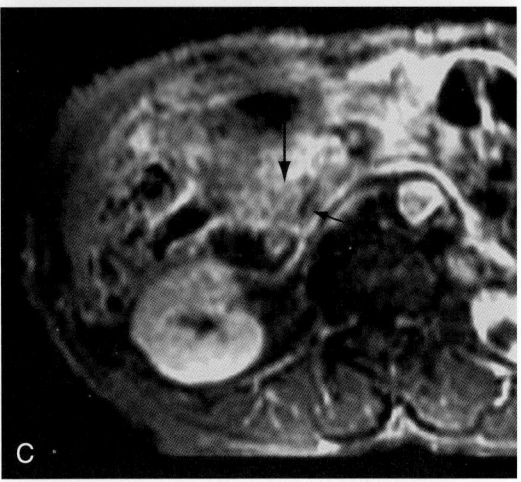

FIGURE 79-26

A, B and **C,** Ampullary fibrosis secondary to passage of stone. **A,** 10 mm coronal SSFSE RARE SLAB MRCP (TE 969) demonstrates a dilated common bile duct (CBD). There is a smooth stricture of the distal CBD (*arrow*). **B,** 5 mm transverse fat-suppressed FSE T2 MRCP (TE 140) demonstrates hypointensity around the narrowed distal CBD (*large arrow*). **C,** 5 mm transverse fat-suppressed postgadolinium T1-weighted image at the level of ampulla. There is no enhancement in the region of bile duct narrowing (*large arrow*) consistent with fibrosis. (*Small arrow*: pancreatic duct).

bile duct dilatation to the level of the ampulla and nonvisualization of sphincteric relaxation, conventional MR imaging with contrast enhancement is necessary to improve detection of ampullary or periampullary carcinoma and plan appropriate biliary intervention.[82]

Primary Sclerosing Cholangitis

Primary sclerosing cholangitis (PSC) is an idiopathic, chronic, fibrosing, inflammatory disease of the bile ducts. PSC eventually gives rise to intra- and extrahepatic bile duct strictures, and ultimately leads to bile duct obstruction, cholestasis and liver cirrhosis. It is more common in men than in women with a ratio of 2:1.[42] PSC may be related to an auto-immune process since it is often associated with other auto-immune diseases such as mediastinal fibrosis, retroperitoneal fibrosis and Sjögren's syndrome. Another hypothesis is that toxic bacterial products entering the portal venous bloodstream by way of an inflamed colonic mucosa result in

a pericholangitic inflammatory process. Up to 70% of patients will have inflammatory bowel disease; approximately 85% of these patients have ulcerative colitis and 15% have Crohn's disease.[127,128] Although 25% to 70% of patients with PSC have ulcerative colitis, only 1% to 4% of patients with ulcerative colitis have PSC.[129-136] An association exists between the risk for developing PSC and the extent of colitis.[130] However, there is no correlation between the length of time a patient has had ulcerative colitis and the time of onset of PSC. As the disease progresses to biliary cirrhosis and liver failure, liver transplantation is often necessary. Orthotopic liver transplantation is a curative therapy for PSC, which is now the fourth leading indication for liver transplantation in adults in the USA.[127,137]

The diagnosis of PSC is challenging and necessitates a multi-modality approach as no specific diagnostic test is available to date. The presence of PSC is established by certain diagnostic criteria which include: 1. appropriate clinical, biochemical, and histological findings; 2. characteristic imaging findings; and 3. exclusion of secondary causes of sclerosing cholangitis. Cirrhosis, hepatic metastases, polycystic liver disease, bacterial and parasitic cholangitis, multi-focal hepatoma, and cholangiocarcinoma are other varieties of nonsclerosing processes that can also mimic PSC. Clinical and laboratory data must be considered to achieve an accurate cholangiographic interpretation in these instances.[67] ERCP is still considered the standard of reference for diagnosing PSC because of its high spatial resolution and because the pressure applied with contrast injection optimizes visualization of multiple strictures even when subtle. However, as discussed earlier in this chapter, ERCP is an invasive procedure and can cause serious complications such as hemorrhage, sepsis, pancreatitis, bowel perforation, and cholangitis. The rate of these complications is higher and progression to cholestasis is faster in patients with PSC compared to patients without PSC.[4,138,139]

MR Considerations

MRCP is a noninvasive modality which can be used to diagnose and follow patients with PSC.[140,141] In a prospective comparative study with ERCP, MRCP achieved a sensitivity of 85% to 88% and a specificity of 92% to 97% to depict PSC.[140] MRCP is also ideal for diagnosing the complications of PSC. However, MRCP may be negative in the early stages of PSC, and therefore, should be reserved for diagnosing patients with more advanced disease and for following known cases of PSC. One limitation of MRCP in the diagnosis of early PSC is its lower spatial resolution compared to ERCP. In addition, because MRCP is performed in the physiologic nondistended state, the peripheral ducts are more difficult to visualize. Still, in patients with more advanced disease, MRCP depicts the intrahepatic bile ducts better than ERCP (69% vs. 52%) and can depict more strictures, especially of the peripheral intrahepatic ducts.[18,67,140-144] These findings can be explained by the fact that conditions which impede contrast opacification of the proximal ducts on ERCP, such as stones, strictures and thick bile, do not limit visualization of these ducts by MRCP. In fact, good visualization on MRCP of the peripheral intrahepatic ducts should alert to the possible presence of strictures. Conversely, MRCP may over- or underestimate the extent of a stricture of the extrahepatic duct, especially in the setting of multiple strictures where the duct downstream from a stricture may be collapsed.[140,142,143] In comparison, the full extent of focal strictures are readily assessed with ERCP since injection of contrast medium causes dilatation of the ducts above and below the area of narrowing.

The most common findings, in order of decreasing frequency, on MR imaging in patients with PSC include: intrahepatic bile duct dilatation (77%), enhancement of the extrahepatic bile duct wall (67%), intrahepatic bile duct strictures (64%), extrahepatic bile duct wall thickening (50%) and stenosis (50%), and intrahepatic bile duct beading (36%).[145] The key MRCP feature of PSC is the characteristic beaded appearance produced by randomly distributed short annular strictures alternating with slightly dilated segments (Fig. 79-27). These strictures are usually located at the bifurcation and are

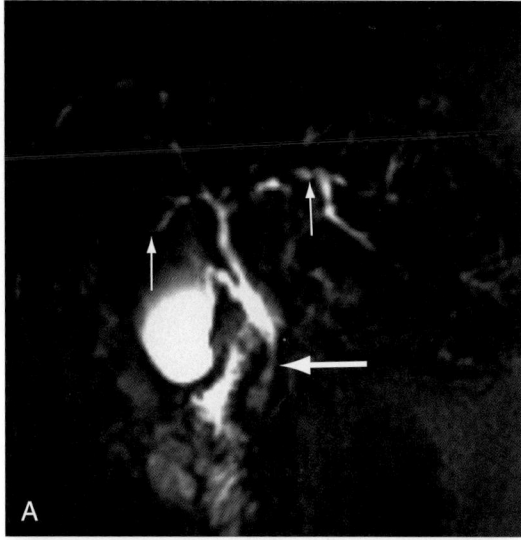

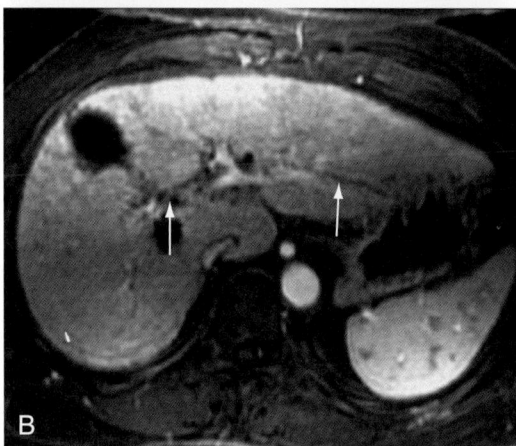

FIGURE 79-27

A and **B,** Primary sclerosing cholangitis (PSC): advanced disease. **A,** 40 mm coronal SSFSE RARE SLAB MRCP (TE 969) demonstrates multifocal strictures involving the intra- (*small arrows*) and extrahepatic (*long arrow*) bile ducts. **B,** 5 mm transverse postgadolinium fat-suppressed SPGR T1-weighted image demonstrates dilated intrahepatic bile ducts (*small arrows*) with irregularity. There is no ductal enhancement.

out of proportion to upstream ductal dilatation. The region of the right and left hepatic duct confluence is a common area for strictures of PSC (Fig. 79-28). When peripheral ducts become obliterated they are not visualized to the periphery of the liver and thus produce a pruned-tree appearance. As well, the normal acute angles that are formed with the central ducts become more obtuse.[144] Essentially in all patients with PSC, the intrahepatic ducts are involved. However, in 20% to 25% of patients there is selective involvement of only the intrahepatic ducts with sparing of the cystic duct and extrahepatic ducts (Fig. 79-29).[42] Intrahepatic bile duct dilatation occurs in about 80% of patients and is considered present if the intrahepatic ducts have a greater diameter than the more central ducts, or if they measure more than 3 mm.[144-148] For the differentiation of

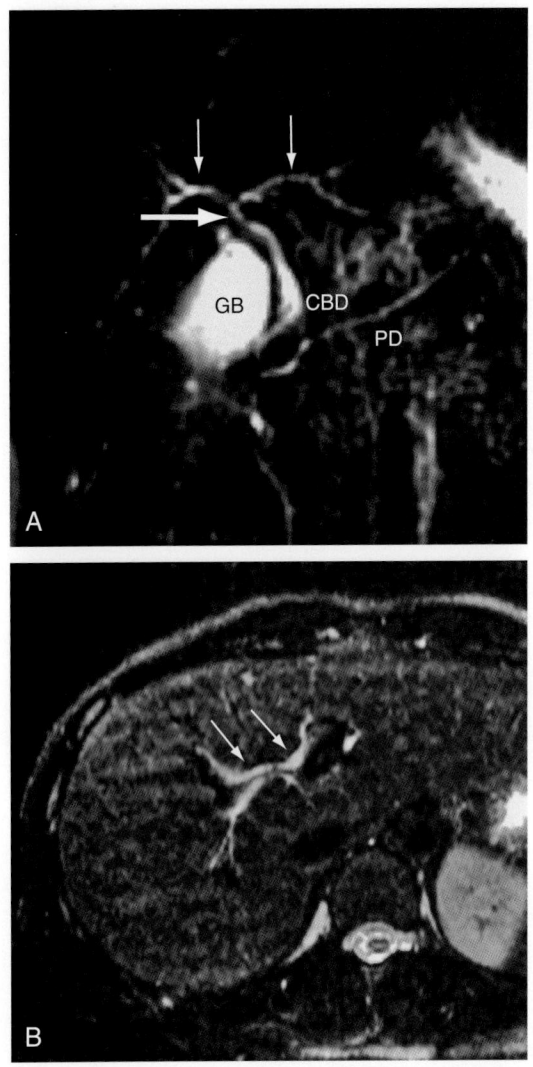

FIGURE 79-28

A and **B,** PSC: early disease. **A,** 40 mm coronal SSFSE RARE SLAB MRCP (TE 969) and **B,** 5 mm transverse fat-suppressed FSE T2 MRCP (TE 140) demonstrate mild dilatation of the central hepatic ducts (*small arrows*). There is a smooth narrowing (*arrow,* **A**) of the common hepatic duct. GB, gallbladder; PD, pancreatic duct.

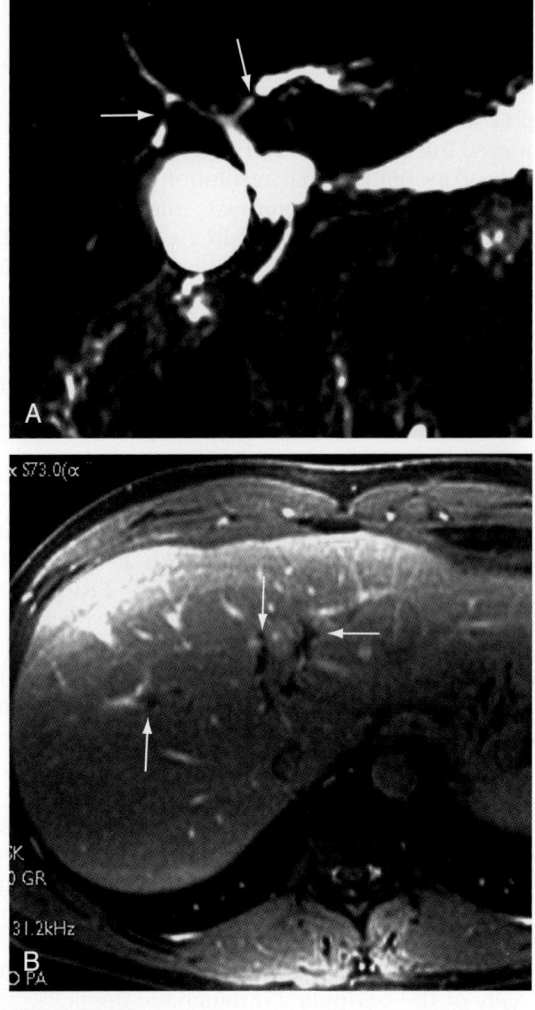

FIGURE 79-29

A and **B,** PSC: intraductal strictures. **A,** 40 mm coronal SSFSE RARE SLAB MRCP (TE 969) demonstrates focal strictures involving the left main and right posterior segmental ducts (*arrows*). **B,** 5 mm transverse fat-suppressed postgadolinium SPGR T1-weighted image demonstrates dilated segmental ducts (*arrows*). There is no ductal enhancement.

normal from strictured central intrahepatic and extra-hepatic bile ducts, coronal oblique thick-slab (40 mm) MRCP is the best technique and provides an excellent anatomic overview.[143]

Early strictures of the peripheral intrahepatic bile ducts are better depicted with a transverse, thin section, high-resolution multislice MRCP technique. Bile duct wall thickening and enhancement is present in 50% and 67% of patients, respectively.[145] Bile duct wall thickening is optimally visualized with breath-hold fat-suppressed gradient-echo (GRE) images acquired 2 minutes after gadolinium administration.[145] Periportal inflammation is seen on T1-weighted images as regions of low-signal intensity and on T2-weighted images as intermediate-signal intensity.[149] Gd-enhancement permits the distinc-tion from nonenhancing periportal edema. Additional cholangiographic findings of PSC which may be seen but are not pathognomonic include webs, stones, and diver-ticula.[144,150] Biliary webs present as 1 to 2 mm focal areas of circumferential and incomplete narrowing of the bile ducts. Pigmented stones occur in 30% of patients with PSC secondary to bile stasis. Diverticula occur in 27% of patients and present as a focal eccentric saccular dilatation of the bile ducts.

A number of different MR imaging patterns of the liver parenchyma can be seen in patients with PSC. Patients who have progressed on to develop liver cirrhosis typically develop a large macronodular pattern of cirrhosis with nodules larger than 3 cm and less commonly a diffuse pattern of cirrhosis, with or without nodules smaller than 3 cm.[148] Large regenerative macronodules of more than 3 cm are rare in the common type of cirrhosis, such as alcohol-related or viral cirrhosis. These large nodules are typically confined to the central portion of the liver in more than 67% of patients. Periportal lymphadenopathy (77%) and secondary findings of liver cirrhosis and portal hypertension have also been reported.[145]

Other MR imaging findings of PSC are abnormal hyperintensity of the liver parenchyma on T1-weighted images and increased enhancement of the liver parenchyma on dynamic arterial phase imaging. These areas of increased enhancement occur primarily in the peripheral areas of the liver and are seen in 56% of patients.[145] Peripheral wedge-shaped areas of increased signal intensity on T2-weighted images are seen in 72% of patients and are pathologically correlated to underlying perfusion changes and inflammation of the bile ducts.[127]

One of the most significant complications of PSC is the development of cholangiocarcinoma, which occurs in 10% to 15% of patients.[132,144] Cholangiocarcinoma in this setting is more likely to be multifocal, and has a poor prognosis with a median survival of 7 months and a 5-year survival ranging from 0% to 10%.[140,142,144,150,151] Treatment of coexistent ulcerative colitis does not change the subsequent risk of developing cholangiocarcinoma.[152] After liver failure, it is the second most common cause of death in patients with PSC. The diagnosis of superimposed cholangiocarcinoma by imaging is difficult. A comprehensive MR examination is required, consisting of MRCP images as well as conventional MR sequences with and without gadolinium administration. There are several cholangiographic findings that suggest the presence of a superimposed cholangiocarcinoma, such as: 1. rapid progression of strictures; 2. high-grade irregular ductal narrowing with shouldering; 3. marked dilatation of ducts proximal to strictures (Fig. 79-30); and 4. the development of polypoid or mass lesions. The MR imaging findings of cholangiocarcinoma are discussed in greater detail later in this chapter.

Secondary Sclerosing Cholangitis

Several other sclerosing processes mimic the cholangiographic findings of PSC, including acquired immune deficiency syndrome (AIDS)-related cholangitis, ascending cholangitis, oriental cholangiohepatitis, and ischemia due to intra-arterial chemotherapy, iatrogenic injury, or postliver transplantation.

AIDS-related Cholangiopathy

Involvement of the pancreaticobiliary tract is an early feature in human immunodeficiency virus (HIV)-positive patients. The hallmark of AIDS cholangiopathy is inflammation and edema of the biliary mucosa, resulting in imaging findings that resemble primary sclerosing cholangitis.[153-156] Clinical features of AIDS-related cholangiopathy are right upper quadrant pain, nausea, vomiting, and fever. Jaundice is not common, and only

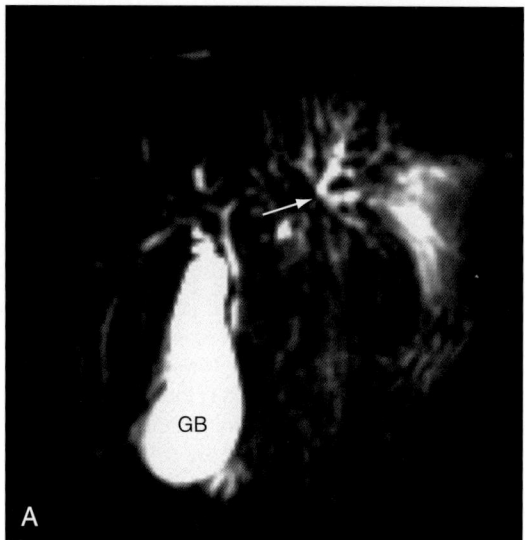

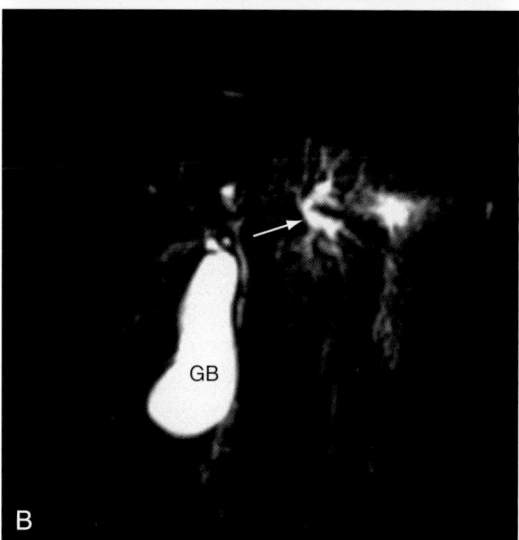

FIGURE 79-30

A and **B,** Cholangiocarcinoma complicating PSC. 40 mm coronal SSFSE RARE SLAB MRCP (TE 969) images. **A,** There are multifocal strictures and irregularity of the intrahepatic bile ducts consistent with PSC. There is a paucity of ducts in the right lobe of the liver. There is focal ductal dilatation of segments 2 and 3 (*arrow*). **B,** MRCP performed at 1-year follow-up demonstrates progressive dilatation of the ducts draining segments 2 and 3 (*arrow*) from development of cholangiocarcinoma. GB, gallbladder.

mild elevation of bilirubin and hepatic transaminases occurs, however marked elevation of alkaline phosphate is typically present.[153-155]

The infectious organisms in AIDS-related cholangiopathy (such as *cytomegalovirus, Mycobacterium avium-intracellulare, cryptosporidium* and *microsporida*) inhabit the duodenum and proximal small intestine and gain access to the biliary system via the major papilla. In 50% of patients an opportunistic organism can be isolated from the bile ducts.[144,157,158] Another mechanism of the disease is direct infiltration of the biliary tree with the human immunodeficiency virus.[154,158-160]

The cholangiographic findings in AIDS-related cholangiopathy can be difficult to distinguish from PSC and include: 1. focal strictures with irregular dilatations; 2. pruning of the peripheral intrahepatic bile ducts; 3. uniform and long dilatations of the extrahepatic bile ducts (up to 2.5 cm); 4. thickening and irregularity of the bile duct walls; and 5. papillary stenosis. Long, tapering strictures of the distal common bile duct, with or without intrahepatic sclerosing cholangitis, are more commonly seen in AIDS patients and less frequently in patients with PSC.[161] Intrahepatic sclerosing cholangitis can also occur alone.[18] Diverticular outpouchings and high-grade segmental common bile duct strictures are not a common feature of AIDS-related cholangiopathy and are more commonly seen in patients with PSC.[42,162] Ampullary stenosis with common bile duct dilatation results when the papilla of Vater is also involved.

Gallbladder wall thickening, acalculus cholecystitis and Kaposi sarcoma of the gallbladder wall are additional manifestations in patients with AIDS-related cholangiopathy.[154,156]

Postliver Transplant Ischemic Cholangitis

Bile duct strictures are the second leading cause of liver failure in transplant recipients. These may be caused by iatrogenic injury, prolonged preservation time, hepatic arterial thrombosis or stenosis, chronic rejection, recurrence of primary liver disease, cholangitis, or cholangiocarcinoma.[144] Between 10% and 33% of postliver transplant patients develop bile duct complications after liver transplantation and about 1% of grafts are lost secondary to technical failure.[163-168] Using standardized transplantation techniques, serious bile duct complications were found by Greif et al[168] in 11.5% of patients with liver transplants, with bile duct strictures being the most common complication.[163]

Post-transplantation strictures are classified into anastomotic and nonanastomotic strictures. Anastomotic strictures occur more frequently. Most anastomotic strictures occur at the level of the extrahepatic bile ducts (Fig. 79-31), and are caused by iatrogenic trauma with resultant ischemia and scar formation.[163,169-171] If the diagnosis is not made, ascending cholangitis can develop, resulting in intrahepatic bile duct strictures that simulate PSC.[144]

Nonanastomotic strictures may be multiple and typically develop at the hepatic hilum and progress peripherally into the intrahepatic bile ducts.[172] Nonanastomotic strictures are usually unrelated to iatrogenic bile duct injury.[144] These are most frequently caused by ischemic injury from prolonged cold ischemia time, or are secondary to arterial insufficiency due to hepatic artery stenosis or thrombosis.[163,171,173,174]

Thrombosis of the hepatic artery occurs in 4% to 8% of liver transplants and causes up to 50% of nonanastomotic strictures.[144,175-177] In the transplanted liver the parabiliary collateral arteries from the hepatic, celiac, gastroduodenal and superior mesenteric arteries are absent. Therefore, the hepatic artery provides the only arterial supply to the transplanted liver. Occlusion or stenosis of the hepatic artery thus results in significant ischemia, leading to bile duct or hepatocyte necrosis and subsequent nonanastomotic bile duct stricture formation.[144] Other causes of nonanastomotic bile duct strictures in a liver transplant must also be excluded, such as prolonged preservation time, rejection, bacterial or viral cholangitis, recurrent PSC and cholangiocarcinoma.[144,178]

Surgical revision is the definitive treatment for bile duct strictures.[168] Surgery should be performed soon after the onset of symptoms to avoid secondary cholangitis and further stricturing. A timely and accurate diagnosis is crucial, and requires visualization of the entire biliary tree.[163]

MR cholangiography can be used to screen for biliary strictures post liver transplantation.[179] The bile ducts proximal to the obstruction are well depicted and the extent of biliary involvement is well delineated. In a study by Ito et al,[172] MRCP completely demonstrated first-order intrahepatic bile ducts in 92%, the recipient extrahepatic bile duct in 94%, the donor extrahepatic bile duct in 100% and anastomosis in 96% of patients. Fulcher et al achieved an accuracy of 100% for detecting biliary dilatation and strictures in transplant patients using MRCP.[179]

A limitation of MRCP is that it tends to overestimate the length of a stricture because the duct immediately distal to the stricture may be collapsed.[163,180,181] This overestimation should be reduced by careful analysis of the source images.

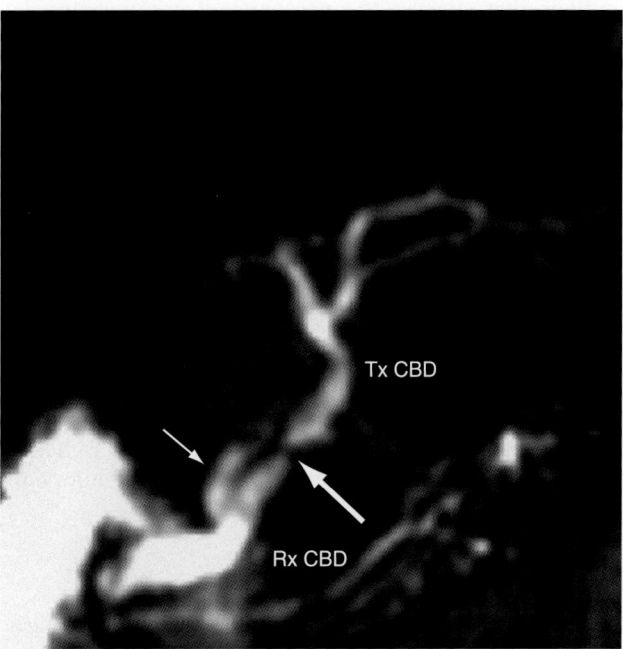

FIGURE 79-31

Post-transplant biliary stricture: 40 mm coronal SSFSE RARE SLAB MRCP (TE 969) demonstrates narrowing at the anastomotic site (*large arrow*). There is intrahepatic bile duct dilatation. *Small arrow* depicts the recipient remnant cystic duct. Tx CBD, transplant bile duct; Rx CBD, recipient bile duct.

Chemotherapy-related Cholangitis

Hepatic arterial infusion of certain chemotherapeutic agents, such as 5-flourodeoxyuridine, is a treatment option in patients with metastatic liver disease from colorectal cancer. These chemotherapeutic agents result in inflammatory changes, endarteritis and fibrosing processes around the portal triad due to a high rate of extraction on the first pass through the liver and biliary excretion.[182-184] These changes may simulate PSC at imaging.[144,185] In up to 15% of treated patients, bile duct strictures occur as early as 2 months after therapy.[185] However, the average time to development of chemotherapy-induced bile duct strictures is approximately 12 months.[184,186] Discontinuation of the chemotherapy agent can arrest the progression of the bile duct abnormalities.[184,186]

Strictures occur due to ischemic changes secondary to thrombosis of the intrahepatic arterial branches, or as a direct toxic effect of the treatment.[187,188] Segmental strictures at the bifurcation of the common hepatic duct with sparing of the intrahepatic and distal common bile ducts is the most common MRCP finding in chemotherapy-induced cholangitis.[133,144,185,186]

CONGENITAL ANOMALIES OF BILE DUCTS

Congenital anomalies of the bile ducts are uncommon and typically consist of cystic dilatation of the extrahepatic bile duct with or without dilatation of the intrahepatic bile ducts. Clinically, patients present with a triad of jaundice, abdominal pain and a palpable right upper quadrant mass.[189,190] These symptoms usually appear before the age of 10 years in two thirds of cases. Only 20% of patients are diagnosed in adulthood and it is 3 to 4 times more common in female than in male patients.[190,191]

There are several causes proposed for cystic anomalies of the bile ducts, which include sequelae of an anomalous junction of the pancreatic and distal common bile ducts.[192] An anomalous pancreaticobiliary junction results in chronic reflux of pancreatic enzymes, causing inflammation and weakness of the common bile duct wall, and subsequent scarring, dilatation, and stricture formation. This anomalous junction is found in 10% to 58% of patients with choledochal cysts.[189] Craig et al suggested that sphincter of Oddi dysfunction may also be related to choledochal cyst formation.[193]

Todani et al[194] modified the original classification of Alonzo-Lej into five types of choledochal cystic disease. Type 1, classified as choledochal cyst, accounts for 77% to 90% of cysts of the biliary tree and is subdivided into: 1a—cystic dilatation of the common bile duct, 1b—focal segmental dilatation of the distal CBD, and type 1c—fusiform dilatation of both the common hepatic duct and the common bile duct. Type 2 choledochal cysts are true diverticulae, arising from the common bile duct and account for 2% of bile duct cysts. Type 3 includes choledochoceles. Type 4 includes type 4a, with multiple intra- and extrahepatic cysts; and type 4b, with multiple extrahepatic cysts only; Type 4 accounts for approximately 10% of bile duct cysts. Type 5 is Caroli's disease.

Choledochal Cyst

Choledochal cyst is the most common type of cystic congenital biliary anomaly (77% to 90%). Choledochal cyst manifests as aneurysmal segmental dilatation of the CBD alone, or dilatation of both the CBD and common hepatic duct (CHD) (Fig. 79-32). It may also coexist with multiple segmental intrahepatic bile duct cysts (Fig. 79-33). The standard treatment of choledochal cysts is complete excision of the extrahepatic bile duct. It is beneficial to evaluate the distance between the site of dissection and the main pancreatic duct preoperatively, to avoid iatrogenic injury of the main pancreatic duct. There are several complications associated with choledochal cysts, which include: choledocholithiasis, pancreatitis, gallbladder stones, ascending cholangitis, strictures of the bile duct, biliary cirrhosis, portal hypertension, hepatic abscesses, and hepatobiliary malignancy. The incidence of malignancy is reported to range from 3% to 40% with a tendency for multicentricity, extensive local spread and a poor prognosis.[189-191,195] The risk increases if the patients are not treated until after the age of 20 years.[152] To decrease the risk of malignancy, the cyst must be removed by complete excision and subsequent biliary enteric anastomosis. If only internal drainage of the cyst is attempted, the risk of malignancy is not reduced.[190,195,196]

Ultrasonography is usually the initial modality of choice for evaluating choledochal cysts, but cannot depict the anomalous pancreaticobiliary ductal union. Other modalities, such as computed tomography (CT), radionuclide scintigraphy and percutaneous transhepatic cholangiography (PTC) are also helpful. ERCP has traditionally been used to confirm the anatomy of the cyst, exclude the presence of tumor masses, and diagnose the presence of an anomalous pancreaticobiliary junction.[90,197]

The role of MRCP is to display the anatomy of the cysts in multiple planes, delineate the relationship of the cysts to the rest of the intra- and extrahepatic biliary tree, and diagnose associated findings such as an anomalous pancreaticobiliary junction (Fig. 79-34). In addition, MRCP can diagnose the presence of complications including stones, strictures and malignancy (Fig. 79-35).[190,198] MRCP offers noninvasive diagnostic information that is equivalent to that of invasive ERCP for the assessment of choledochal cysts in adults.[90,199-206]

Coronal MR imaging displays a cystic dilated tubular structure running in the expected course of the CBD. Other cystic lesions in this region must be differentiated from choledochal cysts such as pancreatic pseudocysts and enteric duplication cysts.[190,195] The presence of wall thickening, enhancement or mural irregularities raises the suspicion of a complicating cholangiocarcinoma.[191]

Single-shot, thick-slice images are generally of better quality than MIPs from lengthier multislice, multi-shot 2D FSE acquisitions in adults with suspected congenital biliary anomalies.[207] A study by Chan et al[201] showed that a multislice 2D FSE sequence with the MIP technique

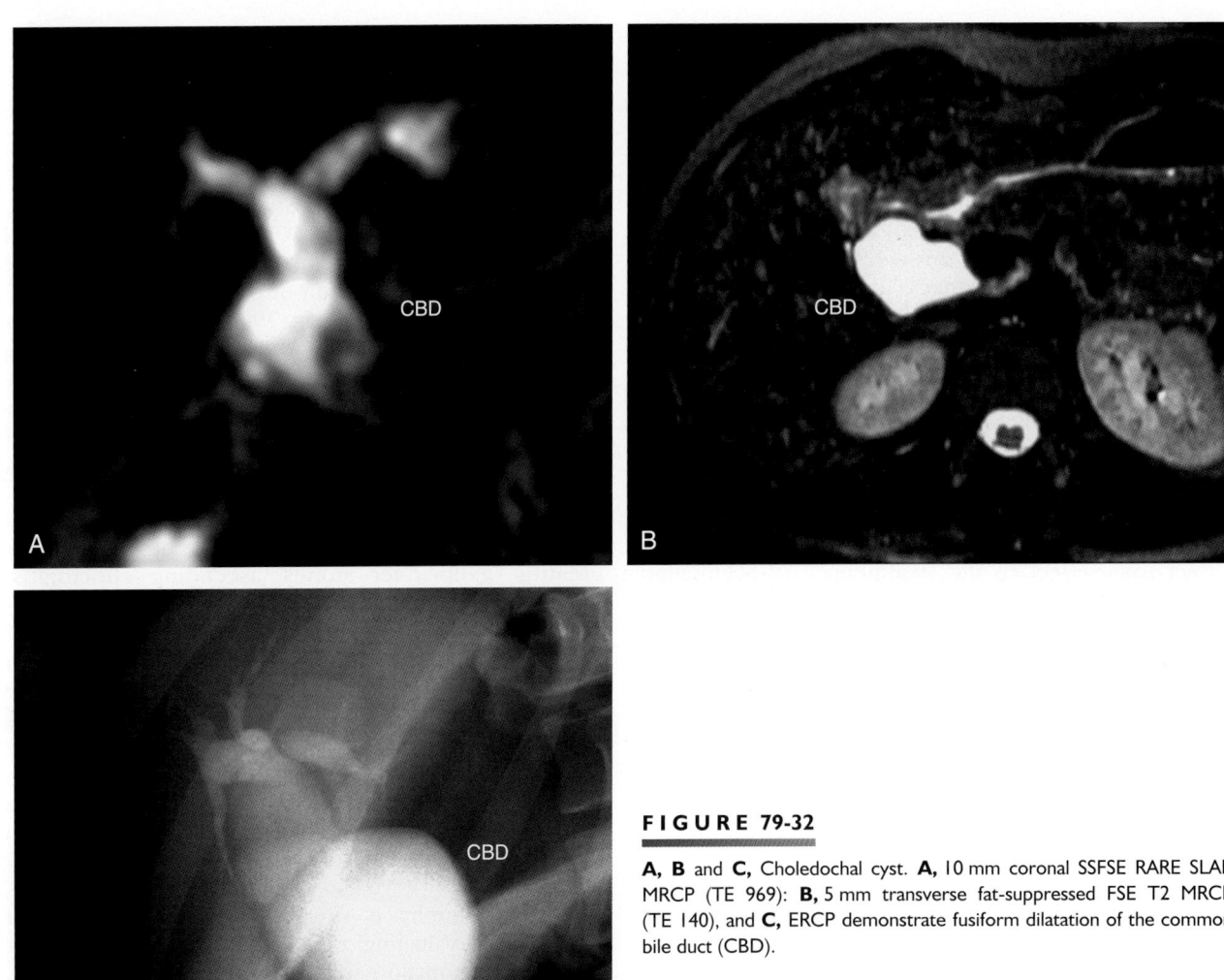

FIGURE 79-32

A, B and **C,** Choledochal cyst. **A,** 10 mm coronal SSFSE RARE SLAB MRCP (TE 969): **B,** 5 mm transverse fat-suppressed FSE T2 MRCP (TE 140), and **C,** ERCP demonstrate fusiform dilatation of the common bile duct (CBD).

failed to reliably depict the anomalous pancreaticobiliary ductal union, whereas MRCP using a HASTE sequence visualized the presence of an anomalous junction correctly in all adult patients.[203,205,206,208]

However, it has been found that the HASTE sequence, with a maximum in-plane spatial resolution of approximately 1 mm, may not be adequate for pediatric patients. The main pancreatic duct could not be visualized reliably and MRCP was only able to depict the anomalous junction of the pancreaticobiliary duct in 40% of patients.[200-205] Additionally, it was shown that when large stones occupied almost the entire portion of the bile ducts, the stones were hard to detect on MRCP since they were outlined only partially or not at all by hyperintense fluid.[90,199] The location of the common channel is another reason for the false-negative findings in pediatric cases, since the common channel is adjacent

to the ampulla of Vater and stones located in that area are often mistaken for stenoses. Another drawback is that large choledochal cysts may obscure the common channel or the anomalous pancreaticobiliary ductal union.[90,199] Therefore, further refinement in MRCP techniques is required before the method can be considered entirely reliable for pediatric patients with choledochal cysts.

Choledochocele

This lesion accounts for 1% to 5% of bile duct cysts and is defined as cystic dilatation isolated to the intra-duodenal portion of the common bile duct. Choledochoceles appear as fluid-filled mass lesions that protrude into the duodenal wall (forming what is called a

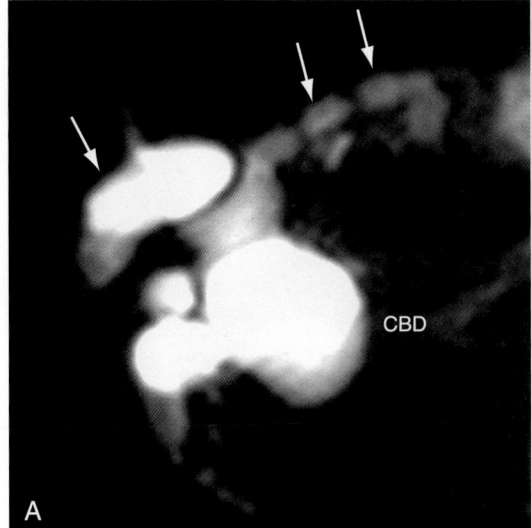

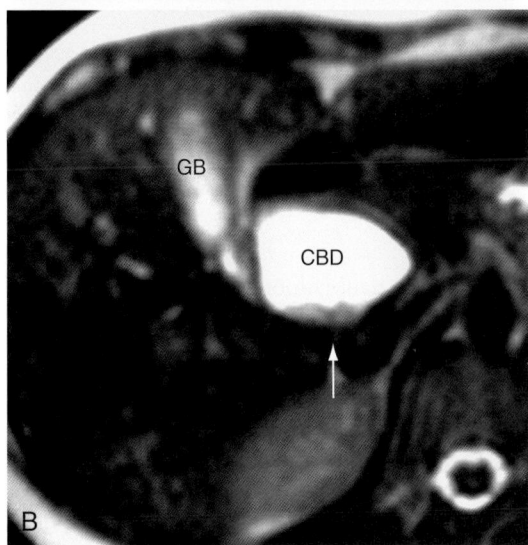

FIGURE 79-33

A and **B,** Choledochal cyst: intra- and extrahepatic involvement. **A,** 70 mm coronal SSFSE RARE SLAB MRCP (TE 969) and **B,** 5 mm transverse SSFSE T2 MRCP (TE 90) demonstrate cystic dilatation of the common bile duct (CBD) with sludge layering dependently (*small arrow,* **B**). There are multiple cystic dilatations of the intrahepatic bile ducts (*arrows,* **A**). GB, gallbladder.

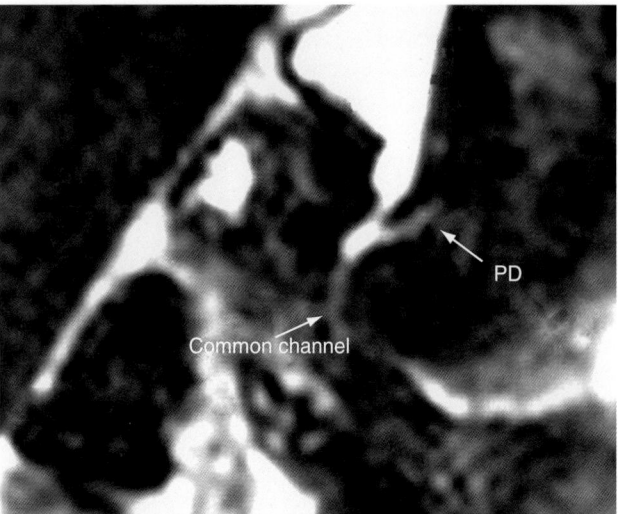

FIGURE 79-34

Common channel in a choledochal cyst. 5 mm coronal SSFSE T2 MRCP (TE 90) zoomed to the distal common bile duct (CBD). There is fusiform dilatation of the CBD consistent with a choledochal cyst. There is a common channel draining both the pancreatic (PD) and common bile ducts.

cobrahead appearance of the duct) (Fig. 79-36), do not fill with gastointestinal (GI) tract oral contrast but will fill with oral biliary contrast agents.[209,210] Unlike other types of choledochal cysts, choledochoceles have no predilection for increased risk of hepatobiliary malignancy, and therefore can be treated without complete surgical excision by unroofing the cyst or by internal drainage.[211]

Caroli's Disease

Caroli's disease is a rare autosomal recessive disorder also called communicating cavernous ectasia of the intrahepatic bile ducts. It involves only the intrahepatic

ducts with single or multiple cysts.[189,190,212] The communicating cystic dilatations of the intrahepatic bile ducts form a spectrum of congenital anomalies. Caroli's disease involves the large intrahepatic bile ducts. However, if predominantly the small interlobular bile ducts are involved, then congenital hepatic fibrosis results. If all levels of the biliary tree are involved, Caroli's syndrome results, and includes the features of both congenital hepatic fibrosis and Caroli's disease.[213] The sex predilection of Caroli's disease is equal and it is usually diagnosed in children and young adults. The patients generally present with fever and jaundice, episodic abdominal pain, ascending cholangitis, liver abscesses or signs and symptoms of portal hypertension.[214]

The extrahepatic bile ducts in patients with Caroli's disease can be slightly dilated (53%), stenotic, associated with a choledochal cyst, or can appear normal.[213]

Caroli's disease is frequently complicated by bile duct stones, ascending cholangitis, and liver abscesses. Caroli's disease is also associated with renal cystic disease, most commonly medullary sponge kidney, as well as hepatic fibrosis.[212,214-216]

The MRCP features of Caroli's disease are characteristic and include saccular or fusiform dilatation of varying sizes of the intrahepatic bile ducts (Fig. 79-37).[213] Additional imaging features include strictures or irregular bile duct walls and intrahepatic bile duct stones. These findings are best demonstrated with thin-section T1- or T2-weighted images where Caroli's disease is diagnosed by showing multiple, round cystic dilatations with signal intensity compatible with bile (dark on T1- and bright on T2-weighted images), and communicating with the biliary tree.[217]

Since the abnormality in Caroli's disease is primarily intrahepatic, it is not treatable by surgical resection and

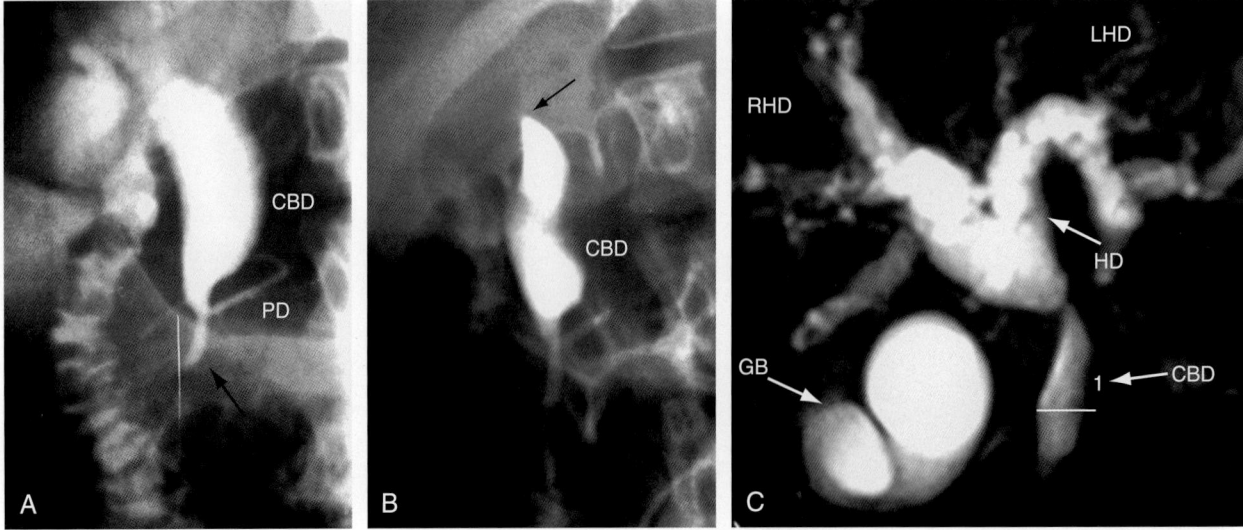

FIGURE 79-35

A, B and **C,** Chlangiocarcinoma complicating choledochal cyst. **A,** Remote ERCP demonstrates fusiform dilatation of the common bile duct (CBD). Note the presence of a common channel (*arrow*). The intrahepatic bile ducts are not opacified by contrast. **B,** Follow-up ERCP on development of jaundice demonstrates an obstruction (*small arrow*) at the level of the proximal CBD. **C,** 70 mm coronal SSFSE RARE SLAB MRCP (TE 969) demonstrates dilated intrahepatic bile ducts (RHD, LHD, and HD). There is a new stricture involving the choledochal cyst from development of cholangiocarcinoma. GB, gallbladder; PD, pancreatic duct. (*Figures 79-33, 79-34 and 79-35: courtesy of Dr Srinivas B. Desai, Joslok Hospital, Mumbai, India.*)

the treatment is directed towards its associated complications. The reported incidence of malignancy in Caroli's disease ranges from 7% to 24%, thus MRCP may also be useful in the evaluation of suspected malignancy.[196,212,213]

It is important to demonstrate that the multiple cystic spaces do communicate with the biliary tree to accurately differentiate Caroli's disease from cystic disease of the liver, since polycystic liver disease is one of the most important differential diagnoses. Other differential diagnoses of Caroli's disease include primary sclerosing cholangitis, obstructive bile duct dilatation, choledochal cyst, recurrent pyogenic cholangitis, liver abscesses, and biliary papillomatosis. The ductal dilatation in primary sclerosing cholangitis is rarely saccular and appears more isolated and fusiform, unlike that of Caroli's disease. In patients with biliary obstruction, the dilatation is most marked centrally and tapers towards the periphery in an organized pattern. There are no focal areas of cystic dilatation as in Caroli's disease, where the dilated bile ducts have a random and bizarre pattern with focal areas of cystic ectasia.[218]

Cystic Fibrosis

There are several pancreatic and hepatobiliary manifestations of cystic fibrosis. Exocrine insufficiency of the pancreas is demonstrated in 85% to 90% of patients, whereas endocrine pancreatic insufficiency is less common and occurs in 30% to 50% of patients with cystic fibrosis.[219,220] There is an increased prevalence of chronic liver disease, occurring in up to 24% of patients.[219-221] Features of hepatobiliary involvement in patients with cystic fibrosis include fatty change, focal

biliary cirrhosis, gallbladder wall thickening, cholelithiasis, and abnormalities of the intra- and extrahepatic bile ducts with choledocholithiasis.[219,220]

MRCP is useful in the assessment of patients with cystic fibrosis who present with hepatobiliary symptoms, especially if ultrasound findings are equivocal. Therefore, assessment of disease progression, establishing the presence and severity of biliary complications, and monitoring response to therapy can be performed with MRCP.

In one study, 65% of patients demonstrated abnormalities of the intra- or extrahepatic ducts by MRCP.[219] Typical appearances include beading with strictures or dilatation of the intrahepatic ducts, diffuse narrowing or focal strictures of the common bile duct, and stones in the intra- and extrahepatic bile ducts. The presence of intrahepatic duct calculi is similar to that described in sclerosing cholangitis. MRCP also showed gallbladder abnormalities such as contraction or calculi.[219,221-224] Atresia or stenosis of the cystic duct has also been described in patients with cystic fibrosis, perhaps resulting from inspissated mucus or mucosal hyperplasia.

Abnormalities of the pancreas demonstrated on MR include: 1. fat deposition, best seen as high signal on T1-weighted images; 2. pancreatic fibrosis demonstrated as low signal on both T1- and T2-weighted images; 3. pancreatic cysts; and 4. pancreatic duct abnormalities.

Biliary Atresia

Early and accurate diagnosis of neonatal extrahepatic biliary atresia (EHBA) is important for successful clinical outcome, since it is surgically amenable in infants

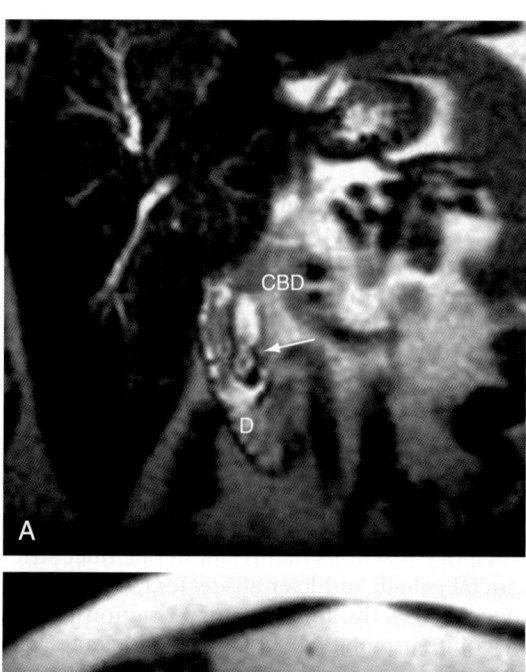

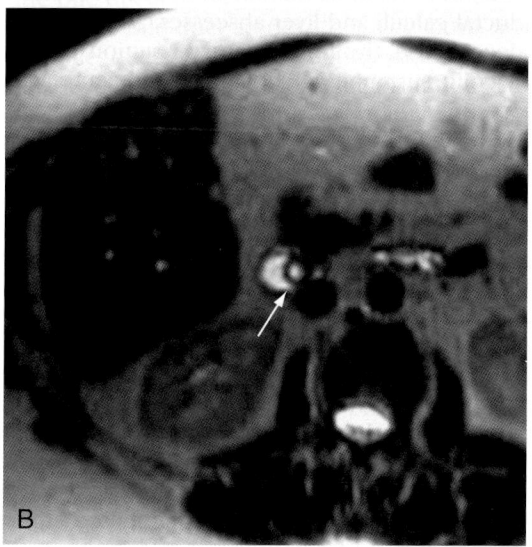

FIGURE 79-36

A and **B,** Choledochocele. **A,** Coronal and **B,** transverse 5 mm SSFSE T2 MRCP (TE 90) demonstrate a cystic dilatation (*arrow*) of the distal common bile duct (CBD) protruding within the wall of the duodenum (D).

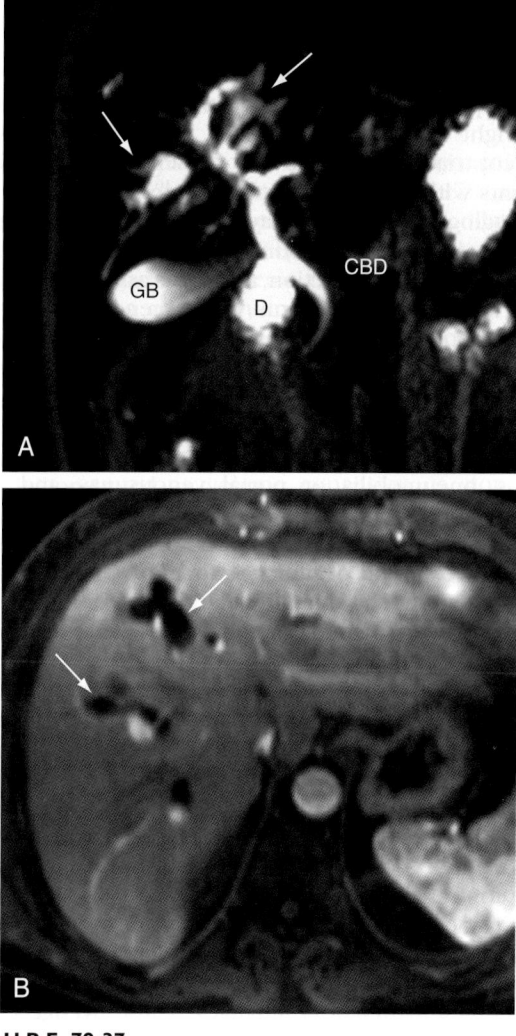

FIGURE 79-37

A and **B,** Caroli's disease. **A,** 40 mm coronal SSFSE RARE SLAB MRCP (TE 969) and **B,** 5 mm transverse fat-suppressed postgadolinium SPGR T1-weighted image demonstrate multiple cystic dilatations (*arrows*) of the intrahepatic bile ducts. CBD, common bile duct; GB, gallbladder; D, duodenum.

younger than 3 months of age.[225,226] Ultrasound has been used for diagnosis, however it only allows limited anatomic delineation of the biliary tree and is often not diagnostic.[227]

ERCP is invasive and subject to substantial morbidity and mortality.[228,229] Liver biopsy is supportive of the clinical diagnosis, but alone is not diagnostic.[230]

MRCP has markedly contributed to the avoidance of exploratory laparotomy and its associated risks.[231] Previous reports showed that MR imaging can reliably diagnose EHBA on the basis of nonvisualization of the CHD or CBD.[232,233] However, another recent study showed that these criteria cannot be relied upon alone since the disease may involve only the proximal extra-hepatic biliary ducts. By using expanded criteria, this study found MRCP to be 82% accurate, 90% sensitive and

77% specific for diagnosing EHBA.[231] The documentation of an intact biliary system is sufficient to exclude EHBA by MRCP.

INFECTIONS OF BILIARY TREE

Ascending Cholangitis

Ascending cholangitis is the infection of either a completely obstructed or partially obstructed biliary tree by gram-negative enteric bacteria. Common causes of obstruction are choledocholithiasis, bile duct strictures and papillary stenosis.[144] In severe cases, the increased pressure within the ducts causes necrosis of the duct wall and reflux of infected bile into the portal triad. This

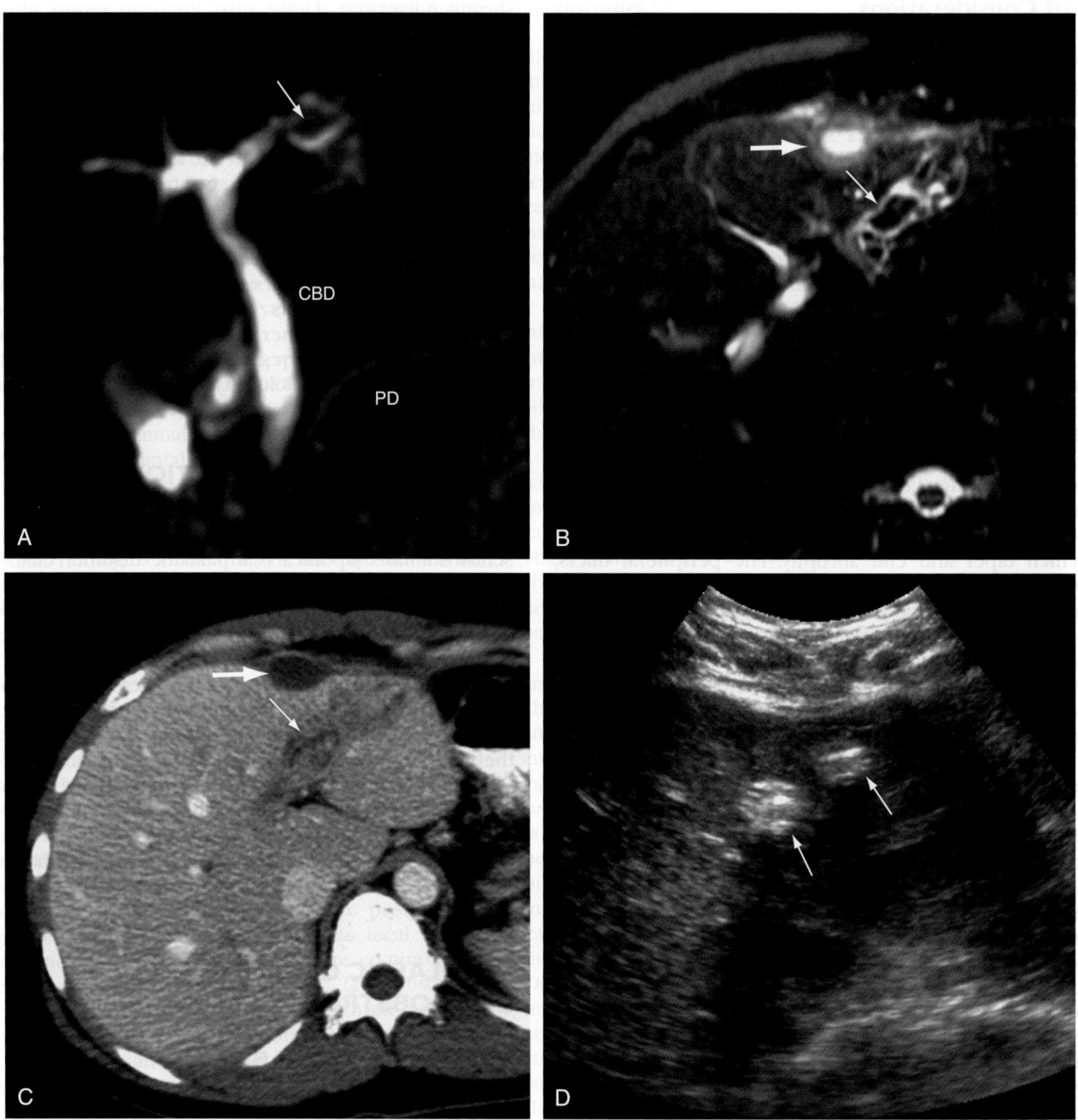

FIGURE 79-38

A, B, C, and **D,** Recurrent pyogenic cholangitis (Oriental cholangiohepatitis). **A,** 40 mm coronal SSFSE RARE SLAB MRCP (TE 969) and **B,** 5 mm transverse fat-suppressed FSE T2 MRCP (TE 140) demonstrate focal dilatation of a segment II duct. There is a focal hypointensity within the lumen consistent with a calculus (*small arrow*). *Large arrow* in **B** and **C** delineates a cholangitic abscess. **C,** Intraductal stone (*small arrow*) is difficult to visualize on 5 mm transverse contrast-enhanced CT scan. **D,** Ultrasound demonstrates the echogenic intrahepatic stones (*small arrows*) with posterior acoustic shadowing. CBD, common bile duct; PD, pancreatic duct.

Cholangiocarcinoma is associated with several predisposing factors, which include: primary sclerosing cholangitis, recurrent pyogenic cholangitis, ulcerative colitis, intrahepatic stone disease, choledochal cysts, clonorchiasis, polyposis syndromes of the colon, choledochoenteric anastomosis and ductal plate malformations (e.g., biliary hamartoma, polycystic disease, congenital hepatic fibrosis, Caroli's disease).[159,258] Several chemical carcinogens are also associated with an increased risk of cholangiocarcinoma such as thorium, radon, nitrosamines and asbestos.

Various histologic types of cholangiocarcinoma are seen at microscopy: ductal (well, moderately or poorly differentiated), papillary, mucinous, signet-ring cell, mucoepidermoid, adenosquamous, squamous, and cystadenocarcinoma.[256,259] Most intra- and extrahepatic cholangiocarcinomas are ductal adenocarcinomas.[256,259]

Cholangiocarcinomas can be classified based on their location as intra- or extrahepatic. A tumor that arises peripheral to the secondary bifurcation of the left or right hepatic duct is considered a peripheral intrahepatic cholangiocarcinoma, whereas a tumor that arises from one of the hepatic ducts or from the bifurcation of the common hepatic duct is considered to be a hilar intrahepatic cholangiocarcinoma (Klatskin tumor). Tumors that originate more distally are referred to as extrahepatic cholangiocarcinomas.[260] The three types of cholangiocarcinoma, i.e., peripheral intrahepatic, hilar intrahepatic, and extrahepatic, are distinct disease entities clinically, therapeutically and radiologically. Peripheral intrahepatic cholangiocarcinoma accounts for 10% of all cholangiocarcinomas, hilar cholangiocarcinoma for 25% and extrahepatic cholangiocarcinoma for 65%.[256] The Liver Cancer Study Group of Japan recently proposed a new classification for intrahepatic cholangiocarcinomas as follows: 1. mass forming; 2. periductal infiltrating; and 3. intraductal intrahepatic cholangiocarcinoma.[261] Periductal infiltrating intrahepatic cholangiocarcinomas are radiologically and pathologically identical to infiltrating hilar cholangiocarcinomas (Klatskin tumor). Intraductal intrahepatic cholangiocarcinomas have a better prognosis and demonstrate a superficial mucosal growth that results in segmental or lobar dilatation of the intrahepatic bile ducts. Cholangiocarcinomas arising in the cystic duct constitute a small percentage of cholangiocarcinomas.[262,263]

MR Considerations

The role of MRI and MRCP in the work-up of patients with suspected cholangiocarcinoma is to establish the diagnosis, assess tumor extension, determine resectability and help in planning the optimal approach for palliative biliary drainage.[264,265] Neither ERCP nor transhepatic cholangiography are accurate in the evaluation of tumors that extend beyond the porta hepatis, since multiple stenoses that isolate the segmental ducts from each other make it difficult to map the entire biliary tree.

For the preoperative evaluation of cholangiocarcinoma, it is important to determine the extent of tumor within the biliary tree, the presence of vascular invasion, hepatic lobar atrophy and metastatic disease. The presence of hepatic lobar atrophy implies portal venous involvement and compels the surgeon to perform a partial hepatectomy. The modified Bismuth/Corlette classification stratifies patients according to the extent of biliary duct involvement by the tumor as follows:

1. Type I involves only the distal common bile duct.
2. Type II involves the confluence of the left and right hepatic duct.
3. Type III involves the confluence and either the right (type IIIA) or the left (type IIIB) hepatic duct.
4. Type IV involves both the left and right secondary confluence.[86,266]

MRCP has a high accuracy for predicting the Bismuth grade of biliary ductal involvement.[265] MRCP provides a complete map of the biliary tree anatomy and a three-dimensional overview with multiplanar imaging capability on both sides of the stricture. Complete tumor staging and assessment of liver involvement, portal nodes, portal veins, and/or hepatic arteries can be obtained from additional MR pulse sequences including fat-suppressed contrast-enhanced T1-weighted gradient-echo sequences.[31]

Peripheral Intrahepatic Cholangiocarcinoma

Peripheral intrahepatic cholangiocarcinomas, as discussed earlier in this section, are further classified into three fundamental subtypes: 1. mass forming; 2. periductal infiltrating; and 3. intraductal intrahepatic cholangiocarcinomas. The mass-forming type presents as a definite tumor mass located in the liver parenchyma. The periductal-infiltrating type extends longitudinally along the bile duct, often resulting in dilatation of the peripheral intrahepatic bile ducts. The intraductal intrahepatic type proliferates toward the lumen of the bile duct, giving the appearance of a papillary projection or tumor thrombus.[267]

The peripheral mass-forming intrahepatic cholangiocarcinoma is the most common type of intrahepatic cholangiocarcinoma and is the second most common primary liver tumor after hepatocellular carcinoma.[260] It constitutes approximately 10% of all cholangiocarcinomas. Peripheral mass-forming cholangiocarcinoma manifests as a large tumor mass at diagnosis, because it is rarely symptomatic early on in its course. There is a propensity of the tumor to invade the adjacent peripheral branches of the portal vein.[268-270] Significant biliary obstruction only results in the late stage, when the tumor causes obstruction of the common hepatic duct by direct invasion or by metastases to hilar lymph nodes.[271] Peripheral cholangiocarcinomas are sclerosing tumors with variable degrees of differentiation. Most are well differentiated, forming ducts and dense fibrous stroma.[272]

The MR imaging appearance of peripheral mass-forming cholangiocarcinomas is influenced by the amount of fibrosis, necrosis and mucinous material within the tumor.[273] Peripheral mass-forming intrahepatic cholangiocarcinoma most frequently presents as a large tumor mass with a circumscribed and lobulated appearance. The tumor is hypointense on T1-weighted images and hyperintense on T2-weighted images. T2-weighted images may show areas of hypointensity, corresponding to fibrosis. On dynamic MR imaging studies, enhancement patterns frequently vary by size of the tumor. Small tumors (2 to 4 cm) may enhance homogeneously and simulate a hepatocellular carcinoma.[274] Larger tumors show peripheral enhancement, followed by progressive and concentric filling in of the tumor with contrast material.[275,276] Delayed enhancement with areas of incomplete fill-in is characteristic of peripheral cholangiocarcinoma. The enhancement pattern likely reflects the peripheral neovascularity and large amount of fibrous tissue within the lesion.[273,277,278] The central scar may show enhancement on delayed images and becomes isointense with the tumor rather than hyperintense, as is seen in focal nodular hyperplasia.[275] Ancillary findings in the peripheral mass-forming cholangiocarcinoma include dilatation with thickening of the peripheral intrahepatic ducts and capsular retraction.[260,279,280]

The periductal infiltrating intrahepatic cholangiocarcinoma is radiologically and pathologically identical to infiltrating hilar cholangiocarcinoma (Klatskin tumor), but is located peripherally. The periductal infiltrating cholangiocarcinoma is small and grows along the bile ducts. There is irregular narrowing of the involved bile duct, leading to obstruction. It tends to spread along the bile duct wall via the nerve and perineural tissues of the Glisson capsule toward the porta hepatis. During the later stage the tumor may invade the hepatic parenchyma, as well as the hilum, and transform into an exophytic hilar cholangiocarcinoma.[259,281]

Intraductal intrahepatic cholangiocarcinoma has a better prognosis than other types of cholangiocarcinoma. At histological analysis, this type of tumor is generally considered to be a papillary cholangiocarcinoma and constitutes 8% to 18% of resected cholangiocarcinomas.[273] This tumor has a superficial mucosal growth that results in segmental or lobar dilatation of the intrahepatic bile ducts. The intraductal mass can appear as an enhancing soft-tissue mass. The mass is confined within the bile ducts and thus the wall of the bile duct remains intact.

Hilar Cholangiocarcinoma

Hilar cholangiocarcinoma accounts for more than 50% of all large bile duct malignancies.[260,282,283] These tumors are usually small at diagnosis since they typically present early with biliary obstruction, jaundice or cholangitis. The most common type of hilar cholangiocarcinoma (Klatskin tumor) is an infiltrating cholangiocarcinoma in 70% of cases. On MRCP, hilar cholangiocarcinoma appears as a moderately irregular thickening of the bile duct wall (3 to 5 mm), with dilation of the intrahepatic bile ducts (Fig. 79-39).[284] High-grade obstruction disproportionate to the degree of duct wall thickening may be a feature of cholangiocarcinoma. On MR imaging, the lesion appears hypointense on T1-weighted images and has moderately high-signal intensity on T2-weighted images. Hilar cholangiocarcinomas do not show any typical enhancement pattern. However, these

are typically hypovascular tumors compared with the adjacent liver parenchyma and show a heterogeneous enhancement that peaks on delayed images.[285] This pattern is consistent with the fibrous nature of the tumor. Other findings may also include periductal enhancement. Increased intrahepatic duct wall enhancement has been observed proximal to the tumor, however, as an isolated finding may not be a predictor of tumor involvement. The increased enhancement of the duct wall may be due to fibrosis, or inflammation resulting from obstruction, and may be particularly prominent following placement of biliary stents.[286]

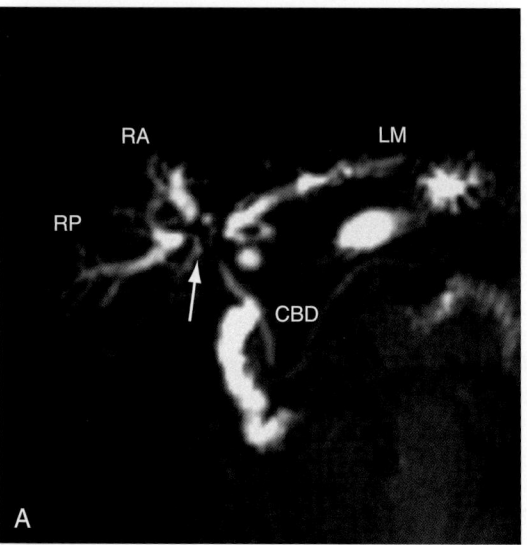

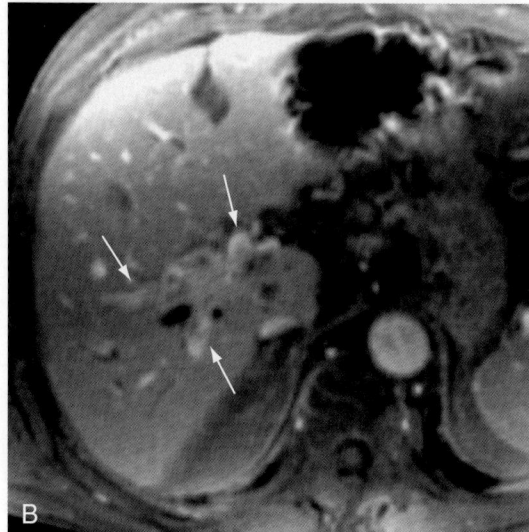

FIGURE 79-39

A and **B,** Hilar cholangiocarcinoma: periductal-infiltrating type. **A,** 40 mm coronal SSFSE RARE SLAB MRCP (TE 969) depicts intrahepatic bile duct dilatation from hilar obstruction (*large arrow*). The right and left main ducts are noncommunicating. RA, right anterior; RP, right posterior; LM, left main. **B,** 5 mm transverse fat-suppressed postgadolinium SPGR T1-weighted image demonstrates infiltrating, periductal tumoral enhancement at the level of the hilum and intrahepatic bile ducts (*small arrows*). CBD, common bile duct.

Additional MR imaging findings include segmental/lobar atrophy of the liver secondary to portal vein invasion, or secondary to right or left ductal obstruction (Fig. 79-40).

The prognosis of hilar cholangiocarcinoma is worse than a tumor close to the papilla. The radiological criteria for unresectability are:

1. Hepatic duct involvement up to secondary biliary radicals bilaterally.
2. Encasement or occlusion of the main portal vein, proximal to the bifurcation.
3. Atrophy of one hepatic lobe with encasement of contralateral portal vein branch.
4. Atrophy of one hepatic lobe with contralateral involvement of secondary biliary radicals.
5. Distal metastasis to the peritoneum, liver or lungs.

Unilateral portal vein or hepatic artery occlusion, unilateral hepatic metastasis, vascular compression or infiltration of fat planes adjacent to nonvascular structures are not considered contraindications to curative resection.[287-290] Most cholangiocarcinomas extend beyond the porta hepatis at the time of diagnosis and result in unresectability. Patients who undergo complete resection of the tumor have a 5-year survival rate of 10% to 50%. There is better prognosis in the postoperative period if the primary tumor is in the distal bile duct, compared to the hilar region or middle third of the duct.[159,290]

Extrahepatic Cholangiocarcinoma

Extrahepatic cholangiocarcinoma can present with three different morphological patterns: 1. infiltrating stenotic

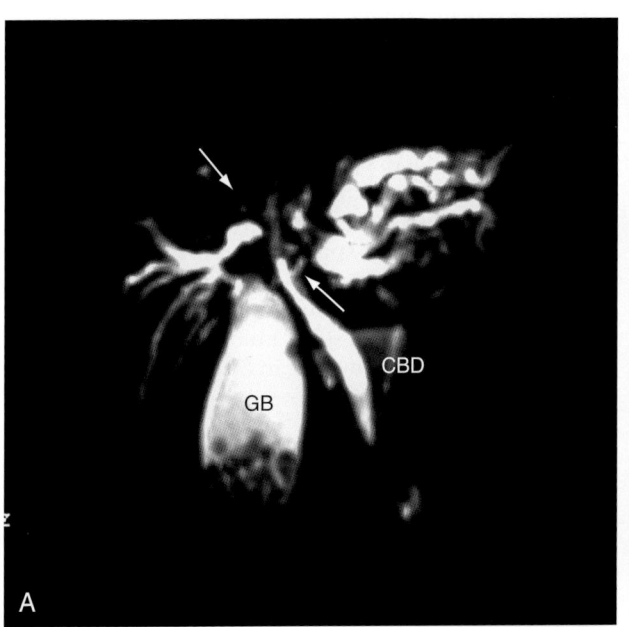

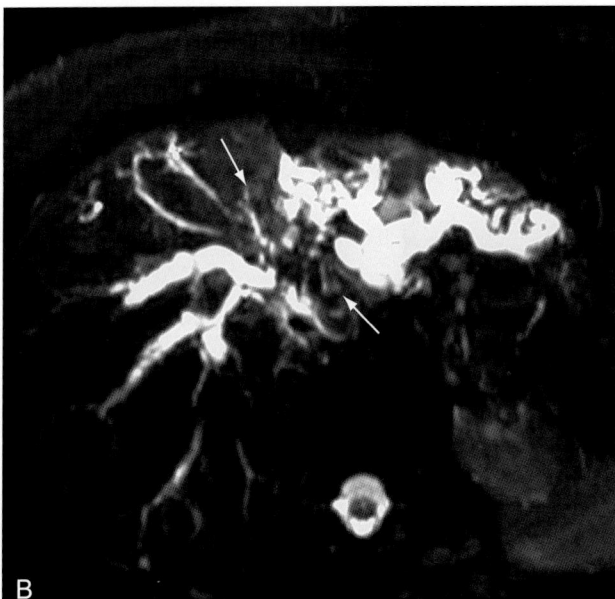

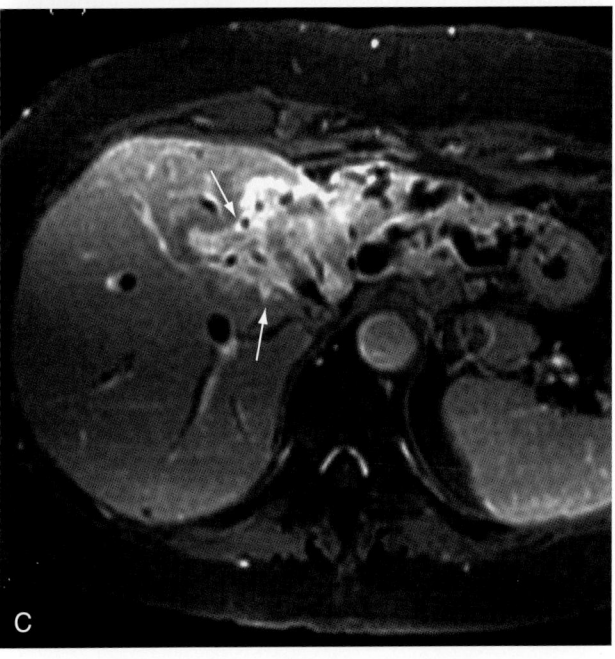

FIGURE 79-40

A, B and **C,** Hilar cholangiocarcinoma: lobar atrophy. **A,** 40 mm coronal SSFSE RARE SLAB MRCP (TE 969) and **B,** 5 mm fat-suppressed transverse FSE T2 MRCP (TE 140) demonstrate a malignant stricture (*arrows*) involving the hepatic hilum. The left and right ducts are noncommunicating and there is intrahepatic bile duct dilatation. In addition, there is atrophy of the left lobe of the liver. Incidentally, there are multiple gallstones. **C,** 5 mm transverse fat-suppressed postgadolinium SPGR T1-weighted image demonstrates diffuse and delayed enhancement (*arrows*) of the hilar cholangiocarcinoma. CBD, common bile duct; GB, gallbladder.

type; 2. bulky exophytic type; and 3. intraluminal polypoid or papillary type.[133,263,290] The infiltrating extrahepatic type manifests as a mass lesion or wall thickening (Fig. 79-41) with lumen replacement. This is the most common type of extrahepatic cholangiocarcinoma occurring in up to 75% of cases. At times, it is very difficult to assess the true extent of the tumor, even with high-quality MRCP; therefore, biopsy is often necessary before curative resection is performed. On magnetic resonance imaging (MRI), ductal tumors arising from the intrapancreatic portion of the CBD are seen as low-signal intensity masses against the high-

signal intensity background of the pancreas on unenhanced and enhanced T1-weighted fat-suppressed images.[291]

Polypoid Cholangiocarcinoma

Polypoid cholangiocarcnioma is an uncommon subtype and can arise from both intra- and extrahepatic bile ducts. Histologically these tumors are papillary adenocarcinomas that present as intraluminal growth.[258] On MRCP, this may present as a polypoid filling defect within the dilated lumen of the involved hepatic segment or hepatic lobe. The tumor may also demonstrate superficial spreading with diffuse involvement, and may be depicted as multiple polypoid filling defects (papillomatosis).[292] On post-gadolinium fat-suppressed T1-weighted images, there is enhancement of the intraductal mass. The mass is confined within the bile ducts, and thus the wall of the bile duct remains intact.

Mucin-hypersecreting Cholangiocarcinoma

There are two histological types (papillary and biliary), which can produce significant amounts of mucin, and result in bile stasis and obstructive jaundice.[293] At imaging, the tumor can present either as an intraluminal, polypoid lesion or can spread along the mucosal surface of the bile ducts. There can be diffuse dilatation of the intra- and extrahepatic ducts, both proximal and distal to the tumor, due to excessive mucin production. Mucin within the dilated bile ducts can be seen as filling defects at MRCP.

Squamous Cell Carcinoma

Squamous cell carcinoma is considered to be adenocarcinoma that is entirely replaced by a squamous element.[258] This subtype of tumor is prone to develop into an advanced stage of cholangiocarcinoma. They present with large tumor size and aggressive intrahepatic spreading.[256] The imaging findings resemble peripheral cholangiocarcinomas.

Differential Diagnosis of Cholangiocarcinoma

Hepatocellular carcinoma typically shows heterogeneous enhancement on the immediate postgadolinium images and early washout due to its hypervascularity.[284] Another differentiating feature is that hepatocellular carcinoma is associated with vascular invasion and cirrhotic livers, whereas choloangiocarcinoma usually is not. Hepatocellular carcinoma occasionally invades and grows within the bile duct as a polypoid mass expanding the bile duct, and in this setting may be difficult to differentiate from polypoid cholangiocarcinoma.

Cholangiohepatocellular carcinoma (combined hepatocellular carcinoma and cholangiocarcinoma) is a rare primary liver cancer that contains unequivocal elements of both hepatocellular carcinoma and cholangiocarcinoma.[294,295] Findings resemble those of hepatocellular carcinoma or cholangiocarcinoma, depending on the dominant component.

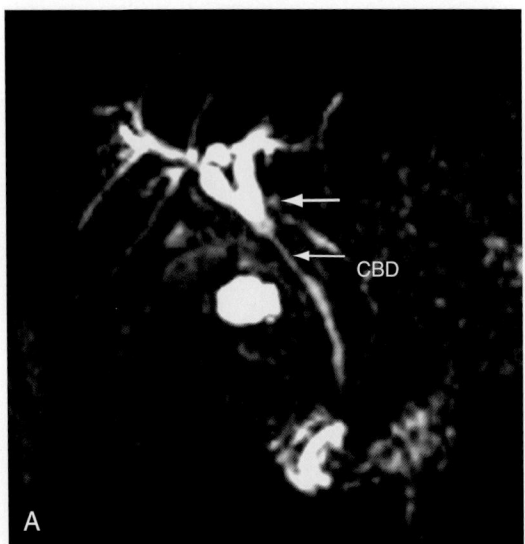

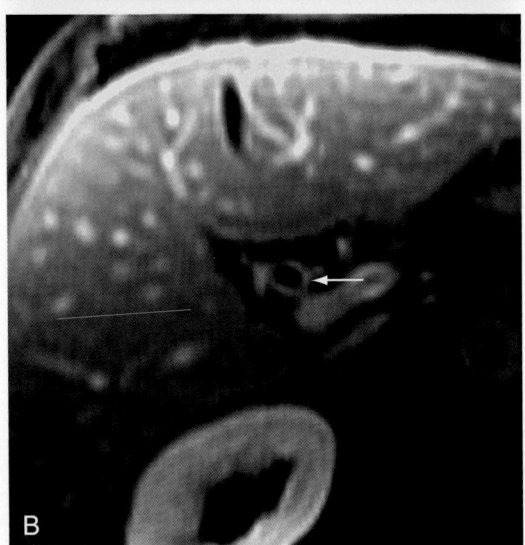

FIGURE 79-41

A and **B,** Extrahepatic cholangiocarcinoma. **A,** 40 mm coronal SSFSE RARE SLAB MRCP (TE 969) demonstrates dilatation of the common hepatic (*large arrow*) and intrahepatic bile ducts. There is a smooth stricture (*small arrow*) in the proximal common bile duct (CBD). **B,** 5 mm transverse fat-suppressed postgadolinium SPGR T1-weighted image obtained at the level of the common hepatic duct (CHD) proximal to the stricture demonstrates enhancement. This is consistent with proximal tumor extension in the dilated segment of the CHD.

Hilar cholangiocarcinoma can have a similar appearance to gallbladder carcinoma, Mirizzi syndrome and idiopathic benign focal stenosis (malignant masquerade). Exploration is indicated in all patients with suspicious hilar lesions, since relying only on biliary brush cytology or percutaneous liver biopsy may be misleading.

Metastatic adenocarcinoma to the liver can mimic exophytic peripheral cholangiocarcinoma. Ancillary findings, which indicate the presence of underlying bile duct disease such as clonorchiasis, recurrent pyogenic cholangitis, and primary sclerosing cholangitis are helpful in differentiating the two conditions.

Benign biliary tumors, such as papillomas and adenomas, may be difficult to distinguish from malignancy. In the presence of benign-appearing strictures from recurrent pyogenic cholangitis and sclerosing cholangitis, for example, underlying malignancy may be difficult to exclude. Other causes of benign strictures to consider are posttraumatic, and post-surgical sequelae, strictures secondary to chronic pancreatitis (Fig. 79-42) and papillary stenosis.

Periampullary and Ampullary Carcinoma

Periampullary carcinoma comprises carcinomas of the ampulla of Vater, distal common bile duct, head and uncinate process of the pancreas, and the duodenum. Recent reports have advocated that ampullary carcinoma should be classified as duodenal cancers, rather than cancers of the distal common bile duct.[296] A

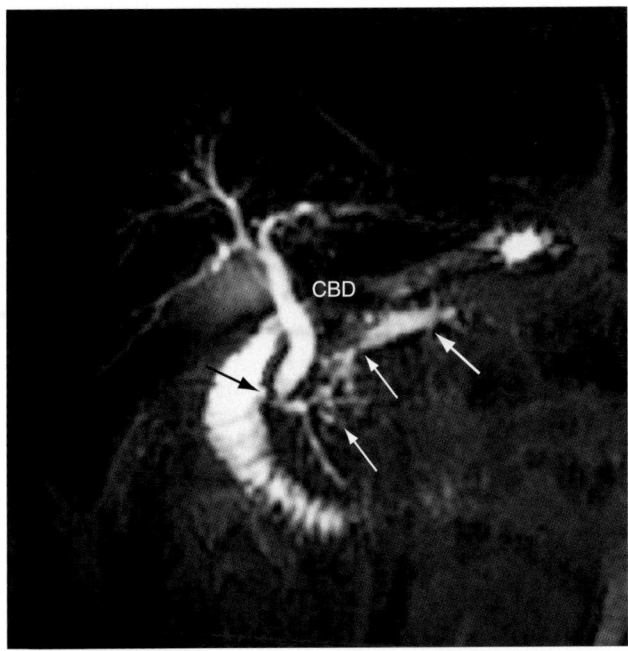

FIGURE 79-42

Stricture of distal CBD in chronic pancreatitis. 40 mm coronal RARE SSFSE SLAB MRCP (TE 969) demonstrates dilatation of the pancreatic duct (*large arrow*) in the distal body. There are strictures involving the pancreatic duct at the level of the head and proximal body (*small white arrows*), and also involving the distal common bile duct (CBD) (*black arrow*).

common ampulla is not present in 40% of the population, but the biliary and pancreatic ducts drain separately into the duodenum. Therefore, it is often difficult to discern the origin based on clinical findings, results of preoperative imaging, and in some cases, even surgical specimens are nonconclusive.[297]

Predisposing factors include ulcerative colitis, Gardner's syndrome and chronic inflammatory changes secondary to congenital choledochocele. *Ascaris* infection also increases the risk of ampullary carcinoma. An indication for the presence of cancer in these patients is a sudden change in clinical course or sudden development of jaundice. Periampullary tumors share similar clinical presentations and can become clinically symptomatic even when they are only a few millimeters in size. Dilatation of the biliary tree and the pancreatic duct are observed; this occurs relatively early in the course of these tumors, which probably accounts, in part, for their better prognosis.

Periampullary carcinoma has a 5-year survival rate of up to 85%.[298] Overall survival is highest for ampullary and duodenal cancers, intermediate for bile duct cancers and lowest for those with pancreatic cancers.[299,300] It has been shown that distal bile duct cancers are more often resectable and less frequently demonstrate tumor spread to adjacent lymph nodes compared to pancreatic cancers.[301,302] For this reason, aggressive surgical resection is indicated in ampullary or periampullary cancers, even in the presence of positive lymph nodes at preoperative staging.

Ampullary carcinomas are usually adenocarcinomas and account for approximately 4% of periampullary tumors.[42] Papillary or polypoid cancers occur more commonly as ampullary and duodenal carcinomas, and these tend to have a better prognosis than invasive or infiltrative cancers. Lymphatic spread and perineural invasion occur infrequently in ampullary cancers.

Transabdominal ultrasound, CT, MRI and endoscopy are used in the investigation of periampullary masses. CT was found to detect the primary tumor in only 64% of cases.[303] The most reliable technique for detection and staging of these tumors is endoscopic ultrasound. ERCP provides a direct endoscopic view of the ampulla in all cases and allows a biopsy of suspicious lesions, whereas the major papilla is visualized on MRCP in only 40% of patients.[88]

MR Considerations

A reasonable approach for the noninvasive evaluation of biliary obstruction due to periampullary disease is the combination of MRCP and conventional MR imaging (Fig. 79-43).[83,304-306] On T1-weighted fat-suppressed images, periampullary carcinomas typically appear as small low-signal intensity masses. Periampullary carcinomas enhance minimally on early postgadolinium images, because of their hypovascularity, compared to the increased enhancement of the surrounding pancreatic parenchyma.[305] A relatively specific finding on the 2-minute postgadolinium fat-suppressed images is a thin rim of enhancement along the periphery of these tumors.[88]

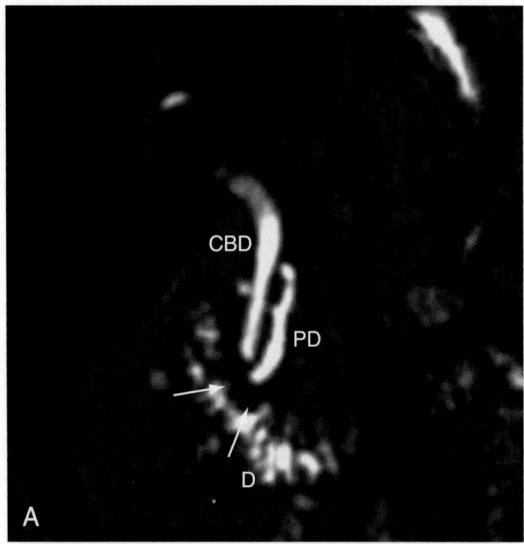

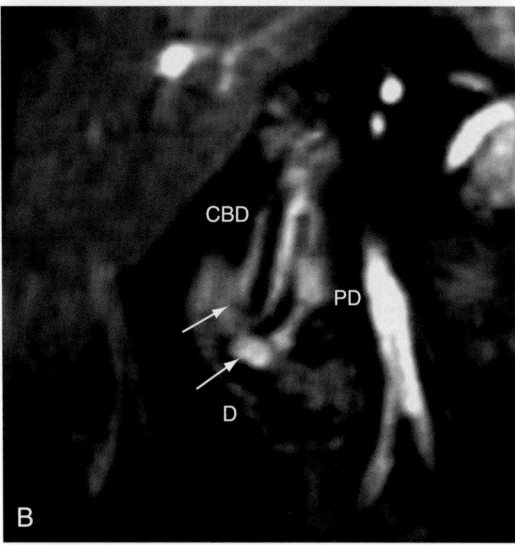

FIGURE 79-43

A and **B,** Periampullary tumor: duodenal carcinoid. **A,** 10 mm coronal SSFSE RARE SLAB MRCP (TE 969) demonstrates a plaque-like infiltrating hypointense lesion in the periampullary region (*arrows*). There is mild dilatation of both the common bile duct (CBD) and pancreatic duct (PD). **B,** 5 mm coronal fat-suppressed postgadolinium SPGR T1-weighted image demonstrates the enhancing tumor (*arrows*) involving the periampullary region. D, duodenum.

Approximately 60% of patients with ampullary carcinoma have a discrete nodular mass with an irregular filling defect at the distal portion of the pancreatico-biliary junction at MR imaging (Fig. 79-44). Irregular periductal thickening can be seen around the pancreaticobiliary junction in 20% of ampullary carcinomas.[83,304-306] However, MR imaging cannot reliably indicate malignancy by changes in signal intensity, and differentiation of ampullary carcinomas from rare benign tumors is difficult. In some patients, the only sign of ampullary carcinoma is a prominence, or bulging appearance of the duodenal papilla formed by protrusion of the dilated biliary or pancreatic duct. In this situation, it is difficult

to differentiate ampullary carcinoma from biliary dyskinesia, benign ampullary stenosis, choledochocele or pancreatitis.[307] Enlargement of the ampulla is a non-specific sign and can be seen in benign inflammatory changes such as choledocholithiasis (Fig. 79-25).[40] Marked and abrupt dilatation of the distal common bile duct or the pancreatic duct at MRCP is suggestive of ampullary carcinoma in the absence of stone disease or pancreatitis. In patients with reduced signal intensity of the pancreas on the precontrast T1-weighted images due to pancreatic duct obstruction, the conspicuity of periampullary carcinomas is diminished.

In patients with distal bile duct carcinoma, MRCP may demonstrate abrupt tapering of the common bile duct (Fig. 79-45). At kinematic MRCP, certain configurations of the distal bile and pancreatic ducts are more predictive of malignancy including a beak sign (most common), followed by a blunted, and rat-tail appearance. In patients with periampullary carcinomas of bile duct origin, the distal segment of the bile duct below the obstructive lesion may also be seen. This results in the "three-segment sign" (the proximal and distal segments of the bile duct and the main pancreatic duct), as opposed to the "four-segment sign", which relates to pancreatic carcinoma, (two bile duct segments and two pancreatic duct segments) (Fig. 79-46).[61] In addition to luminal obliteration, 90% of patients with distal bile duct cancer demonstrate ductal wall thickening.[61] A narrow lumen is well-depicted on MRCP or T2-weighted SSFSE images. However, a thickened ductal wall is best seen on Gd-enhanced dynamic MR images. A polypoid-type carcinoma is well visualized on MRCP and T2-weighted images as an intraductal polypoid mass. Distal common bile duct carcinomas that invade the surrounding pancreatic parenchyma are difficult to differentiate from pancreatic carcinoma. These cancers have a prognosis similar to that of pancreatic carcinoma.[61,297]

Kinematic MRCP plays a useful role in differentiating between pathologic stenosis and physiologic narrowing of the sphincteric segment.[59,65] On kinematic MRCP images, the lack of visualization of sphincteric relaxation has a sensitivity of 88% and a specificity of 100% for the diagnosis of periampullary lesions. In a study by Kim et al, biliary intervention at the sphincter level was required in most patients whose images did not show sphincteric relaxation.[59]

In summary, for differentiation of periampullary tumors, MRCP and conventional MR imaging are useful in determining the mass location, shape and pattern of biliary and pancreatic ductal dilatation. MRCP may show the effects of the tumor mass on the adjacent bile duct and pancreatic duct, however, it frequently fails to demonstrate the actual tumor mass. Endoscopic ultrasound is still the most reliable technique for detecting and staging ampullary and periampullary tumors.[308]

Miscellaneous Bile Duct Tumors

Other reported primary tumors of the bile ducts are rare and include lymphoma, mucus-secreting papillary adenocarcinoma, carcinoid and squamous cell carcinoma.[309-311] Secondary malignant involvement by

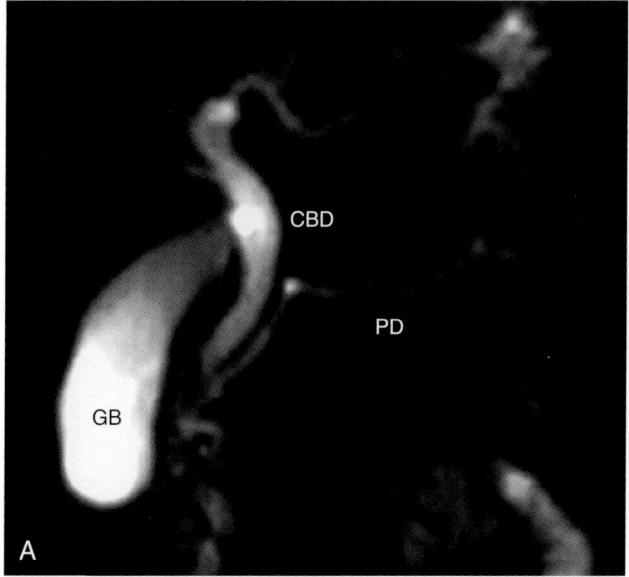

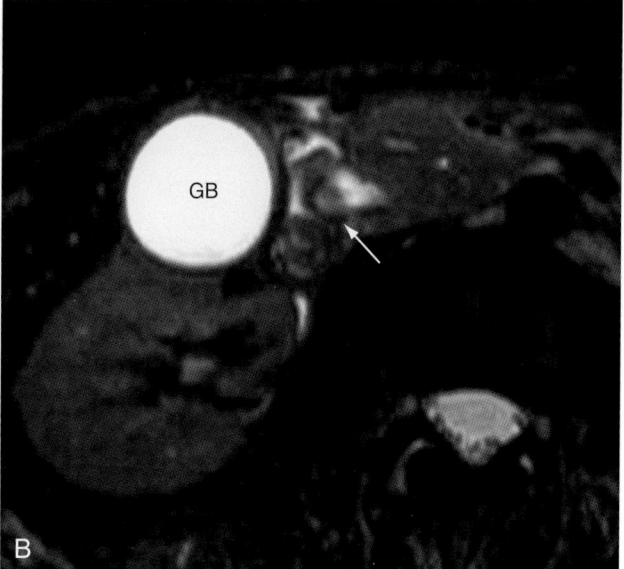

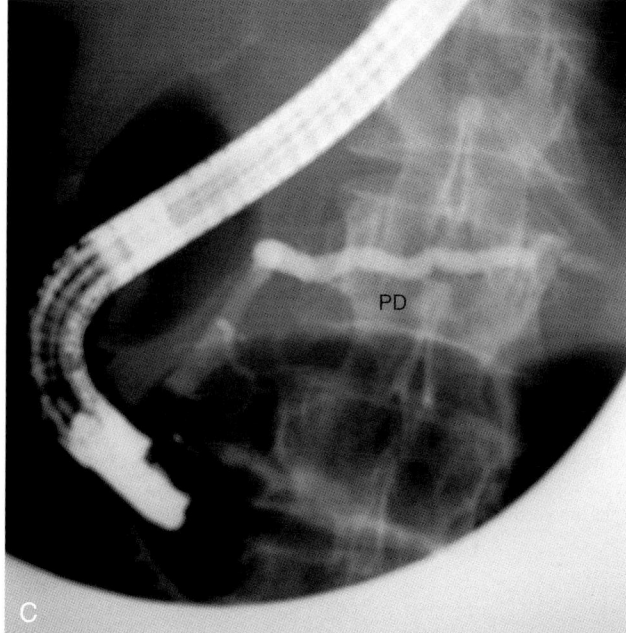

FIGURE 79-44

A and **B,** Periampullary carcinoma. **A,** 40 mm coronal SSFSE RARE SLAB MRCP (TE 969) demonstrates a stricture involving both the distal common bile duct (CBD) and pancreatic duct (PD). **B,** 5 mm transverse fat-suppressed FSE T2 MRCP (TE 140) demonstrates a hypointense, infiltrating periampullary tumor (*arrow*). **C,** There was failed cannulation of the CBD at ERCP. The PD is mildly dilated and filled with contrast. GB, gallbladder.

FIGURE 79-45

Distal bile duct carcinoma. 70 mm coronal SSFSE RARE SLAB MRCP (TE 969) demonstrates marked biliary dilatation secondary to a malignant stricture of the intrapancreatic portion of the common bile duct (CBD) Note the abrupt margin. PD, pancreatic duct.

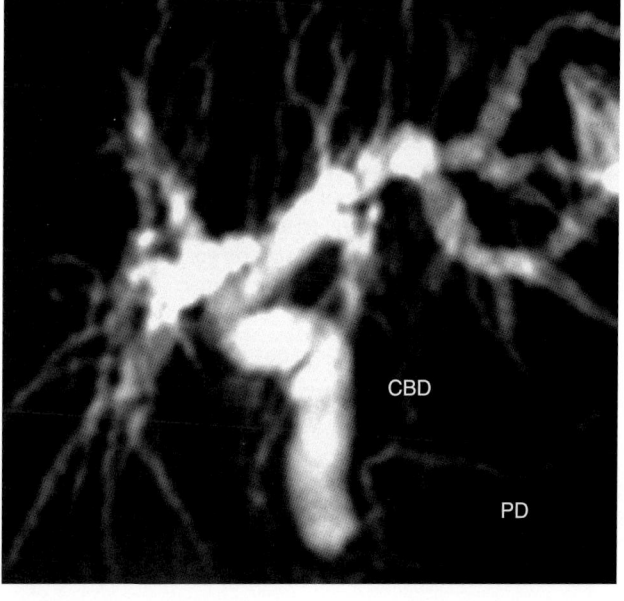

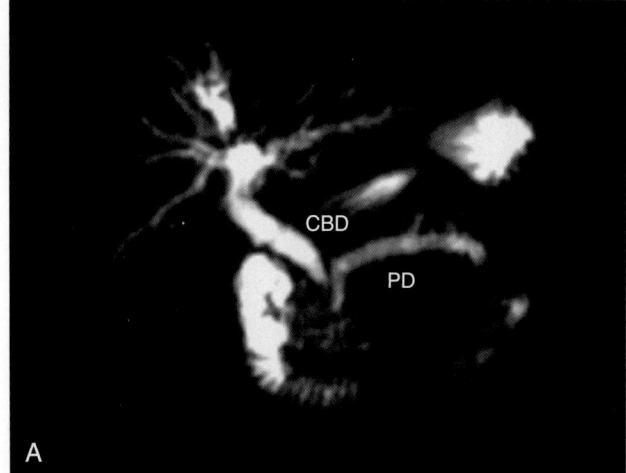

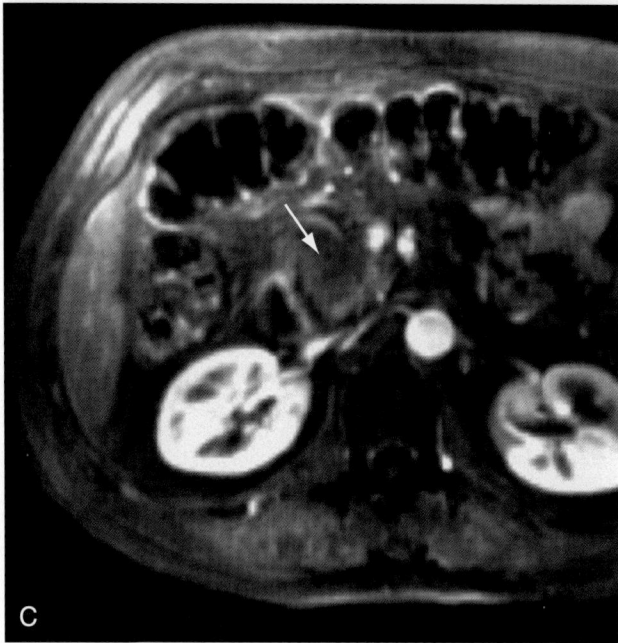

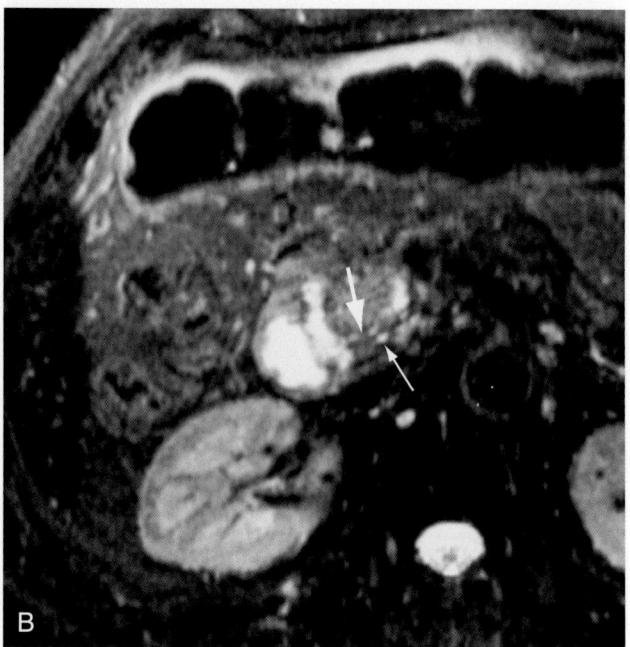

FIGURE 79-46

A, B and **C,** Periampullary tumor: pancreatic carcinoma. **A,** 40 mm coronal SSFSE RARE SLAB MRCP (TE 969) demonstrates a dilated common bile duct (CBD) and pancreatic duct (PD). There is a stricture involving the distal aspect of both ducts. **B,** 5 mm transverse fat-suppressed FSE T2 MRCP (TE 140) demonstrates a hypointense tumor in the head of the pancreas resulting in a stricture of the intrapancreatic portion of CBD (*large arrow*) and ventral PD (*small arrow*). **C,** 5 mm transverse fat-suppressed postgadolinium SPGR T1-weighted image demonstrates poor enhancement of the tumor mass (*arrow*) compared to the normal pancreatic parenchyma.

metastases to the bile ducts results from direct invasion by hepatocellular, gallbladder, or pancreatic carcinoma, or rarely from hematogenous spread by other tumors such as malignant melanoma. Metastases to the bile ducts do not have a specific appearance on MRCP, but may simulate findings of PSC. Bile duct obstruction by extrinsic compression from lymph node metastasis to the porta, hepatoduodenal, or gastrohepatic ligaments is another rare neoplastic cause of bile duct obstruction.[312]

Benign Tumors and Tumor-like Lesions of Bile Ducts

Benign tumors and tumor-like lesions of the bile ducts may mimic the more ominous malignant neoplasms that can develop in the same locations. These can be solitary or multiple. Benign epithelial tumors include extra-

hepatic bile duct adenomas, biliary papillomatosis and biliary cyst adenomas. Nonepithelial tumors include granular cell tumors, neurofibromas and neurofibromatosis.[313] An example of a tumor-like lesion is heterotopia caused by heterotopic gastric, hepatic or pancreatic mucosa. Adrenal heterotopia has also been reported in the literature.[313] Within the bile ducts, gastric heterotopia has a smooth intraluminal polypoid appearance with proximal ductal dilatation.[313]

Extrahepatic Bile Duct Adenomas

Extrahepatic bile duct adenomas are relatively rare. An increased prevalence is seen in patients with familial adenomatous polyposis, Gardner's syndrome and Peutz-Jeghers syndrome.[313] Patients typically present early with signs and symptoms of biliary obstruction. These tumors may involve both the intra- and extrahepatic bile

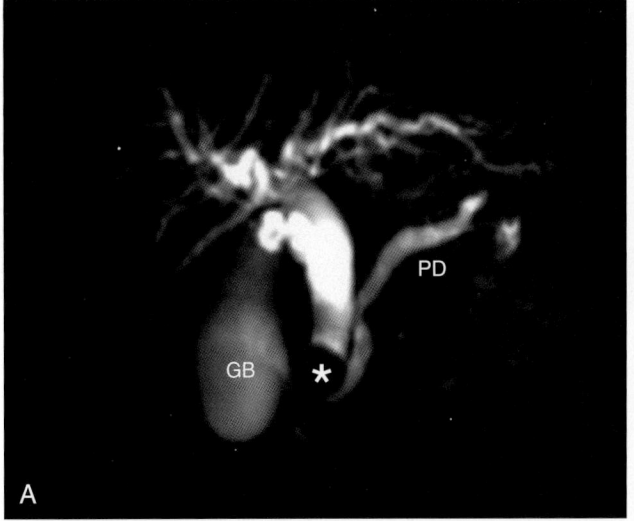

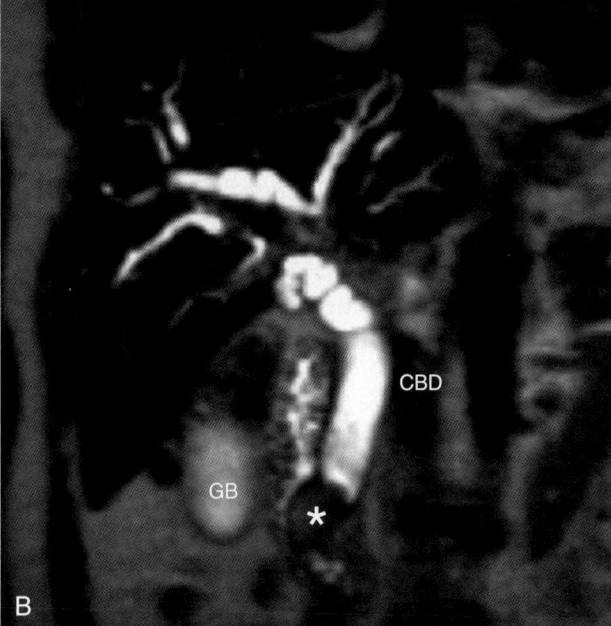

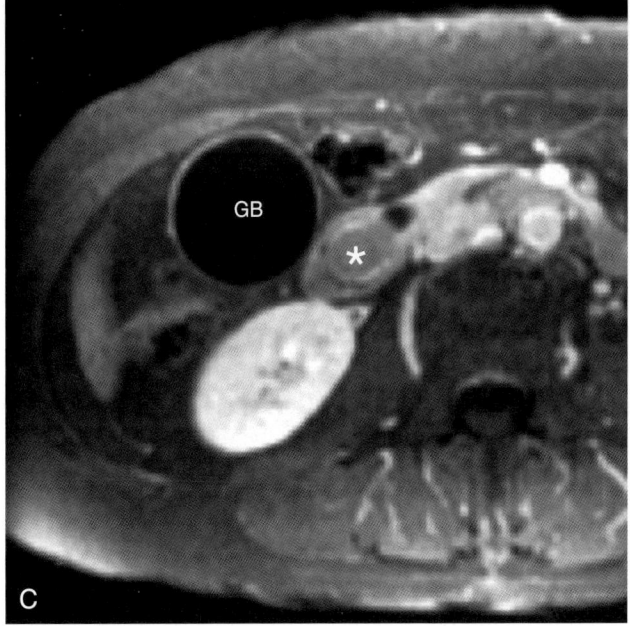

FIGURE 79-47

A, B and **C,** Periampullary tumor: villous adenoma with high-grade dysplasia. **A,** 40 mm coronal SSFSE RARE SLAB MRCP (TE 969) and **B,** 5 mm coronal SSFSE (TE 180) demonstrate dilatation of the intra- and extrahepatic bile ducts to the level of the ampulla. There is also dilatation of the pancreatic duct (PD). There is a polypoid hypointense lesion(*) at the ampulla. **C,** 5 mm transverse fat-suppressed postgadolinium SPGR T1-weighted image demonstrates a mildly enhancing tumor mass. (*) CBD, common bile duct; GB, gallbladder.

ducts. They are most commonly located in the common bile duct, with the majority being tubular adenomas. The papillary tumor of the bile duct is an intraductal tumor with innumerable frond-like papillary projections that are friable and slough easily. The sloughed tumor fragments may float within the bile ducts and result in intermittent partial biliary obstruction or may mimic bile duct stones at cholangiography. Occasionally, this tumor spreads superficially along the mucosa, forming multiple tumors (papillomatosis).[314,315] Papillary adenomas may develop into papillary adenocarcinoma, which involves the mucosa and penetrates the bile duct wall in its late phase.[270,316]

On CT, the tumors are either enhancing or nonenhancing depending on whether the tumor is fixed or detached from the wall. At times it may be difficult to differentiate these tumors from intrahepatic bile duct stones. On cholangiogram, these tumors manifest as single or multiple nodular filling defects with ragged or serrated bile duct walls over a variable length. Tumor fragments may drain through the orifice of the papilla of Vater and then disappear.[316]

On MRCP, the tumor manifests as: 1. thickening or irregularity of the bile duct wall; and 2. as a fixed or sloughed intraductal mass within the bile duct. The filling defect may have a smooth or lobular contour (in tubular adenomas) (Fig. 79-47), or a cauliflower contour (in papillary adenomas). In patients with papillary neoplasms, the extrahepatic bile ducts are typically dilated to the level of the ampulla, irrespective of the location of the papillary tumor. Papillary adenocarcinomas produce profuse amounts of mucus and this may manifest as a mucus cast on MRCP.[270,317] On rare occasions in the appropriate clinical setting, the differential diagnosis includes hepatocellular carcinoma that can grow intraductally and detach from the bile duct wall.[318]

Biliary Papillomatosis

Biliary papillomatosis is a rare disorder that was first described in 1959 by Caroli.[319] Patients present with signs and symptoms of biliary obstruction, often complicated by cholangitis. Biliary papillomatosis is characterized by bile duct dilatation and multiple mucin-secreting papillary adenomas. Biliary papillomatosis mainly involves the extrahepatic bile ducts; however, the intrahepatic bile ducts, cystic duct, gallbladder and pancreatic duct may also be affected. Papillomatosis has a greater potential for malignant transformation than a solitary adenoma.[313] There is a paucity of literature on the MR imaging findings of biliary papillomatosis.[320,321] These lesions typically are hypointense on T1-weighted images, slightly hyperintense to adjacent liver parenchyma on T2-weighted images, and do not show significant enhancement on postgadolinium sequences.[313,315]

Biliary Cystadenomas

Biliary cystadenomas are uncommon, benign tumors that present either as unilocular, or multilocular cystic lesions in the liver, extrahepatic bile ducts or gallbladder.[322,323] In a series reported by Devaney et al,[324] it was shown that 83% of biliary cystadenomas were located within the liver, 13% in the extrahepatic bile ducts and only one case (0.02%) in the gallbladder. Complete surgical excision is necessary for accurate diagnosis and treatment. Although biliary cystadenomas are benign tumors, they may recur after excision and also have the potential to transform into biliary cystadenocarcinoma.[325]

The MR signal intensity of biliary cystadenoma varies on both T1- and T2-weighted images depending on the content of the cyst fluid.[326,327] In general, mucinous fluid within a biliary cystadenoma appears hypointense on T1-weighted and markedly hyperintense on T2-weighted images.[322,326] However, as the protein concentration increases within the cyst, the signal intensity becomes hyperintense on T1-weighted images and may become markedly hypointense on T2-weighted images.[328] Similar changes can occur secondary to hemorrhage within the cyst. However, usually fluid/fluid levels are present in this setting.[329,330]

In a small percentage of cases, communication between the biliary cystadenoma and the biliary tree exists.[313] In these cases, the mucus secreted by these tumors gives rise to filling defects within the biliary tree and may result in bile duct obstruction. Other causes of bile duct obstruction in the setting of a biliary cystadenoma are extrinsic compression of the bile duct or the presence of an intraductal component. It is not possible to reliably differentiate between a biliary cystadenoma and cystadenocarcinoma. Nevertheless, cystadenocarcinomas tend to be thick-walled and may contain thick septations or polypoid masses. The only reliable sign of malignant transformation is the presence of metastases or lymphadenopathy.[67]

The differential diagnosis of cystadenoma includes: hepatic abscess, hemorrhagic bile duct cyst, hepatic echinococcal cyst, and in rare instances mesenchymal hamartoma, cystic hepatocellular carcinoma, and cystic metastases.

Granular Cell Tumors

Granular cell tumors can occur anywhere in the body. The most common site is the tongue; however, 1% of these tumors occur in the biliary tract.[313] Of patients with these tumors, 90% are women, 76% of whom are of African-American origin.[331] Granular cell tumors account for 10% of nonbiliary tumors. Half of granular cell tumors occur in the common bile duct, while 37% occur in the cystic duct. Because granular cell tumors are so small, they are difficult to depict with imaging. At ERCP, a granular cell tumor manifests as a segmental, annular stricture, which is usually short (1 to 3 cm), or as abrupt obstruction of the extrahepatic bile duct. Symmetric or eccentric narrowing of the extrahepatic duct typically results from intramural growth of the tumor. The added benefit of MR imaging is the ability to demonstrate both the intra- and extraluminal extent of disease in patients presenting with bile duct obstruction.

Neurofibromatosis

Neurofibromas of the gallbladder and bile ducts are very uncommon and usually are associated with neurofibromatosis. Biliary involvement is secondary to periampullary neuroendocrine tumors and obstructing duodenal tumors.[332] There are no specific radiological findings of neurofibroma of the bile duct. Rarely, plexiform neurofibroma may result in diffuse involvement of the extra- and intrahepatic bile ducts.[313]

Juxtapapillary Diverticulum

Juxtapapillary diverticulum is defined as a diverticulum of the duodenum within close proximity to the duodenal papilla. It is hypothesized that juxtapapillary diverticulum formation is related to motility disorders of the sphincter of Oddi.[333,334] They are commonly associated with concomitant bile duct dilatation, choledocholithiasis and pancreatitis. Cannulation of the papilla at ERCP can be altered by a juxtapapillary diverticulum; therefore prior detection with MRCP can aid management planning.[335]

Juxtapapillary diverticula are usually located in the medial wall of the second portion of the duodenum. On T1-weighted images, an air-fluid level is visualized as hypointense fluid layering dependently relative to the signal void of air; while on T2-weighted images the fluid layering dependently is hyperintense. If oral gadolinium is given, these diverticula are not visualized on T2-weighted fast spin-echo images, due to the T1 and T2 shortening effect of the oral contrast agent.[336] T2-weighted true FISP and HASTE images best demonstrate the diverticula and its relationship to the papilla.[337] In some cases, the communication between the duodenal wall and diverticulum is clearly shown. These MR

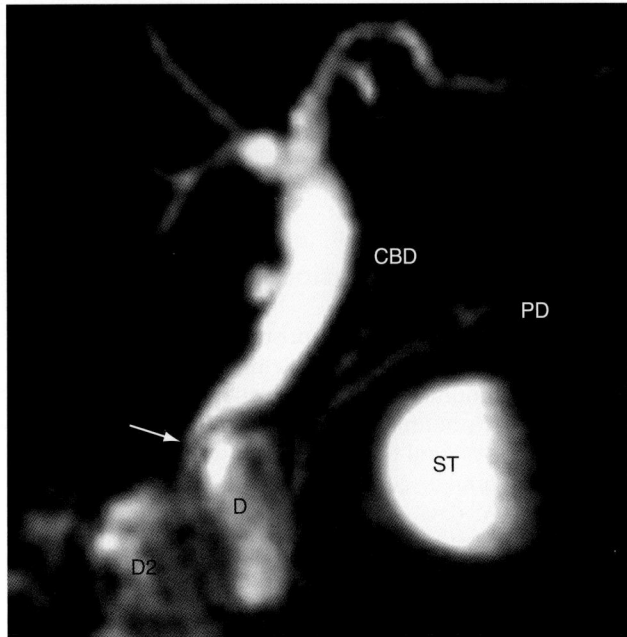

FIGURE 79-48

Extramural compression of distal CBD by a duodenal diverticulum: 70 mm coronal SSFSE RARE SLAB MRCP (TE 969) demonstrates a duodenal diverticulum (D) producing mass effect (*arrow*) on the distal common bile duct (CBD). There is intra- and extrahepatic bile duct dilatation. ST, stomach; PD, pancreatic duct; D2, second stage of duodenum.

imaging features distinguish juxtapapillary diverticula from pancreatic pseudocysts and cystic neoplasms. The complications associated with juxtapapillary diverticula can also be demonstrated on MR imaging, and include findings of pancreatitis, dilatation of the common bile duct (Fig. 79-48) and choledocholithiasis.[338]

Chronic Inflammatory Pseudotumor of Hepaticobiliary System

Inflammatory pseudotumor (also called inflammatory myofibroplastic pseudotumor or plasma cell granuloma) is a benign disease producing laboratory, clinical and radiologic findings suspicious for neoplastic disease. Inflammatory pseudotumors are usually focal and are described in most organ types.[339] Documented myofibroblastic disease of the biliary tree is exceedingly rare. Increased awareness by radiologists of the presence of this entity is important in the differential diagnosis of cholangiocarcinoma, since it may show aggressive behavior with potential for local, regional and systemic extension of disease.[340]

Portal Cavernoma

Another rare benign entity resulting in abnormalities of the biliary tree is portal cavernoma. Patients are usually asymptomatic or may present with cholestasis. Three

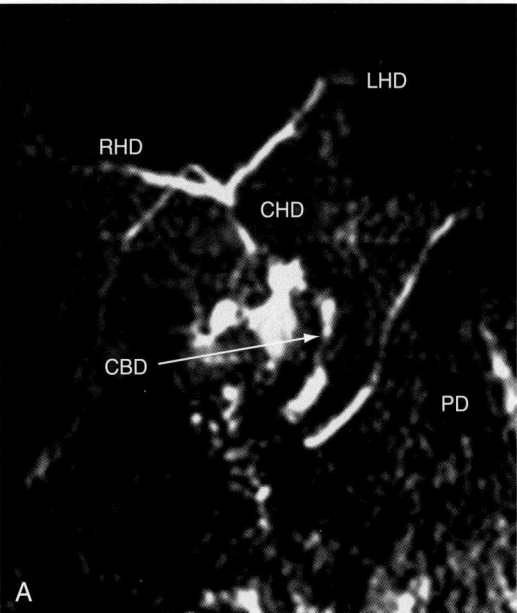

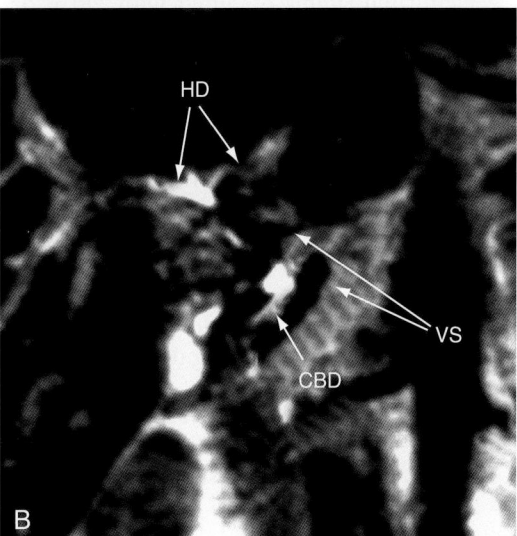

FIGURE 79-49

A, and **B,** Portal cavernoma. **A,** 20 mm coronal SSFSE RARE SLAB MRCP demonstrates multiple areas of narrowing at the level of the common bile duct (CBD). **B,** 6 mm coronal SSFSE T2 MRCP (TE 90) demonstrates multiple vascular impressions (VS) corresponding to the areas of narrowing. HD, hepatic duct; LHD, left hepatic duct; RHD, right hepatic duct; CHD, common hepatic duct; PD, pancreatic duct.

different types of common bile duct abnormalities have been described in patients with portal cavernoma on MR imaging: 1. multiple smooth extrinsic impressions; 2. findings mimicking cholangiocarcinoma; and rarely 3. an irregular narrowing of the common bile duct mimicking chronic cholangitis (Fig. 79-49). The diagnosis can be suggested by identifying the periductal collateral vessels, which demonstrate low-signal intensity on T2-weighted images. In addition, fibrosis can be identified on delayed contrast-enhanced sequences in some cases.[341-343]

PRE- AND POST-SURGICAL EVALUATION OF BILIARY TREE

Preoperative Evaluation

The number of cholecystectomies performed in the USA since the development of laparoscopic surgery has increased to more than 500,000 annually.[344] Biliary anatomy is less well seen with laparoscopic surgery compared to open surgery. The incidence of major bile duct injury varies from 0% to 0.5% for open chole-cystectomy and from 0% to 1.2% for laparoscopic cholecystectomy.[345,346] In the absence of any clinical, biochemical or radiological signs of choledocholithiasis, between 1% to 14% of all patients with gallbladder stones will have common bile duct stones.[36,347,348] Asymptomatic choledochal stones may remain unde-tected in up to 80% of cases.[349,350] Therefore, preopera-tive evaluation of the biliary tract to detect the presence of choledocholithiasis, duct abnormalities, or anatomic variants would aid in surgical planning.

Direct cholangiograms obtained with ERCP or IOC, have an accuracy ranging from 92% to 98% for detecting choledochal stones.[351,352] However, IOC may be tech-nically unsuccessful in 5% to 45% of cases.[347] In addition, IOC has a 4% false-negative and a 4% to 10% false-positive rate for diagnosing choledocholithiasis.[353,354] Finally, IOC lengthens the procedure time of endoscopic biliary surgery.[346,355,356]

To overcome these drawbacks, MRCP has been proposed as a noninvasive imaging modality to evaluate the biliary tree preoperatively. As discussed earlier, MRCP has been shown to be highly accurate in diagnosing choledocholithiasis and in detecting extra-hepatic biliary variants.[79,88,346,357] However, whether anticipation of duct abnormalities prevents iatrogenic injury to the common bile duct is yet to be determined. Currently MRCP is not used to determine which patients should undergo conventional cholecystectomy vs. laparoscopic cholecystectomy. A further limitation of MRCP is the inadequate detection of intrahepatic anatomic anomalies, particularly in nondilated systems.[55] This is a setting where fMRC using a hepatobiliary con-trast agent may be useful.

Although useful, MRCP is not considered an estab-lished screening method for patients undergoing laparoscopic cholecystectomy, given the high cost and limited availability. Several authors have advocated the principle of risk stratification to select patients who would benefit most from undergoing preoperative MR imaging.[27,347] For example, Liu et al[27] classified patients undergoing LC according to their risk of harboring CBD stones into one of four groups:

1. An extremely high-risk group of patients who under-went preoperative ERCP.
2. A high-risk group who underwent MRCP.
3. A moderate-risk group who underwent LC with IOC.
4. A low-risk group who underwent LC without IOC.

Overall, ERCP was performed in 8.9% of patients and MRCP was performed in 9.4%. This stratification resulted in the diagnosis of CBD stones during preoperative ERCP in 92.3% of the patients, while unsuspected CBD stones were found in only 1.4% of patients.

In summary, currently ERCP or IOC remains the standard of practice in this clinical setting.[358] MRCP may have added value in the subgroup of patients undergoing laparoscopic cholecystectomy with a moderate to high risk of choledocholithiasis.

Postoperative Evaluation

There are several expected postoperative findings after laparoscopic cholecystectomy, including the presence of small amounts of fluid in the gallbladder fossa, pneumoperitoneum, adynamic ileus, subcutaneous emphysema, pleural effusion, and lower lobe atelectasis. All these findings generally resolve within the first 7 postoperative days. Ascites most often resolves by the 12th postoperative day.[359,360] Patients whose postopera-tive course is complicated by persistent or increasing ascites, fluid collections, or bile duct obstruction may have suffered injury to the bile ducts at the time of surgery.

Injury to the bile ducts can result from a variety of operative procedures, such as laparoscopic cholecystec-tomy and liver transplantation. Additional complications associated with laparoscopic cholecystectomy include retained common bile duct stones, incomplete resection of the gallbladder and infection.[361]

Most bile duct injuries result from mistaking the common hepatic duct for the cystic duct, so that a portion of the common hepatic duct is resected or ligated (Fig. 79-50). There is often associated injury of

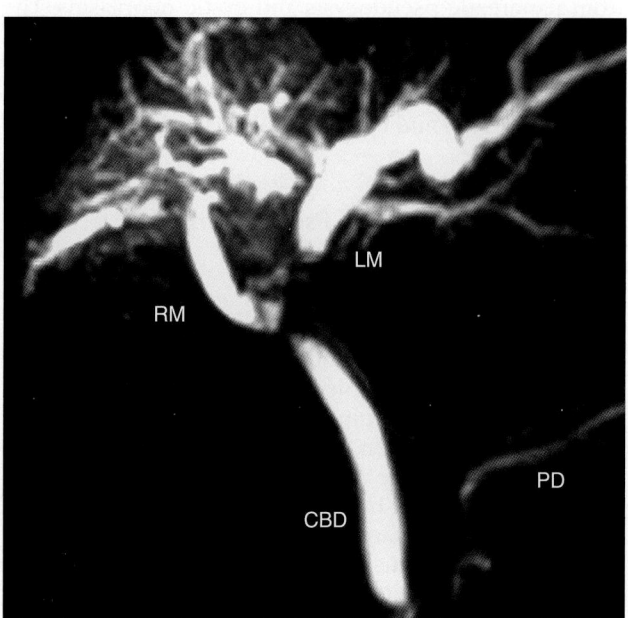

FIGURE 79-50

Iatrogenic bile duct injury during laparoscopic cholecystectomy. 3D MIP demonstrates complete obstruction secondary to a clipped common hepatic duct (*arrow*). The clip results in magnetic susceptibility artifact. CBD, common bile duct; PD, pancreatic duct; RM, right main intrahepatic duct; LM, left main hepatic duct.

the right hepatic artery. An aberrant right hepatic duct may also be mistaken for the cystic duct and be accidentally ligated. It has been shown that anatomic variations of the extrahepatic biliary tree are present in up to 25% of the population.[212]

Ductal injury can be caused by inadvertently misplaced clips, erroneous cutting of bile ducts, periductal leakage with resultant fibrosis, or thermal injury associated with laser or cautery use.[344,345,362-364] The diagnosis of bile duct strictures due to ductal injury is usually made 2 weeks to 4 months after surgery.[365]

Bile leaks appear in 0.5% to 3% of all laparoscopic cholecystectomies (typically manifesting 1 to 2 weeks after cholecystectomy), and account for 30% of bile duct injuries associated with laparascopic cholecystectomy.[366,367] Abdominal pain, distention and fever are the most common symptoms related to bile leaks and result from bile peritonitis or infected bilomas. Gallbladder fossa, or perihepatic fluid collections (bilomas) and often ascites result from bile leaks originating from the cystic duct stump or gallbladder remnant. A bile leak is suspected if free fluid is present on the right side of the abdomen with or without the presence of a fluid collection adjacent to the injured bile duct.

MR Considerations

MR imaging can play an important role in the initial evaluation of patients with suspected bile duct injury. MR imaging can be safely performed in the immediate postoperative period as metallic surgical clips made of titanium are not a contraindication to MR imaging. A study by Khalid showed that MRCP accurately distinguished transection injuries from focal strictures, predicted an intact biliary tree and detected the presence of bile leaks.[362] Although the sensitivity of MRCP in detecting common bile duct stones or strictures preoperatively ranges from 95% to 100%, false-positive findings at postoperative MRCP may be caused by pneumobilia (Fig. 79-51), hematobilia or protein plugs.[347,368] In addition, magnetic susceptibility artifacts from surgical clips projected over the bile ducts may interfere with image interpretation and produce false filling defects or strictures.[66]

MRCP is highly accurate at detecting excluded bile duct segments in patients with ligation of an aberrant right hepatic duct (Fig. 79-52). The Bismuth classification is helpful for surgical planning in patients with complications following laparoscopic cholecystectomy. For optimal planning the entire biliary anatomy must be displayed. For example, the length of the intact common duct distal to the bifurcation, in the presence of a postoperative stricture, determines whether a choledochojejunostomy or hepaticojejunostomy is performed. If disruption of the confluence is present, it requires reconstruction in addition to a hepaticojejunostomy.[345,362] A limitation of MRCP is that the differentiation between biliary strictures and transections may not be distinguished, but rather grouped together as occlusion. To evaluate the extent of a high-grade stenosis in these cases, thin-section source images must be used.[41]

Heavily T2-weighted images are extremely sensitive for the detection of unbound fluid associated with bile leaks (Fig. 79-53). However, fMRC is required to detect the actual bile leak (Fig. 79-54). A prospective study by Vitellas showed that mangafodipir-enhanced fMRC was 86% sensitive and 83% specific for the diagnosis of bile duct leaks.[369] However, bile duct leaks from peripheral intrahepatic bile ducts may be more difficult to characterize due to limited opacification. Finally, hematomas and iodinated contrast agents both show increased T1 signal and thus mimic contrast agent extravasation on mangafodipir-enhanced gradient-echo images.[369]

Biliary Endoprostheses

MRCP can be used to evaluate the biliary tract in patients with biliary endoprostheses to document stent position and provide measurements of luminal stent diameter. However, the internal stent lumen can only be visualized in patients who have indwelling polyethylene stents, but not in patients with cobalt alloy or nitinol base stents (Fig. 79-55).[370] Another indication for MRCP is to assist in determining the placement of unilateral metallic stents for selectively targeted drainage procedures in patients with malignant hilar biliary obstruction.[371]

Liver Transplantation

Orthotopic liver transplantation is the treatment of choice for irreversible advanced liver disease, such as cholestatic liver disease, parenchymal liver disease, congenital errors of metabolism and hepatic tumors.[372] The increased frequency of orthotopic liver transplantation necessitates that radiologists become familiar with the MRCP appearance of normal anatomic variants for preoperative planning, as well as with the expected postoperative changes associated with this procedure (see Chapter 83). Biliary complications are seen in 25% of patients following a liver transplant, but are more frequent in the pediatric population.[179,373-375] The most common complications manifest themselves within several weeks; however, they have been reported to occur in the immediate postoperative period and as long as 4 years after transplantation.[42]

There are a variety of biliary complications related to liver transplant surgery, which include bile duct strictures, obstruction, leaks, bilomas, choledocholithiasis and cystic duct remnant mucoceles. The most common complication is bile duct strictures (Fig. 79-31), which occur in 4% to 17% of patients as a late complication.[168] Bile duct strictures in association with liver transplantation have been discussed earlier in this chapter, in the section on "Postliver Transplant Ischemic Cholangitis".

MRCP can accurately depict the location, length and degree of a stricture with direct projectional imaging (Fig. 79-56). A study by Fulcher et al[179] demonstrated that MRCP was able to demonstrate first-order intrahepatic bile ducts in 92% of patients, the donor extrahepatic bile duct in 100%, recipient extrahepatic bile duct in 94%,

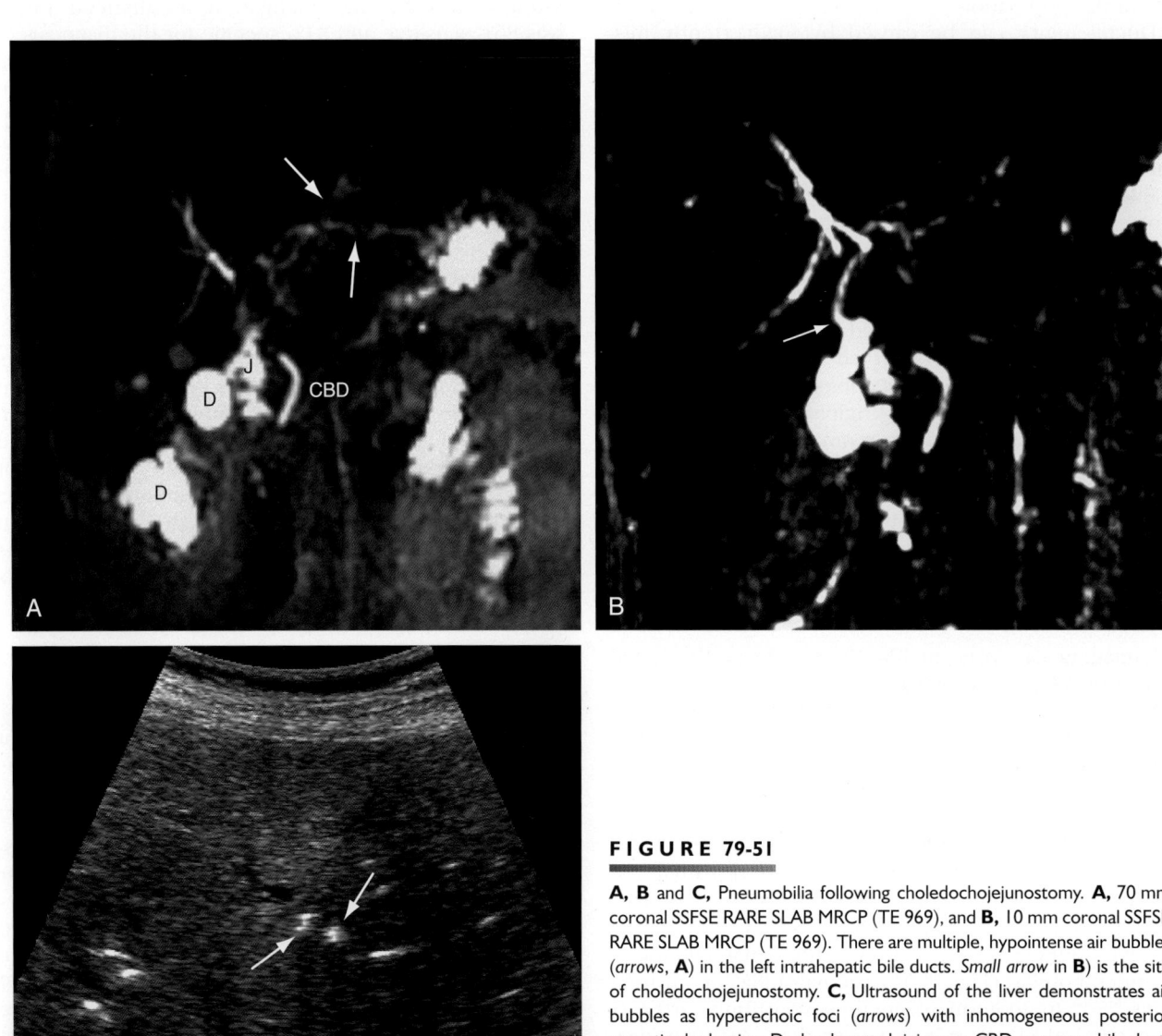

FIGURE 79-51

A, B and **C,** Pneumobilia following choledochojejunostomy. **A,** 70 mm coronal SSFSE RARE SLAB MRCP (TE 969), and **B,** 10 mm coronal SSFSE RARE SLAB MRCP (TE 969). There are multiple, hypointense air bubbles (*arrows*, **A**) in the left intrahepatic bile ducts. *Small arrow* in **B**) is the site of choledochojejunostomy. **C,** Ultrasound of the liver demonstrates air bubbles as hyperechoic foci (*arrows*) with inhomogeneous posterior acoustic shadowing. D, duodenum; J, jejunum; CBD, common bile duct.

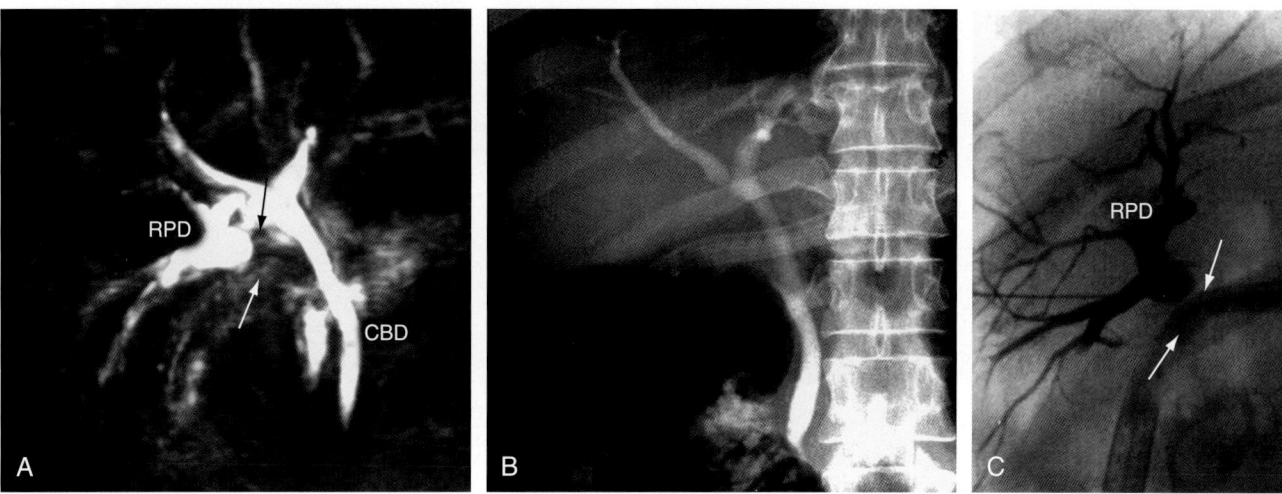

FIGURE 79-52

A, B and **C,** Transection of anomalous bile duct during laparoscopic cholecystectomy. **A,** 40 mm coronal SSFSE RARE SLAB MRCP (TE 969) demonstrates an amputated (*arrows*) and dilated aberrant right posterior hepatic duct (RPD). **B,** ERCP does not demonstrate the isolated anomalous duct. **C,** Selective PTC demonstrates the obstructed (*arrows*) right posterior hepatic duct.

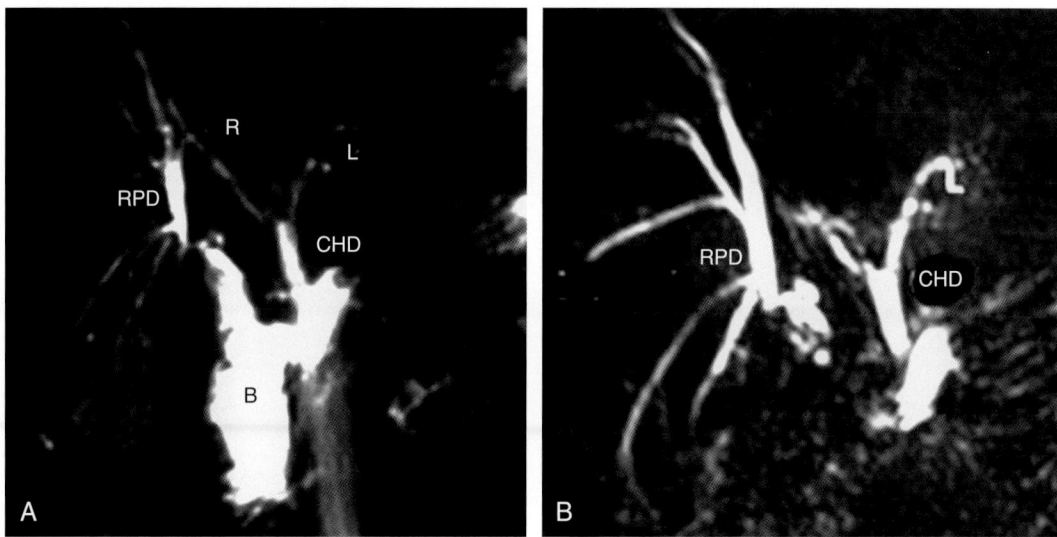

FIGURE 79-53

A, and **B,** Bilioma formation after injury to anomalous right posterior intrahepatic bile duct during laparoscopic cholecystectomy. **A,** 40 mm and **B,** 10 mm coronal SSFSE RARE SLAB MRCP (TE 969) demonstrate an amputated anomalous right posterior bile duct (RPD). There is adjacent bilioma formation (B) from a bile leak. CHD, common bile duct; R, right main intrahepatic duct; L, left main intrahepatic duct.

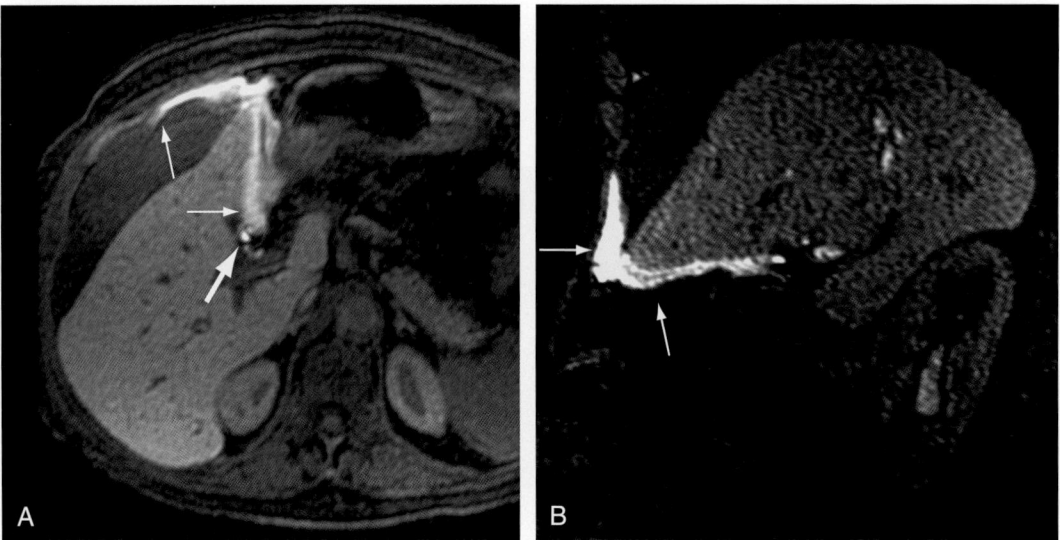

FIGURE 79-54

A, and **B,** Biliary contrast agent: demonstration of bile leak. **A,** Transverse and **B,** sagittal 5 mm fat-suppressed T1-weighted images obtained following administration of IV mangafodipir trisodium (Tesla scan) in a patient with suspected biliary leak following laparoscopic cholecystectomy. The actual bile leak (*small arrows*) can be demonstrated to originate from the cystic duct remnant (*large arrow*). (*Courtesy of Dr Masoom Haider, University of Toronto, Canada.*)

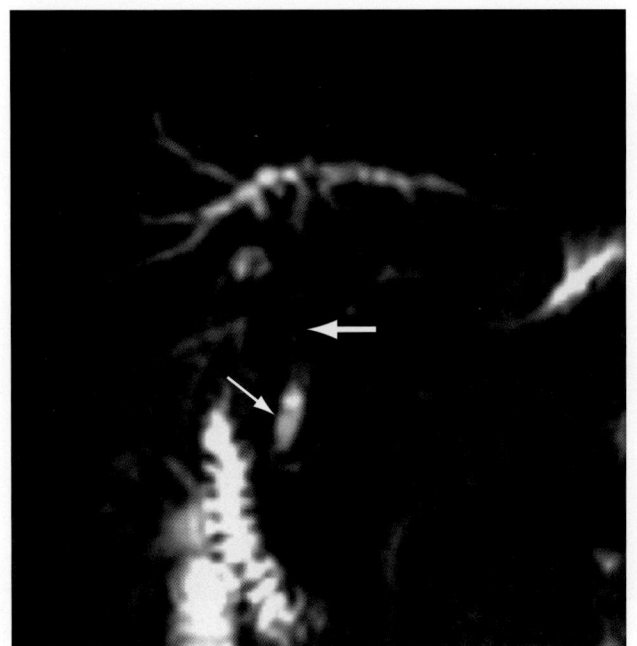

FIGURE 79-55

Susceptibility artifact with biliary endoprosthesis. 70 mm coronal RARE SSFSE SLAB MRCP (TE 969) in a patient with a hilar cholangiocarcinoma and metallic biliary stent. The stent lumen as such is not visualized due to susceptibility artifact and only a thin streak (*large arrow*) of bile is seen coursing through the lumen. The lumen of the intra-pancreatic portion of the bile duct is well visualized (*small arrow*), as the stent does not extend within it.

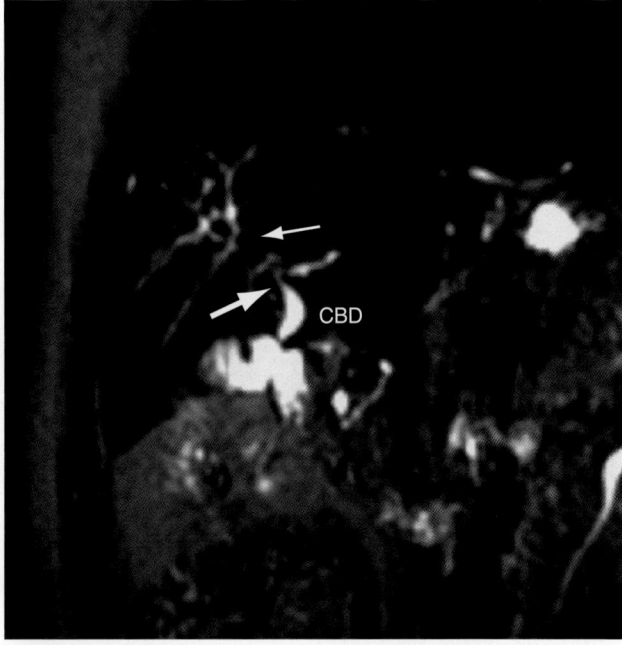

FIGURE 79-56

Recurrent sclerosing cholangitis involving a liver transplant in a patient with Crohn's disease. 40 mm coronal SSFSE RARE SLAB MRCP (TE 969) demonstrates strictures involving the common hepatic duct (*arrow*) and intrahepatic bile ducts (*small arrow*). CBD, common bile duct.

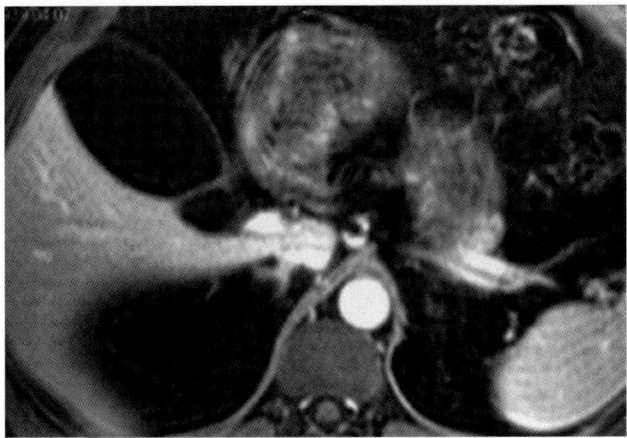

FIGURE 80-3

Normal enhancement of the gallbladder on gadolinium-enhanced axial fat-suppressed TI-weighted images. The enhancement is well appreciated on fat-suppressed images. The portion of the gallbladder wall adjacent to the liver is not well appreciated, as the enhancement is similar in liver parenchyma and gallbladder wall.

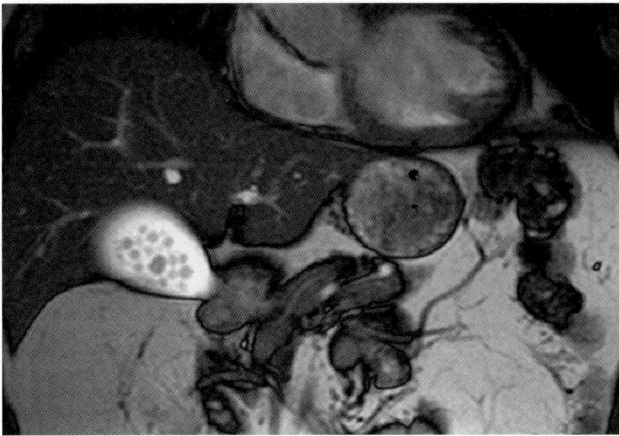

FIGURE 80-4

Coronal T2-weighted image (half-Fourier sequence—SSFSE). Multiple gallstones are well appreciated on this sequence due to the high contrast between hyperintense bile and hypointense gallstones.

cavity. Variations in number are rare but include agenesis and duplication. Anomalies of form include septations within the gallbladder lumen. A septation within the distal fundus of the gallbladder gives the appearance of a "Phrygian cap". Recognition of variations in the cystic duct is clinically important to minimize complications and injury to the extrahepatic bile ducts during laparoscopic surgery. These include abnormally low or medial insertion or parallel course of the duct and common hepatic duct and short cystic duct.

DISEASES OF THE GALLBLADDER

Gallstones

Ultrasound is the modality most commonly used to assess gallstone disease. It has very high sensitivity for the detection of gallstones. Although MR has no established role in the diagnosis of gallstones, it is important to check for the occurrence of gallstones on MR as they often appear incidentally. Gallbladder stones and cystic duct stones are best appreciated on T2-weighted images and on MRCP (Fig. 80-4). Most gallstones appear as signal voids on both T1- and T2-weighted images (Fig. 80-5) because of restricted motion of water and cholesterol molecules in the crystalline lattice of the stone.[1] Occasionally, gallstones have central hyperintensity with a peripheral rim of hypointensity on T1- or T2-weighted images or may appear largely hyperintense on T1-weighted images[2,3] (Fig. 80-6). The central hyperintensity does not correspond to fat or cholesterol within the gallstones[4] and may be related to the presence of protein macromolecules with shorter T1 relaxation times.[5]

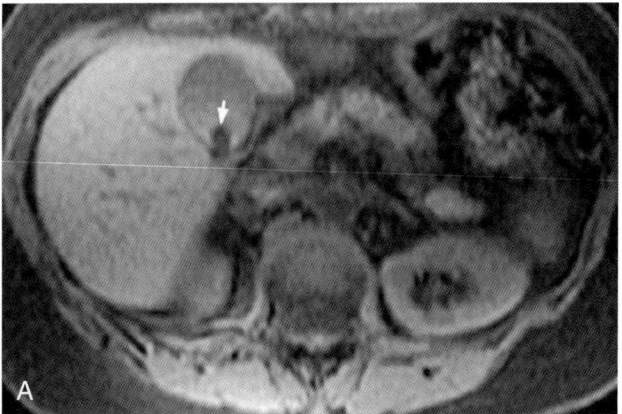

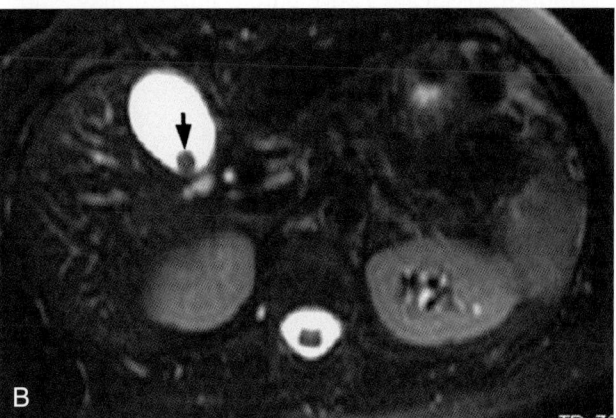

FIGURE 80-5

Axial fat-suppressed TI-weighted (**A**) and T2-weighted (**B**) images. Gallstone appears as a hypointense focus on TI- and T2-weighted images (*arrow*) due to few free protons.

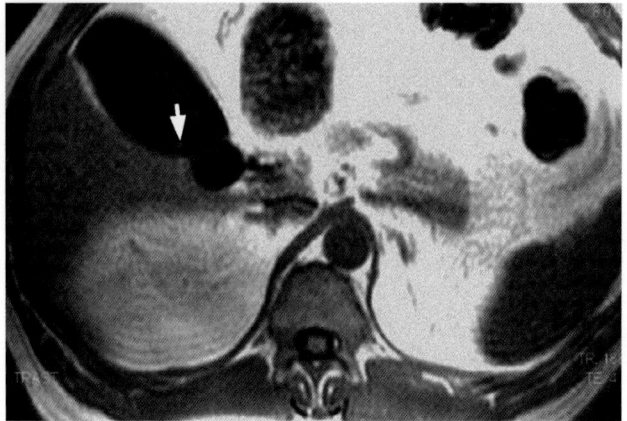

FIGURE 80-6

Axial T1-weighted image of gallbladder. Gallstone appears as a hyperintense focus (*arrow*) with surrounding hypointensity.

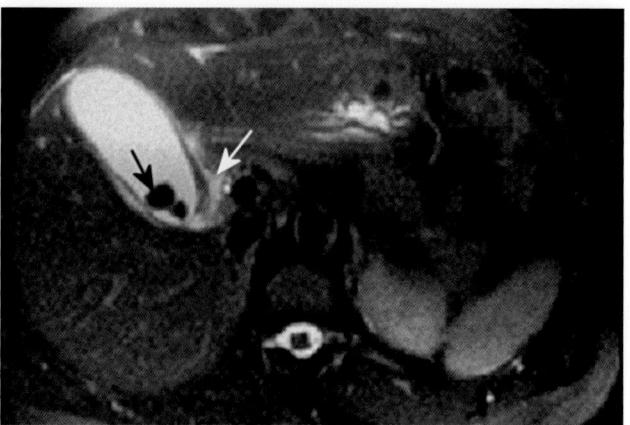

FIGURE 80-7

Acute cholecystitis. Axial T2-weighted (HASTE) image of gallbladder shows gallstones (*black arrow*) with gallbladder wall thickening and increased signal intensity and minimal pericholecystic fluid collection (*white arrow*). (*Image courtesy of Robert Edelman MD.*)

Acute Cholecystitis

Acute cholecystitis typically results from the obstruction of the cystic duct with a gallstone. Ultrasound is usually the first modality of choice for the diagnosis of acute cholecystitis.

When ultrasound is equivocal, MR may be helpful in detecting gallstones in the neck of the gallbladder and the cystic duct[6] and in demonstrating the associated gallbladder wall abnormalities. In a recent study, limited MR of the liver and gallbladder was found to be equivalent to ultrasound in evaluating patients with symptoms of acute right upper quadrant pain and this modality may be used in sonographically challenging patients.[7]

Contrast-enhanced fat-suppressed images are very sensitive in demonstrating inflammatory changes in the gallbladder wall, pericholecystic fat, and intrahepatic periportal tissues.[8] T2-weighted images may show thickening of the gallbladder wall (>3 mm), increased signal intensity, and pericholecystic fluid collection

(Fig. 80-7). The pericholecystic high signal may appear as a linear high signal or band-like or radiating high signal. According to Ito et al, the pericholecystic radiating high signal correlated with necrotic cholecystitis on histology and required percutaneous drainage.[9] In addition, periportal hyperintensity, a nonspecific finding, may be observed on T2-weighted images.[10] Due to the lack of concentrating ability during acute inflammation, the bile appears hypointense, similar to cerebrospinal fluid, on T1-weighted images. However, associated increase in protein content may result in varying signal intensity to bile. Contrast-enhanced fat suppressed images demonstrate increased enhancement of gallbladder wall and adjacent fat (Fig. 80-8). The enhancement is marked in the mucosal surface in the earlier scans and the enhancement spreads to the entire wall in delayed scans.

The interrupted rim sign—patchy enhancement of the gallbladder mucosa—was found to represent areas of necrosis and may be helpful in identifying gangrenous

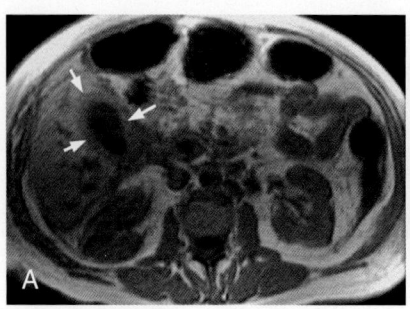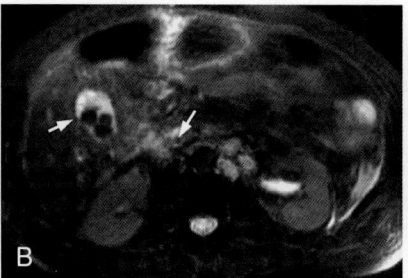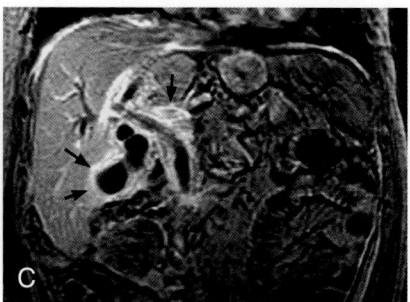

FIGURE 80-8

Acute cholecystitis with cholangitis. Axial T1-weighted image (**A**) shows diffuse gallbladder wall thickening and axial fat-suppressed T2-weighted image (**B**) shows increased signal intensity of gallbladder wall (*left arrow*), gallstones, and a stone in the distal common bile duct (*right arrow*). Contrast-enhanced coronal image (**C**) shows diffuse enhancement of gallbladder wall and bile duct walls (*arrows*).

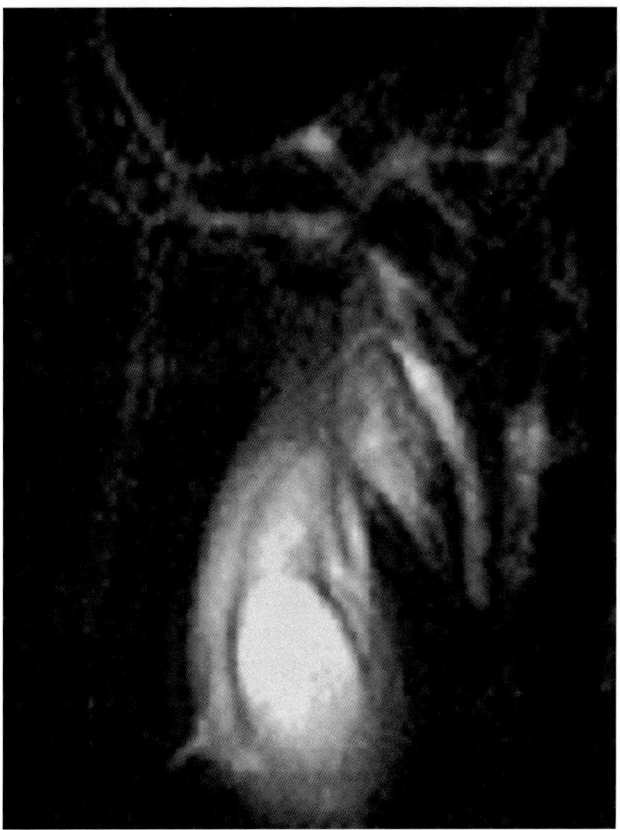

FIGURE 80-9

Acute cholecystis due to cytomegalovirus infection. Thick-slab MRCP demonstrates thickening of the gallbladder wall with high signal intensity within the gallbladder wall.

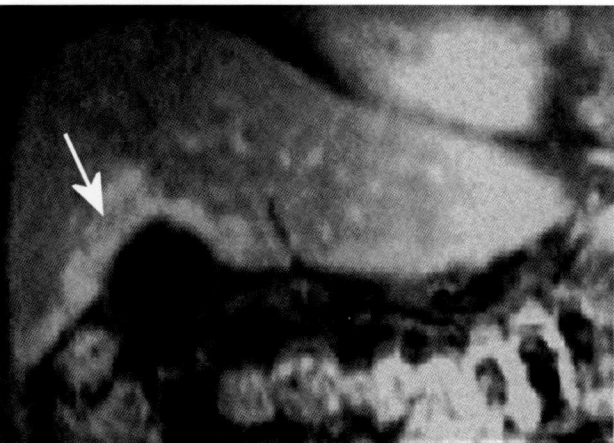

FIGURE 80-10

Acute cholecystitis. Gadolinium-enhanced coronal 3D GRE T1-weighted image of liver shows focal area of enhancement of liver adjacent to gallbladder secondary to hyperemic response in liver parenchyma (arrow) due to acute cholecystitis. (Image courtesy of Robert Edelman MD.)

tissue on MR.[11] Similarly, demonstration of defects in the gallbladder wall on contrast-enhanced MRI was found to correlate with perforation of the gallbladder.[12] In addition, asymmetric gallbladder wall thickening, due to microabscesses, intramural hemorrhage, and the presence of complex pericholecystic fluid collections containing debris, may indicate gangrenous cholecystitis. Viral cholecystitis can have similar appearances (Fig. 80-9). Emphysematous cholecystitis, best diagnosed with computed tomography (CT), may show intraluminal or intramural gas. Pericholecystic abscesses result from perforation of the gallbladder and appear as localized fluid collections with rim enhancement on contrast administration. Associated abnormalities in the adjacent liver include patchy areas of transient increased enhancement in the hepatic parenchyma during capillary phase images, caused by a hyperemic response in the liver due to the adjacent inflammation (Fig. 80-10).[13] Hemorrhagic cholecystitis is unusual but is common in acalculous cholecystitis. MR can accurately diagnose this entity due to the high sensitivity of MR to blood breakdown products.

Torsion of the gallbladder may have a similar presentation to that seen with acute cholecystitis. MRCP findings in gallbladder torsion include V-shaped distortion of the extrahepatic bile ducts due to traction by the cystic duct, tapering and twisting interruption of the cystic duct, distended and enlarged gallbladder that deviates to the midline of the abdomen, and a difference in intensity between the gallbladder and the extrahepatic bile ducts and the cystic duct.[14]

Chronic Cholecystitis

The gallbladder appears small and irregular with a thickened wall and gallstones. On gadolinium-enhanced MR, the wall enhances less intensely compared to acute cholecystitis (Fig. 80-11). The gallbladder wall enhancement in chronic cholecystitis is usually smooth unlike gallbladder carcinoma, which shows irregular enhancement of the wall.[15] Yoshimitsu et al showed that in patients with diffuse gallbladder wall thickening, dynamic MRI was useful in differentiating benign from malignant gallbladder lesions.[16] Early prolonged enhancement was observed in the malignant lesions as opposed to slow, prolonged enhancement in the benign lesions. In addition, the inflammatory diseases do not affect the three-layer structure of the gallbladder wall but gallbladder carcinoma destroys the wall structure[17] and may extend outside the muscular layer.

Mirizzi Syndrome

First described by Pablo Mirizzi in 1948, this syndrome encompasses a rare benign cause of obstructive jaundice caused by a stone impacted in either Hartmann's pouch or the cystic duct, leading to obstruction of the common hepatic duct by extrinsic compression.[18] This may result in simple obstruction of the common hepatic duct (type 1 Mirizzi syndrome) or formation of a cholecysto-choledochal fistula due to erosion of the wall of the common hepatic duct (type 2 Mirizzi syndrome).[19] This

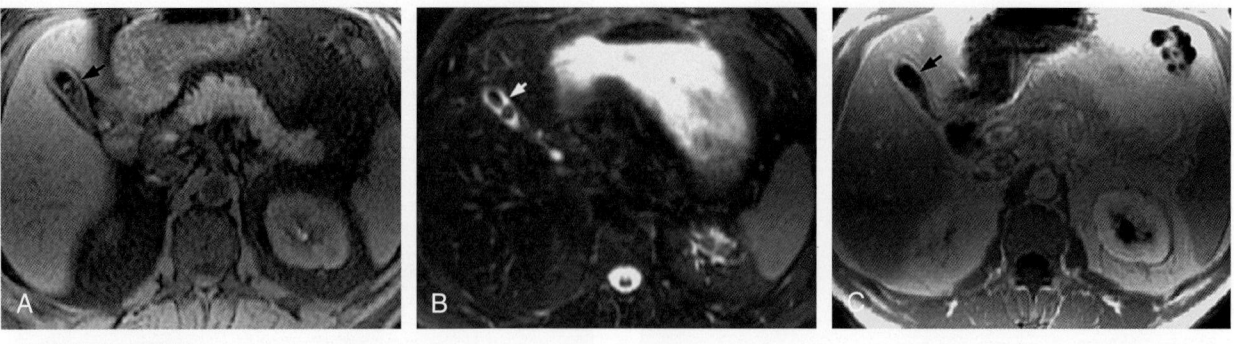

FIGURE 80-11

Chronic cholecystitis. Axial fat-suppressed T1-weighted (**A**) and T2-weighted (**B**) images show small gallbladder with wall thickening (*arrow*) and gallstones. Contrast-enhanced T1-weighted image (**C**) shows diffuse enhancement of gallbladder wall (*arrow*).

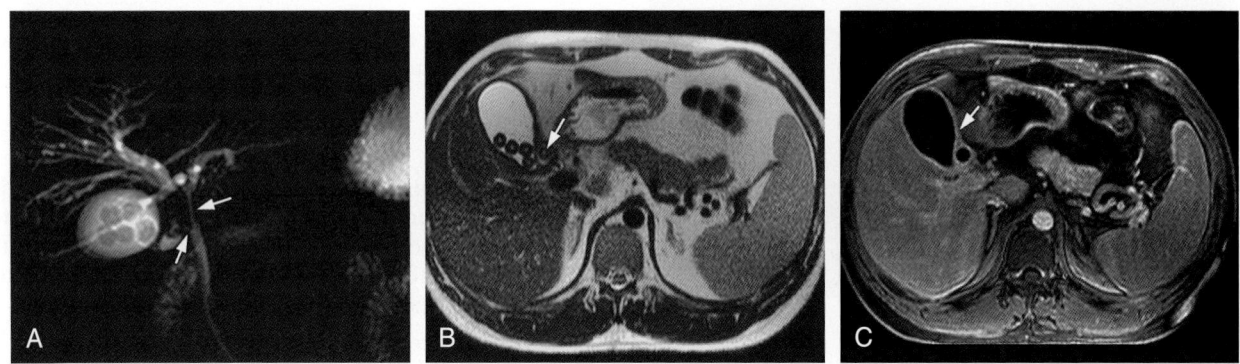

FIGURE 80-12

Mirizzi syndrome. Thick-slab MRCP (**A**) demonstrates dilated intrahepatic biliary ducts and the level of obstruction at the common hepatic duct due to extrinsic impression (*top arrow*). The lower arrow points to the cystic duct as it joins the common hepatic duct. **B,** Respiratory triggered T2-weighted axial FSE image demonstrates multiple gallstones with a cystic duct stone (*arrow*). **C,** Contrast-enhanced axial fat-suppressed T1-weighted image shows diffuse enhancement of gallbladder and cystic duct due to associated inflammation (*arrow*). (*Image courtesy of Jeffrey Brown MD.*)

condition can also occur following cholecystectomy due to impacted stone in the cystic duct remnant.

Mirizzi syndrome is further classified based on the presence of a parallel cystic duct with stones (type IA) or the obliteration of the cystic duct (type IB) and the size of the defect in the common hepatic duct (a defect of <33% of the common hepatic duct circumference is type II, a defect of 33% to 66% is type III, and a defect of >66% is type IV).[20] The original classification has been expanded to include hepatic duct stenosis caused by a stone at the junction of the cystic duct and hepatic ducts or as a result of cholecystitis even in the absence of an obstructing cystic duct stone.[21] The preoperative recognition of this entity is important because of the increased incidence of bile duct injury when a standard cholecystectomy is performed.[22] The Mirizzi syndrome is treated with cholecystectomy in patients without fistula and in patients with fistula, primary closure of the fistula to biliary-enteric bypass with cholecystectomy is performed.[21]

Mirizzi syndrome can be diagnosed by demonstrating the gallstone at the junction of the common hepatic duct and cystic duct with associated biliary ductal dilatation and/or gallbladder inflammation.[23] Ultrasound can demonstrate the gallstone with biliary ductal dilatation; however, the associated gallbladder inflammation cannot be reliably assessed. Similarly, demonstration of the gallstones may be difficult on CT.[24] Endoscopic retrograde cholangiopancreatography (ERCP) may not visualize the gallstone causing obstruction in patients with Mirizzi syndrome but MRCP can demonstrate the biliary dilatation, the level of biliary obstruction, and gallstones. Contrast-enhanced MR can demonstrate the gallbladder inflammation associated with Mirizzi syndrome. MR is also useful in identifying the long parallel cystic duct or low insertion of the cystic duct, which predisposes to the development of this syndrome. The findings on MRCP include a dilated biliary system with obstruction at the junction of the cystic duct and common hepatic duct and the presence of a gallstone in the cystic duct or gallbladder neck. After contrast administration, thickening of the gallbladder wall with a smooth contour and minimal or variable enhancement are usually observed (Fig. 80-12).[25]

Xanthogranulomatous Cholecystitis

Xanthogranulomatous cholecystitis is an uncommon inflammatory process affecting the gallbladder wall. Histologically, the gallbladder wall is thickened by the infiltration of round cells, lipid-rich histiocytes, and multinucleated giant cells with associated fibroblast proliferation in the muscularis propria. This disease presents with diffuse mural thickening or soft-tissue mass in the gallbladder fossa with extension into the liver or adjacent bowel. Sometimes chemical shift imaging may demonstrate fat in the mass. However, this is not diagnostic of xanthogranulomatous cholecystitis, as gallbladder carcinoma may co-exist.[26] The mass shows variable signal intensity on T1- and T2-weighted images. The xanthogranulomas appear as areas of isointensity to slight hyperintensity on T2-weighted images, showing slight enhancement on early-phase and strong enhancement on late-phase images of a dynamic study.[27] Areas of very high signal intensity on T2-weighted images without enhancement represent necrosis or abscesses. It is difficult to differentiate this entity from gallbladder carcinoma on imaging.

Gallbladder Polyp

Polyps in the gallbladder are usually cholesterol polyps and appear as non-mobile 1 cm masses arising from the gallbladder wall. They do not have malignant potential. They demonstrate low to intermediate signal intensity on T1- and T2-weighted images and show moderate enhancement with gadolinium.

Adenomyomatosis of the Gallbladder

Adenomyomatosis of the gallbladder represents a distinctive non-inflammatory benign degenerative condition. It is characterized by proliferation of the gallbladder wall mucosa with a thickened muscular layer and mucosal-submucosal diverticula (Rokitansky-Aschoff sinuses).[28] Grossly, it may present as diffuse, segmental or focal disease. Diffuse adenomyomatosis presents as diffuse mural thickening. In the segmental form, there is mural thickening in the midportion of the gallbladder (waist), producing an "hour-glass" appearance. The localized form of adenomyomatosis presents as a focal solid mass usually in the fundus of the gallbladder. MR demonstrates the mural thickening and multiple intramural cystic components—the Rokitansky-Aschoff sinuses.[29]

MR with half-Fourier RARE sequence was found to be most accurate for diagnosing adenomyomatosis[28] and the demonstration of Rokitansky-Aschoff sinuses differentiates this condition from gallbladder carcinoma.[30] On contrast study, the diffuse type shows early mucosal and subsequent serosal enhancement.[29]

Gallbladder Carcinoma

Gallbladder carcinoma is the fifth most common malignancy of the gastrointestinal tract, with a high rate of mortality in the United States. Risk factors include gallstones, chronic cholecystitis, and porcelain gallbladder. This tumor is common during the sixth and seventh decades and females are more often affected than males.[31]

Gallbladder cancer can present in three different ways: focal or diffuse mural thickening, intraluminal polypoidal mass, and soft-tissue mass replacing the gallbladder with invasion of the liver. Focal or diffuse mural thickening of more than 1 cm is highly suggestive of the diagnosis.[32]

On T2-weighted images, the tumor is usually hyperintense relative to the liver. On T1-weighted images, it is isointense or hypointense to the adjacent liver. Gadolinium-enhanced dynamic imaging may be useful in differentiating benign mural thickening from malignant causes. Malignant lesions cause irregularly delineated, early and prolonged enhancement, as opposed to benign lesions that cause smoothly delineated, slow and prolonged enhancement.[15,16] However, these characteristics may overlap and it may be difficult to differentiate benign mural thickening from gallbladder carcinoma.

Gallbladder carcinoma presenting as an intraluminal polypoid mass occurs in 25% of patients and has a better prognosis.[33] On T1-weighted images, it is seen as an intermediate signal intensity mass arising from the wall of the gallbladder and protruding into the lumen. On T2-weighted images, the mass exhibits increased signal intensity. Necrosis and calcification are rare in this type of tumor.[30] These tumors enhance moderately with gadolinium. Malignant polypoid lesions demonstrate early and prolonged enhancement as opposed to benign lesions that demonstrate early enhancement with subsequent washout.[16]

A large soft-tissue mass in the gallbladder fossa obscuring the gallbladder with extension into the liver or the adjacent organs is the most common presentation of gallbladder carcinoma. The clues to diagnosis include non-visualized gallbladder with mass engulfing gallstones. The mass demonstrates intermediate signal intensity on T1-weighted images and hyperintense signal on T2-weighted images. These tumors demonstrate early and prolonged enhancement after gadolinium administration[34] (Figs. 80-13 and 80-14). Gadolinium-enhanced T1-weighted fat-suppressed sequences are useful in diagnosing the extent of the tumor and direct invasion of the liver, duodenum, colon, and pancreas. MRCP helps in identifying the site of biliary obstruction. Invasion of the liver or the adjacent organs and the presence of lymph node metastases in the gastrohepatic ligament are the criteria for unresectable cancer. MR has been shown to have very high sensitivity and specificity in diagnosing tumor invasion into the bile ducts and periportal and hepatic vasculature and moderate to high sensitivity with high specificity for hepatic invasion and lymph node metastases.[35,36] Metastases to liver can also be reliably detected on contrast-enhanced MR.

Lymphoma of the gallbladder is rare and may be primary non-Hodgkin's lymphoma from the mucosa-associated lymphoid tissue[37,38] or secondary as a part of systemic disease. MR features of gallbladder lymphoma are not well described in the literature. On MR, it is

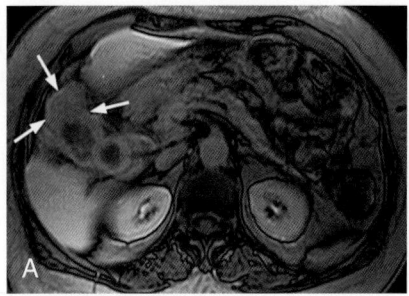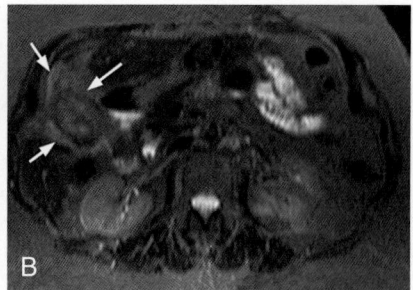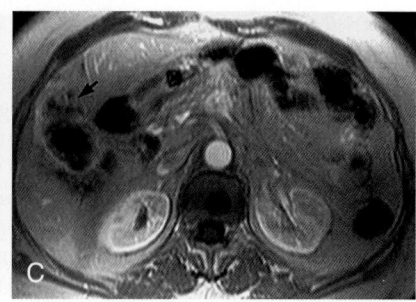

FIGURE 80-13

Gallbladder carcinoma. Axial fat-suppressed T1-weighted image (**A**) shows irregular gallbladder wall thickening with focal mass at the fundus (*arrows*). The mass exhibits intermediate signal intensity on T1-weighted images. On axial fat-suppressed T2-weighted image (**B**), the mass is heterogeneously hyperintense (*arrows*) and shows variable enhancement on contrast-enhanced T1-weighted images (**C**). The tumor interface with the liver is ill defined (*arrow*) and this suggests infiltration of liver by the tumor.

difficult to differentiate primary gallbladder cancer from lymphoma of the gallbladder. The MR findings include thickening of the gallbladder wall, mass in the gallbladder fossa with extension into the liver, biliary obstruction, and lymph nodes in the porta hepatis (Fig. 80-15).

Metastases to the Gallbladder

Metastases to the gallbladder are often reported from malignant melanoma[39] and renal cell carcinoma.[40] The metastatic tumor presents as a focal polypoidal mass within the gallbladder.[41] It is not possible to differentiate primary gallbladder carcinoma from metastatic tumor. Rarely endometrial implants may occur on the surface of the gallbladder. MRI demonstrates the presence of blood products on T1- and T2-weighted images with variable enhancement after contrast administration (Fig. 80-16).

FUNCTIONAL EVALUATION OF THE GALLBLADDER

Functional evaluation of the gallbladder has been a domain of nuclear medicine, using technetium-labeled radionuclides to assess gallbladder volume and contractility and patency of the cystic duct. Similar information regarding the gallbladder function in terms of volume and ejection fraction can be performed with MR cholangiography following a fatty meal or infusion of cholecystokinin. Using MRCP, Inoue et al showed a decreased ejection fraction in patients with gallstones after a fatty meal.[42] Similarly, the gallbladder ejection fraction following the infusion of cholecystokinin was assessed in normal volunteers (Fig. 80-17) and was found to correlate with that obtained with hepatobiliary scintigraphy using ^{99m}Tc mebrofenin.[43] It is possible to assess the segment of biliary duct covered by the sphincter of Oddi with pharmacodynamic MRCP, using a fatty meal and secretin to assess its patency and range of contractions.[44]

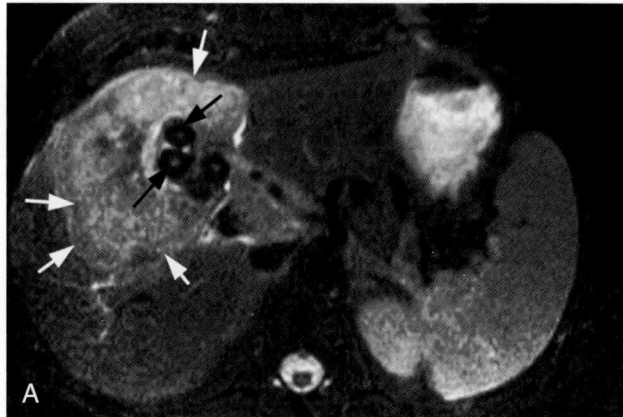
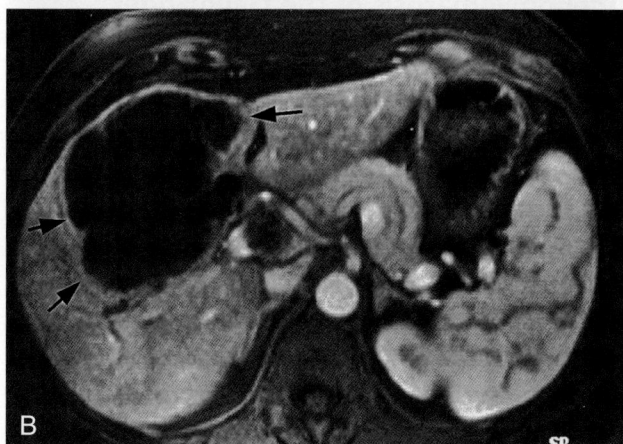

FIGURE 80-14

Gallbladder cancer. Fat-suppressed axial T2-weighted image (**A**) demonstrates large heterogeneous hyperintense mass (*white arrows*) in the gallbladder fossa with infiltration into the liver with extension along the porta hepatis. Associated gallstones (*black arrows*) are also seen. Contrast-enhanced fat-suppressed T1-weighted image (**B**) demonstrates minimal peripheral enhancement of the tumor (*black arrows*). (*Image courtesy of Jeffrey Brown MD.*)

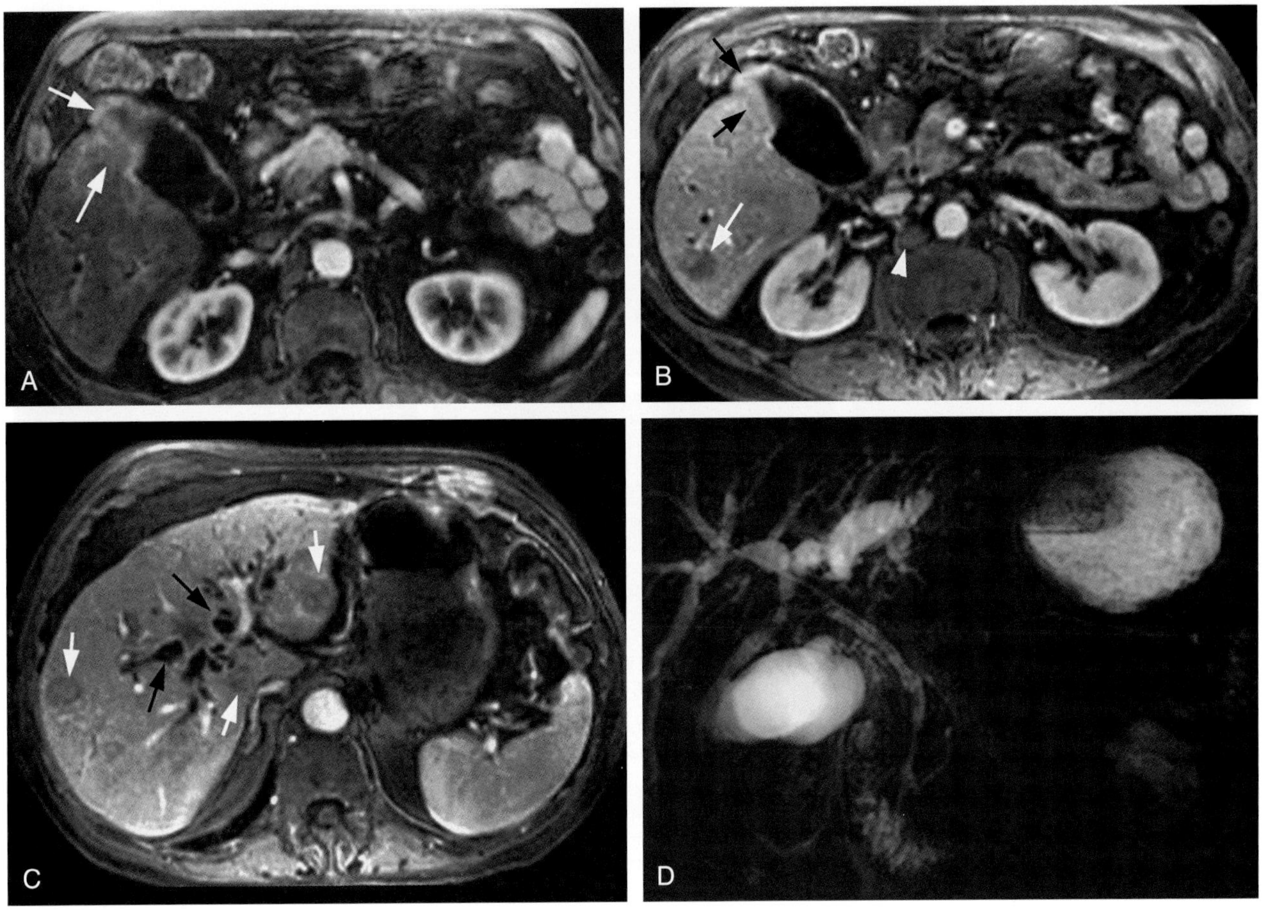

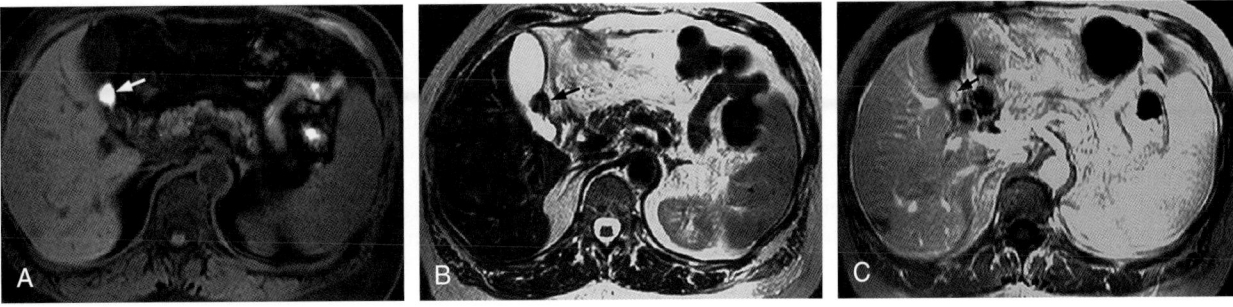

FIGURE 80-15

Lymphoma of gallbladder. Contrast-enhanced fat-suppressed T1-weighted images during arterial phase (**A**) and portal venous phase (**B**) demonstrate irregular thickening of the gallbladder wall in the fundus of the gallbladder with associated soft-tissue mass (*arrows*) infiltrating the liver. A single retroperitoneal lymph node is also seen (*arrowhead*). **C,** Image at a higher level demonstrates biliary ductal dilatation and liver lesions. Focal lesions in liver due to widespread deposits of lymphoma are also seen (*white arrows* in B,C). MRCP (**D**) demonstrates irregular contour of the gallbladder with biliary ductal dilatation. *(Image courtesy of Jeffrey Brown MD.)*

FIGURE 80-16

Endometrial implant on the surface of the gallbladder. Axial fat-suppressed T1-weighted image (**A**) shows hyperintense mass (*arrow*) on the medial surface of the gallbladder, which is hypointense on the T2-weighted axial image (**B**), suggesting subacute blood. On contrast study, the mass exhibits mild to moderate enhancement (**C**).

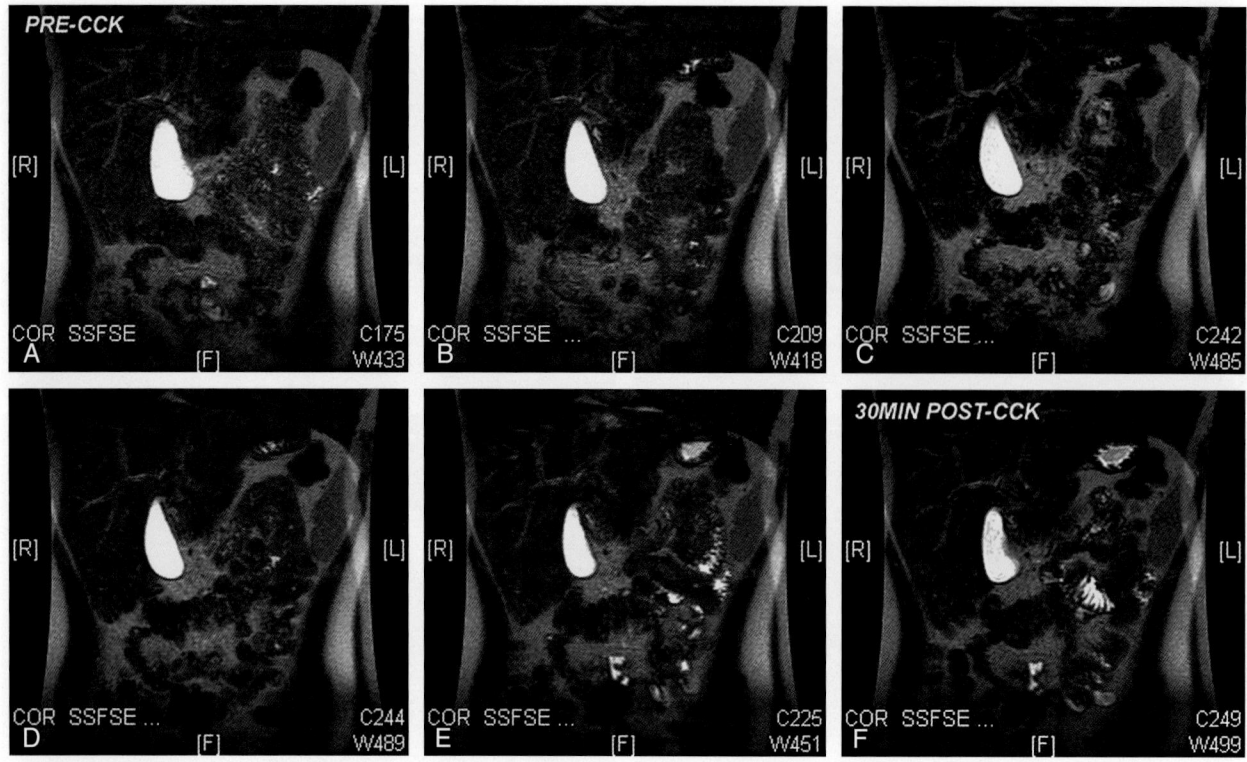

FIGURE 80-17

Functional evaluation of gallbladder with MR utilizing cholecystokinin. **A,** Baseline coronal SSFSE image of gallbladder demonstrates good distention. Following the administration of cholecystokinin, there is progressive contraction of gallbladder (**B-F**) demonstrated at various time points. By noting the change in the volume of the gallbladder, we can derive the ejection fraction and rate of contractility. *(Images courtesy of Robert Silvers MD.)*

Contrast-enhanced MRCP with mangafodipir trisodium or other hepatobiliary MR contrast agents can be used to assess gallbladder function as well as biliary obstruction (Fig. 80-18). In a recent study, contrast-enhanced functional MRCP was found to have better positive predictive value than conventional MRCP in the diagnosis of acute cholecystitis.[45] However, further studies are required to determine the role of contrast agents in functional evaluation of the gallbladder.

Postoperative Imaging

It is important to be familiar with the expected changes on MRI of the biliary tree and gallbladder following papillotomy and bilio-intestinal anastomoses and immediately following ERCP. The presence of air in the biliary system is common after these procedures. As the air is non-dependent in the gallbladder or in the biliary tree, it is seen as a signal void with a fluid-air level on T2-weighted images (Fig. 80-19).

Following surgical interventions for gallbladder diseases, imaging plays an important role in the evaluation of postoperative complications. Laparoscopic cholecystectomy is routinely performed for gallbladder disease and subsequent complications include gallstones

dropped in the peritoneal cavity, biliary leak, bilioma, vascular complications leading to hemobilia, and postoperative infection. Following biliary enteric anastomosis, biliary leak and anastomotic strictures are the main concern.

MR is not routinely used for the evaluation of these postoperative complications. However, it is useful in specific circumstances, such as locating dropped gallstones, as CT may fail to detect non-calcified gallstones. The dropped gallstones appear as focal well-defined signal voids on T2-weighted sequences and variable signal on T1-weighted sequences with inflammatory tissue that is hyperintense on T2-weighted images with variable enhancement on contrast study (Fig. 80-20). An inflammatory response and subsequent abscess can form surrounding the dropped stones. On MR, abscess appears as a relatively well-defined fluid collection with rim enhancement.

MRCP is useful in identifying postoperative biliary leaks and strictures. Cystic duct leaks following laparoscopic injury can also be identified on MRCP.[46] MRCP has been found to be comparable to percutaneous transhepatic cholangiogram (PTC) for the detection and assessment of biliary strictures following cholecystectomy.[47] MRCP can reliably assess biliary enteric anastomotic strictures; in a series of 24 patients, it correctly identified anastomotic strictures in 19 patients.[48]

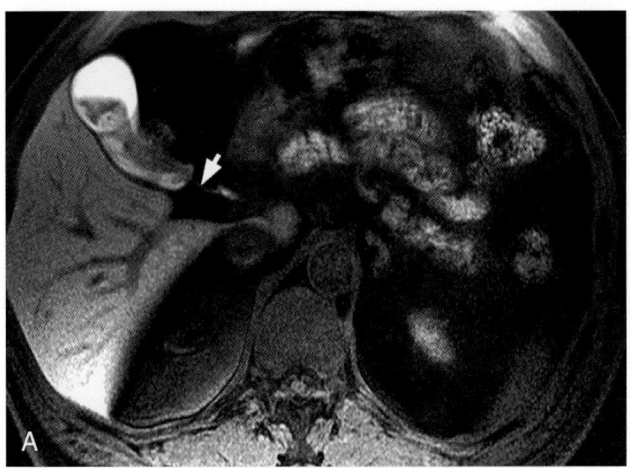

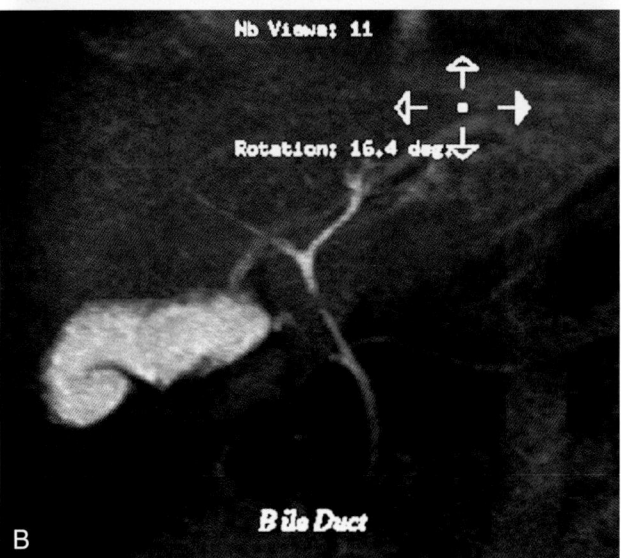

FIGURE 80-18

T1 MR cholangiography after intravenous administration of mangafodipir trisodium. The contrast is excreted into the bile and results in increased signal intensity of bile. Axial fat-suppressed T1-weighted image demonstrates the gallbladder with bright bile and cystic duct (*arrow*). The heterogeneous signal within the gallbladder is due to poor mixing of the contrast and bile. The maximum intensity projection of gallbladder and liver demonstrates the normal intra- and extrahepatic bile ducts and gallbladder.

FIGURE 80-19

Biliary ductal and gallbladder air following papillotomy. Axial fat-suppressed T2-weighted HASTE image demonstrates air-fluid levels in the common bile duct (*two vertical arrows*) and in the gallbladder (*single vertical arrow*) following papillotomy. Air appears as a signal void on MRI and rises to non-dependent location. (*Image courtesy of Robert Edelman MD.*)

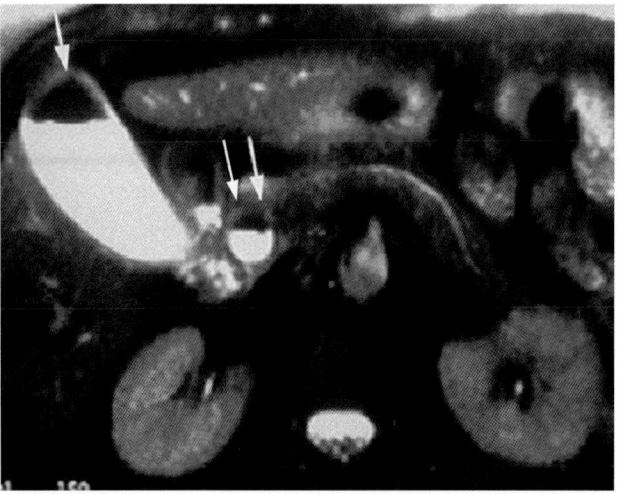

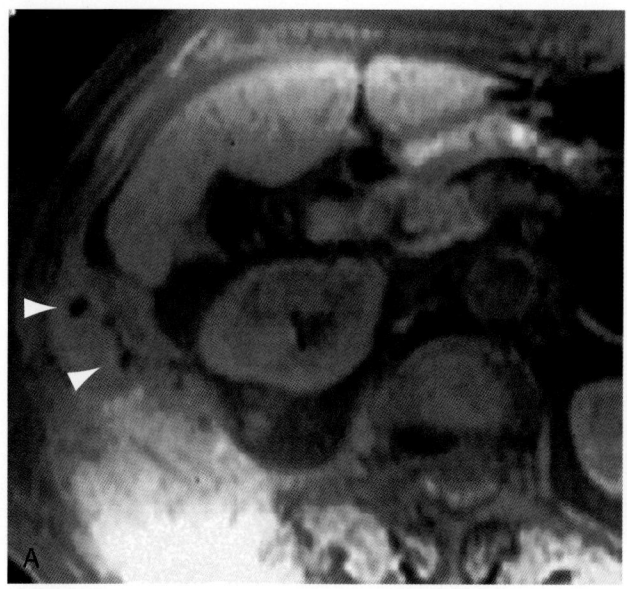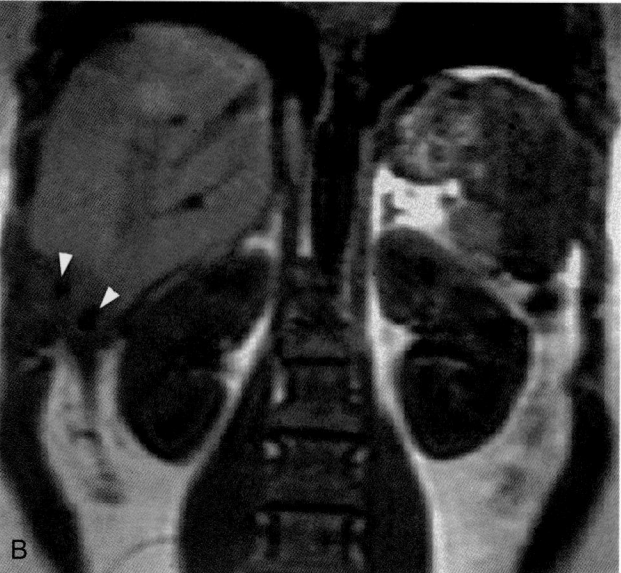

FIGURE 80-20

Abscess due to dropped gallstone following laparoscopic cholecystectomy. **A,** Fat-suppressed FLASH T1-weighted axial image demonstrates multiple dropped gallstones (*arrowheads*) near the inferior edge of the liver with surrounding inflammatory tissue and abscess. **B,** Coronal T1 FLASH image demonstrates the same findings. (*Image courtesy of Robert Edelman MD.*)

Contrast-enhanced MRCP following intravenous administration of hepatobiliary contrast agents can also help to identify biliary leaks.[49] In a series of 11 patients evaluated for suspected biliary leaks following cholecystectomy, mangafodipir trisodium-enhanced MRCP had a sensitivity of 86% with a specificity of 83% compared to direct cholangiography.[49] Similarly, contrast-enhanced MRCP is also useful in differentiating anastomotic strictures at biliary enteric anastomoses from functional obstruction.

REFERENCES

1. Gore RM, Yaghmai V, Newmark GM, et al: Imaging benign and malignant disease of the gallbladder. Radiol Clin North Am 40:1307-1323, 2002.
2. Moeser PM, Julian S, Karstaedt N, Sterchi M: Unusual presentation of cholelithiasis on T1-weighted MR imaging. J Comput Assist Tomogr 12:150-152, 1988.
3. Moriyasu F, Ban N, Nishida O, et al: Central signals of gallstones in magnetic resonance imaging. Am J Gastroenterol 82:139-142, 1987.
4. Baron RL, Shuman WP, Lee SP, et al: MR appearance of gallstones in vitro at 1.5T: correlation with chemical composition. Am J Roentgenol 153:497-502, 1989.
5. Reinold C, Bret PM, Semelka RC: Gallbladder and biliary system. In Semelka RC, Ascher SM, Reinhold C (eds): MRI of the Abdomen and Pelvis. A Text-Atlas. Hoboken, NJ: Wiley-Liss, 1997.
6. Park MS, Yu JS, Kim YH, et al: Acute cholecystitis: comparison of MR cholangiography and US. Radiology 209:781-785, 1998.
7. Oh KY, Gilfeather M, Kennedy A, et al: Limited abdominal MRI in the evaluation of acute right upper quadrant pain. Abdom Imaging 28:643-651, 2003.
8. Hakansson K, Leander P, Ekberg O, et al: MR imaging in clinically suspected acute cholecystitis. A comparison with ultrasonography. Acta Radiol 44:32-38, 2000.
9. Ito K, Fujita N, Noda Y, et al: The significance of magnetic resonance cholangiopancreatography in acute cholecystitis. Nippon Shokakibo Gakkai Zasshi 97:1472-1479, 2000.
10. Matsui O, Kadoya M, Takashima T, et al: Intrahepatic periportal abnormal intensity on MR images: an indication of various hepatobiliary diseases. Radiology 17:335-338, 1989.
11. Pedrosa I, Guarise A, Goldsmith J, et al: The interrupted rim sign in acute cholecystitis: a method to identify the gangrenous form with MRI. J Magn Reson Imaging 18:360-363, 2003.
12. Sood B, Jain M, Khandelwal N, et al: MRI of perforated gallbladder. Australas Radiol 46:438-440, 2002.
13. Loud PA, Semelka RC, Kettritz U, et al: MRI of acute cholecystitis: comparison with normal gallbladder and other entities. Magn Reson Imaging 14:349-355, 1996.
14. Usui M, Matsuda S, Suzuki H, Ogura Y: Preoperative diagnosis of gallbladder torsion by magnetic resonance cholangiopancreatography. Scand J Gastroenterol 35:218-222, 2000.
15. Demachi H, Matsui O, Hoshiba K, et al: Dynamic MRI using a surface coil in chronic cholecystitis and gallbladder carcinoma: radiologic and histopathologic correlation. J Comput Assist Tomogr 21:643-651, 1997.
16. Yoshimitsu K, Honda H, Kaneko K, et al: Dynamic MRI of the gallbladder lesions: differentiation of benign from malignant. J Magn Reson Imaging 7:696-701, 1997.
17. Takashima T, Nakazawa S, Yoshino J, et al: Diagnosis of the wall-thickened lesions of the gallbladder with dynamic MRI. Nippon Shokakibyo Gakkai Zasshi 95:424-431, 1998.
18. Mirizzi PL: Syndrome del conducto hepatico. J Int Chir 8:731-737, 1948.
19. McSherry CK, Fertenberg H, Virshup M: The Mirizzi syndrome: suggested classification and surgical therapy. Surg Gastroenterol 1:219-225, 1982.
20. Fan ST, Lan WY, Lee MJR, Wong KK: Cholecysto-hepaticodochal fistula: the value of pre-operative recognition. Br J Surg 72:743-744, 1985.
21. Nagakawa T, Ohta T, Kayahara M, et al: A new classification of Mirizzi syndrome from diagnostic and therapeutic viewpoints. Hepatogastroenterology 44:63-67, 1997.
22. Bapr JH, Batthews JH, Scheweizer WP, et al: Management of the Mirizzi syndrome and the implications of cholecyst-choledochal fistula. Br J Surg 77:743-745, 1992.
23. Koehler RE, Melson GL, Lee JKT, et al: Common hepatic duct obstruction by cystic duct stone: Mirizzi syndrome. Am J Roentgenol 132:1007-1009, 1979.
24. Becker CD, Hassler H, Terrier F: Preoperative diagnosis of the Mirizzi syndrome: limitations of sonography and computed tomography. Am J Roentgenol 43:591-596, 1984.
25. Kim PN, Outwater EK, Mitchell DG: Mirizzi syndrome: evaluation by MR imaging. Am J Gastroenterol 94:2546-2550, 1999.
26. Nakayama T, Yoshimitsu K, Irie H, et al: Fat detection in gallbladder carcinoma with extensive xanthogranulomatous change demonstrated by chemical shift MR imaging. Abdom Imaging 28:684-687, 2003.

27. Shuto R, Kiyosue H, Komatsu E, et al: CT and MR imaging findings of xanthogranulomatous cholecystitis: correlation with pathologic findings. Eur Radiol 14:440-446, 2004.

28. Yoshimitsu K, Honda H, Aibe H, et al: Radiologic diagnosis of adenomyomatosis of gallbladder: comparative study among MRI, helical CT, and transabdominal US. J Comput Assist Tomogr 25:843-850, 2002.

29. Kim MJ, Oh YT, Park YN, et al: Gallbladder adenomyomatosis: findings on MRI. Abdom Imaging 24:410-413, 1999.

30. Yoshimitsu K, Honda H, Jimi M, et al: MR diagnosis of adenomyomatosis of gallbladder and differentiation from gallbladder carcinoma: importance of showing Rokitansky-Aschoff sinuses. Am J Roentgenol 172:1535-1540, 1999.

31. Sheth S, Bedford A, Chopra S: Primary gallbladder cancer: recognition of risk factors and the role of prophylactic cholecystectomy. Am J Gastroenterol 95:1402-1410, 2000.

32. Rooholamini SA, Tehrani NS, Razavi MK, et al: Imaging of gallbladder carcinoma. Radiographics 14:291-306, 1994.

33. Wilbur AC, Sagireddy PB, Aizestein RI: Carcinoma of the gallbladder: color Doppler ultrasound and CT findings. Abdom Imaging 22:187-189, 1997.

34. Tseng JH, Wan YL, Hung CF, et al: Diagnosis and staging of gallbladder carcinoma: evaluation with dynamic MR imaging. Clin Imaging 26:177-182, 2002.

35. Kim JH, Kim TK, Eun HW, et al: Preoperative evaluation of gallbladder carcinoma: efficacy of combined use of MR imaging, MR cholangiography, and contrast enhanced dual phase three dimensional MR angiography. J Magn Reson Imaging 16:676-684, 2002.

36. Schwartz LH, Black J, Fong Y, et al: Gallbladder carcinoma: findings at MR imaging with MR cholangiography. J Comput Assist Tomogr 26:405-410, 2002.

37. Bickel A, Eitan A, Tsilman B, Cohen HI: Low-grade B cell lymphoma of mucosa-associated lymphoid tissue (MALT) arising in the gallbladder. Hepatogastroenterology 46:1643-1646, 1999.

38. Chim CS, Liang R, Loong F, Chung LP: Primary mucosa-associated lymphoid tissue lymphoma of the gallbladder. Am J Med 112:505-507, 2002.

39. Gogas J, Mantas D, Gogas H, et al: Metastatic melanoma in the gallbladder: report of a case. Surg Today 33:135-137, 2003.

40. Sparwasser C, Krupienski M, Radomsky J, Pust RA: Gallbladder metastasis of renal cell carcinoma. A case report and review of the literature. Urol Int 58:257-258, 1997.

41. De Simone P, Mainente P, Bedin N: Gallbladder melanoma mimicking acute acalculous cholecystitis. Surg Endosc 14:593, 2000.

42. Inoue Y, Komatsu Y, Yoshikawa K, et al: Biliary motor function in gallstone patients evaluated by fatty-meal MR cholangiography. J Magn Reson Imaging 18:196-203, 2003.

43. Vyas PK, Vesy TL, Konez O, et al: Estimation of gallbladder ejection fraction utilizing cholecystokinin-stimulated magnetic resonance cholangiography and comparison with hepatobiliary scintigraphy. J Magn Reson Imaging 15:75-81, 2002.

44. Koike S, Ito K, Honjo K, et al: Oddi sphincter and common channel: evaluation with pharmacodynamic MR cholangiopancreatography using fatty meal and secretin stimulation. Radiat Med 18:115-122, 2000.

45. Fayad LM, Holland GA, Bergin D, et al: Functional magnetic resonance cholangiography (fMRC) of the gallbladder and biliary tree with contrast-enhanced magnetic resonance cholangiography. J Magn Reson Imaging 18:449-460, 2003.

46. Khalid TR, Casillas VJ, Montalvo BM, et al: Using MR cholangiopancreatography to evaluate iatrogenic bile duct injury. Am J Roentgenol 177:1347-1352, 2001.

47. Chaudhary A, Negi SS, Puri SK, Narang P: Comparison of magnetic resonance cholangiography and percutaneous transhepatic cholangiography in the evaluation of bile duct strictures after cholecystectomy. Br J Surg 89:433-436, 2002.

48. Pavone P, Laghi A, Catalano C, et al: MR cholangiography in the examination of patients with biliary-enteric anastomoses. Am J Roentgenol 169:807-811, 1997.

49. Vitellas KM, El-Dieb A, Vaswani KK, et al: Using contrast-enhanced MR cholangiography with IV mangafodipir trisodium (Teslascan) to evaluate bile duct leaks after cholecystectomy: a prospective study of 11 patients. Am J Roentgenol 179:409-416, 2002.

CHAPTER 81

FOCAL LIVER LESIONS

Till Bader ● Ahmed Ba-Ssalamah ● Richard C. Semelka

Focal liver lesions can grossly be divided into benign and malignant disease. The variety of lesions, however, is abundant owing to the complex histologic structure of the liver. All three cellular components of the hepatic parenchyma (i.e., hepatocytes, biliary epithelium, and mesenchymal tissue) can give origin to benign and malignant disease. MRI has shown excellent capability not only in detecting but also in differentiating focal lesions in the liver.

The imaging protocol comprises T1-weighted gradient-echo sequences in phase and out of phase, T2-weighted sequences (preferably with fat suppression in order to increase the signal-to-noise ratio), and serial T1-weighted post-gadolinium images. Fat suppression is especially important with T2-weighted echo-train sequences because fatty liver has relatively high signal intensity on non–fat-suppressed images which may obscure high signal liver lesions (e.g., metastases).

Contrast agents for liver imaging are based on gadolinium, iron oxide, or manganese. They can be categorized as: 1. nonspecific gadolinium chelates; 2. hepatocyte-targeted contrast agents; 3. contrast agents with extracellular and hepatocyte distribution; and 4. reticuloendothelial (RES)-specific contrast agents.[1]

Nonspecific gadolinium chelates have an excellent safety profile.[2,3] They shorten T1 relaxation times so that signal intensity is increased on T1-weighted images. Following bolus injection, they render information about the arterial and portal venous perfusion on immediate and 45-second post-gadolinium images, respectively. After 90 to 120 seconds post injection, the contrast agent has diffused into the interstitial space, rendering information about the amount and composition of the interstitium.[4]

Currently, there are only two hepatocyte-targeted contrast agents on the market, manganese-DPDP (mangafodipir trisodium or Teslascan) and Gd-BOPTA (gadobenate dimeglumine or Multihance). Gd-BOPTA is excreted by the kidneys (75-90%) and, to a lesser extent, the biliary system (10-25%). Mn-DPDP must be applied as a short infusion and can cause mild adverse effects like flushing.[5] After 15 to 20 minutes up to several hours, T1-weighted images can be acquired. The contrast agent is taken up by hepatocytes and pancreatic parenchyma and thus, they have increased signal intensity while other tissues are left nonenhanced. It is partly excreted by bile which causes a positive biligraphic effect.[6]

Contrast agents with extracellular and hepatocyte distribution are gadolinium based (e.g., Gd-BOPTA, Gd-EOB-DTPA). Akin to nonspecific gadolinium chelates, they are given as a bolus injection, and cause enhancement on serial T1-weighted images reflecting the arterial and portal venous perfusion and the amount and composition of the interstitium. In addition, they are specifically taken up by hepatocytes. Delayed-phase images (acquired approximately 1 hour after injection of Gd-BOPTA or 20 minutes after injection of Gd-EOB-DTPA) show enhancement of normal liver parenchyma and of lesions that contain hepatocytes.[7-10]

Superparamagnetic iron oxides (SPIOs) are RES-specific contrast agents that are taken up by Kupffer cells in the liver and by RES cells in the spleen and lymph nodes. Depending on particle size, these contrast agents are subdivided into SPIOs (particle size >50 nm; e.g., AMI-25) and ultra superparamagnetic iron oxides (USPIOs) (particle size <50 nm; e.g., SHU 555A). Both have a T2 shortening effect, leading to signal loss on T2- or T2*-weighted images acquired 10 to 40 minutes post application.[11] SPIOs can cause severe back pain during application and must, therefore, be applied as a slow drip infusion.[12,13] USPIOs cause much fewer side-effects and can be injected as a bolus. Owing to the fact that they also have a T1 shortening effect, they cause enhancement on dynamic T1-weighted images.[14,15] This effect, however, is weaker than with gadolinium-based agents. Normal liver parenchyma and lesions that contain Kupffer cells show signal loss on post-contrast T2- or T2*-weighted images; all other tissues remain unchanged and appear relatively hyperintense compared to liver.[16]

Hepatocyte- and RES-specific contrast agents have proven to be helpful for the detection of metastases. The general problem with these agents, however, is that they do not clearly distinguish between benign and malignant lesions. Well-differentiated hepatocellular carcinoma (HCC), for instance, can take up hepatocyte- and RES-specific contrast agents. In liver cirrhosis, on the other hand, the uptake of both groups of contrast agents can be greatly diminished. Metastases, hemangiomas, and cysts do not take up hepatocyte- or RES-specific agents. Hemangiomas, however, can show a so-called "blood pool effect" with RES-specific contrast agents which can lead to some degree of enhancement. Therefore, these contrast agents seem to be most beneficial for carefully preselected clinical questions. Nonspecific gadolinium chelates can be used without any absolute contraindications and give a wide spectrum of information. Evaluation of the intensity and pattern of enhancement on serial postinjection images allows specific diagnoses to be made and differentiation between benign and malignant disease in most cases.

BENIGN LESIONS

Cysts

Fluid-filled cysts are the most common benign lesions in the liver with a prevalence of about 15% to 25% of all patients. Hepatic cysts are unilocular in about 95% of cases and multilocular in the remainder. They can be differentiated into simple cysts, foregut cysts, cysts in autosomal polycystic kidney disease, and parasitic cysts (hydatid cysts). Parasitic cysts are caused by two main types of echinococcus tapeworms: *Echinococcus granulosus* and *E. alveolaris*.

Simple Cysts

Simple or nonparasitic cysts are lined by a thin layer of fibrous tissue which itself can be lined by a single layer of epithelium. The latter lesions have been termed bile duct cysts. Despite the fact that these types of cysts are so common, their origin is not entirely clear. Developmental and acquired causes leading to retention of bile are postulated.[17] On MR imaging, these cysts are sharply marginated, usually oval-shaped, lesions. Their signal intensity is homogeneously low on T1-weighted images and high on T2-weighted images. Due to the very long T2 time of fluid, cysts retain signal on sequences with very long echo time (e.g., >120 ms) (Fig. 81-1). The fluid content shows no enhancement with contrast agents on early or delayed images, a finding which can be useful to differentiate cysts from poorly vascularized solid lesions. Rarely, cysts can become complicated and hemorrhagic, rendering high signal on T1-weighted images. The wall of simple cysts can, at most, only marginally be depicted on MR images. Abutting cysts may give the impression of thin septations; however, most cysts are unicameral. Occasionally, several small simple cysts are located closely together resembling a multicystic tumor.

In autosomal-dominant polycystic kidney disease (Fig. 81-2), the liver is the primary site for extrarenal cysts. These cysts tend to be multiple and of varying size. However, the cysts in the liver are usually smaller than in the kidneys (<2 cm), do not distort the hepatic architecture, and show no hemorrhage. Extensive replacement of hepatic parenchyma with large cysts has been described.[18]

Hepatic Foregut Cyst

Hepatic foregut cysts are congenital lesions and are believed to arise from the embryonic foregut. Their wall consists of four layers: ciliated epithelium with mucous cells, subepithelial connective tissue, smooth muscle, and a surrounding fibrous capsule. These cysts show a predilection to be located in the anterosuperior margin of the liver or in intersegmental locations. They are almost exclusively situated superficially, bulging the contour of the liver. The signal of foregut cysts is homogeneously high on T2-weighted images. On T1-weighted images, however, it can be anywhere between low and high owing to a variable concentration of mucinous contents.[19,20] Unlike simple cysts, foregut cysts have a much thicker and perceptible wall that enhances on post-gadolinium images. Although the image of a bulging cyst with an enhancing wall is suggestive of a foregut cyst, it can also be observed in some forms of metastases (e.g., ovarian cancer). For this reason, it is advisable to make a diagnosis of foregut cyst only in the absence of a history of malignancy and other indications for malignant disease.

Echinococcal Cyst

Echinococcus granulosus is the parasite that causes hydatid cysts. These are typically round and have a fibrous capsule. Within the periphery of the cyst, smaller daughter cysts can frequently be observed, giving the appearance of a multicystic lesion. Satellite cysts in the adjacent liver parenchyma outside of the fibrous capsule of the main cyst can be found in as many as 16% of hydatid cysts.[21] The fibrous capsule and internal septae can best be visualized on T2-weighted images and on T1-weighted interstitial phase post-gadolinium images (Fig. 81-3). The internal signal of the cysts is typically low on T1-weighted and high on T2-weighted sequences. Due to debris within the cysts, the signal is often moderately inhomogeneous. Capsular calcifications are a typical finding on CT but are not well depicted on MRI.

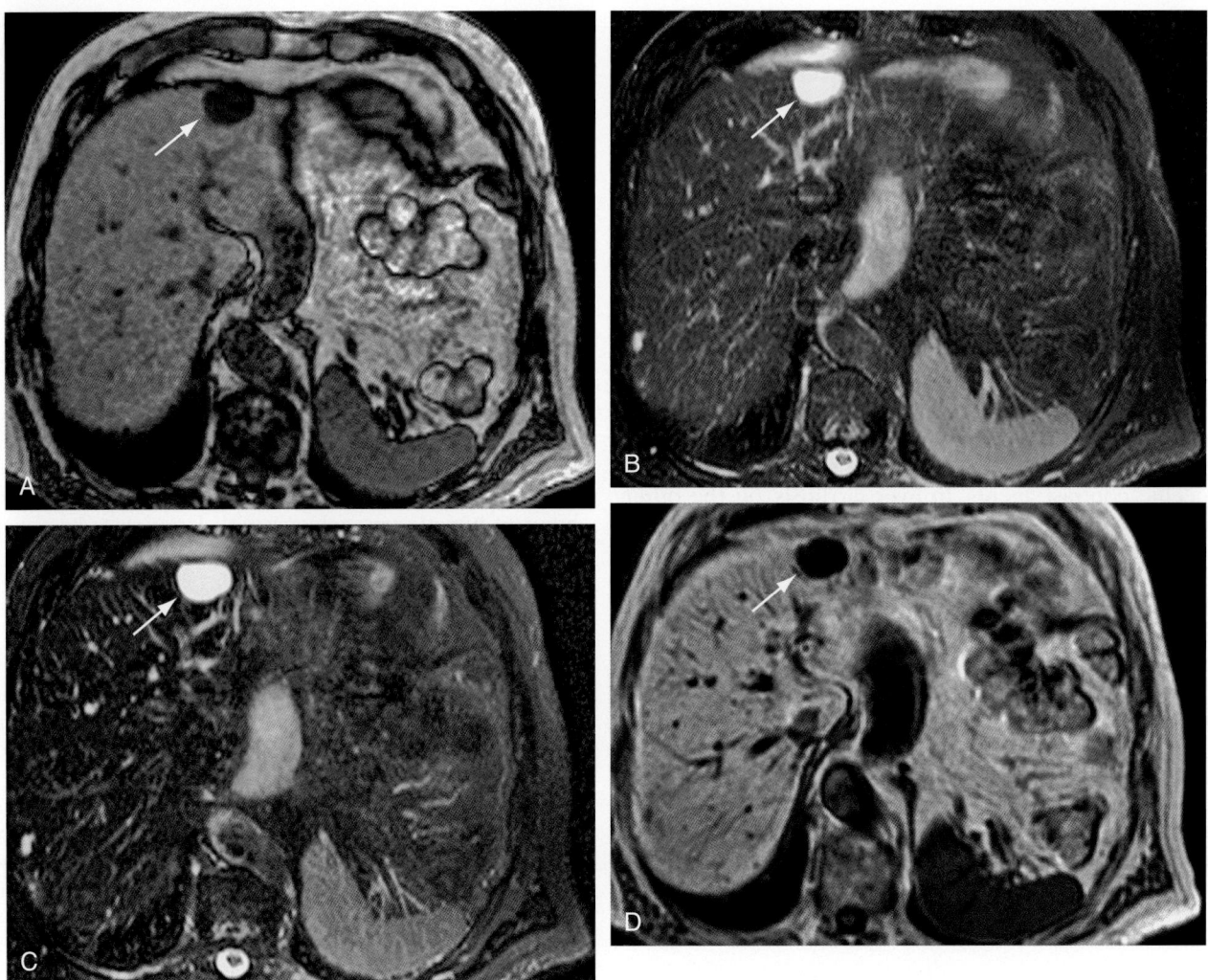

FIGURE 81-1

Liver cyst. **A,** T1-weighted gradient-recalled echo opposed-phase image; **B,** T2-weighted TSE fat-suppressed image; **C,** T2-weighted fat-suppressed turbo spin-echo image with long echo time; and **D,** T1-weighted GRE after administration of mangafodipir trisodium. In the T1-weighted image (**A**) the cyst appears homogeneously hypointense (*arrow*). In the T2-weighted image (**B**) the cyst shows high signal intensity due to fluid content (*arrow*). Due to the very long T2 time, the cyst remains significantly hyperintense on the T2-weighted image with a very long echo time (**C**, *arrow*). The cyst shows no contrast agent uptake after the administration of mangafodipir trisodium (*arrow*) and remains markedly hypointense (**D**).

Echinococcus alveolaris causes hepatic alveolar echinococcosis (HAE) which has a different appearance from hydatid cysts. HAE is composed of multilocular or confluent small cystic lesions that represent necrotic cavities but not true cysts. The MRI findings are typically large (mean 10 cm), solitary lesions with irregular margins lacking a fibrous capsule.[22] The entire lesion has a heterogeneous tumorous appearance due to the small size of the multiple cystic components. Signal intensities are also heterogeneous on T1- and T2-weighted images and on post-gadolinium images. HAE tends to involve extensive regions of the liver with a propensity for the porta hepatic. As a sequel, stenoses of bile ducts, portal veins, and hepatic veins are frequent and can cause portal hypertension. Calcifications, as in hydatid cysts, are better visualized on CT than on MRI.

Biliary Hamartoma

Biliary hamartomas, also known as biliary micro-hamartomas or von Meyenburg complexes, are benign, cystic, biliary malformations that are currently considered to arise from ductal plate malformations of small interlobular bile ducts. Due to their biliary origin, they have also been described as bile duct cysts. Biliary hamartomas are common with an estimated prevalence of approximately 3% of patients. The histologic appearance is a mass containing a collection of small, sometimes dilated, irregular and branching bile ducts embedded in a fibrous stroma.[23,24] In general, biliary hamartomas are poorly vascularized, they may be solitary or multiple, and are usually less than 1 cm. On MRI, they are well-defined cystlike lesions of low signal on T1-weighted images and high signal on T2-weighted

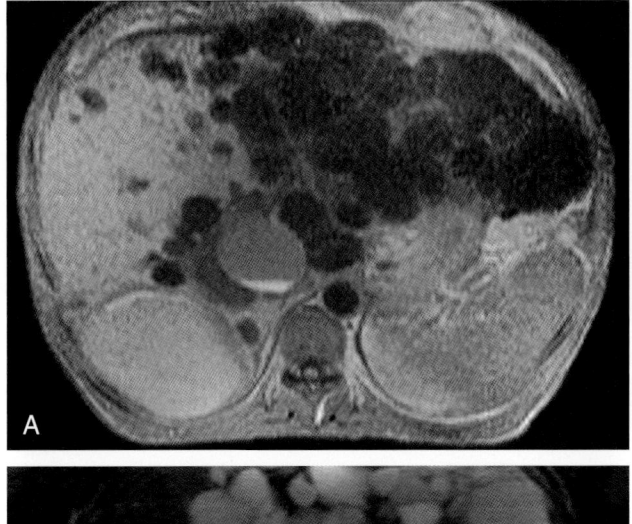

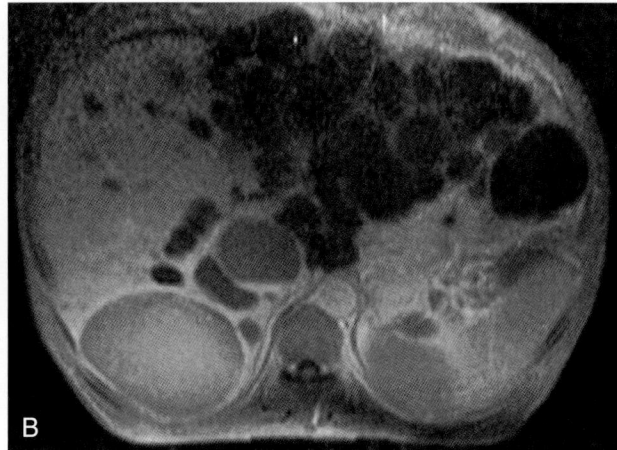

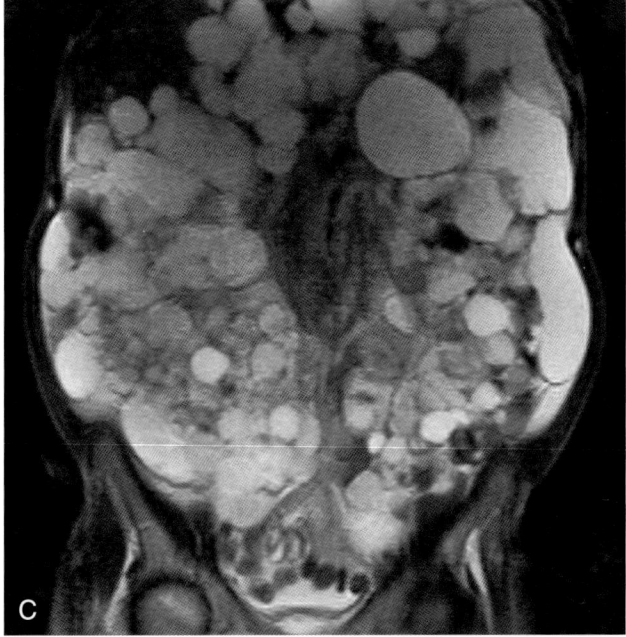

FIGURE 81-2

Multiple cysts in autosomal-dominant polycystic kidney disease. **A,** Nonenhanced and **B,** after administration of gadolinium chelate T1-weighted gradient-recalled echo images; and **C,** coronal T2-weighted fat-suppressed turbo spin-echo image. The multiple cysts are sharply demarcated hypointense lesions on the nonenhanced T1-weighted image (**A**) and do not show enhancement after the administration of gadolinium chelate (**B**). The cysts in the liver and both kidneys appear hyperintense on the T2-weighted image (**C**).

images (Fig. 81-4). On early and late post-gadolinium images, a thin rim of enhancement is a typical finding.[23,24] This rim is composed of compressed abutting hepatic parenchyma and not a fibrous capsule. Biliary hamartomas can be misclassified as metastases due to their ring enhancement. However, unlike metastases, biliary hamartomas do not show perilesional enhancement or progressive centripetal enhancement on late-phase post-gadolinium images.

Hemangioma

Hemangiomas are the most common benign neoplasm of the liver, with a prevalence of up to 20%, and are five times more common in women than in men. They are often multiple and very rarely cause clinical symptoms. They are thought to be hamartomatous lesions and are histologically characterized as well-circumscribed, spongelike, blood-filled mesenchymal tumors. The vast majority are cavernous hemangiomas that are composed of numerous large vascular channels separated by thin fibrous septae and are lined by a single layer of epithelium. Small areas of thrombosis or calcification or areas of extensive fibrosis may be present.[25] Telangiectatic hemangiomas are rare. Hemangiomas are usually round when they are small and tend to show lobular borders when they are bigger. On MRI, hemangiomas present as sharply delineated lesions that are typically of homogeneous low signal intensity on T1-weighted images and of high signal intensity on T2-weighted images (Fig. 81-5). Due to their very long T2 time they retain signal on heavily T2-weighted images (TE >120 ms).[26,27] Hemangiomas demonstrate three typical enhancement patterns on post-gadolinium images.

1. Type 1: Uniform, intense enhancement on arterial phase post-gadolinium images. Isointense or slightly hyperintense signal compared to normal liver on later post-gadolinium images.

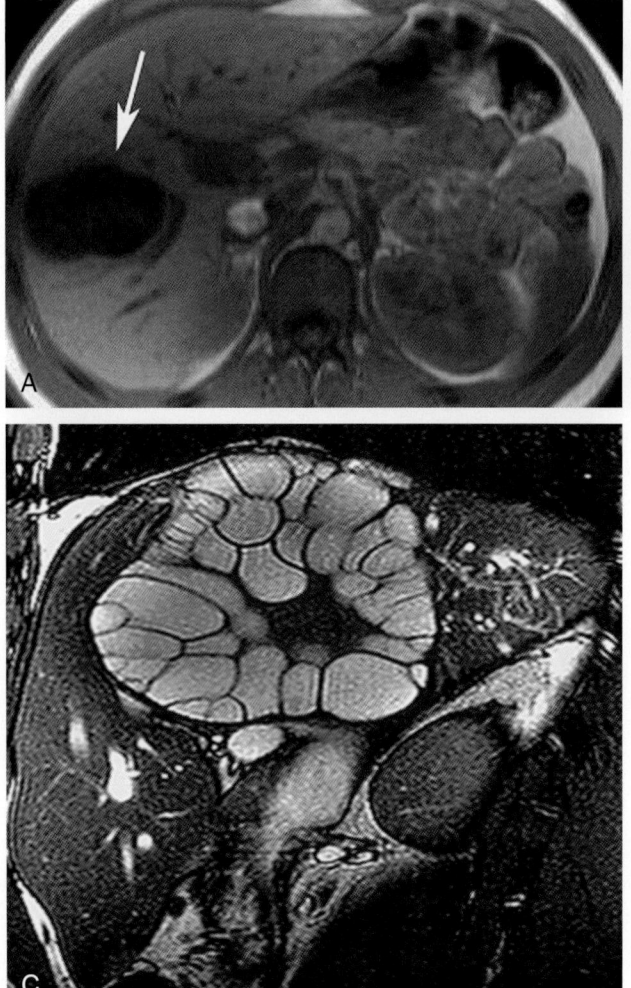

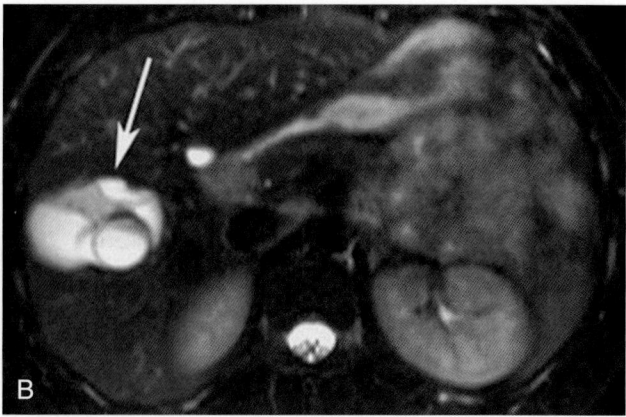

FIGURE 81-3

Echinococcal cyst. **A,** T1-weighted gradient-recalled echo, and **B,** T2-weighted fat-suppressed turbo spin-echo images. A fibrous capsule can be seen on the T1-weighted image (*arrow*, **A**) and on the T2-weighted image internal septae are noted (*arrow*, **B**). **C,** True fast imaging with steady-state precession (FISP) image in a different patient shows a large lesion with multiple internal septations.

2. Type 2: Peripheral, nodular enhancement in a discontinuous ring fashion on arterial phase post-gadolinium images. Centripetal progression of enhancement and confluence of enhancing nodules on later images with, finally, homogeneous fill-in (see Fig. 81-5).

3. Type 3: Peripheral, nodular enhancement in a discontinuous ring fashion on arterial phase post-gadolinium images. Centripetal progression with sparing of enhancement of a central scar, even on much delayed images (up to 15 minutes after contrast infusion) (Fig. 81-6).

These types of enhancement patterns can be related to the size of the hemangioma. In a multi-institutional study, 53% of 154 hemangiomas were less than 1.5 cm, 36% were of medium size (1.5-5 cm), and 11% were greater than 5 cm.[28] Multiple hemangiomas were found in 68% of patients. The most common type of enhancement of small hemangiomas (<1.5 cm) is type 2 enhancement (see Fig. 81-5) and the second most common is type 1 enhancement. Medium size hemangiomas generally demonstrate type 2 enhancement, sometimes type 3 enhancement, and exceedingly rarely type 1 enhancement.

Giant hemangiomas (>5 cm) almost always show type 3 enhancement (Fig. 81-6). On T2-weighted images, these lesions frequently show a central area of bright, dark, or mixed signal intensity and a network of multiple fibrous septa of low signal intensity (Fig. 81-6).[29] Histologically, the bright central area represents hypocellular myxoid tissue. Giant hemangiomas greater than 10 cm in diameter can also show central enhancement and an irregular flame-shaped peripheral pattern of enhancement.[29] Central enhancement is caused by early filling of a large central lake by narrow feeding vessels and is extremely rare in smaller hemangiomas. On rare occasions, hemorrhage may occur in large hemangiomas (Fig. 81-7).

The speed and completeness of enhancement of hemangiomas is quite variable.[30] Fast-enhancing hemangiomas can demonstrate perilesional high signal on T2-weighted images and perilesional hyperenhancement on post-gadolinium images (likely reflecting high flow in efferent veins) which can resemble other tumors (e.g., metastases). Compared to metastases (e.g., colorectal), however, such findings in hemangiomas are generally less pronounced and rare. Hemangiomas may fade in

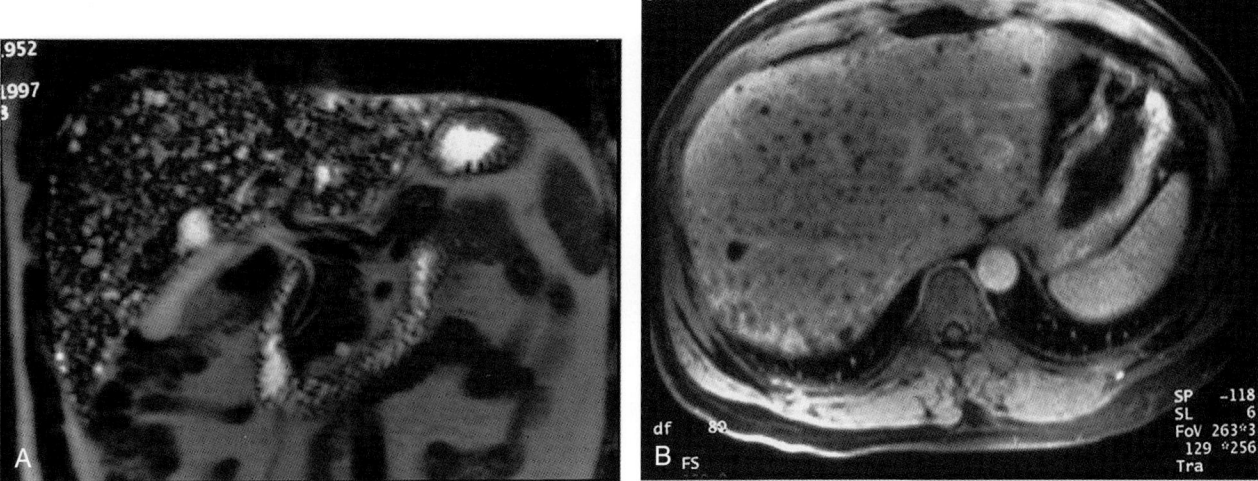

FIGURE 81-4

Biliary hamartoma. **A,** T2-weighted turbo spin-echo image and **B,** T1-weighted fat-suppressed gradient-recalled echo image after administration of gadolinium. Similar to cysts, biliary hamartomas present as high signal lesions on T2-weighted images (**A**) and with low signal on T1-weighted images without enhancement (**B**).

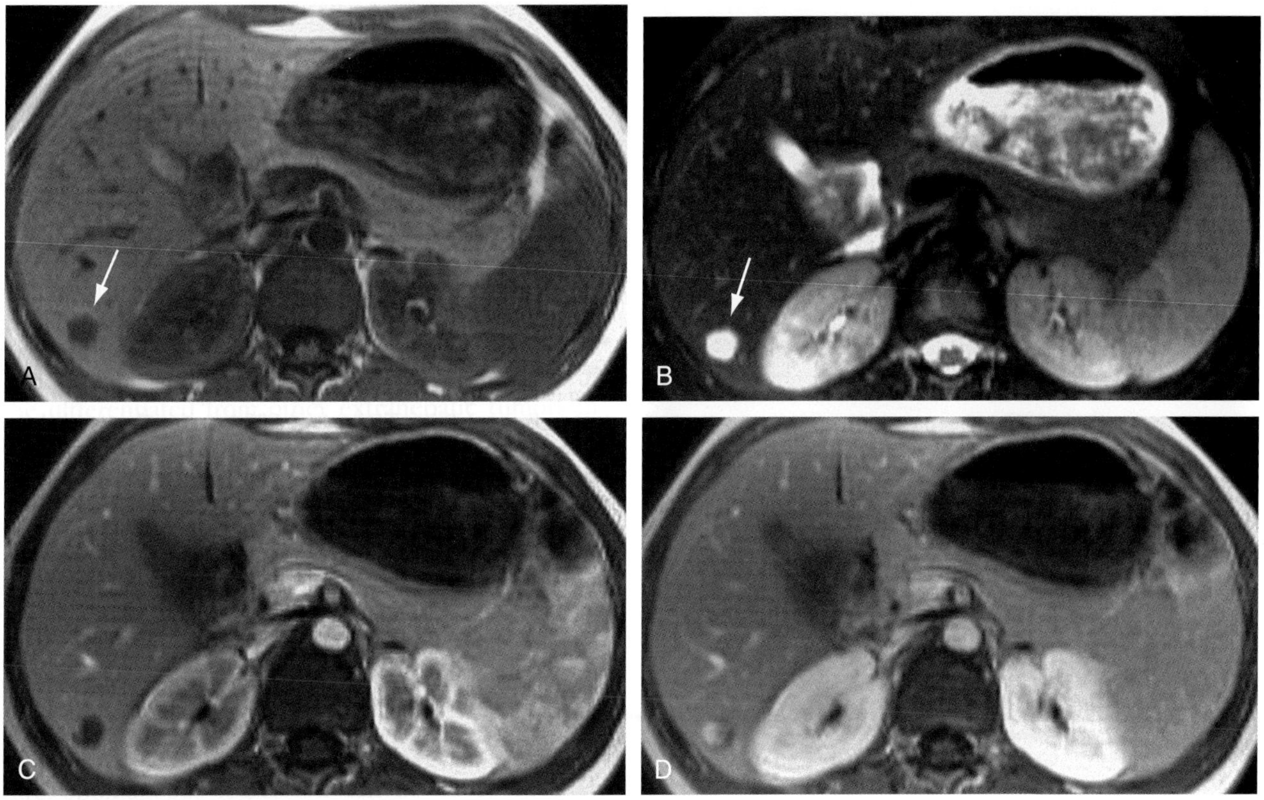

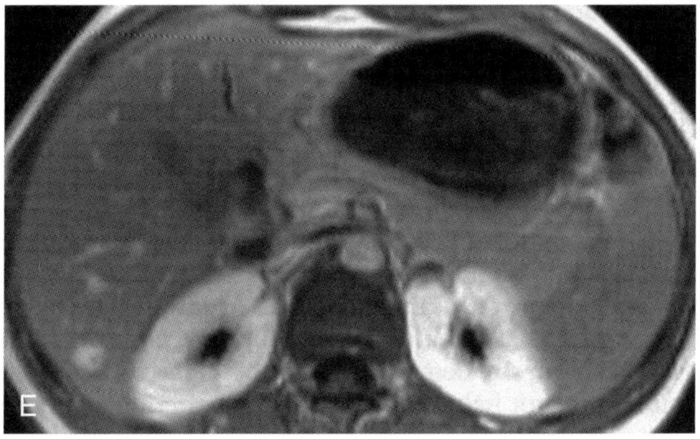

FIGURE 81-5

Small hemangioma. **A,** Nonenhanced T1-weighted gradient-recalled echo (GRE) image and **B,** T2-weighted fat-suppressed turbo spin-echo images. Post-gadolinium T1-weighted GRE images: **C,** immediate, **D,** in the portal venous phase, and **E,** in the late phase. Low signal intensity on the T1-weighted image (*arrow*, **A**) and fairly high signal intensity on the T2-weighted image (*arrow*, **B**) are typical of the type 2 enhancement pattern in hemangioma. These images (**C-E**) demonstrate the most frequent hemangioma enhancement seen on dynamic post-gadolinium images. Note the peripheral nodular enhancement (**C**), which progresses towards the center (**D**) and finally shows homogeneous fill-in (**E**).

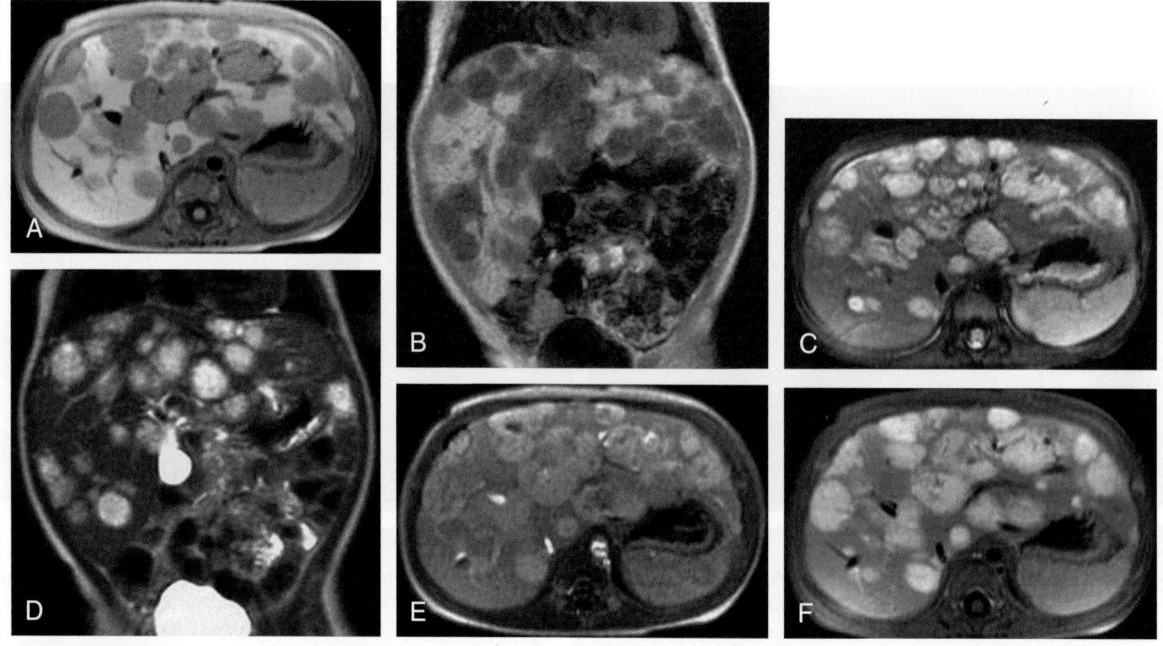

FIGURE 81-8

Infantile hemangioendothelioma. **A,** Axial and **B,** coronal T1-weighted turbo-SGE images; **C,** axial and **D,** coronal T2-weighted echo-train spin-echo images; **E,** axial immediate post-gadolinium T1-weighted turbo-SGE image; and **F,** axial 2-minute post-gadolinium SGE. Multiple round lesions can be observed throughout the entire liver with hypointense signal on T1-weighted sequences (**A** and **B**) and hyperintense signal on T2-weighted images (**C** and **D**). After gadolinium application, they show intense rim enhancement (**E**) with centripetal progression and homogeneous enhancement on 2-minute post-gadolinium images (**F**).

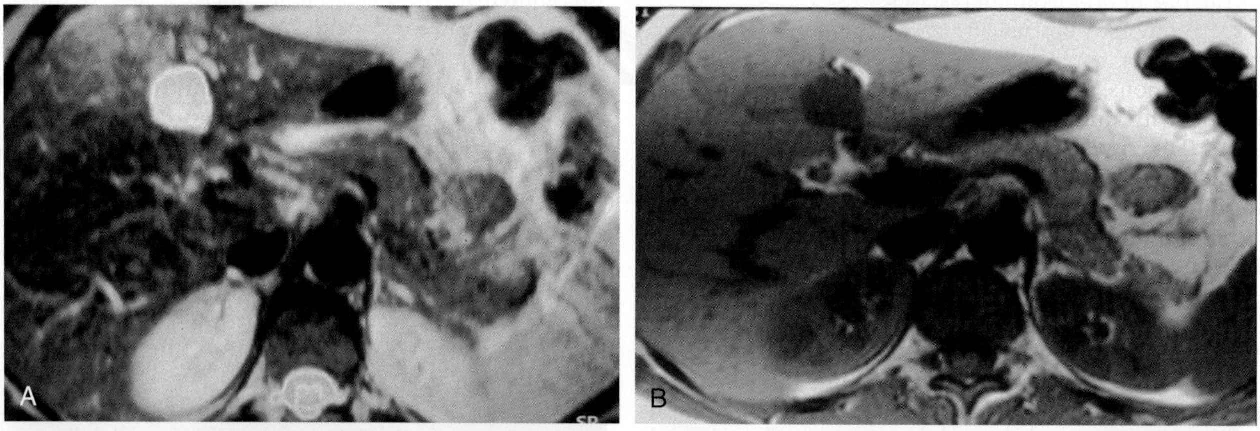

FIGURE 81-9

Coexisting focal nodular hyperplasia (FNH) and cavernous hemangioma. **A,** T2-weighted image shows a nearly isointense peripheral lesion (FNH) and a bright lesion more medially (hemangioma). **B,** T1-weighted image. **C,** Early-phase post-gadolinium image shows intense enhancement of the FNH with only minimal peripheral nodular enhancement of the hemangioma. **D,** Delayed-phase image shows near isointensity of the FNH with enhancement of the central scar, and filling in of the hemangioma. *(Courtesy of Robert Edelman, MD.)*

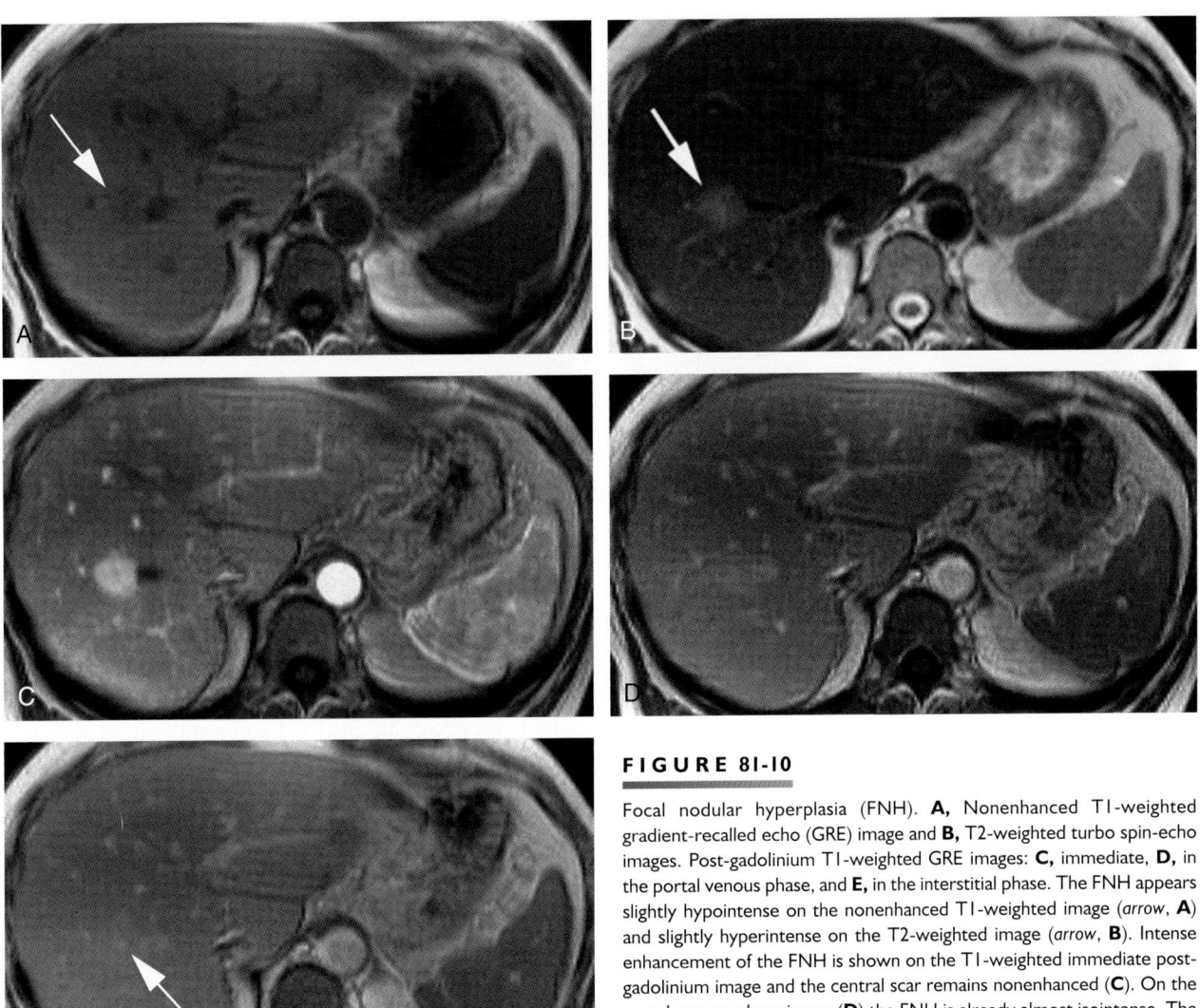

FIGURE 81-10

Focal nodular hyperplasia (FNH). **A,** Nonenhanced T1-weighted gradient-recalled echo (GRE) image and **B,** T2-weighted turbo spin-echo images. Post-gadolinium T1-weighted GRE images: **C,** immediate, **D,** in the portal venous phase, and **E,** in the interstitial phase. The FNH appears slightly hypointense on the nonenhanced T1-weighted image (*arrow,* **A**) and slightly hyperintense on the T2-weighted image (*arrow,* **B**). Intense enhancement of the FNH is shown on the T1-weighted immediate post-gadolinium image and the central scar remains nonenhanced (**C**). On the portal venous phase image (**D**) the FNH is already almost isointense. The central scar shows accumulation of the contrast agent on the interstitial phase image (*arrow,* **E**), whereas the FNH is isointense.

The multiple FNH syndrome is an entity of its own, comprising multicentric lesions, liver hemangiomas, meningioma, astrocytoma, telangiectasia of the brain, berry aneurysm, dysplastic systemic arteries, and portal vein atresia.[50] Although FNH may appear in all age groups and both genders, it is most frequently observed in women between the third and fourth decades but has no association with oral contraceptives. It is usually clinically silent and discovered only as an incidental finding. A palpable mass and abdominal pain can be the symptoms in large lesions. FNH does not show malignant transformation and hemorrhage is exceedingly rare, also only encountered in large lesions.[51]

On noncontrast MRI, FNH usually presents as well-demarcated, slightly hypointense lesions on T1-weighted images and as slightly hyperintense lesions on T2-weighted images. However, near isointensity on both of these sequences is not uncommon (Fig. 81-10). Unlike adenoma, FNH does not contain fat and has no propen-sity for hemorrhage and, therefore, rarely shows hyper-intense signal on T1-weighted images. Fatty liver is quite frequently associated with FNH, resulting in isointense signal of the tumor on in-phase images and hyperintense signal on out-of-phase images (Fig. 81-11). Depicting a hyperintense central scar on T2-weighted images is a characteristic finding. It is, however, present in only 10% to 49% of cases.[44-46,52] This hyperintensity is histologically attributable to the presence of vascular channels, bile duct, edema, chronic inflammation, and fibrosis. The scar is relatively small with sharp angular margins aiding differentiation from other lesions that may exhibit scarlike areas (e.g., fibrolamellar carcinoma).

On immediate post-gadolinium images, FNH shows very intense enhancement. The central scar may remain nonenhanced on these images and be more con-spicuous. On later-phase images, the enhancement of the tumor fades rapidly to near isointensity at about 1 minute after contrast. The central scar, however, shows slow

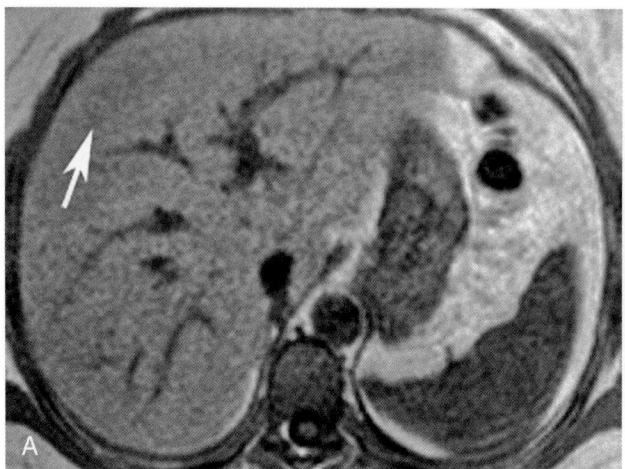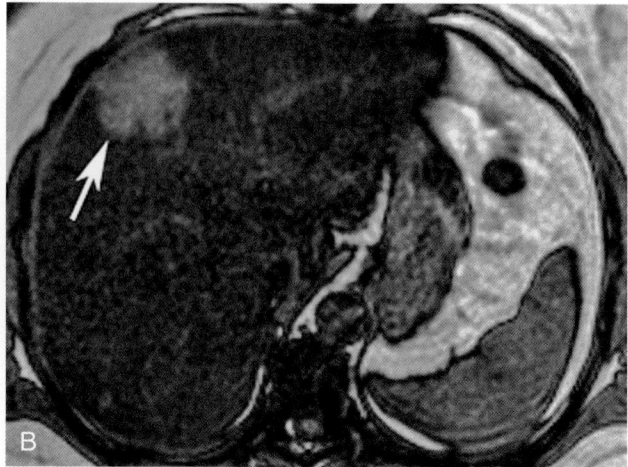

FIGURE 81-11

Focal nodular hyperplasia (FNH) in a fatty liver. T1-weighted gradient-recalled echo **A,** in-phase and **B,** out-of-phase images. FNH can hardly be identified on the T1-weighted in-phase image (*arrow,* **A**). The FNH demonstrates hyperintensity on the T1-weighted out-of-phase image (*arrow,* **B**) due to the signal loss of the fatty liver.

progressive enhancement to hyperintensity on interstitial phase images. This pattern of enhancement is very typical even in exophytic lesions that may be connected to the liver only by a thin stalk.[53] Immediate postgadolinium images are most important, especially for detecting lesions that are isointense on nonenhanced images. Small FNHs (<1.5 cm, lacking a central scar) tend to show homogeneous enhancement on these images. A uniform early blush, however, is also typical for adenoma and HCC and must be interpreted cautiously. HCC, however, tends to show gadolinium washout to hypointensity on late-phase images, a finding that is atypical for FNH or adenoma. An atypical feature of FNH is lack of capillary blush. After application of hepatocyte-specific contrast agents (e.g., Mn-DPDP, Gd-BOPTA, Gd-EOB-DTPA) and acquisition of delayed-phase images, FNHs will often appear slightly hyperintense, reflecting impaired biliary drainage within the lesion (Fig. 81-12).[54,55] FNH contains Kupffer cells, leading to uptake of SPIO contrast agents and signal loss on T2- or T2*-weighted images (Fig. 81-13).[54] The signal loss is usually substantial and can be equal to normal liver. However, Kupffer cells in FNH may suffer lack of function causing reduced SPIO uptake and only minimal decrease of signal resembling adenoma or well-differentiated HCC.[42]

Adenoma

Hepatocellular adenomas are benign epithelial neoplasms usually encountered in patients who are using estrogen- or androgen-containing medication or who suffer from abnormal carbohydrate metabolism (e.g., glycogen storage disease, familial diabetes mellitus, galactosemia).[56] Adenomas, however, can occur in patients without any predisposing risk factors. In women who have never used oral contraceptives, the annual incidence of hepatic adenoma is about 1 per million, which increases to 30 to 40 per million in long-term users of oral contraceptives.[57] Withdrawal from birth control pills usually leads to spontaneous involution of the lesions. Adenomas are solitary in 70% to 80% of cases.[58] If more than 10 lesions are present, this condition is called adenomatosis, which occurs predominantly in glycogen storage diseases and has an elevated complication rate.[59] Although the adenomas in adenomatosis are histologically similar to solitary lesions, they are not steroid dependent. Clinically, most patients with fewer than five adenomas are asymptomatic. Larger or multiple lesions can cause right upper quadrant fullness or discomfort. When adenomas grow large, they show central degenerative changes that can lead to

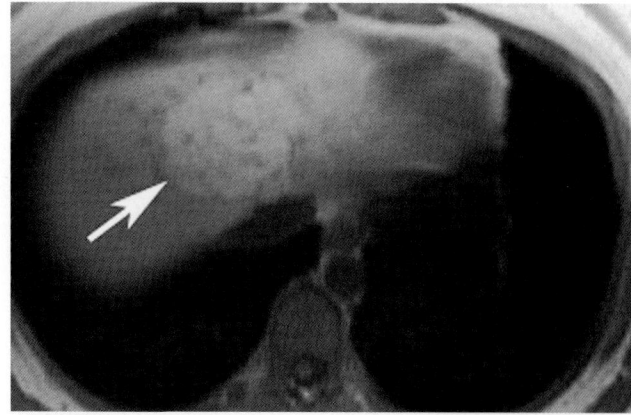

FIGURE 81-12

Focal nodular hyperplasia (FNH). Mangofidipir trisodium–enhanced T1-weighted gradient-recalled echo delayed-phase image. This image renders the FNH hyperintense, due to impaired biliary drainage (*arrow*).

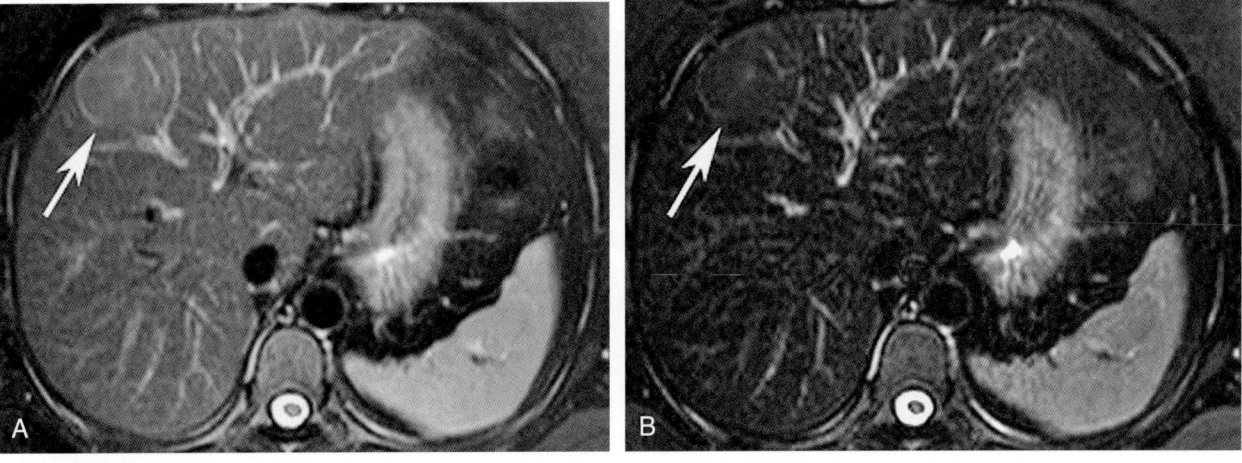

FIGURE 81-13

Focal nodular hyperplasia (FNH). T2-weighted fat-suppressed turbo spin-echo images **A,** nonenhanced and **B,** after administration of a superparamagnetic iron oxide (SPIO) agent. The FNH appears slightly hyperintense on the T2-weighted nonenhanced image (*arrow,* **A**). Due to the Kupffer cell content, the FNH also decreases in signal intensity (slightly less than normal liver parenchyma) after the administration of an SPIO agent (*arrow,* **B**).

hemorrhage, which causes sudden abdominal pain.[60] Rupture in the peritoneal cavity is extremely rare and requires emergency intervention.[61] Histologically, hepatic adenomas are composed of clusters of benign hepatocytes that are separated by dilated sinusoids. Accumulation of lipids is the reason for the yellow color of gross specimens. Adenomas are solely vascularized by hepatic arteries whereas portal veins and bile ducts are absent. Liver cell adenomas are usually encapsulated by a fibrous capsule that may be thin and incomplete or prominent.[60]

Malignant transformation of adenomas is regarded as rare, though the exact incidence is difficult to assess from the literature.

On MRI, adenomas may exhibit substantial fat which can best be visualized on out-of-phase T1-weighted gradient-echo sequences where fatty tissue causes signal drop compared to in-phase images (Fig. 81-14). HCC may also contain fat. In adenomas, however, the distribution of fat and the correlated signal drop on fat-suppressed sequences is usually homogeneous as opposed to HCC

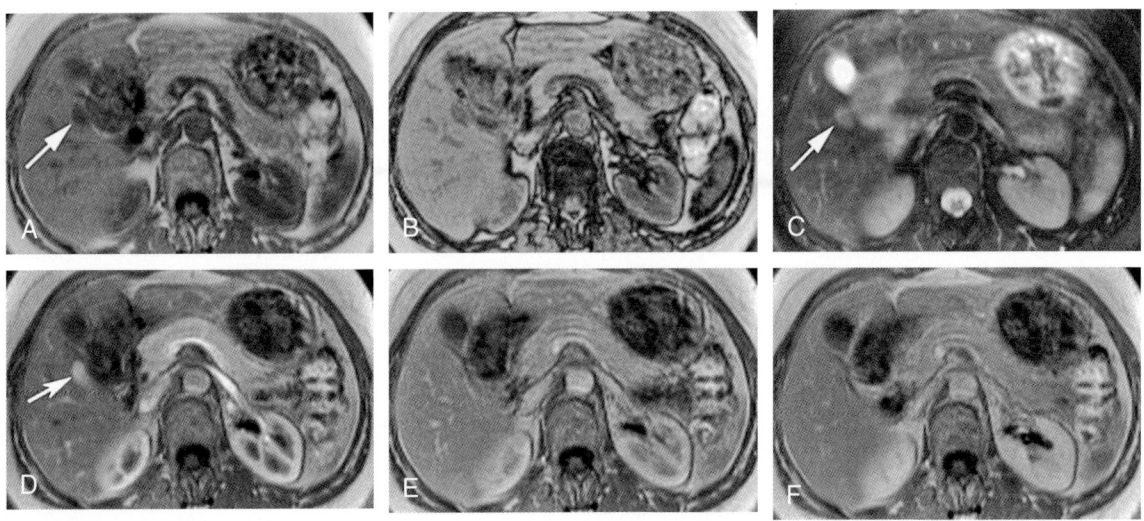

FIGURE 81-14

Small adenoma. Nonenhanced T1-weighted gradient-recalled echo (GRE) **A,** in-phase and **B,** out-of-phase images. **C,** Nonenhanced T2-weighted fat-suppressed turbo spin-echo image. The adenoma (*arrow*) is slightly hyperintense on the T2-weighted image. Post-gadolinium T1-weighted GRE images in the **D,** arterial phase, **E,** portal venous, and **F,** delayed phase. The small adenoma situated below the gallbladder is not as well depicted on the in-phase T1-weighted nonenhanced image (*arrow,* **A**) as in the out-of-phase image (**B**). The adenoma is slightly hyperintense on the T2-weighted image. Uniform blush is seen in the adenoma on the immediate post-gadolinium T1-weighted image (*arrow,* **D**), which fades to isointensity in later phases (**E** and **F**).

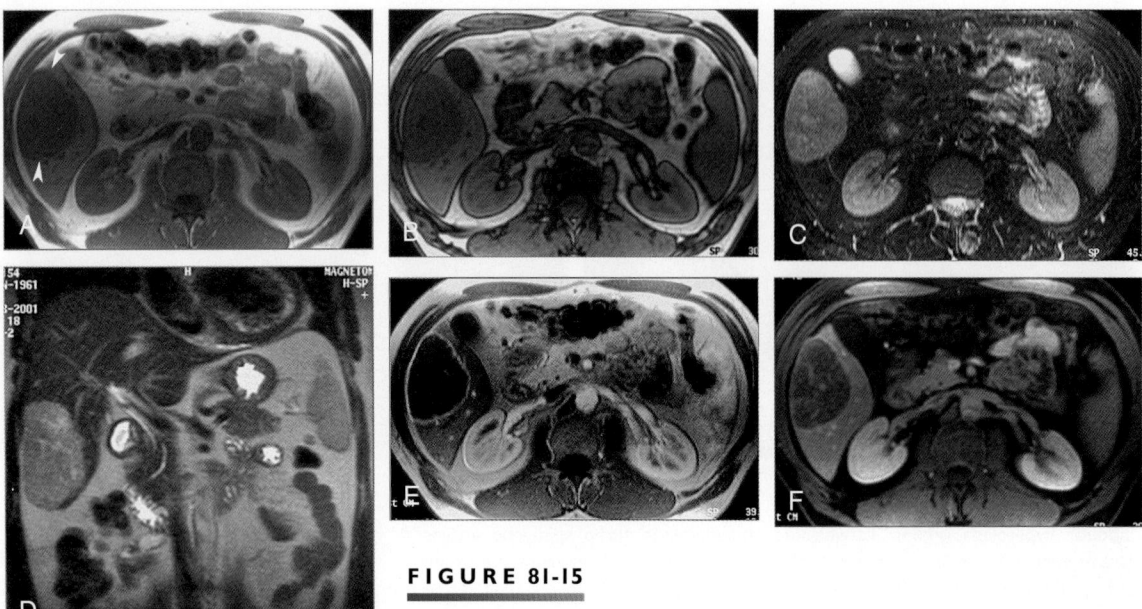

FIGURE 81-15

Angiomyolipoma. Axial T1-weighted SGE **A,** in-phase and **B,** out-of-phase images. **C,** Axial short tau inversion recovery (STIR) image. **D,** Coronal T2-weighted echo-train spin-echo image. **E,** Immediate post-gadolinium T1-weighted SGE image and **F,** 2-minute post-gadolinium T1-weighted fat-suppressed SGE image. A large tumor is observed in the right hepatic lobe with homogeneous low signal on the T1-weighted in-phase SGE image (*arrowhead,* **A**) and hyperintense signal on the T2-weighted image (**C**). The tumor shows insignificant signal drop on the out-of-phase SGE image (**B**) consistent with only minimal fat content. On the immediate post-gadolinium image (**E**), the adjacent liver parenchyma shows a thin rim of hyperenhancement, consistent with compressed liver parenchyma. The tumor itself is not hyperenhancing, which is rare in angiomyolipoma and may be consistent with a high content of fiber and muscle tissue. Note the orderly internal structure of the tumor, containing vessels of normal course and appearance, best depicted on post-gadolinium images (**E** and **F**).

which can show focal or heterogeneous areas of fat. The signal intensity of hepatic adenoma on T1-weighted images varies from mildly hypointense to isointense to moderately hyperintense.[58,62,63] On T2-weighted images, they are generally mildly hyperintense but can also be isointense to normal liver parenchyma. A capsule, if present, can be hyperintense on T2-weighted images. Hemorrhage causes mixed signal intensity on T1- and T2-weighted images. Adenomas may show a central, degenerative, scarlike hypointense area which can mimic FNH. On immediate post-gadolinium images, adenomas characteristically show a uniform blush that fades to near isointensity after 1 minute. The fibrous capsule may appear hyperintense on interstitial phase images. Very large adenomas can show a more heterogeneous enhancement due to internal degenerative changes.

Adenomas can have normal or decreased counts of Kupffer cells. Following the administration of superparamagnetic iron oxide contrast agents (SPIOs, USPIOs), adenomas can, therefore, show isointense signal drop compared to liver parenchyma or remain hyperintense on T2- or T2*-weighted images. In most cases, however, the uptake of iron oxides is moderate at most.[64] Hepatocyte-specific Mn-DPDP is taken up by adenomas in a fashion similar to that in FNH, usually rendering them isointense or slightly hyperintense to normal liver. After application of Gd-BOPTA, adenomas usually appear slightly hypointense on T1-weighted delayed-phase images due to the absence of bile ducts.[42]

Angiomyolipoma

Angiomyolipomas of the liver are benign mesenchymal tumors containing mature fat, blood vessels, and smooth muscle. The association with tuberous sclerosis is much weaker compared to renal angiomyolipomas.[65] On MRI, they present as well-defined masses and are frequently of moderately high signal on T1-weighted images owing to their fatty component and of moderately high signal on T2-weighted images. They drop in signal on fat-suppressed sequences. The content of fat, however, can be low and angiomyolipomas may appear hypointense on T1-weighted images in such instances (Fig. 81-15). On immediate post-gadolinium images, angiomyolipomas enhance strongly in a diffuse heterogeneous fashion.[66] This enhancement pattern may be confused with well-differentiated HCC. Angiomyolipomas, however, tend to enhance in a much more orderly fashion than HCC and do not show washout with hypointense signal on late-phase images.

Lipoma

Hepatic lipomas are rare tumors composed of mature fat and are commonly multiple. Their signal intensity on MRI reflects the characteristics of fat, rendering high signal on T1- and T2-weighted images with signal drop on fat-suppressed images. On T1-weighted out-of-phase images,

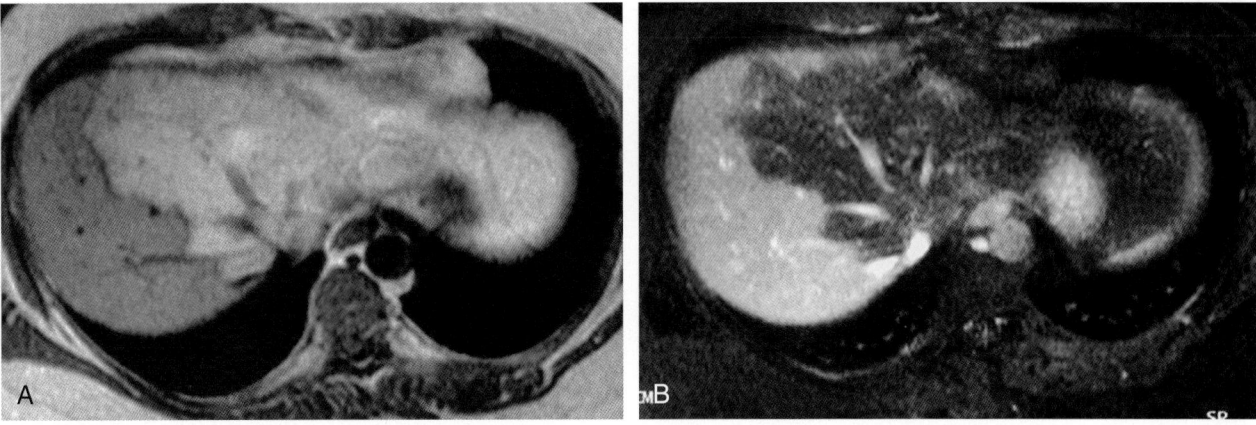

FIGURE 81-16

Extensive focal hepatic fat. **A,** On a T1-weighted image, the fat appears bright. **B,** With chemical shift-selective fat suppression, the fatty areas appear dark. There is no displacement of the hepatic veins, excluding a mass lesion. *(Courtesy of Robert Edelman, MD.)*

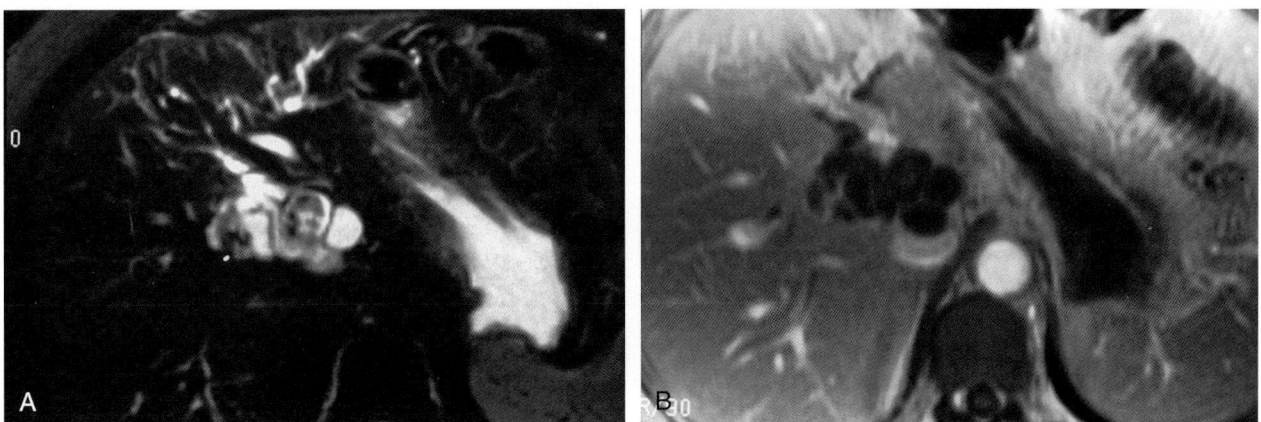

FIGURE 81-17

Biliary cystadenoma. **A,** Axial T2-weighted and **B,** gadolinium-enhanced T1-weighted image show a heterogeneous, multiloculated intrahepatic mass anterior to the inferior vena cava. Low signal regions in **A** may represent mucin-containing components. *(Courtesy of Robert Edelman, MD.)*

they demonstrate a hypointense rim caused by fat cancellation artifact at the border of the lesion.

Focal fat is well assessed on out-of-phase images. However, if present in sufficient amounts, it may be well assessed with chemical shift-selective fat suppression (Fig. 81-16).

Extramedullary Hematopoiesis

In hereditary disorders of hematopoiesis, long-standing anemia, or hematologic malignancies, hematopoiesis may take place in extramedullary locations. This is a compensatory phenomenon for insufficient blood cell production in the bone marrow.[67] The most common sites for extramedullary hematopoiesis are the liver, spleen, and lymph nodes, whereas other locations in the body are very rare. Extramedullary hematopoiesis is usually microscopic and only rarely macroscopic and masslike.[67] Focal hepatic lesions can be solitary or multiple. On MRI, they tend to be homogeneous and moderately low signal on T1-weighted images and moderately high signal on T2-weighted images.[68] On immediate post-gadolinium images, they enhance in a homogeneous to slightly heterogeneous fashion and are almost isointense on late-phase images.[68] For diagnosis, biopsy is usually required.

Biliary Cystadenoma

Biliary cystadenoma is a very rare benign tumor with its peak incidence in the fifth decade and a female predominance. Tumors typically consist of large cystic

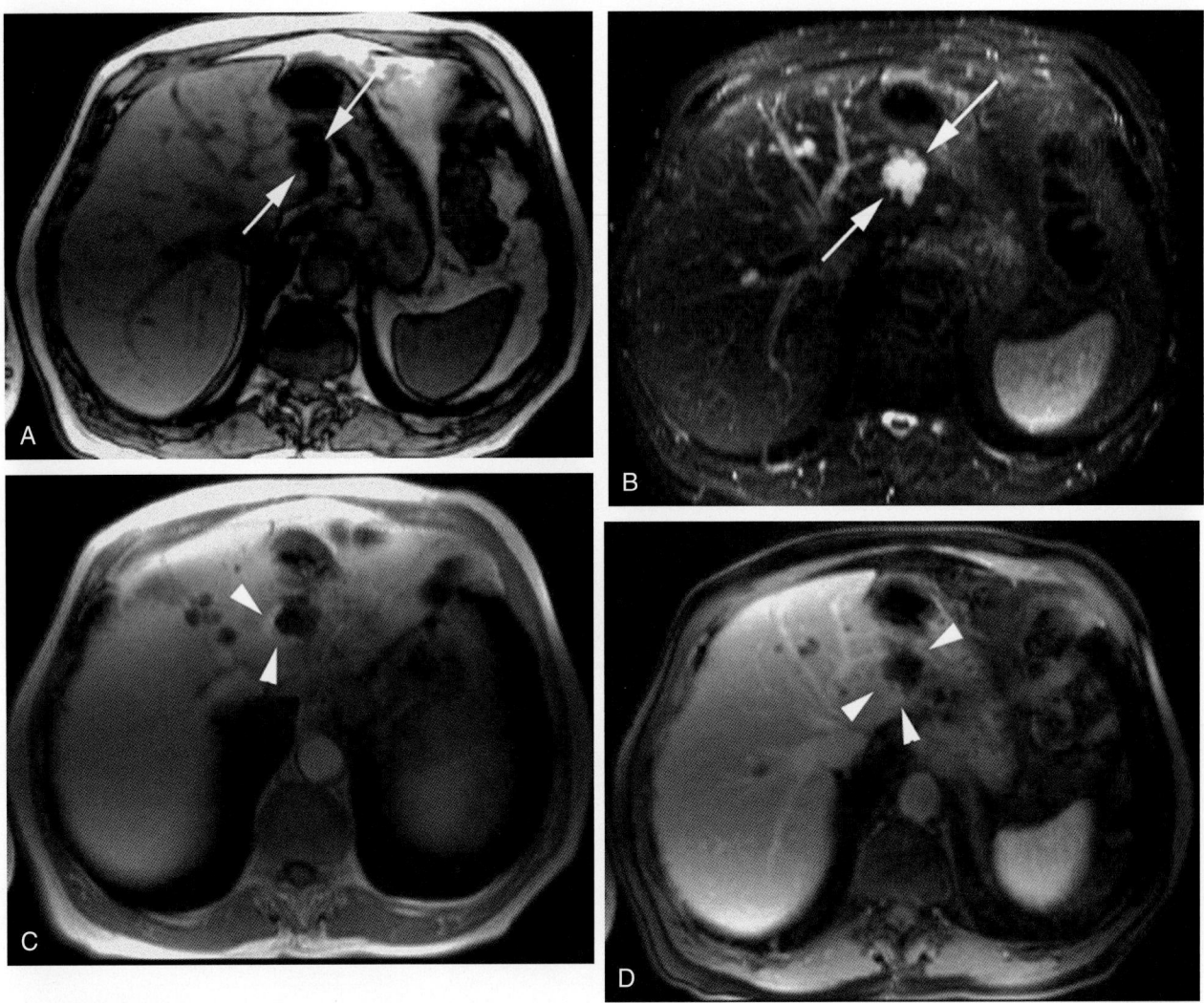

FIGURE 81-18

Biliary cystadenoma. **A,** Axial T1-weighted SGE image and **B,** axial short tau inversion recovery (STIR) image. **C,** Immediate post-gadolinium T1-weighted SGE and **D,** 2-minute post-gadolinium T1-weighted fat-suppressed SGE image. A multiloculated cystic lesion is depicted in the left lobe of the liver (*arrows,* **A** and **B**). The lesion shows hypointense signal on the T1-weighted image (**A**) and hyperintense signal on the T2-weighted images (**B**), due to its fluid content. After administration of gadolinium, a thin rim of enhancement can be seen (*arrowheads,* **C** and **D**). Additional solitary biliary cysts are depicted more laterally, showing similar signal intensities.

spaces which, in contrast to simple cysts, are multiloculated (Fig. 81-17) and are filled with clear or mucinous fluid. The tumor stroma may only be a thin rim but may also comprise mural nodules. Cystic and solid components may be present to variable degrees.[62,69]

On nonenhanced MR images, the cystic component of these tumors shows homogeneous very low signal on T1-weighted and high signal on T2-weighted images. High protein mucin content may render these tumors hyperintense on T1-weighted images. Solid components are of moderately low and high signal on T1- and T2-weighted images, respectively. Solid components of the tumor demonstrate early heterogeneous gadolinium enhancement which is usually not very intense, distinguishing it from the extensive enhancement of HCC (Fig. 81-18).[62,70]

MALIGNANT LESIONS

Liver Metastases

Metastases are the most common hepatic malignancy in Western countries. The impact of detecting or ruling out liver metastases is tremendous on therapeutic strategies and prognosis. Demonstration that malignant disease has limited hepatic involvement may allow more rigorous therapeutic approaches, including partial hepatectomy or metastasectomy which have been shown to be beneficial for patients with colorectal cancer.[71,72] MRI is a highly efficient modality for imaging liver metastases and has been shown to be more sensitive and more specific than sonography, spiral CT, and CT arterial portography (CTAP).[73-76] Another study showed that MRI not only has

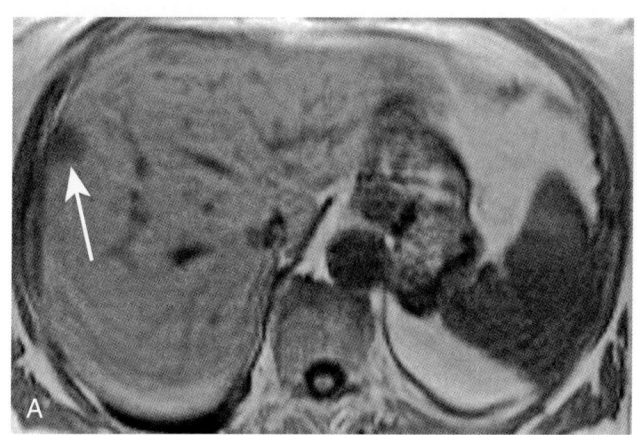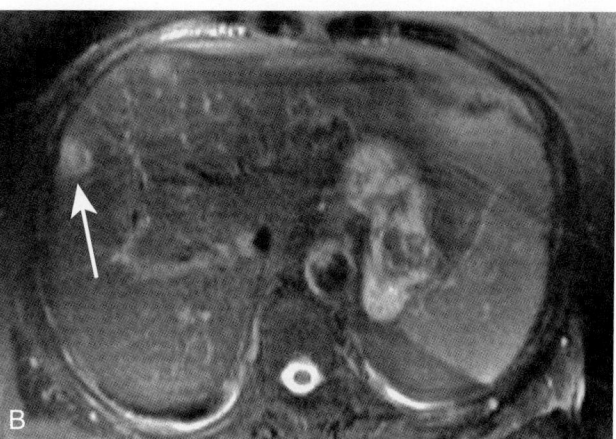

FIGURE 81-19

Metastases. **A,** Nonenhanced T1-weighted gradient-recalled echo image and **B,** nonenhanced T2-weighted fat-suppressed turbo spin-echo image. The metastases appear inhomogeneous and mildly hypointense on the T1-weighted image (*arrow,* **A**) and moderately hyperintense on the T2-weighted image (*arrow,* **B**).

higher accuracy than CTAP but also greater cost-effectiveness.[77] Characterizing focal liver lesions as benign or malignant has paramount importance because patients with known primary malignancies commonly have benign liver lesions (e.g., cysts, hemangiomas) which must not be mistaken for metastases. A study by Jones et al[78] showed benign liver lesions less than 1.5 cm in 51% of 254 cancer patients. Another large study showed that 41.8% of liver lesions in patients with a known primary tumor were benign.[79]

The shape of liver metastases may vary from round and sharply demarcated to irregular and ill defined. On nonenhanced MR images, most liver metastases present with moderately hypointense signal on T1-weighted images and moderately hyperintense signal on T2-weighted images (Fig. 81-19). Particularly high signal on T2-weighted images can be observed in very vascular metastases from islet cell tumors, leiomyosarcoma (Fig. 81-20), pheochromocytoma, and renal cell carcinoma, or in necrotic metastases, or cystic metastases (Fig. 81-21) (e.g., ovarian cancer, gastrinoma). This makes distinction from benign lesions such as hemangioma, cysts, or biliary hamartoma difficult on nonenhanced images alone.[4,80-82] The presence of central hemorrhage, fibrosis, or calcification may decrease the signal on T2-weighted images. Fatty liver is frequently associated with liver metastases either as a response to chemotherapy or to the metastases. Fat suppression of T2-weighted spin-echo images is particularly helpful because it decreases the signal of fatty liver parenchyma and thereby increases the contrast of metastases. Out-of-phase T1-weighted gradient-echo images causes signal drop of fatty parenchyma and may render metastases as hyperintense lesions. This may facilitate lesion detection if metastases are intrinsically high in signal (e.g., melanoma); in most cases, however, lesion conspicuity will be greater on in-phase images. The perilesional liver parenchyma may show compression and atrophy of hepatocytes with concomitant inflammatory changes. In the setting of the fatty liver, this can lead to local fat sparing which will appear as a bright rim on out-of-phase images. This finding is common in colorectal metastases but may also be encountered in other lesions, including hemangioma.

Contrast enhancement on serial post-gadolinium images is most helpful for distinguishing between benign and malignant disease and may display distinct features to suggest a histologic diagnosis. A homogeneous capillary tumor blush is commonly observed in hypervascular metastases less than 2 cm in diameter.[4,83] The most common enhancement pattern of liver metastases, however, is peripheral rim enhancement on immediate post-gadolinium images with slow progressive centripetal filling in on late-phase images. Peripheral washout rendering a bulls-eye appearance on interstitial phase images is common in hypervascular metastases.[4,84]

Certain histologic types of metastases may exhibit specific patterns of signal intensity and enhancement. Metastases from colorectal carcinoma typically are moderately hypointense on T1-weighted images and moderately hyperintense on T2-weighted images. They are generally hypovascular and can be well depicted as hypoenhancing lesions on portal venous phase post-gadolinium images. However, during the hepatic arterial phase of enhancement, they usually show a cauliflower-type appearance with more or less intense peripheral arches of enhancement. This can be observed with regularity when lesions are large (>3 cm) (Fig. 81-22). Smaller lesions tend to show peripheral ring enhancement which can also be quite intense. Perilesional enhancement of adjacent liver parenchyma is also a common finding in colorectal metastases as well as in pancreatic adenocarcinoma metastases. Colorectal metastases have a tendency to show more ill-defined perilesional enhancement, whereas pancreatic metastases tend to show wedge-shaped, sharply demarcated enhancement of adjacent liver parenchyma. These enhancement phenomena are believed to be caused by

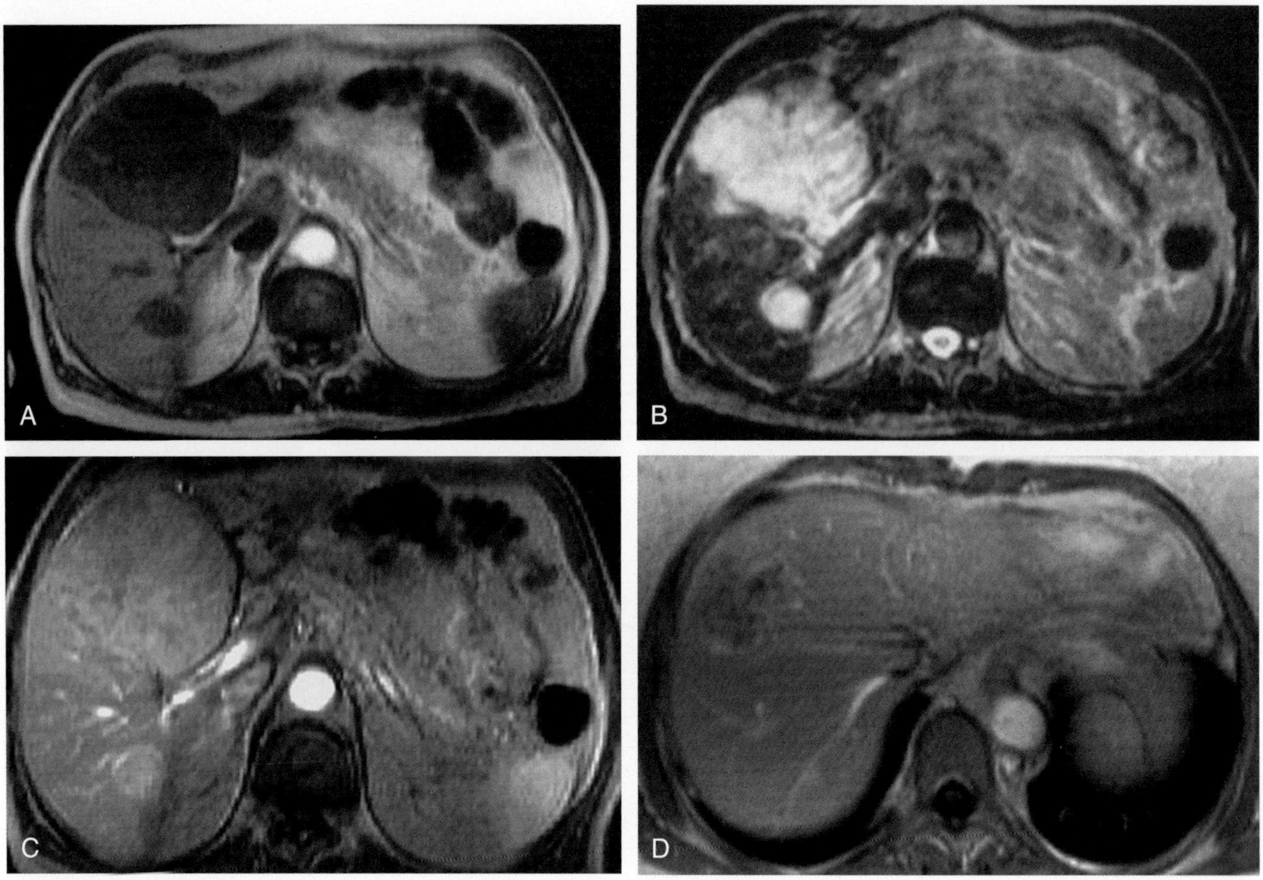

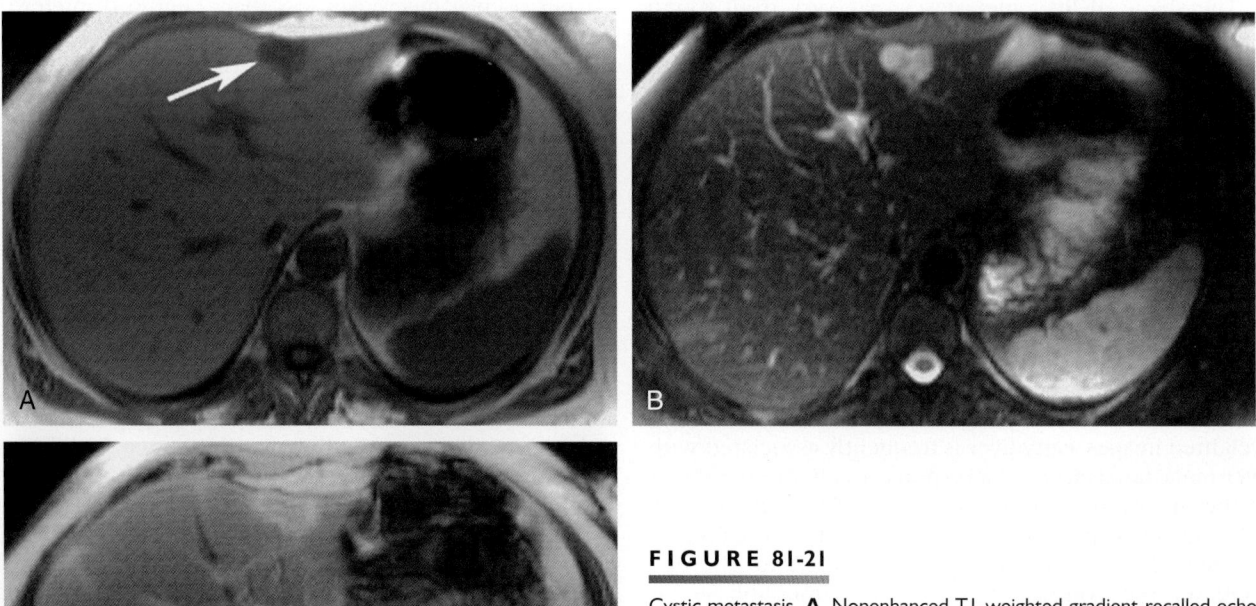

FIGURE 81-20

Sarcoma metastases. **A,** T1-weighted image. **B,** T2-weighted image shows multiple bright lesions, mimicking cavernous hemangiomas. **C,** Immediate post-gadolinium image shows rapid lesion enhancement, not consistent with hemangiomas. **D,** Delayed post-gadolinium image shows a pattern of contrast agent washout consistent with malignancy. *(Courtesy of Robert Edelman, MD.)*

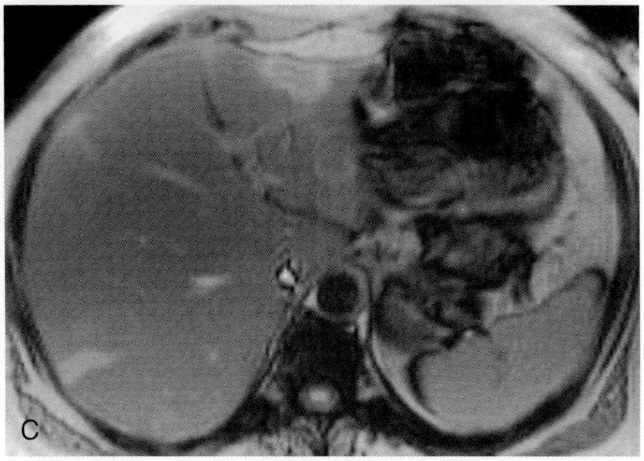

FIGURE 81-21

Cystic metastasis. **A,** Nonenhanced T1-weighted gradient-recalled echo (GRE) image; **B,** nonenhanced T2-weighted fat-suppressed turbo spin-echo image; and **C,** post-gadolinium T1-weighted GRE image. On the T1-weighted image, the metastasis shows low signal intensity (*arrow,* **A**). The diagnosis of metastasis is difficult on the T2-weighted image (**B**) due to cystic content appearing very bright. On the post-gadolinium T1-weighted image (**C**), the metastasis shows rim enhancement.

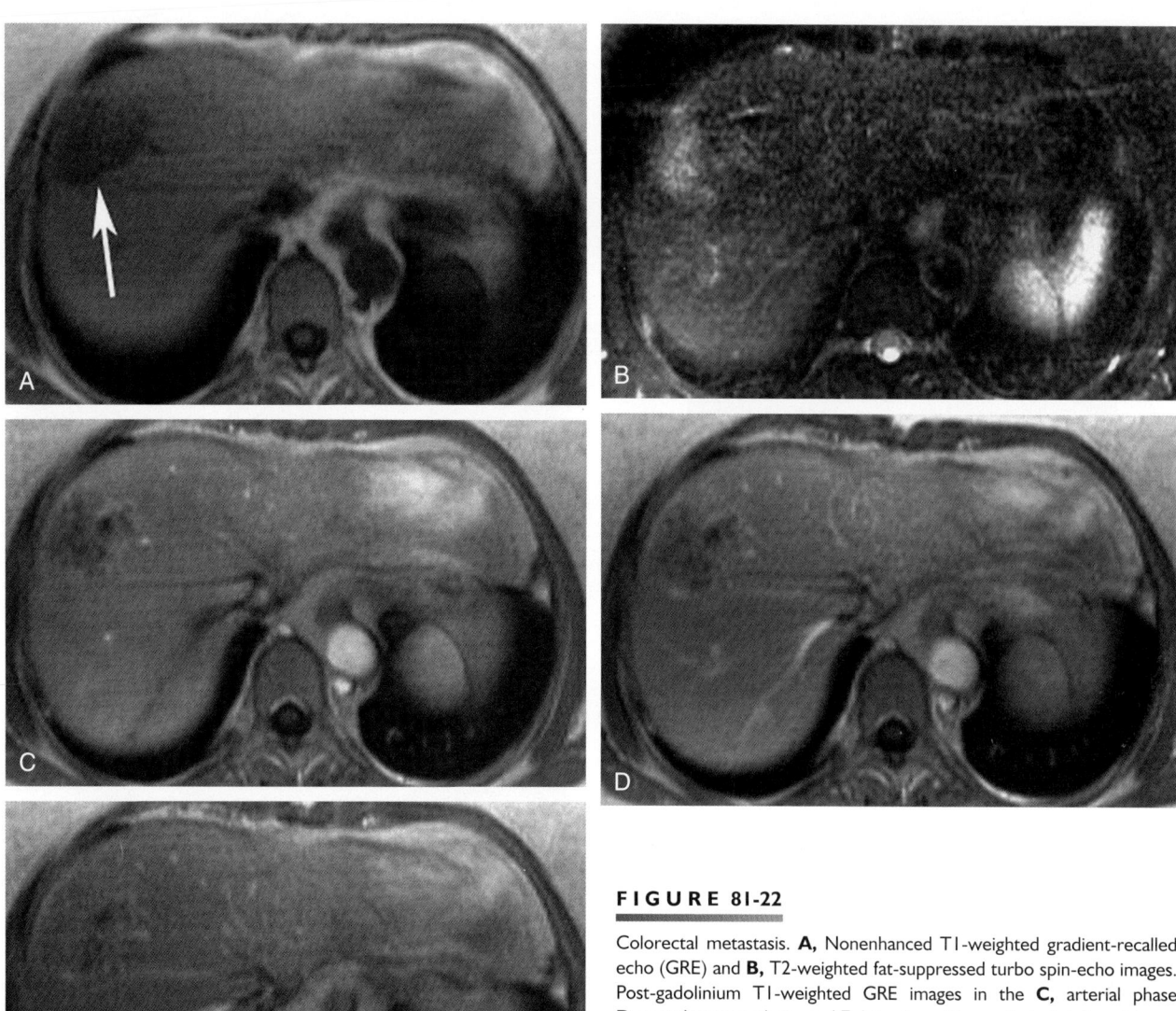

FIGURE 81-22

Colorectal metastasis. **A,** Nonenhanced T1-weighted gradient-recalled echo (GRE) and **B,** T2-weighted fat-suppressed turbo spin-echo images. Post-gadolinium T1-weighted GRE images in the **C,** arterial phase **D,** portal-venous phase, and **E,** late phase. The metastasis is hypointense on the T1-weighted image (*arrow*, **A**), and moderately hyperintense on the T2-weighted image (**B**). After administration of gadolinium, the metastasis shows cauliflower-type enhancement with progressive centripetal filling in (**C-E**).

compression of perilesional parenchyma, inflammatory infiltrates, neovascularization, and desmoplastic changes.[85] Some colorectal metastases may contain mucin, which appears dark on T2-weighted images (Fig. 81-23).

Squamous cell lung cancer generally causes liver metastases that are round and well defined. On T1-weighted images, they are hypointense. On T2-weighted images they typically have a bright peripheral zone and a hypointense center. The outer rim shows intense enhancement on immediate post-gadolinium images, a pattern which is also typical for squamous cell metastases from other origins.

Poorly differentiated adenocarcinomas tend to show multiple metastases not greater than 2 cm. They are typically hyperintense on T2-weighted images and

hypointense on T1-weighted images, and show peripheral ring enhancement on immediate post-gadolinium images. However, the enhancement of these metastases can vary from hypovascular to very hypervascular. These patterns can equally be observed in small cell lung cancer and aggressive nonsquamous cell lung cancer.

Melanoma metastases may show mixed signal intensity on T1- (Fig. 81-24) and T2-weighted images. This can be due to a variable content of melanin, which has paramagnetic property, or to hemorrhage. High signal intensity in other metastases can also be due to hemorrhage (Fig. 81-25).

Ovarian cancer and mucinous cystadenocarcinoma of the pancreas result in metastases of cystlike appearance with a high protein mucinous content that may render

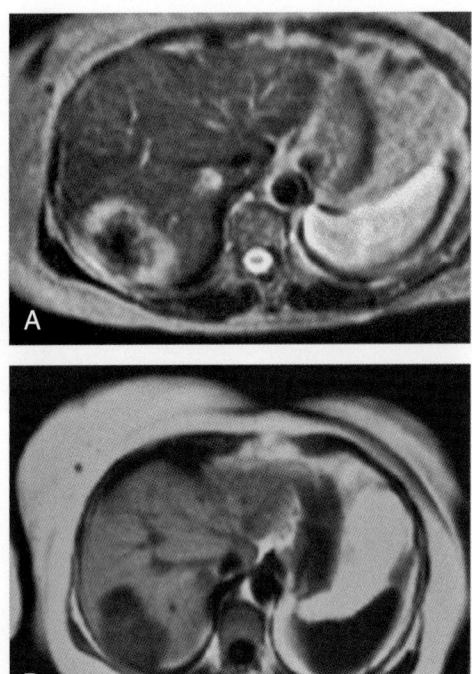

FIGURE 81-23

Mucin-containing metastasis from colon adenocarcinoma. **A,** The T2-weighted image shows low signal intensity in the mucin-containing core with bright perilesional signal intensity. **B,** T1-weighted gradient-echo image shows moderate low signal intensity throughout lesion. *(Courtesy of Robert Edelman, MD.)*

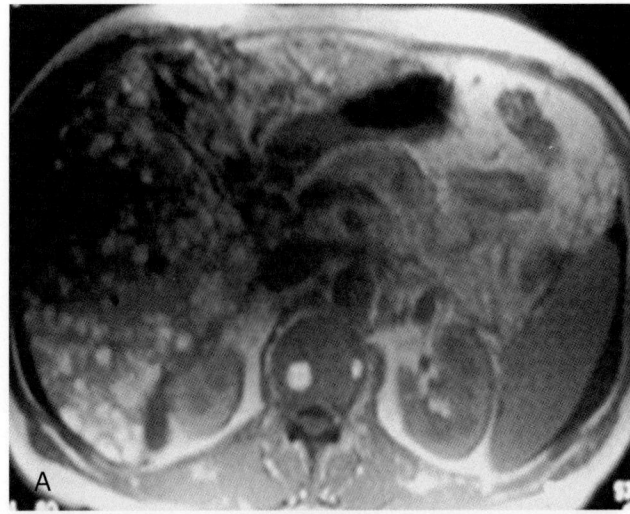

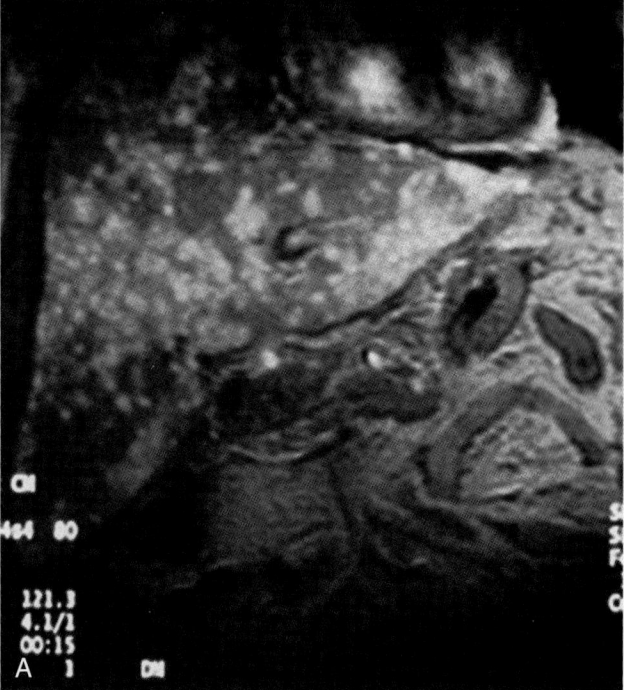

FIGURE 81-24

Melanoma metastases. **A,** Axial precontrast T1-weighted image shows numerous bright metastases within the liver and vertebral body. **B,** Coronal post-gadolinium image shows extensive lesion enhancement. *(Courtesy of Robert Edelman, MD.)*

them hyperintense on T1-weighted images. Furthermore, ovarian cancer has a tendency for capsule-based metastases. However, this location is also frequent with colorectal cancer metastases and can be observed in other tumors. The signal intensity and enhancement characteristics of these tumors can mimic benign liver cysts. Meticulous observation of suspicious features such as ill-defined borders on interstitial phase post-gadolinium images or peripheral enhancement will help to make the distinction.

Metastases with endocrine activity, such as carcinoid, may also show high signal on T1-weighted images due to high protein content owing to production of hormones or enzymes (Fig. 81-26).

Metastases from renal cell cancer, carcinoid, islet cell tumor, leiomyosarcoma, and malignant melanoma are hypervascular and quite hyperintense on T2-weighted images. They are intensely hyperenhancing on arterial phase post-gadolinium images. When lesions are small (<1.5 cm), they are round and their enhancement may be homogeneous and may fade to isointensity after 1 minute, which makes the arterial phase post-gadolinium images most important for detection.[4,83] Larger metastases can be more irregular and tend to show ring enhancement with progressive fill-in.[83] Gastrinoma metastases have a propensity to show peripheral washout on interstitial phase images, giving them a bulls-eye appearance.[86]

Breast carcinoma has the highest variability of appearances of metastases. They can be miliary, ring enhancing, or confluent segmental. They are typically hypervascular and hyperenhancing but to a lesser degree than the hypervascular tumors described earlier (Fig. 81-27).

Hepatocellular-specific contrast agents are usually not taken up by metastases, rendering them hypointense compared to liver parenchyma on delayed-phase images.[87] In some cases, a hyperenhancing rim can be observed which can be useful for the discrimination from cysts.[88] However, metastases from endocrine tumors take up Mn-DPDP which renders them isointense and, thus, is improper for their detection.[89]

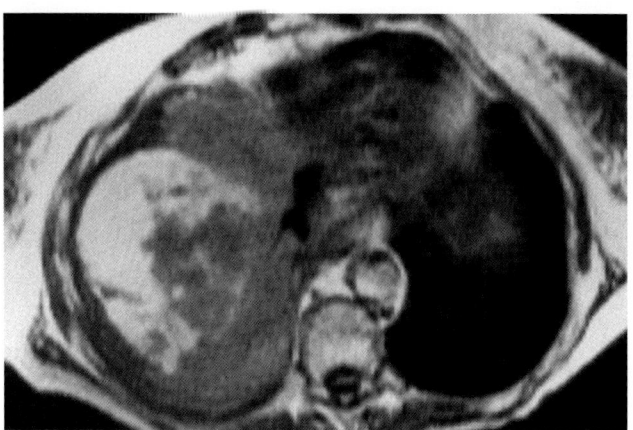

FIGURE 81-25

Hemorrhage within sarcoma metastasis. T1-weighted image shows an inhomogeneous lesion with high signal intensity components representing blood products.

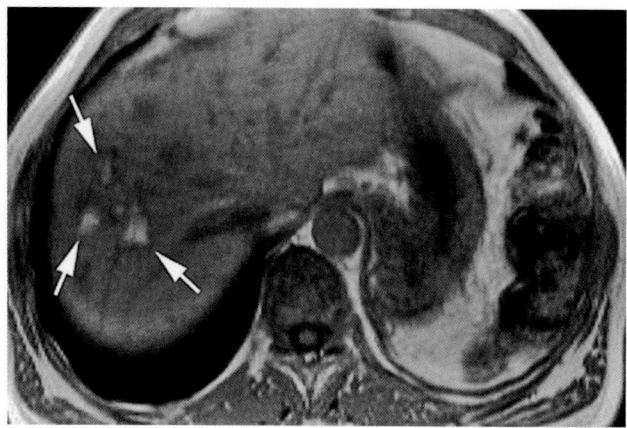

FIGURE 81-26

Metastases with endocrine activity. Nonenhanced T1-weighted gradient-recalled echo image. The metastases show foci of high signal (*arrows*) on the T1-weighted image due to high protein content.

Superparamagnetic iron oxides (SPIOs) are not taken up by metastases because they do not contain Kupffer cells. Metastases appear hyperintense on T2- or T2*-weighted post-contrast images (Fig. 81-28). It has been shown that the sensitivity of MR for the detection of liver metastases can be improved with SPIO contrast agents.[90]

Dual contrast agents (i.e., Gd-BOPTA, Gd-EOB-DTPA) are helpful for detection of metastases as they appear hypointense on delayed-phase images.[91] Earlier-phase post-contrast images are useful for lesion differentiation, much like nonspecific gadolinium chelates.

Lymphoma

Involvement of the liver by lymphoma can either be primary or secondary. Primary lymphoma (Fig. 81-29) is rare with the majority being non-Hodgkin lymphomas. Tumors can be large solitary masses but they can also appear as multiple nodules or diffuse infiltration. Tumors are moderately hypointense on T1-weighted images and moderately hyperintense on T2-weighted images. Gadolinium enhancement is heterogeneous on immediate post-gadolinium images, much like the pattern of other primary malignant tumors of the liver.

Secondary lymphoma of the liver is much more common and occurs in advanced Hodgkin and non-Hodgkin disease.[92] Focal involvement is more frequent in non-Hodgkin than in Hodgkin lymphoma. Lesions are moderately hypointense on T1-weighted images. On T2-weighted images the signal intensity is variable from hypointense to moderately hyperintense. Enhancement on arterial phase post-gadolinium images tends to parallel the signal characteristics on T2-weighted images: hypointense lesions on T2-weighted images enhance minimally, hyperintense lesions enhance substantially.[93] Enhancement is typically peripheral and transient. Perilesional enhancement may occur independent of the

intensity of enhancement of the lesion itself. Invasion of vessels is a finding that can also be rarely observed in lymphoma.

Hepatocellular Carcinoma

Hepatocellular carcinoma (HCC) is the most common primary malignant tumor of the liver. In countries where the incidence is high, the mean age of detection is between 20 and 30 years of age, whereas in other countries it usually appears in the elderly population. HCC in children is rare and typically associated with hepatitis B infection or metabolic diseases.[94] In general, HCC is more common in men and tends to arise in parenchyma that has previously been damaged by alcohol- or non–alcohol-related cirrhosis, viral hepatitis (B or C), or hemochromatosis. In Asia, HCC almost exclusively occurs in patients with these risk factors. In Western countries, however, many patients develop the tumor without any known underlying disease.[95] Alpha-fetoprotein levels are elevated in greater than 50% of patients. Although de novo occurrence of HCC is possible, typically a stepwise progression of cellular atypia is considered to be causative for the development of the malignancy. It starts with low-grade dysplastic nodules that are clearly benign focal hepatic lesions. As cellular atypia progresses, high-grade dysplastic nodules and early HCC are the next steps in malignant transformation.[96] The two latter stages can be difficult to discriminate on histopathology specimens and MR imaging with timely follow-up can play a vital role in the management of these patients. Three types of liver involvement with HCC can be observed. It is solitary in about one half of cases, multifocal in approximately 40%, and diffuse in less than 10%. Tumors possess a pseudocapsule of compressed tissue in 50% to 80% of cases.[97]

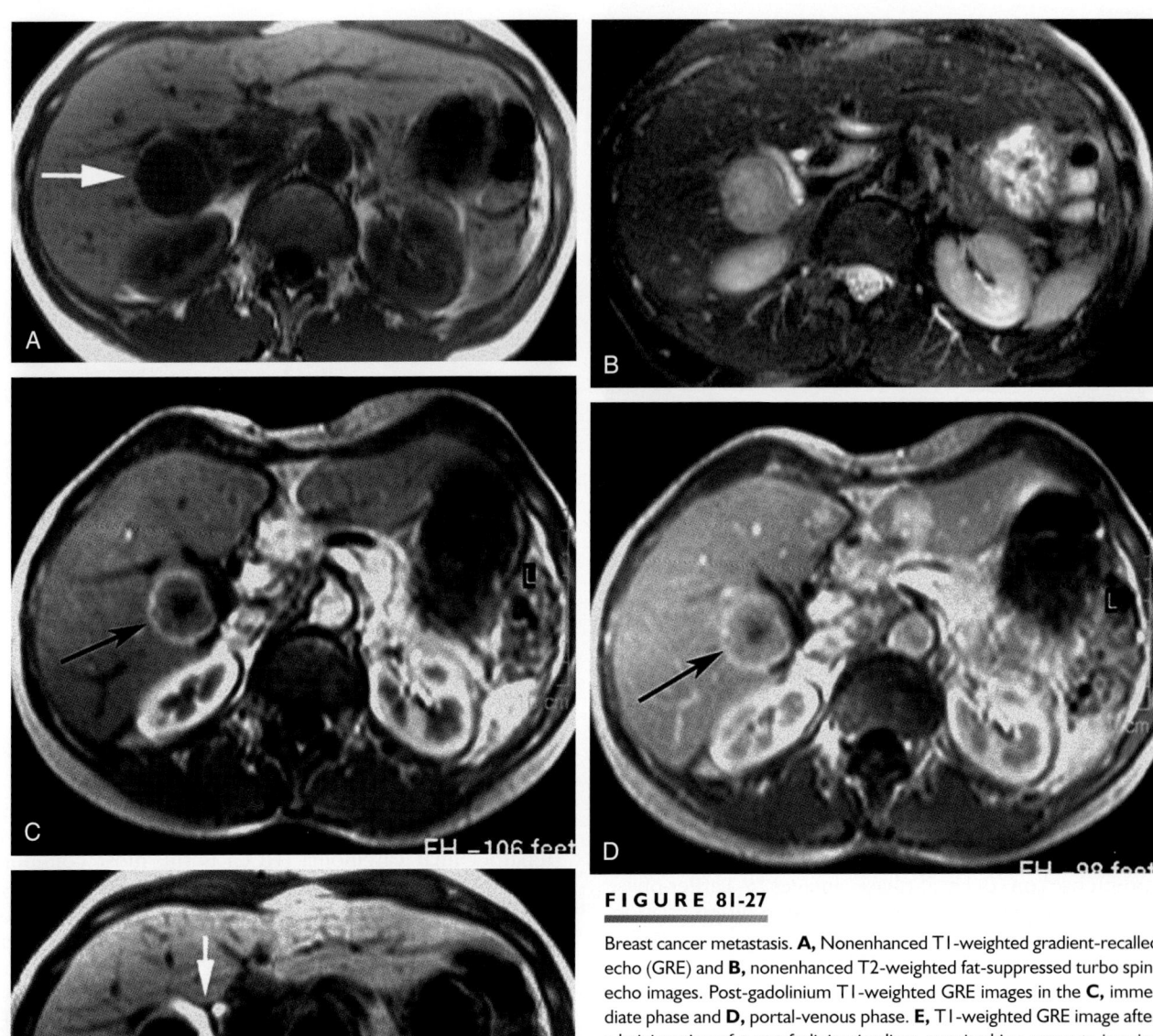

FIGURE 81-27

Breast cancer metastasis. **A,** Nonenhanced T1-weighted gradient-recalled echo (GRE) and **B,** nonenhanced T2-weighted fat-suppressed turbo spin-echo images. Post-gadolinium T1-weighted GRE images in the **C,** immediate phase and **D,** portal-venous phase. **E,** T1-weighted GRE image after administration of mangafodipir trisodium, acquired in a separate imaging session. The tumor is well marginated and hypointense on the T1-weighted nonenhanced image (*arrow,* **A**). On the T2-weighted image the metastasis is moderately hyperintense (**B**). On the immediate T1-weighted post-gadolinium–enhanced image the metastasis shows peripheral ring enhancement (*arrow,* **C**) which progresses towards the center on the portal venous phase (*arrow,* **D**). The metastasis does not show any uptake of the liver-specific contrast agent (mangafodipir) on the delayed-phase image (**E**). The gallbladder and common bile duct are filled with excreted contrast agent (mangafodipir) and are hyperintense (*arrow,* **E**).

On MRI, focal HCC is typically moderately hypointense on T1-weighted images and mildly hyperintense on T2-weighted images (Fig. 81-30). However, tumors may be moderately hyperintense on T1-weighted images or isointense on T1- and/or T2-weighted images, respectively, findings that are frequently observed in early HCC.[98] Hyperintensity on T1-weighted images correlates with well-differentiated HCC that has a more favorable prognosis and is thought to be caused by elevated protein content. Internal fat or hemorrhage are other causes for high signal on T1-weighted images but

occur less frequently.[99,100] Hyperintensity on T2-weighted images correlates more with moderately and poorly differentiated HCC.[101] Isointensity on both T1- and T2-weighted images is frequent in small HCC (<1.5 cm) and requires serial post-gadolinium images for detection (Fig. 81-31).[102] The pseudocapsule, if present, may be visible as a thin hypointense rim on T1-weighted images with mild hyperintensity on T2-weighted images.[102]

HCCs are usually hypervascular and enhance strongly on arterial phase post-gadolinium images. Enhancement is homogeneous in small lesions whereas tumors

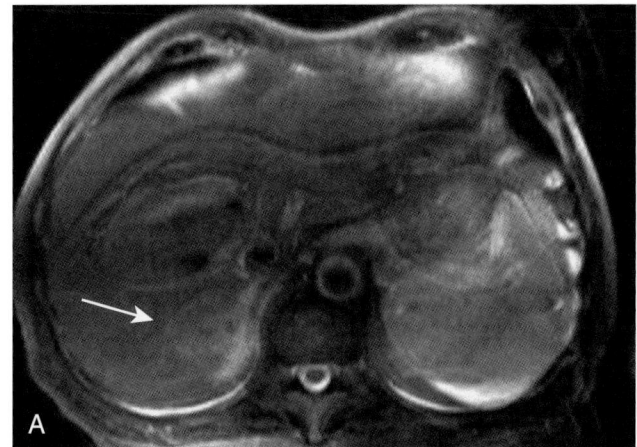

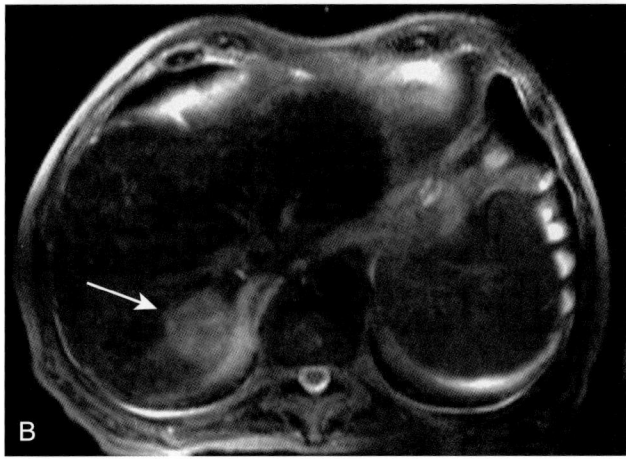

FIGURE 81-28

Colorectal metastasis. Nonenhanced T2-weighted fat-suppressed turbo spin-echo images **A,** before and **B,** after administration of a super-paramagnetic iron oxide (SPIO) contrast agent. The metastasis is mildly hyperintense on the T2-weighted nonenhanced image (*arrow*, **A**). After the administration of an SPIO contrast agent, normal liver parenchyma shows a drop in signal intensity, whereas the metastasis does not show any change in signal intensity and is more conspicuous (*arrow*, **B**).

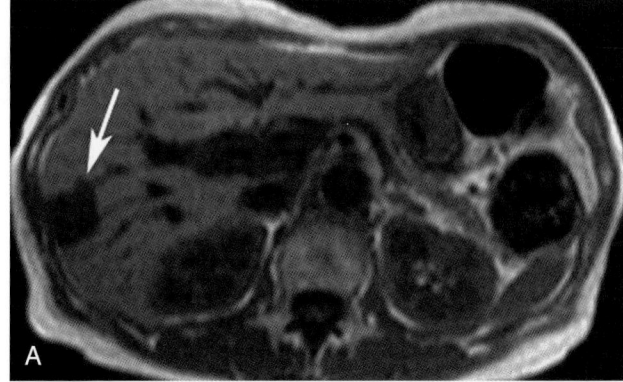

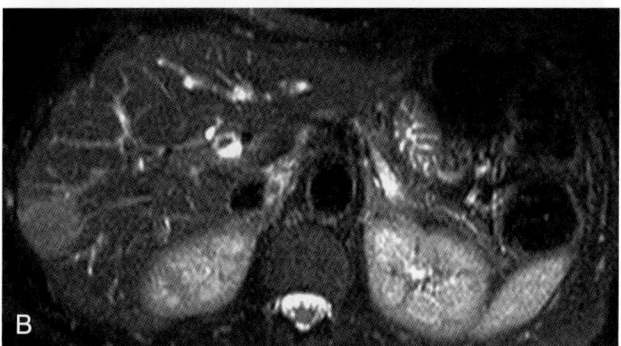

FIGURE 81-29

Primary lymphoma of the liver. **A,** T1-weighted gradient-recalled echo and **B,** T2-weighted fat-suppressed TSE images. On the T1-weighted image the lesion appears hypointense (*arrow*, **A**) and on the T2-weighted image the lymphoma is mildly hyperintense (**B**).

larger than 2 cm enhance in a diffuse heterogeneous fashion.[102,103] Severely dysplastic nodules, however, may also show intense early enhancement and may mimic early HCC. A typical feature of HCC, however, is washout of contrast agent on interstitial phase images (2 minutes post contrast), rendering signal intensity below that of the surrounding liver parenchyma (Fig. 81-32). Severely dysplastic nodules, on the other hand, may become isointense but not hypointense on interstitial phase images. Late enhancement of the pseudocapsule, if present, is another typical finding. The larger HCCs are, the more heterogeneous they tend to be in signal intensity and enhancement. Minimal or no enhancement of HCC can be observed in small, well-differentiated tumors. Especially in patients with severe liver cirrhosis, such hypovascular tumors may be most conspicuous on 2-minute post-gadolinium images as hypointense lesions with a thin hyperenhancing pseudocapsule. Ancillary findings of HCC are tumor invasion of hepatic vessels.

Extension into portal vein branches is most common but invasion into hepatic veins also occurs. Intravascular thrombi are slightly hyperintense on T1-weighted images compared to signal-void perfused vessels. Gadolinium enhancement of feeding vessels within the thrombus is conclusive for tumor invasion of vessels.

Diffuse HCC may simulate the appearance of acute on chronic hepatitis or pronounced liver cirrhosis and may be difficult to detect. Due to the extensive hepatic parenchymal involvement, the MR imaging appearance is mottled with punctuate high intensity on T2-weighted images. On arterial phase post-gadolinium images, mottled enhancement is typical. Diffuse HCC may also present as irregular strands of hypointense or isointense signal on T1-weighted images and iso- to moderately hyper-intense signal on T2-weighted images. These strands enhance in a variable fashion on arterial phase images and may show late enhancement reflecting considerable amounts of fibrous stroma. Ancillary findings that are associated with diffuse HCC and that are helpful for diagnosis are venous tumor thrombus and elevated alpha-fetoprotein levels.

The amount of hepatocyte- and RES-specific contrast agent uptake by HCCs depends on the grade of differentiation of the tumor and the number of functional hepatocytes and Kupffer cells present in the HCC. Mn-DPDP is taken up by many HCCs, especially when they are moderately or well differentiated, and the

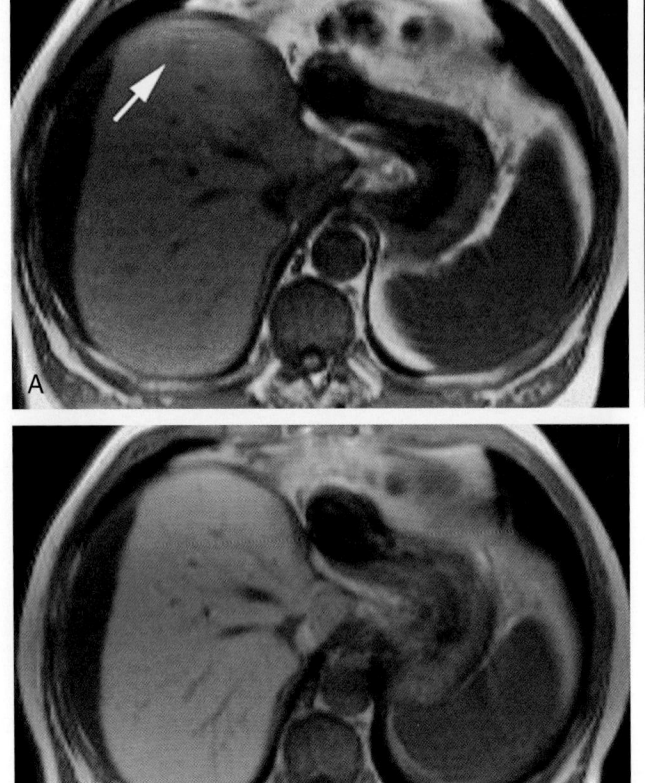

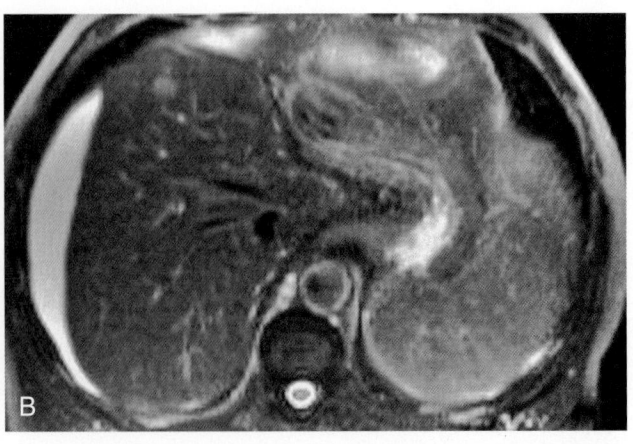

FIGURE 81-30

Well-differentiated focal hepatocellular carcinoma (HCC). **A,** Non-enhanced T1-weighted gradient-recalled echo (GRE) image; **B,** T2-weighted fat-suppressed TSE image; and **C,** T1-weighted GRE image after administration of mangafodipir trisodium. On the T1-weighted image the lesion is slightly hypointense (*arrow*, **A**) and on the T2-weighted image the lesion is slightly hyperintense (**B**). After the administration of mangofidipir trisodium the HCC shows uptake of the agent and cannot be seen anymore. Note the small amount of perihepatic ascites.

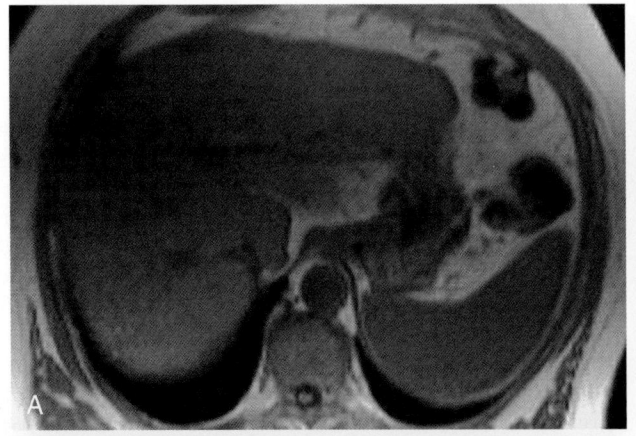

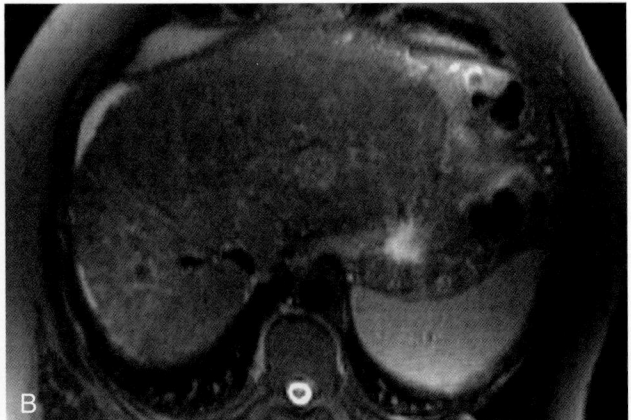

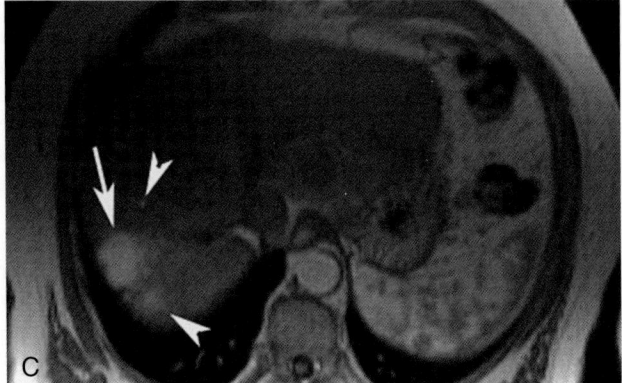

FIGURE 81-31

Poorly differentiated hepatocellular carcinoma. **A,** Nonenhanced T1-weighted gradient-recalled echo (GRE) image; **B,** T2-weighted turbo spin-echo image; and **C,** post-gadolinium T1-weighted GRE image in the arterial phase. The lesion is isointense in both T1- (**A**) and T2-weighted (**B**) images. After the administration of gadolinium chelate the lesion shows intense enhancement on the immediate phase (**C**) and can be easily seen (*arrow*). Tiny satellite lesions can be depicted in the vicinity of the main lesion (*arrowheads*).

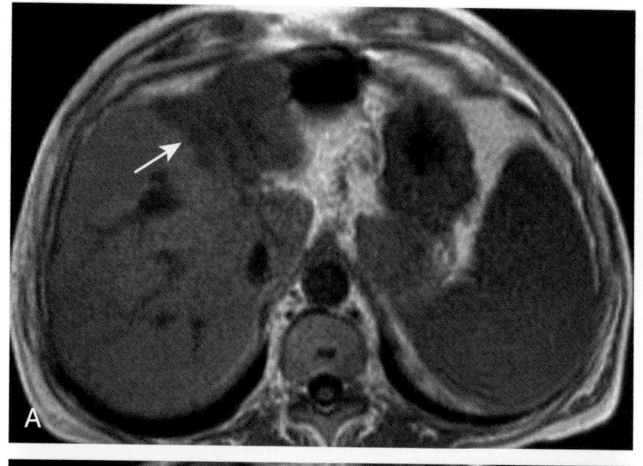

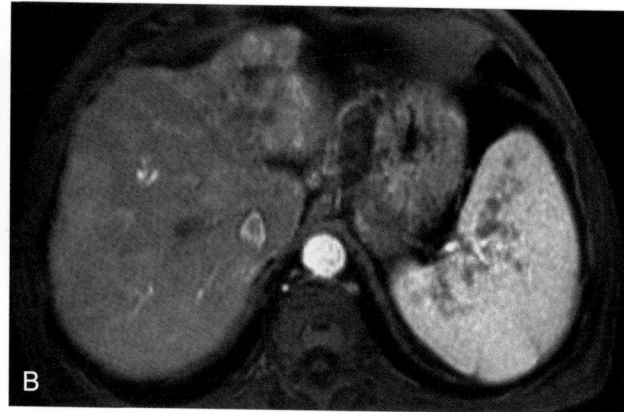

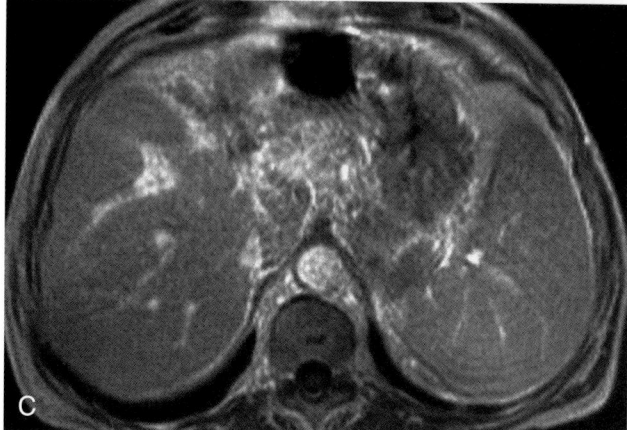

FIGURE 81-32

Hepatocellular carcinoma (HCC). **A**, Nonenhanced T1-weighted gradient-recalled echo (GRE) image; and **B** immediate and **C**, 2-minute post-gadolinium T1-weighted GRE images. HCC in the left liver lobe. On the nonenhanced T1-weighted image (*arrow*, **A**) the tumor is hypointense. On the immediate post-gadolinium image (**B**) the tumor shows heterogeneous intense enhancement and partial washout on the late-phase image (**C**).

enhancement is frequently inhomogeneous.[104] These HCCs may even retain more contrast agent than adjacent liver parenchyma on delayed-phase images owing to impaired biliary clearance. The Kupffer cell count within HCC is variable and tumors may take up SPIOs in a variable fashion. Thus, distinction of well-differentiated HCC from benign tumors such as adenoma or FNH is problematic with both Mn-DPDP and SPIO.

Fibrolamellar Carcinoma

Fibrolamellar carcinoma (FCC) is a distinct subtype of HCC and is sometimes considered a separate pathologic entity. It occurs predominantly in young adults with no underlying liver disease.[100] This tumor shows a lobular histologic architecture and slow growth, and is associated with a favorable prognosis.[105] FCCs are usually solitary lesions and detected when they are large (5-20 cm). Their appearance is similar to that of FNH, showing a central stellate scar with radiating fibrous strands. Calcification of the scar is present in up to approximately one half of cases.[105]

On MRI, FCC is heterogeneous and moderately hypo- or iso-intense on T1-weighted images and moderately hyperintense on T2-weighted images. The central scar is hypointense on both T1- and T2-weighted images. The tumor shows intense heterogeneous enhancement on arterial phase post-gadolinium images. Some parts of the tumor may demonstrate late enhancement rendering the tumor more homogeneous. On 2-minute post-gadolinium images, FCC may be isointense or slightly hypointense to liver parenchyma due to contrast agent washout (Fig. 81-33).[106] The central scar typically demonstrates late enhancement on 2-minute post-gadolinium images but may show minimal or no enhancement. Compared to FNH, the central scar is generally much larger, more irregular, and more heterogeneous in signal intensity and contrast enhancement.

With hepatocyte- or RES-specific contrast agents, FCC usually does not show significant enhancement. This may be helpful for distinguishing this tumor from FNH in very large lesions but is not helpful in smaller lesions.[107]

Cholangiocarcinoma

Intrahepatic or peripheral cholangiocarcinoma originates from bile ducts proximal from the hilum. Risk factors include primary sclerosing cholangitis, choledochal cysts, familial polyposis, congenital hepatic fibrosis, a history of exposure to thorotrast, and infection with *Clonorchis sinensis*. This tumor occurs predominantly after the age of 60 years and is much rarer than HCC. Patients with risk factors, however, may get this tumor at a younger age. Histologically, cholangiocarcinoma

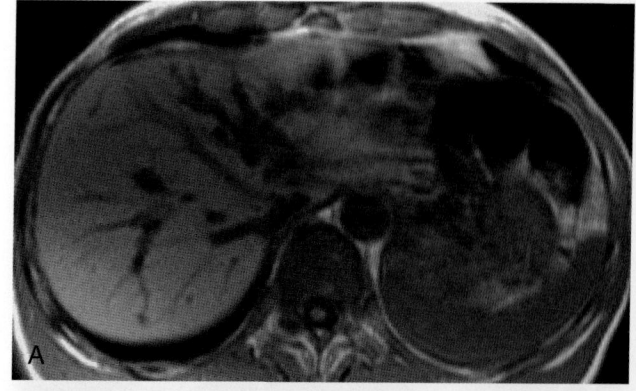

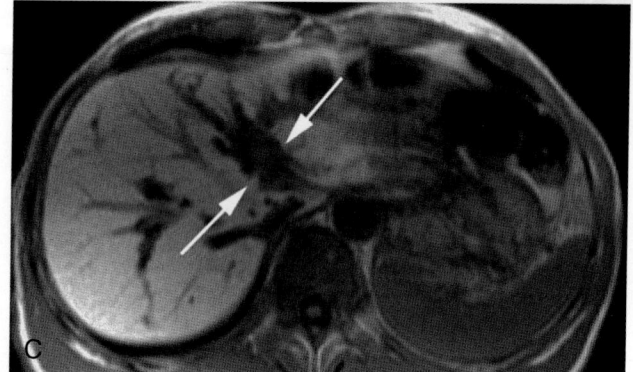

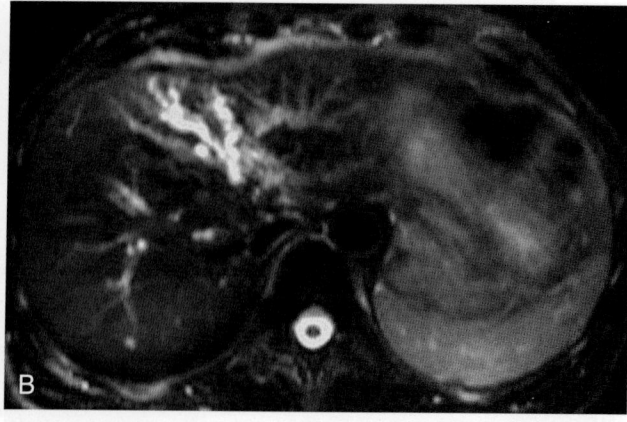

FIGURE 81-35

Cholangiocarcinoma. **A,** Nonenhanced T1-weighted gradient-recalled echo (GRE) image; **B,** T2-weighted turbo spin-echo image; and **C,** T1-weighted GRE image after the administration of mangafodipir trisodium (hepatobiliary contrast agent). The tumor is hypointense on the T1-weighted image (**A**). Dilatation of the left and right main bile duct with segment stenoses is demonstrated on the T2-weighted image (**B**). After the administration of mangofodipir trisodium the tumor remains hypointense in comparison to the enhanced liver parenchyma (*arrows,* **C**).

previous exposure to vinyl chloride, thorotrast, arsenic, radium, or steroids.[118] However, in 60% of cases, no definitive causation can be elucidated. The tumor usually occurs in the fifth decade, has a male predominance, and dismal prognosis.[117] Intra-abdominal massive hemorrhage is a common complication. Histologically, angiosarcoma is composed of clusters of vascular channels lined by malignant endothelial cells forming sinusoid-like structures that can vary from capillary to cavernous. Angiosarcoma typically presents as multifocal nodules diffusely involving the liver. Solitary tumors, however, do occur, are not encapsulated, and contain cystic spaces that are filled with blood and blood products.

On MRI, angiosarcoma is generally hypointense on T1-weighted images and hyperintense on T2-weighted images. Central areas of hemorrhage may present with high signal on T1-weighted images and low signal on T2-weighted images. On arterial phase post-gadolinium images, angiosarcoma typically shows intense, peripheral, nodular enhancement with centripetal progressive enhancement over time, mimicking the appearance of hemangioma (Fig. 81-37).[119,120] Distinguishing findings of angiosarcoma are irregular borders and intratumoral hemorrhage with heterogenous signal on T1- and T2-weighted images.

Epithelioid Hemangioendothelioma

Epithelioid hemangioendothelioma is a very rare malignant tumor of vascular origin. It develops in middle-aged adults and has a female predominance. No typical risk

factors have been defined. The tumor usually presents as a nodular lesion that is typically multifocal with nodules measuring 1 to 3 cm. Nodules have a propensity for the periphery of the liver, can be confluent, and may cause contraction of the liver capsule. Invasion of hepatic and portal veins can be observed.[121] Another appearance is diffuse infiltration of the liver, which is usually observed in the later stages of the disease.[122,123]

On MRI, tumors are typically heterogeneous. They are hypointense on T1-weighted images and moderately to markedly hyperintense on T2-weighted images.[124] After administration of gadolinium chelates, they show moderate peripheral irregular rim enhancement or diffuse heterogenous enhancement, similar to HCC.[125] Peripheral washout can also be observed (Fig. 81-38). Tumors generally do not show uptake of hepatocyte- or RES-specific contrast agents. Epithelioid hemangioendothelioma typically presents hypointense on delayed-phase images after administration of Gd-BOPTA and hyperintense after administration of SPIO on T1- and T2-weighted images, respectively.[111,124]

INFECTIOUS PARENCHYMAL LESIONS

Pyogenic Abscess

Pyogenic abscesses are the most frequent form of focal hepatic infections. Pathologically, pyogenic liver abscesses result from an infectious process of bacterial origin and may occur as solitary or multiple lesions ranging in size from millimeters to several centimeters. Microscopically,

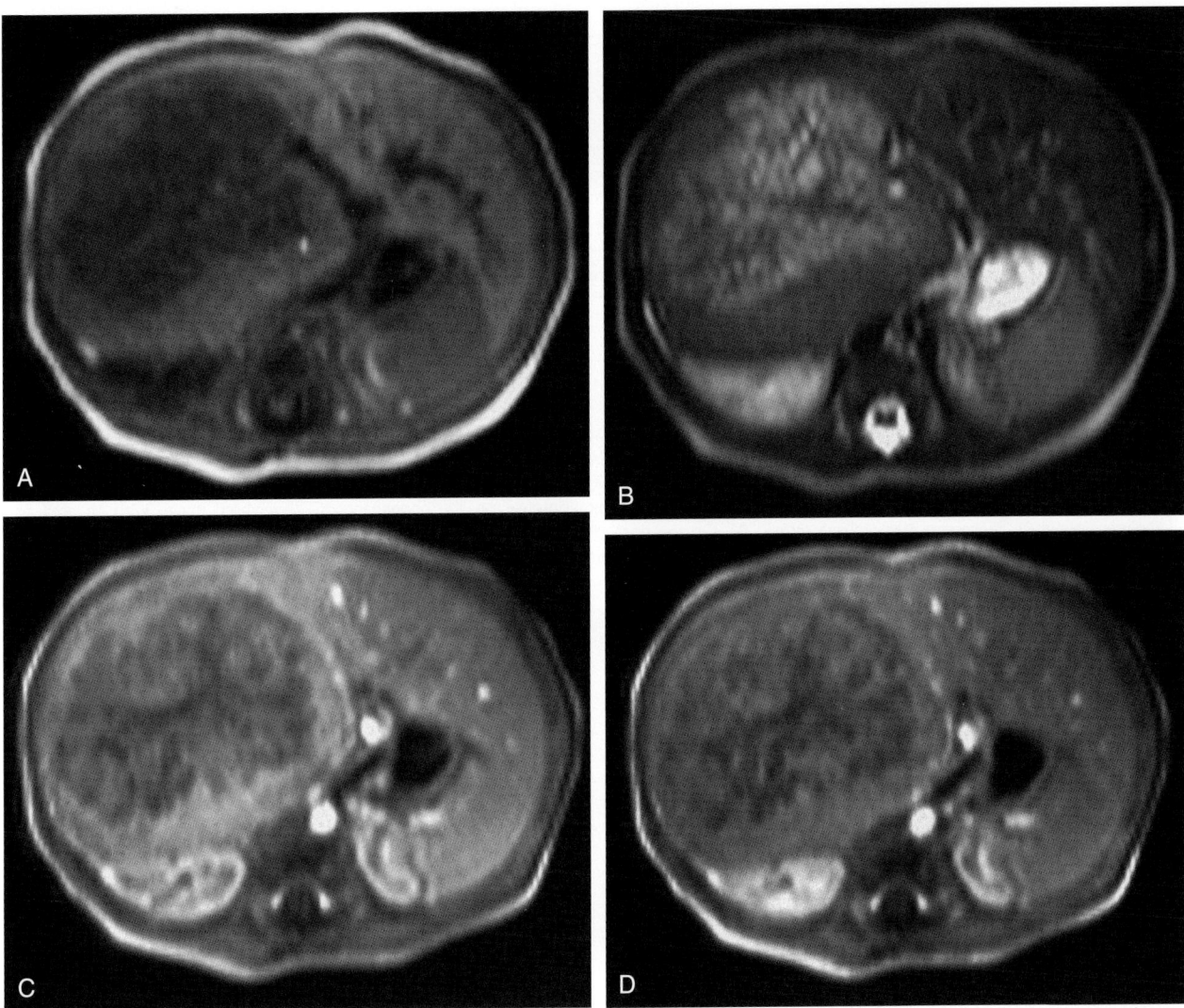

FIGURE 81-36

Mixed form of hepatoblastoma. **A,** Nonenhanced T1-weighted gradient-recalled echo (GRE) image and **B,** T2-weighted turbo spin-echo image. Post-gadolinium T1-weighted GRE in the **C,** arterial and **D,** delayed phase. The tumor appears heterogenous on T1- (**A**) and T2-weighted (**B**) images. After the administration of gadolinium chelate, the hepatoblastoma demonstrates early heterogenous enhancement (**C**) and shows slight washout on the delayed phase (**D**).

in early stages, lesions are ill defined with intense acute inflammation, purulent debris, and devastation of hepatic parenchyma and stroma. In later stages, the abscesses become circumscribed, surrounded by a shell of granulation tissue consisting of abundant, newly formed blood vessels, fibroblasts, and chronic inflammation. Endstages show complete fibrous encapsulation. The pathways of infectious agents are via the biliary tract, portal vein, hepatic artery, and direct extension from contiguous organs. Blunt or penetrating injuries can also cause infection in the liver with abscess formation.[126] Abscesses may occur in the context of recent surgery, Crohn's disease, appendicitis, and diverticulitis. On gadolinium-enhanced MRI, lesions are low signal with enhancing capsules. Typically, the abscess wall reveals intense enhancement on immediate post-gadolinium images, which persists on intermediate- and late-phase images (Fig. 81-39). Some pyogenic abscesses contain internal septations, which enhance early and demonstrate persistent enhancement on serial post-gadolinium images.[126,127] Abscesses typically have perilesional enhancement (Fig. 81-40) with indistinct outer margins on immediate post-gadolinium spoiled gradient-echo (SGE) images caused by a surrounding rim of granulation tissues and a hyperemic inflammatory response in the adjacent liver.[128] The higher sensitivity of MRI to gadolinium chelates than of CT imaging to iodinated agents renders dynamic gadolinium-enhanced MRI a useful technique for patients in whom a distinction between simple cysts and multiple abscesses cannot be made on the basis of CT imaging. Metastases may mimic the appearance of hepatic abscesses because both may

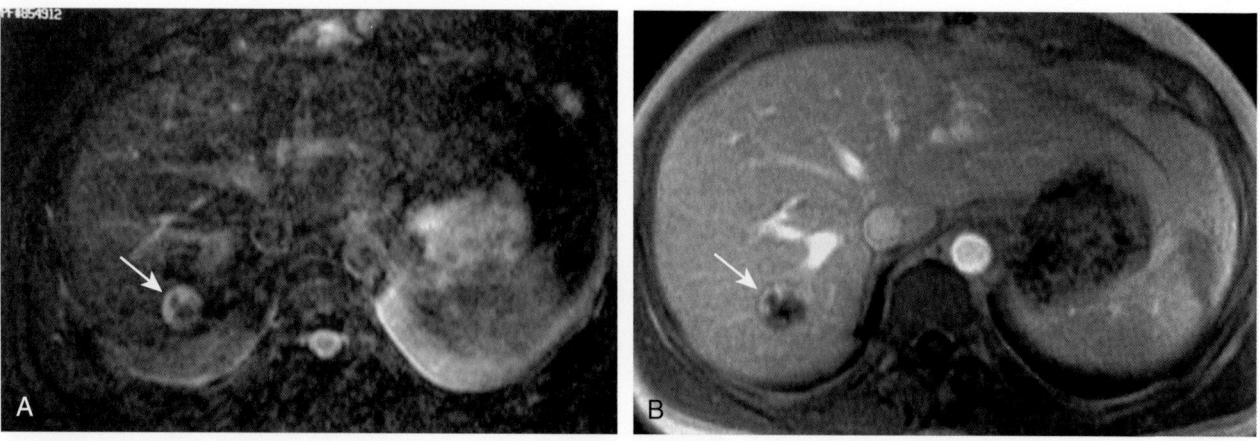

FIGURE 81-37

Angiosarcoma. **A,** Nonenhanced T2-weighted fat-suppressed turbo spin-echo image and **B,** post-gadolinium T1-weighted fat-suppressed gradient-recalled echo image in the parenchymal phase. The lesion appears hyperintense on the nonenhanced T2-weighted image with an area of hypointensity, which represents hemorrhage (*arrow,* **A**). On the post-gadolinium T1-weighted image the lesion shows intense, peripheral, and somewhat nodular enhancement with a centripetal progressive appearance (*arrow,* **B**). Note that the central hemorrhage does not take up any contrast agent and remains hypointense.

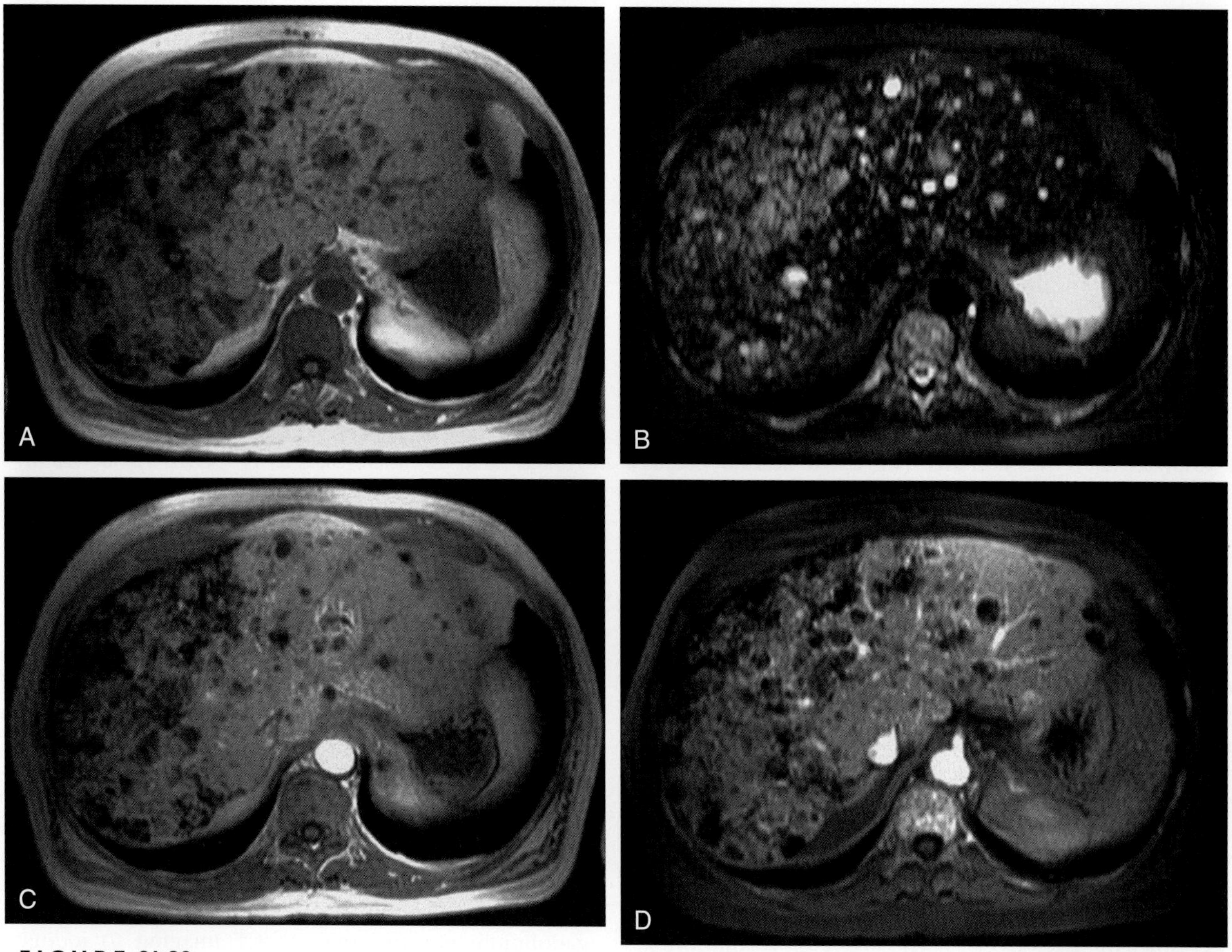

FIGURE 81-38

Epithelioid hemangioendothelioma. **A,** Axial T1-weighted SGE image; **B,** axial short tau inversion recovery (STIR); and **C,** immediate and **D,** 2-minute post-gadolinium T1-weighted fat-suppressed SGE images. The right lobe of the liver is infiltrated by multiple round lesions that are confluent in the periphery of the liver. The left hepatic lobe shows scattered round lesions. The lesions are of low signal intensity on the T1-weighted image (**A**) and hyperintense on the T2-weighted image (**B**). The lesions show no significant gadolinium enhancement (**C** and **D**).

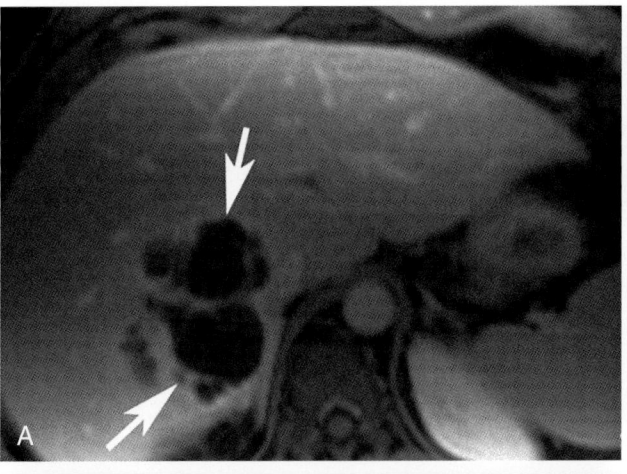
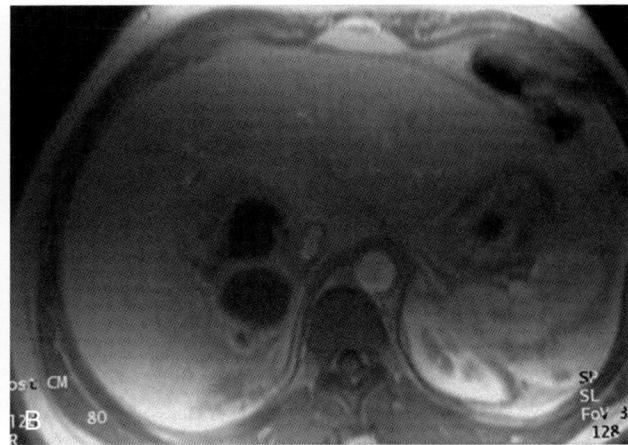
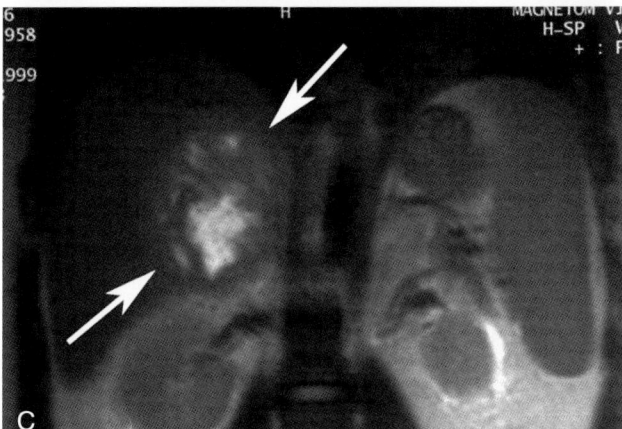

FIGURE 81-39

Pyogenic abscess. **A,** Axial post-gadolinium T1-weighted gradient-recalled echo (GRE) image in the arterial phase; **B,** post-gadolinium T1-weighted GRE image in the parenchymal phase; and **C,** coronal T2-weighted turbo spin-echo image. On the post-gadolinium T1-weighted arterial image (**A**), the abscess (*arrow*) shows strong rim enhancement which persists on the parenchymal phase (**B**). Note the internal septations which are better visualized on the parenchymal phase and which are also depicted on the T2-weighted image (*arrows*, **C**).

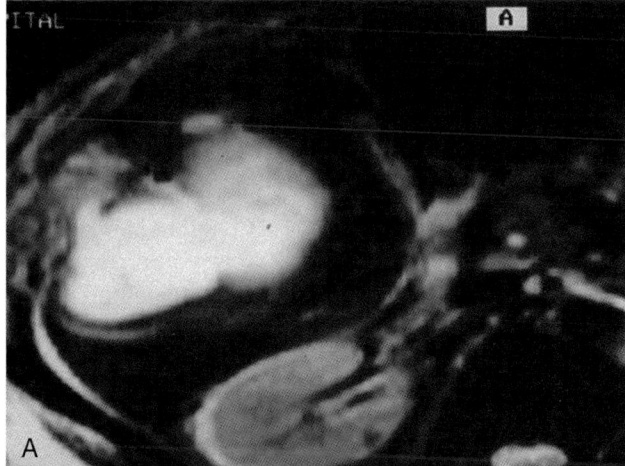
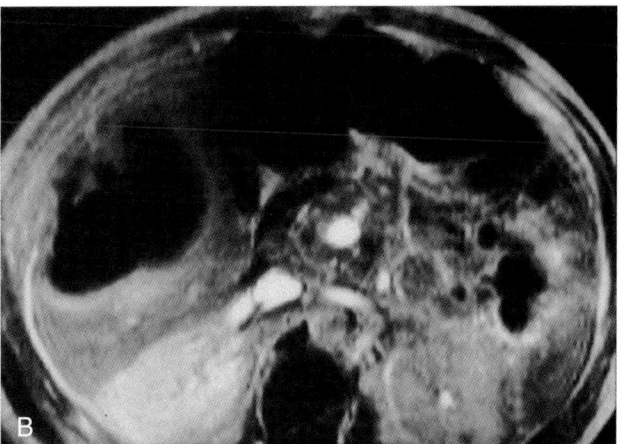

FIGURE 81-40

Actinomycosis. **A,** T2-weighted and **B,** post-gadolinium T1-weighted images show perilesional edema and enhancement and penetration through the liver capsule into the abdominal wall.

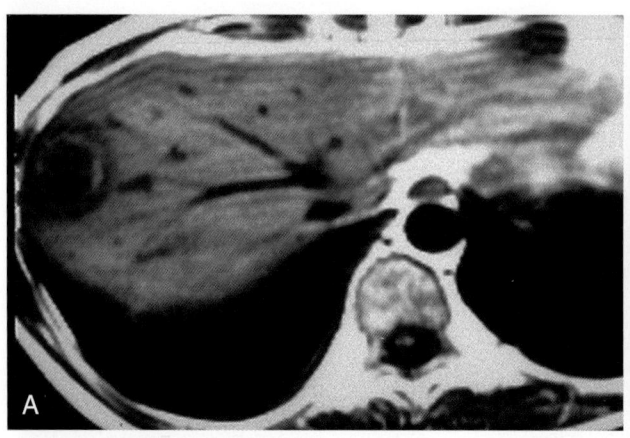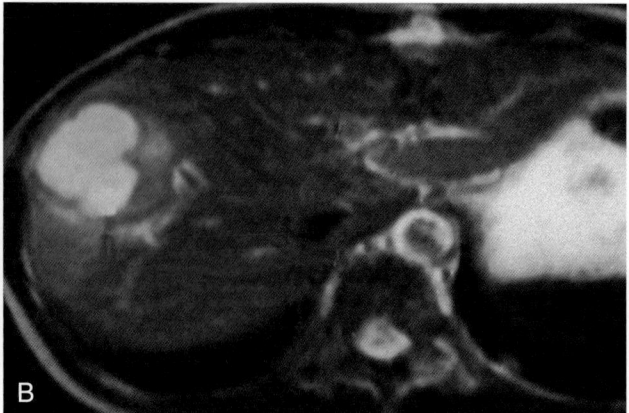

FIGURE 81-41

Amebic abscess. **A,** T1- and **B,** T2-weighted images show a solitary right lobe lesion.

have prominent rim enhancement. Metastases may also mimic abscesses clinically if they become secondarily infected. The diagnosis of infected metastases should be considered when the lesion wall is thicker than 5 mm and has nodular components. Bacterial abscesses commonly are associated with portal vein thrombosis. In contrast to metastases, pyogenic abscesses reveal moderate enhancement of stromal and fibrous elements on immediate post-gadolinium images with persistent enhancement on hepatic venous images and no enhancement of additional stroma or progressive fill-in of the lesion over time. This feature of abscesses is distinctly different from the appearance of the vast majority of metastases, which show progressive internal enhancement on late-phase post-gadolinium images.[128]

Amebic Abscess

Amebic abscesses are caused by a protozoan (*Entamoeba histolytica*) and are not uncommon in tropical countries. They may develop secondary to small ischemic and/or necrotic areas caused by obstruction of small venules by the trophosites and their byproducts.[126] Presenting features include pain, fever, weight loss, nausea and vomiting, diarrhea, and anorexia. Lesions are usually solitary (Fig. 81-41), affect the right lobe more often than the left lobe,[128] and are prone to invade the diaphragm with development of pulmonary consolidation and empyema.[126,129] Lesions are encapsulated and thick walled (5-10 mm) and demonstrate substantial enhancement of the capsule on gadolinium-enhanced images, which permits differentiation from liver cysts.

Mycobacterial Infection

Mycobacterium tuberculosis is the most common cause of infectious hepatic granulomas.[126] The incidence of hepatic infection caused by tuberculosis is increasing, reflecting in part an increase in the numbers of patients who are immunocompromised, such as patients with HIV infection. Abdominal tuberculosis mainly involves abdominal lymph nodes and the ileocecal junction. Hepatic tuberculosis occurs secondary to dissemination of the bacilli. Focal hepatic lesions are typically small and multiple with an appearance similar to that of fungal lesions (see "Fungal Infection"). Infection has a propensity to involve the portal triads and spreads in a superficial infiltrating fashion. This can be visualized as periportal high signal intensity on T2-weighted fat-suppressed images and gadolinium-enhanced T1-weighted fat-suppressed images. Associated porta hepatis nodes are common.

Mycobacterium avium intracellulare (MAI) is the cause of nontuberculous mycobacterial hepatic infections which are common and represent the most frequent hepatic infection in AIDS.[130] MAI infection is found in 50% of livers of patients dying with AIDS.[131] Microscopically, hepatic MAI lesions may show a spectrum of appearances ranging from loose aggregates of histiocytes to tight, well-formed granulomas. CT findings reported to be suggestive of disseminated MAI infection include enlarged mesenteric and/or retroperitoneal lymph nodes, hepatosplenomegaly, and diffuse jejunal wall thickening.[132] Low-density centers of involved lymph nodes are considered a characteristic feature on CT images. Similar findings may be appreciated on MR images.

Fungal Infection

The most common infecting organism is *Candida albicans*. Hepatosplenic or visceral candidiasis is a form of invasive fungal infection that is a serious complication in the immunocompromised patient, especially patients with AIDS on medical therapy for acute myelogeneous leukemia (AML), and patients with bone marrow transplantation.[133,134] Prolonged duration of neutropenia

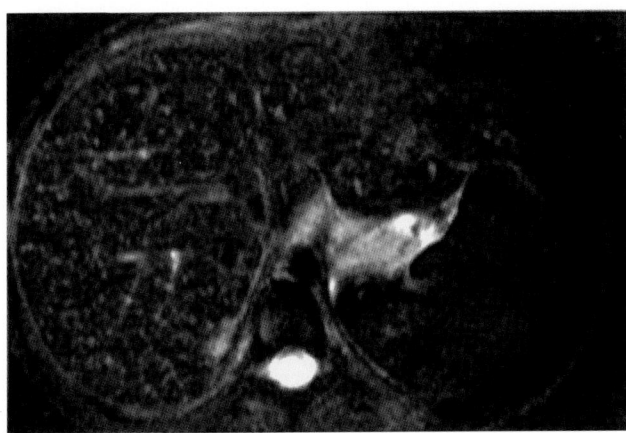

FIGURE 81-42

Hepatosplenic candidiasis. Axial nonenhanced T2-weighted fat-suppressed turbo spin-echo image. The multifocal microabscesses, located throughout the parenchyma, are conspicuous on T2-weighted fat-suppressed sequences.

is thought to be the most important risk factor for hepatosplenic candidiasis.[134] Acute hepatosplenic candidiasis involves the liver and spleen, with renal involvement occurring in less than 50% of patients. Disseminated *C. albicans* infects the liver in a high proportion of cases, leading to development of multifocal microabscesses or granulomas. Although definitive diagnosis requires microbiologic or histologic evidence of infection, the absence of organisms on liver biopsy tissue or negative culture findings in the presence of clinical suspicion does not rule out the diagnosis. Therefore, cross-sectional imaging is necessary for diagnosis.[135] Patient survival depends on early diagnosis. Liver lesions are frequently less than 1 cm and subcapsular in location. The small size and peripheral nature of these lesions make them difficult to detect with CT imaging or standard spin-echo MR sequences. Patients with AML undergo multiple blood transfusions, so the liver and spleen are low in signal intensity on T1-and T2-weighted images.[136,137] T2-weighted fat-suppressed spin-echo sequences are effective at demonstrating these lesions because of the high conspicuity of this sequence for small lesions and the absence of chemical shift artifact that may mask small peripheral lesions (Fig. 81-42). Short tau inversion recovery (STIR) images also show these lesions well because of the fat-nulling effect of this sequence.[136] MRI employing T2-weighted fat suppression and dynamic gadolinium-enhanced SGE images has been shown to be more sensitive for the detection of hepatosplenic candidiasis than contrast-enhanced CT imaging.[135,138]

Because acute lesions of fungal disease are abscesses, they are high in signal intensity on T2-weighted images. They also may be seen on gadolinium-enhanced T1-weighted images as signal-void foci with no appreciable abscess wall enhancement. It has been observed that patients with hepatosplenic candidiasis who are immunocompetent possess abscesses that demon-strate mural enhancement. The absence of abscess wall enhancement may reflect the patient's neutropenic state. Overall sensitivity of MRI is 100%, and specificity is 96%.[135]

After institution of antifungal antibiotics, successful response may be demonstrated. Central high signal develops within lesions on T1- and T2-weighted images that enhances with gadolinium, representing granuloma formation. In addition, a distinctive dark perilesional ring is observed on all sequences, representing collections of iron-laden macrophages throughout the granulation tissue at the periphery of the lesions.[139] This represents the subacute treated phase, which may be a good prognostic finding, reflecting the patient's ability to mount an immune response. MRI also demonstrates chronic healed lesions that have responded to antifungal therapy.[138] These lesions are irregularly shaped and low in signal. Chronic, healed lesions are hypointense on T1-weighted images and are generally isointense and poorly shown on T2-weighted images. The lesions are most conspicuous as low signal intensity defects with angular margins on immediate post-gadolinium SGE images. Capsular retraction may also be observed adjacent to the lesions. This constellation of imaging features is consistent with chronic scar formation.

CONCLUSION

MRI is an excellent modality for the detection and characterization of focal liver lesions. It is safe, lacks ionizing radiation, and is highly sensitive and specific. Especially for the evaluation of hypervascular lesions such as HCC or hypervascular metastases, MRI has been shown to have greater impact on patient management than CT. Gadolinium-based contrast agents have an undisputed role for both detection and characterization of focal liver lesions. The advent of hepatocyte- and RES-specific contrast agents has further enhanced the capabilities of MRI. The benefits and limitations of these contrast agents, however, have to be observed to take advantage of their specific features.

REFERENCES

1. Semelka RC, Helmberger TKG: Contrast agents for MR imaging of the liver. Radiology 218:27-38, 2001.
2. Low RN: Contrast agents for MR imaging of the liver. J Magn Reson Imaging 7:56-67, 1997.
3. Runge VM: Safety of approved MR contrast media for intravenous injection. J Magn Reson Imaging 12:205-213, 2000.
4. Larson RE, Semelka RC, Bagley AS, et al: Hypervascular malignant liver lesions: Comparison of various MR imaging pulse sequences and dynamic CT. Radiology 192:393-399, 1994.
5. Federle MP, Chezmar JL, Rubin DL, et al: Safety and efficacy of mangafodipir trisodium (MN-DPDP) injection for hepatic MRI in adults: results of the U.S. multicenter phase III clinical trials (safety). J Magn Reson Imaging 12:186-197, 2000.
6. Bernardino ME, Young SW, Lee JK, Weinreb JC: Hepatic MR imaging with Mn-DPDP: safety, image quality, and sensitivity. Radiology 183:53-58, 1992.
7. Bartolozzi C, Spinazzi A: Multi-Hance: help or hype? J Comput Assist Tomogr 23(Suppl 1):S151-S159, 1999.
8. Pirovano G, Vanzulli A, Marti-Bonmati L, et al: Evaluation of the accuracy of gadobenate dimeglumine-enhanced MR imaging in the detection and characterization of focal liver lesions. Am J Roentgenol 175:1111-1120, 2000.

9. Reimer P, Rummeny EJ, Shamsi K, et al: Phase II clinical evaluation of Gd-EOB-DTPA: dose, safety aspects, and pulse sequences. Radiology 199:177-183, 1996.

10. Vogl TJ, Kummel S, Hammerstingl R, et al: Liver tumors: comparison of MR imaging with Gd-EOB-DTPA and Gd-DTPA. Radiology 200:59-67, 1996.

11. Fretz CJ, Elizondo G, Weissleder R, et al: Superparamagnetic iron oxide-enhanced MR imaging: pulse sequence optimization for detection of liver cancer. Radiology 172:393-397, 1989.

12. Ros PR, Freeny PC, Harms SE, et al: Hepatic MR imaging with ferumoxides: a multicenter clinical trial of the safety and efficacy in the detection of focal hepatic lesions. Radiology 196:481-488, 1995.

13. Bluemke DA, Weber TM, Rubin D, et al: Hepatic MR imaging with ferumoxides: multicenter study of safety and effectiveness of direct injection protocol. Radiology 228:457-64, 2003.

14. Reimer P, Muller M, Marx C, et al: T1 effects of a bolus-injectable superparamagnetic iron oxide, SH U 555 A: dependence on field strength and plasma concentration—preliminary clinical experience with dynamic T1-weighted MR imaging. Radiology 209:831-836, 1998.

15. Reimer P, Balzer T: Ferucarbotran (Resovist): a new clinically approved RES-specific contrast agent for contrast-enhanced MRI of the liver: properties, clinical development, and applications. Eur Radiol 13:1266-1276, 2003.

16. Vogl TJ, Hammerstingl R, Schwarz W, et al: Magnetic resonance imaging of focal liver lesions. Comparison of the superparamagnetic iron oxide resovist versus gadolinium-DTPA in the same patient. Invest Radiol 31:696-708, 1996.

17. Rossai J: Ackerman's Surgical Pathology, vol.1, 8th ed. St Louis, Mosby, 1995, p 898.

18. Itai Y, Ebihara R, Eguchi N, et al: Hepatobiliary cysts in patients with autosomal dominant polycystic kidney disease: Prevalence and CT findings. Am J Roentgenol 164:339-342, 1995.

19. Kadoya M, Matsui O, Nakanuma Y, et al: Ciliated hepatic foregut cyst: Radiologic features. Radiology 175:475-477, 1990.

20. Shoenut JP, Semelka RC, Levi C, Greenberg H: Ciliated hepatic foregut cysts: US, CT, and contrast-enhanced MR imaging. Abdom Imaging 19:150-152, 1994.

21. Ralls PW, Henley DS, Colletti PM, et al: Amebic liver abscess: MR imaging. Radiology 165:801-804, 1987.

22. Balci NC, Tunaci A, Semelka RC, et al: Hepatic alveolar echinococcosis: MRI findings. Magn Reson Imaging 18:537-541, 2000.

23. Semelka RC, Hussain SM, Marcos HB, Woosley JT: Biliary hamartomas: solitary and multiple lesions shown on current MR techniques including gadolinium enhancement. J Magn Reson Imaging 10:196-201, 1999.

24. Mortele B, Mortele K, Seynaeve P, et al: Hepatic bile duct hamartomas (von Meyenburg complexes): MR and MR cholangiography findings. J Comput Assist Tomogr 26:438-443, 2002.

25. Mitsuodo K, Watanabe Y, Saga T, et al: Nonenhanced hepatic cavernous hemangioma with multiple calcifications: CT and pathologic correlation. Abdom Imaging 20:459-461, 1995.

26. Li KC, Glazer GM, Quint LE, et al: Distinction of hepatic cavernous hemangioma from hepatic metastases with MR imaging. Radiology 169:409-415, 1988.

27. Lombardo DM, Baker ME, Spritzer CE, et al: Hepatic hemangiomas vs. metastases: MR differentiation at 1.5 T. Am J Roentgenol 155:55-59, 1990.

28. Semelka RC, Brown ED, Ascher SM, et al: Hepatic hemangiomas: A multi-institutional study of appearance on T2-weighted and serial gadolinium-enhanced gradient-echo MR images. Radiology 192:401-406, 1994.

29. Danet IM, Semelka RC, Braga L, et al: Giant hemangioma of the liver: MR imaging characteristics in 24 patients. Magn Reson Imaging 21:95-101, 2003.

30. Semelka RC, Sofka CM: Hepatic hemangiomas. Magn Reson Imaging Clin N Am 5:241-253, 1997.

31. Low RN: MRI of the liver using gadolinium chelates. Magn Reson Imaging Clin N Am 9:717-743, 2001.

32. McFarland EG, Mayo-Smith WW, Saini S, et al: Hepatic hemangiomas and malignant tumors: improved differentiation with heavily T2-weighted conventional spin-echo MR imaging. Radiology 193:43-47, 1994.

33. Saini S, Edelman RR, Sharma P, et al: Blood pool MR contrast material for detection and characterization of focal hepatic lesions: initial clinical experience with ultrasmall superparamagnetic iron oxide (AMI-227). Am J Roentgenol 164:1147-1152, 1995.

34. Bader TR, Braga L, Semelka RC: Exophytic benign tumors of the liver: Appearance on MRI. Magn Reson Imaging 19:623-628, 2001.

35. Selby DM, Stocker JT, Waclawiw MA, et al: Infantile hemangioendothelioma of the liver. Hepatology 20(1 Pt 1):39-45, 1994.

36. Klatskin G, Conn HO: Histopathology of the Liver. New York, Oxford University Press, 1993, p 368.

37. Buetow PC, Rao P, Marshall H: Imaging of pediatric liver tumors. Magn Reson Clin N Am 5:397-413, 1997.

38. Kasahara M, Kiuchi T, Haga H, et al: Monosegmental living-donor liver transplantation for infantile hepatic hemangioendothelioma. J Pediatr Surg 38:1108-1111, 2003.

39. Ben-Haim M, Roayaie S, Ye MQ, et al: Hepatic epithelioid hemangio-endothelioma: resection or transplantation, which and when? Liver Transpl Surg 5:526-531, 1999.

40. Chen CC, Kong MS, Yang CP, Hung IJ: Hepatic hemangioendothelioma in children: analysis of thirteen cases. Acta Paediatr Taiwan 44:8-13, 2003.

41. Mortele KJ, Vanzieleghem B, Mortele B, et al: Solitary hepatic infantile hemangioendothelioma: dynamic gadolinium-enhanced MR imaging findings. Eur Radiol 12:862-865, 2002.

42. Schneider G, Grazioli L, Saini S: Imaging of benign focal liver lesions. In Schneider G, Grazioli L, Saini S (eds): MRI of the Liver. New York: Springer, 2003, pp 144-145.

43. Craig JR, Peters RL, Edmondson HA: Tumors of the Liver and Intrahepatic Bile Ducts, Fasc 26, 2nd ser. Washington, DC, Armed Forces Institute of Pathology, 1989.

44. Nguyen BN, Flejou JF, Terris B, et al: Focal nodular hyperplasia of the liver: a comprehensive pathologic study of 305 lesions and recognition of new histologic forms. Am J Surg Pathol 23:1441-1454, 1999.

45. Lee MJ, Saini S, Hamm B, et al: Focal nodular hyperplasia of the liver: MR findings in 35 proved cases. Am J Roentgenol 156:317-320, 1991.

46. Mortele KJ, Praet M, Vlierberghe HV, et al: CT and MR imaging findings in focal nodular hyperplasia of the liver: Radiologic-pathologic correlation. Am J Roentgenol 175:687-692, 2000.

47. Wanless I, Mawdsley C, Adams R: On the pathogenesis of focal nodular hyperplasia of the liver. Hepatology 5:1194-1200, 1985.

48. Bioulac-Sage P, Balabaud C, Wanlees IR: Diagnosis of focal nodular hyperplasia. Not so easy. Am J Surg Pathol 25:1322-1325, 2001.

49. Ndimbie O: Hemangiomas with localized nodular proliferation of the liver: a suggestion on the pathogenesis of focal nodular hyperplasia. Am J Surg Pathol 14:142-150, 1990.

50. Wanless IR, Albrecht S, Bilbao J, et al: Multiple focal nodular hyperplasia of the liver associated with vascular malformations of various organs and neoplasia of the brain: A new syndrome. Mod Pathol 2:456-462, 1989.

51. Shortell CK, Schwartz SI: Hepatic adenoma and focal nodular hyperplasia. Surg Gynecol Obstet 173:426-431, 1991.

52. Vilgrain V, Flejou JF, Arrive L, et al: Focal nodular hyperplasia of the liver: MR imaging and pathologic correlation in 37 patients. Radiology 184:699-703, 1992.

53. Bader TR, Braga L, Semelka RC: Exophytic benign tumors of the liver: appearance on MRI. Magn Reson Imaging 19:623-628, 2001.

54. Ba-Ssalamah A, Schima W, Schmook MT, et al: Atypical focal nodular hyperplasia of the liver: imaging features of non-specific and liver-specific MR contrast agents. Am J Roentgenol 179:1447-1456, 2002.

55. Grazioli L, Morana G, Federle MP, et al: Focal nodular hyperplasia: morphologic and functional information from MR imaging with gadobenate dimeglumine. Radiology 221:731-739, 2001.

56. Soe KL, Soe M, Gluud S: Liver pathology associated with the use of anabolic-androgenic steroids. Liver 12:73-79, 1992.

57. Reddy KR, Schiff E: Approach to a liver mass. Semin Liver Dis 13: 423-435, 1993.

58. Paulson EK, McClellan JS, Washington K, et al: Hepatic adenoma: MR characteristics and correlation with pathologic findings. Am J Roentgenol 163:113-116, 1994.

59. Flejou JF, Barge J, Menu Y, et al: Liver adenomatosis: an entity distinct from liver adenoma? Gastroenterology 83:1132-1138, 1985.

60. Craig JR, Peters RL, Edmondson HA: Atlas of Tumor Pathology: Tumors of the Liver and Intrahepatic Bile Ducts, Fasc 27, 2nd ser. Washington, DC, Armed Forces Institute of Pathology, 1989, pp 19-41.

61. Meissner K: Hemorrhage caused by ruptured liver cell adenoma following long-term oral contraceptives: a case report. Hepatogastroenterology 45:224-225, 1998.

62. Powers C, Ros PR, Stoupis C, et al: Primary liver neoplasms: MR imaging with pathologic correlation. Radiographics 14:459-482, 1994.

63. Semelka RC, Shoenut JO, Kroeker MA, et al: Focal liver diseases: comparison of dynamic contrast-enhanced CT and T2-weighted fat-suppressed, FLASH, and dynamic gadolinium-enhanced MR imaging at 1.5 T. Radiology 184:687-694, 1992.

64. Vogl TJ, Hammerstingl R, Schwarz W, et al: Superparamagnetic iron oxide-enhanced versus gadolinium-enhanced MR imaging for differential diagnosis of focal liver lesions. Radiology 198:881-887, 1996.

65. Nonomura A, Mizukami Y, Cadoya M: Angiomyolipoma of the liver: a collective review. J Gastroenterol 29:95-105, 1994.

66. Worawattanakul S, Kelekis NL, Semelka RC, Woosley JT: Hepatic angiomyolipoma with minimal fat content: MR demonstration. Magn Reson Imaging 14:687-689, 1996.

67. Wong Y, Chen F, Tai KS, et al: Imaging features of focal intrahepatic extramedullary haematopoiesis. Br J Radiol 72:906-910, 1999.

68. Warshauer DM, Schiebler ML: Intrahepatic extramedullary hematopoiesis: MR, CT, and sonographic appearance. J Comput Assist Tomogr 15:683-685, 1991.

69. Choi BI, Lim JH, Han MC, et al: Biliary cystadenoma and cystadenocarcinoma: CT and sonographic findings. Radiology 171:57-61, 1989.

70. Palacios E, Shannon M, Solomon C, Guzman M: Biliary cystadenoma: Ultrasound, CT, and MRI. Gastrointest Radiol 15:313-316, 1990.

71. Sugarbaker PH, Kemeny N: Management of metastatic cancer to the liver. Adv Surg 22:1-56, 1989.
72. Hughes KS, Rosenstein RB, Songhorabodi S, et al: Resection of the liver for colorectal carcinoma metastases: A multi-institutional study of long-term survivors. Dis Colon Rectum 31:1-4, 1988.
73. Lencioni R, Donati F, Cioni D, et al: Detection of colorectal liver metastases: prospective comparison of unenhanced and ferumoxides-enhanced magnetic resonance imaging at 1.5 T, dual-phase spiral CT, and spiral CT during arterial portography. MAGMA 7:76-87, 1998.
74. Semelka RC, Cance WG, Marcos HB, Mauro MA: Liver metastases: comparison of current MR techniques and spiral CT during arterial portography for detection in 20 surgically staged cases. Radiology 213:86-91, 1999.
75. Kinkel K, Lu Y, Both M, et al: Detection of hepatic metastases from cancers of the gastrointestinal tract by using noninvasive imaging methods (US, CT, MR imaging, PET): a meta-analysis. Radiology 224:748-756, 2002.
76. Vogl TJ, Schwarz W, Blume S, et al: Preoperative evaluation of malignant liver tumors: comparison of unenhanced and SPIO (Resovist)-enhanced MR imaging with biphasic CTAP and intraoperative US. Eur Radiol 13:262-272, 2003.
77. Semelka RC, Schlund JF, Molina PL, et al: Malignant liver lesions: Comparison of spiral CT arterial portography and MR imaging for diagnostic accuracy, cost, and effect on patient management. J Magn Reson Imaging 6:39-43, 1996.
78. Jones EC, Chezmar JL, Nelson RC, Bernardino ME: The frequency and significance of small (less than or equal to 15 mm) hepatic lesions detected by CT. Am J Roentgenol 158:535-539, 1992.
79. Bruneton JN, Raffaelli C, Maestro C, Padovani B: Benign liver lesions: Implications of detection in cancer patients. Eur Radiol 5:387-390, 1995.
80. Li KC, Glazer GM, Quint LE, et al: Distinction of hepatic cavernous hemangioma from hepatic metastases with MR imaging. Radiology 169:409-415, 1988.
81. Semelka RC, Cumming MJ, Shoenut JP, et al: Islet cell tumors: Comparison of dynamic contrast-enhanced CT and MR imaging with dynamic gadolinium enhancement and fat suppression. Radiology 186:799-802, 1993.
82. Soyer P, Riopel M, Bluemke DA, Scherrer A: Hepatic metastases from leiomyosarcoma: MR features with histopathologic correlation. Abdom Imaging 22: 67-71, 1997.
83. Bader TR, Semelka RC, Chiu VCY, et al: MRI of carcinoid tumors: spectrum of appearances in the gastrointestinal tract and liver. J Magn Reson Imaging 14:261-269, 2001.
84. Mahfouz AE, Hamm B, Wolf KJ: Peripheral washout: a sign of malignancy on dynamic gadolinium-enhanced MR images of focal liver lesions. Radiology 190:49-52, 1994.
85. Semelka RC, Hussain SM, Marcos HB, Woosley JT: Perilesional enhancement of hepatic metastases: correlation between MR imaging and histopathologic findings—initial observations. Radiology 215:89-94, 2000.
86. Semelka RC, Worawattanakul S, Kelekis NL, et al: Liver lesion detection, characterization, and effect on patient management: comparison of single-phase spiral CT and current MR techniques. J Magn Reson Imaging 7:1040-1047, 1997.
87. Wang C, Ahlstrom H, Ekholm S, et al: Diagnostic efficacy of MnDPDP in MR imaging of the liver. A phase III multicentre study. Acta Radiol 38(4 Pt 2):643-649, 1997.
88. Rofsky NM, Earls JP: Mangafodipir trisodium injection (Mn-DPDP). A contrast agent for abdominal MR imaging. Magn Reson Imaging Clin N Am 4:73-85, 1996.
89. Wang C, Ahlstrom H, Eriksson B, et al: Uptake of mangafodipir trisodium in liver metastases from endocrine tumors. J Magn Reson Imaging 8:682-686, 1998.
90. Ba-Ssalamah A, Heinz-Peer G, Schima W, et al: Detection of focal hepatic lesions: comparison of unenhanced and SHU 555A-enhanced MR imaging versus biphasic helical CTAP. J Magn Reson Imaging 11:665-72, 2000.
91. Runge VM, Lee C, Williams NM: Detectability of small liver metastases with gadolinium BOPTA. Invest Radiol 32:557-565, 1997.
92. Scheimberg IB, Pollock DJ, Collins PW, et al: Pathology of the liver in leukemia and lymphoma. A study of 110 autopsies. Histopathology 26:311-322, 1995.
93. Kelekis NL, Semelka RC, Siegelman ES, et al: Focal hepatic lymphoma: MR demonstration using current techniques including gadolinium enhancement. J Magn Reson Imaging 15:625-636, 1997.
94. Kew MC: Hepatic tumors and cysts. In Feldman M, Scharschmidt BF, Sleisenger MH, eds: Sleisenger and Fordtran's Gastrointestinal and Liver Disease, 6th ed. Philadelphia: WB Saunders, 1998, pp 1364-1387.
95. Nzeako UC, Goodman ZD, Ishak KG: Hepatocellular carcinoma in cirrhotic and noncirrhotic livers. A clinico-histopathologic study of 804 North American patients [see comments]. Am J Clin Pathol 105:65-75, 1996.
96. International Working Party: Terminology of nodular hepatocellular lesions. Hepatology 22:983-993, 1995.
97. Grazioli L, Olivetti L, Fugazzola C, et al: The pseudocapsule in hepatocellular carcinoma: correlation between dynamic MR imaging and pathology. Eur Radiol 9:62-67, 1999.
98. Muramatsu Y, Nawano S, Takayasu K, et al: Early hepatocellular carcinoma: MR imaging. Radiology 181:209-213, 1991.
99. Kadoya M, Matsui O, Takashima T, Nonomura A: Hepatocellular carcinoma: Correlation of MR imaging and histopathologic findings. Radiology 183:819-825, 1992.
100. Kelekis NL, Semelka RC, Woosley JT: Malignant lesions of the liver with high signal intensity on T1-weighted MR images. J Magn Reson Imaging 6:291-294, 1996.
101. Krinsky GA, Lee VS: MR imaging of cirrhotic nodules. Abdom Imaging 25:471-482, 2000.
102. Mahfouz AE, Hamm B, Wolf KJ: Dynamic gadopentetate dimeglumine-enhanced MR imaging of hepatocellular carcinoma. Eur Radiol 3:453-458, 1993.
103. Yoshida H, Itai Y, Ohtomo K, et al: Small hepatocellular carcinoma and cavernous hemangioma: Differentiation with dynamic FLASH MR imaging with Gd-DTPA. Radiology 171: 339-342, 1989.
104. Grazioli L, Morana G, Caudana R, et al: Hepatocellular carcinoma. Correlation between gadobenate dimeglumine enhanced MRI and pathologic findings. Invest Radiol 35:25-34, 2000.
105. Craig JR, Peters RL, Edmondson HA, Omata M: Fibrolamellar carcinoma of the liver: A tumor of adolescents and young adults with distinctive clinico-pathologic features. Cancer 46:372-379, 1980.
106. Corrigan K, Semelka RC: Dynamic contrast-enhanced MR imaging of fibrolamellar hepatocellular carcinoma. Abdom Imaging 20:122-125, 1995.
107. McLarney JK, Rucker PR, Bender GN, et al: Fibrolamellar carcinoma of the liver: radiologic-pathologic correlation. Radiographics 19:453-471, 1999.
108. Marcos-Alvarez A, Jenkins RL: Cholangiocarcinoma. Surg Oncol Clin North Am 5:301-316, 1996.
109. Hamrick-Turner J, Abbitt PL, Ros PR: Intrahepatic cholangiocarcinoma: MR appearance. Am J Roentgenol 158:77-79, 1992.
110. Worawattanakul S, Semelka RC, Noone TC, et al: Cholangiocarcinoma: spectrum of appearances on MR images using current techniques. Magn Reson Imaging 16:993-1003, 1998.
111. Schneider G, Grazioli L, Saini S: Imaging of malignant focal liver lesions. In Schneider G, Grazioli L, Saini S (eds): MRI of the Liver. New York: Springer, 2003, pp 171-242.
112. Carceller A, Blanchard H, Champagne J, et al: Surgical resection and chemotherapy improve survival rate for patients with hepatoblastoma. J Pediatr Surg 36:755-759, 2001.
113. Buetow PC, Rao P, Marshall H: Imaging of pediatric liver tumors. Magn Reson Clin N Am 5:397-413, 1997.
114. Helmberger TK, Ros PR, Mergo PJ, et al: Pediatric liver neoplasms: a radiologic-pathologic correlation. Eur Radiol 9:1339-1347, 1999.
115. Siegel MJ: MR imaging of pediatric abdominal neoplasms. Magn Reson Imaging Clin N Am 8: 837-851, 2000.
116. Ishak KG: Mesenchymal tumors of the liver. In Okuda K, Peter RL, eds: Hepatocellular Carcinoma. New York, John Wiley, 1976, pp 228-587.
117. Molina E, Hernandez A: Clinical manifestations of primary hepatic angiosarcoma. Dig Dis Sci 48:677-682, 2003.
118. Rossai J: Ackerman's Surgical Pathology, vol.1, 8th ed. St Louis, 1995, p 918.
119. Worawattanakul S, Semelka RC, Kelekis NL, Woosley JT: Angiosarcoma of the liver: MR imaging pre- and post-chemotherapy. Magn Reson Imaging 15:613-617, 1997.
120. Koyama T, Fletcher JG, Johnson CD, et al: Primary hepatic angiosarcoma: findings at CT and MR imaging. Radiology 222:667-673, 2002.
121. Van Beers B, Roche A, Mathieu D, et al: Epithelioid hemangioendothelioma of the liver: MR and CT findings. J Comput Assist Tomogr 16:420-424, 1992.
122. Furui S, Itai Y, Ohtomo K, et al: Hepatic epithelioid hemangioendothelioma: report of five cases. Radiology 171:63-68, 1989.
123. Buetow PC, Buck JL, Ros PR, Goodman ZDLC: Malignant vascular tumors of the liver: Radiologic-pathologic correlation. Radiographics 14:153-166, quiz 167-158, 1994.
124. Kehagias DT, Moulopoulos LA, Antoniou A, et al: Hepatic epithelioid hemangioendothelioma: MR imaging findings. Hepatogastroenterology 47:1711-1713, 2000.
125. Leonardou P, Semelka RC, Mastropasqua M, et al: Epithelioid hemangio-endothelioma of the liver. MR imaging findings. Magn Reson Imaging 20:631-633, 2002.
126. Oto A, Akhan O, Ozmen M: Focal inflammatory diseases of the liver. Eur J Radiol 32:61-75, 1999.
127. Mendez RJ, Schiebler ML, Outwater EK, Kressel HY: Hepatic abscesses: MR imaging findings. Radiology 190:431-436, 1994.
128. Balci NC, Semelka RC, Noone TC, et al: Pyogenic hepatic abscesses: MRI findings on T1- and T2-weighted and serial gadolinium-enhanced gradient-echo images. J Magn Reson Imaging 9:285-290, 1999.
129. Landay MJ, Setiawan H, Hirsch G, et al: Hepatic and thoracic amaebiasis. Am J Roentgenol 135: 449-454, 1980.
130. Lebovics E, Thung SN, Schaffner F: The liver in the acquired immuno-deficiency syndrome: a clinical and histologic study. Hepatology 5:293-298, 1995.

131. Schneiderman DJ, Arenson DM, Cello JP: Hepatic disease in patients with acquired immune deficiency syndrome (AIDS). Hepatology 7:925-930, 1987.

132. Pantongrag-Brown L, Krebs TL, Daly BD, et al: Frequency of abdominal CT findings in AIDS patients with M. avium complex bacteraemia. Clin Radiol 53:816-819, 1998.

133. Lewis JH, Patel HR, Zimmerman HJ: The spectrum of hepatic candidiasis. Hepatology 2:479-487, 1982.

134. Sallah S, Semelka RC, Kelekis N, et al: Diagnosis and monitoring response of treatment of hepatosplenic candidiasis in patients with acute leukemia using magnetic resonance imaging. Acta Haematol 100:77-81, 1998.

135. Semelka RC, Kelekis NL, Sallah S, et al: Hepatosplenic fungal disease: diagnostic accuracy and spectrum of appearance on MR imaging. Am J Roentgenol 169:1311-1316, 1997.

136. Cho JS, Kim EE, Varma DG, Wallace S: MR imaging of hepatosplenic candidiasis superimposed on hemochromatosis. J Comput Assist Tomogr 14:774-776, 1990.

137. Lamminen AE, Anttila VJ, Bondestam S, et al: Infectious liver foci in leukemia: Comparison of short-inversion-time inversion-recovery, T1-weighted spin-echo, and dynamic gadolinium-enhanced MR imaging. Radiology 191:539-543, 1994.

138. Semelka RC, Shoenut JP, Greenberg HM, Bow EJ: Detection of acute and treated lesions of hepatosplenic candidiasis: Comparison of dynamic contrast-enhanced CT and MR imaging. J Magn Reson Imaging 2:341-345, 1992.

139. Kelekis NL, Semelka RC, Jeon HJ, et al: Dark ring sign: Finding in patients with fungal liver lesions and transfusional hemosiderosis undergoing treatment with antifungal antibiotics. Magn Reson Imaging 14:615-618, 1996.

CHAPTER 82

DIFFUSE LIVER DISEASE

Katsuyoshi Ito ● Shahid M. Hussain ● Donald G. Mitchell ● Richard C. Semelka

During the past two decades MR imaging has emerged as an important imaging modality for assessing diffuse liver diseases, such as fatty liver, iron overload, cirrhosis, portal hypertension, Wilson's disease, primary sclerosing cholangitis, and hepatic vascular diseases. MR imaging is better able to provide comprehensive information about diffuse liver diseases than any other imaging modality currently available. Even biopsy only provides information limited to a particular location within this large organ. Additionally, the specificity of findings on MR imaging is sufficient to obviate the need for histologic examination in certain circumstances. This chapter will describe and illustrate the MR imaging findings of diffuse liver diseases.

FATTY LIVER

Hepatocellular accumulation of fat results from increased delivery of dietary fat or fatty acids and impaired export of triglycerides out of the liver. Common causes of fatty liver include excessive alcohol intake, diabetes mellitus, obesity, nutritional imbalance, drugs, and hyperalimentation. Fatty liver in most patients can be recovered by weight reduction, adequate nutritional intake, removal of alcohol or other toxins, and correction of any associated metabolic disorders without progressing to other liver disease.

Although fat has high signal intensity on T1-weighted spin-echo MR images, conventional spin-echo imaging is relatively insensitive to mild-to-moderate fatty infiltration of the liver. Chemical shift MR imaging, such as by comparing opposed- and in-phase gradient-echo images obtained during breath-holding, is the most effective technique for detecting regions of fatty liver.[1-4] In nonfatty livers, the signal intensity of the liver parenchyma is unchanged between in- and opposed-phase images. Conversely, in fatty livers there is a notable reduction of signal intensity on the opposed-phase images due to cancellation of opposing signals from water and fat tissues, confirming the presence of fatty infiltration (Fig. 82-1). The spleen is generally used as the organ of reference for signal reduction, although the right kidney or other nearby organs may be substituted if necessary. Subtraction from in- and opposed-phase images obtained simultaneously during a single breath-hold[5] is effective for detecting mild fatty infiltration or a small focus of fatty deposition (Fig. 82-2). Fat-saturation images may also be helpful in cases of moderate or severe fatty infiltration, but the signal from fatty liver is not reduced as much as on opposed-phase images. It should be remembered that on opposed-phase MR images, tissues containing predominantly fat have a paradoxical decrease in signal intensity after the injection of gadolinium chelate, since gadolinium increases water signal, thereby increasing intravoxel cancellation of fat signal.[6]

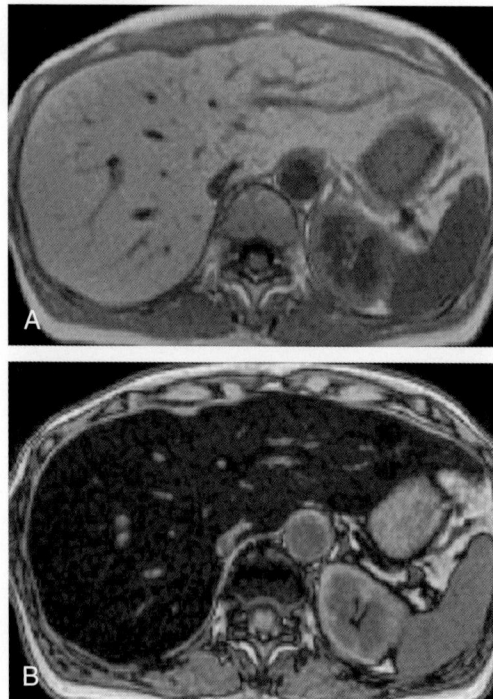

FIGURE 82-1

Severe fatty liver. **A,** In-phase and **B,** opposed-phase T1-weighted gradient-echo images. The liver shows marked homogeneous drop in signal on the opposed-phase image compared with the in-phase image. A black rim at the fat-water boundary around the kidney and the spleen is well seen in the opposed-phase image.

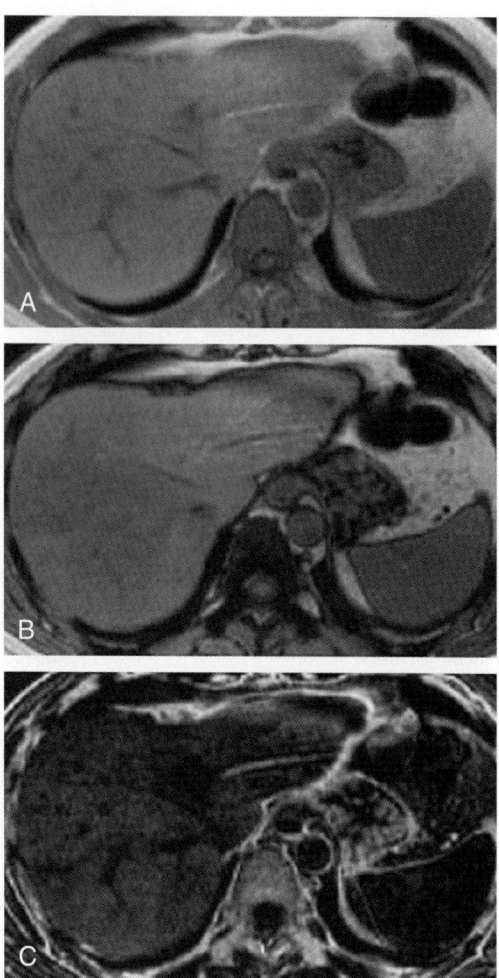

FIGURE 82-2

Mild fatty liver. Simultaneously obtained **A,** in-phase and **B,** opposed-phase images during a single breath-hold; and **C,** subtracted image. There is a slight decrease in signal intensity of the liver on the opposed-phase image compared with the in-phase image. The subtracted image without misregistration clearly shows signal difference of the liver between in- and opposed-phase images, consistent with fatty infiltration.

The distribution of fatty infiltration can be quite variable, ranging from focal to multifocal or diffuse. Diffuse involvement can be either uniform or patchy and nonuniform. Lobar distribution differences in nutritional fatty liver may be related to intrahepatic portal flow distribution created by streamlined flow from the superior mesenteric vein and splenic vein (Fig. 82-3) because nutritional fatty liver is principally induced by excessive transports of nutrient-rich content from the small bowel (e.g., fatty acid and cholesterol) in the superior mesenteric vein. Focal distribution differences in fatty change may be due to regional differences in perfusion. Areas of decreased portal venous flow tend to accumulate less fat than better portal-perfused areas. This is commonly seen near the gallbladder or the hepatic hilum (typically posterior parts of segment IV) caused by replacement of portal venous flow by venous drainage from the cystic vein and the peribiliary venous system or aberrant gastric venous drainage (Figs. 82-4 and 82-5).[7-11] These "focally spared areas" are usually roundish to semicircular, or are in contact with the hepatic capsule, and have a direct splanchnic "nonportal" venous supply rather than through the portal trunk. Areas of hyperplasia near the gallbladder can also be related to relative sparing due to aberrant gastric venous drainage.[12] When focal sparing with round configuration shows an unusual location far from the hepatic capsule, diagnostic confusion may occur (Fig. 82-6). Focal sparing can also be caused by anterioportal shunting from any cause.[13] Peritumoral fatty sparing, seen as a hyperintense rim on opposed-phase MR images, can be caused by impaired portal perfusion of hepatic parenchyma surrounding liver metastases (Fig. 82-7).[14]

Focal fatty infiltration of the liver is commonly seen at the anteromedial edge of the medial segment adjacent to the falciform ligament (Fig. 82-8). Focal fat in this area may be induced by deficient perfusion of systemic venous blood, although the precise mechanism of focal fat deposition has not been clarified. Areas of focal fat deposition as well as focal fatty sparing can be confused with focal liver masses. Differential aspects include the typical location and shape (triangular or wedge-shaped margins), the lack of surrounding mass effect, homogeneity of the signal intensity in the abnormal area, and

FIGURE 82-13, cont'd

Multiple hepatocellular carcinoma (HCC) in a patient under treatment for genetic hemochromatosis. **A,** T2-weighted fat-saturated fast spin-echo (FSE) image shows at least three larger lesions with predominantly high signal intensity within a cirrhotic liver. Note that the liver (L) is darker that usual on T2-weighted FSE sequences. The spleen (S) has normal bright signal intensity. **B,** In-phase T1-weighted gradient-echo (GRE) image shows two lesions with a higher signal intensity compared to the liver; one lesion becomes almost isointense to the liver, except the central part of this lesion which is very bright, indicating the presence of hemorrhage (*arrow*). Note also an additional bright lesion (*curved arrow*) that is not clearly visible on the T2-weighted image (**A**). The liver is almost isointense to the spleen with multiple siderotic nodules due to hemochromatosis. **C,** Opposed-phase T1-weighted GRE image shows that one of the lesions drops its signal intensity and becomes predominantly isointense to the liver, indicating the presence of lipid in this lesion (*arrow*). **D,** Arterial phase of the dynamic contrast-enhanced (DCE) T1-weighted GRE image shows an intense heterogeneous enhancement of the lesions. Note an additional small lesion, not clearly visible on the T2-weighted and nonenhanced T1-weighted images. **E,** Portal phase of the DCE T1-weighted GRE image shows washout of contrast material within the lesions, rendering them more heterogeneous. **F,** Delayed phase of the DCE T1-weighted GRE image shows further washout in most lesions with enhancement of a capsule surrounding two larger lesions (*arrows*). The patient had been successfully under treatment for genetic hemochromatosis for many years but still developed multiple HCC in the course of the disease.

---

elevated ratio between the transverse width of the caudate lobe and the right lobe can be used to differentiate normal and cirrhotic livers, specifically alcoholic cirrhosis (Fig. 82-14).[37] In this original series, a ratio equal to or greater than 0.65 was 90% specific for distinguishing severe cirrhotic from noncirrhotic livers. In the early stages of cirrhosis, however, morphologic changes of the liver are seen less frequently or are very subtle, impairing diagnosis by MRI. The caudate-to-right lobe ratio, particularly using the main portal vein bifurcation to divide caudate from right lobes, cannot predict the presence or absence of early cirrhosis.[38] Conversely, MR depiction of medial segment atrophy is an earlier sign of cirrhosis. For example, an enlarged hilar periportal space has considerable potential impact for detecting patients in the early stage of cirrhosis (Fig. 82-15). Enlargement of the hilar periportal space was visible in 98% of patients with early cirrhosis who did not have conventional signs of cirrhosis (e.g., splenomegaly, portosystemic collateral vessels, ascites, or surface nodularity), while this finding was seen in only 11% of patients with normal livers.[38] In a normal liver, the hilar portal space (the space between the anterior edge of the right portal vein and the posterior edge of the left medial segment) on axial MR images is narrow, containing minimal fatty tissue. In patients with early cirrhosis, however, the hilar periportal space was enlarged and filled with increased fatty tissues due to atrophy of the medial segment of the left hepatic lobe. It should be noted that the progression from chronic hepatitis to cirrhosis is a continuous process so that definitive distinction between these two transitional conditions may not be possible by any method. Expansion of the major interlobar fissure is also seen frequently in these patients with early cirrhosis, causing extrahepatic fat to fill the space between the left medial and lateral segments (Fig. 82-16).

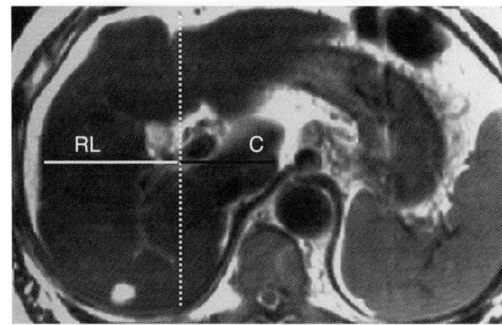

FIGURE 82-14

Ratio of the transverse width of the caudate lobe (C) and right lobe (RL). The ratio calculated by using the bifurcation of the main portal vein as a landmark is 0.71, indicating cirrhosis. The vertical dashed line drawn through the right lateral wall of the main portal vein was used to determine the border between the caudate lobe and right lobe. The diameter of the caudate lobe (*black line*) and right lobe (*white line*) was measured on the horizontal line between the portal vein and inferior vena cava.

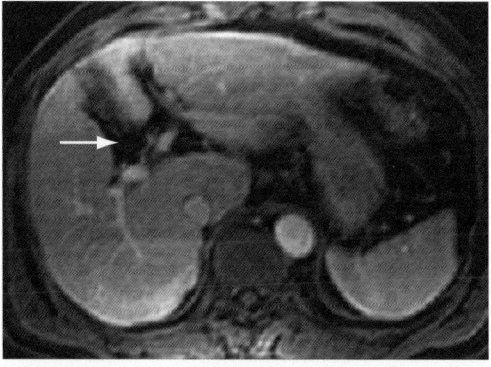

FIGURE 82-15

Early cirrhosis. Gadolinium-enhanced T1-weighted MR image with fat suppression shows enlargement of the hilar periportal space (*arrow*). Note the increased fat tissue (areas of decreased signal intensity due to fat suppression) between the left medial segment of the liver and portal vein.

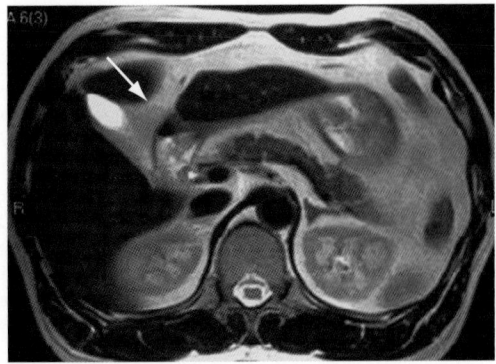

FIGURE 82-16

Early cirrhosis. T2-weighted fast spin-echo image shows expansion of the major interlobar fissure (*arrow*). Note the increased extrahepatic fat between the left medial and lateral segments. *(Reproduced with permission from Ito K, Mitchell DG, Siegelman ES: Cirrhosis: MR imaging features. Magn Reson Imaging Clin North Am 10:75-92, 2002.)*

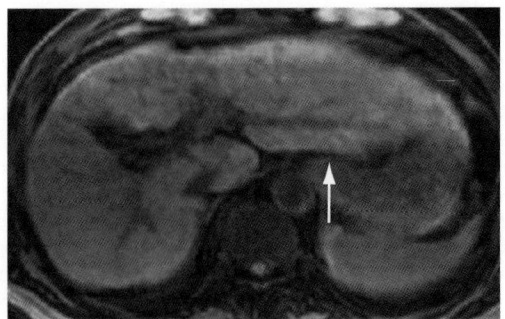

FIGURE 82-17

Advanced hepatitis C-induced cirrhosis. T1-weighted gradient-echo image with fat suppression demonstrates marked hypertrophy of the left lateral segment (*arrow*).

Advanced Cirrhosis

During its course from early compensated to advanced decompensated states, cirrhosis gives rise to progressive lobar or segmental changes of hepatic morphology. Characteristic MR imaging features of advanced cirrhosis include atrophy of the right hepatic lobe and the left medial segment, with compensatory hypertrophy of the caudate lobe and the left lateral segment.[39] The patterns of hepatic morphologic change overlap among different causes of cirrhosis, preventing identification of the specific cause of cirrhosis. However, there are some etiologic tendencies in their appearances. Enlargement of the lateral segment, accompanied by shrinkage of the right lobe and left medial segment, occurs frequently in patients with viral-induced cirrhosis (Fig. 82-17). Conversely, marked caudate lobe enlargement is more frequently associated with alcoholic cirrhosis (Fig. 82-18), although the reasons for these findings are not

understood. Occasionally, only the lateral or posterior segments may be atrophic, seen most commonly in patients with primary sclerosing cholangitis, probably secondary to segmental biliary strictures of these segments (Fig. 82-19).[40,41] The liver in patients with endstage cirrhosis caused by primary biliary cirrhosis occasionally is diffusely hypertrophic. It is important to distinguish between viral and other cirrhosis because HCC occurs more frequently in the former condition.

In normal subjects, there is little fatty tissue anterolateral to the surface of the right anterior and left medial segments. In patients with advanced cirrhosis, atrophy of these segments frequently leads to increased intra-abdominal fat between the diaphragm and the liver surface (Fig. 82-20), sometimes with intrusion of the gallbladder and small intestine into this space.

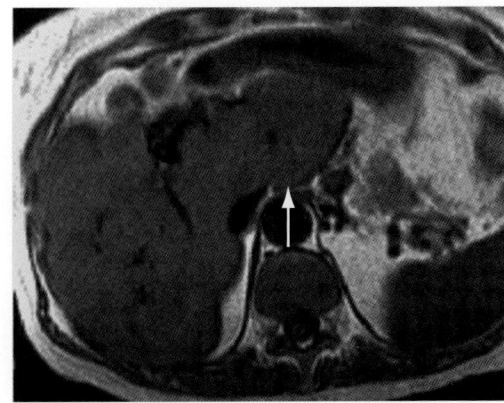

FIGURE 82-19

Cirrhosis due to primary sclerosing cholangitis. T1-weighted conventional spin-echo image shows marked hypertrophy of the caudate lobe of the liver (*arrow*) and atrophy of the lateral and medial segment of the left hepatic lobe. *(From Ito K, Mitchell DG, Outwater EK, Blasbalg R: Primary sclerosing cholangitis: MR imaging features. Am J Roentgenol 172:1527-1533, 1999. Reproduced with permission of Wiley-Liss, Inc., a subsidiary of John Wiley & Sons, Inc.)*

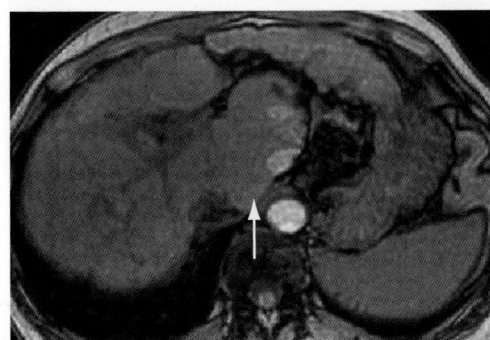

FIGURE 82-18

Advanced alcoholic cirrhosis. Opposed-phase gradient-echo image shows marked enlargement of the caudate lobe (*arrow*).

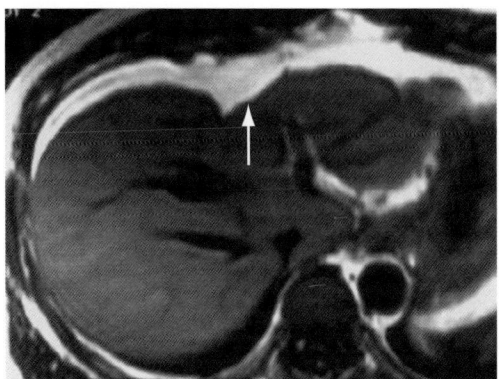

FIGURE 82-20

Increase of intra-abdominal fat in cirrhosis. T1-weighted spin-echo image shows an increase of intra-abdominal fat anterolateral to the liver surface (*arrow*).

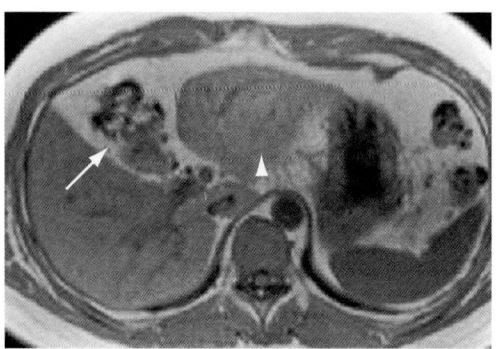

FIGURE 82-21

Cirrhosis with the expanded gallbladder fossa (GBF) sign. In-phase T1-weighted gradient-echo image demonstrates the enlarged pericholecystic space (GBF) filled with increased fat tissue and intrusion of intestines into the space, presenting the expanded GBF sign (*arrow*). Note the slight enlargement of the left lateral segment (*arrowhead*) and the atrophy of the right hepatic lobe. The left medial segment is not seen in this level because of its atrophic change.

Expanded Gallbladder Fossa Sign

The diagnostic value of hepatic measurements, including the ratio of the transverse caudate to right lobe widths and multidimensional caudate lobe indexes at ultrasound and CT have been evaluated.[37,42] However, simple visual criteria for diagnosing cirrhosis would be more helpful. The expanded gallbladder fossa (GBF) sign is one such visual sign. The gallbladder normally fits into a fossa between the right hepatic lobe and the left medial segment, with little fatty tissue in the plane of the major interlobar fissure. At its caudate level, the gallbladder is still covered by a part of the left medial segment. In patients with cirrhosis, however, the pericholecystic space (GBF) is often enlarged and filled with increased fat tissue (Fig. 82-21).[43] The expanded GBF sign had high specificity and positive predictive value (both 98%) for diagnosing cirrhosis,[43] although the sensitivity is relatively low (68%). The expanded GBF sign is defined as enlargement of the pericholecystic space (i.e., GBF), bounded laterally by the edge of the right hepatic lobe, medially by the edge of the lateral segment of the left hepatic lobe, and occasionally by the anterior edge of the caudate lobe, with nonvisualization of the medial segment of the left hepatic lobe on the same axial image. The expanded GBF sign in cirrhotic livers may be dependent on a combination of factors: 1. atrophy of the medial segment of the left hepatic lobe; 2. hypertrophy of the caudate lobe; 3. atrophy of the right hepatic lobe (mainly the anterior segment) with counterclockwise rotation of the major interlobar fissure; and 4. enlargement of the lateral segment of the left hepatic lobe, especially in the cephalocaudal direction.

Right Posterior Hepatic Notch Sign

A smooth hepatic curvature is normally observed on the posteroinferior surface of the right posterior segment due to the right renal impression at the level of the right kidney. Conversely, in patients with cirrhosis, a sharp indentation often develops on the posteroinferior surface of the hepatic right posterior segment, presenting the "right posterior hepatic notch" sign. There are some degrees in severity of the right posterior hepatic notch sign (e.g., deep versus shallow notch), depending on the distortion of the posteroinferior liver surface (Fig. 82-22). The right posterior hepatic notch

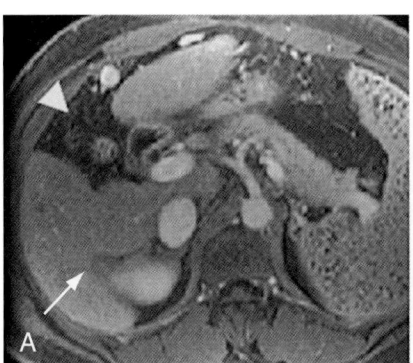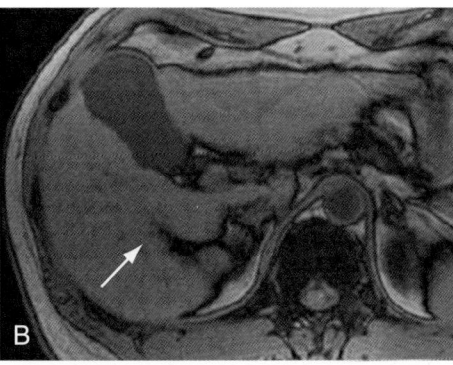

FIGURE 82-22

Right posterior hepatic notch sign. **A** and **B**, MR images obtained from two different patients show a sharp "notch" at the posterior surface of the right hepatic lobe (*arrows*), indicating the presence of the right posterior hepatic notch sign. The caudate lobe mainly enlarges laterally. In one of the patients (**A**), the expanded gallbladder fossa sign is also seen (*arrowhead*).

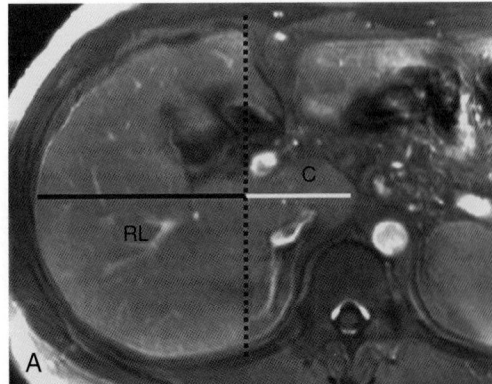

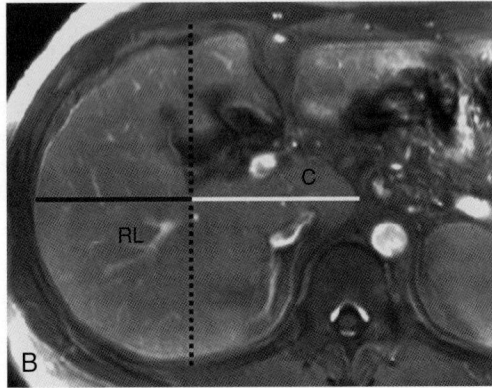

FIGURE 82-23

Modified transverse width of the caudate lobe to the right lobe (C/RL) ratio in cirrhosis. **A,** Classic C/RL ratio. The ratio was calculated using the bifurcation of the main portal vein as a landmark. The classic C/RL ratio is 0.50 and fails to diagnose cirrhosis. **B,** Modified C/RL ratio. The ratio was calculated using the bifurcation of the right portal vein as a landmark. The modified C/RL ratio is 1.10, consistent with a diagnostic criterion of cirrhosis.

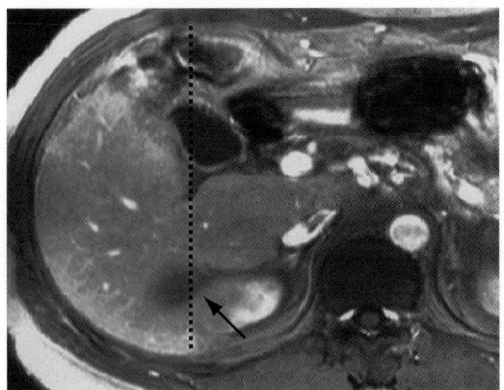

FIGURE 82-24

Modified transverse width of the caudate lobe and the right lobe (C/RL) ratio and right posterior hepatic notch sign. The right posterior hepatic notch (*arrow*) seen in the same patients as in Figure 82-23 corresponds to the location of the right portal vein bifurcation as a landmark for the lateral boundary of the caudate lobe. The modified C/RL ratio and the right posterior hepatic notch sign may represent the same morphologic changes of the cirrhotic liver between the hypertrophied caudate lobe and the atrophied right posterior segment.

sign is highly indicative of cirrhosis with 98% specificity and 99% positive predictive value.[44] Additionally, the combination of the expanded GBF sign with the right posterior hepatic notch sign improves the sensitivity (86%) and overall accuracy (90%) for diagnosing cirrhosis. The right posterior hepatic notch may represent distortion of the liver surface at the segmental border caused by the hypertrophied caudate lobe and the atrophied right posterior segment.[45] Conversely, the expanded GBF sign may be mainly associated with atrophy of the left medial segment and with enlargement of the left lateral segment in the cephalocaudal direction. Thus, each sign is dependent on different types of segmental morphologic changes of the liver, resulting in the improved diagnostic performance for cirrhosis with the combined use of these two signs.

On cross-sectional imaging, the lateral boundary between the caudate lobe and posterior segment of the right hepatic lobe has been unclear, with the bifurcation of the right portal vein, or a line connecting the main portal vein to the inferior vena cava, arbitrarily chosen. The right posterior hepatic notch may represent a functional landmark between the hypertrophied caudate lobe and the atrophied right posterior segment in the

cirrhotic liver. Additionally, this finding implies that the caudate lobe in cirrhotic patients can often enlarge prominently to the lateral (right) side rather than just to the medial (left) side.

Modified Caudate-to-Right Lobe Ratio

The ratio of the transverse diameter of the caudate lobe to the transverse diameter of the right lobe (C/RL ratio > 0.65) has been reported to be a reliable parameter for the diagnosis of alcoholic cirrhosis.[37] However, patients with viral-induced cirrhosis often have a C/RL ratio less than 0.65. For calculating the C/RL ratio, the border between the caudate lobe and right hepatic lobe was determined by the right lateral wall of the main portal vein bifurcation as an easily recognizable boundary landmark. However, the hypertrophied area of the liver usually extends further to the right, which more closely corresponds to the bifurcation of the right portal vein or lateral edge of the ligamentum venosum. Recently, it has been reported that a modified C/RL ratio, using the bifurcation of the right portal vein as a landmark to define a more lateral boundary for the caudate lobe, appears to better represent the division between the hypertrophied caudate lobe and the atrophied right lobe (Fig. 82-23). This modified C/RL ratio is more sensitive and accurate for diagnosing cirrhosis than the previously used C/RL ratio.[46] Additionally, a ratio of 1.0 or greater provides an easy criterion for identifying livers with caudate hypertrophy and right lobe atrophy. The results of Awaya et al[46] indicate that the hypertrophied caudate lobe extends further to the lateral (right) side. In fact, the right posterior hepatic notch usually corresponds to the location of the right portal vein bifurcation as a landmark for the lateral boundary of the caudate lobe (Fig. 82-24). Therefore, the modified C/RL ratio and the

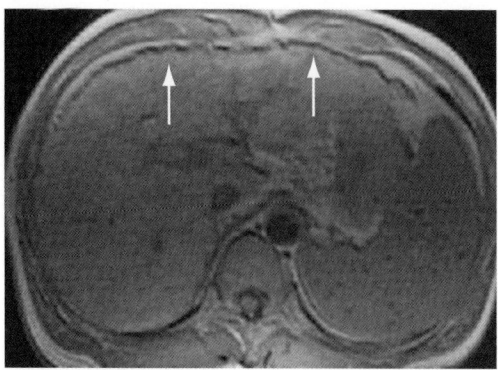

FIGURE 82-25

Nodular liver surface. T1-weighted gradient-echo image shows irregularity of the liver surface of the left lateral and medial segment (*arrows*) caused by regenerative nodules.

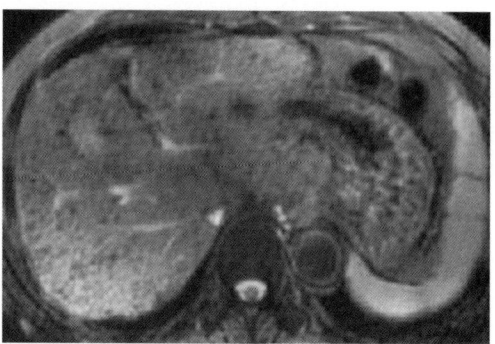

FIGURE 82-26

Micronodular regenerative nodule. Gradient-echo MR image of a patient with alcoholic cirrhosis demonstrates fine hypointense nodules less than 3 mm in diameter, representing micronodular regenerative nodules.

right posterior hepatic notch sign represent the same morphologic changes of the cirrhotic liver: a more lateral division than conventionally considered between the hypertrophied caudate lobe and atrophied right posterior segment.

Liver Surface Nodularity and Regenerative Nodules

Distortion of the hepatic parenchyma in cirrhosis can often cause nodularity of the liver surface.[47] This sign can be identified on MR imaging as irregularity of the liver surface, commonly seen at the anterior surface of the left lateral segment (Fig. 82-25) or the inferior edge of the right hepatic lobe. Liver surface nodularity is an objective finding that directly correlates with the gross appearance of the cirrhotic liver due to the development of regenerative nodules, enabling differentiation between micro- and macro-nodular cirrhosis. A surface

that is smooth or deformed by multiple small nodules is common in micronodular cirrhosis, while a coarse nodularity of the surface implies macronodular cirrhosis.

Micronodular cirrhosis, common in alcohol-related disease or hemochromatosis, has diffuse nodules less than 3 mm in size with thin fibrous septa (Fig. 82-26). Viral hepatitis tends to result in macronodular cirrhosis, characterized by nodules greater than 3 mm in size. In hepatitis B cirrhosis, the size of regenerative nodules is irregular, but there are more macro- than micro-nodules (Fig. 82-27). In hepatitis C cirrhosis, the nodules are smaller and the septa thicker, with frequently active inflammation (Fig. 82-28). Regenerative nodules are commonly isointense, but they may appear relatively hyperintense on T1-weighted images and hypointense on T2-weighted images. This appearance may be related to infiltration of inflammatory cells and development of pseudo bile ducts in the fibrous septa surrounding the regenerative nodules.[48-50]

Some regenerative nodules accumulate iron more than the surrounding hepatic parenchyma. These siderotic regenerative nodules have low signal intensity

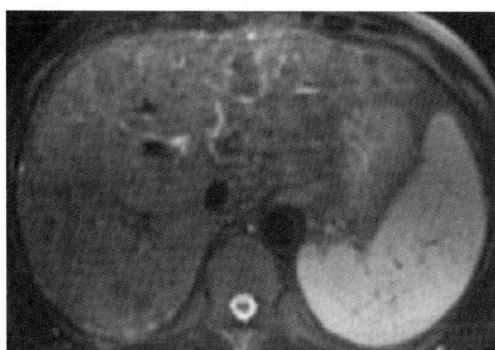

FIGURE 82-27

Macronodular regenerative nodule. T2-weighted fast spin-echo image with fat suppression in a patient with viral hepatitis B-induced cirrhosis shows macronodular regenerative nodules 3 to 15 mm in diameter with low signal intensity relative to the high signal intensity inflammatory fibrous septa or damaged liver.

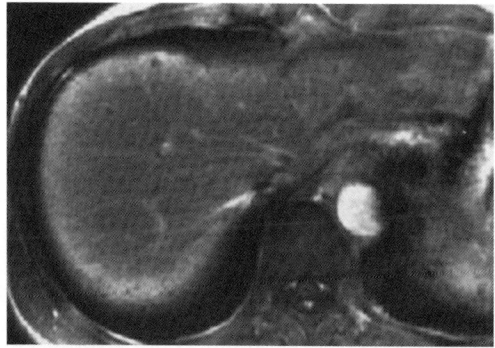

FIGURE 82-28

Regenerative nodules in a patient with viral hepatitis C-induced cirrhosis. Contrast-enhanced gradient-echo image demonstrates fine hypointense nodules in the liver, representing small regenerative nodules.

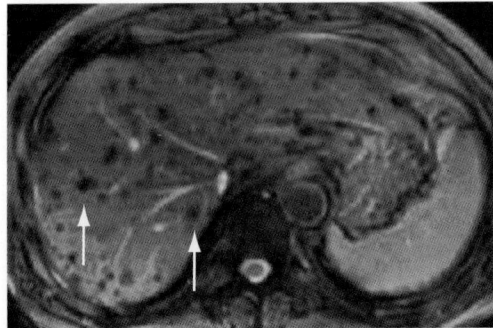

FIGURE 82-29

Siderotic regenerative nodules. T1-weighted gradient-echo image with long echo time (TR/TE 200/18 ms) shows multiple hepatic nodules with markedly low signal intensity (*arrows*), representing siderotic regenerative nodules.

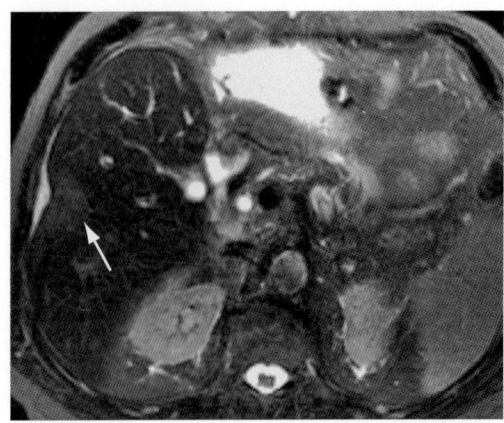

FIGURE 82-30

Confluent fibrosis. T2-weighted fast spin-echo image with fat suppression shows a wedge-shaped lesion with high signal intensity (*arrow*) located in the anterior segment, corresponding to focal confluent fibrosis. Note the characteristic retraction of the liver surface. (*Reproduced with permission from Ito K, Mitchell DG, Siegelman ES: Cirrhosis: MR imaging features. Magn Reson Imaging Clin North Am 10:75-92, 2002.*)

on T2-weighted and gradient-echo (especially long TE) images because of their susceptibility effects (Fig. 82-29). As T2*-weighted gradient-echo MR imaging is particularly susceptible to magnetic field heterogeneity, siderotic regenerative nodules may cause artifactual enlargement of regenerative nodules.[51] An increased probability of developing HCC has been reported in viral hepatitis patients with persistently elevated serum ferritin levels, related to the tumor-stimulating effects of iron,[52] evidence that hepatic iron overload is a risk factor for developing HCC. It is controversial whether the detection of siderotic regenerative nodules at MR imaging should be considered a significant risk factor for HCC.[20,22] However, pathologic observations suggest a role for siderotic regenerative nodules in carcinogenesis. Pathologic studies have suggested that the presence of iron in large (>8 mm) regenerative nodules is a significant risk factor for dysplastic or frank malignant changes.[53,54] Therefore, iron concentration within regenerative nodules that are large enough to be visible on MR images may be related to the occurrence of HCC, and MR imaging can be used to depict these siderotic regenerative nodules as a potential premalignant marker of HCC.

Fibrosis

When the liver is severely damaged, hepatic fibrosis or scar develops. Intrahepatic fibrosis can occur diffusely or focally in the cirrhotic liver. Most fibrosis appears as regions of low signal intensity on T1-weighted MR images and high intensity on T2-weighted MR images, and shows mild enhancement on contrast-enhanced MR images. Diffuse fibrosis is categorized on T2-weighted MR images as: 1. patchy, poorly defined regions of high signal intensity; 2. thin perilobular bands of high signal intensity; 3. thick bridging bands of high signal intensity that surround regenerative nodules; and 4. diffuse fibrosis that causes perivascular (bull's-eye) cuffing.[55] Although most forms of diffuse fibrosis can occur in any type of cirrhosis, thin perilobular bands and perivascular cuffing appear most commonly in primary biliary cirrhosis.

Focal confluent fibrosis is commonly located in the anterior and medial segments of the liver with a wedge-shaped appearance radiating from the hepatic hilum, but in some patients the entire segment may be involved.[56] Focal confluent fibrosis may resemble HCC on MR imaging with abnormal signal intensity and abnormal enhancement. However, T2-weighted MR images depict the lesions as regions of high signal intensity with characteristic retraction of the overlying liver capsule (Fig. 82-30). Prolonged enhancement on late-phase gadolinium-enhanced MR images is also a useful finding for the differentiation between focal confluent fibrosis and HCC.

Abdominal Lymphadenopathy

Enlarged, benign abdominal lymph nodes are a common finding in all types of endstage cirrhosis. It has been reported that enlarged lymph nodes were seen in 253 (50%) of 507 patients who underwent liver transplantation, although the frequency varied with the type of cirrhosis.[57] Enlargement of abdominal lymph nodes is most common in patients with primary biliary cirrhosis (87%) or other forms of biliary cirrhosis, and less common in patients with alcohol-induced cirrhosis (37%). In viral-induced cirrhosis, lymph node enlargement can be seen in the stage of chronic hepatitis or precirrhosis. Lymphadenopathy in viral-induced cirrhosis is more common in C than in B cirrhosis. Their size in C cirrhosis correlates with active inflammation.[58] The most common location of enlarged lymph nodes is around the porta hepatis, hepatoduodenal ligament, portacaval space, gastrohepatic ligament, celiac axis, and peripancreatic regions (Fig. 82-31). The size of enlarged lymph nodes is sometimes greater than 2 cm on the largest axis, usually

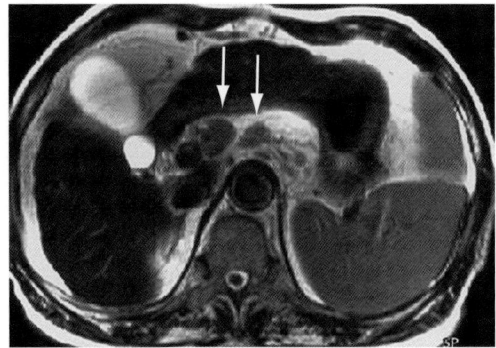

FIGURE 82-31

Lymphadenopathy in a patient with viral-induced cirrhosis. Axial T2-weighted fast spin-echo image demonstrates multiple enlarged, benign lymph nodes in the porta hepatis (*arrows*).

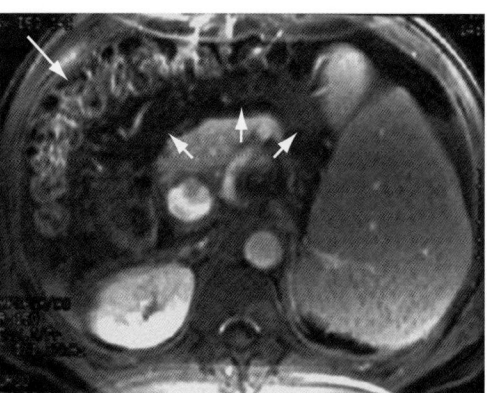

FIGURE 82-32

Colonic wall thickening in cirrhosis. Contrast-enhanced MR image with fat suppression shows diffuse wall thickening of the transverse colon (*long arrow*) and widespread diffuse, infiltrative mesenteric edema (*short arrows*).

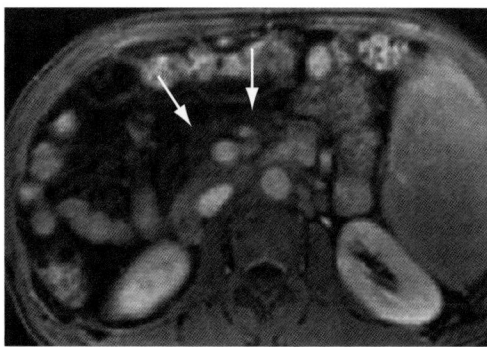

FIGURE 82-33

Mesenteric edema. Contrast-enhanced MR image with fat suppression shows well-marginated, masslike mesenteric edema around the superior mesenteric vessels (*arrows*). Splenomegaly is also noted.

with a flat or oval configuration, but the portal vein and other structures usually maintain their shape and are not compressed. This type of lymphadenopathy may be secondary to dynamic changes in hepatic and intestinal lymph production and flow.

Gastrointestinal Wall Thickening

Gastrointestinal wall thickening is often seen in patients with cirrhosis, probably caused by edema due to hypoproteinemia and/or portal hypertension. Isolated or predominantly right-sided colonic wall thickening is observed in as many as 25% of patients with endstage cirrhosis (Fig. 82-32), probably related to changes in superior mesenteric blood flow circulation and hydrostatic pressures caused by portal hypertension.[59] Specific patterns of gastrointestinal wall thickening in patients with cirrhosis are reported; if the jejunum is normal, no wall thickening is seen in the duodenum or ileum; if the ascending colon is normal, no wall thickening is seen in the transverse or descending colon.[60] Observation of atypical patterns of wall thickening in patients with cirrhosis should prompt a search for additional potential causes, including inflammatory, ischemic, and neoplastic diseases. Haustral thickening of the colon is also seen commonly in patients with cirrhosis, although nodular haustral thickening has been described as a specific feature of pseudomembranous colitis.

Mesenteric, omental, and retroperitoneal edema also occur commonly in patients with cirrhosis, and are well visualized on gadolinium-enhanced MR imaging with fat suppression as increased fat signal (Fig. 82-33). The appearance of mesenteric edema varies from a mild infiltrative haze to a severe masslike sheath that engulfs the mesenteric vessels. Increasing severity, diffuse distribution, masslike appearance, and recruitment of omental and retroperitoneal sites are parameters of mesenteric edema severity and generally correlate with severe ascites, subcutaneous edema, and low serum albumin levels.[61]

Changes of Portal Vein and its Tributaries

In patients with cirrhosis, several hemodynamic changes of the liver are induced. Portal venous flow into the liver is reduced, probably due to increased intrahepatic resistance caused by hepatic fibrosis. Additionally, cirrhosis is usually accompanied by intestinal vascular vasodilatation and increased splanchnic blood flow. The combination of increased splanchnic flow and increased portal pressure leads to increased diameters of the splenic and superior mesenteric veins in cirrhotic patients compared with those in noncirrhotic subjects, a finding first documented by angiographic measurements. At MR measurement, a superior mesenteric vein diameter larger than 13 mm and a splenic vein larger than 11 mm were relatively specific findings for patients with cirrhosis.[62] Dilatation of colic veins due to increased colonic venous flow secondary to portal hypertension may be seen in cirrhotic patients with colonic wall thickening at CT or MR evaluation. Therefore, recognition of dilated portal vein tributaries may be

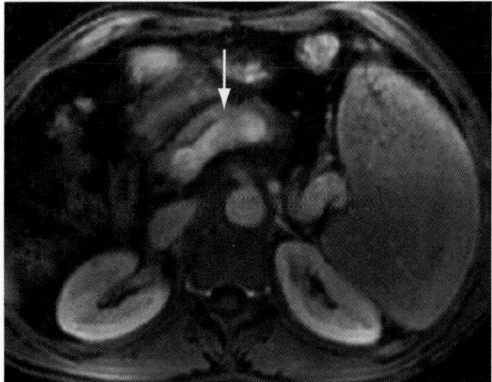

FIGURE 82-34

Enlarged splenic vein in cirrhosis. Contrast-enhanced MR image with fat suppression shows the enlarged splenic vein (*arrow*) larger than 11 mm in diameter, consistent with cirrhosis. Splenomegaly is also noted.

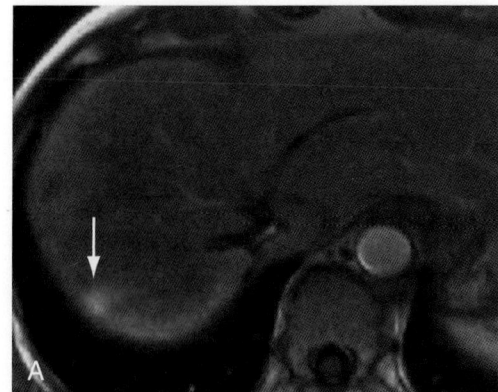

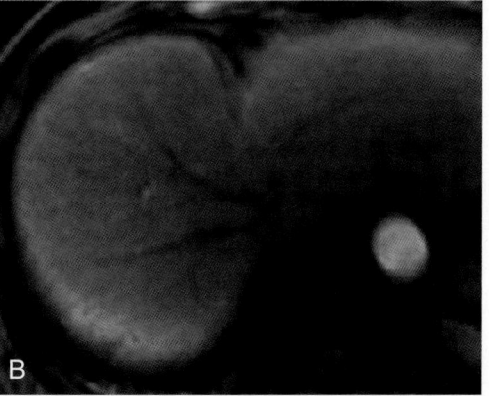

FIGURE 82-35

Small early-enhancing hepatic pseudolesion. **A,** Arterial-phase contrast-enhanced dynamic MR image obtained at the initial MR examination shows a small early-enhancing round lesion (*arrow*) in the right posterior segment of the liver. **B,** Arterial-phase contrast-enhanced dynamic MR image obtained 16 months later shows that the lesion seen in **A** has disappeared, which is indicative of an early-enhancing pseudolesion.

an additional secondary sign of cirrhosis (Fig. 82-34), although there was a considerable overlap in the distribution of the diameter between cirrhotic and noncirrhotic patients. This sign should therefore be used in conjunction with other intra- and extra-hepatic findings for cirrhosis.

Small Early-Enhancing Pseudolesions

Multiphasic contrast-enhanced dynamic MR imaging of the whole liver has been reported to be a highly sensitive method for detecting hypervascular HCC in chronic hepatitis or cirrhosis because they show as early-enhancing lesions on arterial-phase images.[63-65] However, small nodular early-enhancing hepatic lesions that disappear or decrease in size during the clinical course are frequently observed at serial MR examinations (Fig. 82-35).[66] These lesions may be considered to be hypervascular "pseudolesions" due to small arterioportal shunts or other etiologies.[67] The focally increased arterial inflow and decreased portal perfusion caused by a small arterioportal shunt may induce early enhancing pseudolesions. It is important to recognize that subcentimeter early-enhancing round or oval hepatic lesions in patients with cirrhosis or chronic hepatitis can often be pseudolesions, thereby avoiding unnecessary liver biopsy or treatment.

Prediction and Signs of Clinical Progression in Compensated Cirrhosis

During the disease course, compensated cirrhosis slowly progresses to decompensated or endstage cirrhosis with several complications. In the clinical setting, it is important to identify prognostic imaging features at the initial MR examination in patients with cirrhosis because the ability to predict clinical progression (i.e., whether compensated cirrhosis will be stable or progress to

decompensated cirrhosis in the near future) facilitates early management of cirrhotic patients. In patients with compensated cirrhosis (Child A), evaluation of multiple MR features suggested that MR findings of a large spleen, the presence of varices or collaterals, and high C/RL ratio can be used to help predict the clinical progression to decompensated cirrhosis (Child B and C) during long-term follow-up. Conversely, direct findings of cirrhosis, including nodular surface of the liver and presence of regenerative nodules, do not necessarily correlate with clinical progression.[32] The presence of a large spleen, multiple varices or collaterals, and high C/RL ratio at initial MR imaging are important findings since they indicate the need for close follow-up and early medical intervention (Fig. 82-36).

In patients with clinically progressive cirrhosis in whom the clinical stage deteriorates from Child A (compensated) to Child B or C (decompensated) cirrhosis, the volume of anterior, posterior, and medial segments decreases significantly (Fig. 82-37), whereas the volume of the caudate lobe and left lateral segment do not change.[33] Conversely, in patients with clinically stable Child A cirrhosis, the volume of the caudate lobe and left

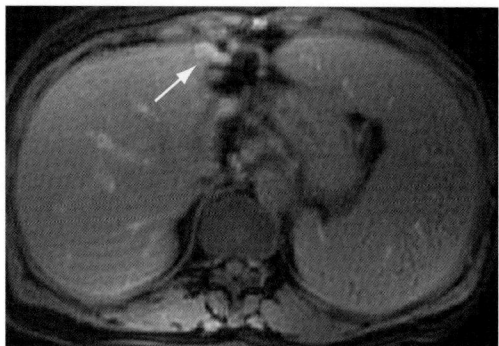

FIGURE 82-36

Cirrhotic patient who clinically progressed during 20 months of follow-up. At the initial MR examination of a Child A cirrhotic patient, the contrast-enhanced gradient-echo image demonstrates marked enlargement of the spleen with multiple small hypointense nodules (Gamna-Gandy bodies) and dilatation of the paraumbilical vein (*arrow*). The clinical stage of this Child A cirrhotic patient progressed to Child C cirrhosis 20 months later.

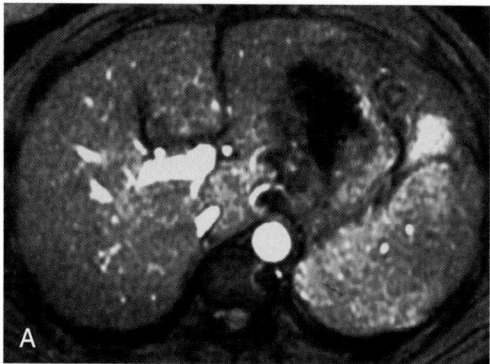
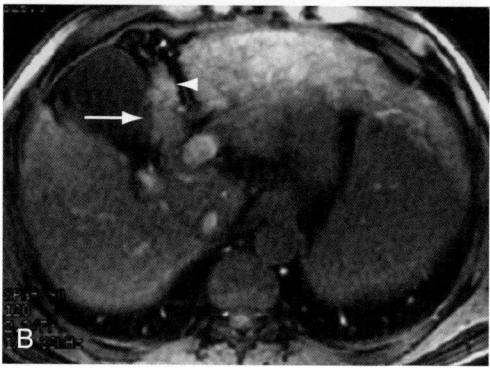

FIGURE 82-37

Progressive cirrhosis that has progressed from Child A to C during 53 months of follow-up. **A,** Initial MR image shows slight enlargement of the caudate lobe of the liver (*arrow*). However, atrophy of the medial segment and the right lobe of the liver is not apparent. **B,** MR image obtained 53 months later shows marked atrophy of the medial segment of the left hepatic lobe (*arrow*). The falciform ligament (*arrowhead*) has rotated counterclockwise relative to the earlier examination due to the atrophy of the left medial segment. (*Reproduced with permission from Ito K, Mitchell DG, Hann HW, et al: Progressive viral-induced cirrhosis: serial MR imaging findings and clinical correlation. Radiology 207:729-235, 1998.*)

lateral segment significantly increases, and there is no significant change in the anterior, posterior, and medial segment volumes.[33] These results indicate that in compensated (stable) cirrhosis, hypertrophy of the lateral segment and caudate lobe are the predominant findings on serial MR imaging, whereas atrophy of the medial segment and right lobe are findings of progressive cirrhosis.

In compensated cirrhosis, substantial hepatic function is preserved by continued compensatory hypertrophy of the lateral segment and caudate lobe, even though cirrhosis might slowly and gradually progress throughout the liver. However, when hepatic fibrosis proceeds further, with increased atrophy of the medial segment and right lobe, the hypertrophied lateral segment and caudate lobe exceed the upper limit for liver function preservation. At this point, the cirrhotic liver cannot compensate any more, resulting in progression to clinically decompensated cirrhosis. These findings are helpful for understanding disease progression in patients with cirrhosis.

Although the causes of lateral segment hypertrophy and right lobe atrophy are unclear, they may be attributed to altered portal blood inflow to these liver segments. The right portal vein directly enters into the liver parenchyma of the right hepatic lobe. In cirrhosis, hepatic fibrosis causes compression and irregular stenosis of the intrahepatic portal vein branches. Therefore, the right portal flow will decrease. Conversely, the left portal vein runs through the falciform ligament which is still outside of the liver parenchyma before entering the left hepatic lobe, resulting in a relatively greater blood supply to the left lateral segment. Thus, it is likely that the ratio of effective blood reaching the left lateral segment to that reaching the right hepatic lobe may be greater in cirrhotic livers, causing atrophy of the right hepatic lobe and hypertrophy of the left lateral segment. Similarly, hypertrophy of the caudate lobe can be explained by its unique portal supply. The caudate

lobe is vascularized by several portal branches, most of which (78%) arise from the left branch of the bifurcation of the portal vein, and thus have a shorter intrahepatic course than the vessels of the right lobe.

Portal Hypertension

Portal hypertension can result from obstruction of post-sinusoidal, sinusoidal, or presinusoidal levels. In the cirrhotic liver, the portal vascular bed is markedly diminished and portal veins are narrowed by fibrosis, increasing the intrahepatic portal resistance, and causing the post-sinusoidal–type portal hypertension. Portal hypertension causes or exacerbates complications of cirrhosis, such as variceal bleeding, ascites, and splenomegaly. During the early stages of portal hypertension, the portal system dilates but hepatopetal flow is maintained. At the next stage, hepatofugal flow starts in some portions of the portal venous system, and this vessel may become enlarged in preference to other veins. The venous anatomy may determine which vein or veins become the major collaterals, although the exact mechanism is still not well understood. As a result, numerous portosystemic collateral pathways from the high-pressure portal system to the low-pressure systemic circulation develop, reducing the volume of flow to the liver and decreasing the size of the main portal vein (unless its size is maintained by predominant shunting through a paraumbilical collateral). With advanced portal hypertension, the main portal vein flow continues to decrease and is sometimes even reversed.

Once a few portosystemic collateral pathways have developed, they become huge shunting routes, not allowing other shunting veins. Collaterals shunt portal blood into systemic veins, bypassing hepatic parenchyma. Nutrients absorbed from the gastrointestinal tract are metabolized less effectively, and toxic metabolites such as ammonia accumulate in the blood, producing hepatic encephalopathy.

MR angiography (MRA) makes it possible to image portal blood flow, identify collateral pathways, and determine flow direction.[68] The two-dimensional (2D) time-of-flight (TOF) method exploits the signal enhancement effects of flowing blood so that vessels are highlighted. However, this technique is less sensitive to slow flow, resulting in poor visualization of the portal venous system, especially when it contains stagnant flow. Flow direction in the portal vein can be evaluated by using 2D phase-contrast techniques.[69] Recently, gadolinium-enhanced 3D MR angiography (portography) has become the most popular and valuable method for imaging the portal vein and its branches.[70,71] Its primary advantages are the elimination of in-plane flow saturation effects of blood resulting from the T1-shortening property of the contrast agent, and minimized respiratory motion because of short acquisition times (single breath-hold). These factors improve the contrast between blood and tissue, permitting exquisite detail of the portal vascular anatomy. Fat-suppression and subtraction techniques are helpful: 1. to eliminate high signal from background, such as adipose tissue, systemic vascular enhancement, and normal liver, renal, and bowel enhancement; and 2. to overcome the insufficient separation of arteries and portal veins in which the arteries overlap the desired portal vessels (Fig. 82-38).

Major sites of portosystemic collaterals include the gastroesophageal junction (from the coronary and short gastric veins to the systemic esophageal vein), paraumbilical veins (from the left portal vein through the paraumbilical veins to the systemic epigastric vein), retroperitoneal regions (from veins of the duodenum, ascending and descending colon, and liver to the systemic lumbar, phrenic, gonadal, and renal veins), gastro- or spleno-renal regions (from the coronary, short gastric, and splenic veins to the systemic left renal vein), and hemorrhoidal veins (from the superior hemorrhoidal vein to the systemic middle and inferior hemorrhoidal veins).[72,73]

The most prevalent and clinically important portosystemic collaterals are gastroesophageal varices. Esophageal varices may rupture through the esophageal mucosa and produce life-threatening hemorrhage. Esophageal and gastric varices frequently coexist, and they are usually

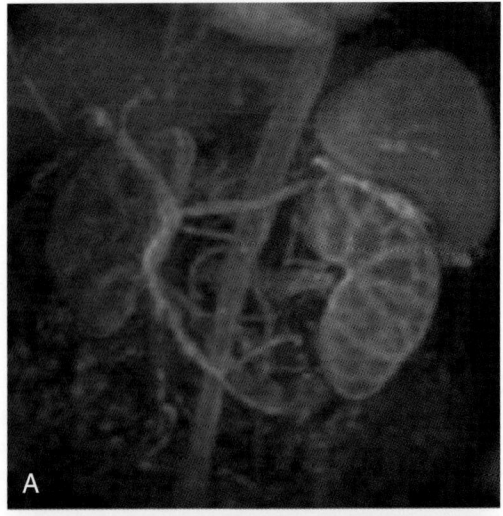
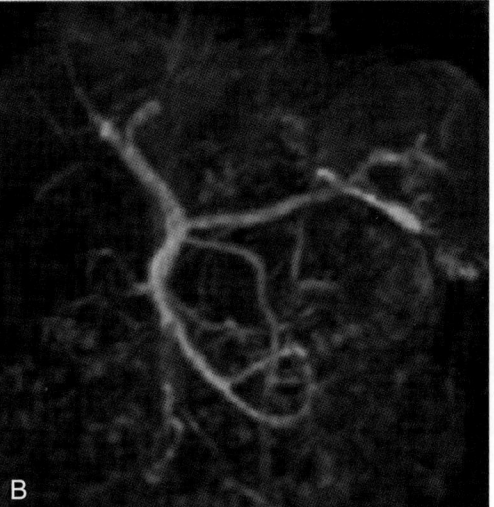

FIGURE 82-38

Subtraction technique for MR angiography of the portal vein. **A,** Portal-phase maximum intensity projection (MIP) MR angiogram with precontrast subtraction shows poor visualization of the portal vein due to superimposition of the aortic and renal venous enhancement and the increased signal of the background structures. **B,** Portal-phase MIP MR angiogram with early arterial-phase subtraction clearly demonstrated the portal venous system. High signal from arteries and background signals are eliminated by the subtraction.

supplied by a dilated coronary gastric vein, which in normal subjects drains inferiorly towards the confluence of the splenic and superior mesenteric veins. In patients with gastroesophageal varices, the flow in this vein reverses. Gastroesophageal varices can be seen as enlarged, tortuous veins within the wall of the gastric fundus and fornix and the lower esophagus (Figs. 82-39 and 82-40) on MR imaging. Esophageal varices are usually supplied by the anterior branch of the left gastric vein, and commonly drain into the azygos vein. Blood flow from esophageal varices may also enter the left subclavian and brachiocephalic veins. Paraesophageal varices are frequently associated with esophageal

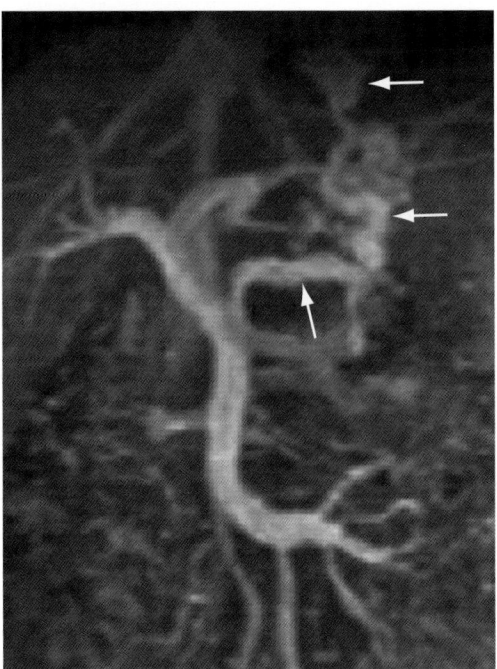

FIGURE 82-39

Gastroesophageal varices. Portal-phase MIP MR portography with early arterial-phase subtraction demonstrates a dilated left gastric vein, gastric varices, and esophageal varices (*arrows*).

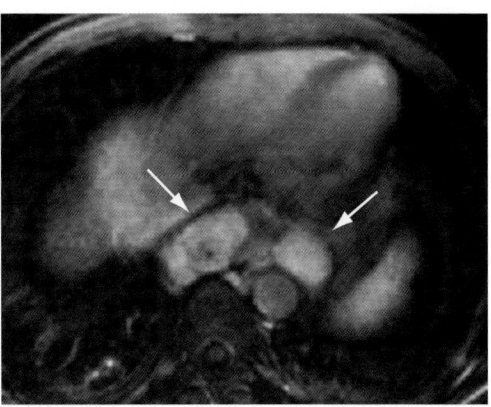

FIGURE 82-40

Massive paraesophageal varices. Contrast-enhanced axial MR image with fat suppression demonstrates enlarged paraesophageal veins (*arrows*), showing masslike appearances.

varices, supplied by the posterior branch of the left gastric vein, and situated outside the wall of the esophagus in the mediastinum not flowing in the wall of the esophagus.

The paraumbilical vein, once mistakenly thought to be a recanalization of the umbilical vein, can develop as a collateral vein in 10% to 43% of patients with portal hypertension.[74-76] The dilated paraumbilical veins originate at the left portal vein near its bifurcation, traverse the falciform ligament (Fig. 82-41) or nearby hepatic

parenchyma, and drain into the veins of the anterior abdominal wall, sometimes producing a Caput medusae (dilated veins radiating from the umbilicus). If it runs farther downward subcutaneously, it may enter the iliac or femoral veins. The paraumbilical vein becomes quite large and functions as a desirable route of natural decompression without gastrointestinal bleeding in portal hypertension, also maintaining flow through the main portal vein.

A spleno- or gastro-renal shunt often occurs through an enlarged, left-sided retroperitoneal channel that arises from preexisting, small, normal portosystemic communications (Fig. 82-42). Splenorenal shunts typically originate from the splenic hilum, course medial to the enlarged spleen toward the left renal hilum, and anastomose with the left renal vein. The dilated, tortuous

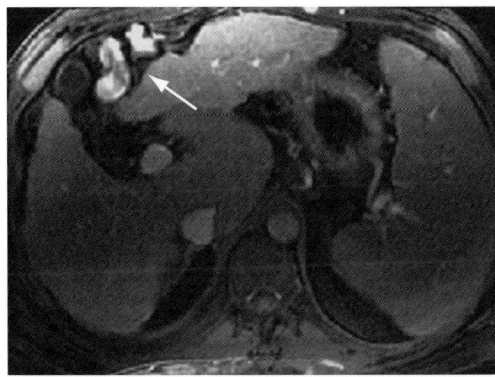

FIGURE 82-41

Paraumbilical vein. Contrast-enhanced axial MR image with fat suppression shows a paraumbilical vein (*arrow*) originating from the left portal vein and passing anteriorly through the falciform ligament.

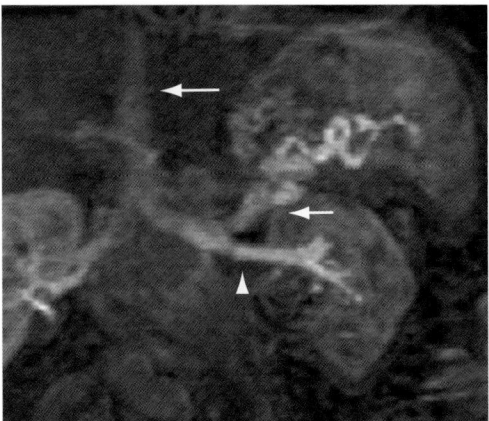

FIGURE 82-42

Splenorenal shunt. Portal-phase MIP MR portography with early arterial-phase subtraction shows collaterals originating from the splenic vein (*short arrow*) and communicating with the left renal vein (*arrowhead*). The long arrow shows the inferior vena cava.

vessels between the splenic hilum and left kidney on MR imaging represent splenorenal shunts. Fusiform dilatation of the left renal vein is also seen frequently. Portosystemic drainage by way of the right renal vein is also possible but uncommon.

HEPATIC NODULES ASSOCIATED WITH CIRRHOSIS

The cirrhotic liver contains regenerative nodules and may also contain dysplastic nodules as well as HCC.[77-79] By understanding the transition between benign through dysplastic to malignant nodules, sense can be made more easily of the complex nodularity depicted in cirrhotic livers on multiple MRI pulse sequences.[80-82]

Etiology

Except for focal nodular hyperplasia (FNH), hepatic nodules usually develop in previously damaged livers. Damage to the liver can be caused by several factors[83]:

- Endemic: aflatoxin, a product of the fungus *Aspergillus flavus*, which grows on improperly stored grain and nuts (including peanuts), is considered an important cause of HCC in Africa and Asia.
- Metabolic and genetic disorders, including hemochromatosis (increased hepatocellular iron deposition), Wilson's disease (increased hepatocellular copper deposition), and α_1-antitrypsin deficiency, can lead to cirrhosis, hepatic nodules, and HCC.
- Dietary: obesity, diabetes (type II), and alcoholism can lead to fatty infiltration of the liver (steatosis), steatohepatitis, and cirrhosis.
- Viral: viral hepatitis, mainly caused by hepatitis B and C viruses, is currently the most important etiologic factor leading to liver fibrosis and cirrhosis in North America.

Terminology

Since 1995, a modified nomenclature has been used to categorize hepatic nodules into two groups, i.e., the regenerative and the dysplastic or neoplastic lesions.[84]

Regenerative nodules result from a localized proliferation of hepatocytes and their supporting stroma. Regenerative lesions include monoacinar regenerative nodules, multiacinar regenerative nodules, cirrhotic nodules, lobar or segmental hyperplasia, and FNH.

A mono- or multi-acinar regenerative nodule is a well-defined region of parenchyma that has enlarged in response to necrosis, altered circulation, or other stimuli. It may contain one (monoacinar) or more than one (multiacinar) portal tracts. The diameter of monoacinar nodules is usually between 0.1 and 10 mm, and that of multiacinar nodules should be at least 2 mm. Large multiacinar nodules are usually between 5 and 15 mm in diameter. Cirrhotic nodules are regenerative and are largely or completely surrounded by fibrous septa.

Cirrhotic nodules can be mono- or multi-acinar. Macronodular cirrhosis contains nodules greater than 3 mm.[84]

Dysplastic or neoplastic lesions are composed of hepatocytes which show histologic characteristics of abnormal growth caused by presumed or proved genetic alteration. Dysplastic or neoplastic nodules include hepatocellular adenoma, dysplastic focus, dysplastic nodule, and HCC.

Dysplastic focus is defined as a cluster of hepatocytes less than 1 mm in diameter with dysplasia but without definite histologic criteria of malignancy. Dysplasia indicates the presence of nuclear and cytoplasmic changes, such as minimal-to-severe nuclear atypia and increased amount of cytoplasmic fat or glycogen, within the cluster of cells that compose the focus. Dysplastic foci are common in cirrhosis and uncommon in non-cirrhotic livers. Dysplasia can be small- or large-cell type.[84]

The dysplastic nodule is a nodular region of hepatocytes at least 1 mm in diameter with dysplasia but without definite histologic criteria of malignancy. These nodules are usually found in cirrhotic livers. Dysplastic nodules can be low or high grade.[84] Nodules with low-grade dysplasia may show an altered liver parenchymal structure as well as an increased number of cells with an increased nuclei-to-cytoplasm ratio. High-grade dysplasia shows increased thickness of the layers of hepatocytes containing nuclei that are variable in size and shape.

HCC is a malignant neoplasm composed of cells with hepatocellular differentiation. A small HCC is defined as measuring less than or equal to 2 cm in diameter. The criteria used to distinguish HCC from high-grade dysplastic nodules are not clearly defined. Criteria favoring malignancy include: 1. prominent nuclear atypia; 2. high nuclear-to-cytoplasmic ratio with nuclear density twice that of normal; 3. plates three or more cells thick, numerous unaccompanied arteries; 4. mitoses in moderate numbers; 5. invasion of stroma or portal tracts. Most small HCC cannot be distinguished histologically from dysplastic nodules with certainty. In addition, foci of carcinoma can be found in otherwise benign dysplastic nodules. These and other findings support the theory of stepwise carcinogenesis of HCC.[84]

Stepwise and De Novo Pathways of Carcinogenesis

A stepwise carcinogenesis of HCC has been proposed based on a gradually increasing size and cellular density among the following lesions: regenerative nodules (RN), adenomatous nodules (AN), atypical AH (AAH), early HCC (eHCC I), and early advanced HCC (eHCC II).[85,86] According to current terminology, the earlier mentioned stepwise sequence of events (RN → AH → AAH → eHCC I → eHCC II) can be translated as follows: regenerative nodule, low-grade dysplastic nodule, high-grade dysplastic nodule, small HCC, and large HCC (Fig. 82-43). Several authors have proposed a de novo pathway for HCC in cirrhotic as well as noncirrhotic livers.[77,85,86] According to the de novo pathway, a single cell or group of hepatocytes may give rise to a focus of small HCC that will grow into a large HCC.[77,78]

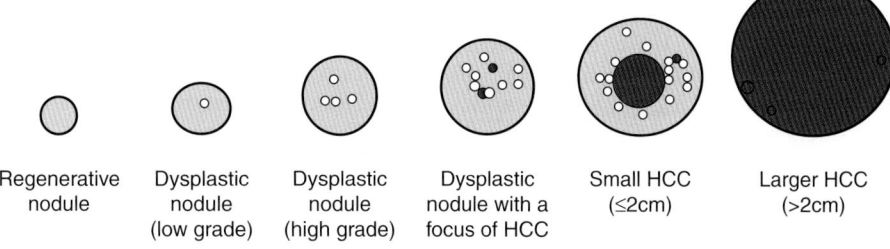

Regenerative nodule | Dysplastic nodule (low grade) | Dysplastic nodule (high grade) | Dysplastic nodule with a focus of HCC | Small HCC (≤2cm) | Larger HCC (>2cm)

FIGURE 82-43

Stepwise pathway for the carcinogenesis of hepatocellular carcinoma (HCC) in cirrhosis. One or more regenerative nodules may show signs of atypia (o) and change into dysplastic nodules. Atypia indicates a number of changes in shape and size of the nuclei and cytoplasm of the hepatocytes. These changes often result in an increased number of cells (increased cellularity) present in groups of small (small cell dysplasia) or large (large cell dysplasia) cells. Atypia within dysplastic nodules can progress further and give rise to small and large HCC. In addition to the cellular changes, the liver parenchymal structure will often be distorted in HCC. *(Modified with permission from Hussain SM, Semelka RC, Mitchell DG: MR imaging of hepatocellular carcinoma. In Semelka RC (ed): MR Imaging of the Liver II: Diseases. Magn Reson Imaging Clin North Am 10:31-52, 2002.)*

At some point during the process of carcinogenesis of HCC (most likely when regenerative nodules become dysplastic nodules), formation of new tumor vessels (tumor angiogenesis, neovascularity) takes place.[77,78] The appearance of new tumor vessels is important in the transformation of regenerative nodules into dysplastic nodules and small HCC. Neoangiogenesis is also important for sustained growth of HCC. In addition, neovascularity within HCC can be used for early detection and characterization of these lesions with imaging.

Histology and Gross Pathology

The histologic grade of tumor differentiation is assigned using the Edmondson Grading System.[87,88] At histology, it may be difficult to differentiate among hepatocellular nodules. Depending on tumor differentiation, one hepatocellular lesion may contain one or more clonelike cell populations and these cell populations can be graded I to IV.

● Grade I: cells that are similar in size to normal hepatocytes and are arranged in relatively thin trabeculae. Acini containing bile are rare.
● Grade II: cells that are larger than normal hepatocytes with more hyperchromatic nuclei, which occupy a higher proportion of cells. The trabeculae are thicker and acini with bile are common.
● Grade III: cells of hepatocytes with larger nuclei, occupying more than 50% of the cytoplasm. The trabeculae are still dominant but solid areas and isolated cells may also be present. In addition, giant and bizarre cells are common. Bile is present rarely.
● Grade IV: cells with nuclei occupying most of the cytoplasm, and the cytoplasm may not be eosinophilic.

Mostly solid areas are found. Bile is rarely found. Intravascular and intrasinusoidal growth is commonly present.

Based on this grading system, grade I cell populations may be difficult to distinguish from hepatocellular adenomas, and grade IV cell populations may be difficult to recognize from tumors of nonhepatocellular origin.[87] The classic macroscopic classification of HCC by Eggle has been used since 1901. According to this classification, Edmondson et al identified 70 HCCs in their series as nodular (81%), massive (23%), or diffuse (3%). This classification is mainly based on autopsy cases of HCC. Compared to the massive lesions, the nodular tumors are smaller and more distinct with sharper margins to the liver.[87] The massive lesions are either composed of confluent smaller tumors or consist of predominantly one large lesion that often occupies almost the entire liver. The diffuse lesions consist of multiple infiltrating lesions that occupy a large part of the liver.[87]

MR Imaging Appearance

Focal Nodular Hyperplasia

FNH is a benign liver tumor that occurs predominantly in women during their reproductive years, but cases have been reported in men and children.[89-91] FNH is lobulated and well circumscribed, although unencapsulated.[90] The pathognomonic macroscopic feature in the presence of a central stellate scar with radiating septa, thereby dividing the lesion into numerous nodules of normal hepatocytes that are abnormally arranged.[90,92] The central scar contains thick-walled vessels with its sources from the hepatic artery that provides excellent arterial blood supply to the lesion.[93] The most characteristic microscopic features of FNH are the fibrous septae and the areas of hepatocellular proliferation.[93] The nodules within FNH lack normal central veins and portal tracts. The bile ducts seen within the central scar do not connect to the biliary tree.[93] According to the International Working Party, FNH is considered as a regenerative benign nodule.[84] FNH is often an incidental finding on imaging studies and needs to be differentiated from other focal liver lesions, such as HCC, hepatocellular adenomas, and hypervascular metastases.[77-79,94] The majority of FNH do not need any treatment.[94]

At MR imaging, FNH is slightly hypointense on T1-weighted and slightly hyperintense on T2-weighted images.[79] FNH may also be nearly isointense on both T1-and T2-weighted sequences. Unlike liver cell adenomas, FNH rarely has higher signal intensity than liver on T1-weighted images.[77-79] The central scar is usually high on T2-weighted images.[91] FNH shows very intense homogeneous enhancement during the arterial phase of the dynamic contrast-enhanced sequence.[77-79,91] The central scar and radiating septa in FNH show enhancement on delayed images (Fig. 82-44).[91]

Hepatocellular Adenoma

Liver adenomas typically occur in young women using oral contraceptives. These tumors were rarely reported in the medical literature before the introduction of oral contraceptives in the early 1960s. Association with other conditions or hepatocellular stimulating agents, such as familial diabetes mellitus, galactosemia, glycogen storage disease type 1, and anabolic steroids, has been reported. Liver cell adenomas are composed of sheets of cells that may resemble normal hepatocytes.[84,95,96] Unlike FNH, liver cell adenomas lack the central scar and radiating septa. Necrosis and hemorrhage are frequent causes of pain. In addition, according to currently used terminology, hepatocellular adenomas are classified as premalignant nodules.[84] Due to their potential for hemorrhage and malignant degeneration, hepatocellular adenomas are preferably treated surgically.[94]

At MR imaging, liver adenomas typically do not differ much in their signal intensity from the surrounding liver parenchyma on T1- and T2-weighted images. The lesions are mildly hypointense to moderately hyperintense on T1-weighted images, and mildly hyperintense on T2-weighted images.[78] They show a blush of

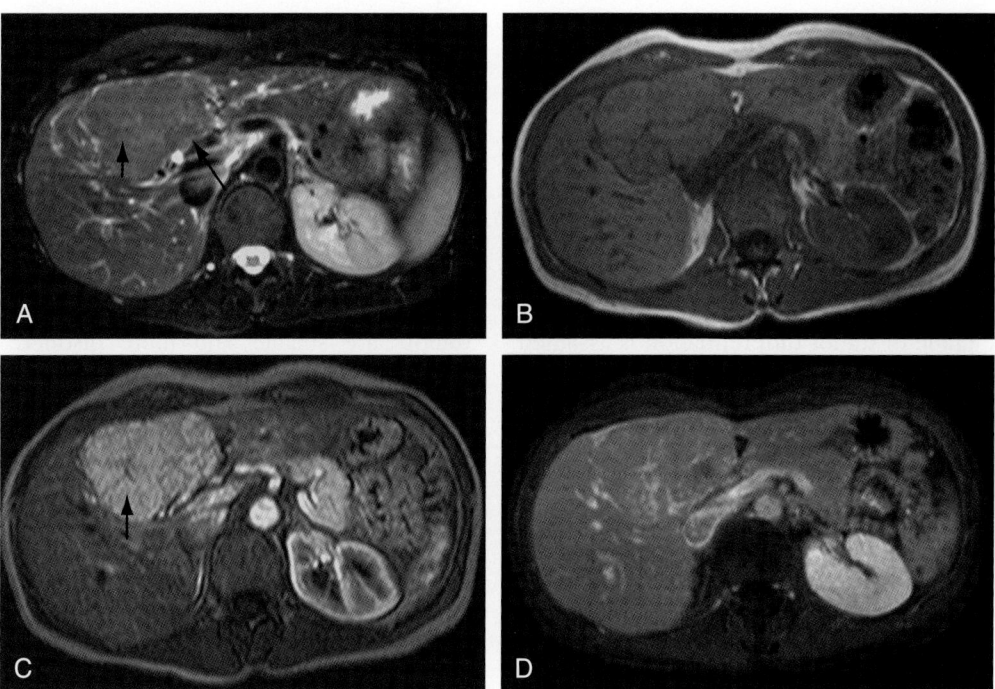

FIGURE 82-44

Focal nodular hyperplasia. **A,** T2-weighted fat-saturated fast spin-echo image shows a lesion that is slightly hyperintense to the liver (*long arrow*) with a bright central scar (*short arrow*). **B,** T1-weighted two-dimensional gradient-echo (2D GRE) (in-phase) image shows the lesion predominantly isointense to the liver with a lower signal intensity central scar. **C,** On the arterial phase of the dynamic contrast-enhanced 2D GRE image, the lesion shows very intense homogeneous enhancement without enhancement of the central scar (*arrow*). **D,** On the delayed contrast-enhanced GRE image, the lesion becomes isointense to the liver with enhancement of the central scar.

homogeneous enhancement on arterial phase and fade to near isointensity on later phases of dynamic gadolinium-enhanced images (Fig. 82-45).

Regenerative Nodules, Dysplastic Nodules, and Hepatocellular Carcinoma

Typically, regenerative nodules have low signal intensity on T2-weighted images, variable signal intensity on T1-weighted images, and do not enhance in the arterial phase of the dynamic gadolinium-enhanced images (Fig. 82-46).[77,96-98]

HCC is a focal liver lesion with high signal intensity on T2- and a variable signal intensity on T1-weighted images, which shows intense enhancement during the arterial phase of dynamic gadolinium-enhanced MR images (Fig. 82-47).[77,96,97,99]

The signal intensity and enhancement characteristics of dysplastic nodules are not well established. Due to a gradual stepwise transition from a regenerative nodule into a low-grade dysplastic nodule, a high-grade dysplastic nodule, and eventually into a small and a large HCC, the hepatocytes within hepatic nodules undergo numerous changes that might not be reflected in their signal intensity or vascularity. So, current MRI sequences might not be able to distinguish regenerative nodules from dysplastic nodules with certainty. Previously, some MR imaging features of high-grade dysplastic nodules and small HCC have been described.[77,80,96-98] A majority

of high-grade dysplastic lesions (formerly adenomatous hyperplastic) and well-differentiated small HCC (Edmondson grade I or II) have high signal intensity on T1-weighted images.[96-98]

Small Hepatocellular Carcinoma

Recent MR imaging techniques allow thinner slices with higher matrices in combination with high intrinsic soft-tissue contrast. In addition, faster imaging sequences allow imaging with sufficiently higher temporal resolution to capture distinct arterial and other phases of enhancement of liver lesions during gadolinium-enhanced imaging.[77,78] This facilitates detection of small HCCs.[80] The definition of small tumors has changed from a solitary lesion of diameter less than 4.5 cm to a tumor less than or equal to 2 cm.[80] High-grade dysplastic nodules and small HCC (≤2 cm) may have a nodule within a nodule appearance on MR images, especially if a focus of HCC originates within a siderotic regenerative nodule.[100] On T2-weighted images, this appearance may consist of low intensity of a large nodule, with one or more internal foci of higher signal intensity. On T1-weighted gradient-echo images, such lesions typically show markedly low intensity of a large nodule, with internal foci that are isointense to the liver. At MR imaging, the recognition of HCC while still small is important because the tumor is aggressive and has a fast doubling time.[101] Small HCC may also appear as small areas of slightly higher signal intensity than the

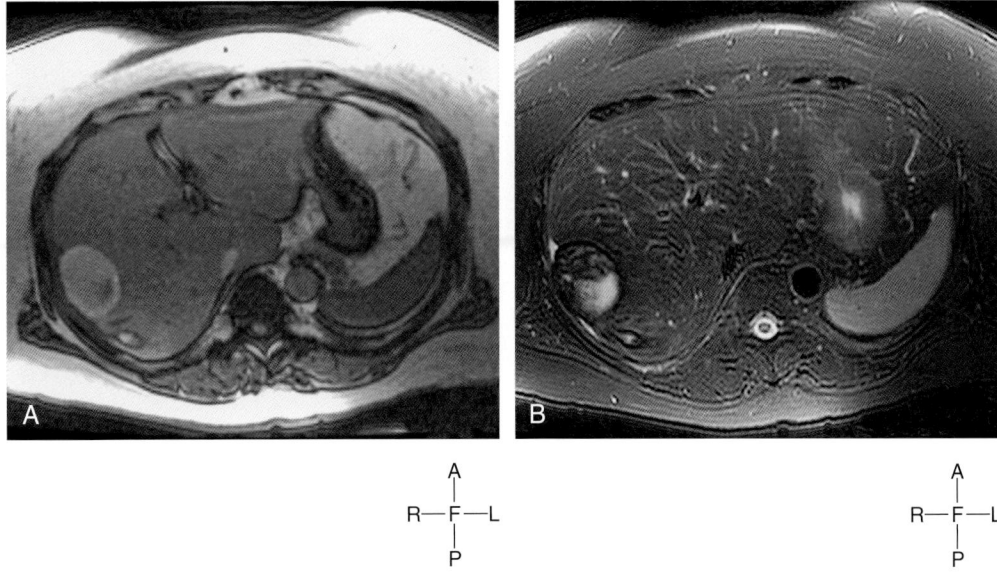

FIGURE 82-45

Hepatocellular adenoma. **A,** T1-weighted opposed-phase gradient-echo (GRE) image shows an elongated subcapsular lesion with predominantly high signal intensity compatible with a hemorrhage from a presumed ruptured hepatocellular ademona in a young woman. There was no direct visualization of adenoma in the vicinity of the hemorrhage. **B,** T2-weighted fat-saturated fast spin-echo (FSE) image shows the hemorrhage with heterogeneous signal intensity without evidence of a focal lesion.   *Continued*

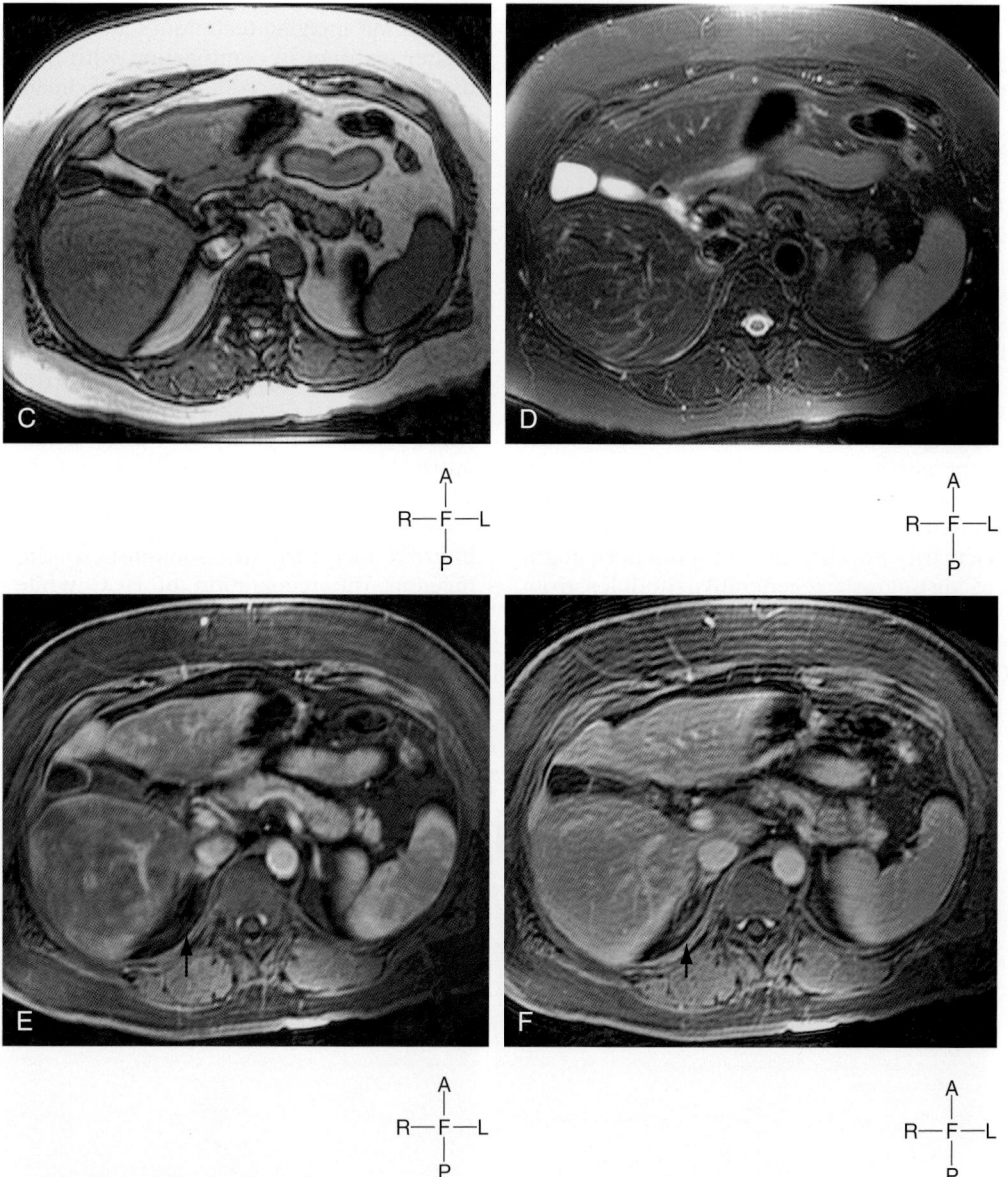

FIGURE 82-45, cont'd

Hepatocellular adenoma. **C,** T1-weighted opposed-phase GRE image at a lower level through the liver shows a small focal lesion that is slightly hyperintense to the liver with mild-to-moderate fatty infiltration. **D,** T2-weighted fat-saturated FSE image at this level does not show the lesion with high signal intensity. **E,** On the arterial phase of the dynamic contrast-enhanced three-dimensional GRE image, the lesion shows homogeneous enhancement with moderate intensity (*arrow*). **F,** On the delayed contrast-enhanced GRE image the lesion (*arrow*) becomes isointense to the liver. These findings are compatible with a ruptured hepatocellular adenoma in segment 7 and a second small adenoma in segment 6 of the liver in a young woman with a long-standing contraceptive use.

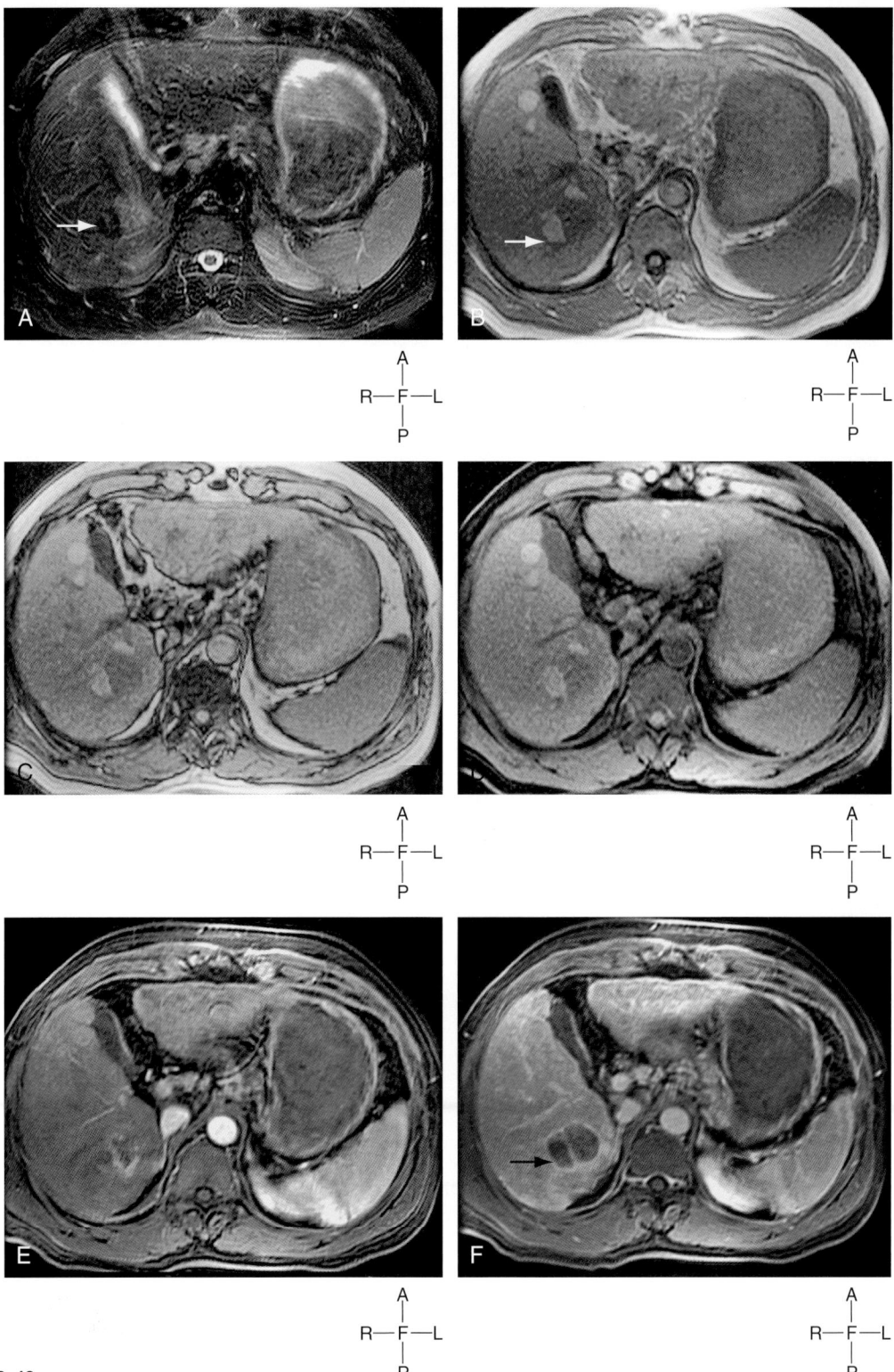

FIGURE 82-49

Large hepatocellular carcinoma (HCC) with a mosaic pattern and a tumor capsule. **A,** T2-weighted fat-saturated fast spin-echo image shows a lesion with areas of low and high signal intensity (*arrow*) indicating the mosaic pattern. **B,** In-phase T1-weighted gradient-echo (GRE) image shows the lesion with high and low signal intensities, i.e., areas that are of high signal intensity on the T2-weighted image are darker, whereas areas that are low in signal intensity are brighter (*arrow*). Note also the additional smaller bright nodules visible on this image. **C,** Opposed-phase T1-weighted GRE image shows no change in the signal intensity of the nodules or the liver, indicating no fatty infiltration. **D,** Fat-saturated T1-weighted GRE image shows that the bright nodules are not composed of a large amount of fatty tissue. **E,** Arterial-phase 3D GRE image shows a heterogeneous enhancement of the part of the lesion that was bright on the T2-weighted image (**A**), indicating an increased vascularity of this part of the lesion. **F,** Portal-phase 3D GRE image shows almost complete washout of the contrast medium within the lesion with enhancement of a tumor capsule (*arrow*). These findings are compatible with a large HCC with a mosaic pattern and tumor capsule.

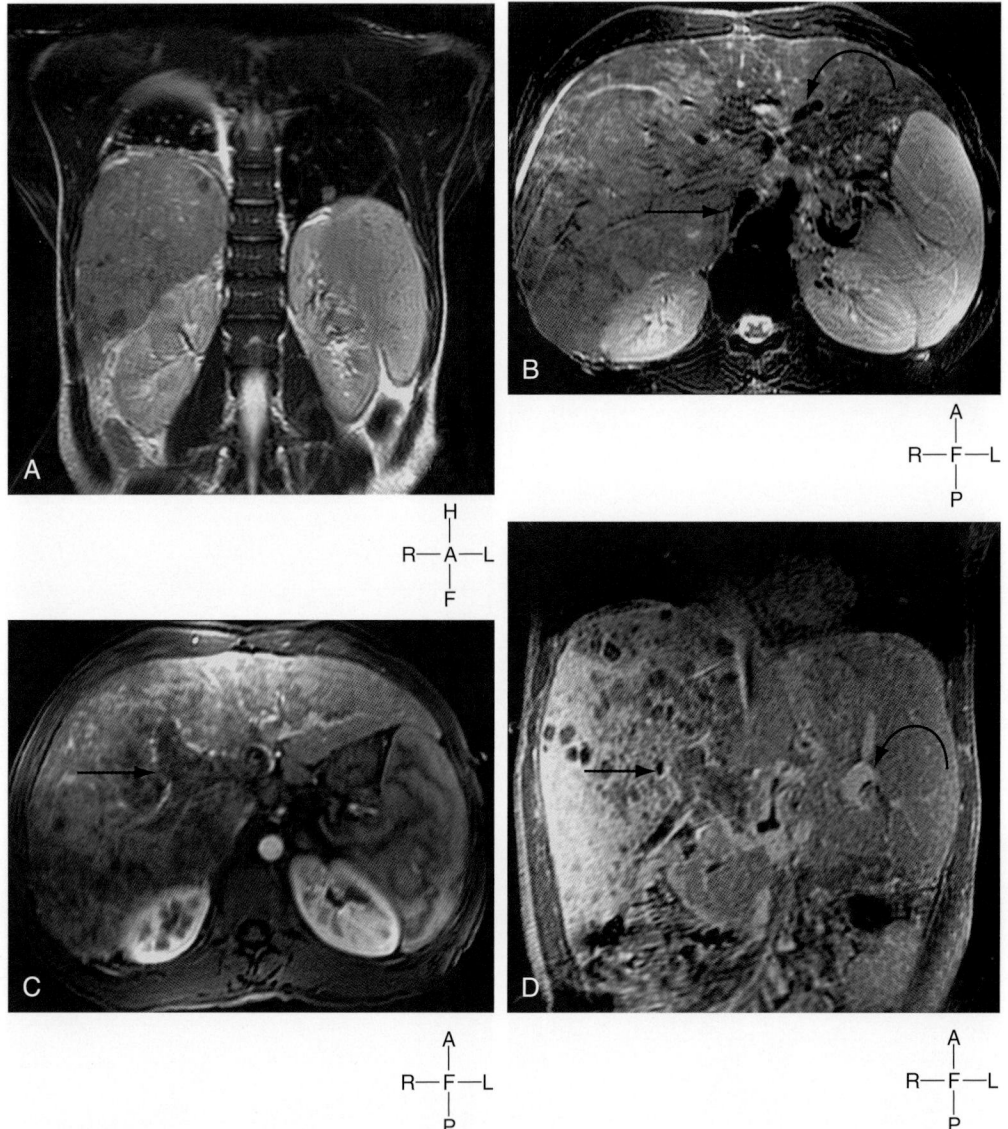

FIGURE 82-50

Large hepatocellular carcinoma with vascular invasion and lung metastases. **A,** Coronal single-shot fast spin-echo (FSE) image shows the liver to be of abnormally high signal intensity due to the presence of a large HCC with multiple lung nodules, indicating lung metastases of HCC. Note that the liver is almost as bright as the spleen. **B,** Axial fat-saturated FSE image shows a large mass with high signal intensity compared to the liver. Note that there is signal void within the inferior vena cava (*arrow*) and the left liver vein (*curved arrow*). At this level, the portal vein should be visible with signal void at least in part. **C,** Axial arterial-phase 3D GRE image shows intense heterogeneous enhancement of almost the entire liver except the left lateral segment. Note also the portal vein with intraluminal heterogeneous enhancement indicating the presence of a tumor thrombus (*arrow*). **D,** Coronal delayed-phase 3D GRE image shows washout of contrast in most parts of the liver mass. Note the normal homogeneous enhancement of the splenic vein (*curved arrow*), whereas the portal vein with tumor thrombus still shows heterogeneous enhancement (*arrow*).

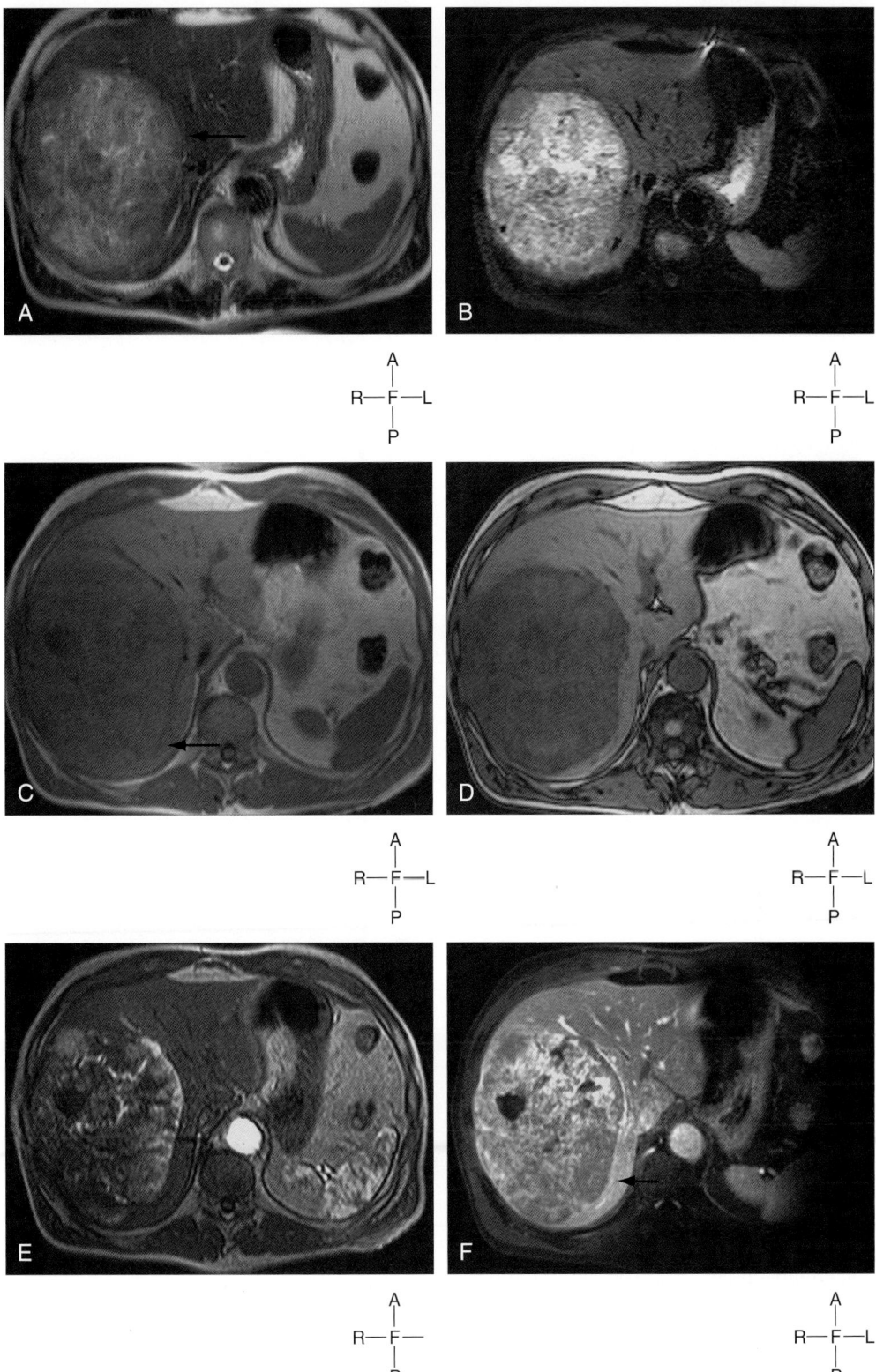

FIGURE 82-51

Large hepatocellular carcinoma (HCC) in a noncirrhotic liver. **A,** Axial single-shot fast spin-echo image shows a large tumor (*arrow*) with predominantly high signal intensity as compared to the normal low signal intensity of the surrounding liver. Note that the liver has smooth edges without evidence of any other nodules. **B,** T2-weighted fat-suppressed black-blood echo planar image shows the bright tumor containing multiple variable sized intratumoral vessels. **C,** In-phase T1-weighted gradient-echo (GRE) image shows the tumor with high and low signal intensity compared to the liver. Note that the tumor is surrounded by a thin tumor capsule of low signal intensity (*arrow*). **D,** Opposed-phase T1-weighted GRE image shows a marked decrease in signal intensity of the tumor, indicating the presence of fatty infiltration within the tumor. **E,** Arterial-phase 2D GRE image shows a very intense heterogeneous enhancement of the entire lesion with enhancement of the intratumoral vessels. **F,** Delayed-phase 2D fat-suppressed GRE image shows washout of contrast within the lesion with enhancement of the tumor capsule (*arrow*). In this patient, a CT examination (not shown) was inconclusive. Based on MR imaging findings the patient was operated on and the diagnosis of a large HCC in a noncirrhotic liver was confirmed at pathology.

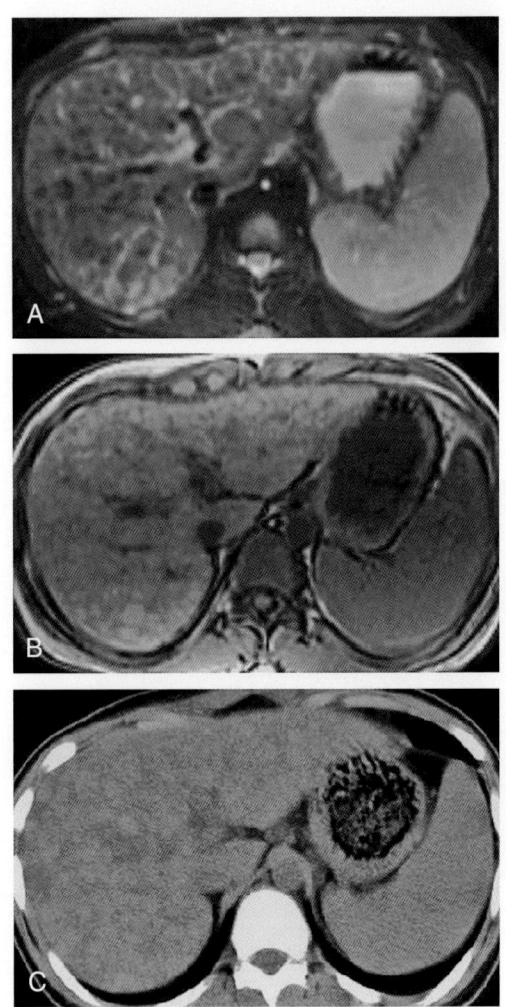

FIGURE 82-52

Wilson's disease. **A,** T2-weighted fast spin-echo image with fat suppression shows a large number of regenerative nodules with low signal intensity surrounded by a hyperintense reticular structure. **B,** On the T1-weighted GRE image, these nodules associated with cirrhosis in Wilson's disease show hyperintensity relative to the surrounding hypointense septa. **C,** Nonenhanced CT shows multiple hyperdense nodules secondary to copper deposition with associated cirrhotic change.

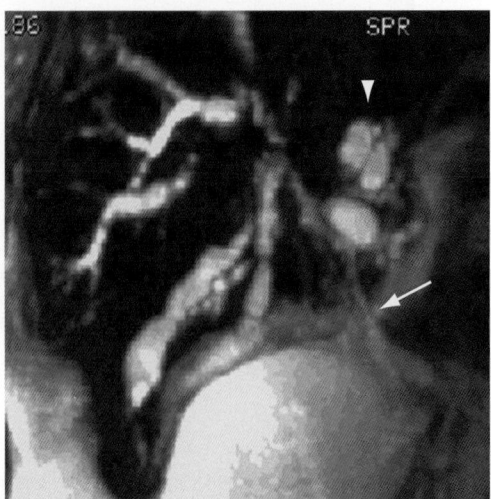

FIGURE 82-53

Primary sclerosing cholangitis. MR cholangiopancreatography image shows a long stricture in the extrahepatic bile duct (*arrow*) and diffuse intrahepatic bile duct dilatation with segmental stenosis, causing a beading appearance. Note the saccular dilatation of the intrahepatic left bile duct (*arrowhead*). *(From Ito K, Mitchell DG, Outwater EK, Blasbalg R: Primary sclerosing cholangitis: MR imaging features. Am J Roentgenol 172:1527-1533, 1999. Reproduced with permission of Wiley-Liss, Inc., a subsidiary of John Wiley & Sons, Inc.)*

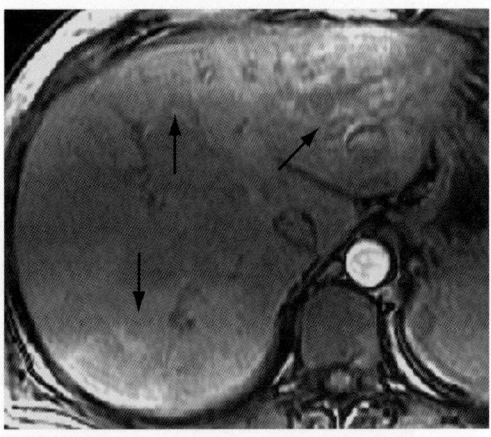

FIGURE 82-54

Primary sclerosing cholangitis. Contrast-enhanced dynamic MR image obtained during the arterial phase shows increased enhancement of the liver parenchyma (*arrows*), predominantly in peripheral areas of the liver. *(From Ito K, Mitchell DG, Outwater EK, Blasbalg R: Primary sclerosing cholangitis: MR imaging features. Am J Roentgenol 172:1527-1533, 1999. Reproduced with permission of Wiley-Liss, Inc., a subsidiary of John Wiley & Sons, Inc.)*

dynamic contrast enhancement.[112,113] The most common MR findings[41] are abnormalities of the intrahepatic bile ducts, including ductal dilatation, stenosis, beading, and pruning, best seen on MR cholangiography (Fig. 82-53). Wall thickening and enhancement of the extrahepatic bile duct, best seen on contrast-enhanced dynamic images, are also common findings. Early enhancement of portions of liver parenchyma is observed during arterial-phase dynamic imaging in over 50% of patients, probably due primarily to a compensatory increase in the arterial blood flow caused by decreased portal flow secondary to impaired biliary drainage (Fig. 82-54). An abnormal segmental or subsegmental high signal of the liver parenchyma on T1-weighted images is occasionally seen, associated with cholestasis caused by impaired drainage

of intrahepatic bile. Abnormal high signal with segmental distribution can be observed in patients with intrahepatic biliary obstruction by any cause (Fig. 82-55), and this finding is reversible when the obstruction is recovered.[114] With severe long-standing biliary obstruction, atrophy and scarring of affected portions of liver occur, leading to reduced volume, decreased signal

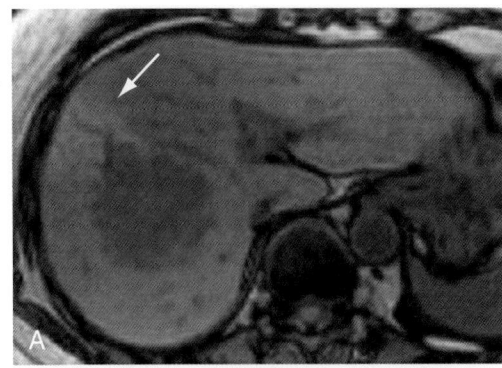

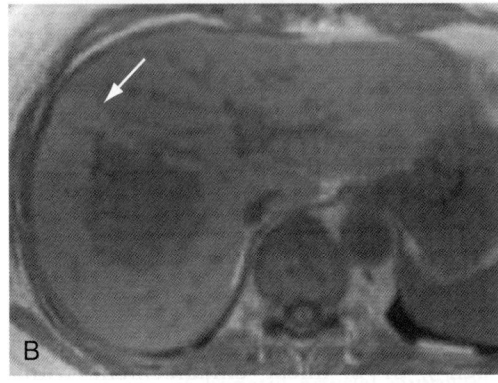

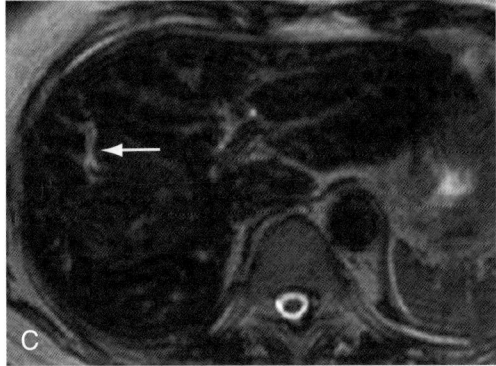

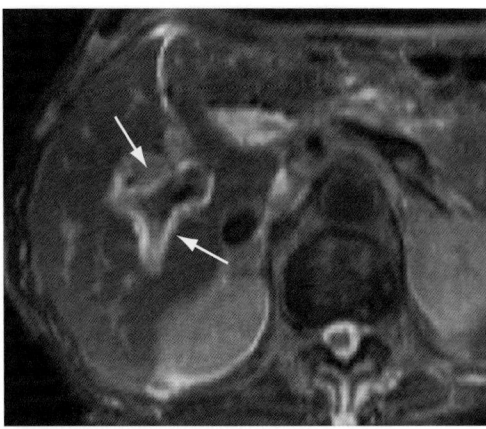

FIGURE 82-56

Primary sclerosing cholangitis. T2-weighted fast spin-echo image shows periportal abnormally high signal intensity seen as a periportal tramline (*arrows*).

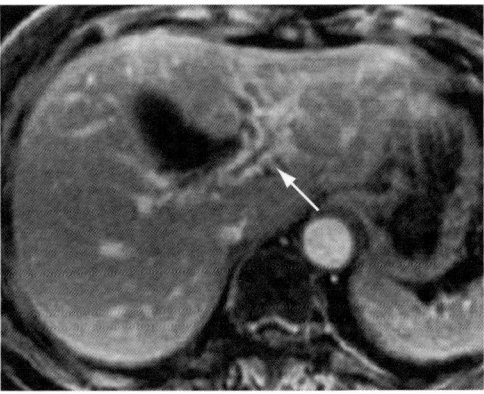

FIGURE 82-57

Benign portal vein thrombus. Contrast-enhanced gradient-echo image shows a low intensity filling defect within the left portal vein (*arrow*), representing an intraluminal thrombus. A high intensity rim represents contrast enhancement of the vessel wall.

FIGURE 82-55

Subsegmental high signal of liver parenchyma in a patient with intrahepatic cholangiocarcinoma. **A,** Opposed-phase and **B,** in-phase T1-weighted gradient-echo images. Subsegmental high signal intensity of liver parenchyma (*arrows*) on T1-weighted images is seen in the peripheral region of the tumor, due to cholestasis caused by impaired drainage of intrahepatic bile. **C,** On the heavily T2-weighted fast spin-echo image, dilatation of the intrahepatic bile ducts (*arrow*) in the corresponding area is observed.

intensity on T1-weighted images, increased signal on T2-weighted images, and increased enhancement on delayed post–gadolinium-enhanced images. Intrahepatic periportal abnormal high intensity on T2-weighted images due to periportal inflammation and enlarged portal lymph nodes[115] are common findings, although these are nonspecific (Fig. 82-56). Hypertrophy of the caudate lobe is frequently seen, especially in patients with endstage PSC (see Fig. 82-19).[40] Severe multifocal peripheral atrophy and marked caudate hypertrophy often lead to bizarre liver shape, resembling a potato.

HEPATIC VASCULAR DISEASE

Portal Vein Obstruction and Thrombosis

Portal vein thrombosis can result from slow flow secondary to cirrhosis, obstruction by enlarged periportal lymph nodes, direct invasion by cancer, inflammatory changes secondary to pancreatitis, or abdominal infection.[116] Chronic, benign thrombus with fibrous organization appears as a low intensity filling defect within the portal vein on contrast-enhanced MR imaging. A high intensity rim representing contrast enhancement of the vessel wall accentuates the presence of intraluminal clot (Fig. 82-57). Fresher thrombus caused by blood clotting shows high signal intensity on T1-weighted MR images (Fig. 82-58). The caliber of benign portal vein thrombus branches is similar to normal (nonoccluded) portal vein diameters without venous expansion.

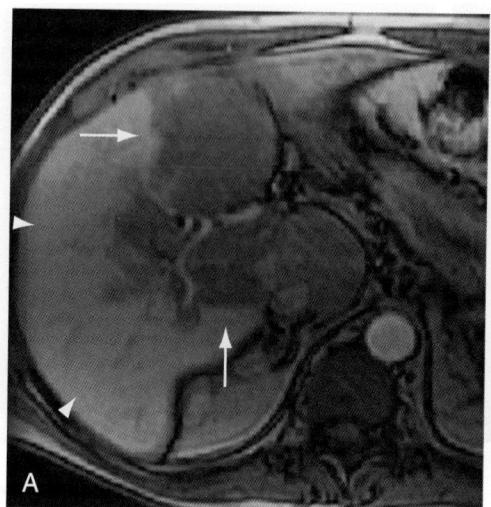
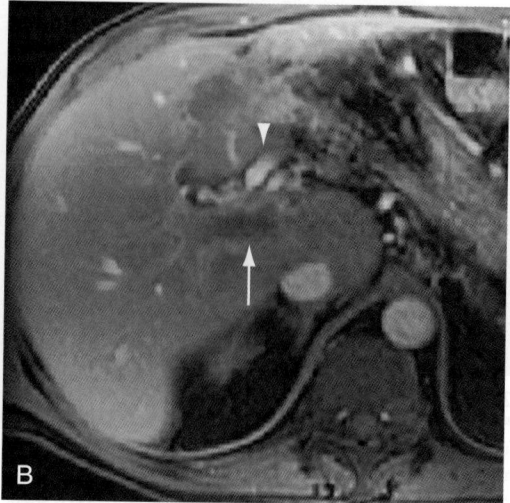

FIGURE 82-63

"Central zone" and "peripheral zone" in a patient with cavernous transformation. **A,** Contrast-enhanced dynamic MR image obtained during the arterial phase shows early enhancement in the peripheral parts of the liver (peripheral zone, *arrowheads*), compared with the central parts of the liver (central zone, *arrows*). **B,** On delayed-phase MR images, thrombi of the right (*arrow*) and main portal veins, and cavernous transformation (*arrowhead*) are noted.

shunts, portal flow is reduced or reversed by high-pressure arterial flow. Contrast-enhanced dynamic MR findings related to arterioportal shunts include early enhancement of the affected portal vein and transient increased hepatic parenchymal enhancement with lobar, segmental or subsegmental distribution (Fig. 82-64).[122,130] Arterioportal shunts can be a cause of focal sparing within diffuse fatty infiltration of the liver due to increased perfusion by non–lipid-rich arterial blood flow.[13] Arterioportal shunts can also cause segmental iron deposition in the corresponding liver parenchyma, most pronounced on T2*-weighted gradient-echo MR images.[131]

Hepatic Perfusion Anomalies

Normal Vascular Variants

There are some variations in communication between the portal venous system and its tributaries, such as cystic veins or coronary gastric veins, which frequently cause intrahepatic perfusion anomalies at contrast-enhanced dynamic MR imaging. An aberrant gastric or cystic vein sometimes communicates directly with the peripheral portal vessels in the left medial or lateral segment of the liver rather than draining directly into the right or main portal veins. Under this condition, on the arterial phase of contrast-enhanced dynamic MR imaging, an early-enhancing hepatic pseudolesion is observed in this area (typically segment 4)[10] because contrast material flows more rapidly to this area through these aberrant veins than to the surrounding hepatic parenchyma, which receives contrast material mainly from the portal veins (superior mesenteric and splenic

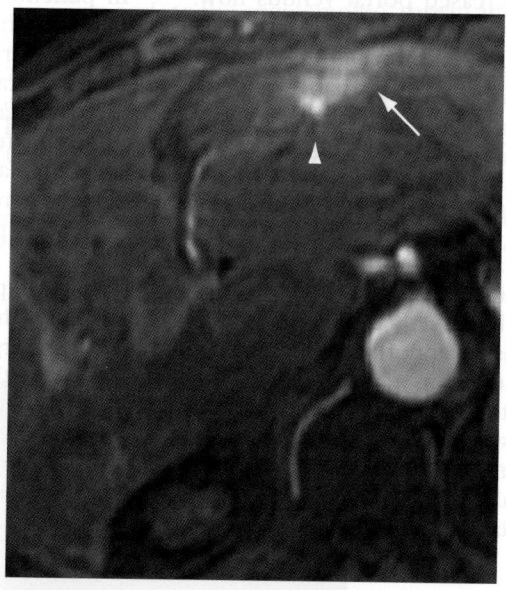

FIGURE 82-64

Intrahepatic arterioportal shunt. Contrast-enhanced dynamic MR image obtained during the arterial phase shows a wedge-shaped early enhancement of the liver with straight boundaries (*arrow*). Early enhancement of the peripheral portal venous branch (*arrowhead*) is noted.

veins) (Fig. 82-65). Conversely, on CT arterial portography, a perfusion defect is seen in this area because of dilution or reversal of the portal flow by the aberrant venous drainages.[8,12] Normal variants in the portal venous tributaries should be recognized when interpreting cross-sectional images because these perfusion anomalies may be misinterpreted as pathologic entities.

cystic vein into the liver parenchyma through the direct communication with peripheral portal branches, compared with the blood flow from the vessels of the portal venous system. Areas of transient increased hepatic enhancement, especially those with a round configuration, may be confused with intrahepatic metastases from gallbladder carcinoma. Homogenous features (isointensity compared with surrounding liver parenchyma) on the portal- or late-phase MR images can help differentiate such areas from true lesions.

Cardiac Dysfunction

In patients with congestive heart failure and passive congestion of the liver, inhomogeneous early enhancement of hepatic parenchyma with a diffusely mottled pattern can be seen on the arterial phase of contrast-enhanced dynamic MR imaging. An alteration in intrahepatic hemodynamics may be a cause of this abnormal enhancement. Hepatic venous outflow is impaired in passive congestion, producing relative stasis of blood in hepatic sinusoids. This impedes antegrade blood flow from the portal and hepatic arterial circulation and delays uniform enhancement in the liver.[133,134] In these patients, retrograde flow of contrast material from the right atrium into the hepatic veins on arterial-phase images is common, indicating elevated right heart pressure (Fig. 82-67).[123]

Budd-Chiari Syndrome

The Budd-Chiari syndrome results from obstruction of hepatic venous outflow at the level of the large hepatic veins.[135] In most cases, hepatic venous outflow is not completely eliminated, because a variety of accessory hepatic veins may drain above or below the principal site of obstruction. It is classified as primary or secondary, depending on the cause and pathophysiologic manifestations. Membranous occlusion of the inferior vena cava (IVC) is most common in Asian patients.

Characteristic findings of the Budd-Chiari syndrome include a striking reduction in caliber or the complete absence of visualized hepatic veins, marked constriction of the intrahepatic IVC, thrombosis of the hepatic veins and/or IVC, arcuate-shaped and transversely oriented intrahepatic collateral vessels,[136] extrahepatic collateral vessels,[137] morphologic changes of the liver, such as central hypertrophy (mainly caudate lobe) and peripheral atrophy (mainly right lobe) in chronic stages,[116] and heterogenous enhancement of hepatic parenchyma at contrast-enhanced CT or MRI (Fig. 82-68).[116,138-141]

In chronic stages of Budd-Chiari syndrome, several pathways of collateral vessels develop and provide hepatic venous drainage. Accessory hepatic veins may drain above or below the principal site of obstruction. Other collaterals connecting with systemic veins include left renal hemiazygos, vertebrolumbar azygos, and inferior phrenic-pericardiacophrenic pathways. Morphologic changes of the liver in Budd-Chiari syndrome may participate in alterations in hepatic circulation. Regions with completely obstructed hepatic venous flow drain via shunting to portal veins, producing

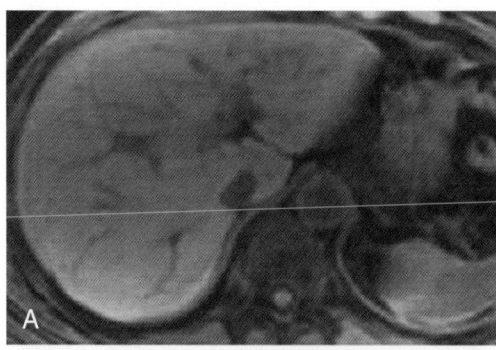
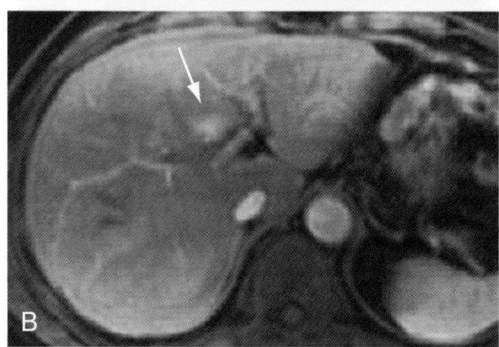
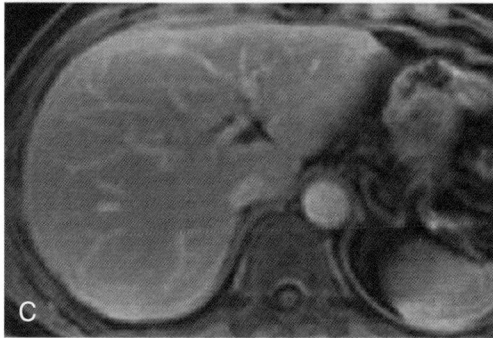

FIGURE 82-65

Early-enhancing pseudolesion in the medial segment of the left hepatic lobe. **A,** Precontrast MR image shows no lesion in the liver. **B,** Contrast-enhanced dynamic MR image obtained during the arterial phase shows an early-enhancing area (*arrow*) in the posterior aspect of the medial segment of the left hepatic lobe, probably due to the aberrant right gastric venous drainage. **C,** Early-enhancing area is isointense relative to the surrounding liver parenchyma on the delayed-phase MR images.

Transient Increased Hepatic Enhancement Caused by Increased Cystic Venous Drainage

In patients with hypervascular gallbladder diseases, including acute cholecystitis, adenomyomatosis, or gallbladder cancers, areas of transient increased hepatic enhancement are frequently seen without invasion or inflammatory changes of the liver parenchyma at contrast-enhanced dynamic arterial-phase CT or MR imaging.[11,132] Although curvilinear areas adjacent to the gallbladder fossa are most common, lobar or segmental areas and focal areas seen as pseudolesions are also noted (Fig. 82-66). The transient increased enhancement in the liver will be caused by the relatively rapid, direct return of the increased blood flow from the dilated

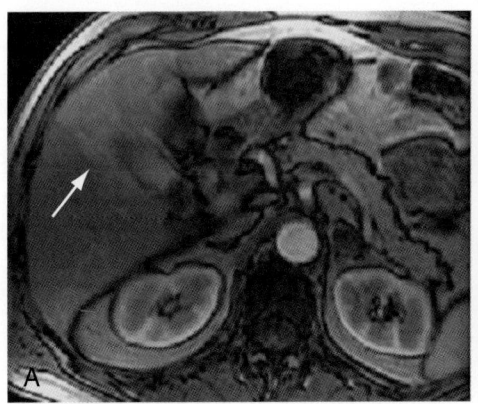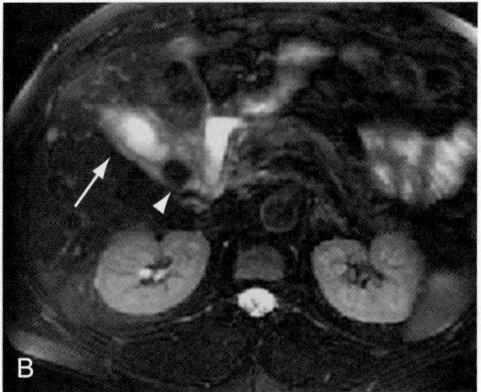

FIGURE 82-66

Transient increased hepatic enhancement caused by increased cystic venous drainage in a patient with acute cholecystitis. **A,** Contrast-enhanced dynamic MR image obtained during the arterial phase shows early enhancement of the left hepatic lobe and a part of segment V adjacent to the gallbladder bed (*arrow*). **B,** On the T2-weighted fast spin-echo image, edematous change of the gallbladder wall is noted (*arrow*). Gallstone is seen as a low intensity structure (*arrowhead*).

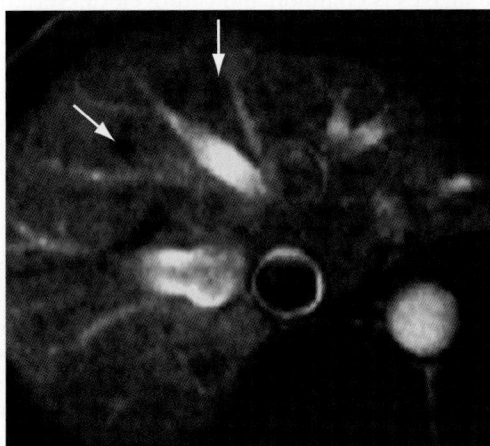

FIGURE 82-67

Retrograde hepatic venous opacification in a patient with poor cardiac function. Contrast-enhanced dynamic MR image obtained during the arterial phase (25 seconds after the start of intravenous administration of contrast material) shows reflux of contrast medium into the hepatic veins. Intrahepatic portal veins are not opacified (*arrows*). Note the signal loss in the inferior vena cava due to dense gadolinium concentration. (*Reproduced with permission from Ito K, Mitchell DG, Honjo K, et al: Biphasic contrast-enhanced multisection dynamic MR imaging of the liver: potential pitfalls. RadioGraphics 17:693-705, 1997.*)

FIGURE 82-68

Budd-Chiari syndrome. Contrast-enhanced MR image shows enhancement in the central portion of the liver (*arrow*), compared with the peripheral parts of the liver which show decreased enhancement. Note the hypertrophy of the caudate lobe of the liver and collateral vessels in the abdominal wall (*arrowheads*).

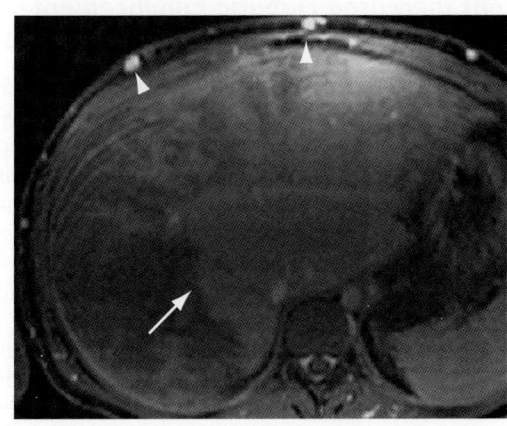

regional reversal of portal venous flow in the peripheral areas, although main portal venous flow may remain antegrade. This decreased portal blood flow induces the atrophy of the peripheral hepatic parenchyma. Conversely, in most cases, the caudate lobe and central part of the right lobe maintain hepatic outflow due to the development of collateral venous pathways, and therefore retain hepatorenal portal flow. As a result, compensatory hypertrophy occurs in these regions.

REFERENCES

1. Mitchell DG: Focal manifestations of diffuse liver disease at MR imaging [review]. Radiology 185:1-11, 1992.
2. Mitchell DG, Kim I, Chang TS, et al: Fatty liver, chemical shift saturation and phase-difference MR imaging techniques in animals, phantoms and humans. Invest Radiol 46:1041-1052, 1991.
3. Wehrli FW, Perkins TG, Shimakawa A, Roberts F: Chemical shift induced amplitude modulations in images obtained with gradient refocusing. Magn Reson Imaging 5:157-158, 1987.
4. Venkataraman S, Braga L, Semelka RC: Imaging the fatty liver. Magn Reson Imaging Clin North Am 10:93-103, 2002.
5. Taupitz M, Deimling M, Malcher R, et al: A new rapid T1-weighted multiplanar spoiled gradient-echo sequence for simultaneous acquisition of in-phase and opposed-phase images (SINOP) [abstract]. Proceedings of ISMRM, 1998, p 103.
6. Mitchell DG, Stolpen AH, Siegelman ES, et al: Fatty tissue on opposed-phase MR images: paradoxical suppression of signal intensity by paramagnetic contrast agents. Radiology 198:351-357, 1996.
7. Itai Y, Matsui O: Blood flow and liver imaging. Radiology 202:306-314, 1997.
8. Matsui O, Takahashi S, Kadoya M, et al: Pseudolesion in segment IV of the liver at CT during arterial portography: correlation with aberrant gastric venous drainage. Radiology 193:31-35, 1994.
9. Matsui O, Kadoya M, Takahashi S, et al: Focal sparing of segment IV in fatty livers shown by sonography and CT: correlation with aberrant gastric venous drainage. Am J Roentgenol 164:1137-1140, 1995.
10. Ito K, Choji T, Fujita, et al: Early-enhancing pseudolesion in medial segment of left hepatic lobe detected with multisection dynamic MR. Radiology 187:695-699, 1993.
11. Ito K, Awaya H, Mitchell DG, et al: Gallbladder disease: Appearance of associated transient increased attenuation in the liver at biphasic, contrast-enhanced dynamic CT. Radiology 204:723-728, 1997.
12. Matsui O, Kadoya M, Yoshikawa J, et al: Aberrant gastric venous drainage in cirrhotic livers: imaging findings in focal areas of liver parenchyma [see comments]. Radiology 197:345-349, 1995.
13. Arita T, Matsunaga N, Honma Y, et al: Focally spared area of fatty liver caused by arterioportal shunt. J Comput Assist Tomogr 20:360-362, 1996.
14. Taupitz M, Schroeter T, Malcher R, et al: MR imaging of focal lesions in fatty degeneration of the liver: Visualization of a hyperintense peritumoral rim on opposed-phase gradient-echo images [abstract]. Radiology 209:677, 1998.
15. Andrews NC: Disorders or iron metabolism. N Engl J Med 341:1986-1995, 1999.
16. Pomerantz S, Siegelman ES: MR imaging of iron depositional disease. In Semelka RC (ed): MR Imaging of the Liver II: Disease. Magn Reson Imaging Clin North Am 10:105-120, 2002.
17. Olynk JK: Hereditary haemochromatosis: diagnosis and management in the gene era. Liver 19:73-90, 1999.
18. Powell LW, George DK, McDonnell SM, Kowdley KV: Diagnosis of hemochromatosis. Ann Intern Med 129:925-931, 1998.
19. Gandon Y, Guyader D, Heautot JF, et al: Hemochromatosis: diagnosis and quantification of liver iron with gradient-echo MR imaging. Radiology 193:533-538, 1994.
20. Ito K, Mitchell DG, Gabata T, et al: Hepatocellular carcinoma: association with increased iron deposition in the cirrhotic liver at MR imaging. Radiology 212:235-240, 1999.
21. Chapoutot C, Esslimani M, Joomaye Z, et al: Liver iron excess in patients with hepatocellular carcinoma developed on viral C cirrhosis. Gut 46:711-714, 2000.
22. Krinsky GA, Lee VS, Nguyen MT, et al: Siderotic nodules in the cirrhotic liver at MR imaging with explant correlation: no increased frequency of dysplastic nodules and hepatocellular carcinoma. Radiology 218:47-53, 2001.
23. Niederau C, Erhardt A, Haussinger D, Strohmeyer G: Haemochromatosis and the liver. J Hepatol 30(Suppl 1):6-11, 1999.
24. Siegelman ES, Mitchell DG, Semelka RC: Abdominal iron deposition: metabolism, MR findings, and clinical importance. Radiology 199:13-22, 1996.
25. Siegelman ES, Mitchell DG, Rubin R, et al: Parenchymal versus reticuloendothelial iron overload in the liver: distinction with MR imaging. Radiology 179:361-366, 1991.
26. Siegelman ES, Mitchell DG, Outwater E, et al: Idiopathic hemochromatosis: MR imaging findings in cirrhotic and precirrhotic patients. Radiology 188:637-641, 1993.
27. Ernst O, Sergent G, Bonvarlet P, et al: Hepatic iron overload: diagnosis and quantification with MR imaging. Am J Roentgenol 168:1205-1208, 1997.
28. Clark PR, St Pierre TG: Quantitative mapping of transverse relaxivity (1/T(2)) in hepatic iron overload: a single spin-echo imaging methodology. Magn Reson Imaging 18:431-432, 2000.
29. Papakonstantinou O, Kostaridou S, Maris T, et al: Quantification of liver iron overload by T2 quantitative magnetic resonance in thalassemia: impact of chronic hepatitis C on measurements. J Pediatr Hematol Oncol 21:142-148, 1999.
30. Waxman S, Eustace S, Hartnell GG: Myocardial involvement in primary hemochromatosis demonstrated by magnetic resonance imaging. Am Heart J 128:1047-1049, 1994.
31. Torres E, Whitmire LF, Gedgauda-McClees K, Bernardino ME: Computed tomography of hepatic morphologic changes in cirrhosis of the liver. J Comput Assist Tomogr 11:47-50, 1986.
32. Ito K, Mitchell DG, Hann HWL, et al: Compensated cirrhosis due to viral hepatitis: using MR imaging to predict clinical progression. Am J Roentgenol 169:801-805, 1997.
33. Ito K, Mitchell DG, Hann HWL, et al: Progressive viral-induced cirrhosis: serial MR imaging findings and clinical correlation. Radiology 207:729-735, 1998.
34. Brown JJ, Naylor MJ, Yagan N: Imaging of hepatic cirrhosis. Radiology 202:1-16, 1997.
35. Ito K, Mitchell DG: MR imaging of cirrhosis and its complications. Contemp Diag Radiol 23:1-6, 2000.
36. Ito K, Mitchell DG, Siegelman ES: Cirrhosis: MR imaging features. Magn Reson Imaging Clin North Am 10:75-92, 2002.
37. Harbin WP, Robert NJ, Ferrucci JT Jr: Diagnosis of cirrhosis based on regional changes in hepatic morphology: a radiological and pathological analysis. Radiology 135:273-283, 1980.
38. Ito K, Mitchell DG, Gabata T: Enlargement of hilar periportal space: a sign of early cirrhosis at MR imaging. J Magn Reson Imaging 11:136-140, 2000.
39. Ito K, Mitchell DG: Hepatic morphologic changes in cirrhosis: MR imaging findings. Abdom Imaging 25:456-461, 2000.
40. Dodd GDI, Baron RL, Oliver JHI, Federle MP: End-stage primary sclerosing cholangitis: CT findings of hepatic morphology in 36 patients. Radiology 211:357-362, 1999.
41. Ito K, Mitchell DG, Outwater EK, Blasbalg R: Primary sclerosing cholangitis: MR imaging features. Am J Roentgenol 172:1527-1533, 1999.
42. Giorgio A, Amoroso P, Lettieri G, et al: Cirrhosis: value of caudate to right lobe ratio in diagnosis with ultrasound. Radiology 161:443-445, 1986.
43. Ito K, Mitchell DG, Gabata T, Hussain SM: Expanded gallbladder fossa: simple MR imaging sign of cirrhosis. Radiology 211:723-726, 1999.
44. Ito K, Mitchell DG, Kim MJ, et al: Right posterior hepatic notch sign: a simple diagnostic MR finding of cirrhosis. J Magn Reson Imaging 18:561-566, 2003.
45. Okazaki H, Ito K, Fujita T, et al: Discrimination of alcoholic from virus-induced cirrhosis on MR imaging. Am J Roentgenol 175:1677-1681, 2000.
46. Awaya H, Mitchell DG, Kamishima T, et al: Cirrhosis: modified caudate-to-right lobe ratio. Radiology 224:769-774, 2002.
47. DiLelio A, Cestari C, Lomazzi A, Beretta L: Cirrhosis: diagnosis with sonographic study of the liver surface. Radiology 172:389-392, 1989.
48. Ohtomo K, Itai Y, Ohtomo Y, et al: Regenerating nodules of liver cirrhosis: MR imaging with pathologic correlation. Am J Roentgenol 154:505-507, 1990.
49. Kita K, Kita M, Sato M, et al: MR imaging of liver cirrhosis: role of fibrous septa in visualization of regenerating nodules. Acta Radiol 37:198-203, 1996.
50. Itai Y, Ohnishi S, Ohtomo K, et al: Regenerating nodules of liver cirrhosis: MR imaging. Radiology 165:419-425, 1987.
51. Murakami T, Kuroda C, Marukawa T, et al: Regenerating nodules in hepatic cirrhosis. MR findings with pathologic correlation. Am J Roentgenol 155:1227-1231, 1990.
52. Hann HWL, Kim CY, London WT, Blumberg BS: Increased serum ferritin in chronic liver disease: a risk factor for primary hepatocellular carcinoma. Int J Cancer 43:376-379, 1989.
53. Terada T, Nakanuma Y: Survey of iron-accumulative macroregenerative nodules in cirrhotic livers. Hepatology 10:851-854, 1989.
54. Terada T, Kadoya M, Nakanuma Y, Matsui O: Iron-accumulating adenomatous hyperplastic nodule with malignant foci in the cirrhotic liver. Cancer 65:1994-2000, 1990.
55. Dodd GDI, Baron RL, Oliver JHI, Federle MP: Spectrum of the liver in end-stage cirrhosis: Part I, gross morphology and diffuse abnormalities. Am J Roentgenol 173:1031-1036, 1999.
56. Ohtomo K, Baron RL, Dodd GD, et al: Confluent hepatic fibrosis in advanced cirrhosis: evaluation with MR imaging. Radiology 189:871-874, 1993.
57. Dodd GDI, Baron RL, Oliver JHI, et al: Enlarged abdominal lymph nodes in end-stage cirrhosis: CT-histopathologic correlation in 507 patients. Radiology 203:127-130, 1997.
58. Zhang XM, Mitchell DG, Shi H, et al: Chronic hepatitis C activity: correlation with lymphadenopathy on MR imaging. Am J Roentgenol 179:417-422, 2002.

SECTION **VI** ■ **BODY**

59. Guingrich J, Kuhlman JE: Colonic wall thickening in patients with cirrhosis: CT findings and clinical implications. Am J Roentgenol 172:919-924, 1999.

60. Karahan OI, Dodd GDI, Chintapalli KN, et al: Gastrointestinal wall thickening in patients with cirrhosis: frequency and patterns at contrast-enhanced CT. Radiology 211:737-742, 1999.

61. Chopra S, Dodd GDI, Chintapalli KN, et al: Mesenteric, omental, and retroperitoneal edema in cirrhosis: frequency and spectrum of CT findings. Radiology 211:737-742, 1999.

62. Ito K, Blasbalg R, Hussain SM, Mitchell DG: Portal vein and its tributaries: evaluation with thin-section three-dimensional contrast-enhanced dynamic fat-suppressed MR imaging. Radiology 215:381-386, 2000.

63. Ito K, Choji T, Nakada T, et al: Multislice dynamic MRI of hepatic tumors. J Comput Assist Tomogr 17:390-396, 1993.

64. Yamashita Y, Mitsuzaki K, Yi T, et al: Small hepatocellular carcinoma in patients with chronic liver damage: prospective comparison of detection with dynamic MR imaging and helical CT of the whole liver. Radiology 200:79-84, 1996.

65. Tang Y, Yamashita Y, Arakawa A, et al: Detection of hepatocellular carcinoma arising in cirrhotic livers: comparison of gadolinium- and ferumoxides-enhanced MR imaging. Am J Roentgenol 172:1547-1554, 1999.

66. Shimizu A, Ito K, Koike S, et al: Cirrhosis or chronic hepatitis: Evaluation of small (<2 cm) early-enhancing hepatic lesions with serial contrast-enhanced dynamic MR imaging. Radiology 226:550-555, 2003.

67. Jeong Y, Mitchell DG, Kamishima T: Small (<20 mm) enhancing hepatic nodules seen on arterial phase MR imaging of the cirrhotic liver: clinical implications. Am J Roentgenol 178:1327-1334, 2002.

68. Edelman RR, Zhao B, Liu C, et al: MR angiography and dynamic flow evaluation of the portal venous system. Am J Roentgenol 153:755-760, 1989.

69. Nghiem HV, Freeny PC, Winter TR, et al: Phase-contrast MR angiography of the portal venous system: preoperative findings in liver transplant recipients. Am J Roentgenol 163:445-450, 1994.

70. Shirkhoda A, Konez O, Shetty AN, et al: Contrast-enhanced MR angiography of the mesenteric circulation: a pictorial essay. RadioGraphics 18:851-861, 1998.

71. Yamashita Y, Mitsuzaki K, Miyazaki T, et al: Gadolinium-enhanced breath-hold three-dimensional MR angiography of the portal vein: value of the magnetization-prepared rapid acquisition gradient-echo sequence. Radiology 201:283-288, 1996.

72. Pieters PC, Miller WJ, DeMeo JH: Evaluation of the portal venous system: complementary roles of invasive and non-invasive imaging strategies. RadioGraphics 17:879-895, 1997.

73. Kim M, Mitchell DG, Ito K: Portosystemic collaterals of the upper abdomen: review of anatomy and demonstration of MR imaging. Abdom Imaging 25:462-470, 2000.

74. McCain AH, Bernardino ME, Sones PJ, et al: Varices from portal hypertension: correlation of CT and angiography. Radiology 154:63-69, 1985.

75. Lebrec D, Fleury PD, Rueff B, et al: Portal hypertension, size of esophageal varices, and risk of gastrointestinal bleeding in alcoholic cirrhosis. Gastroenterology 79:1139-1144, 1980.

76. Cho KC, Patel YD, Wachsberg RH, Seeff J: Varices in portal hypertension: evaluation with CT. RadioGraphics 15:609-622, 1995.

77. Hussain SM, Semelka RC, Mitchell DG: Hepatocellular carcinoma. In Semelka RC (ed): Imaging of the Liver II: Diseases. Magn Reson Imaging Clin North Am 10:31-52, 2002.

78. Hussain SM, Zondervan PE, Izermans JNM, et al: Benign versus malignant hepatic nodules: MR imaging findings with pathologic correlation. RadioGraphics 22:1023-1036, 2002.

79. Hussain SM, Terkivatan T, Zondervan PE, et al: Focal nodular hyperplasia: a spectrum of findings at state-of-the-art MR imaging, US, CT and pathologic analysis. RadioGraphics 24:3-17, 2004.

80. Choi BI, Takayasu K, Han MC: Small hepatocellular carcinoma and associated lesions of the liver: pathology, pathogenesis, imaging findings. Am J Roentgenol 160:1177-1187, 1993.

81. Mitchell DG: Liver I: Currently available gadolinium chelates. Magn Reson Imaging Clin North Am 4:37-51, 1996.

82. Katyal S, Oliver JH, Peterson MS, et al: Extrahepatic metastases of hepatocellular carcinoma. Radiology 216:698-703, 2000.

83. Schalm SW: The diagnosis of cirrhosis: clinical relevance and methodology. J Hepatol 27:118-1119, 1997.

84. International Working Party: Terminology of nodular hepatocellular lesions. Hepatology 22:983-993, 1995.

85. Sakamoto M, Hirohashi S, Shimosato Y: Early stages of multistep hepatocarcinogenesis: adenomatous hyperplasia and early hepatocellular carcinoma. Hum Pathol 22:172-178, 1991.

86. Okuda K: Hepatocellular carcinoma: recent progress. Hepatology 15:948-963, 1992.

87. Edmondson HA, Steiner PE: Primary carcinoma of the liver: a study of 100 cases among 18,900 necropsies. Cancer 7:462-503, 1954.

88. Kanai T, Hirohashi S, Upton MP, et al: Pathology of small hepatocellular carcinoma: a proposal for a new gross classification. Cancer 60:810-819, 1987.

89. Pain JA, Gimson AES, Willims R, Howard ER: Focal nodular hyperplasia of the liver: results of treatment and options in management. Gut 32:524-527, 1991.

90. Mathieu D, Vilgrain V, Mahfouz AE, et al: Benign liver tumors. Magn Reson Imaging Clin North Am 5: 255-288, 1997.

91. Mortele KJ, Praet M, Van Vlierberghe H, et al: CT and MR imaging findings in focal nodular hyperplasia of the liver: radiologic-pathologic correlation. Am J Roentgenol 174:705-712, 2000.

92. Shirkhoda A, Farah MC, Vernacki E, et al: Hepatic focal nodular hyperplasia: CT and sonographic spectrum. Abdom Imaging 19:34-38, 1994.

93. Nguyen BN, Flejou JF, Terris BG, et al: Focal nodular hyperplasia of the liver: a comprehensive pathologic study of 305 lesions and recognition of new histologic forms. Am J Surg Pathol 23:1441-1454, 1999.

94. Terkivatan T, de Wilt JH, de Man RA, et al: Indications and long-term outcome of treatment for benign hepatic tumors: a critical appraisal. Arch Surg 136:1033-1038, 2001.

95. Shortell CK, Schwartz SI: Hepatic adenoma and focal nodular hyperplasia. Surg Gynecol Obstet 173:426-431, 1991.

96. Earls JP, Theise ND, Weinreb JC, et al: Dysplastic nodules and hepatocellular carcinoma: thin-section MR imaging of explanted cirrhotic livers with pathologic correlation. Radiology 201:207-214, 1996.

97. Matsui M, Kadoya M, Kameyama T, et al: Adenomatous hyperplastic nodules in the cirrhotic liver: differentiation from hepatocellular carcinoma with MR imaging. Radiology 173:123-126, 1989.

98. Muramatsu Y, Nawano S, Takayasu K, et al: Early hepatocellular carcinoma: MR imaging. Radiology 181:209-213, 1991.

99. Matsui O, Kadoya M, Kameyama T, et al: Benign and malignant nodules in cirrhotic livers: distinction based on blood supply. Radiology 178:493-497, 1991.

100. Mitchell DG, Rubin R, Siegelman ES, et al: Hepatocellular carcinoma within siderotic regenerative nodules: appearance as a nodule within a nodule on MR images. Radiology 178:101-103, 1991.

101. Sadek AG, Mitchell DG, Siegelman ES, et al: Early hepatocellular carcinoma that develops within macroregenerative nodules: growth rate depicted at serial MR imaging. Radiology 195:753-756, 1995.

102. Kadoya M, Matsui O, Takashima T, Nonomra A: Hepatocellular carcinoma: correlation of MR imaging and histopathologic findings. Radiology 183:819-825, 1992.

103. Imaeda T, Kanematsu M, Mochizuki R, et al: Extracapsular invasion of small hepatocellular carcinoma: MR and CT findings. J Comput Assist Tomogr 18:755-760, 1994.

104. Tsai TJ, Chau GY, Lui WY, et al: Clinical significance of microscopic tumor venous invasion in patients with resectable hepatocellular carcinoma. Surgery 127:603-608, 2000.

105. Lee YT, Geer DA: Primary liver cancer: pattern of metastasis. J Surg Oncol 36:26-31, 1987.

106. Williams R, Rizzi P: Treating small hepatocellular carcinomas. N Engl J Med 334:728-729, 1996.

107. Bismuth H, Chiche L, Castaing D: Surgical treatment of hepatocellular carcinoma in non-cirrhotic liver: experience in 68 liver resections. World J Surg 19:35-41, 1995.

108. Winston CB, Schwartz LH, Fong Y, et al: Hepatocellular carcinoma: MR imaging findings in cirrhotic livers and noncirrhotic livers. Radiology 210:75-79, 1999.

109. Craig JR, Peters RL, Edmondson HA, et al: Fibrolamellar carcinoma of the liver: a tumor of adolescents and young adults with distinctive clinico-pathologic features. Cancer 46:372-379, 1980.

110. McLarney JK, Rucker PT, Bender GN, et al: Fibrolamellar carcinoma of the liver: radiologic-pathologic correlation. RadioGraphics 19:453-471, 1999.

111. Mortele KJ, Ros PR: MR imaging in chronic hepatitis and cirrhosis. Semin Ultrasound CT MRI 23:79-100, 2002.

112. Majoie CBLM, Huibregtse K, Reeders JWAJ: Primary sclerosing cholangitis. Abdom Imaging 22:194-198, 1997.

113. Ernst O, Asselah T, Sergent G, et al: MR cholangiography in primary sclerosing cholangitis. Am J Roentgenol 171:1027-1030, 1998.

114. Gabata T, Matsui O, Kadoya M, et al: Segmental hyperintensity on T1-weighted MRI of the liver: indication of segmental cholestasis. J Magn Reson Imaging 7:855-857, 1997.

115. Outwater EK, Kaplan MM, Bankoff MS: Lymphadenopathy in sclerosing cholangitis: pitfall in the diagnosis of malignant biliary obstruction. Gastrointest Radiol 17:157-160, 1992.

116. Mitchell DG, Nazarian LN: Hepatic vascular diseases: CT and MRI. Semin Ultrasound CT MRI 16:49-68, 1995.

117. Mathieu D, Grenier P, Larde D, Vasile N: Portal vein involvement in hepatocellular carcinoma: dynamic CT features. Radiology 152:127-132, 1984.

118. Araki T, Suda K, Seikiawa T, et al: Portal venous tumor thrombosis associated with gastric adenocarcinoma. Radiology 174:811-814, 1990.

119. Tublin ME, Dodd GDI, Baron RL: Benign and malignant portal vein thrombosis: differentiation by CT characteristics. Am J Roentgenol 168:719-723, 1997.

120. Ito K, Higuchi M, Kada T, et al: CT of acquired abnormalities of the portal venous system. RadioGraphics 17:897-917, 1997.

121. Okuda K, Musha H, Yoshida T, et al: Demonstration of growing casts of hepatocellular carcinoma in the portal vein by celiac angiography: the thread and streaks sign. Radiology 117:303-309, 1975.

122. Ito K, Honjo K, Fujita T, et al: Hepatic parenchymal hyperperfusion abnormalities detected with multisection dynamic MR imaging: appearance and interpretation. J Magn Reson Imaging 6:861-867, 1996.
123. Ito K, Mitchell DG, Honjo K, et al: Biphasic contrast-enhanced multisection dynamic MR imaging of the liver: potential pitfalls. RadioGraphics 17:693-705, 1997.
124. Tyrrel RT, Kaufman SL, Bernardino ME: Straight line sign: appearance and significance during CT portography. Radiology 173:635-637, 1989.
125. Nelson RC, Thompson GH, Chezmar JL, et al: CT during arterial portography: diagnostic pitfalls. RadioGraphics 12:705-718, 1992.
126. Itai Y, Hachiya J, Makita K, et al: Transient hepatic attenuation differences on dynamic computed tomography. J Comput Assist Tomogr 11:461-465, 1987.
127. Ito K, Honjo K, Fujita T, et al: Enhanced MR imaging of the liver after ethanol treatment of hepatocellular carcinoma: evaluation of areas of hyperperfusion adjacent to the tumor. Am J Roentgenol 164:1413-1417, 1995.
128. Mathieu D, Vasile N, Dibie C, Grenier P: Portal cavernoma: dynamic CT features and transient differences in hepatic attenuation. Radiology 154:743-748, 1985.
129. Itai Y, Murata S, Saida Y, Minami M: Central zone and peripheral zone of the liver based on portal and hepatic arterial blood supply: imaging approach to deformity of cirrhotic liver. Jpn J Clin Radiol 39:1553-1559, 1994.
130. Itai Y, Frui S, Ohtomo K, et al: Dynamic CT features of arterioportal shunts in hepatocellular carcinoma. Am J Roentgenol 146:723-727, 1986.
131. Kadoya M, Matsui O, Kitagawa K, et al: Segmental iron deposition in the liver due to decreased intrahepatic portal perfusion: findings at MR imaging. Radiology 193:671-676, 1994. [Erratum 194:915, 1995]

132. Yamashita K, Jin MJ, Hirose Y, et al: CT finding of transient focal increased attenuation of the liver adjacent to the gallbladder in acute cholecystitis. Am J Roentgenol 164:343-346, 1995.
133. Moulton JS, Miller BL, Dodd III GD, Vu DN: Passive hepatic congestion in heart failure: CT abnormalities. Am J Roentgenol 151:939-942, 1988.
134. Holley HC, Koslin DB, Berland LL, Stanley RJ: Inhomogenous enhancement of liver parenchyma secondary to passive congestion: contrast-enhanced CT. Radiology 170:795-800, 1989.
135. Stanley P: Budd-Chiari syndrome. Radiology 170:625-627, 1989.
136. Soyer P, Rabenandrasan A, Barge J, et al: MRI of Budd-Chiari syndrome. Abdom Imaging 19:325-329, 1994.
137. Cho OK, Koo JH, Kim YS, et al: Collateral pathways in Budd-Chiari syndrome. CT and venographic correlation. Am J Roentgenol 167:1163-1167, 1996.
138. Mathieu D, Vasile N, Menu Y, et al: Budd-Chiari syndrome: dynamic CT. Radiology 165: 409-413, 1987.
139. Vogelzang RL, Anschuetz SL, Gore RM: Budd-Chiari syndrome. CT observations. Radiology 163:329-333, 1987.
140. Van Beers B, Pringot J, Trigaux JP, et al: Hepatic heterogenicity on CT in Budd-Chiari syndrome: Correlation with regional disturbances in portal flow. Gastrointest Radiol 13:61-66, 1988.
141. Noone TC, Semelka RC, Siegelman ES, et al: Budd-Chiari syndrome: spectrum of appearances of acute, subacute, and chronic disease with magnetic resonance imaging. J Magn Reson Imaging 11:44-50, 2000.

vascular and biliary anatomy of the donor must be meticulously mapped prior to performing a partial liver transplantation.

MR IMAGING EVALUATION OF POTENTIAL LIVER TRANSPLANT RECIPIENTS

Techniques

The goals of pretransplantation imaging of the liver with MRI are typically: 1. to aid in determining the severity of liver disease; 2. to detect or exclude the presence of HCC; and 3. to define the vascular and biliary anatomy of relevance to the transplant surgeon. The minimal components of a preliver transplant protocol designed to accomplish these aims are presented in Box 83-1.

Ideally, the above sequences should be performed during suspended respiration, or using a form of respiratory compensation or triggering and a surface coil capable of large field-of-view imaging. The dual-echo in- and opposed-phase sequence aids in identifying areas of hepatic steatosis and iron or fat within nodules and tumors. Axial fat-suppressed T2-weighted images are helpful for tumor detection and lesion characterization. The dynamic gadolinium-enhanced sequence is the most sensitive of the sequences listed for the detection of HCC. When possible, dynamic scanning should be performed using a three-dimensional (3D) fat-suppressed sequence. By performing the dynamic sequence using sufficiently high resolution to allow isotropic voxel size, high quality multiplanar reformations (MPRs) and maximum intensity projections (MIPs) can be created in any plane that best demonstrates the anatomy of interest. Some preliminary evidence suggests that double arterial phase dynamic MRI, made possible through the use of parallel imaging, may increase the sensitivity for detection of small HCC.[7] If desired, biliary anatomy can be evaluated with MRCP, though the presence of ascites and soft-tissue edema often have a significant adverse effect on the heavily T2-weighted scans used for static MRCP. Liver volumes can be estimated using MRI with acceptable accuracy.[8] Recipient liver volumes are helpful in assessing the severity of liver disease and assigning priority to transplant candidates when used in conjunction with clinical and laboratory data.[9,10]

Box 83-1 | MRI Protocol for Potential Liver Transplant Recipients

Coronal single-shot echo-train spin-echo localizer
Axial dual-echo in- and opposed-phase T1-weighted spoiled gradient-echo sequence
Axial fat-suppressed T2-weighted sequence
Axial dynamic gadolinium-enhanced T1-weighted spoiled gradient-echo sequence (precontrast, arterial, portal, and equilibrium phases)

Findings of Endstage Liver Disease

Cirrhosis

Most potential liver transplant recipients suffer from cirrhosis induced by chronic hepatocellular injury. Cirrhotic livers may display several abnormalities visible on MRI, including segmental atrophy and hypertrophy, a variety of nodules ranging from benign to malignant, and fibrosis that may appear as a fine diffuse reticular pattern, thick periportal bands, or confluent mass-like areas.

Atrophy

The liver is of normal size in up to one-quarter of end-stage cirrhotics, is diffusely diminished in volume in approximately one-third of patients, or may demonstrate areas of atrophy and hypertrophy.[11] The pattern of hepatic atrophy and hypertrophy demonstrated on MRI of the cirrhotic liver may, in part, depend upon the underlying cause. In the case of focal atrophy, the right lobe and medial segment of the left lobe are most commonly involved. This pattern of atrophy is often associated with hypertrophy of the caudate lobe and lateral segment of the left lobe, though other combinations of atrophy and hypertrophy can occur.

Nodules

A cirrhotic liver consists of regenerative nodules surrounded by bands of fibrosis. The regenerative nodules may be large, resulting in significant contour deformity of the liver, or they may be small and barely perceptible. Regenerative nodules consist of benign hepatocytes and demonstrate variable signal intensity on MRI. Often, regenerative nodules are of intermediate signal intensity on T1-weighted images. However, regenerative nodules may range in signal intensity from hypo- to hyper-intense on T1-weighted images depending upon their composition (Fig. 83-2). For example, siderotic nodules tend to be quite low in signal intensity as a result of their iron content. On dual-echo gradient-echo sequences, siderotic nodules lose signal intensity relative to the rest of the hepatic parenchyma on the second (in-phase) echo time. Alternatively, lipid-containing nodules appear relatively bright on in-phase images and lose signal on the opposed-phase images. For reasons poorly understood, some non–lipid-containing nodules may also demonstrate increased signal intensity on T1-weighted images; however, they do not lose signal on opposed-phase images. On T2-weighted images, regenerative nodules range from hypo- to iso-intense.

Dysplastic regenerative nodules are considered an intermediate step toward the development of HCC. Histopathology of dysplastic nodules reveals cellular atypia without frank malignancy. These nodules can be classified histologically as low- or high-grade dysplastic nodules, depending on the degree of cellular atypia. Classically, dysplastic nodules have been described as appearing relatively bright on T1-weighted images and of intermediate-to-low signal intensity on T2-weighted

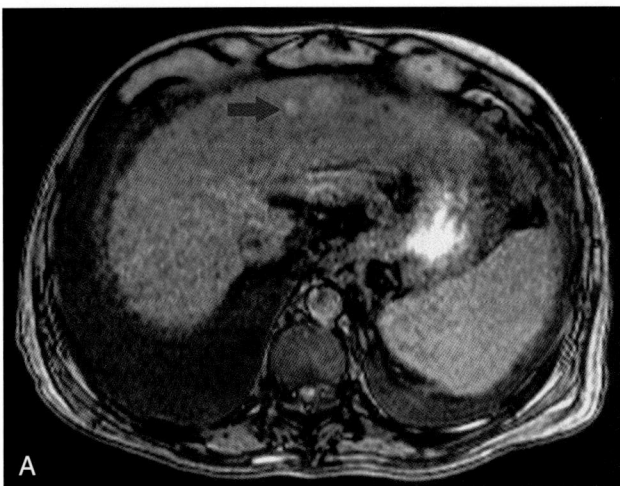

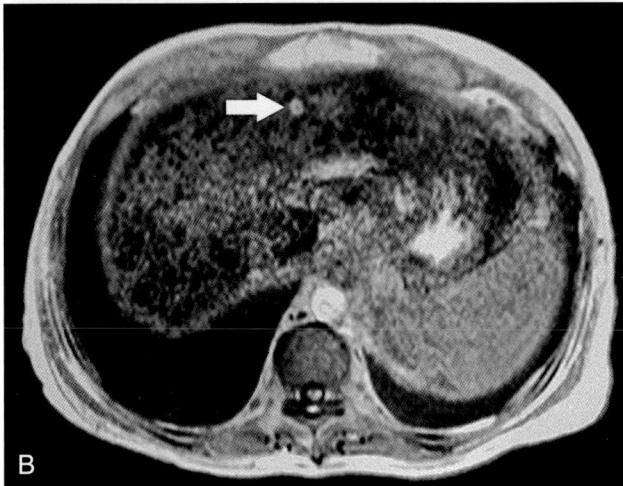

FIGURE 83-2

Cirrhotic nodules. **A,** Axial opposed-phase T1-weighted gradient-echo sequence demonstrates innumerable small low signal intensity nodules and a single high signal intensity nodule (*arrow*) in the liver of a patient with cirrhosis awaiting liver transplantation. **B,** In-phase image from same study as **A** shows the low signal intensity nodules to have decreased in signal intensity with the longer echo time, consistent with iron content. The solitary high signal intensity nodule (*arrow*) remains unchanged. This latter nodule did not demonstrate high signal intensity on T2-weighted images or significant enhancement with gadolinium (not shown). A decision was made to follow this lesion with MRI.

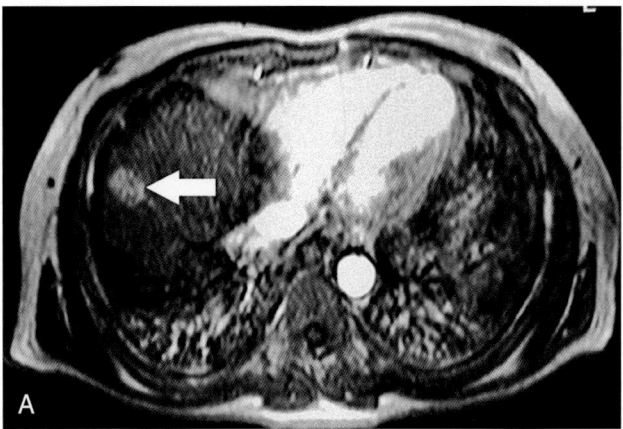

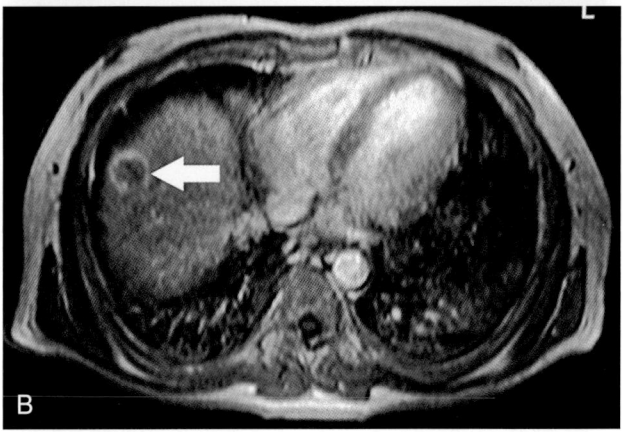

FIGURE 83-3

Small hepatocellular carcinoma (HCC) in a patient awaiting liver transplantation. **A,** Axial arterial phase gradient-echo image through the liver dome demonstrates enhancing focus of HCC (*arrow*). **B,** Same lesion as in **A** demonstrates washout of the lesion with enhancement of the pseudocapsule (*arrow*) on equilibrium-phase image.

images. However, nondysplastic hyperintense regenerative nodules are not unusual on T1-weighted gradient-echo imaging.[12]

The most important distinction that must be made within the cirrhotic liver is between benign cirrhotic nodules and nodules of HCC. In the setting of cirrhosis, nodules that exhibit transient arterial phase enhancement relative to background liver, areas of high signal intensity on T2-weighted images, or a pseudocapsule should be considered malignant until proven otherwise (Fig. 83-3). Because it may be difficult to biopsy or treat suspicious nodules smaller than 1 cm, and because many small arterially enhancing nodules are actually benign, it is reasonable to follow such small lesions with serial imaging examinations at 3- to 4-month intervals.[13,14] Lesions that demonstrate interval growth are highly suspicious for malignancy (Fig. 83-4).

Several studies have reported MRI, using a variety of techniques, to be as good or better than CT for the detection of HCC.[15-22] However, the sensitivity and specificity of MRI for detecting HCC depends greatly on tumor size, pulse sequence, and the contrast agent utilized. The sensitivity of MRI for HCC using a multiphase gadolinium-enhanced technique has been reported to be between 70% and 77%.[15,16,18] The sensitivity deteriorates significantly as lesion size decreases, with MRI probably detecting fewer than a third of HCCs smaller than 1 cm. In fact, Krinsky et al detected only three of 72 HCC lesions under 1 cm in cirrhotic livers in a study comparing MRI with a dynamic gadolinium-enhanced sequence to thin-section liver explant pathology.[23]

The failure of gadolinium-enhanced MRI to detect the majority of small (<1 cm) HCCs has led investigators to evaluate other hepatic contrast agents. One of the most extensively studied hepatic agents for detection of HCC is superparamagnetic iron oxide or ferumoxides. Superparamagnetic iron oxide particles are taken up by

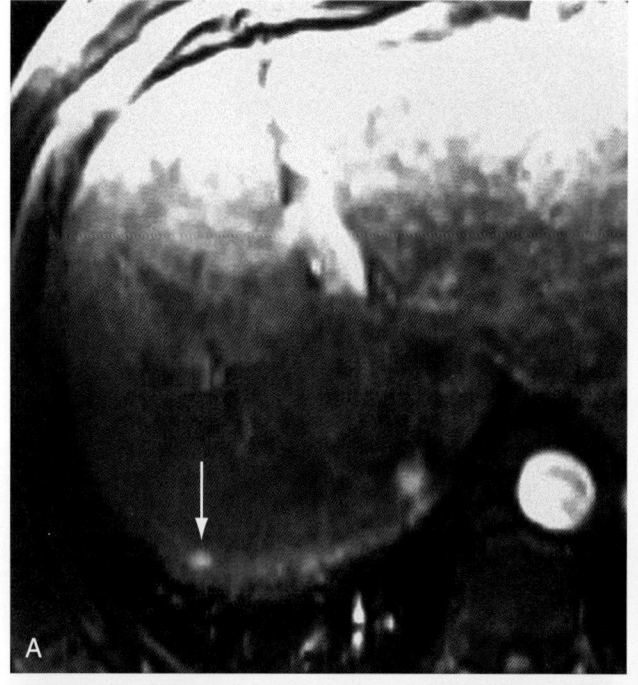

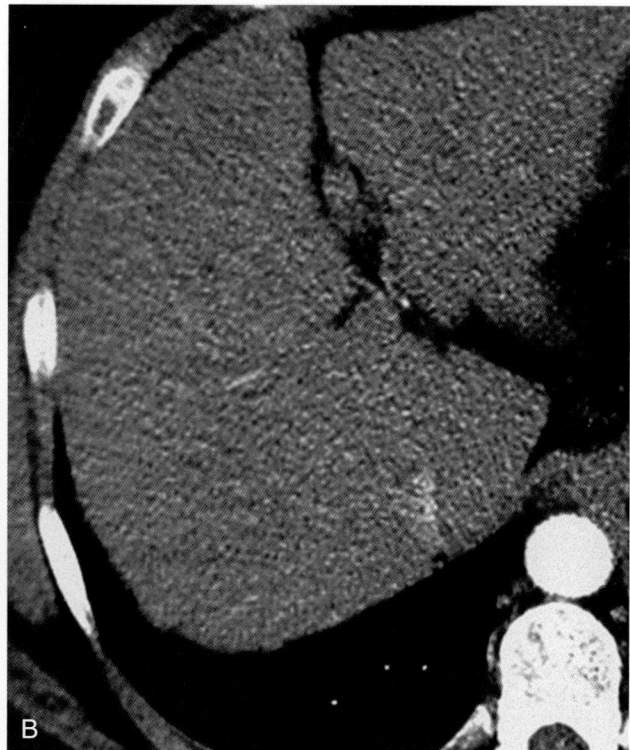

FIGURE 83-4

Interval growth of arterially enhancing nodule detected with MRI but not visualized with multiphase CT. **A,** Axial arterial phase gradient-echo image through the liver of a patient with hepatitis C demonstrates a tiny enhancing focus within the right lobe (*arrow*). **B,** Follow-up dual-phase CT scan performed approximately 4 months later was interpreted as negative. **C,** Follow-up axial arterial phase gradient-echo image performed 9 months after **A** demonstrates interval growth of the lesion (*arrow*), a finding of concern for malignancy.

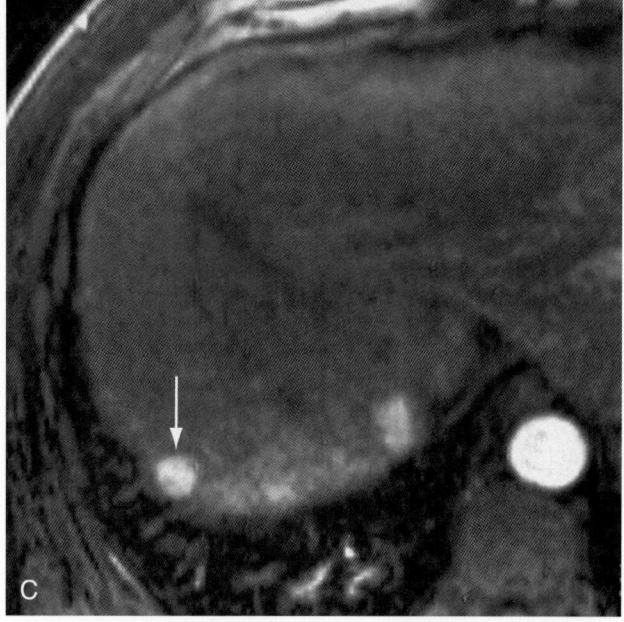

functioning Kupffer cells found in normal liver but rarely present in malignant tumors. MR imaging of the liver following ferumoxides administration employs T2- or T2*-weighted techniques, which demonstrate signal loss of normal liver, increasing the conspicuity of high signal intensity foci of HCC. Ferumoxides-enhanced MRI has a reported per patient sensitivity of 85% for the detection of malignant hepatic lesions in patients awaiting liver transplantation.[24] However, several studies directly comparing ferumoxides-enhanced MRI to dynamic gadolinium-enhanced imaging reported higher sensitivity and lesion conspicuity for the latter technique.[25-27] Ferumoxides-enhanced imaging may be performed in addition to dynamic gadolinium-enhanced imaging with

sensitivity for detection of HCC of greater than 90% for tumors larger than 1 cm. However, as with gadolinium-enhanced imaging alone, sensitivity drops considerably for lesions smaller than 1 cm in diameter.[28] Smaller HCC lesions may be relatively well differentiated and contain sufficient numbers of Kupffer cells to limit the utility of ferumoxides-enhanced imaging.[29]

The imaging features of HCC in the setting of cirrhosis are quite variable.[30] Many smaller lesions are only visible on the arterial phase of a dynamic gadolinium-enhanced examination, remaining isointense on all other images. Larger lesions are typically mildly hyperintense on T2-weighted images, though they range from very hypointense (due to iron content) to very hyperintense

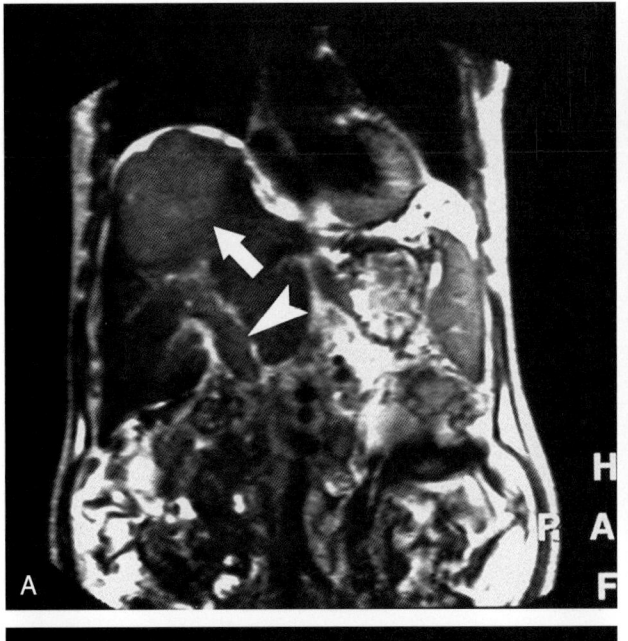

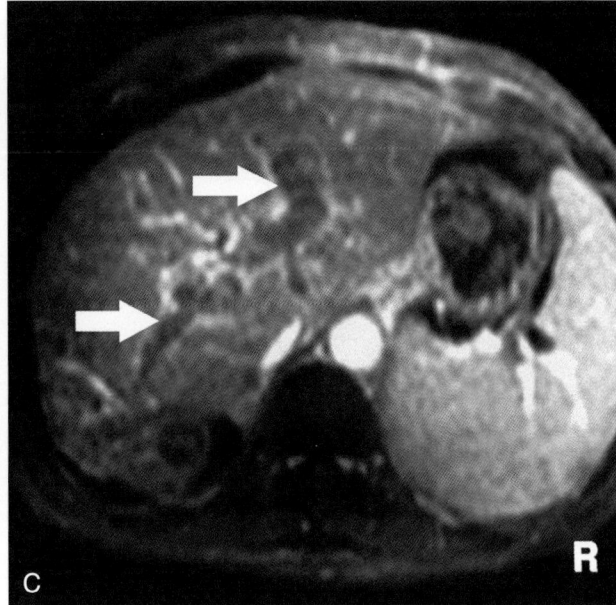

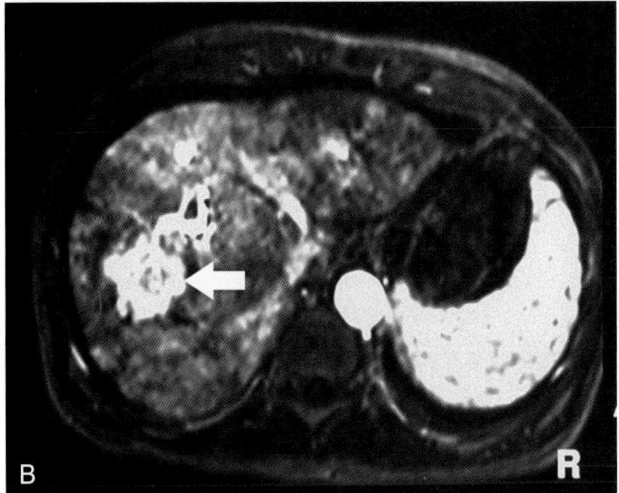

FIGURE 83-5

Hepatocellular carcinoma with invasion of the portal vein. **A,** Coronal T2-weighted single-shot turbo spin-echo sequence shows a large hyperintense mass in the dome of the liver (*arrow*). The portal vein demonstrates abnormally increased signal intensity (*arrowhead*). **B,** Axial arterial phase gradient-echo image through the liver demonstrates brisk arterial enhancement of the inferior portion of the mass (*arrow*). Note the diffusely heterogeneous enhancement of the remainder of the liver due to multifocal disease. **C,** Delayed gadolinium-enhanced image shows the tumor filling the intrahepatic portal veins (*arrows*).

(due to necrosis). On nonenhanced T1-weighted images, HCC is usually hypo- to iso-intense, though high signal intensity lesions may occur. Intracytoplasmic lipid may be present within foci of HCC, manifesting as signal loss on opposed-phase gradient-echo images. Following administration of intravenous gadolinium, lesions of HCC tend to enhance during the arterial phase, with larger lesions enhancing heterogeneously. HCC tends to fade rapidly during subsequent vascular phases, though an enhancing pseudocapsule may persist (see Fig. 83-3). Vascular invasion is common with HCC (Fig. 83-5), typically involving the portal vein and less often the hepatic veins or IVC. Occasionally, confluent hepatic fibrosis may be confused with HCC, as fibrosis demonstrates increased signal intensity relative to liver on T2-weighted images and enhances following gadolinium administration. Although, the enhancement of fibrosis tends to be more conspicuous on delayed images, focal fibrosis may mimic HCC sufficiently to require biopsy.

Additional Findings

Varices are common in patients awaiting liver transplantation and are particularly well demonstrated on gadolinium-enhanced portal phase images (Fig. 83-6). Portal vein thrombosis manifests as an intravascular filling defect when acute or nonocclusive (Fig. 83-7) and may be associated with heterogeneous parenchymal enhancement on dynamic gadolinium-enhanced images. In chronic portal vein thrombosis, often referred to as cavernous transformation of the portal vein, the normal portal vein cannot be identified. Instead, numerous tortuous periportal collateral veins are present in the expected location of the portal vein (Fig. 83-8). Lymphadenopathy is common in the setting of viral hepatitis and cirrhosis and does not necessarily imply metastatic disease, even in the presence of intrahepatic HCC. Lymph nodes are well demonstrated as high signal intensity structures on fat-suppressed T2-weighted images and are commonly present in the region of the

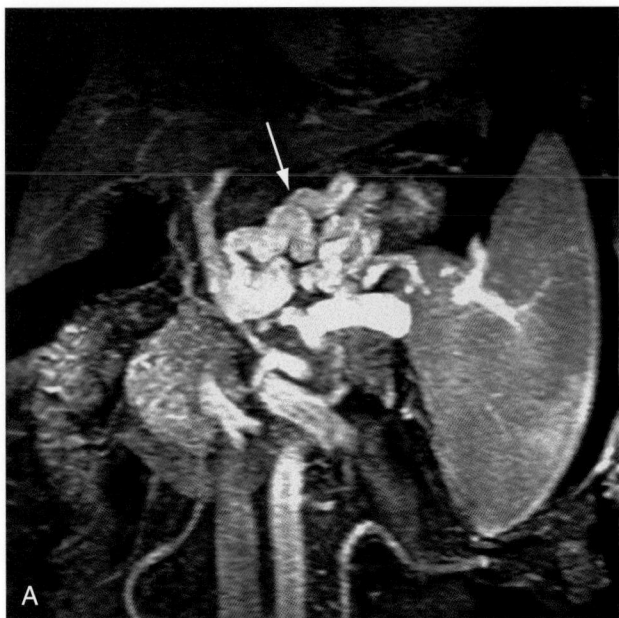 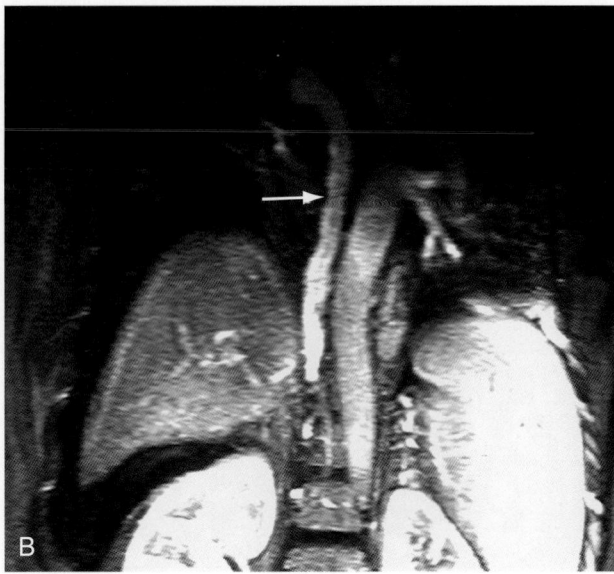

FIGURE 83-6

Varices in a patient awaiting liver transplantation. **A,** Coronal image during the portal phase of a dynamic 3D gadolinium-enhanced gradient-echo acquisition demonstrates large gastroesophageal varices supplied predominantly by the left gastric vein (*arrow*). **B,** More posterior image from the same study as **A** shows a dilated azygous vein (*arrow*) draining the varices.

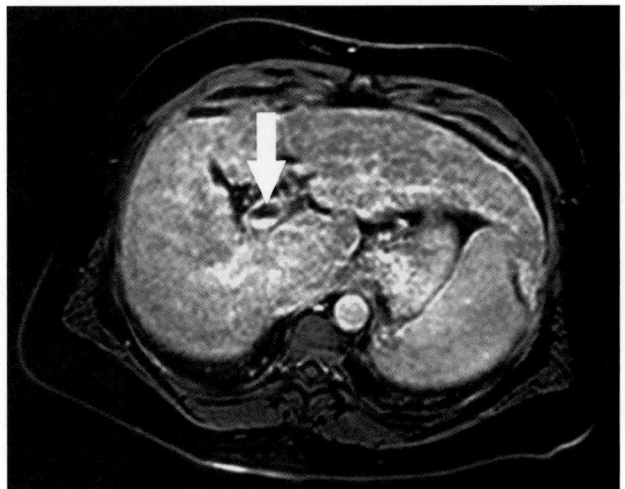

FIGURE 83-7

Portal vein thrombus. Axial fat-suppressed gadolinium-enhanced image through the portal hepatic vein demonstrates a low signal intensity thrombus (*arrow*) within the portal vein.

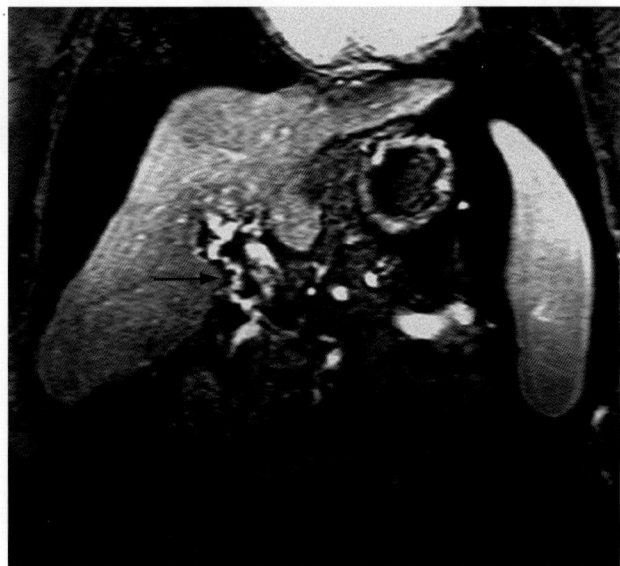

FIGURE 83-8

Chronic portal vein thrombosis. Coronal gadolinium-enhanced gradient-echo image demonstrates periportal collateral veins (*arrow*) in the expected location of the portal vein.

portal vein or portocaval space. Many patients awaiting liver transplantation require transjugular intrahepatic portosystemic shunting (TIPS) to control variceal bleeding or intractable ascites until a new liver becomes available. The appearance of TIPS on MR imaging depends in part on the composition of the stent. Stainless steel stents are currently most prevalent and create a characteristic signal void between the portal vein and IVC (Fig. 83-9). TIPS may complicate liver transplantation when the stent extends into the right atrium or far into the main portal vein, since the surgeon usually will need to have access to and adequate vessel length of normal (non-TIPS) vessel above and below the stent itself for vascular reconstruction. Therefore, the precise location of the stent(s) relative to the right atrium and portal vein should be reported to the transplant surgeon.

Vascular Anomalies

Vascular anomalies are often encountered during MR imaging of liver transplant candidates. Common arterial anomalies include replaced or accessory right (Fig. 83-10) and left hepatic arteries. Occasionally, there may be an unsuspected arterial abnormality present in a transplant recipient that may compromise blood flow to the transplanted liver, such as compression of the celiac artery origin by the median arcuate ligament (Fig. 83-11). Therefore, the entire arterial supply should be closely scrutinized. Venous anomalies may also complicate liver transplantation surgery. They are particularly common in patients with biliary atresia, a condition that may be associated with azygous continuation of the IVC or a preduodenal portal vein.

MR IMAGING EVALUATION OF POTENTIAL LIVING LIVER DONORS

There were over 17,000 waiting-list candidates for liver transplants at the end of 2003 (based on Organ Procurement and Transplantation Network data, December 27, 2003). Unfortunately, the number of patients awaiting new livers far exceeds the number of available organs at any given time. Therefore, several novel methods of expanding the liver donor pool have recently been developed to narrow this gap. Among these is live donor liver transplantation, during which the graft is obtained from a healthy live volunteer donor. Typically, the right hemiliver serves as the graft for an adult recipient. Alternatively, the left lateral segment may be used for a pediatric patient. Living donor transplantation offers the additional benefits of elective timing and shorter ischemia times. To ensure survival of both donor and recipient, careful mapping of the vascular and biliary anatomy and exclusion of significant parenchymal abnormalities in the donor are critical. A recent study demonstrated surgically important hepatic vascular variants in 65% of 107 donor and recipient living liver transplant candidates.[31]

While either CT or MRI can theoretically evaluate the hepatic vessels in sufficient detail to determine the suitability of a potential liver donor, MRCP provides superior evaluation of the biliary tree compared with a standard multiphase contrast-enhanced CT scan. As a result, MRI has been proposed as a comprehensive preoperative imaging modality capable of replacing CT, catheter angiography, and endoscopic retrograde choledochopancreatography (ERCP) for the evaluation of living adult liver donors.[32-35]

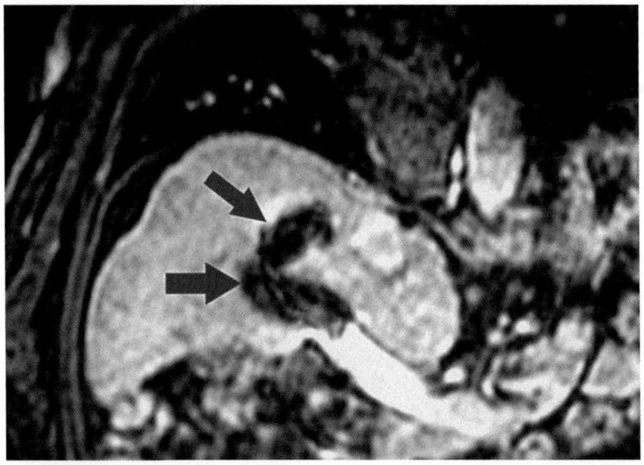

FIGURE 83-9

Transjugular intrahepatic portosystemic shunting (TIPS) artifact. Oblique coronal reformation of gadolinium-enhanced gradient-echo acquisition of a patient with TIPS created using a stent composed of stainless steel alloy demonstrates signal void (*arrows*) extending from the portal vein toward the inferior vena cava.

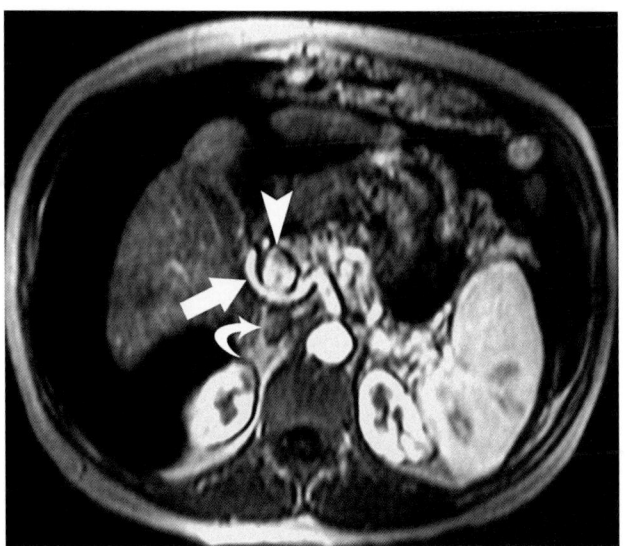

FIGURE 83-10

Replaced right hepatic artery arising from the superior mesenteric artery in a patient awaiting liver transplantation. Axial gadolinium-enhanced gradient-echo image demonstrates the replaced right hepatic artery (*arrow*) coursing between the portal vein (*arrowhead*) and the inferior vena cava (*curved arrow*).

Vascular Anatomy

Evaluation of the arterial anatomy has traditionally been accomplished with a gadolinium-enhanced coronal 3D gradient-echo sequence performed during the arterial phase. However, as 3D gradient-echo sequences improve, allowing acquisitions with isotropic voxel size, there is likely to be a trend toward axial acquisition with

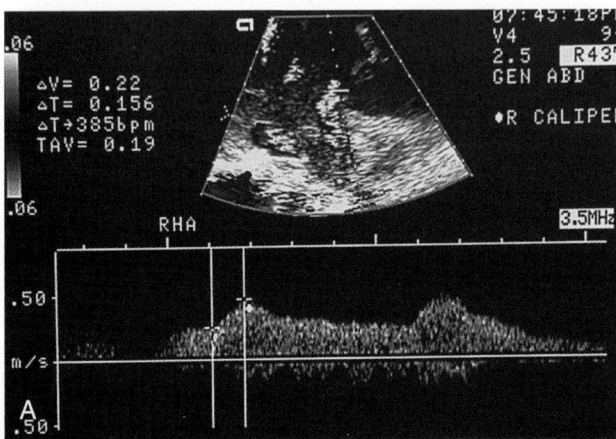
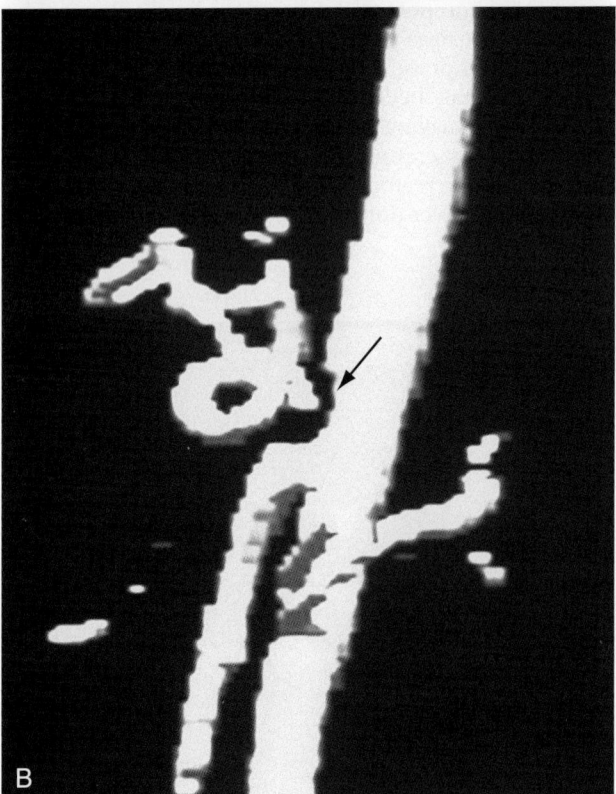

FIGURE 83-11

Unsuspected median arcuate ligament compression. **A,** Duplex sonography image demonstrates abnormal hepatic artery waveform with prolonged systolic acceleration time in a patient recently status post orthotopic liver transplantation. **B,** Shaded surface display of gadolinium-enhanced MR angiogram performed the same day as **A** demonstrates severe stenosis of celiac origin (*arrow*) and a widely patent anastomosis (not shown). Median arcuate ligament compression was confirmed at surgery.

reconstruction of the arterial anatomy in other planes. Therefore, the MR imaging protocol used to evaluate potential living, related liver donors resembles that for recipients with the necessary addition of high-quality MRCP images to identify bile duct variants that would exclude or complicate hemiliver donation. The inclusion of in- and opposed-phase gradient-echo images is essential to detect the presence of hepatic steatosis in the proposed liver donor. Such a finding is an indication for donor liver biopsy at many centers and may necessitate dietary alterations on the part of the proposed donor.

Successful living liver donation depends upon finding a relatively avascular plane of transection in the donor. This is important to ensure that both the portion of remaining liver in the donor and the transplanted graft have sufficient blood supply and drainage to prevent postoperative ischemia and venous congestion. The usual hepatectomy plane for right hemiliver donation in adults is just to the right of the middle hepatic vein (Fig. 83-12). Segments 4, 5, and 8 border the typical hepatectomy plane between the right and left lobes of the liver. Therefore, it is critical to carefully note the arterial supply and venous drainage of these segments for every potential liver donor.

In a study with multidetector row CT it was found that only 31 of 100 consecutive potential living liver donors had conventional hepatic vascular anatomy.[36] In this study, an artery supplying segment 4 arose from the right hepatic artery and traversed the proposed hepatectomy plane in 7% of patients. Extrahepatic hepatic artery variants are also common. The most

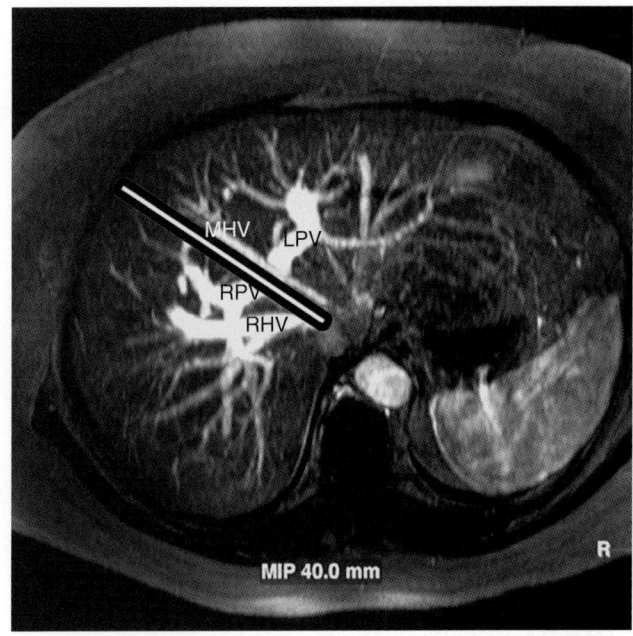

FIGURE 83-12

Transection plane for living liver donation. Axial partial volume maximum intensity projection (MIP) image demonstrates the typical transection plane in a patient with standard venous anatomy. LPV, left portal vein; MHV, middle hepatic vein; RHV, right hepatic vein; RPV, right portal vein.

common variations are a replaced or accessory right hepatic artery arising from the superior mesenteric artery, a replaced or accessory left hepatic artery arising from the left gastric artery, or a combination of these variants. A replaced or accessory right hepatic artery is easily located, passing between the portal vein and IVC on axial images (see Fig. 83-10). A replaced or accessory left hepatic artery is typically found coursing in the fissure for the ligamentum venosum on axial MR images. On coronal images, a replaced or accessory left hepatic artery has a characteristic course as it arises from the left gastric artery which resembles the number "7" (Fig. 83-13).

Because the hepatectomy plane in living liver donation is to the right of the middle hepatic vein, the venous drainage of segments 5 and 8 is of particular interest on preoperative imaging studies. One study examining the anatomy of the middle hepatic vein on multidetector row CT found that a right hepatectomy would avoid transecting major branches of the middle hepatic vein in only one third of patients.[37] Failure to recognize sizeable veins draining from these segments into the middle hepatic vein may result in significant postoperative venous congestion in the graft. To prevent this complication, large tributaries of the middle hepatic vein draining the right lobe of the liver may require reimplantation in the recipient (Fig. 83-14). A surgeon can determine the hemodynamic significance of middle hepatic vein tributaries intraoperatively by temporarily clamping the hepatic artery and looking for discoloration of the liver surface or Doppler ultrasound abnormalities.[38] In a series of 30 adult patients receiving right liver grafts, middle hepatic vein reconstruction was considered prudent in 18 grafts based on intraoperative findings of paramedian sector congestion.[39] As with

middle hepatic vein tributaries, large accessory hepatic veins draining the right hepatic lobe may require implantation in the recipient (Fig. 83-15). Nakamura et al reported such accessory hepatic veins (>5 mm) in 30% of 120 right lobe grafts they examined.[40]

Following hemiliver transplantation, hepatic congestion may manifest as increased signal intensity on T2-weighted images, a finding reported in segments 5 and 8 in 88% and 85%, respectively, of right lobe grafts implanted without anterior segment venous drainage reconstruction.[41] In most cases, this signal intensity abnormality, thought to result from tissue edema, resolves spontaneously. Accessory hepatic veins and middle hepatic vein tributaries less than 5 mm in diameter are typically sacrificed at the time of graft harvest.

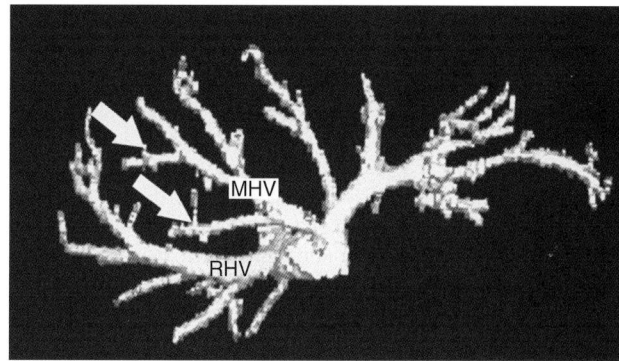

FIGURE 83-14

Middle hepatic vein tributaries. Shaded surface display of venous phase MR angiography shows two large middle hepatic vein tributaries (*arrows*) draining portions of the right lobe. MHV, middle hepatic vein; RHV, right hepatic vein.

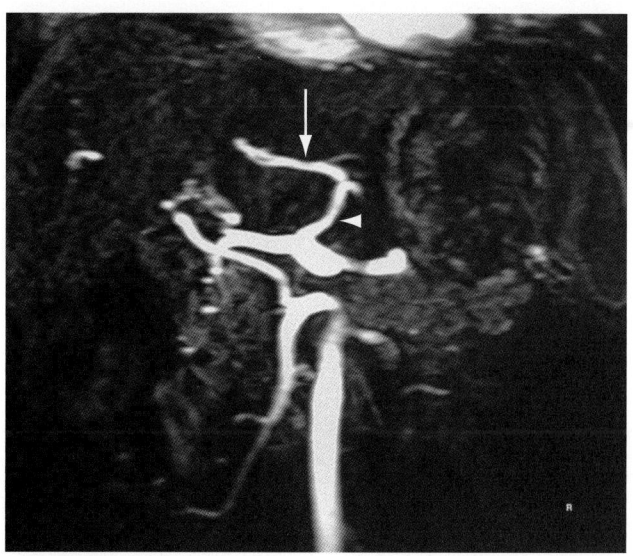

FIGURE 83-13

Accessory left hepatic artery. Partial volume maximum intensity projection MR angiography image through the celiac vessels shows typical appearance of the left hepatic artery (*arrow*) arising from the left gastric artery (*arrowhead*).

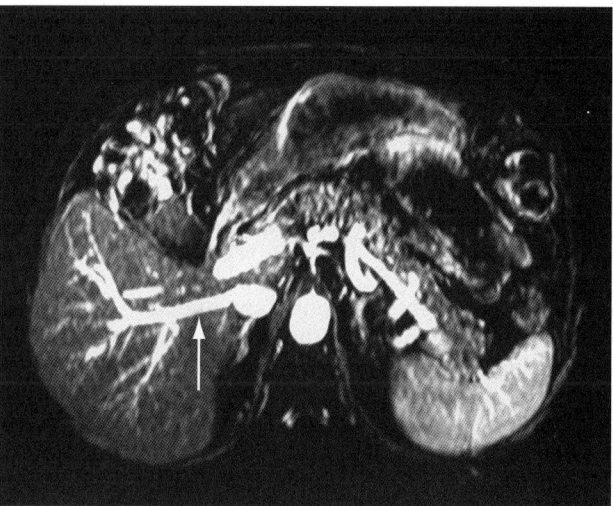

FIGURE 83-15

Large accessory right hepatic vein. Axial partial volume maximum intensity projection of venous phase gadolinium-enhanced image through the caudal right lobe of the liver demonstrates a large right inferior accessory hepatic vein (*arrow*) draining into the inferior vena cava.

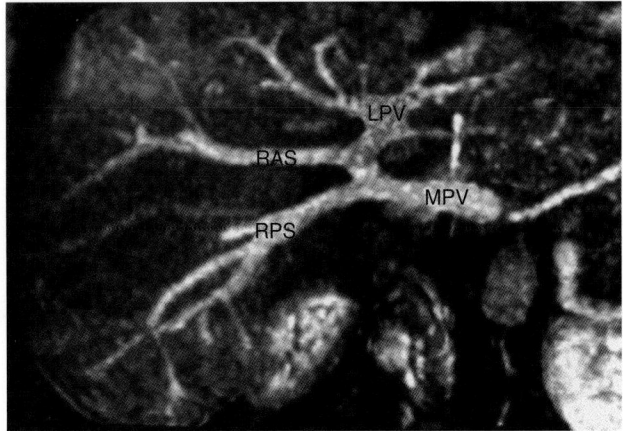

FIGURE 83-16

Anomalous portal vein branching. Oblique axial maximum intensity projection gadolinium-enhanced image shows separate origins of the right anterior and posterior segmental veins. LPV, left portal vein; MPV, main portal vein; RAS, right anterior segment portal branch; RPS, right posterior segment portal branch.

Anomalous portal venous branching may also complicate living donor liver transplantation. Division of the main portal vein into separate right posterior, right anterior, and left branches is referred to as a trifurcation. Alternately, the right anterior branch and left branch may share a common trunk, with the right posterior branch having a separate, more proximal origin (Fig. 83-16). Both of these variants may complicate graft harvest and require back table reconstruction to permit a single portal anastomosis in the recipient. Uncommonly, some or all of the portal venous supply to segment 4 may arise from the right portal vein and traverse the hepatectomy plane. Other portal venous branching variations may occur but are much less common.

Biliary Anomalies

Biliary variants are commonly encountered on MRCP images and may have important implications for living hemiliver donation. In most individuals, the common hepatic duct is formed from separate right and left hepatic ducts, with the right duct formed by the confluence of anterior and posterior segment tributaries. A large number of potential bile duct variations exist, though the more common variants are defined by the site of drainage of the right posterior segment duct.[40] In approximately 9% of individuals, the common hepatic duct is formed by a triple confluence of the anterior segment, posterior segment, and left hepatic ducts (Fig. 83-17). The right posterior segment duct may also drain into the left hepatic duct in approximately 16% of individuals (Fig. 83-18). Somewhat less commonly, the right posterior segment duct may drain into the right lateral wall of the common hepatic duct. Accessory right or left hepatic ducts may also be present and have variable sites of insertion. When the orifices for the right anterior and posterior segment ducts are far apart, separate biliary anastomoses are required in the recipient.

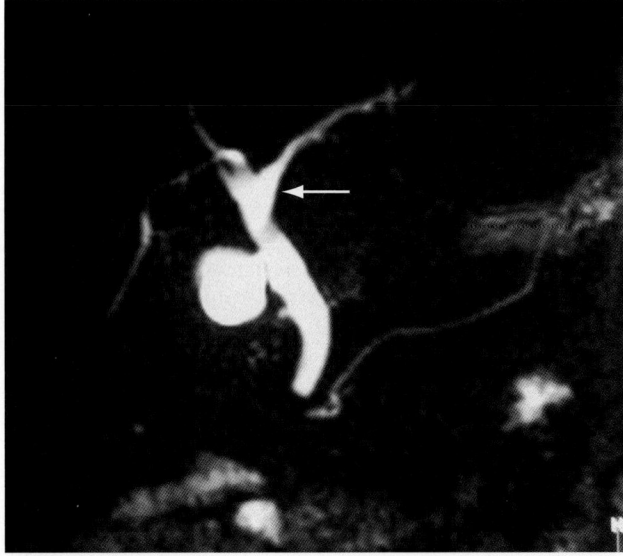

FIGURE 83-17

Biliary triple confluence. Thick-slab MR cholangiopancreatography image shows the posterior segment duct, anterior segment duct, and left duct converging at a single location (*arrow*).

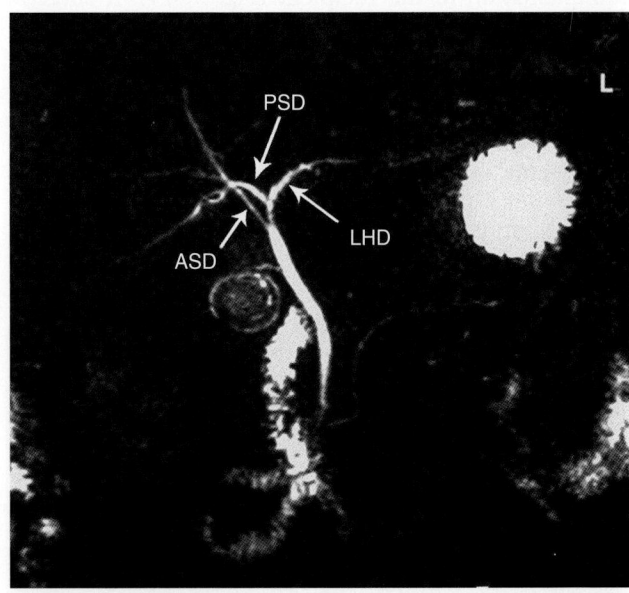

FIGURE 83-18

Variant biliary anatomy. Thick-slab MR cholangiopancreatography image shows the right posterior segment bile duct draining into the left hepatic duct. ASD, anterior segment duct; LHD, left hepatic duct; PSD, posterior segment duct.

Failure to recognize biliary anomalies preoperatively may endanger the donor or recipient by impairing critical biliary drainage from a portion of the remaining liver or graft. Therefore, the bile ducts must be clearly visualized on MRCP images. While heavily T2-weighted sequences typically used for MRCP are excellent for visualizing the static fluid within dilated obstructed bile

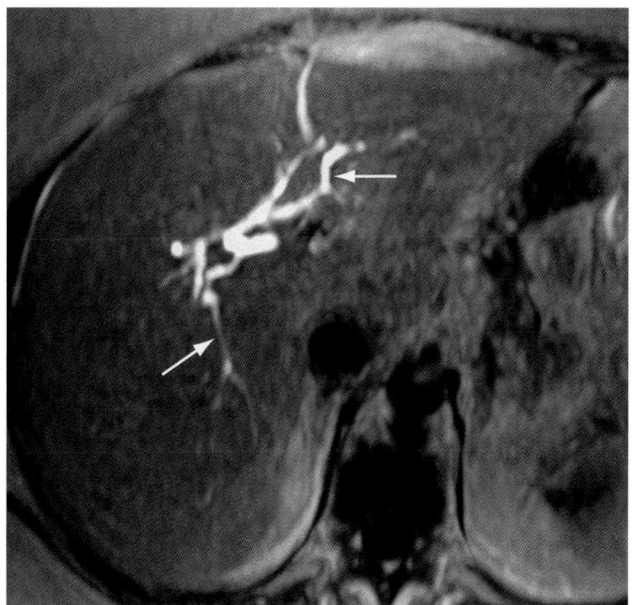

FIGURE 83-19

MR cholangiography utilizing hepatobiliary agent. Axial maximum intensity projection image from a 3D gradient-echo acquisition performed 30 minutes after intravenous administration of mangafodipir trisodium. Note the non-distended high signal intensity intrahepatic ducts (*arrows*).

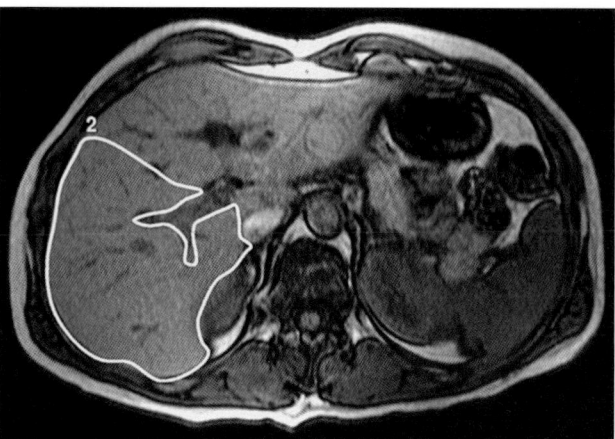

FIGURE 83-20

Example of region of interest for calculation of right hemiliver volume. Note that the major vascular structures are omitted. On some images, it may be necessary to extrapolate the course of the middle hepatic vein.

ducts, visualization of normal caliber intrahepatic ducts may be suboptimal with these techniques. This has led to interest in the use of hepatobiliary MR contrast agents for visualizing normal intrahepatic ducts in living hemiliver donors. Limited data support the use of mangafodipir trisodium, a manganese-based paramagnetic MR contrast agent, to evaluate nondistended bile ducts in potential living hemiliver donors.[42,43] The manganese is taken up by normal hepatocytes and excreted in the bile, resulting in high signal intensity bile ducts on T1-weighted images (Fig. 83-19).

Hepatic Lobe Volumes

Accurate determination of the volumes of the right and left hepatic lobes is an important part of every preoperative hemiliver donor evaluation. Liver volumes are critical in determining whether the graft and the remaining liver will have sufficient functional capacity to sustain life in the recipient and donor, respectively. While the precise minimum necessary graft size to proceed with living hemiliver donation varies slightly by institution, grafts that are less than 1% of the recipient's body weight have been reported to have a lower success rate than larger grafts.[44] For donors, approximately 30% of the total liver volume must remain to ensure adequate residual function.[45] Volume and mass measurements obtained with MRI correlate reasonably well with operative findings.[46,47] Differences of greater than 20% are uncommon and may result from the need to extrapolate the course of the middle hepatic vein on some axial images. Based on serial MRI measurements,

both donor and recipient liver regenerate after living liver transplantation, with the greatest percentage increase in mass occurring in the first postoperative week.[48] In this study, a calculated graft-to-recipient bodyweight ratio of 0.8% was found to be adequate for right lobe living donor liver transplantation.

Volumetric analysis of the right and left hepatic lobes may be performed on any sequence that clearly depicts the relevant vasculature and liver boundaries. To simplify calculation, one sequence may be performed with a slice thickness and gap totaling 1 cm, allowing the areas determined on axial images (in cm^2) to be added together to yield the volume. Any slice gap must be taken into consideration when calculating the volume. Regions of interest are drawn assuming the middle hepatic vein to be the boundary between the right and left lobes, and major vessels and the gallbladder are excluded (Fig. 83-20). The caudate lobe typically remains with the donor.

Several series have demonstrated the potential of MRI to serve as the sole preoperative imaging examination for potential living liver donors.[46,47,49,50] In such studies, MRI assessment of the vascular and biliary systems has correlated well with intraoperative findings and other imaging studies (e.g. intraoperative cholangiography and catheter angiography).

FOLLOW-UP OF LIVER TRANSPLANT RECIPIENTS

Because sonography is relatively inexpensive, readily available, and sensitive for detecting abnormalities of the blood vessels, bile ducts, and hepatic parenchyma, it will likely remain the initial imaging technique of choice for the postoperative evaluation of liver transplants for the foreseeable future. However, sonography is highly operator dependent, often relies on secondary signs

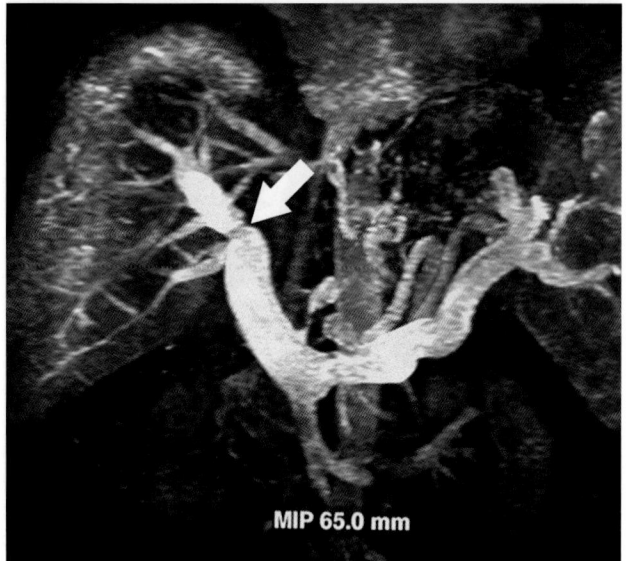

FIGURE 83-25

Normal portal venous anastomosis. Coronal maximum intensity projection portal phase gadolinium-enhanced MR angiography image shows mild focal narrowing (*arrow*) at the portal vein anastomosis in a patient status post right hemiliver transplantation.

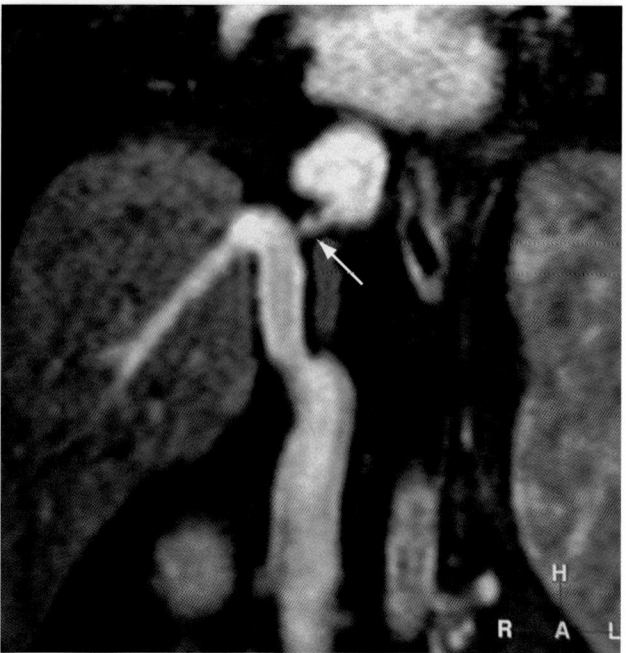

FIGURE 83-26

Stenosis of inferior vena cava anastomosis. Coronal gadolinium-enhanced MR angiography image demonstrates severe narrowing of the superior anastomosis (*arrow*).

hemodynamic significance is frequently present at the portal anastomosis and should not be confused with significant stenosis (Fig. 83-25).

Systemic Venous Complications

Anastomotic stricture and thrombosis within the IVC and hepatic veins are relatively uncommon following liver transplantation.[62] Often, the locations of the IVC anastomoses can be identified by the presence of subtle susceptibility artifacts related to the suture material. Flow-sensitive or gadolinium-enhanced MRA techniques can be used to demonstrate intracaval thrombus or stenosis. Stenosis is well demonstrated on coronal or sagittal images (Fig. 83-26).

Biliary Complications

Biliary complications may occur in 11.5% to 30% of patients following liver transplantation.[63-66] Heavily T2-weighted MRCP sequences are highly sensitive and accurate for evaluation of biliary complications after liver transplantation.[56,57,59] Biliary strictures occur most often at anastomotic sites and may result in dilatation of the proximal bile ducts (Fig. 83-27). However, proximal biliary dilatation may be absent in some cases of anastomotic stricture.[53,67] Nonanastomotic strictures may result from biliary ischemia secondary to hepatic artery thrombosis (Fig. 83-28). Severe biliary ischemia results in bile duct necrosis, which may be associated with bile leaks and biloma formation (Fig. 83-29). Bile leaks may also occur adjacent to the anastomotic site. While standard heavily T2-weighted MRCP images may

suffice for evaluation of some bile leaks, there is evidence to support the use of hepatobiliary agents such as mangafodipir trisodium for this purpose.[68] Bile leaks are usually clinically evident within the first few months after liver transplantation; however, fibrotic strictures may take months to years to develop. Choledocholithiasis may occasionally be diagnosed following liver transplantation (Fig. 83-30). Mucocele of the cystic duct remnant is easily identified on MRCP sequences as cystic dilatation of the cystic duct and may cause obstruction of the common hepatic duct through mass effect. Occasionally, the transplant recipient's extra-hepatic bile duct remnant is also incidentally visible on MRCP images.

Other Complications

In addition to its utility in diagnosing complications of the vascular and biliary systems, MRI is useful for evaluating the liver parenchyma and perihepatic structures following liver transplantation. Hepatic or splenic infarction, hematoma or abscess formation, post-transplant lymphoproliferative disorder, and recurrent malignant tumor may be detected with MRI. Areas of infarction may appear as wedge-shaped or peripheral nonenhancing regions on contrast-enhanced images. Hematomas will often demonstrate areas of increased signal intensity on T1-weighted images resulting from the presence of methemoglobin. Abscess may be difficult to distinguish from sterile biloma or hematoma with certainty, but the presence of a thick enhancing wall common.[70,71] Within the liver, PTLD may occur as a focal parenchymal mass, an ill-defined area of parenchymal infiltration, or as infiltrating periportal soft-tissue.[71,72]

Transplant recipients with a history of chronic viral hepatitis are at risk for reinfection of the donor liver after transplantation. Although it may take 30 years for cirrhosis to develop in a reinfected liver, this time course is markedly accelerated in some patients. Periodic imaging can be used in conjunction with clinical and laboratory surveillance to monitor post-transplant patients for recurrence of cirrhosis. Recurrent cirrhosis can sometimes be successfully treated with a second transplant.

Acknowledgment

We thank William C. Chapman, MD, Professor of Surgery at Washington University School of Medicine, for his helpful comments.

REFERENCES

1. Fuster J, Garcia-Valdecasas JC, Grande L, et al: Hepatocellular carcinoma and cirrhosis: results of surgical treatment in a European series. Ann Surg 223:297-302, 1996.
2. Suarez Y, Franca AC, Llovet JM, et al: The current status of liver transplantation for primary hepatic malignancy. Clin Liver Dis 4:591-605, 2000.
3. Figueras J, Ibanez L, Ramos E, et al: Selection criteria for liver transplantation in early-stage hepatocellular carcinoma with cirrhosis: results of a multicenter study. Liver Transpl 7:877-883, 2001.
4. Mazzaferro V, Regalia E, Doci R, et al: Liver transplantation for the treatment of small hepatocellular carcinomas in patients with cirrhosis. N Engl J Med 334:693-699, 1996.
5. Yao FY, Ferrell L, Bass NM, et al: Liver transplantation for hepatocellular carcinoma: expansion of the tumor size limits does not adversely impact survival. Hepatology 33:1394-1403, 2001.
6. Tzakis A, Todo S, Starzl TE: Orthotopic liver transplantation with preservation of the inferior vena cava. Ann Surg 210:649-652, 1989.
7. Yoshioka H, Takahashi N, Yamaguchi M, et al: Double arterial phase dynamic MRI with sensitivity encoding (SENSE) for hypervascular hepatocellular carcinomas. J Magn Reson Imaging 16:259-266, 2002.
8. Caldwell SH, de Lange EE, Gaffey MJ, et al: Accuracy and significance of pretransplant liver volume measured by magnetic resonance imaging. Liver Transpl Surg 2:438-442, 1996.
9. Zoli M, Cordiani MR, Marchesini G, et al: Prognostic indicators in compensated cirrhosis. Am J Gastroenterol 86:1508-1513, 1991.
10. Schiano TD, Bodian C, Schwartz ME, et al: Accuracy and significance of computed tomographic scan assessment of hepatic volume in patients undergoing liver transplantation. Transplantation 69:545-550, 2000.
11. Dodd GD 3rd, Baron RL, Oliver JH 3rd, et al: Spectrum of imaging findings of the liver in end-stage cirrhosis: part I, gross morphology and diffuse abnormalities. Am J Roentgenol 173:1031-1036, 1999.
12. Krinsky GA, Israel G: Nondysplastic nodules that are hyperintense on T1-weighted gradient-echo MR imaging: frequency in cirrhotic patients undergoing transplantation. Am J Roentgenol 180:1023-1027, 2003.
13. Jeong YY, Mitchell DG, Kamishima T: Small (<20 mm) enhancing hepatic nodules seen on arterial phase MR imaging of the cirrhotic liver: clinical implications. Am J Roentgenol 178:1327-1334, 2002.
14. Shimizu A, Ito K, Koike S, et al: Cirrhosis or chronic hepatitis: evaluation of small (≤2 cm) early-enhancing hepatic lesions with serial contrast-enhanced dynamic MR imaging. Radiology 226:550-555, 2003.
15. Burrel M, Llovet JM, Ayuso C, et al: MRI angiography is superior to helical CT for detection of HCC prior to liver transplantation: an explant correlation. Hepatology 38:1034-1042, 2003.
16. Libbrecht L, Bielen D, Verslype C, et al: Focal lesions in cirrhotic explant livers: pathological evaluation and accuracy of pretransplantation imaging examinations. Liver Transplantation 8:749-761, 2002.
17. Stoker J, Romijn MG, de Man RA, et al: Prospective comparative study of spiral computer tomography and magnetic resonance imaging for detection of hepatocellular carcinoma. Gut 51:105-107, 2002.
18. Rode A, Bancel B, Douek P, et al: Small nodule detection in cirrhotic livers: evaluation with US, spiral CT, and MRI and correlation with pathologic examination of explanted liver. J Comput Assist Tomogr 25:327-336, 2001.
19. Noguchi Y, Murakami T, Kim T, et al: Detection of hypervascular hepatocellular carcinoma by dynamic magnetic resonance imaging with double-echo chemical shift in-phase and opposed-phase gradient echo technique: comparison with dynamic helical computed tomography imaging with double arterial phase. J Comput Assist Tomogr 26:981-987, 2002.
20. de Ledinghen V, Laharie D, Lecesne R, et al: Detection of nodules in liver cirrhosis: spiral computed tomography or magnetic resonance imaging? A prospective study of 88 nodules in 34 patients. Eur J Gastroenterol Hepatol 14:159-165, 2002.
21. Hori M, Murakami T, Kim T, et al: Detection of hypervascular hepatocellular carcinoma: comparison of SPIO-enhanced MRI with dynamic helical CT. J Comput Assist Tomogr 26:701-710, 2002.
22. Kang BK, Lim JH, Kim SH, et al: Pre-operative depiction of hepatocellular carcinoma: ferumoxides-enhanced MR imaging versus triple-phase helical CT. Radiology 226:79-85, 2003.
23. Krinsky GA, Lee VS, Theise ND, et al: Transplantation for hepatocellular carcinoma and cirrhosis: sensitivity of magnetic resonance imaging. Liver Transplantation 8:1156-1164, 2002.
24. Mori K, Scheidler J, Helmberger T, et al: Detection of malignant hepatic lesions before orthotopic liver transplantation: accuracy of ferumoxides-enhanced MR imaging. Am J Roentgenol 179:1045-1051, 2002.
25. Tang Y, Yamashita Y, Arakawa A, et al: Detection of hepatocellular carcinoma arising in cirrhotic livers: comparison of gadolinium- and ferumoxides-enhanced MR imaging. Am J Roentgenol 172:1547-1554, 1999.
26. Matsuo M, Kanematsu M, Itoh K, et al: Detection of malignant hepatic tumors: comparison of gadolinium- and ferumoxide-enhanced MR imaging. Am J Roentgenol 177:637-643, 2001.
27. Pauleit D, Textor J, Bachmann R, et al: Hepatocellular carcinoma: detection with gadolinium- and ferumoxides-enhanced MR imaging of the liver. Radiology 222:73-80, 2002.
28. Bhartia B, Ward J, Guthrie JA, et al: Hepatocellular carcinoma in cirrhotic livers: double-contrast thin-section MR imaging with pathologic correlation of explanted tissue. Am J Roentgenol 180:577-584, 2003.
29. Tanaka M, Nakashima O, Wada Y, et al: Pathomorphological study of Kupffer cells in hepatocellular carcinoma and hyperplastic nodular lesions in the liver. Hepatology 24:807-812, 1996.
30. Kelekis NL, Semelka RC, Worawattanakul S, et al: Hepatocellular carcinoma in North America: a multiinstitutional study of appearance on T1-weighted, T2-weighted, and serial gadolinium-enhanced gradient echo images. Am J Roentgenol 170:1005-1013, 1998.
31. Erbay N, Raptopoulos V, Pomfret EA, et al: Living donor liver transplantation in adults: vascular variants important in surgical planning for donors and recipients. Am J Roentgenol 181:109-114, 2003.
32. Fulcher AS, Szucs RA, Bassignani MJ, et al: Right lobe living donor liver transplantation: preoperative evaluation of the donor with MR imaging. Am J Roentgenol 176:1483-1491, 2001.
33. Lee VS, Morgan GR, Teperman LW, et al: MR imaging as the sole preoperative imaging modality for right hepatectomy: a prospective study of living adult-to-adult liver donor candidates. Am J Roentgenol 176:1475-1482, 2001.
34. Cheng YF, Chen CL, Huang TL, et al: Single imaging modality evaluation of living donors in liver transplantation: magnetic resonance imaging. Transplantation 72:1527-1533, 2001.
35. Goyen M, Barkhausen J, Debatin JF, et al: Right-lobe living related liver transplantation: evaluation of a comprehensive magnetic resonance imaging protocol for assessing potential donors. Liver Transplantation 8:241-250, 2002.
36. Guiney MJ, Kruskal JB, Sosna J, et al: Multi-detector row CT of relevant vascular anatomy of the surgical plane in split-liver transplantation. Radiology 229:401-407, 2003.
37. Kamel IR, Lawler LP, Fishman EK: Variations in anatomy of the middle hepatic vein and their impact on formal right hepatectomy. Abdom Imaging 28:668-674, 2003.
38. Sano K, Makuuchi M, Miki K, et al: Evaluation of hepatic venous congestion: proposed indication criteria for hepatic vein reconstruction. Ann Surg 236:241-247, 2002.
39. Sugawara Y, Makuuchi M, Sano K, et al: Vein reconstruction in modified right liver graft for living donor liver transplantation. Ann Surg 237:180-185, 2003.
40. Nakamura T, Tanaka K, Kiuchi T, et al: Anatomical variations and surgical strategies in right lobe living donor liver transplantation. Transplantation 73:1896-1903, 2002.
41. Yamamoto H, Maetani Y, Kiuchi T, et al: Background and clinical impact of tissue congestion in right-lobe living-donor liver grafts: a magnetic resonance imaging study. Transplantation 76:164-169, 2003.
42. Lee VS, Rofsky NM, Morgan GR, et al: Volumetric mangafodipir trisodium-enhanced cholangiography to define intrahepatic biliary anatomy. Am J Roentgenol 176:906-908, 2001.
43. Kapoor V, Peterson MS, Baron RL, et al: Intrahepatic biliary anatomy of living adult liver donors: correlation of mangafodipir trisodium-enhanced MR cholangiography and intraoperative cholangiography. Am J Roentgenol 179:1281-1286, 2002.
44. Kiuchi T, Kasahara M, Uryuhara K, et al: Impact of graft size mismatching on graft prognosis in liver transplantation from living donors. Transplantation 67:321-327, 1999.
45. Fan ST, Lo CM, Liu CL, et al: Safety of donors in live donor liver transplantation using right lobe grafts. Arch Surg 135:336-340, 2000.

46. Fulcher AS, Szucs RA, Bassignani MJ, et al: Right lobe living donor liver transplantation: preoperative evaluation of the donor with MR imaging. Am J Roentgenol 176:1483-1491, 2001.

47. Cheng YF, Chen CL, Huang TL, et al: Single imaging modality evaluation of living donors in liver transplantation: magnetic resonance imaging. Transplantation 72:1527-1533, 2001.

48. Marcos A, Fisher RA, Ham JM, et al: Liver regeneration and function in donor and recipient after right lobe adult to adult living donor liver transplantation. Transplantation 69:1375-1379, 2000.

49. Goyen M, Barkhausen J, Debatin JF, et al: Right-lobe living related liver transplantation: evaluation of a comprehensive magnetic resonance imaging protocol for assessing potential donors. Liver Transpl 8:241-250, 2002.

50. Lee VS, Morgan GR, Teperman LW, et al: MR imaging as the sole preoperative imaging modality for right hepatectomy: a prospective study of living adult-to-adult liver donor candidates. Am J Roentgenol 176:1475-1482, 2001.

51. Ito K, Siegelman ES, Stolpen AH, et al: MR imaging of complications after liver transplantation. Am J Roentgenol 2000; 175: 1145-1149.

52. Glockner JF, Forauer AR, Solomon H, et al: Three-dimensional gadolinium-enhanced MR angiography of vascular complications after liver transplantation. Am J Roentgenol 174:1447-1453, 2000.

53. Pandharipande PV, Lee VS, Morgan GR, et al: Vascular and extravascular complications of liver transplantation: comprehensive evaluation with three-dimensional contrast-enhanced volumetric MR imaging and MR cholangiopancreatography. Am J Roentgenol 177:1101-1107, 2001.

54. Boraschi P, Braccini G, Gigoni R, et al: Detection of biliary complications after orthotopic liver transplantation with MR cholangiography. Magn Reson Imaging 19:1097-1105, 2001.

55. Kim BS, Kim TK, Jung DJ, et al: Vascular complications after living related liver transplantation: evaluation with gadolinium-enhanced three-dimensional MR angiography. Am J Roentgenol 181:467-474, 2003.

56. Fulcher AS, Turner MA: Orthotopic liver transplantation: evaluation with MR cholangiography. Radiology 211:715-722, 1999.

57. Laghi A, Pavone P, Catalano C, et al: MR cholangiography of late biliary complications after liver transplantation. Am J Roentgenol 172:1541-1546, 1999.

58. Stafford-Johnson DB, Hamilton BH, Dong Q, et al: Vascular complications of liver transplantation: evaluation with gadolinium-enhanced MR angiography. Radiology 207:153-160, 1998.

59. Meersschaut V, Mortele KJ, Troisi R, et al: Value of MR cholangiography in the evaluation of postoperative biliary complications following orthotopic liver transplantation. Eur Radiol 10:1576-1581, 2000.

60. Stange BJ, Glanemann M, Nuessler NC, et al: Hepatic artery thrombosis after adult liver transplantation. Liver Transpl 9:612-620, 2003.

61. Wozney P, Zajko AB, Bron KM, et al: Vascular complications after liver transplantation: a 5-year experience. Am J Roentgenol 147:657-663, 1986.

62. Settmacher U, Nussler NC, Glanemann M, et al: Venous complications after orthotopic liver transplantation. Clin Transpl 14:235-241, 2000.

63. Lerut J, Gordon RD, Iwatsuki S, et al: Biliary tract complications in human orthotopic liver transplantation. Transplantation 43:47-51, 1987.

64. Greif F, Bronsther OL, Van Thiel DH, et al: The incidence, timing, and management of biliary tract complications after orthotopic liver transplantation. Ann Surg 219:40-45, 1994.

65. Verran DJ, Asfar SK, Ghent CN, et al: Biliary reconstruction without T tubes or stents in liver transplantion: report of 502 consecutive cases. Liver Transpl Surg 3:365-373, 1997.

66. Rabkin JM, Orloff SL, Reed MH, et al: Biliary tract complications of side-to-side without T tube versus end-to-end with or without T tube choledochocholedochostomy in liver transplant recipients. Transplantation 65:193-199, 1998.

67. Campbell WL, Sheng R, Zajko AB, et al: Intrahepatic biliary strictures after liver transplantation. Radiology 191:735-740, 1994.

68. Vitellas KM, El-Dieb A, Vaswani K, et al: Detection of bile leaks using MR cholangiopancreatography with mangafodipir trisodium (Teslascan). J Comput Assist Tomogr 25:102-105, 2001.

69. Duvoux C, Pageaux GP, Vanlemmens C, et al: Risk factors for lymphoproliferative disorders after liver transplantation in adults: an analysis of 480 patients. Transplantation 74:1103-1109, 2002.

70. Jain A, Nalesnik M, Reyes J, et al: Posttransplant lymphoproliferative disorders in liver transplantation: a 20-year experience. Ann Surg 236:429-436, 2002.

71. Pickhardt PJ, Siegel MJ: Posttransplant lymphoproliferative disorder of the abdomen: CT evaluation in 51 patients. Radiology 213:73-78, 1999.

72. Strouse PJ, Platt JF, Francis IR, et al: Tumorous intrahepatic lymphoproliferative disorder in transplanted livers. Am J Roentgenol 167:1159-1162, 1996.

CHAPTER 84

PANCREAS

Dushyant V. Sahani ● Raul N. Uppot

INTRODUCTION

Increasingly, technical advances in MRI have expanded its role as a problem solver for pancreatic diseases. Comprehensive imaging of the pancreas requires evaluation of the pancreatic parenchyma, the pancreatic ducts, the surrounding soft-tissues, and the pancreatic vascularity. Technical advances in MRI, including high-performance gradient systems, phased-array coils, and faster sequences, have improved spatial resolution and allowed for single breath-hold imaging.[1-9] These advances have improved overall imaging of the entire abdomen, including the pancreas. However, specific developments, including half-Fourier T2-weighted pulse sequences for MR cholangiopancreatography (MRCP), secretin stimulation for MRCP, dynamic contrast imaging, and MR angiography, have improved evaluation of disease entities specifically involving the pancreas.[10-18] The focus of this chapter is MR techniques for imaging the pancreas and the role of MRI in evaluating the pancreas.

TECHNIQUES

MR imaging of the pancreas is optimally performed using a high-performance gradient system (1.5 T) with phased-array torso coils to optimize the signal-to-noise ratio (SNR) and tissue contrast.[10-18] Images acquired of the pancreas should be tailored to the question being addressed. Protocols for pancreatic imaging fall into three general categories: 1. lesion detection and characterization; 2. MRCP and secretin-stimulated MRCP for evaluation of the pancreatic ducts; and 3. MR angiography for tumor staging.

Protocol for Lesion Detection/Characterization

MR imaging is performed for further evaluation of a lesion seen on CT or ultrasound, or for a clinically suspected lesion not detected on other imaging modalities. The MR protocol for lesion detection and characterization includes gradient-echo T1-weighted sequence, fat-saturated T1-weighted sequence, T2-weighted sequence, and dynamic post-contrast sequences (Box 84-1).

T1-Weighted Sequence

T1-weighted images provide a gross morphologic examination of the pancreas, and allow clear depiction of the fat planes surrounding the pancreas. T1-weighted sequences may be spin-echo or gradient-echo. Spin-echo sequences usually require long acquisition times and are degraded by respiratory motion. The standard T1 sequence is a gradient-echo sequence, typically with a flip angle of 90 degrees, a repetition time (TR) of 175 to 200 ms, and a time to echo (TE) of 2 to 4 ms. These sequences can be performed as a breath-hold volume acquisition, usually about 18 seconds long, or as a "single-slice" approach, each approximately 1 second, for patients who cannot hold their breath.[18]

Fat-Saturated T1-Weighted Sequence

Fat suppression in the pancreas causes a relative increase in signal of the pancreatic parenchyma. With fat suppression, there is an increase in signal intensity of the pancreatic parenchyma and improved tissue contrast

---

Box 84-1 | **Disease Detection/Characterization Protocol**

1. Localizer: Scout with T2 single-shot fast spin-echo in coronal plane. Scout obtained first with breath-hold and then with normal breathing. TE 180 ms; slice thickness 8 mm; spacing 2 mm.
2. Axial 2D spoiled gradient recalled ehco (SPGR) T1 in phase. TE in phase; TR 175 ms; flip angle 90 degrees; thickness 4 mm; spacing 0 mm.
3. Axial 2D SPGR T1 out of phase. TE out of phase; TR 175 ms; flip angle 90 degrees; thickness 4 mm; spacing 0 mm.
4. Axial 2D SPGR T1 out of phase fat saturated. TE out of phase; TR 175 ms; flip angle 90 degrees; thickness 4 mm; spacing 0 mm.
5. Coronal SPGR fat saturated. TE in phase; TR 175 ms; flip angle 90 degrees; thickness 6 mm; spacing 0 mm.
6. Axial fast spin-echo T2 fat saturated and respiratory-triggered dual echo. TE 68 ms; effective TE 136 ms; echo train length (ETL) 16; thickness 7 mm; spacing 1 mm; fat saturation 6-8; skip 0-2 (phase field of view 0.75); TR 175-200 ms; contrast administration dynamic gadolinium 20 mL at 2 ml/s.
7. Axial 2D SPGR T1 DYNAMIC (pre, 20, 60, 180 s). TE in phase; TR 175 ms; flip angle 90 degrees; thickness 6 mm; spacing 0 mm.

Box 84-2 | **MRCP Protocol**

● Scout with T2 single-shot fast spin-echo in coronal plane. Scout obtained first with breath-hold and then with normal breathing.
● Axial respiratory-triggered fast spin-echo T2. TE 150 ms; TR 6000 ms; thickness 3 mm; spacing 0 mm; skip 0.
● Axial 2D spoiled gradient recalled ehco (SPGR) T1 in phase. TR 175 ms; thickness 5 mm; spacing 0 mm.
● Axial 2D SPGR T1 out of phase. TR 175 ms; thickness 5 mm; spacing 0 mm.
● Axial 2D SPGR T1 out of phase fat saturated. TR 175 ms; thickness 5 mm; spacing 0 mm.
● RADIAL n = 12 if patient can hold breath.
● Coronal thick (60 mm) MRCP.
● Use radials and coronal images to post thin MRCP sequences. Tailor study for common bile duct vs pancreas.

Secretin MRCP
● Administration of 1 mL secretin/10 kg body weight of secretin.
● Thick-slab coronal MRCP images 10-15 minutes after the intravenous administration of secretin. Images are centered on the full length of the pancreatic duct, extrahepatic duct, and duodenum.
● Dynamic acquisition of images at 15-30 second intervals.

---

between the nonfatty parenchymal tissue and the surrounding retroperitoneal fat.[19] Fat suppression increases the tissue contrast between the high signal pancreatic parenchyma and the focal pancreatic masses.[20]

T2-Weighted Sequence

T2-weighted sequences allow for evaluation of fluid and fluid-filled lesions around the pancreas. They demonstrate the pancreatic and common bile ducts and can direct the acquisition of MRCP images. T2-weighted sequences are acquired as breath-hold or respiratory triggered single-shot turbo spin-echo (HASTE) sequences with thin sections (4 mm) with short (40-80 ms) and long (325 ms) TE.[17]

Dynamic Contrast-Enhanced Sequences

Contrast enhancement results in prompt homogenous enhancement of the pancreatic parenchyma.[21] The primary contrast agents used in MRI are extracellular gadolinium chelates.[22] Contrast enhancement improves detection and characterization of pancreatic lesions, allows for the evaluation of pancreatic viability in cases of necrotic or chronic pancreatitis, and allows for the creation of MR angiographic images for the evaluation of tumor resectability.[11] A second hepatobiliary contrast agent, mangafodipir trisodium (MnDPDP), was used for pancreatic imaging but is no longer available.[23]

Gadolinium Chelate

Gadolinium chelate functions as an intravascular agent which increases the signal intensity in target tissues. In the pancreas, gadolinium avidly and rapidly enhances the normal pancreatic parenchyma. Typically, for pancreatic imaging, gadolinium is injected with a power injector at a dose of 0.1 mmol/kg (approximately 20 mL) and rate of 2 mL/second via a peripheral intravenous line. Axial T1-weighted images are obtained in the arterial (20-40 second delay), portal (60-80 second delay), and equilibrium phase (180-200 second delay).

MR Cholangiopancreatography Protocol

MRCP is used for the evaluation of the pancreatic ducts. Ductal dilation, duct strictures, intraluminal filling defects, and duct injury can be evaluated with MRCP. Heavily T2-weighted sequences are used that selectively display static or slow moving fluid structures. MRCP protocols may be performed as part of the standard pancreatic protocol described earlier or as a stand-alone protocol for the exclusive evaluation of the pancreatic ducts (Box 84-2).

MRCP images are obtained as a thick-slab (20-60 mm) single-shot turbo spin-echo T2-weighted sequence, or as a multislice thin-slab single-shot turbo spin-echo T2-weighted sequence.[17] Radial projections along the axis of the common hepatic and common bile ducts may also be helpful in evaluating the entire course of the ducts.

Secretin-Enhanced Dynamic MRCP

Secretin acts as an endogenous contrast agent for pancreatic ducts in MRCP. Exogenous administration of secretin stimulates the secretion of fluid and bicarbonate by the exocrine pancreas,[24] thereby increasing the amount of stationary fluid in the pancreatic ducts. Secretin administration allows for more sensitive evaluation of the ducts and for evaluation of duct flow dynamics into the duodenum.[25-27] Secretin stimulation also may be used to evaluate for chronic pancreatitis and functional duct obstructions.[28,29]

Sectretin-enhanced dynamic MRCP is performed by acquiring thick-slab coronal MRCP images 10 to 15 minutes after the intravenous administration of 1 mL of secretin/10 kg body weight.[17] Images are centered on the full length of the pancreatic duct, extrahepatic duct, and duodenum, and are dynamically acquired at 15 to 30 second intervals.

In normal individuals, the baseline duct size is 1.9 mm (range 1-3 mm) and after administration of secretin there is a 70% to 100% increase in duct size. In patients with chronic pancreatitis, there is no significant increase in duct size.[28,29] In patients with a functional duct obstruction, the pancreatic duct remains dilated 15 to 30 minutes after the administration of secretin.

MR Angiography

MR angiography allows for three-dimensional (3D) rendering of the peripancreatic vessels. It is used for the evaluation of anatomic variations, encasement of tumor, and complications of pancreatitis, such as pseudo-aneurysm formation. MR angiographic images are obtained as coronal three-dimensional (3D) gradient-recalled echo (GRE) breath-hold dynamic contrast-enhanced T1-weighted images with high resolution (Box 84-3). Use of a volume-interpolated breath-hold pulse sequence, which is a modified GRE technique, allows for superior angiographic data, surgical planning, and improved lesion detection.[30]

PANCREATIC ANATOMY

The pancreas lies in the anterior retroperitoneal space in an oblique coronal plane (Fig. 84-1). It extends from the C-loop of the duodenum to the splenic hilum and is surrounded by retroperitoneal fat. The head of the pancreas lies to the right of the portal/superior mesenteric vein and to the left of the superior part of the duodenum. The neck of the pancreas lies directly anterior to the superior mesenteric vessels, whereas the body is situated anterior to the splenic vein and artery. The uncinate process lies inferolateral and posterior to the superior mesenteric vessels. The important anatomic

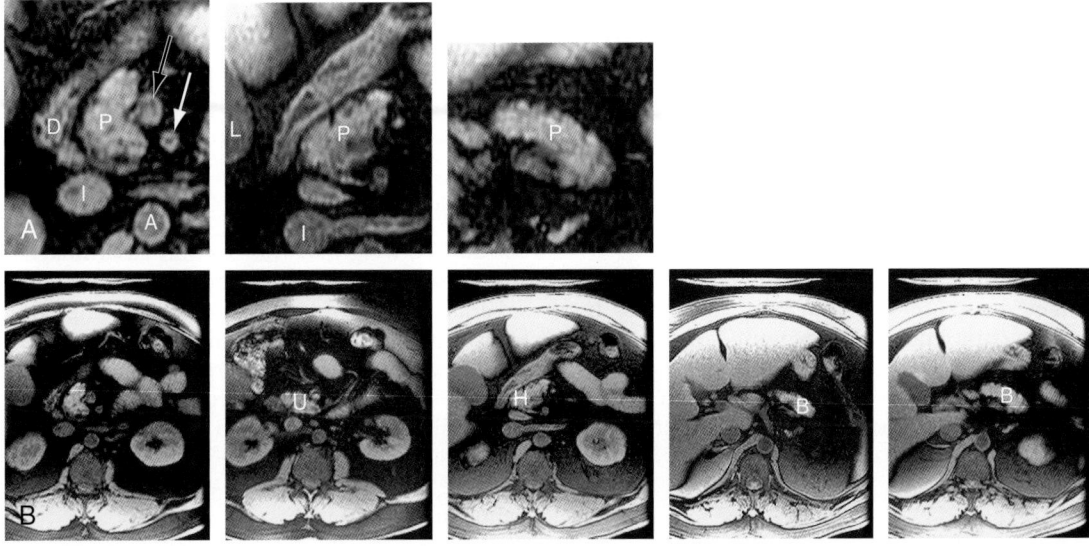

FIGURE 84-1

Normal MR pancreas anatomy. **A,** Series of magnified axial fat-saturated T1-weighted images. **B,** Series of axial fat-saturated T1-weighted images. Pancreas extends from the second portion of the duodenum to the splenic hilum. A, aorta; B, body; D, duodenum; H, pancreas head; I, inferior vena cava; L, liver; P, pancreas; U, uncinate process. Superior mesenteric artery, *white arrow*; superior mesenteric vein, *black arrow*.

structures related to the pancreas include the second part of duodenum that lies to the right of the head of the pancreas, and the third and fourth parts of duodenum, which lie inferior to the uncinate process, and body of the pancreas. The lesser peritoneal space lies between the pancreas and stomach. The tail of the pancreas is intraperitoneal and lies within the splenorenal ligament and extends up to the splenic hilum.

MRI APPEARANCE OF THE NORMAL PANCREAS

Pancreatic Parenchyma

T1-Weighted Images

On in-phase T1-weighted images the pancreas is of intermediate signal intensity similar to or slightly brighter than the liver (Fig. 84-2A). On out-of-phase T1 images, etching artifact from the fat-parenchyma border creates a hypointense rim surrounding the pancreas (Fig. 84-2B).

Fat-Saturated T1-Weighted Images

With fat saturation, the relative signal intensity of the pancreas increases dramatically due to the presence of aqueous protein in the glandular elements of the pancreas (Fig. 84-2C).[31]

T2-Weighted Images

On T2-weighted images, the pancreas is similar in signal intensity or slightly darker than the liver (Fig. 84-2D). T2-weighted sequences are useful for examining the pancreatic duct.

Gadolinium-Enhanced MRI

With the administration of gadolinium there is a prompt homogenous enhancement of the pancreatic parenchyma (Fig. 84-2E). This enhancement persists on delayed images (Fig. 84-2F).

Pancreatic Duct

As a fluid-filled structure, the pancreatic duct may be seen as a thin dark line on T1-weighted images. On T2-weighted images the duct may be more apparent as a linear bright signal along the length of the pancreas (Fig. 84-3). MRCP is useful for evaluating slow moving fluid and can assess the normal pancreatic duct (Fig. 84-4).

Peripancreatic Vessels

Evaluation of the peripancreatic vessels is best accomplished after the administration of intravenous contrast. Evaluation of the superior mesenteric artery, superior and inferior mesenteric veins, splenic artery and vein are accomplished by acquiring contrast-enhanced images in different phases (arterial, portal venous and delayed) (Fig. 84-5).[32] Examination of the peripancreatic vessels is important for the evaluation of tumor staging and to assess for resectability.

DISEASE ENTITIES

MRI has the role of an ancillary imaging modality in the evaluation of pancreatic diseases. Patients present with abnormal laboratory values, CT or ultrasound, or endoscopic retrograde cholangiopancreatography (ERCP) findings that suggest a single or differential diagnosis, and MRI is performed as a focused examination to resolve the clinical question. MRI is used to evaluate congenital, inflammatory, metabolic, neoplastic, and traumatic diseases of the pancreas.

Congenital Anomalies

Pancreatic Divisum

Pancreatic divisum is an anatomic variant that is the result of failure of fusion of the dorsal duct of Wirsung, which drains the head of the pancreas, and the ventral duct of Santorini, which drains the body of the pancreas. It is the most common congenital anomaly of the pancreas, with a prevalence as high as 10%.[33] Although the significance of pancreatic divisum is controversial,[34] clinically patients may present with recurrent episodes of pancreatitis with no other identifiable cause, i.e., alcoholism or gallstones. It is theorized that pancreatitis results from the partial obstruction of the dorsal duct because of its narrow orifice into the duodenum. Although historically ERCP with injection of both pancreatic ducts has been used to confirm the diagnosis, evaluation for pancreatic divisum may now be noninvasively performed with MRCP,[35,36] reserving ERCP for treatment, including dual sphincteroplasty[37] or papillotomy of the minor papilla with short-term stenting in patients with acute recurrent pancreatitis.[38]

MR Imaging

T1- and T2-weighted thin-section axial images centered along the course of the pancreatic duct may depict the separate entry of the duct of Wirsung and duct of Santorini (Fig. 84-6A–C), and this finding should be evaluated in all patients presenting for an MRI and a history of pancreatitis. Coronal and oblique thin- and thick-slab MRCP images can confirm the separate entry of the ducts (Fig. 84-6D, E).[35,36] Secretin stimulation can increase the sensitivity of MRCP in the evaluation for pancreatic divisum.[39,40]

Annular Pancreas

Annular pancreas is a result of the failure of the normal clockwise migration of the ventral pancreas, with normal pancreatic tissue encircling the second portion of the

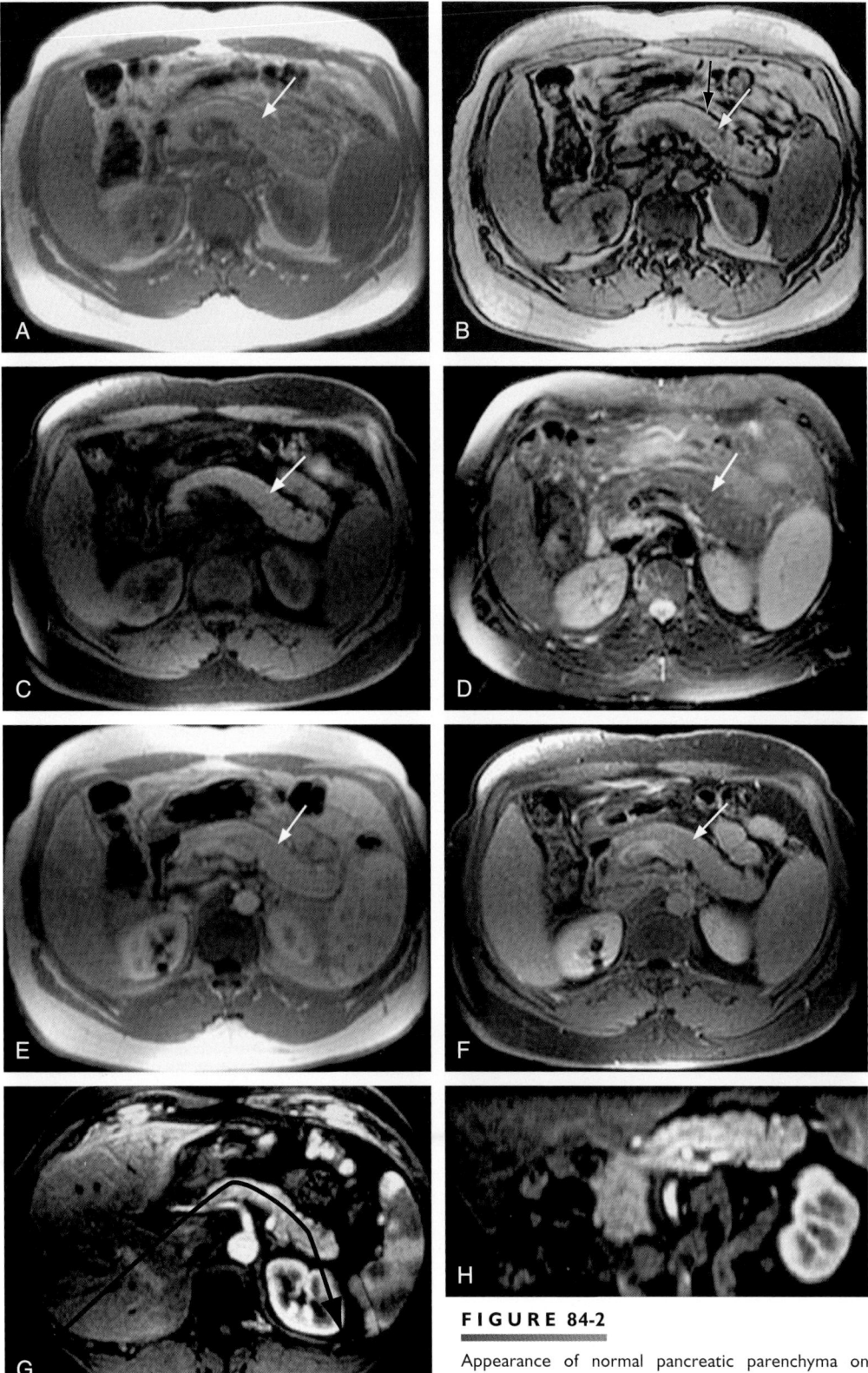

FIGURE 84-2

Appearance of normal pancreatic parenchyma on different MR sequences. Axial MR images of the body and tail of a normal pancreas (*arrow*). **A,** Axial T1-weighted in-phase image. The pancreas is isointense to slightly hyperintense to the liver. **B,** Axial T1-weighted out-of-phase image. Note the etching artifact surrounding the pancreas at the borders between tissues (*black arrow*). **C,** Axial T1-weighted fat-saturated image. Note the relative hyperintensity of the pancreas relative to the surrounding retroperitoneal fat. **D,** Axial T2-weighted image. The pancreas is hypointense and not clearly delineated from the surrounding tissue. **E,** Axial T1-weighted immediate post-gadolinium image shows homogenous enhancement of the pancreatic parenchyma. **F,** Axial T1-weighted delayed post-gadolinium image shows persistent enhancement of the pancreatic parenchyma. **G,** Axial gadolinium-enhanced 3D VIBE or FAME of the pancreas in another subject. **H,** Curved multiplanar reconstruction from **G** showing entire pancreas. *(Figs. 84-2G and 84-2H courtesy of Dr. R. Edelman.)*

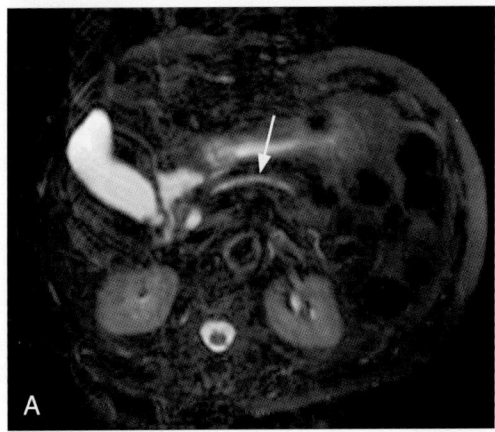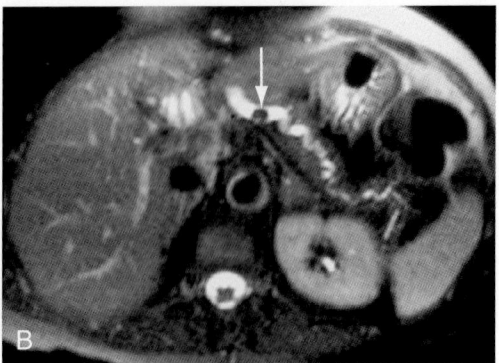

FIGURE 84-3

Normal pancreatic duct. T2-weighted images. **A,** Axial T2-weighted image at the level of the pancreatic body. The normal pancreatic duct is visible as a high signal linear structure (*arrow*) centered along the axis of the pancreas. **B,** Axial T2-weighted single-shot fast spin-echo image of a different patient shows a stone (*arrow*) within a dilated main pancreatic duct. *(Fig. 84-3B courtesy of Dr. R. Edelman.)*

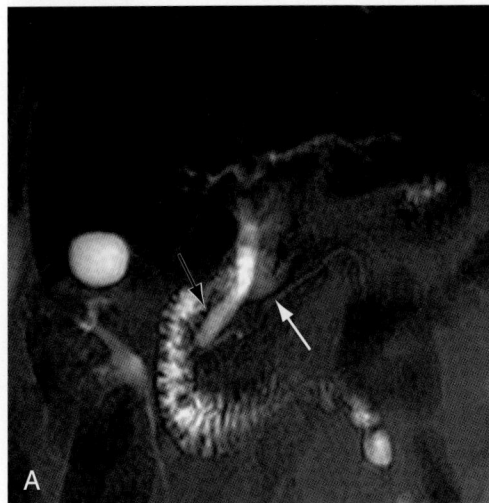

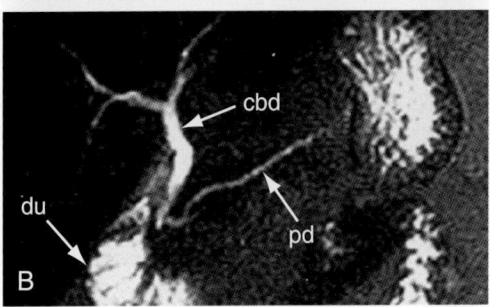

FIGURE 84-4

Normal pancreatic duct. MR cholangiopancreotography (MRCP). **A,** MRCP image shows the pancreatic (*white arrow*) and common bile ducts (*black arrow*). **B,** Oblique MRCP in a different patient shows the common bile duct (cbd), pancreatic ducts (pd) and duodenum (du). *(Fig. 84-4B courtesy of Dr. R. Edelman.)*

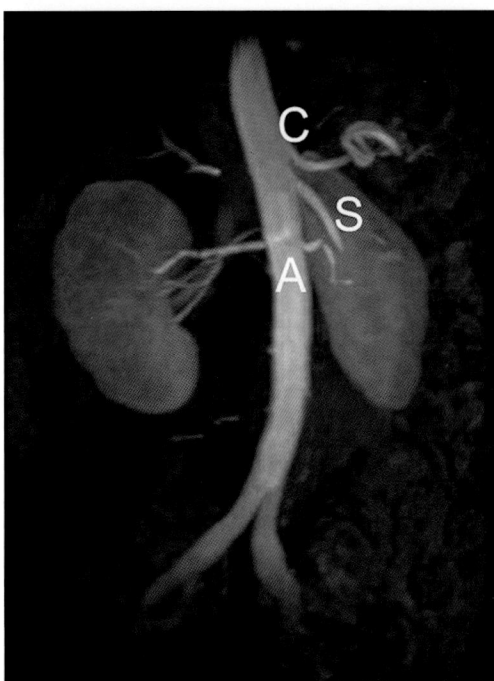

FIGURE 84-5

Peripancreatic vessels. MR angiography. Right anterior oblique and coronal MR angiogram of peripancreatic vessels showing the celiac (C), superior mesenteric artery (S), and aorta (A).

duodenum.[41] Clinically, patients present with varying degrees of duodenal obstruction. In children there is an association with congenital heart defects, Down's syndrome, and intestinal malrotation. Adults present with symptoms of bowel obstruction, pancreatitis, and peptic ulcer disease. Annular pancreas may be seen on ultrasound and CT as contiguous pancreatic soft-tissue surrounding the duodenum. MRI is only a secondary imaging modality which can confirm that the tissue surrounding the duodenum is normal pancreatic parenchyma. Treatment in symptomatic patients is typically operative with a duodenojejonostomy bypass.[34]

MR Imaging

Anatomic evaluation for annular pancreas may be best performed with a fat-suppressed T1-weighted or post-contrast spoiled gradient recalled echo (SPGR) sequence. On both these sequences the normal pancreatic parenchyma has a high signal and can be distinguished from the duodenal and peripancreatic soft-tissues.[42]

Metabolic Disorders

Cystic Fibrosis

Cystic fibrosis is an autosomal-recessive congenital dysfunction of the pancreatic exocrine glands. Clinically, patients present with chronic bronchopulmonary infections, pancreatic insufficiency with associated malabsorption, and increased sodium concentration in sweat. Diagnosis is usually made with a sweat test or by genetic testing for the cystic fibrosis gene, and the role of MRI is to characterize the pancreatic abnormalities. MRI evaluation is useful because it avoids the ionizing radiation of CT, particularly in this young patient population.[43,44] Treatment for cystic fibrosis is medical management with replacement of pancreatic enzymes.

MR Imaging

Three patterns have been described[43]: 1. enlarged, lobulated pancreas with complete fatty replacement; 2. small, atrophic pancreas with partial fatty replacement; and 3. diffusely atrophic pancreas without fatty replacement. Fatty replacement is well seen on T1-weighted images as bright signal replacing the pancreatic parenchyma, which becomes low signal on fat-suppressed image (Fig. 84-7). Fibrotic areas are seen as low signal areas in the pancreatic parenchyma on T1- and T2-weighted images. MRCP is also useful for evaluating complications of cystic fibrosis including[43]: liver—hepatomegaly, diffuse fatty infiltration, cirrhosis with fibrotic changes, regenerative nodules, and portal hypertension; spleen—splenomegaly and siderotic splenic nodules that manifest as multiple focal areas of abnormal low signal intensity within the spleen; biliary—cholelithiasis, stricturization, and narrowing or dilatation of intra- and extra-hepatic bile ducts; and gallbladder—microgallbladder.

Hemochromatosis

Idiopathic hemochromatosis is an hereditary abnormal iron deposition disease. Iron is deposited in the liver, pancreas, and heart. Clinically, patients present with diabetes mellitus due to the iron deposition in the exocrine glands and islet B cells of the pancreas. MRI can evaluate for iron deposition in the pancreas and can noninvasively assess the tissue iron overload.[45] Treatment is by phlebotomy and the use of iron chelators to drain off the excess iron.

MR Imaging

The paramagnetic susceptibility effects of iron cause decreased signal in the liver, spleen, and pancreas on gradient-echo and T2-weighted images (Fig. 84-8). Typically, deposition of iron in the pancreas occurs late in the disease and after liver damage is irreversible.[46]

This pattern of liver, spleen, and pancreas involvement is distinguished from secondary hemochromatosis, due to multiple transfusions, where there is decreased signal in the liver and spleen, but the pancreas is spared and does not have low signal (Fig. 84-9).[47]

Inflammatory Disorders

MR evaluation of the inflammatory pancreatic conditions, acute and chronic pancreatitis, has evolved with the development of dynamic contrast-enhanced imaging

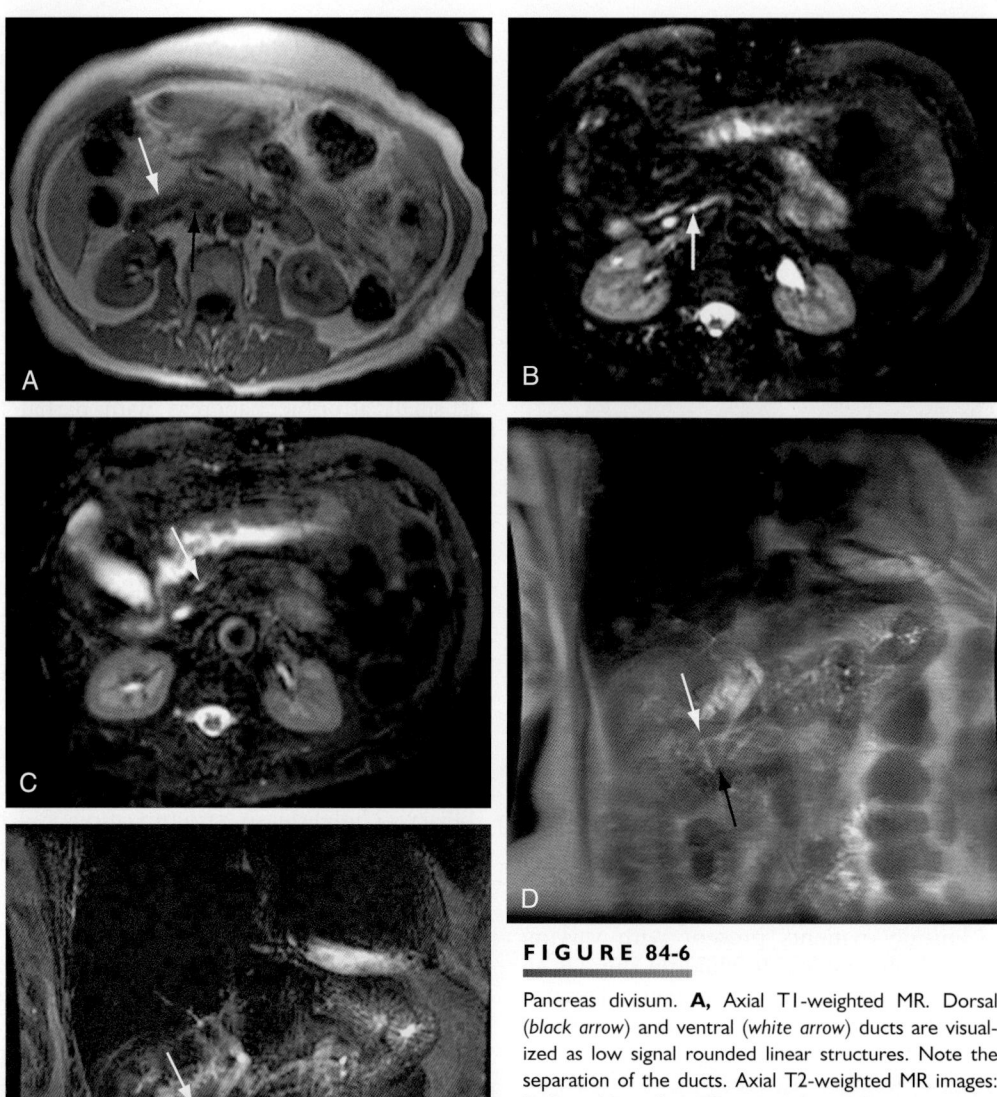

FIGURE 84-6

Pancreas divisum. **A,** Axial T1-weighted MR. Dorsal
(*black arrow*) and ventral (*white arrow*) ducts are visualized as low signal rounded linear structures. Note the
separation of the ducts. Axial T2-weighted MR images:
B, Dorsal (*arrow*) and **C,** ventral (*arrow*) ducts are seen as
two separate high signal structures traveling towards the
duodenum. **D** and **E,** Thick-slab coronal MR cholangio-
pancreotography (MRCP) centered at the insertion of
the pancreatic ducts shows the dorsal pancreatic duct
(*black arrow*) that enters the duodenum at the (Santorini)
minor papilla and is separate from the ventral pancreatic
duct, which joins the common bile duct and enters the
(Wirsung) major papilla (*white arrow*) more inferiorly.

Continued

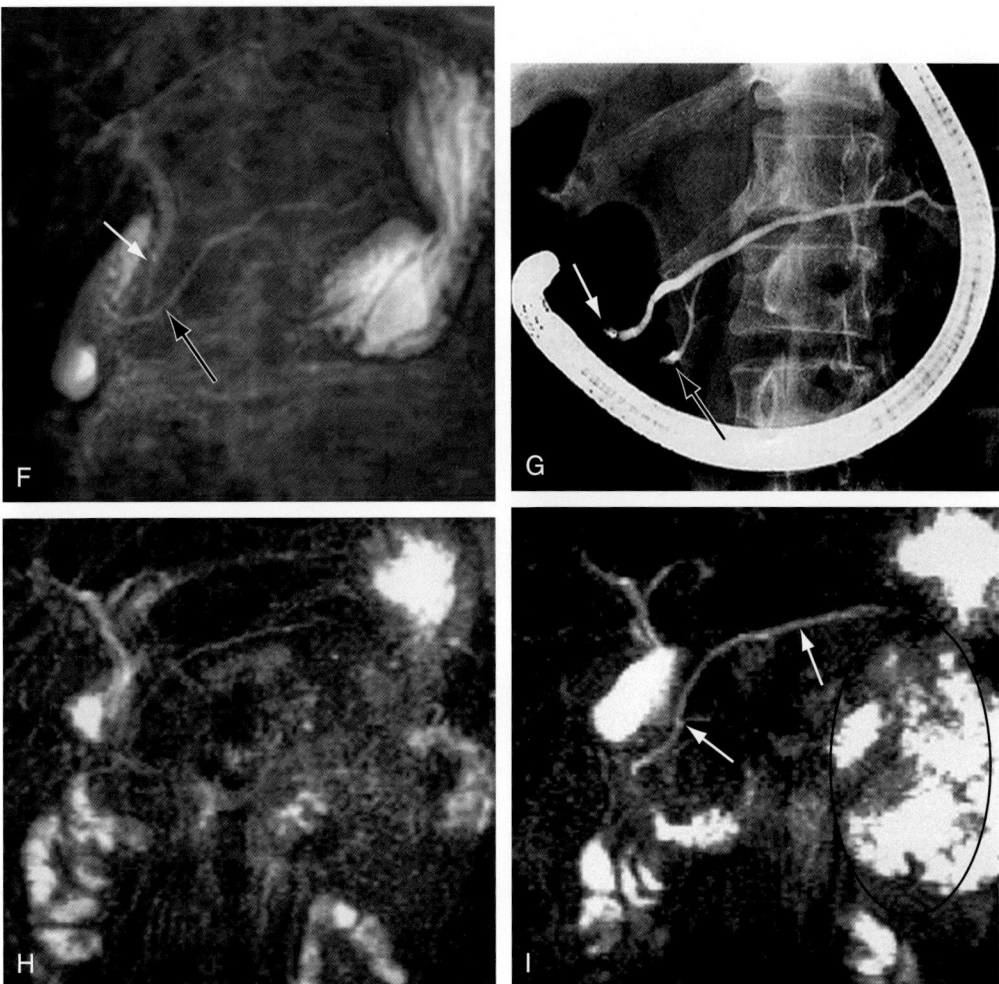

FIGURE 84-6, cont'd

Pancreas divisum. **F,** MRCP shows the dorsal duct (*large arrow*) crossing the common bile duct (*white arrow*). **G,** Endoscopic retrograde cholangiopancreatography shows the dorsal (*large arrow*) and ventral duct (*white arrow*). **H,** MRCP in another subject shows poor visualization of the pancreatic duct. **I,** After secretin administration, there is improved visualization of the pancreatic duct (*arrows*). Note is made of a large amount of fluid in the small bowel (*oval*), indicating normal pancreatic secretory function. A pancreas divisum is now evident. *(Figs. 84-6G-I courtesy of Dr. R. Edelman.)*

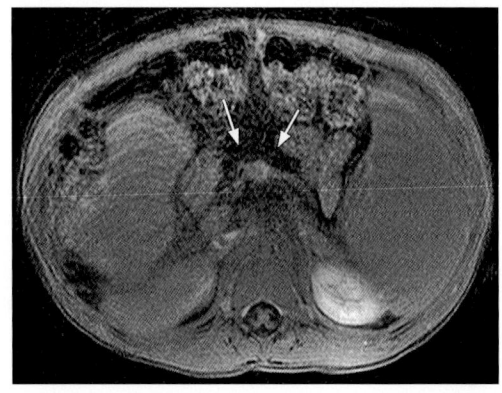

FIGURE 84-7

Cystic fibrosis. Axial fat-saturated T1-weighted image. Retroperitoneal fat is saturated out and is dark signal. The pancreas is not seen in the expected location (*arrows*).

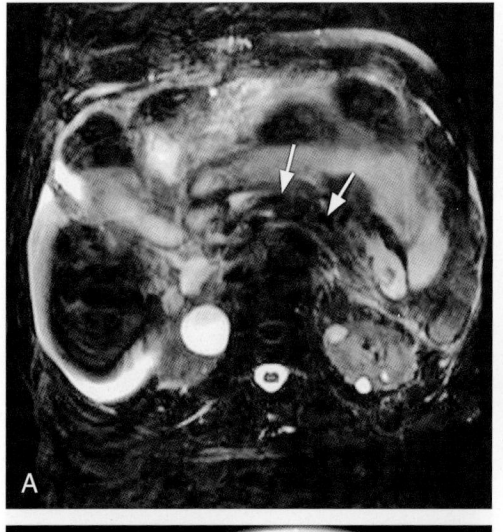
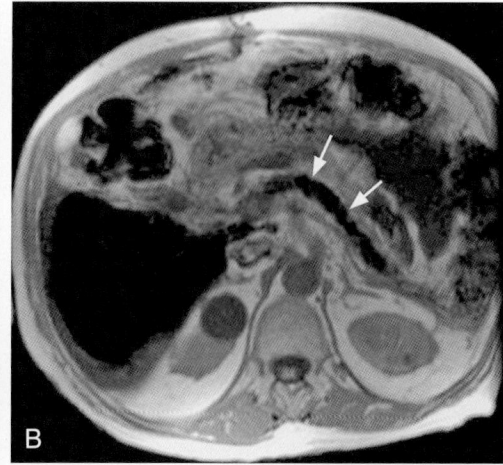
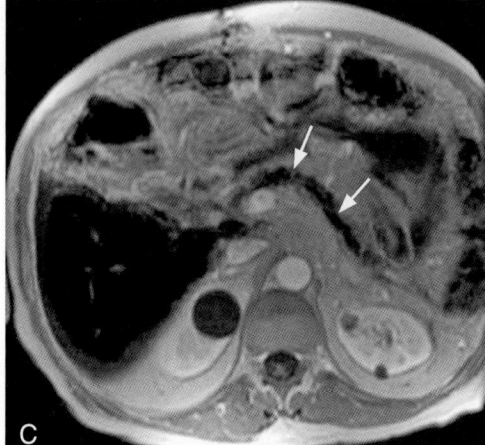

FIGURE 84-8

Idiopathic hemochromatosis. Dark signal is seen in the liver, spleen, and pancreas (*arrows*) on all MR sequences: **A,** axial T2; **B,** axial T1; and **C,** post-gadolinium axial T1.

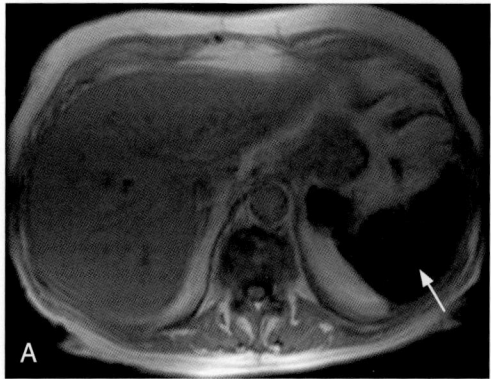
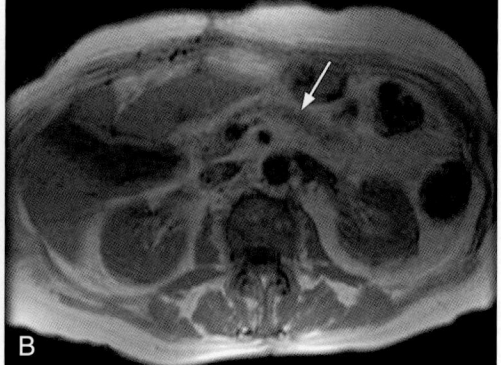

FIGURE 84-9

Iron overload. Sparing of the pancreas from iron overload. Axial T1-weighted images. In contrast to idiopathic hemochromatosis with iron overload, there is dark signal in the **A,** spleen (*arrow*), but the **B,** pancreas (*arrow*) has normal signal.

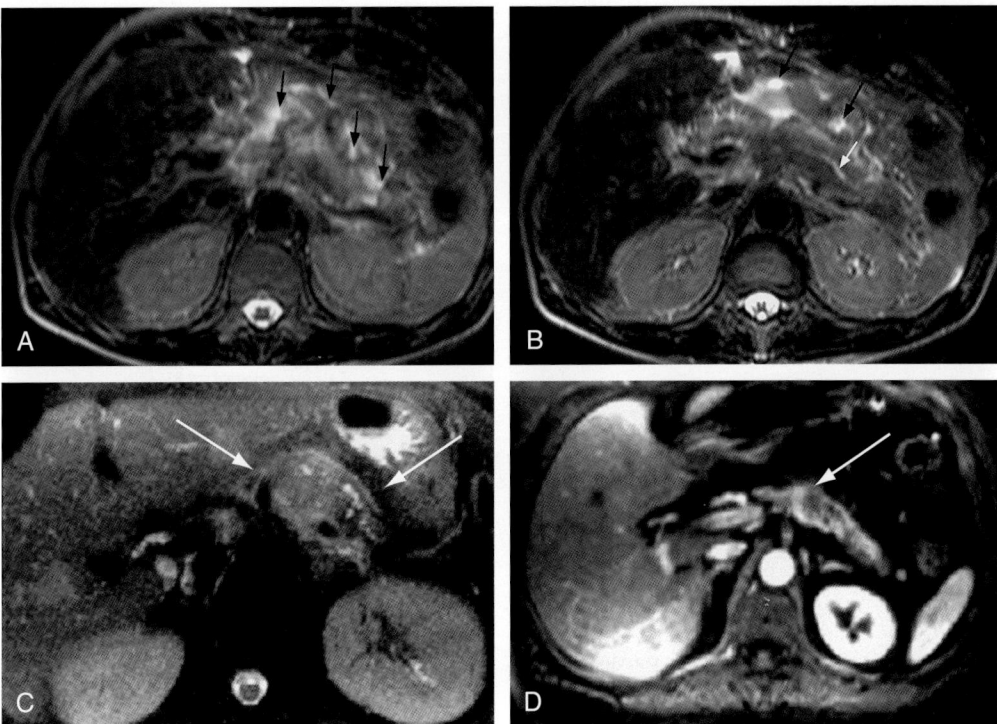

FIGURE 84-I0

Acute pancreatitis. **A,** Axial T2-weighted images. Scattered high signal (*black arrows*) surrounding the pancreas is consistent with peripancreatic edema. **B,** Normal pancreatic duct (*white arrow*). **C,** Axial T2-weighted image of a different patient shows edema of the body of the pancreas and interruption of the duct (*arrows*). **D,** Six weeks later after the acute inflammation had subsided, a gadolinium-enhanced 3D VIBE acquisition demonstrates a small pancreatic carcinoma (*arrow*). (*Figs 84-I0C and 84-I0D courtesy of Dr. R. Edelman.*)

and secretin-enhanced MRCP. Although CT is the standard imaging modality in the evaluation of acute pancreatitis, and for calcifications in chronic pancreatitis, contrast-enhanced MR and MRCP may be used for noninvasive planning prior to therapy.[17] MR can evaluate for choledocholithiasis, ductal distension, or disruption. It can assess the size and location of pseudocyst and peripancreatic fluid collections, and it can evaluate for areas of hemorrhage and necrosis.[48]

Acute Pancreatitis

Inflammation of the pancreas is caused by alcoholism, gallstones, hyperlipidemia, hypercalcemia, familial causes, and trauma.[34] In the United States, the two most common causes of acute pancreatitis are alcoholism and gallstones.[49] Clinically, patients present with mid-epigastric pain, nausea and vomiting, and elevated amylase and lipase serum levels. Contrast-enhanced CT is the standard imaging modality to evaluate for pancreatic inflammatory changes. However, MRI has been proposed as an alternative to CT for the initial staging of acute pancreatitis.[50] MRI can evaluate for early peripancreatic inflammatory changes, complications of acute pancreatitis, including hemorrhage and necrosis, and peripancreatic fluid collections and pseudocysts. MRCP can assess for choledocholithiasis.

MR Imaging

Comprehensive evaluation of acute pancreatitis with MRI includes axial T2-weighted sequence, pre- and post–contrast-enhanced fat-suppressed T1-weighted sequence, and MRCP.

In 15% to 30% of patients with clinical acute pancreatitis, CT examination is normal.[51] T2-weighted MRI, with its ability to detect subtle high signal peripancreatic fluid, can detect the early peripancreatic changes of acute pancreatitis (Fig. 84-10).

MRCP is valuable in evaluating for choledocholithiasis.[52] It can assess for ductal dilatation and filling defects within the pancreatic and common bile ducts. In addition, MRCP may be of value in noninvasively evaluating patients who may be at risk of developing post-ERCP pancreatitis.[17,53]

Complications of acute pancreatitis, including hemorrhage, pseudoaneurysm, parenchymal necrosis, and peripancreatic fluid collections may be evaluated by MR. Hemorrhage and pseudoaneurysm may be evaluated with precontrast T1-weighted fat-saturated imaging. On T1-weighted images, hemorrhage is seen as areas of high signal within the pancreatic parenchyma.

A prognostic factor in pancreatitis is the percent of pancreatic parenchymal necrosis.[54,55] Dynamic gadolinium-enhanced MRI enhances normal parenchyma and can be

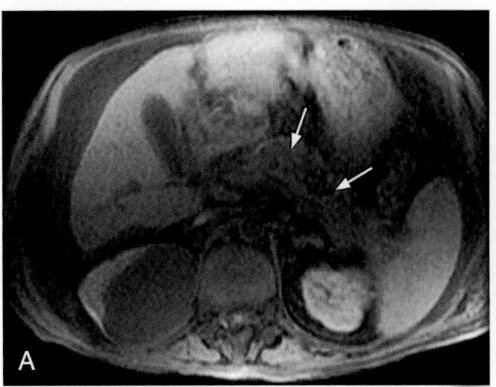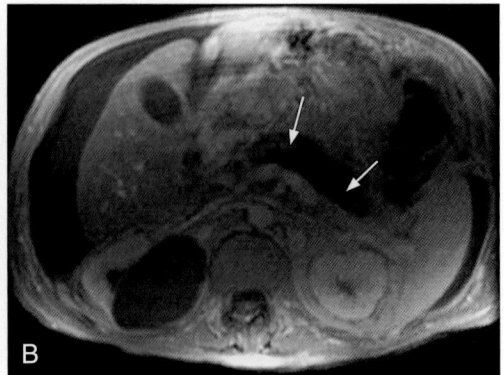

FIGURE 84-11

Acute necrotizing pancreatitis. **A,** Axial T1-weighted image shows an enlarged pancreas (*arrows*). **B,** Post-contrast axial T1-weighted sequence shows lack of enhancement of the pancreatic parenchyma (*arrows*). Ascites and a right renal cyst are visible.

used to assess for necrotic, nonenhancing parenchyma (Fig. 84-11).[56,57]

The improved contrast resolution with T2-weighted MRI for fluid collections may better visualize debris within fluid collections not appreciated on CT.[48,58]

Chronic Pancreatitis

Chronic pancreatitis is associated with alcoholism, hyperparathyroidism, cystic fibrosis, pancreatic divisum, and pancreatic trauma. There is exocrine and endocrine pancreatic insufficiency with irreversible parenchymal destruction, proliferative fibrosis, calcification, and ductal stricturing. Diagnosis of chronic pancreatitis has been based on finding areas of pancreatic enlargement and calcification on CT and evaluating for ductal dilatation and stricturing on ERCP. MRI offers the ability to evaluate the pancreatic parenchyma for areas of fibrosis and the ducts for areas of dilation and stricture.

MR Imaging

Chronic pancreatitis is evaluated by MRI with T1-weighted fat-saturated dynamic contrast-enhanced sequences, and secretin-stimulated MRCP (Figs. 84-12 and 84-13). Areas of pancreatic fibrosis are seen as areas of low signal on T1-weighted fat-saturated images which show diminished contrast enhancement. Focal areas of pancreatic enlargement can be difficult to distinguish from pancreatic adenocarcinoma on CT[59] and some authors have proposed that MRI is useful at making this distinction[60,61]; however, recent reports show that this is difficult even with contrast-enhanced MRI[62] and the distinction may depend on positron emission tomography (PET) imaging.[63] A limitation of MR in the evaluation of chronic pancreatitis is its limited ability to distinguish calcification.

MR has been found to be useful in a subentity of chronic pancreatitis known as "groove pancreatitis." This is a specific form of chronic pancreatitis affecting the groove between the pancreatic head and the duodenum. Fibrous tissue in groove pancreatitis is hypointense relative to pancreatic parenchyma on T1-weighted images and iso- to slightly hyper-intense on T2-weighted images. After administration of gadolinium, the fibrous tissues showed delayed enhancement.[64]

Heavily T2-weighted MRCP may be helpful in the evaluation of chronic pancreatitis by examining the duct for strictures. Administration of secretin may also help evaluation in the early stages of chronic pancreatitis.[65,66] It can show ductal anatomy, degree and level of pancreatic obstruction, bile duct strictures, and exocrine gland functional impairment.[17] Typically, there is transient ductal dilation in normal individuals after the administration of secretin but not in patients with chronic pancreatitis.

Neoplastic Disorders

A comprehensive evaluation of pancreatic masses can be performed with MRI, MRCP, and MR angiography. MR offers excellent tissue contrast. Contrast-enhanced MRI improves detection of pancreatic masses and characterizes their enhancement pattern. MRCP sequences may be used to evaluate for ductal obstruction. MR angiography can evaluate for vascular encasement.

Although MRI may not always distinguish benign from malignant masses, certain characteristics detected on MRI can reliably suggest malignancy (Table 84-1). These include ductal obstruction and dilation, vascular encasement, mural nodular enhancement in a cyst, and arterial enhancement of the lesion.

Benign Masses

Lipoma

Lipoma is the most common benign tumor of the pancreas. On standard MR protocols the lesion follows the signal intensity of retroperitoneal fat on all

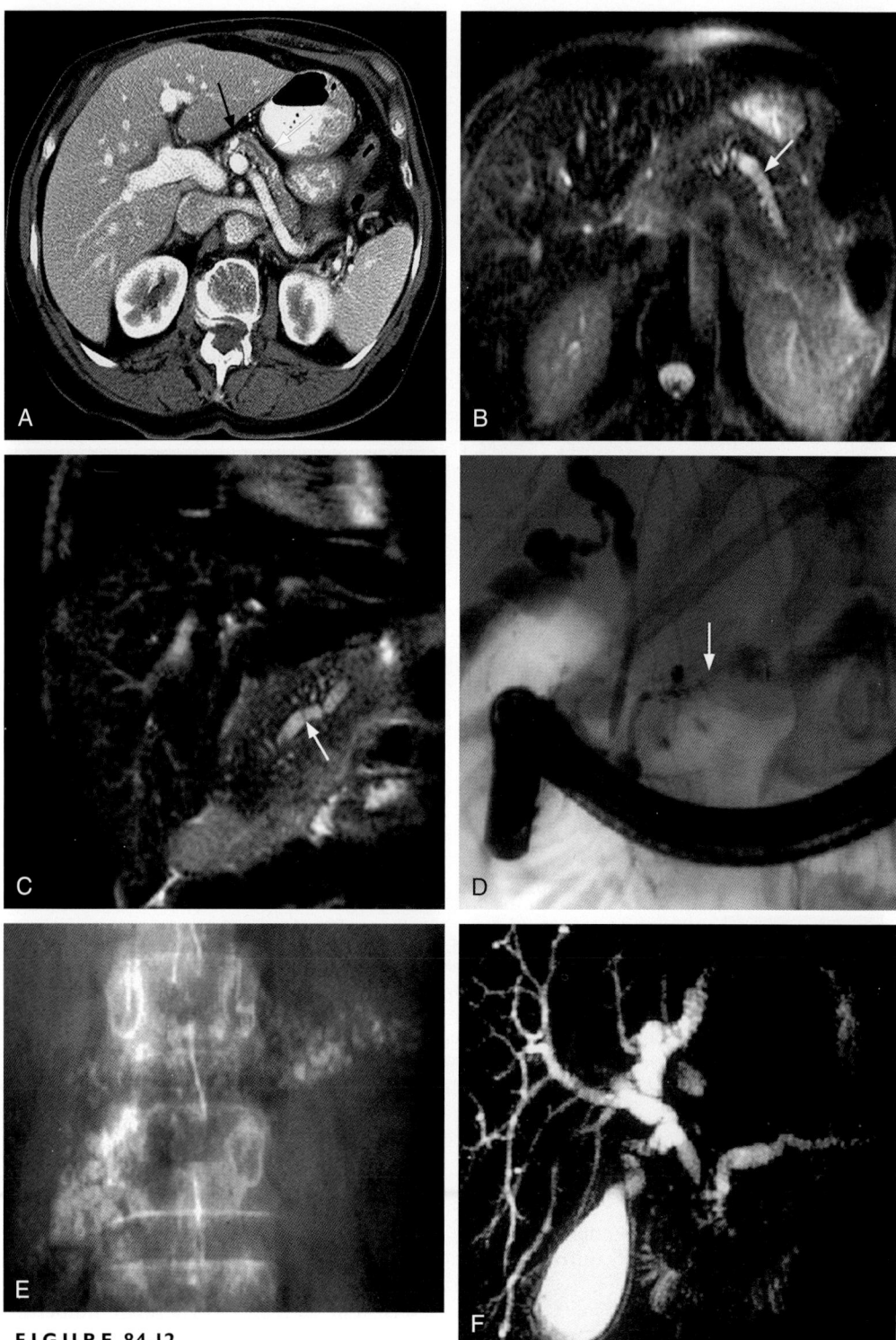

FIGURE 84-12

Chronic pancreatitis. **A,** Axial contrast-enhanced CT showing mild ductal dilation and irregularity (*white arrow*) and calcifications (*black arrow*) consistent with chronic pancreatitis. **B,** Axial and **C,** coronal T2-weighted MR images show ductal dilation and irregularity (*arrow*). **D,** Endoscopic retrograde cholangiopancreatography confirms ductal irregularity (*arrow*). **E,** Plain film in another patient shows extensive pancreatic calcifications. **F,** MR cholangio-pancreotography shows characteristic main duct and side branch dilatation. *(Figs 84-12E and 84-12F courtesy of Dr. R. Edelman.)*

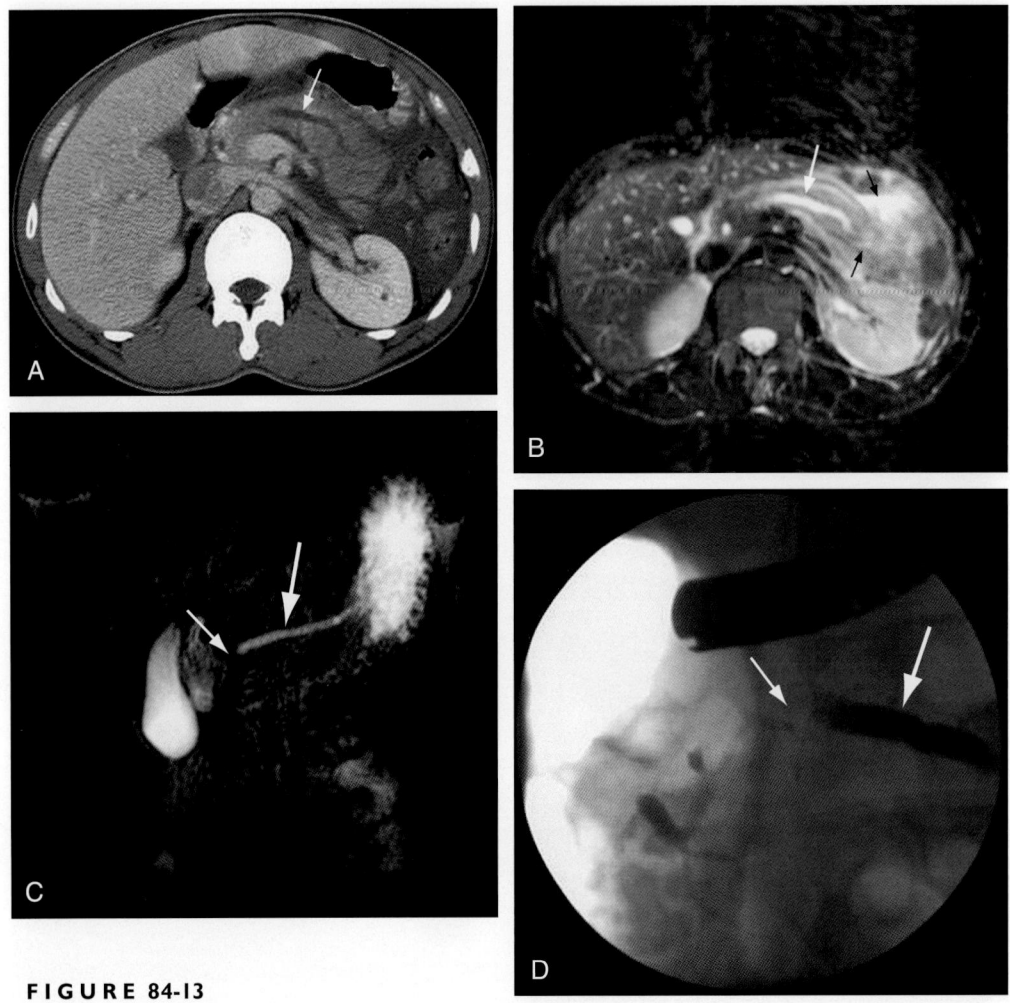

FIGURE 84-13

Acute-on-chronic pancreatitis. Patient with a history of chronic pancreatitis presented with acute pancreatitis. **A,** Axial enhanced CT shows pancreatic enlargement and ductal dilatation (*arrow*), a finding seen with chronic pancreatitis. **B,** Axial T2-weighted MR shows uniformly persistently dilated pancreatic duct (*white arrow*) and peripancreatic edema (*black arrows*) consistent with acute inflammation. **C,** MR cholangiopancreotography (MRCP) shows a dilated duct (*large arrow*) and area of stricture (*small arrow*). **D,** Endoscopic retrograde cholangio-pancreatography confirms findings on MRCP of ductal dilatation (*large arrow*) and stricture (*small arrow*).

sequences, shows fat suppression, has no enhancement, and is larger with a more rounded contour than pancreatic parenchymal fat (Fig. 84-14).

Pseudomasses/Peripancreatic Nodes/Duodenum

Occasionally pancreatic parenchymal bulk variations, contour deformities, and peripancreatic nodes or normal anatomic structures, such as the duodenum, give the appearance of a pancreatic mass on CT. These entities can be distinguished from true pancreatic masses on contrast-enhanced MRI. Using contrast, contour deformities and bulk variations will enhance to the same degree as the pancreatic parenchyma and may be distinguished from peripancreatic structures, which do not enhance.

Cysts

Many complex lesions identified on CT or ultrasound have high T2-weighted signal characteristics on MRI, consistent with a cyst. There are numerous benign cysts in the pancreas including pseudocysts, post-traumatic cysts, cysts associated with Von Hippel-Lindau disease, parasitic cysts, retention cysts, and angiomatous cysts. All have high T2 signal on MRI and distinguishing between them is dependent on the clinical history and associated findings. A pseudocyst is seen in a patient with a prior history of pancreatitis or trauma and who may also have an associated history of elevated amylase and lipase levels (Figs. 84-15, 84-16, and 84-17). Post-traumatic cysts are seen in the setting of trauma. Cysts associated with Von Hippel-Lindau disease may be distinguished by seeing cysts in other locations including the liver and kidneys.

TABLE 84-1 Signal Characteristics of Pancreatic Lesions on MRI

Disease	T1	T2	Gadolinium	MRCP
Acute pancreatitis	Iso- to hypo-intense. Hyperintense areas may represent areas of hemorrhage in hemorrhagic pancreatitis	Occasional peripancreatic hyperintensity from surrounding edema	Areas of nonenhancement may suggest necrotic pancreatitis	Filling defects may suggest cause as gallstone pancreatitis
Chronic pancreatitis	Hypointense	Hypointense	Heterogenous enhancement of the pancreatic parenchyma	Irregular ducts with areas of dilation and stricture
Pseudocyst	Hypointense	Hyperintense cyst indistinguishable from cystic neoplasm except by history of pancreatitis	Possible thick-rim peripheral enhancement in cases of infected pseudocysts	
Serous cystadenoma	Hypointense cyst	Small (<1 cm) hyperintense cystic structure		Normal duct
Mucinous	Hypointense cyst	Large (>1 cm) hyperintense cystic structure	Enhancing septae/enhancing mural nodules	Normal duct
Intraductal papillary mucinous tumor	Hypointense cyst	Hyperintense cyst that communicates with the pancreatic duct		Ductal dilation from overproduction
Adenocarcinoma	Isointense	Isointense	Hypointense to enhancing pancreas	Ductal dilation from obstruction
Islet cell tumors	Isointense	Hyperintense	Strong enhancement in arterial phase	
Metastasis			Vascular metastasis (renal, thyroid, gastrointestinal) enhance during the arterial phase	
Lymphoma	Hypointense parenchyma. Multiple peripancreatic nodes			

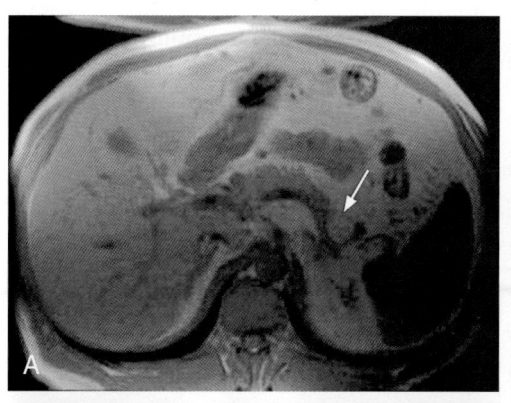
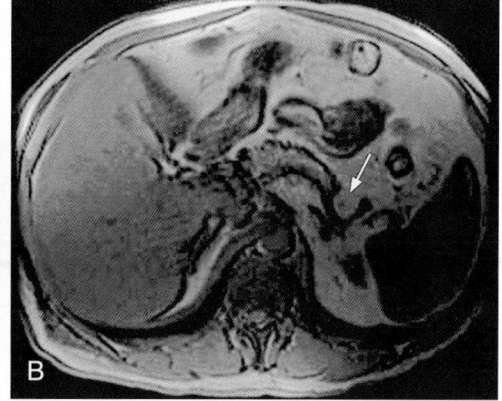
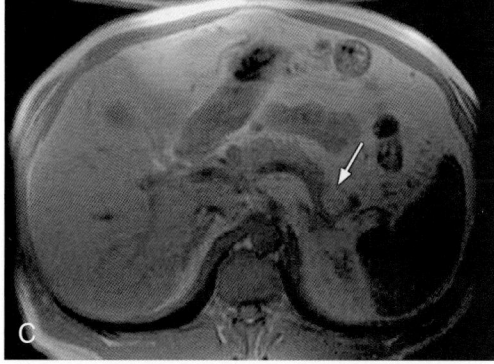

FIGURE 84-14

Lipoma. **A,** Axial T1-weighted in-phase; **B,** axial T1-weighted out-of-phase; and **C,** fat-saturated T1-weighted sequences show a rounded mass in the pancreatic tail (*arrow*) which follows the signal of the surrounding retroperitoneal fat on all sequences.

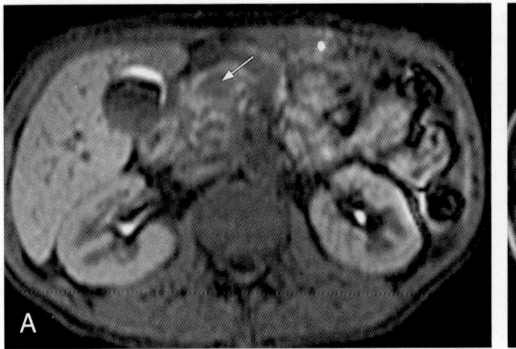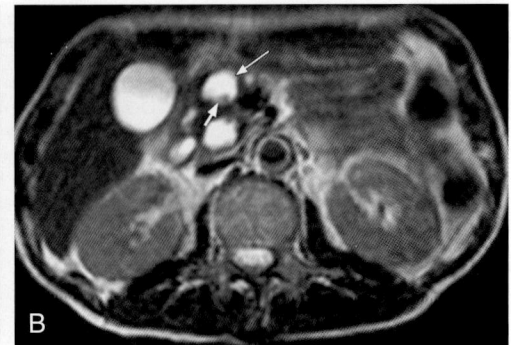

FIGURE 84-15

Chronic pancreatic pseudocyst. **A,** Axial T1-weighted post-gadolinium image shows a low signal collection anterior to the pancreas (*arrow*). **B,** Axial T2-weighted MR image shows high signal collection (*white arrow*). In a patient with a prior history of pancreatitis, this is consistent with a pseudocyst. Debris is noted within the pseudocyst (*small arrow*).

Cystic Neoplasms

Cystic neoplasms constitute 10% of pancreatic cysts. Three primary cystic neoplasms have been identified in the pancreas: serous microcystic adenoma, mucinous macrocystic adenoma, and intraductal papillary mucinous tumors (IPMT). Distinction between these entities is important because the macrocystic adenoma and main-duct type IPMT tumors are malignant and require operative treatment (Fig. 84-18). Secondary cystic neoplasms include cystic degeneration of exocrine (ductal adenocarcinoma) and endocrine neoplasms. Distinction between primary (mucinous cystadenocarcinoma) and secondary (ductal adenocarcinoma) neoplasms is important because the latter has a better prognosis.[67] In most cases differentiating benign from malignant cysts is possible via MRI and clinical/laboratory history.

However, in doubtful cases or when it is important to determine preoperatively the type of cystic neoplasm, endoscopic ultrasound plays a role in cyst fluid analysis and analysis of enzymes, viscosity, cytology, and a variety of tumor markers allows for a better differential diagnosis.[68,69]

Serous Microcystic and Mucinous Macrocystic Adenomas

Serous microcystic adenoma is a benign neoplasm seen in older patients.[70] It has been associated with Von Hippel-Lindau syndrome.[71] There is a slight propensity for the pancreatic head. Serous microcystic adenomas characteristically have multiple tiny cysts with no evidence of peripancreatic fat or vascular invasion.

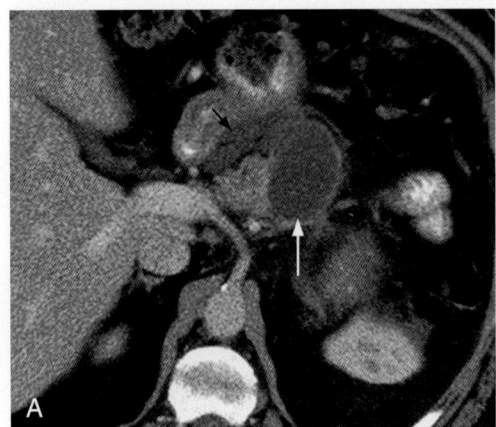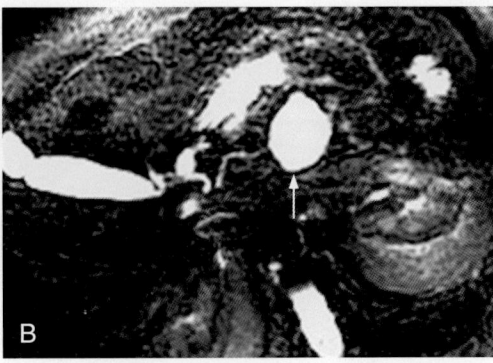

FIGURE 84-16

Pseudocyst. **A,** Axial contrast-enhanced CT shows a low density collection (*white arrow*) in the body of the pancreas. There is peripancreatic inflammation (*black arrow*). **B,** Axial MR cholangiopancreatography image confirms a large cystic collection (*arrow*) abutting the pancreatic duct.

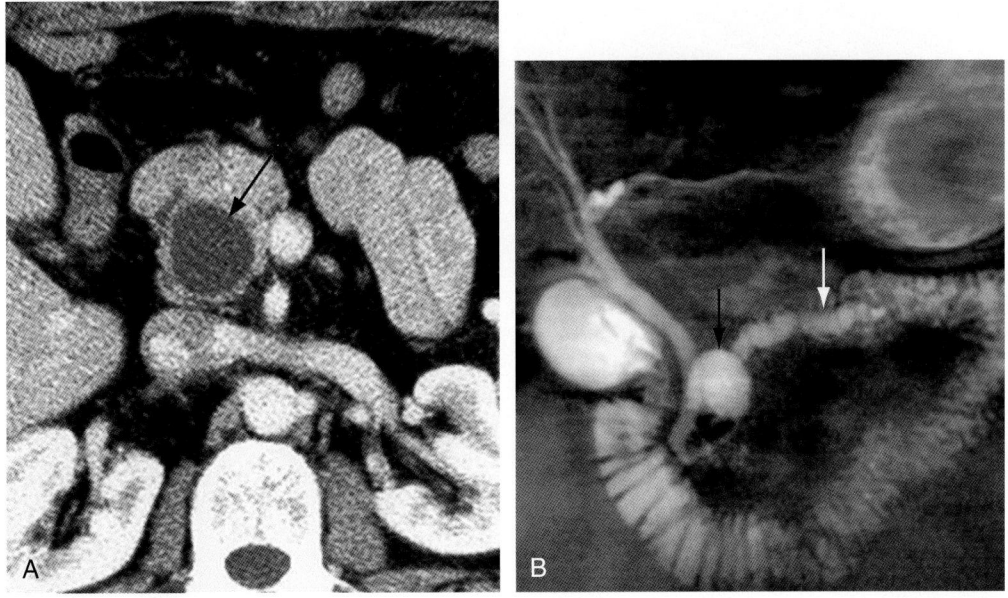

FIGURE 84-17

Pseudocysts. **A,** Axial contrast-enhanced CT shows a large pancreatic pseudocyst (*arrow*). **B,** Coronal plane MR cholangiopancreatography shows a large pancreatic pseudocyst (*black arrow*). There is also ductal dilation (*white arrow*).

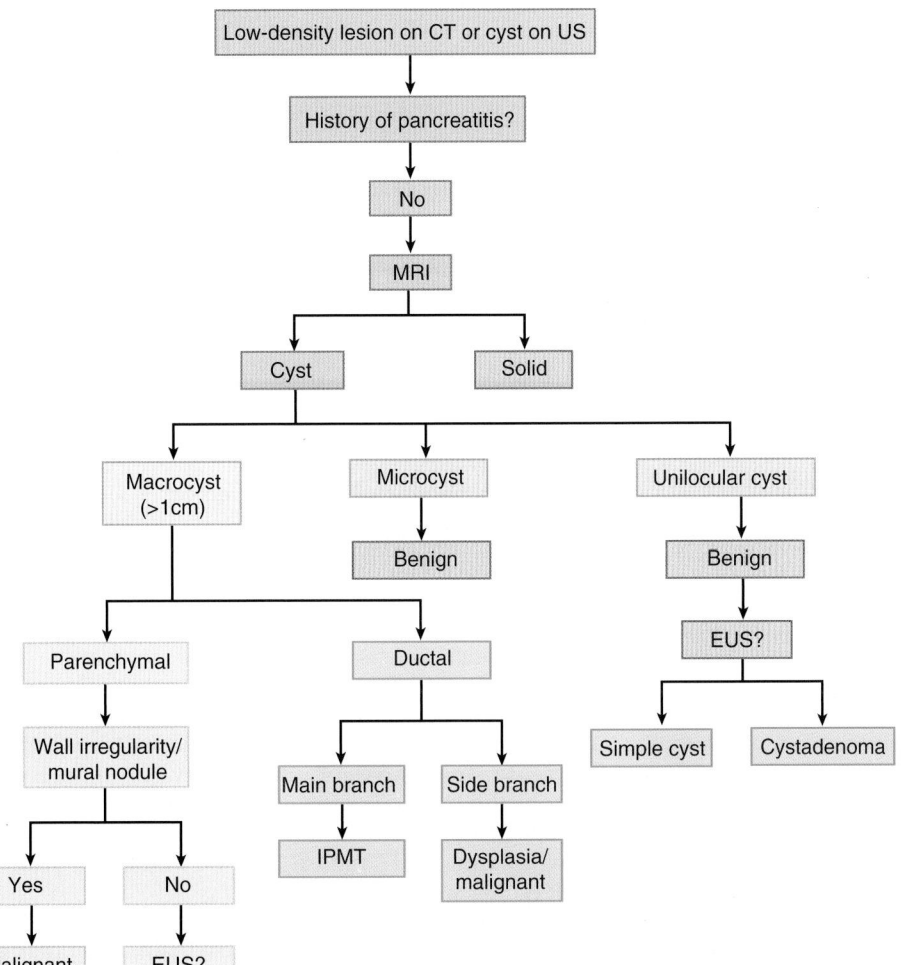

FIGURE 84-18

Algorithm for cystic pancreatic lesions. EUS, endoscopic ultrasound; IPMT, intraductal papillary mucinous tumor.

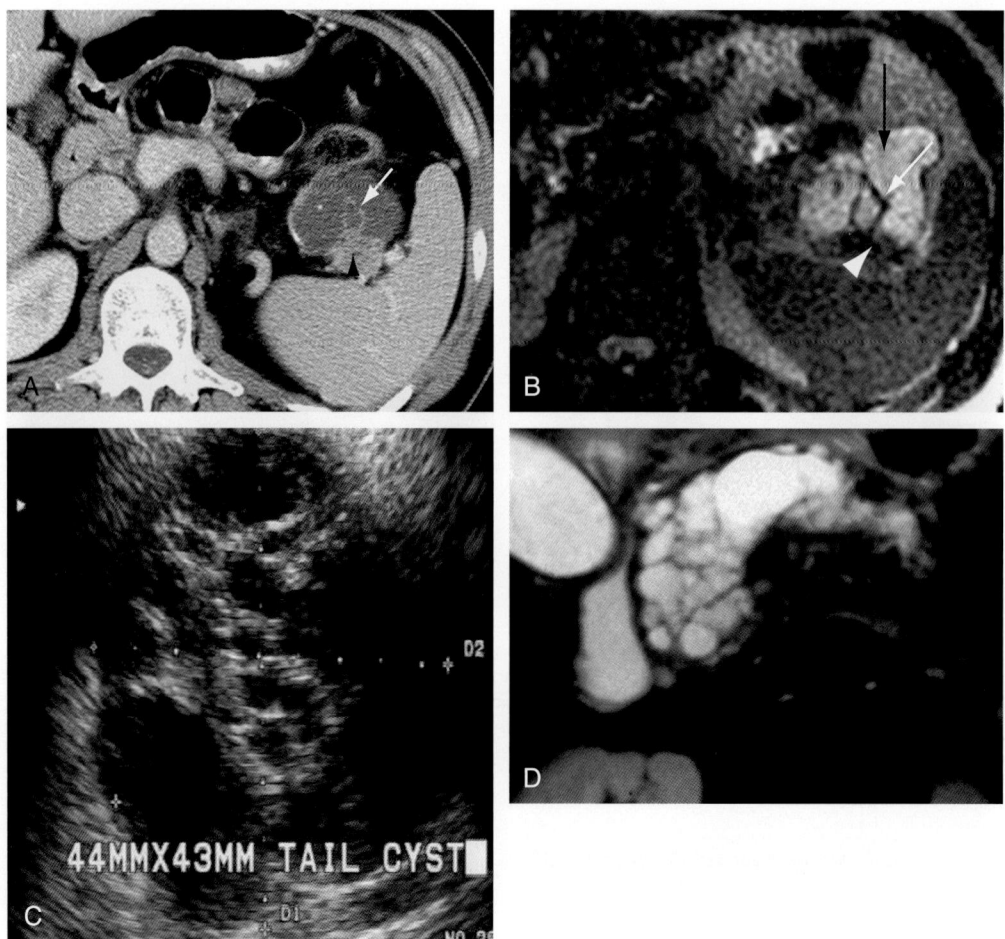

FIGURE 84-19

Cystic pancreatic neoplasms. **A,** Axial contrast-enhanced CT shows a cystic structure in the tail of the pancreas with septations (*white arrow*) and mural nodularity (*arrowhead*). **B,** Axial T2-weighted MR shows a large septated cyst (*black arrow*). There are thickened septations (*white arrow*) and mural nodularity (*arrowhead*) making the lesion suspicious for mucinous cystadenocarcinoma. **C,** Ultrasound confirms the cystic nature of the lesion in the pancreatic tail. **D,** Axial T2-weighted MR image of a different patient shows a lesion in the head of the pancreas with multiple small cysts consistent with serous cystadenoma. (*Fig. 84-19D courtesy of Dr. H. Kressel.*)

Mucinous macrocystic adenomas are malignant or have a malignant potential and need to be resected.[72,73] They are typically found in the body and tail of the pancreas in middle-aged (40-60 years) females (M:F = 6:1).[73,74]

MR IMAGING. Serous and mucinous adenomas both have low signal characteristics on T1- and high signal on T2-weighted sequences. Distinction between the benign serous cystadenoma and malignant mucinous cystadenocarcinoma is based on the size and morphologic features of the cyst.[75] Benign, serous cystadenomas are microcysts measuring less than 1 cm in diameter and have no septations or mural irregularity. Malignant, mucinous, macrocysts are typically greater than 1 cm in diameter and have septations and mural irregularity (Fig. 84-19). In addition, mucinous adenocarcinomas may occasionally have high signal on T1-weighted images due to the protein content of the cysts. Demonstration of communication of a cyst with a duct classifies it as an IPMT.

Intraductal Papillary Mucinous Tumor

IPMT is a rare pancreatic tumor which is a result of papillary proliferation of ductal epithelium. With IPMT there is associated ductal dilation and overproduction of mucin. It may originate from the main pancreatic duct or a side branch and is so classified. Histologically, IPMT can be classified from benign to overtly malignant. In main-duct tumors, a maximum pancreatic duct diameter of 15 mm and diffuse dilation of the main pancreatic duct are suggestive of malignancy. In branch-duct tumors, the presence of main-duct dilation is suggestive of malignancy. This classification is important as some slow growing IPMT tumors may be monitored without undergoing surgery.[75]

Patients with IPMT present in their sixth and seventh decades with recurrent abdominal pain. Although CT is usually performed in the initial evaluation of these

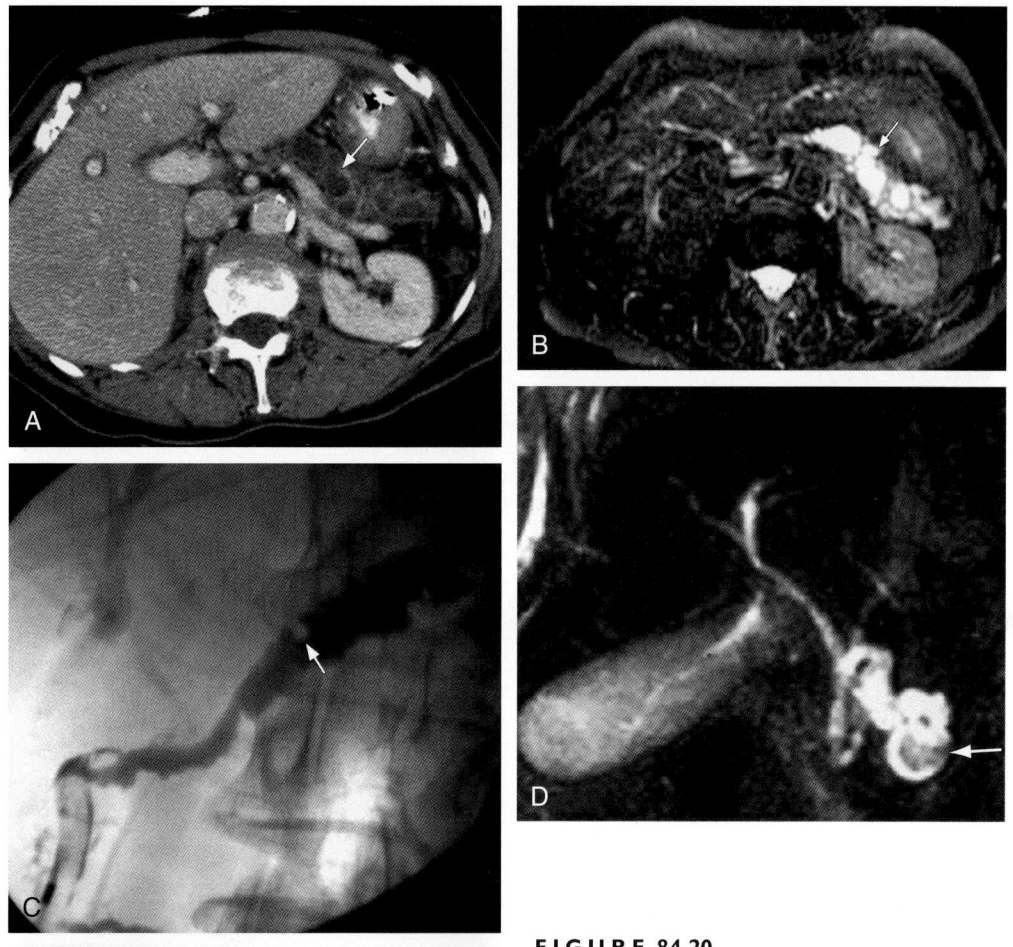

FIGURE 84-20

Intraductal papillary mucinous tumor (IPMT). **A,** Axial contrast-enhanced CT shows the pancreatic body replaced with multiple cysts (*arrow*). **B,** T2-weighted MR image shows multiple cysts occupying the pancreatic body and tail (*arrow*). **C,** Endoscopic retrograde cholangiopancreatography (ERCP) shows a dilated pancreatic duct with filling defects (*arrow*), representing inspissated mucin produced by the IPMT. **D,** MR cholangiopancreatography of a different patient with IPMT shows a characteristic filling defect (*arrow*) consistent with mucin. **E,** ERCP confirms the MR findings. (*Figs. 84-20D and 84-20E courtesy of Dr. R. Edelman.*)

patients, findings can be confused with chronic pancreatitis. ERCP and MRCP are both more definitive in the evaluation of IPMT.

MR IMAGING. MRCP offers noninvasive evaluation for IPMT. Typically, T2-weighted MR and MRCP sequences are performed. With main-duct IMPT, there is diffuse or segmental dilation of the main pancreatic duct (Figs. 84-20 and 84-21). Side-branch IPMT is seen as a cluster of cysts or a single cystic lesion with lobulated or irregular margins with associated dilation of the adjacent pan-

creatic duct. Other MR findings include filling defects with dilated pancreatic ducts and mural nodules within the cysts. MRI has also been found to be useful for postoperative follow-up of IPMT.[76]

Adenocarcinoma

Ductal adenocarcinoma accounts for more than 90% of malignant pancreatic tumors. It is more common in the seventh decade, in males, and in African Americans.

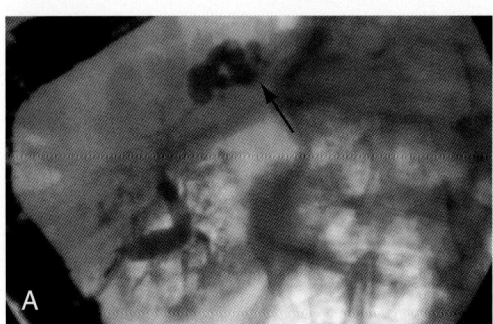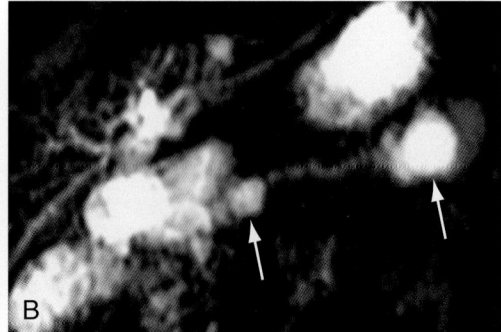

FIGURE 84-21

Main-duct/side-branch intraductal papillary mucinous tumor (IPMT). **A,** Endoscopic retrograde cholangiopancreatography (ERCP) failed to demonstrate the entire main pancreatic duct in a patient with IPMT, likely due to inspissated mucin. On ERCP only side-branch IPMT is noted (*arrow*). **B,** MR cholangiopancreatography delineates the entire main pancreatic duct and also demonstrates that there are two side-branch IPMTs (*arrows*) communicating with the main pancreatic duct.

Pancreatic adenocarcinoma is more frequently seen in the head of the pancreas (60%) versus the body and tail (30%). Patients with periampullary tumors[21] present with jaundice, weight loss, and abdominal pain. Periampullary tumors are treated with Whipple surgery, which has an overall 5-year survival rate of 15% to 25%.[34] Tumors in the body and tail grow to a larger size prior to the development of symptoms, and therefore have a lower resectability rate and present with a more dismal prognosis and poorer mean survival of 5 to 6 months.[34]

Imaging

Detection of pancreatic carcinoma may be performed with contrast-enhanced CT, MR, endoscopic ultrasound, or PET.[77,78] Endoscopic ultrasound uses a high-frequency (7.5-12 MHz) sonographic transducer that is introduced into the gastrointestinal tract. Studies comparing endoscopic sonography to CT have shown the former to be more sensitive for the detection of pancreatic and periampullary tumors, particularly for lesions less than 2 cm, with a sensitivity of 93% to 100%.[79-82] PET traditionally uses ^{18}F-fluorodeoxyglucose (FDG). Images are obtained anywhere between 40 and 180 minutes after injection. The sensitivity of PET for the diagnosis of primary malignant pancreatic tumor is approximately 64%. The use of FDG-PET appears to be limited to the detection of metastases or lymph node involvement distant from the tumor, determining respectability.[83]

In the detection of pancreatic tumors, CT has a sensitivity of 83% to 96% and specificity of 81% to 89%, and MRI of 80% to 95% and 71% to 78%, respectively.[84] The advantage of MRI over the other imaging modalities, in addition to improved tissue contrast and the ability to image in multiple planes, is the ability to evaluate the primary lesion, its effect on the adjacent ducts, its relationship to the vessels, and the presence of any soft-tissue extension with one study.

MRI in pancreatic adenocarcinoma is for lesion detection, staging, and post-treatment surveillance.

TUMOR DETECTION. Adenocarcinoma of the pancreas is most visible on post-gadolinium T1-weighted images as a non-enhancing mass. With contrast enhancement, there is prompt enhancement of the normal parenchyma and no enhancement of the tumor on the arterial or portal venous phases (Figs. 84-22 and 84-23). However, on delayed-phase imaging, because of the desmoplastic reaction of the tumor, there may be variable enhancement of the tumor.[85] The lesion may not be seen on non-enhanced T1-or T2-weighted sequences.

Secondary findings of the tumor are an important part of the MR evaluation. T2-weighted images and MRCP may be used to evaluate for ductal dilatation (Figs. 84-24, 84-25, and 84-26).

The presence of enlarged peripancreatic nodes and liver metastasis seen on fat-saturated T1-weighted, T2-weighted gadolinium-enhanced images may be used to assess for a pancreatic adenocarcinoma.

Occasionally, a small lesion near the pancreatic duct with no associated ductal dilatation may be missed by MRI but seen on endoscopic ultrasound (Fig. 84-27).

STAGING. The second role of MRI in pancreatic adenocarcinoma is to determine whether a lesion is resectable. Findings of nonresectability on MRI include vascular encasement, lymph node involvement, and distant metastasis.

Vascular encasement can be evaluated with gadolinium-enhanced T1-weighted MR sequences. Encasement is defined as:

● Tumor encasing greater than 50% of the vessel lumen (Figs. 84.25 and 84-28)[86,87]
● Decrease in vessel caliber
● Dilated peripancreatic veins
● Tear-drop shape of the superior mesenteric vein.

A recent study of 48 patients that compared MR imaging, MR imaging with MR angiography, and dual-phase CT found comparable accuracies (87%, 90%, and 90%, respectively).[88]

Text continues on page 2675

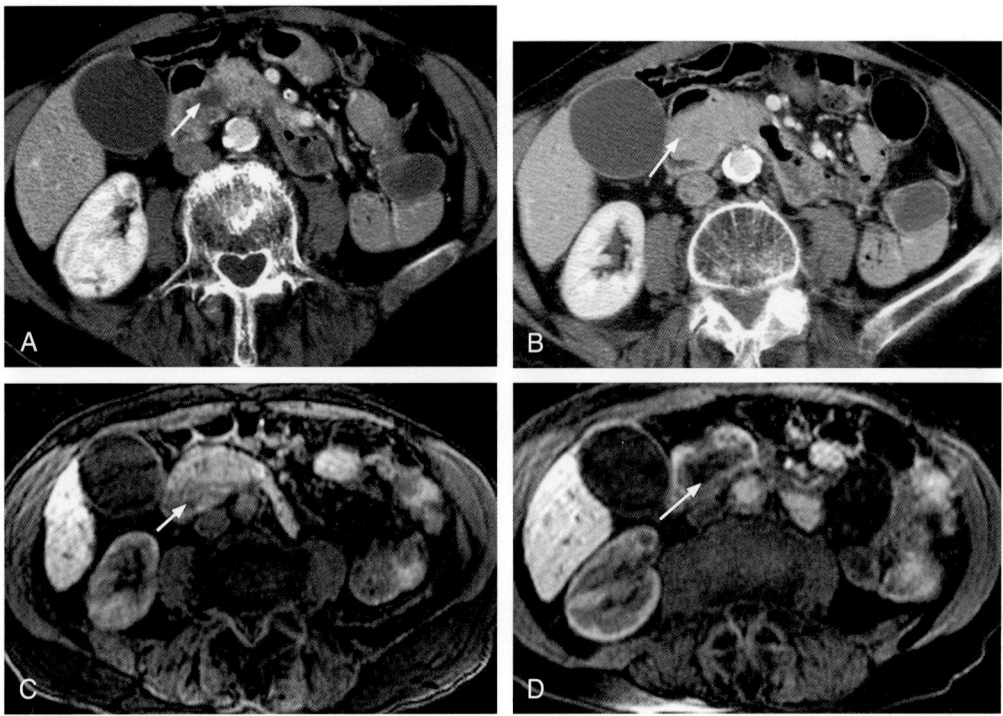

FIGURE 84-22

Ampullary carcinoma. **A** and **B,** Axial contrast-enhanced CT images show a large periampullary mass involving the pancreatic head and duodenum (*arrow*). **C** and **D,** Post-gadolinium T1-weighted MR images show a nonenhancing mass (*arrow*) in the periampullary location.

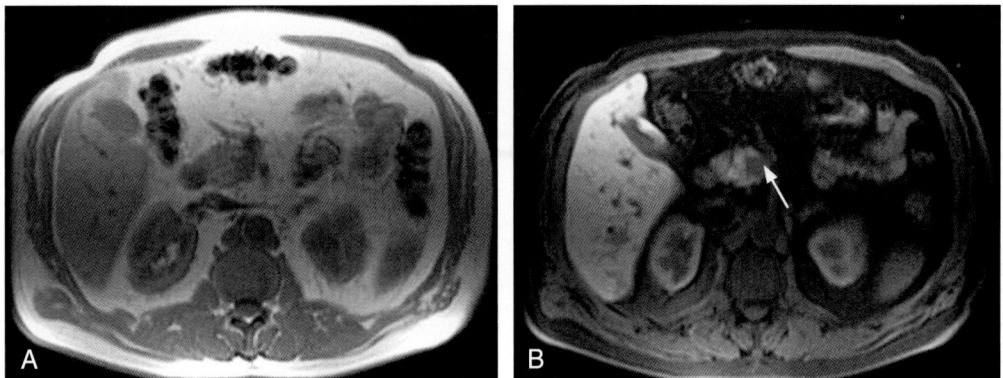

FIGURE 84-23

Small pancreatic cancer. **A,** Axial T1-weighted image of the neck of the pancreas does not definitively identify a pancreatic mass. **B,** Post-gadolinium, axial T1-weighted image in the same area better visualizes a small pancreatic neck mass (*arrow*). With contrast there is homogenous enhancement of the pancreatic parenchyma and nonenhancement of the adenocarcinoma. Gadolinium administration improves tissue contrast and increases the sensitivity of detecting pancreatic tumors.

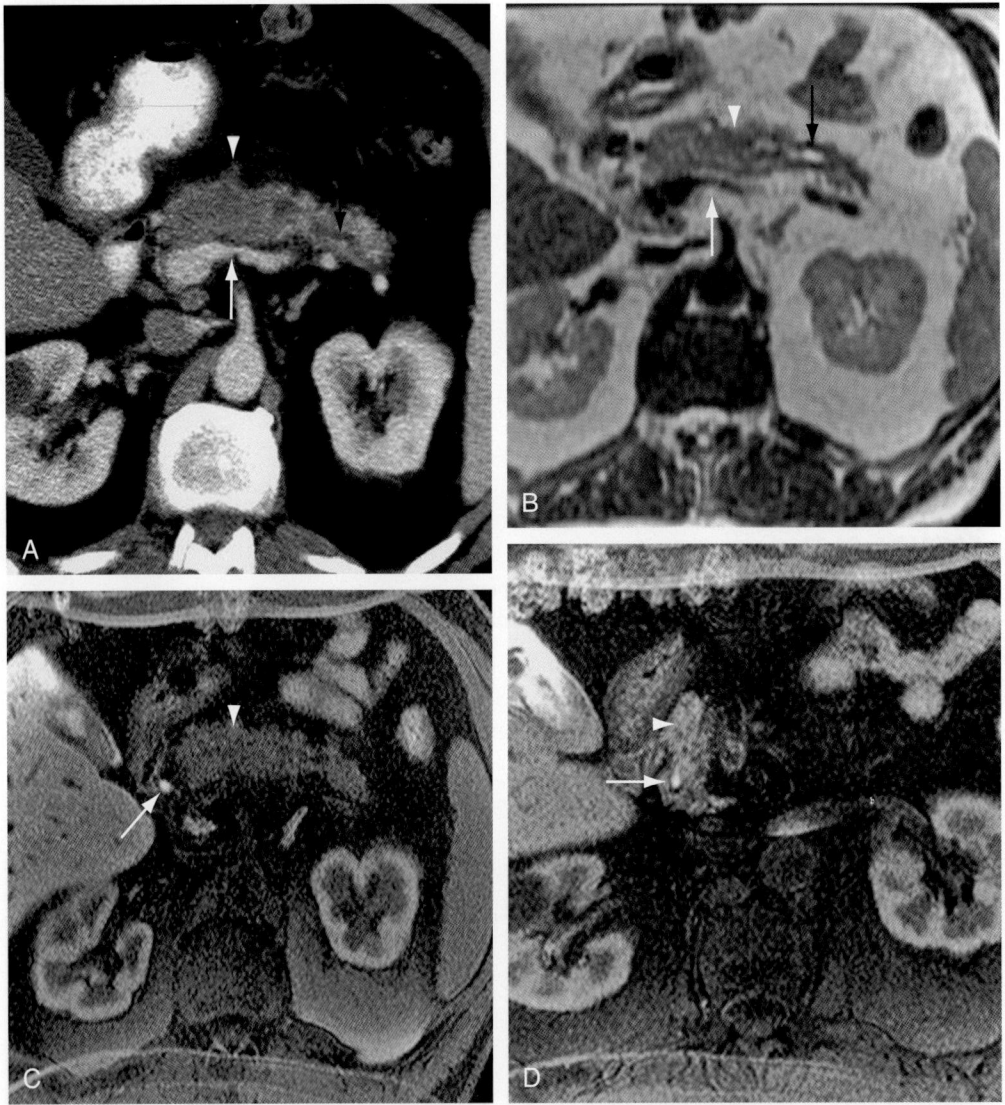

FIGURE 84-24

Pancreatic cancer. **A,** Axial contrast-enhanced CT shows a large pancreatic body mass (*white arrowhead*) with distal ductal dilation (*black arrow*). The splenic vein (*white arrow*) is not invaded. **B,** Axial T1-weighted MR image shows similar findings: pancreatic body mass (*arrowhead*), distal ductal dilation (*black arrow*) and a clear fat plane from the splenic vein (*white arrow*). **C** and **D,** Post-manganese T1-weighted fat-saturated MRI images. The pancreatic mass does not enhance (*arrowhead*). The common bile duct is enhanced and seen as a high signal structure (*arrow*).

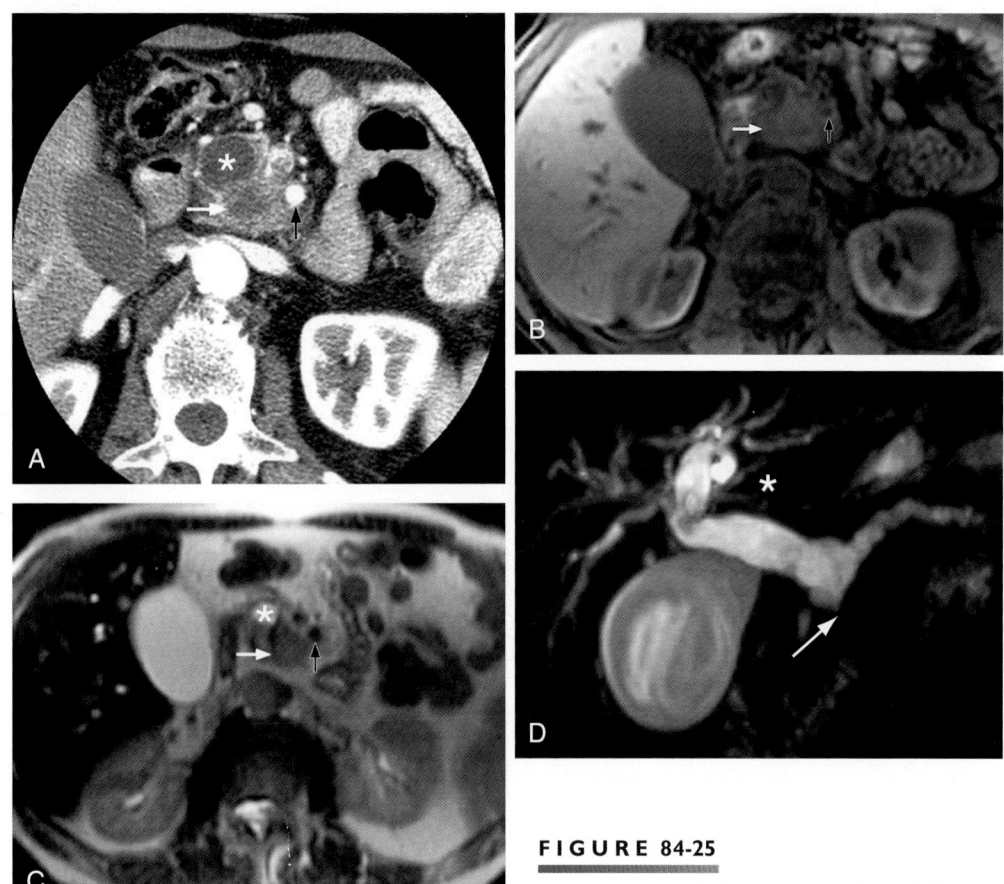

FIGURE 84-25

Adenocarcinoma. **A,** Axial contrast-enhanced CT shows a dilated common bile duct (*). There is a low density mass in the head of the pancreas (*white arrow*) which abuts the superior mesenteric artery (*black arrow*). **B,** Axial T1-weighted MR image suggests that the mass (*white arrow*) abuts only approximately 25% of the superior mesenteric artery (*black arrow*). The dilated duct (*) is visualized. **C,** However, post-gadolinium T1-weighted MR image shows that the mass (*white arrow*) abuts more than 50% of the superior mesenteric artery (*black arrow*) and therefore suggests vascular invasion and nonresectability of the tumor. The dilated common bile duct is visible (*). **D,** MR cholangiopancreatography shows the double-duct sign (*arrow*) with dilated common hepatic and pancreatic ducts. **E,** Endoscopic retrograde cholangiopancreatography confirms distal stenosis (*arrow*).

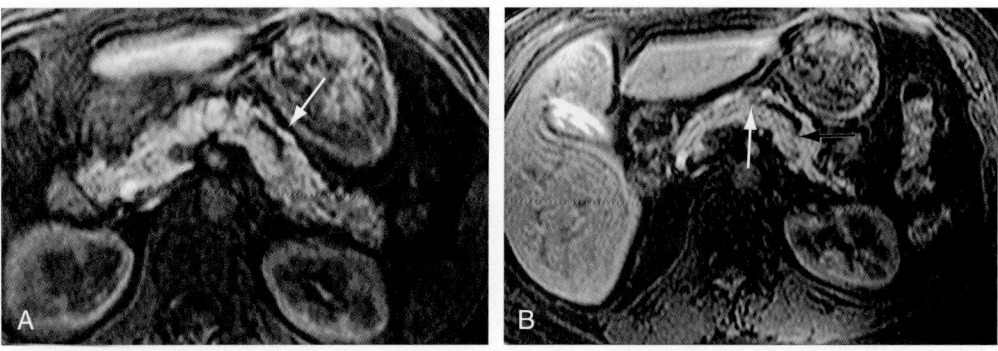

FIGURE 84-26

Mixed duct cancer. **A,** Axial T1-weighed fat-saturated MR image shows a dilated pancreatic duct (*arrow*). **B,** Axial post-gadolinium T1-weighted image shows a small mass in the mid body of the duct (*arrow*) with distal ductal dilation (*black arrow*).

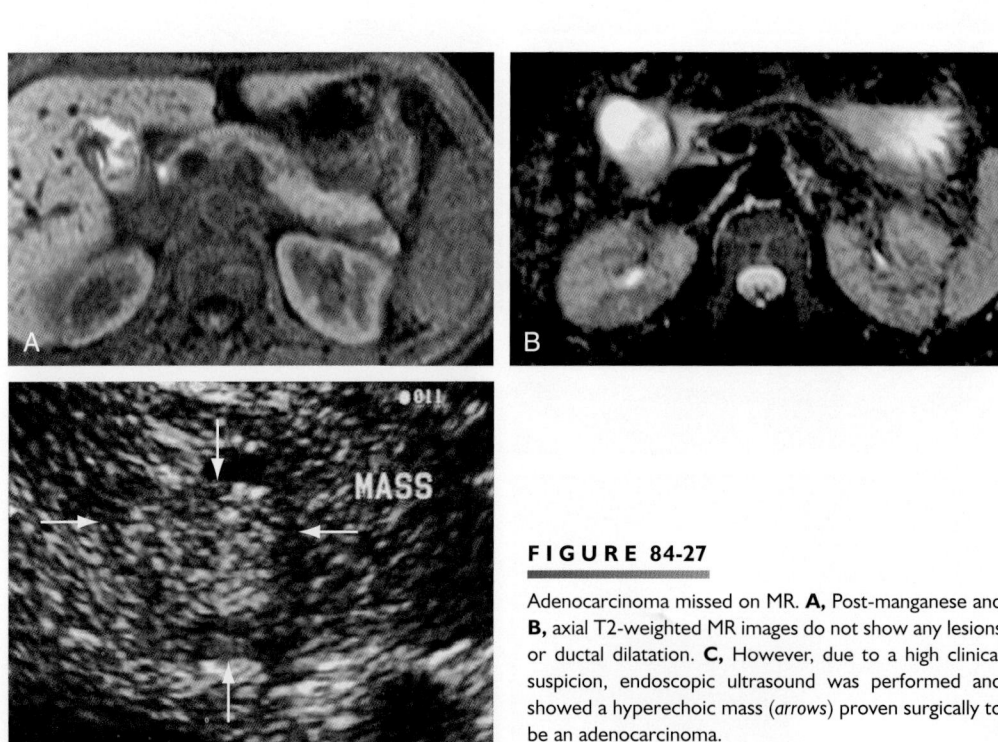

FIGURE 84-27

Adenocarcinoma missed on MR. **A,** Post-manganese and **B,** axial T2-weighted MR images do not show any lesions or ductal dilatation. **C,** However, due to a high clinical suspicion, endoscopic ultrasound was performed and showed a hyperechoic mass (*arrows*) proven surgically to be an adenocarcinoma.

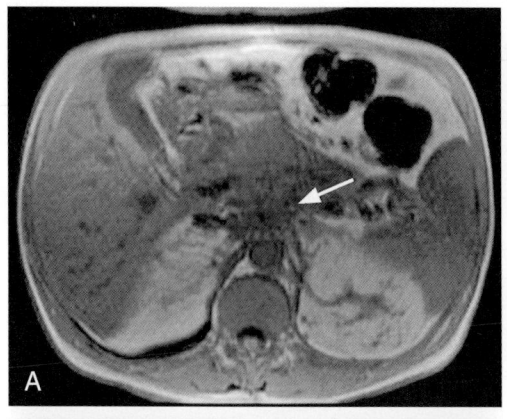

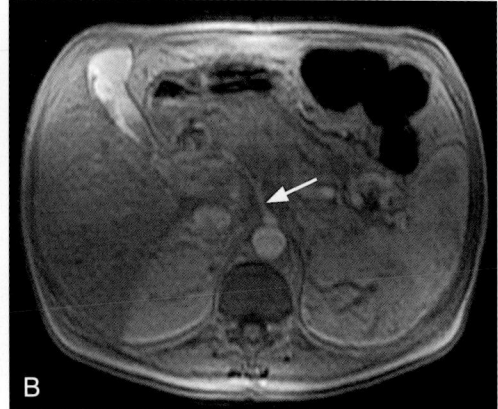

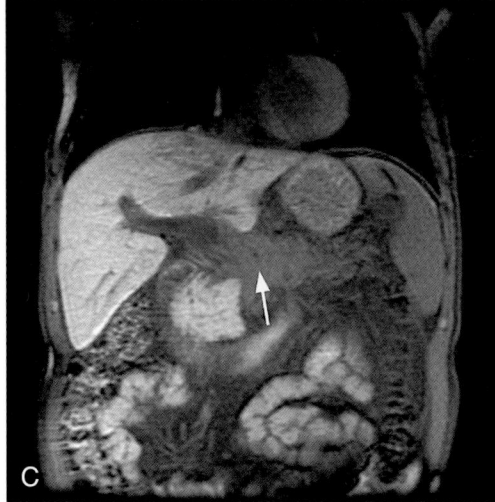

FIGURE 84-28

Nonresectable adenocarcinoma vascular invasion. **A,** Axial T1-weighted image shows a large low signal mass in the pancreatic neck and body (*arrow*). **B,** Axial post-gadolinium image shows the mass surrounds the celiac artery (*arrow*). **C,** Coronal post-gadolinium MR image shows low signal mass (*arrow*).

T1- or post-gadolinium T1-weighted images may be used to evaluate for enlarged peripancreatic nodes. PET imaging may also play a role in the evaluation of malignant peripancreatic nodes.[83] MR lymph-node–specific contrast agents, such as ultrasmall superparamagnetic iron oxide (USPIO) which is in phase III trials for nodal involvement in prostatic colonic endometrial Merkel cell tumor lymphoma and seminoma,[89] may be used in future to evaluate peripancreatic nodes.

Sixty percent of patients who present with pancreatic ductal adenocarcinoma have distant metastasis.[77] MRI has an accuracy of 93.5% for the detection of liver metastases, CT an accuracy of 87%,[90] and PET has been reported to have a sensitivity of 70% and a specificity of 95% for liver metastases.[91] Fat-saturated T1- and T2-weighted, and post-gadolinium sequences imaging the upper abdomen may be used to evaluate for metastases.

POST-TREATMENT SURVEILLANCE. MRI can also be used to noninvasively evaluate the postoperative course and survey for recurrence. It can evaluate for short- and long-term postoperative complications, including hemorrhage, anastomotic leak, and bile duct strictures (Fig.

84-29). MRCP with secretin has also been used to evaluate postoperative pancreaticogastrostomy and pancreaticoduodenectomy anastomosis.[92-94]

Islet Cell Tumors

Islet cell tumors are of neuroendocrine origin. They are rare (<1 per 100,000) and classified as functional or nonfunctional, based on secretion of an active peptide. The types of islet cell tumors include insulinoma, gastrinoma, VIPoma (which secretes a vasoactive intestinal peptide), and somatostatinoma.

MR Imaging

The hallmark of islet tumors, either functional or nonfunctional, on MRI is high signal on T2-weighted images and early arterial enhancement on gadolinium-enhanced sequences (Fig. 84-30).[95] If there is a high clinical suspicion of a neuroendocrine tumor and a negative MRI, a nuclear medicine, ^{111}In-DTPA octreotide study may be performed (Fig. 84-31).[96]

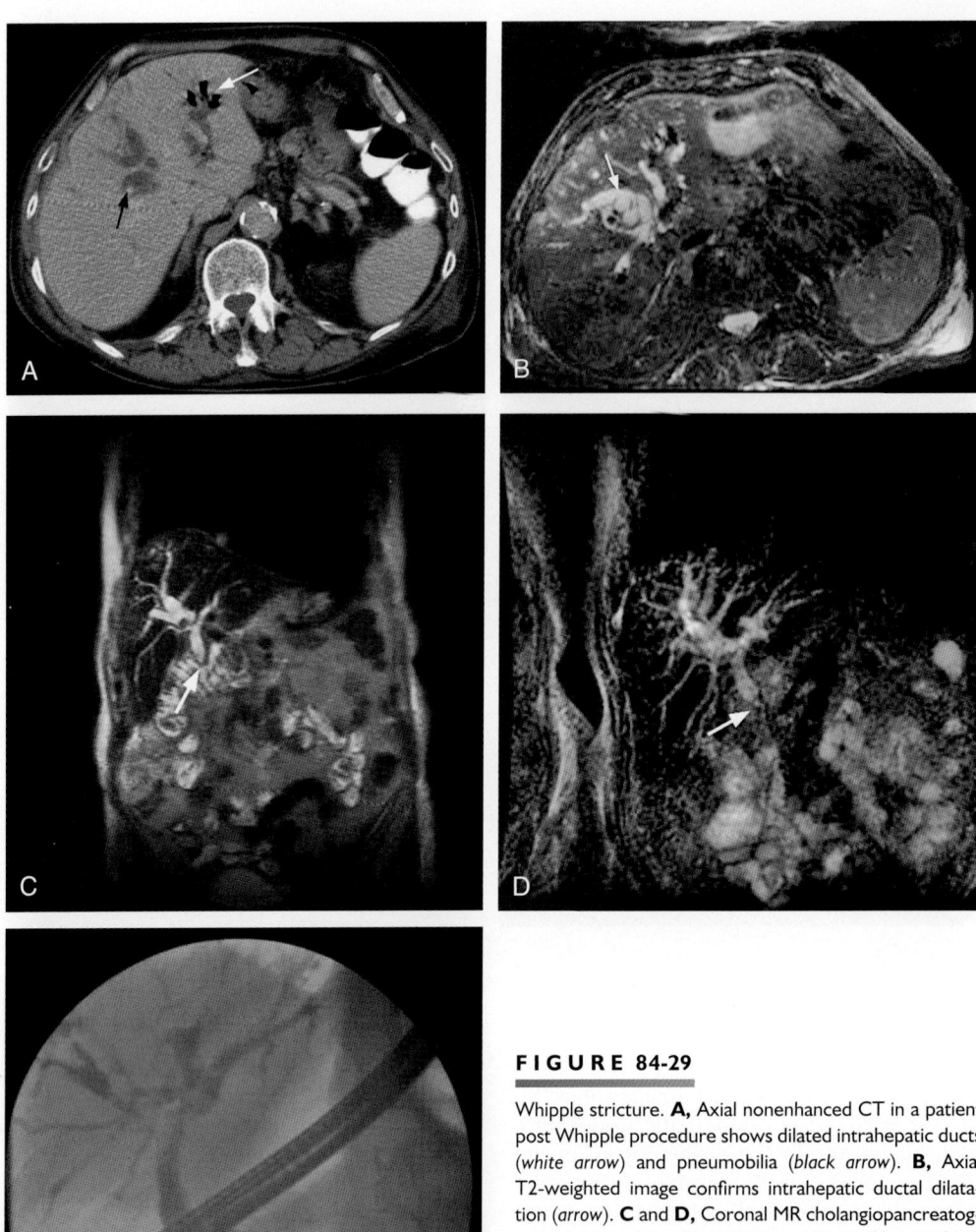

FIGURE 84-29

Whipple stricture. **A,** Axial nonenhanced CT in a patient post Whipple procedure shows dilated intrahepatic ducts (*white arrow*) and pneumobilia (*black arrow*). **B,** Axial T2-weighted image confirms intrahepatic ductal dilatation (*arrow*). **C** and **D,** Coronal MR cholangiopancreatography images show dilated intra- and extra-hepatic ducts extending to the choledochojejunal anastomosis stricture (*arrow*). **E,** Endoscopic retrograde cholangiopancreatography confirms a postoperative stricture (*arrow*).

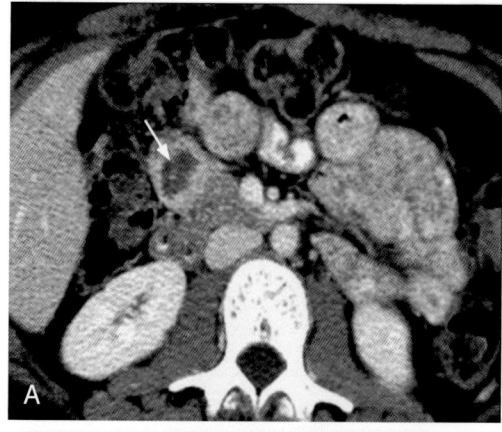
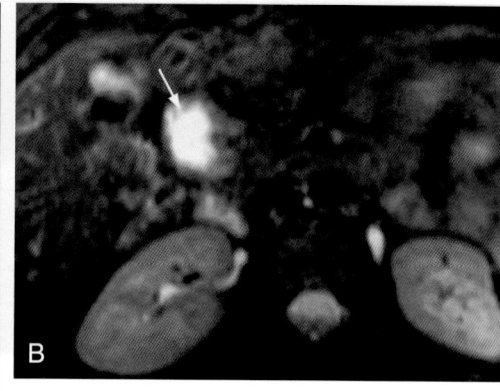
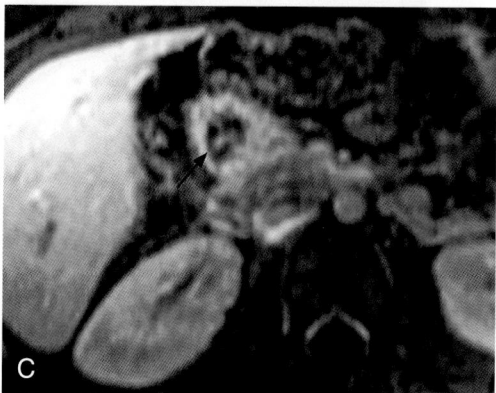

FIGURE 84-30

Islet cell. **A,** Axial contrast-enhanced CT shows a low density mass (*arrow*) in the pancreatic head. **B,** Axial T2-weighted MR image shows a high signal T2- weighted lesion (*arrow*). **C,** Post-gadolinium MR image shows the lesion has slight central enhancement and is not cystic (*arrow*). These findings are consistent with an islet cell tumor.

Solid and Papillary Epithelial Neoplasm

Solid and papillary epithelial tumors have low-grade malignant potential. They are characteristically seen in the body and tail of the pancreas in 20- to 30-year-old females.

MR Imaging

Although the diagnosis can be made on CT, on MRI these tumors are seen as well-demarcated lesions with a central area of high signal on T1-weighted images consistent with hemorrhagic necrosis. There is no enhancement on post-contrast images (Fig. 84-32).[97]

Metastasis

Metastases to the pancreas (including gastrointestinal, breast, kidney, lung, prostate, and melanoma) are rare and may arise hematogenously or by direct invasion.[98] On MRI, most metastasis have low signal on T1-weighted images. The exception to this is melanoma metastasis which has a high signal on T1-weighted images due to its melanin content. Hypervascular metastasis, such as gastrointestinal metastasis, may show rapid enhancement on post-contrast MR images (Fig. 84-33).

Published reports have documented renal cell metastasis identified with chemical shift imaging.[99]

Lymphoma

Non-Hodgkin's lymphoma can involve the pancreas. Nodes can be distinguished due to their intermediate signal intensity on T1-weighted fat-suppressed images adjacent to the normal high signal pancreatic parenchyma. With increased nodal infiltration of the pancreas there will be a corresponding decrease in signal and heterogeneity of the pancreatic parenchyma on T1-weighted fat-suppressed images.

Trauma

Traumatic injury to the pancreas is seen in 2% of abdominal trauma.[34] Although CT can adequately evaluate for injury to the pancreas, MRI is more definitive in assessment for ductal injury. MRCP can examine the entire extent of the duct and look for discontinuity or extravasation (Fig. 84-34).[100]

Post-Transplant Imaging

With increasing use of pancreatic transplantation to treat type 1 diabetes mellitus, imaging is being used more to evaluate for operative complications or graft rejection. Transplanted pancreatic tissue is typically placed in the

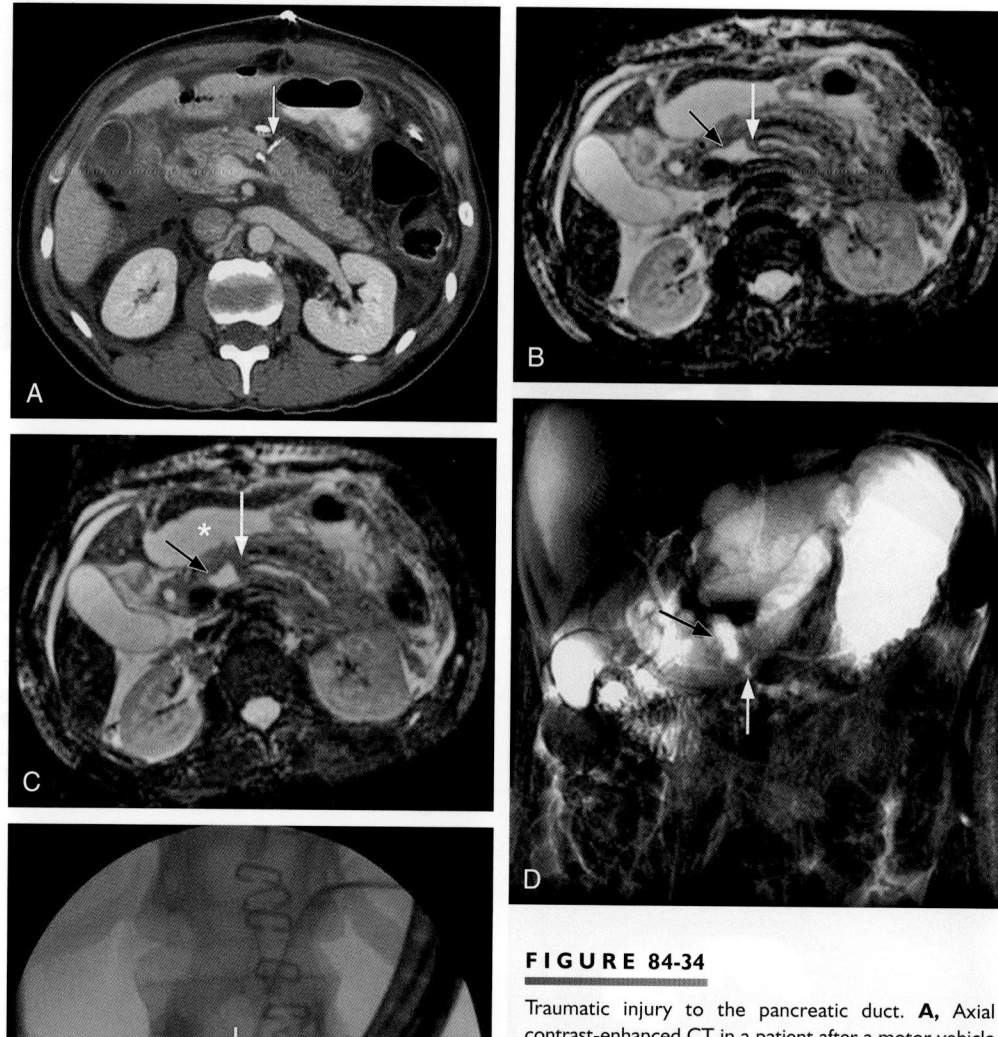

FIGURE 84-34

Traumatic injury to the pancreatic duct. **A,** Axial contrast-enhanced CT in a patient after a motor vehicle accident shows a pancreatic laceration (*arrow*). **B** and **C,** Axial T2-weighted MR images show discontinuity of the pancreatic duct (*white arrow*), small high density collection (*black arrow*), and a slightly larger peripancreatic collection (*). **D,** Coronal MR cholangiopancreatography confirms pancreatic duct disruption (*white arrow*) and extravasation (*black arrow*). **E,** Endoscopic retrograde cholangiopancreatography also shows disruption of the pancreatic duct (*white arrow*) and extravasation (*black arrow*).

secretin-stimulated MRCP and has advanced the imaging of chronic pancreatitis. Current indications for MR include:

- To evaluate pancreatic masses suspected of being adenocarcinoma for detection and staging
- To evaluate suspected islet cell tumors
- Noninvasive evaluation of IPMT
- To evaluate for chronic pancreatitis
- To evaluate for early acute pancreatitis not seen on CT and survey for possible complications
- To image patients with pancreatic diseases and with renal dysfunction and dye allergy.

REFERENCES

1. Mitchell DG: Fast MR imaging techniques: impact in the abdomen. J Magn Reson Imaging. 6:812-821, 1996.
2. Roberts TPL: Fast scan techniques. In Higgins CB, Hricak H, Helms CA (eds): Magnetic Resonance Imaging of the Body, 3rd ed. Philadelphia, Lippincott-Raven, 1996, pp 71-86.
3. Keogan MT, Edelman RR: Technological advances in abdominal MR imaging. Radiology 220:310-320, 2001.
4. Chen Q, Stock KW, Prasad PV, Hatabu H: Fast magnetic resonance imaging techniques. In Hatabu H, Imhof H (eds): Fast Magnetic Resonance Body Imaging. New York, Elsevier Science, 2000, pp 1-12.
5. Ferrucci JT: Advances in abdominal MR imaging. RadioGraphics 18:1569-1586, 1998.
6. Petersein J, Saini S: Fast MR imaging: Technical strategies. Am J Roentgenol. 165:1105-1109, 1995.

7. Haacke EM, Tkach JA: Fast MR imaging: Techniques and clinical applications. Am J Roentgenol 155:951-964, 1995.

8. Chien D, Edelman RR: Fast magnetic resonance imaging. In Higgins CB, Hricak H, Helms CA (eds): Magnetic Resonance Imaging of the Body, 2nd ed. New York, Lippincott-Raven, 1992, pp 175-198.

9. Wehrli FW: Fast-scan imaging: Principles and contrast phenomenology. In Higgins CB, Hricak H (eds): Magnetic Resonance Imaging of the Body. New York, Raven Press, 1987, pp 23-38.

10. Outwater EK, Siegelman ES: MR imaging of pancreatic disorders. Top Magn Reson Imaging 8:265-289, 1996.

11. Outwater EK. Mitchell DG: MR imaging techniques for evaluation of the pancreas. Top Magn Reson Imaging 8:248-264, 1996.

12. Takehara Y: Fast MR imaging for evaluating the pancreaticobiliary system. Eur J Radiol 29:211-232, 1999.

13. Ly JN, Miller FH: MR imaging of the pancreas: a practical approach. Radiol Clin North Am 40:1289-1306, 2002.

14. Mortele KJ, Ros PR: Magnetic resonance imaging of the exocrine pancreas. Rays 26:117-126, 2001.

15. Bartolozzi C, Lencioni R, Donati F, Cioni D: Abdominal MR: liver and pancreas. Eur Radiol 9:1496-1512, 1999.

16. Lee JKT, Sagel SS, Stanley RJ, Heiken JP (eds): Computed Body Tomography with MRI Correlation, 3rd ed. Philadelphia, Lippincott Williams & Wilkins, 1998, pp 873-953.

17. Matos C, Cappeliez O, Winant C, et al: MR imaging of the pancreas: A pictorial tour. RadioGraphics 22:e2, 2002.

18. Megibow AJ, Lavelle MT, Rofsky NM: MR imaging of the pancreas. Surg Clin North Am 81:307-320, ix-x, 2001.

19. Mitchell DG, Winston CB, Outwater EK, Ehrlich SM: Delineation of pancreas with MR imaging: multiobserver comparison of five pulse sequences. J Magn Reson Imaging 5:193-199, 1995.

20. Chan TW, Listerud J, Kressel HY: Combined chemical-shift and phase-selective imaging for fat suppression: theory and initial clinical experience. Radiology 181:41-47, 1991.

21. Kettritz U, Semelka RC: Contrast-enhanced MR imaging of the pancreas. Magn Reson Imaging Clin North Am 4:87-100, 1996.

22. Low RN: Current uses of gadolinium chelates for clinical magnetic resonance imaging examination of the liver. Top Magn Reson Imaging 9:141-166, 1998.

23. Wang C, Johansson L, Western A, et al: Sequence optimization in mangafodipir trisodium-enhanced liver and pancreas MRI. J Magn Reson Imaging 9:280-284, 1999.

24. Dreiling DA, Messer J: The secretin story. Am J Gastroenterol 70:455-479, 1978.

25. Matos C, Metens T, Deviere J, et al: Pancreatic duct: morphologic and functional evaluation with dynamic MR pancreatography after secretin stimulation. Radiology 203:435-441, 1997.

26. Takehara Y: MR pancreatography. Semin Ultrasound CT MR 20:324-339, 1999.

27. Varghese JC, Masterson A, Lee MJ: Value of MR pancreatography in the evaluation of patients with chronic pancreatitis. Clin Radiol 57:393-401, 2002.

28. Manfredi R, Costamagna G, Brizi MG, et al: Severe chronic pancreatitis versus suspected pancreatic disease: dynamic MR cholangiopancreatography after secretin stimulation. Radiology 214:849-855, 2000.

29. Cappeliez O, Delhaye M, Deviere J, et al: Chronic pancreatitis: evaluation of pancreatic exocrine function with MR pancreatography after secretin stimulation. Radiology 215:358-364, 2000.

30. Rofsky NM, Lee VS, Laub G, et al: Abdominal MR imaging with a volumetric interpolated breath-hold examination. Radiology 212:876-884, 1999.

31. Ascher SM, Semelka RC, Brown JJ: Pancreas, spleen, bowel and peritoneum. In Edelman R, Hesselink JR, Zlatkin MB, eds: Clinical Magnetic Resonance Imaging, 2nd ed. Philadelphia, WB Saunders, 1996, pp 1564-1577.

32. Kanematsu M, Shiratori Y, Hoshi H, et al: Pancreas and peripancreatic vessels: effect of imaging delay on gadolinium enhancement at dynamic gradient-recalled-echo MR imaging. Radiology 215:95-102, 2000.

33. Delhaye M, Engelholm CM: Pancreas divisum: congenital anatomic variant or anomaly? Contributions of endoscopic retrograde dorsal pancreatography. Gastroenterology 89:951-958, 1995.

34. Yeo CJ, Cameron JL: The pancreas. In Sabiston DC, Lyerly HK (eds): Sabiston Textbook of Surgery The Biological Basis of Modern Surgical Practice, 15th ed. Philadelphia, WB Saunders, 1997, pp 1152-1186.

35. Bret PM, Reinhold C, Taourel P, et al: Pancreas divisum: evaluation with MR cholangiopancreatography. Radiology 199:99-103, 1996.

36. Arcement CM, Meza MP, Arumanla S, Towbin RB: MRCP in the evaluation of pancreaticobiliary disease in children. Pediatr Radiol 31:92-97, 2001.

37. Madura JA, Fiore AC, O'Connor KW, et al: Pancreas divisum. Detection and management. Am Surg 51:353-357, 1985.

38. Neuhaus H: Therapeutic pancreatic endoscopy. Endoscopy 36:8-16, 2004.

39. Manfredi R, Costamagna G, Brizi MG, et al: Pancreas divisum and "santorinicele": diagnosis with dynamic MR cholangiopancreatography with secretin stimulation. Radiology 217:403-408, 2000.

40. Matos C, Metens T, Deviere J, et al: Pancreas divisum: evaluation with secretin-enhanced magnetic resonance cholangiopancreatography. Gastrointest Endosc 53:728-733, 2001.

41. Baggott BB, Woods AC: Annular pancreas. Am J Gastroenterol 86:224-226, 1991.

42. Desai MB, Mitchell DG, Monoz SJ: Asymptomatic annular pancreas: detection by magnetic resonance imaging. Magn Reson Imaging 12:683-685, 1994.

43. King LJ, Scurr ED, Murugan N, et al: Hepatobiliary and pancreatic manifestations of cystic fibrosis: MR imaging appearances. RadioGraphics 20:767-777, 2000.

44. Tham RT, Heyerman HG, Falke TH, et al: Cystic fibrosis: MR imaging of the pancreas. Radiology 179:183-186, 1991.

45. Jensen PD, Jensen FT, Christensen T, Ellegaard J: Non-invasive assessment of tissue iron overload in the liver by magnetic resonance imaging. Br J Haematol 87:171-184, 1994.

46. Siegelman ES, Mitchell DG, Rubin R, et al: Parenchymal versus reticuloendothelial iron overload in the liver: distinction with MR imaging. Radiology 179:361-366, 1991.

47. Yoon DY, Choi BI, Han JK, et al: MR findings of secondary hemochromatosis: transfusional vs. erythropoietic. J Comput Assist Tomogr 18:416-419, 1994.

48. Morgan DE, Baron TH, Smith JK, et al: Pancreatic fluid collections prior to intervention: evaluation with MR imaging compared with CT and US. Radiology 203:773-778, 1997.

49. Steinberg W, Tenner S: Acute pancreatitis. N Engl J Med 330:1198-1210, 1994.

50. Lecesne R, Taourel P, Bret PM, et al: Acute pancreatitis: interobserver agreement and correlation of CT and MR cholangiopancreatography with outcome. Radiology 211:727-735, 1999.

51. Balthazar EJ: CT diagnosis and staging of acute pancreatitis. Radiol Clin North Am 27:19-37, 1989.

52. Soto JA, Barish MA, Alvarez O, Medina S: Detection of choledocholithiasis with MR cholangiography: comparison of three-dimensional fast spin-echo and single- and multisection half-Fourier rapid acquisition with relaxation enhancement sequences. Radiology 215:737-745, 2000.

53. Loperfido S, Angelini G, Benedetti G, et al: Major early complications from diagnostic and therapeutic ERCP: a prospective multicenter study. Gastrointest Endosc 48:1-10, 1998.

54. Balthazar EJ, Robinson DL, Megibow AJ, Ranson JH: Acute pancreatitis: value of CT in establishing prognosis. Radiology 174:331-336, 1990.

55. Johnson CD, Stephens DH, Sarr MG: CT of acute pancreatitis: correlation between lack of contrast enhancement and pancreatic necrosis. Am J Roentgenol 156:93-95, 1991.

56. Saifuddin A, Ward J, Ridgway J, Chalmers AG: Comparison of MR and CT scanning in severe acute pancreatitis: initial experiences. Clin Radiol 48:111-116, 1993.

57. Piironen A, Kivisaari R, Pitkaranta P, et al: Contrast-enhanced magnetic resonance imaging for the detection of acute haemorrhagic necrotizing pancreatitis. Eur Radiol 7:17-20, 1997.

58. Ward J, Chalmers AG, Guthrie AJ, et al: T2-weighted and dynamic enhanced MRI in acute pancreatitis: comparison with contrast enhanced CT. Clin Radiol 52:109-114, 1997.

59. Lammer J, Herlinger H, Zalaudek G, Hofler H: Pseudotumorous pancreatitis. Gastrointest Radiol 10:59-67, 1985.

60. Kelekis NL, Semelka RC: Carcinoma of the pancreatic head area. Diagnostic imaging: magnetic resonance imaging. Rays 20:289-303, 1995.

61. Brown ED, Semelka RC: Magnetic resonance imaging of the spleen and pancreas. Top Magn Reson Imaging 7:82-89, 1995.

62. Johnson PT, Outwater EK: Pancreatic carcinoma versus chronic pancreatitis: dynamic MR imaging. Radiology 212:213-218, 1999.

63. Higashi T, Saga T, Nakamoto Y, et al: Diagnosis of pancreatic cancer using fluorine-18 fluorodeoxyglucose positron emission tomography (FDG PET)—usefulness and limitations in "clinical reality". Ann Nuclear Med 17:261-279, 2003.

64. Irie H, Honda H, Kuroiwa T, et al: MRI of groove pancreatitis. J Comput Assist Tomogr 22:651-655, 1998.

65. Manfredi R, Costamagna G, Brizi MG, et al: Severe chronic pancreatitis versus suspected pancreatic disease: dynamic MR cholangiopancreatography after secretin stimulation. Radiology 214:849-855, 2000.

66. Khalid A, Peterson M, Slivka A: Secretin-stimulated magnetic resonance pancreaticogram to assess pancreatic duct outflow obstruction in evaluation of idiopathic acute recurrent pancreatitis: a pilot study. Digest Dis Sci 48:1475-81, 2003.

67. Compagno J, Oertel JE: Mucinous cystic neoplasms of the pancreas with overt and latent malignancy (cystadenocarcinoma and cystadenoma). A clinicopathologic study of 41 cases. Am J Clin Pathol 69:573-580, 1978.

68. Gress F, Gottlieb K, Cummings O, et al: Endoscopic ultrasound characteristics of mucinous cystic neoplasms of the pancreas. Am J Gastroenterol 95:961-965, 2000.

69. Fernandez-del Castillo C, Warshaw AL: Cystic neoplasms of the pancreas. Review. Pancreatology 1:641-647, 2001.

70. Ros PR, Hamrick-Turner JE, Chiechi MV, et al: Cystic masses of the pancreas. RadioGraphics 12:673-686, 1992.

71. Sahdev A, Monson JP, Besser GM, et al: Pancreatic lesions in von Hippel-Lindau disease. Clin Endocrinol 57:603-608, 2002.

72. Sarr MG, Kendrick ML, Nagorney DM, et al: Cystic neoplasms of the pancreas: benign to malignant epithelial neoplasms. Surg Clin North Am 81:497-509, 2001.

73. Fernandez-del Castillo C, Warshaw AL: Current management of cystic neoplasms of the pancreas. Adv Surg 34:237-248, 2000.

74. Buetow PC, Rao P, Thompson LD: From the Archives of the AFIP. Mucinous cystic neoplasms of the pancreas: radiologic-pathologic correlation. RadioGraphics 18:433-449, 1998.

75. Sahani D, Prasad S, Saini S, Mueller P: Cystic pancreatic neoplasms evaluation by CT and magnetic resonance cholangiopancreatography. Gastrointest Endosc Clin North Am 12:657-672, 2002.

76. Sugiyama M, Abe N, Tokuhara M, et al: Magnetic resonance cholangio-pancreatography for postoperative follow-up of intraductal papillary-mucinous tumors of the pancreas. Am J Surg 185:251-255, 2003.

77. Tamm E, Silverman P, Charnsangavej C, Evans D: Diagnosis, staging and surveillance of pancreatic cancer. Am J Roentgenol 180:1311-1323, 2003.

78. Mertz HR, Sechopoulos P, Delbeke D, Leach SD: EUS, PET, and CT scanning for evaluation of pancreatic adenocarcinoma. Gastrointest Endosc 52:367-371, 2000.

79. Legmann P, Vignaux O, Dousset B, et al: Pancreatic tumors: comparison of dual-phase helical CT and endoscopic sonography. Am J Roentgenol 170:1315-1322, 1998.

80. Habr F, Akerman P: Role of endoscopic ultrasound in the diagnosis and staging of pancreatic cancer. Front Biosci 5:E30-35, 2000.

81. Harewood GC, Wiersema MJ: Endosonography guided fine needle aspiration biopsy in the evaluation of pancreatic masses. Am J Gastroenterol 97:1386-1391, 2002.

82. Wiersema MJ: Accuracy of endoscopic ultrasound in diagnosing and staging pancreatic carcinoma. Pancreatology 1:625-632, 2001.

83. Valinas R, Barrier A, Montravers F, et al: 18F-fluorodeoxyglucose positron emission tomography for characterization and initial staging of pancreatic tumors [French]. Gastroenterologie Clinique et Biologique 26:888-892, 2002.

84. Nishiharu T, Yamashita Y, Abe Y, et al: Local extension of pancreatic carcinoma: assessment with thin-section helical CT versus with breath-hold fast MR imaging—ROC analysis. Radiology 212:445-452, 1999.

85. Mitchell DG, Semelka RC: The pancreas and spleen. In Higgins CB, Hricak H, Helms CA (eds): Magnetic Resonance Imaging of the Body, 3rd ed. Philadelphia, Lippincott-Raven, 1996, pp 639-665.

86. Loyer E, David C, DuBrow RA. Vascular involvement in pancreatic adeno-carcinoma: reassessment by thin-section CT. Abdom Imaging 21:202-206, 1996.

87. Lu DS, Reber HA, Krasny RM, et al: Local staging of pancreatic cancer: criteria for unresectability of major vessels as revealed by pancreatic-phase, thin-section helical CT. Am J Roentgenol 168:1439-1443, 1997.

88. Arslan A, Buanes T, Geitung JT: Pancreatic carcinoma: MR, MR angiography and dynamic helical CT in the evaluation of vascular invasion. Eur J Radiol 38:151-159, 2001.

89. Harisinghani MG, Saini S, Weissleder R, et al: MR lymphangiography using ultrasmall superparamagnetic iron oxide in patients with primary abdominal and pelvic malignancies: radiographic-pathologic correlation. Am J Roentgenol 172:1347-151, 1999.

90. Trede M, Rumstadt B, Wendl K, et al: Ultrafast magnetic resonance imaging improves the staging of pancreatic tumors. Ann Surg 226:393-405, 1997.

91. Diederichs CG, Staib L, Vogel J, et al: Values and limitations of 18F-fluorodeoxyglucose-positron emission tomography with preoperative evaluation of patients with pancreatic masses. Pancreas 20:109-116, 2000.

92. Sho M, Nakajima Y, Kanehiro H, et al: A new evaluation of pancreatic function after pancreatoduodenectomy using secretin magnetic resonance cholangiopancreatography. Am J Surg 176:279-282, 1998.

93. Pessaux P, Aube C, Lebigot J, et al: Permeability and functionality of pancreaticogastrostomy after pancreaticoduodenectomy with dynamic magnetic resonance pancreatography after secretin stimulation. J Am Coll Surg 194:454-462, 2002.

94. Aube C, Lebigot J, Pessaux P, et al: Evaluation of the permeability of pancreaticogastric anastomoses (PGA) with dynamic magnetic resonance pancreatography after secretin stimulation (secretin MRCP). Abdom Imaging 28:563-570, 2003.

95. Semelka RC, Custodio CM, Cem Balci N, Woosley JT: Neuroendocrine tumors of the pancreas: spectrum of appearances on MRI. J Magn Reson Imaging 11:141-148, 2000.

96. Shi W, Johnston CF, Buchanan KD, et al: Localization of neuroendocrine tumours with [111In] DTPA-octreotide scintigraphy (Octreoscan): a comparative study with CT and MR imaging. Q J Med 91:295-301, 1998.

97. Cantisani V, Mortele KJ, Levy A, et al: MR imaging features of solid pseudopapillary tumor of the pancreas in adult and pediatric patients. Am J Roentgenol 181:395-401, 2003.

98. Merkle EM, Boaz T, Kolokythas O, et al: Metastases to the pancreas. Br J Radiol 71:1208-1214, 1998.

99. Carucci LR, Siegelman ES, Feldman MD: Pancreatic metastasis from clear cell renal carcinoma: diagnosis with chemical shift MRI. J Comput Assist Tomogr 23:934-936, 1999.

100. Fulcher AS, Turner MA, Yelon JA, et al: Magnetic resonance cholangio-pancreatography (MRCP) in the assessment of pancreatic duct trauma and its sequelae: preliminary findings. J Trauma Injury Infect Crit Care 48:1001-1007, 2000.

101. Eubank WB, Schmiedl UP, Levy AE, Marsh CL: Venous thrombosis and occlusion after pancreas transplantation: evaluation with breath-hold gadolinium-enhanced three-dimensional MR imaging. Am J Roentgenol 175:381-385, 2000.

102. Krebs TL, Daly B, Wong JJ, et al: Vascular complications of pancreatic transplantation: MR evaluation. Radiology 196:793-798, 1995.

CHAPTER 85

BOWEL, PERITONEUM, MESENTERY, AND OMENTUM

Russell N. Low

Over the last decade abdominal magnetic resonance imaging (MRI) has evolved to become a vital and integral component of the diagnostic radiology practice. Its successful application for evaluating solid abdominal organs such as the liver, kidneys, pancreas, and spleen is well documented.[1-5] In these areas, the superior soft tissue contrast of MRI is a critical element that facilitates excellent depiction and characterization of benign and malignant abdominal diseases.

However, the use of MRI to evaluate the non-solid abdominal and pelvic structures, such as the bowel, peritoneum, mesentery, and omentum is less well understood.[6-9] Imaging these structures presented many challenges to early abdominal MR imagers. Long acquisition times on early scanners coupled with the normal physiologic motion from breathing and bowel peristalsis often degraded image quality, making it difficult to depict subtle disease of the bowel and peritoneum.

Continuing advances in MRI hardware and software have overcome these initial limitations. Faster pulse sequences have made breath-hold abdominal imaging a routine part of our imaging protocols, eliminating artifacts from physiologic motion.[10,11] High-performance gradient systems have made high-resolution MRI feasible. Finally, by combining intravenous and intraluminal contrast agents with breath-hold high-resolution imaging, one can produce MR images with excellent detail and soft tissue contrast.[6,8,9] On currently available scanners, MRI of the gastrointestinal tract and peritoneum offers many unique advantages that have moved MRI to the forefront of abdominal imaging in our practice. In this chapter I will review imaging protocols and techniques for MR evaluation of the bowel and peritoneum and will then describe their application in defining benign and malignant diseases affecting these structures.

GASTROINTESTINAL TRACT

ANATOMY

The gastrointestinal (GI) tract extends from the mouth to the anus, serving the purposes of ingestion, digestion, and elimination of food. As ingested material passes from the mouth to the anus it traverses a distance of 20 to 30 feet (6-9 m). The wall of the GI tract is composed of four distinct layers: the mucosa, submucosa, muscularis externa, and the adventitia or serosa.[12] The mucosa is the layer closest to the lumen and is composed of an epithelium, lamina propria, and a thin layer of smooth muscle known as the muscularis propria. Beneath the mucosa is the submucosa containing fibrous connective tissue. The submucosa separates the mucosa from the muscularis externa. The muscularis externa contains an inner circular layer and an outer longitudinal layer. The muscularis externa of the proximal esophagus is composed of two layers of striated muscle. In the rest of the GI tract the muscularis externa is composed of layers of smooth muscle. The outermost layer of the intestinal wall is covered by connective tissue, known as the serosa or adventitia.

The esophagus is a muscular tube measuring 22 to 30 cm in length that connects the pharynx with the stomach. Peristaltic contractions propel the bolus of food through the esophagus and into the stomach.

The stomach, in the left upper quadrant of the abdomen, connects the distal esophagus with the first part of the small intestine, the duodenum. The stomach is divided into five parts: the cardia, fundus, body, antrum, and pylorus. The muscularis externa of the stomach is composed of three layers of smooth muscle unlike the remainder of the GI tract wall, which is composed of two layers of smooth muscle. The three layers of the gastric muscularis externa are oriented in oblique, circular, and longitudinal directions. Acidic gastric secretions begin the process of chemical digestion.

The small intestine measures approximately 20 feet (6 m) in length, accounting for 70% of the length and 90% of the surface area of the GI tract. It is divided

into the duodenum, jejunum, and ileum. The duodenum extends from the gastric pylorus to the ligament of Treitz, where it connects with the jejunum. The duodenum is a retroperitoneal structure that is the site of drainage of the common bile duct and pancreatic duct. The remainder of the small intestine is composed of the jejunum, beginning in the left upper quadrant, and the ileum, which terminates at the ileocecal valve in the right lower quadrant of the abdomen. Receiving bile acids from the hepatobiliary system and digestive enzymes from the pancreas, the small intestine serves to break down ingested food into nutrients that are absorbed through its extensive surface area.

The colon is 5 to 6 feet (1.5-1.8 m) in length and begins in the right lower quadrant at the ileocecal valve. The colon is composed of the ascending colon on the right, the transverse colon extending horizontally across the mid abdomen, the descending colon on the left, and the rectosigmoid colon in the left lower quadrant. The colon thus frames the abdomen and small bowel. The ascending and descending colon are attached to the posterior abdominal wall by peritoneal folds or mesenteries. As ingested material passes through the colon, water and electrolytes are absorbed leaving formed stool that is stored in the rectum prior to elimination.

TECHNIQUES AND PROTOCOLS

The unique ability of MRI to directly visualize the bowel wall is the foundation of its power for evaluating inflammatory, infectious, ischemic, and malignant gastrointestinal tract diseases. Mural involvement of the GI tract is the common denominator for all of these varied diseases. By combining breath-hold MRI with intravenous gadolinium, and readily available intraluminal agents, MRI can consistently depict mural diseases of the GI tract as areas of bowel wall thickening and enhancement that can be difficult to depict on other imaging studies[6,13,14] (Fig. 85-1).

Intraluminal Contrast Agents

Adequate distension of the stomach, small intestine, and colon is essential for MRI of the GI tract. Incomplete intestinal distention may mask important findings or may mimic an inflammatory or neoplastic mass. Fortunately, there are many different intraluminal contrast agents available.[16-20] Intraluminal contrast agents may be positive agents that produce high signal on MR images. Examples of positive intraluminal agents include manganese-containing agents and gadolinium chelates diluted in water. Negative agents produce low signal on MR images. Examples of negative intraluminal agents include iron-containing oral agents. Biphasic agents produce intraluminal signal that is high signal on T2-weighted images and low signal on T1-weighted images. Examples of biphasic oral contrast agents include dilute barium sulfate and tap water.

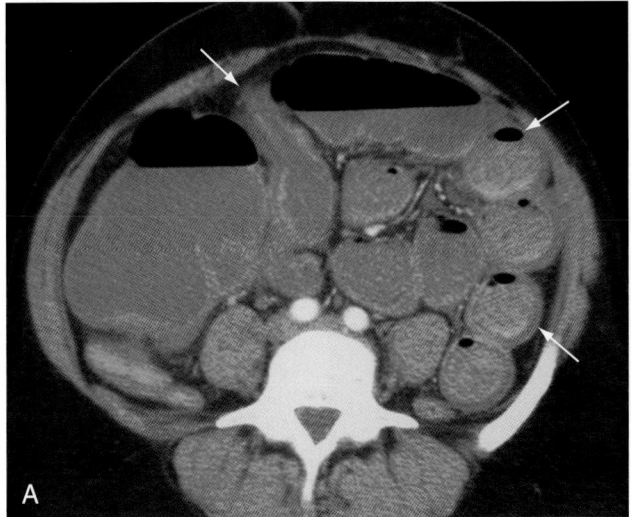

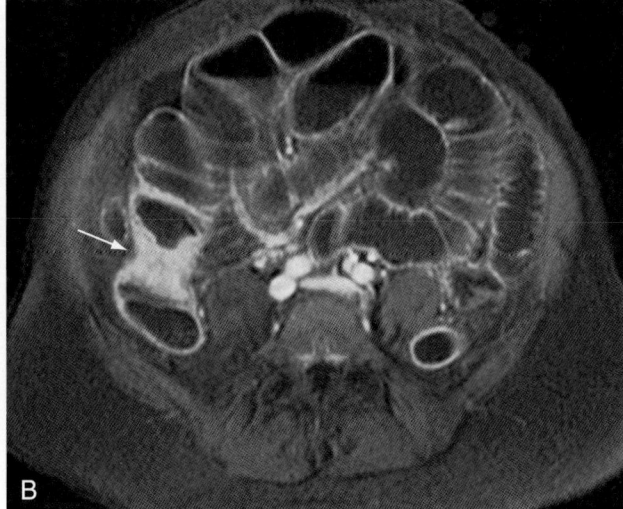

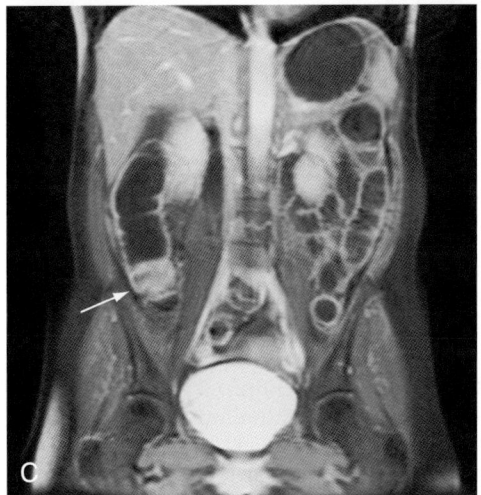

FIGURE 85-1

Colon cancer in a 40-year-old patient presenting with bowel obstruction. Helical CT (**A**) shows dilated colon and small bowel with mural thickening involving bowel loops *(arrows)*. An obstructing mass was not depicted. Axial (**B**) and coronal (**C**) gadolinium-enhanced SGE MR image depicts an enhancing annular cancer *(arrow)* in the ascending colon. The superior contrast conspicuity of enhanced MRI facilitates depiction of mural disease of the GI tract.

While there are clearly many approaches to the use of oral contrast for MRI, our experience has shown the benefits of a biphasic intraluminal agent that is bright on T2-weighted images and dark on T1-weighted images[6,13,14] (Fig. 85-2). A dark or low signal intraluminal agent on gadolinium-enhanced spoiled gradient-echo (SGE) T1-weighted images is very useful as it helps to accentuate enhancement of the adjacent diseased bowel wall. Use of a positive intraluminal oral agent producing high signal on T1-weighted images could obscure subtle mural enhancement.

At our institution, we use either water or dilute barium sulfate, which is 98% water. Either agent demonstrates a biphasic appearance on T2- and T1-weighted images (see Fig. 85-2). Both are well tolerated and readily available. Dilute barium sulfate is iso-osmolar so it will stay in the GI tract and not be reabsorbed. On the other hand, water is reabsorbed, making adequate distension of the distal small bowel unpredictable. One may add agents to the water, such as mannitol or Psyllium husk (Ispaghula husk), to increase its osmolarity and reduce intestinal reabsorption.[20] We have patients ingest 1400 ml of oral contrast material beginning 30 to 45 minutes before exam. Rectal water can be administered through a balloon-tipped barium enema catheter. The balloon should be filled with water to avoid the susceptibility artifact generated by the air in the balloon. Alternative routes of administration have been suggested, including MR enteroclysis via a nasojejunal tube.[21-24]

Intravenous Contrast Agents

Intravenous gadolinium (0.2 mmol/kg) is administered for the gadolinium-enhanced SGE images. Although not essential to the technique, we use a power injector with a bolus injection at a rate of 2 ml/s. The nonspecific extracellular gadolinium chelates will enhance inflammatory, infectious, and malignant disease of the GI tract and peritoneum, markedly increasing their conspicuity. Glucagon (1 mg IV) is preloaded into the IV tubing and is administered at the time of gadolinium injection to decrease bowel peristalsis.

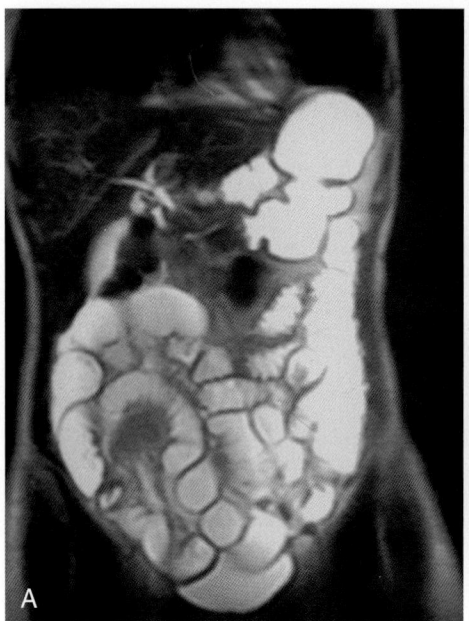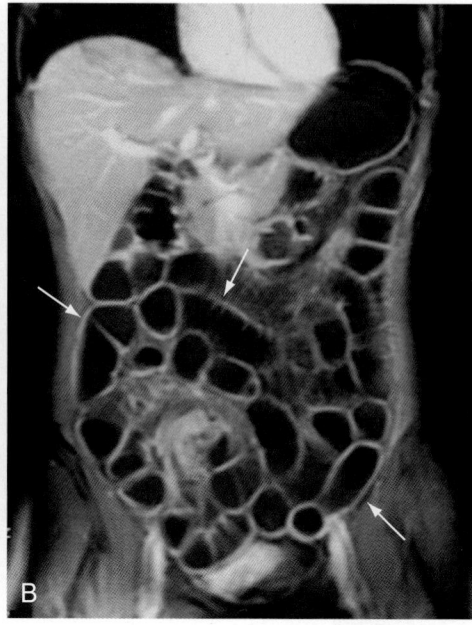

FIGURE 85-2

Biphasic intraluminal contrast material. Coronal single-shot fast spin-echo (SSFSE) image (**A**) shows the bowel distended with high signal intensity water-soluble contrast material. On the coronal fat-suppressed gadolinium-enhanced SGE image (**B**) the water-soluble intraluminal contrast material is low signal intensity. The combination of a dark intraluminal contrast agent, fat suppression, and IV gadolinium facilitates depiction of the bowel wall (*arrows*) shown as white lines and rings.

Pulse Sequences

MRI of the GI tract requires rapid imaging to minimize the effects of respiratory motion and peristalsis.[10,11,25,26] Gastrointestinal tract disease can be subtle so that normal physiologic motion can obscure important findings. Rapid, breath-hold MRI is clearly essential for effective GI tract imaging. Selection of pulse sequences will depend upon the type of gastrointestinal disease one is imaging.

For inflammatory GI tract diseases we utilize coronal and axial breath-hold single-shot rapid relaxation enhancement (SSRARE), and breath-hold, fat-suppressed SGE imaging following IV gadolinium administration[13,1425,26] (Fig. 85-3). Two sets of axial images are obtained through the abdomen and pelvis, followed by a coronal and sagittal acquisition. This combination produces SSRARE T2-weighted, and gadolinium-enhanced SGE T1-weighted images that are relatively insensitive to motion artifact.

For malignant GI tract diseases it is essential to optimally evaluate the liver and other abdominal organs for metastatic tumor. In these patients, we also perform unenhanced T1-weighted and fat-suppressed T2-weighted axial images combined with SSRARE imaging and dynamic gadolinium-enhanced SGE images.

For the gadolinium-enhanced images, one may alternatively perform volumetric imaging with a 3D gradient-echo pulse sequence (THRIVE, VIBE, FAME, etc) (Fig. 85-4). Improvements in 3D pulse sequences when combined with high-performance gradient systems allows one to obtain thin-section, high-resolution images during suspended respiration. Inversion recovery fat suppression is added to the 3D acquisition to improve the conspicuity of enhancing mural disease. Imaging parameters are highly variable depending upon the MR imager used. Typical acquisitions will acquire 56 to 100 sections in one breath hold. The slice thickness is chosen to optimize anatomic coverage during the period of suspended respiration. Typical slice thickness might be 4 to 6 mm with a 50% overlap. As the efficiency and image quality of these 3D images improves, they will likely replace 2D SGE imaging for gadolinium-enhanced MRI.

Specific imaging parameters depend upon the particular MR imager and software one has available. On our current scanner we use the following imaging parameters:

SSRARE—Relaxation time (TR), infinite; Echo time (TE), 90 msec; matrix, 256×192; flip angle, 90 degrees; number of excitations (NEX), 0.5; bandwidth (BW), 62 kHz; slice thickness, 8 mm, 2 mm gap; echo train length (ETL), >100.

Gadolinium-enhanced SGE T1—TR, 160 msec; TE, 2.1 msec; matrix 256×192, 512 zero fill interpolation processing (ZIP); flip angle, 70 degrees; 1 NEX; BW, 20 kHz; slice thickness, 8 mm; fat suppression; 3/4 field of view (FOV).

Gadolinium-enhanced 3D gradient echo—TR, 4 msec; TE, 0.9 msec; matrix 256×201, interpolated 512×201; flip angle, 10 degrees; 1 NEX; slice thickness, 6 mm, 3 mm overlap; spectral presaturation inversion recovery (SPIR) fat suppression; 80% FOV.

The entire abdomen and pelvis is imaged in the axial and coronal planes for both the SSRARE and the 2D or 3D gadolinium-enhanced gradient-echo images. For the gadolinium-enhanced images, we obtain two sets of axial images. This requires multiple breath-holds to cover the abdomen and pelvis. We typically obtain 12 to 24 slices per breath-hold, so the abdomen and pelvis may be covered with 2 to 4 breath-holds per acquisition.

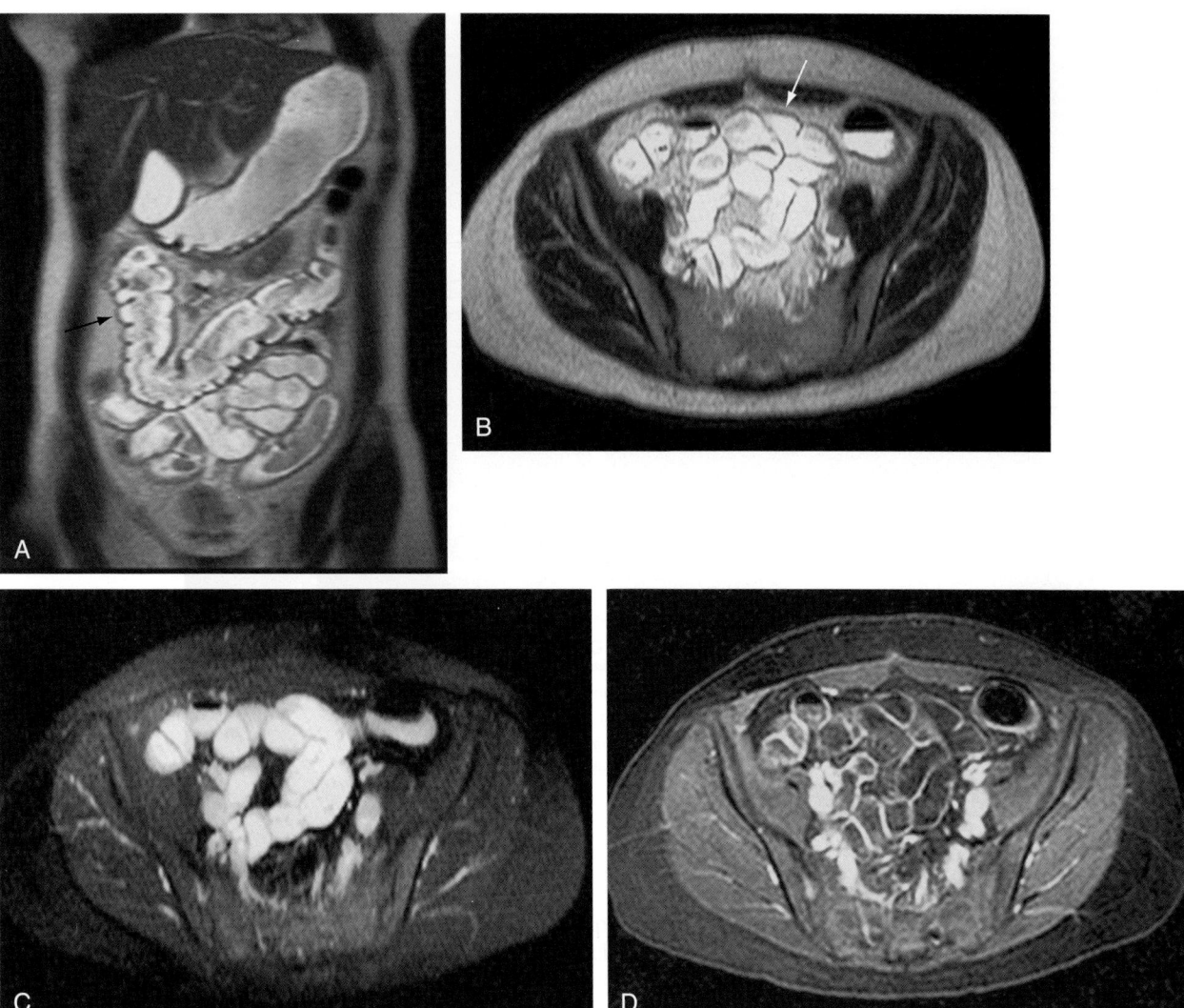

FIGURE 85-3

Examples of MR pulse sequences. Single-shot rapid relaxation enhancement (SSRARE) images in the coronal (**A**) and axial (**B**) planes show excellent definition of the bowel wall *(arrow)* seen as a thin dark line surrounding the bowel lumen distended with water-soluble contrast material. Fat-suppressed T2-weighed images (**C**) can be obtained to assess for edema in the bowel wall or to look for metastatic tumor in a patient with malignant gastrointestinal disease. Fat-suppressed gadolinium-enhanced images (**D**) are obtained in the axial plane twice as well as in the coronal and sagittal plane.

Alternative imaging sequences include true fast imaging with steady precession (FISP) for the T2-weighted images (Fig. 85-5). On these images, there is excellent contrast between the high-signal lumen distended with water or dilute barium sulfate and the adjacent bowel wall. A MR hydrogram can be generated by modifying the SSRARE acquisition to create an image that has the appearance of a GI barium examination (Fig. 85-6). The MR hydrogram is created by obtaining a single-slice thick-slab (>10 cm) coronal acquisition with a long TE (900 msec). This water-sensitive acquisition will show the high signal intensity intraluminal contrast within the stomach, small bowel, and colon.

MAGNETIC RESONANCE ENTEROCLYSIS

Magnetic resonance enteroclysis (MRE) is a new technique for the evaluation of small bowel abnormalities.[20-24] Distention of the small bowel lumen is achieved by the administration of 1.5 to 2 liters of iso-osmotic water solution of polyethylene glycol through a nasojejunal catheter at a rate of 80 to 150 ml/min. Other authors have proposed using orally administered iso-osmotic solution of 2.5% mannitol with 2% locust bean gum solution in water to achieve adequate small bowel distention without the use of a nasojejunal tube.

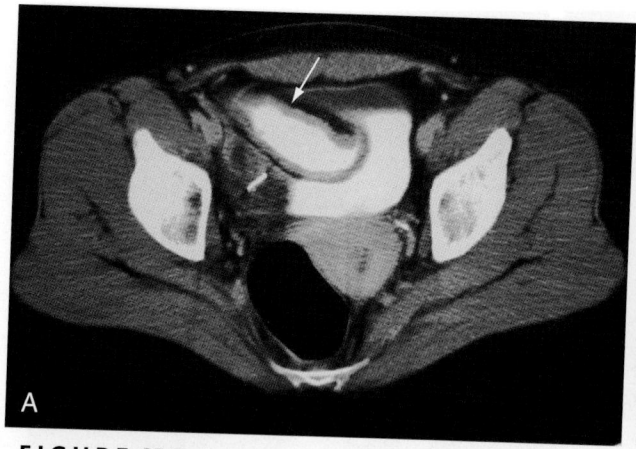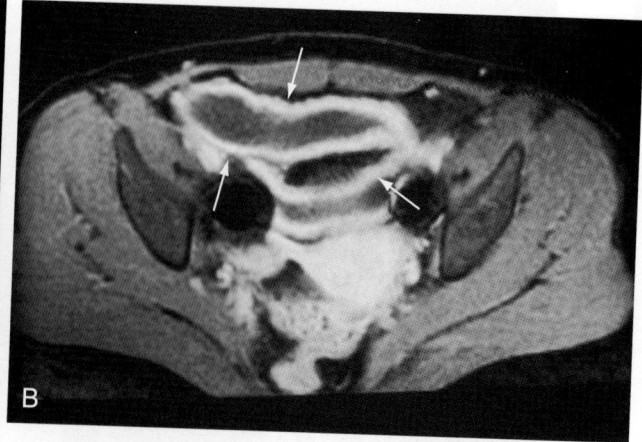

FIGURE 85-7

Crohn's disease. Helical CT (**A**) depicts ileal mural thickening *(arrow)*. Fat-suppressed gadolinium-enhanced SGE MR image (**B**) shows marked enhancement of the thickened ileum *(arrows)*. Enhancement of the diseased small-bowel wall facilitates depiction of inflammatory changes of Crohn's disease.

MRI of Crohn's Disease

Inflammatory diseases of the GI tract such as Crohn's disease or ulcerative colitis are exquisitely depicted with MRI.[7,13-15,29-39] By combining a negative oral contrast agent with fat-suppressed gadolinium-enhanced MRI, one may show bowel wall thickening and enhancement[6,13-15] (Fig. 85-7). Both the T2-weighted SSRARE images and the gadolinium-enhanced SGE images are useful for depicting mural thickening (Fig. 85-8). Marked gadolinium enhancement of the inflamed bowel wall in patients with Crohn's disease facilitates depiction of diseased bowel segments.[13-15] In our experience, compared with helical computed tomography (CT), MRI is much more sensitive to earlier or milder forms of inflammatory bowel disease (Fig. 85-9). In a study of 26 patients with Crohn's disease,[14] depiction of mural thickening and/or enhancement was superior on the MR images, which showed 55 (85%) and 52 (80%) of 65 abnormal bowel segments for the two observers, compared with helical CT, which showed 39 (60%) and 42 (65%) of bowel segments affected by Crohn's disease.

MRI is useful to assess the disease activity and response to treatment in patients with Crohn's disease. Disease activity shows a highly significant correlation with gadolinium enhancement of the diseased bowel wall, and mural hyperintensity on T2-weighted fat-suppressed images[35] (Fig. 85-10). With treatment, both the degree of gadolinium enhancement and its signal on T2-weighted images decreases[36] (Fig. 85-11). The important distinction between an actively inflamed stenosis and a chronically scarred, fibrotic stenosis can be accurately determined on MRI.

The degree of bowel wall enhancement correlates with the activity of the inflammatory process.[13] On the first set of gadolinium-enhanced SGE images, the enhancement of the normal bowel wall is equal to or less than that of the liver parenchyma. Bowel wall enhancement that is more than the liver is mild and enhancement that is equal to intravascular gadolinium is marked in intensity. Bowel that is actively inflamed from Crohn's disease will show a gadolinium enhancement more than that of the liver parenchyma.[13] On the other hand, thickened bowel that does not enhance correlates with non-acute disease (see Fig. 85-10). A layered pattern of mural enhancement with mucosal hyperemia and non-enhancing submucosal edema also indicates active Crohn's disease.

On T2-weighed images, an acutely inflamed bowel wall shows high signal intensity, while a chronically thickened bowel wall without active inflammation shows low signal intensity for fibrosis. This assessment requires the use of fat suppression on the T2-weighted images.[35] The ability to determine disease activity on MR images provides clinically important information that can affect patient management.

Endoscopic findings have shown good correlation with MRI in assessing the degree and extent of changes of Crohn's disease.[13,14,29-39] The spectrum of findings in Crohn's disease can include focal ulceration (Fig. 85-12), discontinuous linear ulcers (Fig. 85-13), pseudopolyps (Fig. 85-14), stricture formation (Fig. 85-15), and an end-stage cobblestone appearance (Fig. 85-16).

It is equally important to be able to accurately depict complications of Crohn's disease.[13,14,35,38,39] MRI and helical CT are equivalent for depicting fistulas (Figs. 85-17 to 85-19), abscesses (Fig. 85-20), and phlegmons.[14] Gadolinium enhancement of extraintestinal abscesses and phlegmons facilitates their detection on MRI. Fistulas are depicted directly as fluid- or air-filled tracts between adjacent bowel loops, viscera, and/or the abdominal wall. More commonly, one may see distortion and tethering of bowel loops at the site of fistulous connection. Abnormal thickening and enhancement of the adjacent bladder wall or skin surface may be indirect evidence for an enterovesicle or enterocutaneous fistula.

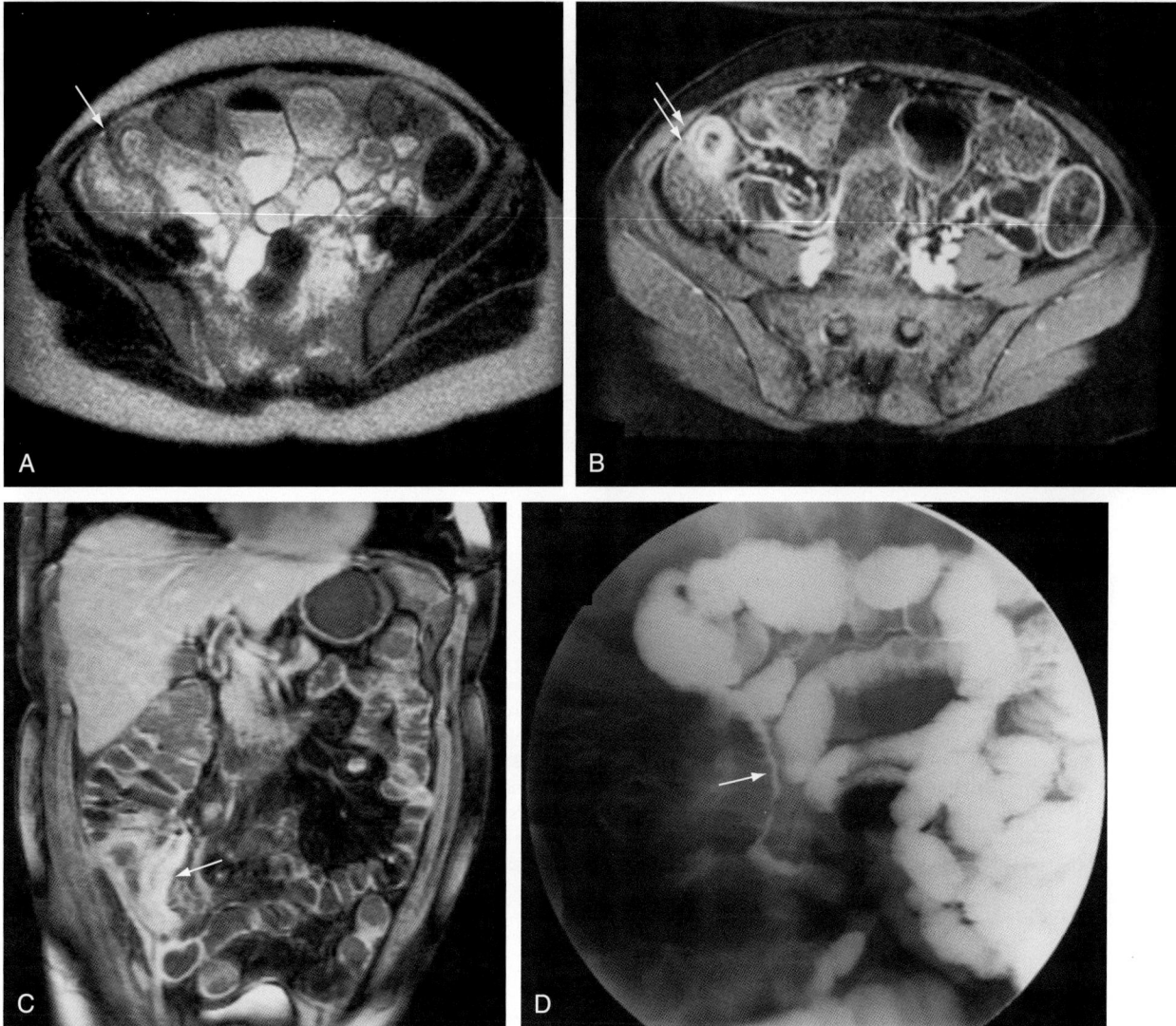

FIGURE 85-8

Crohn's disease SSFSE versus gadolinium-enhanced MRI. Single-shot fast spin-echo (SSFSE) image (**A**) shows mural thickening *(arrow)* involving the terminal ileum. Axial (**B**) and coronal (**C**) gadolinium-enhanced MRI shows marked enhancement of the thick wall terminal ileum *(arrow)*. Small bowel barium examination (**D**) shows a "string sign" *(arrow)* with marked luminal narrowing of the distal ileum due to Crohn's disease.

Thin section 3D gadolinium-enhanced images are particularly useful to depict enhancing fistulous tracts in Crohn's disease. Biliary complications of inflammatory bowel disease including sclerosing cholangitis (Fig. 85-21) can be depicted on enhanced MR images with abnormal peribiliary enhancement on delayed gadolinium-enhanced images.

The MR depiction of mural changes in Crohn's disease and other inflammatory intestinal diseases requires adequate distension of the bowel. Collapsed bowel may enhance and mimic abnormal bowel. In addition, subtle bowel wall changes may be hidden by inadequately distended bowel. Optimal intestinal distension can be achieved by combining orally and rectally administered water-soluble contrast material.[13,14,20] MR enteroclysis has been effectively used in patients with Crohn's disease to maximally distend the small bowel via a nasojejunal catheter.[23,31] Compared with conventional enteroclysis, MR enteroclysis has been shown to demonstrate similar accuracy in determining the severity and extent of disease.[31]

Ulcerative Colitis

Ulcerative colitis is a chronic inflammatory disease of unknown etiology that affects the mucosa of the colon and rectum.[40-43] It most commonly affects the distal

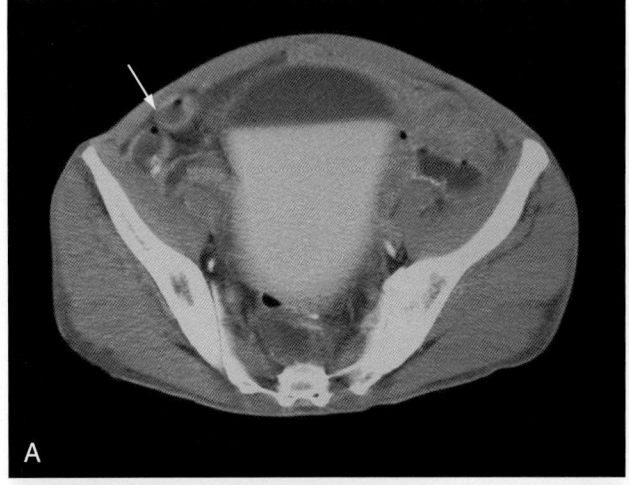

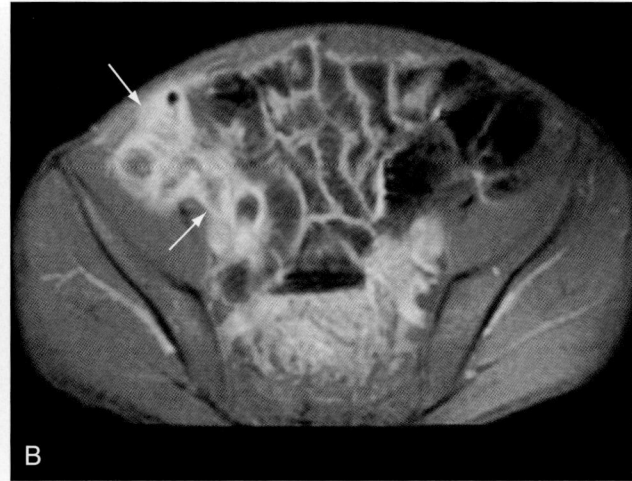

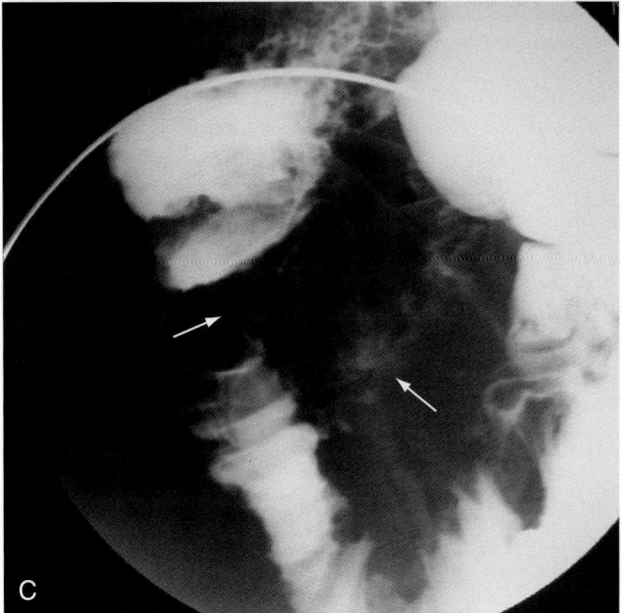

FIGURE 85-9

Mild Crohn's disease. Helical CT scan (**A**) shows possible distal ileal mural thickening *(arrow)* versus incomplete distension. Gadolinium-enhanced MRI (**B**) depicts marked enhancement *(arrows)* of the diseased distal ileum. Small-bowel barium examination (**C**) confirms changes of active Crohn's disease involving the distal ileum *(arrows)*. The extent of the disease and confidence in diagnosis is better on the gadolinium-enhanced MR examination.

colon and rectum but can progress in a retrograde fashion to produce a pancolitis and proctitis (Fig. 85-22). Unlike the skip lesions of Crohn's disease, ulcerative colitis is a continuous and symmetric process. Patients present with abdominal pain, bloody diarrhea, weight loss, and fatigue. Intestinal complications include toxic megacolon, strictures, and colon cancer. Extraintestinal complications include uveitis, liver disease, primary sclerosing cholangitis, arthritis, rashes, anemia, and osteoporosis.

Ulcerative colitis progresses through acute, subacute, and chronic stages. Mucosal granularity, submucosal ulceration, collar button ulcers, thumb printing, and eventual pseudopolyp formation characterize the acute stage. In the subacute stage, one sees inflammatory polyps and a coarse granular mucosa. An ahaustral burned-out colon that can assume a "lead-pipe" appearance characterizes chronic ulcerative colitis.

Treatment of ulcerative colitis is similar to that for Crohn's disease and includes aminosalicylates containing 5-ASA. Sulfasalazine is a combination of sulfapyridine and 5-ASA and is used to induce and maintain remission. As with Crohn's disease corticosteroids and immuno-modulators play an important role in medical manage-ment. Surgery is eventually performed in 25% to 40% of ulcerative colitis patients for refractory disease, bowel perforation or obstruction, or risk of cancer. Approx-imately 5% of patients with ulcerative colitis develop colon cancer, with the risk of cancer increasing with the extent and duration of colitis.

MRI of Ulcerative Colitis

MRI of patients with ulcerative colitis is accomplished with the same double contrast MR techniques used in Crohn's disease.[40-43] During the acute phase of ulcerative

Text continues on page 2700

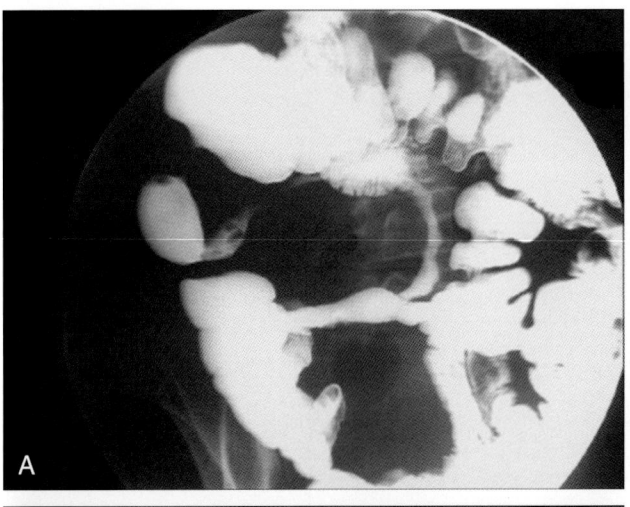

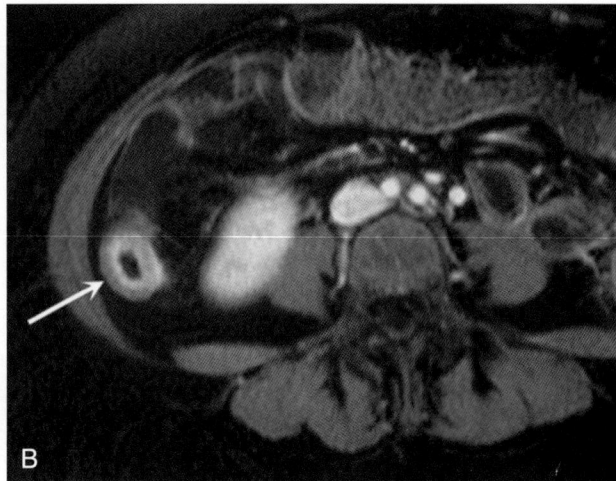

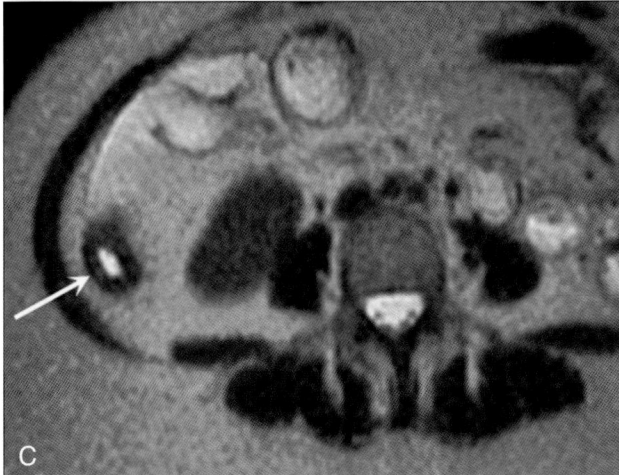

FIGURE 85-10

Chronic Crohn's disease stricture. Barium small bowel examination (**A**) shows a long segment high-grade stricture of the distal ileum. The activity of the underlying Crohn's disease cannot be determined from the barium examination. First pass from a gadolinium-enhanced SGE MRI (**B**) shows absence of significant mural enhancement *(arrow)* in the thickened terminal ileum. Some mucosal enhancement is present. Single-shot fast spin-echo (SSFSE) image (**C**) shows low signal intensity within the thickened wall of the terminal ileum *(arrow)*. Findings correlate with a chronic stricture. Endoscopy confirmed a smooth mucosa without active inflammation.

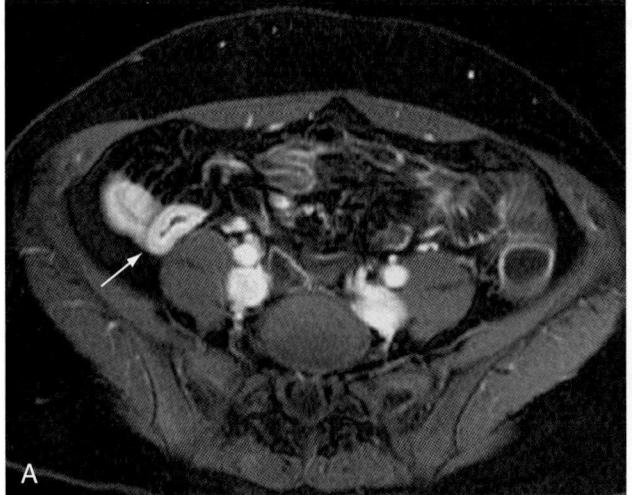

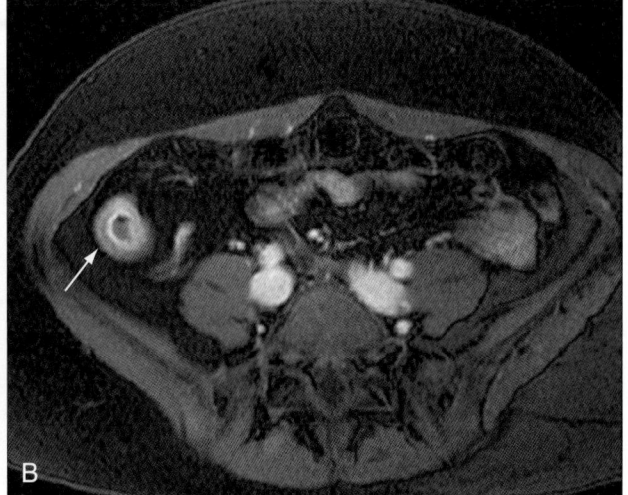

FIGURE 85-11

Crohn's disease response to treatment. Gadolinium-enhanced spoiled gradient-echo (SGE) image before treatment (**A**) shows ileal mural thickening and marked enhancement *(arrow)* indicating active inflammation. Gadolinium-enhanced SGE image obtained following interval treatment for Crohn's disease (**B**) shows marked decrease in mural enhancement. Decreased mural enhancement correlates with response to treatment.

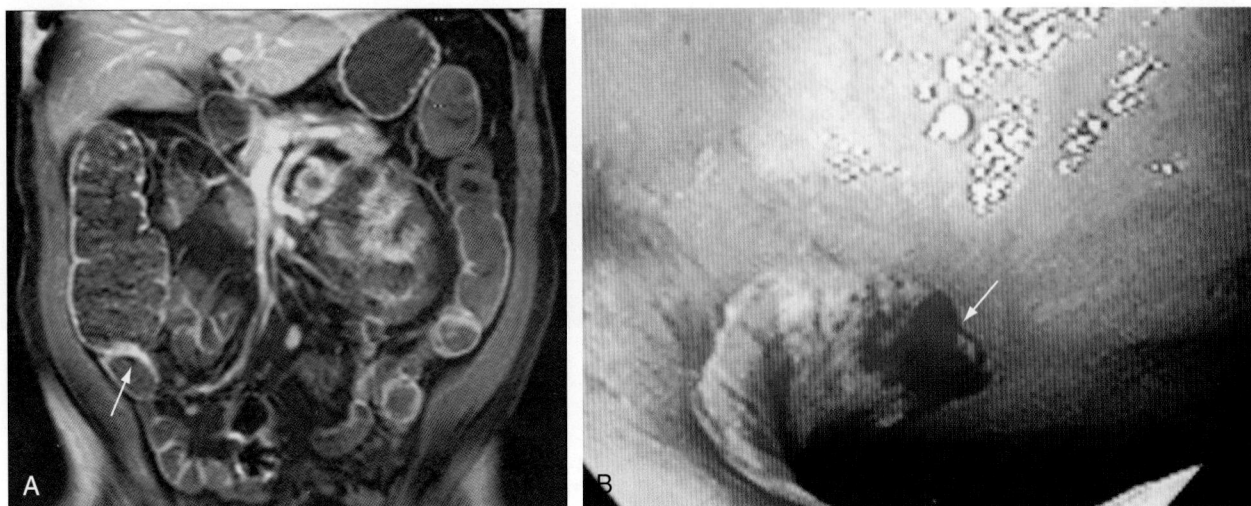

FIGURE 85-12

Focal ulceration from recurrent Crohn's disease. Coronal gadolinium-enhanced spoiled gradient-echo (SGE) image (**A**) shows a focal area of mural thickening and enhancement *(arrow)* near the ileocecal valve. Endoscopic view (**B**) confirms a focal ulceration *(arrow)* at the ileocecal valve.

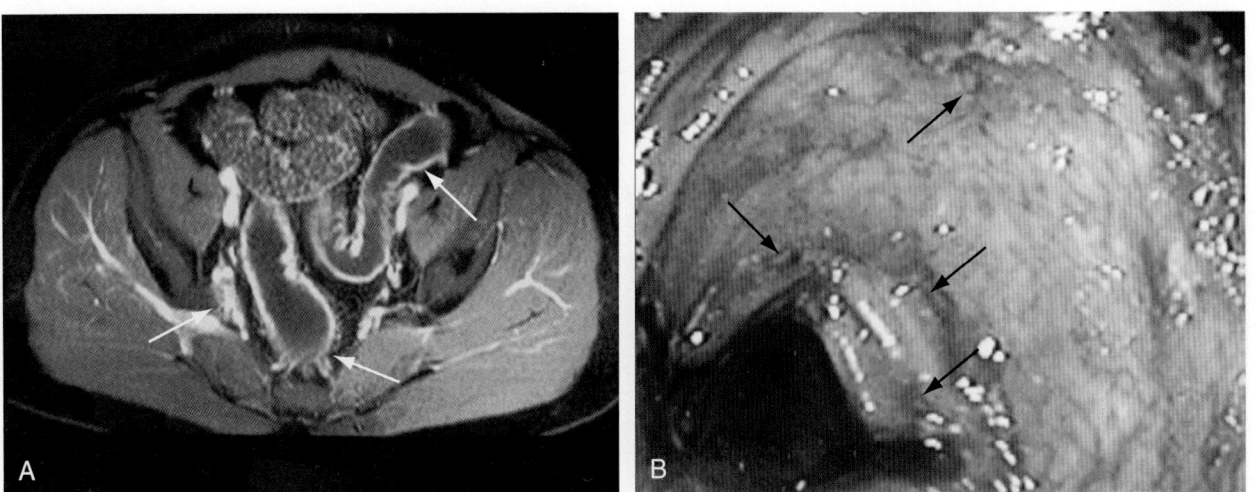

FIGURE 85-13

Crohn's linear skip ulcerations. Axial gadolinium-enhanced spoiled gradient-echo (SGE) image (**A**) with rectal water shows mild colonic mural thickening and marked diffuse mural enhancement. Endoscopic view (**B**) shows scattered colonic linear ulcerations *(arrows)* from newly diagnosed Crohn's disease.

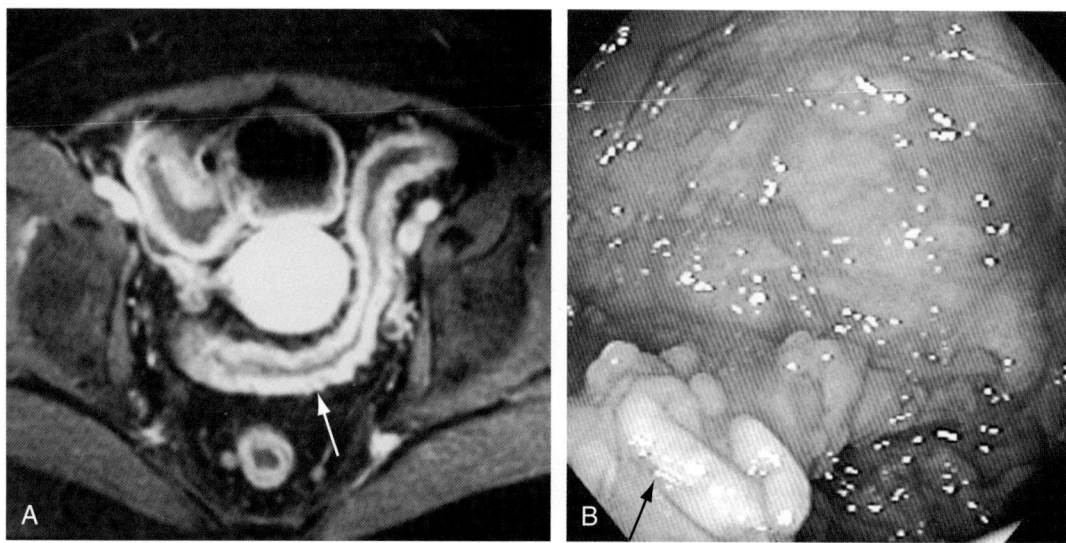

FIGURE 85-14

Crohn's disease with pseudopolyps. Gadolinium-enhanced spoiled gradient-echo (SGE) image (**A**) shows moderate colonic and terminal ileal mural thickening *(arrow)* and marked mural enhancement. Endoscopic view (**B**) shows markedly inflamed mucosa with pseudopolyps *(arrow)*.

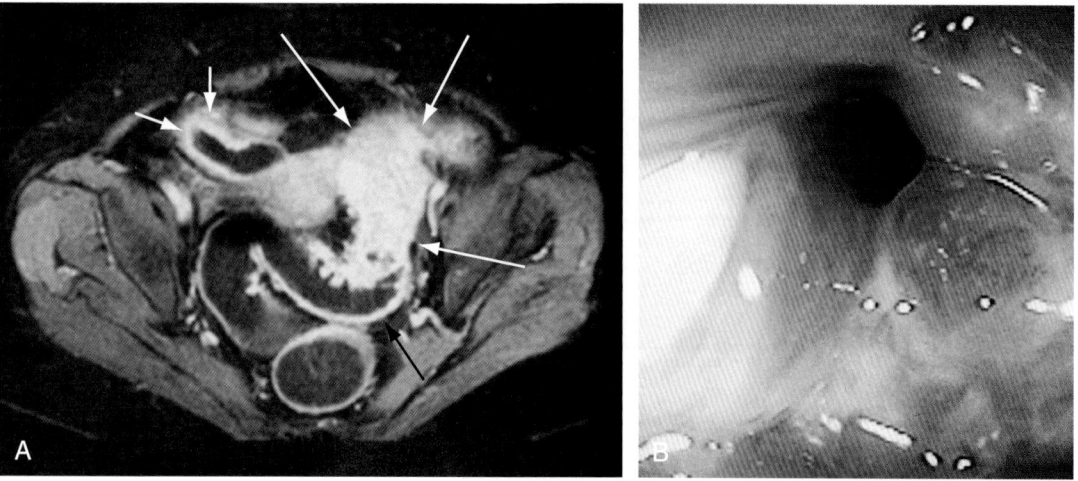

FIGURE 85-15

Crohn's inflammatory mass with stricture. Gadolinium-enhanced spoiled gradient-echo (SGE) image (**A**) shows a large enhancing inflammatory sigmoid colon mass *(long arrows)* with luminal narrowing. Terminal ileal disease is also present *(short arrows)*. Endoscopic view (**B**) shows a stricture with adjacent mucosal inflammation.

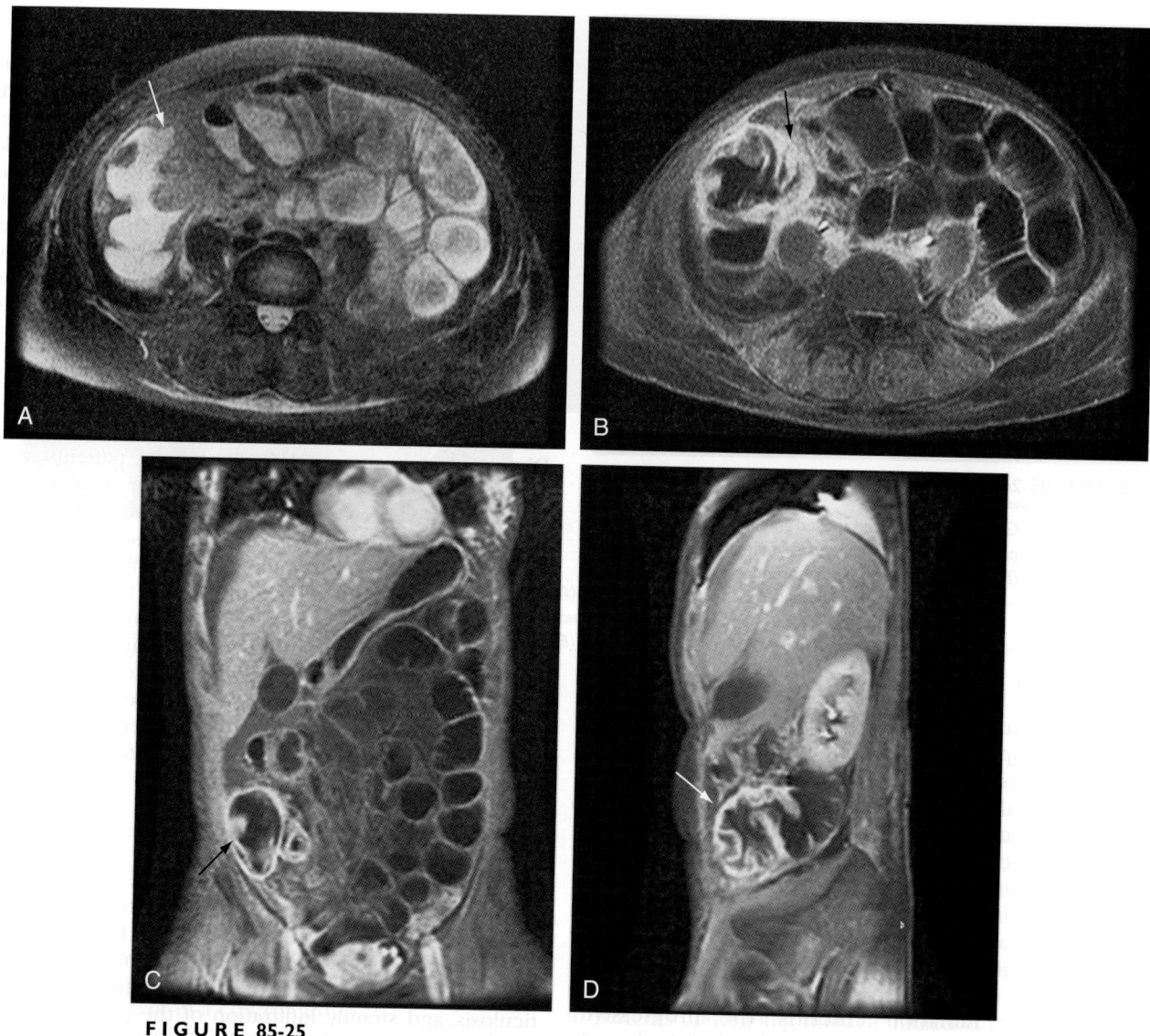

FIGURE 85-25

Typhlitis. Axial single-shot fast spin-echo (SSFSE) (**A**) image shows moderate mural thickening of the cecum (*arrow*). Axial (**B**), coronal (**C**), and sagittal (**D**) gadolinium-enhanced spoiled gradient-echo (SGE) images show marked enhancement of the irregularly thickened cecum (*arrow*) and terminal ileum correlating with typhlitis.

MRI in patients with chemotherapy-related enteritis demonstrate focal or diffuse small-bowel mural thickening and abnormal enhancement. The appearance may be difficult to distinguish from infectious or inflammatory GI diseases.

FUNCTIONAL DISEASES

Irritable Bowel Syndrome

Irritable bowel syndrome is a common functional disorder of the bowel that affects 10% to 20% of the general population. It is the disease most commonly diagnosed by gastroenterologists. Irritable bowel syndrome is also known as mucous colitis, spastic colon, spastic colitis, or irritable colon. It is caused by physiological or functional abnormalities of the bowel rather than by an anatomic or structural change. A functional abnormality in the contractility of the bowel results in pain and altered bowel movements. Patients with irritable bowel syndrome present with abdominal pain associated with a change in bowel habits, such as increased frequency, diarrhea, or constipation. Other symptoms include cramps, urgency, and abdominal distention. Diagnosis is made by exclusion of other organic GI diseases. Laboratory work-up and upper and lower endoscopy are normal in patients with irritable bowel syndrome.[51,52]

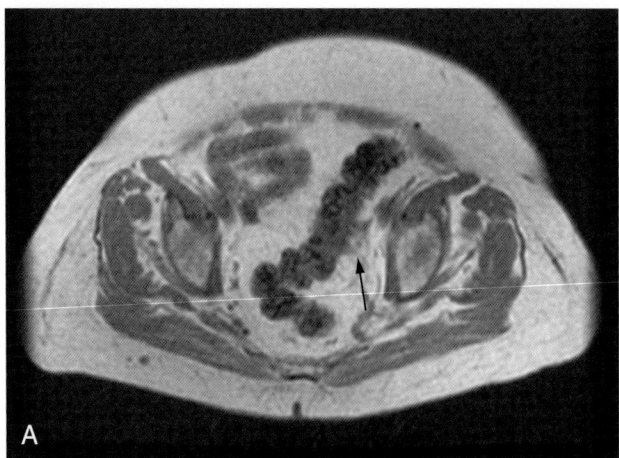

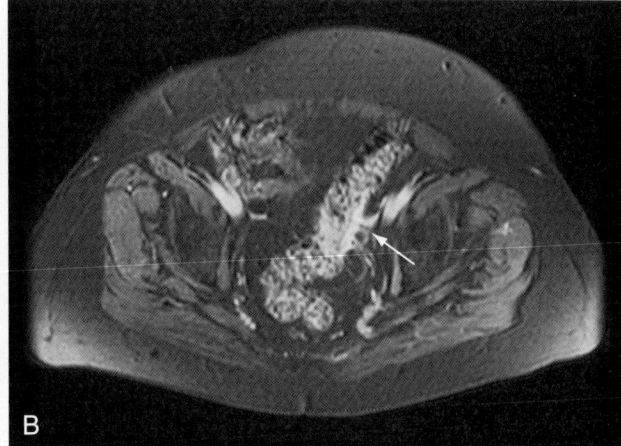

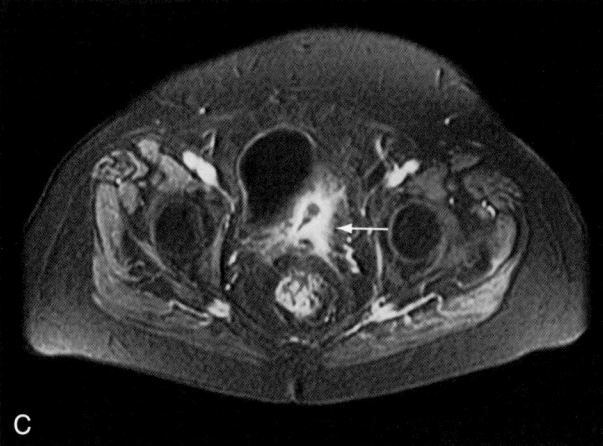

FIGURE 85-26

Diverticulitis. T1-weighted image (**A**) shows strandy infiltration *(arrow)* of the pericolonic fat. Gadolinium-enhanced spoiled gradient-echo (SGE) image (**B**) demonstrates abnormal enhancement of the sigmoid wall and surrounding tissues *(arrow)*. Gadolinium-enhanced image (**C**) at a level caudal to **B** depicts a small abscess *(arrow)* with enhancement of the abscess wall. Findings are those of diverticulitis with abscess formation.

FIGURE 85-27

Chemotherapy-related enteritis. Gadolinium-enhanced spoiled gradient-echo (SGE) image demonstrates abnormal segmental small bowel with mural thickening and enhancement *(arrows)*.

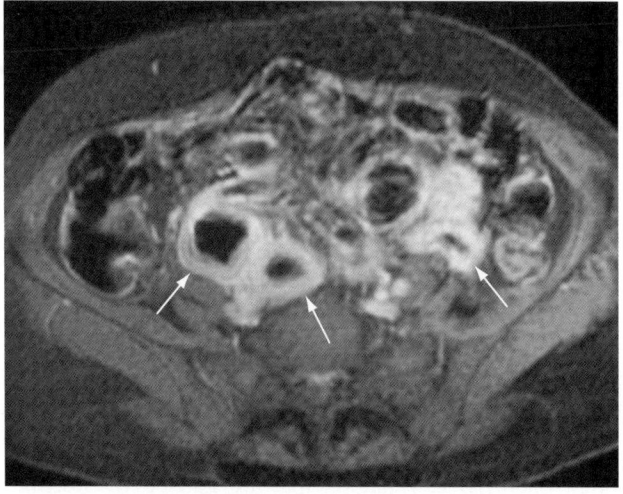

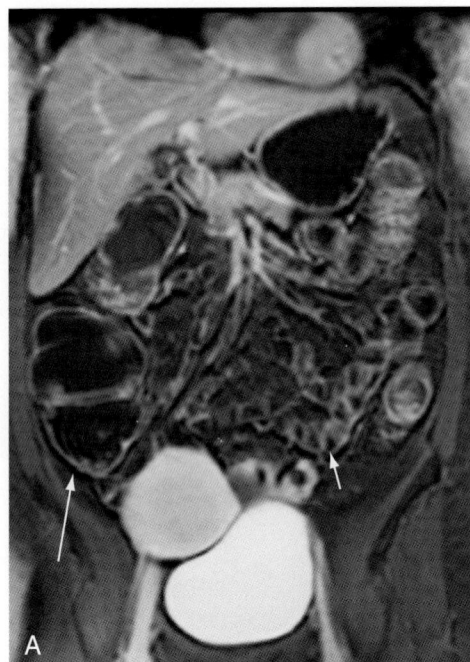
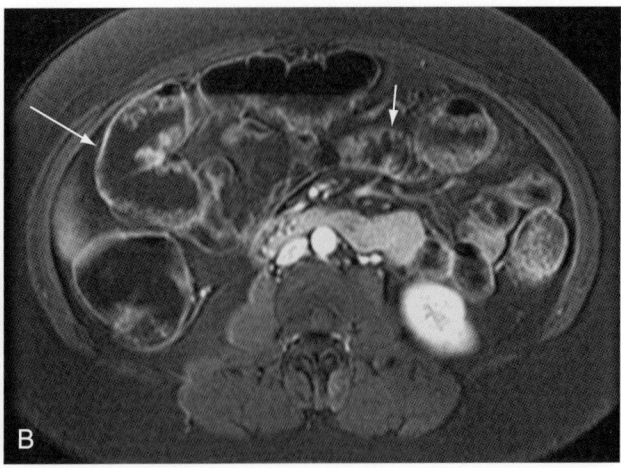

FIGURE 85-28

Irritable bowel syndrome in patient with chronic abdominal pain. Coronal (**A**) and axial (**B**) gadolinium-enhanced spoiled gradient-echo (SGE) images show normal colon (*long arrows*) and small bowel (*short arrows*). Absence of mural thickening or enhancement excludes inflammatory bowel disease. Endoscopy was normal and confirmed the diagnosis of irritable bowel syndrome.

MRI of Irritable Bowel Syndrome

MRI performed in the patient with suspected irritable bowel syndrome reveals normal stomach, small intestine, and colon (Fig. 85-28). There is a notable absence of mural thickening or abnormal mural enhancement. MRI is a useful adjunct to other tests in order to exclude infectious, inflammatory, or ischemic bowel disease. Many of the patients referred for MRI may have inflammatory bowel disease as an alternate diagnosis. In these patients MRI can confidently exclude organic intestinal disease.

INFECTIOUS DISEASES OF THE GASTROINTESTINAL TRACT

Esophagitis

Esophagitis may be due to infectious etiology, gastroesophageal reflux, ingestion of corrosive agents, or radiation therapy. Infectious esophagitis is common in immunocompromised patients but is also seen in healthy individuals. The causative organism may be viral, such as cytomegalovirus, Epstein-Barr virus, varicella-zoster, or herpes simplex virus. Fungal esophagitis may be caused by *Candida albicans*, and less common non-candidal fungi. Bacterial esophagitis may be caused by normal esophageal flora or may be due to secondary infections from organisms such as *Mycobacterium tuberculosis* or *Mycobacterium avium-intracellulare* (MAI). Symptoms of infectious esophagitis include dysphasia, odynophagia, retrosternal pain, nausea, and vomiting.[53-55]

MRI of Esophagitis

While MRI is not typically ordered to evaluate esophagitis, changes of esophageal inflammation are commonly seen on MR examinations performed for other indications. On unenhanced T1-weighted and T2-weighted images, the esophagus appears thickened. However, the most sensitive MR images for depicting esophagitis are the gadolinium-enhanced SGE images, which show marked abnormal enhancement of the inflamed esophagus (Fig. 85-29). Long segments of the esophagus are typically involved and are well demonstrated on sagittal gadolinium-enhanced images.

Peptic Ulcer Disease

Peptic ulcer disease involving the stomach or duodenum affects 4.5 million people annually in the United States. The lifetime prevalence is approximately 10%. Peptic ulcer disease is caused by the bacterium *Helicobacter pylori*, which is associated with 90% of duodenal ulcers and 70% to 75% of gastric ulcers. Other causes of peptic ulcer disease include nonsteroidal anti-inflammatory drugs, acid, and pepsin. Patients present with postprandial epigastric pain, nausea, vomiting, hematemesis, or melena. Treatment of peptic ulcer disease is directed at the *H. pylori* infection using triple drug therapy for 2 weeks. Proton pump inhibitor triple drug therapy consists of a proton pump inhibitor combined with two antibiotics. Bismuth-based triple dose therapy includes a bismuth subsalicylate and two antibiotics.[56-59]

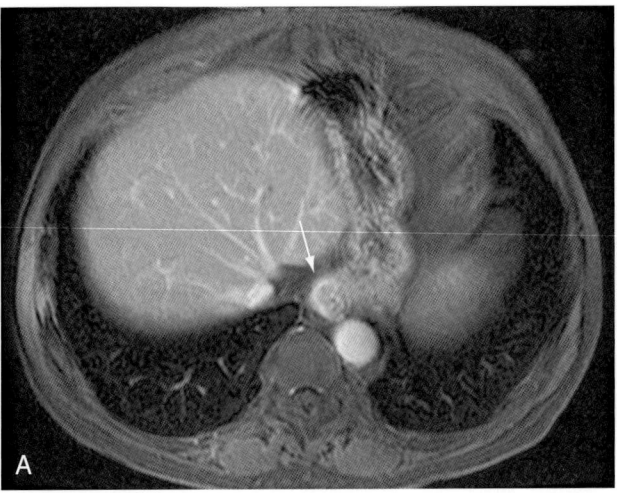

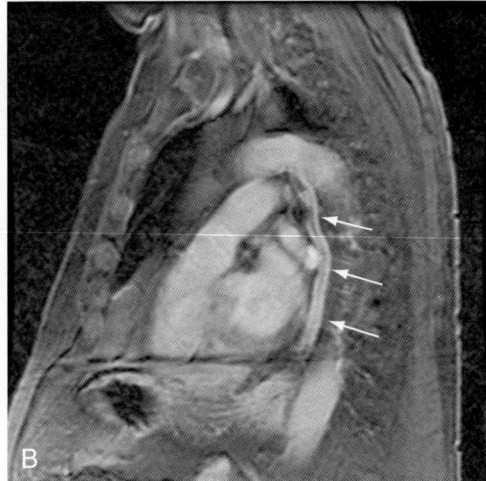

FIGURE 85-29

Esophagitis. Axial (**A**) and coronal (**B**) gadolinium-enhanced spoiled gradient-echo (SGE) images show abnormal esophageal mural thickening and enhancement *(arrows)*. Findings correlate with esophagitis.

MRI of Peptic Ulcer Disease

MRI in patients with peptic ulcer disease depicts gastric or duodenal mural thickening with a central ulceration (Fig. 85-30). Adequate luminal distension with oral contrast material is essential. An inadequately distended stomach or duodenum may mask mural thickening or may produce a false-positive interpretation of mural thickening. Patients are asked to drink large volumes of water just prior to the MR examination. Distention of the

gastric antrum and duodenal bulb may be improved by placing the patient in a prone position. Surface coil imaging combined with SSRARE images obtained in axial, sagittal, and coronal planes will show the thickened gastric or duodenal wall. Fat-suppressed gadolinium-enhanced images are useful to demonstrate the marked enhancement of the inflamed and ulcerated intestinal wall. Complications of peptic ulcer disease, including perforation and abscess or phlegmon formation, can be shown on MRI. An abscess is depicted as an extraintestinal fluid collection with an enhancing wall, while a inflammatory phlegmon is seen as an enhancing soft tissue mass adjacent to the diseased stomach or duodenum. In the patient with peptic ulcer disease secondary to Zollinger-Ellison syndrome, the gastrin-secreting gastrinoma can be shown on MR images.[60] These islet cell tumors occur within or near the pancreatic head, duodenum, distal stomach and adjacent lymph nodes. They may be solitary or multiple and are typically less vascular than insulinomas. They show high signal on T2-weighted images and peripheral, ring-like enhancement on immediate gadolinium-enhanced images.

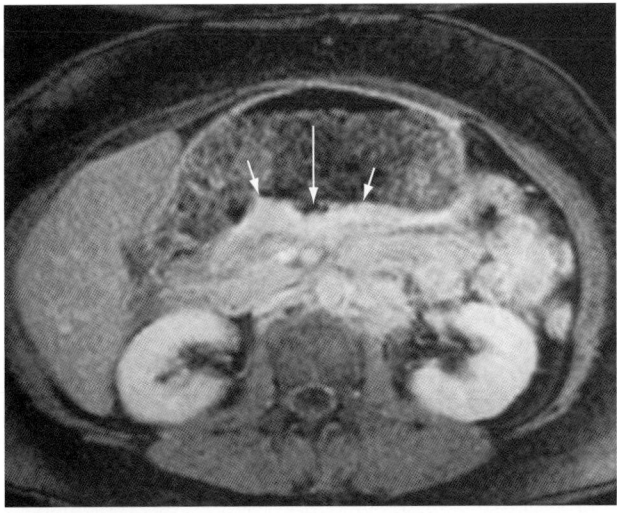

FIGURE 85-30

Peptic ulcer disease. Gadolinium-enhanced spoiled gradient-echo (SGE) image through the upper abdomen demonstrates a gastric ulcer *(long arrow)* in the body of the stomach with surrounding mucosal edema *(short arrows)*. Peptic ulcer disease was confirmed by endoscopy.

Gastritis

Gastritis or inflammation of the gastric mucosa is a non specific entity that may be caused by a number of etiologic agents including: bacterial or viral infections, non steroidal anti-inflammatory drugs, bile reflux, allergies, ischemia, and autoimmunity. Chronic gastritis can be exacerbated by smoking and alcohol ingestion. Patients present with abdominal pain, cramping, nausea and vomiting, and loss of appetite. *H. pylori* infection is the most common cause of chronic gastritis; it may

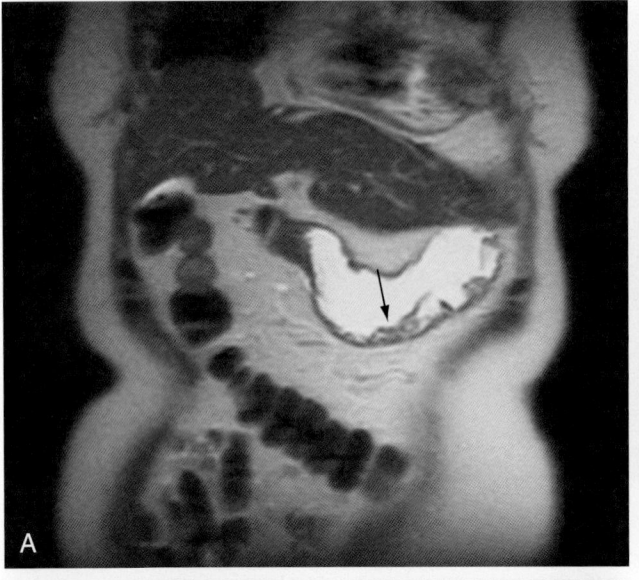
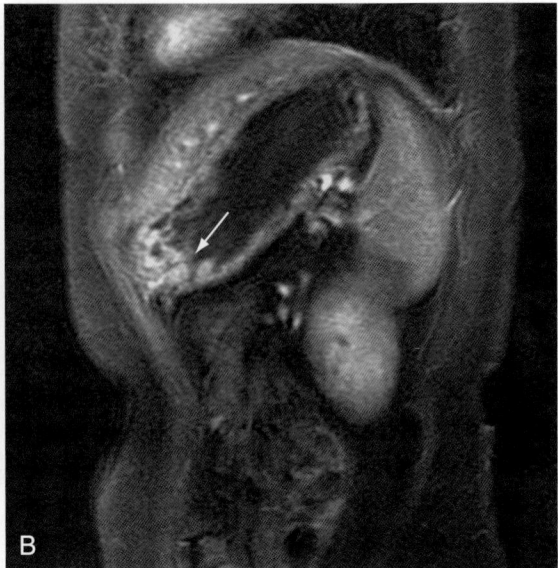
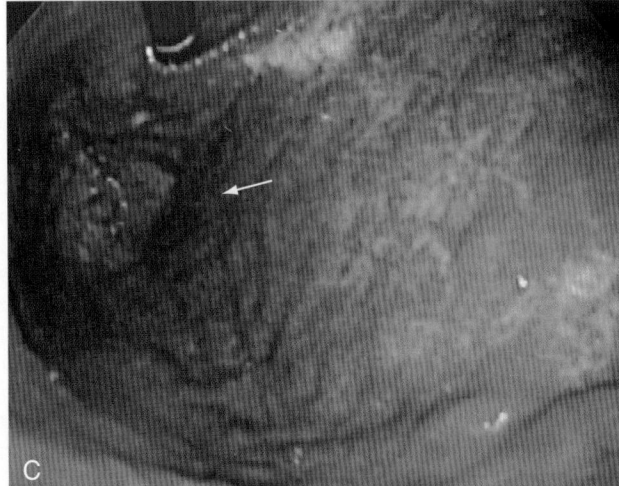

FIGURE 85-31

Gastritis. Coronal single-shot fast spin-echo (SSFSE) image (**A**) depicts gastric mural thickening (*arrow*) along the greater curvature. Sagittal gadolinium-enhanced spoiled gradient-echo (SGE) image (**B**) shows corresponding mural thickening and enhancement (*arrow*) in the gastric body. Endoscopic view (**C**) confirms gastric mucosal erythema (*arrow*) and atrophic gastritis.

lead to antral gastritis or to a multifocal atrophic gastritis with loss of the normal gastric glands in the gastric body and antrum. Intestinal metaplasia with replacement gastric glands in patients with atrophic gastritis can lead to gastric cancer in a small percentage of patients. Mucosa-associated-lymphoid-tissue (MALT) lymphomas also occur in association with *H. pylori* chronic gastritis.[61,62]

MRI of Gastritis

The MR findings of gastritis include gastric mural thickening and enhancement. (Fig. 85-31). Multiplanar SSRARE images combined with fat-suppressed gadolinium-enhanced SGE images depict the normal gastric wall and the portions of the stomach with mural thickening and enhancement. Gastric distention with water is essential for optimal evaluation of the stomach wall (Fig. 85-32).

Gastroenteritis

Gastroenteritis is a nonspecific GI disease characterized by watery diarrhea, abdominal pain, nausea, and vomiting. An infectious etiology is most common and may be secondary to viral, bacterial, or parasitic GI infections. Viral agents cause 50% to 70% of gastroenteritis cases and include coronavirus, adenovirus, rotovirus, parovirus, and calcivirus. Bacterial agents account for 15% to 20% of cases and include *Salmonella, Shigella, Yersinia nterocolitica, Escherichia coli, Campylobacter jejuni, Vibrio cholerae,* and *Clostridium perfringens.* Parasitic infections produce 15% to 20% of gastroenteritis cases and include *Giardia lamblia, Cryptosporidium,* and *Entamoeba histolytica.* The infectious agent may invade the mucosa or produce toxins or enterotoxins that lead to increased fluid secretion or decreased absorption. This leads to increased luminal fluid contents, electrolyte loss, and watery diarrhea. The diarrhea in gastroenteritis may

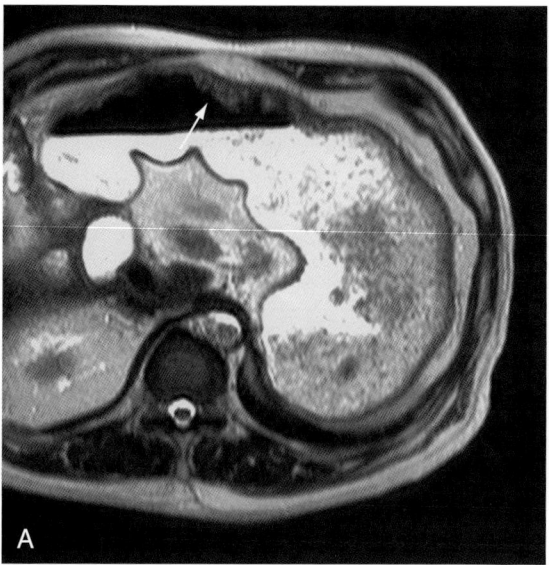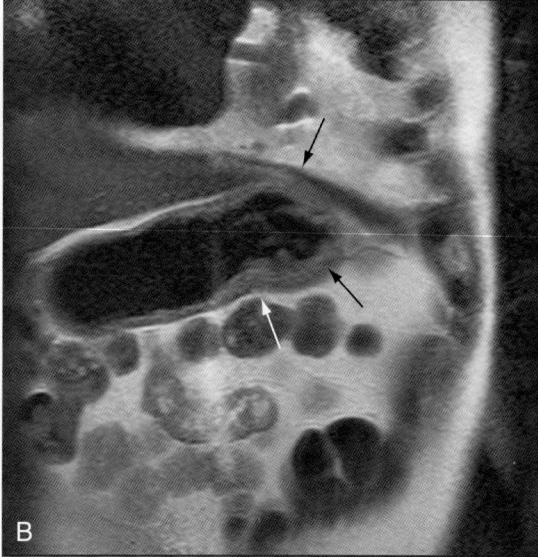

FIGURE 85-32

Gastritis. Axial (**A**) and coronal (**B**) single-shot fast spin-echo (SSFSE) images show gastric mural thickening *(arrows)* corresponding with endoscopically proven gastritis. Optimal distention of the stomach with water facilitates depiction of the thickened gastric wall.

be classified as osmotic, inflammatory, or secretory, or it may be due to altered intestinal motility. Since the small intestine is the primary site for absorption in the GI tract, this is the site typically involved in gastroenteritis.[63,64]

MRI of Gastroenteritis

On MR images the patient with gastroenteritis demonstrates intestinal mural thickening and enhancement with intravenous gadolinium. These findings are best depicted on fat-suppressed gadolinium-enhanced SGE MR images and are typically more conspicuous than on helical CT scans; SSRARE images are useful to confirm small intestinal mural thickening. Extraintestinal complications including abscess formation are depicted on MR images as an extraluminal fluid collection with a thick or thin enhancing rim. An extraintestinal phlegmon is shown as a solid enhancing extraluminal soft tissue mass with infiltration of the adjacent mesenteric fat. The location of the small-bowel findings may provide clues as to the specific infectious etiology. The proximal small bowel may be involved by the protozoa *G. lamblia* and *Strongoloides stercoralis*. The terminal ileum is involved by *Y. enterocolytica*, and *C. jejuni*, often mimicking Crohn's disease or acute appendicitis. Ultimately, the final diagnosis needs to be established by clinical, laboratory, and/or histopathologic findings.

Infectious Colitis

Colitis may be caused by numerous bacteria including *Shigella* and *Salmonella* species, *Y. enterocolitica, E. coli,*

and *C. jejuni*. Viral infections can cause infectious colitis. Infection with the protozoa *E. histolytica* causes colonic amebiasis. Immunocompromised patients may develop colitis secondary to infections with cytomegalovirus or MAI.[65,66] Patients present with frequent loose bowel movements with or without blood, abdominal pain, cramps, fever, and leukocytosis.

MRI of Infectious Colitis

MRI in patients with infectious colitis show focal or diffuse mural thickening and strandy infiltration of the pericolonic fat (Fig. 85-33). These findings are depicted on T1-weighted and SSRARE images. On fat-suppressed gadolinium-enhanced SGE images, there is marked enhancement of the thickened colonic wall. Complications of infectious colitis, including pericolic abscess or phlegmon formation are depicted as adjacent fluid collections or soft tissue inflammatory masses. The use of intraluminal and rectal contrast material will help to distend the colon and allow for optimal visualization of the thickened and inflamed colonic wall.

Antibiotic-Associated Colitis

Pseudomembranous colitis is caused by *Clostridium difficile*, an anaerobic gram-positive bacillus. Use of various antibiotics including clindamycin, broad spectrum penicillins, and cephalosporins, alter the normal colonic flora, allowing for overgrowth of *C. difficile*. Toxins produced by pathogenic strains of *C. difficile* produce diarrhea and pseudomembranous colitis. Onset

imaging studies are equivocal, non-diagnostic, or do not match the clinical findings.[69] In these cases MRI can provide valuable information that may confirm or exclude the diagnosis of appendicitis. Fat-suppressed gadolinium-enhanced SGE are the most useful MR images to evaluate patients with suspected appendicitis. The inflamed appendix shows marked enhancement with intravenous gadolinium (Fig. 85-35). Mural thickening may also be evident. Unenhanced SSRARE, T1-weighted, and fat-suppressed T2-weighted imaging show mural thickening and edema in the appendiceal wall and periappendiceal tissues. A periappendiceal abscess or phlegmon will also be depicted as an adjacent fluid collection with an enhancing wall or as an enhancing soft tissue mass. Unenhanced MRI may also be used in pregnant patients in whom appendicitis is a diagnostic consideration. In these patients SSRARE, unenhanced T1-weighted, and fat-suppressed T2-weighted imaging may show appendiceal mural thickening and inflammation in the right lower quadrant.

DEPOSITION DISEASES AND MISCELLANEOUS DISEASES

Hemorrhage

Intramural hemorrhage can occur within the wall of the stomach, small intestine, or colon as a complication of ischemia, trauma, infections, or tumors, or in the anticoagulated patient.[70,71] Spontaneous intramural hemorrhage occurs in the setting of excessive anti-coagulation. Patients present with circumferential mural thickening producing luminal narrowing and small bowel obstruction. The involved segment of bowel is typically longer, averaging 23 cm in one study.[71] The most common site of spontaneous intramural hemorrhage is the jejunum (69%) followed by the ileum (23%).[71] Duodenal intramural hematoma can be complicated by biliary obstruction. In a clinical setting other than hypercoagulation, intramural hematoma may involve shorter segments of bowel with less prominent mural thickening.[72]

MRI of Intramural Hemorrhage

On T1-weighted images, intramural hemorrhage is seen as high signal intensity within the thickened bowel wall due to the presence of extracellular methemoglobin. Heterogeneous high signal is present on T2-weighted images. On immediate fat-suppressed gadolinium-enhanced images, the intramural hemorrhage is non-enhancing (Fig. 85-36). This may help to distinguish mural thickening due to intramural blood from that due to infectious, inflammatory, or neoplastic process. Associated small-bowel obstruction is depicted with dilated small-bowel loops proximal to the site of intramural hemorrhage.

Hypoproteinemia

Albumin is the major body's serum binding protein and accounts for 75% to 80% of the normal plasma colloid oncotic pressure. It serves to transport a variety of substances including fatty acids, bilirubin, metals, hormones, and drugs. Normal reference levels of albumin are in the range of 3.5 to 4.5 g/dL. Hypoalbuminemia may be caused by protein malnutrition, inadequate production in patients with liver disease, extra vascular protein loss—which may be via massive proteinuria in patients with nephritic syndrome, or via the gut in

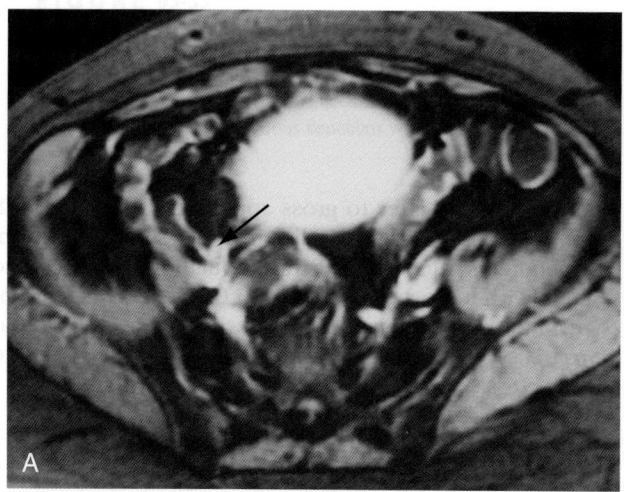
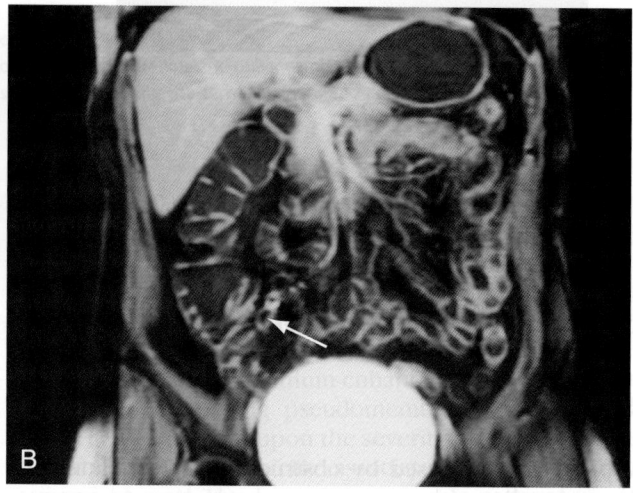

FIGURE 85-35

Appendicitis. Axial (**A**) and coronal (**B**) gadolinium-enhanced spoiled gradient-echo (SGE) image shows an inflamed appendix *(arrows)* with abnormal enhancement. Acute appendicitis was confirmed.

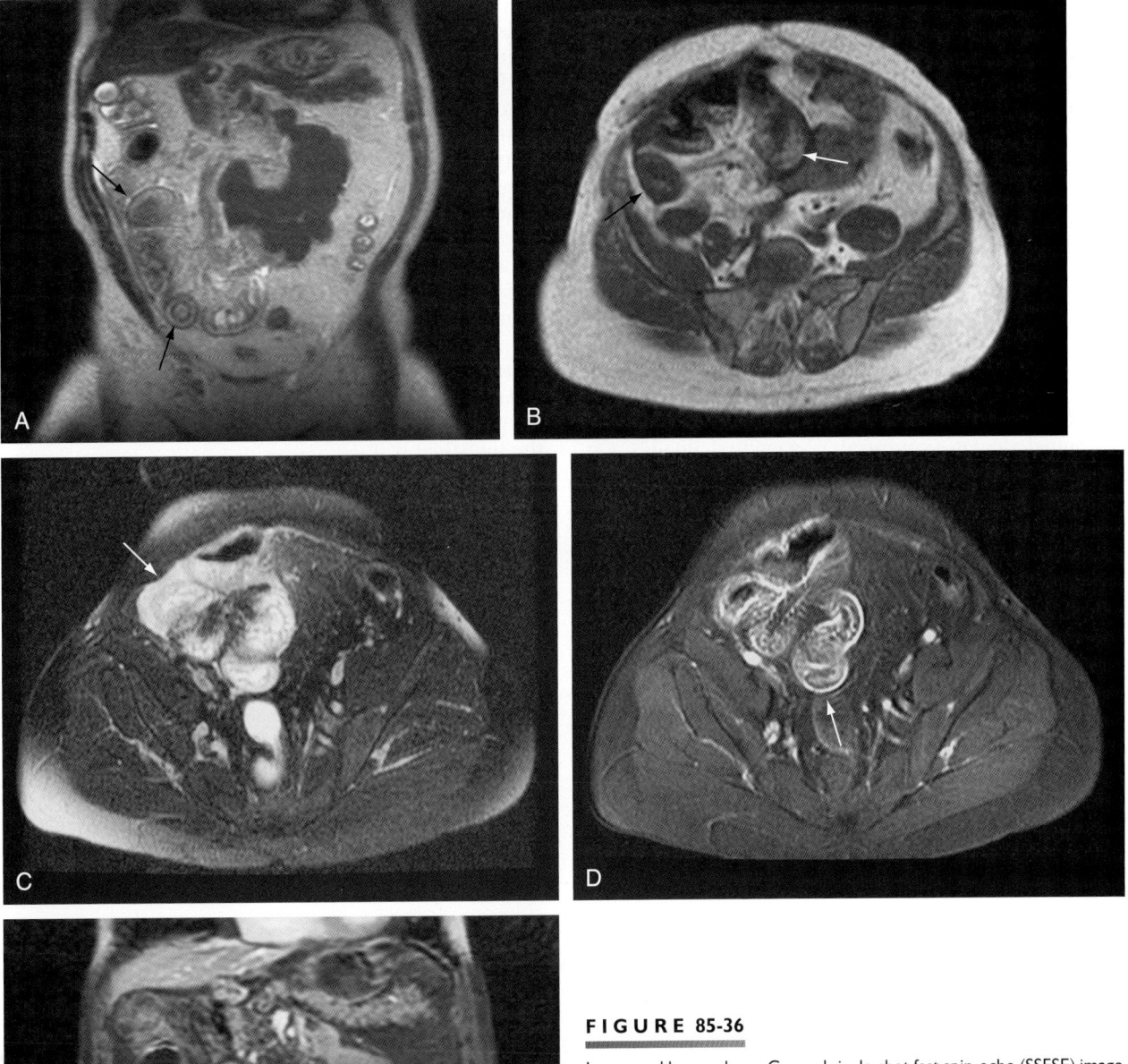

FIGURE 85-36

Intramural hemorrhage. Coronal single-shot fast spin-echo (SSFSE) image (**A**) shows abnormal segments of bowel in the middle and right side of the abdomen *(arrows)* with mural thickening. T1-weighted image (**B**) shows mural thickening *(black arrow)*. One segment of bowel *(white arrow)* shows mural thickening with high signal indicating methemoglobin from intramural hemorrhage. T2-weighted image (**C**) shows bowel loops with mural thickening *(arrow)*. Axial (**D**) and coronal (**E**) gadolinium-enhanced spoiled gradient-echo (SGE) images show abnormal bowel loops *(arrows)* with serosal enhancement but no mural enhancement. Absence of mural enhancement excludes active infectious and inflammatory diseases.

protein-losing enteropathy—and hemodilution in patients with ascites and congestive heart failure. Hypoalbuminemia results in diminished colloid osmotic pressure with resultant subcutaneous edema, ascites, and pulmonary edema. Diffuse bowel wall edema occurs with an albumin level less than 1.5 g/dL.[73]

MRI of Bowel Wall Edema in Hypoalbuminemia

In patients with marked hypoalbuminemia, MRI shows diffuse, marked, and concentric bowel wall edema (Fig. 85-37). These findings are most marked in the small bowel. Marked mural thickening and thickening of small-bowel folds is present. The thickened wall appears edematous with low signal on T1-weighted images and high signal on fat-suppressed T2-weighted images. On immediate fat-suppressed gadolinium-enhanced SGE images, there is little enhancement of the edematous bowel wall. Interstitial enhancement is typically present on delayed equilibrium phase images due to leak of the contrast into the bowel wall. Associated findings of ascites and anasarca are depicted on unenhanced T1-weighted and T2-weighted images.

Intestinal Lymphangiectasia

Intestinal lymphangiectasia is a disorder in which lymphatics within the wall of the small intestines become enlarged and obstructed.[74-76] Lymphatic fluid

leaks into the wall of the small intestine leading to malabsorption of fat and protein. As one of the causes of protein-losing enteropathy, intestinal lymphangiectasia leads to marked hypoalbuminemia, which further exacerbates interstitial fluid accumulation. Intestinal lymphangiectasia may be congenital or may occur secondary to a number of different diseases. These acquired causes of intestinal lymphangiectasia include pancreatitis, constrictive pericarditis, inferior vena cava thrombosis, retroperitoneal tumors or fibrosis, lymphoma, Whipple disease, Crohn's disease, and sclerosing mesenteritis. Patients present with signs and symptoms of malabsorption including steatorrhea, nausea, vomiting, and abdominal pain. Hypoproteinemia leads to accumulation of ascites and peripheral edema. Diagnosis is established by small-bowel biopsy showing dilated lymphatic spaces within the mucosa and submucosa of the intestinal wall.

MRI of Intestinal Lymphangiectasia

MRI in patients with intestinal lymphangiectasia shows diffuse small intestinal mural thickening (Fig. 85-38). Thickening of the small bowel wall and valvulae conniventes is concentric, uniform, and diffuse in distribution. Small-bowel dilatation is present along with infiltration and the small bowel mesentery and ascites. These finding are well visualized on SSRARE images and on fat-suppressed gadolinium-enhanced SGE images. The accumulated fluid within the thickened small bowel wall shows only mild delayed enhancement that is less than is seen with inflammatory enteritis.

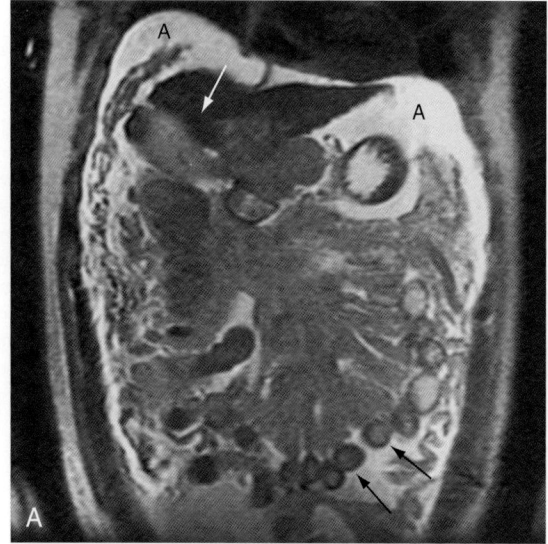
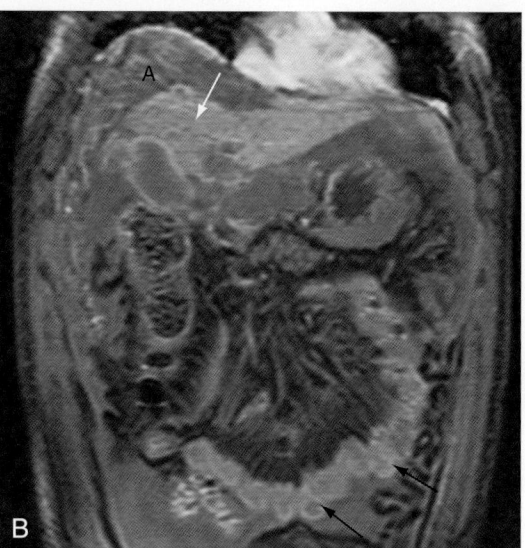

FIGURE 85-37

Hypoalbuminemia in a patient with end-stage cirrhosis. Coronal single-shot fast spin-echo (SSFSE) (**A**) and gadolinium-enhanced spoiled gradient-echo (SGE) (**B**) MR images depict a cirrhotic liver *(white arrow)*, ascites (A), and concentric small bowel mural thickening *(black arrows)*. Findings correlate with mural thickening due to hypoproteinemia secondary to liver disease.

Eosinophilic Gastroenteritis

Eosinophilic gastroenteritis is an uncommon intestinal disease characterized by infiltration of the wall of the esophagus, stomach, and small intestine with eosinophils.[77-79] The disease is limited to the GI tract without involvement of extraintestinal organs. A local inflammatory response to food allergens, infections, or other immunologic stimuli is thought to trigger accumulation of eosinophils with resultant tissue damage. The eosinophils may infiltrate the mucosa and submucosa. Less commonly the muscularis layer of the bowel wall is involved, producing gastric outlet obstruction or small-bowel obstruction. In the least common form of eosinophilic gastroenteritis, involvement of the bowel serosa produces eosinophilic ascites and peritonitis. Patients present with nonspecific symptoms including abdominal pain, nausea, vomiting, bloating, dysphagia, steatorrhea, and weight loss. Only 50% of patients have a history of atopy. Peripheral blood eosinophilia is present in 20% to 80% of patients. Diagnosis is established by endoscopy and biopsy of the intestinal wall showing >20 eosinophils per high-powered field. At endoscopy, the mucosa of bowel affected by eosinophilic gastroenteritis is inflamed, nodular, and often ulcerated. To establish the diagnosis, other causes of eosinophilia first need to be excluded.

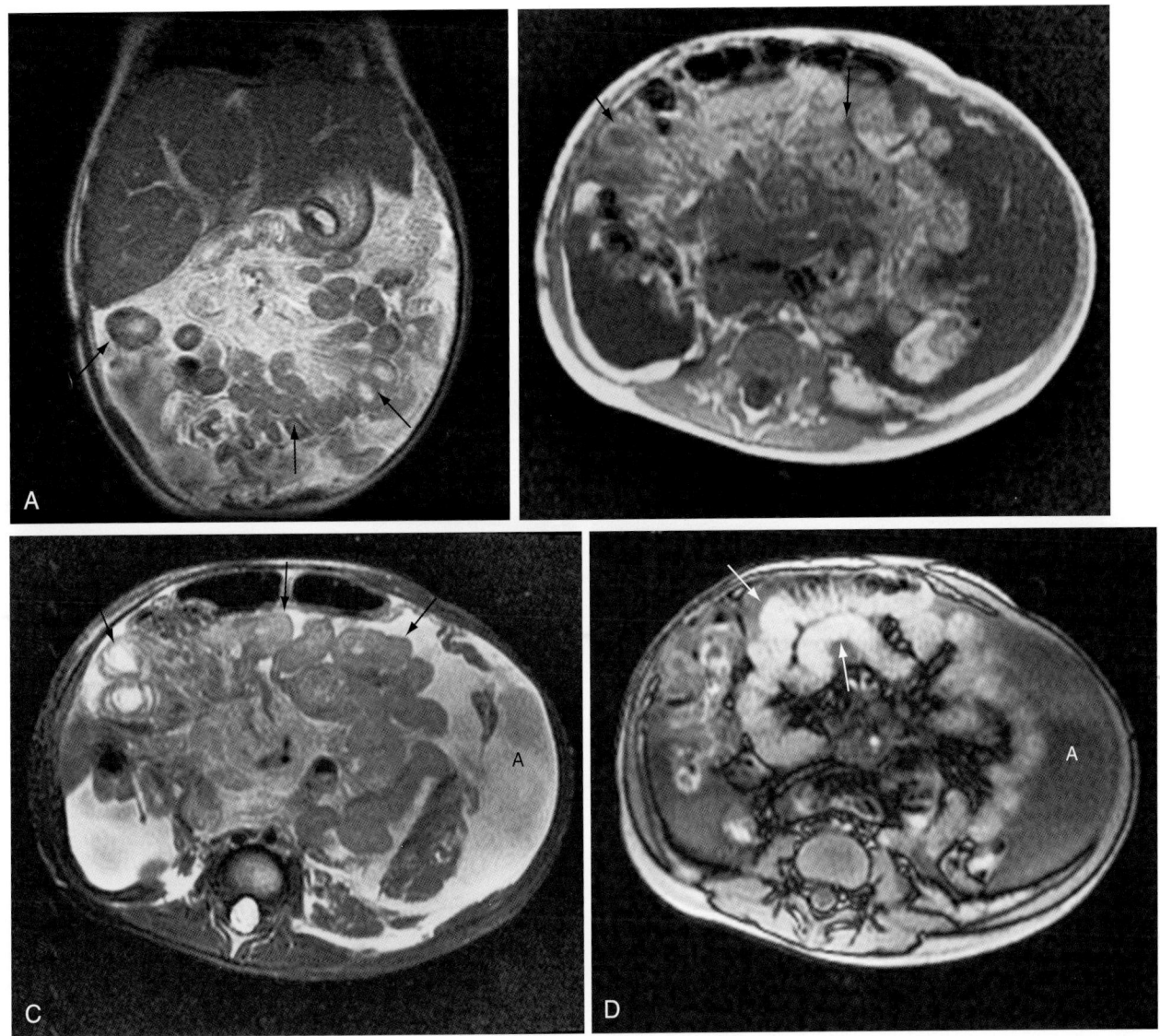

FIGURE 85-38

Intestinal lymphangiectasia in pediatric patient. Coronal single-shot fast spin-echo (SSFSE) image (**A**) shows diffuse mural thickening *(arrows)*. T1-weighted (**B**), T2-weighted (**C**), and gadolinium-enhanced spoiled gradient-echo (SGE) (**D**) images confirm diffuse mural thickening *(arrows)* and ascites (A). Note the high signal intensity of the abnormal bowel loops on **B** and **D**. Endoscopy and biopsy confirmed dilated mucosal and submucosal lymphatic spaces and intestinal lymphangiectasia.

MRI of Eosinophilic Gastroenteritis

Areas of the intestine affected by eosinophilic gastroenteritis show nonspecific mural thickening, best depicted on SSRARE and fat-suppressed gadolinium-enhanced MR images (Fig. 85-39). Involvement of the stomach produces mural and rugal thickening. Gastric outlet obstruction may develop with infiltration of the muscularis layer of the gastric antrum and pylorus. Small-bowel involvement produces mural thickening and thickened valvulae conniventes. Small-bowel luminal narrowing and strictures may lead to dilated proximal small bowel and obstruction. When eosinophilic infiltration extends to the intestinal serosa, MRI demonstrates associated ascites and peritonitis. The MR findings of peritonitis are best appreciated on fat-suppressed gadolinium-enhanced SGE images, in which there are abnormal enhancement of the peritoneum. Adjacent abdominal lymphadenopathy may be depicted on MR images in patients with eosinophilic gastroenteritis.

Celiac Disease

Celiac disease is a genetic inheritable disease characterized by immune-mediated damage to the jejunal mucosa producing villous atrophy and malabsorption. Loss of intestinal villi produces malabsorption of fat, carbohydrates (especially lactose), and proteins. The disease, also known as gluten-sensitive enteropathy, is exacerbated by ingestion of gliadin proteins (gluten) found in wheat, barley, rye, and oats. Onset of symptoms

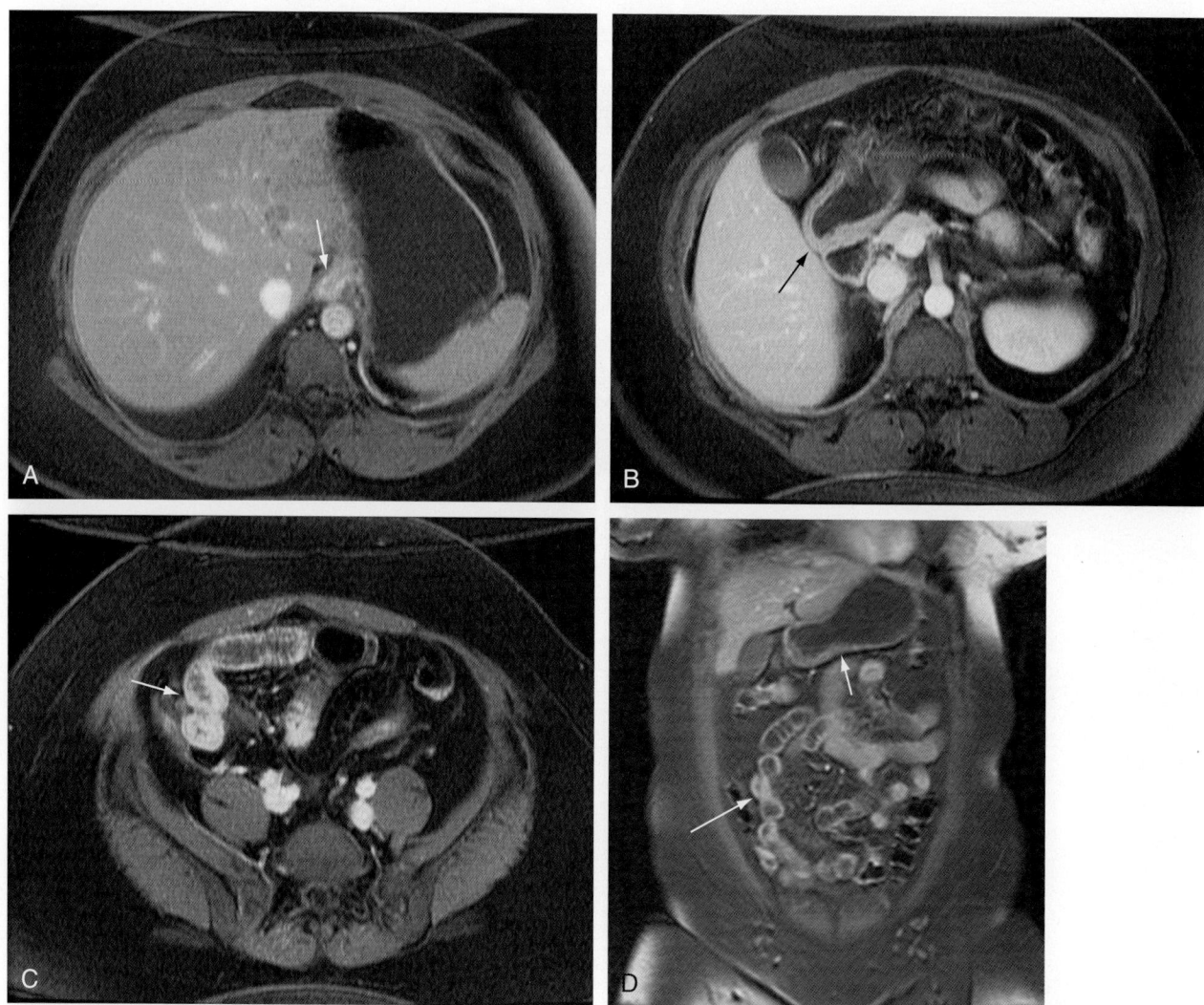

FIGURE 85-39

Eosinophillic enteritis. Axial gadolinium-enhanced spoiled gradient-echo (SGE) image (**A**) shows distal esophageal mural thickening *(arrow)*. Image through the upper abdomen (**B**) shows mural thickening in the gastric antrum *(arrow)*. Image through the right lower quadrant (**C**) depicts similar mural thickening *(arrow)* involving the distal ileum. Coronal gadolinium-enhanced SGE image (**D**) confirms gastric antral *(short arrow)* and ileal *(long arrow)* mural thickening. Endoscopy and biopsy confirmed eosinophillic gastroenteritis with eosinophillic infiltration of the mucosa and submucosa.

may occur immediately following ingestion of gluten or may be a delayed insidious response to chronic ingestion of small amounts of gluten. Patients may present with diarrhea, crampy abdominal pain, bloating, flatus, steatorrhea, and fatigue. Diagnosis is established by endoscopic jejunal biopsy. Treatment is by strict adherence to a gluten-free diet.[80]

MRI of Celiac Disease

MRI of celiac disease may show small-bowel dilatation >3 cm, ileal "jejunization" with an increase in the number of ileal mucosal folds (>5 folds/inch; >2 folds/cm), mural thickening of the proximal small bowel, and a reversal of jejuno-ileal fold pattern[80] (Fig. 85-40). In one study of 27 patients with celiac disease, SSRARE MRI suggested the correct diagnosis in 70.4% of patients. These authors also noted that in 29% of patients with biopsy-proven celiac disease, no small-bowel findings were present. Complications of celiac disease, including jejunal intussusception, ulcerations, and small-bowel neoplasms may also be demonstrated. Extra intestinal findings in celiac disease include mesenteric adenopathy and splenic atrophy.

BENIGN MASSES

Polyposis Syndromes

Familial Adenomatous Polyposis

Familial adenomatous polyposis is an autosomal dominant premalignant condition caused by a germline mutation of the *APC* tumor suppressor gene (adenomatous polyposis coli). It is characterized by the presence of hundreds to thousands of adenomas in the rectum and colon (Fig. 85-41). Patients have a mean age of 16 years at the time of diagnosis with familial polyposis. Familial polyposis is typically asymptomatic until patients develop colon cancer, which occurs in 100% of patients who do not undergo colectomy. The mean age of diagnosis of colon cancer is 39 years, at which time patients present with lower GI bleeding and abdominal pain. Associated duodenal and periampullary adenocarcinomas occur in 4% to 12% of patients with familial polyposis.[81-86]

Gardner syndrome is considered an allelic variant of familial adenomatous polyposis, in which there is a combination of polyposis coli and bone and soft tissue tumors. These extraintestinal manifestations include osteomas, and soft tissue tumors such as fibromas and epidermoid cysts, and dental anomalies, including supernumerary teeth, odontomas, and dentigerous cysts. Turcot syndrome is the combination of polyposis coli and CNS tumors, usually medulloblastomas.

Peutz-Jeghers Syndrome

Peutz-Jeghers syndrome is a rare autosomal dominant condition associated with GI hamartomas and muocutaneous melanocytic macules.[82] It is caused by a germline mutation of the *STK11* gene. The frequency of Peutz-Jeghers syndrome is 1 in 10 that of familial adenomatous polyposis. The hamartomas in Peutz-Jeghers syndrome occur in the small intestine in 95% of cases, while the stomach and colon may be involved in up to 25% of cases (Fig. 85-42). The hamartomas are benign and are not premalignant. There is a 15-fold increased risk of cancer in patients with Peutz-Jeghers syndrome with associated gastric, small intestine, and colon adenocarcinoma, as well as cancers of the pancreas, lung, breast, testes, ovary, and cervix. Fifty percent of patients with Peutz-Jeghers syndrome die from malignancy by 57 years of age.

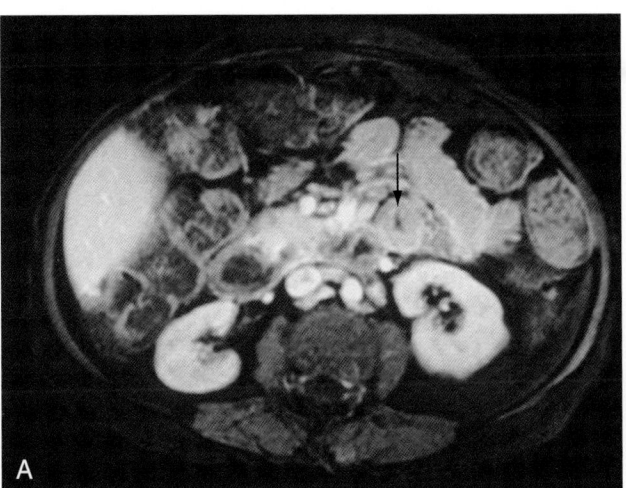 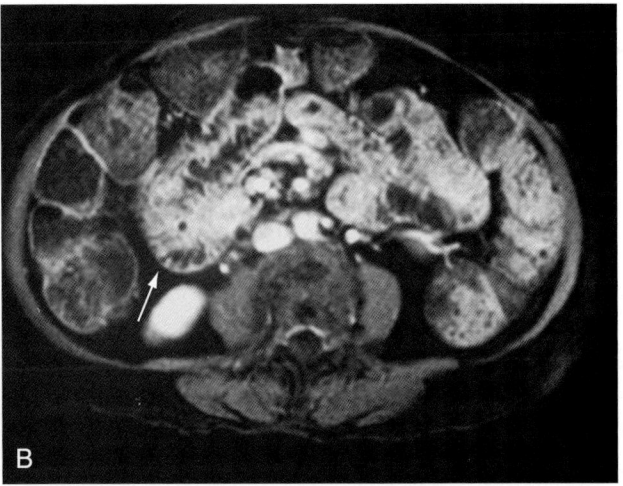

FIGURE 85-40

Celiac disease. Gadolinium-enhanced spoiled gradient-echo (SGE) image through the upper abdomen (**A**) shows jejunal mural thickening *(arrow)*. Image through the right lower quadrant (**B**) demonstrates "jejunization" of the ileum *(arrow)* with an increased number of ileal folds.

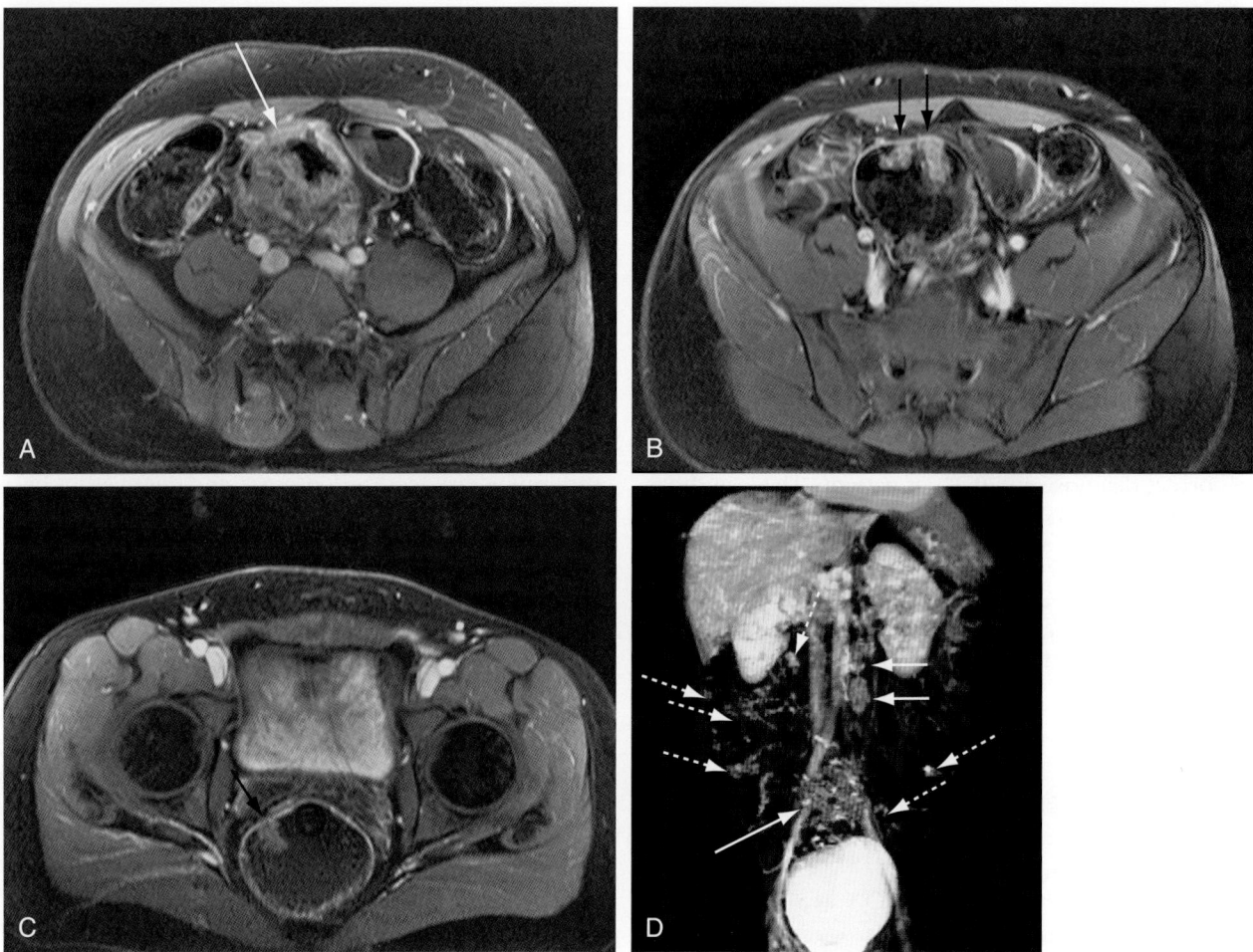

FIGURE 85-41

Familial adenomatous polyposis. Gadolinium-enhanced spoiled gradient-echo (SGE) images (**A-C**) depict multiple scattered rectal and colonic polyps *(short black arrows)* and a sigmoid cancer *(long white arrow)*. Three dimensional color volume model (**D**) generated from the gadolinium-enhanced MR images shows scattered polyps *(dotted arrows)*, nodal metastases *(short solid white arrows)*, and the sigmoid adenocarcinoma *(long white arrow)*.

Juvenile Polyposis

Juvenile polyposis is a rare condition characterized by the development of hamartomatous polyps in the stomach, small intestine, or colon.[84] The term juvenile refers to the type or histology of the polyp and not to the age of the patient at the time of diagnosis. While malignant transformation of the hamartomas is rare, the risk of associated intestinal malignancy is estimated at 9% to 50%. The most common associated malignancy is colon cancer.

Cronkhite-Canada Syndrome

Cronkhite-Canada syndrome is a very rare nonfamilial condition characterized by intestinal hamartomatous polyps and marked cutaneous changes.[85] Dermatological manifestations include alopecia and altered pigmentation of the skin and nail beds. The polyps involve the stomach and small bowel with patterns of polyposis varying from innumerable small polyps carpeting large

areas, scattered varying-size polyps, and sparse involvement with few small polyps.[85] Extensive intestinal polyposis with abnormal intervening mucosa can lead to severe diarrhea and a protein losing enteropathy.

MRI of Polyposis

Intestinal polyposis can be depicted on MRI using routing breath-hold T1-weighed, SS-RARE T2-weighted, and fat-suppressed gadolinium-enhanced SGE MRI.[86] Polyps demonstrate signal intensity similar to the normal bowel wall on T1-weighed and T2-weighted images and enhance to a degree similar to the normal bowel wall with gadolinium injection.[86] Larger polyps may show mild heterogeneous enhancement on delayed gadolinium-enhanced images. The presence of polyp enhancement on delayed images helps to differentiate a polyp from non-enhancing bowel contents. In patients with more extensive polyposis, the sheets of polyps

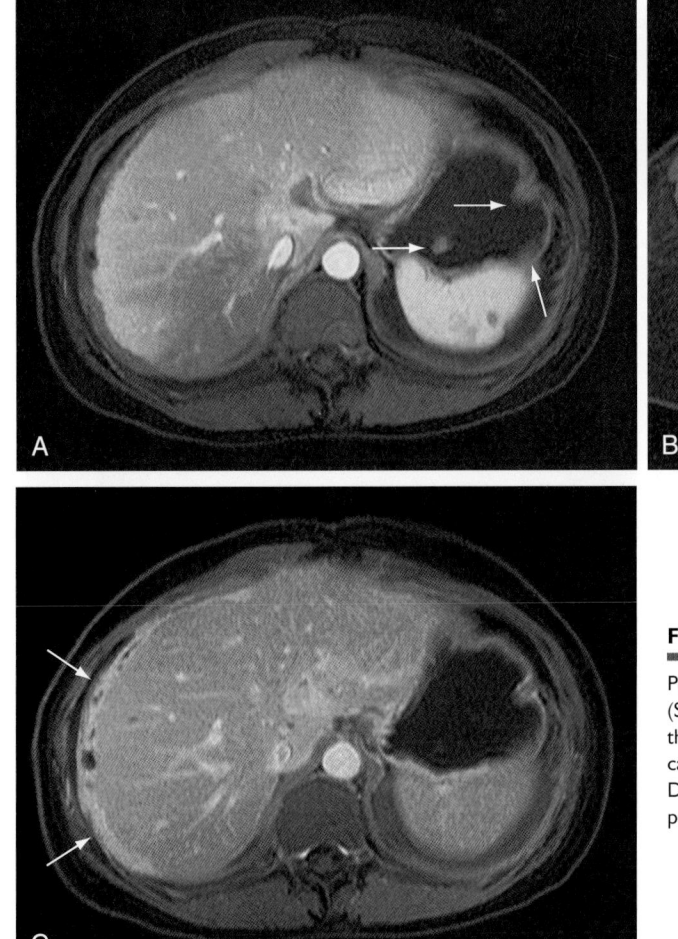
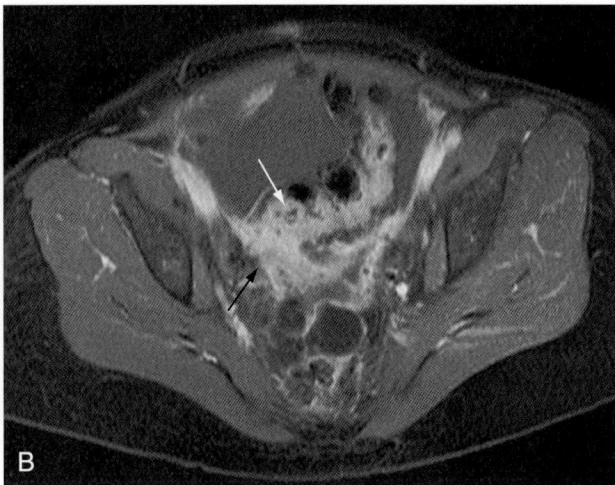

FIGURE 85-42

Peutz-Jeghers polyposis. Gadolinium-enhanced spoiled gradient-echo (SGE) MR image (**A**) depicts multiple gastric polyps *(arrows)*. Image through the pelvis (**B**) demonstrates an associated sigmoid adeno-carcinoma *(white arrow)* with transmural tumor spread *(black arrow)*. Delayed image through the upper abdomen (**C**) shows enhancing perihepatic peritoneal metastases *(arrows)*.

may appear as mural thickening rather than as discrete polyps. Malignant transformation of polyps or associated intestinal cancers will be depicted on MRI as heterogeneous masses, or mural thickening. The distinction between extensive polyposis and intestinal malignancy is incomplete, and ultimately tissue diagnosis is required to establish the correct diagnosis.

Leiomyoma

See Gastrointestinal Stromal Tumors (GIST)

Diverticulum

Diverticula are outpouchings of the mucosa through weak points in the intestinal wall. They occur in the stomach, small intestine, and colon. Gastric diverticula occur most commonly in the proximal stomach involving the posterior gastric cardia. Small intestinal diverticula occur most commonly in the duodenum. Periampullary duodenal diverticula can result in biliary

obstruction. The frequency of jejunal diverticula is one fifth that of duodenal diverticula. Although most diverticula are asymptomatic, multiple jejunal diverticula can lead to bacterial overgrowth and malabsorption. Numerous jejunal diverticula are seen in patients with scleroderma and Ehlers-Danlos syndrome. A Meckel's diverticulum occurs in the distal ileum and is a remnant of the omphalomesenteric duct. Colonic diverticula are acquired and occur most commonly in the sigmoid colon, but can affect any portion of the colon.

MRI of Diverticulum

Diverticula are depicted on SSRARE images as fluid- or air-filled outpouchings arising from the adjacent stomach, small intestine, or colon. The wall of the diverticulum is thin. An MR cholangiopancreaticograph (MRCP) is a useful examination to demonstrate the presence of a periampullary diverticulum and its relationship to the common bile duct insertion into the duodenum (Fig. 85-43). On fat-suppressed gadolinium-enhanced SGE images the wall of the non-inflamed diverticulum is thin

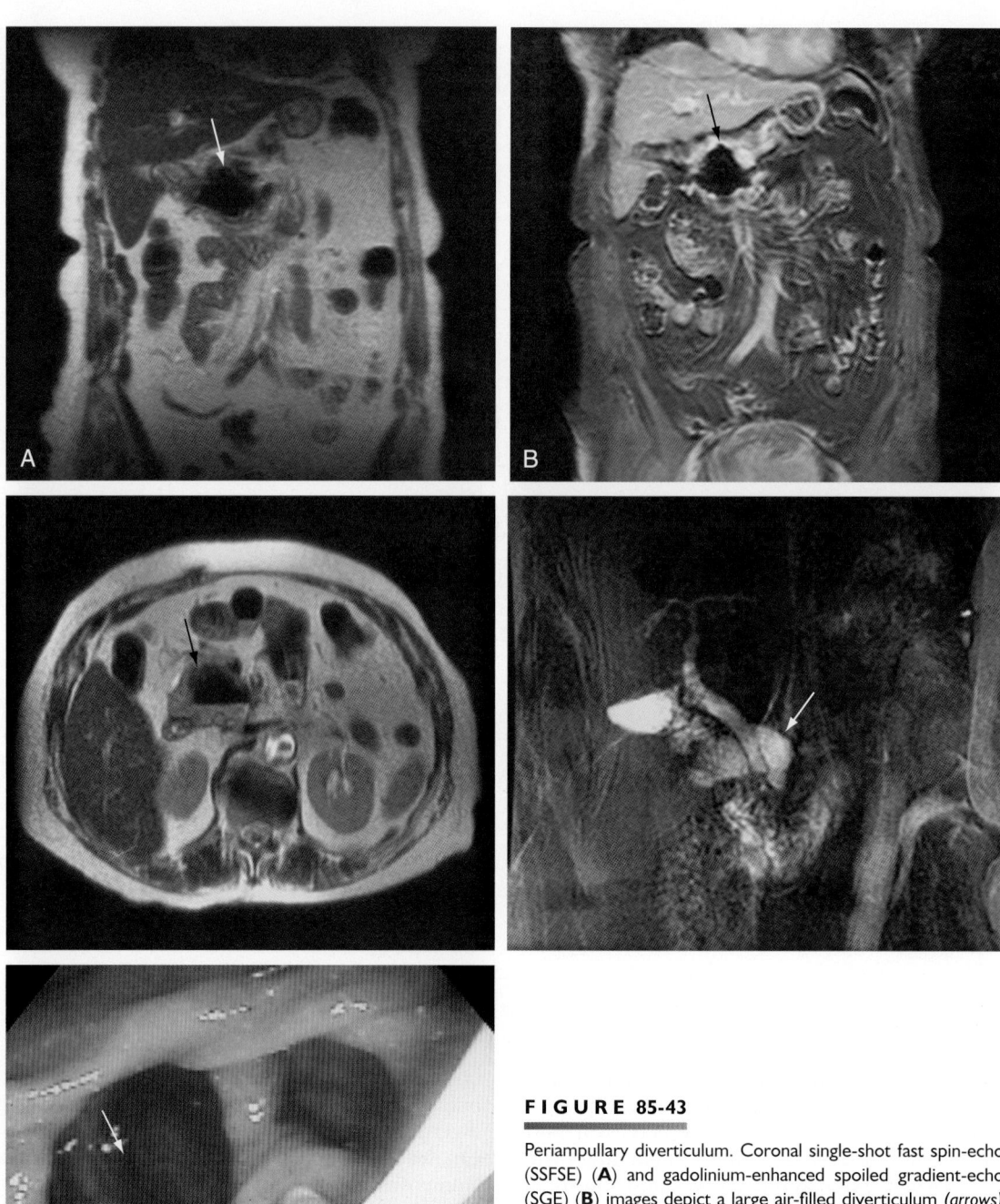

FIGURE 85-43

Periampullary diverticulum. Coronal single-shot fast spin-echo (SSFSE) (**A**) and gadolinium-enhanced spoiled gradient-echo (SGE) (**B**) images depict a large air-filled diverticulum *(arrows)* in the right upper quadrant. Axial SSFSE image (**C**) shows an air-fluid level within the diverticulum *(arrow)*. MR cholangio-pancreaticograph (MRCP) (**D**) shows the relationship of the diverticulum *(arrow)* to the common bile duct. Endoscopic retrograde choledochopancreatography (ERCP) (**E**) shows the large periampullary diverticulum *(arrow)*.

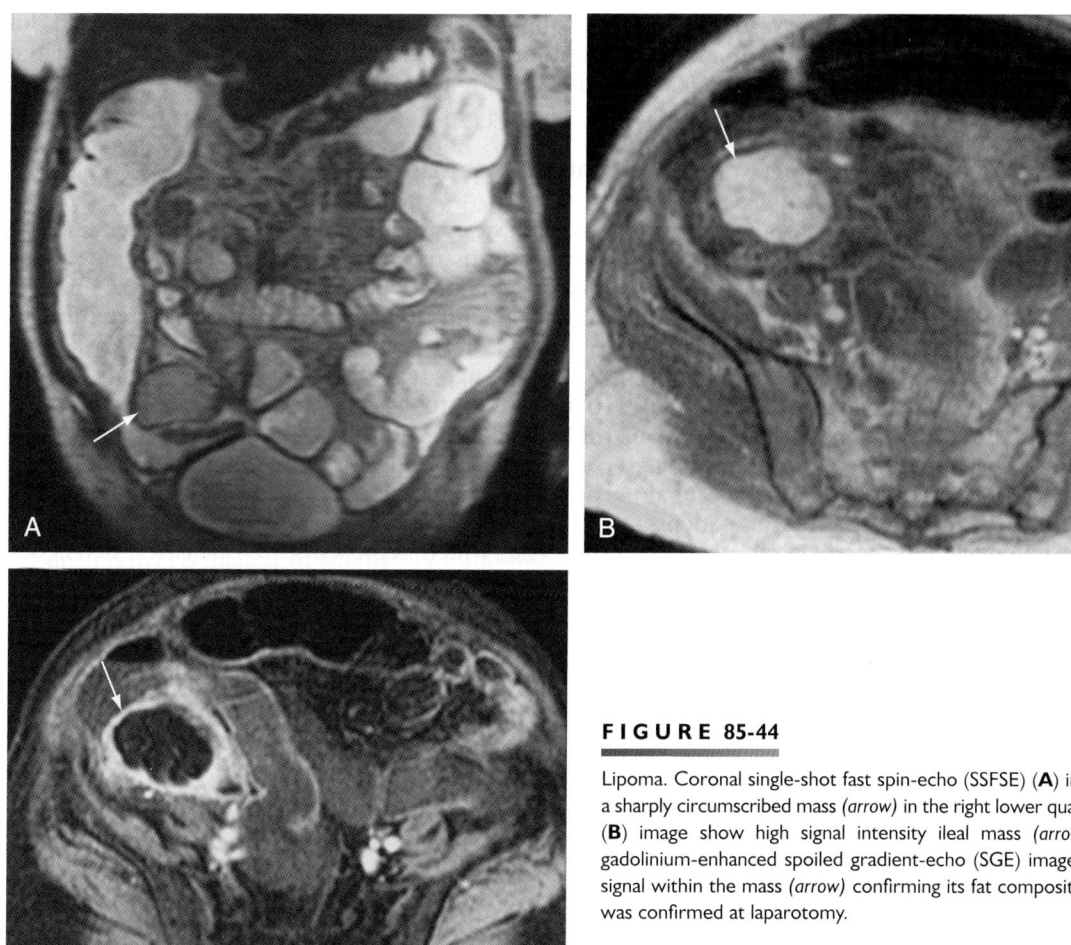

FIGURE 85-44

Lipoma. Coronal single-shot fast spin-echo (SSFSE) (**A**) image demonstrates a sharply circumscribed mass *(arrow)* in the right lower quadrant. T1-weighted (**B**) image show high signal intensity ileal mass *(arrow)*. Fat-suppressed gadolinium-enhanced spoiled gradient-echo (SGE) image (**C**) shows loss of signal within the mass *(arrow)* confirming its fat composition. An ileal lipoma was confirmed at laparotomy.

and shows enhancement similar to the adjacent bowel wall. With inflammation, the wall of the diverticulum shows thickening and abnormal enhancement with infiltration of the surrounding fat.

Lipoma

Lipomas are benign submucosal tumors of mesenenchymal origin.[87] They may occur in the small intestine or colon. In the small bowel, lipomas are found preferentially in the duodenum and ileum, while in the colon lipomas occur in the cecum, ascending colon, and sigmoid colon. Most lipomas are asymptomatic. Symptoms may occur with ulceration and GI hemorrhage or may be due to intermittent obstruction with colicky abdominal pain. A lipoma can act as the lead point of an intussusception.

MRI of Lipoma

On MRI, lipomas have a characteristic appearance with high signal on T1-weighted images (Fig. 85-44). Loss of signal on fat-suppressed imaging confirms the diagnosis. On fat-suppressed gadolinium-enhanced SGE imaging, the mass has low signal intensity. Some peripheral surrounding enhancement may be present. Ulcerated or necrotic lipomas will have a more complicated appearance, with areas of higher signal on T2-weighted images and some enhancement with intravenous gadolinium.

Mucocele

A mucocles occurs as a result of obstruction of the appendix with resultant accumulation of mucinous material within the distended appendiceal lumen.[88]

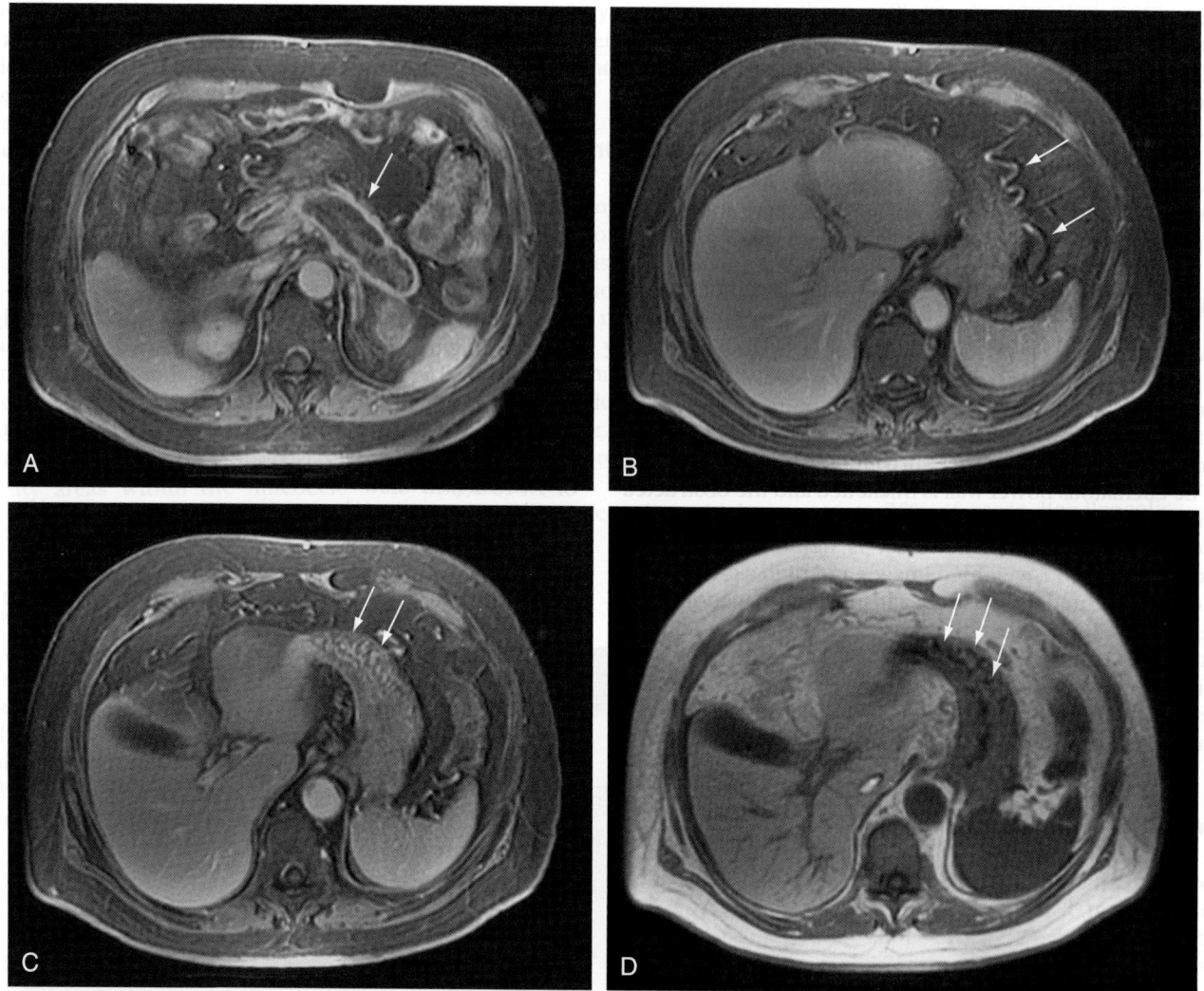

FIGURE 85-46

Varices. Gadolinium-enhanced spoiled gradient-echo (SGE) image (**A**) demonstrates necrosis of the pancreatic body and tail *(arrow)*. Gadolinium-enhanced image (**B**) cephalad to **A** shows perigastric varices *(arrows)* due to associated splenic vein thrombosis (not shown). Gadolinium-enhanced image through the gastric body (**C**) shows enhancing intramural gastric varices *(arrows)*. T1-weighted image through the gastric body (**D**) confirms gastric varices depicted as flow voids *(arrows)*.

MRI of Esophageal Cancer

Preoperative imaging of patients with esophageal cancer should include the chest and abdomen. Oral water is administered to distend the stomach, optimizing depiction of the gastroesophageal junction. Surface coil images of the distal esophagus and stomach can be obtained with thin section SSRARE images in multiple planes combined with routine T1-weighted, and T2-weighted imaging and fat-suppressed gadolinium-enhanced imaging. The direct multiplanar capabilities of MRI facilitate depiction of esophageal cancers. Coronal and sagittal images excel at demonstrating tumors at the gastroesophageal junction and their extension into the stomach.[97-100]

In vitro studies have shown very good correlation between high-resolution MR images and histopathologic determination of the depth of tumor penetration.[97]

However, in general, endoscopic ultrasound is more accurate in determining the depth of tumor penetration[100] compared with helical CT and MRI. MRI is useful to evaluate more extensive tumor with mediastinal invasion or distant metastases. Invasion of the pericardium, aorta, and tracheobronchial tree can be depicted with MRI with moderate accuracy. However, the depiction of nodal tumor in normal sized lymph nodes remains problematic. The presence of multiple normal sized para-esophageal nodes is suspicious for nodal tumor involvement.

The MR appearance of a primary esophageal cancer shows a segment of the esophagus with mural thickening or a mural mass (Fig. 85-47). The tumor can be depicted on unenhanced T1-weighed and T2-weighted images, or SSRARE images. On fat-suppressed gadolinium-enhanced images the esophageal cancer will show

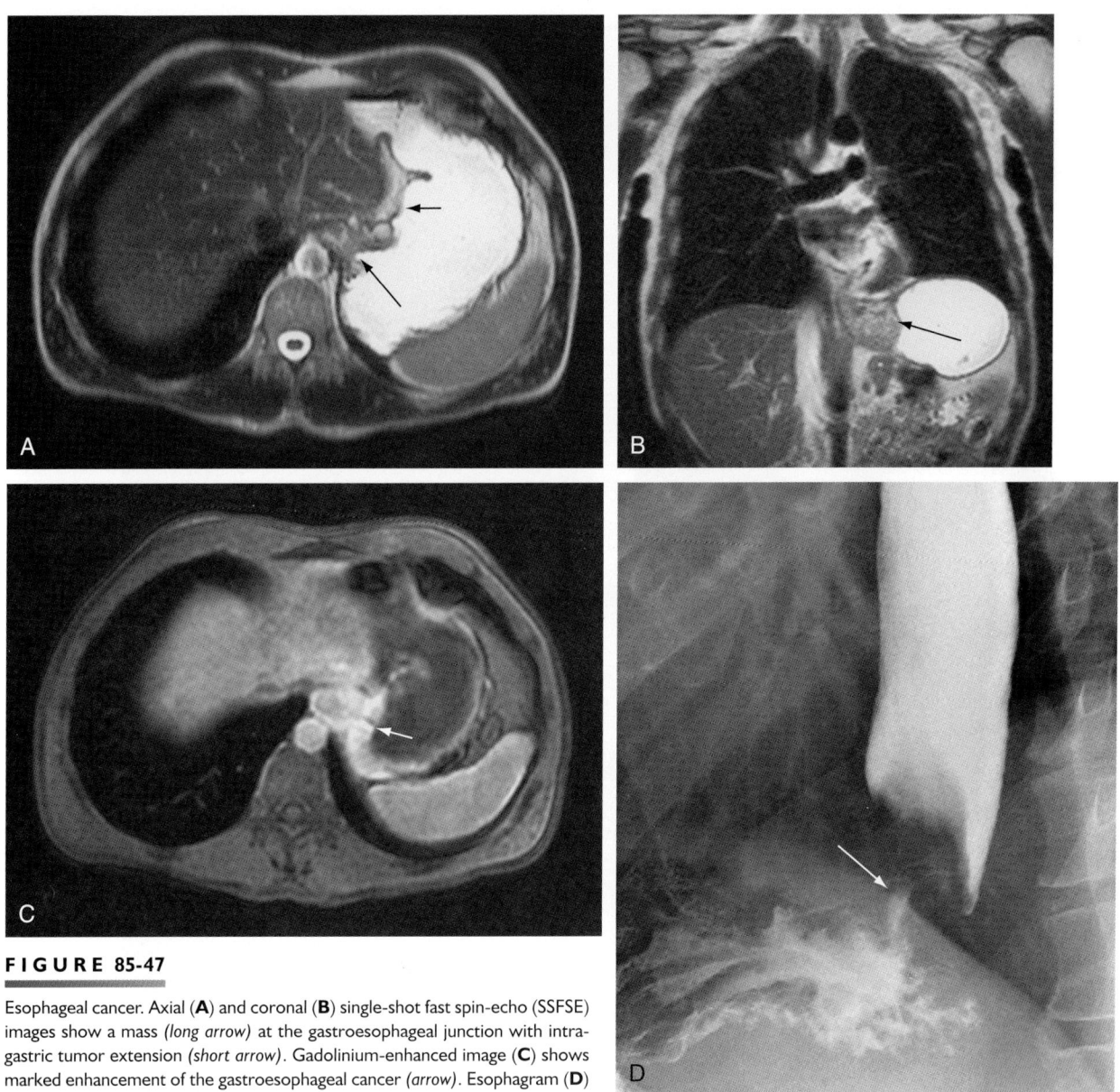

FIGURE 85-47

Esophageal cancer. Axial (**A**) and coronal (**B**) single-shot fast spin-echo (SSFSE) images show a mass *(long arrow)* at the gastroesophageal junction with intragastric tumor extension *(short arrow)*. Gadolinium-enhanced image (**C**) shows marked enhancement of the gastroesophageal cancer *(arrow)*. Esophagram (**D**) depicts a large mass *(arrow)* in the distal esophagus with mucosal destruction.

marked enhancement, improving its conspicuity. Transmural tumor extension is indicated by a nodular outer contour to the thickened wall or by gross extramural tumor extension. A complete examination of the chest and abdomen is performed to assess for distant metastases and the degree of local invasion by the esophageal cancer (Fig. 85-48).

Gastric Cancer

Gastric cancer is the 14th most common malignancy in the United States. The American Cancer Society estimates that in 2003, about 22,400 new cases will be diagnosed in the United States and 12,100 people will die of the disease. Worldwide, gastric cancer is the second most common incident malignancy, second only to lung cancer in 1996. There is an increased incidence of gastric cancer in South America, Central Europe, and Asia. Risk factors for gastric cancer include *H. pylori* gastric infection, atrophic gastritis, pernicious anemia, cigarette smoking, Ménétrier's disease, familial polyposis, advanced age, and male gender.[101-103]

Adenocarcinomas account for 90 to 95% of gastric cancers. The location of the tumor within the stomach has changed over the last several decades. In the United States, cancers in the distal half of the stomach are decreasing in frequency while cancers arising in the gastric cardia and gastroesophageal junction have shown a marked increase in frequency. The prognosis of the gastric cancer is related to local tumor extent, nodal metastases, distant metastases, and the site of origin of

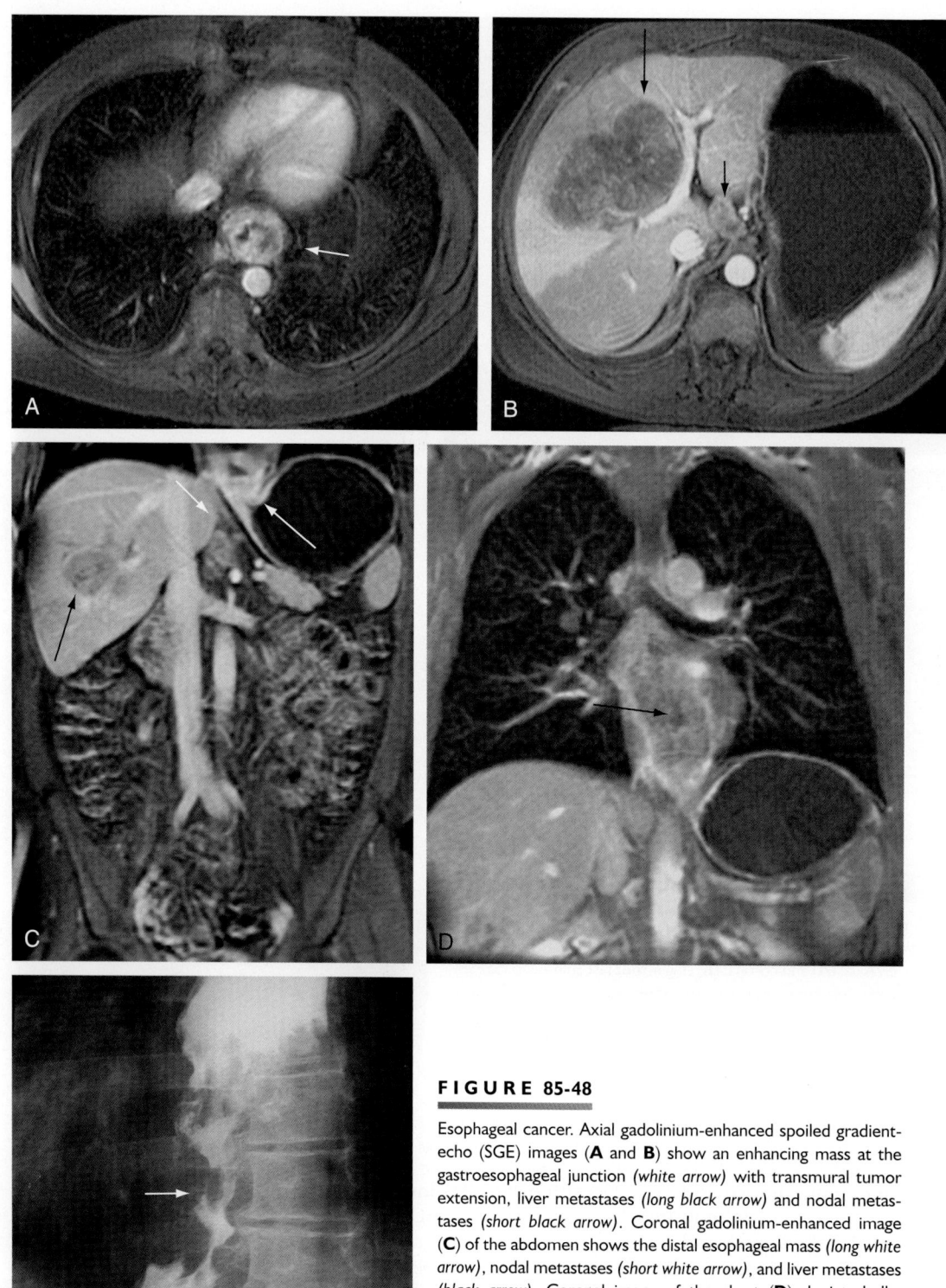

FIGURE 85-48

Esophageal cancer. Axial gadolinium-enhanced spoiled gradient-echo (SGE) images (**A** and **B**) show an enhancing mass at the gastroesophageal junction *(white arrow)* with transmural tumor extension, liver metastases *(long black arrow)* and nodal metastases *(short black arrow)*. Coronal gadolinium-enhanced image (**C**) of the abdomen shows the distal esophageal mass *(long white arrow)*, nodal metastases *(short white arrow)*, and liver metastases *(black arrow)*. Coronal image of the chest (**D**) depicts bulky mediastinal lymphadenopathy *(arrow)*. Esophagram (**E**) confirms the bulky distal esophageal cancer *(arrow)* with mucosal destruction.

Primary Tumor (T)

Tis: Carcinoma in situ—very superficial tumor, without invasion of the stomach wall

T1: Tumor invades only the superficial portions of the stomach wall

T2: Tumor invades the deeper layers of the stomach wall

T3: Tumor extends through the stomach wall into the fat outside of the stomach

T4: Tumor extends outside the stomach wall and invades other organs

Regional Lymph Nodes (N)

N0: No spread to lymph nodes

N1: Tumor spread to 1-6 lymph nodes

N2: Tumor spread to 7-15 lymph nodes

N3: Tumor spread to more than 15 lymph nodes

Distant Metastasis (M)

M0: No tumor spread to other organs

M1: Tumor spread to other organs

Overall Stage

Stage 0   Tis, N0, M0
Stage IA   T1, N0, M0
Stage IB   T1, N1, M0 *or* T2, N0, M0
Stage II   T1, N2, M0 *or* T2, N1, M0 *or* T3, N0, M0
Stage IIIA T2, N2, M0 *or* T3, N1, M0 *or* T4, N0, M0
Stage IIIB T3, N2, M0 *or* T4, N1, M0
Stage IV   T4, N2, M0 *or* T1-3, N3, M0 *or* T4, N2-3, M0 *or* any M1

the cancer within the stomach. The overall 5-year survival for patients with gastric cancer in the United States is 21%. However, survival is clearly related to the site of tumor origin within the stomach. Cancers arising in the distal stomach have an overall better prognosis. With localized cancer in the distal stomach the 5-year survival is up to 50%. Unfortunately, only 10 to 20% of patients in the United States present with localized disease. Most patients will have either local or distant tumor spread at the time of diagnosis. Cancers arising in the proximal stomach have a much worse prognosis. Even with apparent localized disease, the 5-year survival is only 10 to 15%.[101-105]

Staging of Gastric Cancer

Using the TNM system, the overall staging of gastric cancer results in a rather complex set of definitions, described in Box 85-2.

Treatment of Gastric Cancer

Curative treatment for gastric cancer requires surgical resection with a 5-cm tumor-free margin. Smaller tumors may be removed with a partial gastrectomy, while more extensive tumors will require total gastrectomy. Invasive tumors with transmural extension or invasion of adjacent organs will require additional resection of the

surrounding perigastric fat, omentum, spleen, pancreas, and/or intestines. Dissection of adjacent lymph nodes is routinely performed for surgical staging.[105-107]

Neoadjuvant chemotherapy may increase the tumor resectability and reduce the risk of postoperative recurrence. The value of neoadjuvant chemotherapy and radiation therapy was established in a large study, which confirmed a survival benefit for all patients with stage 1B or higher gastric cancers.[106] Current recommendations for treatment of gastric cancer involves complete surgical resection with nodal dissection, followed by radiation therapy 5 days per week for 5 weeks starting between 4 and 6 weeks following surgery. Adjuvant chemotherapy with 5-fuorouracil and leucovorin is routinely administered either before or concurrent with the radiation therapy.

MRI of Gastric Cancer

With adequate distention of the gastric lumen, MRI can provide excellent depiction of the stomach wall and gastric cancers[108-115] (Fig. 85-49). Gastric distention is easily accomplished with ingestion of large volumes of contrast material immediately prior to scanning. Negative intraluminal agents on fat-suppressed gadolinium-enhanced T1-weighted images are desirable, as the dark lumen will help to highlight the adjacent bowel wall and mural tumors. Tap water is an effective gastric intraluminal agent that is well tolerated and readily available.

The wall of the normal, well-distended stomach is depicted on unenhanced T1-weighted, T2-weighted, and SSFSE images as a thin, uniform hypointense line typically measuring 2 to 3 mm in thickness. Prominent gastric rugae can increase the apparent thickness of the stomach wall. Fat-suppressed gadolinium-enhanced T1-weighted images depict the gastric wall as a thin, uniformly enhancing line. The degree of enhancement of the normal stomach wall is equal to or less than that of liver parenchyma. On dynamic gadolinium-enhanced images, the stomach wall will show only mild, uniform, and homogeneous enhancement. The surrounding perigastric fat is maintained without infiltration or enhancement.

Gastric cancers are depicted on MR images as areas of focal mural thickening (Fig. 85-50) or as mural masses. Some superficial gastric cancer may not be visible on cross-sectional imaging. As they grow they will be depicted as areas of focal mural thickening and eventually as a gastric mass. On dynamic gadolinium-enhanced MRI, gastric cancers will show more enhancement than the adjacent normal gastric wall. Extensive gastric cancer with linitis plastica will be depicted on MR images as extensive, marked mural thickening involving most of the stomach wall. Associated narrowing of the gastric lumen and loss of distensibility will be present. As with more focal gastric cancer, the tumor in linitis plastica shows marked enhancement with intravenous gadolinium chelates.

Accurate staging of gastric cancer on MRI requires depiction of the depth of tumor penetration into the stomach wall, as well as an assessment of regional nodal

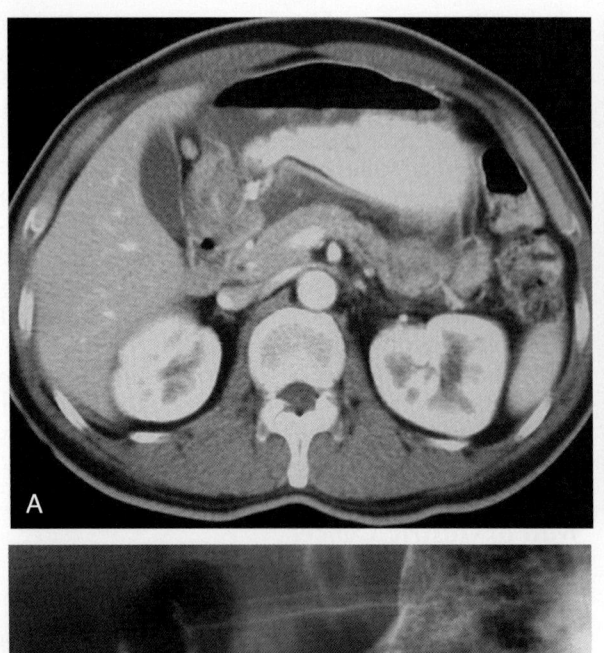

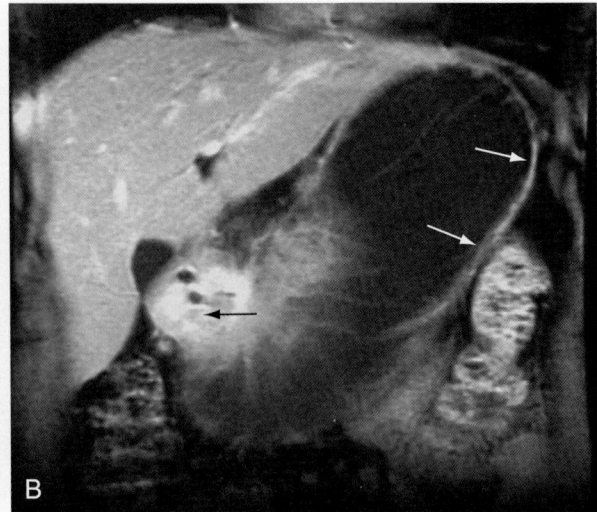

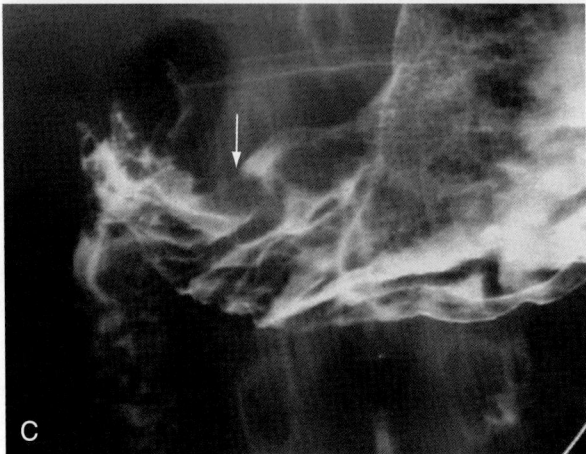

FIGURE 85-49

Gastric cancer Helical CT and MRI. Helical CT (**A**) shows mixture of barium, air, fluid, and soft tissue, or ingested food. Coronal gadolinium-enhanced MR image (**B**) using water as an intraluminal contrast material shows the normal thin gastric wall *(white arrows)* and a bulky, enhancing gastric antral cancer *(black arrow)*. Upper GI barium examination (**C**) confirms the gastric antral cancer *(arrow)*.

and distant metastases. Extraserosal invasion of advanced gastric cancer has been described on unenhanced MRI as disruption of the normal low signal intensity band surrounding the normal stomach on opposed phase gradient-echo images.[108] Transmural tumor invasion by a T3 or T4 tumor is indicated by disruption of this low signal intensity band overlying the mural tumor. Using this sign resulted in an 88% accuracy in determining the depth of tumor penetration.[108]

Dynamic and delayed gadolinium-enhanced MR images are also useful for depicting the depth of penetration for gastric cancers.[109,110] Gastric cancers are depicted as areas of mural thickening with marked gadolinium enhancement on early dynamic and delayed phase images. On dynamic gadolinium-enhanced MR images gastric cancer will enhance more rapidly than the adjacent normal gastric wall. In a study of 46 patients with gastric cancer, Kang et al[109] noted that the mucosa and/or submucosa affected by stomach cancer showed an early enhancement pattern 30 to 90 seconds after Gd-DTPA administration) in 43 of 46 patients (93%). Normal gastric mucosa and submucosa showed a more delayed peak enhancement >90 seconds in 63% of patients and a variable enhancement pattern in 37% of patients.

The presence of focal gastric mural thickening with a pattern of rapid enhancement is suggestive of gastric cancer. The use of subtraction techniques on dynamic gadolinium-enhanced MRI may increase the conspicuity of enhancing tumor, improving depiction and definition of tumor extent.[111]

Invasion of adjacent organs is evaluated by assessing differences in enhancement patterns between the gastric tumor and the adjacent parenchyma. Comparing early and delayed gadolinium-enhanced MR images is useful for depicting extragastric tumor that will show enhancement on delayed images. On these delayed images one may see enhancing soft tissue within the perigastric ligaments or encasing adjacent vascular structures, representing extragastric tumor spread.

Preoperative MR staging of gastric cancer has been shown to be comparable to helical CT scanning.[112,113] In several studies MRI has shown a slightly higher accuracy for T-staging compared with helical CT, although the differences did not always achieve statistical significance. Comparing MRI and helical CT for gastric cancer staging, Kim et al[112] noted a T-staging accuracy of 81% versus 73% (P < .05), while Sohn et al[113] noted T-staging accuracy of 73% versus 67% (P > .05). Both studies

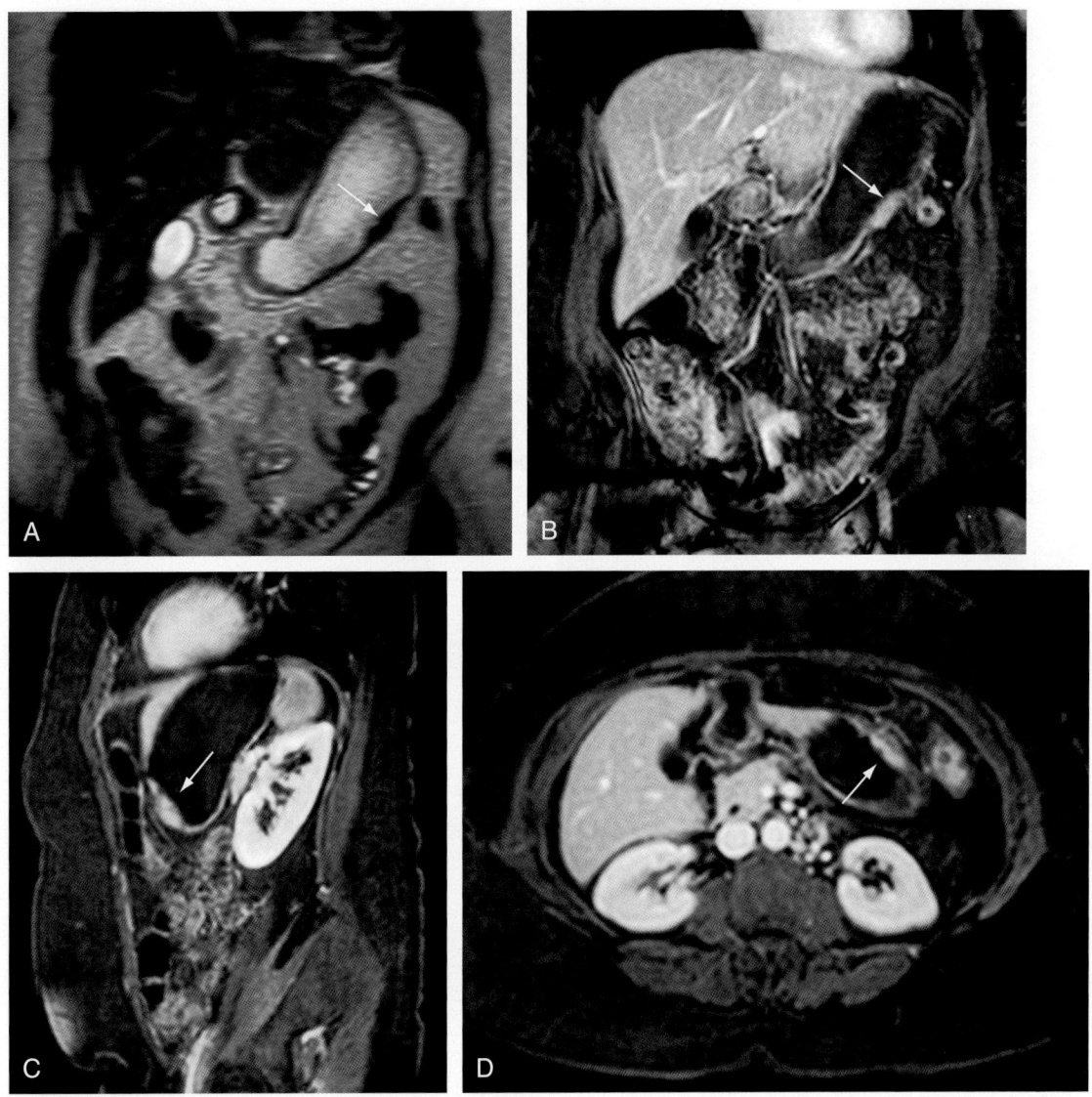

FIGURE 85-50

Gastric cancer. Coronal single-shot fast spin-echo (SSFSE) (**A**) and gadolinium-enhanced spoiled gradient-echo (SGE) (**B**) images depict a small plaque like gastric cancer *(arrow)* along the lesser curve that is confined to the gastric wall. Sagittal (**C**) and axial (**D**) gadolinium-enhanced images demonstrate the focal gastric cancer *(arrow)*. Endoscopy and biopsy confirmed a small gastric cancer.

showed a consistent underestimation of nodal metastases for MRI and helical CT scanning, accuracy of N-staging 65% versus 73%, and 55% versus 58% with no significant difference between the two imaging techniques.

Distant metastases from gastric cancer may involve the liver, peritoneum, or other abdominal and pelvic organs, and lung (Fig. 85-51). Liver metastases are well depicted on combined unenhanced T1- and T2-weighted images and dynamic gadolinium-enhanced MR images. Gastric cancer may also spread by shedding of tumor cells into the peritoneal cavity with subsequent carcinomatosis. Tumor cells may migrate into the pelvis and deposit on the ovaries, producing Krukenberg tumors. MRI excels at depicting peritoneal metastases. Compared with helical CT, subtle peritoneal metas-

tases are much more readily depicted on gadolinium-enhanced MR images. Preoperative depiction of peritoneal tumor spread on MRI will establish the non-resectability of a gastric cancer and obviate unnecessary surgery.

Small-Intestinal Cancer

Cancer arising in the small intestine is an uncommon malignancy occurring in fewer than 2 in 100,000 persons in the United States each year. Cancer arising in the colon is 50 times more common than small-bowel cancer. Small-bowel cancer accounts for 2% of GI cancers and 1% of deaths from intestinal cancer. Adenocarcinoma is the most common cell type accounting for

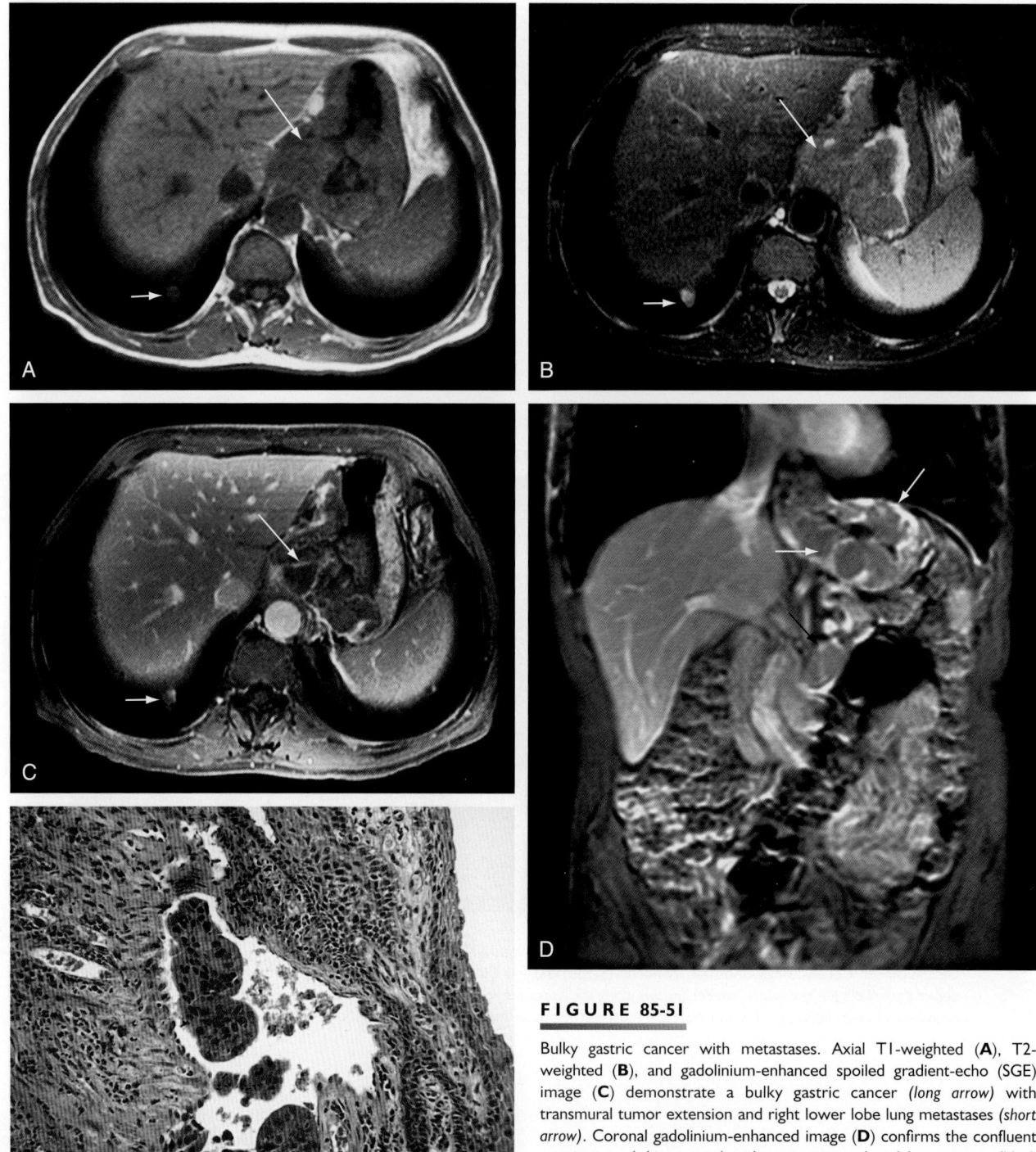

FIGURE 85-51

Bulky gastric cancer with metastases. Axial T1-weighted (**A**), T2-weighted (**B**), and gadolinium-enhanced spoiled gradient-echo (SGE) image (**C**) demonstrate a bulky gastric cancer *(long arrow)* with transmural tumor extension and right lower lobe lung metastases *(short arrow)*. Coronal gadolinium-enhanced image (**D**) confirms the confluent gastric mass *(white arrows)* and retroperitoneal nodal metastases *(black arrow)*. Photomicrograph of the gastric mass biopsy (**E**) confirms gastric adenocarcinoma.

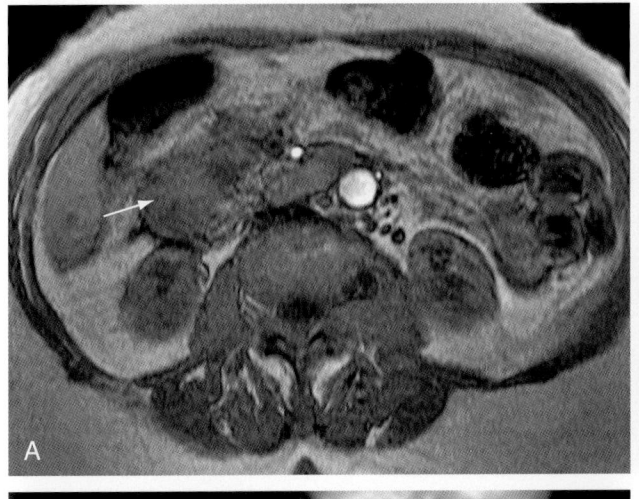

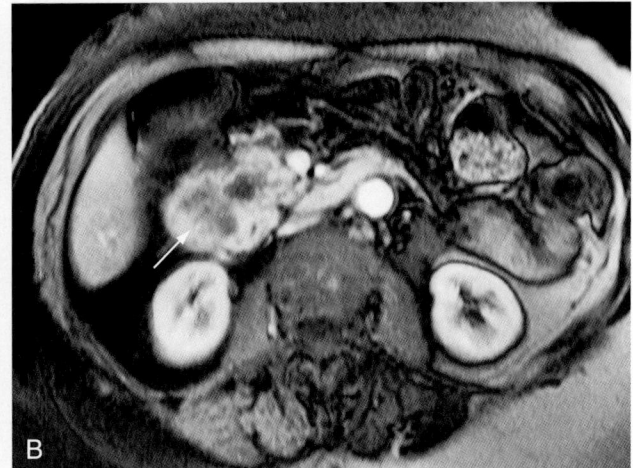

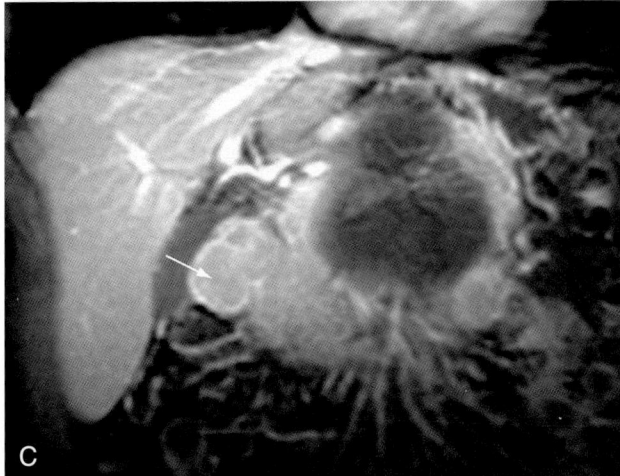

FIGURE 85-52

Small intestinal cancer. Axial T1-weighted image (**A**), and gadolinium-enhanced image (**B**) and coronal gadolinium-enhanced spoiled gradient-echo (SGE) image (**C**) demonstrate a 4-cm duodenal mass *(arrow)*. Tissue diagnosis confirmed a duodenal adenocarcinoma.

approximately half of small-bowel cancers. Other types include carcinoid tumors, leiomyosarcoma, and lymphoma.[116,117]

A review of the National Cancer Database from 1985 to 1995 demonstrated 4995 cases of small bowel adenocarcinoma.[117] The duodenum was the most common location (55%), followed by the jejunum (18%), ileum (13%), and unspecified location (14%). There is a six-fold increased incidence of small bowel cancer in patients with Crohn's disease compared with the general population. Patients with celiac disease, and familial polyposis syndrome also are at increased risk for developing small-bowel adenocarcinoma.

The clinical presentation of patients with small-bowel cancer is often nonspecific, resulting in a delay in diagnosis.[118] Early on patients are typically asymptomatic. Eventually, patients may present with GI bleeding, abdominal pain, distention, vomiting, bowel obstruction, and jaundice. Treatment is by surgical resection. Postoperative chemotherapy or radiation may be useful in patients with widespread disease but may not affect overall survival.[116] The 5-year survival for small intestinal adenocarcinoma is 30%.[117]

MRI of Small-Intestinal Cancer

The advances in MRI hardware and software have been applied to small-bowel imaging.[118-120] Semelka et al described the appearance of small bowel tumors on MRI[119] and noted that small-bowel tumors were isointense to small bowel on T1-weighted images. Malignant tumors showed moderate heterogeneous enhancement greater than adjacent normal bowel on gadolinium-enhanced SGE imaging (Fig. 85-52). The extent of tumor was best depicted on unenhanced T1-weighted and fat-suppressed gadolinium-enhanced imaging (Fig. 85-53).

The techniques of a small-bowel MR enteroclysis have been described and are useful for depicting small-bowel cancer. With maximal small-bowel distention, SSRARE, and fat-suppressed gadolinium-enhanced imaging allows one to obtain diagnostic information about the small-bowel lumen, wall, and extraintestinal structures.[21-24,121] Small-bowel cancers will be depicted as areas of small intestinal mural thickening and masses. Due to their late clinical presentation, small-bowel tumors are typically large tumor masses.

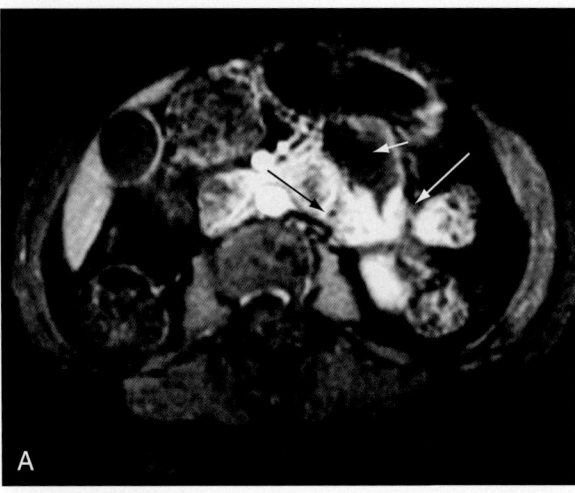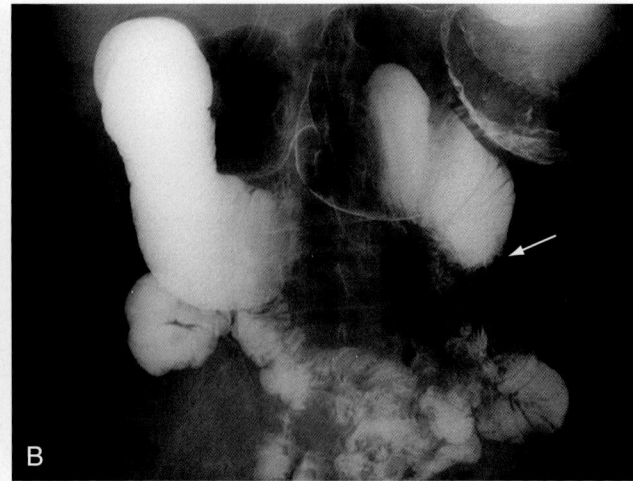

FIGURE 85-53

Jejunal cancer. Gadolinium-enhanced spoiled gradient-echo (SGE) image (**A**) shows an enhancing proximal jejunal mass *(arrows)* with luminal narrowing and proximal small bowel dilatation *(short arrow)*. Upper GI barium examination (**B**) shows jejunal obstruction *(arrow)* with an irregular margin at the point of the jejunal cancer.

Colorectal Cancer

Colorectal cancer is the second most commonly diagnosed malignancy in the United States and is the second leading cause of cancer related death. The American Cancer Society estimates that there will be about 105,500 new cases of colon cancer and 42,000 new cases of rectal cancer in 2003 in the United States. Combined, they will cause about 57,100 deaths.[122,123] Early detection and accurate staging are essential to the long-term survival of colon cancer patients. Overall prognosis is directly related to the depth of tumor penetration through the bowel wall, the presence of nodal metastases, and the presence or absence of distant metastases.

Staging of Colon Cancer

The American Joint Committee on Cancer has designated staging by TNM classification,[124] which should replace the older Dukes' classification system (Box 85-3). Local tumor staging (T staging) is based upon the depth of tumor penetration into the bowel wall (Fig. 85-54). In summary, Stage I colon cancers are any T1 or T2 tumors without nodal or distant metastases. Stage II colon cancers are T3 or T4 tumors without nodal or distant metastases. Stage III colon cancers are any tumor with nodal involvement and Stage IV colon cancers are those with distant metastases (Fig. 85-55).

Treatment Options

Colon Cancer

Standard treatment of colon cancer has been exploratory laparotomy with segmental surgical resection of the primary tumor and regional lymph nodes for localized disease.[123-125] The role of adjuvant chemotherapy in

---

Box 85-3 | TNM Staging of Colorectal Carcinoma

Primary Tumor (T)
TX: Primary tumor cannot be assessed
T0: No evidence of primary tumor
Tis: Carcinoma in situ: intraepithelial or invasion of the lamina propria*
T1: Tumor invades submucosa
T2: Tumor invades muscularis propria
T3: Tumor invades through the muscularis propria into the subserosa, or into non-peritonealized pericolic or perirectal tissues
T4: Tumor directly invades other organs or structures, and/or perforates visceral peritoneum.

Regional Lymph Nodes (N)
NX: Regional nodes cannot be assessed
N0: No regional lymph node metastasis
N1: Metastasis in 1 to 3 regional lymph nodes
N2: Metastasis in 4 or more regional lymph nodes

Distant Metastasis (M)
MX: Distant metastasis cannot be assessed
M0: No distant metastasis
M1: Distant metastasis

Overall Staging
Stage 0   Tis, N0, M0
Stage I   T1, N0, M0 *or* T2, N0, M0
Stage II   T3, N0, M0 *or* T4, N0, M0
Stage III Any T, N1, M0 *or* Any T, N2, M0
Stage IV   Any T, Any N, M1

Stage II disease remains controversial. Patients with Stage III cancer are treated with wide surgical resection and anastamosis plus adjuvant chemotherapy with fluorouracil (5-FU) plus either levamisole hydrochloride or leucovorin for 6 to 12 months. Stage IV cancers are treated with surgical resection/anastamosis or bypass

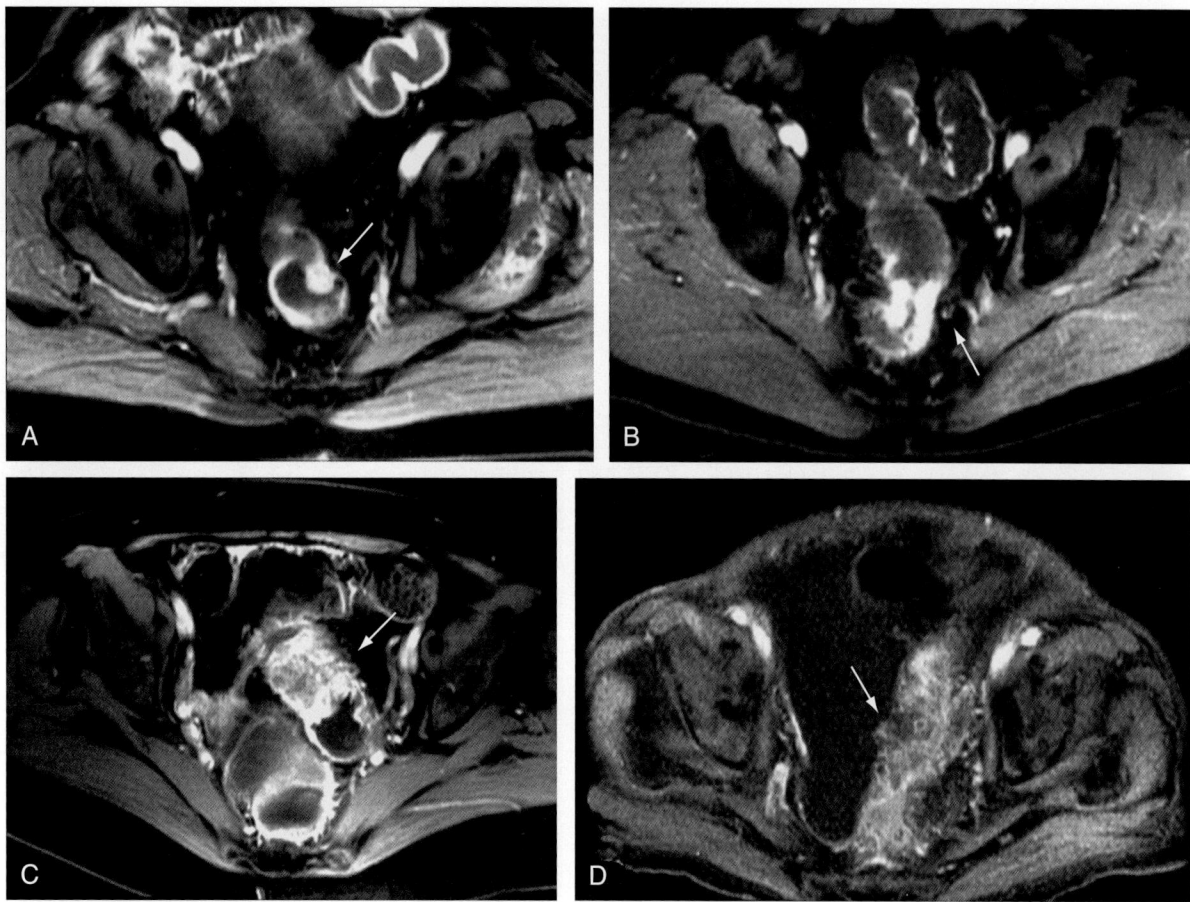

FIGURE 85-54

Rectal cancer T staging. Axial fat-suppressed gadolinium-enhanced spoiled gradient-echo (SGE) image in four patients with rectal cancer. In patient **A,** a small polypoid rectal cancer *(arrow)* correlates with a T1 tumor. In patient **B,** a rectal cancer *(arrow)* is present with full thickness involvement of the rectal wall. Note the smooth outer margin of the rectal wall and absence of tumor extension into the perirectal fat. Findings correlate with a T2 tumor. In patient **C,** the rectal cancer *(arrow)* shows transmural tumor extension with nodular tumor growing into the surrounding perirectal fat, correlating with a T3 tumor. In patient **D,** the bulky rectal cancer *(arrow)* is invading adjacent structures and represents a T4 tumor.

of obstructing primary lesions in selected cases, and post-operative chemotherapy or radiation therapy. Surgical resection of isolated liver metastases (1 to 3 lesions) has resulted in a 5-year survival of 20% to 40%.[126,127]

Rectal Cancer

Treatment of rectal cancer follows the same basic approach with the addition of preoperative chemotherapy and/or radiation therapy for Stage II or III rectal cancers with transmural tumor extension (T3). Preoperative radiation therapy is commonly used in these patients with T3 or T4 rectal tumors to decrease the bulk of tumor and improve the chances for subsequent complete surgical resection.

The primary rectal cancer is resected by a low anterior (LA) resection for tumors in the upper rectum or abdominal perineal (AP) resection for tumors in the lower rectum near the anus. Small stage I rectal cancers may be treated by local full-thickness resection together with chemotherapy and radiation therapy given before

or after surgery. Stage II rectal cancers are usually treated by LA resection or AP resection, followed by both chemotherapy and radiation therapy. When the cancer has spread to nearby organs, pelvic exenteration may be performed in some cases of stage II rectal cancer, local full-thickness rectal resection is done after chemotherapy, with or without radiation therapy. This approach can prevent the need for AP resection and colostomy in some cases. The treatment of stage III rectal cancer is the same as for stage II cancers. For stage IV rectal cancers, surgery may be performed to relieve obstruction combined with chemotherapy and radiation therapy.

Preoperative Imaging of Colon Cancer—Helical CT and MRI

Early reports of the accuracy of CT scanning and MRI in preoperative staging of colon cancer showed an overall staging accuracy of 70% with only an approximately 45% sensitivity for identifying local nodal metastases.[128] In 1996, the Radiology Diagnostic Oncology Group II

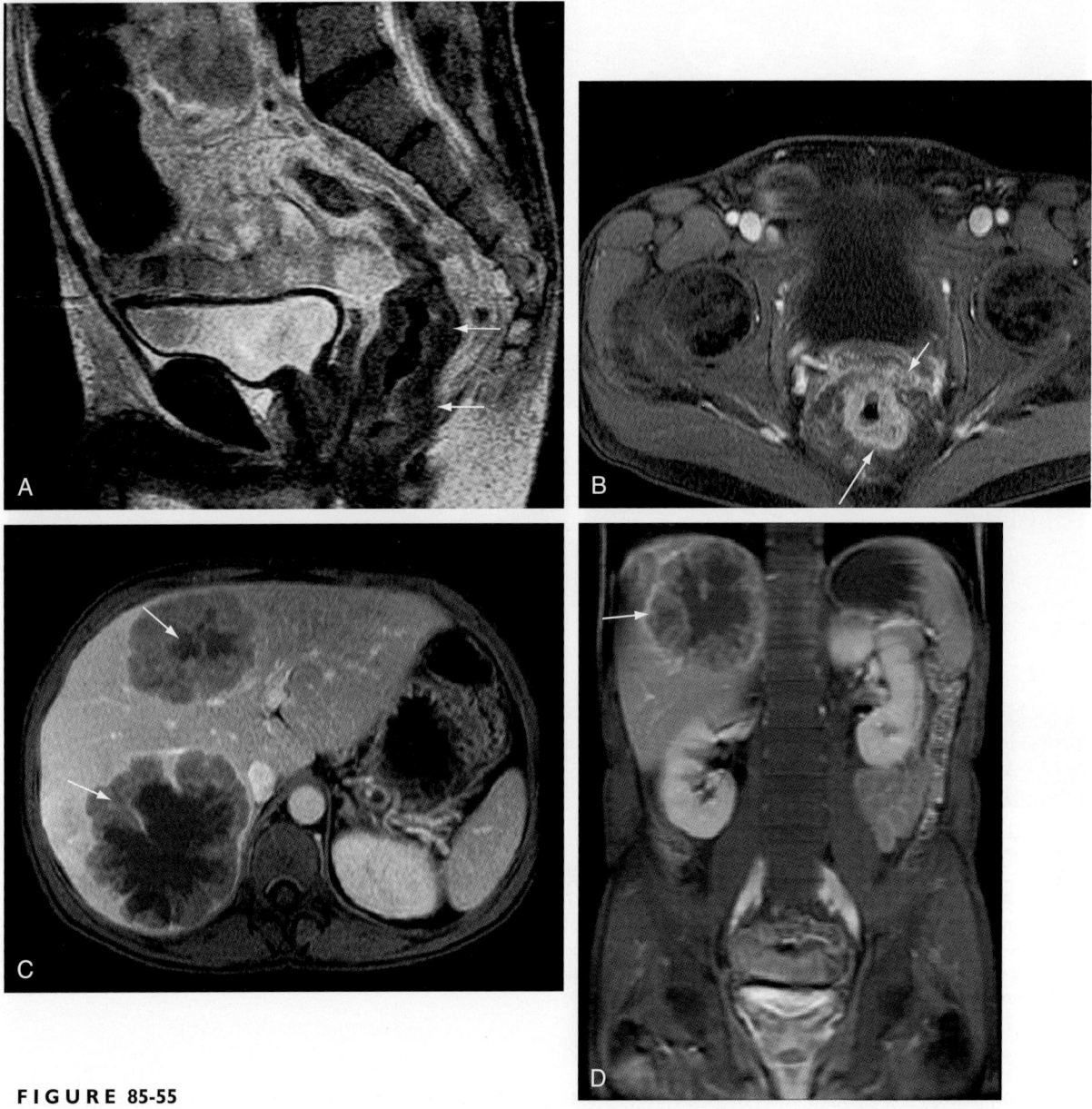

FIGURE 85-55

Stage IV rectal cancer. Sagittal T2-weighted image (**A**) shows a large circumferential rectal cancer (*arrows*). Axial gadolinium-enhanced image (**B**) confirms a T3 rectal cancer with transmural tumor extension (*long arrow*) and perirectal nodes (*short arrow*). Axial (**C**) and coronal (**D**) gadolinium-enhanced images demonstrate multiple liver metastases (*arrows*). Findings are that of a Stage IV (T3N1M1) rectal cancer.

compared older CT scan and MRI techniques for the staging of colorectal cancer in 478 patients.[129] This report found that for rectal cancers, CT scanning (78%) was more accurate for determining the transmural extent than was MRI (58%), while for colon cancer CT scanning (62%) and MRI (64%) were equivalent. Limited depiction of nodal metastases was noted for both CT scanning (sensitivity 48%) and MRI (sensitivity 22%). Notable limitations of the MRI in this study include the lack of images obtained with intravenous, oral, or rectal contrast material.

Many refinements in MRI of colorectal cancer have since occurred, taking advantage of high-performance gradients, faster pulse sequences, and higher resolution MRI. Technical improvements include MRI using an endorectal coil,[12-18] the addition of IV gadolinium chelates,[19-21] and the use of oral and rectal contrast agents to achieve bowel distention.[20,21] High-resolution half-Fourier RARE imaging using an abdominal flex surface coil has also been reported.[22] All of these refinements to MRI have improved image quality facilitating the depiction of primary colorectal cancer.

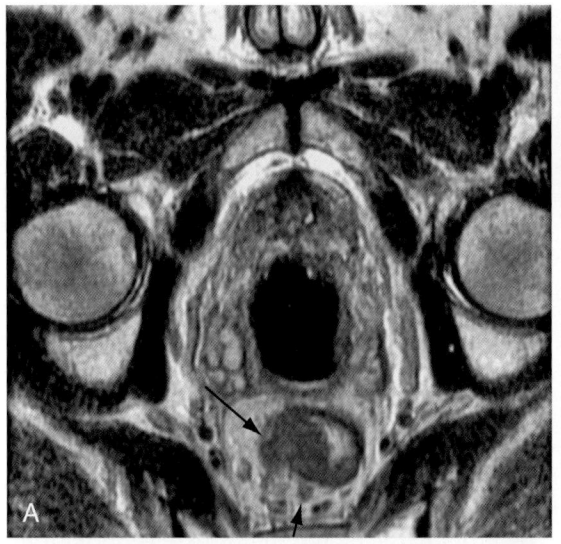
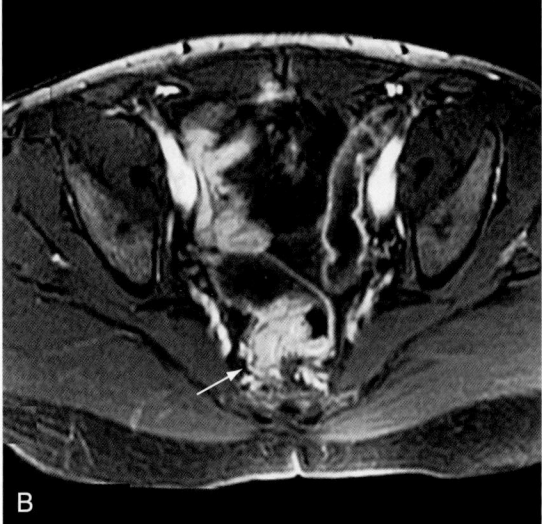
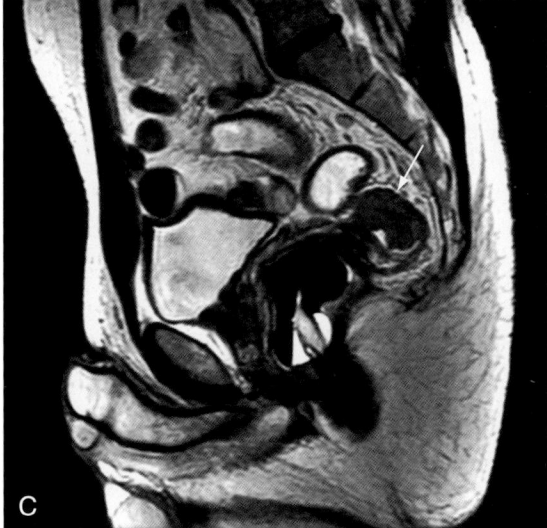

FIGURE 85-56

Thin section surface coil images of Stage III rectal cancer. Fast spin-echo (FSE) T2-weighted image (**A**) angled perpendicular to rectal mass shows a T3 rectal cancer (*long arrow*) with tumor extension through the rectal wall. Perirectal lymph nodes (*short arrow*) are also noted. Fat-suppressed gadolinium-enhanced image (**B**) demonstrates the enhancing rectal cancer (*arrow*) with transmural tumor extension. Sagittal T2-weighted image (**C**) confirms the position of the mass (*arrow*). Findings correlate with a Stage III (T3N1M0) rectal cancer.

In more recent reports, Kim et al[130] demonstrated an 81% accuracy for depth of tumor penetration and 63% accuracy for depicting regional nodal involvement in 217 patients with rectal cancer. Comparing multi-detector helical CT and MRI in 21 patients with rectal cancer, Matsuoka et al[131] found similar accuracy for determining depth of tumor penetration for helical CT (95.2%) and MRI (100%) and for depicting nodal metastases: helical CT (61.9%) and MRI (70%).

Technical Advances in MRI of Colorectal Cancer

Surface Coils

MRI using an endorectal coil allows one to directly visualize the layers of rectal wall.[132-136] Depth of tumor penetration into the wall of the rectum can be accurately assessed. Comparisons of endorectal MRI (ERMRI) and endorectal ultrasound (ERUS) have shown an overall similar accuracy for depicting the transmural extent of the cancer. Hunerbein et al[133] found comparable accuracy's for endorectal US (84%), 3D endorectal US (88%), and endorectal MRI (91%) for predicting rectal tumor invasion. In a comparison of ERUS, ERMRI, and CT scanning in 89 patients with rectal cancer Kim et al[134] found comparable accuracy for ERUS (81%) and ERMRI (81%) for depth of tumor penetration, and that both were superior to CT scanning (65%).

High-resolution MRI of colorectal cancer using external surface coils has also been reported (Fig. 85-56). Beets-Tan et al[137] compared high-resolution MRI with a phased-array surface coil and CT scanning in 26 patients and noted that MRI was superior for predicting tumor infiltration into surrounding structures. The sensitivity and specificity for MRI was 97% and 98% compared with 70% and 85% for CT scanning. The multiplanar capability of MRI and its excellent contrast resolution facilitate depiction of tumor extension into adjacent structures.

Brown et al[138] described the use of preoperative thin-section SSFSE MRI with an external abdominal flex surface coil for evaluation of depth of tumor penetration in 28 patients with rectal cancer. Thin-section MRI correctly indicated local tumor staging in all 25 patients in whom comparison with histopathologic findings was possible. The difference between measurements of extramural tumor extension on MR images and histopathologic specimens varied from −5.0 mm to +5.5 mm (mean +0.13 mm). Accurate depiction of T3 tumors on thin section MRI improves patient management as these patients will be referred for preoperative therapy.

Intraluminal Contrast Agents

The administration of oral and/or rectal contrast material with an intraluminal agent distends the lumen of the colon and rectum facilitating depiction of the wall of the colon. Many different intraluminal contrast materials have been proposed including iron oxide based agents, water with dilute gadolinium chelate, barium sulfate, air, and water.

Solutions containing iron oxide have been administered rectally to distend the rectum during the preoperative MR evaluation of rectal cancer. Wallengren et al[139] found that a double-contrast technique combining an enema of superparamagnetic iron oxide contrast material and an IV gadolinium chelate had a sensitivity 100%, specificity 70%, and accuracy 90% for depicting rectal cancers more advanced than Dukes' A ($T_1N_0M_0$ or $T_2N_0M_0$). The double-contrast MR images were superior to unenhanced MR images and to the MR images obtained only with the rectal enema.

Water and dilute barium sulfate may also be used as intraluminal agents. Dilute barium sulfate is 98% water, which provides the predominant intraluminal signal. This hydro-MRI technique produces a biphasic appearance of the bowel lumen with high signal on T2-weighted images and low signal on T1-weighted images. Intraluminal water has the advantage of being inexpensive, well tolerated, and readily available. In addition, intraluminal water produces no susceptibility artifact that can occur with iron oxide oral or rectal contrast agents.

Double-Contrast MR Staging of Colorectal Cancer

Combining intraluminal agents with intravenous gadolinium facilitates depiction of the wall of the colon or rectum and allows one to estimate the depth of tumor penetration into the bowel wall. Adequate bowel distention is a critical element of this MR technique. A collapsed segment of bowel may obscure a colon or rectal cancer, or alternatively may produce false-positive interpretations of mural thickening or mass. Combining water-soluble oral and rectal contrast material and IV gadolinium produces MR images with good bowel distention and excellent depiction of the enhancing mural tumor.

A combination of thin-section T2-weighted images and double-contrast gadolinium-enhanced SGE MRI can be used to evaluate colon and rectal cancers. Thin-section T2-weighted images provide excellent depiction of the bowel wall and of the mural tumor. On IV gadolinium-enhanced SGE MR images with oral and rectal contrast, the tumor is depicted as an enhancing soft tissue mass or as mural thickening. Partial thickness involvement of the bowel indicates a T1 tumor. Full thickness involvement of the colon correlates with a T2 tumor. A tumor with full thickness involvement and nodular tumor extension into the adjacent pericolonic or perirectal fat indicates a T3 tumor. Strandy enhancement extending from the tumor into the pericolonic fat may represent reactive changes and not direct tumor extension. Nodular enhancing soft tissue or bulky tumor extension into the pericolonic fat is the finding that correlates best with a T3 tumor. A T4 tumor is indicated by gross extracolonic tumor extension with invasion of adjacent organs.

The depiction of nodal metastases is still limited by our inability to detect tumor in normal-sized lymph nodes. In addition, enlarged pericolonic lymph nodes may be inflammatory. This distinction may be simpler for rectal cancers as enlarged perirectal nodes are not typically inflammatory in etiology. Nodal metastases should be suspected with enlarged perirectal nodes. Thin-section, high-resolution surface coil imaging will likely improve the MR depiction of pericolonic and perirectal lymph nodes. Brown et al[140] noted that prediction of nodal involvement in rectal cancer with MRI is improved by using the border contour and signal intensity characteristics of lymph nodes instead of size criteria alone. However, depicting tumor in normal-sized lymph nodes may require the use of additional contrast agents directed at imaging nodal metastatic disease.

Up to one third of patients with stage IV colon cancer may present with isolated liver metastases. MRI performed with a combination of unenhanced T1- and T2-weighted imaging and dynamic gadolinium-enhanced SGE MRI excels at hepatic imaging. Most colon metastases are hypovascular and are best depicted on portal venous phase MR images. However, it is not uncommon for colon metastases to show enhancement on arterial phase images, facilitating their detection on these early dynamic images. Colorectal cancer may also metastasize to the peritoneum, mesentery, omentum, bowel serosa, lymph nodes, osseous structures, and lungs. All of these extrahepatic anatomic sites must be carefully evaluated to assess for possible metastatic tumor. It is my experience that MRI excels at depicting all forms of extrahepatic tumor. In particular, fat-suppressed gadolinium-enhanced SGE MR images are most useful for extrahepatic imaging. In many cases, extrahepatic tumors may be shown to better advantage on MR images than on helical CT scans. In a comparison of helical CT and MRI in 57 patients with malignancy who underwent surgical staging, helical CT scans depicted 101 of 154 (66%) findings of surgically confirmed extrahepatic tumor compared to MRI which depicted 139 sites (90%) (P < .0001).[8]

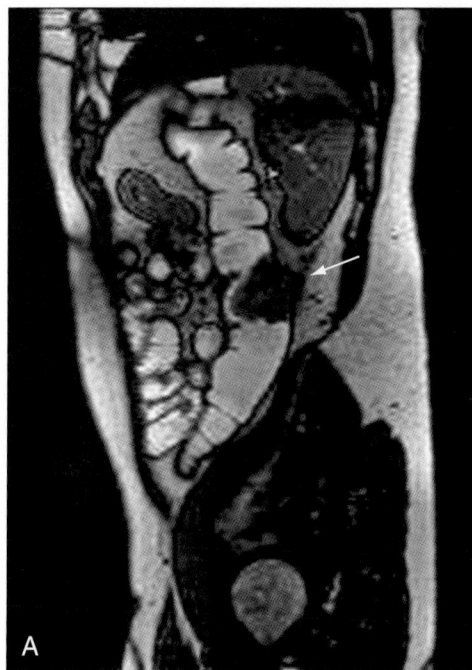
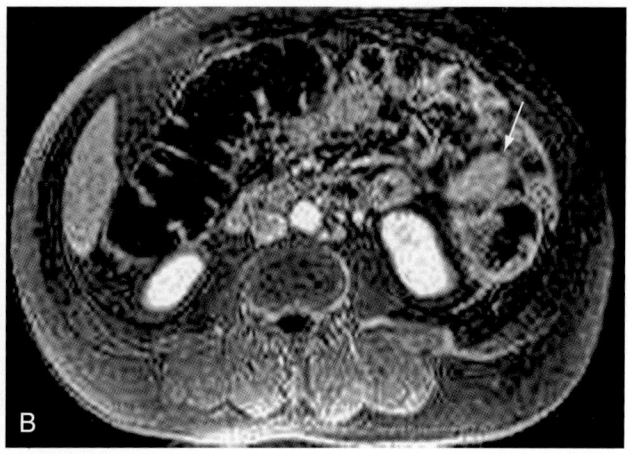

FIGURE 85-57

MR colonography. Patient has undergone bowel preparation and the colon has been distended with water administered via a rectal tube. Sagittal true fast imaging with steady precession (FISP) image (**A**) depicts a mass (arrow) in the descending colon. Gadolinium-enhanced 3D volumetric interpolated breath-hold examination (VIBE) image (**B**) demonstrates the enhancing adenocarcinoma (arrow). (Courtesy of Diego Martin, MD.)

MR Colonography

MR colonography is a new MR technique that may play an important role in the future direction of MRI of colorectal cancer. Clinical studies have shown that it is a non-invasive, safe, and well-tolerated alternative to conventional endoscopy (Fig. 85-57). Compared with CT colonography, MR colonography uses no ionizing radiation, which is a distinct advantage when considering the widespread use of these tests for screening purposes. The role of this innovative MR technique in the evaluation of colon cancer is yet to be determined. In the future it may become routine to provide endoluminal images of colon and rectal cancers in addition to cross-sectional MR images of the bowel wall. MRI and MR colonography imaging techniques can be implemented on currently available commercial MR imagers using high-performance gradient systems and product software.

MR screening for colonic polyps using MR colonography has been described[141-145] using thin section 3D SGE MRI combined with rectal enemas of dilute gadolinium solutions. Other approaches to MR colonography include the use of true FISP imaging and gadolinium-enhanced 3D gradient-echo imaging combined with rectally administered water (Fig. 85-58).[143] MR colonography has been demonstrated to be effective in detecting clinically important colonic polyps greater than 1 cm in diameter with reported sensitivity and specificity greater than 95%. In a study of 132 patients referred for colonoscopy for suspected colonic mass, Luboldt et al[144] found that most small (≤5 mm diameter) masses were overlooked at MR colonography, but 19 of 31 lesions of 6 to 10 mm, and 26 of 27 large lesions (>10 mm), were correctly identified. For larger polyps

and masses, MR colonography had a sensitivity of 93%, specificity of 99%, positive predictive value of 92%, and negative predictive value of 98%.

To improve patient acceptance, it has been proposed that routine bowel preparation prior to MR colonography can be eliminated using fecal tagging. Strategies for fecal tagging have recently been developed that modulate the signal of feces to be identical to the signal of the enema used to distend the colon. With fecal tagging, the signal intensity of the stool is modulated by adding contrast-modifying substances to the patient's meals prior to the MR examination. Fecal tagging renders the residual stool in the colon invisible during the MR examination, obviating the need for bowel cleansing.[145]

Gastrointestinal Lymphoma

The GI tract is the most common primary extranodal site of lymphoma involvement. Primary GI lymphoma comprises a group of distinct clinical and pathologic entities that may be either T-cell or B-cell type (Box 85-4). Primary Hodgkin's GI lymphoma is extremely uncommon. Most lymphomas involving the bowel are non-Hodgkin's lymphomas that arise from lymphoid tissue associated with the GI tract or that secondarily affect the bowel in patients with widespread abdominal and pelvic lymphoma.[146-148]

The lymphoid tissue associated with the GI tract is found in the epithelium, lamina propria mucosa, submucosa, and mesenteric lymph nodes. This lymphoid tissue is collectively described as MALT tissue. Mucosa-associated-lymphoid-tissue lymphomas comprise the

| Box 85-4 | Gastrointestinal Lymphomas |

B Cell Lymphoma
- MALT Lymphoma
- Follicular Lymphoma
- Mantle Cell Lymphoma
- Diffuse B-cell Lymphoma
- Burkitt Lymphoma
- AIDS Related Lymphoma

T Cell Lymphoma
- Celiac Sprue Related Lymphoma

Hodgkin's Lymphoma

majority of low-grade B-cell GI lymphomas and are also known as extranodal marginal zone B-cell lymphomas. They may also occur in the thyroid, lung, breast, and skin. In the GI tract, MALT lymphomas are most commonly found in the stomach, which paradoxically contains very little lymphoid tissue, where they are seen as a reaction to infection with the bacteria *H. pylori*. They are typically low grade with an overall favorable prognosis and clinical course.

Another B-cell GI lymphoma is mantle cell lymphoma, which presents as intestinal polyposis, Burkitt's lymphoma, follicular lymphoma, diffuse large B-cell lymphoma, and immunodeficiency-related GI lymphoma. Gastrointestinal lymphomas of T-cell origin also occur, including the clinically aggressive lymphoma associated with celiac disease.

Treatment of Gastrointestinal Lymphoma

Mucosa-associated-lymphoid-tissue lymphomas show regression with treatment of the underlying *H. pylori* infection. Fifty percent of patients will show endoscopically proven resolution of gastric MALT lymphoma after 3 months of antibiotic therapy. Patients who progress are treated with surgery, radiation therapy, and chemotherapy or combined therapy.

MRI of Gastrointestinal Lymphoma

Cross-sectional imaging with helical CT or MRI can be utilized in patients with GI lymphoma to help determine the extent and distribution of disease and to evaluate associated nodal tumor or marrow involvement.[149-150] The appearance of the intestinal lymphoma will depend upon its location within the gastrointestinal tract and upon the form that the tumor assumes.

The stomach is the intestinal site most commonly involved with non-Hodgkin's lymphoma, accounting for approximately 50% of cases. Gastric lymphoma can be classified as infiltrative, polypoid, ulcerative, or nodular. The infiltrative form of gastric lymphoma will be depicted on MR images as marked concentric mural thickening and rugal thickening (Fig. 85-59). The appearance can be similar to Ménétrier's disease or gastritis. Unlike Ménétrier's disease, which involves the proximal stomach, gastric lymphoma has a predilection for involving the distal stomach or the entire stomach. Anecdotal cases in our experience have shown less enhancement of the thickened gastric wall with gastric lymphoma than is typically seen with gastric cancer and

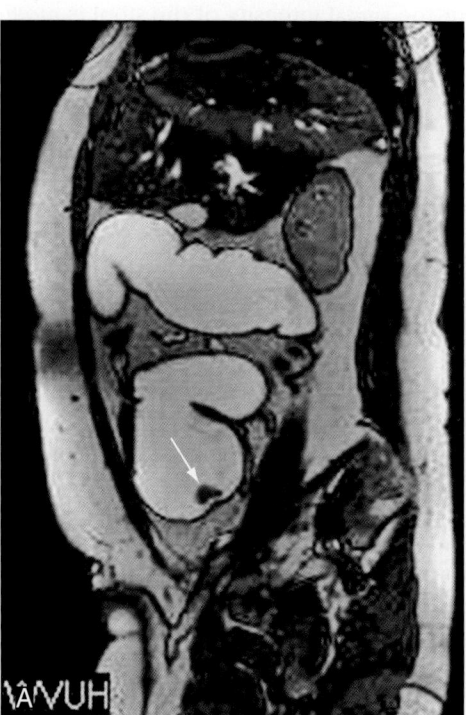
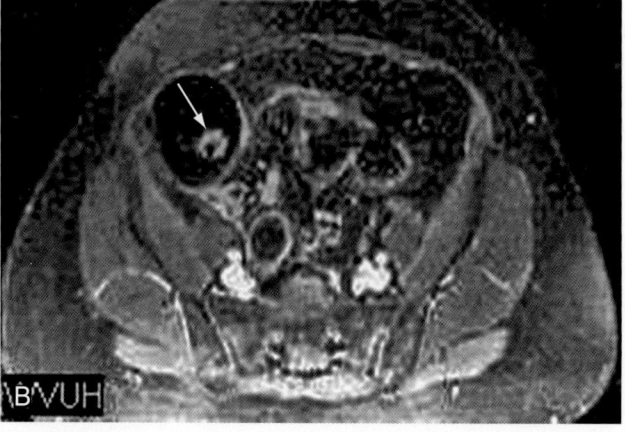

FIGURE 85-58

MR colonography. Patient has undergone bowel preparation and the colon has been distended with water administered via a rectal tube. Sagittal true fast imaging with steady precession (FISP) image (**A**) depicts a small hyperplastic polyp (*arrow*) in the cecum. Gadolinium-enhanced 3D volumetric interpolated breath-hold examination (VIBE) image (**B**) shows the small enhancing cecal polyp (*arrow*). (*Courtesy of Diego Martin, MD.*)

gastritis. Ultimately, tissue diagnosis will be required to confirm the diagnosis of gastric lymphoma.

Gastric lymphoma may also be depicted on MR images as a polypoid or ulcerated gastric mass that can be indistinguishable from gastric adenocarcinoma. The nodular form of gastric lymphoma will present with multiple separate gastric submucosal nodules. On barium examinations, this form is often depicted as classic target lesions due to central ulceration. On cross-sectional examinations one may see discrete or confluent areas of gastric mural thickening.

The small intestine is the next most commonly involved site in patients with GI lymphoma. Classically, the distal ileum is believed to be most frequently involved with non-Hodgkin's lymphoma due to the presence of more lymphoid tissue in this location. In contrast, small-bowel lymphoma associated with celiac disease usually involves the proximal small jejunum as this portion of the small bowel is subject to the most inflammation and villous damage.

Small-bowel lymphoma can present as disseminated disease or as a solitary mass or multiple small bowel masses. Primary small-bowel lymphoma begins in the wall of the small intestine. On MR images, one sees segments of small intestine with mural thickening or mural masses. The tumor may extend beyond the bowel serosa to involve the adjacent mesentery and lymph nodes. The caliber of the small intestinal lumen may be narrowed, although bowel obstruction is uncommon as the wall of the bowel remains pliable. Alternatively, the lumen of the bowel may be focally dilated in patients with GI lymphoma. Dilatation is thought to be due to destruction of the autonomic nerves within the bowel wall and from tumor replacement of the normal muscularis layer of the intestinal wall.

Small bowel lymphoma may also result in a large cavitary mass that communicates with the intestinal lumen. This endoexoenteric form of GI lymphoma begins within the wall of the bowel. As the tumor grows, it may ulcerate through the bowel wall with perforation and formation of a confined extraluminal tumor cavity (Fig. 85-60). On barium studies, communication between the intestinal lumen and the extraluminal cavitary tumor mass can be seen. On MR images, one can see a large tumor with a central cavity and adjacent confluent loops of thickened small bowel involved with non-Hodgkin's lymphoma. Communication between the bowel and the mass is confirmed by documenting the presence of oral contrast material or intestinal fluids extending from the bowel lumen into the tumor cavity. Air-fluid levels or fluid-debris levels may be seen within the mass.

Extensive extraintestinal lymphoma may secondarily involve the GI tract. Large mesenteric nodal masses may extend to the mesenteric border of the bowel and then directly invade the small intestines. Subsequent distortion of bowel loops, angulation, luminal narrowing, or bowel obstruction may develop. On MRI this mesenteric nodal form of bowel lymphoma will be depicted as multiple large mesenteric nodal masses that distort the adjacent bowel loops. Associated mural thickening may be direct evidence of intestinal tumor invasion and spread. Coronal MRI using SSRARE or fat-suppressed gadolinium-enhanced MRI is particularly useful to depict the small bowel mesentery and associated mesenteric tumor. As with all other types of intestinal MRI, the use of oral contrast material to distend the bowel lumen is essential when looking for mural thickening as an indication of tumor involvement.

Colonic lymphoma is much less common than gastric or small bowel lymphoma. When it affects the colon,

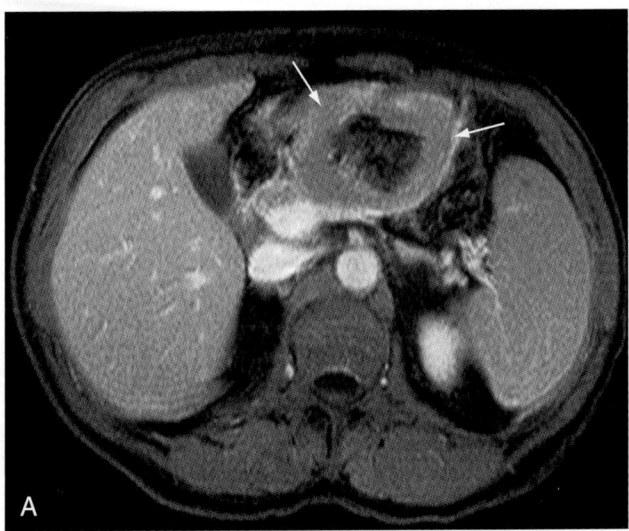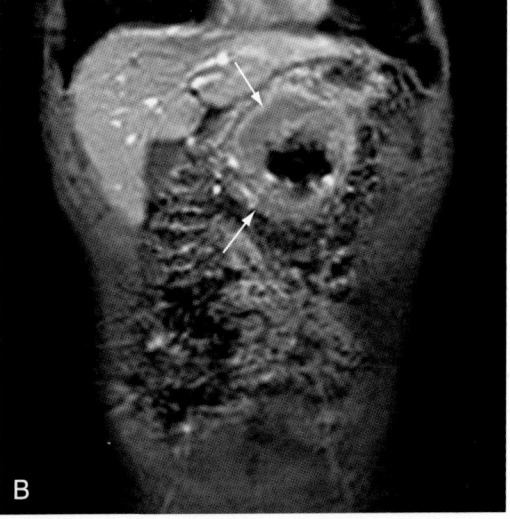

FIGURE 85-59

Gastrointestinal lymphoma. Axial (**A**) and coronal (**B**) fat-suppressed gadolinium-enhanced spoiled gradient-echo (SGE) images show marked concentric gastric mural thickening (*arrows*). Endoscopy and biopsy confirmed gastric lymphoma.

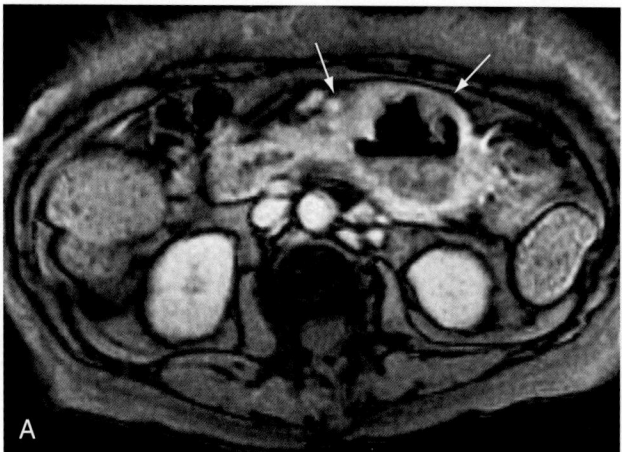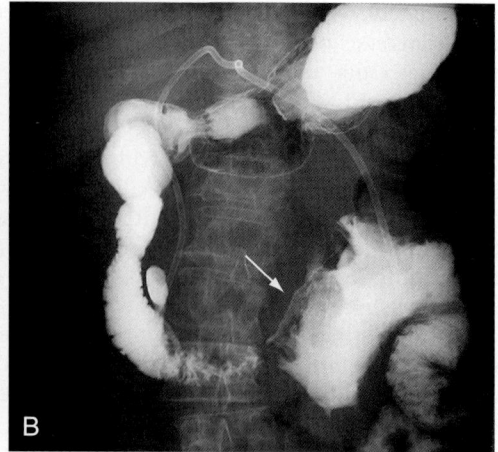

F I G U R E 85-60

Small bowel lymphoma. Gadolinium-enhanced spoiled gradient-echo (SGE) image (**A**) depicts a large abdominal mass *(arrows)* with an air fluid level. Barium small bowel examination (**B**) shows that the large mass *(arrow)* fills with barium, establishing a connection to the small bowel. Findings are that of the endoexoenteric form of intestinal lymphoma with a large extraluminal cavitary mass.

non-Hodgkin's lymphoma most frequently involves the cecum or rectum. There are several forms of colonic lymphoma. Colonic lymphoma may present as a bulky polypoid mass that most commonly occur near the ileocecal valve. These large tumors often extend into the terminal ileum. As the tumor enlarges, erosion through the wall may result in the formation of a large extraintestinal cavitary mass. A diffuse infiltrative form of colonic lymphoma will present with concentric mural thickening involving long segments of the colon. Finally, a multinodular form of colonic lymphoma will demonstrate multiple nodules affecting long segments of the colon. This latter multinodular form of colonic lymphoma can be indistinguishable from familial polyposis.

Immunodeficiency-related GI lymphoma could occur as a complication of acquired immune deficiency syndrome (AIDS). Non-Hodgkin's lymphoma is the second most common neoplasm in patients with AIDS. Compared with non-immunocompromised patients, in AIDS patients non-Hodgkin's lymphoma is characteristically widely disseminated with frequent extranodal involvement of sites of the CNS and GI tract. On MRI, one may depict gastric involvement indicated by concentric mural thickening or mural tumors. Small intestinal lymphoma in AIDS patients will be depicted as a focal or diffuse mural thickening affecting segments of the small intestine. As with non-immunocompromised patients, large cavitated masses may develop as a complication of small bowel lymphoma that has eroded through the wall with formation of a large extraintestinal mass. In the colon, the anus and rectum are the sites most commonly involved in AIDS-related non-Hodgkin's lymphoma. Mural thickening and anorectal masses may be depicted on MR images. In these patients, other associated findings include hepatosplenomegaly, lymphadenopathy, hepatic masses, and hypercellular bone marrow.

Gastrointestinal Stromal Tumors

Gastrointestinal stromal tumors (GISTs) are a subset of intestinal mesenchymal tumors, previously classified as leimomyomas (Fig. 85-61), leiomyosarcomas, leimyoblastomas, or schwanomas.[151] They are rare tumors accounting for 3% of malignant GI tumors. They arise in the muscularis propria layer of the intestinal wall. About 10% to 30% of GISTs are malignant.

Gastrointestinal stromal tumors demonstrate intramural, endoluminal, and exophytic patterns of growth.

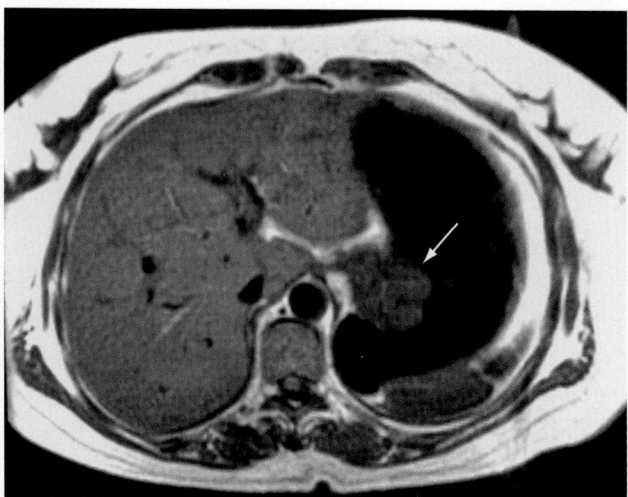

F I G U R E 85-61

Gastric leiomyoma (GI stromal tumor; GIST). T1-weighed image demonstrates a sharply circumscribed solid gastric mass *(arrow)* with intramural and endoluminal growth. Tissue diagnosis revealed a benign GIST or gastric leiomyoma.

Within the GI tract they occur most frequently in the stomach, where they represent 1% of gastric malignant tumors; they also occur in the small bowel (33%), rectum and colon (5% to 15%), and esophagus (1% to 5%).[151] Malignant GISTs are characterized by direct spread to involve adjacent organs, peritoneum, and mesentery (21% to 43%). Hematogenous metastases to liver (50 to 65%), lungs, and osseous structures (10%) occur. Nodal metastases are rare (<10%).

Most GISTs are large at the time of diagnosis with extraintestinal tumor extension and invasion of adjacent organs. Their size, however, can vary from a few centimeters to 30 cm in diameter. Central necrosis is common in larger tumors. Symptoms at clinical presentation include a palpable abdominal mass, GI bleeding, and hemorrhage into the peritoneal cavity. Treatment is by surgical resection combined with chemotherapy. The 5-year survival for malignant GISTs is 29% to 35%.

MRI of Gastrointestinal Stromal Tumors

On MRI, GISTs appear as large, solid, heterogeneous abdominal masses. They are isointense to muscle on T1-weighted images and heterogeneously hyperintense on T2-weighted images. The tumors show moderate heterogeneous enhancement following intravenous gadolinium administration. Larger tumors show non-enhancing areas central necrosis (Fig. 85-62). Associated calcification will appear as focal low signal intensity areas on all MR images. The multiplanar capabilities of MRI are particularly useful to evaluate larger GISTs,

depicting invasion of adjacent organs. MRI also excels at depicting associated liver, peritoneal, and osseous metastases.

Intestinal Metastases

Metastatic tumor may spread to the GI tract via hematogenous and intraperitoneal routes, or by direct spread from an adjacent tumor.[152,153] Tumors that may undergo hematogenous spread to the intestinal tract include malignant melanoma, Kaposi's sarcoma, breast cancer, lung cancer, parotid cancer, testicular cancer, and carcinoid tumor. Intraperitoneal dissemination with involvement of the bowel serosa occurs in tumors arising in the stomach, colon, ovary, pancreas, and endometrium. Tumors arising in any abdominal or pelvic organ may enlarge and spread to directly involve adjacent bowel. Patients with GI metastases can present with bowel obstruction, visceral perforation, or GI bleeding.

MRI of Intestinal Metastases

Gastrointestinal metastases are depicted on MR images as mural nodules, masses, eccentric or concentric mural thickening, or as a large abdominal mass invading adjacent bowel loops (Fig. 85-63). Adequate bowel distention is essential to depict subtle mural thickening or masses that may be obscured by collapsed bowel. Mural nodules or masses are shown as focal, solid enhancing soft tissue masses arising from the intestinal

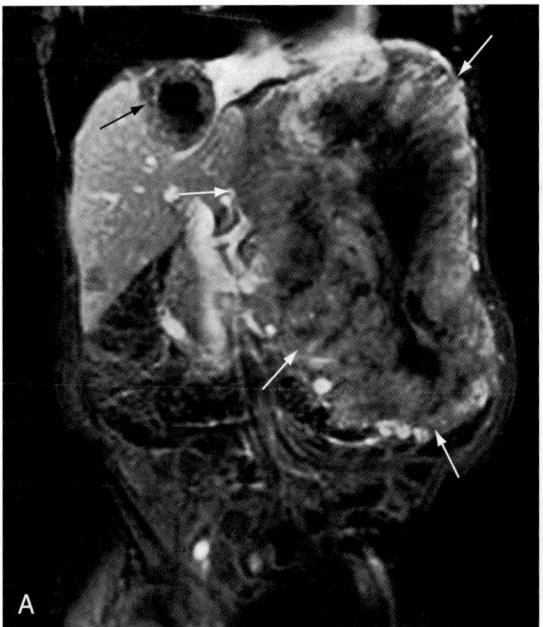
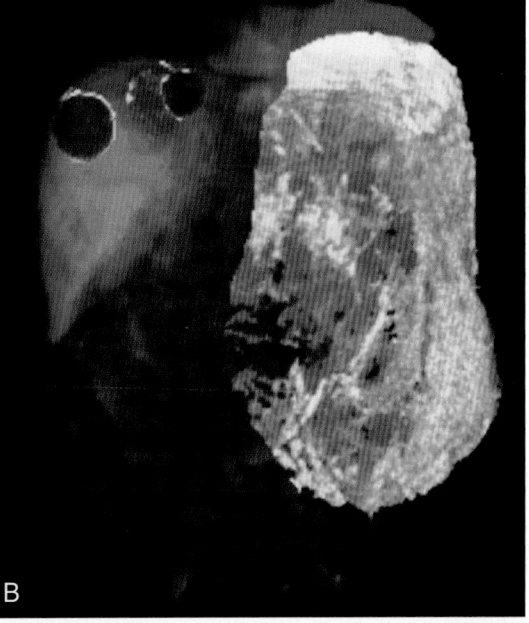

FIGURE 85-62

Coronal gadolinium-enhanced image (**A**) demonstrates a large left-sided abdominal mass (*white arrows*) with central necrosis and liver metastases (*black arrow*). Three dimensional color model (**B**) shows the relationship of the mass to the liver metastases and other organs.

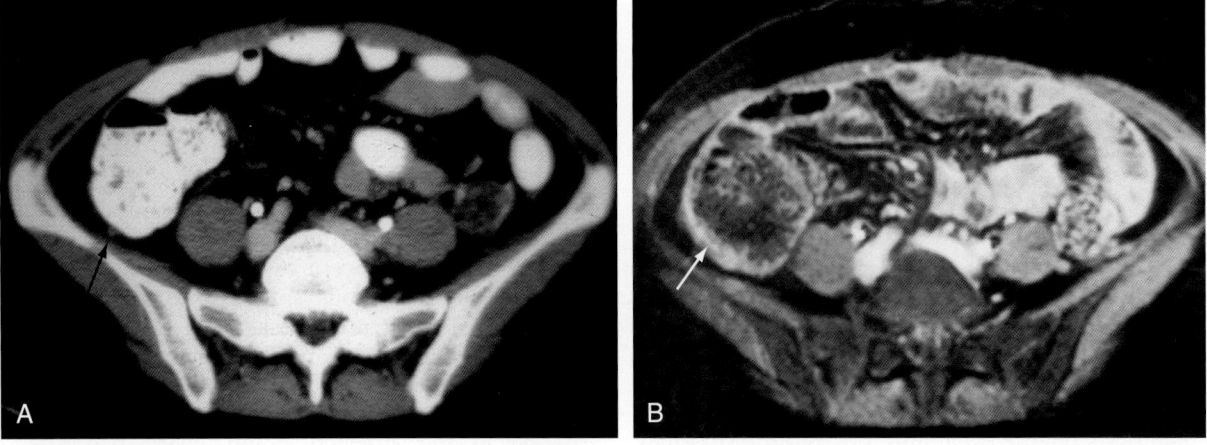

FIGURE 85-63

Intestinal metastases in patient with ovarian cancer. Helical CT (**A**) shows a small nodule *(arrow)* adjacent to the cecum. Gadolinium-enhanced spoiled gradient-echo (SGE) image (**B**) shows a rind of enhancing serosal tumor involving the cecum *(arrow)*. The extent of the serosal metastases is better defined on the MR image. Serosal tumor was confirmed at laparotomy.

wall. Serosal and mural tumor may also be depicted as segments of bowel with concentric or eccentric mural thickening. This appearance may be identical to inflammatory bowel disease. However, the patient's history of malignancy and absence of inflammatory symptoms should suggest the possibility of intestinal metastases. Initially serosal metastases often involve short segments of bowel. However, with more extensive intra-abdominal tumor, long segments of the intestines become involved with metastatic tumor, showing mural thickening and enhancement. There is typically other evidence of disseminated abdominal tumor with bulky abdominal masses and peritoneal carcinomatosis. Patients with tumor extending directly to involve adjacent bowel will demonstrate bulky abdominal and pelvic tumors invading the stomach, small intestine, or colon.

Bowel Obstruction in Patients with Malignancy

Bowel obstruction is a common complication in the patient with advanced stage cancer, occurring in 5% to 42% of patients with advanced ovarian cancer[154-156] and 4% to 24% of patients with advanced colorectal cancer.[157-159] Distinguishing benign from malignant bowel obstruction in a patient with malignancy is a critical diagnostic and imaging challenge that confronts radiologists and clinicians on a daily basis. Diagnosing benign or malignant bowel obstruction profoundly affects management decisions and has significant prognostic implications. Benign bowel obstruction may occur from postsurgical adhesions, radiation enteritis, abscess, phlegmon, or other infectious or inflammatory GI diseases. Malignant bowel obstruction may be due to an obstructing primary tumor, local tumor recurrence, or metastases involving the bowel and adjacent mesentery. Following abdominal surgery for cancer, non-malignant adhesions account for 21% to 38% of intestinal obstructions, while malignant obstruction accounts for the remaining 62% to 79% of patients. It has been reported that in patients with colorectal cancer nearly half of the cases of bowel obstruction are due to benign conditions.[160]

MRI of Bowel Obstruction

MRI is an effective imaging tool in the patient with bowel obstruction.[26,46] Oral contrast material may not be necessary since the patient with acute high-grade bowel obstruction will present with dilated fluid-filled bowel. In the patient with partial bowel obstruction, limited additional oral contrast material can be administered, as tolerated by the patient. Useful imaging pulse sequences include T2-weighted breath-hold SSRARE, which provides an excellent depiction of the dilated fluid filled bowel showing a zone of transition at the point of obstruction. The dilated bowel will have very high signal intensity due to its fluid content (Fig. 85-64). The SSRARE images are also useful to assess intestinal wall thickening and the presence of large abdominal or pelvic masses. Fat-suppressed gadolinium-enhanced images obtained with 2D SGE imaging or 3D SGE imaging show the distended bowel filled with low signal intensity fluid. The gadolinium-enhanced images are useful to depict intestinal mural thickening, an enhancing obstructing mass (Fig. 85-65), and associated disseminated abdominal tumor.

Malignant bowel obstruction is indicated by the presence of an obstructing mass, focal mural thickening (<10 cm), or evidence of disseminated tumor and carcinomatosis. The presence of an obstructing mass is the most accurate indicator of malignant bowel obstruction (Fig. 85-66). Due to the high soft tissue contrast of gadolinium-enhanced MRI, the obstructing mass is often more conspicuous on MR examinations. The distribution

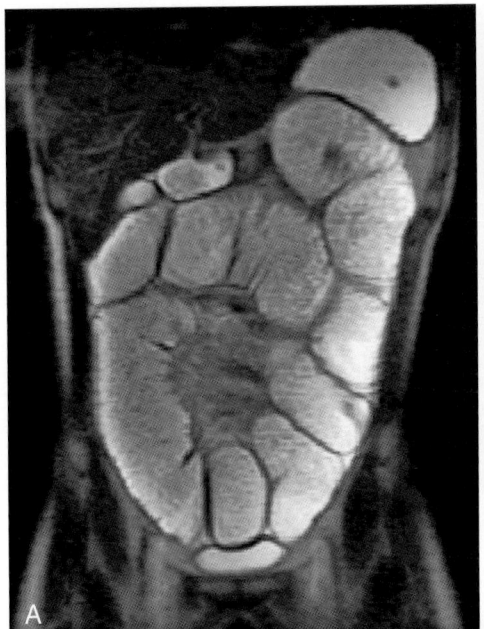

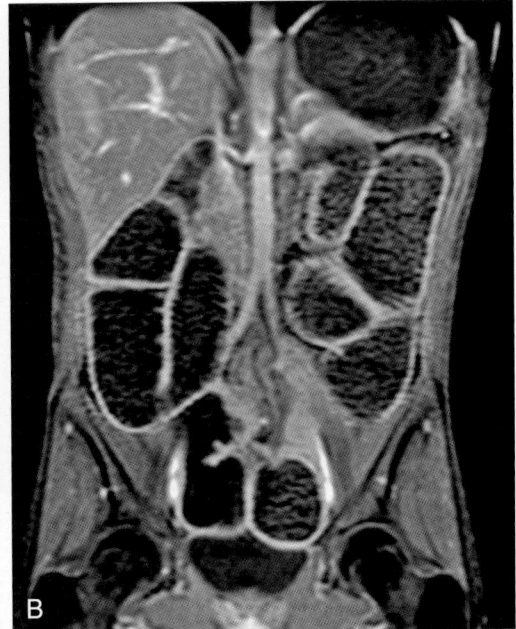

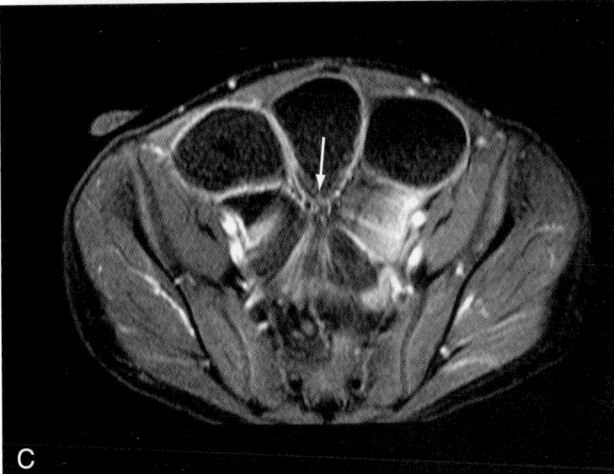

FIGURE 85-64

Benign bowel obstruction in a patient status post colon cancer resection. Coronal single-shot fast spin-echo (SSFSE) (**A**) and gadolinium-enhanced spoiled gradient-echo (SGE) (**B**) images demonstrate bowel obstruction with markedly dilated fluid-filled bowel loops. Axial gadolinium-enhanced SGE MR image (**C**) shows tethering of bowel loops at the site of adhesion *(arrow)*, but no evidence of an obstructing mass. Benign bowel obstruction due to adhesions was confirmed at laparotomy.

FIGURE 85-65

Malignant bowel obstruction in a patient with prior resection of cervical cancer. Gadolinium-enhanced spoiled gradient-echo (SGE) image shows bowel obstruction with dilated fluid-filled bowel loops and an enhancing obstructing mass *(arrow)* in the right lower quadrant. Malignant bowel obstruction was confirmed at laparotomy.

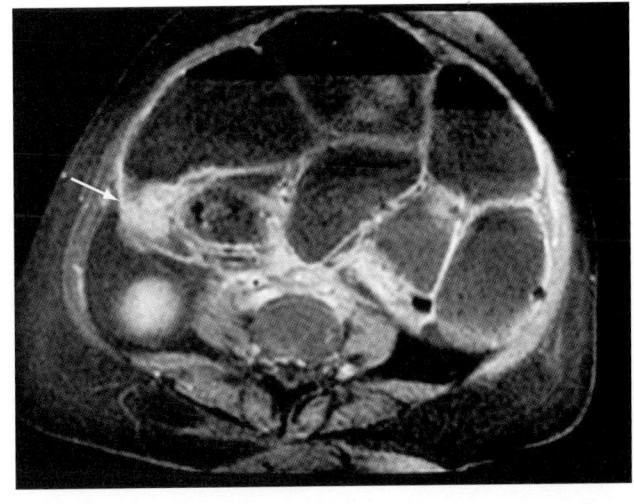

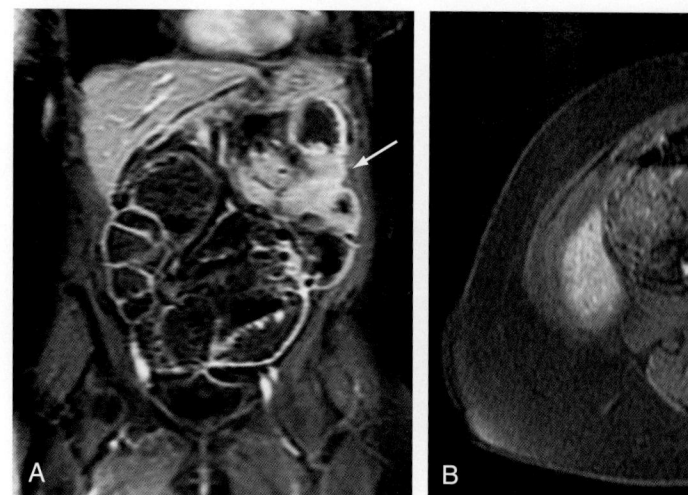

FIGURE 85-66

Malignant bowel obstruction in a patient with treated ovarian cancer. Coronal gadolinium-enhanced spoiled gradient-echo (SGE) image (**A**) demonstrates an irregular enhancing mass (*arrow*) in the left side of the abdomen producing obstruction of small bowel and colon. Axial gadolinium-enhanced image (**B**) confirms the enhancing tumor (*long arrow*) and focal mural thickening (*short arrow*) of adjacent bowel loops. Malignant bowel obstruction was confirmed at laparotomy.

of mural thickening can provide important clues in distinguishing benign and malignant obstruction. Focal mural thickening is an important sign that indicates malignant obstruction, most commonly from serosal metastases (Fig. 85-66).

Benign bowel obstruction is indicated by absence of an obstructing mass, diffuse mural thickening (>50% of bowel), and absence of disseminated tumor or carcinomatosis. Patients with benign bowel obstruction may show enhancement of thin and smooth peritoneum. However, the MR finding of marked, bulky peritoneal carcinomatosis in the setting of bowel obstruction indicates a malignant etiology.[46]

Segmental mural thickening may be due to either benign or malignant intestinal obstruction. Within the segmental category, benign segmental obstruction due to radiation enteritis, postoperative changes, or adhesions often involves longer segments of bowel, may be bilateral, and can be in the distribution of a radiation port. Malignant mural thickening from serosal metastases is generally more localized, unilateral, and involves shorter segments of bowel. Patients with disseminated abdominal tumor may show serosal metastases involving longer segments of bowel when associated with bulky abdominal metastases.

THE PERITONEUM, MESENTERY, AND OMENTUM

The depiction of small peritoneal implants and carcinomatosis is a challenge for cross-sectional imaging studies, including CT scanning and unenhanced MRI. However, with gadolinium-enhanced MRI, small peritoneal tumors are routinely depicted with a level of

conspicuity that is unmatched by other imaging studies tumor (Fig. 85-67). Marked enhancement of small peritoneal implants with IV gadolinium on MR images facilitates detection of metastases to free peritoneal surfaces and bowel serosa.[8,9,160-162] Following the injection of gadolinium, peritoneal implants slowly accumulate the contrast material and are, therefore, most conspicuous on images obtained 5 minutes following the IV injection of the gadolinium chelate. The addition of fat suppression reduces the competing high signal of the adjacent fat and is an important element in this technique.

Several studies have shown that gadolinium-enhanced fat-suppressed MRI is superior to CT scanning in depicting peritoneal tumors.[8,9,160-162] The superior performance of enhanced MRI compared with CT scanning is most noticeable in the depiction of small (<1 cm) tumor implants and carcinomatosis. In one study, gadolinium-enhanced MRI detected 75% to 80% of small tumor implants (<1 cm) compared with 22% to 33% for CT scans (P < .0001).[160]

ANATOMY

The peritoneum is a serous lining of mesothelial cells that lines the abdominal cavity and covers the abdominal organs. It consists of a parietal layer lining the inner surface of the abdominal and pelvic cavity and the visceral peritoneum that covers the organs. The parietal and visceral peritoneum contains a rich vascular and lymphatic capillary network. Peritoneal reflections form the ligaments and mesenteries that connect organs and secure organs to the abdominal wall. In the anterior abdomen, the omentum is composed of four layers of peritoneum.[163-166]

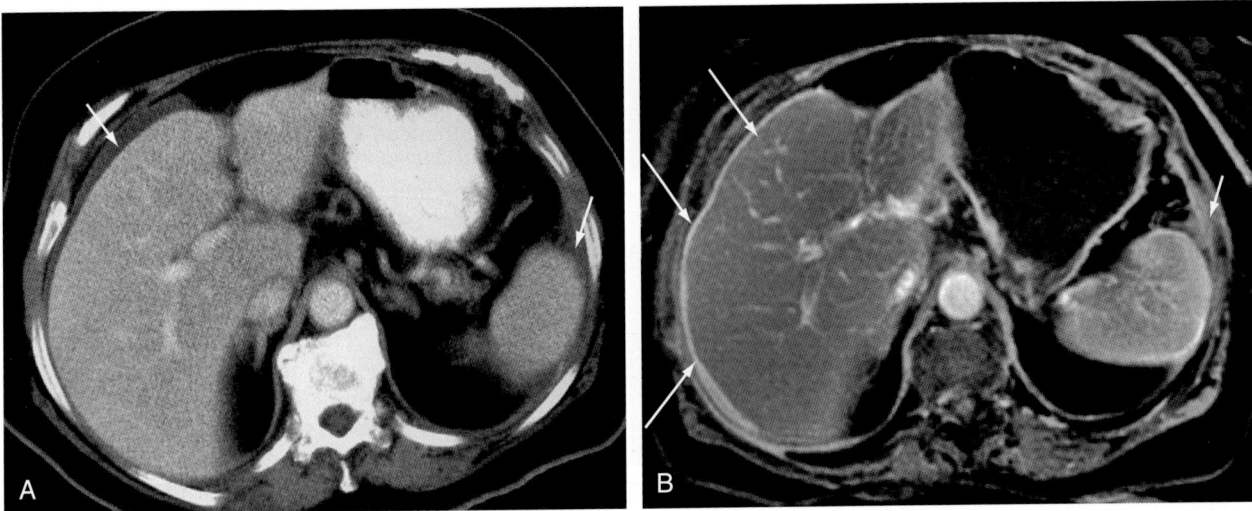

FIGURE 85-67

Comparison of Helical CT and MRI for peritoneal metastases in a patient with treated ovarian cancer. Helical CT scan (**A**) shows perihepatic and perisplenic ascites *(arrows)*. Delayed gadolinium-enhanced spoiled gradient-echo (SGE) MRI image (**B**) shows a rim of enhancing perihepatic *(long arrows)* and perisplenic *(short arrow)* peritoneal tumor. Also note the enhancing tumor *(short arrow)* in the left intersegmental fissure.

Peritoneal Mesenteries

A mesentery is a double layer of peritoneum that results from the invagination of an organ into the peritoneum. Mesenteries contain the neurovascular network connecting the organ to the abdominal wall. Examples of mesenteries include:

Small-bowel mesentery. The small-bowel mesentery connects the jejunum and ileum to the posterior abdominal wall. It extends from the left upper quadrant to the right lower quadrant.

Transverse mesocolon. This horizontally oriented mesentery connects the transverse colon to the posterior abdominal wall. Inferior to the transverse colon, it fuses with the posterior wall of the omentum.

Sigmoid mesentery. This mesentery in the left lower quadrant attaches the sigmoid colon to the posterior abdominal wall.

Mesoduodenum. The mesoduodenum attaches the duodenum to the posterior abdominal wall.

Mesoappendix. This mesentery attaches the cecum and the proximal appendix.

Mesenteric Vascular Anatomy

Branches of the celiac artery, superior mesenteric artery (SMA), and inferior mesenteric artery (IMA) supply the GI tract.

CELIAC ARTERY. This supplies the foregut, liver, and spleen. It arises from the anterior abdominal aorta and gives rise to the left gastric artery, the common hepatic artery, and the splenic artery.

SUPERIOR MESENTERIC ARTERY. This artery arises from the anterior abdominal aorta at the L1 vertebral body 1 cm below the origin of the celiac artery. The SMA supplies the duodenum, the jejunum, the ileum, ascending colon, and usually the transverse colon. The branches of the SMA forming the pancreatoduodenal arcade supply blood to the duodenum. The SMA gives rise to between 4 and 6 jejunal branches arising from its left side. The ileocolic artery arises from the right side of the SMA, marking the transition from the jejunal to the ileal arteries. The ileocolic artery supplies the terminal ileum, cecum, and ascending colon. Between 9 and 13 ileal arteries supply blood to the ileum. The right colic artery is absent in 80% of people. When present, it assists the ileocolic and middle colic arteries to supply blood to the ascending colon. The middle colic artery arises from the right side of the SMA just before it enters the small-bowel mesentery. The middle colic artery has branches that descend to anastomose with the ileocolic artery and a branch that ascends to anastomose to the left colic artery from the IMA.

INFERIOR MESENTERIC ARTERY. This artery arises from the anterior abdominal aorta seven centimeters below the SMA origin at the L3 vertebral body level. The IMA gives rise to the left colic artery that anastomoses with the middle colic artery from the SMA to supply the transverse colon. The left colic artery is absent in 12% of people. The colosigmoid artery supplies blood to the descending colon and the sigmoid colon. The rectosigmoid artery and superior rectal arteries arise from the IMA to supply the sigmoid colon and rectum.

Collateral Pathways

CELIAC ARTERY TO SUPERIOR MESENTERIC ARTERY. Collateral pathways exist between the celiac artery and the SMA to form the anterior and posterior pancreatoduodenal arcades and the arc of Buehler, which is an embryonic remnant.

enhancement of the gallbladder wall and surrounding peritoneal reflections should be considered to represent peritoneal tumor spread.

TRANSVERSE FISSURE AND PERIPORTAL SPACE. The peritoneal reflections surrounding the hepatic pedicle as it enters the liver parenchyma form the transverse fissure. The transverse fissure contains the horizontal portions of the right and left portal veins. The fissure is continuous with the periportal space, which is a potential space surrounding the intrahepatic portal vein branches. The periportal space is a common site for direct tumor spread in patients with ovarian carcinoma or pancreatic carcinoma. Tumor involving the periportal space will be depicted as enhancing periportal soft tissue on delayed gadolinium-enhanced SGE MR images or as a collar of high signal tumor adjacent to the portal vein on T2-weighted images. The immediate gadolinium-enhanced images show only the enhancing portal vein, while the delayed images depict the portal vein and enhancing periportal tumor.

RIGHT SUBPHRENIC SPACE. The right subphrenic space is a large, continuous space separating the right lobe of the liver from the adjacent right hemidiaphragm. It is lined by the visceral peritoneum covering the liver surface and the parietal peritoneum lining the under surface of the diaphragm. This large space is delimited posteriorly and inferiorly by the right coronary ligament and medially by the falciform ligament. It is continuous inferiorly with the right subhepatic space or Morrison's pouch. The right subphrenic space is the most common site for peritoneal tumor involvement in patients with peritoneal carcinomatosis. Peritoneal tumor typically deposits on the parietal peritoneum lining the under surface of the right hemidiaphragm. Metastatic tumor in the right subphrenic space is depicted as enhancing soft tissue along the surface of the liver on delayed gadolinium-enhanced SGE MR images.

LEFT SUBPHRENIC SPACE. The anatomic spaces in the left upper quadrant form one continuous space that freely communicates. The perihepatic spaces surrounding the left lobe of the liver freely communicate with the adjacent perigastric and perisplenic spaces in the left upper quadrant of the abdomen. When involved by inflammation or tumor, this large potential space in the left upper abdomen may be compartmentalized by the splenorenal ligament, gastrosplenic ligament or lesser omentum.

THE LESSER SAC. The lesser sac is bounded anteriorly by the stomach, lesser omentum, and gastrocolic ligament, and posteriorly by the pancreas. Inferiorly the lesser sac is delimited by the transverse colon and the mesocolon. On the left, the lesser sac is delimited by the splenorenal ligament and the gastrosplenic ligament. On the right the lesser sac communicates with the greater sac via the foramen of Winslow, an opening behind the free edge of the lesser omentum.

RIGHT SUBHEPATIC SPACE. The right subhepatic space is separated into an anterior right subhepatic space and a posterior right subhepatic space. The anterior compartment is delimited inferiorly by the transverse mesocolon. The posterior right subhepatic space separates the right lobe of the liver and the right kidney

and is known as Morrison's pouch or the hepatorenal fossa. The superior extension of the posterior compartment is the right coronary ligament. When the body is a supine position, Morrison's pouch is the most dependent site of the peritoneal cavity. It is, therefore, an important anatomic site for localization of inflammatory and neoplastic diseases. Careful inspection of Morrison's pouch for enhancing soft tissue is important in patients with disseminated tumor or infection. The right subhepatic space communicates with the adjacent right subphrenic space and the right paracolic gutter. In addition to axial images, coronal and sagittal MR images are particularly useful for depicting the right subhepatic space.

Middle Abdominal Peritoneal Anatomy

The parietal and visceral peritoneum extends inferiorly into the middle abdomen to cover the inner surface of the abdominal wall and the small intestine and colon. Tumor and inflammation of the parietal peritoneal surfaces will be depicted as peritoneal thickening or enhancement along the inner surface of the abdominal wall. The thickening may be nodular and mass-like or may be smooth and regular (Fig. 85-69). Bowel serosal tumor and inflammation will be depicted as mural thickening and enhancement (Fig. 85-70A).

In the middle abdomen, the four-layered greater omentum arises from the greater curvature of the stomach and drapes over the small bowel, colon, and other abdominal viscera. Tumor involving the omentum may be depicted as mild infiltration of omental fat on T1-weighted images and gadolinium-enhanced SGE images, or as a bulky thick omental cake several centimeters in thickness (Fig. 85-71A).

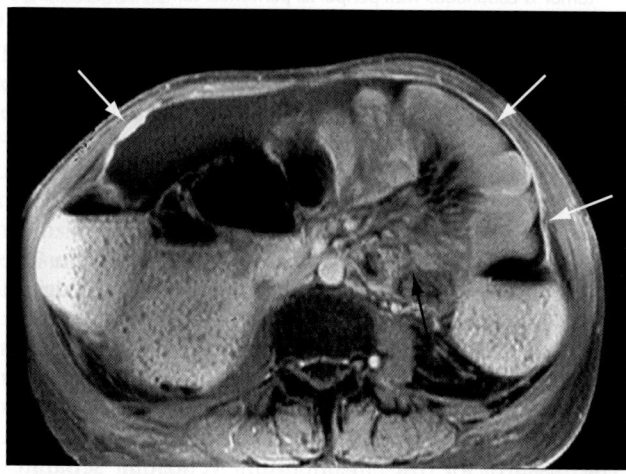

FIGURE 85-69

Parietal peritoneal metastases. Fat-suppressed gadolinium-enhanced spoiled gradient-echo (SGE) image through the middle abdomen demonstrates enhancing parietal peritoneal metastases *(arrows)*. In the right anterior abdomen the tumor is slightly nodular and irregular, while on the left side of the abdomen the tumor is smooth and regular in contour. Mesenteric infiltration *(black arrow)* indicates mesenteric peritoneal metastases.

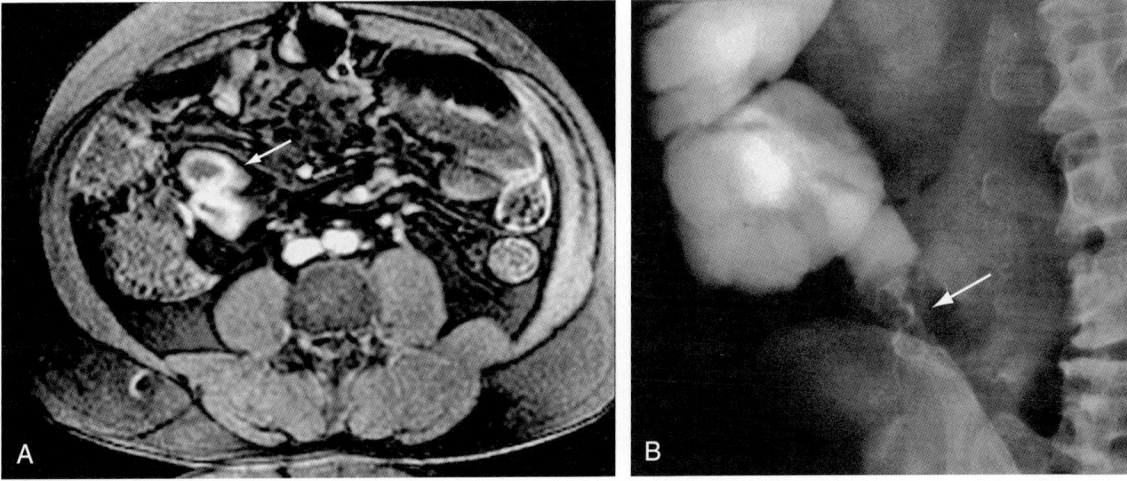

FIGURE 85-70

Serosal metastases in a patient with colon cancer. **A,** Gadolinium-enhanced spoiled gradient-echo (SGE) image shows moderate mural thickening and marked enhancement involving the terminal ileum *(arrow)* without an obstructing mass. **B,** Barium examination shows mucosal destruction *(arrow)* involving the terminal ileum confirming serosal and mural metastases.

The transverse mesocolon, attaching the transverse colon to the posterior abdominal wall is best depicted on sagittal MR images. Below its colonic attachment the transverse mesocolon fuses with the posterior portion of the omentum inferiorly, forming the posterior two layers of the four-layered omentum.

Much of the middle abdomen is dominated by small intestine and the small bowel mesentery that attaches the jejunum and the ileum to the posterior abdominal wall. The fan-shaped folds of the small-bowel mesentery are well depicted on axial, coronal, or sagittal MR images. The small-bowel mesentery is a common site for peritoneal tumor deposition. As ascites pools in the folds of the small-bowel mesentery, it flows to the most dependent section, which is the mesentery of the distal ileum in the right lower quadrant. The mesentery of the terminal ileum is, therefore a common first site of peritoneal tumor deposition. Small-bowel mesenteric tumor may be depicted as large bulky tumor masses (Fig. 85-72) or as subtle soft tissue infiltration and enhancement of the small-bowel mesenteric fat (Fig. 85-73).

The colon is positioned around the periphery of the middle abdomen and pelvis. The attachments of the ascending and descending colon to the posterior abdominal wall define the paracolic gutters and serve to

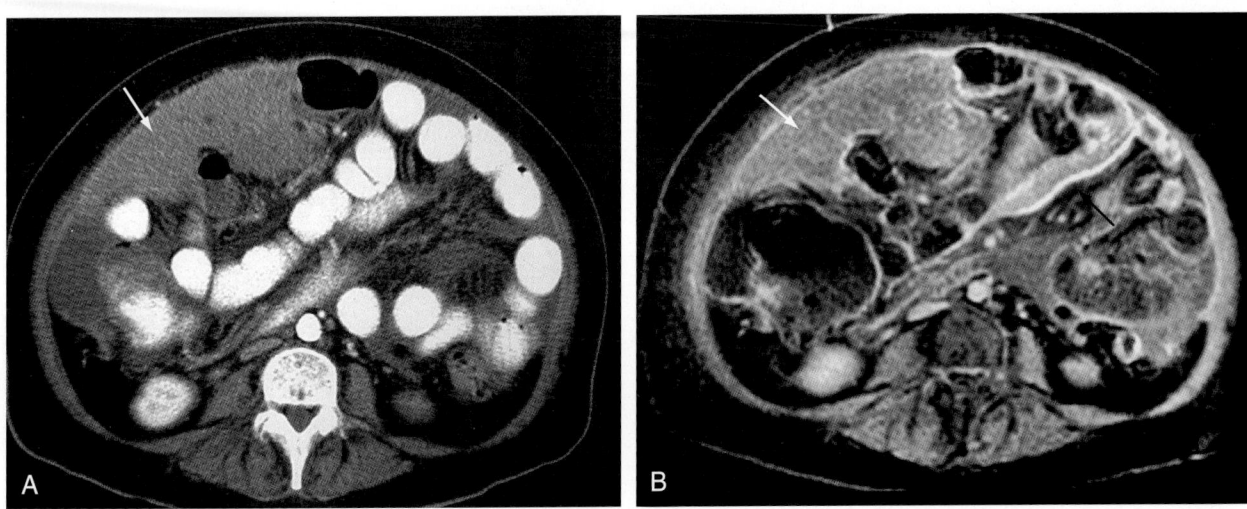

FIGURE 85-71

Omental metastases. **A,** Helical CT scan shows a thick omental cake of tumor *(arrow)* in the anterior abdomen. **B,** Gadolinium-enhanced spoiled gradient-echo (SGE) MR image shows a thick enhancing omental mass *(white arrow)* and mesenteric tumor *(black arrow)*.

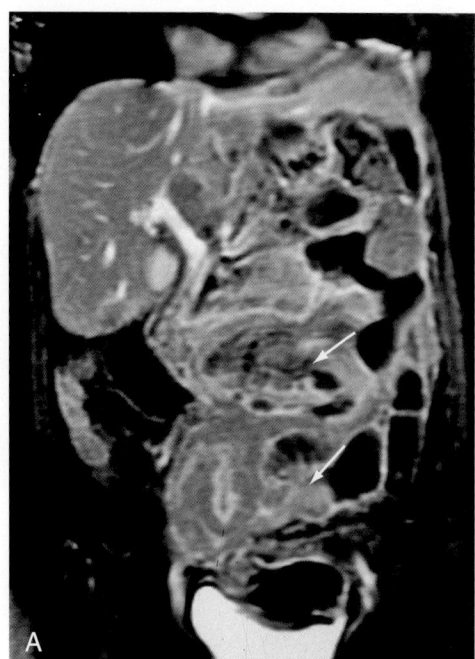

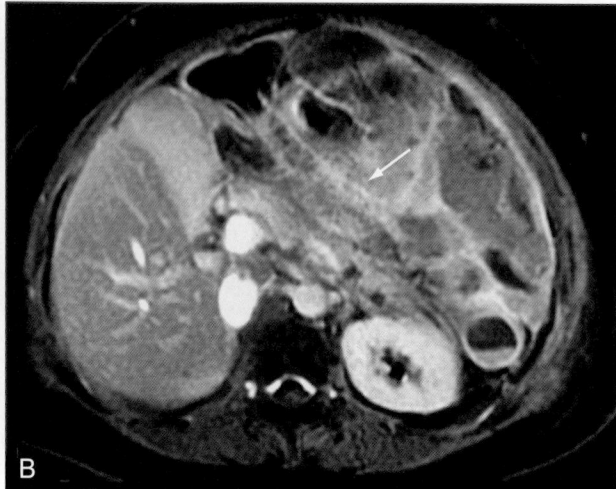

FIGURE 85-72

Small bowel mesenteric metastases. Coronal (**A**) and axial (**B**) gadolinium-enhanced spoiled gradient-echo (SGE) MR images show large bulky tumor masses *(arrows)* replacing the small bowel mesentery and producing partial small bowel obstruction.

help direct the flow of ascites and peritoneal tumor deposition (Fig. 85-74). Because the phrenicocolic ligament blocks flow of ascites up the left paracolic gutter, there is preferential flow of ascites and disseminated peritoneal tumor cells up the wider right paracolic gutter. From the right paracolic gutter the peritoneal tumor cells will freely flow into the right subhepatic space, right subphrenic space and the other perihepatic spaces described above.

Pelvic Peritoneal Anatomy

Within the pelvis, the parietal peritoneum covers the inner surface and the abdominal and pelvic wall. The parietal peritoneum lining the pelvis is a common site of peritoneal tumor deposition or involvement by pelvic inflammation. The peritoneum reflects over the bladder, rectum, and uterus placing these structures in an extra-peritoneal location. The inferior extent of the pelvic

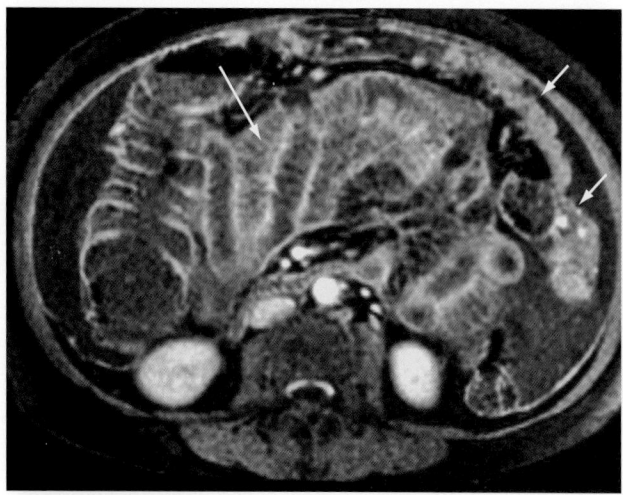

FIGURE 85-73

Subtle small bowel mesenteric metastases. Gadolinium-enhanced spoiled gradient-echo (SGE) MR image show infiltration and enhancement *(long white arrow)* of the terminal ileal mesentery. Enhancing omental tumor *(short white arrows)* is also depicted. Findings were confirmed at laparotomy.

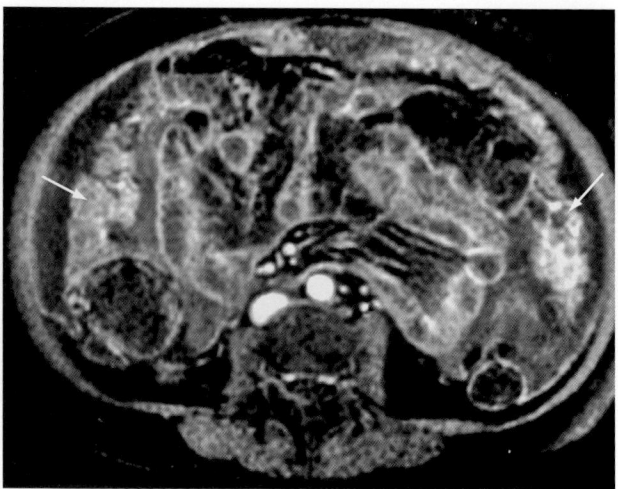

FIGURE 85-74

Paracolic metastases. Gadolinium-enhanced spoiled gradient-echo (SGE) MR image shows enhancing paracolic peritoneal metastases *(arrows)* adjacent to the ascending and descending colon.

peritoneal reflections forms the pouch of Douglas or rectovaginal pouch in the female and the rectovesical pouch in the male. As the most dependent portions of the peritoneal cavity, the rectovaginal pouch and rectovesical pouch are the first sites to accumulate ascitic fluid. Seeding of disseminated intraperitoneal tumor cells in these pelvic recesses is common. Increasing amounts of ascites will then fill the bilateral paravesical recesses. These anatomic sites should be carefully examined on pelvic MR images in patients with suspected peritoneal tumor. Sagittal MR images are particularly useful in depicting nodular peritoneal metastases interposed between the rectum and vagina or uterus in the female and the rectum and bladder in the male.

The dome of the bladder is covered by the visceral peritoneum and may be involved by peritoneal tumor or inflammation. Adequate distention of the bladder combined with sagittal and coronal imaging can facilitate depiction of peritoneal metastases to the bladder dome. Typically axial images are less useful for showing small bladder-dome masses.

The sigmoid mesentery is another important site of peritoneal tumor deposition (Fig. 85-75). This mesentery attaches the sigmoid colon to the posterior abdominal wall. Peritoneal tumor first involves the upper margin of the sigmoid colon and is depicted as mural thickening or scalloping of the sigmoid colonic wall. Tumor then progresses to form a circumferential mass with annular luminal narrowing. Subsequent left-sided colonic obstruction may ensue as the mass envelops and obstructs the sigmoid colon. Rectal water administered through a barium enema tube can be useful to distend the rectosigmoid colon, improving depiction of sigmoid mesenteric and serosal tumor.

TECHNIQUES AND PROTOCOLS

The MR protocols and techniques used for evaluating peritoneal disease are very similar to those that are used for MRI of the GI tract. Breath-hold acquisitions are employed to reduce motion artifact. The abdomen and pelvis are covered in the axial and coronal planes with a breath-hold fat-suppressed T2-weighted FSE acquisition and then with the same gadolinium-enhanced fat-suppressed SGE acquisition described for GI tract imaging. Because peritoneal tumor tends to enhance slowly, it is often more conspicuous on delayed gadolinium-enhanced MR images obtained 3 to 5 minutes following injection of the gadolinium chelate (Fig. 85-76). For this reason, it is essential to obtain a second, delayed set of axial gadolinium-enhanced images. Applying fat suppression will facilitate depiction of subtle enhancing peritoneal or serosal tumor by suppressing the high signal of adjacent fat. Alternatively, one can use thin-section 3D gradient-echo acquisitions for the gadolinium-enhanced imaging (Fig. 85-77).

Image homogeneity is an essential element of peritoneal MRI. Image inhomogeneity from poor fat suppression or from surface coil artifact may mask peritoneal tumor or may falsely create an appearance of peritoneal enhancement. One should optimize image quality on each MR scanner to obtain high-resolution homogeneous images. For this reason we often use the body coil instead of surface coils in patients with suspected peritoneal tumor. The body coil provides maximum coverage for imaging the abdomen and pelvis and provides the most homogeneous images with the least variation in signal intensity across the image. In the future, development of larger and more homogeneous surface coils for abdominal and pelvic imaging may alter this approach.

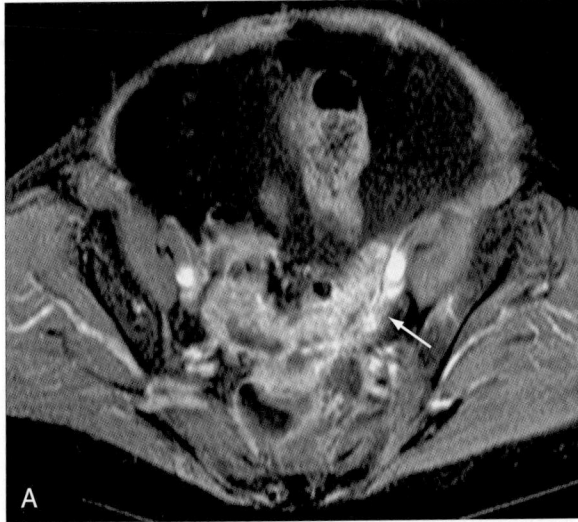
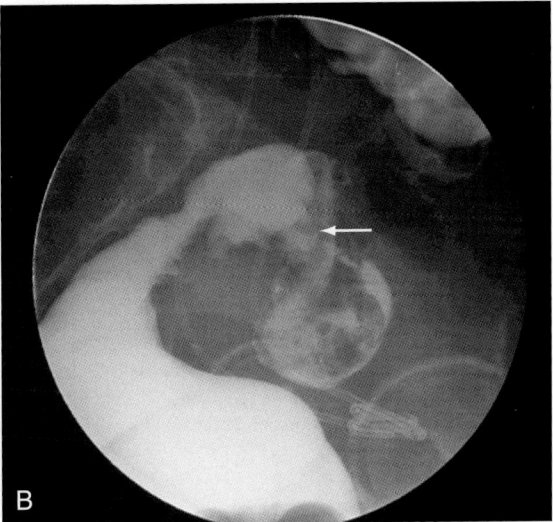

FIGURE 85-75

Sigmoid peritoneal metastases from ovarian cancer. Gadolinium-enhanced spoiled gradient-echo (SGE) MR image (**A**) shows bulky enhancing tumor (*arrow*) encasing the sigmoid colon. Barium enema (**B**) confirms mucosal destruction (*arrow*) and obstruction of the sigmoid colon.

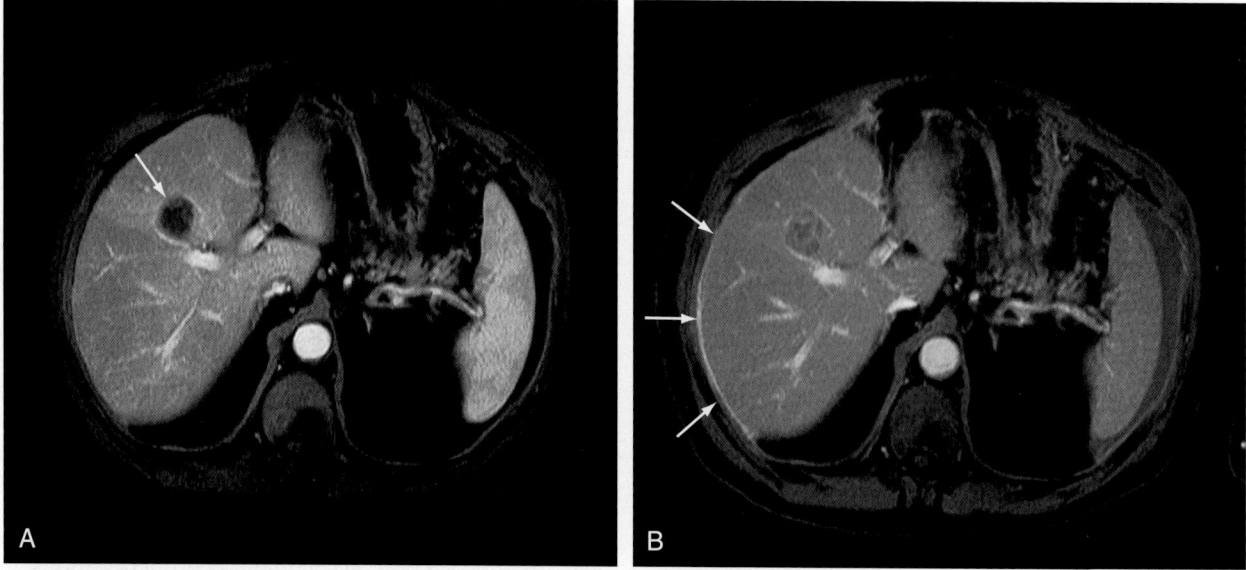

FIGURE 85-76

Timing for peritoneal imaging. Immediate gadolinium-enhanced spoiled gradient-echo (SGE) MR image (**A**) shows a liver metastasis *(arrow)* from colorectal cancer. Delayed gadolinium-enhanced SGE image (**B**) shows a thin enhancing rim of perihepatic peritoneal tumor *(arrows)*. Peritoneal tumor enhances slowly and is typically most conspicuous on delayed equilibrium phase images.

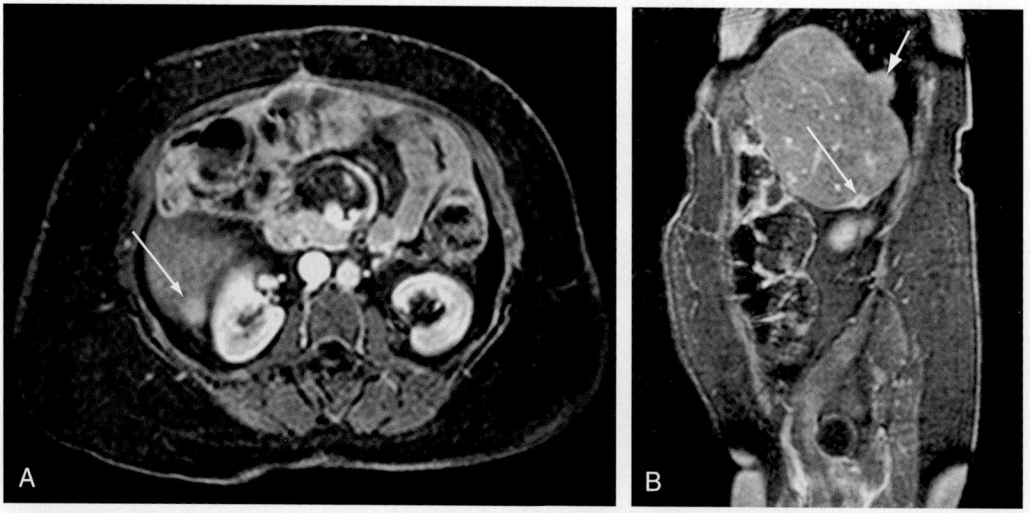

FIGURE 85-77

Three-dimensional T1W high resolution isotropic volume examination (THRIVE) MR images. Gadolinium-enhanced axial (**A**) and sagittal (**B**) thin-section 3D-THRIVE images obtained in a patient with ovarian cancer show a small right subhepatic metastases *(long arrows)*. An additional 2.5 cm right subphrenic metastases *(short arrow)* is also noted on the sagittal image. Thin-section 3D images may provide an advantage for depicting small peritoneal metastases.

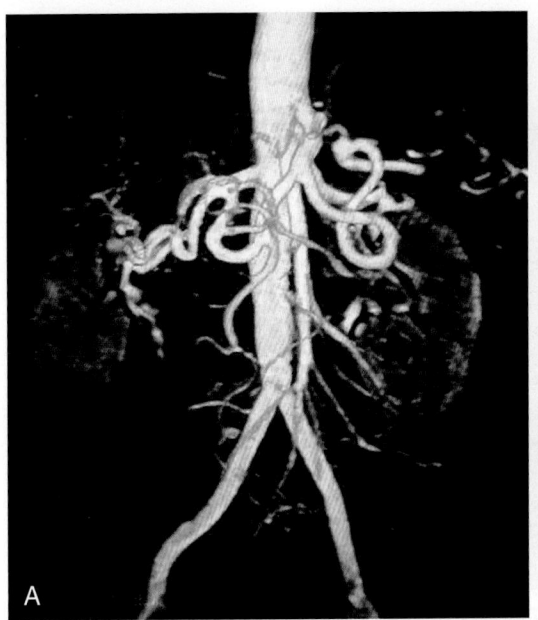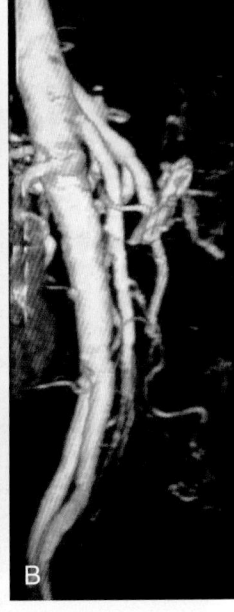

FIGURE 85-83

Magnetic resonance angiogram. Three-dimensional color volume models generated from a gadolinium-enhanced MR angiogram demonstrate the mesenteric arterial anatomy in the antero-posterior (**A**) and lateral (**B**) projections.

ischemia account for 75% of cases and is due to acute arterial embolus (50%), or atheromatous plaques with acute thrombosis (25%). Secondary arterial occlusion may be due to dissecting abdominal aortic aneurysms involving the SMA. Less common mechanical causes of intestinal ischemia include adhesions, small bowel herniation, intussception, or a volvulus.

Embolic acute mesenteric ischemia is most commonly from a cardiac origin. Precipitating factors include myocardial infarction, atrial fibrillation, or vegetative endocarditis. Noncardiac sources include a mycotic aneurysm. The embolus most commonly involves the SMA, 6 to 8 cm from its origin near the take off of the middle colic artery. Due to the sudden onset of the embolic occlusion, there is an acute presentation with no time for collateral circulation to develop. These patients typically have a worse prognosis than those with thrombotic acute mesenteric ischemia.

The pathophysiology of acute mesenteric ischemia is well described. Insufficient perfusion of the colon or small bowel produces hemorrhagic infarction. Damage may be reversible or may progress to transmural infarction of the bowel wall. The intestinal wall becomes cyanotic and edematous. Sepsis and shock may develop as the mucosa is disrupted with release of toxins and vasoactive substances into the blood stream. Bowel necrosis may occur within 8 to 12 hours from the onset of symptoms. Eventual bowel wall perforation leads to peritoneal signs and an acute abdominal presentation.

Chronic Mesenteric Ischemia

Chronic mesenteric ischemia is a gradual occlusive process in which the mesenteric vessels remain patent but have insufficient reserves to meet the increased metabolic demands of digestion. Due to the rich collateral arterial network supplying the GI tract, chronic mesenteric ischemia is relatively uncommon. Diffuse atherosclerotic disease is the cause of chronic mesenteric ischemia in 95% of cases, producing stenosis or occlusions of at least two of the three mesenteric arteries. Typically, the celiac artery, the SMA, and the IMA are all involved in the diffuse vascular disease. Compared with acute mesenteric ischemia, patients with chronic mesenteric ischemia have a low mortality.

With chronic mesenteric ischemia, patients present with the classical clinical triad of post-prandial abdominal pain, food aversion, and weight loss. The abdominal pain is typically vague and diffuse, beginning 15 to 30 minutes following a meal. Risk factors for chronic mesenteric ischemia include diabetes mellitus, hypertension, hypercholesterolemia, and smoking. Patients often have symptoms of vascular disease involving other territories, with a history of myocardial infarction, cerebral infarction, and peripheral vascular disease.

Once the diagnosis of chronic mesenteric ischemia is established, treatment is aimed at revascularizing the affected bowel. This may be achieved surgically with endarterectomy or bypass grafting. Noninvasive endovascular treatment with percutaneous angioplasty and placement of arterial stents is an alternative treatment that can successfully open critically stenotic mesenteric arteries. Additional treatment must be directed at correcting the severe malnutrition that is common in patients with long stating chronic mesenteric ischemia.

MRI of Mesenteric Ischemia

By combining gadolinium-enhanced MR angiography (MRA)[175] (Fig. 85-83) and anatomic MRI of the abdomen and pelvis,[176,177] one can perform a comprehensive exam

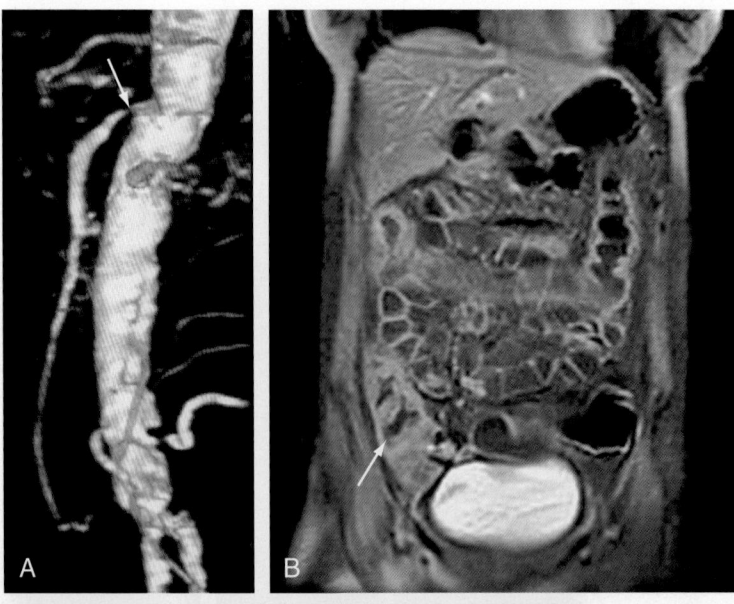

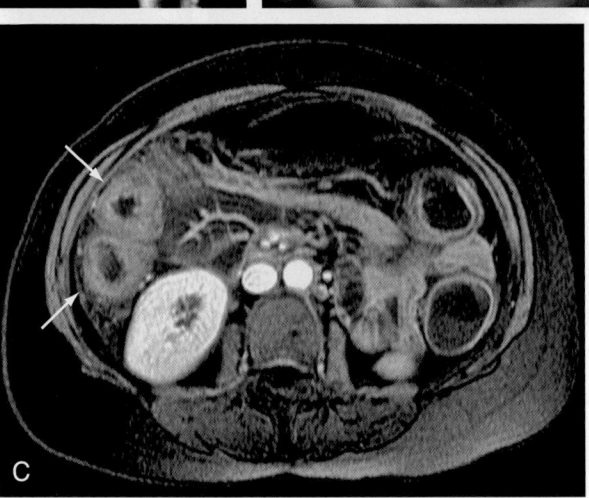

FIGURE 85-84

Mesenteric ischemia. Color volume model (**A**) from a gadolinium-enhanced MR angiogram shows high-grade stenosis *(arrow)* of the proximal superior mesenteric artery. Coronal (**B**) and axial (**C**) gadolinium-enhanced spoiled gradient-echo (SGE) image shows colonic mural thickening *(arrows)* with diminished mural enhancement.

in the patient with suspected intestinal ischemia. The MRA will evaluate possible occlusive disease of the SMA and IMA, while the anatomic images will show mural thickening of the involved bowel segments. Our current approach involves administering the intraluminal contrast agents described previously, followed by gadolinium-enhanced MR angiograms of the abdominal aorta and mesenteric vessels. This is followed by the breath-hold SSFSE and gadolinium-enhanced fat-suppressed SGE images of the abdomen and pelvis.

Findings of mesenteric ischemia include stenosis or occlusion of the SMA (Fig. 85-84), IMA, or, rarely, of the celiac artery branches. Due to collateral circulation, typically two of the three mesenteric vessels must be involved to produce symptoms of mesenteric ischemia. It is important to realize that distal small-vessel occlusion may produce focal ischemia. Such distal occlusions are beyond the resolution of current MRA techniques. For this reason we always assess the bowel wall for secondary changes of mural thickening.

On the anatomic SSFSE or true FISP images and the gadolinium-enhanced SGE images, one will see focal mural thickening in a vascular distribution. In patients with acute arterial insufficiency, there will be diminished or absent enhancement within the thickened segments of ischemic bowel (Fig. 85-85). A target appearance with enhancement of the mucosal and serosal surrounding a non-enhancing muscularis layer can be seen. This assessment of lack of enhancement should be made on the initial gadolinium-enhanced images. On delayed images, bowel wall enhancement may be evident from leakage of the contrast from the capillaries into the damaged bowel wall. In the non-acute setting the pattern of enhancement will be variable depending upon the degree of revascularization, fibrosis, or tissue necrosis. In our experience the findings on MRI can resolve very rapidly following spontaneous revascularization of the ischemic segment of bowel.

Chronic mesenteric ischemia can also be evaluated with a combination of gadolinium-enhanced 3D MR

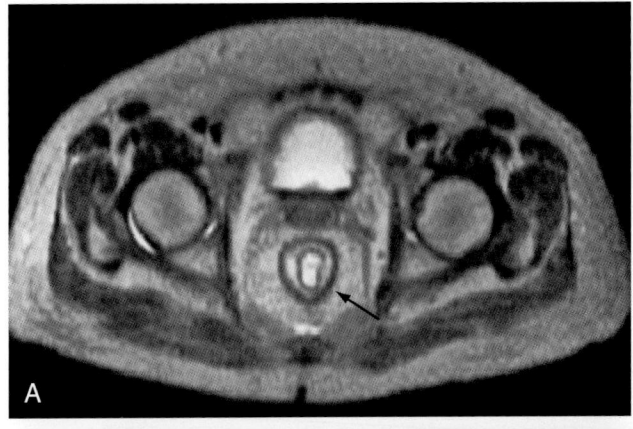

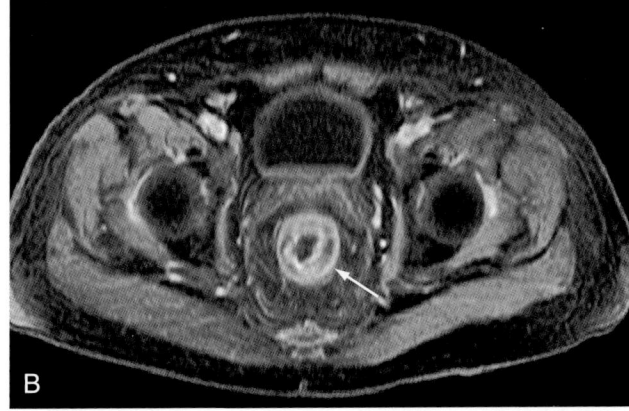

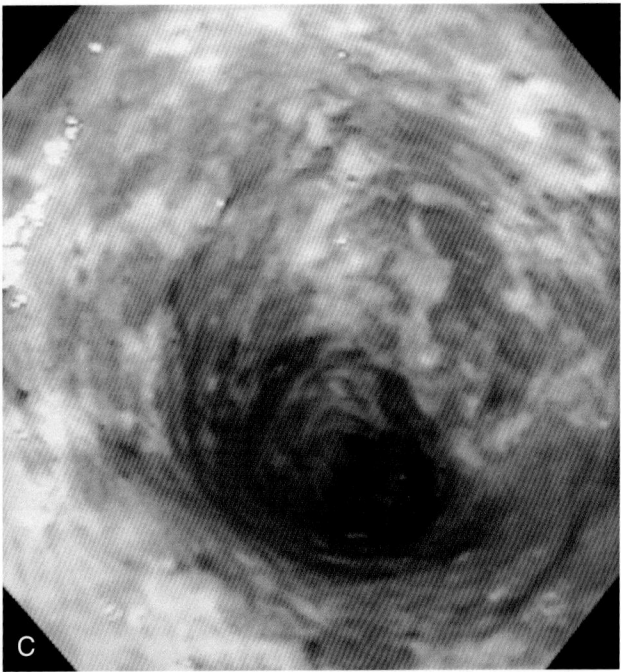

FIGURE 85-85

Rectal ischemia. Axial single-shot fast spin-echo (SSFSE) image (**A**) shows rectal wall thickening *(arrow)* and edema. Gadolinium-enhanced image (**B**) shows a target pattern with mucosal and serosal enhancement but absent muscularis enhancement. Endoscopy (**C**) and biopsy confirmed changes of rectal ischemia.

angiography and cine phase contrast MRI to quantify mesenteric blood flow. MR oximetry has been proposed as a technique to assess oxygenation of mesenteric venous blood.[178]

Mesenteric venous thrombosis may be depicted on MRI with non-enhancing filling defects visualized in the superior mesenteric vein and portal vein. Secondary venous congestion with bowel wall edema and mural thickening will be present (Fig. 85-86). In the chronic setting patients with venous thrombosis will demonstrate collateral veins and persistent mural thickening or ischemic strictures.

BENIGN MASSES

Mesenteric and Omental Cysts

A mesenteric or omental cyst is an rare abnormal fluid collection lined by epithelium located in the mesentery or omentum[171] (Fig. 85-87). The cell of origin is most commonly lymphatic producing a chylous cyst. They are thought to arise from benign ectopic lymphatic tissue that lacks communication with the lymph system. Mesenteric cysts can arise anywhere along the GI tract with the most common locations in the lower small-bowel mesentery and the sigmoid mesentery. In one series of 162 patients, 60% of mesenteric cysts occurred

in the small-bowel mesentery, 24% in the large-bowel mesentery, and 14.5% in the retroperitoneum.[171] A mesenteric cyst may present as a painless slowly growing mid-abdominal mass that is mobile. A presentation with acute or recurrent abdominal pain may be due to torsion, hemorrhage into the cyst, or superimposed infection.

MRI of Mesenteric and Omental Cysts

MRI of mesenteric and omental cysts shows a sharply circumscribed fluid containing mass that is hypointense on T1-weighted images and hyperintense on T2-weighted images. With gadolinium injection, the thin cyst wall and thin septations will enhance. With superimposed hemorrhage or infection, the cysts will show increased signal on T1-weighted images and more heterogeneous increased signal on T2-weighted images. Thickened cyst wall or septations will show enhancement with gadolinium chelates.

Endometriomas and Endometriosis

Endometriosis arises from ectopic endometrial tissue. When located outside of the uterus, the ectopic endometrium may be located on the surface of the ovaries, bladder, pelvic peritoneum, mesenteries, or bowel

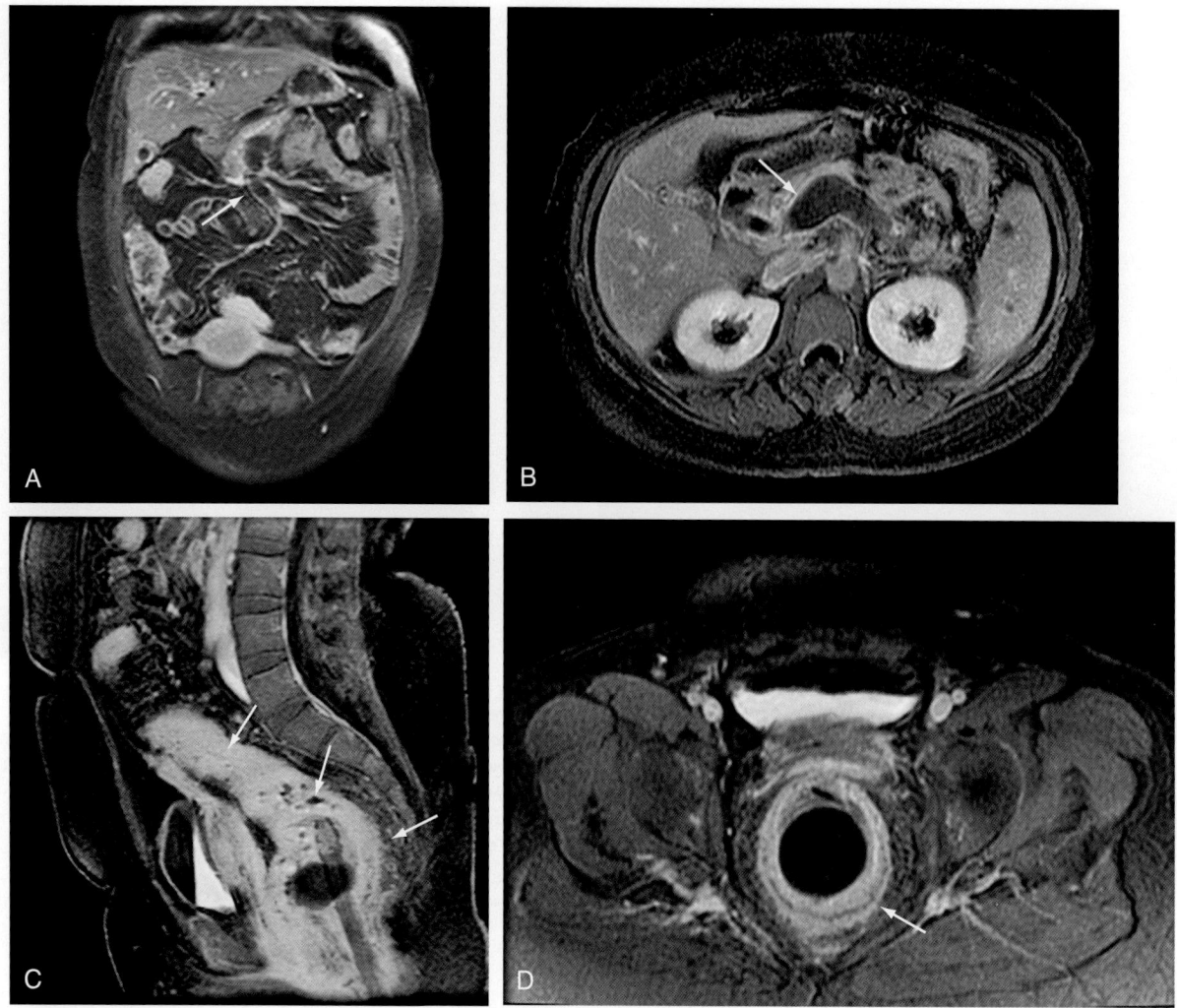

FIGURE 85-86

Mesenteric venous ischemia. Coronal (**A**) and axial (**B**) gadolinium-enhanced spoiled gradient-echo (SGE) images demonstrate thrombosis of the superior mesenteric vein and portal vein *(arrows)*. Sagittal (**C**) and axial (**D**) gadolinium-enhanced images through the pelvis show marked rectal mural edema and thickening *(arrows)*.

serosa. These endometrial implants may form masses or endometriomas (Fig. 85-88). Alternatively, small endometrial implants may coat the peritoneal and serosal surfaces. Patients with endometriosis present with pelvic and abdominal pain that occurs with menses or ovulation. Other symptoms include abdominal bloating, back pain, hip pain, pain with urination, and painful intercourse. Large endometriomas may produce bowel obstruction.[179-181]

MRI of Endometriosis

MRI of endometriosis may show well-defined masses or endometriomas that have variable signal intensity.[179-181] Endometriomas are typically high signal intensity on T1-weighted images and heterogeneous low signal intensity on T2-weighted images due to the presence of blood products. Endometriomas show enhancement with gadolinium chelates. Small endometrial implants can be difficult to depict on cross-sectional imaging. Fat-suppressed gadolinium-enhanced MRI may show abnormal peritoneal and serosal enhancement at the sites of endometrial implants. This appearance may be identical to peritoneal carcinomatosis or peritonitis. The addition of fat suppression will increase the conspicuity of the enhancing peritoneum by suppressing the competing high signal intensity from fat. Rectal water is also useful to distend the rectosigmoid colon, improving the depicting of serosal implants.

Desmoids

Desmoids tumors are benign slowly growing myelofibro-blastic neoplasms that can occur in the abdominal wall and intra-abdominally within the intestinal mesentery or

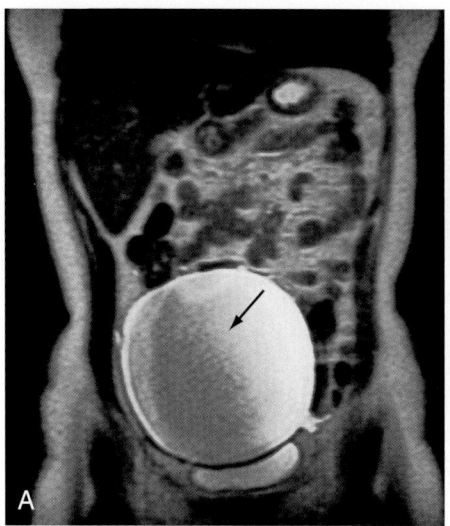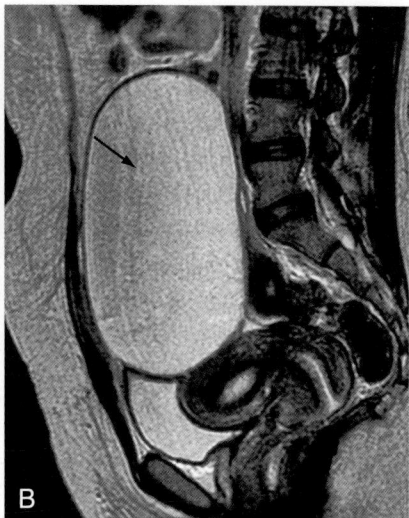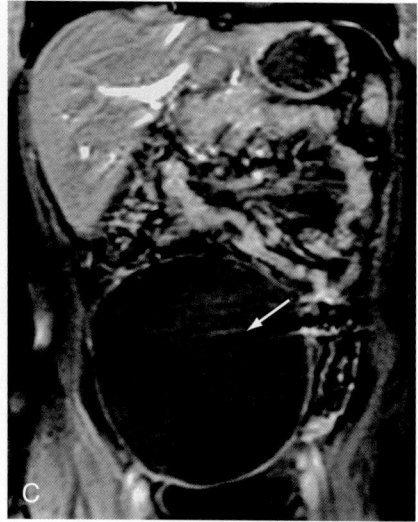

FIGURE 85-87

Mesenteric cyst. Axial (**A**) and coronal (**B**) T2-weighted images depict a large simple cystic abdominal mass *(arrows)*. Coronal gadolinium-enhanced spoiled gradient-echo (SGE) image (**C**) confirms the non-enhancing mesenteric cyst *(arrow)*.

pelvis.[182-185] Less commonly, they can occur in the chest wall, retroperitoneum, or within surgical scars. They arise from fascia and muscle aponeurosis. Desmoids can occur in isolation, but in 45% of cases they are associated with Gardner syndrome. Although desmoids are benign tumors without metastatic potential, they are locally invasive and aggressive neoplasms with a high recurrence rate of up to 45%.[182] As intra-abdominal desmoids slowly enlarge, they compress adjacent organs eventually leading to bowel obstruction and/or hydronephrosis. Treatment is by surgical resection.

MRI of Intra-Abdominal Desmoids

MRI of intra-abdominal desmoids is useful to depict the location and extent of the tumor. A desmoid is a solid mass that may be sharply circumscribed (Fig. 85-89) or ill defined and infiltrative. Chronic desmoids will be hypointense on T1-weighted and T2-weighted images, and will show little enhancement with gadolinium. Acute phase desmoids will show areas of increased signal intensity on T2-weighted images and will show heterogeneous slow enhancement with gadolinium chelates.

INFLAMMATION

Pancreatitis

In acute pancreatitis, extra-pancreatic fluid collections and inflammation may extend from the retroperitoneum into the peritoneal cavity. Inferior extension often involves the transverse mesocolon and small bowel mesentery. Superiorly the inflammation may involve the hepatoduodenal ligament and lesser omentum to reach the porta hepatis and liver. Associated pancreatic

ascites within the peritoneal cavity is commonly depicted. The exudative ascites produces a chemical peritonitis shown as abnormal peritoneal enhancement on gadolinium-enhanced MR images (Fig. 85-90). Fluid also commonly accumulates around the gallbladder with abnormal enhancement of the gallbladder wall. Lesser sac fluid collections are depicted interposed between the pancreas and stomach.

Extra-pancreatic fluid collections may form pseudocysts with well-defined, loculated collections of fluids within the retroperitoneum or the peritoneal cavity. MRI will show simple pseudocysts as well-defined thin-walled fluid collections. Associated hemorrhage of pseudocysts will be depicted on MR images as fluid with high signal on T1-weighted images. Superimposed infection of a pancreatic pseudocysts or pancreatic abscess will be depicted as a complicated fluid collection with a thick enhancing wall or with thick enhancing septations.

MRI of Pancreatitis

MRI of acute pancreatitis includes routine unenhanced T1-weighted, fat-suppressed T1-weighted, T2-weighted, and fat-suppressed gadolinium-enhanced SGE imaging. An MRCP may also be performed for depiction of the bile ducts, pancreatic duct, and pseudocysts. The extra-pancreatic extension of acute pancreatitis is well depicted on MRI. The coronal and sagittal fat-suppressed gadolinium-enhanced SGE images are particularly useful to show extension of inflammation into the transverse mesocolon and small bowel mesentery (Fig. 85-91). These mesenteries will show infiltration and abnormal enhancement with gadolinium.

Extra-pancreatic fluid collections are shown best on SSRARE images due to their intrinsic high signal

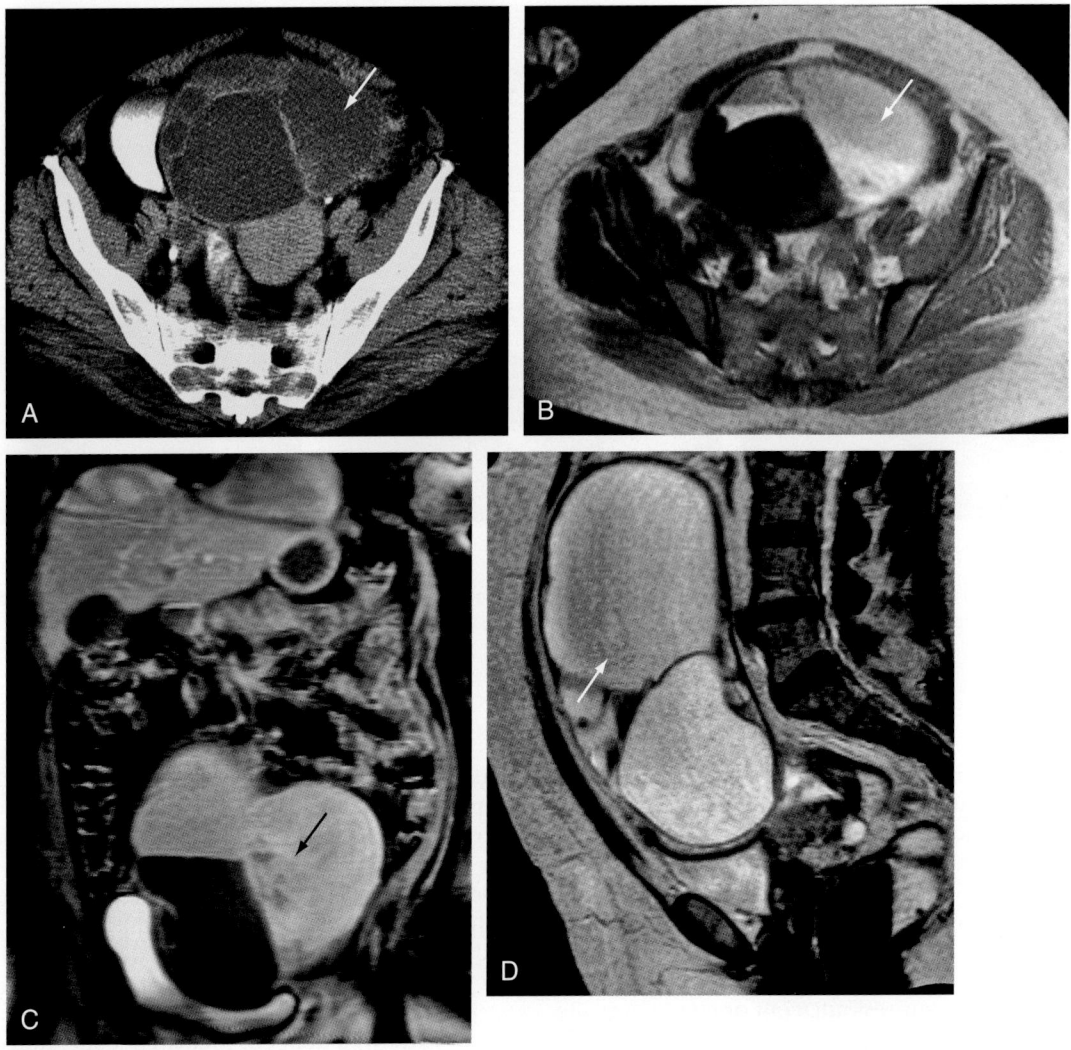

FIGURE 85-88

Endometrioma. Helical CT scan (**A**) shows a complex cystic pelvic mass *(arrow)* that is incompletely characterized. Axial T1-weighted MR image (**B**) shows the complex mass *(arrow)* with areas of high and low signal intensity. Coronal fat-suppressed gadolinium-enhanced spoiled gradient-echo (SGE) image (**C**) shows the high signal intensity methemoglobin *(arrow)*. Sagittal T2-weighted MR image (**D**) shows the complex cystic hemorrhagic mass *(arrow)* representing an endometriomas.

intensity. An MRCP can also be useful to depict extra-pancreatic pseudocysts (Fig. 85-92). In patients with acute pancreatitis, the additional extra-pancreatic fluid and inflammation may obscure detail on an MRCP. The presence of pancreatic ascites and associated chemical peritonitis is shown on fat-suppressed gadolinium-enhanced SGE images. On these images, the ascites does not enhance, while the adjacent inflamed peritoneum, mesenteries, and gallbladder wall will show abnormal enhancement. Bowel serosal inflammation is commonly seen involving the duodenum with mural thickening and enhancement. In more extensive cases of acute pancreatitis, jejunal, ileal, and colonic serosal inflammation will also be depicted on fat-suppressed gadolinium-enhanced images.

Mesenteric Panniculitis

Mesenteric panniculitis is an inflammatory and fibrotic disease involving the fatty tissues of the mesentery. Histopathologically, one sees a combination of mesenteric fibrosis, inflammation, and fat necrosis.[186-189] The term *retractile mesenteritis* has been used when the fibrotic reaction predominates. *Mesenteric lipodystrophy* is the term used when the mesenteric fat necrosis is the predominant feature. Mesenteric panniculitis is usually idiopathic. The clinical presentation includes long-standing abdominal pain, nausea, vomiting, fever, and weight loss. The small-bowel mesentery is involved most frequently by a solitary large dominant mass averaging 10 cm in diameter.[186] Less commonly, one may see

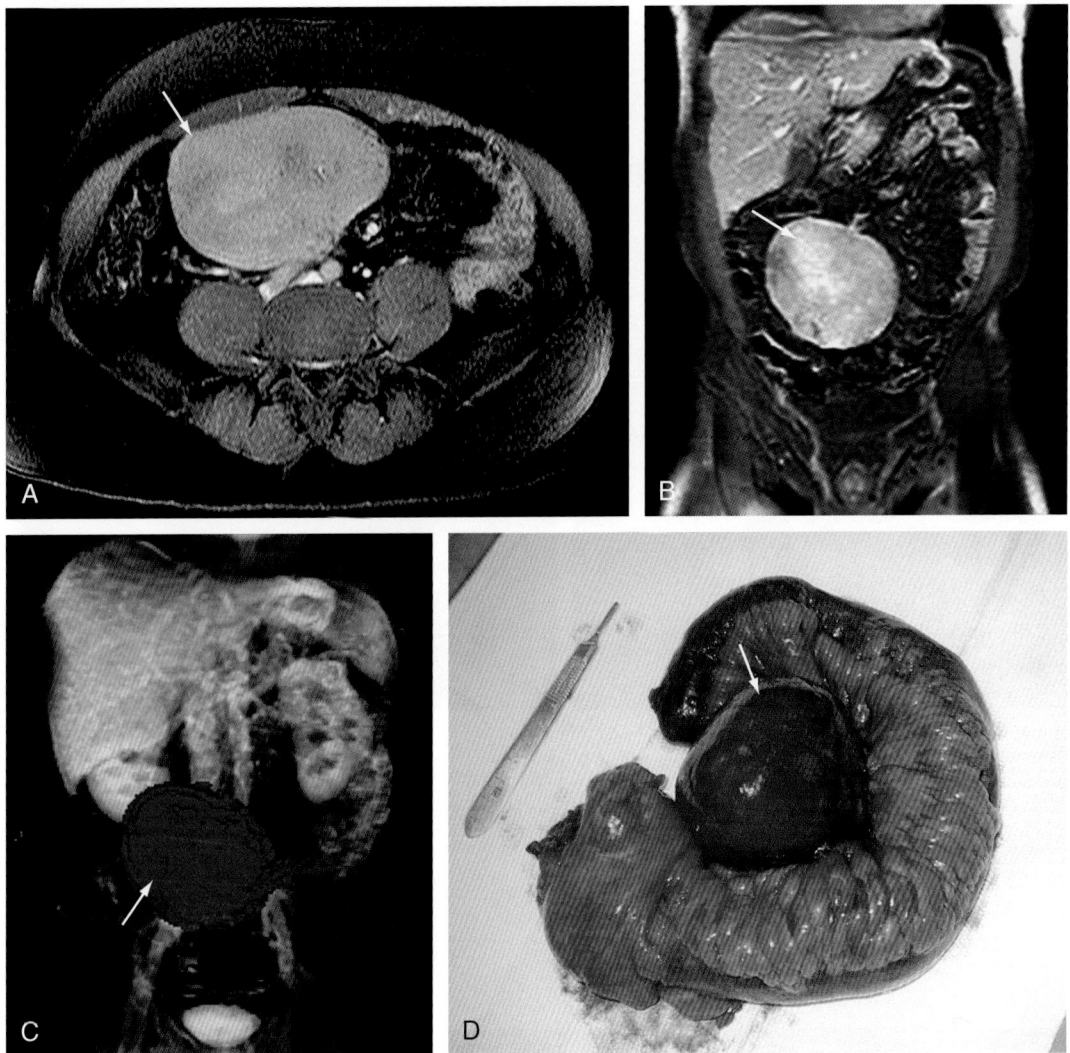

FIGURE 85-89

Desmoid. Axial (**A**) and coronal (**B**) fat-suppressed gadolinium-enhanced spoiled gradient-echo (SGE) images demonstrate a large, sharply circumscribed abdominal mass *(arrow)*, centered in the small bowel mesentery. Color volume 3D model of the mass (**C**) generated from the MR images shows the relationship of the mass *(arrow)* to adjacent abdominal and pelvic organs. Surgical specimen (**D**) depicts the mesenteric desmoid tumor *(arrow)*.

multiple smaller mesenteric masses or diffuse mesenteric thickening. Other inflammatory and infectious diseases can lead to mesenteric inflammation and retractile mesenteritis.

MRI of Mesenteric Panniculitis

MRI may demonstrate single or multiple enhancing soft tissue masses in the small-bowel mesentery with tethering and distortion of adjacent bowel loops. The mass may contain regions of fat, demonstrated as high signal on T1-weighted images or as areas of low signal on fat-suppressed images. In the diffuse form of mesenteric panniculitis one will see ill-defined areas of soft tissue infiltration of the mesentery representing inflammation

and fibrosis. (Fig. 85-93) On T1-weighted MR images, this will be depicted as low signal intensity strands infiltrating the small-bowel mesentery. On fat-suppressed gadolinium-enhanced images, the mesentery will be infiltrated with enhancing soft tissue.

Mesenteric Adenitis

Mesenteric adenitis is an uncommon inflammatory process involving the mesenteric lymph nodes. It most commonly involves the lymph nodes near the terminal ileum and is, therefore, often misdiagnosed as acute appendicitis. It is a self-limited disease that presents with right lower quadrant abdominal pain, nausea, vomiting, fever, and occasionally diarrhea.

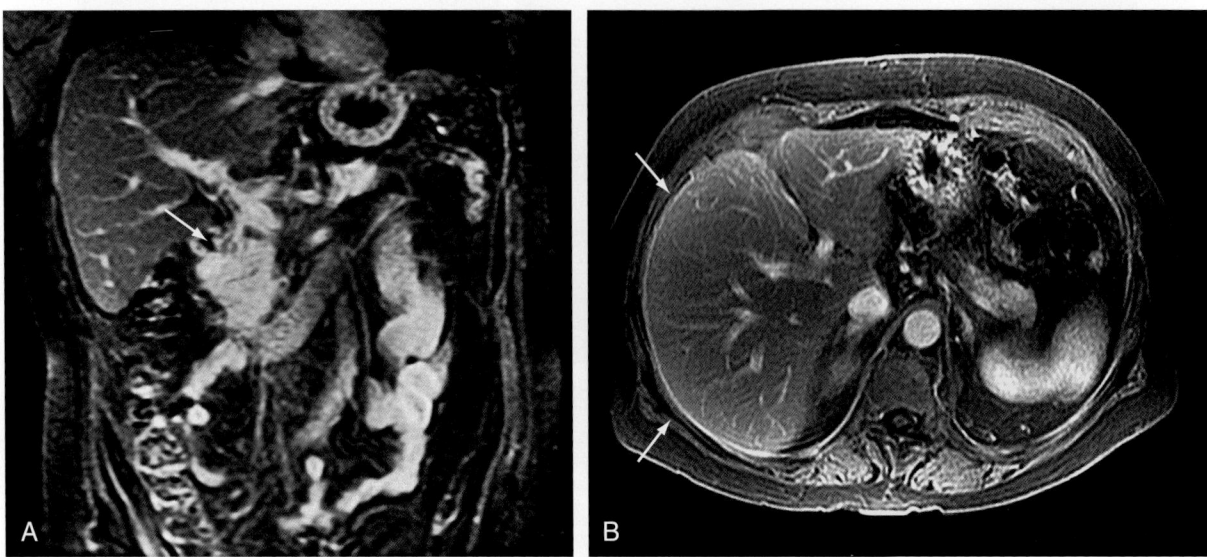

FIGURE 85-90

Mild pancreatitis. Coronal gadolinium-enhanced spoiled gradient-echo (SGE) image (**A**) shows mild focal enlargement of the pancreatic head (*arrow*) in a patient with clinical pancreatitis. Axial gadolinium-enhanced image (**B**) shows chemical peritonitis with a abnormal enhancement (*arrows*) of the perihepatic peritoneum.

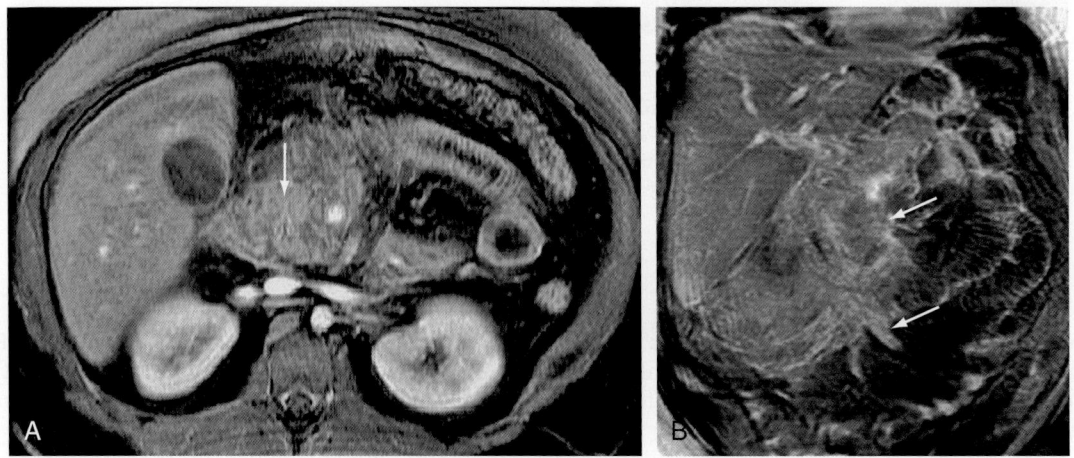

FIGURE 85-91

Severe pancreatitis. Axial gadolinium-enhanced spoiled gradient-echo (SGE) image (**A**) shows findings of acute pancreatitis with enlargement of the pancreatic head (*arrow*) and infiltration of the peripancreatic fat. Coronal image (**B**) shows inferior extension of the inflammatory process with marked infiltration and enhancement of the small-bowel mesentery (*arrows*).

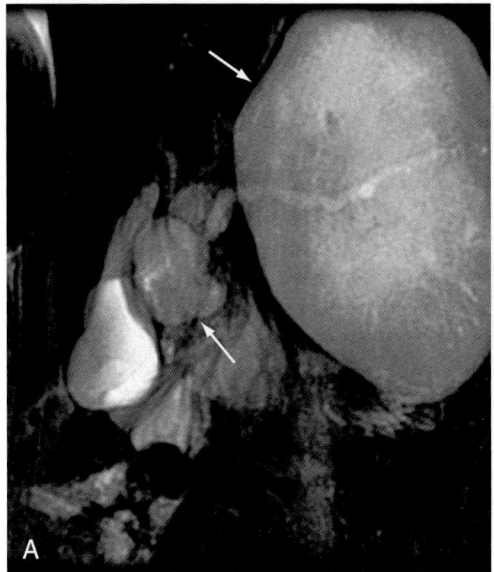
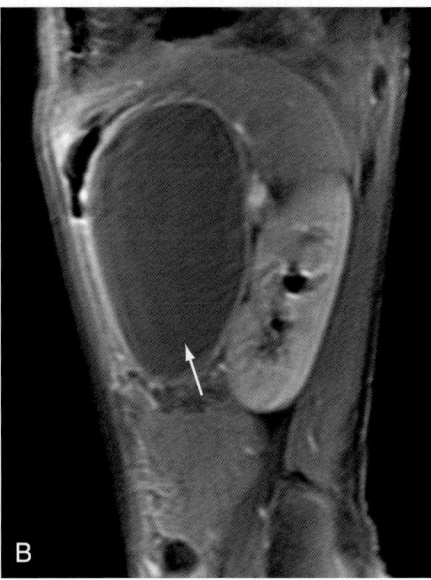

FIGURE 85-92

Pancreatic pseudocysts. MR cholangi-opancreaticography (MRCP) image (**A**) and sagittal gadolinium-enhanced SGE (**B**) MR images depict two traumatic pseudocysts (arrows). The larger pseudocyst is located in the lesser sac.

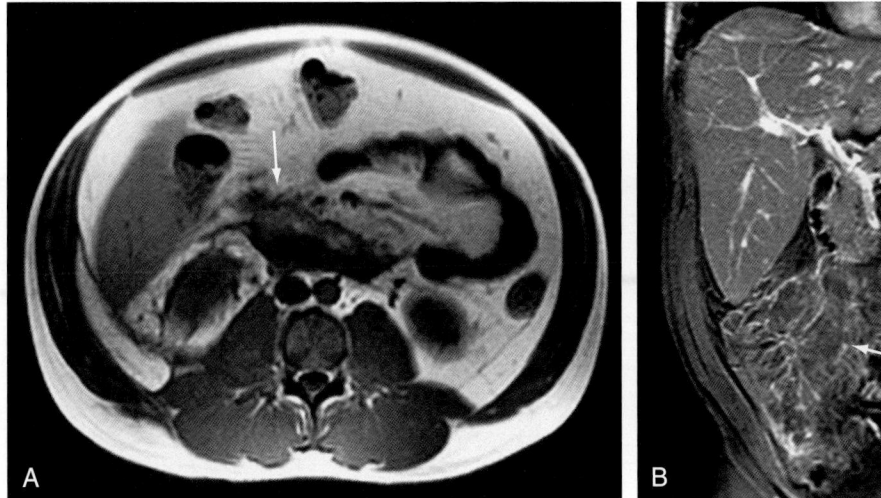

FIGURE 85-93

Mesenteric panniculitis. Axial T1-weighted (**A**) and coronal, fat-suppressed gadolinium-enhanced spoiled gradient-echo (SGE) image (**B**) demonstrate abnormal diffuse infiltration and enhancement of the small-bowel mesentery (arrows).

MRI of Mesenteric Adenitis

The MR features of mesenteric adenitis include enlarged mesenteric lymph nodes in the right lower quadrant. Strandy infiltration and enhancement of the adjacent mesentery may also be seen. Absence of an enlarged and inflamed appendix excludes the diagnosis of acute appendicitis.

Peritonitis

Peritonitis is an inflammation of the peritoneal lining of the abdomen cavity.[190,191] Peritonitis may be spontaneous, secondary, or a complication of catheter peritoneal dialysis. Spontaneous bacterial peritonitis is seen in patients with chronic liver disease or renal failure in which ascites accumulates in the peritoneal cavity. Infection of the ascitic fluid may occur as a result of hematogenously borne bacteria that spread to the peritoneal cavity (Fig. 85-94). Secondary peritonitis may occur as a result of bowel perforation with subsequent leak of intestinal fluids and bacteria into the peritoneal cavity. Causes of secondary peritonitis include a perforated gastric ulcer, perforated appendicitis, and colonic perforation due to an underlying malignancy, or diverticulitis. Bowel perforation as a complication of trauma or surgical intervention may also produce secondary peritonitis. A chemical peritonitis will develop in patients with pancreatitis or a biliary leak due to the release of pancreatic enzymes or bile into the peritoneal cavity. Dialysis-associated peritonitis occurs from skin bacteria that are introduced into the peritoneal cavity by the dialysis catheter (Fig. 85-95).

Autoimmune diseases such as lupus erythematosus can develop a diffuse serositis and associated peritonitis (Fig. 85-96).

Patients with peritonitis present with abdominal pain and tenderness, distension, nausea, vomiting, fever, chills, and leukocytosis. Due to the nonspecific nature of these symptoms, patients with peritonitis may be misdiagnosed with other infectious or inflammatory abdominal diseases (Fig. 85-97). Complications of peritonitis include development of an intra-abdominal abscess and sepsis. Treatment will depend upon the cause of the peritonitis. Intravenous antibiotics are used to control the bacterial infection. Secondary peritonitis due to bowel perforation will require laparotomy and bowel resection. Chemical peritonitis due to a biliary leak is treated by placement of a biliary stent or surgical intervention. In the setting of dialysis-associated peritonitis, the infected dialysis catheter is removed with subsequent antibiotic therapy.

MRI of Peritonitis

MRI is an effective and very sensitive examination in patients with suspected peritonitis.[190,191] Compared with helical CT, gadolinium-enhanced MRI is superior for depicting the changes of peritonitis. Inflammation of the peritoneum leads to increased vascularity and subsequent abnormal enhancement with intravenous gadolinium. As with peritoneal carcinomatosis, peritonitis shows slow gradual enhancement of the peritoneum. For this reason, the findings of peritonitis are most evident on delayed gadolinium-enhanced SGE images. The presence of delayed enhancement of ascitic fluid has been noted in patients with peritoneal disease.

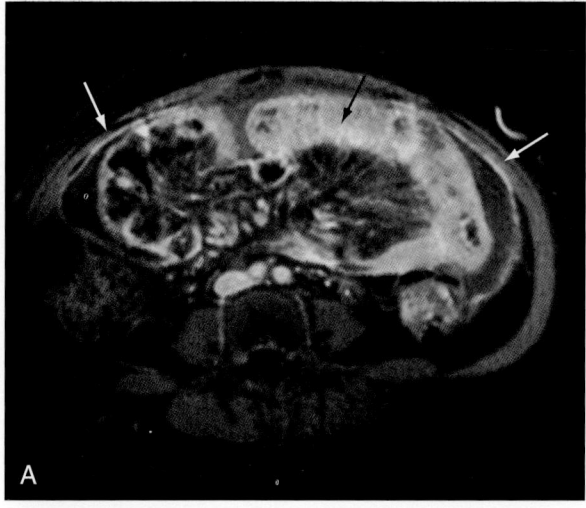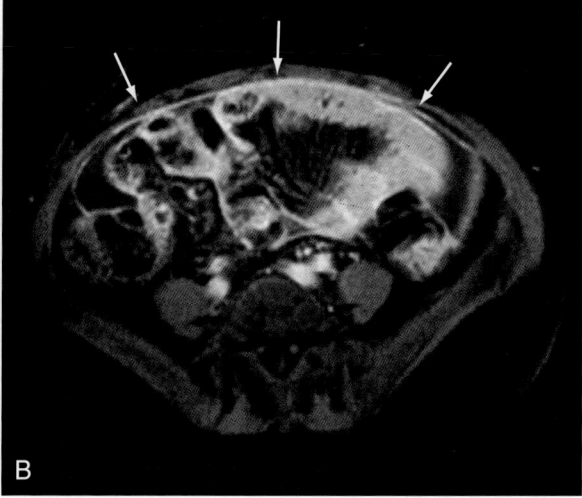

FIGURE 85-94

Bacterial peritonitis. Axial gadolinium enhanced spoiled gradient-echo (SGE) images through the lower abdomen (**A**) and pelvis (**B**) show diffuse marked peritoneal (*white arrows*) and serosal (*black arrow*) enhancement in this patient with pseudomonas peritonitis.

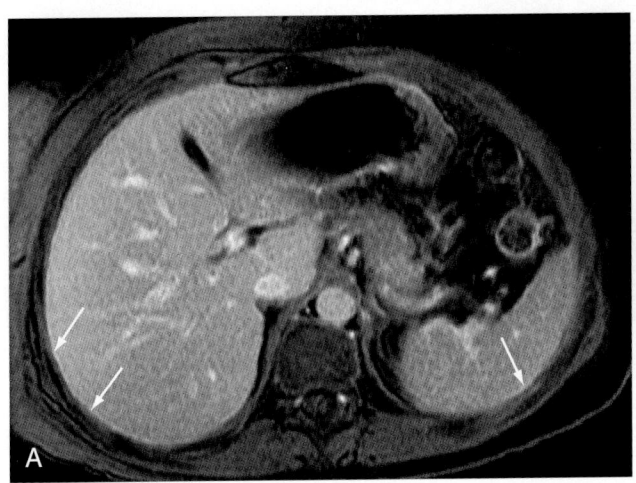
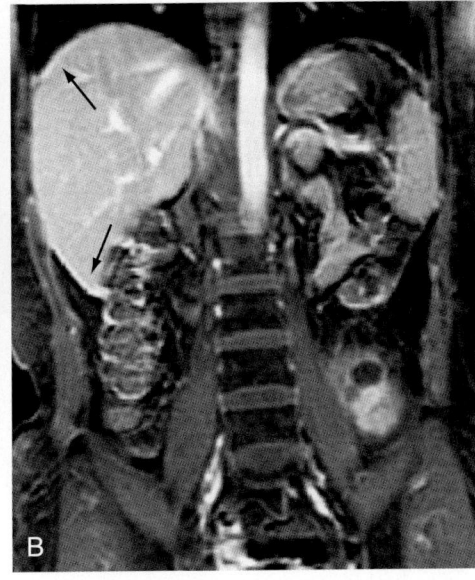

FIGURE 85-95

Dialysis peritonitis. Axial (**A**) and coronal (**B**) fat-suppressed gadolinium-enhanced spoiled gradient-echo (SGE) images demonstrate moderate abnormal peritoneal enhancement *(arrows)* in this dialysis patient presenting with abdominal pain and fever. The changes of dialysis-related peritonitis can be very subtle.

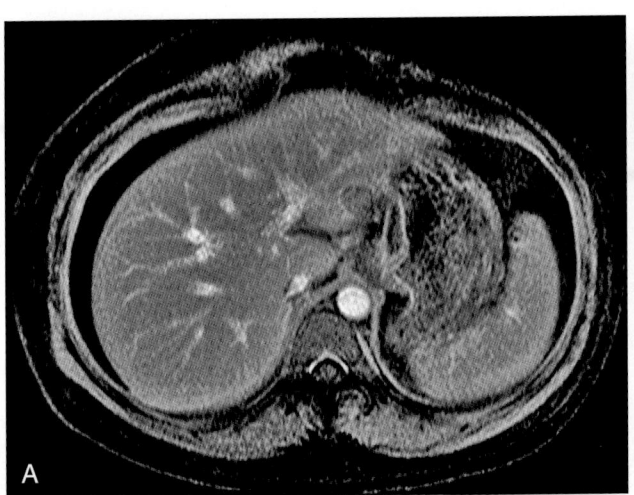
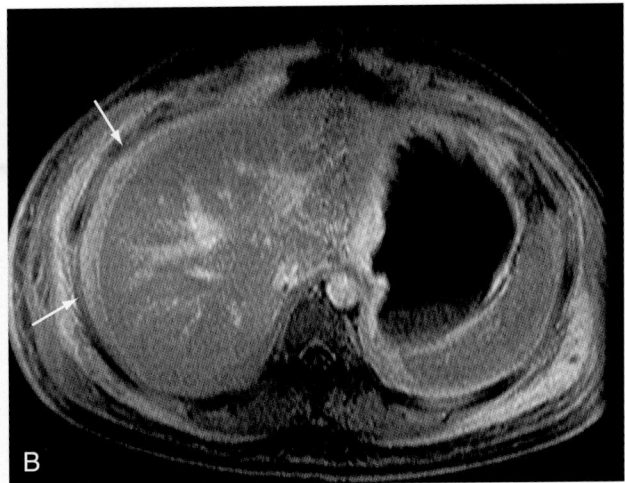

FIGURE 85-96

Lupus peritonitis. Immediate (**A**) and delayed (**B**) gadolinium-enhanced images in a patient with systemic lupus erythematosus. The immediate image (**A**) shows ascites, while the delayed image (**B**) shows marked diffuse enhancement of ascites and peritoneum *(arrows)*.

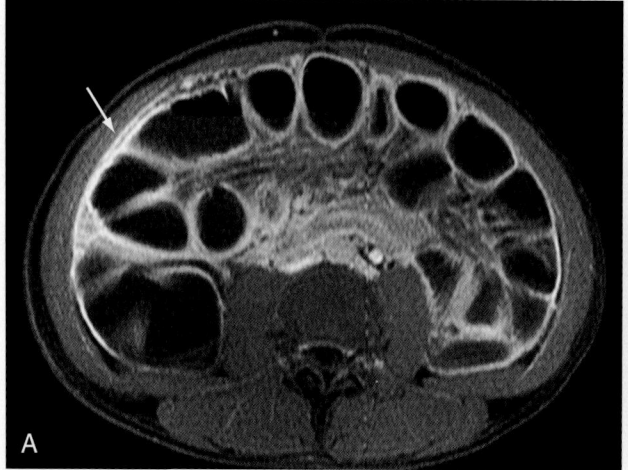

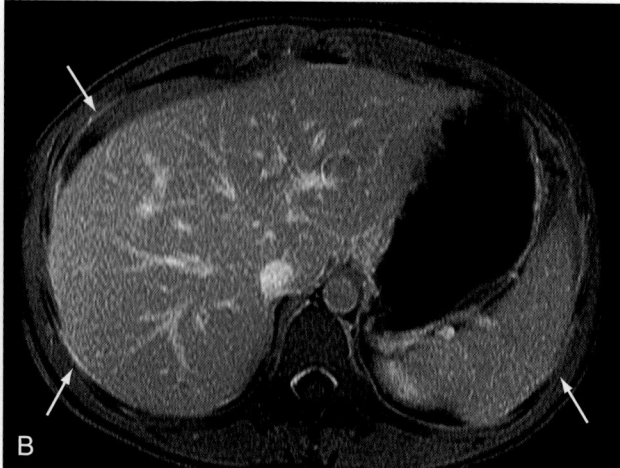

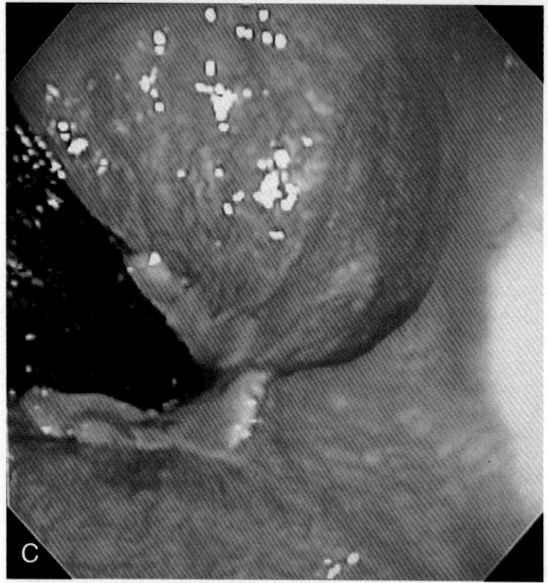

FIGURE 85-97

A 19-year-old with abdominal pain was referred for MRI after helical CT scan suggested Crohn's disease of the terminal ileum. Axial fat-suppressed gadolinium-enhanced spoiled gradient-echo (SGE) images through the middle abdomen (**A**) and liver (**B**) show normal bowel wall with abnormal peritoneal enhancement (*arrow*) indicating peritonitis. Colonoscopy (**C**) was performed, which confirmed normal appearance of the mucosa in the terminal ileum. Peritonitis was confirmed and the patient's symptoms responded to antibiotics.

Kanematsu et al[190] noted delayed gadolinium enhancement of ascites in spontaneous bacterial peritonitis. Other authors have noted that delayed enhancement of ascites on MRI is a nonspecific finding that correlates with the presence of exudative ascites and increased peritoneal permeability, which may be due to benign or malignant peritoneal disease.[191]

Fat suppression is used to eliminate the competing high signal of adjacent abdominal or pelvic fat. On these gadolinium-enhanced images, one may see abnormal peritoneal enhancement with peritoneal thickening. In some mild cases of peritonitis, the abnormally enhancing peritoneum may be normal in thickness. In my experience, the degree of thickening of the peritoneum with peritonitis is less than that often seen with peritoneal tumor. Also the peritoneum tends to be smoothly thickened without the nodular thickening and peritoneal masses seen with carcinomatosis. Fat-suppressed T2-weighted images or SSRARE images are also useful to depict associated ascites. In order to

depict serosal inflammation, the addition of oral contrast material can be used to distend and separate loops of intestine.

Tuberculous Peritonitis

Peritoneal involvement by tuberculosis may rarely occur in isolation, but, more commonly, it is present in association with GI tuberculosis[192-194] (Fig. 85-98). Three forms of tuberculous peritonitis have been described[193]: 1. The wet type is characterized by large volume ascites and is the most common form. 2. The fibrotic-mixed type is characterized by large omental masses, with matted intestines and mesentery. 3. The dry or plastic type is uncommon and is characterized by caseous nodules and fibrous peritoneal reaction. This latter form is indistinguishable from peritoneal carcinomatosis. Features that favor the presence of tuberculous peritonitis include the presence of associated

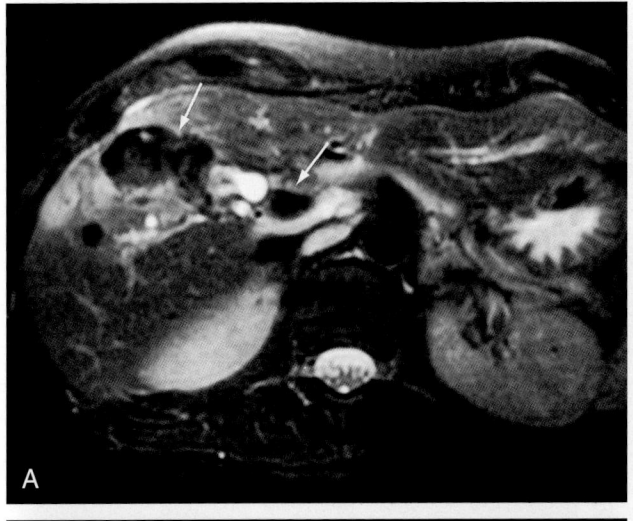

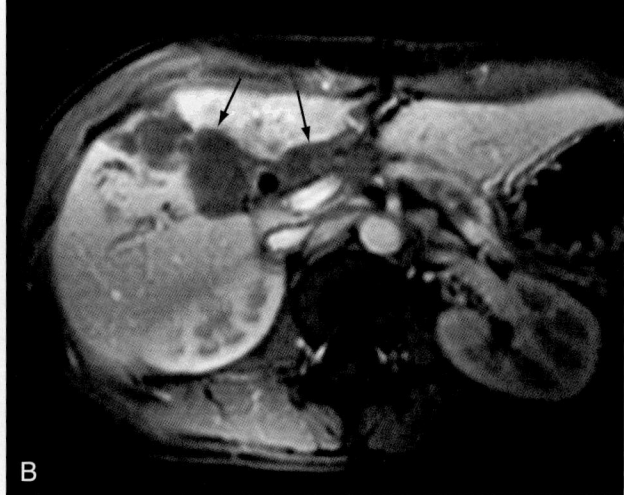

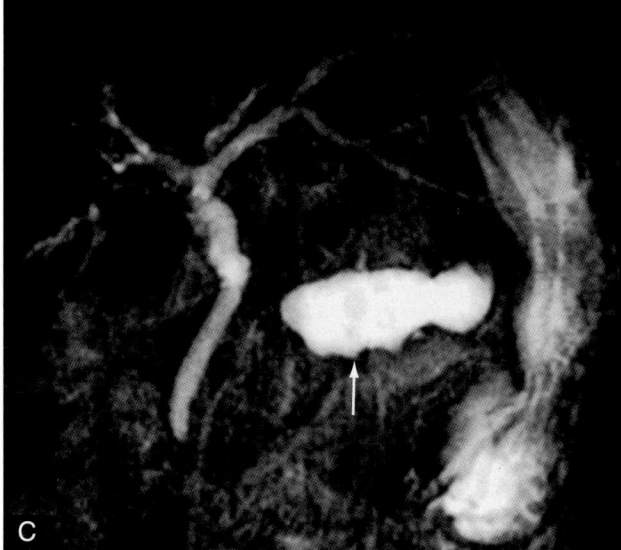

FIGURE 85-98

Abdominal tuberculosis. T2-weighted (**A**) and gadolinium-enhanced spoiled gradient-echo (SGE) (**B**) images depict calcified intraperitoneal masses (arrows) in the porta hepatis and main interlobar fissure. MR cholangiopancreaticography (MRCP) image (**C**) shows marked dilatation of the pancreatic duct (arrow) from associated pancreatic duct obstruction. Abdominal tuberculosis with intraperitoneal tuberculomas was confirmed.

abdominal and retroperitoneal tuberculous lymphadenitis. Nodal masses will show peripheral enhancement with low signal intensity centers on gadolinium enhanced MRI. This appearance is due to lymph nodes with peripheral inflammation and central caseous necrosis and corresponds with the low-density lymph nodes seen on helical CT in patients with abdominal tuberculosis. Other authors have noted mass-like cystic lesions in patients with tuberculous lymphadenitis.[194] Inflammation that extends through the peritoneum to involve the abdominal wall has also been described as a feature of abdominal tuberculosis.

Intra-Abdominal Abscess

An intra-abdominal abscess is an infected localized collection of fluid within the abdominal cavity.[195,196] It may arise in any of the abdominal and pelvic organs with subsequent spread to the peritoneal cavity. Inflammatory diseases arising in the liver, biliary tree, pancreas,

GI tract, bladder, gynecologic organs, or peritoneum may extend outside of the organ with development of an intra-abdominal abscess. Possible causes include appendicitis, diverticulitis (Fig. 85-99), peptic ulcer disease, inflammatory bowel disease, infectious enteritis, bowel perforation, cholecystitis, pancreatitis, or peritonitis. An intra-abdominal abscess may also be seen as a complication of malignancy, trauma, as a postsurgical complication (Fig. 85-100), or in the setting of a retained foreign body (Fig. 85-101).

The clinical presentation of a patient with an intra-abdominal abscess includes abdominal pain, tenderness, nausea, vomiting, fever, and leukocytosis. Treatment is percutaneous or surgical drainage of the abscess followed by antibiotic therapy.

MRI of an Intra-Abdominal Abscess

MRI of an intra-abdominal abscess will demonstrate a localized fluid collection that has a low signal intensity on T1-weighted images and may show homogeneous or

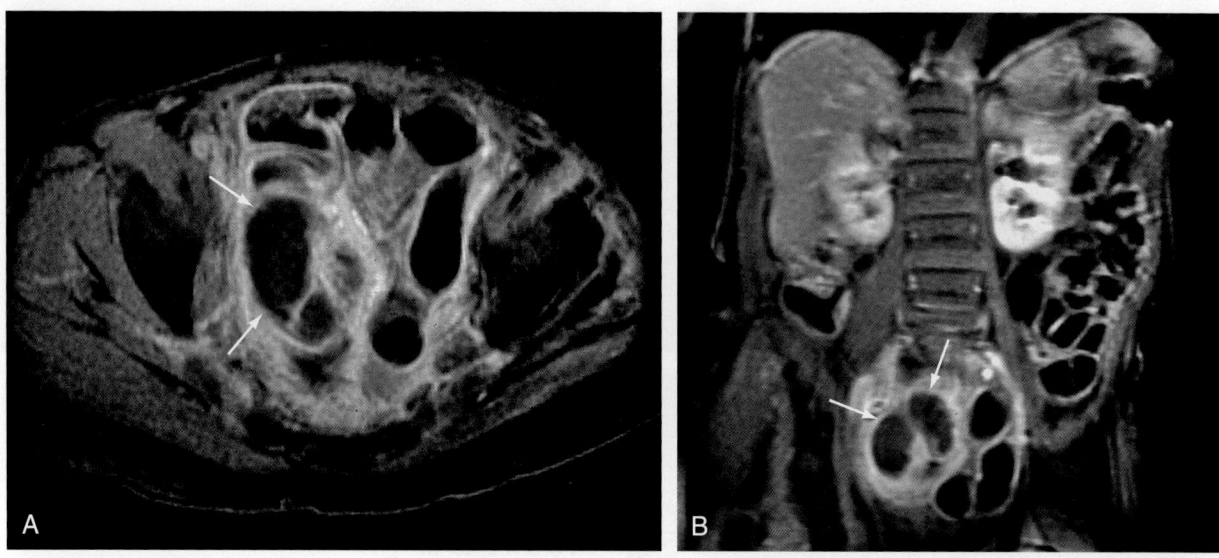

FIGURE 85-99

Diverticular abscess. Axial (**A**) and coronal (**B**) fat-suppressed gadolinium-enhanced spoiled gradient-echo (SGE) images demonstrate a complex pelvic mass *(arrows)* representing an abscess in this patient with diverticulitis. The wall and septations within the abscess show marked enhancement with gadolinium.

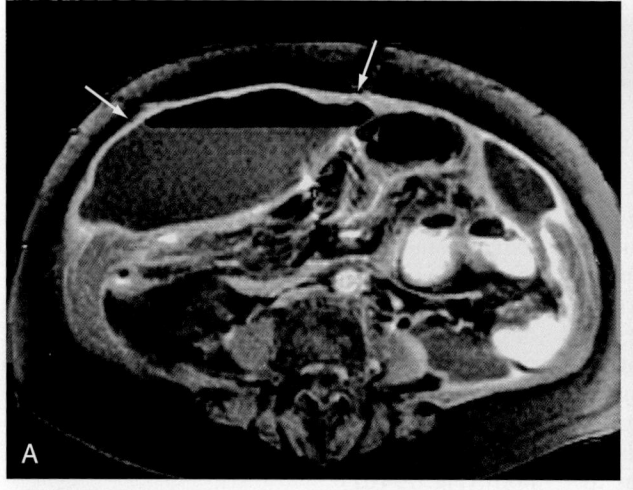

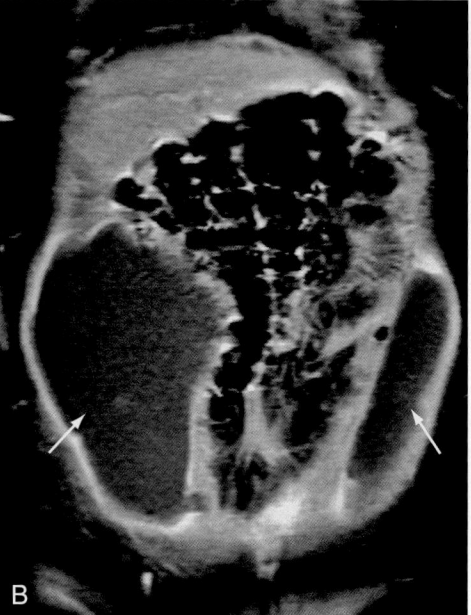

FIGURE 85-100

Postoperative intra-abdominal abscess. Axial (**A**) and coronal (**B**) gadolinium enhanced spoiled gradient-echo (SGE) images show a large intra abdominal abscess *(arrows)* with an air-fluid level. Note the non-enhancing liquefied portion of the abscess and the enhancing surrounding abscess wall.

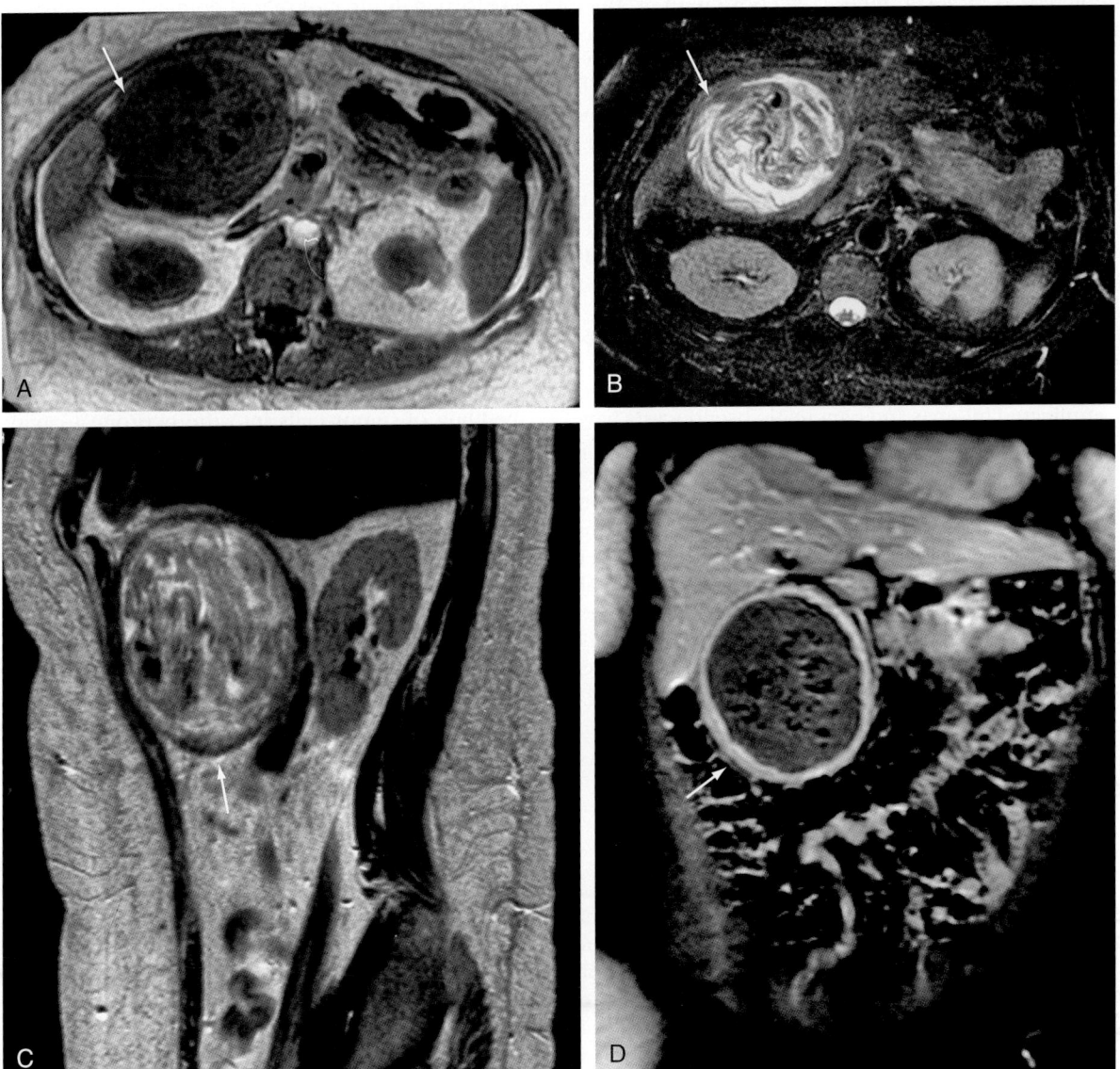

FIGURE 85-101

Intra-abdominal abscess from a retained foreign body. Axial T1-weighted (**A**) and fat-suppressed T2-weighted (**B**) MR images depict a large complex fluid collection *(arrow)* in the right middle abdomen. The location of the mass *(arrow)* is well depicted on sagittal T2-weighted (**C**) and coronal gadolinium-enhanced (**D**) images. The internal matrix within the abscess cavity represents a retained lap sponge.

heterogeneous increased signal intensity on T2-weighted images.[195,196] In an evaluation of 67 patients with suspected intra-abdominal abscess, Noone et al[195] found that fat-suppressed gadolinium-enhanced MR images were most useful. On gadolinium-enhanced images an abscess is depicted as a focal fluid collection with a thick enhancing rim. The central portion of the abscess does not enhance, while the surrounding soft tissue rim shows marked enhancement with gadolinium. Noone et al[195] found that MRI has high diagnostic accuracy in the evaluation of acute intraperitoneal abscesses with 100% sensitivity, 94% specificity, and 96% accuracy.

The degree of enhancement of the abscess wall is typically more marked than is seen with helical CT scanning. On MRI, associated inflammation of the adjacent peritoneum and bowel is seen with thickening and abnormal enhancement of these tissues.

Differential considerations include a sterile loculated fluid collection, a biloma, pancreatic pseudocysts, and a liquefying intra-abdominal hematoma. In my experience, uncomplicated bilomas and pancreatic pseudocysts have thin walls, unlike an abscess, which is thick walled. A liquefying hematoma, however, often has an appearance very similar to an abscess. A hematoma may show a non-enhancing center surrounded by an irregular enhancing rim of soft tissue. A clue to the correct diagnosis is often found on the T1-weighted images that can show high signal from methemoglobin in a subacute hemorrhage. The similar appearance between an abscess and a liquefying hematoma on the gadolinium-enhanced images should be kept in mind.

MALIGNANT DISEASES

Mesothelioma

Mesothelioma is a rare tumor that can affect the pleura, pericardium, or peritoneal surfaces of the abdomen and pelvis.[197-200] They may be benign or malignant. Mesotheliomas are associated with asbestos exposure, with a long latency period of several decades between the exposure and the development of the malignant tumor. Pleural involvement by mesothelioma is more frequent, however, peritoneal involvement by mesothelioma is seen in between one fifth and one third of cases of mesothelioma. The incidence of peritoneal mesothelioma is one per 1,000,000. Presenting symptoms include abdominal pain (60%), anorexia (27%), weakness (12%), and nausea (11%). Two patterns of clinical presentation have been described. Either patients present with abdominal pain from a large tumor mass without ascites or they present with painless abdominal distention from large volume ascites. Bowel obstruction is a common complication. Traditionally, mesotheliomas have been treated with a combination of surgical cytoreduction, chemotherapy, and radiation therapy. The role of other treatments for peritoneal mesothelioma including heated intraperitoneal chemotherapy and immunotherapy is being evaluated.

MRI of Mesothelioma

On MRI, peritoneal mesothelioma may be depicted as abnormal peritoneal thickening and enhancement with or without associated ascites. Later in the course of the disease, single or multiple abdominal and pelvic tumor masses will be demonstrated involving the peritoneum, omentum, or mesentery. With complicating bowel obstruction, MR images will show focally dilated loops of bowel and an obstructing tumor mass. A desmoplastic effect with encasement of bowel and mesenteric vessels has also been described with peritoneal mesotheliomas involving the mesentery.

Peritoneal Metastases

The extensive surface area of the peritoneum can be involved by metastases from numerous primary tumors. The peritoneum is most commonly involved by direct shedding of tumor cells into the peritoneal cavity as is seen in ovarian cancer. However, other extra-abdominal tumors can metastasize hematogenously with spread to the peritoneal surfaces of the abdomen and pelvis. Finally, lymphatic dissemination to involve the mesentery commonly occurs in non-Hodgkin's lymphoma.

Intraperitoneal Seeding

Tumors that spread by shedding tumor cells into the peritoneal cavity include gynecologic and GI malignancies, including tumors arising in the stomach, colon, ovary, pancreas, and endometrium (SCOPE). Once the tumor cells gain access to the peritoneal cavity, they will spread according to the patterns of the flow of ascites described by Myers. The transverse mesocolon, small-bowel mesentery, sigmoid mesocolon, and peritoneal attachments of the ascending and descending colon direct the flow of ascites. For ovarian cancer, tumor cells arising in the pelvis spread to the mid and upper abdomen via the right paracolic gutter. The phrenico-colic ligament blocks the flow of ascites up the smaller left paracolic gutter. Subsequent involvement of the right subhepatic space and right subphrenic space is commonly seen. Due to the effects of gravity, tumor cells will predictably deposit in dependent recesses defined by peritoneal reflections and mesenteries. These common sites of tumor deposition include the pouch of Douglas in the pelvis, the lower small-bowel mesentery at the terminal ileum and cecum in the right lower quadrant, the superior surface of the sigmoid colon, and the right subphrenic space.

Ovarian Cancer

Ovarian cancer is the fifth most common malignancy among women. The American Cancer Society estimates that there will be 25,400 new cases of ovarian cancer diagnosed in the United States in 2003. Ovarian cancer is the fifth leading cause of cancer-related deaths with

24,300 deaths in 2003. It is the leading cause of deaths from gynecologic malignancies.[201-204]

The overall prognosis for women with ovarian cancer is related to the tumor stage at the time of diagnosis. Patients with Stage I ovarian cancer, which is confined to the ovary at the time of diagnosis, have a 5-year survival rate of 95%. Unfortunately, 60% to 70% of patients have widespread abdominal metastases at the time of diagnosis with Stage III or IV disease. Ovarian cancer tumor cells shed into the peritoneal cavity and spread via intraperitoneal dissemination. This insidious tumor spread is clinically silent. Late stage presentation is with nonspecific symptoms such as abdominal distention or pain, bloating, indigestion, cramps, pelvic pain, loss of appetite, change in bowel or bladder habits, or change in weight. Other factors that negatively affect prognosis in ovarian cancer include the presence of ascites, poorly differentiated tumor, mucinous and clear cell histology, and inadequate debulking following initial surgical cytoreduction.

Risk factors for ovarian cancer include patient age; the mean age at the time of initial diagnosis of sporadic ovarian cancer is 61 years. The next most important risk factor is a family history of ovarian cancer, particularly a close family member (mother, sister, or daughter), who is diagnosed with ovarian cancer at an early age. It is estimated that 7% to 10% of ovarian cancers occur as the result of a hereditary genetic syndrome. There are three genetic syndromes that can lead to an increased risk of developing ovarian cancer: 1. ovarian cancer associated with colon and endometrial cancer called hereditary nonpolyposis colorectal cancer syndrome (HNPCC); 2. breast and ovarian cancer syndrome that is associated with mutations in the *BRCA1* or *BRCA2* genes; and 3. site-specific ovarian cancer syndrome that produces an increased risk for ovarian cancer alone.[202]

Staging and Histopathology

The staging of ovarian cancer is based upon surgical and imaging findings that describe the location of the tumor (Box 85-5). In summary, Stage I cancers are confined to one or both ovaries. Stage II cancers have spread beyond the ovary but are confined to the pelvis. Stage III cancers have spread into the abdomen via intraperitoneal dissemination or via lymphatics with nodal metastases. Stage IV cancers have distant metastases to other organs including the liver, lungs, and brain.

Ninety percent of ovarian cancers arise from the surface epithelium of the ovary (Fig. 85-102). Five percent of ovarian cancers arise from the germ cells that produce ova, and 5% arise from the ovarian stromal tissues. Epithelial ovarian cancers are those that spread by intraperitoneal tumor dissemination. Cellular classification divides ovarian cancers into 1. serous; 2. mucinous; 3. endometrioid; and 4. clear cell histologic classifications.[201]

Box 85-5 | Ovarian Cancer Staging

Stage I

Stage I ovarian cancer is limited to the ovaries.

● Stage IA: Tumor limited to one ovary; capsule intact, no tumor on ovarian surface. No malignant cells in ascites or peritoneal washings.*
● Stage IB: Tumor limited to both ovaries; capsules intact, no tumor on ovarian surface. No malignant cells in ascites or peritoneal washings.*
● Stage IC: Tumor limited to one or both ovaries with any of the following: capsule ruptured, tumor on ovarian surface, malignant cells in ascites or peritoneal washings.*

Stage II

Stage II ovarian cancer is tumor involving one or both ovaries with pelvic extension and/or implants.

● Stage IIA: Extension and/or implants on the uterus and/or fallopian tubes. No malignant cells in ascites or peritoneal washings.*
● Stage IIB: Extension to and/or implants on other pelvic tissues. No malignant cells in ascites or peritoneal washings.*
● Stage IIC: Pelvic extension and/or implants (stage IIA or IIB) with malignant cells in ascites or peritoneal washings.*

Stage III

Stage III ovarian cancer is tumor involving one or both ovaries with microscopically confirmed peritoneal implants outside the pelvis. Superficial liver metastasis equals stage III. Tumor is limited to the true pelvis but with histologically verified malignant extension to small bowel or omentum.

● Stage IIIA: Microscopic peritoneal metastasis beyond pelvis (no macroscopic tumor).
● Stage IIIB: Macroscopic peritoneal metastasis beyond pelvis 2 cm or less in greatest dimension.
● Stage IIIC: Peritoneal metastasis beyond pelvis more than 2 cm in greatest dimension and/or regional lymph node metastasis.

Stage IV

Stage IV ovarian cancer is tumor involving one or both ovaries with distant metastasis. If pleural effusion is present, there must be positive cytologic test results to designate a case to stage IV. Parenchymal liver metastasis equals stage IV.

Note: malignant ascites is not classified. The presence of ascites does not affect staging unless malignant cells are present.

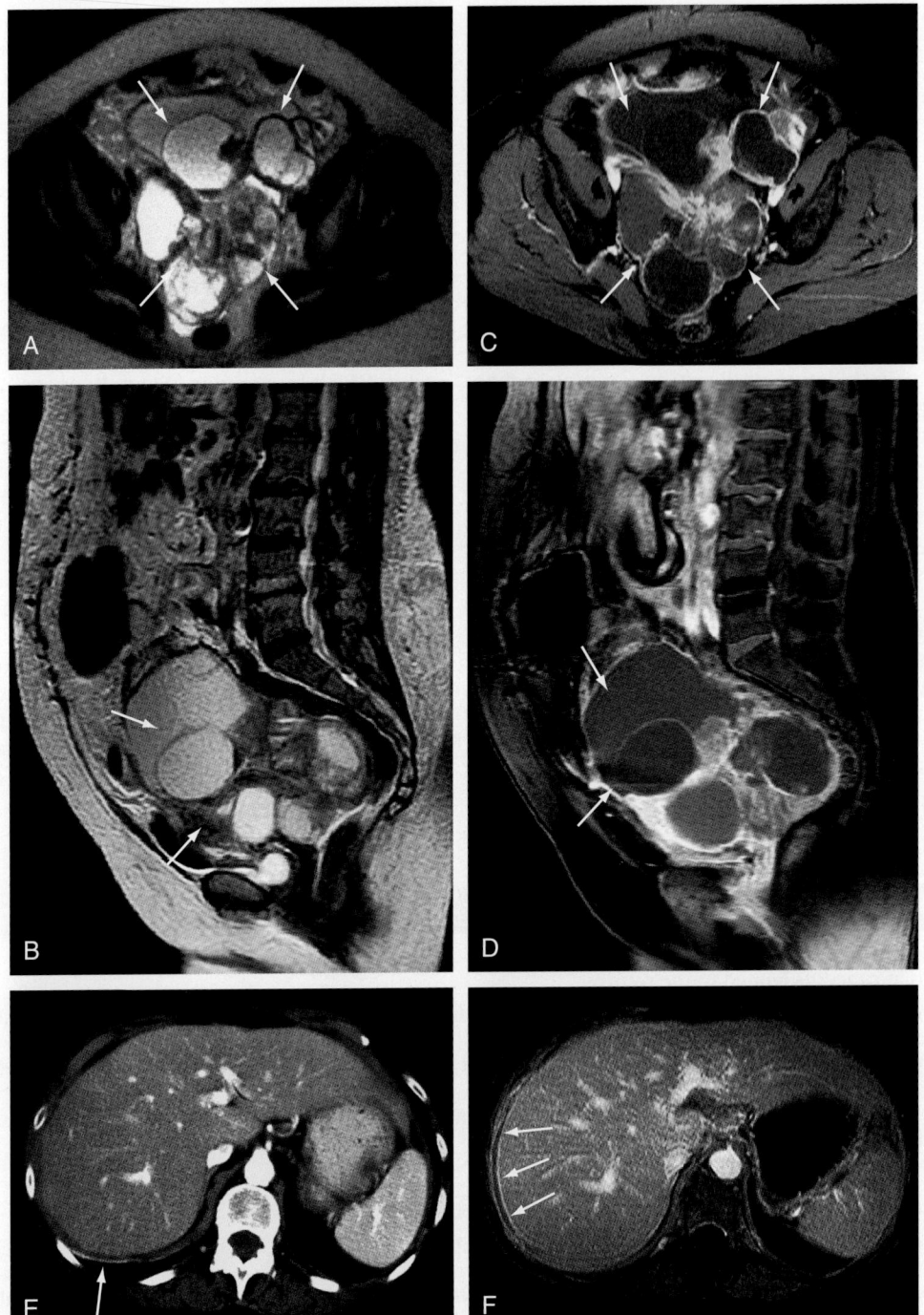

FIGURE 85-102

Primary ovarian cancer. Axial (**A**) and sagittal (**B**) T2-weighted images demonstrate a complex cystic and solid pelvic mass (*arrows*). Axial (**C**) and sagittal (**D**) gadolinium-enhanced images demonstrate the enhancing septations and solid components within the mass (*arrows*). Helical CT (**E**) scan through the upper abdomen in this patient showed perihepatic ascites (*arrow*) without evidence of peritoneal metastases. Delayed gadolinium-enhanced spoiled gradient-echo (SGE) MR image (**F**) shows a thin rim of enhancing right subphrenic parietal and visceral peritoneal tumor (*arrows*). Surgery confirmed Stage III primary epithelial ovarian cancer with spread to the upper abdomen.

Treatment

Stage IA and IB ovarian cancer are treated surgically with total abdominal hysterectomy, bilateral oophorectomy and omentectomy. Peritoneal biopsies and peritoneal washings are obtained. For densely adherent tumor or Stage IC tumor, one may add adjuvant chemotherapy or pelvic radiation, because of the increased incidence of relapse.

Stage II ovarian cancer is treated with hysterectomy, bilateral oophorectomy, omentectomy, and tumor debulking. Surgical cytoreduction is combined with multi drug adjuvant chemotherapy. Combinations of taxol, cisplatin or carboplatin, and cyclophosphamide are commonly utilized.

Stages III and IV ovarian cancer are treated with surgical tumor debulking, with hysterectomy and bilateral oophorectomy. As much of the tumor is removed as is possible at the initial surgical cytoreduction. In patients with large volume peritoneal tumor (>2 cm), surgery may be deferred until after initial rounds of chemotherapy have been performed. In either case, long-term prognosis is directly related to the volume of residual tumor left following surgical debulking. Chemotherapeutic agents are the same as those listed above for Stage II ovarian cancer.

In the past, second-look laparotomy (SLL) was routinely performed after the patient underwent systemic chemotherapy.[205] The role of the SLL was to assess the extent of residual tumor and to perform additional tumor debulking. It was traditionally reserved for patients in complete clinical and imaging remission. Several studies have shown that SLL does not change the long-term outcome of the patient and does not confer a survival benefit when compared with patients who do not undergo SLL.[205] Currently, fewer SLLs are being performed, which increases the importance of accurate cross-sectional imaging.

The role of intraperitoneal chemotherapy in patients with ovarian cancer is reserved for those patients with small volume or microscopic residual tumor following systemic chemotherapy and surgical cytoreduction.

MRI of Ovarian Cancer

Gadolinium-enhanced MRI is useful in women with primary ovarian cancer to characterize the pelvic mass and to detect intraperitoneal abdominal spread[160-172] (see Fig. 85-102). MR is used in patients who have been treated for ovarian cancer to monitor response to therapy by depicting residual peritoneal tumor. Detecting clinically occult tumor is critical in determining appropriate patient management. Following chemotherapy, declining serum cancer antigen 125 (CA 125) values indicated tumor response to treatment. Unfortunately, a normal CA 125 value does not exclude residual tumor, as up to 50% of women with a normal CA 125 value following chemotherapy still have residual tumor.[206,207]

As fewer second-look surgeries are being performed,[205] oncologists depend upon the results of cross-sectional imaging exams to determine clinical response to chemotherapy. In order to establish the accuracy of MRI in depicting tumor in women with treated ovarian cancer a 5-year longitudinal study was performed comparing the results of MRI with serum CA 125 level and physical examination in 69 women with treated ovarian cancer.[161] Gadolinium-enhanced MRI successfully detected clinically occult tumor in women with treated ovarian cancer who were in clinical remission (Fig. 85-103). Twenty-three patients, who were in clinical remission with a normal CA 125 level and physical examination, had residual subclinical tumor confirmed by laparotomy or clinical follow-up. Gadolinium-enhanced MRI correctly showed residual tumor in 20 of these 23 patients.[161]

For all 69 patients, MRI had an 91% sensitivity, 87% specificity, 90% accuracy, and 72% negative predictive value, and was superior to serum CA 125 level (53%, 94%, 63%, and 38%) (P < .0001) for depicting residual tumor. Second-look laparotomy was performed in 34 patients. There was no significant difference between SLL and MRI, each of which had an 87% sensitivity, 75% specificity, and 85% accuracy.[161]

The improved sensitivity of gadolinium-enhanced MRI in depicting small volume tumor, compared with CA 125 levels alone, can provide oncologists with information critical to patient management; providing a more accurate means of monitoring responses to adjuvant chemotherapy and detecting recurrence after initial response. In my experience, gadolinium-enhanced MRI often shows residual tumor in patients following adjuvant chemotherapy, indicating a need for additional treatment. MRI is also useful in depicting recurrent ovarian cancer in women with a rising serum CA 125 value (Fig. 85-104). In these patients, MRI is used to show the extent and distribution of the recurrent tumor.

Residual or recurrent ovarian cancer typically presents as peritoneal carcinomatosis, which may involve the free peritoneal surfaces, bowel serosa, omentum, or pelvic peritoneum. Findings vary from mild peritoneal thickening and enhancement to large bulky abdominal and pelvic tumor masses. As with other forms of peritoneal disease, the delayed gadolinium-enhanced images are most sensitive for depicting peritoneal metastases in ovarian cancer.

A common site for residual or recurrent peritoneal tumor is in the right subphrenic space. Peritoneal thickening and enhancement along the surface of the liver is abnormal and represents peritoneal metastases. Even with prior surgery, there should not be peritoneal enhancement in the right subphrenic space. After a simple and uncomplicated laparotomy for ovarian cancer, there is minimal postsurgical peritoneal enhancement except for the anterior abdominal wall near the incision. However, in the setting of intraperitoneal chemotherapy combined with a peritonectomy and peritoneal stripping, it is common to see enhancement in the right subphrenic space from the prior intervention. Also patients with a postsurgical course complicated by abscesses and peritonitis often show peritoneal thickening and enhancement with matted bowel loops.

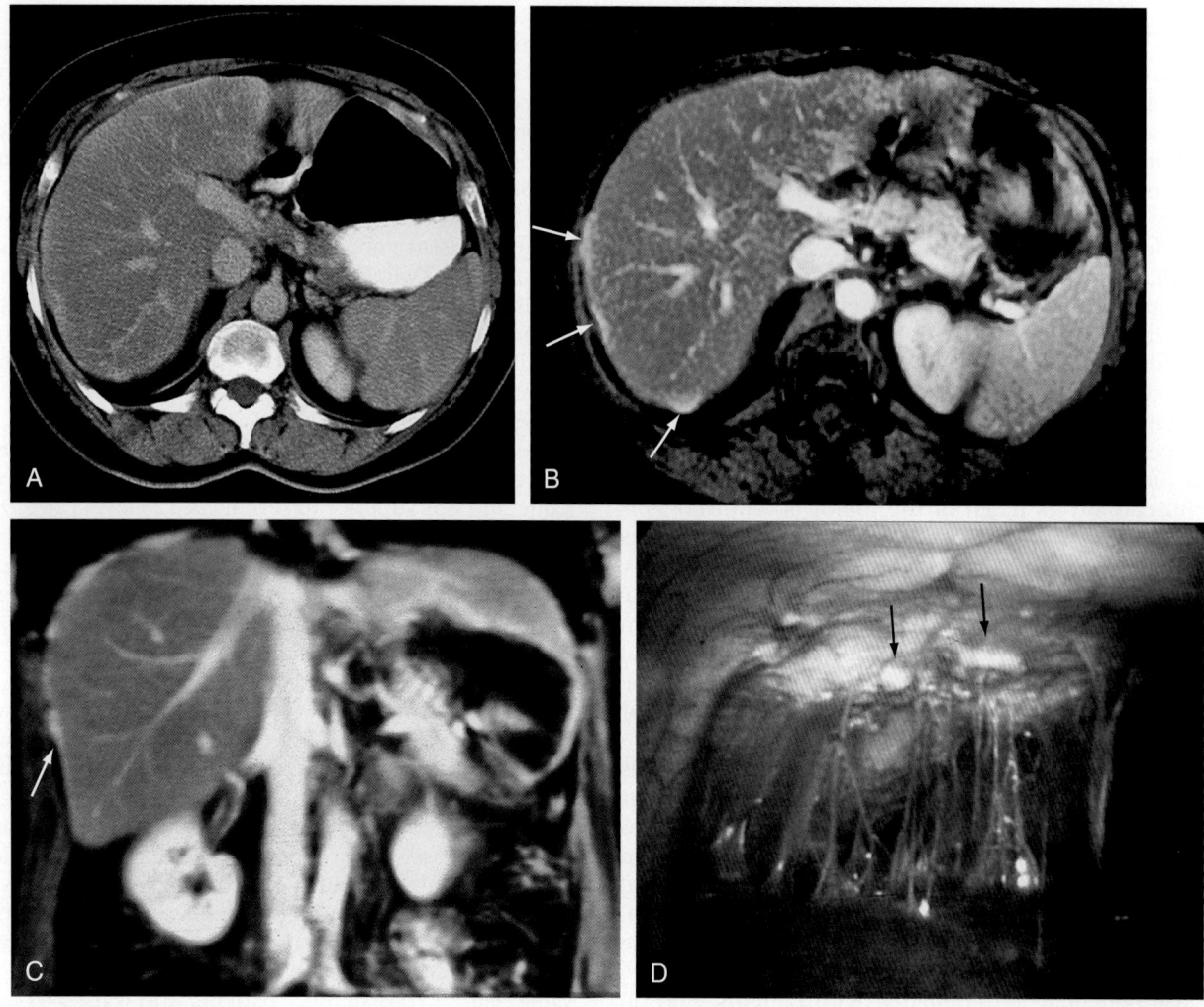

FIGURE 85-103

Treated ovarian cancer. Patient is in clinical remission following multiple rounds of chemotherapy with a normal serum CA 125 value. Compared with the helical CT (**A**), the delayed gadolinium-enhanced spoiled gradient-echo (SGE) MR image (**B**) more convincingly shows enhancing right subphrenic peritoneal tumor *(arrows)*. Coronal gadolinium-enhanced SGE MR image (**C**) shows a rim of right subphrenic tumor *(arrow)*. Laparoscopic view (**D**) shows multiple small tumor nodules *(arrows)* on the under surface of the right hemidiaphragm.

Other common sites of peritoneal tumor in patients with ovarian cancer are the sigmoid mesentery, where tumor envelops the sigmoid colon (Fig. 85-105), and the right lower quadrant near the terminal ileum (Fig. 85-106). Serosal tumor from ovarian cancer may be depicted as mural thickening or focal masses involving the small intestine or colon (Fig. 85-107). Adequate bowel distension with a negative intraluminal contrast agent improves the depiction of serosal metastases. Ultimately, any peritoneal or serosal site may be involved with metastases from ovarian cancer. In end stage carcinomatosis from ovarian cancer, the peritoneal reflections around the liver, spleen, and stomach are often encased in confluent peritoneal tumor.

Nodal metastases from ovarian cancer occur less commonly but are also well depicted on MR images. Enlarged pelvic or retroperitoneal lymph nodes are best depicted on fat-suppressed FSE T2-weighted images or on immediate and delayed fat-suppressed gadolinium-enhanced images.

Peritoneal Metastases from Other Tumors

The extensive surface area of the visceral and parietal peritoneum can be involved by metastases from tumors arising in many other abdominal and pelvic organs. Tumors of the stomach (Figs. 85-108 and 85-109), pancreas (Fig. 85-110), bile ducts (Fig. 85-111), colon (Fig. 85-112), and uterus (Fig. 85-113) often shed tumor cells into the peritoneal cavity. These tumor cells will deposit on local or distant peritoneal sites producing peritoneal metastases and carcinomatosis. The incidence

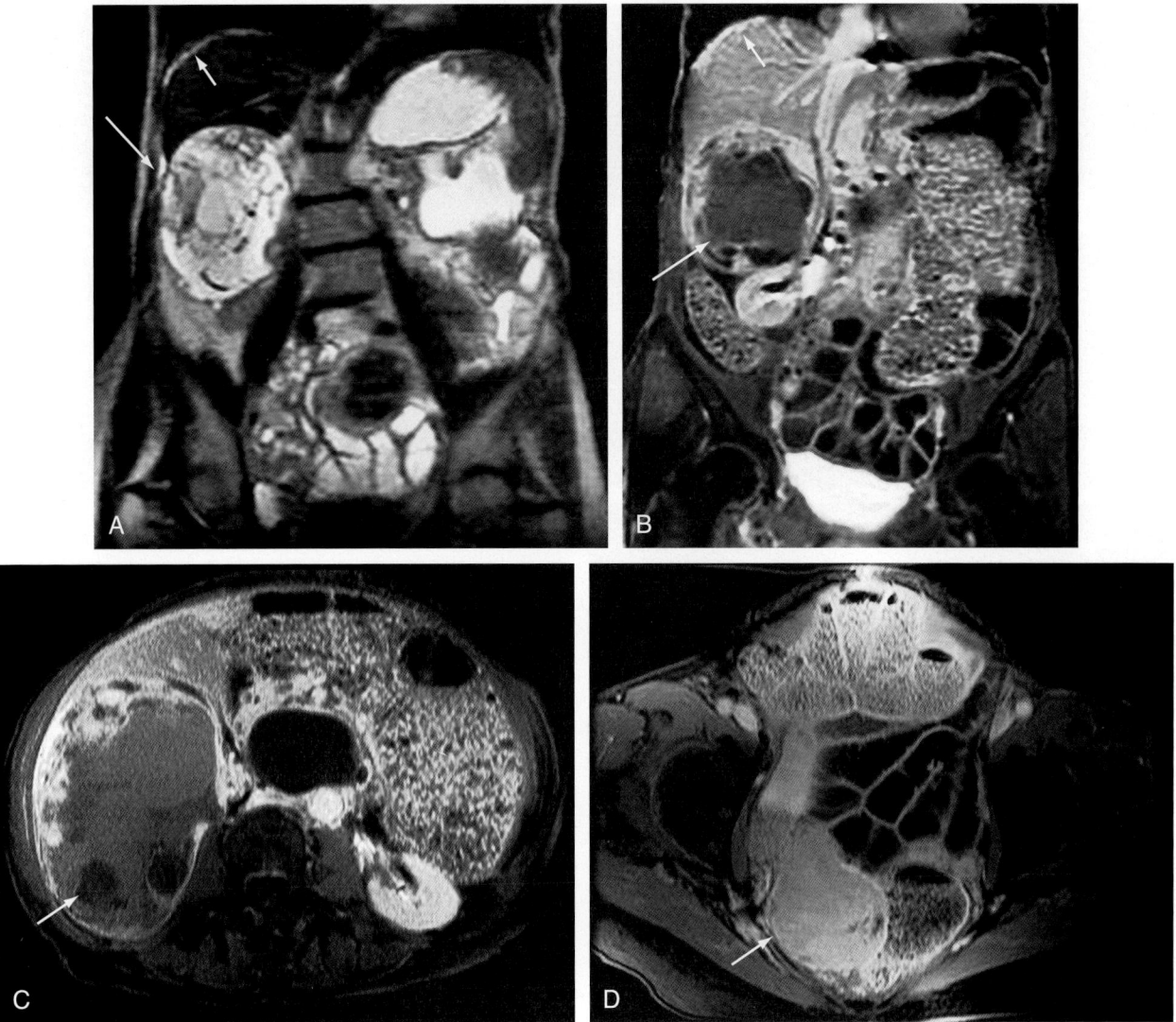

FIGURE 85-104

Recurrent ovarian cancer in patient with a rising serum CA 125 value. Coronal single-shot fast spin-echo (SSFSE) (**A**) and gadolinium-enhanced spoiled gradient-echo (SGE) (**B**) MR images show a large tumor mass in the right subhepatic space *(long arrows)*. Enhancing right subphrenic tumor *(short arrows)* is also noted. Axial gadolinium-enhanced SGE MR image (**C**) depicts the large right sided abdominal mass *(arrow)*. Axial gadolinium enhanced image (**D**) through the pelvis depicts a tumor mass *(arrow)* to the right of the rectum.

of peritoneal carcinomatosis is much greater than is appreciated on helical CT scanning, which underestimates subtle peritoneal tumor. Accurate preoperative imaging depicting peritoneal tumor spread may obviate unnecessary surgical exploration for a nonresectable cancer.

Alternatively, these tumors may spread directly into the adjacent peritoneal reflection, using them as conduits to reach adjacent structures and organs. For example, a pancreatic cancer may easily spread cephalad through the hepatoduodenal ligament to involve the porta hepatis and liver. With advanced tumor dissemination, one will often see spread through all of the perihepatic ligaments, spaces, and fissures. Gastric cancers often spread into the adjacent gastrohepatic

ligament or gastrosplenic ligament. The four-layered omentum forms the peritoneal connection between the greater curvature of the stomach and the transverse colon. Using this route, a gastric cancer can spread inferiorly through the layers of the omentum to reach the transverse colon. Colon cancers may also extend into the omentum, transverse mesocolon, sigmoid mesentery, and peritoneal reflections, attaching the ascending and descending colon to the posterior abdominal wall.

Treatment for peritoneal metastases is by chemotherapy and surgical debulking of a potentially obstructing mass. Interventional therapy aimed at stenting GI masses are now being employed. The role of intraperitoneal therapy combined with surgical cytoreduction is being explored.

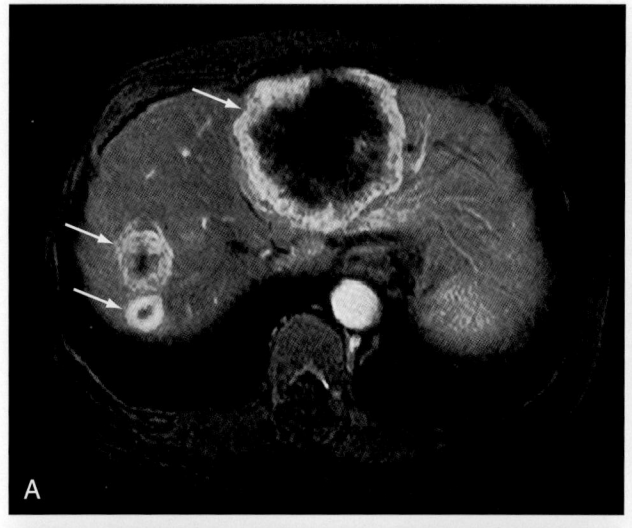

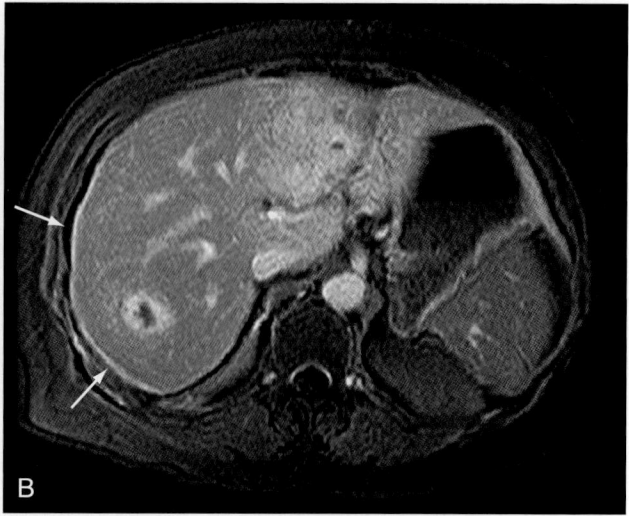

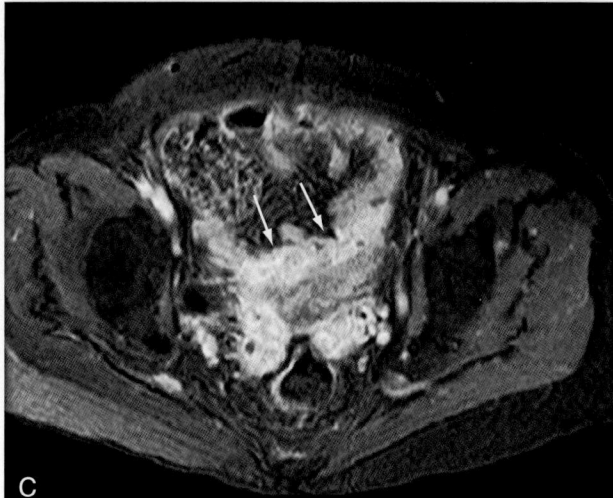

FIGURE 85-105

Ovarian cancer with liver metastases. Axial arterial phase gadolinium-enhanced spoiled gradient-echo (SGE) image (**A**) shows liver metastases *(arrows)* from ovarian cancer. Delayed gadolinium-enhanced SGE image (**B**) shows enhancing right subphrenic peritoneal metastases *(arrows)*. Gadolinium-enhanced image through the pelvis (**C**) depicts confluent tumor *(arrows)* encasing the sigmoid colon.

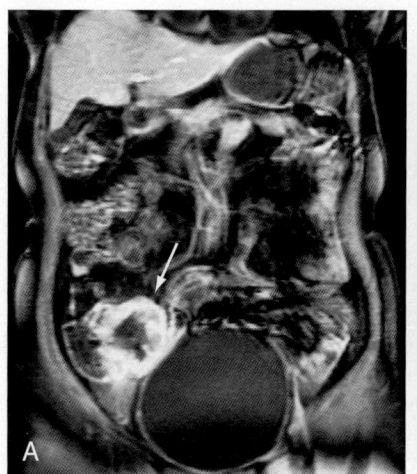

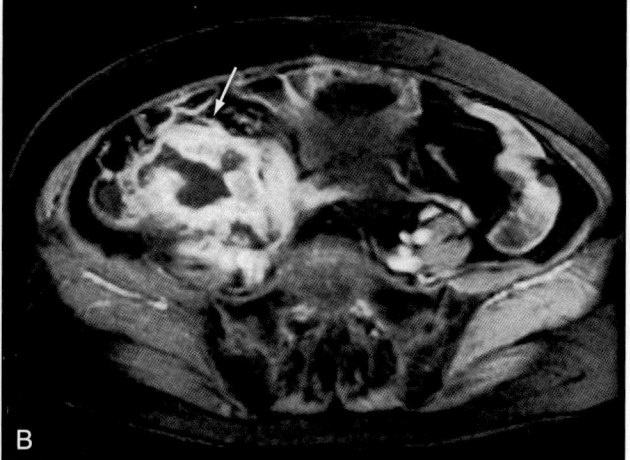

FIGURE 85-106

Ovarian cancer with metastases to terminal ileum. Coronal (**A**) and axial (**B**) gadolinium-enhanced spoiled gradient-echo (SGE) MR images depict a large enhancing mass *(arrows)* encasing the terminal ileum.

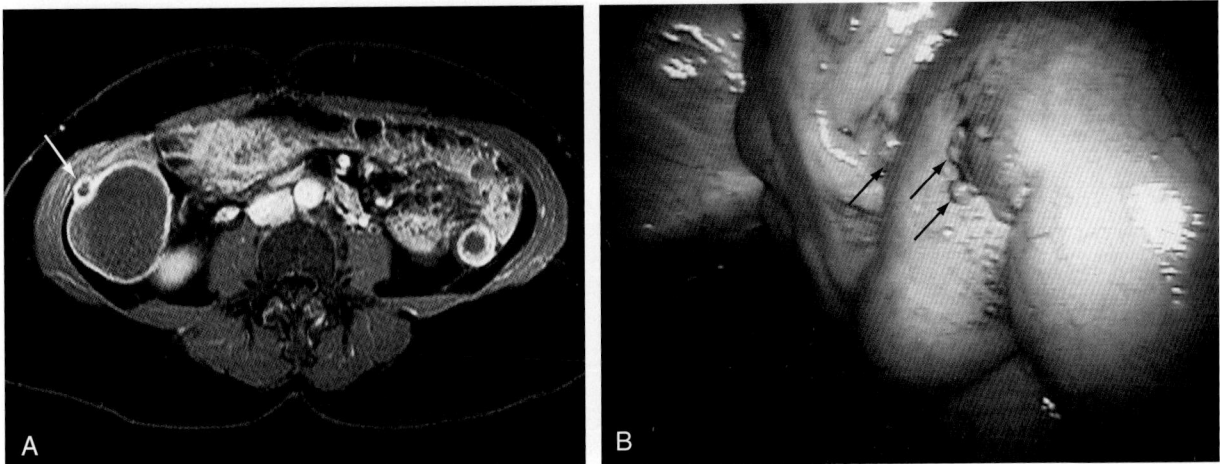

FIGURE 85-107

Ovarian cancer with serosal metastases. Axial gadolinium-enhanced spoiled gradient-echo (SGE) MR image (**A**) with intraluminal water soluble contrast material, shows an enhancing serosal metastasis *(arrow)* involving the ascending colon. Laparoscopic view (**B**) shows multiple small serosal implants on the bowel surface *(arrows)*.

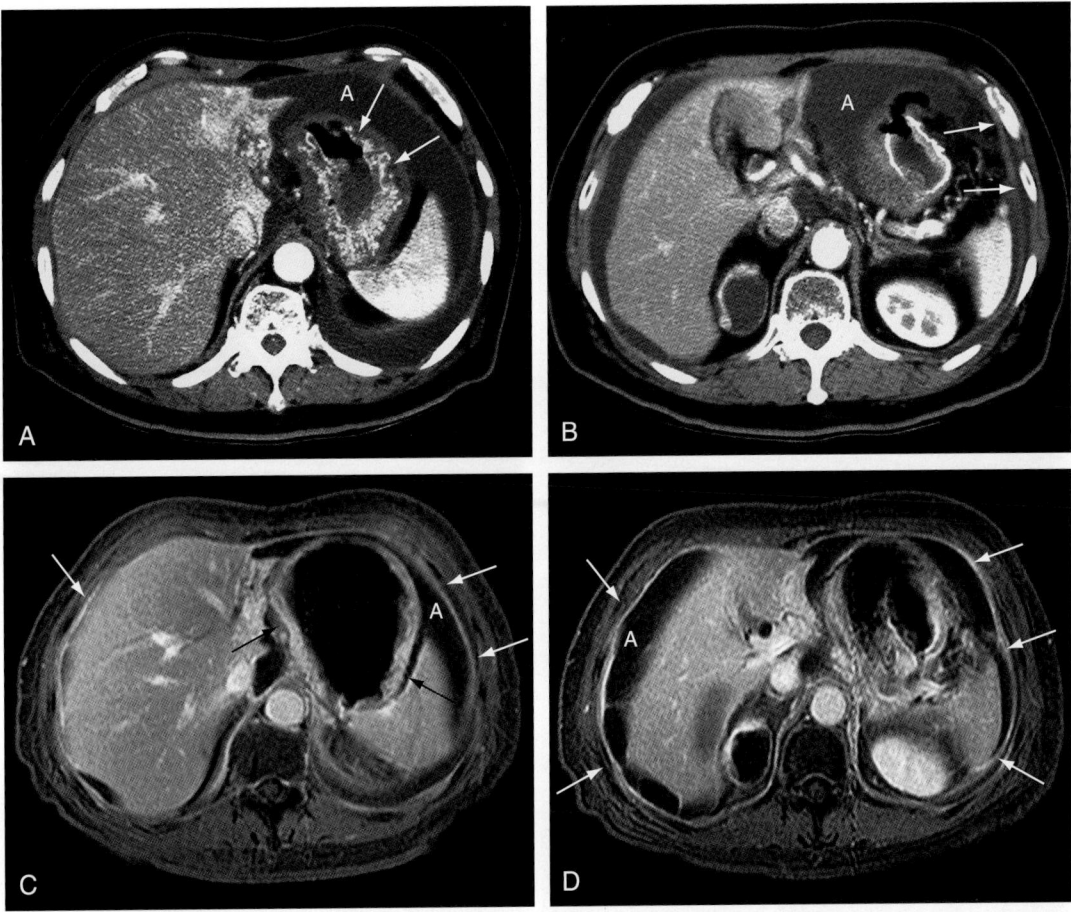

FIGURE 85-108

Gastric cancer. **A** and **B,** Helical CT shows gastric mural thickening *(arrows in **A**)*, ascites (A), and mild thickening of peritoneum in the left side of the abdomen *(arrows in **B**)*. **C** and **D,** Axial gadolinium-enhanced spoiled gradient-echo (SGE) MR images confirm the thickened gastric wall *(black arrows)* and ascites (A). MR images also show diffuse carcinomatosis with marked enhancement *(white arrows)* of all peritoneal surfaces. The conspicuity of the enhancing peritoneal tumor on MR images leads to greater confidence in the diagnosis and more accurate depiction of the extent of metastases.

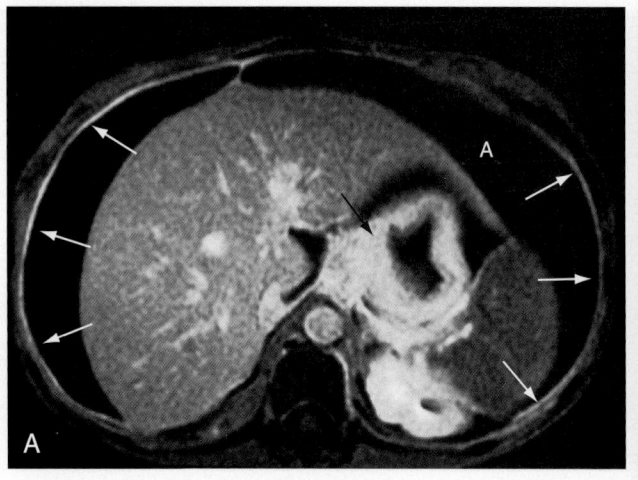

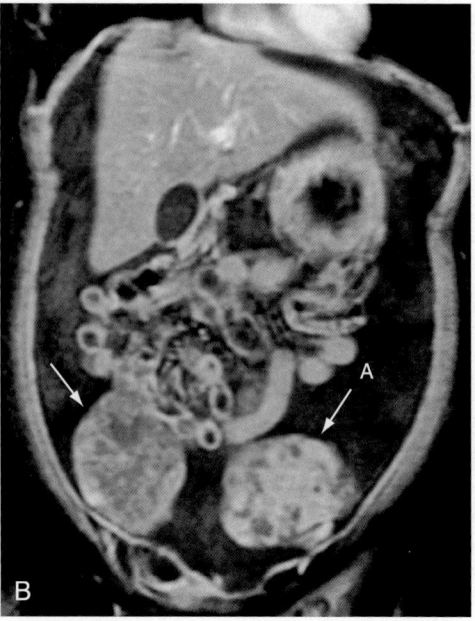

FIGURE 85-109

Gastric cancer with bilateral Krukenberg tumors. **A,** Axial gadolinium-enhanced spoiled gradient-echo (SGE) MR image through the upper abdomen shows gastric cancer with marked thickening and enhancement of the stomach wall *(black arrow).* Ascites (A) and peritoneal carcinomatosis *(white arrows)* is also present. **B,** Coronal image shows bilateral pelvic masses *(arrows)* representing drop metastases to the ovaries or Krukenberg tumors.

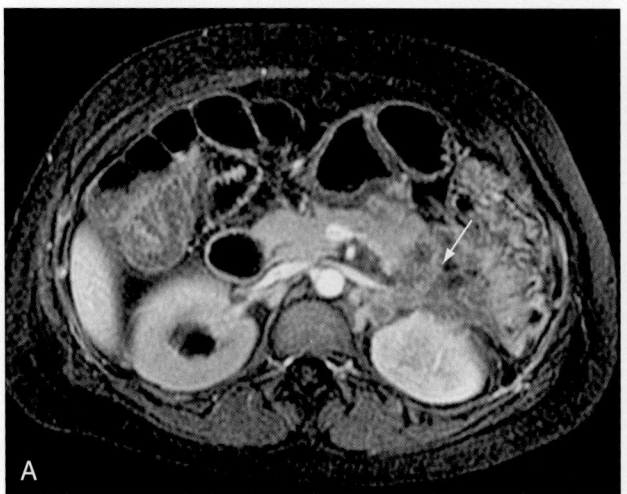

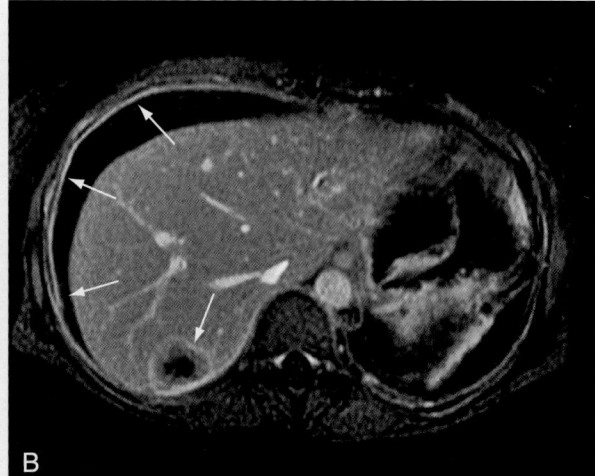

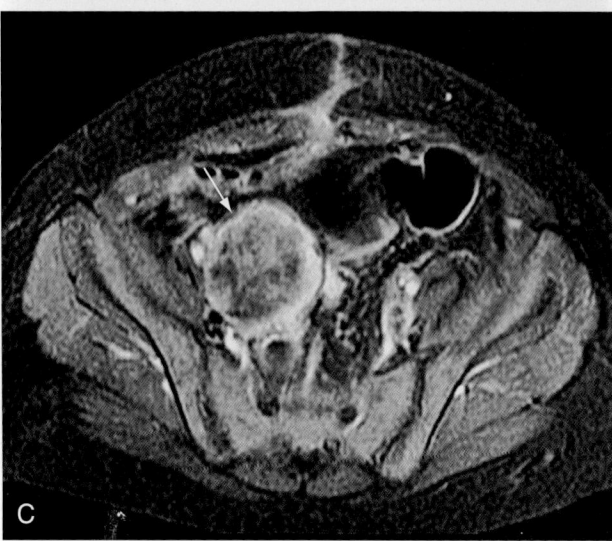

FIGURE 85-110

Pancreatic cancer with carcinomatosis. **A,** Gadolinium-enhanced image through the middle abdomen shows an infiltrative hypointense mass *(arrow)* in the pancreatic tail. **B,** Gadolinium-enhanced image through the upper abdomen shows a rim of right subphrenic peritoneal tumor *(arrows).* **C,** Image through the pelvis demonstrates a solid right-sided pelvic mass *(arrow)* representing a drop metastases to the right ovary.

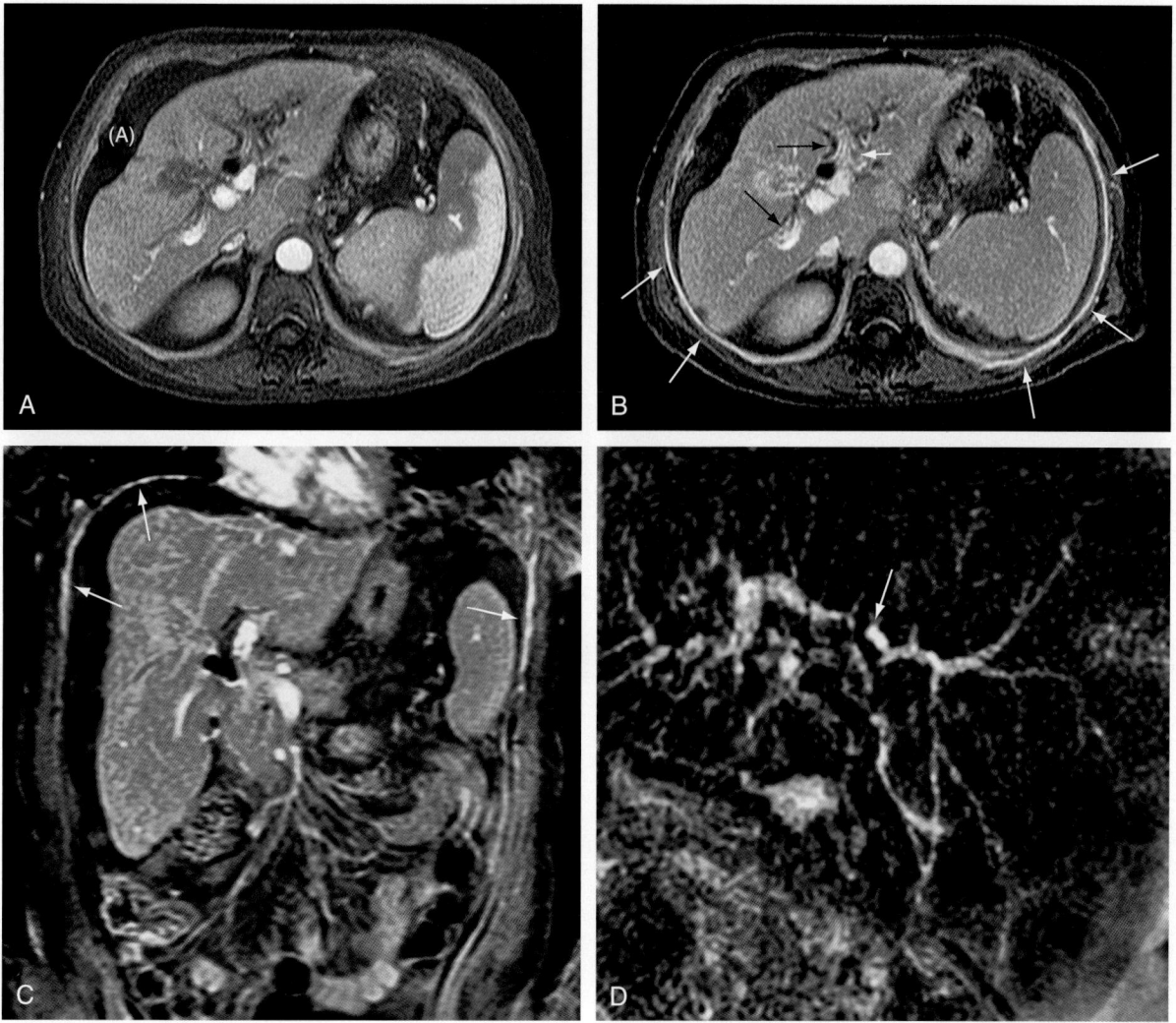

FIGURE 85-111

Cholangiocarcinoma. **A,** Arterial gadolinium-enhanced spoiled gradient-echo (SGE) MR image shows ascites (A). **B,** Portal venous phase gadolinium-enhanced SGE image shows dilated intrahepatic bile ducts *(black arrows)*, enhancing periportal tumor *(short white arrow)* representing a Klatskin tumor, and enhancing peritoneal carcinomatosis *(long white arrows)*. **C,** Coronal gadolinium-enhanced SGE image confirms the peritoneal metastases. **D,** MR cholangiopancreaticograph (MRCP) shows central biliary stricture *(arrow)* due to the Klatskin tumor.

MRI of Peritoneal Metastases

MRI of peritoneal metastases follows the same techniques and protocols outlined above. Peritoneal tumor typically enhances slowly, becoming most conspicuous on delayed fat-suppressed gadolinium-enhanced images. High-resolution gadolinium-enhanced images obtained with perfect breath holding will optimize one's ability to depict subtle enhancing peritoneal metastases. Careful inspection of the parietal and visceral peritoneum, and the peritoneal reflections and ligaments is essential in the patient with possible carcinomatosis.

Hematogenous Peritoneal Metastases

Blood-borne metastases to the peritoneum can occur with end stage extra-abdominal tumors. Widely disseminated tumors of the breast, lungs, and other primary tumors may metastasize to the parietal or visceral peritoneum. There is typically other evidence of widespread metastases, which may involve the liver, osseous structures, and lymph nodes (Fig. 85-114). The MR appearance of hematogenous peritoneal metastases from extra-abdominal tumors will show peritoneal, mesenteric, and omental tumor masses combined with other evidence of widely disseminated tumor.

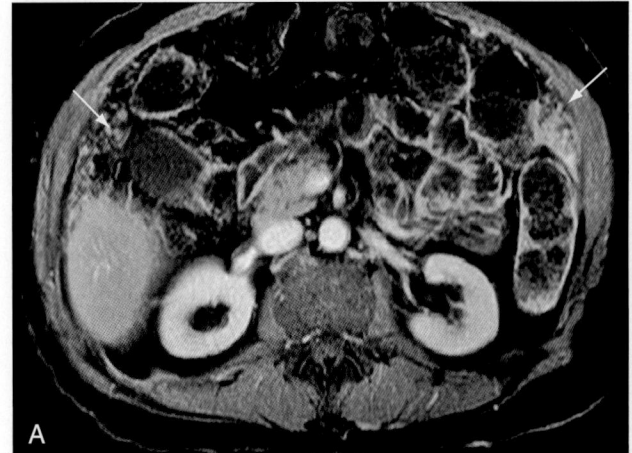

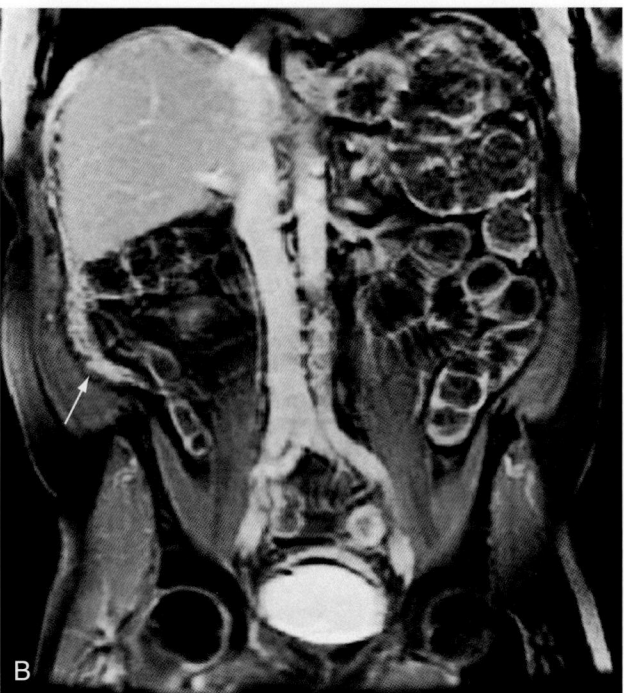

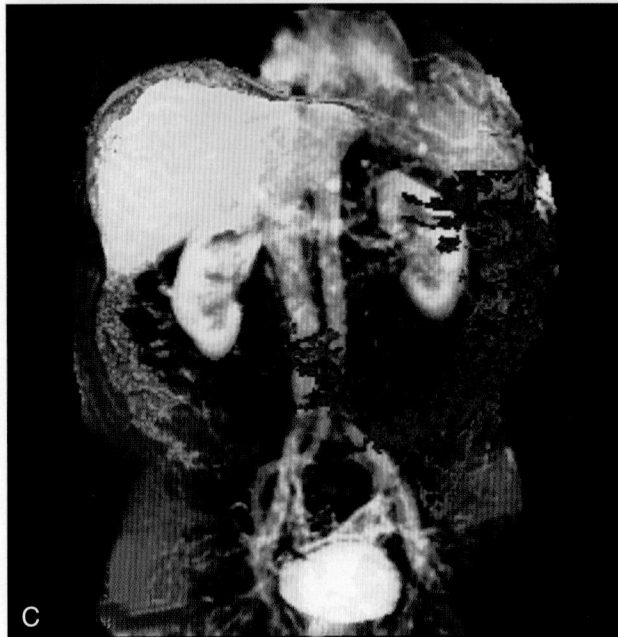

FIGURE 85-112

Recurrent rectal cancer with carcinomatosis. Axial (**A**) and coronal (**B**) gadolinium-enhanced spoiled gradient-echo (SGE) MR images show heterogeneous enhancing peritoneal and omental metastases *(arrows)* from recurrent rectal cancer. Three dimensional color model (**C**) generated from the coronal gadolinium-enhanced images shows the distribution of peritoneal and omental tumor shown in purple.

Lymphatic Metastases Involving the Peritoneum

The lymphatics within the peritoneum may be a source of tumor spread in patients with non-Hodgkin's lymphoma and other tumors with diffuse metastasis (Fig. 85-115). These patients will present with enlarged lymph nodes or nodal masses involving the mesentery and omentum. Confluent nodal masses may produce the "sandwich sign," in which the mesenteric vessels are encased in a large nodal mass. Progressive omental tumor involvement will lead to the formation of an "omental cake" with bulky tumor in the anterior abdomen.

MRI of Lymphatic Metastases

MRI of the mesentery and omentum is facilitated by the addition of fat suppression to the T2-weighted and

gadolinium-enhanced SGE MR images. On MR images, lymphatic tumor dissemination is depicted as numerous mesenteric lymph nodes that may progress to confluent mesenteric masses. Early omental tumor involvement is depicted as mild infiltration of the omental fat. With progressive tumor involvement, the omentum will become thickened, forming a sheet of tumor in the anterior abdomen. Direct coronal and sagittal MRI is useful to confirm mesenteric and omental tumor and to clarify the relationship of the tumor to adjacent structures. Associated retroperitoneal, abdominal, and pelvic enlarged lymph nodes are helpful in establishing the correct diagnosis.

On MR images, one may assess the activity of the nodal tissue by examining the signal intensity of the nodal masses on T2-weighted images and their enhancement with gadolinium. With treatment, the nodal masses will decrease in size. Low signal intensity of the

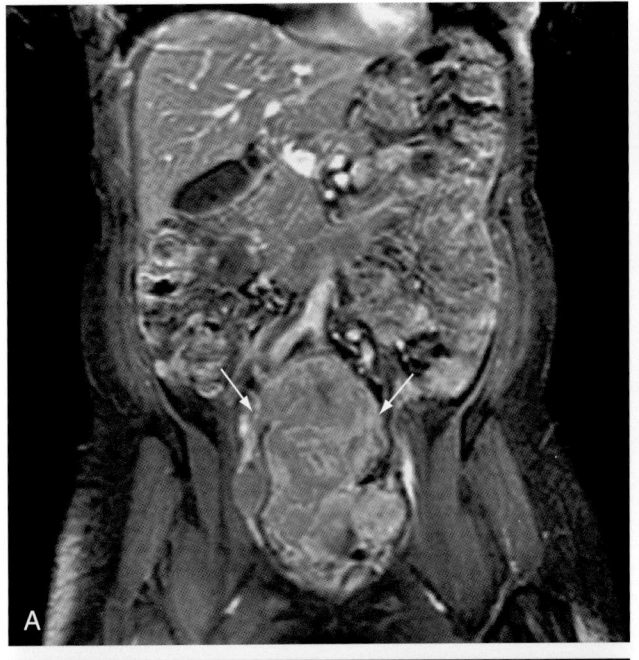

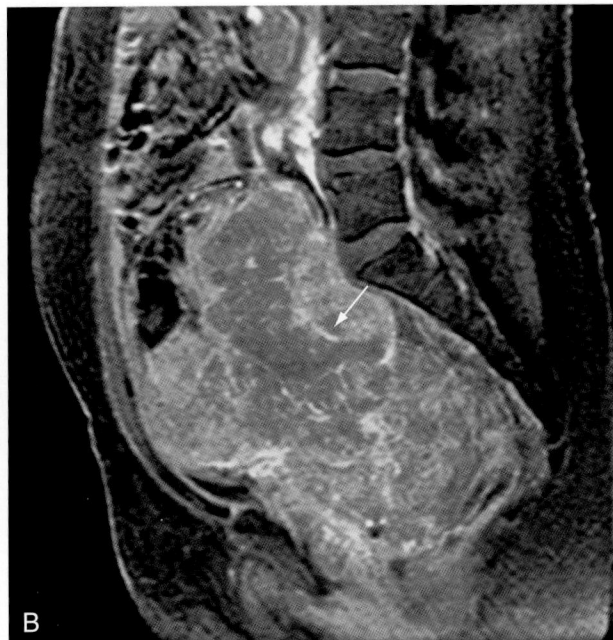

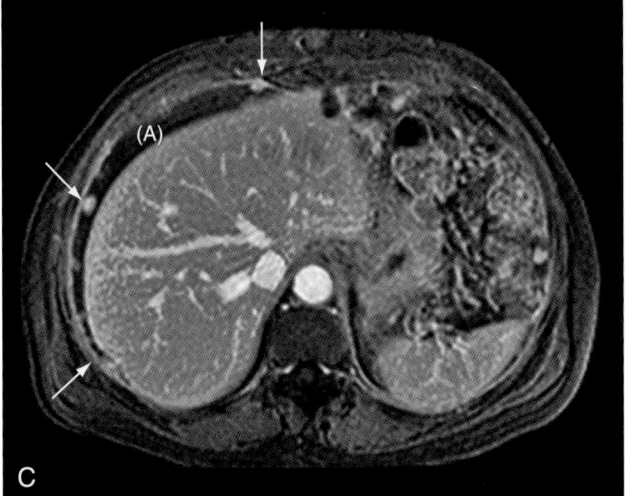

FIGURE 85-113

Leiomyosarcoma with carcinomatosis. Coronal (**A**) and sagittal (**B**) gadolinium-enhanced spoiled gradient-echo (SGE) MR images show a large solid pelvic mass *(arrows)* representing a uterine leiomyosarcoma. Axial gadolinium-enhanced image (**C**) through the upper abdomen shows ascites (A) and enhancing right subphrenic peritoneal metastases *(arrows)*.

residual nodal mass on T2-weighted images and lack of enhancement with gadolinium suggest fibrosis and lack of viable tumor in the remaining nodes. Residual or recurrent lymphoma has a high signal intensity on T2-weighted images and demonstrates enhancement with gadolinium.

Primary Peritoneal Cancer

Extraovarian primary peritoneal cancer is a rare cancer that arises in the peritoneal lining of the abdomen and pelvis[208] (Fig. 85-116). It is notable that the mesothelial cells of the peritoneum and the germinal epithelial cells of the ovary have the same embryologic origin. These peritoneal cells may later undergo malignant degeneration to form papillary and serous tumors that are

histopathologically identical to epithelial ovarian cancer. The presentation, pattern of spread, treatment, and prognosis of primary ovarian cancer mimics that of advanced epithelial ovarian cancer. The staging system used for primary peritoneal cancer is identical to that used for ovarian cancer. Patients with primary peritoneal cancer generally present with stage III or stage IV disease. It is well described that a small number of women who undergo prophylactic oophorectomy may later develop primary peritoneal cancer. In the past, numerous names have been used to describe this tumor including: extraovarian peritoneal serous papillary carcinoma, serous surface papillary carcinoma, multiple focal extraovarian serous carcinoma, primary peritoneal papillary serous adenocarcinoma, serous surface carcinoma of the peritoneum, and papillary serous carcinoma of the peritoneum.

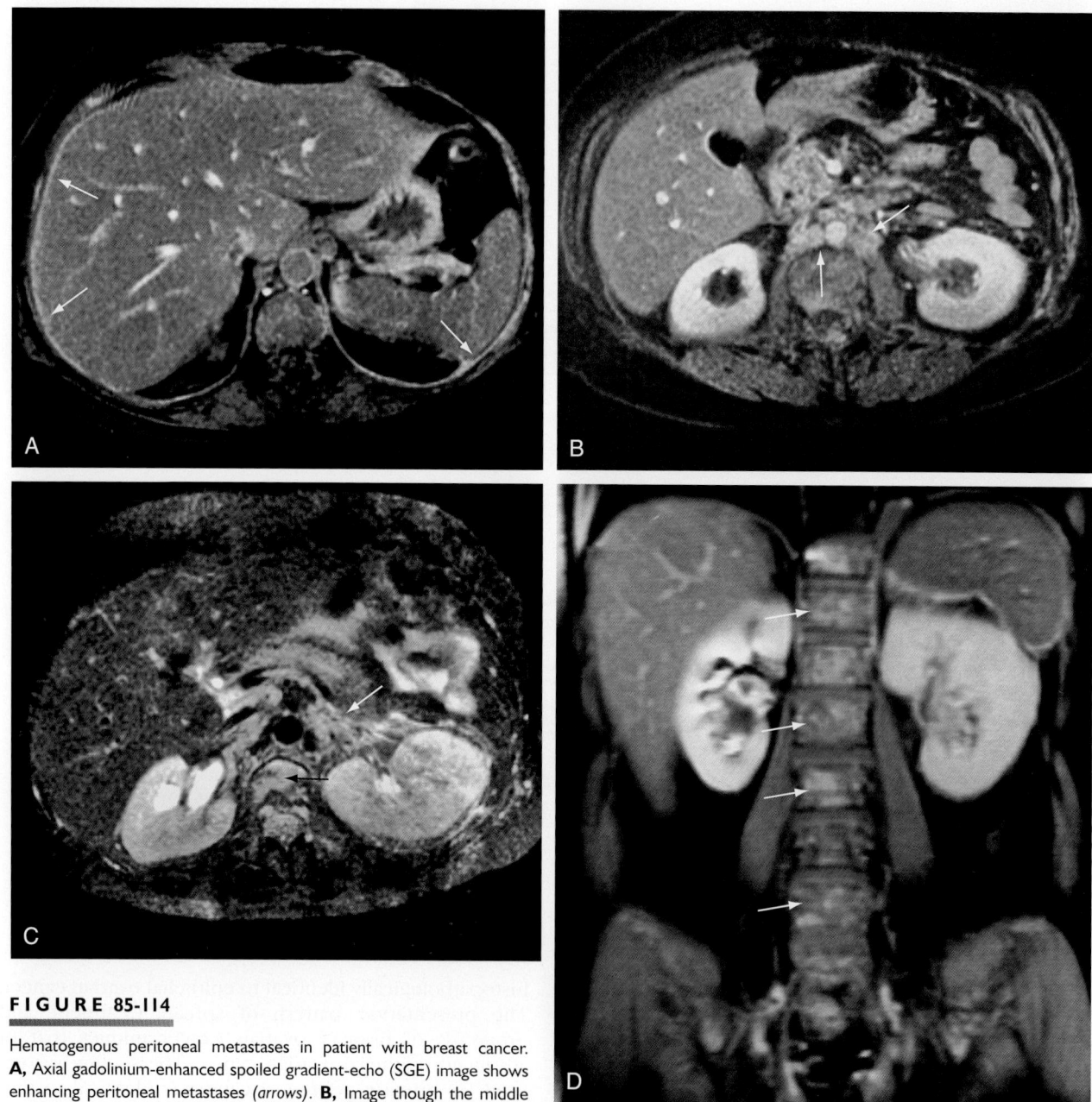

FIGURE 85-114

Hematogenous peritoneal metastases in patient with breast cancer. **A,** Axial gadolinium-enhanced spoiled gradient-echo (SGE) image shows enhancing peritoneal metastases *(arrows).* **B,** Image though the middle abdomen depicts retroperitoneal nodal metastases *(arrows).* **C,** Fat-suppressed T2-weighted image confirms the retroperitoneal lymphadenopathy *(white arrow)* and also shows vertebral body metastases *(black arrow).* **D,** Coronal gadolinium-enhanced image demonstrates diffuse enhancing osseous metastases *(arrows).*

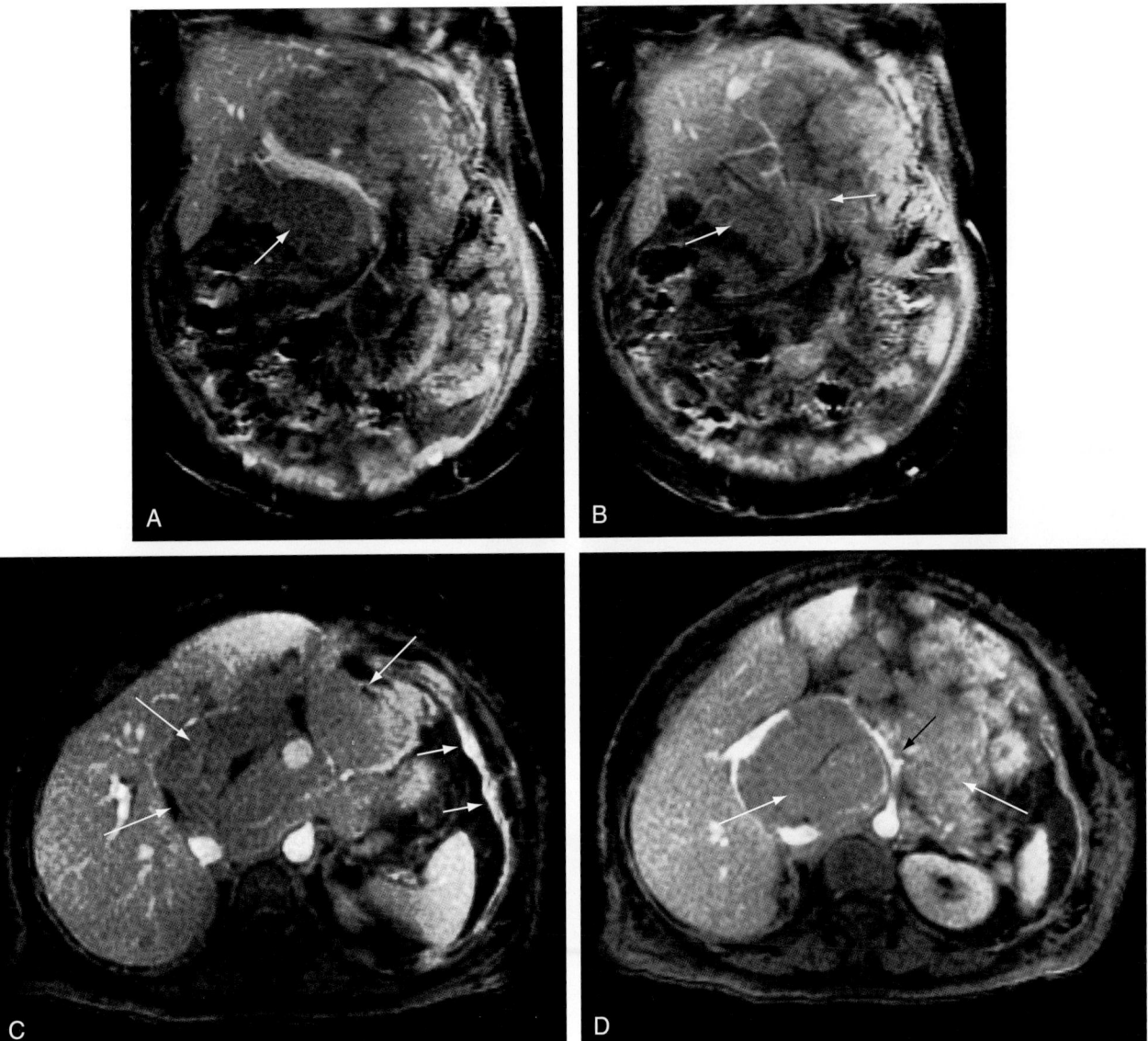

FIGURE 85-115

Lymphatic peritoneal metastases. Patient with diffusely metastatic breast cancer. Coronal gadolinium-enhanced MR images (**A** and **B**) demonstrate a bulky mesenteric mass *(arrows)* encasing the mesenteric vessels. Axial gadolinium-enhanced images (**C** and **D**) show the mesenteric mass *(long white arrows)* encasing the superior mesenteric artery *(black arrow)*. Also note the left-sided peritoneal metastases *(short white arrows)*.

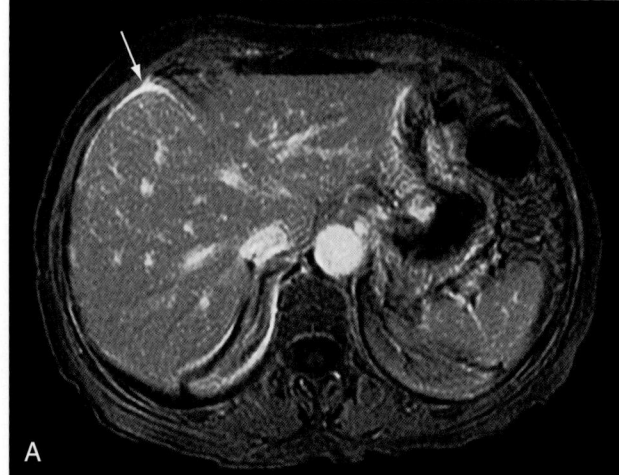

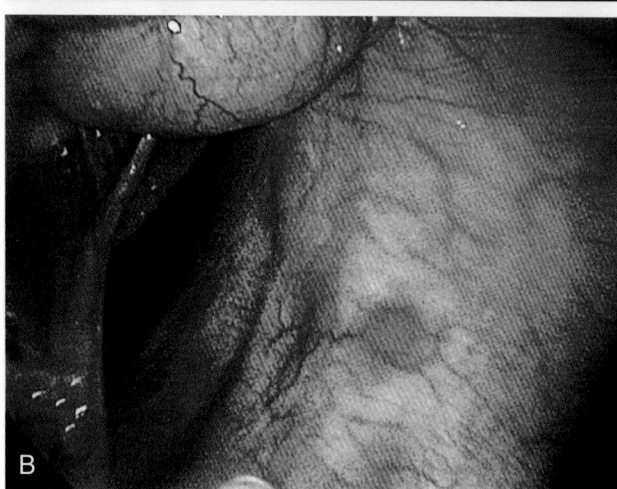

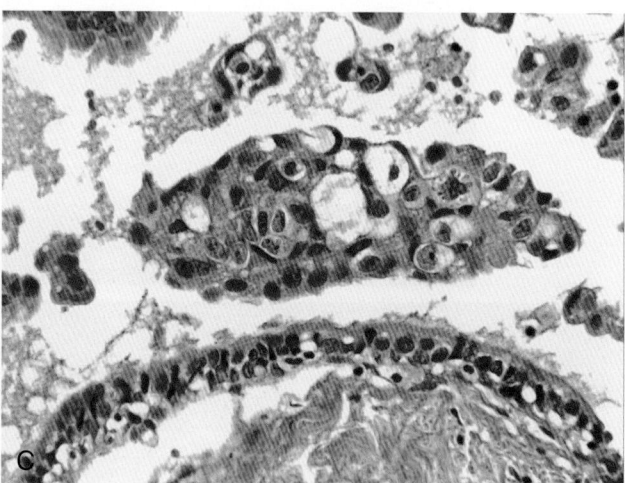

FIGURE 85-116

Primary peritoneal cancer. Gadolinium-enhanced image MR image (**A**) depicts enhancing perihepatic peritoneal tumor (arrow). Laparoscopic view (**B**) of the peritoneal cavity was unremarkable. However, microscopic evaluation (**C**) of peritoneal washings confirmed tumor cells in the peritoneal fluid from primary peritoneal cancer.

MRI of Primary Peritoneal Cancer

MRI of primary peritoneal cancer is identical to that for epithelial ovarian cancer. Fat-suppressed gadolinium-enhanced MR images will show abnormal peritoneal thickening and enhancement. With chemotherapy, the peritoneal thickening and enhancement will diminish as the tumor responds to therapy (Fig. 85-117). Associated ascites and larger abdominal and pelvic masses can also be seen with primary peritoneal cancer. Gadolinium-enhanced MR images shows greater enhancement and conspicuity of the primary peritoneal cancer compared with helical CT (Fig. 85-118). Excluding the presence of an ovarian mass is essential in establishing the diagnosis of primary peritoneal cancer.

Pseudomyxoma Peritonei

Pseudomyxoma peritonei is a rare condition characterized by the accumulation of copious gelatinous masses throughout the peritoneal cavity.[209-211] Pseudomyxoma peritonei may be associated with appendiceal mucin-producing tumors or may occur as a complication of ovarian mucinous cystadenoma. The classification and nomenclature of mucinous tumors of the appendix is confusing and controversial. In the past, classification has included simple mucoceles, adenomas and cyst-adenomas, mucinous tumors of uncertain malignant potential, and adenocarcinoma of the appendix. In particular, confusion existed regarding terminology for mucinous tumors of the appendix without malignant features, but with associated intraperitoneal spread.

A recently devised classification scheme separates these tumors into low-grade appendiceal mucinous neoplasms (LAMNs), mucinous adenocarcinomas of the appendix (MACAs), and discordant tumors.[210] Low-grade appendiceal mucinous neoplasms are characterized by villous or flat proliferation of mucinous epithelium with low-grade atypia. They may be confined to the appendix or may spread into the peritoneal cavity. Pools of mucin-containing low-grade mucinous epithelial cells characterize intraperitoneal spread of LAMNs. Those that are confined to the appendix are considered benign with a good prognosis, whereas LAMNs with intraperitoneal spread have a worse prognosis, with 50% survival at 10 years.[209] While their clinical course is more aggressive, histopathologically, LAMNs with intraperitoneal spread are identical to LAMN's confined to the appendix and do not warrant the term adenocarcinoma.

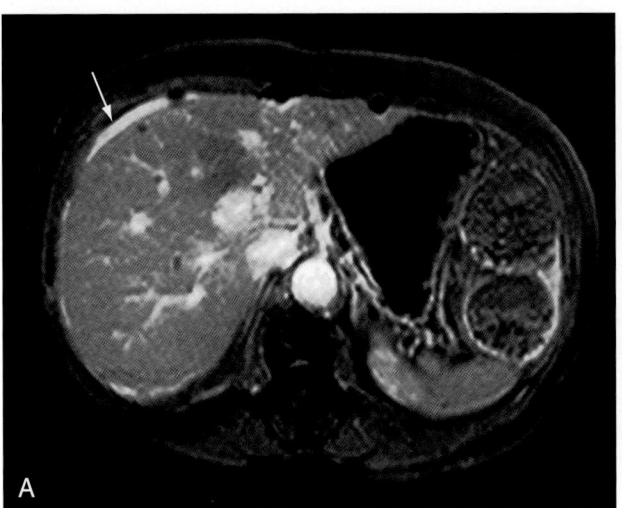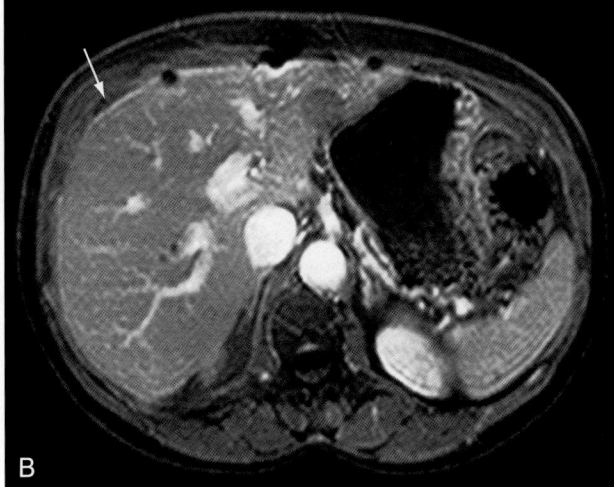

FIGURE 85-117

Primary peritoneal tumor response to chemotherapy. Gadolinium-enhanced spoiled gradient-echo (SGE) MR image (**A**) shows a moderately thick rind of enhancing right subphrenic tumor *(arrow)*. Following multiple cycles of chemotherapy, follow up MRI (**B**) shows marked decrease in the thickness of the peritoneal tumor *(arrow)*.

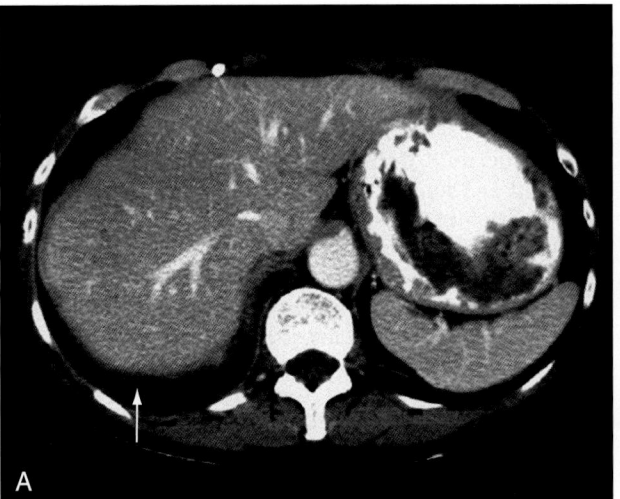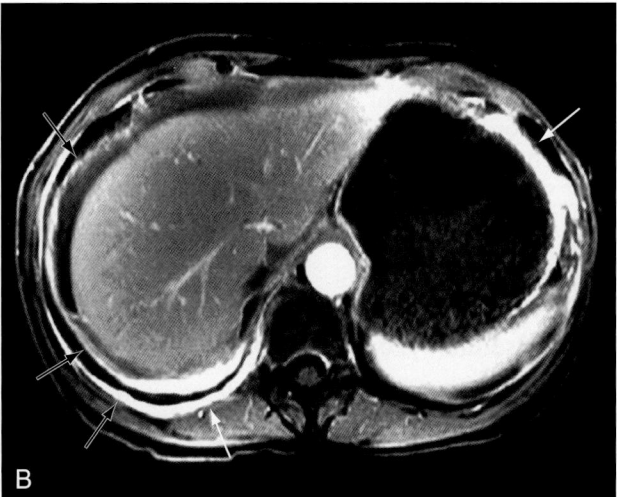

FIGURE 85-118

Primary peritoneal tumor comparison of helical CT and MRI. **A,** Helical CT scan shows perihepatic ascites *(arrow)*. **B,** Gadolinium-enhanced MRI demonstrates diffuse peritoneal thickening and enhancement *(white arrow)* representing primary peritoneal cancer. Pleural metastases *(black arrows)* are also present.

On the other hand, appendiceal tumors with destructive mural invasion, complex epithelial proliferations, or high-grade atypia are classified as MACAs. They may show invasion of the appendiceal wall or may be confined to the appendix. Extraintestinal spread of MACAs may show mucinous pools containing mucinous epithelium with high-grade atypia and, in some cases, increased cellularity compared with LAMNs These tumors are clinically aggressive with a 5-year survival rate of approximately 50%. Discordant tumors are appendiceal LAMNs with high-grade intraperitoneal tumor spread. Their behavior is the same as adenocarcinomas.

Pseudomyxoma peritonei is typically a slowly progressive disease in which patients present with increasing abdominal girth, an inguinal hernia, or a palpable ovarian mass. While pseudomyxoma does not metastasize via the lymphatics or blood stream, it is a progressive disease that, if untreated, eventually leads to death by replacement of the peritoneal cavity by mucinous tumor.

The primary tumor of the appendix or ovary is typically inconspicuous at the time of diagnosis. Mucin-producing tumor cells escape from the appendix or ovary and distribute throughout the peritoneal cavity. The eventual deposition of the tumor cells is determined

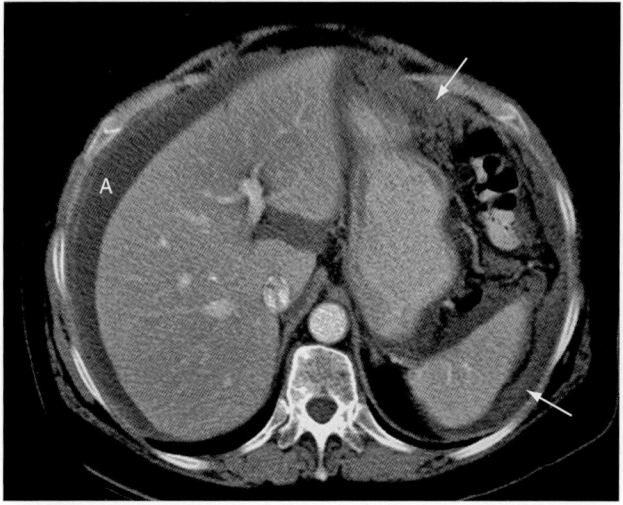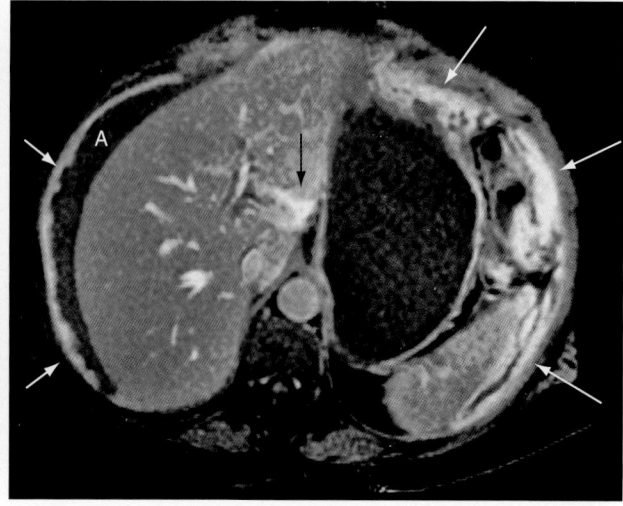

FIGURE 85-119

Pseudomyoma peritonei. **A,** Helical CT scan shows perihepatic ascites (A) and ascites or soft tissue in the left side of the abdomen (arrows). The distinction between ascites and tumor can be difficult on CT scans. **B,** Gadolinium-enhanced MRI shows ascites (A) as well as right subphrenic peritoneal tumor (short white arrows) and bulky confluent peritoneal tumor (long white arrows) encasing the stomach and spleen. Enhancing peritoneal tumor (black arrow) is also present in the superior recess of the lesser sac.

by pathways of flow of peritoneal fluid and by gravity. Bulky tumor deposits in the omentum and right and left subphrenic spaces are most common. Deposition of tumor cells on bowel surfaces is uncommon except at the ileocecal region, the rectosigmoid regions, and the gastric antrum.

MRI of Pseudomyxoma Peritonei

MRI techniques for evaluating patients with pseudomyxoma peritonei are identical to those used for evaluating other forms of peritoneal disease. Unenhanced T1-weighted, fat-suppressed T2-weighted, and immediate and delayed fat-suppressed gadolinium-enhanced SGE MRI are performed. Intraluminal contrast material is useful to distend and separate bowel loops, facilitating depiction of adjacent peritoneal and serosal tumor.

On gadolinium-enhanced MRI, pseudomyxoma peritonei is depicted as thick and heterogeneously enhancing peritoneal tumor masses (Fig. 85-119). As with other types of peritoneal tumor, the tumor masses of pseudomyxoma peritonei enhance slowly, becoming more conspicuous on delayed images. Careful comparison of immediate and delayed gadolinium-enhanced images will show enhancing mucinous tumor implants involving free peritoneal surfaces, omentum, mesentery, and bowel serosa. The peritoneal implants are typically less homogeneous in appearance than in ovarian cancer. This more heterogeneous appearance may reflect various amounts of nonenhancing mucinous material versus enhancing cellular tumor in the pseudomyxoma peritonei implants. As in ovarian cancer, eventually all of the peritoneal surfaces become encased in tumor.

By comparing the T2-weighted images and the gadolinium-enhanced SGE images, one may distinguish the associated peritoneal fluid from the enhancing peritoneal tumor. On the T2-weighted images, both the ascitic fluid and the solid peritoneal tumor will be depicted as areas of heterogeneous high signal in the peritoneal cavity. However, on the fat-suppressed gadolinium-enhanced images, only the solid cellular tumor will enhance. In my experience low-grade appendiceal neoplasms with intraperitoneal spread will show less enhancement than the more cellular mucinous adenocarcinomas.

Complications of pseudomyxoma peritonei, including bowel obstruction, can be depicted on MR images. Typically, multiple large abdominal and pelvic masses are seen, encasing the small bowel and colon with associated obstruction. Multiple sites of bowel involvement are typical. Other complications such as postoperative abscess can be evaluated with MRI. Intraabdominal abscesses will be shown as focal fluid collections with a thick enhancing wall.

Carcinoid Tumor

Carcinoid tumor is a rare, slowly growing neuroendocrine tumor that arises from enterochromaffin cells widely distributed in the body.[212-215] Enterochromaffin cells are found in greatest amounts in the small intestine and less commonly in the appendix, rectum, lung, and pancreas, and very rarely in the ovaries, testes, liver, and bile ducts. Two thirds of carcinoid tumors arise in the GI tract with 39% occurring in the small intestine, 26% in

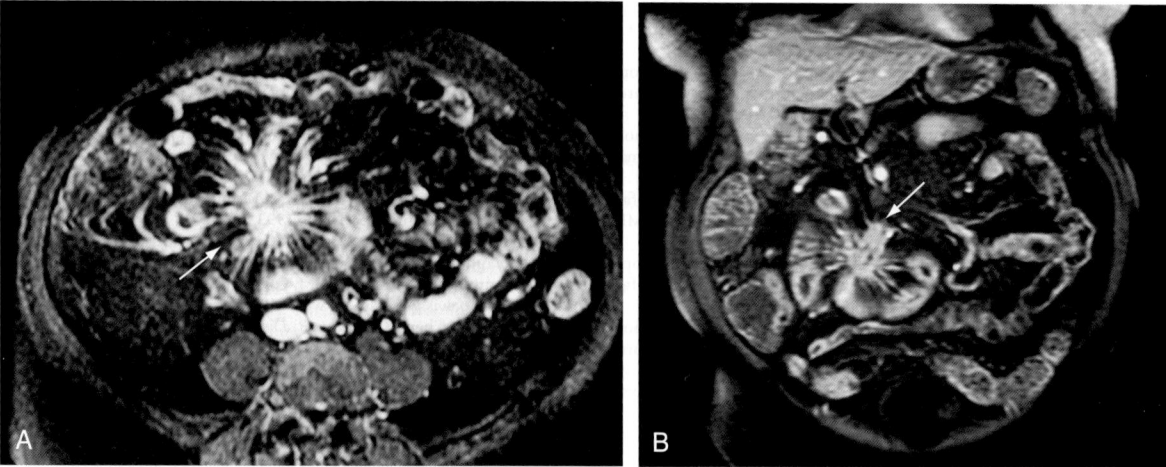

FIGURE 85-120

Carcinoid tumor. Axial (**A**) and coronal (**B**) fat-suppressed gadolinium-enhanced spoiled gradient-echo (SGE) MR images demonstrate a spiculated mesenteric mass (*arrows*) representing a mesenteric metastasis from a small-bowel carcinoid tumor.

the appendix, 15% in the rectum, 5% to 7% in the colon, and 2% to 4% in the stomach. Carcinoid tumors arising in the distal ileum often extend into the adjacent small-bowel mesentery, where they present as a speculated mesenteric mass.

Twenty percent of carcinoid tumors will metastasize and one third of these will develop carcinoid syndrome. Due to efficient hepatic metabolism of vasoactive amines, carcinoid syndrome rarely occurs in the absence of liver metastases. Carcinoid syndrome is due to tumor secretion of vasoactive substances such as 5-hydroxytryptamine (serotonin), histamine, bradykinin, and chromogranin A, and is characterized by facial flushing, diarrhea, abdominal cramps, hypertension, and wheezing. Cardiac complications, including tricuspid regurgitation and pulmonic valve stenosis occur with long-standing untreated carcinoid syndrome. The more common non-functioning carcinoid tumor grows slowly, presenting only after the tumor has grown large enough to cause abdominal distension, pain, or bowel obstruction.

The diagnosis of carcinoid syndrome is established by confirming elevated urine levels of 5-HIAA, the main break down product of serotonin. Most carcinoid tumors are small (<1 cm). The risk of metastasis increases as the tumor enlarges. Tumors >1 cm in diameter have a 50% incidence of metastases while those >2 cm have a 90% incidence of metastases. Treatment for carcinoid tumors includes surgical resection and multidrug chemotherapy.

MRI of Carcinoid Tumor

On MRI the primary GI carcinoid tumor may be depicted as a nodular mass arising from the bowel wall or as localized concentric GI mural thickening.[216,217] In some cases, the primary tumor may be too small to be depicted. Mesenteric metastases or direct tumor extension into

the mesentery will be seen as an enhancing speculated tumor mass within the small bowel mesentery (Fig. 85-120). Typically, the primary GI carcinoid tumor and any metastases show marked enhancement with intravenous gadolinium.

Metastases from carcinoid tumors involving regional or distant lymph nodes, liver parenchyma, or peritoneum are well depicted on a comprehensive MR examination of the abdomen and pelvis.

In a study of 29 patients with carcinoid tumor, Bader et al[216] found that MRI depicted the primary tumor in 8 of 12 patients with presurgical MR imaging, while in four patients the primary tumor was not depicted. The primary tumor was best seen on fat-suppressed gadolinium-enhanced images. Mesenteric metastases were present in eight patients. Liver metastases were hypervascular in 94% of 156 lesions, and 15% of liver metastases were only visualized on immediate gadolinium-enhanced MR images.

REFERENCES

1. Chezmar JL, Rumanick WM, Megibow AJ, et al: Liver and abdominal screening in patients with cancer: CT versus MRI. Radiology 168:43-47, 1988.
2. Semelka RC, Schlung JF, Molina RL, et al: Malignant liver lesions: comparison of spiral CT arterial portography and MRI for diagnostic accuracy, cost, and effect on patient management. J Magn Reson Imag 6:39-43, 1996.
3. Yamashita Y, Mitsuzaki K, Yi T, et al: Small hepatocellular carcinoma in patients with chronic liver damage: prospective comparison of detection with dynamic MRI and helical CT of the whole liver. Radiology 200:79-84, 1996.
4. Semelka RC, Shoenut JP, Magro CM, et al: Renal cancer staging: comparison of contrast-enhanced CT and gadolinium-enhanced fat suppressed spin-echo and gradient-echo MRI. J Magn Reson Imag 3:597-602, 1993.
5. Ichikawa T, Hardrome H, Hachiya J, et al: Pancreatic ductal adenocarcinoma: preoperative assessment with helical CT versus dynamic MRI. Radiology 202:655-662, 1997.
6. Low RN, Francis IR: MRI of the gastrointestinal tract with IV gadolinium and diluted barium oral contrast media compared with unenhanced MRI and CT. Am J Roentgenol 169:1051-1059, 1997.
7. Kettritz U, Isaacs K, Warshauer DM, Semelka RC: Crohn's disease. Pilot study comparing MRI of the abdomen with clinical evaluation. J Clin Gastroenterol 21:249-253, 1995.

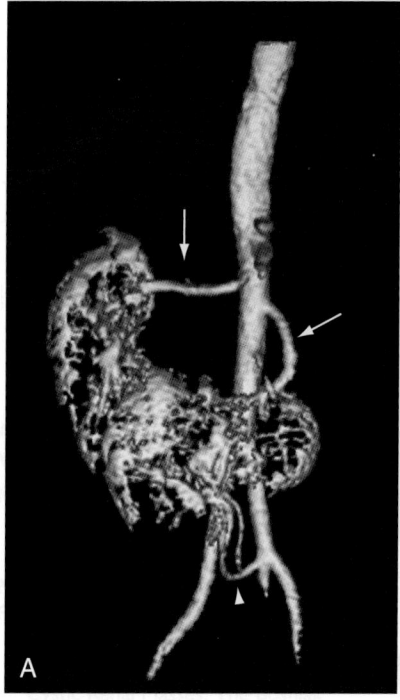
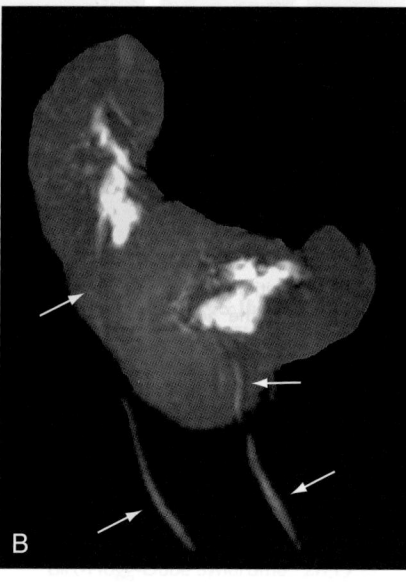

FIGURE 86-2

Cross-fused ectopia. **A,** Shaded surface display of a coronal contrast-enhanced 3D fat-saturated T1-weighted gradient-recalled echo (GRE) acquisition during the arterial phase shows the left kidney located in the midline with fusion of its upper pole to the inferior pole of the right kidney. There is one main renal artery for each kidney (*arrows*). In addition, two smaller accessory arteries (*arrowhead*) are noted arising from a common trunk off the left distal common iliac artery and supplying the mid portion of the left kidney. **B,** Maximum intensity projection from a coronal gadolinium-enhanced 3D fat-saturated T1-weighted GRE image during the excretory phase shows the independent collecting system and ureters (*arrows*) for each kidney.

breath out" yield good results. If the patient is unable to sustain a breath-hold during the coaching session, a nasal cannula to administer oxygen is provided and this greatly increases the individual's breath-hold ability.[7] Alternatively, end inspiration with or without oxygen supplementation can be used. For ventilated patients, temporary suspension of the respirator allows breath-hold protocols to be utilized and often yields motion-free images. Finally, if these strategies fail, a non–breath-hold MR protocol may be used.

Non–breath-Hold Imaging

Fast acquisitions, single-shot imaging and/or respiratory correction techniques can be used in patients with poor breath-hold capacity. The kidneys have somewhat restricted motion during respiration due to their retroperitoneal location. For this reason, renal images are frequently insensitive to subtle movements.

Multislice single-shot acquisitions are typically obtained in a sequential fashion with each slice acquired in approximately 1 second. This strategy provides motion-insensitive images of the kidneys. While the use of suspended respiration is not required to assure image quality, a breath-hold acquisition is recommended when feasible because it facilitates anatomic co-registration of slices. Extreme respiratory motion can result in slice misregistration and can inadvertently lead to incomplete and/or nonsequential anatomic coverage.

Single-shot half-Fourier turbo spin-echo (HASTE; Siemens Medical Systems, Erlangen, Germany) images or single-shot fast spin-echo (SSFSE; GE Medical Systems, Milwaukee, WI) images provide rapid breath-hold–independent, T2-weighted evaluations of the abdomen, including the kidneys. These acquisitions are similar to those obtained during the breath-hold examination of the kidneys. Fat suppression can be used with these acquisitions to augment image contrast and reduce artifacts caused by respiration and other bulk motions. This can also help with the identification of fat in a lesion.

Magnetization-prepared gradient-recalled echo (MagPrepGRE) imaging provides fast acquisitions for motion-insensitive T1-weighted images. Similarly to the single-shot T2-weighted images, this strategy allows for very fast acquisition times with each slice obtained in less than 1.5 seconds; suspended respiration is not necessary to achieve motion-free images. Pulsation and motion artifacts are largely eliminated using this sequence.[8,9] Since these images are acquired sequentially on a per slice basis, anatomic misregistration among data sets is common without breath-holding. This may potentially limit the comparison of in- and out-of-phase images when acquired as separate image data sets. Similarly, comparison of pre- and post-contrast images can be challenging since the anatomic misregistration makes subtraction post-processing virtually impossible. In that case, direct measurement of signal intensity before and after contrast administration is used to assess the presence and degree of enhancement in a suspicious renal lesion. Despite its limitations, MagPrepGRE imaging is a vital strategy for obtaining diagnostic quality T1-weighted images in patients unable to maintain a breath-hold examination. Other strategies to compensate for respiratory motion artifacts add considerable time to the acquisition, thus risking subsequent image degradation; simple averaging strategies, respiratory gating, and respiratory triggering represent alternatives. The latter two approaches are particularly valuable in patients with an erratic respiratory pattern.[10,11]

T2-Weighted Imaging

The normal kidney has a relatively long T2 time. The renal parenchyma is hyperintense relative to liver and close in signal intensity to the spleen. The renal medulla is typically hyperintense to the renal cortex on T2-weighted images of normal kidneys. T2-weighted images are most helpful in distinguishing simple renal cysts from other lesions. Simple cysts display homogeneous high signal intensity due to their long relaxation time. Septations and solid nodules can be readily seen within cysts on T2-weighted images. Complicated renal cysts with hemorrhagic and/or proteinaceous contents may show heterogeneous or low signal intensity on T2-weighted images. Solid tumors can have variable signal intensity on T2-weighted images.[12] Solid neoplasms are not reliably distinguished from complicated cysts based on their T2-weighted imaging features. Definitive characterization depends on the demonstration of enhancement within a lesion on post-contrast images. Renal cysts lack vascular supply and therefore, demonstration of enhancement within a renal lesion excludes this diagnosis.

Conventional spin-echo imaging should be avoided since it requires long acquisition times that far exceed breath-hold capabilities. Echo-train imaging, generically referred to as rapid acquisition with relaxation enhancement (RARE),[13] is preferred for evaluation of renal pathology since it allows for substantial reductions in acquisition times. Echo-train imaging is associated with vendor-specific acronyms, such as fast spin-echo (FSE) and turbo spin-echo (TSE) imaging. Breath-hold T2-weighted images are feasible with the use of longer echo trains and have been shown to improve results.[14,15] Fat suppression augments image contrast and reduces blurring and ghost artifacts caused by respiration.

Echo-train imaging with half-Fourier reconstruction (e.g., HASTE, SSFSE), as described above, can further decrease the acquisition time. All the data for a single image can be acquired in less than a second and a multislice acquisition is performed on a per slice basis. Thus, HASTE is very helpful in patients unable to breath-hold or when a rapid survey for hydronephrosis, focal lesions, or collecting system defects is needed. In addition, simple renal cysts can be readily characterized with this technique when a uniform, markedly hyperintense lesion without mural nodularity or complicated internal septations is seen. Drawbacks of half-Fourier imaging include signal-to-noise limitations and some blurring to the images.

T1-Weighted Imaging

The normal renal cortex is slightly higher in signal intensity than the medulla on adequately T1-weighted sequences and the medulla has a similar signal intensity compared with muscle. Most renal cysts are low in signal intensity on T1-weighted images compared to the normal renal parenchyma due to their long relaxation time. Increased signal intensity within cysts can be seen when they are complicated by hemorrhage or contain proteinaceous fluid. Heterogeneous signal features or

fluid-fluid levels can also be found. Most of the solid renal lesions, other than angiomyolipoma (AML), demonstrate slightly lower signal intensity than that of the renal cortex on T1-weighted images. AML and other fat-containing lesions demonstrate high signal intensity compared to the renal cortex on T1-weighted images. The signal intensity of AML on T1-weighted images may vary depending on the amount of fat. Macroscopic fat within AML is best confirmed with the use of frequency-selected fat-saturated T1-weighted images. AML can also be reliably diagnosed on in- and opposed-phase T1-weighted GRE imaging.

The presence of an "India ink" artifact at the interface between the mass and the kidney is typically seen on opposed-phase images. In addition, chemical shift imaging allows for detection of minimal amounts of fat when a drop in signal intensity is noted within the mass on opposed-phase images compared to in-phase images (Fig. 86-3). While this finding can be the only clue for the diagnosis of an AML containing minimal amounts of fat, this is not specific because clear-cell type RCCs and, rarely, other renal neoplasms can demonstrate similar findings (Fig. 86-4). High signal intensity within a renal lesion can also be secondary to paramagnetic effects. These can be seen in intralesional hemorrhage cyst, AML and RCC, melanin-containing lesions (metastases from malignant melanoma), and proteinaceous mucin-containing lesions (complicated cyst and abscess).

Spin-echo T1-weighted sequences, formerly the standard for body imaging, should be relegated to those systems unable to achieve good quality breath-hold imaging. Breath-hold T1-weighted imaging of the kidneys can be obtained using multishot spoiled GRE techniques, including fast spoiled gradient-echo sequences (FSPGR; GE Medical Systems, Milwaukee, WI) and fast low-angle shot sequences (FLASH; Siemens Medical Systems, Erlangen, Germany). Typically, a short repetition time (TR 120-200 ms) and a flip angle of 70 to 90 degrees are used to allow full coverage of the kidney in one breath-hold. These acquisitions offer good signal-to-noise ratio and regular section spacing, and minimize respiratory-related artifacts. These sequences can also be used for dynamic contrast-enhanced MR imaging with or without fat suppression.[16,17] Again, magnetization-prepared GRE imaging is an excellent alternative in patients with a limited breath-hold capacity.

In- and Opposed-Phase Imaging

GRE images can be obtained with protons from fat and water either in- or out-of-phase with one another by selecting specific time to echo (TE) values.[18] When fat and water are present within a voxel, there is loss of signal intensity in the opposed-phase images compared with the in-phase images. While frequency-selected fat-suppression techniques allow for detection of bulk fat, the opposed-phase technique is sensitive for detecting intracellular lipid. Renal masses may contain focal bulk fat (AMLs), intracellular lipid (clear-cell renal carcinomas) or scant amounts of lipid (lipid-poor AML).[19,20] The latter two circumstances can each result in a relative focal or diffuse loss of signal intensity on opposed-phase images,

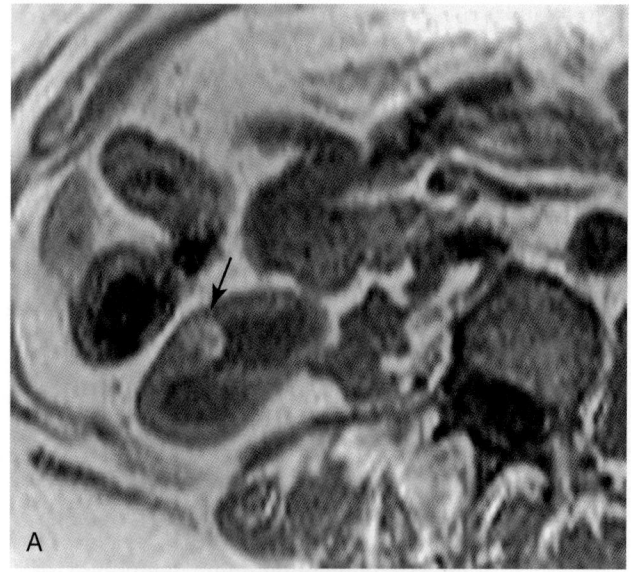

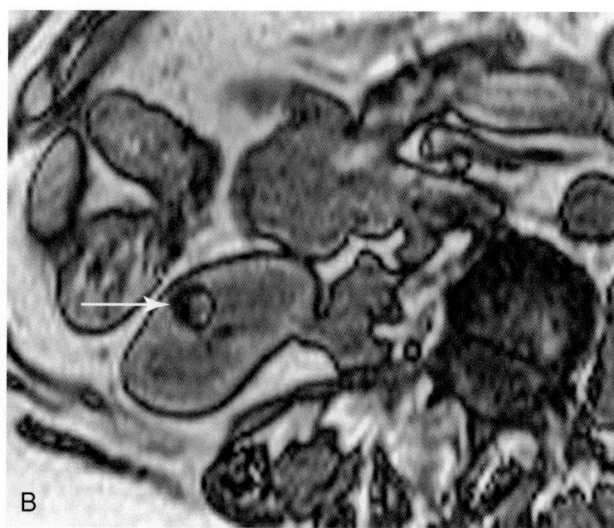

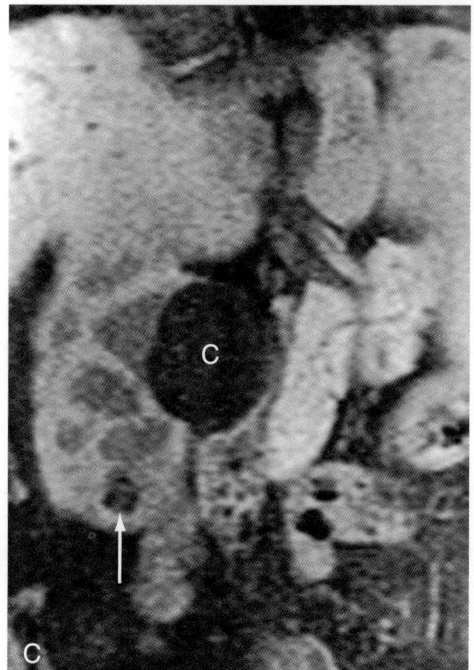

FIGURE 86-3

Angiomyolipoma (AML). **A,** Axial T1-weighted in-phase gradient-recalled echo (GRE) image demonstrates a small renal mass in the lower pole of the right kidney of diffuse high signal intensity (*arrow*). **B,** Axial T1-weighted opposed-phase image shows a drop in signal intensity in the lateral aspect of the lesion (*arrow*) due to the intravoxel coexistence of fat and water. The medial aspect of the lesion does not show a drop in signal intensity, which is similar to that of the in-phase image. This is consistent with a significant amount of bulk fat within the lesion and, therefore, the diagnosis of AML can be made with confidence. Note the presence of the India ink artifact at the fat-water interface between the mass and the normal renal parenchyma, which is characteristic of AML. **C,** Sagittal frequency selective fat-saturated T1-weighted noncontrast GRE image confirms the presence of bulk fat by showing saturated areas within the mass (*arrow*). A large cyst (C) is also noted in the interpolar region of the right kidney.

making such a finding nonspecific.[21,22] A boundary chemical shift artifact or India ink artifact can be seen on opposed-phased GRE images at the interface between bulk fat and water. Identification of this artifact between the fatty component of the mass and the normal kidney can help characterize many AMLs. This effect is not visualized at the interface of the mass and the retroperitoneal fat when an exophitic fatty component exists (Fig. 86-5).

At 1.5 T, GRE images obtained at TEs of approximately 2.2 ms and 4.4 ms yield features of opposed- and in-phase effects, respectively. A single multislice acquisition can be obtained for the in- and opposed-phase images by acquiring two echoes per excitation at different echo times and reconstructing the data as separate image sets. The acquisition of both echoes in a single breath-hold eliminates respiratory misregistration between in- and opposed-phase images and facilitates a comparison of the two image sets.

Contrast-Enhanced Dynamic Imaging

The presence of enhancement within a renal lesion after administration of an intravenous contrast agent is the most reliable criterion for distinguishing solid masses from cysts. MR images should be acquired in various vascular phases after intravenous administration of a single bolus of gadolinium-based contrast agent. The ideal MR imaging protocol includes nonenhanced MR images followed by imaging during the cortico-medullary (timed to the arterial phase), nephrographic (20 seconds after the corticomedullary phase), and

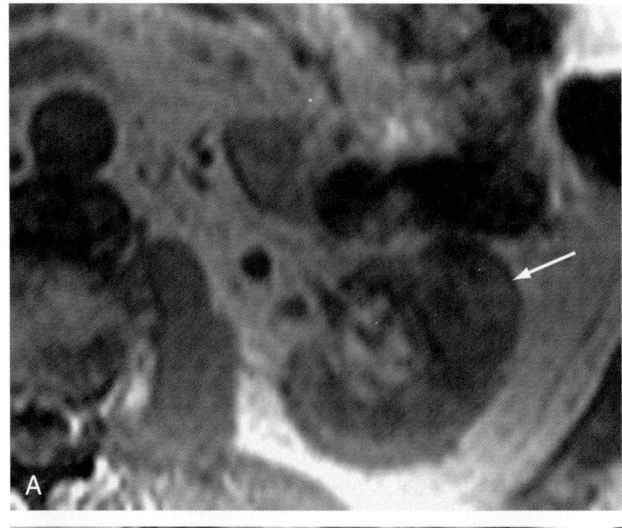

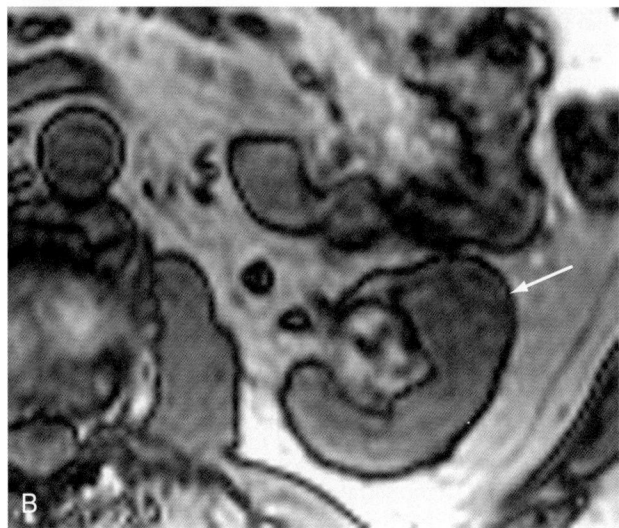

FIGURE 86-4

Intracellular fat in clear-cell carcinoma. **A,** Axial T1-weighted in-phase gradient-recalled echo (GRE) image shows a heterogeneous mass in the inferior pole of the left kidney with areas of high signal intensity (*arrow*). **B,** Axial T1-weighted opposed-phase GRE image demonstrates a subtle drop in signal intensity in those areas of high signal intensity on **A** due to the coexistence of intravoxel fat and water (*arrow*). A partial nephrectomy was performed and pathology analysis confirmed clear-cell type renal cell carcinoma (RCC). Clear-cell RCC can demonstrate a drop in signal intensity on opposed-phase imaging compared to in-phase imaging due to its intracellular fat content. A clear distinction between lipid-poor angiomyolipoma and clear-cell RCC is not possible based on current MR techniques.

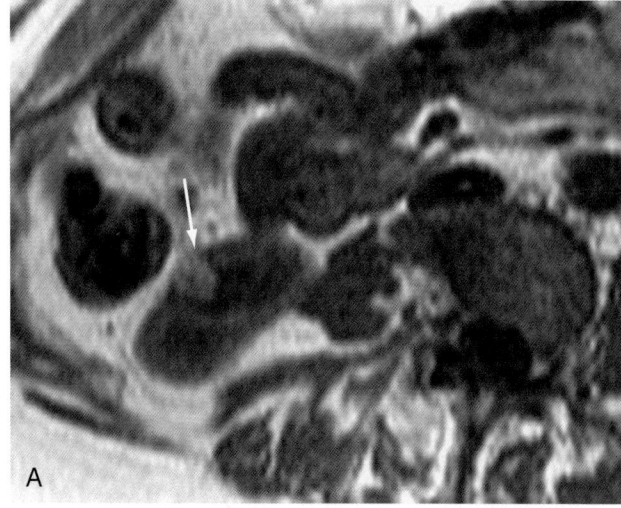

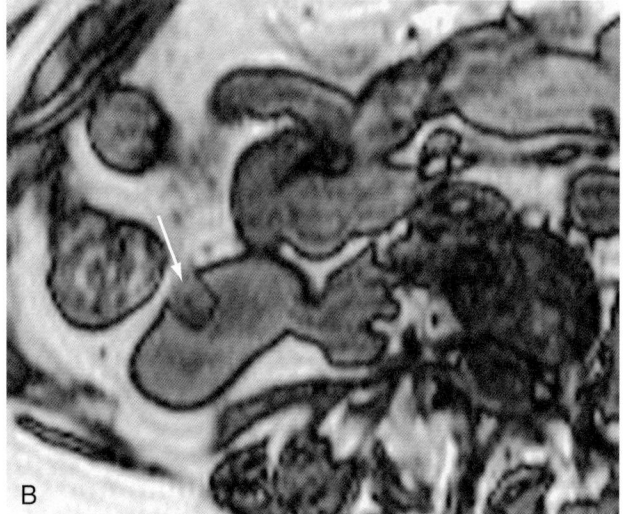

FIGURE 86-5

Angiomyolipoma (AML). **A,** Axial T1-weighted in-phase gradient-recalled echo (GRE) image demonstrates a small hyperintense right renal mass (*arrow*). **B,** Axial T1-weighted opposed-phase image shows the characteristic India ink artifact interface between the mass and the normal renal parenchyma due to the intravoxel coexistence of fat and water. Note the lack of India ink artifact at the fat-fat interface between the AML and retroperitoneal fat (*arrow*).

delayed venous phases (30 seconds after the previous phase). The corticomedullary phase allows for delineation of the arterial anatomy and helps identify hypertrophied columns of Bertin as pseudotumors. The nephrographic phase is the most sensitive for tumor detection and it is essential for imaging the renal veins for possible tumoral extension, as well as the rest of the intra-abdominal organs for potential metastases.

Fast T1-weighted imaging with GRE sequences is the cornerstone of renal imaging. Two-dimensional (2D) breath-hold imaging of the kidneys is constrained by the need to acquire enough sections to cover a relatively large anatomic area within a single breath-hold (usually <25 seconds). Typically, a 160 to 200 mm region is covered with relatively thick sections (8-10 mm) separated by an interslice gap (1-2 mm). With this approach, smaller lesions and/or small enhancing foci within larger lesions can be missed or insufficiently characterized because of partial volume averaging.

Three-dimensional (3D) Fourier transform imaging has advantages over 2D imaging. Compared with 2D GRE acquisitions, properly structured 3D T1-weighted GRE sequences have the capacity to provide thinner contiguous sections without interslice gaps, with fat saturation, higher signal-to-noise ratios, and comparable image contrast in the same breath-hold time frame.[23] Volumetric 3D sequences used for gadolinium-enhanced MR angiography can be optimized for combined parenchymal and vascular imaging by reducing the flip angle to 10 to 15 degrees and using a symmetric or full echo for readout.[23] Optimization of the scan parameters using these techniques provides nearly isotropic resolution, which combined with an accurate timing method can be used to generate high quality images of the parenchyma as well as MR angiograms from a single data set. Volumetric acquisitions with thin sections can also be used to create meaningful multiplanar reconstructions in any plane, facilitating characterization of lesions that may be difficult to evaluate on axial images.

MR Urography

A tailored MR protocol can be helpful in the evaluation of pathology in the collecting system.[24-27] MR may be particularly helpful when the use of iodinated contrast media or radiation is undesirable (e.g. allergic or pregnant patients, and young adults).[28] MR evaluation of the collecting system is based on heavily T2-weighted images and gadolinium-enhanced T1-weighted images.

Heavily T2-weighted MR images allow for rapid, safe, and noninvasive evaluation of the collecting system.[27,28] Breath-hold imaging of the urinary tract can be obtained with HASTE and RARE sequences without the need of contrast media.[26,27] Thin-slice images (thickness, 3-6 mm) with a half-Fourier T2-weighted sequence (HASTE or SSFSE) are typically obtained in the coronal plane in one breath-hold, though two breath-holds may be required to include the desired anatomy in patients with large body habitus. Fat saturation improves the visualization of the collecting system. These images can be reconstructed using a maximum intensity projection (MIP) algorithm which, in general, does not offer additional diagnostic information but provides urographic-like images that are better accepted by urologists.[27]

A 20 to 60 mm thick slab can be obtained in the coronal plane in a short breath-hold with a RARE sequence that includes the entire collecting system in a single image that resembles the conventional excretory urography. However, an acquisition of multiple thin slices tends to provide better image quality than a single thick-slab technique because the background tissues are usually better delineated and there are fewer partial volume effects.[36] An MR protocol that combines both approaches, including multiple thin-slice HASTE and thick-slab RARE images, can increase the confidence of the radiologist in the evaluation of urinary obstruction.[24]

Gadolinium-enhanced MR urography (MRU) is a valuable addition to the T2-weighted images for evaluation of the collecting system.[25,28] MRU examinations can be performed using a high-resolution 3D T1-weighted sequence after administration of gadolinium contrast media. A low dose of furosemide (0.1 mg/kg bodyweight, maximum dose 10 mg) is administered approximately 30 to 60 seconds prior to the administration of gadolinium. This provides good distension of the collecting system with homogenous distribution of the gadolinium inside the entire urinary tract.[25] Since furosemide increases

urine volume, there is dilution of the concentrated gadolinium within the collecting system which leads to homogeneous high signal intensity by decreasing the T2* effects.[25] MRU can be performed with a respiratory-gated T1-weighted spoiled gradient-echo sequence,[25] though a breath-hold 3D fat-saturated T1-weighted gradient-echo sequence is much faster and decreases the artifacts related to respiratory motion.[24] The latter approach requires a cooperative patient capable of performing typical breath-holds of 18 to 25 seconds, though with parallel imaging shorter acquisitions are possible. The background signal can be partially saturated when a high flip angle (>45°) is selected. This helps to create better MIP reconstructions that provide excretory urography-like images with better spatial resolution than thin-slice HASTE or thick-slab RARE images.[24] A potential limitation of gadolinium-enhanced MRU examinations is delayed excretion of the contrast in the presence of high-grade obstruction.[28] Delayed MR acquisitions can be obtained once the contrast has reached the level of obstruction, though this can be quite time consuming.

Contrast Media

Gadolinium-based contrast agents that distribute in the extracellular fluid (ECF) spaces have been proven safe in patients with renal failure.[29-31] Allergic reactions to gadolinium chelates are extremely rare.[32] These characteristics make gadolinium an excellent contrast agent in the evaluation of renal pathology, including patients with a contraindication to the administration of iodinated contrast media due to known allergy or renal insufficiency, as first demonstrated in 1991.[29-31]

For renal imaging, we use gadopentetate dimeglumine (Magnevist; Berlex Laboratories, Wayne, NJ) at the standard dose of 0.1 mmol/kg, though no efficacy difference among the Food and Drug Administration (FDA)-approved ECF gadolinium chelate contrast agents has been demonstrated.[33] Another contrast agent, gadobenate dimeglumine (MultiHance; Braco, Milan, Italy), has been shown to produce higher signal-to-noise ratios at 0.1 mmol/kg when compared to gadopentetate dimeglumine at the same dose[34]; the possible impact on diagnostic efficacy awaits further study.

In our practice it is routine to administer contrast at a rate of 2 mL/second for dynamic contrast-enhanced MR images using an antecubital vein for access. The bolus of contrast should be flushed with 20 mL saline at the same rate of 2 mL/second. When the intravenous catheter is placed in the hand, 30 mL saline flush is recommended to ensure that a tight bolus of contrast reaches the heart.

Precise timing of image acquisition during selected periods of enhancement is recommended for detection and characterization of renal pathology. While the use of fixed-image delays is effective in the majority of patients, up to 20% of patients have different circulatory dynamics that result in failure to capture the arterial phase appropriately.[35] Gradient-echo imaging with a timing bolus of as little as 0.5 to 1 mL gadolinium can be injected,[36,37] but 2 mL gadolinium is currently our routine. The imaging delay for the acquisition of the corticomedullary phase is determined in each patient on the basis of the results of the timing examination and has been described elsewhere.[37] MR-compatible power injectors are recommended to yield reliable and reproducible contrast delivery for optimized results.

MR CHARACTERIZATION OF RENAL MASSES

Detection of Tumor Enhancement

The presence of enhancement within a renal lesion on gadolinium-enhanced MR images is the most reliable criterion for distinguishing solid masses from cysts on MR examinations. Comparison of precontrast and delayed post-contrast T1-weighted images is the key to the detection and characterization of renal lesions.[29,38,39] Dynamic contrast-enhanced MR imaging using fast GRE sequences with or without fat suppression can be used to characterize renal lesions by means of quantitative analysis of signal intensity changes over time.[16,17]

Renal cysts do not show enhancement after administration of intravenous contrast. A 15% increase in signal intensity within a renal lesion at 2 to 4 minutes after administration of contrast material has been proposed as an optimal threshold for distinguishing malignancies from benign cysts.[16,17] However, quantitative criteria should be used with caution in the characterization of renal masses since no standardized scale for signal intensity values exists. Furthermore, changes in the signal intensity scale occur from scanner to scanner, as well as among different sequences within the same MR scanner. For quantitative evaluations it is important that the receiver gain and attenuation values be held constant for the identical sequences obtained prior to and after contrast. Qualitative assessment of enhancement can be used when identical sequences for pre- and post-contrast imaging are employed.[40,41] Determination of subtle enhancement in hypovascular lesions can be challenging. A quantitative approach or subtraction imaging can be helpful in these cases.[42]

Subtraction Technique

Subtraction of the nonenhanced data set from the contrast-enhanced data sets can be performed for better detection of subtle enhancement. Each data set acquired during the dynamic contrast-enhanced MR examination can be used as a template from which the nonenhanced data set is subtracted. Subtraction can help in the detection of a small enhancing component within a cystic renal lesion. This is particularly helpful in the evaluation of complicated cystic lesions, when hemorrhagic or proteinaceous contents account for high signal intensity within the lesion on nonenhanced images. In this situation, detection of subtle areas or even moderate-sized foci of enhancement within the lesion can be challenging (Fig. 86-6).

The degree of misregistration must be taken into account when subtraction imaging is used for the qualitative assessment of renal lesion enhancement. Misregistration of the nonenhanced and contrast-enhanced data sets occurs when the patient's breath-hold varies from one acquisition to another. Ghosting artifact around the renal contour can be used as an index of the degree of misregistration. End-expiratory breath-hold imaging is recommended since it is more easily replicated and typically eliminates or minimizes misregistration concerns.

The subtraction technique also benefits the image contrast between vessels and background tissue. Thus, ancillary imaging processing with MIP and volume rendering algorithms is facilitated.[43]

Cystic Renal Masses: The Bosniak Classification

Simple renal cysts are easily diagnosed based on their appearance on cross-sectional imaging. However, cystic lesions with complicated appearance can present a dilemma regarding their management. Bosniak[44] proposed a classification that has served as a guideline for the management of these lesions and it is well accepted among urologists. This classification was initially developed for CT evaluation of cystic renal lesions and it has recently been applied to MR examinations.[45]

The Bosniak classification includes five categories[45]:

- Category I lesions are benign simple cysts defined as well-marginated lesions with hairline-thin walls, no septa, calcifications, or solid components. These lesions do not show enhancement after intravenous contrast material administration.
- Category II masses are benign cystic lesions that may contain hairline-thin septa and fine calcification in the walls or septa. A short segment of slightly thickened calcification can be present. Hairline-thin septae can demonstrate minimal enhancement after contrast administration. This category also includes cysts with uniform high attenuation contents (high-attenuation cysts) on CT that are less than 3 cm in diameter and show no enhancement after contrast administration.
- Category IIF lesions include complex cysts that cannot be clearly classified within category II or III. An increased number of hairline-thin septa or minimal but smooth thickening of the wall or septa can be seen. There may be thick and nodular calcifications in the wall and/or septa. Minimal perceived enhancement of hairline-thin smooth septae or wall can be appreciated, though no enhancing soft-tissue component should be present. The "F" in this category indicates the need for follow-up imaging. Hyperdense cysts (see category II) that are 3 cm or larger are also included in this category.
- Category III lesions are indeterminate cystic renal masses. Differentiation between the benign or malignant nature of the lesion cannot be established based on radiologic findings. These lesions have thickened irregular enhancing walls or septa.

the Robson's classification has poor correlation with prognosis. While the TNM system was initially considered complex relative to the Robson's classification due to its large number of categories, it was simplified in 1992 and it is now considered the superior evaluation for tumor extent and prognosis.[48-51]

The latest revision of the TNM classification in 1997 modified the tumor size cut-off of the T1 stage to 7 cm versus the previously used 2.5 cm because the smaller cut-off does not change the prognosis.[48-50] The presence of tumor thrombus within the inferior vena cava (IVC), previously T3c, was changed to T3b (similar to renal vein thrombosis).[48] Tumor thrombus above the diaphragm, previously T4, was changed to T3c.

The overall 5-year survival based on the 1997 TNM stage groupings is 91% to 100%, 69% to 95%, 59% to 76%, and 16% to 32% for stages I through IV, respectively.[48-51]

Tumor size is an independent predictor of outcome.[52] Accurate presurgical measurement of tumor size is possible by means of cross-sectional imaging studies, particularly CT and MR imaging. The multiplanar capability of MR and the excellent quality of multiplanar reconstructions of CT examinations (especially multidetector CT) allow for precise measurement in virtually any plane.

The presence of a pseudocapsule surrounding the tumor predicts the absence of perinephric fat involvement.[53,54] At MR, this pseudocapsule is seen as a linear hypointensity on T1- and T2-weighted images in 66% of patients with RCC equal to or smaller than 4 cm in diameter.[53] Histologically, those patients with a visible pseudocapsule on MR imaging tend to have low-grade neoplasms (Fig. 86-8).[54] Aggressive tumors are usually poorly marginated and a pseudocapsule is not visualized. T2-weighted MR images are superior to CT for the detection of this pseudocapsule.[55] Furthermore, the pseudocapsule is usually invisible on contrast-enhanced CT.[54] This finding may be useful to better select cases for partial versus radical, and laparoscopic versus open, nephrectomy. Perinephric extension of tumor can also be detected using opposed-phase GRE images. The renal contour is artificially accentuated by the black line at the renal-retroperitoneal fat interface caused by chemical shift artifact in these images.[19] In our experience, the preservation of this black line or India ink artifact at the tumor boundaries has excellent negative predictive value for contiguous organ invasion and correlates with the presence of an intact fat plane around the tumor. The absence of this black line does not necessarily correlate with tumor invasion. A renal mass that extends beyond the renal capsule and abuts an adjacent organ can cause obscuration of this black line *without* invasion of that adjacent organ.

In patients with venous tumor thrombus, the significance of the level of extension remains controversial.[48] While some authors have found a clear correlation between the extension of the thrombus and the prognosis,[56] others believe that the extension of tumor thrombus is much less important than the presence of capsular invasion, regional lymph node involvement, or distant metastases.[57,58] At our institution, the surgical approach in patients with RCC in the left kidney and tumor thrombus within the left renal vein is decided

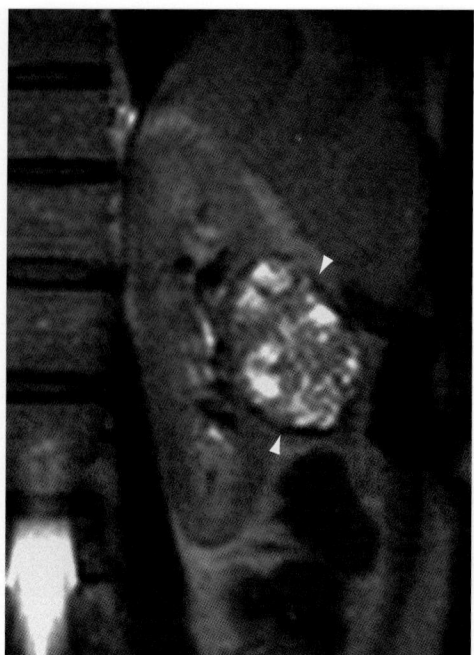

FIGURE 86-8

Pseudocapsule in renal cell carcinoma (RCC). Coronal T2-weighted half-Fourier turbo spin-echo (HASTE) image demonstrates an exophytic hyperintense mass in the interpolar region of the left kidney well demarcated by a hypointense pseudocapsule (*arrowheads*). Histopathologic analysis revealed a low grade (I-II) clear-cell RCC with clear margins and no evidence of perirenal extension.

based on the MR findings. In those patients where the tumor thrombus does not extend beyond the level of the superior mesenteric artery (SMA) (midline), a left flank incision is usually sufficient for complete resection of the thrombus (Fig. 86-9). A midline laparotomy incision is used in those patients with thrombus extending beyond the level of the SMA in the left renal vein and/or IVC because this approach provides superior access to the distal thrombus.

The IVC is involved in 4% to 15% of patients with RCC.[59] MR has been shown to be superior to CT in the detection of tumor extension within the renal vein and IVC based on data prior to the multidetector era.[60] Thrombus of the IVC is not a contraindication for surgical resection. In the absence of distal metastases, patients with RCC and venous thrombus extending into the IVC have survival rates as high as 68% 5 years after resection.[59] Extension of the IVC thrombus above the level of the hepatic veins into the right atrium has direct implications for the surgical approach. In these situations, cardiopulmonary bypass with deep hypothermic cardiac arrest should be considered to allow for close visual examination of the atrium and caval lumen, which can decrease the risk of sudden, life-threatening hemorrhage.[47,61]

Necrosis occurs in approximately one third of RCCs.[48] Recently, the histologic presence of tumor necrosis has been correlated with a poor prognosis.[62] Any degree of microscopic tumor necrosis has an impact

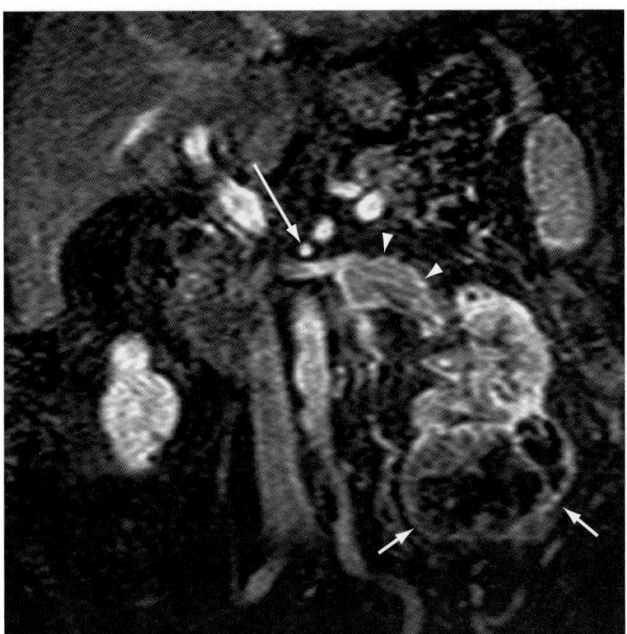

FIGURE 86-9

Renal vein thrombosis. Coronal 3D contrast-enhanced fat-saturated T1-weighted gradient-recalled echo (GRE) subtracted (delayed venous phase minus precontrast) image demonstrates enlargement of the left renal vein by enhancing tumor thrombus (*arrowheads*) that extends beyond the superior mesenteric artery (*long arrow*). A large enhancing partially necrotic mass is noted in the inferior pole of the left kidney (*short arrows*). A left flank incision at the top of the 12th rib provided good surgical access to remove the thrombus within the left renal vein.

on prognosis. Macroscopic necrosis can be seen on contrast-enhanced imaging studies but obviously some necrotic features will be beyond the resolution of current imaging techniques.[48] While microscopically tumor necrosis has been associated with a worse prognosis in clear-cell and chromophobe RCC, this correlation has not been found in papillary RCC.[62]

Lymph node involvement occurs in approximately 10% to 20% of patients with RCC without evidence of metastases.[47] Preoperative diagnosis of lymph node involvement is currently based on detection of lymph node enlargement. This approach has known false negatives (micrometastasis in lymph nodes <1 cm) and false positives (enlarged lymph nodes due to follicular hyperplasia). Studer et al[63] found a sensitivity of 95% for detection of enlarged lymph nodes in patients with RCC using CT and a cut-off of 1 cm in short diameter. However, follicular hyperplasia was found in 58% of the enlarged lymph nodes. Retroperitoneal lymph node enlargement can be secondary to inflammatory changes, particularly in the presence of tumor necrosis,[63] and other non-neoplastic conditions.

Ipsilateral adrenal gland involvement occurs in approximately 4% of patients with RCC, most commonly associated with direct extension of a neoplasm in the upper pole or with hematogenous metastatic disease.[47] Surgical resection of the adrenal gland should be reserved for those patients with abnormal-appearing glands on imaging studies or in patients with large upper pole masses.[47]

MALIGNANT RENAL MASSES

Renal Cell Carcinoma

RCC is the most common renal neoplasm accounting for 80% to 85% of all malignant renal masses and 2% of all cancers.[46,47] The incidence of RCC varies substantially between different regions of the world. RCC occurs nearly twice as often in men as in women.[47] It generally occurs in people older than 40 years of age and is most common among those in their 50s and 60s. RCC can occur in younger patients with familial forms of the disease. Its incidence has increased steadily in recent years. This has been accompanied by a significant improvement in 5-year survival from 52% (between 1974 and 1976) to 58% (between 1983 and 1989).[47] This is likely related to the improvement in imaging technology that allows early diagnosis of RCC and an increased number of incidentally detected neoplasms.

Cigarette smoking contributes to the development of RCC in one third of cases.[47] Other risk factors associated with the development of RCC include obesity (particularly in women), hypertension, treatment for hypertension, unopposed estrogen therapy, and occupational exposure to petroleum products, heavy metals, or asbestos. Patients with endstage renal disease are also at risk.[64,65]

The histopathologic classification of renal tumors was reviewed in 1986.[66] Based on morphologic, histochemical, and electron-microscopic data, renal carcinomas are now classified into clear-cell, chromophilic (papillary), chromophobic, oncocytic, and collecting duct (Bellini's duct) tumors. While ultrasound and CT imaging characteristics have been described for these subtypes, the MR appearance is not discussed for all of them in the literature. A discussion of the pathologic, clinical, and imaging findings in these tumors is presented in the following sections.

Conventional (Clear-Cell) Carcinoma

Clear-cell RCC is the most common type of RCC (65-80%).[67] Tumors are characterized by a deletion of one or both copies of chromosome 3p.[68] Microscopically, clear-cell RCC is composed of cells with optically clear cytoplasm arranged in sheets, acini, or alveoli.[62] Prominent thin-wall vasculature is characteristic.[62] Dissolved lipids and cholesterol account for the appearance of the clear cytoplasm.[62] Hyalinization and fibrosis are common, as well as coagulative tumor necrosis in high-grade tumors.[62] Cystic degeneration occurs in 4% to 15% of RCCs.[69,70] Clear-cell carcinoma has a worse prognosis than papillary and chromophobe RCCs.[62,71] Clear-cell RCC can undergo varied cell differentiations, including sarcomatoid and rhabdoid; these features are associated with poor prognosis.[62] Renal vein thrombosis is common in patients with advanced RCC.

The MR appearance of clear-cell carcinoma is variable depending on the presence of hemorrhage and necrosis. Central necrosis is typically of homogeneous low signal intensity on T1-weighted imaging and of high signal intensity on T2-weighted imaging.[39] A solid rim of viable tumor is commonly seen in the periphery of the mass of intermediate signal intensity on T1- and T2-weighted imaging. Hemorrhage may have different appearances depending on the stage of degradation of the blood products. While subacute-to-chronic hemorrhage usually demonstrates high signal intensity on both T1- and T2-weighted imaging, long-standing hemorrhage predominantly formed by hemosiderin is typically of low signal intensity.[72] The latter is better seen on T2-weighted imaging due to increased susceptibility effects. Hemosiderin deposition usually occurs in a rim configuration, though occasionally iron deposition may be responsible for the diffuse low signal intensity of some RCCs.[72,73]

Hyperintense areas within a RCC can also be secondary to the presence of bulk fat. This situation occurs when retroperitoneal fat is engulfed by the tumor mass. Bulk fat can be recognized by saturation of the signal intensity in these areas with chemical selective fat-suppression sequences. This is supplemented by a morphologic assessment to differentiate RCC-related engulfed fat from the fat seen with AML. Clear-cell carcinomas can accumulate fat in vacuoles within the cytoplasm. The presence of this microscopic (intracellular) form of fat usually does not correlate with high signal intensity on T1-weighted imaging and can only be detected when there is a drop in signal intensity in those areas on out-of-phase images (Fig. 86-10). This phenomenon has been observed in up to 60% of clear-cell RCCs.[21]

Cystic degeneration of RCC is common and can be detected on MR images as areas of low signal intensity on T1-weighted imaging, high signal intensity on T2-weighted imaging, and lack of enhancement. Occasionally, RCC can be predominantly cystic or can originate within a cyst. In these cases only small areas of solid tumor are appreciated in the wall of the cyst or within the septations. This should be distinguished from the more "benign" multilocular RCC. In the latter case, tumor cells extend along the septae within the cyst but there is no expansile or solid tumor growth. RCC with extensive cystic degeneration is more likely to have a diffusely irregular inner wall.[69]

Clear-cell RCC usually demonstrates avid enhancement during the arterial phase after administration of contrast media on both CT and MR imaging. However, these neoplasms are almost always hypovascular relative to the renal cortex during the arterial phase with some rare exceptions (Fig. 86-11). Masses with central coagulative necrosis and/or hemorrhage typically show a central area of high signal intensity on precontrast T1-weighted images. This area shows no enhancement after contrast administration. An enhancing thick rim of solid viable tumor is typically seen in the periphery of the mass. The solid component of the RCC can demonstrate heterogeneous enhancement (Fig. 86-12).

While small, low-grade carcinomas tend to be well circumscribed on MR imaging, large, aggressive tumors

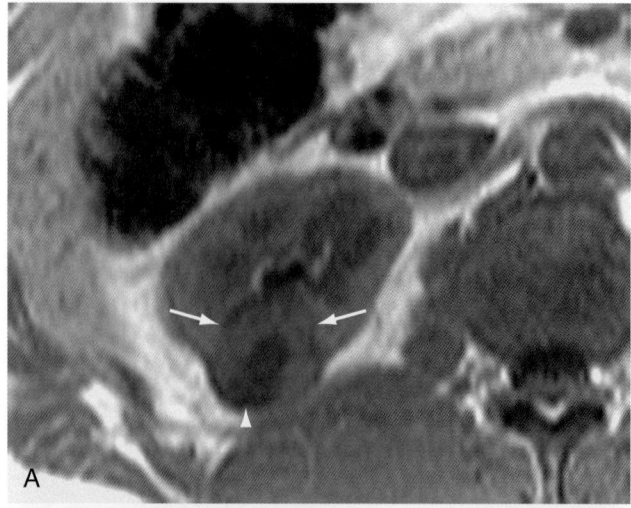

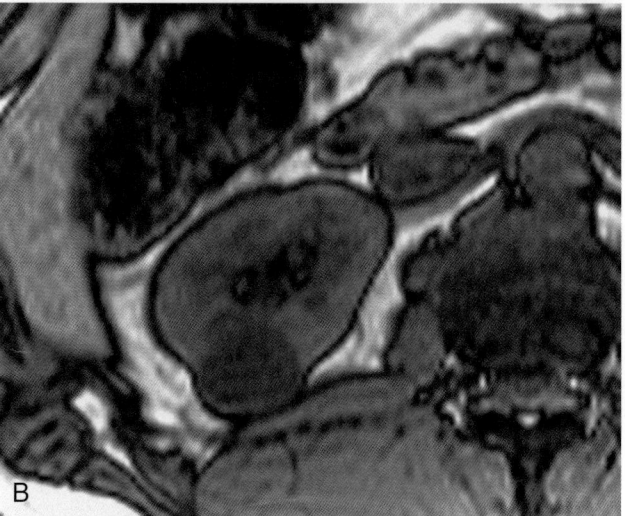

FIGURE 86-10

Intracellular fat in conventional (clear-cell) carcinoma. **A,** Axial T1-weighted in-phase gradient-recalled echo (GRE) image demonstrates a mass in the posterior aspect of the right kidney. There is low signal intensity in the center of the mass due to necrosis (*arrowhead*) and a thick rim of tumor is noted at the periphery of the lesion with signal intensity similar to that of the muscle (*arrows*). **B,** Axial T1-weighted opposed-phase GRE image (from dual echo acquisition in **A**) now demonstrates homogeneous signal intensity throughout the mass. Due to the presence of intracellular fat in the peripheral rim, the signal of this tissue has become isointense with the necrotic center. Clear-cell renal cell carcinoma with central necrosis was confirmed after nephrectomy.

are usually poorly marginated. A pseudocapsule has been described on MR imaging as a rim of low signal intensity on both T1- and T2-weighted imaging and corresponds to compressed renal parenchyma. Low-grade tumors usually demonstrate a pseudocapsule. Interruption of this pseudocapsule has been correlated with advanced stage (invasion of perirenal fat) and higher nuclear grade.[55] After administration of gadolinium, there is decreased conspicuity in the visualization of the enhancing pseudocapsule due to poor contrast relative to the surrounding tissue.[54]

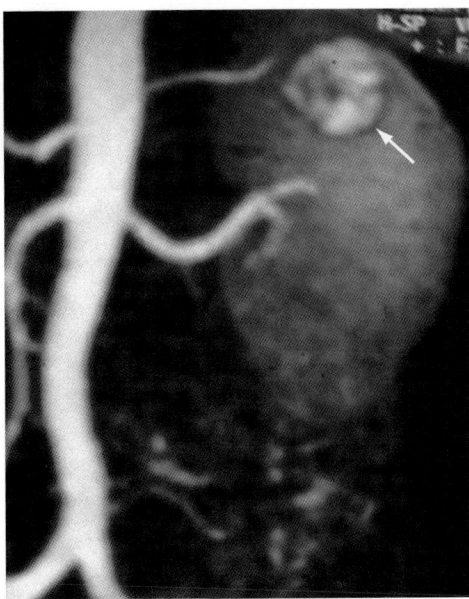

FIGURE 86-11

Hypervascular renal cell carcinoma (RCC). Maximum intensity projection from a coronal contrast-enhanced 3D fat-saturated T1-weighted gradient-recalled echo acquisition obtained during the arterial phase demonstrates a mass in the upper pole of the left kidney (arrow) that enhances to a greater degree than the adjacent renal parenchyma. At pathology, a conventional RCC was found.

Calcifications are present in approximately 10% of clear-cell RCC.[74] While calcifications in solid renal masses have been traditionally considered a sign of malignant process,[75] both benign and malignant renal cysts can demonstrate calcifications as well.[46] CT is clearly superior to MRI for the demonstration of calcifications. However, a recent report has found no advantage for their characterization in demonstrating calcification in cystic lesions.[46] Identification of enhancing solid tumor in the wall or septa of these lesions (Bosniak category III) requires surgical management in most cases, though some of these lesions will prove to be benign.[46]

Sarcomatoid features can be seen in approximately 5% of RCCs and are associated with poor prognosis. Any histologic subtype of RCC can present with spindle cell growth characteristic of sarcomatoid differentiation. Although this diagnosis cannot be made based on imaging findings, MR imaging can demonstrate a locally aggressive infiltrating mass in these patients (Fig. 86-13).

Papillary Renal Cell Carcinoma

Papillary RCC is the second most common malignant renal neoplasm in adults and accounts for 10% to 15% of all RCCs.[76] Papillary RCC has a better prognosis than clear-cell carcinoma.[62] Papillary tumors are composed of fibrovascular cores lined by a single layer of tumor cells. Two types of papillary tumors have been recently recognized.[77] Type I papillary RCC is characterized by a small cuboidal cell covering thin papillae with a single

line of uniform nuclei and small nucleoli.[77] Type II neoplasms have large eosinophilic cells with pleomorphic nuclei and prominent nucleoli covering the papillae. This distinction is important since type II papillary neoplasms are associated with a higher Fuhrman grade and poorer prognosis.[78,79] Papillary RCC is multifocal in 20% to 40% of patients with two to three tumors in 78% of them.[79] Bilateral tumors are also common.[47,49] Multifocal tumors in these patients frequently represent small adenomas (<5 mm) or small papillary RCC, which probably accounts for the low reported detection rate using contrast-enhanced CT.[79] Multifocality is not associated with stage, grade, or histologic type of tumors and, therefore, is not a contraindication of nephron-sparing surgery.[79] Presurgical diagnosis of papillary RCC can help in the selection of the best surgical approach in these patients.

On contrast-enhanced CT, papillary neoplasms tend to enhance homogeneously and less than conventional (clear-cell) carcinoma due to their relative hypovascularity.[80,81] Herts at al[81] reported that a high (>25%) tumor-to-aorta enhancement ratio on contrast-enhanced CT during the vascular phase or tumor-to-parenchyma enhancement ratio during the nephrographic phase excludes the possibility of a papillary RCC. Calcification is more common than in conventional (clear-cell) RCC.[80,82] Heterogeneous enhancement of papillary tumors on contrast-enhanced CT has also been described.[82] Calcifications can be seen in approximately 30% of papillary RCCs.[74] Recently, CT identification of "bulk" fat within papillary RCCs has been reported and it seems to be secondary to cholesterol clefts and foam cells producing cholesterol necrosis.[83] In these cases, the diagnosis should be suspected when the tumor demonstrates a homogeneous (except for the fat-containing foci), low (<25%) tumor-to-aorta enhancement ratio during the vascular phase.[83]

To our knowledge, the MR appearance of papillary neoplasms has not been previously described. In our experience, two different patterns can be found and these correlate with the histologic type. Low-grade (type I) papillary neoplasms tend to demonstrate homogeneous low signal intensity on T2-weighted images and low-grade homogeneous enhancement (Fig. 86-14). Detection of enhancement in low-grade papillary RCC can be challenging. Subtraction imaging can help to recognize subtle tumor enhancement (Fig. 86-15). This pattern of enhancement correlates with the reported enhancing characteristics of these neoplasms on CT.[81] When these findings are present the diagnosis of low-grade papillary tumor is suggested, though other hypovascular masses, including mesenchymal tumors (e.g. fibroma, leiomyoma) or oncocytomas, can have similar appearance. Necrosis and hemorrhage can be present even in low-grade neoplasms, making their appearance heterogeneous on pre- and post-contrast images. High-grade (type II) neoplasms are typically heterogeneous due to the presence of central hemorrhage and necrosis. Enhancing papillary projections are typically seen in the periphery of the tumor. In contrast to low-grade neoplasms, the solid component of high-grade neoplasms can demonstrate avid contrast

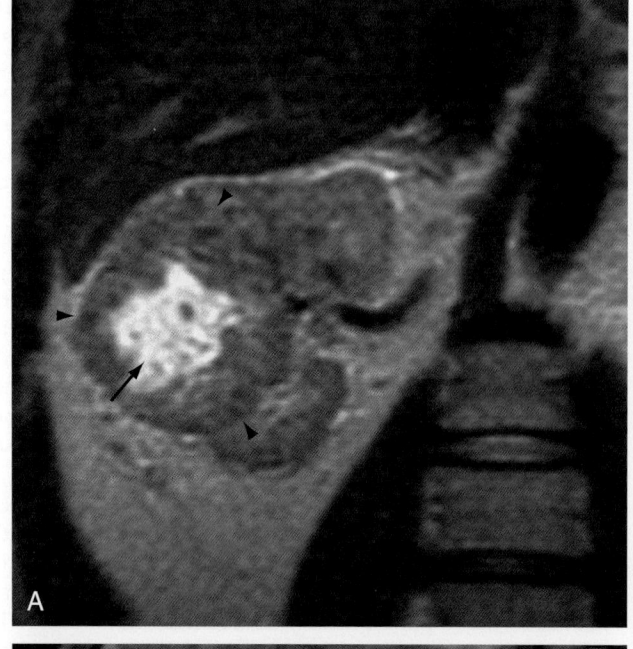

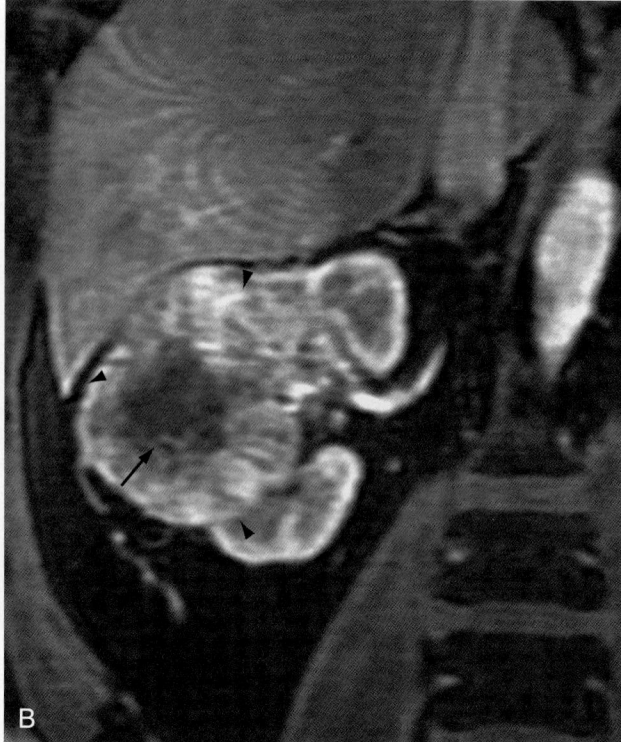

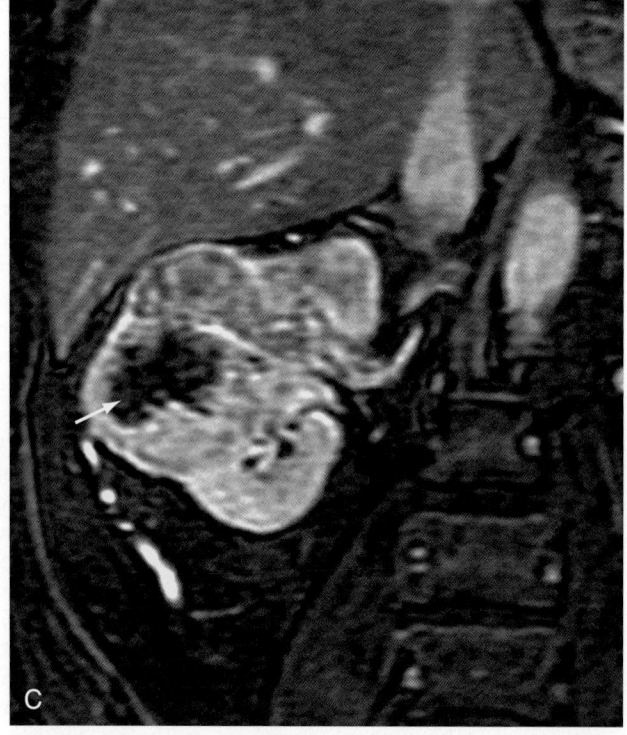

FIGURE 86-12

Conventional (clear-cell) carcinoma. **A,** Coronal T2-weighted half-Fourier turbo spin-echo (HASTE) image demonstrates a large heterogeneous mass in the right kidney. The mass has a thick rim of intermediate signal intensity similar to that of the renal parenchyma (*arrowheads*) and a large central area of high signal intensity consistent with necrosis (*arrow*). **B,** Coronal contrast-enhanced 3D fat-saturated T1-weighted gradient-recalled echo (GRE) image obtained during the corticomedullary phase demonstrates avid heterogeneous enhancement of the peripheral rim of tumor (*arrowheads*) and no apparent enhancement of the central necrosis (*arrow*). **C,** Coronal contrast-enhanced 3D fat-saturated T1-weighted GRE subtracted image (delayed venous phase minus precontrast) confirms the lack of enhancement in the central necrotic region (*arrow*).

enhancement. In the presence of extensive hemorrhagic contents within the mass, visualization of enhancing papillary projections can be challenging (Fig. 86-16).

Chromophobe Renal Cell Carcinoma

Chromophobe RCC represents approximately 4% of all RCCs.[47] It is composed of broad sheets of cells with eosinophilic and clear cytoplasm and tumor cells arranged along vascular septae.[62] A perinuclear halo is a characteristic feature and binucleate cells are common.[62] Necrosis and hemorrhage are uncommon.[62] Patients with these tumors tend to have excellent prognosis.[47]

The MR imaging findings in chromophobe carcinomas have not been described in the literature. A homogenous enhancement pattern can be found on contrast-enhanced CT examinations in up to 69% of these tumors and calcifications are present in up to 38%.[74] Perinephric tumor spread and renal vein invasion are rare.[74] On MR imaging, chromophobe RCC can demonstrate diffuse high signal intensity on T2-weighted images (Fig. 86-17).

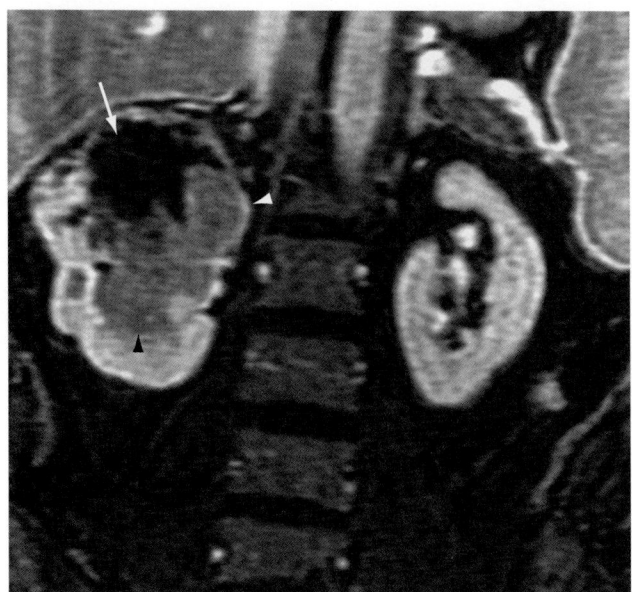

FIGURE 86-13

Sarcomatous differentiation in renal cell carcinoma. Coronal contrast-enhanced 3D fat-saturated T1-weighted gradient-recalled echo subtracted (delayed venous phase minus precontrast) image shows an infiltrating enhancing mass centered in the upper half of the right kidney that extends inferiorly into the lower pole (*black arrowhead*) and medially into the renal hilum (*white arrowhead*). Large areas without enhancement (*arrow*) are due to tumor necrosis.

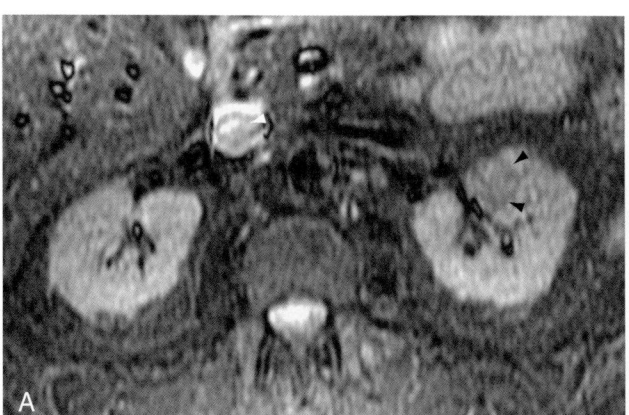

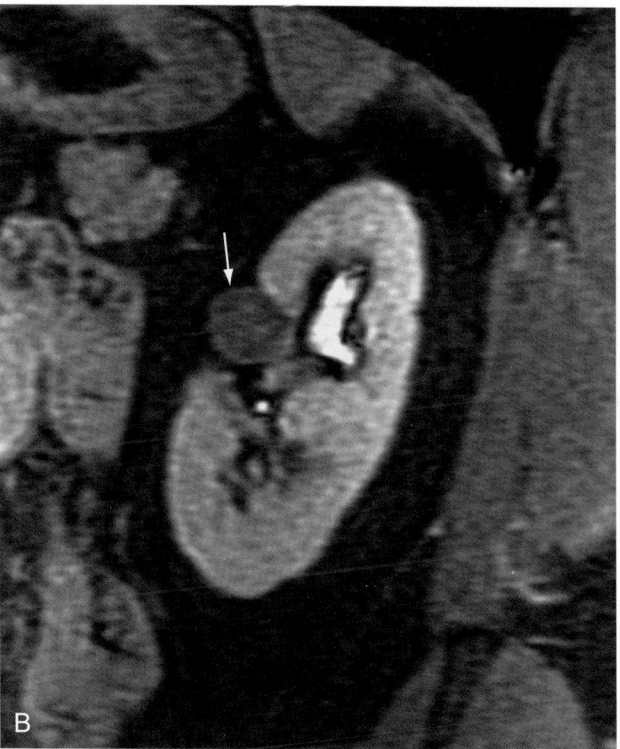

FIGURE 86-14

Low-grade papillary renal cell carcinoma (RCC). **A,** Axial short-tau inversion recovery (STIR) image at the level of the renal hilum shows a small left anterior renal mass (*arrowheads*) with homogenous signal intensity that is slightly lower than that of the normal renal parenchyma. **B,** Sagittal contrast-enhanced 3D fat-saturated T1-weighted gradient-recalled echo image during the delayed venous phase reveals homogeneous low signal intensity in the mass (*arrow*) compared to that of the enhancing renal parenchyma. Quantitative evaluation of the signal intensity within the mass was consistent with low level enhancement. Low-grade (I-II) papillary RCC was found at histopathologic analysis.

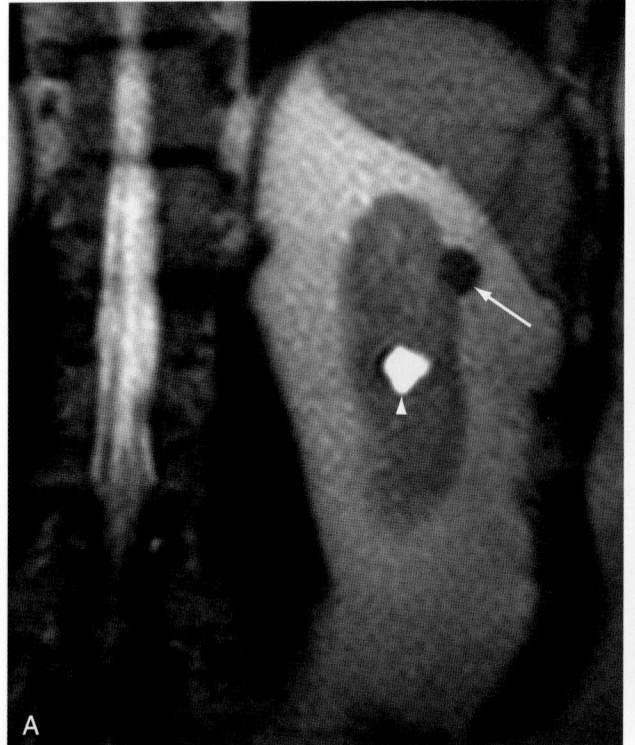

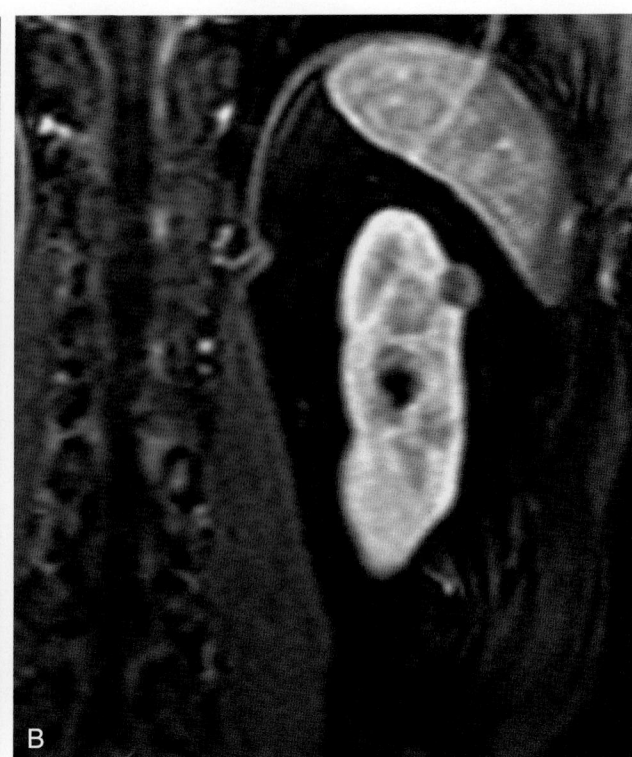

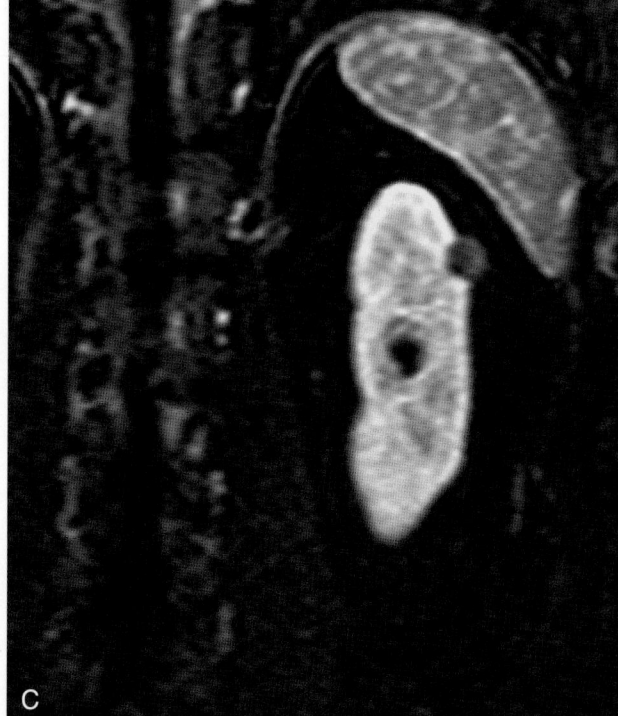

FIGURE 86-15

Subtraction imaging in papillary renal cell carcinoma (RCC). **A,** Coronal T2-weighted half-Fourier turbo spin-echo (HASTE) image shows a renal lesion in the upper pole with homogeneous low signal intensity (*arrow*). A second lesion in the interpolar region with homogenous very high signal intensity is also visualized (*arrowhead*). **B,** Coronal 3D contrast-enhanced fat-saturated T1-weighted gradient-recalled echo (GRE) image during the nephrographic phase shows homogeneous signal intensity within the lesion in the upper pole. Determination of enhancement within this lesion is difficult based on these findings. The inferior lesion demonstrates no obvious enhancement. **C,** Coronal 3D contrast-enhanced fat-saturated T1-weighted GRE subtracted (**B** minus precontrast) image during the nephrographic phase confirms the presence of enhancement within the mass. Papillary RCC was confirmed after partial nephrectomy. The inferior lesion is not enhancing and, therefore, consistent with a simple cyst.

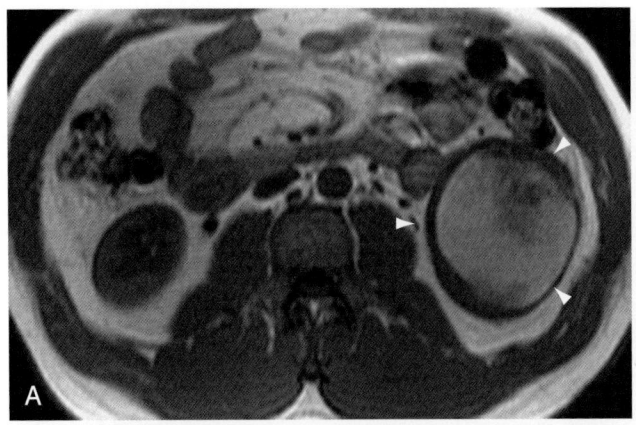

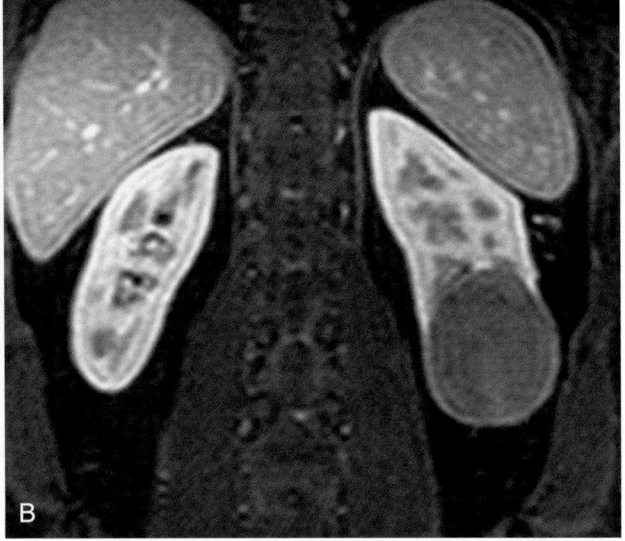

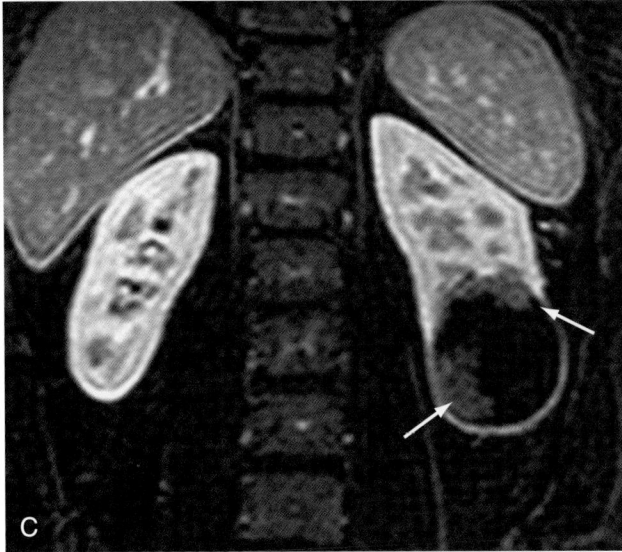

FIGURE 86-16

High-grade papillary renal cell carcinoma (RCC). **A,** Axial T1-weighted in-phase gradient-recalled echo (GRE) image shows a large left renal mass with predominantly hyperintense contents consistent with hemorrhage (*arrowheads*). **B,** Coronal 3D contrast-enhanced fat-saturated T1-weighted GRE image during the nephrographic phase demonstrates homogeneous signal intensity within the mass. Since the lesion is hyperintense on precontrast images, detection of enhancing components within the lesion is challenging. **C,** Coronal subtracted image (**B** minus precontrast) better confirms the presence of enhancing elements within the wall of the lesion (*arrows*). A high-grade (III-IV) papillary RCC was found after nephrectomy.

Collecting Duct (Bellini's Tumor) Carcinoma

Collecting duct carcinomas are extremely rare neoplasms that account for less than 1% of all renal neoplasms.[84] These neoplasms have aggressive clinical behavior and poor prognosis.[47,85] The mean age at presentation is 55 years with a 2:1 male predominance.[86] A variety of histologic appearances are described with different sized tubules and papillae.[62] Approximately 80% of patients have lymph node involvement at the time of presentation; 25% have lung or adrenal metastases, and 20% hepatic metastases.[85]

Cross-sectional imaging studies frequently demonstrate a large infiltrating mass with an average diameter of 7.7 cm.[87] The tumor originates in the renal medulla, though cortical and exophitic components are present in 88% and 59%, respectively; the reniform shape of the kidney can be preserved in smaller tumors.[87] An infiltrative appearance is seen in 65% of these tumors and cystic degeneration is present in one third of cases.[87]

At MR imaging, collecting duct carcinomas can demonstrate low signal intensity on T2-weighted images. Although the enhancement pattern at MR has not been described, these tumors tend to be hypovascular

at angiography.[86] Differentiation of collecting duct carcinoma from an invasive pelvic urothelial tumor based on imaging findings may not be possible.[86] Since the latter has a high incidence of synchronous urothelial tumors and is much more common than the former, collecting duct carcinomas are treated presumptively as urothelial tumors with nephroureterectomy.

Multilocular Cystic Renal Cell Carcinoma

Cystic changes occur in up to 15% of RCCs[69] and are mainly secondary to degenerative processes within the neoplasm.[88] Multilocular cystic RCC (MCRCC) must be distinguished from RCC with cystic degeneration and multilocular cystic nephroma because its natural history seems to be different. MCRCC is a rare tumor that accounts for 1% to 4% of all RCCs; approximately 250 cases have been reported in the literature with rare cases of bilateral synchronous tumors described.[88] Patients with MCRCC are usually asymptomatic and these tumors are most commonly discovered incidentally on imaging studies performed for unrelated abdominal conditions.[88] MCRCC has a better prognosis than unilocular cystic RCC. While tumor progression and metastases can occur

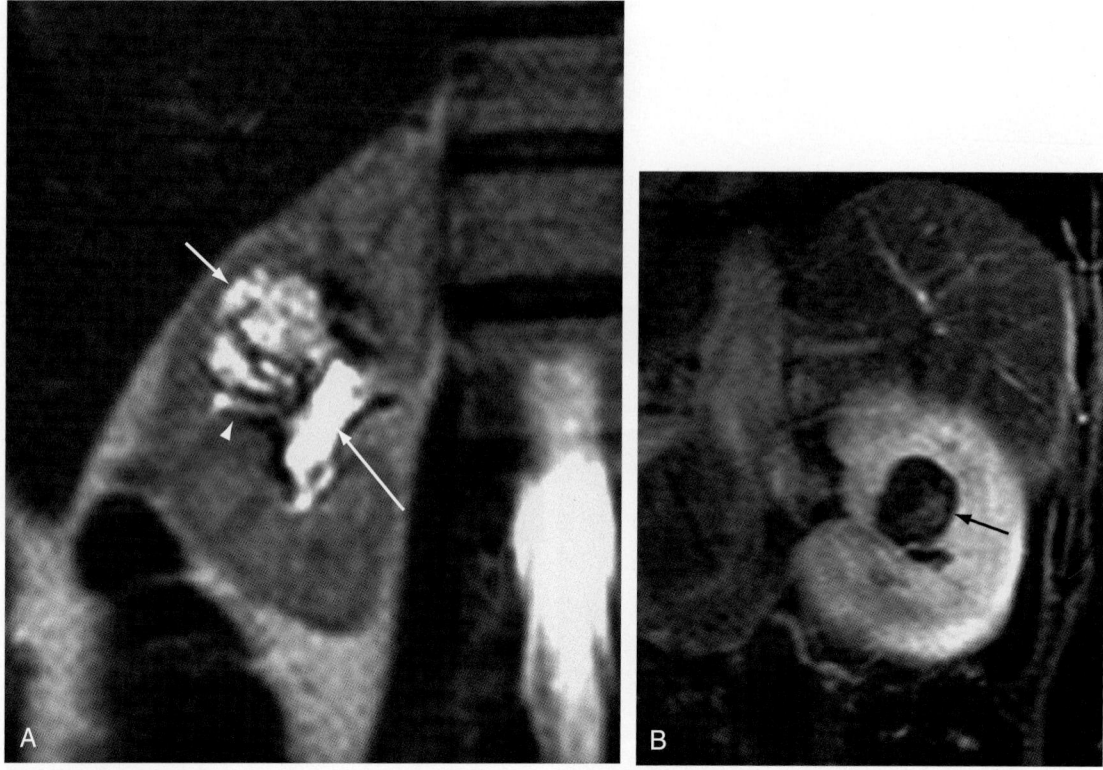

FIGURE 86-17

Chromophobe renal cell carcinoma (RCC). **A,** Coronal T2-weighted half-Fourier turbo spin-echo (HASTE) image shows a heterogeneous, predominantly hyperintense, well-circumscribed mass in the interpolar region of the right kidney (*arrow*). The mass is causing a mass effect upon the middle calyx (*arrowhead*) and mild hydronephrosis (*long arrow*). **B,** Sagittal subtracted (post-minus pre-contrast) 2D fat-saturated T1-weighted gradient-recalled echo image shows diffuse subtle enhancement with a slightly more vascular area in the posterior aspect of the mass (*arrow*). Chromophobe RCC was diagnosed at pathology after nephrectomy.

with the latter, these features are uncommon in MCRCC.[89] The 5-year disease-specific survival rates for MCRCC versus RCC with cystic necrosis are 100% and 80%, respectively.[89] Reported specific 10-year survival rate and nonrecurrence rate for MCRCC are 97.3% and 90.3%, respectively.[90]

Histologically, the MCRCCs are well-demarcated multicystic lesions that contain variable-sized aggregates of neoplastic clear cells showing grade 1 nuclear features and little or no mitotic activity.[91] As a diagnostic criterion some authors have proposed a threshold (varying from <10% to <25%[91,92]) for the amount of solid component in these lesions. Eble at al[93] have suggested three diagnostic criteria for the diagnosis of MCRCC: 1. expansile mass surrounded by a fibrous wall; 2. tumor entirely composed of cysts and septa with no expansile solid nodules; and 3. septa containing aggregates of epithelial cells with clear cytoplasm. MCRCC probably represents a low-grade variant of RCC that has little malignant potential due to its relatively low epithelial tumor volume.[88,91]

Given the subtleties at histopathology in making the diagnosis of MCRCC it is no surprise that a specific diagnosis is difficult to render with MR imaging. MCRCC shows a predominantly hyperintense mass on T2-weighted images with a signal intensity similar to that of other fluid-filled structures in the abdomen (e.g. gallbladder). Multiple thin internal septations are frequently seen. After administration of gadolinium, there is enhancement of the internal septa but no obvious nodular component is seen (Fig. 86-18). MR imaging is superior to CT in distinguishing hemorrhagic cysts from multiloculated cystic masses.[94] The diagnosis can be difficult in small-sized MCRCC because these lesions may appear as solid neoplasms with heterogeneous enhancement after administration of gadolinium.[95]

Transitional Cell Carcinoma

Transitional cell carcinoma (TCC) of the upper urinary tract accounts for 5% of all TCCs and 10% of all renal tumors and is much less common than primary TCC of the urinary bladder.[96,97] However, TCC accounts for 90% of all tumors that arise from the renal pelvic urothelium.[86] Patients are typically in their sixth or seventh decade of life with a mean age of 68 years.[86] Upper tract TCCs are bilateral in up to 4.5% of patients.[98] Up to 31% of patients with unilateral TCC of the upper

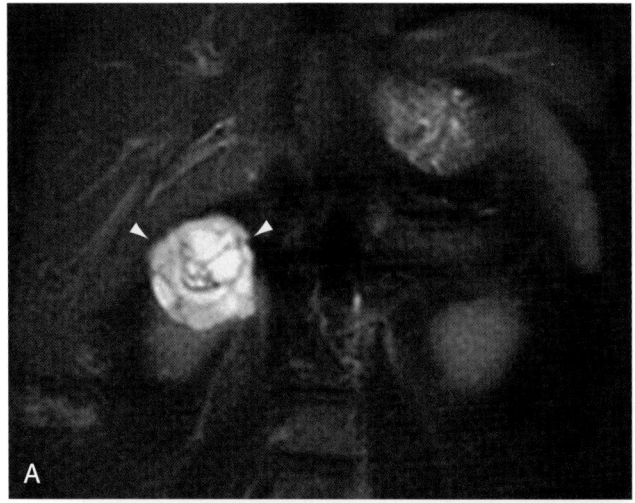

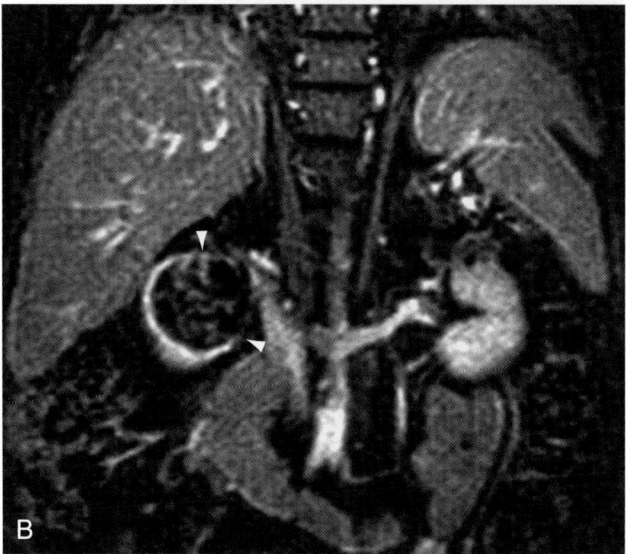

FIGURE 86-18

Multilocular cystic renal cell carcinoma. **A,** Coronal fat-saturated T2-weighted half-Fourier turbo spin-echo (HASTE) image shows a cystic mass arising from the upper pole of the right kidney (*arrowheads*) with multiple internal hairline-thin septations. **B,** Coronal 3D contrast-enhanced fat-saturated T1-weighted gradient-recalled echo subtracted (delayed venous phase minus precontrast) image shows enhancement within the internal septations (*arrowheads*) without evidence of solid components.

urinary tract without metastases will develop TCC of the bladder at some point.[98] This risk increases in patients with multiple tumors in the upper tract at presentation.[98] TCC is frequently multiple, involving any part or all of the collecting system, though most of the tumors in the upper tract occur in the renal pelvis.[97] Papillary TCC is the most common cellular type. Lung, lymph nodes, and liver are the most common locations of metastatic disease in patients with TCC, with lymphatic metastasis occurring early in these patients. Hematogenous spread is less common than in patients with RCC. Patients with tumors that do not invade the muscularis mucosa of the urothelial epithelium have a 5-year survival rate of 77% to 80%.[86] Prognosis in patients

with advanced stage is poor with a 5-year survival rate of 40.5% for T3 tumors and a mean survival of 6 months for T4 neoplasms.[99] Ureteral TCC has a worse prognosis than pelvic TCC at the same stage.[97] TCC with thrombus extending into the IVC is uncommon though it has been reported (Fig. 86-19).[100]

At MR imaging, upper tract TCC usually appears as an irregular, enhancing filling defect within the pelvocalyceal system and/or ureter. Hydronephrosis proximal to the obstructing lesion is common unless the collecting system is completely filled by tumor (Fig. 86-20). Occasionally, identification of upper tract TCC can be challenging with only subtle thickening of the wall of the renal pelvis and/or ureter (Fig. 86-21). High-grade infiltrative tumors invading the renal parenchyma alter the normal renal architecture with loss of the normal corticomedular differentiation. The reniform shape is usually preserved even in the presence of large tumors with extensive infiltration. Dynamic post-contrast images during the corticomedulary and nephrographic phases can help to demonstrate parenchymal infiltration. Heterogeneous enhancement is common in larger, infiltrative tumors (Fig. 86-22). Subtraction images can help to better differentiate enhancing filling defects from the hyperintense urine within the collecting system on post-contrast T1-weighted images. Thickening and enhancement of the wall of the collecting system can also be secondary to non-neoplastic processes (Fig. 86-23).

The entire collecting system must be evaluated in patients with upper tract TCC because there is a high incidence of tumor multiplicity. Gadolinium-enhanced MR urography after administration of 10 mL furosemide (see "MR Techniques") allows for evaluation of the entire collecting system with excellent spatial and contrast resolution. Synchronous foci of ureteral TCC can be demonstrated as enhancing polypoid filling defects within the lumen of the ureter. Enhancement must be interpreted with caution as ureteral calculi can produce inflammatory changes in the wall of the ureter leading to increased enhancement. The goblet sign, also known as the "chalice sign" or "Bergman's sign", was originally described on intravenous urography, though it is better appreciated on retrograde ureterography.[101,102] This sign refers to the presence of a cup-shaped collection of contrast material just distal to an intraluminal filling defect of the ureter.[102] Propulsion of a slow-growing polypoid intraluminal mass distally during ureteral peristalsis causes dilatation of the ureter distal to the tumor.[102] This sign can help to differentiate ureteral tumors from ureteral obstruction caused by calculi with wall spasm, edema, or both.[102] In the presence of a calculus the ureter distal to the level of obstruction is collapsed. The goblet sign can also be seen at MR imaging and may add confidence to the diagnosis of ureteral neoplasm (Fig. 86-24).

Lymphoma

Renal involvement by lymphoma is more typical in patients with known diffuse disease and it is more common in non-Hodgkin's than in Hodgkin's disease

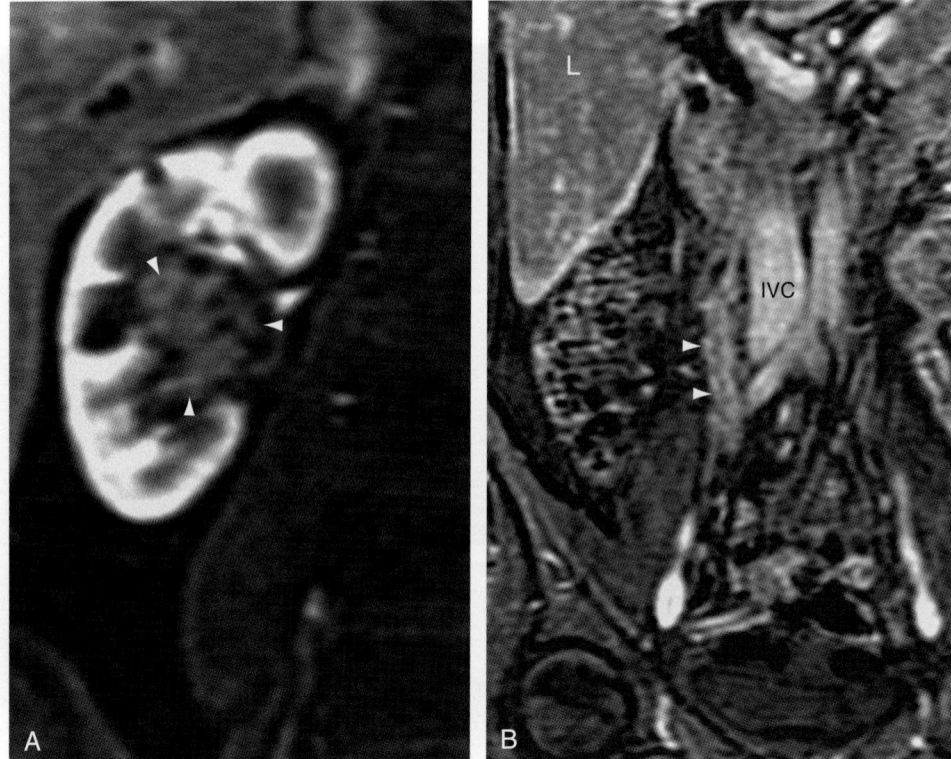

FIGURE 86-22

Transitional cell carcinoma with periureteral extension. **A,** Coronal gadolinium-enhanced 3D fat-saturated T1-weighted gradient-echo image during the corticomedullary phase, when compared with the precontrast image (not shown), revealed enhancement in a large heterogeneous collecting system mass (*arrowheads*). **B,** Coronal gadolinium-enhanced 3D fat-saturated T1-weighted gradient-echo subtracted image (delayed excretory phase minus precontrast) shows irregular enhancing thickening along the wall of the ureter (*arrowheads*), which is suspicious for diffuse urothelial carcinoma. At pathology, a large urothelial tumor was found in the renal pelvis extending inferiorly along the periureteral retroperitoneal fat without involvement of the ureteral mucosa. IVC, inferior vena cava; L, liver.

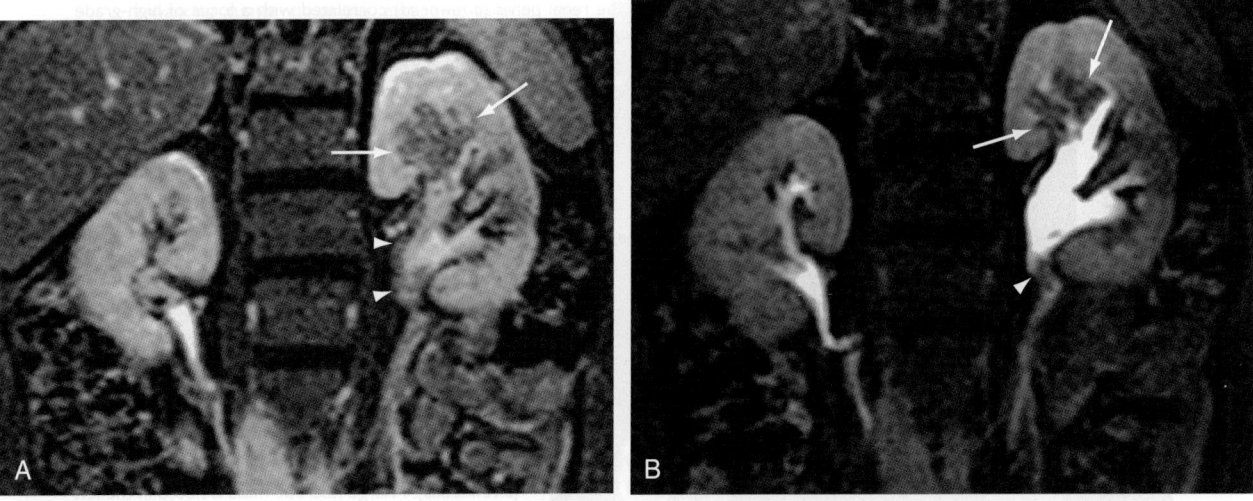

FIGURE 86-23

Transitional cell carcinoma (TCC) and inflammatory changes in the collecting system. **A,** Coronal gadolinium-enhanced 3D fat-saturated T1-weighted gradient-recalled echo (GRE) subtracted (excretory phase minus precontrast) image shows a large enhancing mass infiltrating the calyx for the upper pole of the left kidney (*arrows*). The medial wall of the renal pelvis and ureteropelvic junction (UPJ) is thickened and enhanced (*arrowheads*). **B,** MR urogram from a maximum intensity projection of the coronal gadolinium-enhanced 3D fat-saturated T1-weighted GRE subtracted acquisition (delayed excretory phase minus precontrast) confirms the presence of an enhancing mass in the upper calyx of the left kidney (*arrows*). There is moderate hydronephrosis and a filling defect is noted at the UPJ (*arrowhead*). At pathology, a high-grade TCC was found in the upper pole and extensive inflammatory changes in the wall of the rest of the collecting system were noted and thought to be secondary to the presence of a catheter within the collecting system.

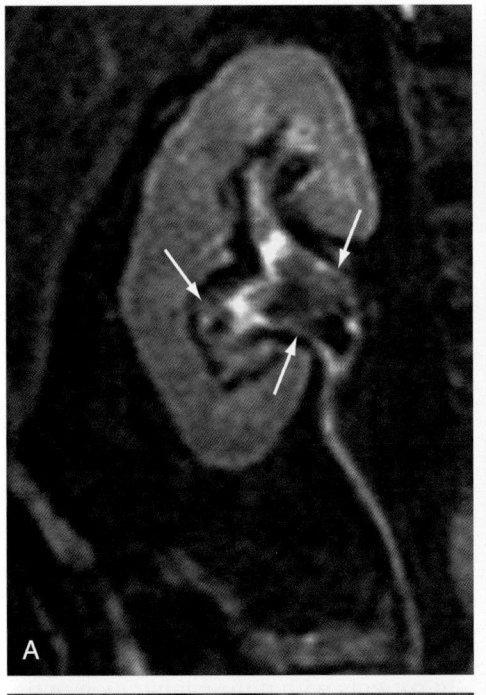

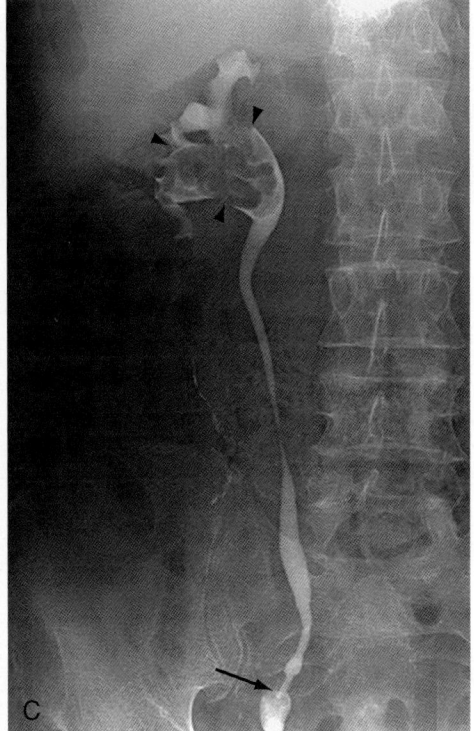

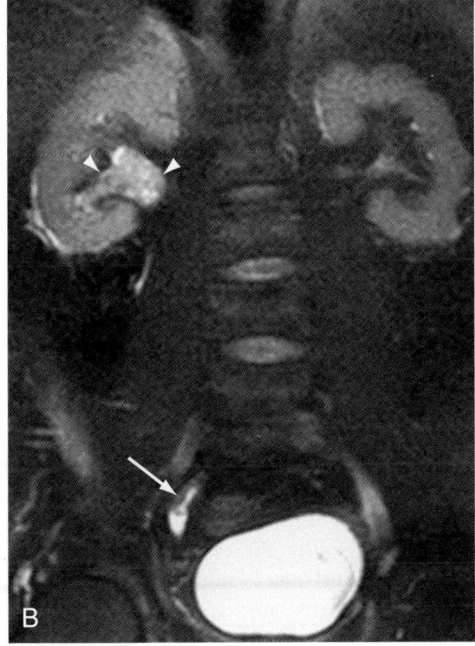

FIGURE 86-24

Multifocal transitional cell carcinoma. **A,** Coronal gadolinium-enhanced subtracted (post-contrast during the delayed venous phase minus precontrast) 3D fat-saturated T1-weighted GRE image shows enhancing filling defects in the renal pelvis (*arrows*). **B,** Coronal fat-suppressed half-Fourier turbo spin-echo (HASTE) image shows a large filling defect in the renal pelvis (*arrowheads*) and a second lesion in the lower ureter (*arrow*) with distal dilatation (goblet sign). **C,** Note the excellent correlation to the retrograde ureterogram showing a large filling defect in the renal pelvis (*arrowheads*) as well as a second lesion in the lower ureter (*arrow*) with distal dilatation. Multifocal tumor in the renal pelvis and distal ureter was confirmed at pathology.

Pathologically, an initial growth of the lymphomatous cells occurs in the interstitium using the nephrons, collecting ducts, and blood vessels as a framework for the tumor growth.[104,106] In the early stages, lymphomatous cells proliferate between nephrons without affecting their function.[106] Since renal function and gross morphology is preserved at this stage, radiologic detection is very difficult.[106] With continuous proliferation, there is parenchymal compression and destruction.[106] In this stage, masslike expansile proliferation occurs, with or without extension beyond the renal capsule; these masses resemble other primary renal neoplasms.[104,106] Complete replacement of the renal parenchyma by lym-

phomatous cells may be evident in advanced stages.[106] Perinephric extension is common and may lead to vascular and ureteral encasement.[106,107]

Patterns of involvement that have been described include multiple renal masses, direct renal invasion from contiguous retroperitoneal disease, diffuse renal infiltration, and perirenal disease.[86,104,105,108-110] The most common pattern is multiple bilateral expansile homogeneous masses, which occurs in approximately 60% of the overall cases and is more common than unilateral involvement (Fig. 86-25).[86,104,108,109] Lymphomatous masses usually range in size from 1 to 3 cm.[104,110] Renal lymphomatous masses are iso- or slightly hypo-intense

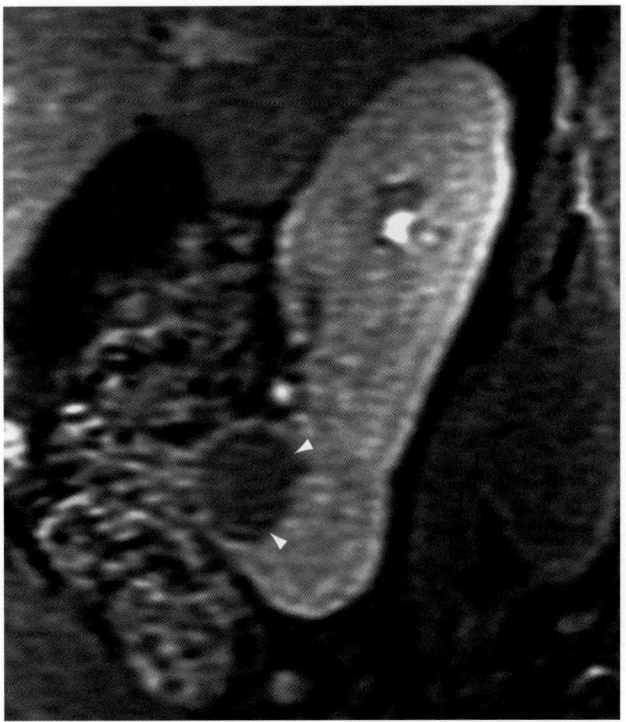

FIGURE 86-25

Renal lymphoma. Sagittal gadolinium-enhanced fat-saturated 2D T1-weighted gradient-recalled echo image obtained during the delayed venous phase shows a homogeneous low level enhancing mass in the lower pole of the right kidney (*arrowheads*). Lymphoma was confirmed after percutaneous CT-guided biopsy.

on T1-weighted images and significantly hypointense on T2-weighted images compared to the signal intensity of the renal cortex.[111] A similar accuracy was reported for the evaluation of the number and extent of lesions when T2-weighted MR images were compared to findings at CT.[111] Following treatment lymphomatous lesions can resolve completely or leave minimal scarring.[108] Abdominal and retroperitoneal lymph nodes in patients with widely extended lymphoma can be readily detected with MR imaging as these are usually enlarged and demonstrate increased signal intensity compared with that of muscle on T2-weighted MR images.[112] However, differentiation of lymphomatous involvement from metastatic disease or inflammatory response based on these findings is not possible.

Direct extension of retroperitoneal masses into the kidney occurs in approximately 25% to 30% of cases.[104,108,110] A large, bulky retroperitoneal mass is usually present in these cases. MR imaging can demonstrate these masses, which commonly show contiguous involvement with extension into the renal hilum.[113] Untreated lymphomatous masses demonstrate slightly hypointense signal intensity on T1-weighted images and heterogenous and slightly hypo- or iso-intense signal intensity on T2-weighted images relative to the renal cortex; heterogenous and minimal enhancement is seen in most cases on early and delayed gadolinium-enhanced MR images.[113] Central necrosis and renal vein thrombus

are not characteristics of this disease, helping to distinguish it from RCC.

Vascular encasement is seen more commonly in those cases where the tumor mass extends to the level of the renal hilum.[113] In this circumstance diminished perfusion to one or both kidneys can be seen on gadolinium-enhanced MR images. However, when there is encasement of the collecting system, obstruction is not uncommon and hydronephrosis is evident.[104,108]

Diffuse infiltration of the kidney manifested as nephromegaly with preservation of its reniform shape and no distinct focal mass is seen in approximately 20% of patients with renal lymphoma and such involvement is almost always bilateral.[104,107] This likely reflects lymphomatous growth that occurs in the interstitium.[86] Detection on cross-sectional imaging studies can be very challenging and frequently requires administration of contrast material.[104,108] Not uncommonly, the diagnosis is made retrospectively when follow-up imaging studies show a return of the kidneys to their normal size after chemotherapy. Focal areas of infiltrative disease can manifest ill-defined interfaces with the renal parenchyma.[104] The collecting system is usually encased in patients with diffuse infiltration of the kidney and can be deformed by the tumor.[114]

Perirenal involvement by lymphoma can be secondary to direct extension of retroperitoneal disease or transcapsular spread of renal lymphoma (Fig. 86-26).[104] Less frequently, the entire kidney can be surrounded by tumor without causing compression or functional impairment and sparing the renal parenchyma. While uncommon, this pattern is virtually pathognomonic.[104] The differential diagnosis for perirenal masses includes malignant causes with direct extension from RCC and metastases (e.g. lung, breast, and melanoma), and a variety of inflammatory non-neoplastic conditions (e.g., infection, xanthogranulomatous pyelonephritis, amyloidosis, retroperitoneal fibrosis and pancreatitis).[104,115,116]

Primary renal lymphoma (PRL) is extremely rare and its existence has been questioned because the kidney does not contain lymphoid tissue. Clear diagnostic criteria for PRL have not been established.[117,118] The disease usually affects adults with an average age of 60 years and has a slight male preponderance.[119] While non-Hodgkin's lymphoma is more commonly described, cases of primary Hodgkin's disease of the kidney have also been reported.[119] The neoplastic lymphoid cells may express both B- and T-immunoblastic phenotypes.[119] For the diagnosis of PRL to be established a total body CT, bone scan, and bone marrow biopsy should be obtained in order to exclude lymphoma elsewhere.[117-119] The prognosis and treatment of choice is controversial.

Primary lymphoma of the renal pelvis and ureter has been reported.[120,121] The MR appearance shows diffuse thickening along the wall of the renal pelvis and proximal ureter with hypointense signal intensity on both T1- and T2-weighted images, and delayed enhancement of the walls following contrast administration (Fig. 86-27). MR imaging can be useful for monitoring the response of tumor after treatment; decrease in the size of the periureteral disease and diminished hydronephrosis can be seen after chemotherapy.[120]

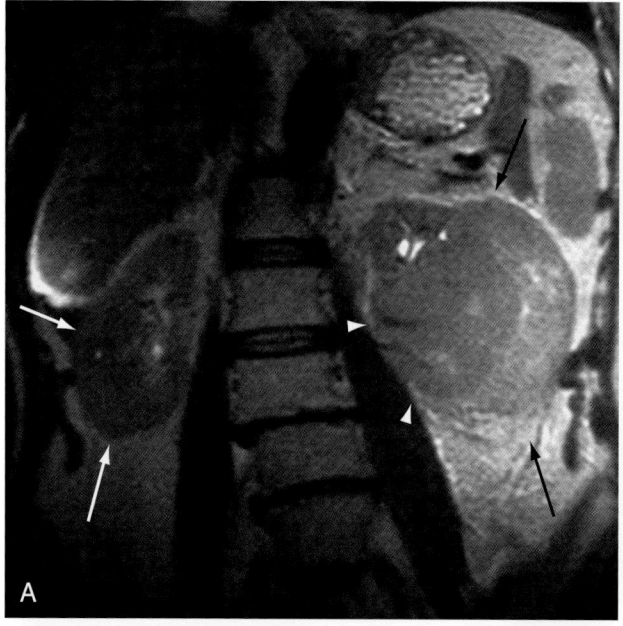

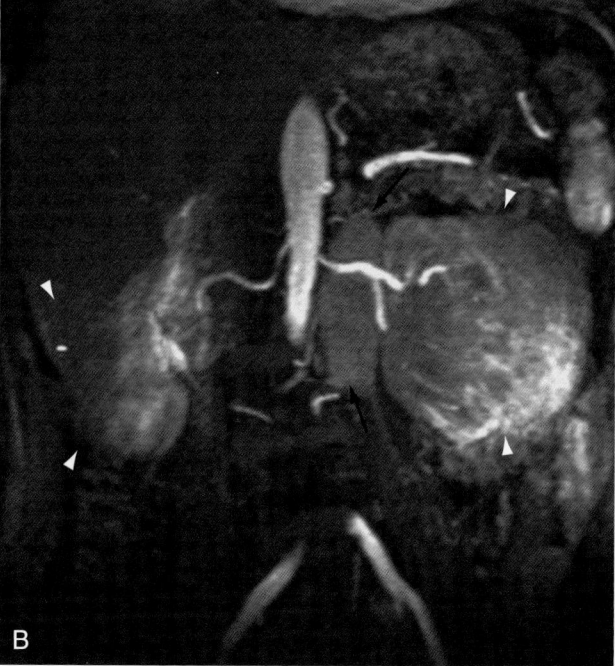

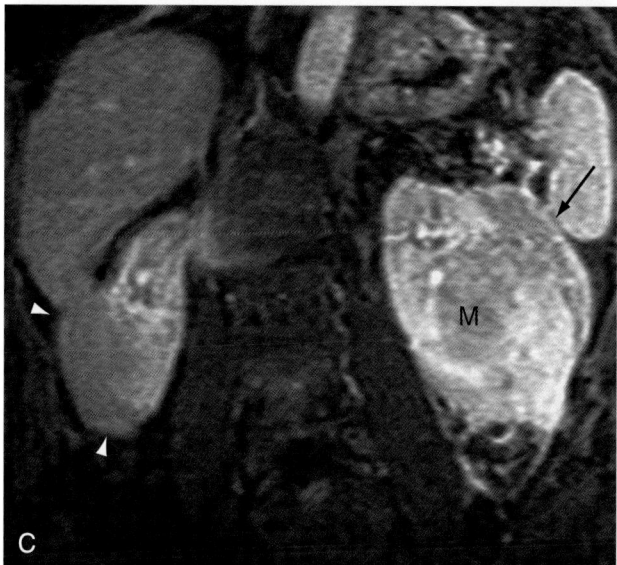

FIGURE 86-26

Renal B-cell lymphoma. **A,** Coronal T2-weighted (HASTE) image demonstrates a large left renal mass (*arrowheads*) extending into the perirenal fat (*black arrows*). A more subtle homogeneous tumor mass is noted in the lateral aspect of the right kidney (*white arrows*). **B,** Volume rendered reconstruction from a coronal gadolinium-enhanced 3D fat-saturated T1-weighted gradient-echo acquisition shows encasement of the left renal artery by a concurrent retroperitoneal tumor mass (*arrows*). A large enhancing left renal mass replacing almost the entire kidney is again noted as well as a smaller right mass (*arrowheads*). **C,** Coronal gadolinium-enhanced fat-saturated 3D T1-weighted GRE image obtained during the delayed venous phase better delineates the infiltrative mass in the mid portion of the left kidney (M) extending into the lateral perirenal fat (*arrow*). The right renal mass is now seen clearly extending into the lateral perirenal fat as well (*arrowheads*).

Metastasis

The incidence of renal metastases found at autopsy varies from 1.5% to approximately 13% of patients.[105] The most common primary tumors that metastasize to the kidney are lung, breast, melanoma, and stomach.[105] Renal metastases are more common in patients with known disseminated primary neoplasm elsewhere. Excluding lymphomatous lesions, only 3% of patients with renal metastases have no other sites of metastatic involvement.[105] Renal metastases typically reach the kidney via hematogenous seeding and they are seen at pathology as multiple cortical nodules; involvement of the urothelial mucosa is uncommon.[105] For this reason, these patients are frequently asymptomatic, even with large lesions, and hematuria is uncommon.[105] Renal metastases are frequently encountered as an incidental finding in cross-sectional imaging examinations performed for initial staging or routine follow-up.

MR is not the routine examination for staging or follow-up of nonrenal neoplasms and, therefore, metastases are rarely found in these studies. The reported imaging findings of renal metastases on CT can be extrapolated to MR imaging. Renal metastases are typically multiple, bilateral, small, and have ill-defined contours.[105] The reniform shape of the kidney is usually preserved.[105] These lesions are frequently hypovascular on contrast-enhanced CT and, therefore, could potentially be confused with cysts.[105] Multifocal low-grade enhancing papillary tumors may have the same appearance. Multifocal inflammatory lesions tend to be poorly defined and may show a peripheral rim enhancement following the administration of intravenous contrast; this feature may help to differentiate

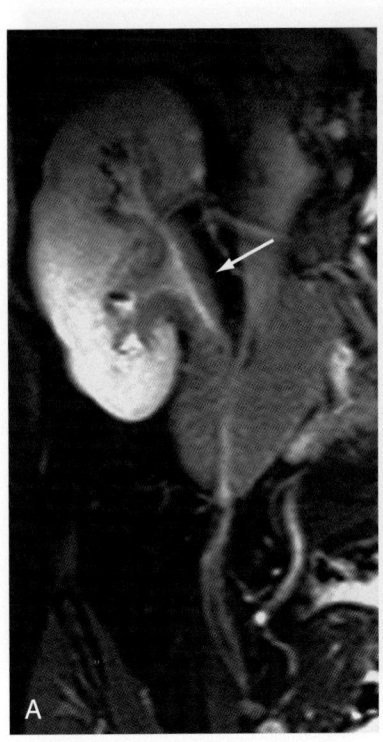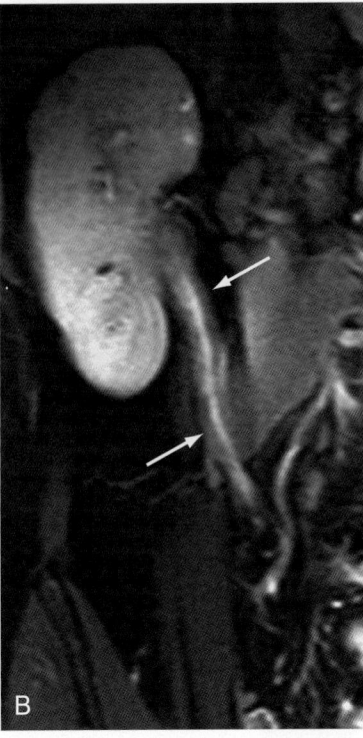

A   B

FIGURE 86-27

Periureteral B-lymphoma. **A** and **B,** Gadolinium-enhanced sagittal 2D fat-saturated T1-weighted gradient-recalled echo images obtained during the delayed excretory phase show diffuse enhancement (versus precontrast, not shown) and thickening of the wall of the renal pelvis (*arrow* in **A**) and ureter (*arrows* in **B**). A percutaneous CT-guided biopsy was nondiagnostic. Non-Hodgkin's follicular B-cell lymphoma of the wall of the collecting system was found after nephroureterectomy.

these lesions from metastases.[122] In addition, renal abscesses should be suspected when there is associated thickening of the Gerota's fascia and/or clinical signs of infection.[105] Renal metastases cannot be distinguished from lymphoma, RCC, or adenoma based on their radiologic appearance alone.[122] Renal infarcts show a wedge shape and thin peripheral rim of cortical enhancement, features not seen in multifocal neoplastic disease.[123,124]

Other Masses

Primary Renal Sarcoma

Primary renal sarcomas are rare neoplasms of mesenchymal origin that account for less than 1% of all malignant renal neoplasms and have an extremely poor prognosis.[86,125] RCC with sarcomatoid differentiation and direct extension of retroperitoneal sarcomas into the kidney are more common than primary sarcomas of the kidney.[86] These two situations must be excluded before the diagnosis of primary renal sarcoma is made.[86]

Leiomyosarcoma is the most common type and accounts for over 50% of all primary sarcomas.[86] Leiomyosarcomas are frequently well-defined expansile tumors.[125] Other primary renal sarcomas include malignant fibrous histiocytoma, hemangiopericytoma, fibrosarcoma, rhabdomyosarcoma, angiosarcoma, and osteosarcoma.[125] Rhabdomyosarcoma and angiosarcoma can present as infiltrative tumors.[86]

At CT and MR, leiomyosarcoma can be seen as well-defined multinodular mass.[126] A heterogeneous appear-

ance with areas of low signal intensity on T2-weighted images has been described. These low signal intensity areas enhanced in a delayed fashion on contrast-enhanced CT[126]; at pathology the enhancing areas showed an extensive fibrous component in comparison with the rest of the tumor where spindle-shaped muscle cells were present.[126]

Squamous Cell Carcinoma

Squamous cell carcinoma accounts for 0.5% of all renal tumors and 5% to 10% of all malignant tumors arising in the renal pelvis epithelium.[86,127] There is increased prevalence among patients with renal calculi, probably due to chronic irritation of the urothelium.[86] There is a slightly increased prevalence among males and it is more common between the sixth and seventh decades of life.[86] Patients typically present with painless hematuria or flank pain secondary to obstruction of the upper urinary tract. Prognosis is poor with mean survival of 5 months after diagnosis.[127]

Pathologically, squamous cell carcinoma is composed of sheets of epithelium that are often keratinized, recapitulating epidermis.[86] These tumors are locally invasive and the kidney may demonstrate extensive infiltration.[86]

Patients with squamous cell carcinoma of the kidney demonstrate urolithiasis in up to 87% of cases.[128] Cross-sectional imaging studies demonstrate an enlarged kidney, though its reniform shape is preserved.[86,114] Not infrequently, the kidney does not excrete contrast due to the obstruction caused by the tumor and existing calculi.[86] The tumor mass is not always apparent as these neoplasms tend to grow directly from the urothelium into the renal sinus and parenchyma.[86,129] The imaging findings can be indistinguishable from those of xanthogranulomatous pyelonephritis.[86] Occasionally, patients with squamous cell carcinoma can present with symptoms and imaging findings that mimic an infectious process.[130] Perirenal extension of the tumor can be confused with perirenal abscesses.[130] Invasion of the IVC from a squamous cell carcinoma of the renal pelvis has been reported.[131]

Renal Leukemia

Renal leukemia occurs in approximately 50% of children and up to 65% of adults who die of generalized leukemia and is more common in acute lymphoblastic forms.[86] Since abdominal imaging is not routinely performed for staging in patients with leukemia, it is difficult to know the true incidence of renal involvement.

Diffuse bilateral infiltration with moderate to massive nephromegaly is the most common finding in cross-sectional imaging studies.[86] While imaging findings may resemble the appearance of renal lymphoma, discrete renal masses are unusual in patients with leukemia.[86]

Plasmacytoma

Neoplasms involving differentiated B lymphocytes or plasma cells typically arise in the bones as a solitary lesion (plasmacytoma) or in multiple locations (multiple myeloma). These account for up to 95% of all plasma cell neoplasms.[86] Plasma cell neoplasms present as a primary extramedullary plasmacytoma in 5% of cases with the upper respiratory tract being the most common location.[86] The kidneys can be secondarily involved in approximately 17% of patients with generalized multiple myeloma. Primary plasmacytomas arising from the renal interstitium have been rarely reported.[86,132]

Renal plasmacytoma can appear as a well-circumscribed mass or as an infiltrative process. This condition cannot be reliably distinguished from other primary renal tumors and infiltrative processes based on imaging findings.[86] The presence of monoclonal immunoglobulin at serum electrophoresis or Bence-Jones proteinuria can establish the diagnosis.[86]

BENIGN RENAL MASSES

Angiomyolipoma

Angiomyolipomas (AML) are renal hamartomas containing varying proportions of fat, smooth muscle, and thick-walled blood vessels.[133] Hamartomas are not truly neoplasms; these lesions are *choristomas,* which represent a disordered arrangement of mature tissue appearing at a site in which that tissue does not normally reside.[134,135] Tumors may contain only two of the tissue elements and thus may represent angiolipomas, angiomyomas, or myolipomas. The vessels of AMLs are tortuous and often develop aneurysms because of a lack of elastic tissue in their walls.

AMLs are round or oval tumors that arise in both the cortex and medulla and elevate the renal capsule. AMLs can grow by expansion and local invasion. Extension into the perirenal space can occur in about 25% of tumors. Involvement of regional lymph nodes is usually due to a separate hamartomatous foci.

AMLs are found in 0.3% of all autopsies and in 0.13% of the population when screened by ultrasonography. Approximately 20% of AMLs are found in patients with tuberous sclerosis syndrome (TS), and 40% to 80% of patients with TS have AMLs.[136] In patients with TS, AMLs tend to be bilateral and multiple, with a mean age at presentation of 30 years, and there is a 2:1 female predominance.[137,138] Multiple renal cysts resembling autosomal-dominant polycystic disease and occasionally RCC may coexist in patients with TS.[137,138]

The great majority of incidentally detected AMLs are found in patients without TS, are asymptomatic, and are relatively small lesions (measuring 1-3 cm). Patients without TS tend to have single tumors and are older at presentation (usually between the fifth and sixth decades of life), and there is a more pronounced female predominance.[137,138] AML is rarely diagnosed before puberty in patients without TS, large masses are more common in women than men, and they can grow rapidly during pregnancy. All these findings suggest that AML growth may be stimulated by hormones.[138] Patients with lymphangiomyomatosis, a "forme fruste" of TS, also have an increased incidence of AML. While these tumors are usually single, up to 23% of patients with lymphangiomyomatosis have multiple AMLs.[136]

AML can cause significant symptoms, including pain, gross hematuria, anemia, and hypertension.[139,140] Symptoms are more common in patients with tumors larger than 4 cm.[140] Tumors larger than 4 cm have an increased risk for potentially life-threatening hemorrhage (Wunderlich's syndrome), which has been reported in up to 10% of these patients.[140,141] The risk of hemorrhage from AML increases during pregnancy.[138] Surgical resection or angiographic embolization is generally recommended in tumors larger than 4 cm.[139] An exophitic noninfiltrating growth pattern is typical of these tumors and allows for nephron-sparing surgical resection even in some larger tumors.[139] Most incidentally detected AMLs, particularly those under 4 cm, can be followed with imaging studies due to their low risk of growth or bleeding.[142,143]

AMLs have been detected with increased frequency in recent years due to the increased utilization of cross-sectional imaging.[144] A reliable diagnosis of AML can be made when fat is unequivocally demonstrated in a renal mass.[35] With ultrasound, AMLs commonly appear as a hyperechoic mass; however, the substantial overlap with mildly or very echogenic RCC is problematic.[145,146] Up to 30% of RCCs equal to or less than 3 cm in size are markedly hyperechoic and, therefore, indistinguishable from AML, necessitating further imaging for characterization.[146] The diagnosis of AML can be easily made with CT when even small amounts of fat are present.[147] However, this diagnosis must be made with caution when tiny amounts of fat are detected in predominantly solid neoplasms. Small amounts of fat can be detected in

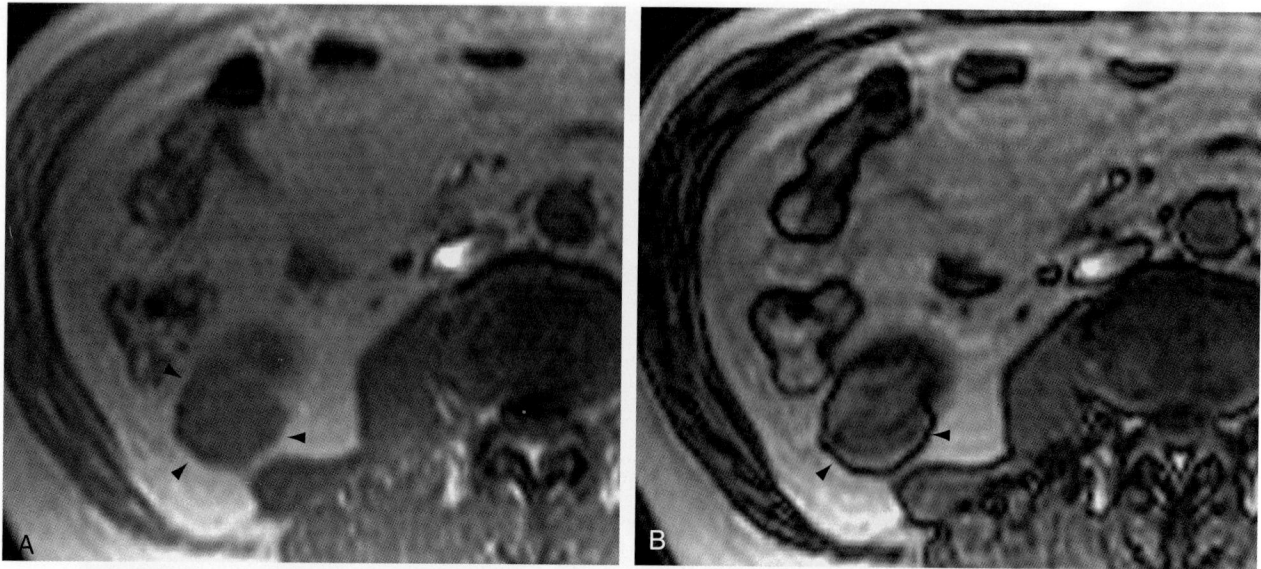

FIGURE 86-30

Lipid-poor angiomyolipoma (AML). **A,** Axial T1-weighted gradient-recalled echo (GRE) in-phase image shows a mass arising from the lower pole of the right kidney (*arrowheads*) with homogeneous signal intensity similar to that of the psoas muscle. **B,** Axial T1-weighted GRE out-of-phase image at the same level as **A** demonstrates only a minimal drop in signal intensity in the posterior aspect of the lesion (*arrowheads*), which is due to the intravoxel coexistence of fat and water. The diagnosis of AML by MRI is virtually impossible in the absence of detectable bulk fat. Since clear-cell renal cell carcinoma should be considered in the differential diagnosis if only intracellular fat is detected, this patient underwent partial nephrectomy. At pathology, a lipid-poor AML was diagnosed.

recognized within large retroperitoneal hematomas which help to make the diagnosis. MR imaging with chemical selective fat suppression can confirm the diagnosis (Fig. 86-31).

Differentiation of large exophitic AMLs from well-differentiated retroperitoneal liposarcomas can also be difficult.[153] A defect in the surface of the kidney and large intratumoral vessels can be seen on contrast-enhanced CT images in patients with AMLs and in almost all cases can help to accurately distinguish these two entities.[153] Similar findings would be expected to aid in this distinction with contrast-enhanced MRI.

Oncocytoma

Renal oncocytomas, also known as proximal tubular adenomas with so-called oncocytic features or as oxyphilic adenomas, account for 3% to 7% of all renal tumors.[154] Oncocytomas are benign neoplasms, believed to have their origin in the proximal tubular epithelium. Their incidence is greater in the sixth decade with a mean age of 62 years.[155,156] There is a male predominance (about 3.1:1).[155] Oncocytomas can be multicentric and bilateral and extrarenal locations have been described, including adrenal, thyroid, parathyroid, and salivary glands. A coexistent RCC is present in approximately 30% of patients with oncocytomas.[157] The chromophobe variant of RCC shares a specific phenotype of intercalated cells of the collecting duct system and mitochondrial DNA alterations with renal oncocytomas.[154]

Macroscopically, the cut surface of these tumors is generally mahogany brown or dark red in color which differentiates these tumors from RCC, which typically show yellow coloration.[154] In general, oncocytomas are more homogeneous than RCCs of similar size mainly due to the absence of necrosis, cystic changes, hemorrhage, and calcification.[72,158] Oncocytomas are typically well defined because they are encapsulated.[72] A stellate central area of fibrosis or hyalinized connective tissue with compressed blood vessels, the so-called central scar, is observed in up to 54% of cases.[72,155] This finding is probably the result of long-standing ischemia in this slowly growing neoplasm.[72]

Histologically, these neoplasms are composed of an exclusive or predominant component of acidophilic cells. By definition, these lesions lack areas of clear-cell carcinoma, significant lesional necrosis, or conspicuous papillary formations.[155]

The value of percutaneous needle aspiration and biopsy for the diagnosis of oncocytoma is controversial. There is a potential for confusing oncocytomas with RCCs, since both may contain eosinophilic granular cytoplasm and a variant of RCC contains oncocytic cells. Furthermore, when considering the sampling errors inherent to percutaneous needle biopsy procedures, an accurate diagnosis without surgery is rarely feasible.[72]

A recent report suggests a reliable method to distinguish renal oncocytoma from RCCs using fine needle aspiration and core biopsy specimens based on the cytologic morphology and immunostaining.[159] If these results are confirmed in larger prospective studies,

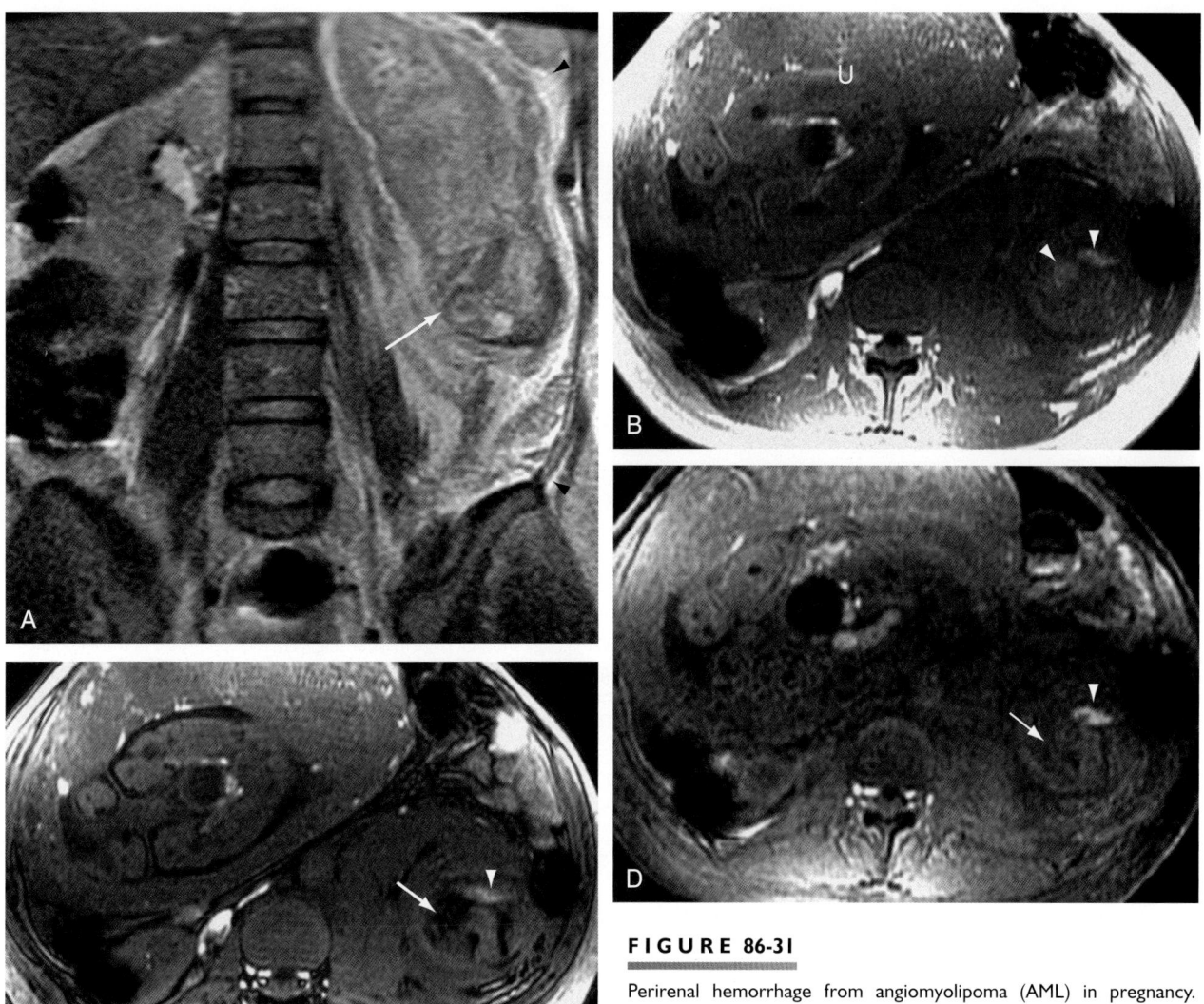

FIGURE 86-31

Perirenal hemorrhage from angiomyolipoma (AML) in pregnancy. **A,** Coronal T2-weighted half-Fourier turbo spin-echo (HASTE) image reveals a large mass arising from the lower pole of the left kidney (*arrow*). A large perirenal hematoma is noted (*arrowheads*). **B,** Axial T1-weighted in-phase gradient-recalled echo (GRE) image from a dual-echo acquisition at the level of the mass demonstrates two areas of high signal intensity (*arrowheads*) which could represent hyperintense hemorrhage or fat contents within the lesion. U, gravid uterus. **C,** Axial T1-weighted opposed-phase GRE image from a dual-echo acquisition at the same level as **B** demonstrates a drop in signal intensity within the medial area of high signal intensity seen in **B** (*arrow*), which is consistent with the intravoxel coexistence of fat and water. The anterior area of signal intensity (*arrowhead*) shows no change and therefore is likely to be an area of hyperintense hemorrhage. **D,** Axial 3D fat-saturated T1-weighted gradient-echo (VIBE) acquisition at the same level as **B** and **C** shows persistent high signal in the hemorrhagic area anteriorly (*arrowhead*) and suppression of the signal of the fatty contents (*arrow*), which confirms the presence of bulk fat within the mass and makes possible the diagnosis of AML.

percutaneous needle aspiration and/or biopsy may be beneficial, particularly in cases in which renal surgery must be avoided because of poor operative risk.

Most renal oncocytomas are asymptomatic and are detected incidentally.[155] Occasionally patients can present with hematuria, flank pain, or a palpable mass, particularly when the tumor is large.[72]

Renal oncocytomas are typically well-demarcated solid renal masses. There are no reported specific imaging findings in studies including intravenous urography, ultrasound, CT, or angiography. Similarly, the MRI appearance of oncocytomas is variable and

nonspecific. Oncocytomas are hypointense relative to the renal cortex on T1-weighted images in approximately 70% of cases.[160] Up to 67% of these lesions can demonstrate high signal intensity compared to the renal cortex on T2-weighted images.[160]

In general, renal oncocytomas have distinct margins between the tumor and remaining kidney and do not invade the pararenal fascia.[161] When a central scar is present, it can be seen on MR imaging as a stellate area of low signal intensity on T1-weighted images and high signal intensity on T2-weighted images.[162] However, this finding is present only in a minority of cases[158] and is not

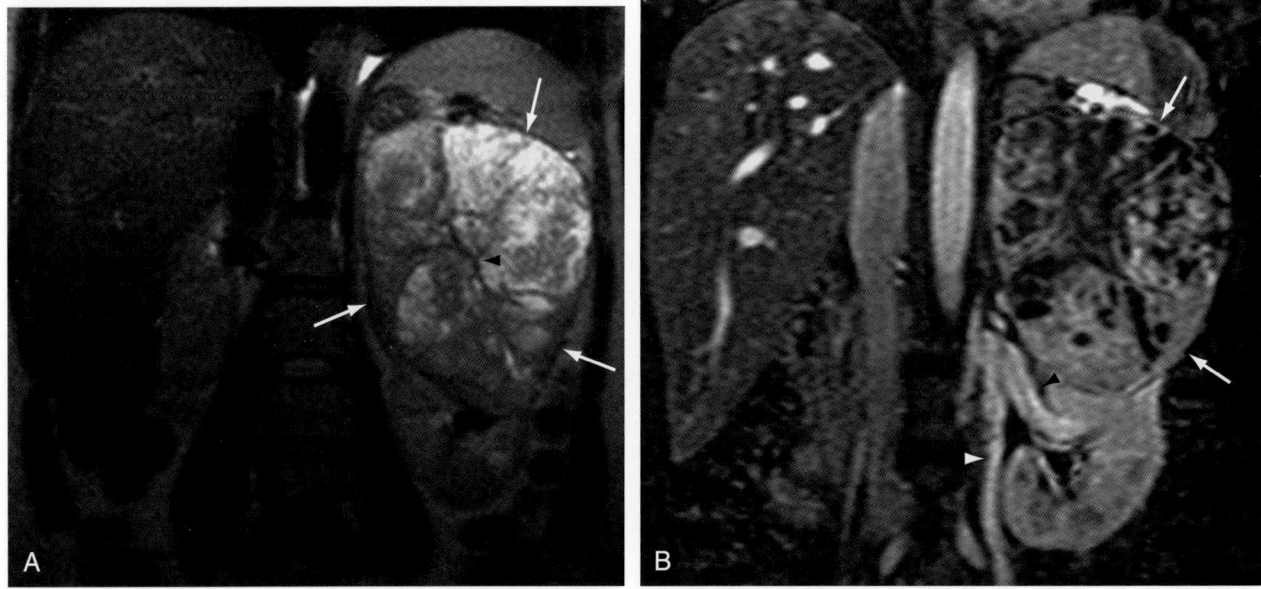

FIGURE 86-32

Oncocytoma. **A,** Coronal T2-weighted half-Fourier turbo spin-echo (HASTE) image shows a large mass arising from the upper pole of the left kidney with predominantly high signal intensity. A well-defined hypointense capsule is noted around the mass (*arrows*). Note the central stellate area suggestive of a scar (*arrowhead*). **B,** Coronal gadolinium-enhanced fat-saturated 3D T1-weighted gradient-recalled echo image obtained during the nephrographic phase demonstrates heterogeneous enhancement (*arrows*). The renal vein (*black arrowhead*) and gonadal vein (*white arrowhead*) are patent.

specific because central scars have been reported in RCC.[162,163] A well-defined capsule of low signal intensity on various pulse sequences can be seen surrounding the tumor in almost half of renal oncocytomas (Fig. 86-32).[160] Similarly, compressed renal parenchyma can appear as a pseudocapsule surrounding 60% of RCCs.[53] Calcification within the tumor is extremely rare, but has been reported.[164]

The experience of conventional angiography has shown that suggestive findings of oncocytoma can be identified but these are insufficient for a reliable distinction from RCC.[165] Similarly, the enhancement patterns on cross-sectional imaging of oncocytomas are not sufficiently specific to distinguish them from RCCs (Fig. 86-33).

Few descriptions of oncoctyomas on contrast-enhanced cross-sectional imaging are available.[53,160,166] Oncocytomas may be hypervascular during the early corticomedullary phase, compared with renal tissue.[167] During the nephrographic phase, oncocytomas usually show enhancement of a lower degree than that of normal renal parenchyma.[167] Homogeneous attenuation and a central, marginated stellate area of low attenuation after administration of contrast material are predictors of oncocytoma on contrast-enhanced CT examinations.[168] Homogeneous enhancement can be seen in small oncocytomas at gadolinium-enhanced MR imaging.[39] However, this can also be seen in small RCCs, especially in low-grade papillary tumors. In the presence of intratumoral hemorrhage and/or necrosis the tumors will appear heterogeneous, in which case a diagnosis of oncocytoma cannot be suggested.

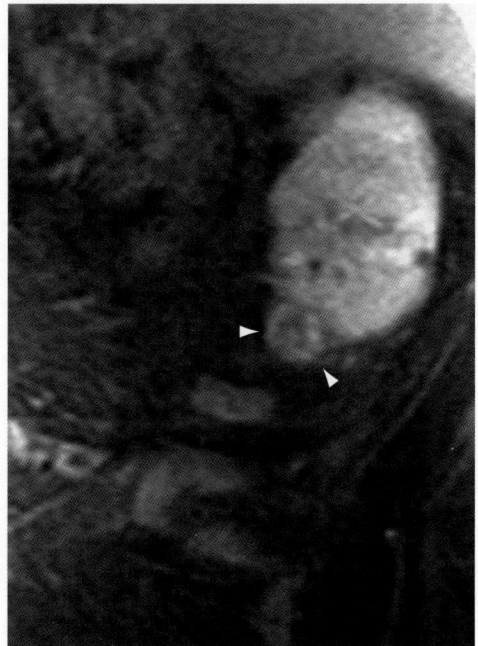

FIGURE 86-33

Oncocytoma. Sagittal contrast-enhanced fat-saturated T1-weighted image when compared to the precontrast image (not shown) demonstrates an enhancing mass with nonspecific features (*arrowheads*). Histopathology revealed oncocytoma after partial nephrectomy.

Juxtaglomerular Cell Tumor (Reninoma)

Juxtaglomerular cell tumors (reninomas) are rare benign tumors which originate, as their name indicates, from the juxtaglomerular cells. First recognized in 1967 by Robertson et al,[169] these tumors actively produce and secrete excessive amounts of renin into the blood stream causing moderate-to-severe hypertension. Patients can present with headache, polyuria, polydipsia, nocturia, and myalgia due to hypertension, hyper-reninemia, and secondary aldosteronism. Hypertensive retinopathy is common.[170] These uncommon tumors represent a form of a surgically correctable hypertension.

Reninomas are most common in children and young adults. They have been described in patients between the ages of 7 and 58 years with a female-to-male ratio of 1.8:1.[170,171] Because these tumors are more common in young females, reninomas can present as uncontrollable hypertension during pregnancy.[172] All patients have elevated plasma renin activity due to aldosteronism, though there is no correlation with tumor size.[170] These patients' hypertension typically shows an effective response to treatment with angiotensin-converting enzyme inhibitors.[170] However, while this is a very sensitive test, it is not specific since similar results can be found in all forms of hypertension when there is activation of the renin angiotensin system.[170]

Renal venous sampling for renin assay can help to localize the tumor in only 40% of patients.[170] False-negative results have been correlated with a peripheral location of the tumor, at the surface of the kidney, with most of the tumoral venous blood collected into the pericapsular veins instead of the renal vein.[170]

Most tumors are small with an average diameter of 2 to 3 cm. Occasionally, larger or even very small tumors, measuring only a few millimeters, can be found. Reninomas are usually well-marginated neoplasms located beneath the renal capsule. On cut section, these masses are tan or gray in color and may show foci of hemorrhage.

Histologically, juxtaglomerular cell tumors show a nodular or trabecular proliferation of polygonal mesenchymal cells.[173] Tubular components are commonly seen.[173] Characteristic renin granules can be demonstrated by Bowie stain or electron microscopy.[174] The ultrastructural characteristics of the cytoplasmic granules are identical to those of the epithelial cells of the normal human juxtaglomerular complex. Rhomboid secretion granules at electron microscopy are characteristic.[175]

Most cases described in the literature have been localized by catheter angiography or found at surgery.[176] Tumors are typically small and located near the renal surface which makes their identification very difficult on catheter angiography.

Reported indications for catheter angiography in the past included detection of reninomas, assessment of the vascularity of these tumors seen on sonography or CT, depiction of the detailed vascular anatomy for possible local resection of the tumor or heminephrectomy, and exclusion of renal artery stenosis as the cause of secondary reninism. With current cross-sectional imaging techniques, specifically CT angiography and MR angiography, a comprehensive evaluation, including morphology and size of tumor, vascularity, and evaluation of the renal arteries, can provide accurate presurgical evaluation of these patients; catheter angiography should not be necessary when state-of-the-art CT angiography or MR angiography are performed.

The MR findings for juxtaglomerular cell tumors include a hypointense well-defined mass on precontrast T1-weighted images. Visualization of the mass on T2-weighted images can be challenging because the lesion may be isointense with the renal parenchyma. Early peripheral enhancement of the tumor has been described at MR after administration of gadolinium.[176] On delayed–post-contrast T1-weighted images, peripheral washout of the contrast with enhancement of the central portion of the tumor can be seen.[176] Lack of enhancement on post-contrast images has been described.[171] In our experience, juxtaglomerular cell tumors can be seen at MR as hypovascular enhancing masses during the corticomedullary and nephrographic phases after administration of gadolinium. Detection of enhancement can be difficult in these lesions due to their inherent hypovascularity. Subtraction imaging can facilitate the demonstration of low level intratumoral enhancement (Fig. 86-34).

Solitary Fibrous Tumor

Solitary fibrous tumors (SFTs) were originally described in the pleura, though they have been found on rare occasions in other organs including the kidney.[177-181] Most cases of SFT are benign and occur in middle-aged and older patients, more often in women.[181] However, up to 12% to 23% of SFTs are malignant.[177] Only a few SFTs have been reported in the urogenital system and most of these were located in the kidney.[177-181] Patients are mostly asymptomatic or have referred pain secondary to a mass effect due to the size of the tumor.[181]

Histologic examination of SFT shows the characteristic spindle cells dispersed among elongated dense collagen fibers in what has been called the "patternless" pattern.[179,182] Regardless of the location of the SFTs, histologically the tumors are identical to those occurring in the pleura.[179] While the diagnosis of extrapleural SFT can be suspected at light microscopy, the diagnosis is confirmed by demonstrating diffuse expression of CD34 antigen in tumor cells at immunohistochemistry and rare mitotic figures.[178]

Renal SFTs present frequently as a large mass.[179] These tumors have been described as homogenous, well circumscribed, and isointense to the renal capsule on T1-weighted images. Areas of very low signal intensity are visible throughout the mass on T2-weighted images (Fig. 86-35). These areas can be attributed to dense collagenization and fibrosis which is characteristic for SFTs. Mixed signal intensity on T2-weighted images has also been observed in SFTs of the pleura[183] and a SFT of the presacral space.[184] Previous reports of SFTs of the kidney have shown the absence of enlarged lymph nodes and local invasion of all of them, including those presenting with very large renal masses.[181]

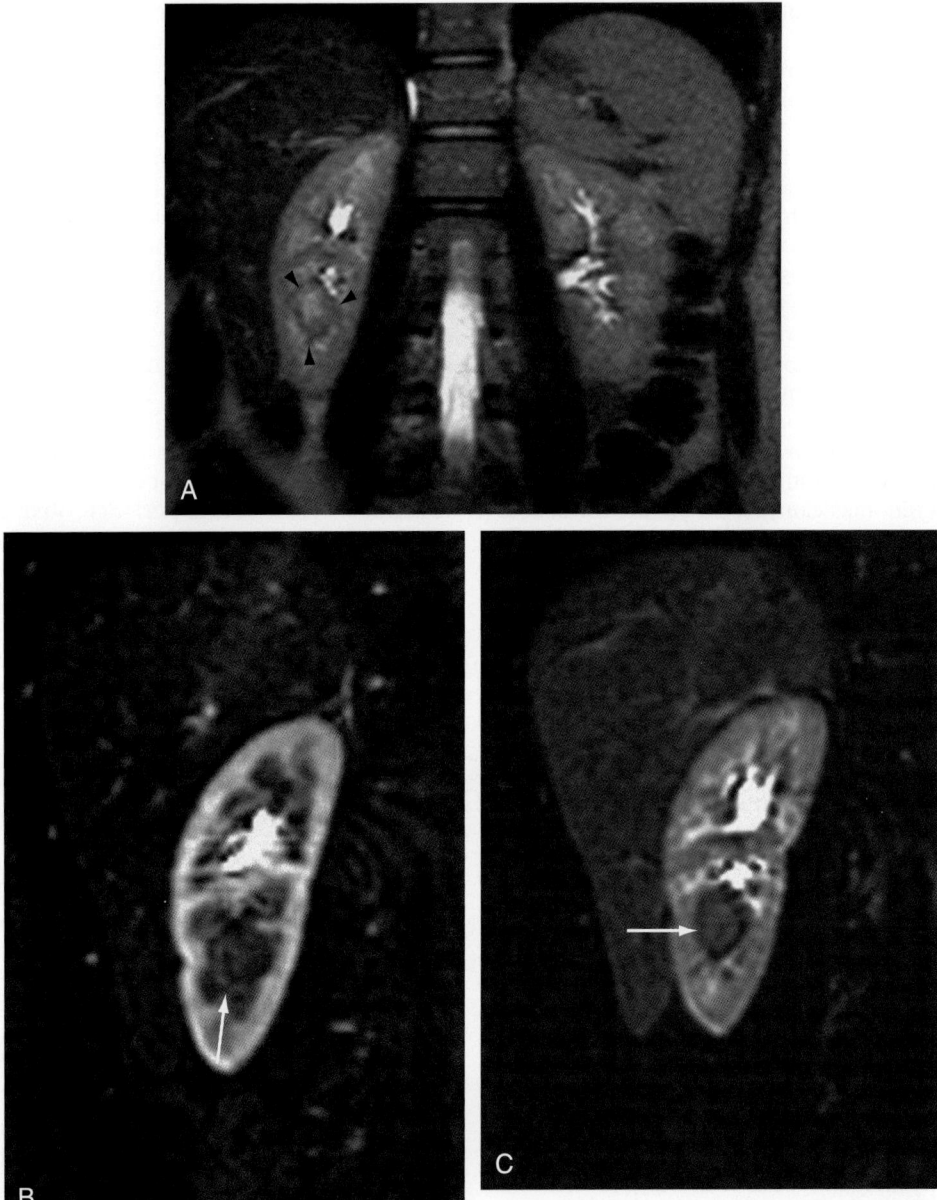

FIGURE 86-34

Reninoma. **A,** Coronal T2-weighted single-shot fast spin-echo (SSFSE) image shows a small mass in the central portion of the lower pole of the right kidney (*arrowheads*). **B,** Coronal gadolinium-enhanced 3D fat-saturated T1-weighted gradient-recalled echo (GRE) image during the arterial phase shows the hypovascular nature of this mass (*arrow*), which enhances similar to the renal medulla and is therefore difficult to detect. **C,** Coronal gadolinium-enhanced 3D fat-saturated T1-weighted GRE image during the nephrographic phase better delineates this hypovascular lesion. The mass shows homogeneous and lower signal intensity compared with the adjacent enhancing renal parenchyma. Histopathologic analysis was consistent with reninoma. While these MR imaging findings are nonspecific, the diagnosis of reninoma should be a consideration in a young patient with a hypovascular central mass and hypertension.

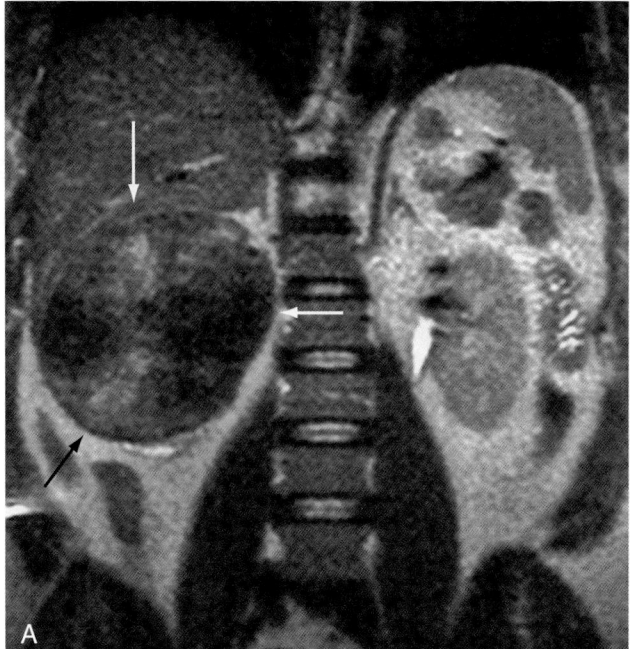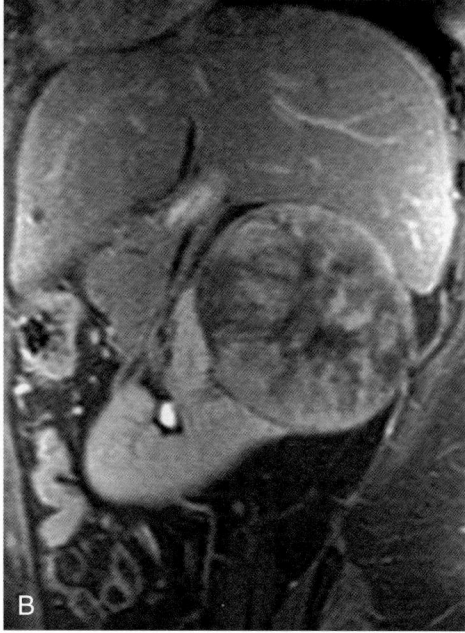

FIGURE 86-35

Solitary fibrous tumor. **A,** Coronal T2-weighted half-Fourier turbo spin-echo (HASTE) image shows a large mass (*arrows*) with areas of very low signal intensity alternating with areas of moderately high signal intensity. **B,** Sagittal 2D fat-saturated T1-weighted gradient-echo image during the delayed venous phase after administration of gadolinium confirms the origin of the mass off the upper pole of the right the kidney. There is heterogeneous enhancement within the mass. Note the lack of necrosis and perirenal collateral vessels despite the large size of the tumor. These findings suggest the possibility of a mesenchymal tumor. At pathology, a benign solitary fibrous tumor of the renal capsule was diagnosed.

The presence of a large solitary enhancing renal mass should be considered consistent with an RCC until proven otherwise. However, lack of central necrosis within a large renal mass, retroperitoneal collateral vessels around the lesion, and enlarged retroperitoneal lymph nodes argue for a benign tumor. In these cases, mesenchymal masses, including SFT, should be considered in the differential diagnosis.

Renal Adenoma

Renal adenomas are one of the most common benign renal tumors, identified in 4% to 37% of all kidneys at autopsy.[185,186] By definition, these lesions are smaller than 5 mm and usually less than 2 mm.[186] Renal adenomas are indistinguishable from low-grade papillary carcinomas at histologic, immunohistochemical, and cytogenetic analysis. The only difference between these two entities is the size of the lesion.[185,186] The great majority of adenomas are generally discovered incidentally at pathology.[186] Renal adenomas occur more frequently in kidneys with RCC and oncocytoma.[185] The incidence of adenomas is particularly high in normal-appearing renal parenchyma in patients with hereditary papillary renal cancer.[187]

Most pathologists believe that renal adenomas are "premalignant" lesions and that papillary renal carcino-mas arise from renal adenomas.[186] However, it is unclear how many of these adenomas grow into a clinically relevant RCC.[186] Few studies have demonstrated progression of small renal tumors into larger carcinomas.[188,189] The implication of the presence of renal adenomas for a patient's management is unclear; specifically, the increased risk for local recurrence after partial nephrectomy in these patients has to be evaluated.[186] While there is an approximately 7% recurrence rate after partial nephrectomy in patients with renal tumors, it is unclear if this affects patient survival.[190]

The imaging features of renal adenomas are non-specific. They have a similar appearance on MR imaging to low-grade papillary carcinomas. While these lesions are by definition smaller than 5 mm, it should be emphasized that the differentiation between an adenoma and a carcinoma cannot be made radiologically.

Miscellaneous Tumors

Lymphangioma

Lymphangiomas are congenital malformations in the development of the lymphatic channels. They are benign tumors that occur more commonly in children in the neck and axillary region; rarely, these lesions occur in the kidneys, with less than 40 reported cases of renal

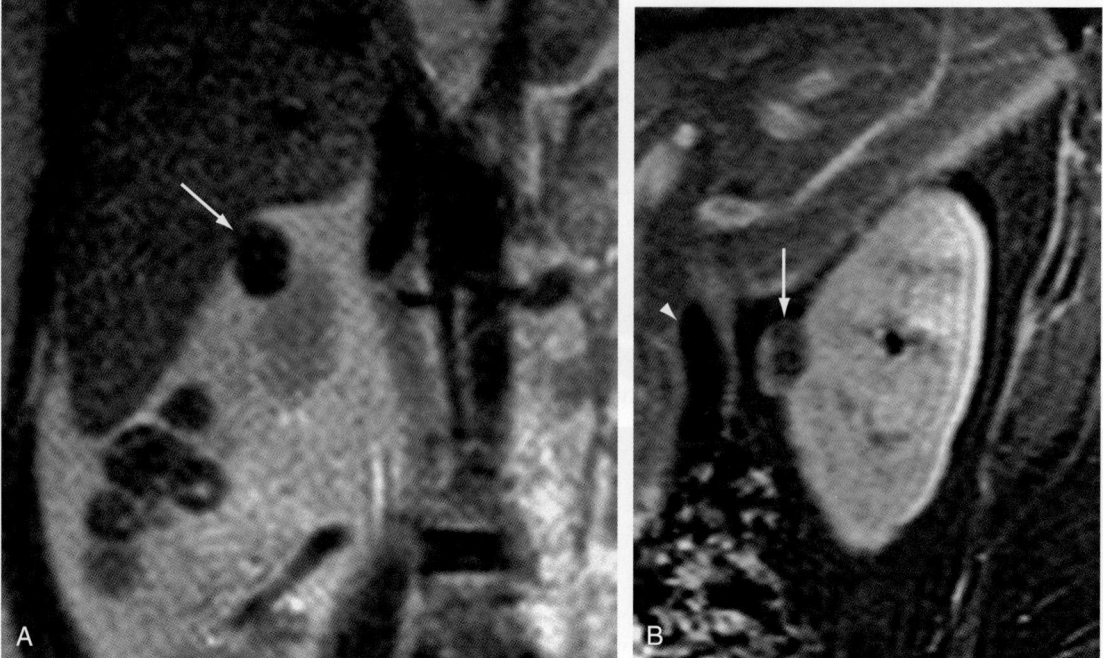

FIGURE 86-37

Leiomyoma. **A,** Coronal T2-weighted half-Fourier turbo spin-echo (HASTE) image shows an exophytic mass in the anterior aspect of the right kidney (not shown) with homogeneous low signal intensity (*arrow*). **B,** Sagittal gadolinium-enhanced 2D fat-saturated T1-weighted subtracted image (delayed venous phase minus precontrast) shows homogenous low level enhancement within the mass (*arrow*). The nonenhancing content of the gallbladder (*arrowhead*) serves as an internal control for lack of enhancement. A benign leiomyoma was diagnosed after partial nephrectomy.

these masses can project into the renal pelvis. Most of these tumors are small, measuring from only a few millimeters to 1 to 2 cm. However, tumors up to 10 cm can be seen.[214] Patients can be asymptomatic or present with hematuria and renal colic due to the passage of blood clots.[213,214] Since spontaneous regression of these tumors has been described, a conservative approach is recommended wherever possible.[213]

Small renal hemangiomas are rarely seen on conventional pyelography, ultrasound, or CT. Larger lesions can be seen as hyperechoic masses on ultrasound.[215] These masses are isodense to the renal cortex during the excretory phase.[214] At catheter angiography a hypovascular mass displacing the collecting system can be seen.[214,216] In addition, irregular and tortuous arteries that typically feed these masses can be demonstrated.[216] Larger hemangiomas may be confused with a vascular RCC at catheter angiography.

The MR findings of renal hemangiomas have been only rarely described.[214] Renal cavernous hemangiomas can be seen on MR as a mass centered in the medulla with low signal intensity on T1-weighted images and high signal intensity on T2-weighted images compared to the renal parenchyma.[214] Ring- or tube-like areas of flow void can be seen on T2-weighted images and reflect the vascular nature of the lesion.[214] The lesion demonstrates delayed enhancement after administration of gadolinium.[214]

Multilocular Cystic Nephroma

Multilocular cystic nephroma (MLCN) is an uncommon cystic renal lesion composed of multiple noncommunicating cysts surrounded by a thick, fibrous capsule. Eighty percent of children with MLCN are aged between 3 and 24 months, and 85% of adults with MLCN are older than 40 years.[217] While approximately 65% of affected children are male, up to 76% of affected adults are female.[217] MLCN is typically discovered incidentally in asymptomatic children. However, symptoms related to the mass are common in adults, including abdominal pain, hematuria, hypertension, or urinary tract infection.[218]

Diagnosis of MLCN is based on the criteria proposed in 1951 by Powell et al[219,220]:

1. Unilateral involvement;
2. Solitary lesion;
3. Multilocular lesion;
4. No communication between individual cysts;
5. No communication between cysts and the renal pelvis;
6. Cysts lined by epithelium
7. No normal nephrons in the septa separating the cysts;
8. Remaining normal parenchyma.

These criteria have been revised to stress an important concept: the only solid tissue present within the multilocular cysts is the thin septa dividing the individual cysts.[220,221] These septa conform to the spherical shape of the cysts and may contain mature renal tubules, though fully developed nephrons should not be present.[220-222] The fluid within the cysts is similar to serum and its cytology is typically normal.[220]

These lesions represent a diagnostic dilemma in children. The differential diagnosis of a multilocular cyst in childhood includes MLCN, multilocular cyst with partially differentiated Wilms' tumor, and a cystic Wilms' tumor.[220] While MLCNs are benign lesions that do not recur or metastasize, multilocular cysts with partially differentiated Wilms' tumor can recur locally; cystic Wilms' tumor is considered a malignant tumor.[220] The distinction between MLCNs and multilocular cysts with partially differentiated Wilms' tumor cannot be made based on radiologic or gross findings.[220] Fibrous tissue with mature tubules compose the fibrous septa in MLCN. Multilocular cysts with partially differentiated Wilms' tumor have blastema with or without embryonic stromal or epithelial cells.[220] Radiologically, the presence of solid components within the lesion excludes the diagnosis of MLCN. These solid portions within the tumor are characteristic in Wilms' tumors.[220]

The masses are located within the renal parenchyma and do not communicate with the renal pelvis, though cysts may herniate into the renal pelvis. The content of the cysts usually is clear fluid but occasionally myxomatous, proteinaceous, or hemorrhagic material is present.

MR imaging demonstrates a well-circumscribed, encapsulated mass consisting of multiple cysts that vary from several millimeters to 4 cm in diameter.[223,224] Cysts have variable signal intensity on T1-weighted images and moderate-to-high signal intensity may be evident in the presence of proteinaceous, myxomatous, or hemorrhagic material within the cysts.[224] Herniation of the lesions into the renal collecting system is characteristic (Fig. 86-38).[218,224] While the signal intensity of the septa may be variable, the tumor capsule tends to show low signal intensity on all MR sequences. Gadolinium-enhanced MR images show variable enhancement of the septations.[224] Plain radiographs and CT may demonstrate calcifications, which usually arise from the capsule or septa.

RENAL NEOPLASMS IN THE PEDIATRIC POPULATION

Renal masses account for approximately 55% of all abdominal masses from birth to 18 years of age.[218] Most renal tumors in the neonatal population are benign, including multicystic dysplastic kidney and polycystic renal diseases.[218]

Benign Renal Masses

The most common benign renal tumors are AML, multilocular cystic nephroma, and mesoblastic nephroma.[218] Renal AMLs are rare in children and approximately 50% occur in patients with tuberous sclerosis.[218] Similarly to

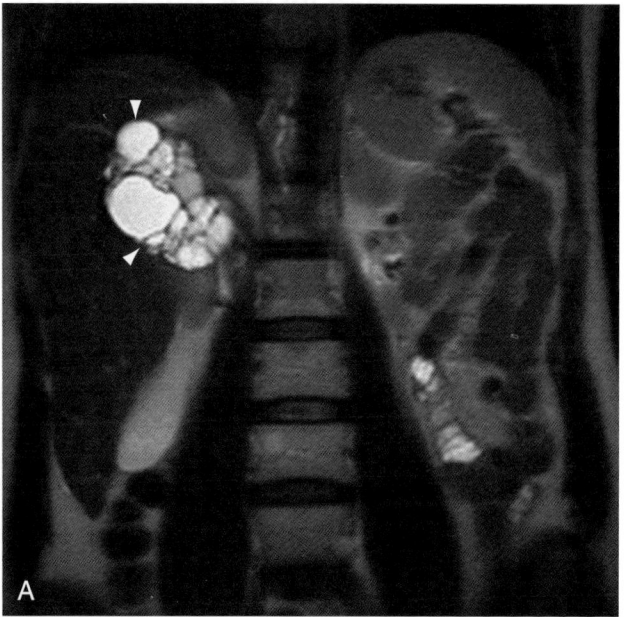
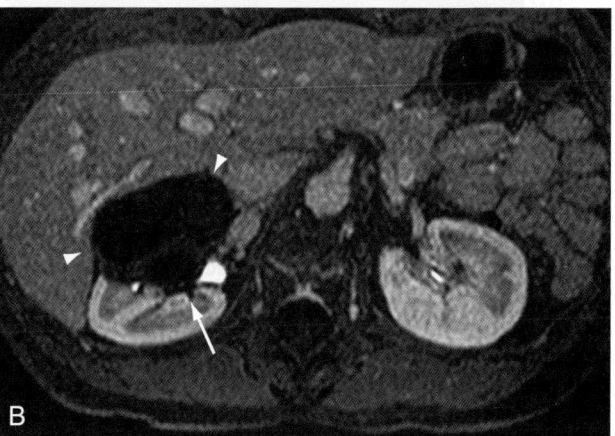

FIGURE 86-38

Multilocular cystic nephroma (MLCN). 50-year–old woman with an unchanged cystic lesion in the right kidney for 4 years and presumptive diagnosis of MLCN. **A,** Coronal T2-weighted half-Fourier turbo spin-echo (HASTE) image demonstrates a cystic lesion with homogeneous high signal intensity (*arrowheads*) and multiple thin septations. **B,** Axial gadolinium-enhanced 3D fat-saturated T1-weighted gradient-recalled echo image during the nephrographic phase demonstrates a nonenhancing mass (*arrowheads*) with the characteristic herniation into the renal pelvis (*arrow*).

AMLs in the adult population, this diagnosis in children is based on the presence of macroscopic fat within the tumor.

MLCN is most common in boys between 3 months and 4 years of age.[218] Typically, this lesion affects only one portion of the kidney. The presence of the remaining normal renal parenchyma helps to distinguish this entity from the multicystic dysplastic kidney.

Mesoblastic nephroma or renal fetal hamartoma is the most common renal tumor in neonates and young infants.[218] The mean age at presentation is 3 months, though it can be present at birth.[218] Patients usually present with a nontender abdominal mass. Hematuria,

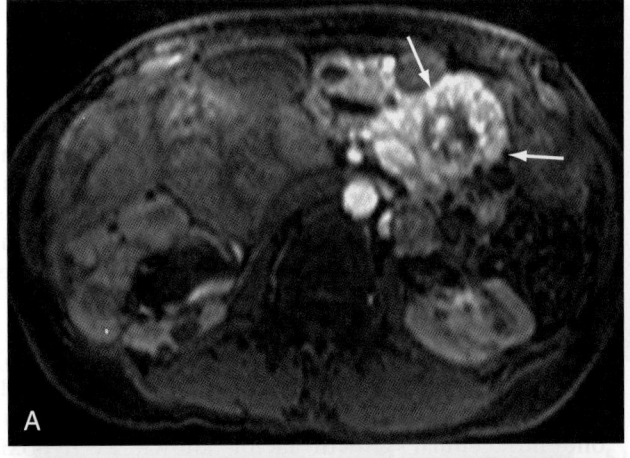
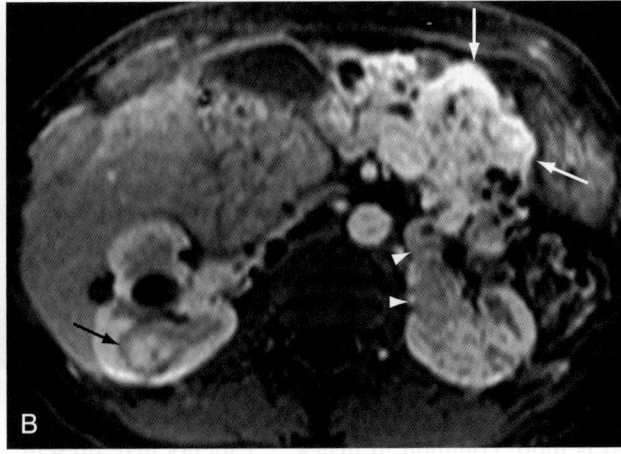
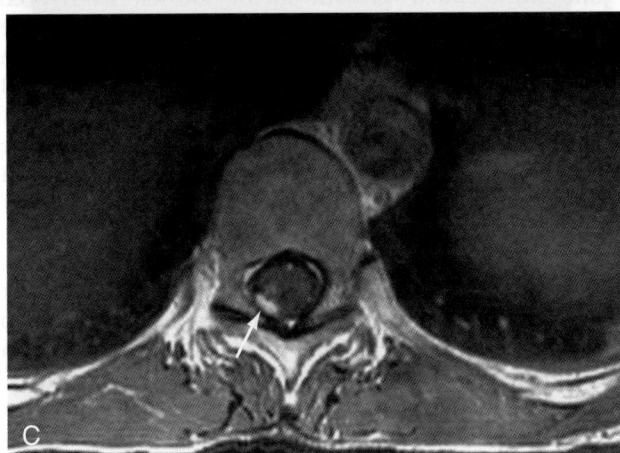

FIGURE 86-40

Metastatic renal cell carcinoma and neuroendocrine pancreatic tumor in a patient with von Hippel-Lindau disease. **A,** Axial 3D contrast-enhanced fat-saturated T1-weighted GRE image during the arterial phase shows an arterial enhancing pancreatic mass consistent with a neuroendocrine neoplasm (*arrows*). **B,** Axial 3D contrast-enhanced fat-saturated T1-weighted GRE image during the portal venous phase shows a right renal mass (*black arrow*) and enhancing tumor thrombus in the left renal vein (*arrowheads*). Other tumors were seen in the both kidneys at different levels (not shown). The pancreatic mass is again noted (*white arrows*). **C,** Axial contrast-enhanced T1-weighted fast spin-echo image at the level of the T9-T10 interspace demonstrates a small enhancing nodule (*arrow*) in the right lateral aspect of the spinal cord consistent with a hemangioblastoma.

intracystic hemorrhage or proteinaceous fluid. Enlargement of any enhancing lesion must be considered to be RCC until proven otherwise.

The risk for metastatic disease has to be balanced with the preservation of renal function in patients with VHL disease. While surgical removal of the renal tumor is considered curative in sporadic disease, patients with VHL disease are exposed to a life-long increased risk for the development of renal neoplasms. In these patients, most RCCs under 3 cm are low-grade neoplasms (Furhman grade I-II).[234] Since metastatic disease is virtually nonexistent in small renal tumors, surgical treatment is generally reserved for lesions that are greater than or equal to 3 cm in diameter.[234,238] This approach, together with nephron-sparing surgical techniques, allows for preservation of the renal function in these patients with minimal risk for metastatic disease.[239]

Hereditary Papillary Renal Cell Carcinoma

Hereditary papillary renal cell carcinoma (HPRCC) is an autosomal-dominant hereditary condition characterized by the development of multiple, bilateral, low-grade (type I) papillary renal cancers. A proto-oncogene located at 7q31.3, *MET*, is responsible for this condition.[240] These patients have overexpression of the *MET* gene, which codes for a transmembrane tyrosine kinase. However, the exact mechanism by which tumors develop is still unknown.[234] *MET* mutations have been shown to play a role in up to 13% of patients with sporadic papillary RCC.[240] Renal tumors with the *MET* genotype, both sporadic and those occurring in patients with HPRCC, show a distinctive papillary RCC type 1 phenotype that is genetically and histologically different from renal tumors seen in other hereditary renal syndromes and most sporadic renal tumors with papillary architecture.[240]

Similar to sporadic type I papillary RCCs, tumors in patients with HPRCC are typically low-grade, slow growing neoplasms with low metastatic potential. The median tumor doubling time is 18 months.[241]

Papillary neoplasms in patients with HPRCC demonstrate low-level homogeneous enhancement on contrast-enhanced CT examinations similar to that of sporadic type I papillary tumors. Similar findings have been described on contrast-enhanced MR images.[241] Careful evaluation of pre- and post-contrast images, as well as subtraction techniques, can help to detect low level enhancement in these hypovascular masses.

Birt-Hogg-Dube Syndrome

Birt-Hogg-Dube syndrome is an autosomal-dominant disorder characterized by fibrofoliculomas in the face and trunk, pulmonary cysts, and a variety of renal tumors.[234,242] The lung involvement can vary from a few scattered cysts to extensive cyst formation complicated by spontaneous pneumothoraces.[234] While an increased incidence of colonic polyps has been described, the increased risk for colon cancer is not clear. The gene responsible for this disease is located at 17p11.2 and codes for a protein named folliculin.[234,244] The mechanism of tumor formation is unclear.

Approximately 15% to 30% of patients with this disorder develop renal cancer.[234] Up to 34% of these tumors are chromophobe carcinomas and 50% are mixed chromophobe-oncocytomas.[245] However, different histologic types of renal tumors have been described in these patients, including clear-cell (9%), oncocytomas (5%), and papillary types (2%).[245]

These patients are typically followed with serial chest and abdomen CT examinations.[234] The clinical management is similar to patients with VHL where surgical treatment is reserved for masses equal to or larger than 3 cm in diameter.[234] Typically, a nephron-sparing surgical removal of these masses is attempted to preserve renal function.

Familial Renal Oncocytoma

Patients with familial renal oncocytoma (FRO) have an increased incidence of renal oncocytomas. A clear hereditary pattern has not yet been established in these patients and no putative genetic locus has been identified for this condition.[234] The term renal oncocytomatosis has been used to describe cases where extensive and confluent oncocytomas are found.[246]

At imaging studies, oncocytomas are indistinguishable from RCCs. For this reason, patients are treated as if these lesions were renal cancers.[168,234] Renal failure is not uncommon in patients with renal oncocytomatosis.[247,248] MR imaging can provide a comprehensive evaluation of these patients, including serial follow-up imaging, without the risk of the iodinated contrast media compromising further the renal function.

Hereditary Leiomyoma Renal Cell Carcinoma

Hereditary leiomyoma renal cell carcinoma (HLRCC) is an autosomal-dominant disorder characterized by the presence of cutaneous and uterine leiomyomas as well as type II papillary cancers.[234,249] The association of cutaneous and uterine leiomyomas is known as the Reed syndrome.[234] Approximately 90% of these patients have uterine leiomyomas and most also have cutaneous leiomyomas.[234,250] There is an increased risk in these patients for malignant transformation of uterine leiomyomas into leiomyosarcomas.[250] A few cases of cutaneous leiomyosarcomas have also been reported.[234,250] The gene responsible for this disorder is at 1q4.3 and codes for the enzyme fumarate hydratase, which is involved in one of the critical steps in the Krebs cycle.[250] The mechanism for tumor formation is not understood.

Approximately 17% of patients with HLRCC have type II papillary renal cancers.[234] In contrast with other hereditary forms of renal cancer, these patients tend to have unilateral solitary masses.[234] These tumors are typically aggressive (Fuhrman nuclear grades 3 or 4) and metastasize in approximately 50% of patients, even those with relatively small tumors.[234]

The reported appearance of type II papillary neoplasms on contrast-enhanced CT is similar to that of low-grade type I papillary neoplasms with patients presenting with a hypovascular renal mass.[234] The MR imaging findings for these tumors have not been described. In our experience, sporadic type II papillary neoplasms tend to be more heterogeneous due to the presence of hemorrhage and necrosis. Typically, enhancing papillary projections are seen in the periphery of the tumor. More studies are needed to evaluate the MR appearance of these tumors in patients with HLRCC.

Tuberous Sclerosis

Tuberous sclerosis (TS) is an autosomal-dominant neurocutaneous disorder characterized by the development of hamartomas in multiple organs. The dermatologic manifestations of TS include adenoma sebaceum or facial angiofibromas, ungual fibromas, hypomelanotic macules, and the shagreen patch.[251] Cortical hamartomas or tubers, focal cortical dysplasia, subependymal nodules, and subependymal giant cell astrocytomas are the characteristic lesions in the central nervous system.[251] Pulmonary cysts (lymphangiomyomatosis), cardiac rhabdomyomas, and renal lesions, including AML, epithelial cysts, and RCC, may also be present in these patients.[251] The incidence of TS in the general population is estimated to be between 1 in 6000 and 1 in 10,000.[251] Approximately 66% to 86% of index cases are related to spontaneous germline mutations, rather than an inherited genetic cause.[252] The classic clinical triad in TS includes epilepsy, mental retardation, and adenoma sebaceum.[253] However, a wide spectrum of phenotypic manifestations has been described in patients with TS.

Two genes have been associated with TS, *TSC1* and *TSC2*, located at 9q34 and 16p13.3, respectively.[252] Both are tumor suppressor genes and inactivation of both copies of the allele is necessary for tumor formation.[251] *TSC1* codes for a protein called hemartin, which mediates cell adhesion, and *TSC2* encodes a protein named tuberin, which is involved in various cellular processes.[251] Most cases of TS are secondary to mutations in these genes.

Approximately 80% of patients with TS develop AMLs.[251] While sporadic AMLs tend to be solitary, unilateral, and have a very high female predilection, most AMLs associated with TS are multiple, bilateral, and have no sex predilection.[254] Enlarging AMLs have potential risk for spontaneous bleed. Clinically, they can present with hematuria, compression of adjacent organs, hypertension, and renal insufficiency.[251] Rarely, AMLs can demonstrate local aggressive behavior with extracapsular extension, local invasion, renal vein invasion, and/or lymph node involvement.[255,256] For these reasons, nephron-sparing nephrectomy or catheter angiography with selective embolization has been advocated in AMLs larger than 4 cm.[141,251] Simple renal cysts are present in up to 15% to 20% of patients with TS and they are usually discovered in childhood.[141] Patients with TS have also a higher risk of developing RCC. RCC occurs in approximately 2% of patients with TS,[251] and typically occurs at a younger age (mean age at presentation, 28 years) than sporadic RCC in the general population.[257] RCC is bilateral in 43% of these patients.[257] In contrast to a male predominance for sporadic RCC (70%), in TS there is a significant female predominance (81%). The most common histologic type in TS is the clear-cell type, though papillary and chromophobe carcinomas also occur.[258] An increased incidence of oncocytomas has also been reported.[259]

Patients with TS are followed up periodically, typically with CT, because of the increased risk of renal malignancy and potential life-threatening complications of large AMLs. MR is an alternative in these patients and can avoid repetitive radiation and exposure to iodinated contrast media. Also, MR imaging can help in selected cases to differentiate between RCC and AMLs with scant fat.

Renal Medullary Carcinoma

Renal medullary carcinoma occurs in relatively young black patients with sickle cell trait.[86] While patients with sickle cell trait develop these tumors, those with sickle cell anemia do not.[86] Age at presentation varies from 11 to 39 years.[86] In younger patients (between 11 and 24 years) there is a 3:1 male predominance, though beyond age 24 years the tumors occur equally in men and women.[86,260] The prognosis is very poor with frequent metastases to lymph nodes, liver, and lung at presentation and a mean survival after surgery of 15 weeks.[86]

Renal medullary carcinomas are large tumors (mean size, 7 cm) that originate in the central portion of the kidney.[86,260] Peripheral satellite lesions in the renal cortex and extension into the pelvic soft-tissues are frequently present.[260] Venous and lymphatic invasion are also common.[260]

At pathology, reticular, yolk-sac–like, or adenoid cystic appearances are described, often with poorly differentiated areas in a highly desmoplastic stroma.[260] Recently, this tumor has been considered as a particularly aggressive form of collecting duct carcinoma.[261]

Radiologically, these tumors present as ill-defined infiltrative masses arising in the central portion of the kidney.[86] Extension into the renal sinus and cortical involvement are characteristic.[86] Caliectasis can be present secondary to renal sinus involvement.[86] Although the kidney can be markedly enlarged, the reniform shape of the tumor tends to be maintained even with large tumors.[86] These tumors are heterogeneous on ultrasound and contrast-enhanced CT.[86] To our knowledge, the MR findings in these tumors have not been described. Iron deposition in the renal cortex, which is a finding in patients with sickle cell disease, is not present in patients with mild disease who have not undergone transfusions.[82,262] Therefore, the MR findings of cortical iron deposition (described later) are probably not present in patients with sickle cell trait and medullary renal carcinomas.

RENAL CYSTIC DISEASES

Genetic Cystic Disease

Autosomal-Dominant Polycystic Kidney Disease

Autosomal-dominant polycystic kidney disease (ADPKD) is characterized by the progressive development of various-sized renal cysts in both kidneys and which leads to progressive renal failure. ADPKD accounts for 8% to 10% of patients with endstage renal disease in the United States and Europe and represents the most common hereditary disorder of the kidneys.[263-265] The *PKD1* gene is responsible for this condition in 85% to 90% of cases and is located on the short arm of chromosome 16.[263,266] Mutations in the *PKD2* gene, located on chromosome 4, account for 15% of affected families.[266] Most cases are inherited in an autosomal-dominant pattern, though up to 10% of cases are secondary to a spontaneous mutation.[263]

Patients with ADPKD develop multiple renal cysts that typically grow over time. Renal failure, hematuria, hypertension, cyst infection, and renal stones are complications of this disease.[263] Not uncommonly, patients have pain related to the renal cysts.

ADPKD is a multisystemic disease affecting multiple organs. Associated extrarenal findings include cardiac valve anomalies, intracranial aneurysms, liver cysts, pancreatic cysts, and colonic diverticula.[267] ADPKD has been associated with an increased incidence of renal cancer, though some studies have failed to demonstrate this association.[267] A higher incidence of concurrent bilateral (12% versus 1-5%), multicentric (28% versus 6%), and sarcomatoid-type (33% versus 1-5%) RCCs have been described in patients with APKD compared to that in the general population.[268]

Ultrasound and CT are the most common imaging modalities used for the evaluation of these patients because of their availability. However, MR imaging has several advantages over other imaging techniques in the diagnosis and follow-up of patients with ADPKD. Gadolinium contrast agents are safe even in the presence of renal failure.[29-31] In addition, patients with ADPKD frequently develop intracystic hemorrhage. These cysts are commonly complex on ultrasound and hyperdense on CT. Detection of a solid component in these lesions can be very challenging using ultrasound and CT. MR imaging has excellent soft-tissue contrast that allows characterization of intracystic hemorrhage and recognition of enhancing components.

Hemorrhagic cysts are typically hyperintense on T1-weighted images and hypointense on T2-weighted images compared to the renal parenchyma.[267] Mural and septal thickening, irregularity, and enhancement can be the only clues for detection of a malignant cystic neoplasm. The enhancing solid component in the lesion can be recognized with careful evaluation of pre- and post-contrast images. In our experience, subtraction imaging facilities the recognition of enhancing lesions in patients with APKD and multiple hemorrhagic cysts. While nonenhancing hyperintense hemorrhagic cysts become black on subtracted images, enhancing lesions are readily obvious due to their higher signal intensity (Fig. 86-41).

Recently, kidney volume and renal hemodynamic parameters measured by MR have been correlated with functional indices of disease severity.[269] Renal blood flow as determined by phase-contrast imaging represented the strongest predictor of renal function in these patients.[269]

Autosomal-Recessive Polycystic Kidney Disease

Autosomal-recessive polycystic kidney disease (ARPKD) is a congenital disorder that affects the kidneys bilaterally and symmetrically and is most frequently seen in neonates.[218] Flank mass, polyuria, congestive heart failure, or pneumothorax are among the variable presenting signs and symptoms.[218] Pulmonary hypoplasia (Potter's syndrome) is associated with severe bilateral

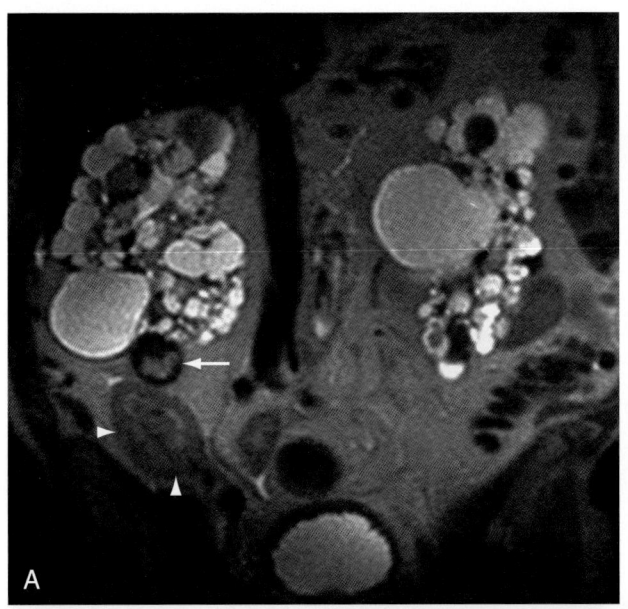

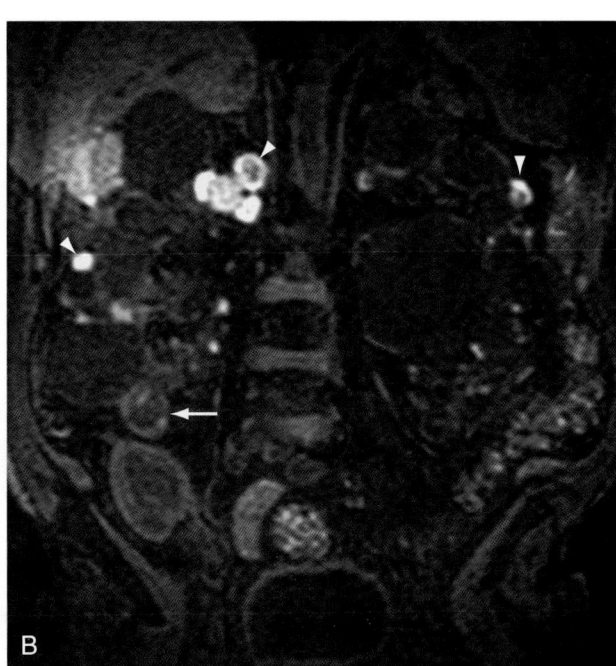

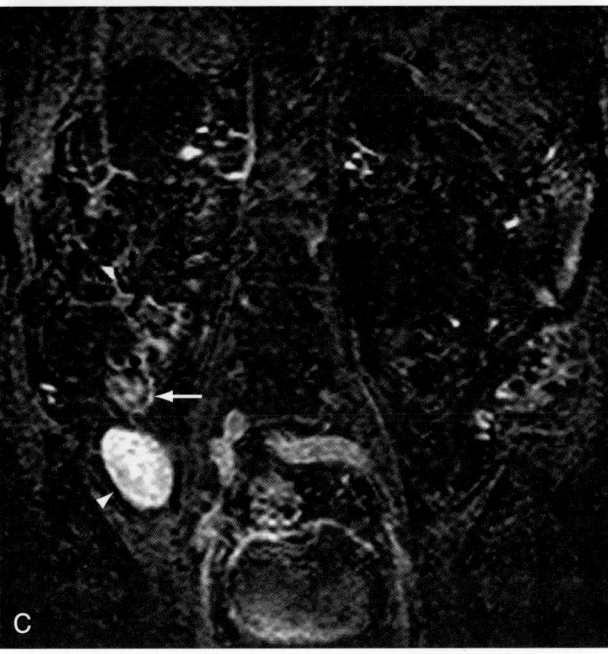

FIGURE 86-41

Polycystic kidney disease (PCKD) and renal cell carcinoma (RCC). **A,** Coronal T2-weighted half-Fourier turbo spin-echo (HASTE) image shows complete replacement of the renal parenchyma by numerous cysts in both kidneys. An exophytic lesion with a hypointense nodular thick wall is noted arising from the lower pole of the right kidney (*arrow*). A renal transplant is partially seen in the right lower quadrant (*arrowheads*). **B,** Coronal nonenhanced 3D fat-saturated T1-weighted gradient-recalled echo (GRE) image shows multiple hyperintense cysts in both kidneys (*arrowheads*). The lesion in the lower pole of the right kidney is again noted and has intermediate signal intensity (*arrow*). **C,** Coronal subtraction image from gadolinium-enhanced 3D fat-saturated T1-weighted GRE sequences shows enhancement in the central portion of this lesion (*arrow*). After nephrectomy, sclerotic RCC was diagnosed at pathology. Note the lack of enhancement of the upper pole lesions. Subtraction imaging facilitates determination of enhancement, including the hyperintense cysts typical of PCKD. Note the segment of the transplanted kidney with expected enhancement (*arrowhead*).

renal disease.[218] Most patients with this condition die due to severe renal impairment. Those patients who survive typically develop hypertension and hepatic fibrosis during adolescence and adulthood.[218] The severity of the hepatic involvement is inversely related to the severity of renal impairment. Patients presenting with hypertension and renal dysfunction later in childhood tend to have a more severe hepatic fibrosis and portal hypertension. However, their overall prognosis is better compared to those presenting with renal impairment in the neonatal period.[218]

Patients with ARPKD have bilaterally enlarged kidneys containing multiple small cysts.[227] These have similar MR imaging findings to those of simple cysts with low signal intensity on T1-weighted images and very high homogeneous signal intensity on T2-weighted images.[227] Some of these cysts may show high signal intensity on T1-weighted images due to hemorrhagic contents.[227] MR imaging can also demonstrate hepatic cysts and fibrosis.[227]

Nephronophthisis and Medullary Cystic Disease Complex

Nephronophthisis/medullary cystic disease complex is an important cause of renal failure in adolescents and young adults.[270] Nephronophthisis is characterized by an autosomal-recessive trait and is responsible for those cases presenting during childhood.[270,271] These patients have an increased risk for associated extrarenal anomalies, including retinal degeneration, hepatic fibrosis, and skeletal anomalies.[270] Patients with medullary cystic disease present during young adulthood and have an autosomal-dominant transmission.[271] Extrarenal manifestations are uncommon.[270]

Refractory anemia, polydispsia, and polyuria are common at presentation.[270] Hypertension is not frequent earlier in the disease because of an abnormal increased urinary excretion of sodium.[270] Urinary sediment is usually normal.[270] The median age for development of chronic renal failure is 13 years in patients with the autosomal-recessive transmission.[271] Patients with medullary cystic disease typically develop endstage renal disease in their third to fourth decade.[271]

Histologically, this condition is characterized by an interstitial sclerosing nephropathy with thickening of the tubular basement membrane, tubular ectasis and atrophy, and Tamm-Horsfald protein deposits.[271] Diverticula/cysts may be seen on microdissection examination communicating with the distal convoluted tubules and collecting ducts.[272]

Imaging plays a primary role in the diagnosis of these conditions. Renal cysts are characteristically seen in the renal medulla and corticomedullary junction.[270,271] The kidneys are usually normal or small in size.[270] Ultrasound is the initial imaging modality of choice and may demonstrate cysts in the characteristic location.[270] Patients with inconclusive ultrasound may benefit from other imaging studies. MR imaging can provide excellent visualization of these cysts due to its inherent soft-tissue contrast. Furthermore, it avoids the use of iodinated contrast radiation exposure in this group of patients which usually includes adolescents and young adults

with renal failure.[270] Multiple cysts can be seen with their characteristic homogenous low signal intensity on T1-weighted images and very high signal intensity on T2-weighted images.[270] The renal cortex and medulla demonstrate normal enhancement after contrast administration.[270] The cysts do not enhance on gadolinium-enhanced MR imaging (Fig. 86-42).[270] While accumulation of contrast within the cysts on delayed images has not been described, this could potentially be due to the existing communication between these cysts and the distal convoluted tubules and collecting ducts.[272]

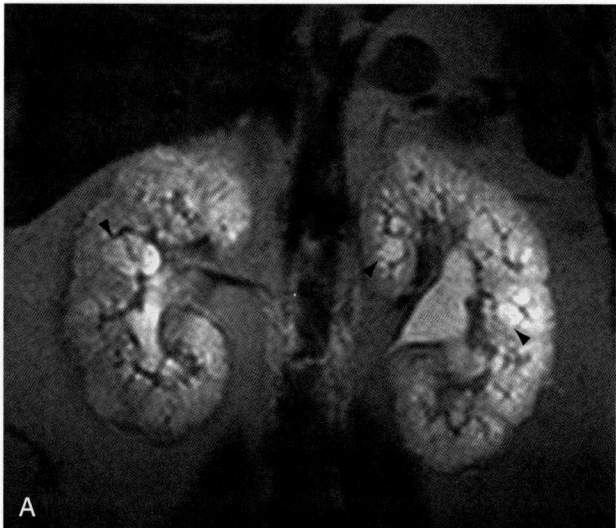

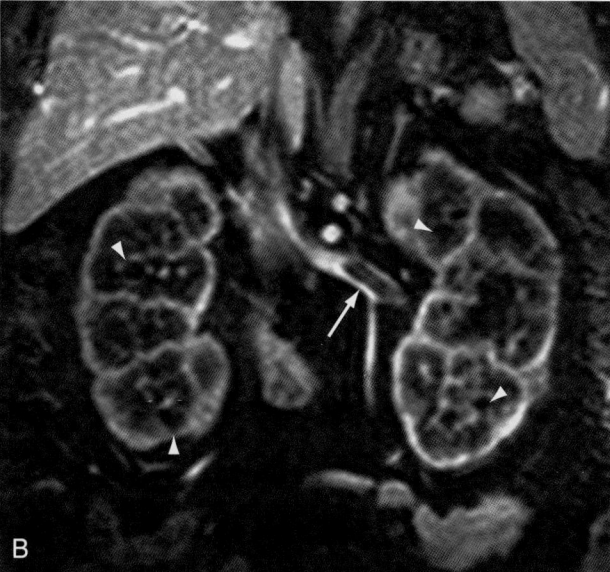

FIGURE 86-42

Medullary cystic kidney disease. **A,** Coronal T2-weighted half-Fourier turbo spin-echo (HASTE) image shows diffuse high signal intensity throughout both kidneys. Several well-demarcated cysts are noted bilaterally within the medullary region (*arrowheads*). **B,** Coronal 3D contrast-enhanced fat-saturated T1-weighted gradient-recalled echo (GRE) image during the nephrographic phase demonstrates bilateral cortical thinning and multiple foci of low signal intensity in the medulla consistent with cysts (*arrowheads*). Incidentally, a thrombus was detected in the left renal vein (*arrow*).

Obstructive Cystic Disease

Multicystic Dysplastic Kidney

Multicystic dysplastic kidney (MCDK) is a developmental, nonhereditary condition characterized by the presence of multiple cysts that may vary in size and number, with little or no normal renal parenchyma.[273] MCDK is also known as renal dysplasia, renal dysgenesis, multicystic kidney, and Potter's type II renal cystic disease.[273] MCDK represents one of the most common abdominal masses in newborns,[273] and is the most common cystic renal disease in infancy.[218] It occurs equally in boys and girls.[273] Most patients are asymptomatic and many cases are detected in utero during a routine ultrasound examination of the fetus.[274] Patients with bilateral forms of MCKD have a higher association with congenital syndromes and almost always a poor outcome.[273]

MCDK is in the same group of congenital anomalies of the kidney and urinary tract as ureteropelvic junction obstruction, hypoplastic kidneys, vesicoureteral reflux, nonobstructed, nonrefluxing primary megaureter, and bladder outlet obstruction (e.g., posterior urethral valves).[275] Different theories have been postulated about the origin of these congenital anomalies. For a long time it has been the general belief that renal dysgenesis is caused by embryonic urinary tract obstruction.[275] Renal dysplasia can present with a spectrum of severity and it is commonly accompanied by poor function in the involved kidney.[275] The most severe form is the multicystic dysplastic kidney, which has no demonstrable function and is accompanied by complete obstruction in some part of the outflow tract.[275] The "bud theory" proposes that these abnormalities in both the kidney and ureter derive from abnormal ureteral budding from the Wolffian duct.[275] Failure of the ureteral bud to induce adequate maturation of the metanephric blastema into nephrons during intrauterine development would be responsible for the abnormal development of the kidney.[275]

While the disease is usually unilateral there is a serious contralateral anomaly in 30% to 80% of cases, with obstruction at the ureteropelvic junction and other ureteral anomalies being the most common.[218,273] There is an increased risk for associated anomalies in other systems; the gastrointestinal tract and heart are the most common locations.[276] This condition has been associated with infection, hypertension, and malignancy.[274] The true incidence of malignant transformation is unknown, though this has been reported rarely, including cases of RCC, Wilms' tumor, and central nephroblastomatosis.[218,273]

The management of patients with MCKD is under debate. Nephrectomy has been proposed for confirmation of the diagnosis, relief of symptoms, avoidance of malignant potential, and treatment of hypertension.[277] However, these criteria have been questioned because the diagnosis can be made reliably before surgery, the malignant potential is extremely low, and the number of patients with hypertension is very low.[273] Furthermore, regression of MCDK changes has been noted on follow-up ultrasound in utero and after birth.[277-279]

The radiologic appearance of MCDK depends on whether there has been a hydronephrotic component during development of the kidney.[273] The MCDK is composed of multiple noncommunicating cysts separated by connective tissue with little or no normal renal parenchyma. The normal reniform shape is typically lost. Microscopically, a reduced number of nephrons and primitive glomeruli can be present.[273] There is atresia or hypoplasia of the ureter and renal pelvis in most cases and the renal artery is very small or absent.[273] A dilated renal pelvis may be seen in cases where an incomplete but severe obstruction occurs early in nephrogenesis.[273] Communication of the renal pelvis with the peripheral cysts, as well as between the cysts, can occur in these cases.

The diagnosis of MCDK is made most often with in utero ultrasound, as early as 15 weeks' gestation, or neonatal ultrasound.[273] A paraspinous mass with multiple cysts that are variable in size and shape and without identifiable communication can be seen, and the ureter and renal pelvis usually are not visible. The presence of oligohydramnios with bilateral MCDK is a poor prognostic sign.[273]

A nonfunctioning kidney can be seen on radiographic studies in older children or adults.[273] Ring calcifications in the renal region may be seen on plain films.[273] Few reports have described the intrauterine diagnosis of MCDK with MR imaging. A large, multicystic mass can be seen in the renal fossa.[280] Multiple noncommunicating cysts are well appreciated with single-shot fast spin-echo sequences and can be reliably differentiated from hydronephrosis (Fig. 86-43).[280]

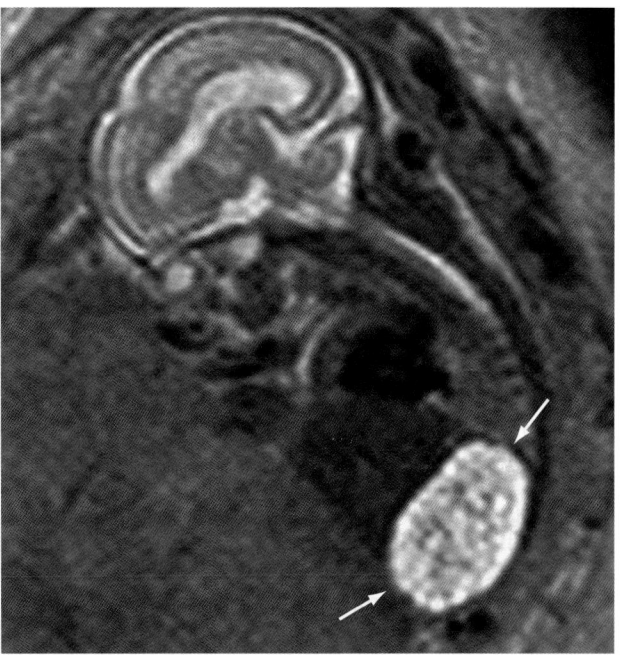

FIGURE 86-43

Multicystic dysplastic kidney in utero. Half-Fourier single-shot fast spin-echo (SSFSE) image of the fetus at 22 weeks' gestation demonstrates multiple hyperintense cysts replacing the right kidney (*arrows*). (*Courtesy of Deborah Levine, MD, Boston.*)

experience, tubular ectasia can be seen on delayed gadolinium-enhanced MR images as tubular accumulations of contrast radiating from the calices into the papillae.

UROLITHIASIS

In the past decade, nonenhanced CT has become the imaging study of choice for demonstrating ureteric obstruction, its cause, level, and size of stones,[28] replacing excretory intravenous urography in many institutions. However, limitations of CT include the lack of information about the excretory function of the kidneys, the use of ionizing radiation, and the difficulty in differentiating pelvic phleboliths from distal stones.[28]

MR is an alternative imaging technique for patients presenting with acute flank pain.[24-27] MR may be particularly helpful when the use of contrast media or radiation is undesirable (e.g., in pregnant patients and young adults).[28] The MR demonstration of ureteric obstruction can be seen with heavily T2-weighted images or gadolinium-enhanced T1-weighted images.

HASTE and RARE sequences provide heavily T2-weighted images to demonstrate the urinary tract without contrast media.[26,27] HASTE thin-slice (thickness, 3-6 mm) images with sufficient anatomic coverage are typically obtained in the coronal plane in one to two breath-holds, depending on body habitus. The use of fat suppression can improve the visualization of the collecting systems. Such images are amenable to further processing with maximum intensity projection (MIP) or volume rendering (VR) algorithms. The MIP or VR images provide a urographic-like appearance that is familiar to the referring physician, but this processing rarely adds to the diagnostic content.[27]

A coronal thick slab (thickness, 20-60 mm) can be obtained in one breath-hold with a RARE sequence commonly referred to as echo-train spin-echo imaging. This approach does not require further post-processing and includes the entire collecting system in a single image that resembles the conventional excretory urogram. Thick-slab RARE can demonstrate both kidneys and ureters in a single image. However, the multislice technique usually provides better image quality than the single thick-slab technique due to the better delineation of background tissues and diminished partial volume effects of the former.[26] A combination of thin-slice HASTE and thick-slab RARE images may increase the confidence of the radiologist in detecting the level of obstruction.[24]

When an obstructed system is identified, the ancillary finding of hyperintense, perirenal fluid on HASTE and RARE images favors an acute process; this probably arises from lymphatic congestion or forniceal rupture.[295] However, perirenal fluid can be secondary to any insult to the kidney and should be considered a nonspecific sign.[28]

A relatively low sensitivity and specificity for small ureteral stones is a known limitation of T2-weighted imaging.[27] Sudah et al[24] found a sensitivity of approximately 54% to 58% in 40 consecutive patients with acute flank pain. Their reported specificity was 100%, though all their patients had ureteral stones as a cause of obstruction. Intraluminal clots, debris, or neoplasms can mimic ureteral stones on T2-weighted images as they appear as filling defects.[24,27] Thin-slice HASTE images are superior to thick-slab RARE images for the detection of small filling defects.[26]

Gadolinium-enhanced MR urography is a valuable addition to the T2-weighted images for evaluation of patients with suspected acute renal colic.[28] As first described by Nolte-Ernsting et al,[25] a high-resolution, respiratory-gated T1-weighted sequence was used after the administration of gadolinium contrast media. A low dose of furosemide (0.1 mg/kg bodyweight, maximum dose 10 mg) immediately before the administration of the contrast media (30-60 seconds) allows for a complete distension of the collecting system with homogenous distribution of the gadolinium inside the entire urinary tract.[25] Furosemide increases urine volume and results in dilution of the concentrated gadolinium within the collecting system; this decreases the T2* effects and maintains increased signal intensity.[25] The use of breath-hold 3D T1-weighted gradient-echo sequences with this technique has become more popular.[24]

The entire urinary tract can be visualized with this approach even in the absence of urinary tract obstruction.[24] An increased flip angle (>30 degrees) allows for excellent visualization of the enhanced collecting systems while the background signal is saturated. MIP reconstructions provide excretory urography-like images with better spatial resolution than thin-slice HASTE or thick-slab RARE images.[24] The review of source images is essential for the diagnosis, particularly for the detection of small urinary stones.[24]

With high-grade obstruction, contrast-enhanced MR urography requires delayed imaging to allow for a sufficient concentration of contrast media in the collecting system and ureters.[28] It is often practical to remove a patient from the MR scanner and allow other examinations to be performed while waiting for the obstructed collecting system to fill with contrast.[28]

The presence of an intraureteral filling defect with smooth margins that shows no enhancement is considered a ureteral stone (Fig. 86-45).[28] A radiograph of the abdomen to identify a calcification at the same level as the obstruction may be helpful in characterizing a stone.[28] The presence or absence of post-contrast enhancement of an intraluminal filling defect can be helpful in characterizing a tumor for the former versus a stone or blood clot for the latter. Enhancement must be interpreted with caution as ureteral calculi can produce inflammatory changes and enhancement in the wall of the ureter. Similarly, increased periureteral high signal intensity on T2-weighted images has been described in patients with ureteral stones as a confounding finding that may mimic or obscure a neoplastic process.[28]

In patients with ruptured fornices, extravasation of contrast can be readily seen on gadolinium-enhanced MR urography; T2-weighted images reveal the extravasation as hyperintense fluid.[28] MR may be more sensitive than conventional excretory urography in demonstrating small extravasations.[28]

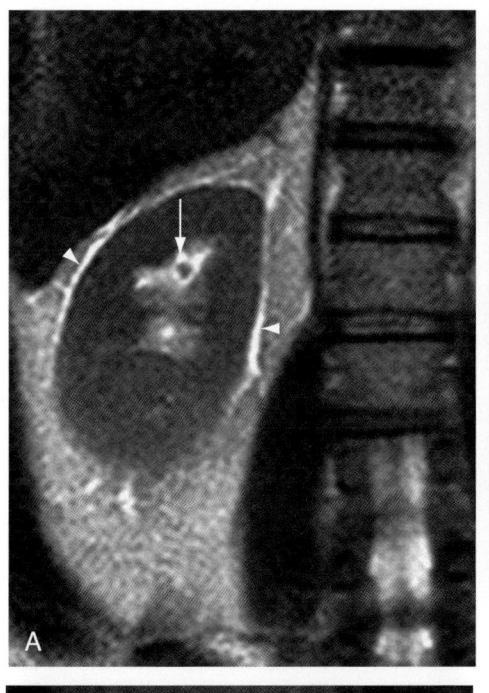

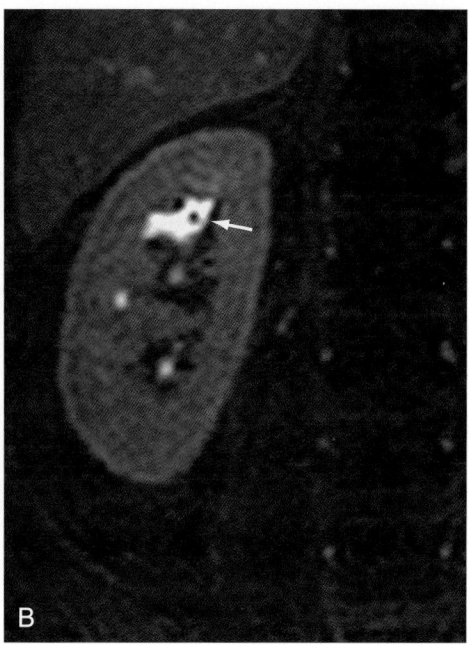

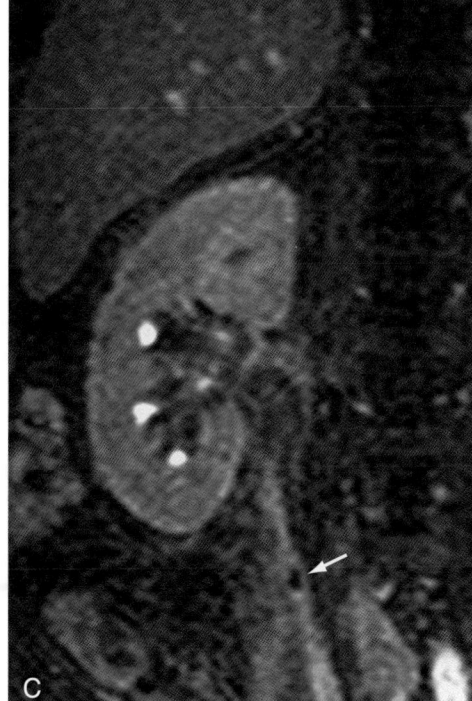

FIGURE 86-45

Calculus in upper calyx. **A,** Coronal half-Fourier turbo spin-echo (HASTE) image demonstrates a small rounded hypointense filling defect (*arrow*) in the mildly hydronephrotic upper pole calyx. The small amount of perinephric fluid (*arrowheads*) suggests acute obstruction. **B,** Delayed post-contrast coronal 3D fat-saturated T1-weighted gradient-recalled echo (GRE) image after administration of 10 mL furosemide demonstrates filling of the collecting system with gadolinium and a hypointense nonenhancing filling defect within an upper pole calyx (*arrow*) consistent with a nonobstructive stone. **C,** Coronal image from same acquisition as B but at a slightly more anterior anatomic level demonstrates an obstructing stone in the mid ureter (*arrow*), which is the cause of the hydronephrosis previously seen.

T1-weighted magnetization-prepared gradient-echo images can provide breath-hold–independent gadolinium urography images. Despite lower spatial resolution compared with 3D T1-weighted images, the presence and degree of obstruction as well as the presence of contrast extravasation can still be evaluated, even in patients unable to hold their breath.

Pregnant patients with suspected acute renal colic and limited ultrasound visualization of the ureters can be assessed with T2-weighted images (HASTE and RARE). This approach enables identification of the presence and level of obstruction in an expeditious manner. Positioning of the patient in the lateral decubitus (with elevation of the affected side) may help to visualize the distal part of the ureter when compression by the gravid uterus limits its visualization. Gadolinium-enhanced MR urography should be avoided whenever possible in these patients.

INFECTIONS

Bacterial Pyelonephritis

Bacterial infection of the renal parenchyma and collecting system (pyelonephritis) can result from urinary tract infections. Imaging studies are usually performed in cases that do not respond to appropriate antibiotic treatment to assess for obstruction, abscess, or emphysematous pyelonephritis.[296]

In clinical practice, CT or ultrasound are typically performed when pyelonephritis is suspected. When multiple imaging techniques were compared in a swine model of pyelonephritis similar sensitivity and specificity values were shown using technetium-99m dimercapto-succinic acid (DMSA) single photon emission CT (SPECT), spiral CT, and MR imaging.[297] The reported specificity and sensitivity values for MR were 89.5% and 87.5%, respectively.[297] Power Doppler ultrasound was less accurate in that study than the other three modalities. In 37 children with fever and urinary infection, MR imaging depicted more pyelonephritic lesions than renal cortical scintigraphy and interobserver agreement for the presence of pyelonephritis was superior for MR imaging.[298]

In pyelonephritis there is renal enlargement with a heterogeneous appearance to the kidneys on MR images. Perirenal edema is usually present and best seen on T2-weighted images as areas of high signal intensity. T2-weighted images can show heterogenous signal intensity with multiple cortical areas of high signal intensity. Post-contrast images of the renal parenchyma show heterogenous striated enhancement, similar to findings described on contrast-enhanced CT.[299] More advanced cases may show multiple nonenhancing cortical defects, which may represent multiple abscesses and/or infarctions. The clinical context is important when interpreting the images since there is an overlap in the findings for infectious and vascular disorders.

A method to distinguish pyonephrosis from hydronephrosis has been proposed based on diffusion MR imaging.[300] In a study of 12 patients, pus in the collecting system (pynephrosis) correlated with marked hyperintense signal, while the pelvicalyceal system was hypointense in the hydronephrotic kidney.[300] Furthermore, the apparent diffusion coefficient (ADC) value of the pyonephrotic kidney was extremely low compared to the hydronephrotic kidney.[300] More studies with larger patient populations are needed to confirm these initial findings.

Candidiasis

Renal candidiasis occurs most frequently as a result of a systemic infection.[301,302] Occasionally, the kidney is involved during the course of candida cystitis or may even be affected primarily without evidence of candidemia. Risks factors for renal candidiasis include diabetes, obstructive uropathy, chronic pyelonephritis, debilitated individuals, and premature babies. The specific diagnosis is made with urine culture.

Similar to the hepatic and splenic involvement, renal candidiasis causes innumerable tiny microabscesses that can be seen as well-defined lesions ranging from 1 to 2 mm in diameter.[301] Increased mucosal and submucosal thickening in the renal pelvis has been described on ultrasound images in patients with renal candidiasis.[303] This finding is most likely secondary to mucosal edema and can be readily seen on T2-weighted MR images as increased thickening of the wall with very high signal intensity similar to that of urine. The presence of fungal balls or mycetomas as filling defects within the collecting system can help recognize this entity. Fungal balls have been reported to be nearly iso- and hyperintense compared to the renal parenchyma on T1- and T2-weighted images, respectively.[301] Associated thickening of the perirenal fascia may also be present in these patients.

Xanthogranulomatous Pyelonephritis

Xanthogranulomatous pyelonephritis (XGP) is a serious, debilitating illness caused by a chronic inflammatory disorder of the kidney that occurs in approximately 1% of all renal infections. Unilaterality is most common, though bilateral involvement has been reported.[304,305] The disease has a female-to-male ratio of 4:1. XGP is most common between the fifth and sixth decades of life. It is caused by a long-term obstruction leading to chronic infection of the kidney, though the exact etiology is not well understood. Abnormal lipid metabolism has been hypothesized as an etiologic factor in patients with XGP. Most patients present with flank pain, fever and chills, and persistent bacteriuria. While *Proteus mirabilis* is the most common causative agent, other bacteria have also been implicated in the pathogenesis, including *Escherichia coli* and pseudomonas species.[305] Partial or complete nephrectomy is the treatment of choice, depending on the extent of renal involvement.[305,306]

Two forms of XGP have been reported: diffuse and focal or "tumefactive." The diffuse form is the most common and is characterized by extensive involvement of the renal parenchyma. The kidney is usually nonfunctional.[305] The focal or "tumefactive" form presents as a focal renal mass mimicking RCC.[307] Nephrolithiasis is present in approximately 80% of patients with staghorn calculi in 50% of them.[305] However, the presence of calculi is not necessary for the diagnosis of XGP. XGP tends to fistulize into adjacent organs. Pyelocutaneous, ureterocutaneous, and pyeloenteric fistulae have been reported.

Massive renal enlargement, lithiasis, peripelvic fibrosis, hydronephrosis, and lobulated yellow masses replacing renal parenchyma are characteristic on gross examination.[308] The focal form is seen as a mass of yellow tissue with regional necrosis and hemorrhage which resembles an RCC.[308] The presence of lipid-laden "foamy" macrophages accompanied by both chronic- and acute-phase inflammatory cells on microscopic examination is pathognomonic.[308] This can be associated with focal abscesses.

XGP is commonly misinterpreted as a renal neoplasm on imaging studies. Involvement of the perinephric and

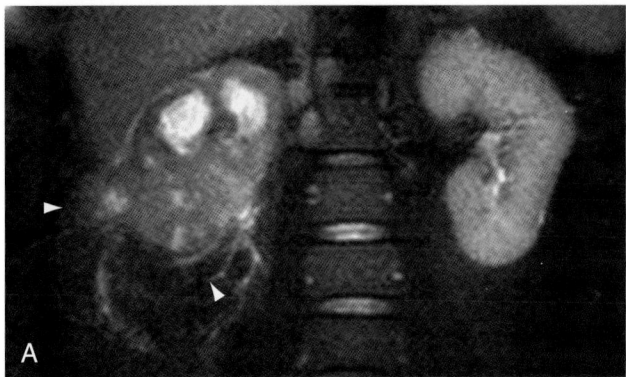

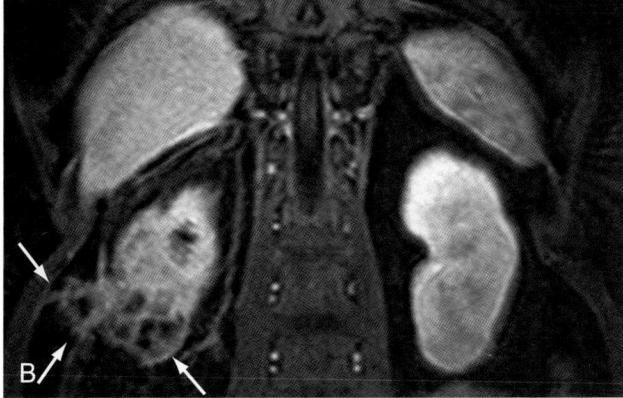

FIGURE 86-46

Xanthogranulomatous pyelonephritis. **A,** Coronal fat-saturated T2-weighted half-Fourier turbo spin-echo (HASTE) image shows a poorly-defined mass in the lower pole of the right kidney (*arrowheads*) and hydronephrosis in the upper pole. **B,** Coronal 3D fat-saturated T1-weighted gradient-recalled echo image in the delayed phase after contrast shows a heterogeneous mass with irregular areas of enhancement extending into the perinephric space (*arrows*).

adjacent structures or organs is common.[309] Several findings have been described as suggestive of XGP, including renal enlargement, perinephric fat stranding, thickening of the Gerota's fascia, and thick enhancing septa separating hypodense areas in the renal parenchyma.[306,310-312] Three stages have been described depending on the extent of involvement: confined to the kidney (stage I), extension into the perinephric fat (stage II), or adjacent retroperitoneal organs (stage III).[313]

The MR findings in XGP have been briefly described in the literature.[314,315] In the focal type, the inflammatory mass demonstrates slight hyperintensity on T2-weighted images and low signal intensity on T1-weighted images.[305] Involvement of the perirenal fat and adjacent organs can be seen (Fig. 86-46). Patients with diffuse XGP demonstrate replacement of the renal parenchyma by multiple water-density masses representing dilated calyces and abscess cavities. Cystic foci of intermediate signal intensity on T1-weighted images and hyperintensity on T2-weighted images can be seen.[315] The cavity walls show prominent enhancement on gadolinium-enhanced MR images. The staghorn calculus can be seen, though it is better seen on CT.

Tuberculosis

Towards the end of the 20th century tuberculosis showed a resurgence due to an expanding pool of immune-suppressed patients, particularly HIV-infected individuals, and the development of drug-resistant tuberculosis.[316] In the 1990s, implementation of control activities has caused a continual decline in the cases of tuberculosis, though the incidence of genitourinary tuberculosis has not reduced.[316]

Genitourinary tuberculosis is caused by *Mycobacterium tuberculosis* and it is the second most common form of extrapulmonary disease after peripheral lymphadenopathy.[316] Genitourinary tuberculosis accounts for up to 30% of patients with nonpulmonary tuberculosis.[316] Although renal tuberculosis is more commonly the result of hematogenous spread of the bacillus from the lungs, less than 5% of patients with genitourinary tuberculosis have active pulmonary disease.[316]

The clinical presentation of tuberculosis of the upper tracts can mimic other renal or urologic conditions, including pyelonephritis, renal colic, stones, sepsis, renal failure, and death.[316] Chronic pyuria and/or hematuria are commonly present. While *M. tuberculosis* is not detected on routine microbiologic studies, concurrent and recurrent *E. coli* urinary infection may be detected in these patients.[316]

Renal tuberculosis is characterized by progressive inflammatory changes within the parenchyma that begin with metastatic dissemination of blood-borne *M. tuberculosis*.[316] Initially, a microscopic foci near the glomeruli develops, followed by an acute, inflammatory response with polymorphonuclear leukocytes.[316] As the infection progresses, a chronic inflammatory response with macrophages leads to the development of granulomas with Langerhans giant cells, lymphocytes, and fibroblasts.[316] Coalescence of the inflammatory foci results in the formation of central caseous necrosis. As the infection continues, there is extension to the renal medulla with involvement and necrosis of the papilla.[316] Renal colic may be the result of sloughed renal papilla.[316] Ulceration of the calyces occurs and extensive parenchymal calcification or renal calculi may develop in 24% of patients.[316] Fibrosis of the collecting system and ureter are late manifestations of this condition that may lead to a clinical picture of obstructive uropathy.[316] The obstruction/stenosis may be at the level calyceal infundibulum and a single or multiple obstructed calyces may be present.[316]

Depending on the stage of the tuberculosis infection, renal involvement may show variable radiologic findings. These include moth-eaten calix, amputated infundibulum, autonephrectomy, urinary tract calcifications, renal parenchymal cavities, and hydrocalycosis, hydronephrosis or hydroureter due to stricture.[317] Multiple strictures in the collecting system are almost pathognomonic for urinary tuberculosis. Renal parenchymal masses and scarring, thick urinary tract walls, and extraurinary tubercular manifestations are also common and can be detected with cross-sectional studies. Multiple strictures are most commonly located at the infundibulum and ureters, and can be seen on excretory urography and CT in 70% and 58% of cases, respectively.[317]

The endstage "autonephrectomized" kidney in patients with genitourinary tuberculosis is typically small in size, though enlargement may be present rarely and can mimic diffuse XGP.[317] Renal tuberculosis and XGP can show thickening of the perirenal fasciae and spread of inflammation into the adjacent organs.[317]

Renal macronodular tuberculomas can appear on MR imaging as a mass with low signal intensity on T1-weighted images.[318] A thick irregular hypointense peripheral wall around the mass and intralesional fluid debris levels can be seen on T2-weighted images.[318] Abdominal tuberculomas without calcification, hemorrhage, or fibrosis at histology frequently show low signal intensity on both T1- and T2-weighted images.[319]

Renal Manifestations in Acquired Immunodeficiency Syndrome

Human immunodeficiency virus (HIV)-associated nephropathy is the most common cause of renal disease in HIV-infected patients undergoing renal biopsies in the United States.[320] Patients with HIV-associated nephropathy develop rapid progressive renal failure without treatment, which often leads to endstage renal disease within 2 to 4 months of diagnosis.[320] Decreased corticomedullary definition, decreased renal sinus fat, parenchymal heterogeneity, and globular renal configuration have been described on ultrasound examinations in these patients.[321] On MR imaging the findings are nonspecific with diffuse enlargement and loss of corticomedullary distinction on T1-weighted images having been reported.[322]

Patients with acquired immunodeficiency syndrome (AIDS) may also have a variety of conditions affecting the kidneys, including pyelonephritis, lobar nephronia, abscesses, lymphoma, parenchymal calcification, hydronephrosis, and infarcts (Fig. 86-47).[323]

REFLUX NEPHROPATHY AND CHRONIC PYELONEPHRITIS

A common sequela of patients with reflux nephropathy is the presence of renal scarring. Renal scars are more commonly located in the polar regions adjacent to the renal calyces. Patients with chronic pyelonephritis typically have a combination of calyceal dilatation and overlying cortical scarring. MR imaging is an excellent imaging modality for the demonstration of cortical thinning and benefits from multisequence, multiplanar options. MR images obtained during the nephrographic phase after administration of gadolinium are especially helpful.

Renal scarring has been associated with parenchymal loss, deterioration of renal function, endstage renal disease, and development of hypertension in children.[324] Up to 17% to 30% of children with renal scarring develop hypertension.[324] For this reason many children are followed with serial studies that may include multiple voiding cystourethrograms, nuclear scans, and ultrasounds.[324] In addition, impairment of renal function is determined by a decrease in differential function or

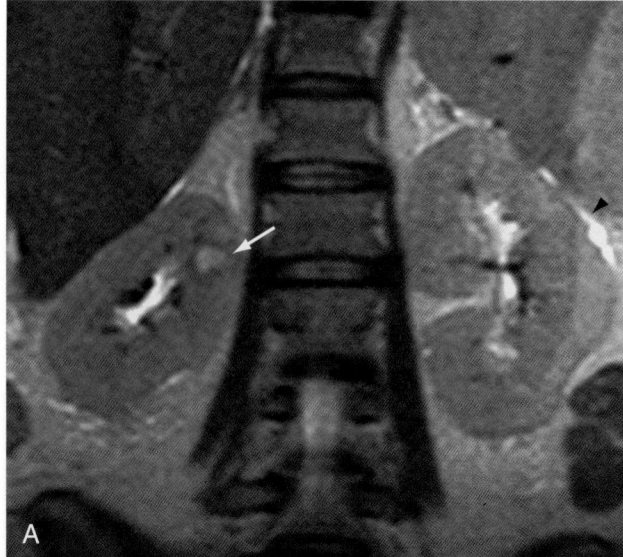
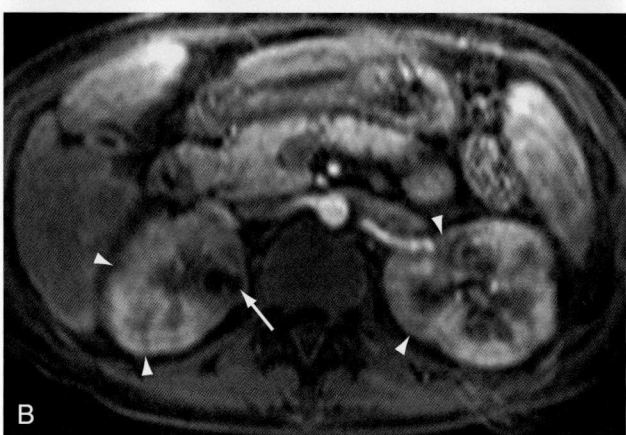

FIGURE 86-47

Methicillin-resistant *Staphylococcus aureus* (MRSA) infection in a patient with AIDS. **A,** Coronal T2-weighted half-Fourier turbo spin-echo (HASTE) image shows a small area of moderately increased signal intensity in the upper pole of the right kidney (*arrow*). There is minimal perirenal fluid adjacent to the left kidney (*arrowhead*). **B,** Axial gadolinium-enhanced 3D fat-saturated T1-weighted gradient-echo acquisition during the corticomedullary phase demonstrates bilateral striated nephrograms in both kidneys with multiple tiny areas of decreased cortical enhancement (*arrowheads*). A large, focal area of decreased enhancement with a fluid center is noted in the upper pole of the right kidney (*arrow*) which correlates with the area of high signal in **A**. These findings are consistent with bilateral pyelonephritis and a right renal abscess.

development of renal scarring, worsening or persistent vesicoureteral reflux, and worsening hydronephrosis.[324] The clinical management of this condition is based on these important prognostic factors.

Patients with the most severe renal scarring can demonstrate caliceal deformity, renal parenchymal thinning, and renal shrinkage on renal ultrasound and intravenous pyelogram (IVP).[324] MR imaging has been proposed as an alternative to the usual battery of diagnostic tests performed in these patients, offering a comprehensive evaluation while avoiding ionizing radiation.[324] MR voiding cystourethrography using the MR fluoroscopy technique after instillation of intravesical contrast material (Gd-DTPA) allows for evaluation of hydronephrosis and vesicoureteral reflux in these children with results comparable to those from conventional voiding cystourethrography.[324] Dynamic MR imaging during administration of a bolus of gadolinium contrast media provides excellent evaluation of renal function and renal scarring.[324] MR appears to be as sensitive as a nuclear scan in identifying renal scars in patients with vesicoureteral reflux but allows better anatomic localization.[324] MR can offer diagnostic information in these children that is comparable to that provided by nuclear scans, ultrasound, and voiding cystourethrography.[324]

HEMORRHAGE AND TRAUMA

Spontaneous retroperitoneal hemorrhage of renal origin can occur secondary to neoplasms, vasculitis, bleeding disorders, infection, and hemodialysis. Blood typically extends into the subcapsular and/or perirenal space.[325] The appropriate treatment for these patients is based on an accurate diagnosis, which often requires a combination of clinical information and radiologic imaging. CT is typically used as the first imaging modality in these cases. The sensitivity and specificity of CT for detection of an underlying renal mass in these patients are 57% and 82%, respectively.[326] The sensitivity and specificity of ultrasound is much lower.[326] MR imaging is generally reserved for those patients with stable hemodynamic conditions and inconclusive CT findings.

In a meta-analysis of 154 cases with spontaneous retroperitoneal hemorrhage (Wunderlich's syndrome), the majority (101 patients) were secondary to renal neoplasms; AML and RCC accounted for 48% and 43% of the cases, respectively.[326] Hemorrhage secondary to metastasis, sarcomas, oncocytomas, and adenomas have also been reported.[326,327] Before cross-sectional imaging studies were widely available, up to 50% of patients with an unknown cause for renal bleeding were associated with a small renal neoplasm.[328] Nowadays, cross-sectional studies allow for detection of small renal masses even in the presence of large perirenal hematomas.

Vascular diseases are the second most common condition leading to spontaneous perirenal hemorrhage and include 17% of these cases, with polyarteritis nodosa the most common disease in this group.[326] Renal artery aneurysm and arteriovenous malformation are relatively uncommon causes.[326]

Rarer etiologies of Wunderlich's syndrome include portal hypertension, Wegener's granulomatosis, infarction, severe pyelonephritis (including the xanthogranulomatous variant), cyst rupture, nephrosclerosis and pre-eclampsia.[326] The underlying cause is not identified in approximately 7% of patients.

MR findings in retroperitoneal hematomas depend upon the age of hemorrhage.[36] For T1-weighted images, sequences with strong T1 weighting are suggested. Hematomas in the acute stage can be hypointense on T1-and T2-weighted images relative to the muscle.[329] MR imaging is particularly helpful in detecting underlying renal masses. Subtraction techniques allow for suppression of the signal from the hyperintense perirenal hematoma and recognition of small enhancing renal masses. Identification of a renal mass with bulk fat is virtually diagnostic of AML. This may be challenging in the presence of extensive hemorrhage and, therefore, lack of identification of fat does not exclude the presence of an underlying AML. Arterial visceral microaneurysms are characteristic of polyarteritis nodosa. Unfortunately, these pseudoaneurysms are unlikely to be seen on MR imaging due to their small size. Patients with retroperitoneal hemorrhage secondary to bleeding renal arteriovenous fistulas may demonstrate perinephric hemorrhage associated with a discrete focal intraparenchymal hematoma.[330] Multiple cortical perfusion defects can be seen in patients with vasculitis on contrast-enhanced MR imaging (Fig. 86-48).

The role of MR imaging in the evaluation of renal trauma is limited. CT offers a rapid and readily available assessment.[331] Similar to contrast-enhanced CT examinations, gadolinium-enhanced MR can demonstrate active urine extravasation into a perinephric urinoma.[332] A more accurate differentiation between intra- and perirenal hematoma has been reported with MR compared to CT.[36] MR may be helpful in the determination of the age of the hematoma based on differences in signal intensity.[36] MR imaging may detect nonviable fragments of renal parenchyma in patients with severe lacerations.[36] MR offers excellent visualization of the collecting system in patients with renal lacerations (Fig. 86-49).

VASCULAR PATHOLOGY

Occlusion or injury to the main renal arteries or its segmental branches results in ischemia and renal infarction.[333] Patients typically present with acute flank pain. In an experimental model it was shown that renal infarcts can demonstrate a variety of signal intensities on T1- and T2-weighted images depending on the time between the onset of the vascular insult and the MR examination.[334] Acute infarcts (<6 hours) had lower signal intensity than the surrounding kidney in the acute stage on both T1- and T2-weighted images. With time, infarcts become hyperintense on T1-weighted images due to interstitial hemorrhage (24 hours) and hyperintense on both T1- and T2-weighted images (3 days) due to coagulative necrosis.[334] After 2 to 4 weeks organizing fibrosis in the infarcted area accounts for the lower signal intensity on both T1- and T2-weighted images.[334] Gadolinium-enhanced MR angiography is useful for visualization of renal artery pathologies as a cause for the ischemic renal insult.

Cholesterol embolism is a potentially fatal complication of endovascular procedures.[335] Patients can present with acute renal failure, eosinophilia, and signs of peripheral ischemia. MR imaging may reveal bilateral renal infarcts and severe atheromatous plaque formation in the abdominal aorta. A diffuse heterogeneous enhancing pattern may be noted on post-contrast MR images.

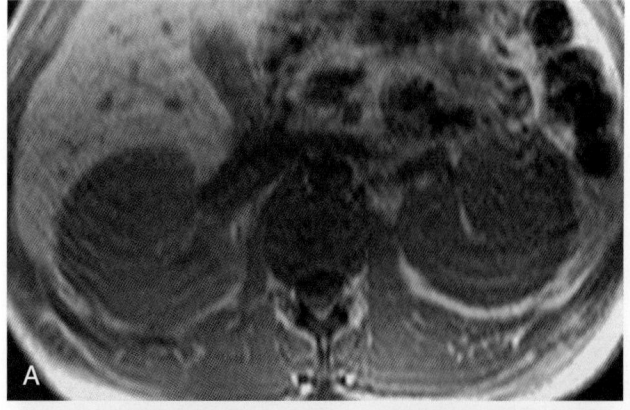

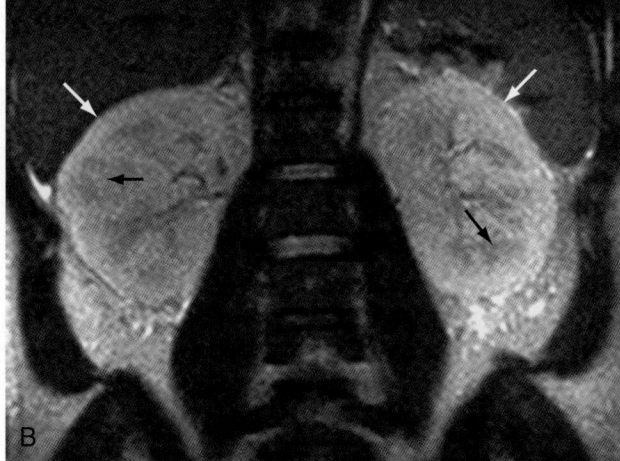

FIGURE 86-50

Acute renal failure from ethylene glycol intoxication. **A,** Noncontrast, axial T1-weighted in-phase image shows bilateral enlargement of both kidneys with loss of corticomedullary differentiation. **B,** Coronal T2-weighted half-Fourier turbo spin-echo (HASTE) image shows enlarged kidneys with reversal of the usual T2-weighted corticomedullary features due to diffuse increased signal of the renal cortex (*white arrows*) compared to the medulla (*black arrows*).

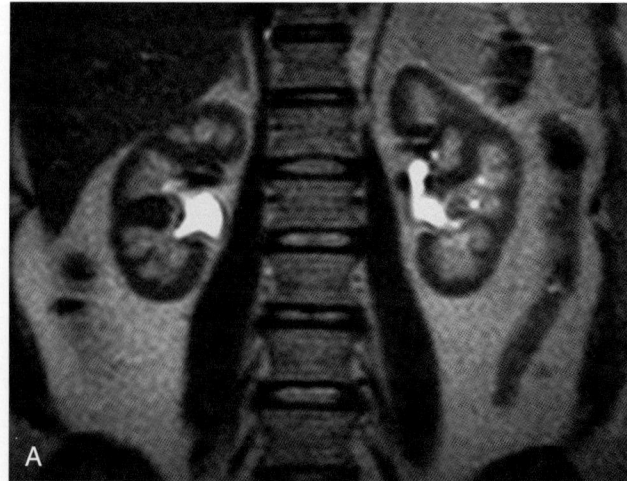

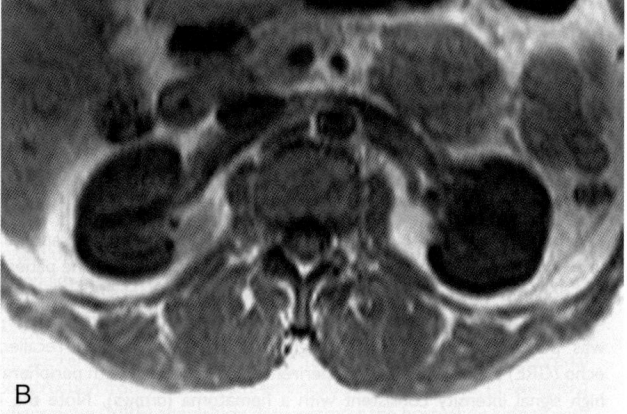

FIGURE 86-51

Iron deposition. **A,** Coronal T2-weighted single-shot fast spin-echo (SSFSE) image shows diffuse bilateral decreased signal intensity of the renal cortex. **B,** Axial T1-weighted in-phase gradient-recalled echo image demonstrates marked bilateral and diffuse decrease in signal intensity of the renal cortex due to iron deposition.

thrombosis and hemosiderin deposition in the renal cortex are characteristics of this condition.

MR imaging is the best imaging technique to demonstrate hemosiderin deposition in the renal cortex.[341] Low signal intensity on T1- and T2-weighted images is noted in the renal cortex.[341] T2-weighted images make this finding more conspicuous because the adjacent medulla (not affected by PNH) is typically hyperintense.[82,341] Dual-echo T1-weighted gradient-echo images obtained in and out of phase in a single acquisition can confirm the presence of hemosiderin in the renal cortex. Drop of signal in the renal cortex on the in-phase (with a longer echo time) compared to the out-of-phase (with a shorter echo time) images is caused by dephasing of the protons secondary to magnetic susceptibility caused by the hemosiderin. Patients with PNH have no evidence of hemosiderin deposition in the liver or spleen except those who have received multiple transfusions.[82,342]

Hemosiderin deposition in the renal cortex may occur in patients with malfunctioning prosthetic cardiac valve replacement. MR findings are identical to those of the PNH with very low signal intensity in the renal cortex on T2-weighted images compared to that of the renal medulla (Fig. 86-51).[82]

Sickle cell disease is a hereditary disorder commonly seen among African Americans.[82] Patients with mild forms of this disease undergo extravascular hemolysis in the reticuloendothelial system and, therefore, do not show iron deposition in the kidney.[82] However, acute hemolytic crises characteristic of this disease are responsible for one third of the hemolysis in these patients and it is an intravascular process.[82] These patients typically show low signal intensity in the renal cortex on T2-weighted images due to hemosiderin deposition.[82] Low signal intensity in the spleen on T2-weighted images is secondary to extravascular hemolysis and may help to distinguish this condition.[82]

Infection

Hemorrhagic fever with renal syndrome or Korean hemorrhagic fever is an acute infectious process caused by the genus Hantavirus. The disease is transmitted by rodents and is characterized by fever, visceral hemorrhage, and variable degrees of renal failure.[82] Low signal intensity along the medulla, either the outer portion or the entire medulla, is noted on T1-weighted images and is more pronounced on T2-weighted images.[82] This causes a reverse pattern of CMD on T2-weighted images with a bright cortex and dark medulla.[82] A well-defined zone of low signal intensity in the outer medulla, possibly representing medullary hemorrhage, is fairly constant and characteristic on MR images of the kidneys in patients with this condition.[343]

Vascular Diseases

Renal vein thrombosis can cause decreased signal intensity in the renal cortex and the outer part of the medulla, while the inner portion is relatively preserved (see "Vascular Pathology").

Renal cortical necrosis is an uncommon form of renal failure that is commonly associated with acute hypovolemic status caused by a variety of conditions, including abruption placentae, severe traumatic and septic shock, transfusion reaction, severe dehydration, venum toxin, and hemolytic uremic syndrome. MR imaging shows low signal intensity in the inner renal cortex and the columns of Bertin on T1- and T2-weighted images.[82] Marked CMD on T2-weighted images instead of T1-weighted images and increased signal intensity in the cortex can also be seen.[82] A thin rim of enhancing subcapsular tissue can be seen surrounding the renal necrotic cortex and it is supplied by capsular collaterals.[82]

Renal infarction may result in areas of low signal intensity on both T1- and T2-weighted images, though the signal intensity varies with time and with the presence of hemorrhage (see "Vascular Pathology").

Acute nonmyoglobinuric renal failure occurs in young healthy individuals after strenuous exercise.[82] A history of taking analgesics prior to exercise is common. MR imaging shows patchy areas of high signal intensity on T1-weighted images with loss of the CMD and variable signal intensity on T2-weighted images.[344]

URETEROPELVIC JUNCTION OBSTRUCTION AND CROSSING VESSELS

Ureteropelvic junction (UPJ) obstruction may be secondary to intrinsic or extrinsic causes. Intrinsic pelviureteral abnormalities seem to be the cause of most cases of UPJ obstruction in the pediatric population.[345] Extrinsic UPJ obstruction may be attributed to fixed kinks or angulations, bands of tissue, and high insertions of the ureter on the renal pelvis.[345] Infection, stones, surgery, ischemia, and iatrogenic injury are reported causes of secondary UPJ obstruction.[345]

It is unclear if the presence of crossing vessels at the location of the UPJ obstruction has functional significance and direct implications for the etiology of the obstruction. It has been postulated that crossing vessels more commonly aggravate rather than cause the obstruction at the UPJ.[346,347] While up to 70% of patients without UPJ obstruction are found to have incidental vessels, approximately 44% of those with UPJ obstruction have crossing vessels at the level of the obstruction.[347] A distinction should be made between crossing vessels that appear to be incidental and those that appear to cause obstruction.[348] Many of the vessels seen during angiography in a close relation to the UPJ are described as anomalous and reported as the cause of the UPJ obstruction. However, many of these vessels represent normal segmental arteries that do not cause UPJ obstruction.[349] Cross-sectional imaging is superior to conventional angiography in the demonstration of the relationship between these vessels and the UPJ. CT has been used to delineate the anatomy in these cases with excellent results.[345] MR imaging offers a comprehensive evaluation of these patients. A combined protocol using MR angiography and MR urography allows for accurate identification of crossing vessels and their relationship with the UPJ without the need for iodinated contrast media or radiation exposure (Fig. 86-52).

Intermittent hydronephrosis has been described as a unique feature of UPJ obstruction caused by a crossing lower-pole renal vessel in children.[350] While patients imaged during episodes of pain may demonstrate marked obstruction at the UPJ, excretory urograms between episodes of pain show no evidence of obstruction.[350]

There is an ongoing debate about the best surgical approach for patients with UPJ obstruction, including open pyeloplasty, endopyelotomy, and laparoscopic pyeloplasty.[351] While Gupta and Smith[348] reported that the presence of a crossing vessel is potentially the cause of endopyelotomy failure in less than 4% of patients undergoing this procedure, most urologists consider the presence of a crossing vessel on preoperative imaging to be an important factor in the choice of surgical procedure.[351] Crossing vessels have a statistically significant negative effect on the outcome of endoureteropyelotomy, reducing the success rate from 82% to 33%.[346] If a crossing vessel is at the level of UPJ obstruction, endopyelotomy without transfer of the crossing vessel and vasculopexy is often unsuccessful.[345,352] Furthermore, iatrogenic complications, including retroperitoneal hemorrhage, hematuria, arteriovenous fistula, and pseudoaneurysm, may result from inadvertent injury of the crossing vessel during surgical UPJ repair.[345,353] For these reasons, accurate preoperative delineation of the relationship between the crossing vessel and the UPJ is mandatory.

RENAL TRANSPLANT

Technical Considerations

Ultrasound is usually the first imaging modality in the evaluation of the renal transplant. MR imaging has been shown to be very useful in cases with suspected arterial

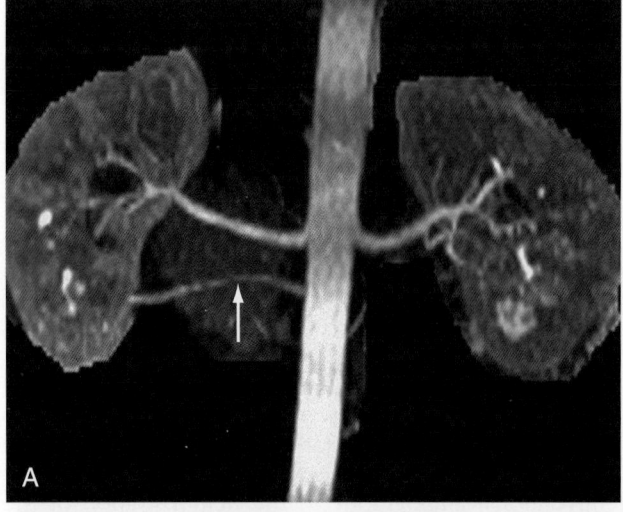
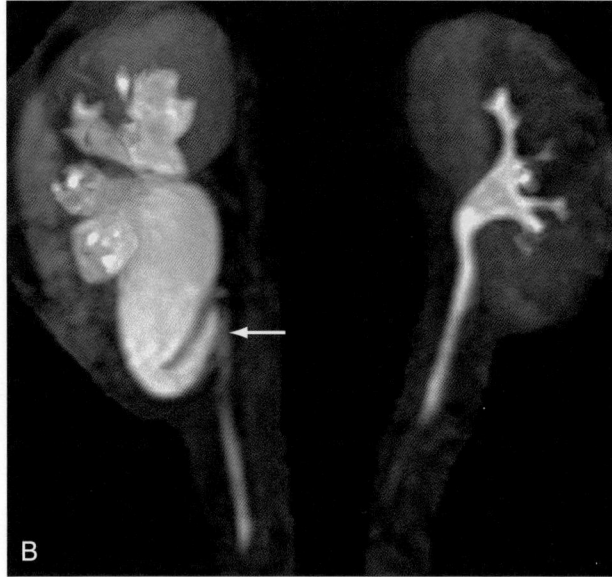
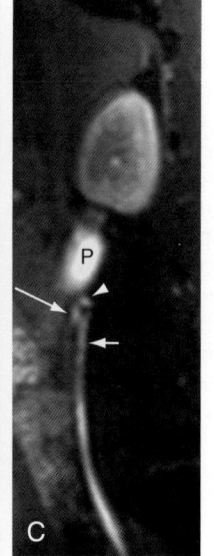

FIGURE 86-52

Ureteropelvic junction obstruction associated with a crossing vessel. **A,** Coronal maximum intensity projection (MIP) reconstruction from a gadolinium-enhanced 3D fat-saturated T1-weighted gradient-recalled echo (GRE) acquisition during the arterial phase shows an accessory renal artery to the inferior pole of the right kidney (*arrow*). **B,** Coronal MIP reconstruction from a coronal gadolinium-enhanced 3D fat-saturated T1-weighted GRE acquisition during the excretory phase after administration of 10 mL furosemide shows marked dilatation of the right collecting system. Note the tortuosity of the proximal ureter and the abrupt change in its caliber with normal appearance after the second turn (*arrow*). **C,** Sagittal reconstruction from the same acquisition as in **B** at the level of the change in caliber of the ureter demonstrates the ureter draped over the accessory artery (*arrowhead*). The artery is seen crossing posterior to the proximal ureter (*long arrow*) and anterior to the distal ureter (*short arrow*). P, renal pelvis. A crossing renal artery was confirmed at surgery.

pathology or unclear diagnosis on ultrasound. From a renal safety perspective, the lack of nephrotoxicity seen with the currently available gadolinium contrast media makes MR imaging a very useful and attractive alternative for evaluating renal transplant patients.[29-31]

The superficial location of the transplanted kidney in the right or left iliac fossa is in close proximity to local phased-array coils and allows for excellent signal-to-noise images. Transplanted kidneys are also less vulnerable to respiratory motion compared with native kidneys. However, we still recommend performing these examinations with suspended respiration whenever possible.

HASTE T2-weighted acquisitions provide a rapid assessment of the anatomy of the renal transplant, the presence of hydronephrosis, and the existence of perirenal collections.

Axial T1-weighted in- and opposed-phase images can be used to distinguish susceptibility artifacts from surgical clips. The longer echo time of the in-phase images compared with that of the opposed-phased images is sensitive to magnetic susceptibility effects caused by surgical clips. A blooming of dark signal is typically seen on the in-phase compared to the opposed-phase images. Recognition of this phenomenom may avoid false-positive diagnosis of vascular stenosis caused by susceptibility artifact. This phenomenom can also be exploited to identify calculi or hemosiderin.

A dynamic MR examination performed with a 3D fat-saturated gradient-echo T1-weighted sequence provides information about the functional status of the renal transplant, and renal and perirenal complications. In addition, these acquisitions can be post-processed to obtain meaningful diagnostic angiographic images of the transplant vasculature, including both arteries and veins.[354,355] A bolus of a single dose of gadolinium (0.1 mmol/kg bodyweight) is given at 2 mL/second in a similar fashion to the MR examinations of the native kidneys. Maximum intensity projections and volume rendering reconstructions are routinely generated using the dynamic acquisitions during the corticomedullary and nephrographic phases.

MR Evaluation of the Renal Transplant

Vascular Complications

Arterial Complications

Renal artery stenosis is reported in approximately 1% to 23% of cases.[356] Atherosclerosis in the donor or recipient arteries, surgical trauma to the vessels, improper or inadequate suture technique, and immunologic causes account for most of these cases.[356,357] Rare cases of fibromuscular dysplasia in a donor transplant renal artery have been reported.[355] Clinically, an arterial complication is suspected any time after transplantation when an abrupt onset of hypertension or unexplained impairment of the renal function is detected.[357]

The location of the stenosis may vary depending of the cause.[358] Technical errors during the surgical procedure are the most common cause of arterial stenosis.[358] These usually occur at the anastomosis, especially an end-to-end anastomosis.[358] Arterial injury caused by the surgical clamp can occur distal to the anastomosis or even at the level of the iliac artery.[359]

Arterial kinking may occur in cases where the transplant donor artery is excessively long.[357] This may result in turbulent flow and decreased perfusion to the renal transplant.[357] In this situation revision is usually necessary.[355]

MR imaging is an excellent modality for screening of arterial inflow stenosis in patients with renal transplant.[354] Normal MR angiography examinations can help avoid unnecessary catheter angiography examinations.[354,355] Patients with abnormal MR findings can be directed to catheter angiography and angioplasty.[355]

Pseudoaneurysms of the transplant renal artery and native iliac artery can be secondary to fungal infection.[360,361] Saccular, irregular dilatation of the affected vessel is usually obvious on MR angiographic images (Fig. 86-53). Hyperintense fluid collections adjacent to the vessel may be seen on T1-weighted images and represent hematomas secondary to rupture of the aneurysm.

Renal transplant arteriovenous fistulas occur most commonly after percutaneous renal biopsies.[362] These can be accurately diagnosed on Doppler US examination.[363] Gadolinium-enhanced MR imaging can show abnormally enlarged vessels in the renal parenchyma that suggest the diagnosis.

Venous Complications

Ultrasound is routinely used for the assessment of flow in the renal vein of the kidney transplant. Lack of venous Doppler signals in the whole kidney is highly suggestive of renal transplant vein thrombosis.[363] MR imaging can be used in cases with unclear ultrasound findings. In addition, MR can help evaluate the extent of the venous thrombosis when present. Coronal gadolinium-enhanced MR images obtained during the delayed venous phase (80-90 seconds after the arterial peak) provide excellent visualization of the transplant renal vein as well as the iliac veins and IVC.

Infarcts

Renal infarcts occurring early in the postoperative period may arise from preservation damage to the renal transplant or arterial complications.[364] Infarction beyond the postoperative period may occur due to embolus, cytomegalovirus infection, and acute rejection.[364] On precontrast images, renal infarction is usually seen as an ill-defined area of signal abnormality. Wedge-shaped areas of decreased parenchymal enhancement are usually more evident in the nephrographic phase of the dynamic MR examination. MR imaging is superior to Doppler ultrasound in the detection of small infarcts.[363] In addition, MR imaging provides accurate visualization of the arterial supply to the renal transplant that may help to identify the cause of the renal infarct.

Obstruction

Ureteric obstruction is a relatively common complication after kidney transplantation, occurring in 2% to 10% of cases 1 year and in up to 9% 5 years post transplantation.[365,366] Ureteral obstruction may lead to organ loss or even death.[365] The most important causes are technical factors during the surgical procedure and ureteral fibrosis secondary to ischemia.[365]

MR has excellent sensitivity for detection of hydronephrosis in the renal transplant, though this diagnosis is typically made with ultrasound.[367] A potential limitation of MR is detection of ureteral stones and misinterpretation of these as ureteral stenosis.[367] Heavily T2-weighted images provide accurate visualization of the collecting system.[368] Maximum intensity projection reconstructions help to visualize the entire collecting system in a single image.[368] A thick-slab T2-weighted RARE acquisition may offer similar images in a single breath-hold. Gadolinium-enhanced MR urography can also delineate the collecting system and offers additional functional information on the transplanted kidney.

Rejection

Acute rejection remains a serious complication affecting renal transplants despite improved protocols for immunosuppression. Furthermore, acute rejection is a major risk factor for chronic rejection, which is currently the most common cause of late graft loss.[369] Early recognition of this condition is crucial to limit the extent and severity of graft damage.[369] Patients with acute allograft rejection may present with graft tenderness, fever, oliguria, proteinuria, lymphocyturia, and deteriorating graft function.[369] However, the diagnosis may be difficult due to the use of newer and more potent immunosuppressive agents that make its clinical course more insidious.[369] Lack of clinical symptoms does not exclude rejection.[369]

Noninvasive diagnostic techniques play an important role in providing early evidence of an ongoing acute rejection and in ruling out other causes of graft dysfunction.[369] Ultrasound is commonly used as the primary imaging modality in the evaluation of patients with suspected allograft rejection. Reported sonographic

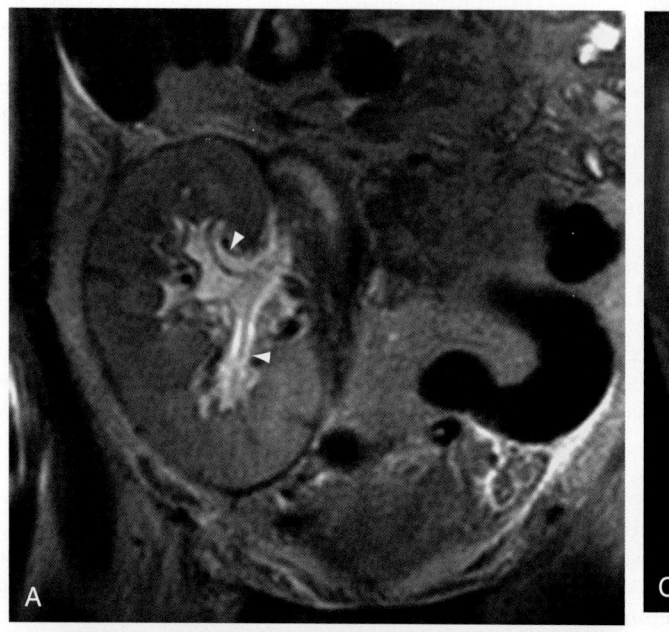

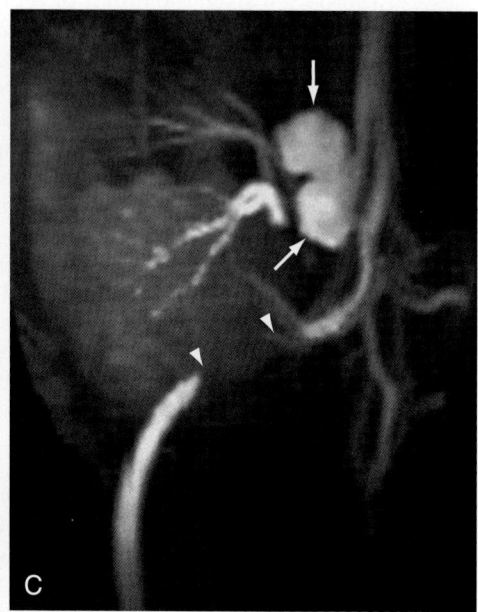

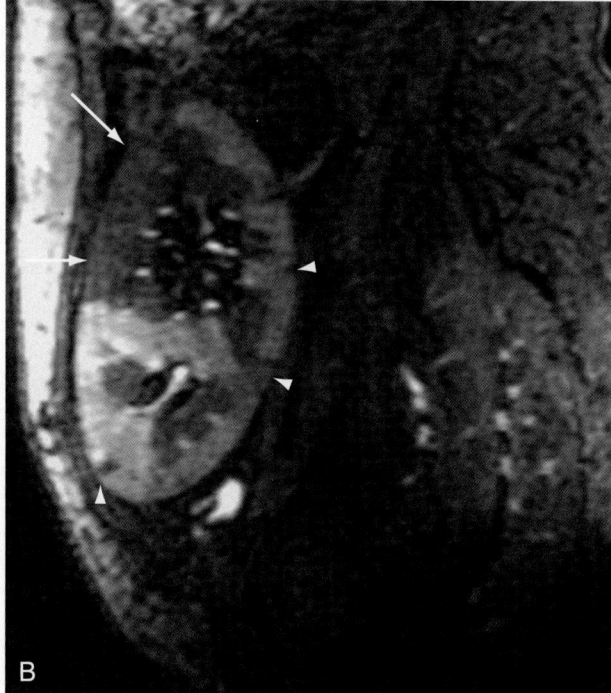

FIGURE 86-53

Candidiasis and infective vasculitis in a transplanted kidney. **A,** Coronal T2-weighted half-Fourier turbo spin-echo (HASTE) image demonstrates thickening and high signal intensity along the wall of the collecting system consistent with diffuse urothelial edema. **B,** Sagittal gadolinium-enhanced 3D fat-saturated T1-weighted gradient-echo image during the cortico-medullary phase demonstrates upper pole renal infarct (*arrows*). Multiple smaller areas of hypoperfusion are also noted throughout the allograft (*arrowheads*) and likely represent infarcts as well. **C,** Maximum intensity projection of the same acquisition as in **B** shows a complex pseudoaneurysm of the renal artery (*arrows*). There is segmental thrombosis of the external iliac artery distal to the anastomosis (*arrowheads*). Surgical excision of the transplant confirmed the findings. At pathology, diffuse parenchymal candidiasis was present as well as infectious arteritis with necrosis in the transplanted renal and external iliac arteries.

findings in these cases include decreased renal sinus area, thickening of the collecting system, prominence of the pyramids, increased graft size, and elevation of Doppler impedance indexes, such as pulsatility or resistive index. However, these findings have been shown not to be specific for acute rejection.[370,371]

A preserved CMD is typically seen in normally functioning renal transplants on T1-weighted images.[372] Decreased or absent CMD on T1-weighted images secondary to decreased signal intensity of the renal cortex can be found in the majority of patients with acute allograft rejection.[372] However, this finding is not specific and can also be seen in allograft infection, cyclosporin nephrotoxicity, and infiltrative or diffuse parenchymal diseases.[372,373] Severe urothelial thickening in the collecting system can occur with transplant rejection, but this finding can also be seen with urinary infection, reflux, or chronic obstruction.[371] High signal intensity within the thickened urothelium, similar to that for fluid on T2-weighted images, is consistent with edema and likely suggests an acute condition affecting the renal transplant. Normal functioning allografts demonstrate a rapid increase and slow decay in signal intensity in the cortex on dynamic gadolinium-enhanced MR imaging; the signal intensity of the normal medulla typically shows a slow rise and equals that of the renal cortex on a delayed venous phase image.[374] A blunted uprise and delayed peak in the cortical signal intensity curves and decreased enhancement in the medulla can be seen in patients with acute rejection.[374] The reported sensitivity of MR imaging for the diagnosis of transplant rejection is 97% versus 80% and 70% for quantitative scintigraphy and ultrasonography, respectively, but MR suffers from limited specificity.[375]

Infection

The prevalence of infections in transplant recipients usually varies from country to country.[376] There are three time frames during which infections of specific types most frequently occur in patients after kidney transplantation: the first month; the second through the sixth month; and the late post-transplant period (beyond the sixth month).[377] During the first month after kidney transplant most infections relate to surgical complications, including bacterial and candidal wound infections, pneumonia, urinary tract infection, and line sepsis. Between the second and the sixth month after kidney transplant, opportunistic infections such as cytomegalovirus, *Pneumocystis carinii,* aspergillus, nocardia, *Toxoplasma gondii,* and *Listeria monocytogenes* develop. After 6 months, most infections are similar to those seen in the general community.[377]

Ultrasound is the modality of choice in the diagnosis of perirenal fluid collections. Occasionally, other cross-sectional imaging modalities, including CT and MR, allow better evaluation of the extension of peritransplant abscesses. MR findings in transplant infection are nonspecific. A heterogeneous nephrogram can be seen on contrast-enhanced MR images and suggests pyelonephritis. Urothelial edema may also be present.

Fluid Collections

Peritransplant fluid collections are usually lymphoceles, hematomas, urinomas, or abscesses. Pelvic lymphoceles occur in up to 18% of patients undergoing renal transplantation.[362] Large collections can cause a mass effect upon the renal parenchyma, collecting system, and vascular supply causing impairment of renal function.[355] These are frequently well visualized on T2-weighted HASTE images due to their high signal intensity. Perirenal abscesses and hematomas demonstrate high signal intensity on T1-weighted images and can be differentiated from the hypointense lymphoceles, urinomas, and post-surgical seromas.[372]

Neoplasms and Renal Transplant

There is a 100-fold increase in the prevalence of cancer in immunosuppressed transplant recipients compared with the age-matched general population, with non-Hodgkin's lymphoma and squamous cell carcinoma of the skin and lips being the most common types of cancer.[378] Patients with known malignant diseases prior to transplantation are prone to develop another malignant tumor and/or progression of existing tumors.[379]

Post-transplantation lymphoproliferative disorder (PTLD) is a lymphoma-like lymphoid proliferation that is associated with Epstein-Barr virus infection.[380] The incidence of PTLD is approximately 2% of all solid-organ transplant recipients.[378] Immunosuppression related to cyclosporin is the main causative factor of PTLD.[381] Regression of PTLD with reduction or cessation of cyclosporin therapy has been reported and PTLD may not respond to conventional antilymphoma chemotherapy.[381] PTLD affects most commonly the brain, lymph nodes, gastrointestinal tract, and lungs.[380] The renal allograft is a relatively uncommon location of involvement by PTLD.[380]

There is a predilection of PTLD to affect the hilum of the renal transplant.[380] MR imaging findings are relatively constant with the presence of a hilar mass that demonstrates low signal intensity on T1- and T2-weighted images.[380] Minimal enhancement is noted after administration of gadolinium and typically, hilar vessels are seen traversing the mass.[380] Nodal involvement in PTLD is readily apparent on MR imaging. Rarely, more than one primary neoplasm may coexist in the same patient, including PTLD.

Renal carcinomas represent 4.6% of post-transplant cancers compared with 3% of tumors in the general population.[382] In the majority of the patients the native diseased kidneys are involved, though tumors arising in the allograft are not infrequent.[382] MR imaging is an excellent technique for the evaluation of masses arising in the kidney transplant. Detection of enhancement on contrast-enhanced MR imaging is virtually diagnostic of renal cancer in a newly detected enhancing mass in the renal transplant. MR imaging can also be useful in the monitoring of patients after nephron-sparing surgery or radiofrequency ablation treatment of these lesions (Fig. 86-54).

82. Jeong JY, Kim SH, Lee HJ, Sim JS: Atypical low-signal-intensity renal parenchyma: causes and patterns. Radiographics 22:833-846, 2002.
83. Lesavre A, Correas JM, Merran S, et al: CT of papillary renal cell carcinomas with cholesterol necrosis mimicking angiomyolipomas. Am J Roentgenol 181:143-145, 2003.
84. Rumpelt HJ, Storkel S, Moll R, et al: Bellini duct carcinoma: further evidence for this rare variant of renal cell carcinoma. Histopathology 18:115-122, 1991.
85. Peyromaure M, Thiounn N, Scotte F, et al: Collecting duct carcinoma of the kidney: a clinicopathological study of 9 cases. J Urol 170(4 Pt 1):1138-1140, 2003.
86. Pickhardt PJ, Lonergan GJ, Davis CJ, Jr, et al: From the archives of the AFIP. Infiltrative renal lesions: radiologic-pathologic correlation. Armed Forces Institute of Pathology. Radiographics 20:215-243, 2000.
87. Pickhardt PJ, Siegel CL, McLarney JK: Collecting duct carcinoma of the kidney: are imaging findings suggestive of the diagnosis? Am J Roentgenol 176:627-633, 2001.
88. Nassir A, Jollimore J, Gupta R, et al: Multilocular cystic renal cell carcinoma: a series of 12 cases and review of the literature. Urology 60:421-427, 2002.
89. Koga S, Nishikido M, Hayashi T, et al: Outcome of surgery in cystic renal cell carcinoma. Urology 56:67-70, 2000.
90. Tosaka A, Yoshida K, Kobayashi N, et al: [A report of two cases of multilocular cystic renal cell carcinoma: review of 51 cases reported and the results of a prognostic survey]. Hinyokika Kiyo 38:1045-1050, 1992.
91. Murad T, Komaiko W, Oyasu R, Bauer K: Multilocular cystic renal cell carcinoma. Am J Clin Pathol 95:633-637, 1991.
92. Corica FA, Iczkowski KA, Cheng L, et al: Cystic renal cell carcinoma is cured by resection: a study of 24 cases with long-term followup. J Urol 161:408-411, 1999.
93. Eble JN, Bonsib SM: Extensively cystic renal neoplasms: cystic nephroma, cystic partially differentiated nephroblastoma, multilocular cystic renal cell carcinoma, and cystic hamartoma of renal pelvis. Semin Diagn Pathol 15:2-20, 1998.
94. Yamazaki Y, Toma H, Nakazawa H, et al: [Evaluation of complicated renal cyst: a comparison of CT and MR imaging]. Hinyokika Kiyo 38:635-640, 1992.
95. Yamashita Y, Miyazaki T, Ishii A, et al: Multilocular cystic renal carcinoma presenting as a solid mass: radiologic evaluation. Abdom Imaging 20:164-168, 1995.
96. Guinan P, Vogelzang NJ, Randazzo R, et al: Renal pelvic cancer: a review of 611 patients treated in Illinois 1975-1985. Cancer Incidence and End Results Committee. Urology 40:393-399, 1992.
97. Park S, Hong B, Kim CS, Ahn H: The impact of tumor location on prognosis of transitional cell carcinoma of the upper urinary tract. J Urol 171:621-625, 2004.
98. Kang CH, Yu TJ, Hsieh HH, et al: The development of bladder tumors and contralateral upper urinary tract tumors after primary transitional cell carcinoma of the upper urinary tract. Cancer 98:1620-1626, 2003.
99. Hall MC, Womack S, Sagalowsky AI, et al: Prognostic factors, recurrence, and survival in transitional cell carcinoma of the upper urinary tract: a 30-year experience in 252 patients. Urology 52:594-601, 1998.
100. Oba K, Suga A, Shimizu Y, et al: Transitional cell carcinoma of the renal pelvis with vena caval tumor thrombus. Int J Urol 4:307-310, 1997.
101. Bergman HFR, Sayegh V: New roentgenologic signs of carcinoma of the ureter. Am J Roentgenol 86:707-717, 1961.
102. Daniels RE, 3rd: The goblet sign. Radiology 210:737-738, 1999.
103. Richmond J, Sherman RS, Diamond HD, Craver LF: Renal lesions associated with malignant lymphomas. Am J Med 32:184-207, 1962.
104. Urban BA, Fishman EK: Renal lymphoma: CT patterns with emphasis on helical CT. Radiographics 20:197-212, 2000.
105. Bailey JE, Roubidoux MA, Dunnick NR: Secondary renal neoplasms. Abdom Imaging 23:266-274, 1998.
106. Hartman DS, David CJ, Jr, Goldman SM, et al: Renal lymphoma: radiologic-pathologic correlation of 21 cases. Radiology 144:759-766, 1982.
107. Reznek RH, Mootoosamy I, Webb JA, Richards MA: CT in renal and perirenal lymphoma: a further look. Clin Radiol 42:233-238, 1990.
108. Heiken JP, Gold RP, Schnur MJ, et al: Computed tomography of renal lymphoma with ultrasound correlation. J Comput Assist Tomogr 7:245-250, 1983.
109. Jafri SZ, Bree RL, Amendola MA, et al: CT of renal and perirenal non-Hodgkin lymphoma. Am J Roentgenol 138:1101-1105, 1982.
110. Cohan RH, Dunnick NR, Leder RA, Baker ME: Computed tomography of renal lymphoma. J Comput Assist Tomogr 14:933-938, 1990.
111. Imai Y, Sone S, Serizawa S, et al: [Magnetic resonance imaging of renal lymphoma with computed tomography correlation]. Nippon Igaku Hoshasen Gakkai Zasshi 55:562-568, 1995.
112. Lee JK, Heiken JP, Ling D, et al: Magnetic resonance imaging of abdominal and pelvic lymphadenopathy. Radiology 153:181-188, 1984.
113. Semelka RC, Kelekis NL, Burdeny DA, et al: Renal lymphoma: demonstration by MR imaging. Am J Roentgenol 166:823-827, 1996.
114. Hartman DS, Davidson AJ, Davis CJ, Jr, Goldman SM: Infiltrative renal lesions: CT-sonographic-pathologic correlation. Am J Roentgenol 150:1061-1064, 1988.
115. Bechtold RE, Dyer RB, Zagoria RJ, Chen MY: The perirenal space: relationship of pathologic processes to normal retroperitoneal anatomy. Radiographics 16:841-854, 1996.
116. Sheeran SR, Sussman SK: Renal lymphoma: spectrum of CT findings and potential mimics. Am J Roentgenol 171:1067-1072, 1998.
117. Stallone G, Infante B, Manno C, et al: Primary renal lymphoma does exist: case report and review of the literature. J Nephrol 13:367-372, 2000.
118. Arranz Arija JA, Carrion JR, Garcia FR, et al: Primary renal lymphoma: report of 3 cases and review of the literature. Am J Nephrol 14:148-153, 1994.
119. Porcaro AB, D'Amico A, Novella G, et al: Primary lymphoma of the kidney. Report of a case and update of the literature. Arch Ital Urol Androl 74:44-47, 2002.
120. Lebowitz JA, Rofsky NM, Weinreb JC, Friedmann P: Ureteral lymphoma: MRI demonstration. Abdom Imaging 20:173-175, 1995.
121. Begara Morillas F, Silmi Moyano A, Hermida Gutierrez J, et al: [Lymphoproliferative pathology of the genitourinary tract. Report of 6 cases and review of the literature]. Arch Esp Urol 49:562-570, 1996.
122. Hauser M, Krestin GP, Hagspiel KD: Bilateral solid multifocal intrarenal and perirenal lesions: differentiation with ultrasonography, computed tomography and magnetic resonance imaging. Clin Radiol 50:288-294, 1995.
123. Glazer GM, Francis IR, Brady TM, Teng SS: Computed tomography of renal infarction: clinical and experimental observations. Am J Roentgenol 140:721-727, 1983.
124. Wong WS, Moss AA, Federle MP, et al: Renal infarction: CT diagnosis and correlation between CT findings and etiologies. Radiology 150:201-205, 1984.
125. Grignon DJ, Ayala AG, Ro JY, et al: Primary sarcomas of the kidney. A clinicopathologic and DNA flow cytometric study of 17 cases. Cancer 65:1611-1618, 1990.
126. Ochiai K, Onitsuka H, Honda H, et al: Leiomyosarcoma of the kidney: CT and MR appearance. J Comput Assist Tomogr 17:656-658, 1993.
127. Blacher EJ, Johnson DE, Abdul-Karim FW, Ayala AG: Squamous cell carcinoma of renal pelvis. Urology 25:124-126, 1985.
128. Lee TY, Ko SF, Wan YL, et al: Renal squamous cell carcinoma: CT findings and clinical significance. Abdom Imaging 23:203-208, 1998.
129. Narumi Y, Sato T, Hori S, et al: Squamous cell carcinoma of the uroepithelium: CT evaluation. Radiology 173:853-856, 1989.
130. Nakamura Y, Tokunaga S, Ito H, et al: [Squamous cell carcinoma of the renal pelvis associated with renal stones in a patient with chronic renal failure: a case report and a review of the Japanese literature]. Hinyokika Kiyo 42:451-455, 1996.
131. Oh SJ, Lim DJ, Cho JY, et al: Squamous cell carcinoma of the renal pelvis with invasion of the infradiaphragmatic inferior vena cava. Br J Urol 82:918-919, 1998.
132. Igel TC, Engen DE, Banks PM, Keeney GL: Renal plasmacytoma: Mayo Clinic experience and review of the literature. Urology 37:385-389, 1991.
133. Dunnick N, Sandler C, Amis E, et al (eds): Textbook of Uroradiology, 2nd ed. Baltimore, Williams & Wilkins, 1997.
134. Bennington J, Beckwith J: In Firminger HI (ed): Atlas of Tumor Pathology. Washington, DC: Armed Forces Institute of Pathology, 1975.
135. Murphy W, Beckwith J, Farrow G: Tumors of the kidney, bladder and related urinary structures. Atlas of Tumor Pathology 3rd series, fascicle 311. Washington, DC, Armed Forces Institute of Pathology, 1994.
136. Avila NA, Kelly JA, Chu SC, et al: Lymphangioleiomyomatosis: abdomino-pelvic CT and US findings. Radiology 216:147-153, 2000.
137. Neumann HP, Schwarzkopf G, Henske EP: Renal angiomyolipomas, cysts, and cancer in tuberous sclerosis complex. Semin Pediatr Neurol 5:269-275, 1998.
138. Eble JN: Angiomyolipoma of kidney. Semin Diagn Pathol 15:21-40, 1998.
139. Clark PE, Novick AC: Exophytic noninvasive growth pattern of renal angiomyolipomas: implications for nephron sparing surgery. J Urol 165:513-514, 2001.
140. Steiner MS, Goldman SM, Fishman EK, Marshall FF: The natural history of renal angiomyolipoma. J Urol 150:1782-1786, 1993.
141. Oesterling JE, Fishman EK, Goldman SM, Marshall FF: The management of renal angiomyolipoma. J Urol 135:1121-1124, 1986.
142. De Luca S, Terrone C, Rossetti SR: Management of renal angiomyolipoma: a report of 53 cases. Br J Urol Int 83:215-218, 1999.
143. Kennelly MJ, Grossman HB, Cho KJ: Outcome analysis of 42 cases of renal angiomyolipoma. J Urol 152(6 Pt 1):1988-1991, 1994.
144. Wills JS: Management of small renal neoplasms and angiomyolipoma: a growing problem. Radiology 197:583-586, 1995.
145. Robbin ML, Lockhart ME, Barr RG: Renal imaging with ultrasound contrast: current status. Radiol Clin North Am 41:963-978, 2003.
146. Forman HP, Middleton WD, Melson GL, McClennan BL: Hyperechoic renal cell carcinomas: increase in detection at US. Radiology 188:431-434, 1993.
147. Bosniak MA, Megibow AJ, Hulnick DH, et al: CT diagnosis of renal angiomyolipoma: the importance of detecting small amounts of fat. Am J Roentgenol 151:497-501, 1988.
148. Strotzer M, Lehner KB, Becker K: Detection of fat in a renal cell carcinoma mimicking angiomyolipoma. Radiology 188:427-428, 1993.
149. Uhlenbrock D, Fischer C, Beyer HK: Angiomyolipoma of the kidney. Comparison between magnetic resonance imaging, computed tomography, and ultrasonography for diagnosis. Acta Radiol 29:523-526, 1988.
150. Metro MJ, Ramchandani P, Banner MP, et al: Angiomyolipoma of the renal sinus: diagnosis by percutaneous biopsy. Urology 55:286, 2000.
151. Rubio-Briones J, Palou Redorta J, Salvador Bayarri J, et al: Incidentally detected renal angiomyolipoma with tumour thrombus into the inferior vena cava. Scand J Urol Nephrol 31:189-191, 1997.

152. Paivansalo M, Lahde S, Hyvarinen S, et al: Renal angiomyolipoma. Ultrasonographic, CT, angiographic, and histologic correlation. Acta Radiol 32:239-243, 1991.
153. Israel GM, Bosniak MA, Slywotzky CM, Rosen RJ: CT differentiation of large exophytic renal angiomyolipomas and perirenal liposarcomas. Am J Roentgenol 179:769-773, 2002.
154. Kuroda N, Toi M, Hiroi M, et al: Review of renal oncocytoma with focus on clinical and pathobiological aspects. Histol Histopathol 18:935-942, 2003.
155. Amin MB, Crotty TB, Tickoo SK, Farrow GM: Renal oncocytoma: a reappraisal of morphologic features with clinicopathologic findings in 80 cases. Am J Surg Pathol 21:1-12, 1997.
156. Monge Mirallas JM, Gutierrez Banos JL, Martin Garcia B, et al: [Renal oncocytoma: report of 14 cases and review of the literature]. Arch Esp Urol 47:564-570, 1994.
157. Licht MR, Novick AC, Tubbs RR, et al: Renal oncocytoma: clinical and biological correlates. J Urol 150(5 Pt 1):1380-1383, 1993.
158. Maatman TJ, Novick AC, Tancinco BF, et al: Renal oncocytoma: a diagnostic and therapeutic dilemma. J Urol 132:878-881, 1984.
159. Liu J, Fanning CV: Can renal oncocytomas be distinguished from renal cell carcinoma on fine-needle aspiration specimens? A study of conventional smears in conjunction with ancillary studies. Cancer 93:390-397, 2001.
160. Harmon WJ, King BF, Lieber MM: Renal oncocytoma: magnetic resonance imaging characteristics. J Urol 155:863-867, 1996.
161. Sohn HK, Kim SY, Seo HS: MR imaging of a renal oncocytoma. J Comput Assist Tomogr 11:1085-1087, 1987.
162. Ball DS, Friedman AC, Hartman DS, et al: Scar sign of renal oncocytoma: magnetic resonance imaging appearance and lack of specificity. Urol Radiol 8:46-48, 1986.
163. Defossez SM, Yoder IC, Papanicolaou N, et al: Nonspecific magnetic resonance appearance of renal oncocytomas: report of 3 cases and review of the literature. J Urol 145:552-554, 1991.
164. Honda H, Bonsib S, Barloon TJ, Masuda K: Unusual renal oncocytomas: pathologic and CT correlations. Urol Radiol 14:148-154, 1992.
165. Ambos MA, Bosniak MA, Valensi QJ, et al: Angiographic patterns in renal oncocytomas. Radiology 129:615-622, 1978.
166. Barth KH, Menon M: Renal oncocytoma. Further diagnostic observations. Diagn Imaging 49:259-265, 1980.
167. Neisius D, Braedel HU, Schindler E, et al: Computed tomographic and angiographic findings in renal oncocytoma. Br J Radiol 61:1019-1025, 1988.
168. Davidson AJ, Hayes WS, Hartman DS, et al: Renal oncocytoma and carcinoma: failure of differentiation with CT. Radiology 186:693-696, 1993.
169. Robertson PW, Klidjian A, Harding LK, et al: Hypertension due to a renin-secreting renal tumour. Am J Med 43:963-976, 1967.
170. Haab F, Duclos JM, Guyenne T, et al: Renin secreting tumors: diagnosis, conservative surgical approach and long-term results. J Urol 153:1781-1784, 1995.
171. Mete UK, Niranjan J, Kusum J, et al: Reninoma treated with nephron-sparing surgery. Urology 61:1259, 2003.
172. Henderson NL, Mason RC: Juxtaglomerular cell tumor in pregnancy. Obstet Gynecol 98(5 Pt 2):943-945, 2001.
173. Kuroda N, Moriki T, Komatsu F, et al: Adult-onset giant juxtaglomerular cell tumor of the kidney. Pathol Int 50:249-254, 2000.
174. Abbi RK, McVicar M, Teichberg S, et al: Pathologic characterization of a renin-secreting juxtaglomerular cell tumor in a child and review of the pediatric literature. Pediatr Pathol 13:443-451, 1993.
175. Hasegawa A, Iwasaki T: Rhomboid secretion granules in a juxtaglomerular cell tumour of the kidney. Br J Urol 79:296-297, 1997.
176. Agrawal R, Jafri SZ, Gibson DP, et al: Juxtaglomerular cell tumor: MR findings. J Comput Assist Tomogr 19:140-142, 1995.
177. Gelb AB, Simmons ML, Weidner N: Solitary fibrous tumor involving the renal capsule. Am J Surg Pathol 20:1288-1295, 1996.
178. Magro G, Cavallaro V, Torrisi A, et al: Intrarenal solitary fibrous tumor of the kidney. Report of a case with emphasis on the differential diagnosis in the wide spectrum of monomorphous spindle cell tumors of the kidney. Pathol Res Pract 198:37-43, 2002.
179. Wang J, Arber DA, Frankel K, Weiss LM: Large solitary fibrous tumor of the kidney: report of two cases and review of the literature. Am J Surg Pathol 25:1194-1199, 2001.
180. Fukunaga M, Naganuma H, Nikaido T, et al: Extrapleural solitary fibrous tumor: a report of seven cases. Mod Pathol 10:443-450, 1997.
181. Yazaki T, Satoh S, Iizumi T, et al: Solitary fibrous tumor of renal pelvis. Int J Urol 8:504-508, 2001.
182. England DM, Hochholzer L, McCarthy MJ: Localized benign and malignant fibrous tumors of the pleura. A clinicopathologic review of 223 cases. Am J Surg Pathol 13:640-658, 1989.
183. Tateishi U, Nishihara H, Morikawa T, Miyasaka K: Solitary fibrous tumor of the pleura: MR appearance and enhancement pattern. J Comput Assist Tomogr 26:174-179, 2002.
184. Chun HJ, Byun JY, Jung SE, et al: Benign solitary fibrous tumour of the pre-sacral space: MRI findings. Br J Radiol 71:677-679, 1998.
185. Grignon DJ, Eble JN: Papillary and metanephric adenomas of the kidney. Semin Diagn Pathol 15:41-53, 1998.
186. Renshaw AA: Subclassification of renal cell neoplasms: an update for the practising pathologist. Histopathology 41:283-300, 2002.
187. Ornstein DK, Lubensky IA, Venzon D, et al: Prevalence of microscopic tumors in normal appearing renal parenchyma of patients with hereditary papillary renal cancer. J Urol 163:431-433, 2000.
188. Bosniak MA, Birnbaum BA, Krinsky GA, Waisman J: Small renal parenchymal neoplasms: further observations on growth. Radiology 197:589-597, 1995.
189. Bosniak MA: Observation of small incidentally detected renal masses. Semin Urol Oncol 13:267-272, 1995.
190. Morgan WR, Zincke H: Progression and survival after renal-conserving surgery for renal cell carcinoma: experience in 104 patients and extended followup. J Urol 144(4):852-857; discussion 857-858, 1990.
191. Honma I, Takagi Y, Shigyo M, et al: Lymphangioma of the kidney. Int J Urol 9:178-182, 2002.
192. Nakai Y, Namba Y, Sugao H: Renal lymphangioma. J Urol 162:484-485, 1999.
193. Zapzalka DM, Krishnamurti L, Manivel JC, DiSandro MJ: Lymphangioma of the renal capsule. J Urol 168:220, 2002.
194. Hartman DS, Davis CJ, Sanders RC, et al: The multiloculated renal mass: considerations and differential features. Radiographics 7:29-52, 1987.
195. Mostofi FK, Davis CJ, Jr: Tumors and tumor-like lesions of the kidney. Curr Probl Cancer 10:53-114, 1986.
196. Davis CJ, Jr, Barton JH, Sesterhenn IA, Mostofi FK: Metanephric adenoma. Clinicopathological study of fifty patients. Am J Surg Pathol 19:1101-1114, 1995.
197. Jones EC, Pins M, Dickersin GR, Young RH: Metanephric adenoma of the kidney. A clinicopathological, immunohistochemical, flow cytometric, cytogenetic, and electron microscopic study of seven cases. Am J Surg Pathol 19:615-626, 1995.
198. Mahoney CP, Cassady C, Weinberger E, et al: Humoral hypercalcemia due to an occult renal adenoma. Pediatr Nephrol 11:339-342, 1997.
199. Renshaw AA, Freyer DR, Hammers YA: Metastatic metanephric adenoma in a child. Am J Surg Pathol 24:570-574, 2000.
200. Brown JA, Anderl KL, Borell TJ, et al: Simultaneous chromosome 7 and 17 gain and sex chromosome loss provide evidence that renal metanephric adenoma is related to papillary renal cell carcinoma. J Urol 158:370-374, 1997.
201. Nonomura A, Mizukami Y, Hasegawa T, et al: Metanephric adenoma of the kidney. Pathol Int 45:160-164, 1995.
202. Imamoto T, Furuya Y, Ueda T, Ito H: Metanephric adenoma of the kidney. Int J Urol 6:200-202, 1999.
203. Araki T, Hata H, Asakawa E: MRI of metanephric adenoma. J Comput Assist Tomogr 22:87-90, 1998.
204. Tsuji M, Murakami Y, Kanayama H, et al: A case of renal metanephric adenoma: histologic, immunohistochemical and cytogenetic analyses. Int J Urol 6:203-207, 1999.
205. Inoue K, Tsukuda S, Kayano H, et al: A case of hypervascular renal capsule leiomyoma. Radiat Med 18:323-326, 2000.
206. Radvany MG, Shanley DJ, Gagliardi JA: Magnetic resonance imaging with computed tomography of a renal leiomyoma. Abdom Imaging 19:67-69, 1994.
207. Steiner M, Quinlan D, Goldman SM, et al: Leiomyoma of the kidney: presentation of 4 new cases and the role of computerized tomography. J Urol 143:994-998, 1990.
208. Xipell JM: The incidence of benign renal nodules (a clinicopathologic study). J Urol 106:503-506, 1971.
209. Uchida K, Shibahara T, Hoshina A, et al: [A case of renal capsular leiomyoma]. Hinyokika Kiyo 45:703-705, 1999.
210. Costello J, Zinman L, Michaud J: The angiography of intrarenal leiomyoma. J Can Assoc Radiol 29:134-135, 1978.
211. Zollikofer C, Castaneda-Zuniga W, Nath HP, et al: The angiographic appearance of intrarenal leiomyoma. Radiology 136:47-49, 1980.
212. Hayasaka K, Amoh K, Hashimoto H, Yachiku S: Evaluation of renal and perirenal leiomyoma on US, CT, and angiography. Radiat Med 11:81-85, 1993.
213. Jahn H, Nissen HM: Haemangioma of the urinary tract: review of the literature. Br J Urol 68:113-117, 1991.
214. Geenen RW, Den Bakker MA, Bangma CH, et al: Sonography, CT, and MRI of giant cavernous hemangioma of the kidney: correlation with pathologic findings. Am J Roentgenol 182:411-414, 2004.
215. Fujii Y, Ajima J, Oka K, et al: Benign renal tumors detected among healthy adults by abdominal ultrasonography. Eur Urol 27:124-127, 1995.
216. Stanley RJ, Cubillo E, Mancilla Jimenez R, et al: Cavernous hemangioma of the kidney. Am J Roentgenol Radium Ther Nucl Med 125:682-687, 1975.
217. Castillo OA, Boyle ET, Jr, Kramer SA: Multilocular cysts of kidney. A study of 29 patients and review of literature. Urology 37:156-162, 1991.
218. Bilal MM, Brown JJ: MR imaging of renal and adrenal masses in children. Magn Reson Imaging Clin N Am 5:179-197, 1997.
219. Powell T, Shackman R, Johnson HD: Multilocular cysts of the kidney. Br J Urol 23:142-152, 1951.
220. Broecker B: Non-Wilms' renal tumors in children. Urol Clin North Am 27:463-469, ix, 2000.
221. Joshi VV, Beckwith JB: Multilocular cyst of the kidney (cystic nephroma) and cystic, partially differentiated nephroblastoma. Terminology and criteria for diagnosis. Cancer 64:466-479, 1989.

222. Joshi VV: Cystic partially differentiated nephroblastoma: an entity in the spectrum of infantile renal neoplasia. Perspect Pediatr Pathol 5:217-235, 1979.
223. Lowe LH, Isuani BH, Heller RM, et al: Pediatric renal masses: Wilms' tumor and beyond. Radiographics 20:1585-1603, 2000.
224. Kettritz U, Semelka RC, Siegelman ES, et al: Multilocular cystic nephroma: MR imaging appearance with current techniques, including gadolinium enhancement. J Magn Reson Imaging 6:145-148, 1996.
225. Wootton SL, Rowen SJ, Griscom NT: Pediatric case of the day. Congenital mesoblastic nephroma. Radiographics 11:719-721, 1991.
226. Kangarloo H, Dietrich RB, Ehrlich RM, et al: Magnetic resonance imaging of Wilms tumor. Urology 28:203-207, 1986.
227. Boechat MI: Magnetic resonance imaging of abdominal and pelvic masses in children. Top Magn Reson Imaging 3:25-41, 1990.
228. Fernbach SK, Feinstein KA, Donaldson JS, Baum ES: Nephroblastomatosis: comparison of CT with US and urography. Radiology 166(1 Pt 1):153-156, 1988.
229. Gylys-Morin V, Hoffer FA, Kozakewich H, Shamberger RC: Wilms tumor and nephroblastomatosis: imaging characteristics at gadolinium-enhanced MR imaging. Radiology 188:517-521, 1993.
230. Weeks DA, Beckwith JB, Mierau GW, Luckey DW: Rhabdoid tumor of kidney. A report of 111 cases from the National Wilms' Tumor Study Pathology Center. Am J Surg Pathol 13:439-458, 1989.
231. El-Galley R: Surgical management of renal tumors. Radiol Clin North Am 41:1053-1065, vii, 2003.
232. Kshirsagar AV, Choyke PL, Linehan WM, Walther MM: Pseudotumors after renal parenchymal sparing surgery. J Urol 159:1148-1151, 1998.
233. Pedrosa I, Naidich JJ, Rofsky NM, Bosniak MA: Renal pseudotumors due to fat necrosis in acute pancreatitis. J Comput Assist Tomogr 25:236-238, 2001.
234. Choyke PL: Imaging of hereditary renal cancer. Radiol Clin North Am 41:1037-1051, 2003.
235. Igarashi H, Esumi M, Ishida H, Okada K: Vascular endothelial growth factor overexpression is correlated with von Hippel-Lindau tumor suppressor gene inactivation in patients with sporadic renal cell carcinoma. Cancer 95:47-53, 2002.
236. Poston CD, Jaffe GS, Lubensky IA, et al: Characterization of the renal pathology of a familial form of renal cell carcinoma associated with von Hippel-Lindau disease: clinical and molecular genetic implications. J Urol 153:22-26, 1995.
237. Choyke PL, Glenn GM, Walther MM, et al: The natural history of renal lesions in von Hippel-Lindau disease: a serial CT study in 28 patients. Am J Roentgenol 159:1229-1234, 1992.
238. Bosniak MA: The small (less than or equal to 3.0 cm) renal parenchymal tumor: detection, diagnosis, and controversies. Radiology 179:307-317, 1991.
239. Herring JC, Enquist EG, Chernoff A, et al: Parenchymal sparing surgery in patients with hereditary renal cell carcinoma: 10-year experience. J Urol 165:777-781, 2001.
240. Lubensky IA, Schmidt L, Zhuang Z, et al: Hereditary and sporadic papillary renal carcinomas with c-met mutations share a distinct morphological phenotype. Am J Pathol 155:517-526, 1999.
241. Choyke PL, Walther MM, Glenn GM, et al: Imaging features of hereditary papillary renal cancers. J Comput Assist Tomogr 21:737-741, 1997.
242. Birt AR, Hogg GR, Dube WJ: Hereditary multiple fibrofolliculomas with trichodiscomas and acrochordons. Arch Dermatol 113:1674-1677, 1977.
243. Khoo SK, Bradley M, Wong FK, et al: Birt-Hogg-Dube syndrome: mapping of a novel hereditary neoplasia gene to chromosome 17p12-q11.2. Oncogene 20:5239-5242, 2001.
244. Nickerson ML, Warren MB, Toro JR, et al: Mutations in a novel gene lead to kidney tumors, lung wall defects, and benign tumors of the hair follicle in patients with the Birt-Hogg-Dube syndrome. Cancer Cell 2:157-164, 2002.
245. Pavlovich CP, Walther MM, Eyler RA, et al: Renal tumors in the Birt-Hogg-Dube syndrome. Am J Surg Pathol 26:1542-1552, 2002.
246. Warfel KA, Eble JN: Renal oncocytomatosis. J Urol 127:1179-1180, 1982.
247. Israeli RS, Wise GJ, Bansal S, et al: Bilateral renal oncocytomatosis in a patient with renal failure. Urology 46:873-875, 1995.
248. Farkas LM, Szekely JG, Karatson A: Bilateral, multifocal renal oncocytomatosis with rapid progression leading to renal insufficiency. Nephrol Dial Transplant 14:2262-2263, 1999.
249. Launonen V, Vierimaa O, Kiuru M, et al: Inherited susceptibility to uterine leiomyomas and renal cell cancer. Proc Natl Acad Sci USA 98:3387-3392, 2001.
250. Tomlinson IP, Alam NA, Rowan AJ, et al: Germline mutations in FH predispose to dominantly inherited uterine fibroids, skin leiomyomata and papillary renal cell cancer. Nature Genet 30:406-410, 2002.
251. Hwang JJ, Uchio EM, Linehan WM, Walther MM: Hereditary kidney cancer. Urol Clin North Am 30:831-842, 2003.
252. Weiner DM, Ewalt DH, Roach ES, Hensle TW: The tuberous sclerosis complex: a comprehensive review. J Am Coll Surg 187:548-561, 1998.
253. Lagos JC, Gomez MR: Tuberous sclerosis: reappraisal of a clinical entity. Mayo Clin Proc 42:26-49, 1967.
254. Torres VE, Zincke H, King BK, Bjornsson J: Renal manifestations of tuberous sclerosis complex. Contrib Nephrol 122:64-75, 1997.
255. Reiff DB, Dow J: Case report: invasive renal angiomyolipoma—sonographic and CT features. Clin Radiol 48:283-285, 1993.
256. Taylor RS, Joseph DB, Kohaut EC, et al: Renal angiomyolipoma associated with lymph node involvement and renal cell carcinoma in patients with tuberous sclerosis. J Urol 141:930-932, 1989.
257. Washecka R, Hanna M: Malignant renal tumors in tuberous sclerosis. Urology 37:340-343, 1991.
258. Al-Saleem T, Wessner LL, Scheithauer BW, et al: Malignant tumors of the kidney, brain, and soft tissues in children and young adults with the tuberous sclerosis complex. Cancer 83:2208-2216, 1998.
259. Jimenez RE, Eble JN, Reuter VE, et al: Concurrent angiomyolipoma and renal cell neoplasia: a study of 36 cases. Mod Pathol 14:157-163, 2001.
260. Davis CJ, Jr, Mostofi FK, Sesterhenn IA: Renal medullary carcinoma. The seventh sickle cell nephropathy. Am J Surg Pathol 19:1-11, 1995.
261. Srigley JR, Eble JN: Collecting duct carcinoma of kidney. Semin Diagn Pathol 15:54-67, 1998.
262. Lande IM, Glazer GM, Sarnaik S, et al: Sickle-cell nephropathy: MR imaging. Radiology 158:379-383, 1986.
263. Gabow PA: Autosomal dominant polycystic kidney disease—more than a renal disease. Am J Kidney Dis 16:403-413, 1990.
264. Perrone RD, Ruthazer R, Terrin NC: Survival after end-stage renal disease in autosomal dominant polycystic kidney disease: contribution of extrarenal complications to mortality. Am J Kidney Dis 38:777-784, 2001.
265. Bogdanova N, Markoff A, Horst J: Autosomal dominant polycystic kidney disease—clinical and genetic aspects. Kidney Blood Press Res 25:265-283, 2002.
266. Rizk D, Chapman AB: Cystic and inherited kidney diseases. Am J Kidney Dis 42:1305-1317, 2003.
267. Mosetti MA, Leonardou P, Motohara T, et al: Autosomal dominant polycystic kidney disease: MR imaging evaluation using current techniques. J Magn Reson Imaging 18:210-215, 2003.
268. Keith DS, Torres VE, King BF, et al: Renal cell carcinoma in autosomal dominant polycystic kidney disease. J Am Soc Nephrol 4:1661-1669, 1994.
269. King BF, Torres VE, Brummer ME, et al: Magnetic resonance measurements of renal blood flow as a marker of disease severity in autosomal-dominant polycystic kidney disease. Kidney Int 64:2214-2221, 2003.
270. Wise SW, Hartman DS, Hardesty LA, Mosher TJ: Renal medullary cystic disease: assessment by MRI. Abdom Imaging 23:649-651, 1998.
271. Neumann HP, Zauner I, Strahm B, et al: Late occurrence of cysts in autosomal dominant medullary cystic kidney disease. Nephrol Dial Transplant 12:1242-1246, 1997.
272. Sherman FE, Studnicki FM, Fetterman G: Renal lesions of familial juvenile nephronophthisis examined by microdissection. Am J Clin Pathol 55:391-400, 1971.
273. Levine E, Hartman DS, Meilstrup JW, et al: Current concepts and controversies in imaging of renal cystic diseases. Urol Clin North Am 24:523-543, 1997.
274. Levine E: Acquired cystic kidney disease. Radiol Clin North Am 34:947-964, 1996.
275. Pope JCt, Brock JW, 3rd, Adams MC, et al: How they begin and how they end: classic and new theories for the development and deterioration of congenital anomalies of the kidney and urinary tract, (CAKUT). J Am Soc Nephrol 10:2018-2028, 1999.
276. Hartman GE, Smolik LM, Shochat SJ: The dilemma of the multicystic dysplastic kidney. Am J Dis Child 140:925-928, 1986.
277. Gordon AC, Thomas DF, Arthur RJ, Irving HC: Multicystic dysplastic kidney: is nephrectomy still appropriate? J Urol 140(5 Pt 2):1231-1234, 1988.
278. al-Khaldi N, Watson AR, Zuccollo J, et al: Outcome of antenatally detected cystic dysplastic kidney disease. Arch Dis Child 70:520-522, 1994.
279. Avni EF, Thoua Y, Lalmand B, et al: Multicystic dysplastic kidney: natural history from in utero diagnosis and postnatal followup. J Urol 138:1420-1424, 1987.
280. Huppert BJ, Brandt KR, Ramin KD, King BF: Single-shot fast spin-echo MR imaging of the fetus: a pictorial essay. Radiographics 19(Spec No):S215-227, 1999.
281. Miller MA, Brown JJ: Renal cysts and cystic neoplasms. Magn Reson Imaging Clin N Am 5:49-66, 1997.
282. Cho C, Friedland GW, Swenson RS: Acquired renal cystic disease and renal neoplasms in hemodialysis patients. Urol Radiol 6:153-157, 1984.
283. Choyke PL: Acquired cystic kidney disease. Eur Radiol 10:1716-1721, 2000.
284. Hughson MD, Buchwald D, Fox M: Renal neoplasia and acquired cystic kidney disease in patients receiving long-term dialysis. Arch Pathol Lab Med 110:592-601, 1986.
285. Matson MA, Cohen EP: Acquired cystic kidney disease: occurrence, prevalence, and renal cancers. Medicine (Baltimore) 69:217-226, 1990.
286. Hoshida Y, Nakanishi H, Shin M, et al: Renal neoplasias in patients receiving dialysis and renal transplantation: clinico-pathological features and p53 gene mutations. Transplantation 68:385-390, 1999.
287. Slywotzky CM, Bosniak MA: Localized cystic disease of the kidney. Am J Roentgenol 176:843-849, 2001.
288. O'Callaghan FJ, Osborne JP: Advances in the understanding of tuberous sclerosis. Arch Dis Child 83:140-142, 2000.
289. Levine E, Collins DL, Horton WA, Schimke RN: CT screening of the abdomen in von Hippel-Lindau disease. Am J Roentgenol 139:505-510, 1982.
290. Farres MT, Ronco P, Saadoun D, et al: Chronic lithium nephropathy: MR imaging for diagnosis. Radiology 229:570-574, 2003.

291. Markowitz GS, Radhakrishnan J, Kambham N, et al: Lithium nephrotoxicity: a progressive combined glomerular and tubulointerstitial nephropathy. J Am Soc Nephrol 11:1439-1448, 2000.

292. Kaver I, Flanders EL, Kay S, Koontz WW, Jr: Segmental medullary sponge kidney mimicking a renal mass. J Urol 141:1181-1183, 1989.

293. Betts CD, O'Reilly PH: Profound haemorrhage causing acute obstruction in medullary sponge kidney. Br J Urol 70:449-450, 1992.

294. Ginalski JM, Schnyder P, Portmann L, Jaeger P: Medullary sponge kidney on axial computed tomography: comparison with excretory urography. Eur J Radiol 12:104-107, 1991.

295. Regan F, Petronis J, Bohlman M, et al: Perirenal MR high signal—a new and sensitive indicator of acute ureteric obstruction. Clin Radiol 52:445-450, 1997.

296. Roberts JA: Management of pyelonephritis and upper urinary tract infections. Urol Clin North Am 26:753-763, 1999.

297. Majd M, Nussbaum Blask AR, Markle BM, et al: Acute pyelonephritis: comparison of diagnosis with ^{99m}Tc-DMSA, SPECT, spiral CT, MR imaging, and power Doppler US in an experimental pig model. Radiology 218:101-108, 2001.

298. Lonergan GJ, Pennington DJ, Morrison JC, et al: Childhood pyelonephritis: comparison of gadolinium-enhanced MR imaging and renal cortical scintigraphy for diagnosis. Radiology 207:377-384, 1998.

299. Saunders HS, Dyer RB, Shifrin RY, et al: The CT nephrogram: implications for evaluation of urinary tract disease. Radiographics 15(5):1069-1085, discussion 1086-1068, 1995

300. Chan JH, Tsui EY, Luk SH, et al: MR diffusion-weighted imaging of kidney: differentiation between hydronephrosis and pyonephrosis. Clin Imaging 25:110-113, 2001.

301. Erden A, Fitoz S, Karagulle T, et al: Radiological findings in the diagnosis of genitourinary candidiasis. Pediatr Radiol 30:875-877, 2000.

302. Wise GJ, Goldberg P, Kozinn PJ: Genitourinary candidiasis: diagnosis and treatment. J Urol 116:778-780, 1976.

303. Bick RJ, Bryan PJ: Sonographic demonstration of thickened renal pelvic mucosa/submucosa in mixed candida infection. J Clin Ultrasound 15:333-336, 1987.

304. Ozcan H, Akyar S, Atasoy C: An unusual manifestation of xanthogranulo-matous pyelonephritis: bilateral focal solid renal masses. Am J Roentgenol 165:1552-1553, 1995.

305. Ramboer K, Oyen R, Verellen S, et al: Focal xanthogranulomatous pyelonephritis mimicking a renal tumor: CT- and MR-findings and evolution under therapy. Nephrol Dial Transplant 12:1028-1030, 1997.

306. Di Tonno F, Capizzi G, Laurini L, et al: Focal xanthogranulomatous pyelonephritis: diagnostic and therapeutic aspects. Urol Int 48:453-456, 1992.

307. Verswijvel G, Oyen R, Van Poppel H, Roskams T: Xanthogranulomatous pyelonephritis: MRI findings in the diffuse and the focal type. Eur Radiol 10:586-589, 2000.

308. Hayes WS, Hartman DS, Sesterbenn IA: From the Archives of the AFIP. Xanthogranulomatous pyelonephritis. Radiographics 11:485-498, 1991.

309. Eastham J, Ahlering T, Skinner E: Xanthogranulomatous pyelonephritis: clinical findings and surgical considerations. Urology 43:295-299, 1994.

310. Goldman SM, Hartman DS, Fishman EK, et al: CT of xanthogranulomatous pyelonephritis: radiologic-pathologic correlation. Am J Roentgenol 142:963-969, 1984.

311. Lopez-Medina A, Ereno MJ, Fernandez-Canton G, Zuazo A: Focal xantho-granulomatous pyelonephritis simulating malignancy in children. Abdom Imaging 20:270-271, 1995.

312. Parker MD, Clark RL: Evolving concepts in the diagnosis of xanthogranu-lomatous pyelonephritis. Urol Radiol 11:7-15, 1989.

313. Malek RS, Elder JS: Xanthogranulomatous pyelonephritis: a critical analysis of 26 cases and of the literature. J Urol 119:589-593, 1978.

314. Soler R, Pombo F, Gayol A, Rodriguez J: Focal xanthogranulomatous pyelonephritis in a teenager: MR and CT findings. Eur J Radiol 24:77-79, 1997.

315. Mulopulos GP, Patel SK, Pessis D: MR imaging of xanthogranulomatous pyelonephritis. J Comput Assist Tomogr 10:154-156, 1986.

316. Wise GJ, Marella VK: Genitourinary manifestations of tuberculosis. Urol Clin North Am 30:111-121, 2003.

317. Wang LJ, Wu CF, Wong YC, et al: Imaging findings of urinary tuberculosis on excretory urography and computerized tomography. J Urol 169:524-528, 2003.

318. Verswijvel G, Janssens F, Vandevenne J, et al: Renal macronodular tuberculoma: CT and MR findings in an asymptomatic patient. Journal Belge de-Belgish Tijdscrift voos: Radiologie 85:203-205, 2002.

319. Murata Y, Yamada I, Sumiya Y, et al: Abdominal macronodular tubercu-lomas: MR findings. J Comput Assist Tomogr 20:643-646, 1996.

320. Olatinwo T, Hewitt RG, Venuto RC: Human immunodeficiency virus-associated nephropathy: a primary care perspective. Arch Intern Med 164:333-336, 2004.

321. Kay CJ: Renal diseases in patients with AIDS: sonographic findings. Am J Roentgenol 159:551-554, 1992.

322. Kuhlman JE, Browne D, Shermak M, et al: Retroperitoneal and pelvic CT of patients with AIDS: primary and secondary involvement of the genitourinary tract. Radiographics 11:473-483, 1991.

323. Miller FH, Parikh S, Gore RM, et al: Renal manifestations of AIDS. Radiographics 13:587-596, 1993.

324. Rodriguez LV, Spielman D, Herfkens RJ, Shortliffe LD: Magnetic resonance imaging for the evaluation of hydronephrosis, reflux and renal scarring in children. J Urol 166:1023-1027, 2001.

325. Reiter WJ, Haitel A, Heinz-Peer G, et al: Spontaneous nontraumatic rupture of a contracted kidney with subcapsular and perirenal hematoma in a patient receiving chronic hemodialysis. Urology 50:781-783, 1997.

326. Zhang JQ, Fielding JR, Zou KH: Etiology of spontaneous perirenal hemorrhage: a meta-analysis. J Urol 167:1593-1596, 2002.

327. Albi G, del Campo L, Tagarro D: Wunderlich's syndrome: causes, diagnosis and radiological management. Clin Radiol 57:840-845, 2002.

328. Novicki DE, Turlington JT, Ball TP, Jr: The evaluation and management of spontaneous perirenal hemorrhage. J Urol 123:764-765, 1980.

329. Balci NC, Sirvanci M, Tufek I, et al: Spontaneous retroperitoneal hemorrhage secondary to subcapsular renal hematoma: MRI findings. Magn Reson Imaging 19:1145-1148, 2001.

330. Beauchamp N, Kuhlman JE: MR features of bleeding renal arteriovenous fistulae. J Comput Assist Tomogr 17:297-299, 1993.

331. Leppaniemi AK, Kivisaari AO, Haapiainen RK, Lehtonen TA: Role of magnetic resonance imaging in blunt renal parenchymal trauma. Br J Urol 68:355-360, 1991.

332. Marcos HB, Noone TC, Semelka RC: MRI evaluation of acute renal trauma. J Magn Reson Imaging 8:989-990, 1998.

333. Tillou A, Romero J, Asensio JA, et al: Renal vascular injuries. Surg Clin North Am 81:1417-1430, 2001.

334. Choo SW, Kim SH, Jeong YG, et al: MR imaging of segmental renal infarction: an experimental study. Clin Radiol 52:65-68, 1997.

335. Thadhani RI, Camargo CA, Jr, Xavier RJ, et al: Atheroembolic renal failure after invasive procedures. Natural history based on 52 histologically proven cases. Medicine (Baltimore) 74:350-358, 1995.

336. Hricak H, Crooks L, Sheldon P, Kaufman L: Nuclear magnetic resonance imaging of the kidney. Radiology 146:425-432, 1983.

337. Marotti M, Hricak H, Terrier F, et al: MR in renal disease: importance of cortical-medullary distinction. Magn Reson Med 5:160-172, 1987.

338. Semelka RC, Corrigan K, Ascher SM, et al: Renal corticomedullary differentiation: observation in patients with differing serum creatinine levels. Radiology 190:149-152, 1994.

339. Chung JJ, Semelka RC, Martin DR: Acute renal failure: common occurrence of preservation of corticomedullary differentiation on MR images. Magn Reson Imaging 19:789-793, 2001.

340. Scalley RD, Ferguson DR, Piccaro JC, et al: Treatment of ethylene glycol poisoning. Am Fam Physician 66:807-812, 2002.

341. Roubidoux MA: MR imaging of hemorrhage and iron deposition in the kidney. Radiographics 14:1033-1044, 1994.

342. Roubidoux MA: MR of the kidneys, liver, and spleen in paroxysmal nocturnal hemoglobinuria. Abdom Imaging 19:168-173, 1994.

343. Kim SH, Kim S, Lee JS, et al: Hemorrhagic fever with renal syndrome: MR imaging of the kidney. Radiology 175:823-825, 1990.

344. Kim SH, Han MC, Han JS, et al: Exercise-induced acute renal failure and patchy renal vasoconstriction: CT and MR findings. J Comput Assist Tomogr 15:985-988, 1991.

345. Mitsumori A, Yasui K, Akaki S, et al: Evaluation of crossing vessels in patients with ureteropelvic junction obstruction by means of helical CT. Radiographics 20:1383-1393, discussion 1393-1385, 2000.

346. Van Cangh PJ, Nesa S, Galeon M, et al: Vessels around the ureteropelvic junction: significance and imaging by conventional radiology. J Endourol 10:111-119, 1996.

347. Sampaio FJ, Favorito LA: Ureteropelvic junction stenosis: vascular anatomical background for endopyelotomy. J Urol 150:1787-1791, 1993.

348. Gupta M, Smith AD: Crossing vessels. Endourologic implications. Urol Clin North Am 25:289-293, 1998.

349. Sampaio FJ: The dilemma of the crossing vessel at the ureteropelvic junction: precise anatomic study. J Endourol 10:411-415, 1996.

350. Hoffer FA, Lebowitz RL: Intermittent hydronephrosis: a unique feature of ureteropelvic junction obstruction caused by a crossing renal vessel. Radiology 156:655-658, 1985.

351. Marcovich R, Jacobson AI, Aldana JP, et al: Practice trends in contemporary management of adult ureteropelvic junction obstruction. Urology 62:22-25, discussion 25-26, 2003.

352. Perlberg S, Pfau A: Management of ureteropelvic junction obstruction associated with lower polar vessels. Urology 23:13-18, 1984.

353. Badlani G, Karlin G, Smith AD: Complications of endopyelotomy: analysis in series of 64 patients. J Urol 140:473-475, 1988.

354. Ferreiros J, Mendez R, Jorquera M, et al: Using gadolinium-enhanced three-dimensional MR angiography to assess arterial inflow stenosis after kidney transplantation. Am J Roentgenol 172:757-757, 1999.

355. Hohenwalter MD, Skowlund CJ, Erickson SJ, et al: Renal transplant evaluation with MR angiography and MR imaging. Radiographics 21:1505-1517, 2001.

356. Fervenza FC, Lafayette RA, Alfrey EJ, Petersen J: Renal artery stenosis in kidney transplants. Am J Kidney Dis 31:142-148, 1998.

357. Amante AJ, Kahan BD: Technical complications of renal transplantation. Surg Clin North Am 74:1117-1131, 1994.

358. Buturovic-Ponikvar J: Renal transplant artery stenosis. Nephrol Dial Transplant 18(Suppl 5):v74-77, 2003.

359. Khankan AA, Maeda M, Osuga K, et al: Post-kidney transplantation iliac artery stenosis due to iatrogenic injury: case report. Cardiovasc Intervent Radiol 26:186-188, 2003.

360. Potti A, Danielson B, Sen K: "True" mycotic aneurysm of a renal artery allograft. Am J Kidney Dis 31:E3, 1998.

361. Garrido J, Lerma JL, Heras M, et al: Pseudoaneurysm of the iliac artery secondary to Aspergillus infection in two recipients of kidney transplants from the same donor. Am J Kidney Dis 41:488-492, 2003.

362. Hobart MG, Streem SB, Gill IS: Renal transplant complications. Minimally invasive management. Urol Clin North Am 27:787-798, 2000.

363. Helenon O, Correas JM, Thervet E, et al: [Imaging of vascular complications of renal transplantation]. J Radiol 75:61-68, 1994.

364. Cosio FG, Pesavento TE, Sedmak DD, et al: Clinical implications of the diagnosis of renal allograft infarction by percutaneous biopsy. Transplantation 66:467-471, 1998.

365. Vennarecci G, Tisone G, Pisani F, et al: [Ureteral obstruction in the kidney transplant patient]. Minerva Urol Nefrol 47:59-64, 1995.

366. Swierzewski SJ, 3rd, Konnak JW, Ellis JH: Treatment of renal transplant ureteral complications by percutaneous techniques. J Urol 149:986-987, 1993.

367. Cohnen M, Brause M, May P, et al: Contrast-enhanced MR urography in the evaluation of renal transplants with urological complications. Clin Nephrol 58:111-117, 2002.

368. Schubert RA, Gockeritz S, Mentzel HJ, et al: Imaging in ureteral complications of renal transplantation: value of static fluid MR urography. Eur Radiol 10:1152-1157, 2000.

369. Salgado O: Noninvasive acute rejection diagnosis in kidney transplantation. Transplant Proc 34:2543-2544, 2002.

370. Hollenbeck M, Hilbert N, Meusel F, Grabensee B: Increasing sensitivity and specificity of Doppler sonographic detection of renal transplant rejection with serial investigation technique. Clin Invest 72:609-615, 1994.

371. Nicolet V, Carignan L, Dubuc G, et al: Thickening of the renal collecting system: a nonspecific finding at US. Radiology 168:411-413, 1988.

372. Hricak H, Terrier F, Demas BE: Renal allografts: evaluation by MR imaging. Radiology 159:435-441, 1986.

373. Liou JT, Lee JK, Heiken JP, et al: Renal transplants: can acute rejection and acute tubular necrosis be differentiated with MR imaging? Radiology 179:61-65, 1991.

374. Sharma RK, Gupta RK, Poptani H, et al: The magnetic resonance renogram in renal transplant evaluation using dynamic contrast-enhanced MR imaging. Transplantation 59:1405-1409, 1995.

375. Hricak H, Terrier F, Marotti M, et al: Posttransplant renal rejection: comparison of quantitative scintigraphy, US, and MR imaging. Radiology 162:685-688, 1987.

376. Tsai MK, Lee PH, Hu RH, Lee CJ: Infectious complications in renal transplant recipients: a 10-year review of cyclosporine-based immunosuppression. Transplant Proc 30:3125-3126, 1998.

377. Patel R: Infections in recipients of kidney transplants. Infect Dis Clin North Am 15:901-952, xi, 2001.

378. Hoover R, Fraumeni JF, Jr: Risk of cancer in renal-transplant recipients. Lancet 2:55-57, 1993.

379. Winter P, Schoeneich G, Miersch WD, Klehr HU: Tumour induction as a consequence of immunosuppression after renal transplantation. Int Urol Nephrol 29:701-709, 1997.

380. Ali MG, Coakley FV, Hricak H, Bretan PN: Complex posttransplantation abnormalities of renal allografts: evaluation with MR imaging. Radiology 211:95-100, 1999.

381. Starzl TE, Nalesnik MA, Porter KA, et al: Reversibility of lymphomas and lymphoproliferative lesions developing under cyclosporin-steroid therapy. Lancet 1:583-587, 1984.

382. Penn I: Primary kidney tumors before and after renal transplantation. Transplantation 59:480-485, 1995.

87

ADRENAL GLANDS

Sridhar R. Charagundla ● Evan S. Siegelman

DEVELOPMENT, ANATOMY, AND APPEARANCE

Development

The adrenal gland is a retroperitoneal organ named because of its intimate anatomic association with the kidney. It is composed of a cortex and medulla, which are physiologically and embryologically distinct. The adrenal cortex arises from mesenchymal cells located near the urogenital ridge,[1] and is formed during the fifth week of gestation. The primitive fetal cortex undergoes necrosis after birth and is replaced by the permanent cortex, which subsequently differentiates into discrete histologic zones that serve a variety of endocrine functions. The adrenal medulla is derived from neural crest cells that migrate from the primitive sympathetic ganglia and penetrate the adrenal cortex during the 10th week of gestation.[2]

Anatomy

The normal weight of the adult adrenal gland is estimated to be 4 to 5 g, although this value can vary greatly depending on the physiologic state of the individual. The adrenal gland has normal dimensions of 4 to 6 cm in length, 2 to 3 cm in width, and 3 to 6 mm in thickness, again with large physiologic variation.[2] Each adrenal gland is contained within the fascia of the adjacent kidney. The arterial vasculature to the adrenal gland is derived from branches of the inferior phrenic artery, abdominal aorta, and renal artery. Venous drainage within the adrenal gland is from a peripheral to central direction, forming a single adrenal medullary vein. The right adrenal vein drains directly into the inferior vena cava, while the left adrenal vein drains into the left renal vein. There is extensive lymphatic drainage of each adrenal gland, ultimately reaching lateral aortic lymph nodes.[2,3]

The right adrenal gland is roughly triangular in shape, while the left is somewhat crescentic or Y-shaped.[2,4] The shape of the adrenal gland is influenced by the presence of the ipsilateral kidney. In patients with renal agenesis, anomalies of adrenal shape have been observed; the gland takes on a rounded, flat, discoid shape that appears linear on cross-sectional imaging.[5] The abnormally shaped adrenal gland can be misinterpreted as hypertrophy at sonography; the gland, despite its abnormal shape, probably has a normal weight.[6]

The kidneys ascend during development to approximate the adrenal glands. The right adrenal gland is located posterior to the inferior vena cava and superior, anterior, and medial to the upper pole of the right kidney. The left adrenal gland is not suprarenal, but is usually located anterior to the upper pole of the left kidney.

state.[33] Thus, some advocate follow-up of adenomas with imaging and biochemical testing, although the appropriate time interval is debatable.[29]

Cortisol-Producing Adrenal Adenomas and Cushing's Syndrome

Cushing's syndrome describes the symptom complex resulting from excess levels of cortisol, due to either endogenous causes or prolonged steroid administration. Approximately 85% of endogenous Cushing's syndrome is caused by overproduction of adrenocorticotropic hormone (ACTH), usually by a pituitary adenoma (Cushing's disease). The remaining causes of endogenous Cushing's syndrome are ACTH-independent, where adrenal production of cortisol is autonomous; about half of these cases are caused by an adrenocortical neoplasm, more commonly an adenoma and less commonly a carcinoma.[31,36] Cortisol-producing adenomas are the most common hyperfunctioning adrenocortical neoplasm.[31] Some overlap may occur in long-standing Cushing's disease, in which prolonged adrenal stimulation by high levels of ACTH can transform adrenal tissue into autonomous cortisol-producing nodules, resulting in a paradoxically low ACTH level by feedback inhibition.[1]

Cushing's syndrome can be a challenging clinical diagnosis, with signs and symptoms that are subtle early in the disease. For this reason, cortisol-producing adenomas can be an incidental finding and may represent 20% of incidentally discovered adrenal masses.[36] Many incidentally discovered cortisol-producing adenomas do so at a low level, causing hypercortisolism without overt signs or symptoms, the so-called "subclinical" Cushing's syndrome. The clinical significance and morbidity of this condition is unclear,[28] but some studies have shown an increased incidence of both impaired glucose tolerance and diabetes in patients with incidentally discovered adrenal masses that were thought to be clinically silent.[27,37] The amount of cortisol production correlates with both the biochemical significance and size of the adenoma.[36,37] Adenomas with sufficient cortisol production can suppress the normal adrenal tissue in a long-lasting fashion, resulting in adrenal insufficiency after adrenalectomy[31]; for this reason, patients scheduled for removal of a cortisol-producing adenoma should receive peri- and post-operative steroid therapy as needed. Suppression of normal adrenal tissue by a hyperfunctioning adenoma may manifest as contralateral adrenal atrophy at MR imaging,[26,27] therefore providing another clue to biochemically significant cortisol production.

Aldosteronomas and Primary Hyperaldosteronism

Excess levels of aldosterone should be suspected in patients who present with hypertension and hypokalemia or in those with hypertension that persists despite conventional therapy. Hypokalemia was once thought to be an essential component of primary hyperaldosteronism. However, new biochemical screening methods have resulted in a dramatic increase in estimated prevalence, with hypokalemia present in only a minority of affected patients. Using the ratio of plasma aldosterone concentration to plasma renin activity as a screening test suggests that primary hyperaldosteronism has a prevalence between 5% and 13% of all hypertensive patients.[38,39]

Approximately 60% of primary hyperaldosteronism is caused by an aldosterone-producing adenoma, or "aldosteronoma," as first described by Conn.[40] Most other cases are idiopathic, with bilateral hypertrophy of the zona glomerulosa and adrenocortical nodules.[1] This distinction is critical to therapy; patients with an aldosteronoma can undergo potentially curative unilateral adrenalectomy, while those with bilateral adrenal hypertrophy and idiopathic hyperaldosteronism do not benefit from unilateral adrenalectomy but instead are treated medically. An additional rare cause of primary hyperaldosterism is unilateral adrenal hyperplasia, also termed primary adrenal hyperplasia (PAH); this entity is also surgically treated.[39]

Cross-sectional imaging can play a useful role in differentiating these subtypes of primary hyperaldosteronism. When an adrenal mass characteristic of an adenoma is discovered in this clinical setting, and the adrenal glands appear otherwise normal, the diagnosis of aldosteronoma can be presumed.[41] When there is bilateral adrenal gland enlargement without nodularity or focal mass, idiopathic hyperaldosteronism can be suggested. However, diagnostic dilemmas can arise for a number of reasons. First, aldosteronomas are often small, frequently measuring less than 1.5 cm,[42] and may not be resolved. Second, the adrenal glands become more nodular with age,[43] and the incidence of non-hyperfunctioning adenomas in the general population may be as high as 2% to 10%,[28,42,43] increasing with age.[31] Therefore, detection of an adrenal adenoma, especially if the adrenal glands are hyperplastic, does not exclude the diagnosis of idiopathic hyperaldosteronism.[44] Third, the adrenal hyperplasia that occurs in idiopathic hyperaldosteronism can appear micro- or macro-nodular.[42] Since an aldosterone-producing adenoma is essentially a surgical lesion, diagnostic criteria with a low false-positive rate, i.e., high specificity, are desired in order to prevent unnecessary adrenalectomy. On the other hand, potentially curative surgery should not be denied to patients on the basis of a misdiagnosis of idiopathic hyperaldosteronism. In cases with equivocal findings, adrenal vein sampling has been advocated as a final diagnostic test,[1,42,45] although it has a recognized, albeit low, complication rate.

Certain clinical data and imaging findings may establish a noninvasive diagnosis and avoid adrenal vein sampling. Aldosteronomas are associated with higher levels of aldosterone, more severe hypokalemia and hypertension, and occur more often in young patients[39]; a patient with these clinical and laboratory findings and an imaging study demonstrating a single adrenal adenoma is likely to have an aldosteronoma. A diagnostic algorithm (incorporating CT imaging rather than MR) is shown in Figure 87-2, as proposed by Young.[39] This type of algorithm could be adapted to MR.

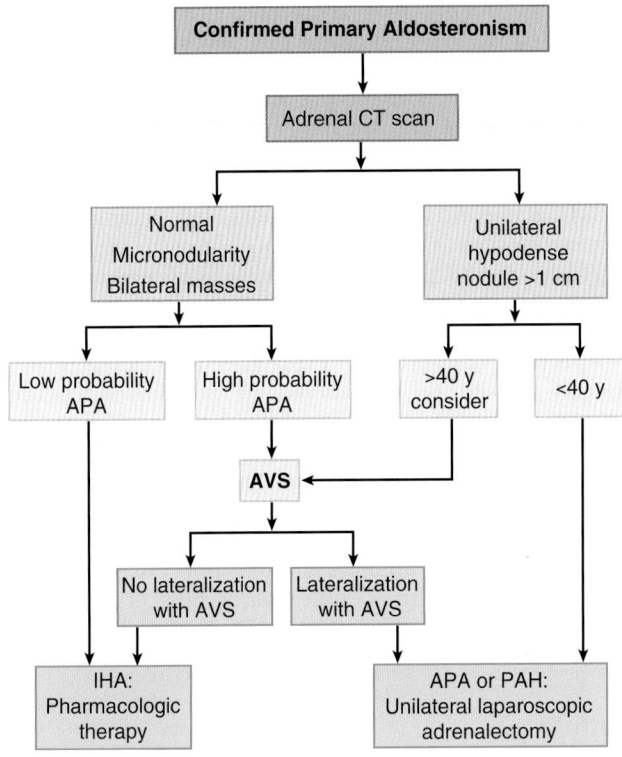

```
        ┌─────────────────────────────────┐
        │  Confirmed Primary Aldosteronism │
        └─────────────────────────────────┘
                        │
                        ▼
              ┌──────────────────┐
              │  Adrenal CT scan │
              └──────────────────┘
```

FIGURE 87-2

Proposed algorithm for management of imaging findings in primary hyper-aldosteronism. APA, aldosterone-producing adenoma; AVS, adrenal vein sampling; IHA, idiopathic hyperaldosteronism; PAH, primary adrenal hyper-plasia. *(Reproduced with permission from Young WF Jr: Minireview: primary aldosteronism—changing concepts in diagnosis and treatment. Endocrinology 144:2208-2213, 2003.)*

Recent studies have sought to establish criteria for adrenal size, so that adrenal hyperplasia (suggesting idiopathic hyperaldosteronism) can be diagnosed with greater sensitivity.[41,46] The size of the adrenal body remains normal in idiopathic hyperaldosteronism, while the adrenal limbs become enlarged, presumably due to the larger proportion of cortex in the adrenal limbs.[47] Using CT, a size threshold of 3 mm has a reported sensitivity of 100%, but a specificity of only 54% for idiopathic hyperaldosteronism, while a threshold of 5 mm has a sensitivity of 47% and a specificity of 100%.[46] The data suggest that if a patient, particularly an older patient, has an adrenal adenoma with contralateral adrenal gland thickening, the diagnosis of idiopathic hyperaldosteronism with an incidental non-hyperfunctioning adenoma should still be considered, and therefore adrenal vein sampling may be necessary.

Sex Hormone-Producing Adrenal Adenomas

Excess levels of sex hormones may result in sexual precocity, hirsutism, gynecomastia, or impotence.[1,31,48] The etiology may be central or peripheral; hyper-functioning adrenal adenomas are a rare peripheral source of excess androgens or estrogens, less common than ovarian sources.[1] Adrenocortical adenomas that overproduce sex hormones comprise less than 10% of incidental adrenal masses,[29] and biochemical screening for this uncommon entity should be predicated on appropriate symptoms. Adrenocortical tumors are rare in children, but when present are more likely to cause an endocrine abnormality. These tumors often secrete androgens, but can secrete a host of other hormones as well, and may cause a mixed clinical picture, combining, for example, features of precocious puberty and Cushing's syndrome.[49,50]

In either gender, adrenal adenomas may secrete androgens or estrogens, causing virilization or feminization.[48,51,52] Rapid progression of symptoms suggests a neoplastic source of hormones, and the ovaries and adrenal glands should be evaluated.[1] The specific pattern of hormone production does not reliably predict the origin of a tumor, although elevated levels of dihydro-epiandrosterone-sulfate (DHEAS) that do not suppress with dexamethasone suggest a virilizing ovarian or adrenal source.[50,53]

MRI Diagnosis of Adrenal Adenoma

Adrenal adenomas are usually slightly hypo- or iso-intense relative to liver on T1-weighted images, iso- to slightly hyper-intense relative to liver on T2-weighted images,[30,54] and show less enhancement and more rapid washout than adrenal metastases and pheochromocytoma.[55,56] However, conventional T1- and T2-weighted images, fat-suppressed images, and gadolinium-enhanced images are not reliable means of diagnosing adrenal adenomas.[54,57-59] The best MR technique to characterize adenomas is chemical shift imaging, accomplished with in- and opposed-phase gradient-echo sequences.[57] The diagnostic power of chemical shift imaging derives from the intracellular lipid content of adrenocortical adenomas. Voxels that contain both fat and water will exhibit signal loss on opposed-phase images relative to in-phase images, due to the destructive interference of the fat and water signals. On the other hand, voxels containing only fat or only water will exhibit similar signal intensity on opposed-phase images relative to in-phase images. Adrenal adenomas usually lose signal on opposed-phase images (see Fig. 87-1), and the degree of signal loss has been correlated with lipid content,[19] and, similarly, with low attenuation measurements on CT.[20] Although normal adrenal cortex also contains lipid, high-resolution in vitro imaging of excised adrenal specimens does not show any signal loss on opposed-phase imaging, presumably related in some way to the biophysical state of the normal cortical lipid.[7]

Quantitative assessment of signal loss within an adrenal mass at chemical shift imaging requires adequately coregistered images, and region-of-interest measurements within the adrenal mass must avoid including "etching" artifact at the interface between the gland and retroperitoneal fat. Since the signal intensity in MRI is a relative quantity, absolute measurements of signal change are of limited value.

A method of quantifying signal loss is the "signal intensity (SI) index," calculated as:

SI index

$$= \frac{SI(adrenal)_{in\text{-}phase} - SI(adrenal)_{opposed\text{-}phase}}{SI(adrenal)_{in\text{-}phase}} \times 100\%$$

(Eq. 87-1)

Adrenal lesions with greater signal loss on opposed-phase images yield a larger SI index. Adenomas have a higher SI index than adrenal metastases.[15,25,60]

Some investigators have advocated using an internal reference within the image to reduce spurious measurements that may arise from T2 decay, changes in receiver gain, or image artifacts. Proposed reference tissues include the liver, spleen, and paraspinal musculature.[24,57,59-66] This method utilizes an SI ratio calculated as:

$$SI\ Ratio = \frac{\dfrac{SI(adrenal)_{opposed\text{-}phase}}{SI(reference)_{opposed\text{-}phase}}}{\dfrac{SI(adrenal)_{in\text{-}phase}}{SI(reference)_{in\text{-}phase}}} - 1 \times 100\%$$

(Eq. 87-2)

where *reference* indicates the reference tissue. Adrenal lesions with greater signal loss on opposed-phase images yield more negative values. Most recent studies consider the spleen to be the most appropriate reference tissue, since fatty infiltration of the liver or muscle can alter the SI ratio in a manner that compromises sensitivity.[60,61] Of course, iron deposition in the spleen can also alter the SI ratio, and attention to such caveats is important if this method of quantitation is to be utilized.

Studies have in general reported excellent sensitivity and specificity of chemical shift MRI in the diagnosis of adrenal adenomas, but have suggested varying values for the SI index or SI ratio as the diagnostic criterion. This variation likely arises from differences in imaging parameters; the studies used varying field strength and echo time for in- and opposed-phase sequences, depending on the availability of the pulse sequence as well as the gradient speed. Commercially available gradients have only recently achieved adequate speed to allow a TE as short as 2.1 to 2.3 ms, i.e., the first time point at which fat and water protons are out of phase at 1.5 T; therefore, only the most recent studies use this particular TE. The results of multiple studies are shown in (Table 87-1). Qualitative comparison of in- and opposed-phase images has a similar accuracy to quantitative measures in the diagnosis of adrenal adenomas.[24,59,60,62] However, quantitative measures probably remain useful for less experienced radiologists or for interdeterminate cases.

Despite the high accuracy of MRI in adrenal mass characterization, there remain small numbers of adrenal adenomas that have an unusually low lipid content. These "lipid-poor" adenomas continue to present a diagnostic challenge (Fig. 87-3). Delayed enhanced CT has been advocated as an accurate means of differentiating adrenal adenomas from metastases,[67,68] even in the case of lipid-poor adenomas.[69,70] This technique should prove a useful adjunct in adrenal imaging, particularly in cases where MRI is indeterminate. Rarely, large, degenerated adenomas can contain hemorrhage, calcification, and fibrosis, and may not be distinguishable from other adrenal neoplasms by imaging, although they do not cause tumor thrombus.[71]

Management of an adrenal mass with indeterminate characterization on MRI varies according to the clinical scenario. In the patient with malignancy undergoing a staging work-up, the mass should be further characterized with delayed enhanced CT if it is the only site of suspected metastasis. If even this is indeterminate, biopsy should be considered to confirm metastatic disease and exclude an atypical adenoma, so that the patient is not unnecessarily deprived of potentially curable surgery. In the patient with no known primary malignancy, biochemical testing to exclude pheochromocytoma or hyperfunctioning adenoma should be performed. Follow-up imaging can support diagnosis of a benign adenoma by documenting a slow growth rate. Tissue sampling is probably not necessary for masses smaller than 3 cm.

Pitfalls

The diagnosis of adrenal adenoma by chemical shift MRI hinges on the presumption that a mass containing microscopic lipid is specific for an adenoma. This leads to certain extremely rare pitfalls in chemical shift MRI, as documented by several case reports. Clear-cell carcinoma of the kidney is known to contain macroscopic lipid, and there are reported cases of metastases to the adrenal gland that lose signal intensity on chemical shift imaging.[72,73] Appropriate clinical and pathologic history can help prevent this pitfall. The pitfall of intratumoral lipid within adrenal cortical carcinoma is discussed later.

The collision tumor is a rare entity in which two histologically distinct tumors are contiguous, without significant mixture of the two cell types.[74,75] This can occur in the adrenal gland, more commonly with adenoma coexisting with a myelolipoma,[75] but occasionally with an adenoma coexisting with a metastasis.[76] The two tumors should exhibit different signal intensities and different behavior at chemical shift imaging. Characterizing the various components of the collision tumor can provide improved guidance for biopsy.

ADRENAL MYELOLIPOMA

Myelolipoma of the adrenal gland is a tumor containing fat and hematopoietic elements.[77] Fatty or myeloid components may predominate.[78] The pathogenesis of this tumor remains uncertain.[79] It is typically not associated with endocrine hyperfunction and is often detected incidentally. The tumor is usually slow growing.[77,80,81] Symptoms may arise from compression of adjacent organs or rarely from tumor hemorrhage.[82] When it occurs, extracapsular hemorrhage has been observed more commonly in males and arising from right-sided masses.[83] The risk of hemorrhage increases

TABLE 87-1   Studies of Chemical Shift MRI in Adrenal Mass Characterization

Study	Sensitivity (%)	Specificity (%)	Number of masses	Equation(s)	Reference tissue(s)	Threshold for diagnosis of adenoma
Mitchell et al (1992)[57]	95	Not given	20	SI ratio	Liver, muscle	Not given
Tsushima et al (1993)[15]	100	100	53	SI index	None	>5% (no reference tissue)
Bilbey et al (1995)[61]	100 (spleen as reference)	100 (spleen as reference)	39	SI ratio	Liver, muscle, spleen	<−20% (spleen as reference)
Mayo-Smith et al (1995)[60]	100 (spleen as reference)	82 (spleen as reference)	46	SI index, SI ratio	None, liver, muscle, spleen	<−25% (spleen as reference)
Outwater et al (1995)[62]	87	92	58	N/A (qualitative)	Spleen	N/A
Korobkin et al (1995)[59]	Liver: 84 Muscle: 26	Liver: 100 Muscle: 100	46	SI ratio	Liver, muscle	<−12% (liver as reference)
Schwartz et al (1995)[63]	80	100	68	SI ratio	Spleen	<−45% (spleen as reference)
McNicholas et al (1995)[64]	Not given	Not given	11	SI ratio	Spleen	<−30% (spleen as reference)
Schwartz et al (1997)[65]	94	100	54	SI ratio	Spleen	<−45% (spleen as reference)
Heinz-Peer et al (1999)[24]	94	95	74 (adenomas)	SI index, SI ratio	None, spleen	Not given
Honigschnabl et al (2002)[66]	96	90	136 (adenomas)	SI index, SI ratio	None, spleen	Not given
Fujiyoshi et al (2003)[25]	100	100	102	SI index, SI ratio	None, liver, muscle, spleen	Adenoma >11.2-16.5% (no reference tissue)

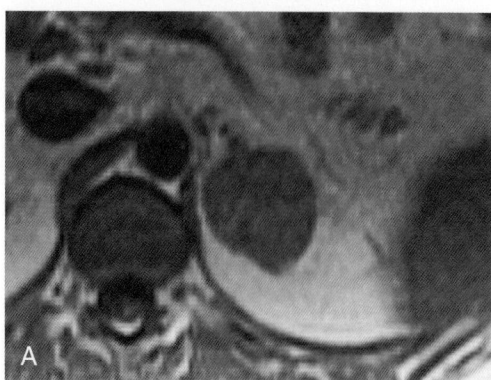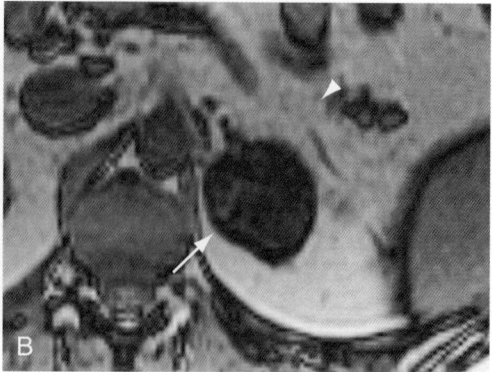

FIGURE 87-3

Adrenal adenoma with a lipid-poor focus in a 44-year-old man. **A,** Axial in-phase and **B,** opposed-phase T1-weighted gradient-echo images. The left adrenal gland contains a smoothly marginated 4.0 cm mass, most of which loses signal on the opposed-phase image, diagnostic of intracellular lipid (*arrowhead*). However, a 0.9 cm lipid-poor focus is present medially (*arrow*); adrenal adenoma remains, by far, the most likely diagnosis, although a collision tumor (e.g., a metastasis to an adenoma) is a possibility. Stability of this lesion over 1 year and very slow growth over 5 years confirmed its benign nature.

with tumors greater than 10 cm in size.[84] Myelolipomas may also occur in extra-adrenal locations, most commonly in the retroperitoneum.[85]

The diagnostic imaging feature of myelolipoma is the demonstration of macroscopic fat. This is best evaluated on MR with the use of T1-weighted images obtained both with and without fat suppression, or T1-weighted images with water saturation.[26] Chemical shift imaging will show an etching artifact within the tumor at interfaces between fatty and myeloid components on opposed-phase imaging (Fig. 87-4). Punctate intratumoral calcification is better revealed on CT[77]; intratumoral hemorrhage may evolve into a more variable pattern of calcification.[75] Average size is approximately 10 cm, but can range from 2.5 to 20 cm.[84] Contrast enhancement may be present, particularly within myeloid components.[83]

ADRENOCORTICAL CARCINOMA

Carcinoma arising from the adrenal cortex is rare, with an estimated incidence of 0.5 to 2 cases per million people. It is more common in children younger than 5 years of age and in adults between the ages of 40 and 50.[1,86] Adrenocortical carcinoma is hyperfunctioning in approximately 60% of patients, with Cushing's syndrome being the most common endocrine abnormality (Table 87-2).[86] Adrenocortical carcinomas occur more frequently in the Li-Fraumeni syndrome (a familial tumor syndrome consisting of adrenocortical carcinoma, breast cancer, leukaemia, sarcoma, and glioma) and the Beckwith-Wiedemann syndrome (adrenocortical carcinoma, Wilms' tumor, rhabdomyosarcoma, hepatoblastoma, and abnormal physical features, including macroglossia, earlobe pits, and gigantism).[87]

Histologically, adrenocortical carcinoma and adrenal adenomas may be difficult to differentiate,[88] particularly in the pediatric population.[49,89] Necrosis, calcification,

and vascular and capsular invasion are features suggesting malignancy.[89] Frequent sites of metastatic disease include the lung, liver, lymph nodes, and bone. Local invasion of the kidneys and inferior vena cava may occur.[86] Treatment often consists of surgery; in such cases, postoperative steroid replacement therapy may be necessary due to suppression of normal adrenal tissue, with recovery of adrenal function taking as long as 22 months.[90] The prognosis is generally poor, with a 5-year survival rate below 20%.[1] Higher survival rates have been suggested in children younger than 5 years of age.[49]

Adrenocortical carcinoma is frequently large at presentation, almost always greater than 6 cm in size,[86] and often greater than 10 cm[30]; approximately 25% of adrenal tumors greater than 6 cm are adrenocortical carcinomas (Fig. 87-5).[28] The tumor occurs bilaterally in 2% to 6% of cases.[86] Hyperfunctioning tumors tend to be smaller at the time of diagnosis due to earlier production of clinical symptoms.[30] The tumor is hypo- or iso-intense to liver on T1-weighted images and hyperintense on T2-weighted images,[30,54,90] and is often hemorrhagic or necrotic; calcification occurs in 30%.[30] This results in considerable heterogeneity in signal intensity.[90]

TABLE 87-2 Frequency of Endocrine Abnormalities Caused by Adrenocortical Carcinoma

Endocrine Abnormality	Frequency (%)
Cushing's syndrome	30-40
Cushing's syndrome with virilization	24
Virilization alone	20-30 (3-5 in adults)
Feminization	6
Hyperaldosteronism	2.5

From Ng L, Libertino JM: Adrenocortical carcinoma: diagnosis, evaluation and treatment. J Urol 169:5-11, 2003.

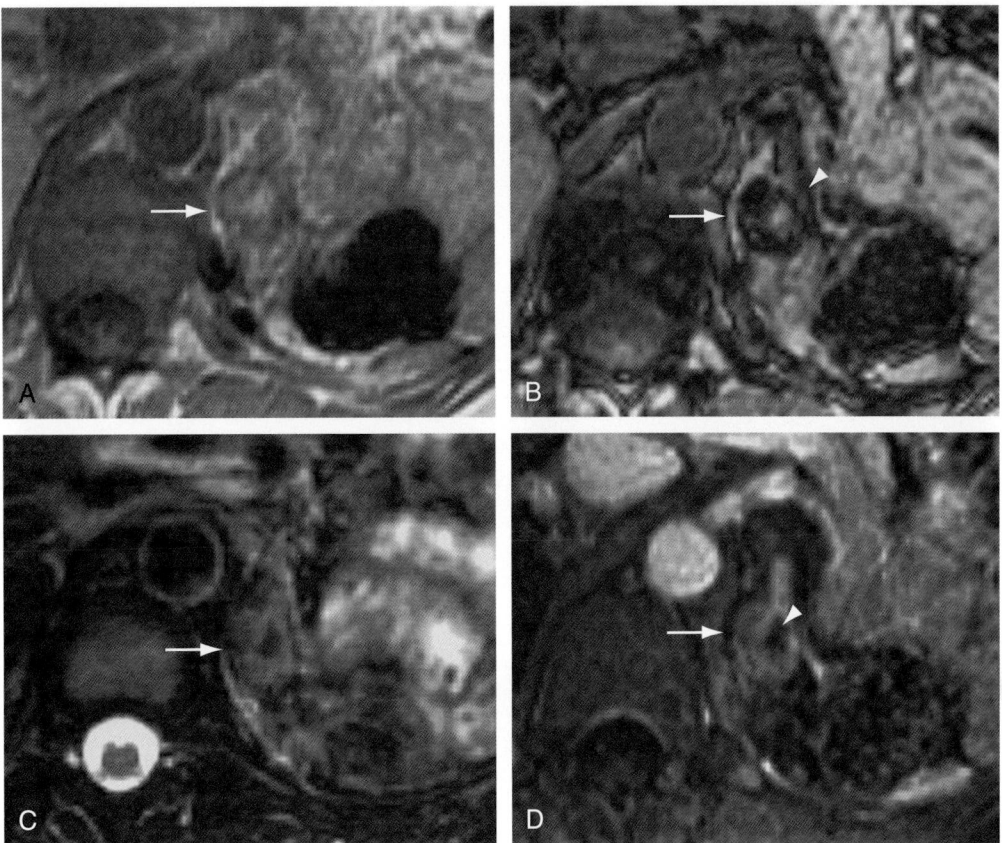

FIGURE 87-4

MR images of an adrenal myelolipoma in a 51-year-old woman. **A,** Axial in-phase and **B,** opposed-phase gradient-echo images; **C,** axial respiratory-triggered fat-suppressed T2-weighted image; and **D,** fat-suppressed three-dimensional gradient-echo image in a delayed phase of enhancement show a 1.4 cm left adrenal mass (*arrow*) with a T1 hyperintense component (*arrowhead*) that does not lose signal on the opposed-phase image, is bounded by chemical shift artifact, and suppresses with fat, representing macroscopic lipid and diagnostic of a myelolipoma. Note the enhancing myeloid components in **D**.

Enhancement is usually nodular with a relatively poorly-enhancing central component; contrast washout may be delayed.[18] MRI is considered the best modality for delineation of vascular involvement and depiction of tumor extension into the inferior vena cava, especially with imaging in the coronal and sagittal planes.[30,54,90,91] In a series including 10 adrenocortical carcinomas, MRI had a sensitivity of 93% and specificity of 100% in the diagnosis of these tumors.[66]

Since adrenocortical carcinoma is derived from the adrenal cortex, it may contain intracellular lipid in the same way that adrenal adenomas can contain lipid. Several cases of lipid-containing adrenocortical carcinomas with signal loss on opposed-phase chemical shift images have been documented.[92,93] In one case report, the area of signal loss corresponded to a portion of the tumor dominated by a clear-cell histology.[93] It is therefore important to note that an adrenal tumor with size, behavior, and morphology suspicious for malignancy should be histologically sampled or resected even if it contains a small lipid-rich focus.[18,88]

PHEOCHROMOCYTOMA

Pheochromocytomas are neuroectodermal tumors, arising from chromaffin cells of the adrenal medulla.[1] They may be sporadic or associated with a genetic syndrome (Table 87-3).[94,95] Sporadic pheochromocytomas are the most common, accounting for approximately 90% of lesions. The remaining 10% of cases occur in association with von Hippel-Lindau (VHL) disease, familial pheochromocytoma, multiple endocrine neoplasia (MEN) type 2, and neurofibromatosis type 1 (NF-1),[96] and are more likely to be bilateral.[88] Advances in molecular genetics may alter estimates of prevalence as germline mutations are found with greater sensitivity. A study of patients with apparent sporadic pheochromocytoma detected germline mutations in 24%.[97] Identification of occult germline mutations has implications for screening and surveillance of the patient and his/her family members.

The incidence of pheochromocytoma ranges from less than 1% in the general population to as high as 1.9% in clinically suspicious scenarios. Younger patients are more

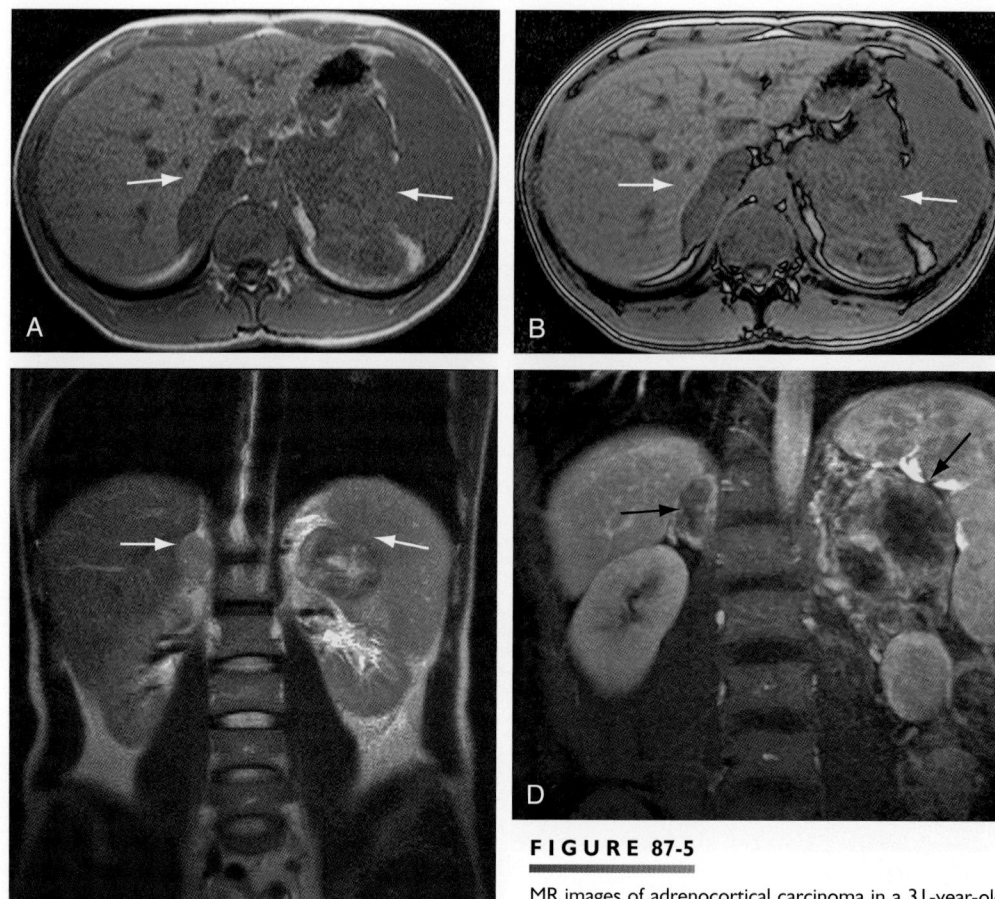

FIGURE 87-5

MR images of adrenocortical carcinoma in a 31-year-old man. The patient initially presented with scrotal swelling and a left-sided varicocele; retroperitoneal ultrasound and CT discovered a mass immediately contiguous to the left kidney. **A,** Axial in-phase and **B,** opposed-phase T1-weighted gradient-echo images; **C,** coronal single-shot fast-spin-echo image; and **D,** coronal oblique section through a post-gadolinium volumetric fat-suppressed three-dimensional gradient-echo data set show bilateral adrenal masses (*arrows*), left larger than right, which do not lose signal on opposed-phase images and enhance with marked heterogeneity. Resection of the left adrenal tumor revealed an adrenocortical carcinoma with extensive regional metastatic adenopathy. The contralateral adrenal mass was presumed to be a metatasis.

TABLE 87-3 Syndromic Associations of Pheochromocytoma

Syndrome	Incidence of pheochromocytoma (%)	Other tumors/conditions
Multiple endocrine neoplasia (MEN) type 2A	50	Medullary thyroid carcinoma Parathyroid adenoma
MEN type 2B	50	Medullary thyroid carcinoma Mucosal neuromas
von Hippel-Lindau disease type 2	25	Renal cell carcinoma Hemangioblastoma Pancreatic microcystic adenoma Pancreatic islet cell tumor
Neurofibromatosis type 1	5	Neurofibroma Glioma

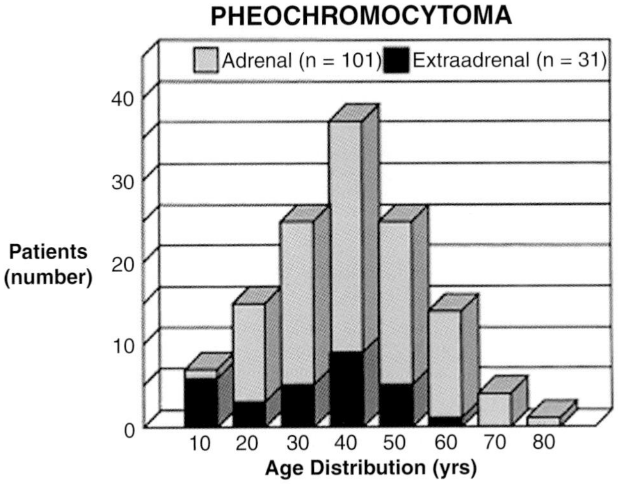

PHEOCHROMOCYTOMA

FIGURE 87-6

Incidence of pheochromocytoma as a function of age, from a retrospective study of 132 patients at the Cleveland clinic. *(Reproduced with permission from Bravo EL, Tagle R: Pheochromocytoma: state-of-the-art and future prospects. Endocrine Rev 24:539-553, 2003.)*

likely to have pheochromocytomas that are syndrome-related, multiple, and extra-adrenal (Fig. 87-6).[98] Approximately 10% of sporadic adrenal pheochromocytomas are malignant,[96] with a higher rate of malignancy in tumors greater than 5 cm in size (76% malignant) and in extra-adrenal paragangliomas (52% malignant).[98] A variety of aberrant genotypes have been identified in sporadic pheochromocytomas, including mutations similar or identical to germline mutations found in syndromic pheochromocytoma.[96]

In VHL disease, a germline mutation of the VHL tumor suppressor gene leaves only one normal allele. Mutation of the remaining normal allele in somatic cells leads to tumor formation, as predicted by Knudson's two-hit hypothesis.[99] Subtypes of VHL disease are categorized by the specific type of mutation that occurs, resulting in either gain or loss of function of the VHL protein and increased risk for certain tumors. Pheochromocytomas occur in only type 2 disease with a 25% incidence.[98,99] In type 2C VHL disease, as well as in variants such as familial pheochromocytoma, only pheochromocytomas occur, without increased risk for other VHL-associated tumors.[99,100] In other types of the disease, pancreatic islet cell tumors occur in association with pheochromocytomas (Fig. 87-7).[101]

Similarly, in MEN type 2, a germline mutation of the rearranged during transfection (RET) proto-oncogene confers increased risk for the development of multiple tumors (see Table 87-3), including pheochromocytoma. Approximately half of patients with MEN type 2 develop pheochromocytoma (Fig. 87-8).[94]

Patients with NF-1 are at increased risk for the development of pheochromocytoma, with an incidence ranging from 0.1% to 5.7,[102] although a concomitant history of hypertension places these patients at greater risk. Pheochromocytomas are present in up to half of patients with hypertension and NF-1.[102]

Histopathologic differentiation of benign from malignant pheochromocytoma remains difficult. Abundant vascularity, invasion of the adrenal capsule, and vascular invasion are present in both benign and malignant disease.[18,96,103] Signs of malignancy include invasion of adjacent organs and metastases. Malignant tumors also tend to be larger and have greater degrees of necrosis (Fig. 87-9).[96] Biochemical markers of malignancy remain an active area of research.[103,104]

Clinical findings of pheochromocytoma most commonly consist of headache, palpitations, diaphoresis, and hypertension.[96,98] However, clinical diagnosis remains challenging because symptoms vary greatly, may be paroxysmal, and may not even be present; the variable presentation is likely related to the wide range of hormone products as well as varying catecholamine sensitivity of the host. Approximately 8% of patients with pheochromocytoma are asymptomatic,[98] and 10% of tumors are discovered incidentally. Hypertension may be sustained (norepinephrine-producing tumors) or paroxysmal (predominantly epinephrine-producing tumors), and is poorly correlated with hormone levels. Hypotension may occur with pure epinephrine-producing tumors.[98] Importantly, pheochromocytomas may sometimes cause hypertensive crisis and death.[28]

MRI is useful in detecting and characterizing pheochromocytomas, with 100% sensitivity and 98% specificity in one study[24] and 93% sensitivity and 98% specificity in another.[66] Since pheochromocytoma is derived from the adrenal medulla, it should not contain lipid and should not lose signal on opposed-phase images (Fig. 87-10). Pheochromocytomas tend to be hyperintense on T2-weighted images due to high intracellular water content; tumors may also have T2 hyperintensity on the basis of central necrosis, cystic change, or hemorrhage (Fig. 87-11).[18,101,105] However, on heavily T2-weighted images (TE on the order of 180 ms), pheochromocytomas are usually hypointense to adrenal cysts. The term "light bulb" sign has been used to describe pheochromocytoma,[106] but is probably more appropriate for the adrenal cyst.[26] Pheochromocytomas usually exhibit avid, early enhancement with delayed washout of contrast[55,56]; enhancement is often uniform, but there may occasionally be a central nonenhancing region.[101] Gadolinium-enhanced images can be useful in differentiating pheochromocytoma from a debris-containing adrenal cyst (with T2 shortening caused by debris). Calcification occurs in approximately 10% of pheochromocytomas and is better depicted with CT.[88] Characteristic imaging features are not always present[107]; "atypical" appearances were seen in 23% of one series of 17 pheochromocytomas.[54] In another series only 60% of pheochromocytomas had the characteristic T2 hyperintensity.[18]

A multitude of plasma and urine tests exist for detection of catecholamines and catecholamine metabolites, with varying sensitivity and specificity. Biochemical testing should precede cross-sectional imaging in the evaluation of patients suspected of having pheochromocytoma,[98] with imaging reserved for anatomic localization. However, with the increased use of cross-sectional imaging, increasing frequency of incidentally

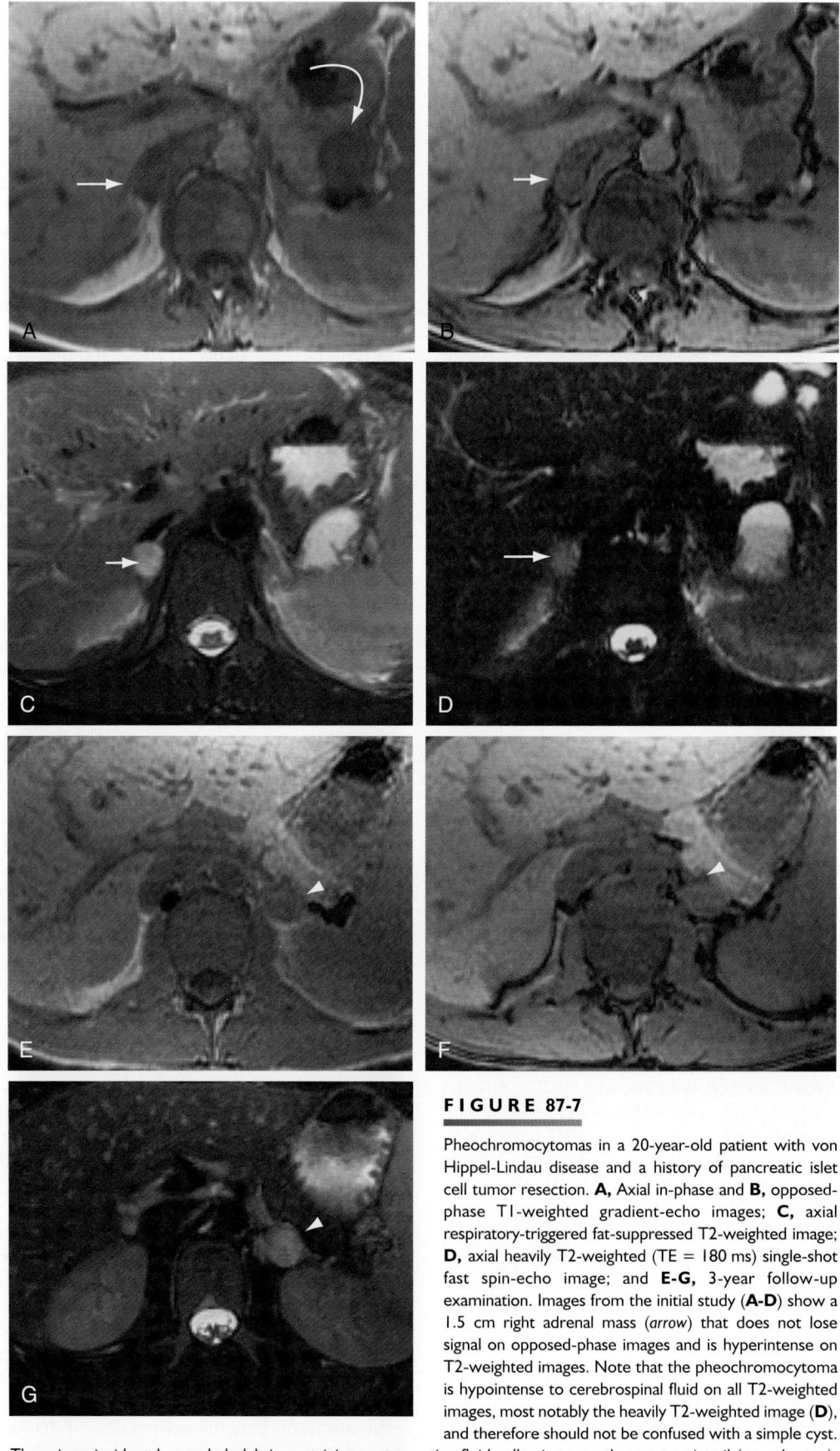

FIGURE 87-7

Pheochromocytomas in a 20-year-old patient with von Hippel-Lindau disease and a history of pancreatic islet cell tumor resection. **A,** Axial in-phase and **B,** opposed-phase T1-weighted gradient-echo images; **C,** axial respiratory-triggered fat-suppressed T2-weighted image; **D,** axial heavily T2-weighted (TE = 180 ms) single-shot fast spin-echo image; and **E-G,** 3-year follow-up examination. Images from the initial study (**A-D**) show a 1.5 cm right adrenal mass (*arrow*) that does not lose signal on opposed-phase images and is hyperintense on T2-weighted images. Note that the pheochromocytoma is hypointense to cerebrospinal fluid on all T2-weighted images, most notably the heavily T2-weighted image (**D**), and therefore should not be confused with a simple cyst. There is an incidental, rounded, debris-containing postoperative fluid collection near the pancreatic tail (*curved arrow*). The patient underwent right adrenalectomy. Follow-up study 3 years later (**E-G**) shows a new 2 cm pheochromocytoma in the left adrenal gland (*arrowhead*). Note the interval resolution of the peripancreatic collection.

FIGURE 87-8

Bilateral pheochromocytoma in a 51-year-old man with multiple endocrine neoplasia (MEN) type 2A. Axial respiratory-triggered fat-suppressed T2-weighted image shows bilateral 0.9 cm T2 hyperintense adrenal masses (*arrows*) that do not lose signal on opposed-phase images and exhibit enhancement on post-gadolinium images (not shown), diagnostic of pheochromocytoma.

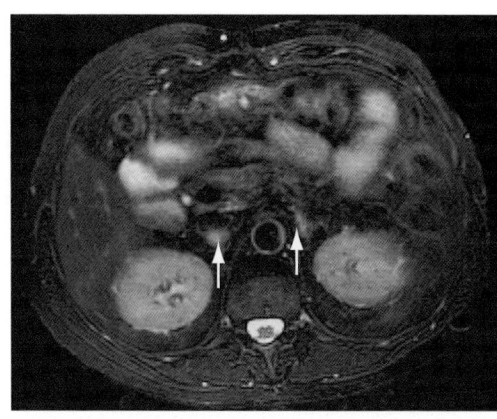

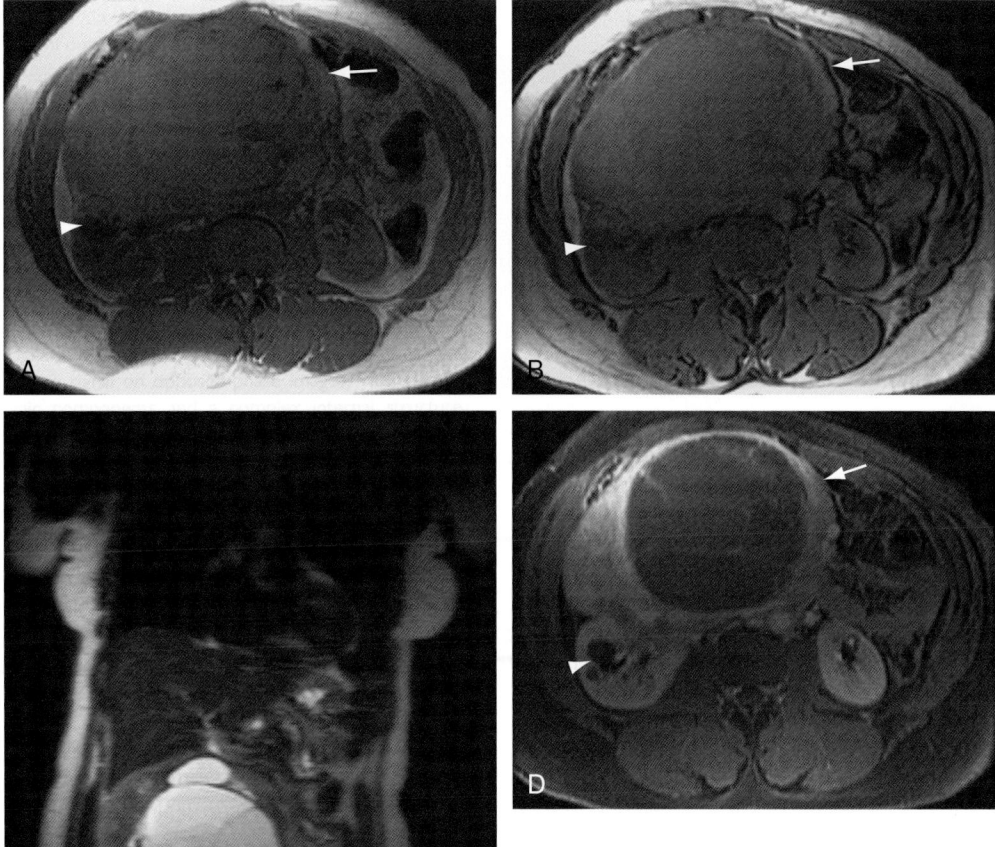

FIGURE 87-9

Malignant extra-adrenal pheochromocytoma (paraganglioma) in a 51-year-old woman. **A,** Axial in-phase and **B,** opposed-phase T1-weighted gradient-echo images; **C,** coronal single-shot fast spin-echo T2-weighted image; and **D,** delayed post-gadolinium axial fat-suppressed two-dimensional gradient-echo image show a large, partially solid, partially cystic, multiseptated 13 cm mass (*arrow*) in the right lower abdomen, compressing the inferior vena cava and displacing the aorta to the left, clearly separate from the liver and kidney. The mass does not lose signal on the opposed-phase image. In comparison to the simple right renal cyst (*arrowhead*), the cystic component of the mass is characterized as complex because it does not follow simple fluid.

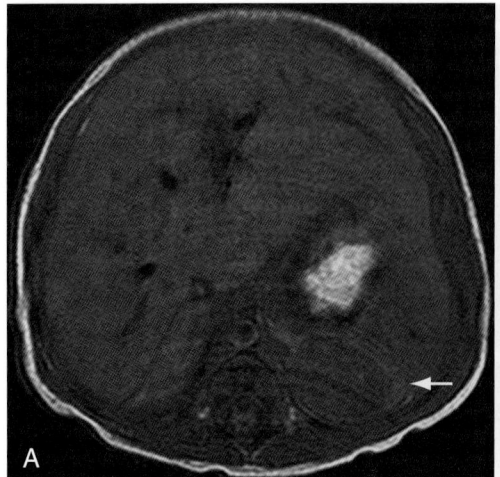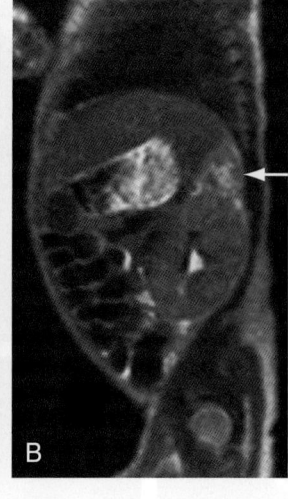

FIGURE 87-12

MR images of a left adrenal neuroblastoma in a 2-day-old girl. **A,** Axial T1-weighted spin-echo and **B,** sagittal T2-weighted single-shot fast spin-echo images reveal a mass (*arrow*) arising from the left adrenal gland with heterogeneous high signal on T2-weighted images. Neuroblastoma has variable signal intensity on MR images. (*Courtesy of Sandra S. Kramer, MD, Department of Radiology, Children's Hospital of Philadelphia, Philadelphia, PA.*)

Adrenal biopsy should be reserved only for lesions that have indeterminate imaging evaluation.

Adrenal metastases can have highly variable imaging features. Most have nonspecific signal intensity, appearing hypointense to liver on T1-weighted images and hyperintense to liver on T2-weighted images (Fig. 87-13).[88,91] Differentiation of benign from malignant adrenal masses with MRI relies heavily on the characterization achieved with chemical shift imaging[57]; adenomas generally lose signal on opposed-phase images, while metastases do not (Fig. 87-14). A rare but important exception to this rule is the possibility of clear-cell renal cell carcinoma (a fat-containing primary tumor) metastasizing to the adrenal gland.[73] Metastases tend to enhance avidly,[55,56] although MR enhancement patterns are not helpful in differentiating benign from malignant disease.[59] Larger metastases are often more heterogeneous (Fig. 87-15).[30] Adrenal gland enlargement in cancer patients has been reported in the absence of adrenal metastases, probably occurring on the basis of adrenal hyperplasia[120]; hyperplastic adrenal tissue that is not involved by metastatic disease should probably lose signal on opposed-phase images. CT evaluation of delayed enhancement may be a useful adjunct in cases where MRI is indeterminate.[69,70]

ADRENAL LYMPHOMA

Autopsy series show that 25% of patients with lymphoma have involvement of the adrenal glands, but only 4% of such cases are prospectively revealed by imaging.[91] Non-Hodgkin's lymphoma is the most frequent subtype to involve the adrenal glands.[18]

Lymphomatous involvement of the adrenal glands may manifest as diffuse adrenal gland enlargement[121] with preservation of adrenal morphology.[105] Solid adrenal masses[122-124] and adrenal nodularity can also

occur.[18] Adenopathy is frequently an associated finding (Fig. 87-16),[125] but is not always present.[88,122] Signal intensity characteristics are entirely nonspecific. However, the adrenal glands would not be expected to lose signal intensity on chemical shift imaging as the normal adrenal cortical cells are replaced by lymphoma.

Primary adrenal lymphoma is extremely rare, and is thought to arise from hematopoietic cells of the adrenal gland itself. Necrotic or hemorrhagic adrenal masses may be present, in contrast to secondary adrenal lymphoma, where adrenal masses tend to be more uniform. Bilateral adrenal involvement can cause adrenal insufficiency.[123]

INFLAMMATORY ADRENAL MASSES

Inflammatory masses of the adrenal glands are most often caused by granulomatous disease, usually due to either tuberculosis or histoplasmosis.[88] Bilateral adrenal involvement is most common,[126-129] although unilateral involvement has been reported.[130] In the subacute phase of illness, the adrenal glands become enlarged and sometimes contain cystic or necrotic masses with peripheral enhancement.[88,128] Calcification occurs later in the disease.[88] Signal intensity of the involved adrenal gland is variable.[129] As the granulomatous process matures, the adrenal glands decrease in size and become more calcified.[131] Granulomas show little enhancement.[56] Pyogenic adrenal abscesses are rare, with most cases occurring in neonates following episodes of adrenal hemorrhage.[132-134]

Granulomatous disease of the adrenal glands is the most common cause of Addison's disease after the idiopathic form.[88] In patients being evaluated for Addison's disease, the presence of bilateral adrenal enlargement should suggest a differential diagnosis that includes granulomatous infection (especially histoplasmosis in endemic areas).[135,136]

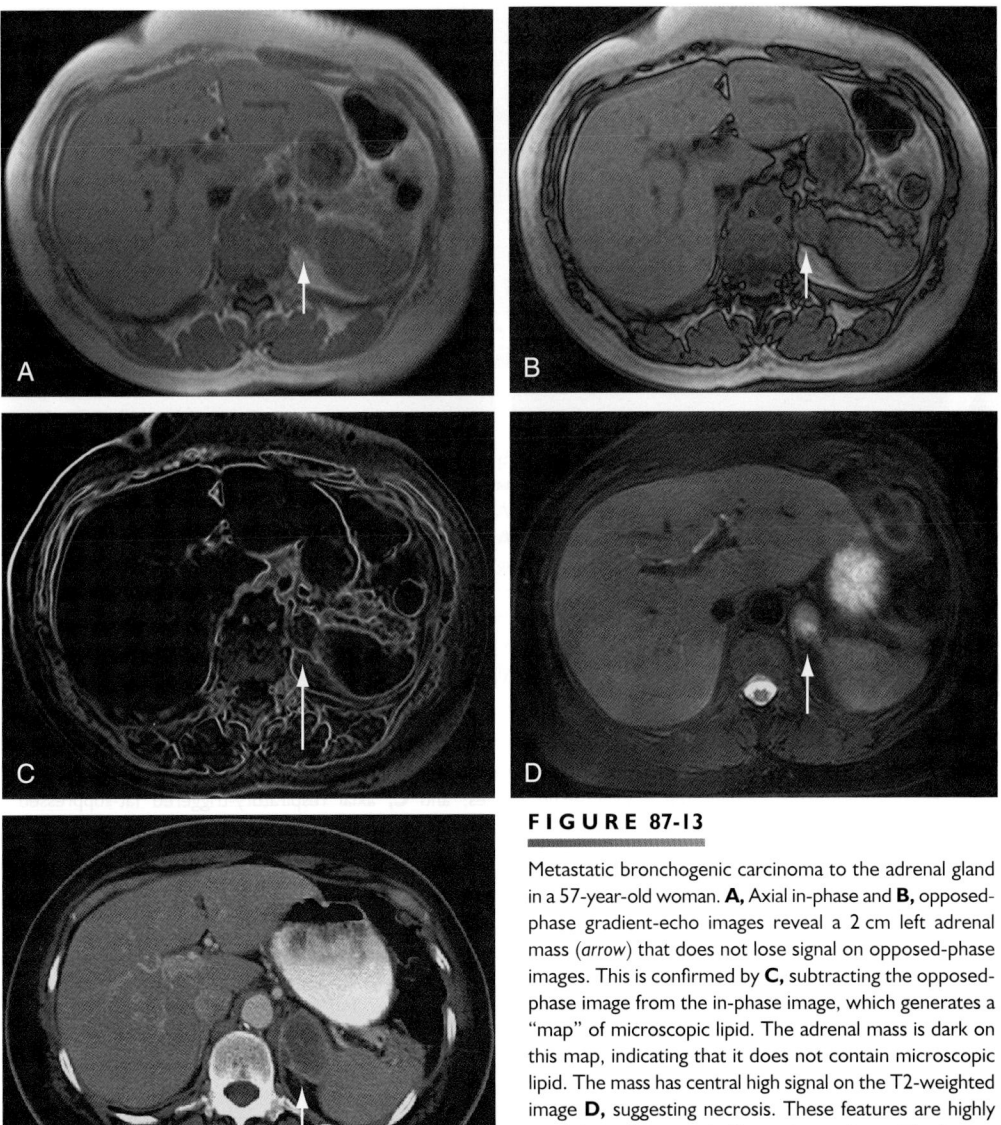

FIGURE 87-13

Metastatic bronchogenic carcinoma to the adrenal gland in a 57-year-old woman. **A,** Axial in-phase and **B,** opposed-phase gradient-echo images reveal a 2 cm left adrenal mass (*arrow*) that does not lose signal on opposed-phase images. This is confirmed by **C,** subtracting the opposed-phase image from the in-phase image, which generates a "map" of microscopic lipid. The adrenal mass is dark on this map, indicating that it does not contain microscopic lipid. The mass has central high signal on the T2-weighted image **D,** suggesting necrosis. These features are highly suspicious of metastatic disease in a patient with a known primary tumor. Metastatic disease is confirmed by **E,** a follow-up CT 4 months later, demonstrating interval growth of the mass and extensive central necrosis.

ADRENAL HEMORRHAGE

Etiology

Anatomic and physiologic features of the adrenal gland predispose it to develop hemorrhage. Within the zona reticularis, an abrupt transition from arteriole to capillary creates a so-called "vascular dam" that can result in vessel rupture if vascular pressure becomes elevated. This may occur in physiologic stress when adrenal blood flow is increased. This may also occur with adrenal vein thrombosis; eccentrically arranged smooth muscle within the walls of draining adrenal veins can lead to turbulent flow and predispose the vessel to thrombo-sis.[137-139] Hypotension can also lead to adrenal hemorrhage by causing necrosis and vascular damage at the corticomedullary junction, with bleeding occurring after reperfusion.[140] Alternatively, a preexisting adrenal mass can also undergo hemorrhage, and is an important consideration in the setting of spontaneous adrenal hemorrhage.

Penetrating or blunt abdominal trauma may cause adrenal injury.[141,142] In the setting of blunt trauma, adrenal hemorrhage is usually unilateral and more commonly on the right side.[143,144] This is speculated to be due to compression of the right adrenal gland between the liver and kidney.[138] There are usually multiple accompanying visceral injuries.[143,144]

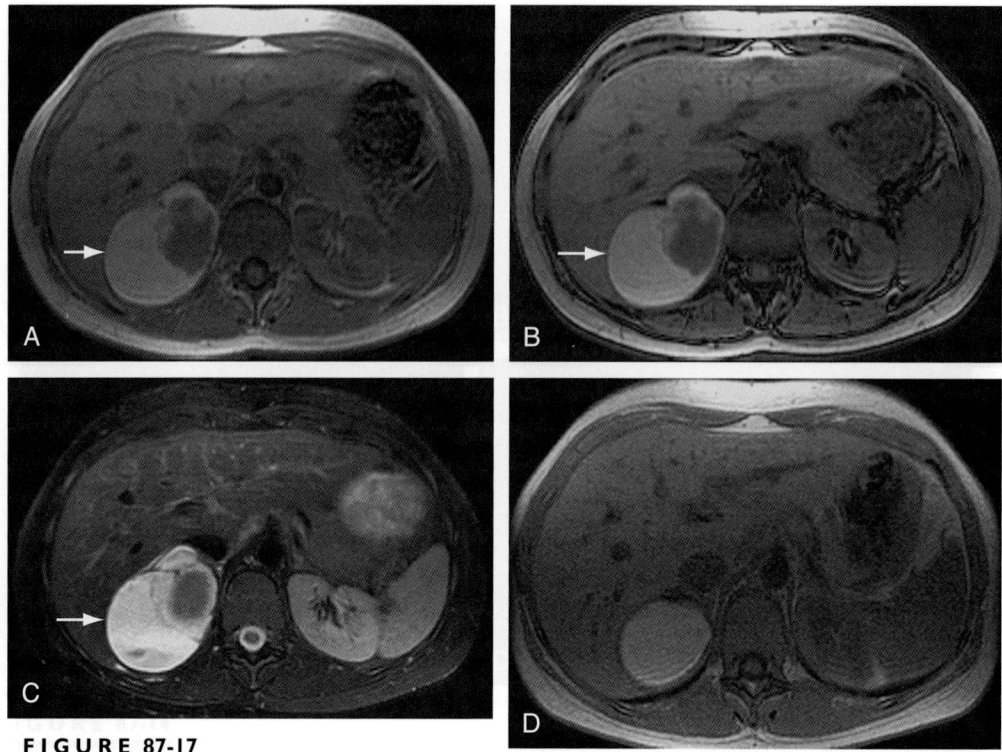

FIGURE 87-17

Adrenal hemorrhage in a 32-year-old woman with an episode of severe right flank pain and possible trauma several weeks previously. **A,** Axial in-phase and **B,** opposed-phase T1-weighted gradient-echo images; and **C,** axial respiratory-triggered fat-suppressed T2-weighted image show a 7 cm right adrenal collection (*arrow*) with T1 and T2 hyperintense components, representing subacute hemorrhage, and central hypointense components probably representing more acute blood products. The lesion showed no enhancement after gadolinium administration, compatible with benign hemorrhage. **D,** Follow-up MRI after 3 months shows a decrease in size and interval maturation of the hematoma *without* depiction of an occult neoplasm.

Imaging

MRI is useful in diagnosing adrenal hemorrhage. Depending on the age of the hematoma, the MR appearance can be variable. Acutely, a hematoma will appear hypo- to iso-intense to liver on T1-weighted images and hypointense on T2-weighted images due to the presence of deoxyhemoglobin. Subacutely, a hematoma becomes hyperintense on T1-weighted images, due to the presence of extracellular methemoglobin, and hyperintense on T2-weighted images, due to the separation of serum from blood products (Fig. 87-17); a fluid-hematocrit level may be present. Chronically, a hematoma should decrease in size and develop a rim of hypointensity on both T1- and T2-weighted images, indicating the presence of hemosiderin. Gradient-echo imaging exhibits "blooming" artifact from susceptibility.[138] Stranding of the periadrenal fat and pararenal hematomas have been described on CT,[143] and similar findings may be present on MR in the acute setting.

Ultimately, adrenal hematomas resolve or develop into a pseudocyst, and follow characteristics of simple fluid. Since a large hematoma can obscure an underlying mass, contrast-enhanced imaging is useful for detecting a causative neoplasm. A hematoma shows no enhancement, whereas a metastasis or primary adrenal tumor should enhance to some degree. Follow-up imaging could be performed in order to document decrease in size (see Fig. 87-17) and maturation of the hematoma, and ensure the absence of an occult neoplasm.

ADRENAL CYST AND PSEUDOCYST

Cysts of the adrenal gland are classified as true cysts if they possess an endothelial lining, or pseudocysts if their capsule consists of only fibrous tissue. Approximately 45% of adrenal cysts are endothelial, while 39% are pseudocysts, 9% are epithelial, and 7% are parasitic.[159] A recent review of the Japanese literature suggests that pseudocysts are in fact the most common adrenal cyst.[160] They represent the sequela of prior hemorrhage.[125] Parasitic adrenal cysts are frequently due to echinococcal infection, and are called hydatid cysts[75]; these are more commonly present in the liver and lung.[161]

Adrenal cysts are usually found incidentally. Symptoms may arise from compression of local organs. Abdominal pain may occur if the cyst becomes hemorrhagic,

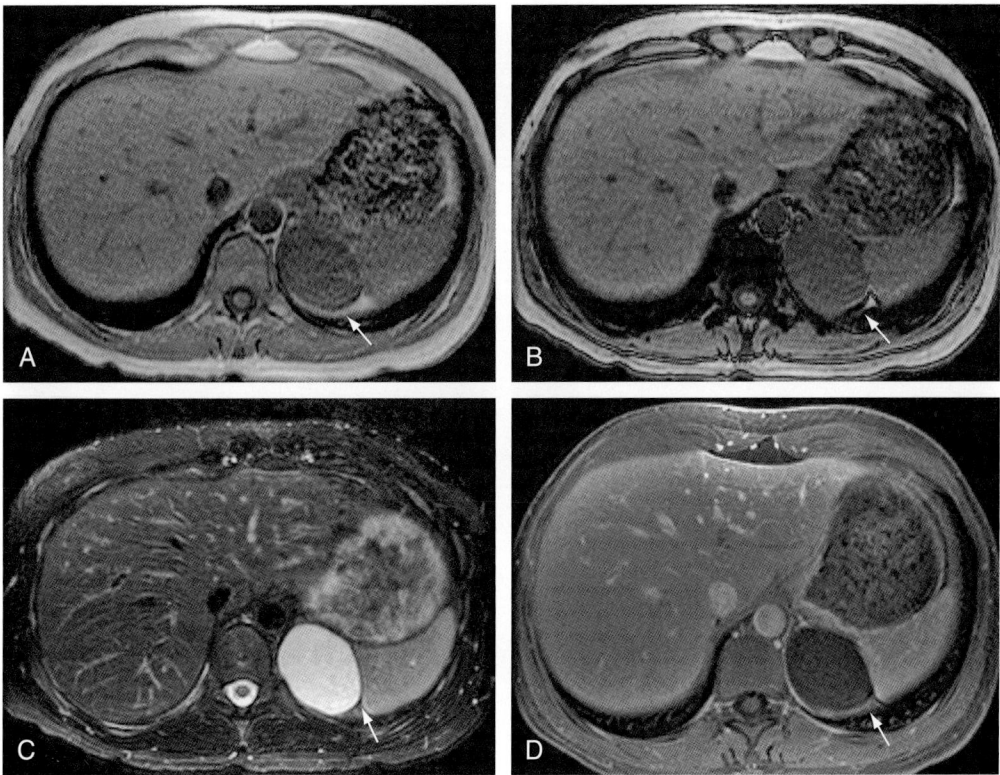

FIGURE 87-18

Adrenal cyst in a 36-year-old woman. **A,** Axial in-phase and **B,** opposed-phase T1-weighted gradient-echo images; **C,** axial respiratory-triggered T2-weighted fast spin-echo image; and **D,** delayed post-gadolinium axial fat-suppressed two-dimensional gradient-echo image show a left adrenal mass (*arrow*) with a smooth, thin wall that does not lose signal on the opposed-phase image, is markedly and homogeneously hyperintense on the T2-weighted image, and does not enhance. The mass remained isointense to cerebrospinal fluid on long TE images (not shown), diagnostic of an adrenal cyst.

infected, or if the cyst ruptures. Rupture of a hydatid cyst can cause spread of parasitic infection or anaphylactic shock.[161] Adrenal hydatid cyst[162] and adrenal pseudocyst[163] are rare causes of hypertension.

MRI can characterize adrenal cysts. Simple cysts are hypointense to liver on T1-weighted images and markedly hyperintense on T2- and heavily T2-weighted images (Fig. 87-18). However, the signal intensity can vary depending on the amount of protein or hemorrhage within the cystic fluid. The wall should be smooth and thin, measuring no more than 3 mm in thickness.[164] Cysts can occasionally be septated. They demonstrate no internal contrast enhancement, but may have enhancement within the cyst wall and septa.

ADRENAL HYPERPLASIA

Congenital Adrenal Hyperplasia

Congenital adrenal hyperplasia is a group of syndromes characterized by deficient biosynthesis of corticosteroids due to an enzymatic defect. The low cortisol level causes increased ACTH secretion, resulting in adrenal hypertrophy.[165] Depending on the specific mutation, the syndrome may include increased or decreased levels of mineralocorticoids and androgens.[1] Adrenal adenomas are also present with increased frequency in patients with congenital adrenal hyperplasia.[165]

Macronodular Adrenal Hyperplasia

The adrenal glands may undergo hyperplasia from primary or secondary causes. Secondary causes, due to elevated levels of ACTH, are far more common and are usually secondary to an ACTH-producing pituitary adenoma (Cushing's disease); another ACTH-producing tumor is a less likely possibility (Fig. 87-19). The adrenal glands in patients with Cushing's disease increase in size,[166] sometimes massively, and may take on a multinodular configuration. Prolonged exposure to ACTH may stimulate the development of autonomous adrenal adenomas. The adrenal cortex interspersed between the nodules is always hyperplastic in this entity. As the adrenal glands become hyperplastic, they secrete greater amounts of cortisol for the same degree of ACTH stimulation. This may finally lead to low levels of ACTH,

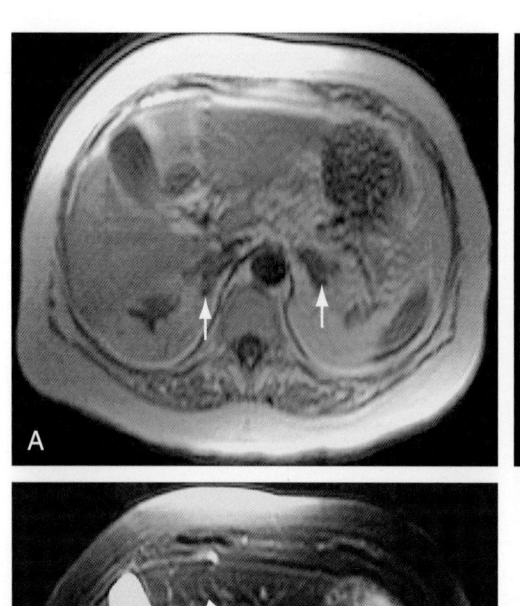
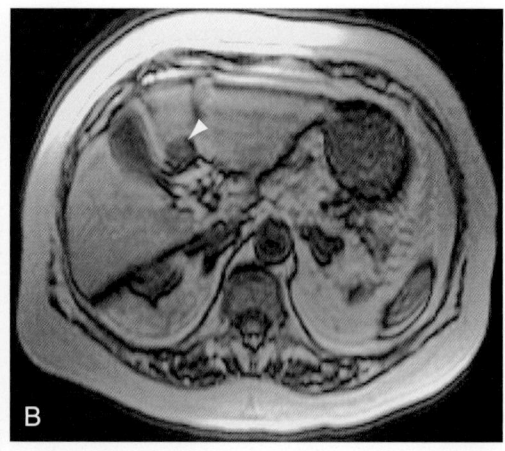
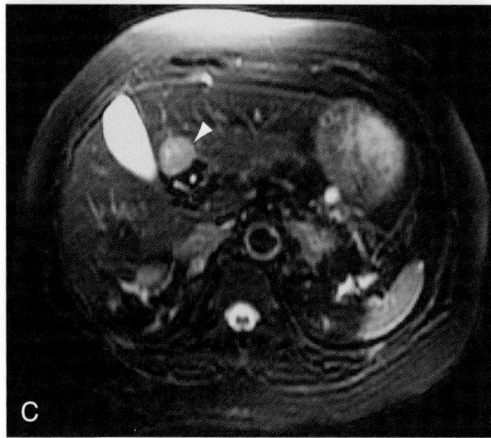

FIGURE 87-19

MR demonstration of adrenocorticotropic hormone (ACTH)-dependent adrenal hyperplasia in a 60-year-old woman with a history of Cushing's syndrome due to an ACTH-secreting metastatic islet cell tumor. **A,** Axial in-phase and **B,** opposed-phase T1-weighted gradient-echo images; and **C,** axial respiratory-triggered fat-suppressed T2-weighted image. The adrenal glands (*arrows*) are markedly thickened and enlarged, without focal mass. The T2 hyperintense liver lesion (*arrowhead*) represents a hepatic metastasis, which artifactually loses signal on opposed-phase images because of partial volume averaging with perihepatic fat.

despite the fact that this is an ACTH-dependent cause of Cushing's syndrome.[1] Normal size of the adrenal glands does not exclude the diagnosis of Cushing's syndrome,[166] presumably because hyperplasia is subtle.

ACTH-independent macronodular adrenal hyperplasia (AIMAH) is an extremely rare cause of Cushing's syndrome. In some patients, the disorder is secondary to mutation of an ACTH-G-protein-coupled receptor, resulting in an "always on" state. In other cases, abnormal receptor expression is speculated.[1] The adrenal glands are massively enlarged, probably more so than in ACTH-dependent hyperplasia,[167] and contain multiple nodules ranging in size from 0.1 to 5.5 cm. The adrenal glands are hypointense to liver on T1-weighted images and only slightly hyperintense to liver on T2-weighted images.[168] Despite its rarity, the diagnosis of AIMAH can be suggested prospectively, as the imaging findings are characteristic, while the patients usually only have mild Cushing's syndrome.[168] Treatment consists of bilateral adrenalectomy.[169]

Primary Pigmented Nodular Adrenocortical Disease

Primary pigmented nodular adrenocortical disease (PPNAD) is a rare cause of ACTH-independent Cushing's syndrome, and in some patients is thought to arise

from mutation of a regulator of protein kinase A, leading to abnormal intracellular signalling and cellular proliferation.[170] Pathologically, the adrenal glands contain numerous pigmented nodules measuring about 2 to 4 mm in diameter,[1] but as large as 3 cm, with variable lipid content.[171] The nodules paradoxically secrete cortisol upon dexamethasone administration.[172] PPNAD is the only known heritable form of Cushing's syndrome[170] and is inherited in an autosomal-dominant fashion.[172] Treatment consists of bilateral adrenalectomy.[1] Unilateral and bilateral adrenal nodularity has been revealed on cross-sectional imaging.[173] Approximately one quarter of patients with PPNAD also have findings of the Carney complex,[174] a multiple endocrine neoplasia consisting of PPNAD, myxomas of the heart, breast, mucosa, and skin, spotty mucocutaneous pigmentation, and calcified Sertoli cell testicular tumors.[170]

McCune-Albright Syndrome

McCune-Albright syndrome consists of café au lait skin lesions, polyostotic fibrous dysplasia, and polyendocrine abnormalities. Affected endocrine organs may include the ovaries and pituitary, thyroid, parathyroid, and adrenal glands. The disease is caused by a G-protein mutation resulting in an "always on" state.[175] At the level of the adrenal gland, this simulates constant stimulation by ACTH and can cause adrenal hyperplasia, sometimes with a nodular configuration. Cushing's syndrome occurs in 5% of cases.[1]

ADRENAL INSUFFICIENCY

Causes of adrenal insufficiency are divided into primary and secondary categories. Primary adrenal insufficiency (Addison's disease) indicates an abnormality of the adrenal glands themselves, while secondary causes arise from abnormal function of the hypothalamus or pituitary gland.[146]

Primary adrenal insufficiency can be caused by extensive loss of adrenal tissue. Over 90% of the adrenal glands must be destroyed for the onset of functional abnormalities.[118] Autoimmune disease of the adrenal glands is now the most common cause of Addison's disease.[146] Gramulomatous disease, particularly due to tuberculosis, was previously considered the most common cause, and continues to be an important etiology of Addison's disease worldwide.[146,176,177] Metastatic disease to the adrenal gland can also result in adrenal insufficiency; several primary tumors have been associated with this, including lung,[178] lymphoma,[179] and hepatocellular carcinoma.[180] Other causes of adrenal gland destruction include adrenal hemorrhage[137,151] and infiltrative disorders, such as sarcoidosis, amyloidosis, and hemochromatosis.[177] Alternatively, primary adrenal insufficiency can arise from an enzyme deficiency causing functional failure, as, for example, in congenital adrenal hyperplasia.[146]

Clinical presentation may be acute or chronic, with somewhat nonspecific symptoms in either scenario. Acutely, Addison's disease may present with hypotension, fever, abdominal pain, and vomiting; chronically, symptoms of fatigue, weakness, and irritability predominate.[177] Mineralocorticoid deficiency occurs only in primary adrenal insufficiency, since secondary causes do not affect the renin-angiotensin-aldosterone system. Additionally, ACTH levels are high only in primary adrenal insufficiency, resulting in hyperpigmentation if the condition is present for a sufficient period of time.[146,147] Biochemical diagnosis of primary adrenal insufficiency can be accomplished with cosyntropin stimulation tests and measurements of cortisol and ACTH levels.[181] Autoimmune adrenalitis can be diagnosed through detection of circulating autoantibodies.[177] The diagnosis of adrenal insufficiency becomes more challenging in the acute setting (e.g., sepsis or the postoperative state), because of wide variation in cortisol and cosyntropin response during stress.

In the patient with clinically established autoimmune adrenalitis, there is little role for imaging. However, imaging can be useful in diagnosing other causes of adrenal failure. MRI is useful in characterizing adrenal size, adrenal masses, and adrenal hemorrhage. Small, atrophic adrenal glands in the setting of primary adrenal insufficiency suggest a late stage of granulomatous disease, particularly if the glands are calcified.[136] Enlarged glands with primary adrenal insufficiency raise the possibility of acute/subacute granulomatous disease, metastatic disease, lymphoma, or hemorrhage.[136] If a patient with adrenal insufficiency presents with unilateral adrenal gland destruction, metastatic disease to the pituitary gland as a cause of secondary adrenal insufficiency should be considered.[118]

REFERENCES

1. Williams RH, Larsen PR: William's Textbook of Endocrinology, 10th ed. Philadelphia, WB Saunders, 2003.
2. Mitty HA: Embryology, anatomy, and anomalies of the adrenal gland. Semin Roentgenol 23:271-279, 1988.
3. Moore KL: Clinically Oriented Anatomy, 3rd ed. Baltimore, Williams & Wilkins, 1992, p 917.
4. Avisse C, Marcus C, Patey M, et al: Surgical anatomy and embryology of the adrenal glands. Surg Clin North Am 80:403-415, 2000.
5. Kenney PJ, Robbins GL, Ellis DA, Spirt BA: Adrenal glands in patients with congenital renal anomalies: CT appearance. Radiology 155:181-182, 1985.
6. Droste S, Fitzsimmons J, Pascoe-Mason J, et al: Size of the fetal adrenal in bilateral renal agenesis. Obstet Gynecol 76:206-209, 1990.
7. Mitchell DG, Nascimento AB, Alam F, et al: Normal adrenal gland: in vivo observations, and high-resolution in vitro chemical shift MR imaging-histologic correlation. Acad Radiol 9:430-436, 2002.
8. Boll DT, Hillenbrand CM, Seaman DM, et al: Assessment of Parallel Acquisition Techniques in Adrenal MR Imaging: Does Increased Temporal Resolution Significantly Improve Characterization of Adrenal Lesions? Toronto, Proceedings of the International Society of Magnetic Resonance Medicine. 2003, p 2333.
9. Ito K, Mitchell DG, Outwater EK, et al: Hepatic lesions: discrimination of nonsolid, benign lesions from solid, malignant lesions with heavily T2-weighted fast spin-echo MR imaging. Radiology 204:729-737, 1997.
10. Blake MA, Jhaveri KS, Sweeney AT, et al: State of the art in adrenal imaging. Current Problems in Diagnostic Radiology 31:67-78, 2002.
11. Dixon WT: Simple proton spectroscopic imaging. Radiology 153:189-194, 1984.
12. Wehrli FW, Perkins TG, Shimakawa A, Roberts F: Chemical shift-induced amplitude modulation in images obtained with gradient refocusing. Magn Reson Imaging 5:157-158, 1987.
13. Namimoto T, Yamashita Y, Mitsuzaki K, et al: Adrenal masses: quantification of fat content with double-echo chemical shift in-phase and opposed-phase FLASH MR images for differentiation of adrenal adenomas [comment]. Radiology 218:642-646, 2001.
14. Martin J, Sentis M, Puig J, et al: Comparison of in-phase and opposed-phase GRE and conventional SE MR pulse sequences in T1-weighted imaging of liver lesions. J Comput Assist Tomogr 20:890-897, 1996.
15. Tsushima Y, Ishizaka H, Matsumoto M: Adrenal masses: differentiation with chemical shift, fast low-angle shot MR imaging. Radiology 186:705-709, 1993.
16. Tsushima Y, Dean PB: Characterization of adrenal masses with chemical shift MR imaging: how to select echo times. Radiology 195:285-286, 1995.
17. Rofsky NM, Lee VS, Laub G, et al: Abdominal MR imaging with a volumetric interpolated breath-hold examination. Radiology 212:876-884, 1999.
18. Krebs TL, Wagner BJ: MR imaging of the adrenal gland: radiologic-pathologic correlation. RadioGraphics 18:1425-1440, 1998.
19. Korobkin M, Giordano TJ, Brodeur FJ, et al: Adrenal adenomas: relationship between histologic lipid and CT and MR findings. Radiology 200:743-747, 1996.
20. Outwater EK, Siegelman ES, Huang AB, Birnbaum BA: Adrenal masses: correlation between CT attenuation value and chemical shift ratio at MR imaging with in-phase and opposed-phase sequences. Radiology 200:749-752, 1996 [erratum 201:880, 1996].
21. Suzuki H, Shibata H, Maruyama T, et al: Significance of steroidogenic enzymes in the pathogenesis of hyperfunctioning and nonhyperfunctioning adrenal tumor. Steroids 60:42-47, 1995.
22. Shibata H, Kobayashi S, Kurihara I, et al: Nuclear receptors and co-regulators in adrenal tumors. Hormone Res 59(Suppl 1):85-93, 2003.
23. Remer EM, Weinfeld RM, Glazer GM, et al: Hyperfunctioning and nonhyperfunctioning benign adrenal cortical lesions: characterization and comparison with MR imaging. Radiology 171:681-685, 1989.
24. Heinz-Peer G, Honigschnabl S, Schneider B, et al: Characterization of adrenal masses using MR imaging with histopathologic correlation [comment]. Am J Roentgenol 173:15-22, 1999.
25. Fujiyoshi F, Nakajo M, Fukukura Y, Tsuchimochi S: Characterization of adrenal tumors by chemical shift fast low-angle shot MR imaging: comparison of four methods of quantitative evaluation. Am J Roentgenol 180:1649-1657, 2003.
26. Siegelman ES: MR imaging of the adrenal neoplasms. Magn Reson Imaging Clin North Am 8:769-786, 2000.
27. Tanabe A, Naruse M, Nishikawa T, et al: Autonomy of cortisol secretion in clinically silent adrenal incidentaloma. Hormone Metab Res 33:444-450, 2001.

28. Grumbach MM, Biller BM, Braunstein GD, et al: Management of the clinically inapparent adrenal mass ("incidentaloma"). Ann Intern Med 138:424-429, 2003.

29. Barzon L, Boscaro M: Diagnosis and management of adrenal incidentalomas. J Urol 163:398-407, 2000.

30. Dunnick NH, Korobkin M, Francis I: Adrenal radiology: distinguishing benign from malignant adrenal masses. Am J Roentgenol 167:861-867, 1996.

31. Vierhapper H: Adrenocortical tumors: clinical symptoms and biochemical diagnosis. Eur J Radiol 41:88-94, 2002.

32. Barry MK, van Heerden JA, Farley DR, et al: Can adrenal incidentalomas be safely observed? World J Surg 22:599-603, 1998.

33. Barzon L, Scaroni C, Sonino N, et al: Risk factors and long-term follow-up of adrenal incidentalomas. J Clin Endocrinol Metab 84:520-526, 1999.

34. Siren J, Tervahartiala P, Sivula A, Haapiainen R: Natural course of adrenal incidentalomas: seven-year follow-up study. World J Surg 24:579-582, 2000.

35. Grossrubatsher E, Vignati F, Possa M, Lohi P: The natural history of incidentally discovered adrenocortical adenomas: a retrospective evaluation. J Endocrinol Invest 24:846-855, 2001.

36. Reincke M: Subclinical Cushing's syndrome. Endocrinol Metab Clin North Am 29:43-56, 2000.

37. Fernandez-Real JM, Engel WR, Simo R, et al: Study of glucose tolerance in consecutive patients harbouring incidental adrenal tumors. Study Group of Incidental Adrenal Adenoma. Clin Endocrinol (Oxf) 49:53-61, 1998.

38. Rossi E, Regolisti G, Negro A, et al: High prevalence of primary aldosteronism using postcaptopril plasma aldosterone to renin ratio as a screening test among Italian hypertensives. Am J Hypertension 15:896-902, 2002.

39. Young WF Jr: Minireview: primary aldosteronism—changing concepts in diagnosis and treatment. Endocrinology 144:2208-2213, 2003.

40. Conn JW: Presidential address. I. Painting background. II: Primary aldosteronism: a new clinical syndrome. J Lab Clin Med 45:3-17, 1955.

41. Sohaib S, Peppercorn PD, Allan C, et al: Primary hyperaldosteronism (Conn syndrome): MR imaging findings. Radiology 214:527-531, 2000.

42. Rossi GP, Sacchetto A, Chiesura-Corona M, et al: Identification of the etiology of primary aldosteronism with adrenal vein sampling in patients with equivocal computed tomography and magnetic resonance findings: results in 104 consecutive cases. J Clin Endocrinol Metab 86:1083-1090, 2001.

43. Hornsby PJ: Aging of the human adrenal cortex. Ageing Res Rev 1:229-242, 2002.

44. Magill SB, Raff H, Shaker JL, et al: Comparison of adrenal vein sampling and computed tomography in the differentiation of primary aldosteronism. J Clin Endocrinol Metab 86:1066-1071, 2001.

45. Doppman JL: The dilemma of bilateral adrenocortical nodularity in Conn's and Cushing's syndromes. Radiol Clin North Am 31:1039-1050, 1993.

46. Lingam RK, Sohaib SA, Vlahos I, et al: CT of primary hyperaldosteronism (Conn's syndrome): the value of measuring the adrenal gland. Am J Roentgenol 181:843-849, 2003.

47. Sternberg SS: Histology for Pathologists, 2nd ed. Philadelphia, Lippincott-Raven, 1997, p 1200.

48. Danilowicz K, Albiger N, Vanegas M, et al: Androgen-secreting adrenal adenomas. Obstet Gynecol 100:1099-1102, 2002.

49. Argrons GA, Lonergan GJ, Dickey GE, Perez-Monte JE: Adrenocortical neoplasms in children: radiologic-pathologic correlation. RadioGraphics 19:989-1008, 1999.

50. Wolthers OD, Cameron FJ, Scheimberg I, et al: Androgen secreting adrenocortical tumors. Arch Dis Child 80:46-50, 1999.

51. Phornphutkul C, Okubo T, Wu K, et al: Aromatase p450 expression in a feminizing adrenal adenoma presenting as isosexual precocious puberty. J Clin Endocrinol Metab 86:649-652, 2001.

52. Bouraima H, Lireux B, Mittre H, et al: Major hyperestrogenism in a feminizing adrenocortical adenoma despite a moderate overexpression of the aromatase enzyme. Eur J Endocrinol 148:457-461, 2003.

53. Derksen J, Nagesser SK, Meinders AE, et al: Identification of virilizing adrenal tumors in hirsute women. N Engl J Med 331:968-973, 1994.

54. Lee MJ, Mayo-Smith WW, Hahn PF, et al: State-of-the-art MR imaging of the adrenal gland. RadioGraphics 14:1015-1029; discussion 1029-1032, 1994.

55. Krestin GP, Steinbrich W, Friedman G: Adrenal masses: evaluation with fast gradient-echo MR imaging and Gd-DTPA-enhanced dynamic studies. Radiology 171:675-680, 1989.

56. Ichikawa T, Ohtomo K, Uchiyama G, et al: Contrast-enhanced dynamic MRI of adrenal masses: classification of characteristic enhancement patterns. Clin Radiol 50:295-300, 1995.

57. Mitchell DG, Crovello M, Matteucci T, et al: Benign adrenocortical masses: diagnosis with chemical shift MR imaging. Radiology 185:345-351, 1992.

58. Semelka RC, Shoenut JP, Lawrence PH, et al: Evaluation of adrenal masses with gadolinium enhancement and fat-suppressed MR imaging. J Magn Reson Imaging 3:337-343, 1993.

59. Korobkin M, Lombardi TJ, Aisen AM, et al: Characterization of adrenal masses with chemical shift and gadolinium-enhanced MR imaging. Radiology 197:411-418, 1995.

60. Mayo-Smith WW, Lee MJ, McNicholas MM, et al: Characterization of adrenal masses (<5 cm) by use of chemical shift MR imaging: observer performance versus quantitative measures. Am J Roentgenol 165:91-95, 1995.

61. Bilbey JH, McLoughlin RF, Kurkjian PS, et al: MR imaging of adrenal masses: value of chemical-shift imaging for distinguishing adenomas from other tumors. Am J Roentgenol 164:637-642, 1995.

62. Outwater EK, Siegelman ES, Radecki PD, et al: Distinction between benign and malignant adrenal masses: value of T1-weighted chemical-shift MR imaging. Am J Roentgenol 165:579-583, 1995.

63. Schwartz LH, Panicek DM, Koutcher JA, et al: Adrenal masses in patients with malignancy: prospective comparison of echo-planar, fast spin-echo, and chemical shift MR imaging. Radiology 197:421-425, 1995.

64. McNicholas MM, Lee MJ, Mayo-Smith WW, et al: An imaging algorithm for the differential diagnosis of adrenal adenomas and metastases. Am J Roentgenol 165:1453-1459, 1995.

65. Schwartz LH, Panicek DM, Doyle MV, et al: Comparison of two algorithms and their associated charges when evaluating adrenal masses in patients with malignancies. Am J Roentgenol 168:1575-1578, 1997.

66. Honigschnabl S, Gallo S, Niederle B, et al: How accurate is MR imaging in characterisation of adrenal masses: update of a long-term study. Eur J Radiol 41:113-122, 2002.

67. Korobkin M, Brodeur FJ, Francis IR, et al: Delayed enhanced CT for differentiation of benign from malignant adrenal masses. Radiology 200:737-742, 1996.

68. Korobkin M, Brodeur FJ, Francis IR, et al: CT time-attenuation washout curves of adrenal adenomas and nonadenomas. Am J Roentgenol 170:747-752, 1998.

69. Caoili EM, Korobkin M, Francis IR, et al: Delayed enhanced CT of lipid-poor adrenal adenomas. Am J Roentgenol 175:1411-1415, 2000.

70. Pena CS, Boland GW, Hahn PF, et al: Characterization of indeterminate (lipid-poor) adrenal masses: use of washout characteristics at contrast-enhanced CT. Radiology 217:798-802, 2000.

71. Newhouse JH, Heffess CS, Wagner BJ, et al: Large degenerated adrenal adenomas: radiologic-pathologic correlation. Radiology 210:385-391, 1999.

72. Elashry OM, Clayman RV, Soble JJ, McDougall EM: Laparoscopic adrenalectomy for solitary metachronous contralateral adrenal metastasis from renal cell carcinoma. J Urol 157:1217-1222, 1997.

73. Shinozaki K, Yoshimitsu K, Honda H, et al: Metastatic adrenal tumor from clear-cell renal cell carcinoma: a pitfall of chemical shift MR imaging. Abdom Imaging 26:439-442, 2001.

74. Schwartz LH, Macari M, Huvos AG, Panicek DM: Collision tumors of the adrenal gland: demonstration and characterization at MR imaging. Radiology 201:757-760, 1996.

75. Otal P, Escourrou G, Mazerolles C, et al: Imaging features of uncommon adrenal masses with histopathologic correlation. RadioGraphics 19:569-581, 1999.

76. Shifrin RY, Bechtold RE, Scharling ES: Metastatic adenocarcinoma within an adrenal adenoma: detection with chemical shift imaging. Am J Roentgenol 167:891-892, 1996.

77. Han M, Burnett AL, Fishman EK, Marshall FF: The natural history and treatment of adrenal myelolipoma. J Urol 157:1213-1216, 1997.

78. Lam KY, Lo CY: Adrenal lipomatous tumours: a 30 year clinicopathological experience at a single institution. J Clin Pathol 54:707-712, 2001.

79. Osborn M, Smith M, Senbanjo T, et al: Adrenal myelolipoma—clinical, radiological, and cytological findings: a case report. Cytopathology 13:242-246, 2002.

80. Hoeffel C, Chelle C, Clement A, Hoeffel JC: Spontaneous retroperitoneal hemorrhage from a giant adrenal myelolipoma (comment). J Urol 158:2251, 1997.

81. Hoeffel C, Kowalski S: Giant myelolipoma of the adrenal gland: natural history. Clin Radiol 55:402-404, 2000.

82. Appetecchia M, Chilelli M, Sciarretta F, Anza M: Bilateral symptomatic adrenal myelolipoma. Urol Int 62:37-39, 1999.

83. Russell C, Goodacre BW, van Sonnenberg E, Orihuela E: Spontaneous rupture of adrenal myelolipoma: spiral CT appearance. Abdom Imaging 25:431-434, 2000.

84. Kenney PJ, Wagner BJ, Rao P, Heffess CS: Myelolipoma: CT and pathologic features. Radiology 208:87-95, 1998.

85. Rao P, Kenney PJ, Wagner BJ, Davidson AJ: Imaging and pathologic features of myelolipoma. RadioGraphics 17:1373-1385, 1997.

86. Ng L, Libertino JM: Adrenocorticol carcinoma: diagnosis, evaluation and treatment. J Urol 169:5-11, 2003.

87. Reincke M: Adrenocortical tumors and oncogenes. In Margioris AN, Chrousos GP (eds): Adrenal Disorders, Contemporary Endocrinology. Totowa, NJ, Humana Press, 2001, pp 219-230.

88. Lockhart ME, Smith JK, Kenney PJ: Imaging of adrenal masses. Eur J Radiol 41:95-112, 2002.

89. Cifci AO, Senocak ME, Tanyel FC, Buyukpamukcu N: Adrenocortical tumors in children. J Pediatr Surg 36:549-554, 2001.

90. Schulick RD, Brennan MF: Adrenocortical carcinoma. World J Urol 17:26-34, 1999.

91. Sohaib SA, Reznik RH: Adrenal imaging. BJU Int 86:95-110, 2000.

92. Schlund JF, Kenney PJ, Brown ED, et al: Adrenocortical carcinoma: MR imaging appearance with current techniques. J Magn Reson Imaging 5:171-174, 1995.

93. Yamada T, Saito H, Moriya T, et al: Adrenal carcinoma with a signal loss on chemical shift magnetic resonance imaging. J Comput Assist Tomogr 27:606-608, 2003.

94. Morrison PJ, Nevin NC: Multiple endocrine neoplasia type 2 B (mucosal neuroma syndrome, Wagenmann-Froboese syndrome). J Med Genet 33:779-782, 1996.

95. Hoff AO, Cote GJ, Gagel RF: Multiple endocrine neoplasias. Annu Rev Physiol 62:377-411, 2000.

96. Pacak K, Chrousos GP, Koch CA, et al: Pheochromocytoma: Progress in diagnosis, therapy, and genetics. In Margioris AN, Chrousos GP (eds): Adrenal Disorders, Contemporary Endocrinology. Totowa, NJ, Humana Press, 2001, pp 379-413.

97. Neumann HP, Bausch B, McWhinney SR, et al: Germ-line mutations in nonsyndromic pheochromocytoma. N Engl J Med 346:1459-1466, 2002.

98. Bravo EL, Tagle R: Pheochromocytoma: state-of-the-art and future prospects. Endocrinol Rev 24:539-553, 2003.

99. Hes FJ, Hoppener JW, Lips CJ: Clinical review 155: Pheochromocytoma in von Hippel-Lindau disease. J Clin Endocrinol Metab 88:969-974, 2003.

100. Ritter MM, Frilling A, Crossey PA, et al: Isolated familial pheochromocytoma as a variant of von Hippel-Lindau disease. J Clin Endocrinol Metab 81:1035-1037, 1996.

101. Tattersall DJ, Moore NR: von Hippel-Lindau disease: MRI of abdominal manifestations. Clin Radiol 57:85-92, 2002.

102. Walther MM, Herring J, Enquist E, et al: von Recklinghausen's disease and pheochromocytomas. J Urol 162:1582-1586, 1999.

103. Salmenkivi K, Heikkila P, Liu J, et al: VEGF in 105 pheochromocytomas: enhanced expression correlates with malignant outcome. Apmis 111:458-464, 2003.

104. Salmenkivi K, Arola J, Voutilainen R, et al: Inhibin/activin β-subunit expression in pheochromocytomas favors benign diagnosis. J Clin Endocrinol Metab 86:2231-2235, 2001.

105. Cirillo RL Jr, Bennett WF, Vitellas KM, et al: Pathology of the adrenal gland: imaging features. Am J Roentgenol 170:429-435, 1998.

106. Beland SS, Vesely DL, Arnold WC, et al: Localization of adrenal and extra-adrenal pheochromocytomas by magnetic resonance imaging. South Med J 82:1410-1413, 1989.

107. Varghese JC, Hahn PF, Papanicolaou N, et al: MR differentiation of phaeochromocytoma from other adrenal lesions based on qualitative analysis of T2 relaxation times. Clin Radiol 52:603-606, 1997.

108. Kudva YC, Sawka AM, Young WF Jr: Clinical review 164: The laboratory diagnosis of adrenal pheochromocytoma: the Mayo Clinic experience. J Clin Endocrinol Metab 88:4533-4539, 2003.

109. Rha SE, Byun JY, Jung SE, et al: Neurogenic tumors in the abdomen: tumor types and imaging characteristics. RadioGraphics 23:29-43, 2003.

110. Brodeur GM: Neuroblastoma: biological insights into a clinical enigma. Nat Rev Cancer 3:203-216, 2003.

111. Siegel MJ: MR imaging of pediatric abdominal neoplasms. Magn Reson Imaging Clin North Am 8:837-851, 2000.

112. Berthold F, Hero B: Neuroblastoma: current drug therapy recommendations as part of the total treatment approach. Drugs 59:1261-1277, 2000.

113. Ikeda H, Iehara T, Tsuchida Y, et al: Experience with International Neuroblastoma Staging System and Pathology Classification. Br J Cancer 86:1110-1116, 2002.

114. Lonergan GJ, Schwab CM, Suarez ES, Carlson CL: Neuroblastoma, ganglio-neuroblastoma, and ganglioneuroma: radiologic-pathologic correlation. RadioGraphics 22:911-934, 2002.

115. Kerbl R, Urban CE, Ambros IM, et al: Neuroblastoma mass screening in late infancy: insights into the biology of neuroblastic tumors. J Clin Oncol 21:4228-4234, 2003.

116. Schilling FH, Spix C, Berthold F, et al: Children may not benefit from neuroblastoma screening at 1 year of age. Updated results of the population based controlled trial in Germany. Cancer Lett 197:19-28, 2003.

117. Westra SJ, Zaninovic AC, Hall TR, et al: Imaging of the adrenal gland in children. RadioGraphics 14:1323-1340, 1994.

118. Lam KY, Lo CY: Metastatic tumours of the adrenal glands: a 30-year experience in a teaching hospital. Clin Endocrinol (Oxf) 56:95-101, 2002.

119. Pope RJ, Hansell DM: Extra-thoracic staging of lung cancer. Eur J Radiol 45:31-38, 2003.

120. Vincent JM, Morrison ID, Armstrong P, Reznek RH: Computed tomography of diffuse, non-metastatic enlargement of the adrenal glands in patients with malignant disease. Clin Radiol 49:456-460, 1994.

121. Paling MR, Williamson BR: Adrenal involvement in non-Hodgkin lymphoma. Am J Roentgenol 141:303-305, 1983.

122. Lee FT Jr, Thornbury JR, Grist TM, Kelcz F: MR imaging of adrenal lymphoma. Abdom Imaging 18:95-96, 1993.

123. Kato H, Itami J, Shiina T, et al: MR imaging of primary adrenal lymphoma. Clin Imaging 20:126-128, 1996.

124. Matsuda T, Okihama Y, Egami K, et al: Complete cure of malignant lymphoma of the stomach with a huge adrenal lesion achieved by preoperative chemotherapy and surgery: report of a case. Surg Today 31:62-67, 2001.

125. Mayo-Smith WW, Boland GW, Noto RB, Lee MJ: State-of-the-art adrenal imaging. RadioGraphics 21:995-1012, 2001.

126. Wilson DA, Muchmore HG, Tisdal RG, et al: Histoplasmosis of the adrenal glands studied by CT. Radiology 150:779-783, 1984.

127. Radin DR: Disseminated histoplasmosis: abdominal CT findings in 16 patients. Am J Roentgenol 157:955-958, 1991.

128. Kawashima A, Sandler CM, Fishman EK, et al: Spectrum of CT findings in non-malignant disease of the adrenal gland. RadioGraphics 18:393-412, 1998.

129. Kumar N, Singh S, Govil S: Adrenal histoplasmosis: clinical presentation and imaging features in nine cases. Abdom Imaging 28:703-708, 2003.

130. Swartz MA, Scofield RH, Dickey WD, et al: Unilateral adrenal enlargement due to *Histoplasma capsulatum*. Clin Infect Dis 23:813-815, 1996.

131. Villabona CM, Sahun M, Ricart W, et al: Tuberulous Addison's disease. Utility of CT in diagnosis and follow-up. Eur J Radiol 17:210-213, 1993.

132. Steffens J, Zaubitzer T, Kirsch W, Humke U: Neonatal adrenal abscesses. Eur Urol 31:347-349, 1997.

133. Midiri M, Finazzo M, Bartolotta TV, Maria MD: Nocardial adrenal abscess: CT and MR findings. Eur Radiol 8:466-468, 1998.

134. Arena F, Romeo C, Manganaro A, et al: Bilateral neonatal adrenal abscess. Report of two cases and review of the literature. Pediatr Med Chir 25:185-189, 2003.

135. Levine E: CT evaluation of active adrenal histoplasmosis. Urol Radiol 13:103-106, 1991.

136. Efremidis SC, Harsoulis F, Douma S, et al: Adrenal insufficiency with enlarged adrenals. Abdom Imaging 21:168-171, 1996.

137. Redd DC, Soulen MC, Crooks GW: Bilateral adrenal hemorrhage resulting in acute adrenal insufficiency as an unusual complication of hepatic arterial chemoembolization. J Vasc Interv Radiol 9:271-274, 1998.

138. Kawashima A, Sandler CM, Ernst RD, et al: Imaging of nontraumatic hemorrhage of the adrenal gland. RadioGraphics 19:949-963, 1999.

139. Vella A, Nippoldt TB, Morris JC 3rd: Adrenal hemorrhage: a 25-year experience at the Mayo Clinic. Mayo Clin Proc 76:161-168, 2001.

140. Kovacs KA, Lam YM, Pater JL: Bilateral massive adrenal hemorrhage. Assessment of putative risk factors by the case-control method. Medicine (Baltimore) 80:45-53, 2001.

141. Gomez RG, McAninch JW, Carroll PR: Adrenal gland trauma: diagnosis and management. J Trauma 35:870-874, 1993.

142. Asensio JA, Rojo E, Roldan G, Petrone P: Isolated adrenal gland injury from penetrating trauma. J Trauma 54:364-365, 2003.

143. Burks DW, Mirvis SE, Shanmuganathan K: Acute adrenal injury after blunt abdominal trauma: CT findings. Am J Roentgenol 158:503-507, 1992.

144. Rammelt S, Mucha D, Amlang M, Zwipp H: Bilateral adrenal hemorrhage in blunt abdominal trauma. J Trauma 48:332-335, 2000.

145. Cozzolino D, Peerzada J, Heaney JA: Adrenal insufficiency from bilateral adrenal hemorrhage after total knee replacement surgery. Urology 50:125-127, 1997.

146. Williams GH, Dluhy RG: Disease of the adrenal cortex. In Harrison TR, Fauci AS (eds): Harrison's Principles of Internal Medicine, 14th ed. New York, McGraw-Hill, 1998, pp 2035-2057.

147. Murphy JF, Purdue GF, Hunt JL: Acute adrenal insufficiency in the patient with burns. J Burn Care Rehabil 14:155-157, 1993.

148. Sheridan RL, Ryan CM, Tompkins RG: Acute adrenal insufficiency in the burn intensive care unit. Burns 19:63-66, 1993.

149. Bowen AD, Keslar PJ, Newman B, Hashida Y: Adrenal hemorrhage after liver transplantation. Radiology 176:85-88, 1990.

150. Bober E, Kovanlikaya A, Buyukgebiz A: Primary antiphospholipid syndrome: an unusual cause of adrenal insufficiency. Hormone Res 56:140-144, 2001.

151. Espinosa G, Santos E, Cervera R, et al: Adrenal involvement in the anti-phospholipid syndrome: clinical and immunologic characteristics of 86 patients. Medicine (Baltimore) 82:106-118, 2003.

152. Warkentin TE: Heparin-induced thrombocytopenia. Curr Hematol Rep 1:63-72, 2002.

153. Yamada AH, Sherrod SE, Boswell W, Skinner DG: Massive retroperitoneal hemorrhage from adrenal gland metastasis. Urology 40:59-62, 1992.

154. Kinoshita A, Nakano M, Suyama N, et al: Massive adrenal hemorrhage secondary to metastasis of lung cancer. Intern Med 36:815-818, 1997.

155. Thompson KE, Willard TB, Kuvshinoff B, Teague JL: Adrenal hemorrhage mimicking an abdominal aortic aneurysm. Urology 61:1260, 2003.

156. Kartsios C, Kaloyannidis P, Yannaki E, et al: Spontaneous adrenal hemor-rhage as a manifestation of isolated relapse of non-Hodgkin's lymphoma. Acta Haematol 110:197-199, 2003.

157. Outwater E, Bankoff MS: Clinically significant adrenal hemorrhage secondary to metastases. Computed tomography observations. Clin Imaging 13:195-200, 1989.

158. Caron P, Chabannier MH, Cambus JP, et al: Definitive adrenal insufficiency due to bilateral adrenal hemorrhage and primary antiphospholipid syndrome. J Clin Endocrinol Metab 83:1437-1439, 1998.

159. Foster DG: Adrenal cysts. Review of literature and report of case. Arch Surg 92:131-143, 1966.

160. Tanuma Y, Kimura M, Sakai S: Adrenal cyst: a review of the Japanese literature and report of a case. Int J Urol 8:500-503, 2001.

161. Schoretsanitis G, de Bree E, Melissas J, Tsiftsis D: Primary hydatid cyst of the adrenal gland. Scand J Urol Nephrol 32:51-53, 1998.

162. Escudero MD, Sabater L, Calvete J, et al: Arterial hypertension due to primary adrenal hydatid cyst. Surgery 132:894-895, 2002.

163. Karayiannakis AJ, Polychronidis A, Simopoulos C: Giant adrenal pseudocyst presenting with gastric outlet obstruction and hypertension. Urology 59:946, 2002.

164. Rozenblit A, Morehouse HT, Amis ES Jr: Cystic adrenal lesions: CT features. Radiology 201:541-548, 1996.

165. Jaresch S, Kornely E, Kley HK, Schlaghecke R: Adrenal incidentaloma and patients with homozygous or heterozygous congenital adrenal hyperplasia. J Clin Endocrinol Metab 74:685-689, 1992.

166. Sohaib SA, Hanson JA, Newell-Price JD, et al: CT appearance of the adrenal glands in adrenocorticotrophic hormone-dependent Cushing's syndrome. Am J Roentgenol 172:997-1002, 1999.

167. Doppman JL, Nieman LK, Travis WD, et al: CT and MR imaging of massive macronodular adrenocortical disease: a rare cause of autonomous primary adrenal hypercortisolism. J Comput Assist Tomogr 15:773-779, 1991.

168. Doppman JL, Chrousos GP, Papanicolaou DA, et al: Adrenocorticotropin-independent macronodular adrenal hyperplasia: an uncommon cause of primary adrenal hypercortisolism. Radiology 216:797-802, 2000.

169. Shinojima H, Kakizaki H, Usuki T, et al: Clinical and endocrinological features of adrenocorticotropic hormone-independent bilateral macronodular adrenocortical hyperplasia. J Urol 166:1639-1642, 2001.

170. Stergiopoulos SG, Stratakis CA: Human tumors associated with Carney complex and germline PRKAR1A mutations: a protein kinase A disease! FEBS Lett 546:59-64, 2003.

171. Travis WD, Tsokos M, Doppman JL, et al: Primary pigmented nodular adrenocortical disease. A light and electron microscopic study of eight cases. Am J Surg Pathol 13:921-930, 1989.

172. Bourdeau I, Lacroix A, Schurch W, et al: Primary pigmented nodular adrenocortical disease: paradoxical responses of cortisol secretion to dexamethasone occur in vitro and are associated with increased expression of the gluocorticoid receptor. J Clin Endocrinol Metab 88:3931-3937, 2003.

173. Doppman JL, Travis WD, Nieman L, et al: Cushing syndrome due to primary pigmented nodular adrenocortical disease: findings at CT and MR imaging. Radiology 172:415-420, 1989.

174. Groussin L, Kirschner LS, Vincent-Dejean C, et al: Molecular analysis of the cyclic AMP-dependent protein kinase A (PKA) regulatory subunit 1A (PRKAR1A) gene in patients with Carney complex and primary pigmented nodular adrenocortical disease (PPNAD) reveals novel mutations and clues for pathophysiology: augmented PKA signaling is associated with adrenal tumorigenesis in PPNAD. Am J Hum Genet 71:1433-1442, 2002.

175. Lania A, Mantovani G, Spada A: G protein mutations in endocrine diseases. Eur J Endocrinol 145:543-559, 2001.

176. Soule S: Addison's disease in Africa—a teaching hospital experience. Clin Endocrinol (Oxf) 50:115-120, 1999.

177. Arlt W, Allolio B: Adrenal insufficiency. Lancet 361:1881-1893, 2003.

178. Potti A, Schell DA: Unusual presentations of thoracic tumors: Case 1. Acute adrenal insufficiency due to metastatic lung cancer. J Clin Oncol 19:3780-3782, 2001.

179. Pimentel M, Johnston JB, Allan DR, et al: Primary adrenal lymphoma associated with adrenal insufficiency: a distinct clinical entity. Leuk Lymphoma 24:363-367, 1997.

180. Takamura T, Nagai Y, Yamashita H, et al: Adrenal insufficiency due to metastatic hepatocellular carcinoma. Endocrine J 46:591-596, 1999.

181. Dorin RI, Qualls CR, Crapo LM: Diagnosis of adrenal insufficiency. Ann Intern Med 139:194-204, 2003.

88

URINARY BLADDER CANCER

Essam Abou-Bieh ● Tarek A. El-Diasty ● Jelle O. Barentsz

INTRODUCTION

Bladder cancer is more common in males than in females with a ratio of approximately 4:1, and is predominantly seen in the sixth and seventh decades of life.[1,2] In countries where schistosomiasis is endemic, like Egypt and other African countries, bladder cancer accounts for 11% of all malignant diseases.[3] These cancers are mostly of the squamous cell type.[4] Elsewhere bladder cancer is rare in the first decade of life but after this age the incidence rises steadily.[3] The most frequent location of urinary bladder cancer is the posterior and lateral wall near the vesicoureteric junction.[5]

Determination of local tumor staging and detection of nodal or bone metastases are extremely important.[1,6,7] Appropriate use of the different techniques is crucial for accurate assessment of prognosis and for the development of appropriate treatment planning. As clinical staging is not reliable for determining tumor extension beyond the bladder wall, imaging techniques are needed.[8]

Among the noninvasive imaging modalities, MRI is the modality of choice for imaging urinary bladder cancer. Multiplaner capabilities and superior soft-tissue make this technique a valuable tool for imaging the urinary bladder. In addition, recent advances, such as high-resolution fast imaging sequences, and the use of pelvic phased-array coils and contrast agents, further improve the imaging quality and thus the diagnostic accuracy for staging urinary bladder carcinoma.[1,9]

This chapter will review the general features of urinary bladder cancer and the role of imaging, especially MRI.

NORMAL ANATOMY

Urinary Bladder Wall

The urinary bladder wall consists of the muscularis and mucosa, and is covered by the pelvic peritoneum which constitutes the serosa. The muscularis is made up of the three layers of smooth muscle that intermingle to such an extent that their boundaries are indistinct.[10] In the outer layer, the smooth muscle bundles are oriented longitudinally along its side and then transversely over its dome. The thin middle layer is discontinuous and its scattered bundles are predominantly circular or oblique. The fibers of the thin inner layer are again primarily longitudinal.[11]

The mucosa lining the bladder is loosely attached to the muscularis and has a transitional epithelium, which is thin in the full bladder but thicker when the wall is contracted.[11]

Lymphatic Drainage of the Urinary Bladder

The pelvic lymph nodes are classified according to the accompanying vessels (Fig. 88-1):[12]

● *Common iliac lymph nodes:* located around the common iliac arteries.
● *External iliac lymph nodes:* these are arranged in three chains—lateral chain on the lateral aspect of the external iliac artery; middle chain anterior and medial

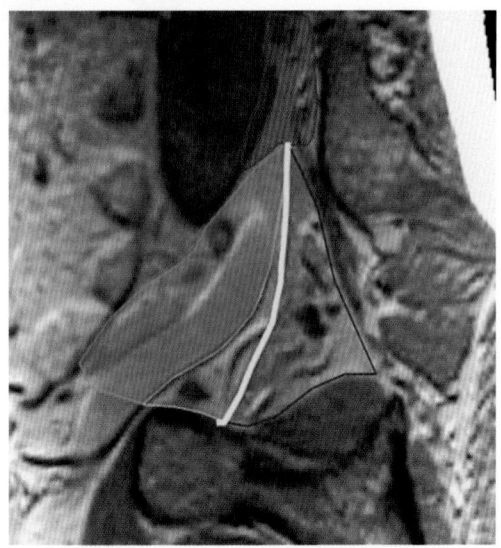

FIGURE 88-1

Lymphatic drainage of the urinary bladder. Common iliac lymph node area (red); external iliac lymph node area (green); "obturator" area (yellow); obturator nerve (yellow line); internal iliac/hypogastric lymph nodes (blue).

to the external iliac vein; medial or "obturator" chain posterior to the external iliac vein against the pelvic sidewall, ventral to the obturator nerve.

- *Internal iliac (or hypogastric) lymph nodes:* located anterior to the piriform muscle, around the inferior gluteal artery and vein, dorsal to the obturator nerve.
- *Superficial inguinal lymph nodes:* lie caudal to the inguinal ligament anterior to the femoral artery and vein.

The lymphatic drainage goes from the anterior bladder wall directly to the obturator nodes, and from the posterior bladder wall to the internal iliac nodes, or occasionally to the presacral nodes.[13]

URINARY BLADDER CANCER

Histologic Types

Transitional Cell Carcinoma

Transitional cell cancer is the most common primary bladder malignancy and arises from the mucosa. The predominant form is the papillary type. It is most frequently located at the lateral wall and less often at the posterior wall.[14] Transitional cell carcinoma of the urinary bladder is classified histologically according to the World Health Organization (WHO) grading system:

- *Grade I:* papillary projections lined by neoplastic transitional epithelial cells that show minimal nuclear polymorphism and mitotic activity; papillae are long and delicate; fusion of papillae is focal and limited.

- *Grade II:* histologic and cytologic features are intermediate between those of grade I (the best differentiated) and grade III (the most poorly differentiated).
- *Grade III:* significant nuclear polymorphism, frequent mitosis, and fusion of papillae are typical. Occasional bizarre cells may be present, and focal sites of squamous differentiation are often seen. Although invasion of the underlying bladder wall muscle may occur with any grade of transitional cell carcinoma, it is most frequently seen in grade III.

Squamous Cell Carcinoma

Squamous cell cancer accounts for 3% to 8% of all bladder malignancies in the Western world, with an age and sex distribution similar to transitional cell carcinoma. Risk factors are urinary tract infection, urolithiasis, chronic indwelling catheter, and schistosomiasis. These tumors are ulcerating and infiltrating rather than exophytic.[15] All patients with squamous cell carcinoma usually have invasion of the bladder wall at the time of initial presentation, and thus have a worse prognosis than those with transitional cell carcinoma.[16]

Adenocarcinoma

Adenocarcinoma is an uncommon type of bladder malignancy. All variants of adenocarcinoma can be seen in the urinary bladder. Its histologic pattern includes papillary, glandular, mucinous, adenoid, cystic, signet ring cell, and clear-cell type. Foci of transitional cell carcinoma with or without areas of squamous cell carcinoma may be observed. An association with cystitis cystica and cystitis glandularis has been reported in the majority of cases.[3]

Mesenchymal Tumors

Leiomyoma, hemangioma, glandular cell tumors, and neurofibroma have been reported to arise within the urinary bladder. Rhabdomyosarcoma commonly occurs in children. This is an edematous mucosal polypoid mass linked to a cluster of grapes.[3] Hemangioma is uncommon in the urinary bladder.[15]

Metastatic Tumors

The urinary bladder can sometimes be involved by direct extension of cancers from adjacent organs.[3]

Staging

A uniform TNM system staging system is used for evaluating bladder cancer (Table 88-1).[16,17] This system addresses the depth of invasion of an epithelial tumor through the mucosa and muscle layer of the bladder, and the presence or absence of penetration into extravesical structures, adjacent organs, and the pelvic and

TABLE 88-1 TNM Classification of Bladder Carcinoma

Stage	Extent of Invasion
PT_x	Extent of invasion cannot be assessed
PT_{is}	Carcinoma in situ
PT_a	Papillary, noninvasive tumor
PT_1	Tumor not extending beyond the lamina propria
PT_2	Superficial muscle invasion, not more than half way through the muscle coat.
PT_3	Deep muscle invasion (more than half way through the muscle coat or invasion of perivesical tissue).
PT_4	Invasion of extravesical structures
N_0	No lymph node involvement
N_1	Involvement of single homolateral lymph node
N_2	Involvement of contralateral or bilateral lymph nodes
N_3	Fixed regional lymph nodes
N_4	Common iliac, aortic, or inguinal lymph nods
M_0	No metastasis
M_1	Distant metastasis

From Macvicar AD: Bladder cancer staging. Br J Urol 86:111-121, 2000.

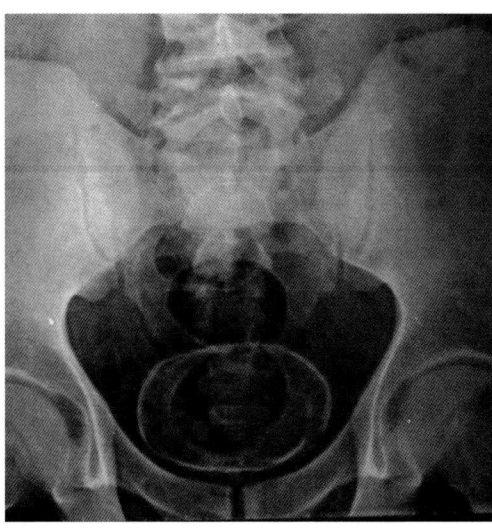

FIGURE 88-2

Plain X-ray of the pelvis showing the calcified bladder wall due to bilharzias.

abdominal walls (T stage). Also, the presence of lymph node (N stage) and distant metastases (M stage) are included in this classification.

Spread

Direct Extension

Invasive bladder cancer initially spreads radially through the inner bladder wall and then circumferentially through the muscular layer. Depending on its point of origin, it may invade perivesical fat, prostate, seminal vesicles, or obturator internus muscle. In women, it rarely invades the uterus or cervix. Invasion of or growth into the ureter or urethra is common when the tumor originates near one of these structures.[18]

Lymphatic Spread

Lymphatic spread in the pelvic chains is found in 25% of invasive tumors, and is seen in the three major lymphatic trunks that drain into the external iliac nodal groups. Although lymphatic spread into the external iliac group is much more common, spread from the posterior bladder wall with drainage into internal (hypogastric) nodes also may occur.[19,20]

Hematogenous Spread

Hematogenous spread of bladder carcinoma is infrequent. If it occurs, these metastases usually appear in the bones, lungs, and liver. Bony metastases predominantly are seen in, in order of frequency, pelvic bones, upper femora, ribs, and skull, and are always osteolytic.[21]

Implantation

Bladder cancer can also spread by implantation in abdominal wounds, denuded urothelium, resected prostatic fossa, or a traumatized urethra.

RADIOLOGIC EXAMINATION

Plain Radiography

In a bladder with bilharzia (schistosomasis) complicated by carcinoma, plain radiography may suggest the correct diagnosis. Calcification of the wall of the bilharzial bladder usually appears as a continuous curved line of calcification, either smooth or irregular in contour depending on the state of distention (Fig. 88-2). If bladder cancer develops the continuity of the linear calcification is usually interrupted.[22]

Dystrophic calcification infrequently may occur in a necrotic bladder tumor, which is visible on the plain film as a finely speckled collection of calcifications, or as a well circumscribed calcification with a dense or even a calcified nodule in the bladder region.[22,23]

Intravenous Urography

Intravenous urography is performed to exclude upper renal tract abnormalities.[24] It is important to have films with the patient both in the prone and supine position. A filling defect is only visible when the lesion is surrounded by opaque urine. Hence, carcinoma of the posterior wall of the bladder is seen best with the patient in the supine position, and carcinoma of the anterior wall with the patient in the prone position. Oblique views of the bladder may also be helpful in the detection and localization of lesions.[24]

If the tumor is located near the ureteral orifice, there may be incomplete or even complete obstruction subsequent to dilatation of the urinary tract or even decreased excretion of the kidney on that side.[5] When one nonexcretory kidney is found in the presence of bladder cancer, an antegrade pyelogram can be helpful.

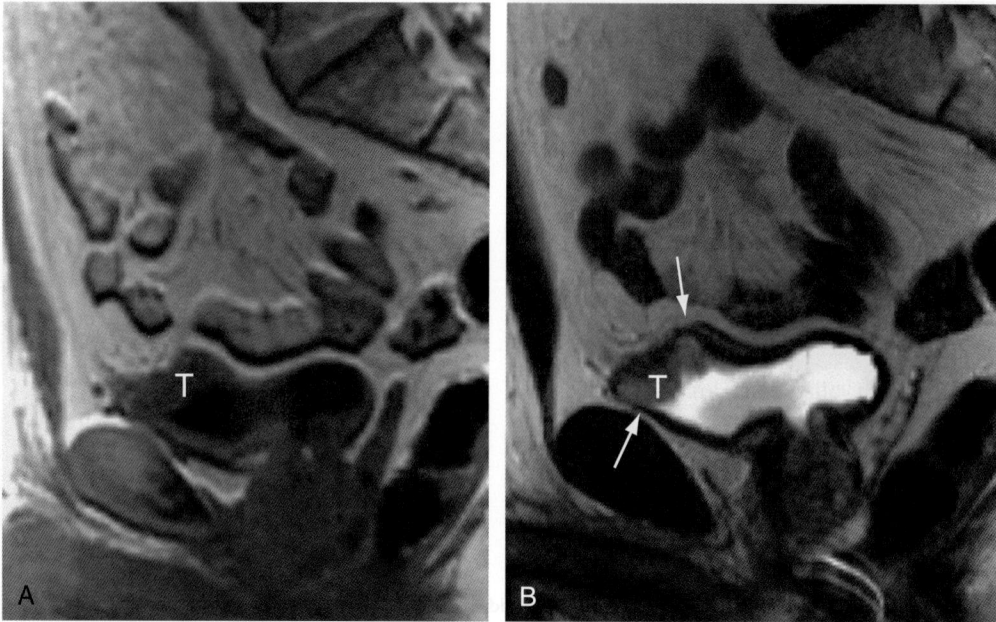

FIGURE 88-4

Stage T2b bladder cancer. **A,** On the T1-weighted MR image, tumor (T) has identical signal intensity to the bladder wall. Urine has lower and perivesical fat has higher signal intensity. **B,** On the T2-weighted MR image, tumor has higher signal intensity than the bladder wall, and lower than urine. It can be seen that the bladder wall is disrupted by tumor (*arrows*), which argues for at least deep muscle invasion (stage T2b).

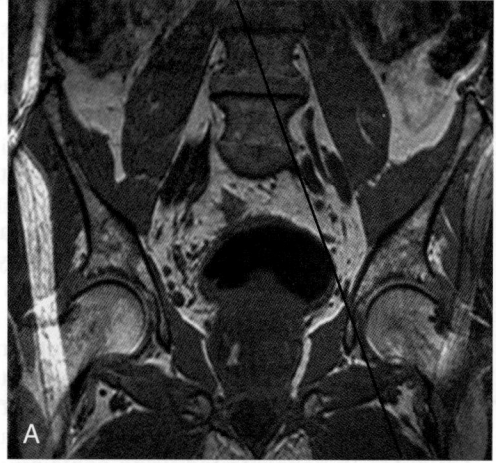

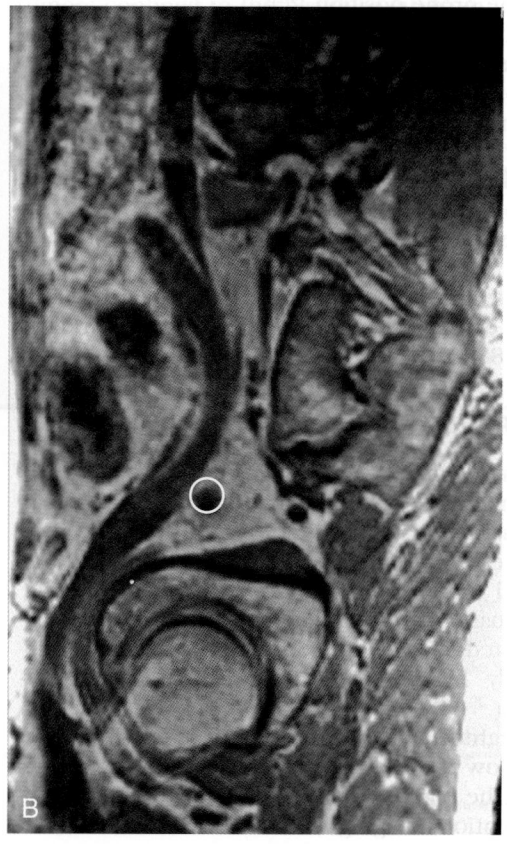

FIGURE 88-5

Normal node. **A,** Coronal T1-weighted image with the imaging plane parallel to the psoas muscle ("obturator" plane) (*black line*). **B,** T1-weighted "obturator" plane image shows a small 3 mm normal node (*circle*) which can easily be separated from the longitudinal running vessels.

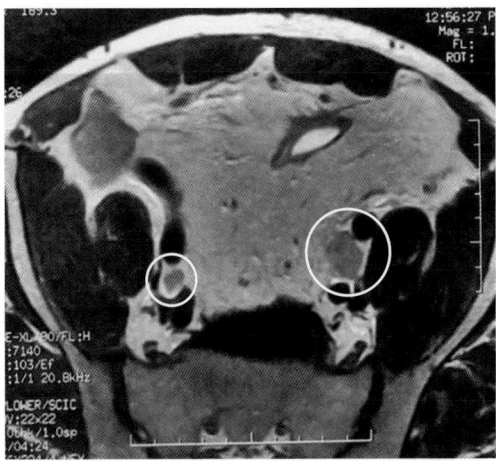

FIGURE 88-6

Metastatic enlarged nodes (*circles*). On the T2-weighted image nodes have higher signal intensity compared to muscle, and identical signal intensity compared to bladder cancer.

higher than that of muscle. T1-weighted images provide the optimal contrast between medium intensity nodes and high intensity fat.[7]

Optimizing MRI of the Urinary Bladder

Several factors, related both to the patient and the technique, must be considered when trying to optimize MRI of the urinary bladder. The most important are motion-artifact reduction,[35] and the degree of bladder filling.[32] Selection of appropriate pulse sequences, and the use of surface coils and contrast agent must also be considered when trying to improve image quality.[1]

Artifact Reduction

Voluntary motion artifacts can be reduced by making the patient feel at ease. Sedatives are effective in claustrophobic patients.[36] Intestinal motion artifacts can be reduced by giving 0.5 mL of glucagon or buscopan intramuscularly before the examination and 1.5 mL of glucagon by an intravenous drip infusion during the examination.[32] Respiratory motion artifacts are not a major problem in pelvic scanning, though a retroperitoneal lymph nodal survey may be affected.[34] These artifacts can be reduced by wrapping an adjustable belt around the patient's abdomen to cause a slight compression.[32] Vascular pulsation artifacts can be reduced by using flow compensation.[37,38]

Bladder Distention

Adequate distention of the bladder will improve evaluation of the wall and allows visualization of focal lesions. However, if the bladder is too distended, small lesions may be stretched and harder to visualize. Also, the patient will be uncomfortable and more likely to move.[32]

Optimal distention of the urinary bladder can be achieved by asking the patient to void 2 hours before the examination and then not again until it is completed.[32]

Imaging Planes

In general, axial images should be acquired using T1- and T2-weighted sequences followed by imaging in other planes. The direction of these planes depends on the site of the tumor.[1,14] For example, coronal images are particularly helpful for visualizing tumors arising from the base, dome, and lateral bladder wall, whereas sagittal images can be used to visualize anterior and cranially located tumors and tumors at the bladder sphincter. In addition, images should be acquired in a plane perpendicular to the wall at the base of the tumor.[39] This allows better delineation of muscle involvement. Use of multiplanar reconstruction with a 3D sequence gives the best results. An important plane direction in evaluating lymph nodes is parallel to the psoas muscle. This so-called "obtutator plane" allows visualization of nodes along its long axis and can locate them in relation to the iliac vessels and obturator nerve (see Fig. 88-5).

Slice Thickness

The slice thickness should be 4 mm at the most, with a maximum gap of 1 mm. A thinner slice thickness produces better anatomic detail and improved partial volume; however, the signal-to-noise ratio (SNR) then decreases. The field of view (FOV) usually ranges from 24 to 36 cm in diameter.

Surface Coils

Image quality in the pelvis should be improved by using surface coils. Phased-array body coils are well suited for pelvic MRI. The high SNR obtained with these coils facilitates excellent image quality with superior spatial resolution.[32]

Pulse Sequences

Since MRI is a highly flexible and versatile system, many different imaging sequences and imaging planes are used for pelvic scanning. The choice will depend largely on the type of the scanner used and its ability to obtain fast images. However, irrespective of the scanner features, T1-and T2-weighted sequences are mandatory.[1]

T1-WEIGHTED IMAGING. For T1-weighted images, turbo or fast spin-echo, or gradient-recalled echo sequences should be used. On these sequences bladder carcinoma has intermediate signal intensity equal to that of the muscle and can be delineated from fat and urine. T1-weighted images are therefore used to determine tumor infiltration into the perivesical fat. As mentioned earlier, these sequences are also most suitable for imaging lymph nodes (see Fig. 88-5). In addition there is a good contrast between the metastasis and surrounding fatty bone marrow. Gradient-echo images are susceptible to motion and therefore may cause motion artifacts. They can be helpful for demonstrating pelvic side-wall infiltration and vessels, and for distinguishing vessels from enlarged lymph nodes. In addition, as these sequences have a short imaging time they can be used for dynamic contrast-enhanced imaging, or for quickly acquiring three-dimensional (3D) data. The combined time saving from turbo or fast spin-echo sequences and excellent image quality has led to the widespread use of this sequence type.

T2-WEIGHTED IMAGING. T2-weighted turbo or fast spin-echo sequences are considered state of the art. On T2-weighted images urine has high signal intensity and the tumor has an intermediate intensity, higher than the bladder wall or fibrosis and lower than the urine (see Fig. 88-4B). The zonal anatomy of the prostate or uterus and vagina can also clearly be recognized on these images.[30] The T2 weighting should, however, not be too strong (TE ≤ 90 ms) or the bladder cancer will have too low a signal intensity, resulting in decreased discrimination from the wall. These sequences allow high-resolution images in a relatively short time and are used for determining depth of tumor infiltration within the bladder wall, for differentiating tumor from fibrosis, for assessment of invasion into the prostate, uterus or vagina, and for confirming bone marrow metastasis seen on T1-weighted images (Fig. 88-7A). For this last purpose, a short tau inversion recovery (STIR) sequence also can be used (Fig. 88-8). Metastases have high and bone marrow low signal intensity on this sequence type (Fig. 88-7b).[40]

DYNAMIC CONTRAST-ENHANCED SEQUENCES. MRI using extracellular gadolinium-based contrast medium can be used to improve visualization of bladder cancer (Fig. 88-9). The success of dynamic contrast-enhanced MRI depends on its ability to demonstrate intrinsic differences between a variety of tissues that affect contrast-medium behavior.[41-44] Gadolinium contrast is given as an intravenous bolus injection with a power injector in the anticubital vein in a dose of 0.1 mmol/kg.[1,45,46] This extracellular contrast agent readily passes from the vasculature into the extravascular, extracellular space and gives rise to enhancement. The contrast medium causes shortening of the T1 relaxation time, and thus causes increased signal intensity on T1-weighted images. The early phase of contrast enhancement—often referred to as the first pass—includes the arrival of contrast medium. In this phase, the increased signal seen on T1-weighted images arises from both the vascular and interstitial component. Also, when a bolus of contrast medium passes through the capillary bed, it produces magnetic field inhomogeneities that decrease in the signal intensity of the surrounding tissues.[47]

Urinary bladder carcinoma develops neovascularization[2,8,48-53]; therefore, after intravenous administration of gadolinium, bladder cancer shows earlier and greater enhancement than the normal bladder wall or other nonmalignant tissues. Urinary bladder cancer starts to enhance 7 seconds after the beginning of arterial enhancement which is at least 4 seconds earlier than most other structures.[2]

Contrast enhancement has many advantages including: improved detection of small bladder tumors, especially those measuring less then 1 cm that may be missed on T2-weighted images because the high signal

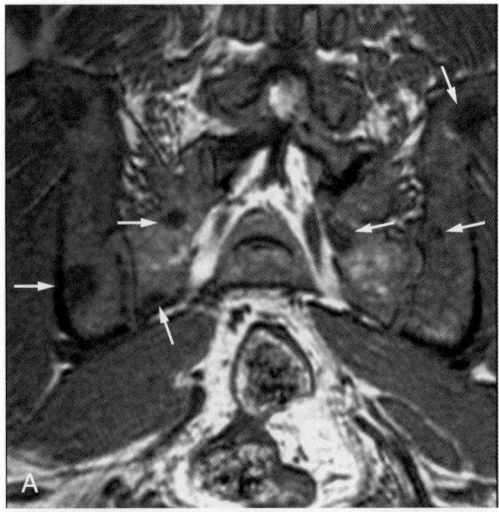
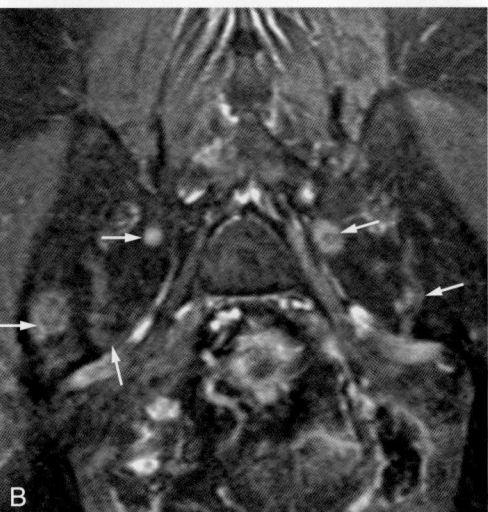

FIGURE 88-7

Bone marrow metastases. **A,** On the T1-weighted MR image metastases (*arrows*) can be seen as low signal intensity round lesions. **B,** On the post-gadolinium fat-saturated T1-weighted image, due to enhancement, bone marrow metastases (*arrows*) can be recognized as high signal intensity lesions.

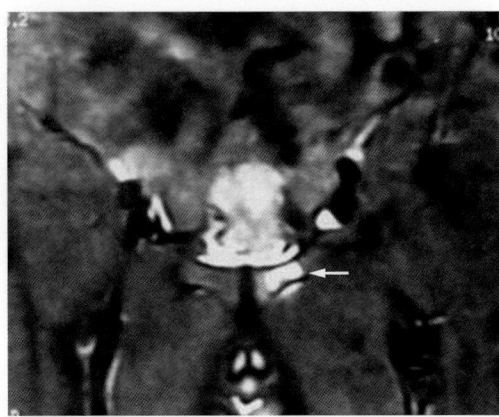

FIGURE 88-8

Bone marrow metastasis in pubic bone. On the STIR image bone marrow metastasis has high signal intensity (*arrow*).

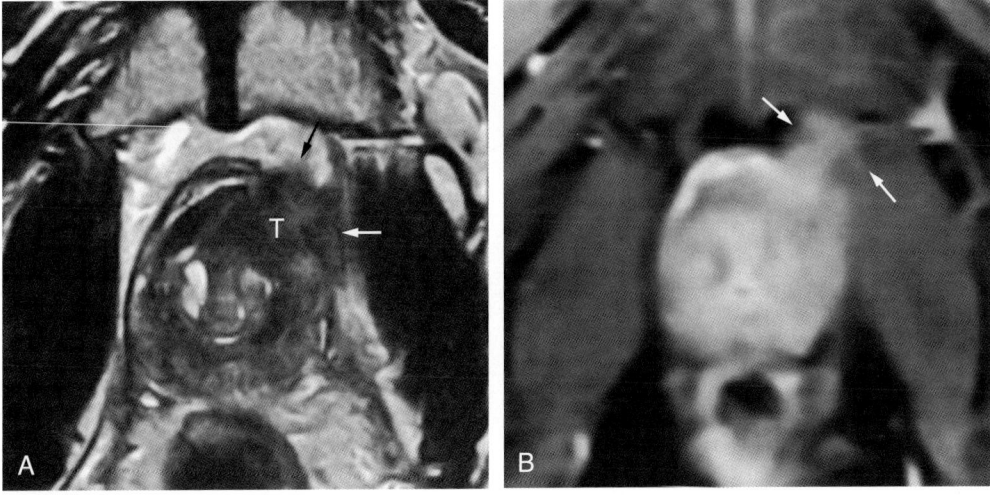

FIGURE 88-9

Stage T4b urinary bladder cancer infiltrating the prostate and pelvic side-wall muscle (*arrows*). **A,** T2-weighted turbo spin-echo image shows bladder cancer (T) infiltrating the prostate and periprostatic fat (*arrows*). **B,** Post-gadolinium fat-saturated T1-weighted image also shows enhancing tumor infiltration in the muscle of the pelvic side wall (*arrows*).

tumor can be obscured by urine; improved differentiation of bladder tumors from blood clot and other debris; improved detection of muscular and perivesical fat invasion[39]; and improved conspicuity of (small) vessels. For contrast-enhanced imaging of bladder cancer T1-weighted sequences with a time resolution of less than 20 seconds should be used. Cancer and the bladder wall or fibrosis are best discriminated in the early (first-pass) phase. Also, this speed avoids the filling of the bladder lumen due to renal excretion. To enhance tumor visualization in the perivesical fat, subtraction or fat saturation must be applied. Usually GRE sequences are used for dynamic MRI. The imaging plane can be preselected based on the previously performed T1- and or T2-weighted sequences.

BLADDER CANCER STAGING

Local tumor extension, the degree of lymph node and distant metastases, and histologic tumor type largely determine treatment and prognosis. Therefore, exact staging is imperative. To determine local tumor extension (T), presence of lymph node (N), and distant metastases (M), the International Union against Cancer proposed a uniform clinical staging method (see Table 88-1). In Table 88-4 a correlation is presented between this TNM system and MRI findings. Patients with superficial tumors, i.e., tumors without muscle invasion (stages Ta and T1), are treated with local endoscopic resection followed by adjuvant intravesical installations. Patients with a tumor invading the muscle layer of the bladder

TABLE 88-4 MRI Staging of Urinary Bladder Cancer

TNM	AUS	Histologic description	MRI criteria
T_{is}	O	Carcinoma in situ	Not applicable
T_a		Noninvasive papillary carcinoma	
T_1	A	Superficial limited to mucosa and submucosa	Stages T_1 and T_2 are diagnosed when the tumor is confined
T_2	B_1	Superficial invasion of the muscle layer	to the bladder wall with the outer bladder wall being of normal low signal intensity on T2-weighted imaging
T_{2b}	B_2	Deep invasion of the muscular wall	Interruption of low signal intensity bladder wall on T2-weighted imaging
T_{3a-b}	C_1	Perivesical fat invasion: 3a: microscopic, 3b: macroscopic	Transmural extension, tumor extension into the perivesical fat
T_4	C2	Invasion of adjacent organs	Direct invasion of adjacent organs
NO	D1	No lymph node involvement	
N_1		Single homolateral side	>1 cm
N_2		Collateral, bilateral regional nodes	>1 cm
N_3		Fixed regional nodes	>1 cm
N_4		Common iliac, aortic, or inguinal nodes	>1cm
M_1	D2	Distant metastasis	Distant metastasis

AUS, American Urologic System.
From Walsh JW, Amendola MA, Konerding KF, et al: Computed tomographic detection of pelvic and inguinal lymph node metastases from primary and recurrent pelvic malignant disease. Radiology 137:157-166, 1980.

wall or with minimal perivesical extension (stages T2a to T3a) are treated for cure by radical cystectomy and lymphadenectomy. However, if the tumor is in a more advanced stage (stages T3b-T4b) or if there are nodal or distant metastases, the patient is given palliative chemo- or radio-therapy.

Local Staging

Bladder tumors demonstrate different patterns of growth: papillary, sessile, infiltrative, or mixed pattern. Papillary tumors are usually superficial (i.e., no muscle wall infiltration, stage T1 or less) and are best demonstrated on T1-weighted images in which the intermediate signal intensity of the intraluminal tumor is outlined by surrounding low signal intensity urine. On T2-weighted images, the signal intensity of both bladder tumor and intravesical urine increases and intraluminal projections of bladder tumors may be less conspicuous than on T1-weighted images.[51] Papillary transitional cell carcinoma of the bladder has a loose connective tissue stalk. On MRI, the stalk is defined as a structure that extends from the bladder wall to the center of the tumor with signal intensity different from that of the tumor.[54] Most stalks show lower signal intensity than tumor on T2-weighted images, less enhancement on dynamic images, and stronger enhancement on delayed-enhanced images (Fig. 88-10). The identification of the stalk of a polypoid tumor may be an important observation to exclude muscle wall invasion of the tumor.[54]

Muscle-wall infiltrative tumors (stages T2a or higher) present as a diffuse or focal thickening of the bladder wall with increased signal intensity on T2-weighted images. This increase is in contrast to the low signal intensity of normal bladder wall.[31] Early contrast-enhanced images may help to recognize muscle wall infiltration. Findings suggesting superficial tumors are:

smooth muscle layer, tenting of the bladder wall, fernlike vasculature, and uninterrupted submucosal enhancement. Findings that suggest muscle invasion are: irregular wall at the base of the tumor, and focal wall enhancement or wall thickening around the tumor.[39]

MRI can differentiate between neoplastic infiltration of the bladder wall and bladder wall hypertrophy secondary to outlet obstruction. In bladder wall hypertrophy, the wall is diffusely thickened (>5 mm) but no alternation of the low signal intensity wall is present on T2-weighted images.[31]

Muscle wall invasion is divided into superficial (stage T2a) and deep (stage T2b). In stage T2b the low signal intensity layer of the bladder wall is disrupted on T2-weighted images by the higher signal tumor (see Figs. 88-3B and 88-4B). Stage T2b cannot be separated on MRI from stage T3a (microscopic fat infiltration). Macroscopic tumor extension through the bladder wall into the perivesical fat (stage T3b) will cause a focal, irregular decrease in fat signal intensity on standard T1- or T2-weighted images (Fig. 88-11A). Contrast-enhanced images with fat saturation also show tumor (enhancement) in the perivesical fat. Invasion of adjacent organs may be inferred from the extension of abnormal tumor signal intensity through fat planes into adjacent structures (Fig. 88-11B). This is well demonstrated with contrast-enhanced images. Invasion of the seminal vesicles can be demonstrated by an increase in vesicular size, decrease in signal intensity on T2-weighted images, and obliteration of the angle between the seminal vesicle and the posterior bladder wall (Fig. 88-12). Invasion of the prostate and rectum is seen as direct tumor extension with an increase in signal intensity. Obliteration of the angle between the bladder and prostate also indicates prostate invasion. Invasion of the pelvic side wall (stage T4b) is seen on T1-weighted images as a loss of the normal fat plane between the bladder wall (tumor) and the vessels or musculature of the side wall, or on T2-weighted images

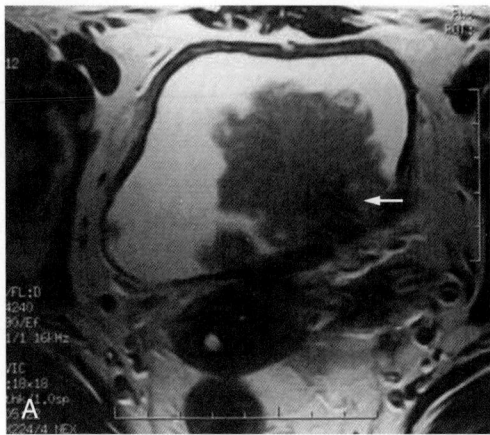 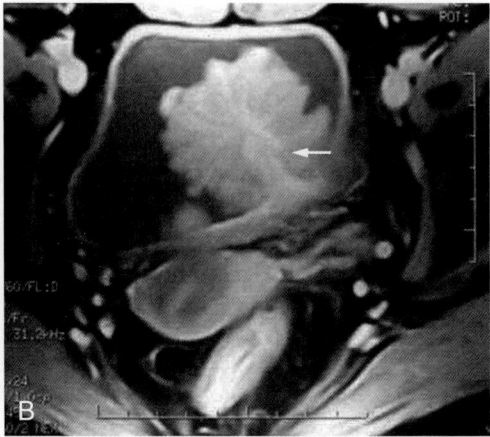

FIGURE 88-10

Papillary stage T1 tumor with stalk. **A,** On the T2-weighted turbo spin-echo image the low signal intensity muscle is not disrupted by the higher signal intensity tumor. In the center of the papillary tumor the low signal intensity stalk (*arrow*) can be seen. **B,** On the post-gadolinium fat-saturated T1-weighted image this stalk shows greater enhancement than the rest of the tumor (*arrow*).

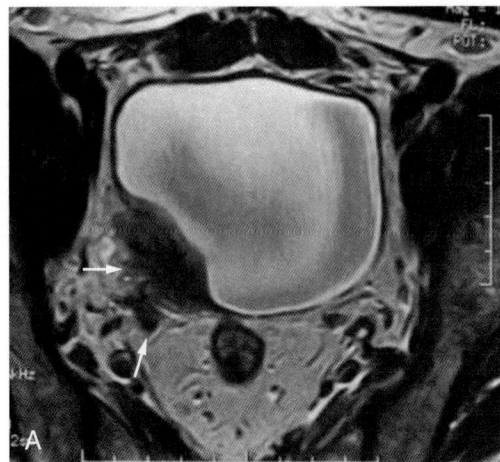

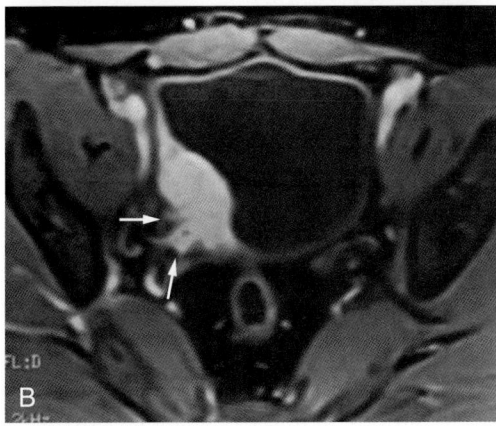

FIGURE 88-11

Stage T3b urinary bladder cancer infiltrating perivesical fat (*arrows*). Bladder cancer can be seen at the right laterodorsal wall with macroscopic infiltration of the perivesical fat (*arrows*) on both the **A,** T2-weighted turbo spin-echo image and **B,** post-gadolinium fat-saturated T1-weighted image.

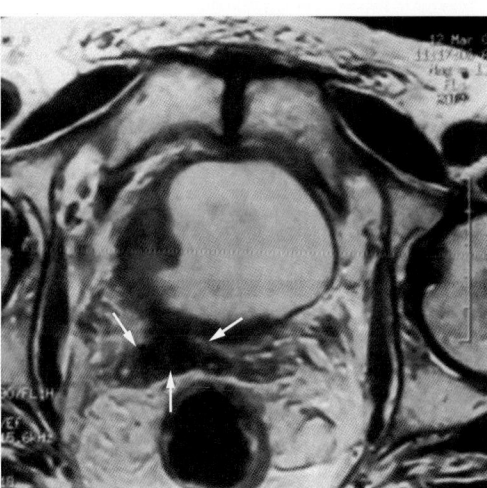

FIGURE 88-12

Stage T4a urinary bladder cancer infiltrating the right seminal vesicle (*arrows*). The T2-weighted turbo spin-echo image shows a hypointense intravesical mass arising from the right lateral wall with obliteration of the fat plain between the bladder and right seminal vesicle, and abnormal signal intensity of the left seminal vesicle denoting invasion by the tumor (*arrows*).

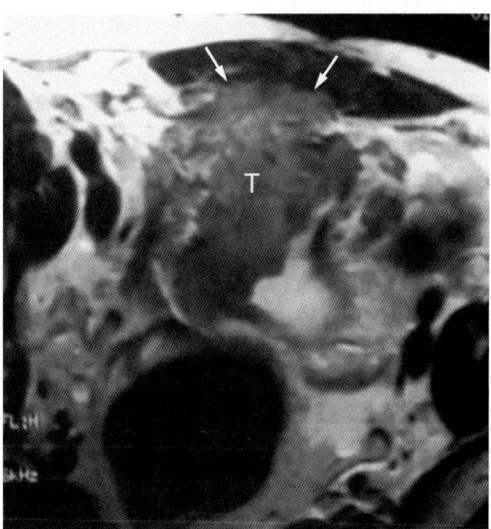

FIGURE 88-13

Stage T4b urinary bladder cancer infiltrating the ventral abdominal wall. The T2-weighted turbo spin-echo image shows a large intravesical mass arising from the anterior bladder wall with abnormal high signal intensity in the muscles of the anterior pelvic wall denoting invasion by the tumor (T) (*arrows*).

as invasion of the side-wall musculature by intermediate-to-high signal intensity tumor (Fig. 88-13).

Bladder diverticula represent an outpouching of the urothelium through the muscular wall, which is usually related to chronic outlet obstruction. Urinary stasis within the poorly contractile diverticulum leads to chronic inflammation and squamous metaplasia in up to 80% of cases. Dysplasia and neoplasm may subsequently develop.[55] The diverticulum may not be opacified on intravenous pyelography because the diverticular neck is inflamed or occluded by tumor, limiting the utility of that examination.[56] CT may fail to demonstrate the connection between the mass and bladder, and the contrast material may also fail to opacify the diverticulum. Some bladder diverticular tumors may be missed on cystoscopy, particularly if the diverticular neck is narrow. So differentiation between diverticular masses and necrotic extravesical tissue or other pelvic soft-tissue masses may be difficult.[56] Multiplaner MRI can demonstrate the presence and precise location of the bladder diverticular neck (Figs. 88-14 and 88-15). Also, the intrinsic tissue contrast of both T1- and T2-weighted images allows

differentiation of urine and tumor, and shows the intraluminal extent of the tumor.[56]

All forms of cystitis can cause diffuse or focal thickening of the bladder wall and in same cases extension into the perivesical fat may be seen. MR findings for cystitis are generally nonspecific and can mimic bladder carcinoma. Contrast-enhanced images demonstrate diffuse or focal enhancement of the bladder mucosa which at times can make it indistinguishable from cancer.[31]

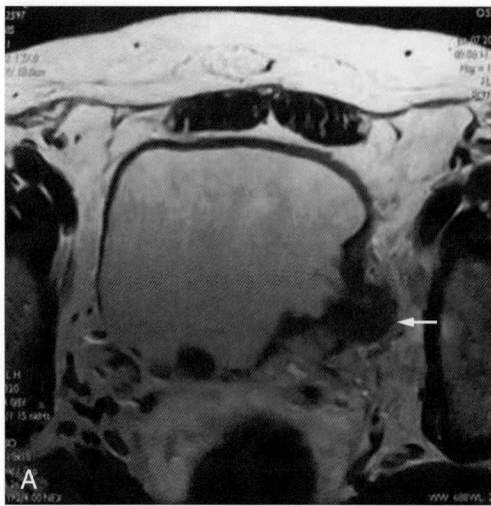

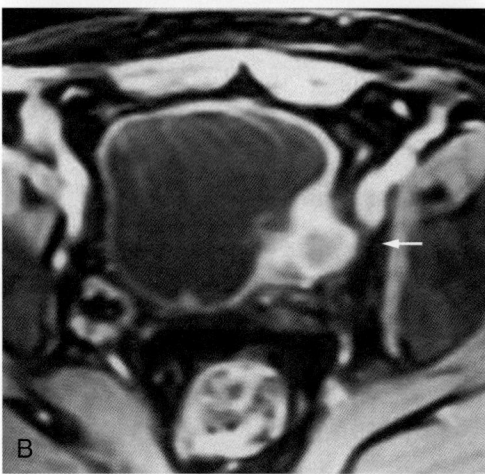

FIGURE 88-14

Stage T3b urinary bladder cancer extending into a diverticulum. **A,** Axial T2-weighted turbo spin-echo image shows thickening of the left lateral wall of the bladder with evidence of a diverticulum that is filled with a soft-tissue mass infiltrating the perivesical fat (*arrow*). **B,** In the post-contrast fat-saturated T1-weighted image, the tumor in the diverticulum is recognized by its enhancement (*arrow*).

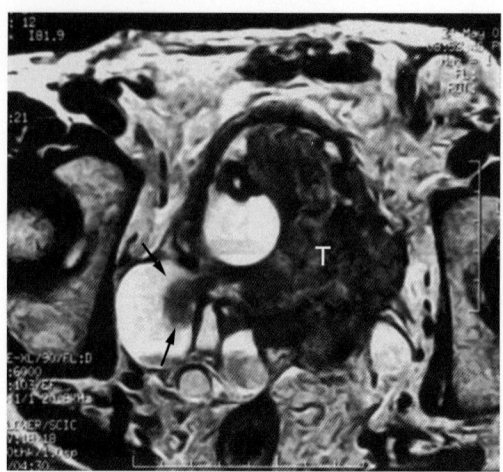

FIGURE 88-15

Large intravesical tumor extending into a diverticulum. T2-weighted turbo spin-echo image shows a large intravesical urinary bladder cancer (T) protruding into a small right lateral wall diverticulum (*arrows*).

As clinical staging is not reliable in determining tumor extension beyond the bladder wall, other methods are needed. CT is a valuable addition, but since the introduction of pelvic MRI in 1983 several reports have shown the superiority of this technique for staging urinary bladder carcinoma.[3,10,11]

MR imaging appears to be superior to CT scanning for staging carcinoma of the urinary bladder. Multiplanar imaging allows better visualization of the bladder dome, trigone, and adjacent structures such as the prostate and seminal vesicles. The accuracy of MR imaging in staging bladder cancer varies from 73% to 96%. These values are 10% to 33% higher than those obtained with CT.[10] Recently several reports have been published[14] on the staging of urinary bladder carcinoma with the use of intravenous gadolinium contrast. A 9% to 14% increase in local staging accuracy has been reported using these contrast agents. Furthermore, when using contrast agent, visualization of small tumors (>7 mm) improves. The most accurate staging results using intravenous gadolinium contrast material are obtained with very fast T1-weighted sequences.[5] This can be explained by the earlier enhancement of tumors compared to surrounding tissues. Although contrast-enhanced MRI has advantages over nonenhanced T2-weighted sequences, such as higher SNR and shorter acquisition time, it is advised not to skip the T2-weighted images. Large prospective studies in this regard are necessary to compare the value of T2-weighted TSE sequences with Gd-enhanced T1-weighted sequences.

Lymph Node Staging

Normal nodes down to a size of 2 mm can be recognized with MRI. With multiplanar imaging both the size and shape of the nodes can be assessed. The maximal length (long axis) and the minimal axial size of the node can be determined. Round nodes can be distinguished from oval nodes with an index obtained by dividing the axial size by the long axis. Lymph nodes are considered rounded when this index is between 1.0 and 0.8 and are spheric or elongated if this index is greater than 0.8. The cut-off value for the minimal axial diameter is 10 mm for a spherical/elongated node and 8 mm for a rounded node. An asymmetric cluster of small lymph nodes also is considered to be pathologic.[7]

Lymph node metastasis in patients with superficial tumors (lower than stage T2) is rare, but if the deep muscle layer is involved (stages T2a and higher) or if extravesical invasion is seen, the incidence of lymph node metastasis rises to 20% to 30% and 50% to 60%, respectively. A noninvasive, reliable method for detecting and staging nodal metastasis would reduce the extent of surgery. Four imaging techniques have been described for nodal staging: lymphangiography, CT, MRI, and 18-fluorodeoxyglucose (^{18}FDG) PET scanning.

Bipedal lymphangiography is no longer used as an imaging method, though it has the capacity to show micrometastases in normal-sized nodes. Its inability to depict internal iliac nodes and its invasiveness are major drawbacks.

CT and MRI

Detection of lymph node metastases has very important clinical consequences. If metastatic disease is present, curative cystectomy usually will not be performed. Current imaging techniques can only show nodal size. Sensitivity and specificity depend on the selection of the cut-off size for lymph nodes.[57] Recently, Jager et al[7] showed that using a 3D high-resolution technique not only nodal size but also nodal shape could be assessed. Assessment of nodal shape in relation to the cut-off size also improved their results. They obtained an accuracy of 90% and a positive predictive value of 94%.[6] This is clinically relevant as a high positive-predictive value in the detection of nodal metastasis can facilitate the indication for (MR-guided) biopsy.[58] This will avoid an invasive pelvic lymph node dissection which is important if the biopsy turns out to be positive. Cross-sectional imaging modalities like CT and (3D) MR imaging have a low sensitivity (76%) as metastases in normal-size lymph nodes are still missed, since both modalities use the nonspecific criterion of size to distinguish between normal and malignant nodes.[7,57] Although fast dynamic MRI has been shown to improve sensitivity by showing fast and high enhancement in metastatic nodes, specificity decreases. In addition, fast dynamic imaging is further limited by its low resolution and pronounced vascular artifacts.[2]

Staging pelvic lymph node dissection still remains the most sensitive method for assessing lymph node metastases and thus continues to be the first step in the management protocol. In a cost-effectiveness analysis, Wolf et al[57] concluded that imaging was superior to no imaging only when the pretest probability of lymph node metastasis was high, which is the case if tumor infiltration is in or beyond the muscular layer of the bladder wall. The most important parameter was the sensitivity of cross-sectional imaging for lymphadenopathy. Pelvic imaging combined with fine needle aspiration has also been investigated. The data of Wolf et al[57] further suggest that only a subset of patients at high risk for lymph node metastasis benefits from cross-sectional imaging and preoperative lymph node sampling.

^{18}FDG PET Scanning

Although very promising in metastatic lung cancer,[59] the role of ^{18}FDG PET scanning is limited in the urinary tract region as ^{18}FDG accumulates as part of the physiologic process in this area and uptake is low in urinary bladder cancer. This makes an evaluation of metastases at this site difficult. In a study using PET in 64 patients with urinary bladder cancer, Bachor et al[61] recorded a sensitivity of 67% and a negative predictive value of 84%. In addition,

their reported specificity of 86% is lower than those obtained with CT and MRI. Heicappell et al[61] recorded a sensitivity of 65% with PET. These figures are not high enough for ^{18}FDG PET scanning to replace pelvic lymph node dissection.

Bone Marrow Metastases

Currently, the mainstay for the detection of bone metastases is a radionuclide bone scan. However, MRI is superior to technetium-99m bone scan in the assessment of bone marrow involvement.[62] The high sensitivity of MRI for evaluating bone marrow metastasis makes it an ideal tool for detecting suspected osseous metastatic disease and determining its extent.[47,63] Osseous metastases are generally hematogenously spread and the vascular bone marrow is usually the earliest site of involvement. For the purpose of screening, T1-weighted and STIR images are adequate to detect foci of abnormal marrow. Therefore, MRI can be useful in the evaluation of patients suspected of having vertebral metastases with equivocal or negative bone scans. Thanks to its high spatial resolution MRI may also guide needle biopsy procedures. Plain radiographs are the least sensitive in evaluating the axial skeleton for metastases: 50% of the bone mineral content must be altered before metastases are visible. The limitation of MRI, however, is the inability to produce "whole-body" images.

Limitations of MRI

MRI has important limitation with regards to staging bladder tumors. Edema and fibrosis cannot be distinguished reliably from tumor within the bladder wall and, as with CT, this may lead to overstaging. Understaging results from the inability to demonstrate microscopic or minimal perivesical spread and early adjacent organ invasion, and from decreased image quality in patients who are unable to tolerate urinary bladder distention which makes delineation of the continuity of the thin black line of the bladder wall less reliable. General disadvantages include the high cost and limited availability, as well as the exclusion of patients with the standard contraindications.

NEW MRI TECHNIQUES

USPIO MRI

Reports have shown that the information about lymph nodes on MR images can be improved by pharmaceutical manipulation of tissue proton relaxation times. Ultrasmall super paramagnetic iron oxides (USPIOs) with a long plasma circulation time have been shown to be suitable as MR contrast agents for intravenous MR lymphangiography (see Chapter 14).[45,47]

After intravenous injection USPIO particles are transported to the interstitial space and from there through the lymph vessels to the lymph nodes. Once within normally functioning nodes the iron particles are taken up by macrophages and reduce the signal intensity of normal lymph node tissue in which they accumulate, due to the T2 and susceptibility effect of iron oxide, thus producing a negative enhancement. In areas of lymph nodes that are involved with malignant cells, macrophages are replaced by cancer cells, which lack reticuloendothelial activity and are unable to take up USPIO particles. Another condition in which uptake may be decreased is inflammatory nodes. In addition, due to the increased vascular permeability and increased diffusion in cancer tissue, there is leakage of USPIO particles into the metastatic areas, which produces a low local concentration and nonclustering of USPIO at these metastatic sites.[46] Through their T1 relaxivity this can induce an increase in signal intensity on T1-weighted images, producing positive enhancement.[64-66]

Thus, the ability of post-USPIO MRI to identify metastatic areas in lymph nodes depends primarily on the degree of uptake of USPIO by the macrophages in normal lymph node tissue and the leakage of USPIO in the metastatic area itself. Twenty-four hours after intravenous injection of USPIO normal lymph node and malignant tissue have different signal intensity on MR images (Fig. 88-16); thus, this noninvasive technique may detect metastatic normal-size nodes.[67]

Papers describing this technique in the evaluation of pelvic malignancies report a sensitivity of 82% to 100%.[67,68] Reported sensitivities using this technique in lymph node evaluation in other areas—predominantly head and neck, and chest—are higher compared to precontrast MRI (mean 91%, variation 84-100%).[69-73] As these authors did not use high-resolution techniques, they had limited visualization of small (<8 mm) lymph nodes. In a study performed at UMC in Nijmegen and Mass General in Boston[68] in 80 patients with histologically proven prostate cancer using high-resolution techniques (at 1.5 T using a body phased-array coil), post-USPIO MRI significantly improved the rate of detection of small nodal metastases in normal 5 to 8 mm nodes (sensitivity 100%, accuracy 98%, and negative-predictive value 100%). This was due to the detection of small 3 to 4 mm metastases in normal-size nodes. In addition, in 9 of 80 patients post-USPIO MRI detected nodes that were found outside the surgical field. During the slow (30 minute) infusion of the USPIO contrast only two patients showed minor side effects (low back pain), due to a too rapid infusion. After slowing down the infusion rate the symptoms decreased, and no further treatment was needed. Similar post-USPIO results in urinary bladder cancer (sensitivity 96%, accuracy 95%, and negative-predictive value 98%) have been reported recently.[74]

Virtual Cystoscopy

Recent studies have reported the feasibility of 3D rendering of the bladder, which provides an imaging format familiar to urologist.[73,75-77] Bernhardt et al[78]

reported no statistically significant difference between findings at MR cystoscopy and at cystoscopy for the detection of the tumors. Compared with axial images, however, CT or MR cystoscopy showed no significant differences in detection of polyps with a diameter of 10 mm or larger and had almost the same sensitivity and specificity as these modalities[75-78]; therefore, the additional role of virtual cystoscopy still needs to be assessed.

SUMMARY AND RECOMMENDATIONS

Table 88-5, which is based on published reports and our experience,[1,14,26,29] offers an overview of the value of several staging techniques for urinary bladder cancer. MRI is superior to CT as CT cannot differentiate between the various layers of the bladder wall and cannot, therefore, distinguish lesions of the lamina propria from those invading the superficial and deep muscle wall. There are also difficulties in assessing tumors at the dome and trigone. The multiplaner and soft-tissue characterization capabilities of MRI make it a valuable diagnostic tool among the noninvasive imaging modalities. Also, MRI is the most promising technique in the detection of nodal and bone marrow metastases. Where MRI is available, CT is no longer needed. In addition, recent advances in MRI, such as fast imaging, fast dynamic gadolinium-enhanced techniques, and the use of specific contrast for assessment of lymph nodes, improve the imaging quality and diagnostic accuracy for staging urinary bladder carcinoma. However, due to finite resources, this technique should only be used to obtain information that directly influences therapeutic management and outcome. To achieve this, urologists need knowledge of MRI and radiologists of clinical handling, and therefore continuous education and communication between these two specialties is a necessity.

Figure 88-17 summarizes the diagnostic management of urinary bladder cancer. Detection of bladder cancer should be performed by cystoscopy. Once bladder cancer is diagnosed, the next step should be staging. For superficial tumors, clinical staging, which includes transuretheral resection, is the best technique. If, however, there is muscle invasion, further staging has to be performed with MRI. To avoid post-biopsy overstaging from edema and fibrosis or the inconvenience of waiting 2 to 3 weeks after transurethral biopsy, we recommend fast dynamic imaging. Superficial tumors without muscle invasion (stages Ta-T1) are treated with local endoscopic resection with or without adjuvant intravesical installations. If cystoscopy reveals large multiple nodular or papillary tumors, a MRI examination can be helpful to provide an overview of the tumor prior to the biopsy.

Patients with muscle invasion (stages T2a-b) and with perivesical infiltration (stages T3a-b) or with invasion into the prostate, vagina, or uterus (stage T4a) will undergo attempted cure by radical cystectomy and lymphadenectomy.

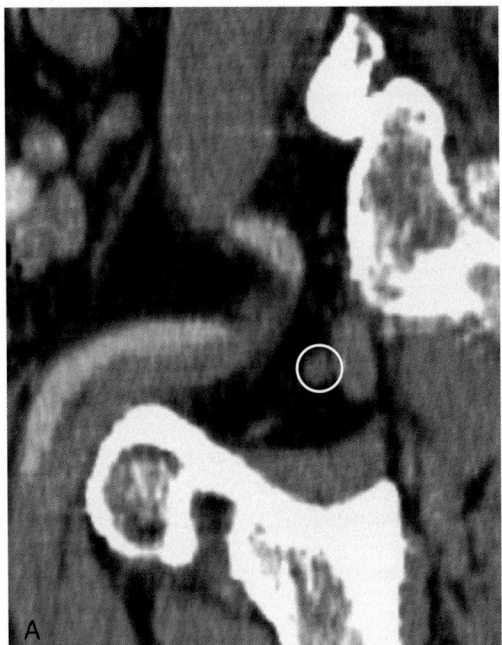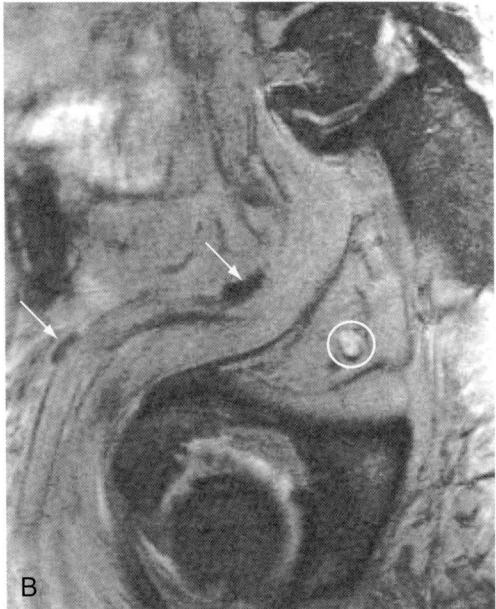

FIGURE 88-16

Normal size metastatic node. **A,** Multi Detector CT reconstruction in the "obturator" plane shows a normal size (5 mm) node (*circle*). **B,** In the T2*-weighted MR image obtained in the identical plane 24 hours post-USPIO this node (*circle*) has high signal intensity which argues for metastasis. Two small normal nodes (*arrows*) are also visible; they have low signal intensity due to accumulation of iron-loaded macrophages in normal nodal tissue. These nodes are not visible on MDCT.

TABLE 88-5 Accuracy of Different Staging Techniques

Stage	Clinical staging including transurethral resection	CT	MRI
T0-T+	++	−	+
Tis-Ta	++	−	−
Ta-T1	++	−	−
T1-T2a	++	−	+
T2a-T2b	0	−	+
T2b-T3a	−	−	−
T3a-T3b	−	++	++
T3b-T4a	−	+	++
T4a-T4b	−	+	++
N0-N+	−	+	+
M0-M+	−	0/+	++

M+, bone marrow infiltration; T0, no malignancy, e.g., scar, fibrosis, granulation tissue, hypertrophy; T+, malignancy; ++, highly accurate; +, accurate; 0 not accurate; − not possible.

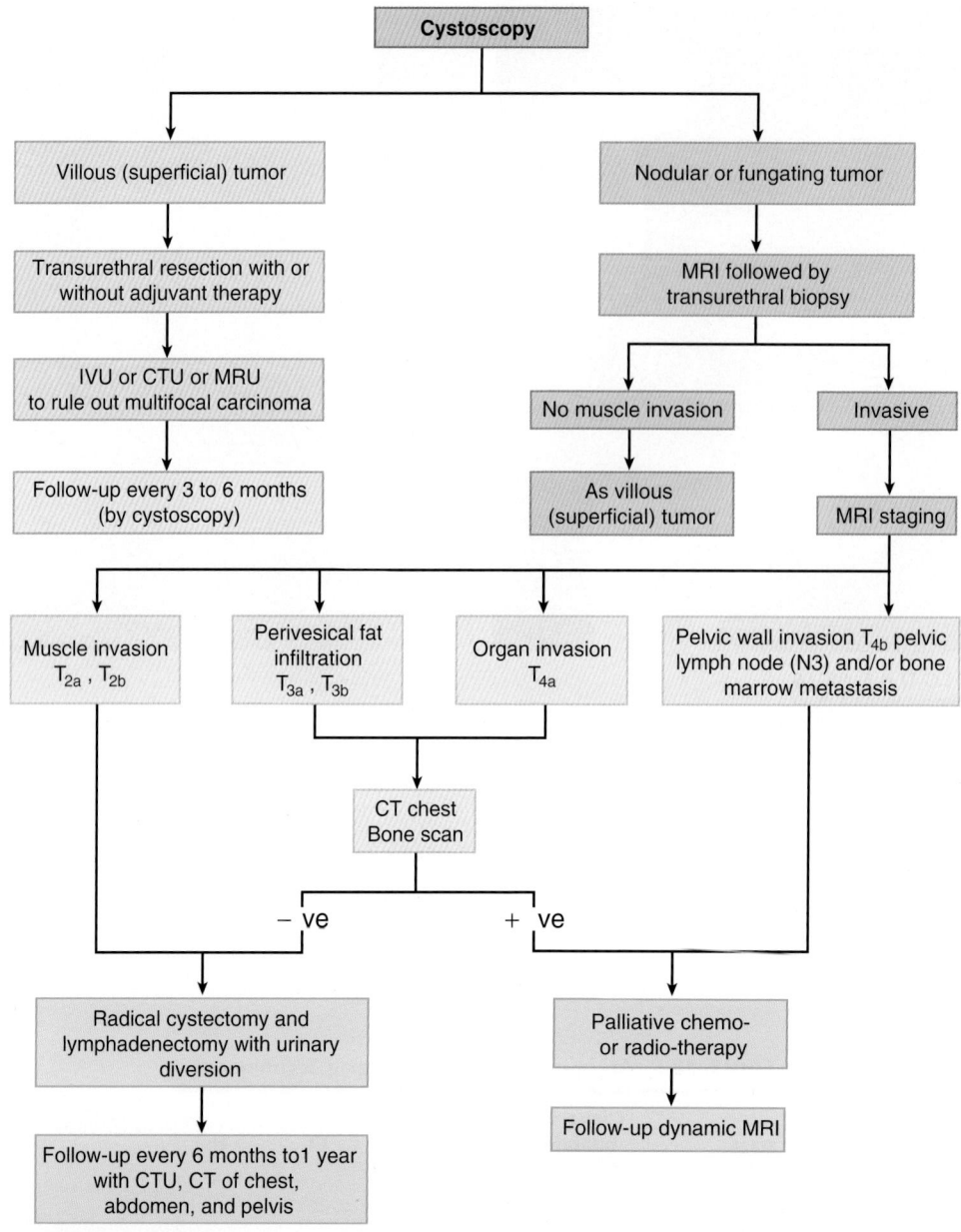

FIGURE 88-17

Diagnostic management of urinary bladder cancer. CTU, CT urography; IVU, intravenous urography; MRU, MR urography.

REFERENCES

1. Barentsz JO, Debruyne FMJ, Ruijs SHJ (eds): Magnetic Resonance Imaging of Carcinoma of the Urinary Bladder. Dordracht, Kluwer Academic Publishers, 1990.
2. Barentsz JO, Jager GJ, van Vierzen PB, et al: Staging urinary bladder cancer after transurethral biopsy: value of fast dynamic contrast-enhanced MR imaging. Radiology 201:185-193, 1996.
3. Woolf N: Urinary bladder. In Woolf N (ed): Pathology Basic and System. Philadelphia, WB Saunders, 1998, pp 713-717.
4. El-Mawla NG, El-Bolkain, Khaled HM: Bladder cancer in Africa: update. Semin Oncol 28:174-178, 2001.
5. Richards D, Jones S: The bladder and prostate. In: Sutton D (ed): Textbook of Radiology and Imaging, 6th ed. London: Churchill Livingstone, 1998, pp 1167-1187.
6. Barentsz JO, Jager GJ, Mugler JP, et al: Staging urinary bladder cancer, value of T1weighted three-dimensional magnetization prepared-rapid gradient-echo two-dimensional spin-echo sequences. Am J Roentegnol 164:109-115, 1995.

7. Jager GJ, Barentsz JO, Oosterhof GO, et al: Pelvic adenopathy in prostatic and urinary bladder carcinoma: MR imaging with a three-dimensional TI-weighted magnetization-prepared-rapid gradient-echo sequence. Am J Roentgenol 167:1503-1507, 1996.
8. Barentsz JO, Berger-Hartog O, Witjes JA, et al: Evaluation of chemotherapy in advanced urinary bladder cancer with fast dynamic contrast-enhanced MR imaging. Radiology 207:791-797, 1998.
9. Maeda H, Kinukawa T, Hottori R, et al : Detection of muscle layer invasion with submillmeter pixel MRI: Staging of bladder carcinoma. Magn Reson Imaging 13:9-19, 1995.
10. Ross MH, Romrell LJ, Kaye GI: Urinary system. In Histology: A Text and Atlas, 3rd ed. Philadelphia, William & Wilkins, 1995, pp 582-583.
11. Fawcett DW, Jensh RP: Histology of the urinary system. Concise Histology. London, Chapman & Hall, 1998, pp 240-251.
12. Castellino RA: Lymph nodes of the posterior iliac crest: CT and lymphgraphic observations. Radiology 175:687-689, 1990.
13. Williams PL, Warwick R: Angiology. In Williams PL, Warwick R, Dysen M, et al: Gray's Anatomy, 37th ed. Edinburgh, Churchill Livingstone, 1989, pp 1416-1421.

14. Barentsz JO: Bladder cancer. In Pollack H, McClennan BL, eds. Clinical Urography, 2nd ed. Philadelphia, WB Saunders, 2000, pp 1642-1668.
15. Damjanov I, Linder J: Diseases of the urogenital and reproductive systems. In Damjanov I, Linder J (eds): Anderson's Pathology, 10th ed. St Louis, Mosby, 1996, pp 2154-2163.
16. Macvicar AD: Bladder cancer staging. Br J Urol 86:111-121, 2000.
17. Husband JE, Reznek RH : Bladder cancer. In Husband JE, Reznek RH (eds): Imaging on Oncology, Vol I. Oxford, ISIS Medical Media, 1998, pp 215-237.
18. Heiken JP, Fofman HP, Brown JJ: Neoplasms of the bladder, prostate and testis. Radiol Clin North Am 32:81-98, 1994.
19. Babaian RJ, Johnson DE, Liamas L, et al: Metastases from transitional cell carcinoma of the urinary bladder. Urology 16:142-145, 1980.
20. Walsh JW, Amendola MA, Konerding KF, et al: Computed tomographic detection of pelvic and inguinal lymph node metastases from primary and recurrent pelvic malignant disease. Radiology 137:157-166, 1980.
21. Elkin M: Tumors of urinary tract. In Elkin M (ed): Radiology of the Urinary System, Vol I. Boston, Little, Brown, 1980, pp 296-426.
22. Hricak H, White S: Radiological evaluation of the urinary bladder and prostate. In Grainger RG, Allison D (eds): Grainger and Allison's Diagnostic Radiology: A Textbook of Medical Imaging, Vol 2, 3rd ed. Edinburgh, Churchill Livingstone, 1997, pp 1427-1438.
23. Sherwood T: Bladder and urethra. In: Sherwood T, Davidson AJ, Talner LB (eds): Uro-Radiology. Oxford, Blackwell Scientific, 1980, pp 255-312.
24. Hatch TR, Barry JM: The value of excretory urography in staging bladder cancer. J Urol 135:49-54, 1986.
25. Dershow PD, Scher HI: Sonography in the evaluation of carcinoma of the bladder. Urology 29:454-457, 1987.
26. Barentsz JO, Jager GJ, Witjes JA, Ruijs JHJ: Primary staging of urinary bladder carcinoma: the role of MR imaging and a comparison with CT. Eur Radiol 6:134-139, 1996.
27. Tsuda K, Narumi U, Nakamura H, et al: Staging urinary bladder cancer with dynamic MRI [abstract]. Hinyokika Kiyo 46:835-859, 2000.
28. Lipson SA, Hricak H: The urinary bladder and female urethra. In Higgins CB, Hricak H, Helms CA (eds): Magnetic Resonance Imaging of the Body, 3rd ed. New York, Lippincott-Raven, 1997, pp 875-900.
29. Barentsz JO, Witjes JA, Ruijs JH: What is new in bladder cancer imaging. Urol Clin North Am 24:583-602, 1997.
30. Takeda K, Kawaguchi T, Shiraishi T, et al: Normal bladder wall morphology in Gd-DTPA-enhanced clinical MR imaging using an endo-rectal surface coil and histological assessment of submucosal linear enhancement using Gd-DTPA auto-radiography in an animal model. Eur J Radiol 26:290-296, 1988.
31. Barentsz JO: Magnetic resonance imaging of urinary bladder carcinoma. In Jafri SH, Diokno AC, Amendola MA (eds): Lower Genitourinary Radiology, Imaging and Intervention. New York, Springer-Verlag, 1998, pp 138-158.
32. Barentsz JO, Ruijs JHJ, Strijk SP: Review article. The role of MR imaging in carcinoma of the urinary bladder. Am J Roentgenol 160:937-947, 1993.
33. Siegelman ES, Schnall MD: Contrast-enhanced MR imaging of the bladder and prostate. Magn Reson Imaging Clin North Am 4:153-169, 1996.
34. Fisher MR: Pelvis. In Runge VM (ed): Clinical Magnetic Resonance Imaging. Philadelphia, JB Lippincott, 1990, pp 385-401.
35. Farahani K, Lufkin RB: Flow motion and artifacts in MRI. In Lufkin RB (ed): The MRI Manual, Part 1 Basic Principles, 2nd ed. USA, Mosby, 1998, pp 101-151.
36. Sallevelt PE, Barentsz JO, Heksler Y: MR imaging and patients with claustrophobia: results of treatment with parental tranxene. Eur Radiol 3:355-356, 1993.
37. Shellock FG, Kanal E: Bioeffects and safety. In Lufkin RB: The MRI Manual, Part 1, Basic Principles, 2nd ed. USA, Mosby, 1998, pp 415-497.
38. Edelman RR, Klieefield J, Wentzk U, et al: Basic principles of magnetic resonance imaging. In Edelman R, Hesselink JR, Newhouse J, et al (eds): Clinical Magnetic Resonance Imaging. Philadelphia, WB Saunders, 1996, pp. 3-51.
39. Narumi Y, Kadota T, Inoue E, et al: Bladder tumors: staging with gadolinium-enhanced oblique MR imaging. Radiology 187:145-150, 1993.
40. Eustase S, Tello R, DeCarvalbo V, et al: A comparison of whole body turbo short tau inversion recovery MR imaging and planar technetium 99m methylene diphosphonate scintigraphy in the evaluation of patients with suspected skeletal metastases. Am J Roentgenol 169:1655-1661, 1997.
41. Padhani AR, Husband JE: Dynamic contrast enhanced MRI studies in oncology with an emphasis on quantification, validation human studies. Clin Radiol 56:607-620, 2001.
42. Lin W, Hoacke EM, Smith AS, et al: Gadolinium enhanced high resolution MRA with adaptive vessel tracking: Preliminary results in the intracranial circulation. Magn Reson Imaging 2:227-284, 1992.
43. Vens S, Hosten N, Ilg J, et al: Pre-operative staging of bladder carcinomas with Gd-DTPA-supported dynamic magnetic resonance tomography. Comparison with plain and Gd-DTTA-supported spin-echo sequences. Rofo Fortschr Ged Rontgenstr Neuen Bilged Verfahr 164:218-225, 1996.
44. Hamm P, Laniado M, Saini S: Contrast-enhanced magnetic resonance imaging of the abdomen and pelvis. Magn Reson 6:108-135, 1990.
45. Weissleder R, Elizondo G, Wittenberg J, et al: Ultrasmall paramagnetic iron oxide: an intravenous contrast agent for assessing lymph nodes with MR imaging. Radiology 175:494-498, 1990.
46. Gerlowski LE, Jain RK: Microvascular permeability of normal and neoplastic tissues. Microvasc Res 31:288-305, 1986.
47. Vassallo P, Matei C, Heston WDW, et al: AMI-227-enhanced MR lymphography: usefulness for differentiating reactive from tumor bearing lymph nodes. Radiology 193:501-506, 1994.
48. El-Diasty T, El-Sobky E, Abou El-Ghar M, et al: Triphasic helical CT of urinary bladder carcinomas correlation with tumour angiogenesis and pathologic types [abstract]. Eur Radiol 12:D1-D25, 2002.
49. Nicolas V, Spielmann R, Mass R, et al: The diagnostic value of MRI tomography following gadolinium-DTPA compared to computed-tomography in bladder tumors. Fortschr Rontgenstr 154:357-363, 1991.
50. Braun RD, Lanzen JL, Dewhirst NW: Fourier analysis of fluctuations of oxygen tension and blood flow in R3230Ac tumors and muscle of rats. Am J Physiol 277:551-568, 1999.
51. Dovark HF, Nagy JA, Feng D, et al: Vascular permeability factor/vascular endothelial growth factor and the significance of micro-vascular hyper-permeability in angiogenesis. Curr Top Microbiol Immunol 237:97-132, 1999.
52. Dewhirst M: Angiogenesis and blood flow in solid tumors. In Teicher B (ed): Drug Resistance in Oncology. New York, Marcel Dekker Inc, 1993, pp 3-24.
53. Neeman M, Provenzale JP, Dewhirst MW: MRI application in evaluation of tumor angiogenesis. Semin Radiol Oncol 11:70-82, 2001.
54. Saito W, Amanuma M, Tanaka J, et al: Histopathological analysis of bladder cancer stalk observed on MRI [abstract]. Magn Reson Imaging 18:411, 2000.
55. Durfee SM, Schwarts LH, Panicek DM, et al: MR imaging of carcinoma within urinary bladder diverticulum. Clin Imaging 21:291-292, 1997.
56. Husband JE: Review of staging bladder cancer. Clin Radiol 46:153-159, 1992.
57. Wolf JS, Cher M, dalla 'Era M, et al: The use and accuracy of cross-sectional imaging and fine needle aspiration cytology for detection of pelvic lymph node metastases before radical prostatectomy. J Urol 153:993-999, 1995.
58. Barentsz JO: MR intervention in the pelvis: an overview and first experiences in MR-guided biopsy in nodal metastases in urinary bladder cancer. Abdom Imaging 22:524-530, 1997.
59. Pieterman RM, Van Putten JWG, Meuzelaar JJ, et al: Preoperative staging of non-small-cell lung cancer with positron-emission tomography. N Engl J Med 343:254, 2000.
60. Bachor R, Kotzerke J, Reske SN, Hautmann R: Lymph node staging of bladder neck carcinoma with positron emission tomography. Urologe 38:46-50, 1999.
61. Heicappell R, Muller Mattheis V, Reinhardt M, et al: Staging of pelvic lymph nodes in neoplasms of the bladder and prostate by positron emission tomography with 2-[(18) F]-2-deoxy-D-glucose. Eur Urol 36:582-587, 1999.
62. Manyak MJ, Hinkle GH, Olsen JO, et al: Immunoscintigraphy with indium-111-capromab penetide: evaluation before definitive therapy in patients with prostate cancer. Urology 54:1058-1063, 1999.
63. Hinkle GH, Burgers JK, Neal CE, et al: Multicenter radioimmunoscintigraphic evaluation of patients with prostate carcinoma using indium-111 capromab pendetide. Cancer 83:739-747, 1998.
64. Bellin MF, Roy C, Kinkel K, et al: Lymph node metastases: safety and effectiveness of MRI with ultrasmall superparamanetic iron oxide particles. Initial clinical experience. Radiology 207:799-808, 1998.
65. Chambon C, Clement O, Le Blanche A: Superparamagnetic iron oxides as positive MR contrast agents: in vitro and in vivo evidence. Magn Reson Imaging 11:509-519, 1993.
66. Guimares R, Clement O, Bittoun J, et al: MR Lymphography with super paramagnetic nanoparticles in rats: pathologic basis for contrast enhancement. Am J Roentgenol 162:201-207, 1994
67. Harisinghani MG, Saini S, Slater GJ, et al: MR imaging of pelvic lymph nodes in primary pelvic carcinoma with ultrasmall superparamagnetic iron oxide (Combidex): preliminary observations. J Magn Reson Imaging 7:161-163, 1997.
68. Harisinghani MG, Barentsz J, Hahn PF, et al: Noninvasive detection of clinically occult lymph-node metastases in prostate cancer. N Engl J Med 348:2491-2499, 2003.
69. Anzai Y, Prince MR: Iron oxide-enhanced MR lymphography: the evaluation of cervical lymph node metatstases in head and neck cancer. J Magn Reson Imaging 7:75-81, 1997.
70. Kerstine KH, Stanford W, Mullan BF, et al: PET, CT, and MRI with Combidex for mediastinal staging in non-small lung carcinoma. Ann Thorac Surg 68:1022-1028, 1999.
71. Hoffman HT, Quets J, Toshiaki T, et al: Functional magnetic resonance imaging using iron oxide particles in characterizing head and neck adenopathy. Laryngoscope 110: 1425-1430, 2000.
72. Nguyen BC, Stanford W, Thompson RH, et al: Multicenter clinical trial of ultrasmall superparamagnetic iron oxide in the evaluation of mediastinal lymph nodes in patients with primary lung cancer. J Magn Reson Imaging 10:468-473, 1999.
73. Pannu HK, Wang KP, Borman TL, Bluemke DA: MR imaging of mediastinal lymph nodes: evaluation using superparamagnetic contrast agent. J Magn Reson Imaging 12:899-904, 2000.
74. Deserno WM, Harisinghani MG, Taupitz M, et al. Urinary bladder cancer: preoperative nodal staging with ferumoxtran-10-enhanced MR imaging. Radiology 233;449-456, 2004.
75. Narumi Y, Kumatani , Sawai Y, et al: The bladder and bladder tumors: imaging with three-dimensional display of helical CT data. Am J Roentgenol 167:1134-1135, 1996.
76. Vining DJ, Zagoria RJ, Liu K, Stelts D: CT cystoscopy. An innovation in bladder imaging. Am J Roentgenol 166: 409-410, 1996.
77. Fenion HM, Bell TV, Ahari HK, Hussain S: Virtual cystoscopy, Early clinical experience. Radiology 205:272-275, 1997.
78. Bernhardt TM, Schmidl H, Philipp C, et al: Diagnostic potential of virtual cystoscopy of the bladder: MRI vs CT. Preliminary report. Eur Radiol 13:305-312, 2003.

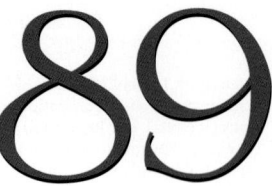

PROSTATE

Fergus V. Coakley ● John Kurhanewicz ● Aliya Qayyum

INTRODUCTION

Epidemiology

Approximately 8% of American men will be diagnosed with prostate cancer during their lifetime, and 20% of these men will die of the disease.[1] The etiology of prostate cancer is unknown, though hereditary, hormonal, racial, and geographic factors all appear to contribute. During the 1990s, the incidence of prostate cancer increased and later decreased, probably due to the emergence of widespread serum prostatic-specific antigen (PSA) level testing resulting in a change in diagnostic sensitivity. However, the age-adjusted mortality increased over the same period, suggesting a possible true increase in disease prevalence or aggressiveness. More recently, the age-adjusted mortality has decreased, which could reflect earlier diagnosis allowing for more effective treatment (Fig. 89-1). Alternatively, these changes in mortality may simply be due to "attribution bias," particularly since the changes have paralleled those of incidence. Given the indolent natural history of prostate cancer, a true improvement in treatment would likely take several years to have an impact on mortality. The absence of a lag between the incidence and mortality changes may support this latter explanation.[2]

Despite this sizeable mortality, many cases of prostate cancer are subclinical, and small foci of incidental prostate cancer can be detected in up to 40% of men at autopsy.[3] Interestingly, the autopsy incidence of histologic prostate cancer appears constant between countries and races, but the clinical incidence of prostate cancer is higher in Western countries and in African-Americans. The management of early-stage prostate cancer is controversial because patients whose disease is indolent and incidental cannot be reliably distinguished from those whose disease is progressive and life threatening. Current methods of prostate cancer evaluation by digital rectal examination (DRE), transrectal ultrasound (TRUS), Gleason score, sextant biopsy, and serum PSA assay can generally only predict behavior for very indolent or aggressive cancers. Most patients fall

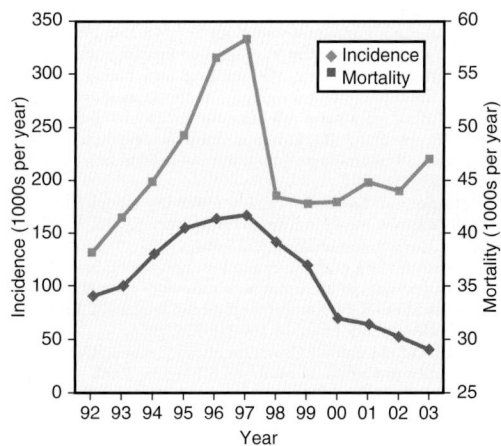

FIGURE 89-1

Epidemiologic trends in prostate cancer incidence and mortality in the United States for the years 1992 to 2003.

TABLE 89-1 Staging Systems for Prostate Cancer

Jewett-Whitmore	TNM	Description
A	I (T1N0M0)	Organ-confined tumor. Clinically and radiologically inapparent
B	II (T2N0M0)	Organ-confined tumor. Clinically or radiologically apparent. T2A: Localized to a quadrant; T2B: localized to one side; T2C: bilateral
C	III (T3N0M0)	Extracapsular extension, or seminal vesicle invasion.* T3A: Unilateral or bilateral extracapsular extension; T3B: seminal vesicle invasion
D1	IV (N1-2)	Locoregional adenopathy. N1: Microscopic nodal metastases; N2: macroscopic nodal metastases
D2	IV (T4 or N3 or M1-2)	Distant spread. T4: Invasion of the bladder, external sphincter or rectum; N3: extraregional nodal metastases; M1: elevated acid phosphatase; M2: distant visceral or bony metastases

*In the fourth edition of the AJCC staging system, unilateral and bilateral extracapsular extension were classified separately as T3A and T3B. This distinction was dropped from the fifth and subsequent editions.

between these extremes, when the techniques are of limited accuracy.[4-6] Because of the prevalence and mortality of prostate cancer and the limitations of current evaluation methods, prostate cancer is a major medical and socioeconomic problem.

Staging

Both the TNM and Jewett-Whitmore staging systems are in common usage, and are based on the local, nodal, and distant extent of disease (Table 89-1).[7,8] Staging of prostate cancer is important because it contributes both to predicting prognosis and planning treatment. A general understanding of prognosis and treatment strategies by stage facilitates clinically relevant radiologic interpretation of prostate MRI and MR spectroscopic imaging (MRSI). Prognosis is closely related to stage. Despite the prevalence of prostate cancer, published studies on prognosis are relatively sparse (Table 89-2).[9-13] Good prognostic studies are lacking because the mortality from unrelated causes is high in elderly men with prostate cancer, available studies often describe outcome only for highly selected patients undergoing specific treatment, and long-term follow-up of 10 to 15 years is required for meaningful evaluation in lower-stage disease. Treatment options are related to stage and are summarized in Table 89-3.[14] Unfortunately, there are many controversies and unanswered questions in the management of prostate cancer, primarily because of an inability to accurately predict the natural history of localized disease.[15] Some recent studies have questioned the validity of watchful waiting or surveillance as an option for those with localized disease and a reasonable life expectancy. A Danish Cancer Registry study showed that patients with clinically localized prostate cancer who are candidates for curative therapy at diagnosis have significant excess mortality when treated expectantly and followed for 10 years or longer.[16] A Scandinavian randomized controlled trial demonstrated improved outcome at 8 years of follow-up and beyond when radical prostatectomy was compared to watchful waiting.[17] However, these results may not be directly applicable to the North American population of men with newly diagnosed prostate cancer, in whom disease is more frequently impalpable and detected by PSA testing alone. Watchful waiting may still be an appropriate option for at least some of these patients with early low-grade or small-volume tumors.

Pathologic Factors

It is important for radiologists interpreting imaging studies of the prostate to have a working knowledge of several relevant pathologic terms, since these terms are likely to appear in biopsy reports or be discussed in clinical conferences. Understanding these terms and their clinical implications will facilitate interpretation of endorectal prostatic MRI and MRSI studies.

Gleason Score

The histology of prostate cancer is variable, ranging from well to poorly differentiated. This variation occurs not only between cases, but also within different parts of the

TABLE 89-2 Prognosis in Prostate Cancer by Stage

Jewett-Whitmore	TNM	2-year mortality (%)	5-year disease-specific mortality (%)	10-year disease-specific mortality (%)
A and B	I/II	—	10	9-22
C	III	—	18	40
D1	IV	—	34	—
D2	IV	42	—	—

TABLE 89-3 Treatment in Prostate Cancer by Stage

Jewett-Whitmore	TNM	TMN	Conventional treatment options
A and B	I/II	T1 and T2	<10-year life expectancy: radiotherapy,* watchful waiting >10-year life expectancy: prostatectomy, radiotherapy
C	III	T3	Radiotherapy, adjuvant hormonal therapy in high-risk patients
D1	IV	N1-2	Hormonal therapy†
D2	IV	N3/M1-2	Hormonal therapy, palliative radiotherapy for bony metastases, second-line agents for hormone refractory cancer

*Includes standard external beam radiotherapy, 3D conformal radiotherapy, intensity-modulated radiotherapy, and brachytherapy.
†Includes subcapsular orchidectomy, estrogens, antiandrogens, and luteinizing hormone-releasing hormone agonists.

same tumor. The evaluation of the dominant histologic pattern is important, because poorly differentiated tumors are more aggressive, and vice versa. The Gleason grading system assigns a grade from 1 (very well differentiated) to 5 (very poorly differentiated) to the dominant and second most dominant histologic patterns, respectively.[18] The sum of these two *grades* is the Gleason *score*, and it ranges from 2 (well differentiated) to 10 (poorly differentiated). The Gleason score is an indicator of disease aggressiveness and stage. In a study of 113 patients undergoing radical prostatectomy,[19] 63% of those with a Gleason score of 6 or less had organ-confined disease, compared to 33% of patients with a Gleason score of 7 and 0% of patients with a Gleason score of 8. Limitations of the Gleason score are clustering of assigned values to 6 and 7, and high interobserver variability.[20]

Extracapsular Extension

Extracapsular extension is the usual histologic feature that identifies a tumor as T3 rather than T2. Its prognostic importance has been closely evaluated in a 10-year follow-up study of 617 men after radical prostatectomy at John Hopkins for T1 to T3A node-negative tumors.[21] This study found the 10-year risk of recurrence (clinical, radiologic, or biochemical) was closely related to extracapsular extension (Table 89-4). An important aspect of the data in Table 89-4 is the high risk of recurrence in patients with extracapsular extension treated by radical prostatectomy. This provides the rationale for managing such patients with definitive radiotherapy rather than surgery; many (but not all) urologists consider the extra morbidity of surgery to be unjustified in patients with extracapsular extension,

given the limited probability of long-term cure; i.e., extracapsular extension is not technically nonresectible, but rather is an indicator that systemic microscopic metastatic spread may have already occurred, precluding curative surgery.

Seminal Vesicle Invasion

Seminal vesicle invasion can occur by spread of tumor along the ejaculatory ducts, by direct extension of tumor at the prostate base through the capsule up into the seminal vesicle, or by skip-metastasis.[22] While these three different mechanisms have been described, our experience suggests that seminal vesicle invasion, at least as detected by MRI, occurs predominantly by direct contiguous spread of tumor from the base of the prostate into the seminal vesicle. Seminal vesicle invasion (T3B) should be distinguished from extracapsular extension at the base that abuts the seminal vesicle, but does not invade it (T3A). Seminal vesicle invasion is an independent predictor of disease progression, and is associated with microscopic nodal metastases in up to 80% of cases.[23]

Central Gland Tumors

In a study of 104 prostatectomy specimens, the zonal cancer origin could be identified in 88 cases. Most (68%) arose in the peripheral zone, while 24% arose in the transition zone and 8% in the central zone.[24] The central and transition zones make up the radiologic central gland, and therefore appear to account for over 30% of all tumors. This is a disturbing result, since it is generally not possible to evaluate the central gland for tumor by TRUS, MRI, or MRSI, because of central gland anatomic and metabolic heterogeneity caused by benign prostatic hyperplasia (BPH). Some degree of BPH is virtually invariable in the population of men who undergo prostate MRI, and in this population the transition zone is essentially equivalent to the radiologic central gland. However, several lines of evidence suggest that such central gland tumors, which are likely to be missed on imaging, are not a major clinical concern. For example, prostate cancer was diagnosed by transition zone biopsy in only 7 of 565 men undergoing routine sextant biopsy, with transition zone biopsy performed as an investigational supplement.[25] Patients with a high PSA and a

TABLE 89-4 Prognosis in Prostate Cancer by Stage

	Recurrence rate (%)	
Stage	4 years	10 years
Organ-confined (T1/T2)	2	15
Focal ECE (T3A)	9	32
Established ECE (T3A)	22	42
SVI (T3B)	60	73

previous negative routine sextant biopsy might be considered likely to harbor transition zone cancer. However, transition zone or transurethral biopsies in these patients have an extremely low yield.[26,27] Cancers diagnosed in the transition zone are usually of lower Gleason score than peripheral zone tumors, and appear to have a lower malignant potential.[28] At least some so-called central gland tumors at pathology may represent peripheral zone tumors invading the central gland, so that the overall fraction of primarily central gland tumors may be less than 30%. In a more recent study, only 7 of 58 (12%) prostate cancer nodules were primarily transition zone tumors.[29]

Perineural Invasion

Perineural invasion refers to prostatic carcinoma that tracks along or around the perineural space of a nerve within the prostate; i.e., the term refers to an intraprostatic finding and not to an extracapsular extension. It is seen in up to 24% of prostate needle biopsies.[30] It has been suggested that perineural invasion is an adverse finding, and is associated with an increased likelihood of extraprostatic disease. However, in a multivariate analysis based on 349 prostatectomy specimens, perineural invasion was not independently predictive of extraprostatic disease or pathologic stage when adjusted for PSA, Gleason score, and tumor extent.[31] Perineural invasion was predictive on univariate analysis, which likely accounts for previous studies suggesting it was a significant prognostic factor.

Prostate Cancer Evaluation

Current methods used to evaluate prostate cancer extent and aggressiveness include DRE, TRUS, sextant biopsy, and serum PSA assay. DRE, historically a primary diagnostic test, only has a sensitivity of 30% and a specificity of 40% for the diagnosis of organ-confined disease.[4] DRE is also inaccurate in staging; 47% of patients with organ-confined disease on DRE have T3 disease pathologically, while 33% of patients with T3 disease on DRE have organ-confined disease pathologically.[4] TRUS has been used to detect extracapsular extension and seminal vesicle invasion, but, in a multiinstitutional prospective study, TRUS was no better than DRE in local staging.[6] Prostate cancer histology varies between cases and between different parts of the same tumor. Sextant biopsy has traditionally been the standard of reference for nonsurgical tumor localization,[32] but suffers from significant limitations.[5,33] In a study of 47 patients, using radical prostatectomy specimens as the standard of reference, the sensitivity and specificity of sextant biopsy for sextant localization of tumor were only 50% and 82%, respectively.[34]

PSA is an enzyme secreted by the epithelial cells of the prostate that probably functions to liquefy the ejaculate.[35] Normal serum PSA level is under 4 ng/L and is raised in prostate cancer.[15] The identification of PSA in the 1980s revolutionized the diagnosis and surveillance of prostate cancer. PSA level also correlates with stage.

In 945 patients undergoing radical prostatectomy, extraprostatic disease was found in 30% of those with a PSA less than 2 ng/L compared to 93% of those with a PSA over 50 ng/L.[36]

Because of the limited accuracy of any single traditional technique in the evaluation of prostate cancer, a number of studies have examined combining information from different techniques. One of the most frequently cited studies used the combination of clinical stage, Gleason score, and PSA level to assign probabilities for extracapsular extension, seminal vesicle invasion, and regional node metastases.[37] The tabulated risk assignments in this study are popularly known as the Partin tables. Unfortunately, many patients have an assigned risk for extracapsular extension that is in the intermediate range, and the Partin tables are therefore of limited practical benefit in choosing treatment. These limitations to the traditional methods for the evaluation of prostate cancer extent and aggressiveness have driven the development of prostate MRI and MRSI.

TECHNIQUE OF PROSTATE MR IMAGING

A number of general introductory points are worth noting. MRI allows a "one-stop shop" detailed evaluation of prostatic, periprostatic, and pelvic anatomy. Neither TRUS nor CT can offer this simultaneous coverage and tissue detail. MRSI is a method of demonstrating normal and altered tissue metabolism, and is therefore fundamentally different from other imaging modalities such as MRI or TRUS that only assess abnormalities of structure. MRI and MRSI are relatively new technologies, and both are in continued evolution. It is too early to judge the true role of these modalities, which may not be established for many years. For example, an early multiinstitutional trial showing no difference between TRUS and MRI in staging accuracy is frequently cited as evidence that MRI has no role in the assessment of prostate cancer,[38] but this study was conducted without the incorporation of MRSI or the use of endorectal coils, and with sequences and equipment that are obsolete by current standards. MRI and MRSI can be performed as a single combined examination that takes about 60 minutes in total. An endorectal coil is essential for performance of MRSI, and, in addition, has been shown to significantly improve the staging accuracy of MRI.[39] It is helpful, but not crucial, to post process to compensate for the reception profile of the endorectal coil.[40]

T1-Weighted MRI

T1-weighted images of the pelvis are helpful in the evaluation of prostate cancer for several reasons. Postbiopsy hemorrhage can be detected on T1-weighted images of the prostate (Fig. 89-2), while lymphadenopathy and bone metastases may be detected on T1-weighted images of the pelvis. Approaches to T1-weighted images vary, with some centers only obtaining relatively thick sections from the iliac crests to the

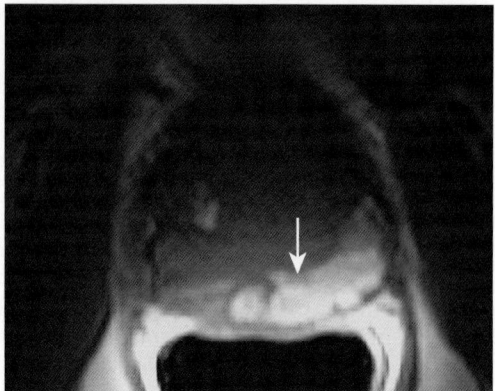

FIGURE 89-2

Axial T1-weighted MR image of the prostate, demonstrating a large area of post-biopsy hemorrhage (*arrow*) in the left side of the prostate gland. Such hemorrhage can mimic tumor on T2-weighted images and can also lower the staging accuracy of MRI.

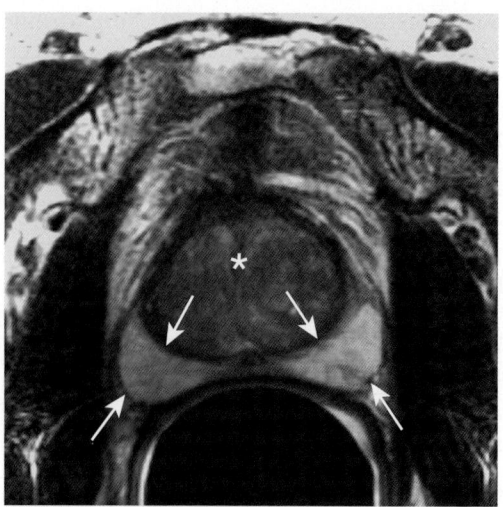

FIGURE 89-3

Axial T2-weighted MR image of the prostate, demonstrating the excellent anatomic detail obtained with endorectal coil images and showing the clear distinction between the transition zone (*) and the peripheral zone (*arrows*).

symphysis pubis, while others also obtain thin-section T1-weighted images through the prostate that correspond to the thin-section T2-weighted images. Spin-echo imaging is a reasonable sequence choice, because of low susceptibility to artifact as compared to gradient-echo sequences. Our protocol utilizes axial spin-echo T1-weighted images obtained from the aortic bifurcation to the symphysis pubis, using the following parameters: TR/TE = 700/8 ms; slice thickness − 5 mm; interslice gap = 1 mm; field of view = 24 cm; matrix 256 × 192; frequency direction transverse (to prevent obscuration of pelvic nodes by endorectal coil motion artifact); and one excitation.

T2-Weighted MRI

T2-weighted images are the cornerstone of MRI in prostate cancer evaluation, since these images clearly distinguish the peripheral zone and central gland, allow the detection of tumor as low T2 signal intensity foci in the peripheral zone, and facilitate staging by demonstration of extracapsular extension and seminal vesicle invasion (Fig 89-3). These features are usually best assessed on thin-section axial images, though the coronal plane is helpful for the sextant localization of tumor in the craniocaudad direction as being in the base, midgland, or apex. The coronal plane may also assist in the assessment of seminal vesicle invasion. Our protocol utilizes thin-section high spatial resolution axial and coronal T2-weighted fast spin-echo images of the prostate and seminal vesicles, which are obtained using the following parameters: TR/effective TE = 5000/96 ms; echo train length = 16; slice thickness = 3 mm; interslice gap = 0 mm; field of view = 14 cm; matrix 256 × 192; frequency direction anteroposterior (to prevent obscuration of the prostate by endorectal coil motion artifact); and three excitations. Fat saturation does not appear to have either a positive or negative effect on staging accuracy,[41] and its use is therefore a matter of preference.

Gadolinium-Enhanced MRI

In the normal prostate, the central gland and peripheral zone enhance homogeneously, with the central gland enhancing more than the peripheral zone.[42-44] Benign prostatic hyperplasia results in marked inhomogeneity of central gland enhancement.[42,43] Some reports suggest that prostate cancer enhances more rapidly than adjacent peripheral zone tissue, and can be demonstrated on early dynamic contrast-enhanced images.[45] Other studies have shown no significant difference between the enhancement pattern of prostate cancer and noncancerous peripheral zone tissue.[46] In clinical practice, gadolinium-enhanced images have not been shown to improve tumor localization or staging,[42,43] with the possible exception of better visualization of seminal vesicle invasion in equivocal cases.[42,44] In general, gadolinium-enhancement is not considered helpful in routine prostate MRI. It should be noted that macromolecular contrast media are in development and may prove more useful, because tumor microvessels are permeable to macromolecular contrast molecules and normal microvessels are not (standard small molecular contrast media pass through the endothelium of both normal and neoplastic microvessels).[47]

TECHNIQUE OF PROSTATE MR SPECTROSCOPIC IMAGING

MRSI uses a strong magnetic field and radiowaves to noninvasively obtain metabolic information (spectra) that illustrate the relative concentrations of various endogenous metabolites in the cytosol of the cell and in the extracellular space. In contrast, MRI uses a strong magnetic field and radiowaves to generate anatomic images based on water and lipid protons. During MRSI, the large tissue water and lipid signals must be actively suppressed in order to detect the prostatic metabolites citrate, choline, creatine, and polyamines that are present in much lower concentrations.[48-53] MRSI is always performed in conjunction with high spatial resolution MRI (Fig. 89-4), because concordant anatomic and metabolic findings provides the most accurate assessment of cancer.[34,54] The resonances for citrate, choline, creatine, and polyamines occur at distinct frequencies or positions in the spectrum, though the peaks for choline, creatine, and polyamines overlap when MRSI is performed at 1.5 T (Fig. 89-5). The areas under these resonances are related to the concentration of the respective metabolites, and changes in these concentrations can be used to identify cancer with high specificity. In particular, prostate cancer, when compared to healthy peripheral zone tissue, is characterized by reduced or absent citrate and polyamines, and elevated choline (Fig. 89-5). The technology required for the robust acquisition of MRSI data from the prostate has just become commercially available and requires very accurate volume selection and efficient outer volume suppression.[48-53]

MRSI Acquisition

Combined MRI and MRSI of the prostate can be performed in less than an hour using a standard clinical 1.5-T MRI scanner and commercially available endorectal

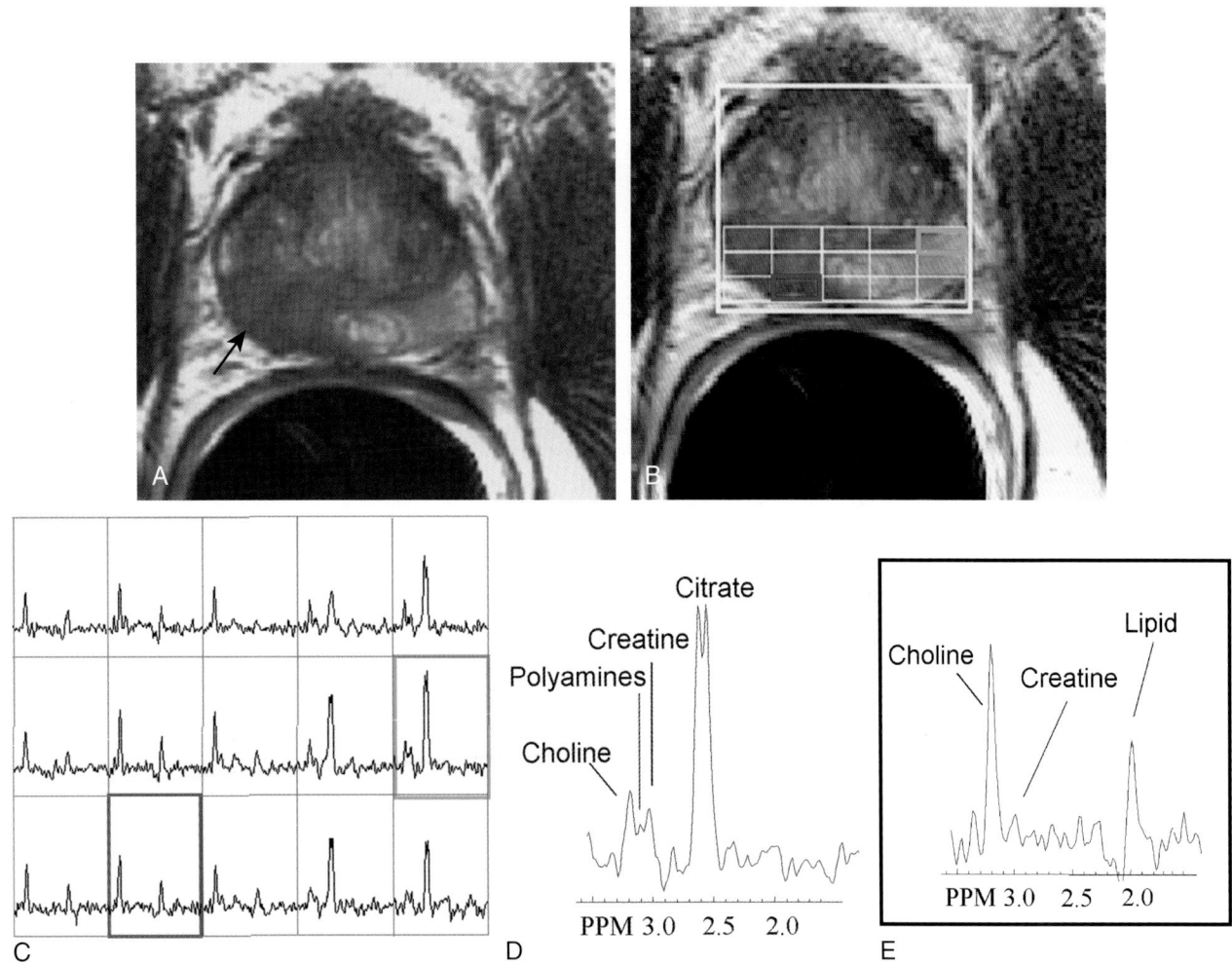

FIGURE 89-4

A, Axial T2-weighted MR image demonstrating a large focus of reduced T2 signal intensity (*arrow*) in the right midgland, suggestive of cancer. **B,** Grid corresponding to the spectroscopic voxels obtained from this section of the prostate has been overlaid on the image in **A**. **C,** Array showing the spectra obtained from the voxels in the grid in **B**. **D,** Spectrum obtained from the single voxel outlined in red in **B** and **C** is shown in greater magnification and detail. Note the dramatically elevated choline peak, absent citrate peak, and prominent "dip" between the choline and creatine peaks (i.e., reduced polyamines) when compared to the spectrum from healthy peripheral zone tissue (see **E**). **E,** Spectrum obtained from the single voxel outlined in green in **B** and **C** is shown in greater magnification and detail. The spectrum demonstrates the characteristic metabolic "fingerprint" of healthy peripheral zone tissue, low choline, high citrate, and polyamine "filling" of the "dip" between choline and creatine.

coils designed for MRI.[48,49,55] The total examination time includes coil placement, patient positioning, and both MRI and MRSI data acquisition. Several vendors are offering or are close to releasing product versions of this combined MRI and MRSI examination. The three-dimensional (3D) MRSI data are acquired using a water and lipid suppressed double–spin-echo PRESS (point-resolved spectroscopy) sequence.[49] Axial T2-weighted images are typically used to graphically select the PRESS volume with the goal of maximizing coverage of the prostate, while minimizing the inclusion of periprostatic fat and rectal air. The volume is often obliqued in the z-axis since the long axis of the prostate is usually angled anteriorly (typically from 0 to 25 degrees) in this direction (Fig. 89-6). The sharpness of the PRESS volume

selection is enhanced through the use of the Shinnar-Le Roux 90- and 180-degree pulses,[56] or through the use of high bandwidth spectral-spatial 180-degree pulses that also reduce chemical shift misregistration errors.[50,52] Even with the use of these optimized pulses, spectroscopic voxels at the edge of the PRESS volume can still be contaminated by residual signal arising in adjacent tissues. To further reduce contamination from tissues surrounding the prostate, the selected volume is automatically over-prescribed by 30% and the recently developed very selective outer volume saturation (VSS) pulses with very sharp transition bands are placed at the edges of the originally selected volume.[53] Subsequently, the MR technologist or spectroscopist graphically places four more of these VSS pulses to better conform the

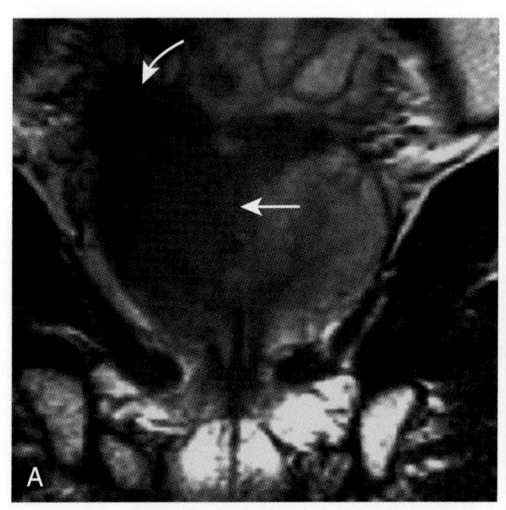
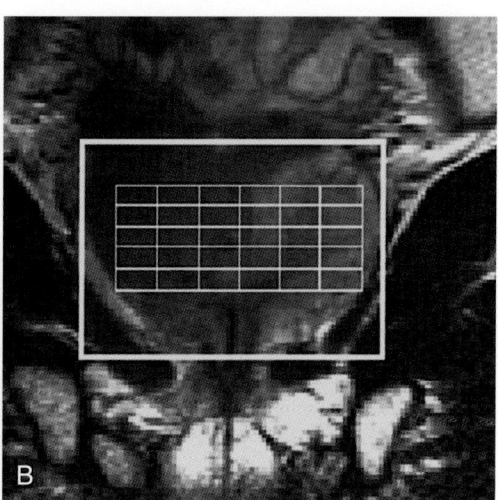
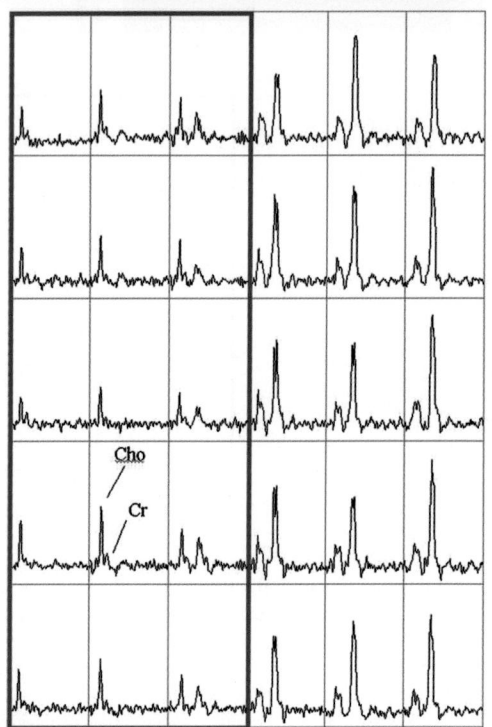

FIGURE 89-5

A, Coronal T2-weighted MR image demonstrating a large focus of reduced T2 signal intensity (*straight arrow*) in the right base, suggestive of cancer. Tumor is seen extending outside the confines of the prostate capsule in the region of the right base (*curved arrow*), consistent with stage T3 disease. **B,** Grid corresponding to the spectroscopic voxels obtained from this section of the prostate has been overlaid on the image in **A**. The spectroscopic-selected volume is indicated by the bold white box, while the spectra from the grid marked by fine white lines is shown in **C. C,** Array showing the spectra obtained from the voxels indicated in **B**. The voxels outlined in red all demonstrate marked elevation of choline and absence of citrate, consistent with a large volume of metabolically aggressive cancer.

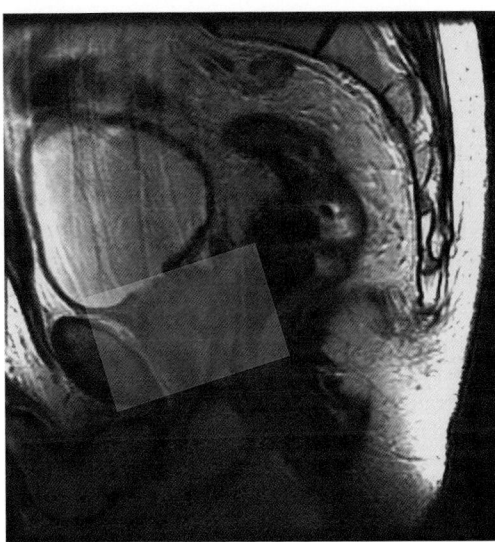

FIGURE 89-6

Sagittal T2-weighted imaging of the prostate, illustrating the typical mild anterior angulation of the long axis of the prostate in this plane. Axial images of the prostate are best obtained perpendicular to this long axis, and so lie at a slight degree of obliquity (opaque rectangle) to the z-axis.

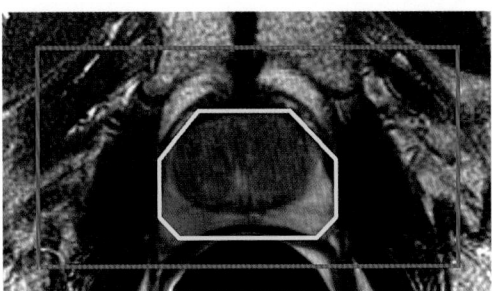

FIGURE 89-7

Spatially-encoded volume, or MRSI volume (orange border), is selected to encompass the prostate with a generous margin. At our institution, we use a volume of $110 \times 55 \times 55$ mm, with the longest dimension in the transverse direction (since this is usually the longest dimension of the prostate). The PRESS volume (yellow border), from which signal is obtained, is chosen to tightly conform to the margins of the prostate in order to reduce spectroscopic contamination from extraprostatic tissues. To further reduce spectral contamination, very selective outer volume saturation (VSS) bands are used to "round off" the corners of the PRESS volume.

rectangular PRESS volume to the shape of the prostate. This often involves placing saturation bands across the corners of the PRESS volume to eliminate periprostatic lipids that normally occupy these regions (Fig. 89-7).

Critical to the acquisition of good quality prostate spectra is optimization of the B_0 homogeneity of the selected PRESS volume. This is achieved through a combination of an automated phase map shimming algorithm and, if necessary, manually touching up the x, y, and z gradients. During manual shimming, the technologist or spectroscopist uses both the magnitude and shape of the free induction decay (FID) and the Fourier-transformed water resonance to assess the quality of the shim.

Water and lipid suppression is achieved using either BASING (band selective inversion with gradient dephasing) pulses placed within the PRESS volume selection[51] or using spectral-spatial pulses capable of both volume selection and frequency selection.[52,54] The influence of chemical shift on the apparent location of the selected box is also greatly reduced due to the higher spectral bandwidth of the spectral spatial pulses.[52,54] Both of these approaches to water and lipid suppression allow for residual water to be left in the spectra to serve as a phase and frequency reference. Residual water also allows for assessment of technical success of the acquisition when there are no metabolite peaks present in prostate spectra due to successful therapy.[55] That is, if there are no metabolic peaks visible, the detection of residual water confirms that this reflects atrophy in the prostate rather than MRSI technical failure, since, in the latter case, residual water would not be detected.

The PRESS-selected volume is subsequently phase encoded to produce 3D arrays of 0.3 mL proton spectra (7 mm on a side) throughout the prostate.[48] Selection of

the appropriate phase-encoding scheme (transverse × anteroposterior × superior inferior, $16 \times 8 \times 8$, and corresponding field of view of $112 \times 56 \times 56$ mm), one acquisition per phase encode, and a repetition time of 1 second is optimized for the dimensions of the prostate and an overall acquisition time of 17 minutes.[48] The echo time used (120-130 ms) is optimized based on the J-modulation of the citrate and polyamine resonances.[48,56]

MRSI Data Processing

Historically, MRSI data were taken off the MR scanner and processed using inhouse research software. In the current commercial MRI and MRSI packages, the MRSI data can be processed and displayed on the MR scanner. For MRSI data, the first processing steps are to construct arrays of spectra by applying time-domain apodization, Fourier transformation, and reconstructing the spatial dependence of the data.[57] For cases where the examination is the initial study on a particular patient, the spectral data may be reconstructed using a discrete Fourier transform on a rectangular grid corresponding to the coordinate system for the reference image. For follow-up examinations alignment parameters from the images may be used to reconstruct the spectra on a point-by-point basis to correspond as closely as possible with the locations from previous studies.

In quantifying prostate spectra it is necessary to correct for constant and spatially-dependent frequency and phase shifts as well as baseline variations due to broad resonances or residual water. Frequency and phase corrections may be achieved using a water reference or by using the spectra themselves to estimate correction parameters. Baseline corrections and estimation of peak parameters are best achieved using prior knowledge of the approximate relative position of the major peaks in the spectrum. Peak areas may be estimated by integration between a range of different frequencies or by fitting baseline-subtracted data as a sum of components with particular line shapes.[58-61] Whichever fitting algorithm is used, the number of spectra involved makes it critical that the procedure is fully automated, as well as robust to low signal-to-noise ratios and missing peaks.

MRSI Data Display

MRSI produces arrays of spectra from contiguous voxels that are approximately 0.3 mL in volume and cover most or all of the prostate. Because MRSI and MRI are acquired within the same examination, the data sets are already in alignment and can be directly overlaid (see Figs. 99-5 and 99-6). In this way, areas of anatomic abnormality (decreased signal intensity on T2-weighted images) can be correlated with the corresponding area of metabolic abnormality (increased choline and decreased citrate and polyamines). Several different approaches have been used to display the combination of anatomic and metabolic information derived from simultaneous MRI and MRSI.[62-66] These include superimposing a grid on the MR image and plotting the corresponding arrays of spectra (see Figs. 89-3 and 89-4), and calculating images of the spatial distribution of metabolites to overlay on the corresponding MR images. These formats provide an excellent summary of the spatial distribution of different metabolites, enabling rapid identification of regions of suspected abnormal anatomy and metabolism. Additionally, since 3D volumetric MRI and MRSI data are collected, the data can be viewed in any plane (axial, coronal, or sagittal) (see Figs. 89-3 and 89-4), and the position of spectroscopic voxels can be retrospectively changed to better examine a region of abnormality on MRI after the data is acquired (Fig. 89-8). This method of interactive analysis will likely be the way that MRI and MRSI data are used in the future and should reduce interpretative errors associated with the overlap of normal and cancerous tissues.

MRSI Interpretation

Interpretation of prostate spectra requires both knowledge of what constitutes a clinically interpretable spectrum and an understanding of the underlying biochemistry and morphology that result in metabolic changes. Prostate MRSI spectra are considered clinically interpretable if they are not contaminated by insufficiently suppressed water or lipid and have resolvable metabolite peaks with peak-area–to-noise ratios of greater than 5:1. The interpretation of prostate spectra requires knowledge of the complex zonal anatomy of the gland, which produces differing metabolic profiles due to the presence of differing tissue types. Of particular importance to the interpretation of prostate spectra is the amount of glandular versus stromal tissue that is present in the voxel, which differs significantly with the different zones of the prostate. High levels of citrate and intermediate levels of choline have been observed

throughout the normal peripheral zone (Fig. 89-9). High levels of citrate in the normal peripheral zone are consistent with the fact that citrate production, secretion, and storage are only associated with prostatic glandular tissues,[67,68] the majority of which (75%) is contained within the peripheral zone.[69] Consistent with the reduction in glandular cell content of the central prostate gland (central zone and transition zones), a significant decrease in citrate in this region relative to the normal peripheral zone has been observed (see Fig. 89-8).[48] Since it is difficult to distinguish between the central (25% of the glandular tissue) and transition zones (5%) based on T2-weighted imaging, these two regions are grouped together when interpreting spectral results. Nonglandular elements of the prostate include the anterior fibromuscular band and periurethral tissues, and these regions demonstrated three-fold lower citrate levels.[48] Additionally, in tissues surrounding the urethra and seminal vesicles, the in vivo choline peak can be elevated due to the presence of high levels of glycero-phosphocholine in the fluid within these structures (see Fig. 89-8). With increasing age the glandular and stromal content of the central gland changes due to the evolution of BPH, which can be predominately glandular, stromal or most often a mixture of glandular and stromal proliferation (see Fig. 89-9). Predominately glandular BPH demonstrates very high citrate levels similar to healthy peripheral zone tissue, while predominately stromal BPH demonstrates dramatically reduced citrate (see Fig. 89-9).[48]

Therefore, the first step in the analysis of the spectral data is to identify whether the spectral voxels arise from the peripheral zone or the central gland and to determine whether the voxels are clinically interpretable. Since at least 68% of all prostate cancers and the most clinically significant cancers arise in the peripheral zone, prior MRI and MRSI research has focused on peripheral zone cancer. The interpretation of central gland voxels is complicated by metabolic overlap between prostate cancer and predominately stromal BPH that is almost always present in the prostate of older men.[70]

The metabolic criteria that are used to identify prostate cancer in the peripheral zone have evolved from an understanding of prostate cancer metabolism and empirical observations in over 4000 clinical MRI and MRSI examinations performed at our institution and from ex vivo high-resolution magic angle spinning spectroscopy of biopsy and surgical tissues that underwent subsequent full pathologic analysis.[55,71] Healthy prostate epithelial cells possess the unique ability to synthesize and secrete enormous quantities of citrate.[68] The decrease in citrate with prostate cancer is due to changes both in cellular function[67,68] and in the organization of the tissue, resulting in a loss of its characteristic ductal morphology.[72,73] Biochemically, the loss of citrate in prostate cancer is intimately linked with changes in zinc levels that are extraordinarily high in healthy prostate epithelial cells and low in prostate cancer.[74,75] In healthy prostatic epithelial cells, the presence of high levels of zinc inhibits the enzyme aconitase, thereby preventing the oxidation of citrate in the Krebs' cycle. Zinc levels are dramatically reduced in prostate cancer and the

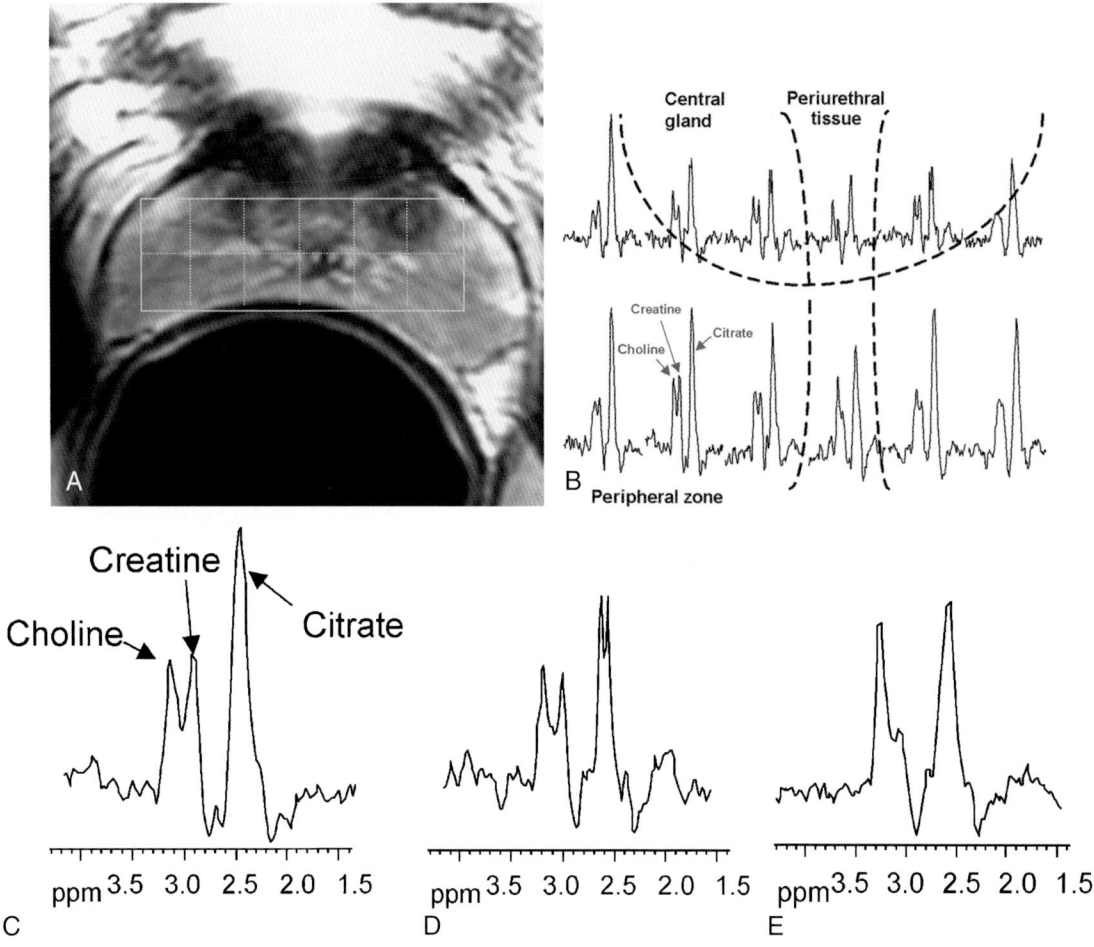

FIGURE 89-8

A, Axial T2-weighted MR image of the mid prostate in a normal 35-year-old volunteer. **B,** Spectra from the normal prostate (grid marked in **A**) demonstrate three distinct metabolic patterns, shown in greater magnification and detail in **C-E**. **C,** Spectrum from normal peripheral zone demonstrates high citrate and intermediate choline and creatine levels. **D,** Spectrum from normal central gland demonstrates lower citrate levels than the peripheral zone, but similar choline and creatine levels. **E,** Spectrum from normal periurethral tissue demonstrates low citrate and mildly elevated choline. The latter presumably reflects choline within the muscular layer of the distal prostatic urethra.

malignant epithelial cells demonstrate a diminished capacity for net citrate production and secretion.[74,75] There exists strong evidence that the loss of the capability to retain high levels of zinc is an important factor in the development and progression of malignant prostate cells.[74-76] Unfortunately, citrate can also be reduced by prostatitis or post-biopsy hemorrhage or any condition that causes a reduction in prostatic ductal morphology and the associated citrate-rich fluids.

As in other human cancers, the elevation of the choline peak in prostate cancer is associated with changes in cell membrane synthesis and degradation that occur with the evolution and progression of cancer.[77,78] Phosphatidylcholine is the most abundant phospholipid in biological membranes and together with other phospholipids, such as phosphatidylethanolamine and neutral lipids, forms the characteristic bilayer structure of cells and regulates membrane integrity and function.[79,80] High-resolution ^{31}P- and ^{1}H-NMR studies

of surgical prostate cancer tissue extracts have demonstrated that many of the compounds involved in phosphatidylcholine and phosphatidylethanolamine synthesis and hydrolysis (choline, phosphocholine, glycerophosphocholine, ethanolamine, phosphoethanolamine, and glycerophosphoethanolamine) contribute to the magnitude of the in vivo "choline" resonance.[81-84] Additionally, changes in epithelial cell density can also contribute to the observed increase in the "in vivo" choline resonance in prostate cancer, since densely packed malignant epithelial cells replace the normal ductal morphology forming prostate cancer nodules that are often palpable by DRE.[72] In more recent high-resolution NMR studies of human prostate cell extracts, elevated phosphocholine and glycerophosphocholine in prostate cancer has been associated with altered phospholipid metabolism.[85]

Recent, high-resolution NMR studies of ex vivo prostatic tissues have identified several new metabolic

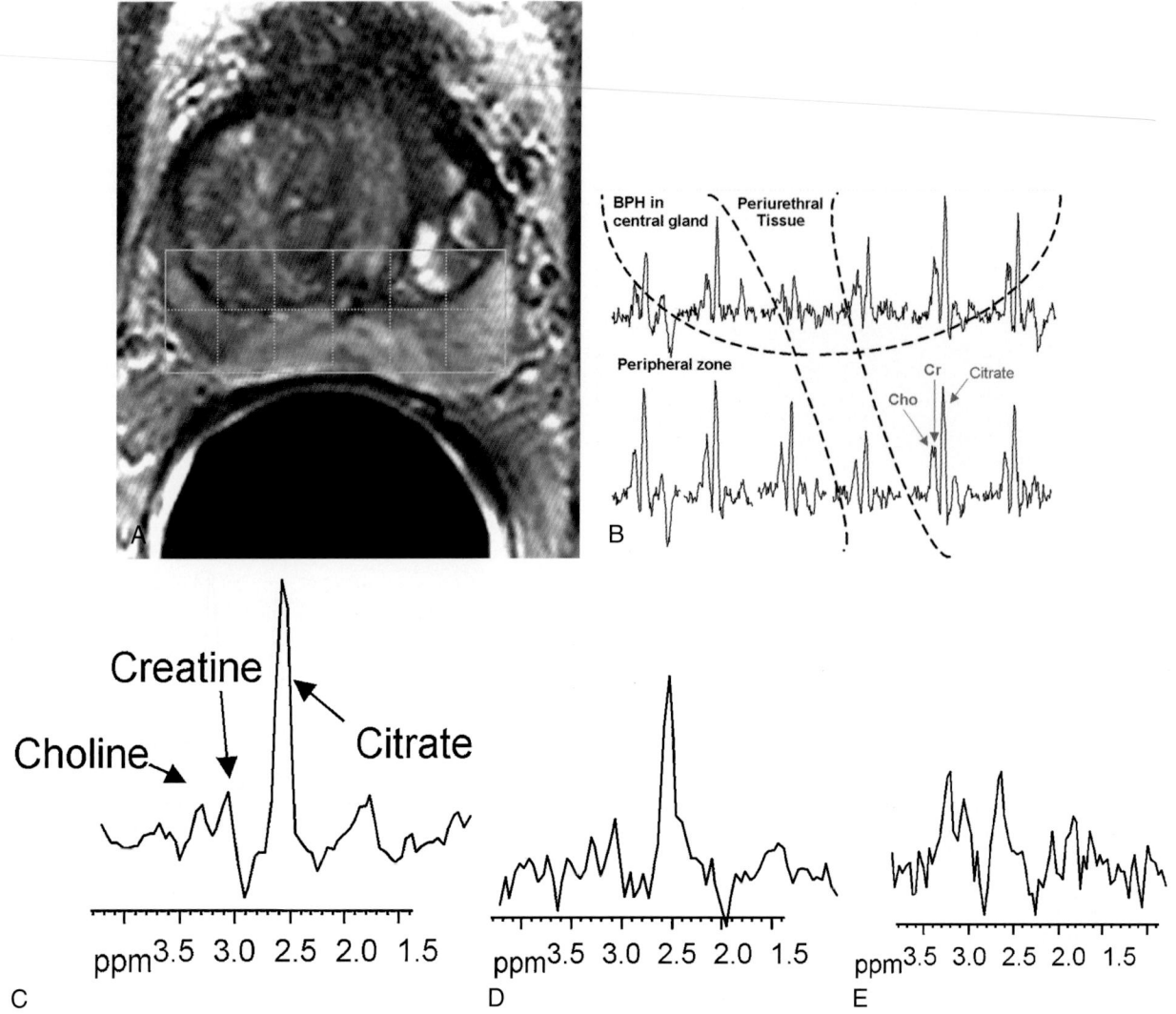

FIGURE 89-9

A, Axial T2-weighted MR image of the mid prostate in a healthy 68-year-old with benign prostatic hyperplasia. **B,** Spectra from the normal older prostate (grid marked in **A**) demonstrate three distinct metabolic patterns, shown in greater magnification and detail in **C-E**. **C,** Spectrum from normal peripheral zone demonstrates high citrate and intermediate choline and creatine levels, similar to the younger prostate. **D,** Spectrum from aging central gland demonstrates higher citrate levels, on average, than the younger central gland. **E,** Spectrum from aging periurethral tissue demonstrates low citrate and mildly elevated choline. The latter presumably reflects choline within the muscular layer of the distal prostatic urethra.

markers for prostate cancer, including polyamines, myo-inositol, scyllo-inositol, and taurine.[71,86,87] Of these, the most promising are the polyamines, which appear very elevated in the spectra of healthy prostatic peripheral zone tissues and predominantly glandular BPH, and dramatically reduced in prostate cancer. Similar to changes in choline-containing compounds, changes in cellular polyamine levels have been associated with cellular differentiation and proliferation.[88,89] Moreover, it has recently been demonstrated that the loss of polyamines in regions of cancer can be detected by MRSI as an improvement in the resolution of the choline and creatine peaks (see Fig. 89-5D).[90]

Based on metabolic changes in choline, polyamines, and citrate in regions of prostate cancer a standardized five-point scale for the interpretation of peripheral zone metabolism in the pretherapy prostate was recently developed and validated.[91] Representative spectra illustrating this scoring system are shown in Figure 89-10. This scoring system proved to be highly accurate (approximately 88% accuracy) in distinguishing benign and malignant tissue with excellent interobserver agreement ($\kappa = 0.80$).

ANATOMY OF THE PROSTATE

The prostate is a pale, firm, exocrine gland shaped like an inverted pyramid that surrounds the urethra between the bladder neck and genitourinary membrane. The

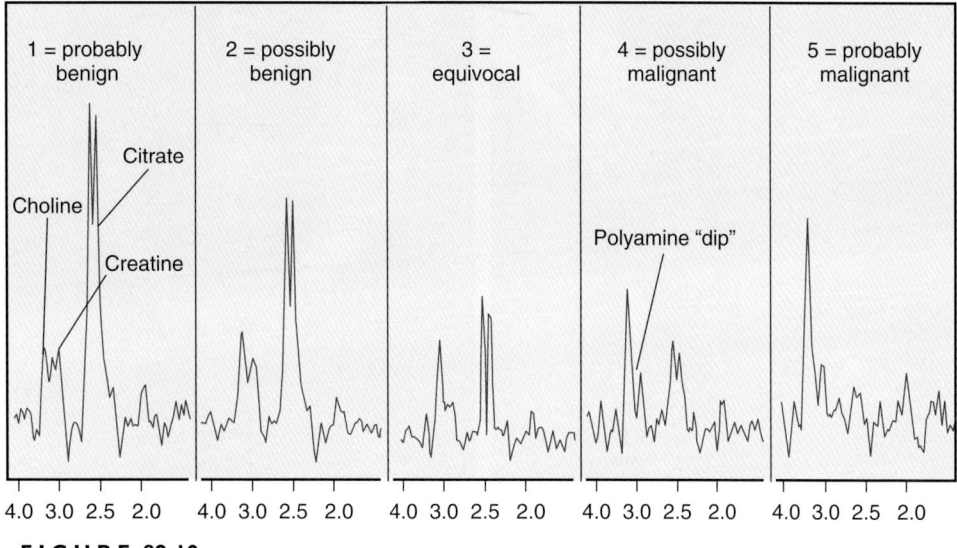

FIGURE 89-10

Representative spectra illustrating the spectral patterns associated with the standardized five-point scale used for the interpretation of peripheral zone metabolism.

ejaculatory ducts pass obliquely through the gland to enter the prostatic urethra at the verumontanum. The normal adult gland is about the size of a walnut, measuring approximately 4 (transverse) × 3 (anteroposterior) × 3 (craniocaudad) cm, and weighing 15 to 20 g. It functions as an accessory sex gland, and contributes approximately 0.5 mL to the normal ejaculate volume of 3.5 mL. The secretions of the prostate are thought to help liquefy semen. The contemporary approach to prostate anatomy describes the internal structure in terms of zones.

Zonal Anatomy

The simplest conceptual approach to the zonal anatomy of the prostate is the two-compartment model, where the prostate is likened to a cone containing a scoop of ice cream.[92] The cone is the peripheral zone and makes up 70% of the prostate gland by volume in young men. The ducts of the peripheral zone glands drain to the distal prostatic urethra. The scoop of ice cream is the central zone and makes up 25% of the prostate gland volume in young men. The ejaculatory ducts traverse the central zone, and the ducts of the central zone drain to the region of the verumontanum clustered around the entry of the ejaculatory ducts. The final 5% of the prostate consists of the transition zone, which is composed of two small bulges of tissue that surround the anterior and lateral parts of the proximal urethra in a horseshoe-like fashion. This two-compartment model is deficient anteriorly, where the peripheral zone is interrupted by the anterior fibromuscular stroma, a band of smooth muscle mixed with fibrous tissue that forms a thick shield over the anterior aspect of the gland. As a result, the peripheral zone lies predominantly lateral and posterior to the central zone.

Confusion regarding the zonal anatomy of the prostate arises because the zonal anatomy changes with age (Fig. 89-11). The transition zone is the portion of the prostate that develops BPH. As a result, the transition zone becomes progressively bigger with age and compresses the surrounding central zone. The latter becomes the surgical pseudocapsule. One approach to incorporate and simplify this age-related complexity is to refer to the transition and central zones collectively as the central gland. Using this terminology, the prostate is composed of the peripheral zone and central gland, such that the central gland is composed mainly of central zone tissue in young men and mainly of transition zone tissue in older men. Given that prostate cancer is largely a disease of older men, in the population that comes to MRI it is reasonable to regard the terms "central gland" and "transition zone" as nearly synonymous.

Anatomy on MRI

The prostate is of uniformly intermediate signal intensity on T1-weighted images, and the zonal anatomy cannot be appreciated.[93] Conversely, the prostatic zones are well demonstrated on T2-weighted images. The anterior fibromuscular stroma is of low T1 and T2 signal intensity.[94] The peripheral zone is of high T2 signal intensity, similar to or greater than the signal of adjacent periprostatic fat. It is surrounded by a thin rim of low T2 signal intensity, which represents the anatomic or true capsule. The central and transition zones are both of lower T2 signal intensity than the peripheral zone, possibly because of more compact smooth muscle and sparser glandular elements.[94] The central and transition zones are of similar T2 signal intensity and cannot be clearly differentiated in normal young men. As previously noted, BPH develops in the transition zone,

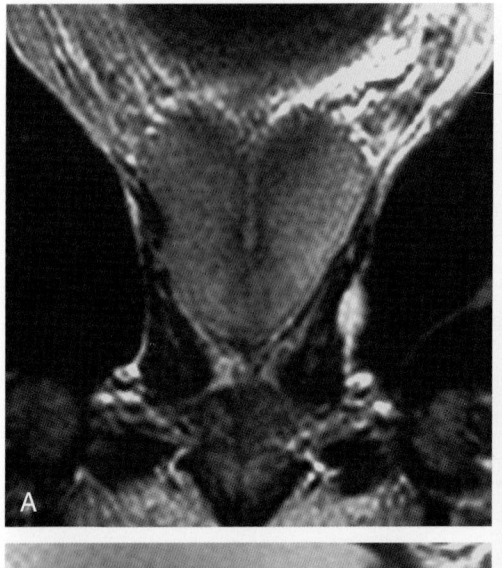

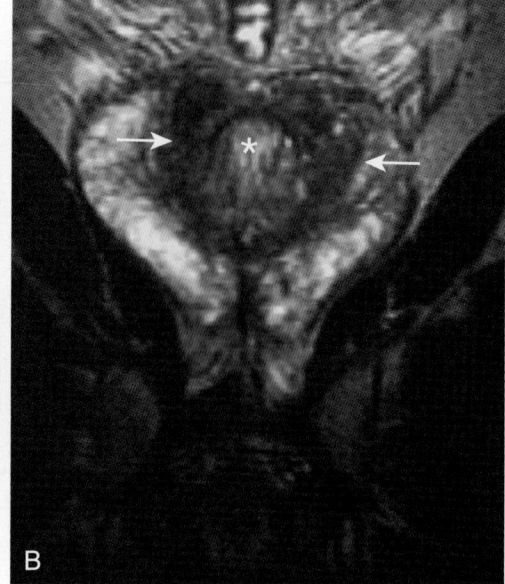

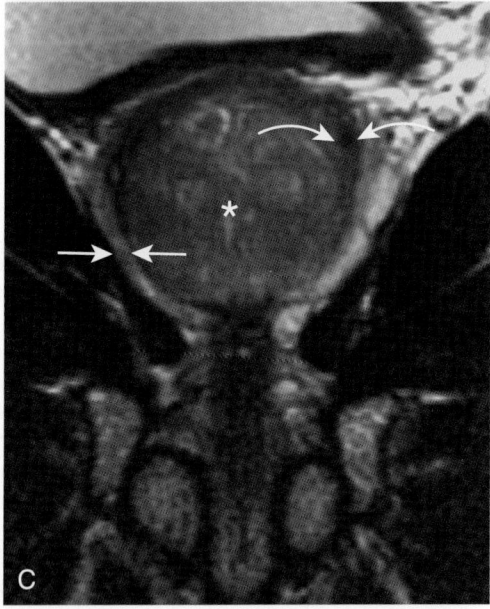

FIGURE 89-11

A, Coronal T2-weighted MR image of the prostate in a healthy 26-year-old man. The prostate is small, of uniform, intermediate T2 signal intensity, and lacking visible zonal differentiation. **B,** Coronal T2-weighted MR image of the prostate in a healthy 50-year-old man. The prostate is of intermediate size due to early changes of benign prostatic hyperplasia, and the hyperplastic transition zone (*) can be seen as a central globular structure, surrounded by the compressed central zone (*arrows*). **C,** Coronal T2-weighted MR image of the prostate in a healthy 78-year-old man. The prostate is enlarged due to marked hyperplastic changes in the transition zone (*). The peripheral zone is compressed to a rim of thin tissue (*straight arrows*) and the central zone is barely visible as a thin "pseudocapsule" (*curved arrows*) between the transition and peripheral zones.

gradually compresses the central zone, and may ultimately compress the peripheral zone as well. The typical changes of BPH often facilitate identification of the transition zone in older men. Ultimately, the central zone becomes compressed to the point of inapparency around the hyperplastic transition zone. The central zone also atrophies with age. A further change that helps distinguish the peripheral zone from the central gland is the age-related increase in the T2 signal intensity of the peripheral zone.[95]

The proximal urethra is rarely identifiable, unless a Foley catheter is present or a transurethral resection has been performed. The verumontanum can usually be visualized as a distinctive structure (Fig. 89-12). The distal prostatic urethra can be seen as a low T2 signal intensity ring in the lower prostate, because it is enclosed by an additional layer of muscle (Fig. 89-13).[93] The ability of MRI to provide multiplanar images of the prostate, with separation of the gland from adjacent structures, makes

it the ideal modality to perform volumetric measurements. Using an ellipsoid formula, the prostate volume is half the product of the maximum craniocaudad, anteroposterior, and transverse dimensions.[96] The vas deferens and seminal vesicles are particularly well seen on axial and coronal images, while the neurovascular bundles can be seen best on axial images (Fig. 89-14). The penile root can be seen inferiorly, separated from the prostatic apex by the urogenital membrane (Fig. 89-15).

While the zonal model of prostatic anatomy can be simplified to a two-compartment model (i.e., the peripheral zone and the central gland), for descriptive purposes further subdivisions are required. Thus, the prostate is conventionally described in terms of sextants, based on division of the gland into thirds in the craniocaudad direction (base, mid gland, and apex), and then into left and right sides. The prostate is shaped like an inverted pyramid, so that the base lies superiorly (just below the bladder) and the apex lies inferiorly (just above the

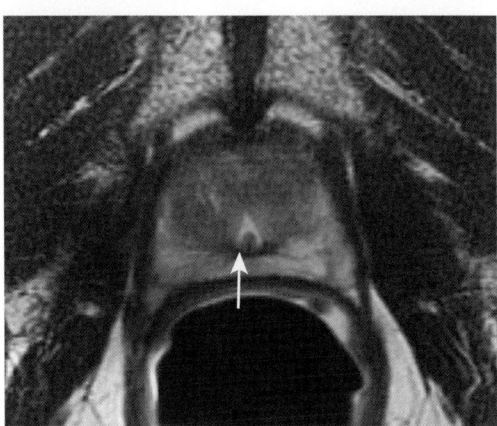

FIGURE 89-12

Axial T2-weighted MR image of the prostate at the level of the verumontanum. The urethra at this level has a distinctive triangular configuration (*arrow*).

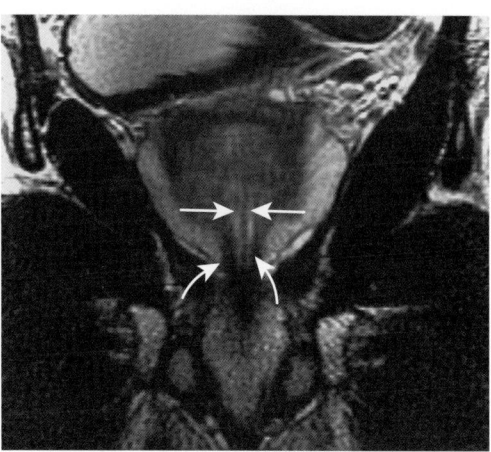

FIGURE 89-13

Coronal T2-weighted MR image of the prostate through the distal prostatic urethra. The distal urethra is seen as two bright lines (*straight arrows*), representing the opposed mucosal layers, and surrounded by an additional layer of low T2 signal (*curved arrows*), representing the additional layer of muscle that encloses this portion of the urethra.

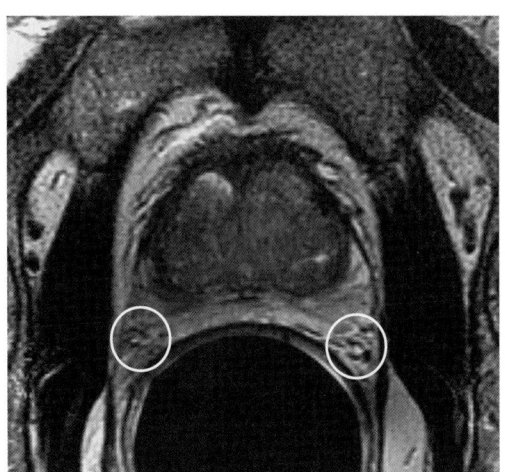

FIGURE 89-14

Axial T2-weighted MR image of the mid prostate. The neurovascular bundles are seen at the lateral aspect of the interface between the rectum and prostate as a cluster (*circles*) of small black dots, representing flow voids within the small vessels of the neurovascular bundles.

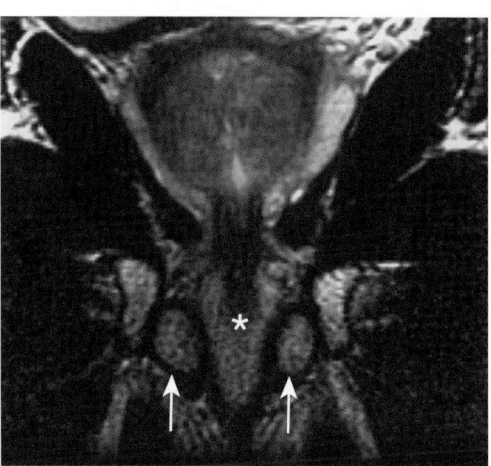

FIGURE 89-15

Coronal T2-weighted MR image of the prostate illustrating the penile root inferior to the prostatic apex and genitourinary diaphragm. The corpus spongiosum is seen as a single midline, high T2 signal intensity structure (*) flanked by the paired corpora cavernosa (*arrows*).

urogenital diaphragm). The mid gland lies between the base and apex. Accordingly, the six sextants are the left base, left mid gland, left apex, right base, right mid gland, and right apex (Fig. 89-16).

Prostate Capsule

The prostate is surrounded by a 2 to 3 mm thick layer of fibromuscular tissue that forms the anatomic or true capsule.[97] The anatomic capsule should not be confused with the surgical or pseudo-capsule that develops around the central gland in the aging hyperplastic prostate. The prostatic capsule comprises the fibromuscular stroma that lies between the glandular components of the prostate and the periprostatic loose connective tissue. The histology of the capsule is particularly complex at the apex, because the fibromuscular band is less well demarcated and because the glandular elements are not as clearly confined. Occasionally, glandular elements are found loose in the apical fibromuscular stroma. These features are relevant to the pathologist attempting to assess extracapsular extension at the prostatic apex, since the apex does not have clearly defined histologic landmarks. At the prostatic base, the periphery of the prostate is composed predominantly of prostatic stroma,

Right   Left

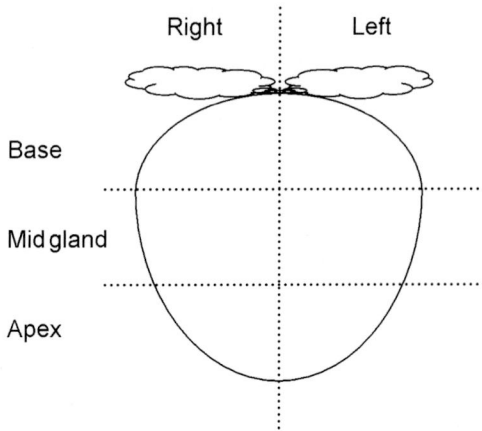

Base

Mid gland

Apex

FIGURE 89-16

Schematic diagram illustrating the six sextants of the prostate: left base, left mid gland, left apex, right base, right mid gland, and right apex.

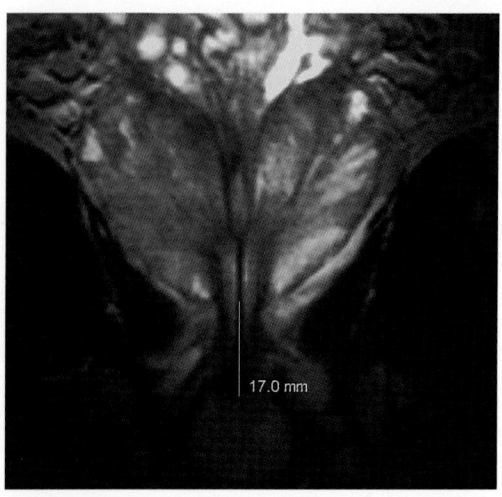

17.0 mm

FIGURE 89-17

Coronal T2-weighted MR image of the prostate illustrating measurement of the membranous urethral length as the distance between the prostatic apex and the corpus spongiosum. Average membranous urethral length is 14 mm. A longer membranous urethral length is associated with more rapid return of urinary continence after radical prostatectomy. *(Reproduced with permission from Coakley FV, Eberhardt S, Kattan MW, et al. Urinary continence after radical retropubic prostatectomy: relationship with membranous urethral length on preoperative endorectal magnetic resonance imaging. J Urol 168:1032-1035, 2002.)*

which merges imperceptibly with the bladder musculature and the stroma of the seminal vesicles. Glandular elements are sparse in this region and usually form epithelial islands surrounded by thick bundles of fibromuscular stroma.

Anatomy of Continence

The posterior urethra, extending from the bladder neck to the distal margin of the membranous urethra, forms a single continence zone, as confirmed by normal urethral pressure profiles.[98] This continence zone can be divided into proximal and distal components, corresponding to the old description of internal and external sphincters. The proximal component consists of two opposed horseshoe-like loops of detrusor muscle.[99,100] These loops are innervated by the autonomic nervous system. They are normally contracted, and urinary continence can be maintained by an intact bladder neck alone.[101-103] Immediately before micturition, the loops relax, and urine enters the prostatic urethra. The continuation of the circular muscle layer of the bladder to the level of the verumontanum as the preprostatic sphincter also contributes to the proximal sphincteric mechanism.

The distal sphincteric mechanism consists of a cone of striated muscle that commences at the prostatic apex and ends at the corpus spongiosum.[98] This cone of muscle increases in diameter from above down. Striated muscle fibers of the upper part of the external sphincter are intermingled with the fibromuscular stroma of the prostatic apex. These findings refute the traditional concept of apical anatomy. The distal sphincteric mechanism has a rich innervation by both autonomic and somatic fibers, from the pelvic plexus and the pudendal nerves, respectively.[104] The longitudinal smooth muscle layer of the membranous urethra probably also contributes to the distal sphincter mechanism, and it is believed that the striated muscle component alone cannot maintain

continence if the smooth muscle component is injured.[105]

A number of factors contribute to incontinence after surgery for prostate cancer. The most important is the extent to which the distal sphincteric mechanism is preserved during radical prostatectomy. The conical shape of the distal sphincter suggests that sacrifice of small amounts of sphincter tissue superiorly at the prostatomembranous junction may not be clinically relevant, provided the inferior bulk of the sphincter is preserved.[98] Other factors that contribute to postoperative continence include age-related sphincteric atrophy and neurophysiologic deterioration.[106] Urinary incontinence is a recognized complication of radiotherapy for prostate cancer, with a reported frequency of 0.5% to 36%,[107,108] depending on the definition of incontinence and the thoroughness of patient assessment. The mechanism is likely radiation damage to the urinary sphincter, either directly or indirectly by neurovascular injury. The relationship between periprostatic anatomy and operative outcomes has been investigated. In a study of 211 consecutive patients with newly diagnosed prostate cancer undergoing radical prostatectomy performed by a single surgeon,[109] membranous urethral length was measured on preoperative endorectal MRI (Fig. 89-17) and correlated with postoperative urinary continence. After controlling for age and surgical technique, multivariate analysis showed that membranous urethral length was related to the time to stable postoperative continence ($P = 0.02$), such that a longer membranous urethra was associated with a shorter time to stable continence.

Anatomy of Potency

The neurovascular bundles and penile root are crucial to erection, and both can be visualized by MRI. These structures are described in turn. Sympathetic nerve fibers from the lumbar sympathetic chain pass inferiorly into the pelvis alongside the aorta and iliac arteries.[93] Parasympathetic fibers enter the pelvis as direct branches of S2 to S4. Both sets of fibers intermix as a mesh of nerves posterior to the bladder, seminal vesicles, and prostate. This mesh is known as the pelvic plexus. The cavernous nerve arises as many fine fibers from the pelvic plexus containing both sympathetic and parasympathetic nerves. The cavernous nerve then runs inferiorly, as one or several large bundles, along the posterolateral aspect of the prostate. In this location, the cavernous nerve is accompanied by arterial and venous prostatic vessels, and together these structures form the neurovascular bundles. The nerve passes through the genitourinary membrane as several fine branches lying 4 to 12 mm lateral to the membranous urethra.[110] These branches end by innervating the corpus spongiosum and corpus cavernosa. The nerves enter the corporeal bodies at the root of the penis, on the undersurface of the urogenital membrane.

The penis arises from the undersurface of the urogenital membrane, inferior to the prostatic apex. This is the penile root, which contains several structures involved in erection: corpora cavernosa, corpus spongiosum, ischiocavernosa, and bulbospongiosus muscles, nerves to these muscles, and arteries to the penis. The paired corpora cavernosa arise as the crura of the penis from the inferior ischiopubic rami and the lateral aspect of the urogenital membrane.[111] They pass anteriomedially to run together in the penile shaft. The single corpus spongiosum arises from the inferior aspect of the urogenital membrane in the midline, and then passes forwards to lie in the anterior groove between the two corpora cavernosa. The posterior part of the corpus spongiosum is expanded, forming the bulb of the penis. The membranous urethra enters the corpus spongiosum from the urogenital membrane, and runs forwards in the center of the corpus spongiosum to reach the external urethral meatus. The crura of the corpora cavernosa are encased by a layer of striated muscle, which arises from the ischial bone around the attachment of the crura and inserts distally into the surface of the corpora. The bulb of the corpus spongiosum is encased by a layer of striated muscle, which arises from the perineal membrane bone around the attachment of the crura and inserts distally into the surface of the corpus. These muscles are known as the ischiocaveronosa and bulbospongiosum muscles, respectively. Both muscles are innervated by somatic fibers from S3 and S4, which reach the muscles from the sacral plexus via the perineal nerve.[93] The nerves enter the corpora near their origins in the penile root.[110] The blood supply to the penis is derived predominantly from the internal pudendal artery, which arises from the internal iliac artery.[98] The internal pudendal artery runs inferiorly along the pelvic side wall, and then divides into the perineal artery and penile artery. The penile artery runs behind the inferior ischiopubic ramus, piercing the urogenital membrane near the membranous urethra, and ends by supplying fine branches to the structures of the penis.

During normal erection, parasympathetic activation through the neurovascular bundles causes relaxation of the arteriolar smooth muscle in the corpora cavernosa and spongiosum.[112] This leads to corporeal engorgement. The bulbocavernosus and bulbospongiosus muscles contract, further increasing corporeal rigidity. These factors act to compress the venous outflow of the penis, further increasing penile rigidity. These complex neurovascular and muscular interactions are referred to as the veno-occlusive mechanism of erectile function.

Potency refers to normal male erectile and sexual function. Impotence is commonly used to refer to impaired erectile function. However, the term is pejorative and imprecise, since it may also be used to refer to orgasmic and ejaculatory dysfunction.[112] The currently preferred term is erectile dysfunction, which is defined as the inability to maintain or achieve an erection sufficient for satisfactory sexual function.[113] Erectile dysfunction is a common side-effect of prostate cancer treatment. Erectile dysfunction after definitive treatment for prostate cancer may arise at several anatomic levels. Excision or manipulation of the neurovascular bundles disrupts the parasympathetic component, and appears to cause erectile dysfunction predominantly by denervation cavernosal dysfunction which results in inadequate veno-occlusion and consequent venous leaking.[114] Nerve-sparing prostatectomy reduces, but does not eliminate, the risk of erectile dysfunction.[115] A tangential but interesting anatomic correlate is the occasional occurrence of erectile dysfunction after therapeutic injection of hemorrhoids; the neurovascular bundles lie anterior to the rectum at the posterolateral margins of the prostate and are therefore liable to injury from inadvertently deep injection of sclerosant agents.[116] A second tangential issue is the occurrence of erectile dysfunction after transurethral resection of the prostate, which is recognized but difficult to explain anatomically. It is possible that there is occasionally damage to the neurovascular bundles.[117] It is also possible that the incidence is overestimated, because patients erroneously equate retrograde ejaculation with erectile dysfunction (retrograde ejaculation occurs after transurethral resection of the prostate because of disruption of the preprostatic sphincter, which is essential for normal antegrade ejaculation).[118] Erectile dysfunction after radiotherapy is predominantly due to arteriolar damage, though cavernosal dysfunction may also contribute.[114] The close relationship of the prostate apex to the penile root provides the anatomic basis for these changes. The arteries to the penis, the nerves to the corpora, and the corporal muscles may all be damaged by inclusion in the radiation field.[119] Imaging can play a role in the elucidation of the complex and multiple factors that contribute to erectile dysfunction after treatment for prostate cancer.[120]

Examination of the region of the neurovascular bundles and the penile root before and after treatment

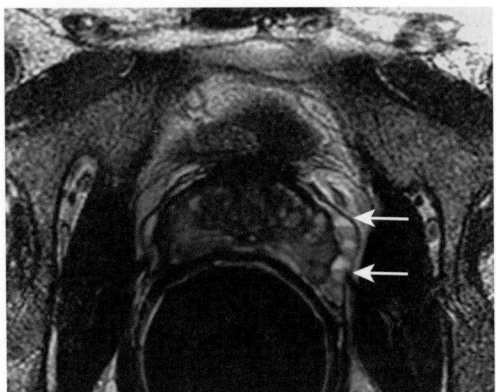

FIGURE 89-18

Axial T2-weighted MR image of the prostate demonstrating prominent periprostatic veins. Hematocrit levels (*arrows*) are visible within many of these veins, presumably related to stasis and slow flow. Prominence of these veins at the prostatic apex is associated with greater blood loss during radical prostatectomy. (*Reproduced with permission from Coakley FV, Eberhardt S, Wei DC, et al. Blood loss during radical retropubic prostatectomy: relationship to morphologic features on preoperative endorectal magnetic resonance imaging. Urology 59:884-888, 2002.*)

may demonstrate changes that could result in erectile dysfunction. Such changes may be visible even after innovative treatments that may be viewed as having low morbidity, such as cryosurgery and seed implantation.

Periprostatic Veins

Blood loss is the most common intraoperative complication of radical retropubic prostatectomy, and predominantly arises from the intercommunicating network of small friable veins that surrounds the prostate.[121] This periprostatic plexus of Santorini receives blood from the prostate and from the deep dorsal vein of the penis, as the latter passes inferior to the symphysis pubis and anterior to the prostatic apex and membranous urethra. The periprostatic plexus drains to the internal iliac veins via the inferior vesical veins. The average volume of blood lost during radical prostatectomy is 700 to 1000 mL,[122,123] even when using techniques that reduce intraoperative hemorrhage, such as early division of the dorsal vein complex and temporary clamping of the internal iliac arteries. In one study, 28 of 200 patients (14%) undergoing radical retropubic prostatectomy required a blood transfusion.[124] A study of 143 patients with newly diagnosed prostate cancer treated by radical retropubic prostatectomy performed by a single surgeon showed that prominence of the periprostatic venous plexus at the prostatic apex (Fig. 89-18) was positively associated with blood loss.[125] However, the correlation was statistical and this observation is of limited clinical utility in an individual patient. Nonetheless, marked prominence of the periprostatic veins at the apex is probably worth noting, particularly in preoperative patients.

MRI AND MRSI OF PROSTATE CANCER

Initial studies in the 1980s established that prostate cancer is characterized at MRI by low T2 signal intensity in the normally high T2 signal intensity peripheral zone.[126-128] Subsequent studies showed that prostate cancer is characterized at MRSI by raised choline (a normal cell membrane constituent that is elevated in many tumors) and/or reduced citrate (a constituent of normal prostatic tissue).[129] The strength of these early studies is that they established morphologic and metabolic MR markers for the diagnosis of prostate cancer. However, these studies merit close scrutiny because of the widespread acceptance of the proposed diagnostic criteria in clinical and scientific practice. Carrol et al[126] studied 12 patients undergoing radical prostatectomy for prostate cancer. All had palpable nodules. Tumor was visible as a hypointense nodule (defined as a discrete well-defined focus of lower signal intensity than the remaining peripheral zone) at T2-weighted MRI in eight cases, based on correlation with histopathologic tumor maps derived from axial sections. However, the authors noted that in only three of these eight cases was "the size of the tumor depicted with MR imaging considered to be relatively accurate." They noted that in the remaining five cases, MRI underestimated the actual tumor volume. Phillips et al[127] found that of 17 patients with biopsy-proven prostate cancer and extracapsular extension (as assessed by DRE) all had a hypointense nodule of at least 1 cm in diameter in the peripheral zone that "correlated with the clinically and pathologically determined location of carcinoma."[127] Tumor maps were not available because the patients had not undergone radical prostatectomy, and the size of the MRI abnormality could not be compared with the true tumor volume. Bezzi et al[128] found discrete T2 hypointense regions in the peripheral zone of the prostate that correlated with tumor based on DRE and biopsy findings in 34 of 37 patients undergoing radical prostatectomy. The authors reported tumor volume as measured by MRI, but did not correlate the MRI tumor volume with the histopathologic volume because "the prostate glands were not serially sectioned for volume reconstruction." The limitations of these studies are important to note, because they indicate the true accuracy of MRI and MRSI with respect to the volumetric localization of prostate cancer has not been well established.

Diagnostic Role

MRI and MRSI are generally performed in patients with histologically confirmed prostate cancer, either in the pretreatment evaluation of disease extent and aggressiveness, or for the assessment of post-treatment recurrence. Occasionally, the test is requested in a patient who has a raised PSA but does not have a histologic diagnosis of prostate cancer, either because the patient is reluctant to undergo biopsy or because a biopsy was performed and was negative (Fig. 89-19). Only a few studies have investigated the accuracy of MRI in the diagnosis of

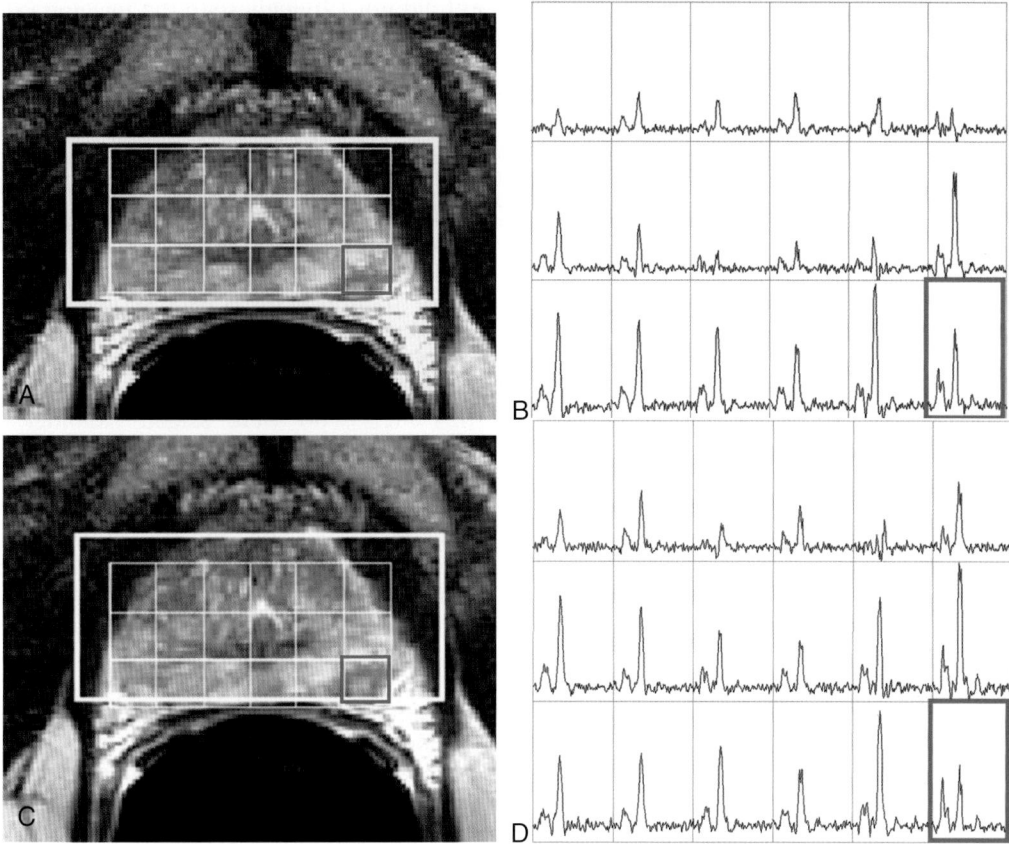

FIGURE 89-19

A, Axial T2-weighted MR image of the apical prostate in a patient who had an elevated prostatic-specific antigen (6.0 ng/mL) but a prior negative biopsy. Note the suspicious focus of low T2 signal in the left apex. **B,** Spectra from the grid marked in **A**. No convincing spectral abnormality is evident in the voxel outlined by red, which corresponds to the voxel partially overlying the focus of low T2 signal and outlined in red in **A**. **C,** The spectral grid has been repositioned so that the voxel outlined in red more precisely corresponds to the focus of low T2 signal intensity. **D,** Spectra from the repositioned grid. After improved alignment, the voxel outlined in red demonstrates a clear-cut metabolic abnormality, with relative elevation of choline and reduction of citrate. A subsequent transrectal ultrasound-guided biopsy confirmed the presence of cancer in this location. Such "voxel shifting" to produce optimal alignment of the spectral voxels is particularly crucial for small tumor foci, since otherwise metabolic abnormalities may be missed due to partial volume averaging between voxels.

prostate cancer in such a setting. In a study of 33 patients with an elevated PSA and at least one negative sextant biopsy prior to MRI,[130] two readers rated the likelihood of malignancy as low, intermediate, or high. Repeat biopsy was positive in 1 of 18 patients considered low likelihood, 1 of 8 patients considered intermediate likelihood, and 5 of 7 patients considered high likelihood. A more recent similar study of 38 patients with prior negative biopsies, 12 of whom had a positive post-MRI biopsy, demonstrated a sensitivity of 83% and a positive predictive value of 50% for the MRI diagnosis of prostate cancer.[131] These results suggest MRI can be used in this setting to stratify patients with a high and low probability of a subsequent positive biopsy. The potential incremental benefit of MRSI in this setting has not been reported, but based on the results for tumor localization (see later), a positive impact would be expected. However, these results also suggest that MRI

would result in an unacceptably large number of false-positive and -negative results if used as a diagnostic tool for prostate cancer in the general population, though such a strategy would, in any case, be impractical for logistic and financial reasons.

Cancer Localization

Sextant biopsy has traditionally been regarded as the standard of reference for nonsurgical tumor localization.[32] However, the limitations of sextant biopsy are being increasingly recognized.[33] In a study with two readers using step-section histopathology as the standard of reference in 53 patients,[54] MRI alone had a sensitivity of 77% to 81% and a specificity of 46% to 61% for the sextant localization of prostate cancer. With the addition of MRSI, sensitivity fell slightly to 68% to 73%, but specificity increased substantially to 70% to 80%. In a different study of 47 patients using step-section histopathologic analysis of radical prostatectomy specimens as the standard of reference,[34] the separate and combined accuracy of preoperative sextant biopsy, MRI, and MRSI were compared. When all three tests were positive for cancer in a sextant, sensitivity was 33% and specificity was 98%. Conversely, a single positive test had a sensitivity of 94% and a specificity of 38%. This suggests that when correct tumor localization is crucial, only sextants that are positive at biopsy, MRI, and MRSI should be considered as definitely cancer containing.

It should be emphasized that these results refer to the sextant localization of prostate cancer, which is not synonymous with volumetric localization. In a recent study,[29] MRI and MRSI were performed in 37 patients prior to radical prostatectomy. Two independent readers recorded peripheral zone tumor nodule location and volume. Results were analyzed using step-section histopathologic tumor volumetry as the standard of reference. The mean volume of all peripheral zone tumor nodules ($n = 51$) was 0.79 mL (range, 0.02-3.70). Readers detected 20 (65%) and 23 (74%) of the 31 peripheral zone tumor nodules greater than 0.5 mL. For these nodules, tumor volume measurements by MRI alone and combined MRI and MRSI were all positively correlated with histopathologic volume (Pearson's correlation coefficients of 0.49 and 0.55, respectively), but only measurements by combined MRI and MRSI reached statistical significance ($P < 0.05$). When all nodules were analyzed, tumor volume measurements were poorly and not statistically significantly correlated with histopathologic tumor volume. These results for prostate cancer tumor volume measurement may appear disappointing, particularly in the context of other studies indicating high accuracy for sextant localization. Two factors probably account for this discrepancy. First, per sextant rather than per nodule analysis does not require size concordance between imaging and pathology, so a very small imaging abnormality counts as a true positive even if the tumor is pathologically much larger, and vice versa. Second, there has been a general downward stage migration of prostate cancer in the era of widespread PSA testing. For example, the rate of organ-confined disease in patients undergoing prostatectomy and MRI at the University of California San Francisco (UCSF) between 1992 and 1995 was 56% (43 of 77),[132] compared to 89% (33 of 37) in 1999.[29] High accuracy is difficult to achieve when imaging smaller tumors.

Cancer Staging

From the inception of prostate MRI, the hope has been that the modality would be more accurate in local staging and detection of extraprostatic disease. Disappointingly, an early multi-institutional study examining the detection of extracapsular extension showed no difference in the area under the receiver operating characteristic (ROC) curve for MRI (0.67) compared to transrectal ultrasound (0.62).[38] However, this study was performed without the use of surface or endorectal coils,

and did not explicitly state the imaging criteria used to diagnose extracapsular extension. Single-institution studies since that time have shown higher overall staging accuracies of 86% to 88%,[133,134] and this is probably a reflection of improving technology and better diagnostic criteria. Multivariate feature analysis has shown the MRI findings that are most predictive of extracapsular extension are a focal irregular capsular bulge, asymmetry or invasion of the neurovascular bundles, and obliteration of the rectoprostatic angle (Fig. 89-20).[132] The addition of MRSI to MRI has been shown to increase staging accuracy for less experienced readers and to reduce interobserver variability.[134] The value of MRI staging has been demonstrated in a 5-year follow-up study of 1025 men who were staged radiologically prior to prostatectomy.[135] The MRI detection of extracapsular extension conferred a significantly worse prognosis in the 39% of patients with moderate- or high-risk tumors. Similarly, a decision analysis model suggested that preoperative MRI was cost effective for men with moderate or high probability of extracapsular disease.[136] Reader variation in the interpretation of prostate MRI remains a barrier to greater acceptance of this technique for preoperative staging. Radiologists who interpret prostate MRI should be aware that high specificity, even if accompanied by low sensitivity, is a more cost-effective approach in patients being considered for surgery.[137]

Extracapsular extension is generally reported as a simple binary observation, either present or absent. This is an oversimplification because extracapsular extension is a continuum that varies in degree. It is instructive to consider how this impacts on prognosis and imaging accuracy. The prognostic importance of the degree of extracapsular extension was evaluated in a 10-year follow-up study of 617 men with T1 to T3A node-negative prostate cancer after radical prostatectomy.[21] The 10-year risk of recurrence (clinical, radiologic, or biochemical) was 32% in patients with microscopic extracapsular extension (defined as the presence of no more than a few malignant cells immediately outside the capsule on no more than two sections) compared to 42% in patients with more established extracapsular extension (see Table 89-4) suggesting microscopic extracapsular extension is nearly as important as macroscopic extracapsular extension with respect to prognosis. This is an important finding, since microscopic extracapsular extension is unlikely to be directly visualized by any currently available radiologic test. The degree of extracapsular extension almost certainly affects MRI staging accuracy. This was directly shown in one study of 34 patients undergoing endorectal MRI prior to radical prostatectomy.[138] The sensitivity of MRI for extracapsular extension of less than 1 mm was only 14% (one of seven sites detected), compared to 71% (five of seven sites detected), for extracapsular extension greater than 1 mm. It is important not to mistake the normally thicker and darker appearance of the ductus deferens at the medial aspect of the seminal vesicles for tumor invasion.[139] Senile amyloidosis of the seminal vesicles is also relatively common as a localized idiopathic phenomenon, and has also been reported as a potential mimic of tumor invasion.[140,141]

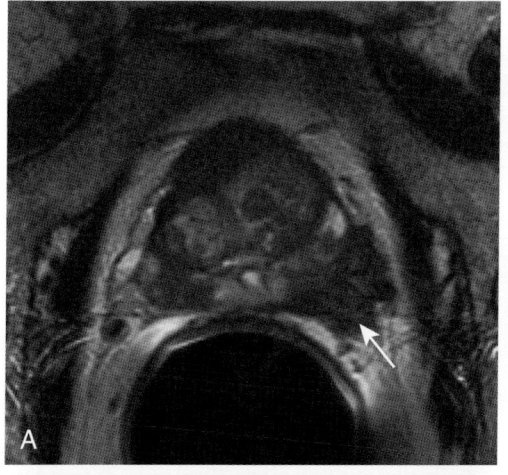

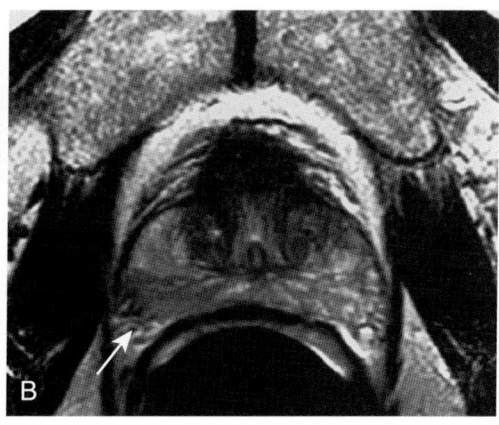

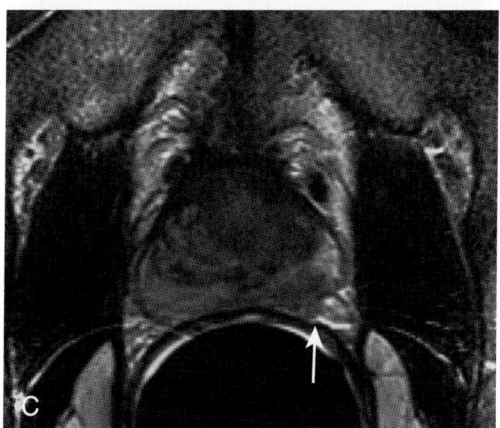

FIGURE 89-20

A, Axial T2-weighted MR image of the prostate showing a focal irregular capsular bulge (*arrow*) consistent with extracapsular extension. **B,** Axial T2-weighted MR image of the prostate showing asymmetry of the neurovascular bundle on the right (*arrow*) consistent with extracapsular extension. **C,** Axial T2-weighted MR image of the prostate showing obliteration of the rectoprostatic angle on the left (*arrow*) consistent with extracapsular extension.

Treatment Planning

Anecdotally, MRI and MRSI results may be of value to patients with prostate cancer who are undecided as to whether to undergo surgery or radiation therapy (Fig. 89-21), though the influence of MRI and MRSI on such decision making is difficult to quantify and has not been systematically reported. We have found that urologists who review the MR images find the depiction of the relationship between the tumors and neurovascular bundles helpful in planning the surgical approach, though this also has not been scientifically validated. Several possible roles for MRI and MRSI have been suggested in radiation treatment planning. Using fiducial markers and image fusion software, it has been shown that CT overestimates the clinical target volume by 34% when compared to MRI,[142] and that dose-volume planning with MRI would decrease radiation dose to the bladder, rectum, and femoral heads. This result is hardly unexpected, given the limited soft-tissue contrast of CT in the prostate and perineum, particularly when CT is performed without intravenous contrast enhancement, as is the usual protocol for radiation planning CT scans. More recently, several groups have reported the use of MRSI to increase the brachytherapy radiation dose in

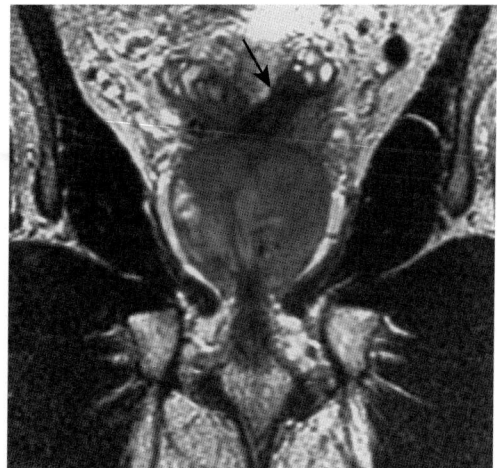

FIGURE 89-21

Coronal T2-weighted MR image of the prostate in a patient with a prostatic-specific antigen of 9.2, Gleason 7 cancer on biopsy, and organ-confined disease on digital rectal examination. The patient was being assessed for radical prostatectomy. Low T2 signal intensity is seen extending into the left seminal vesicle (*arrow*), consistent with T3B disease. In view of this unequivocal finding, the patient opted to undergo radiation treatment instead of surgery.

prostatic locations considered suspicious for cancer.[143,144] Such studies, which suggest that technically successful dose escalation in spectroscopically suspicious locations implies improved clinical outcome, must be viewed with caution given the limited ability of MRI and MRSI to assess tumor volume, as discussed earlier. More convincing evidence of benefit was shown in a study of 390 patients with prostate cancer treated by brachytherapy, either alone (46%) or in combination with external beam radiotherapy (54%), and MRI was used to evaluate stage and guide therapy in 327 of these patients.[145] MRI findings changed the overall treatment recommendation in 60 patients. The majority of these patients were advised to receive combined therapy instead of monotherapy after MRI documented extensive disease. Seed distribution was modified in 183 patients, mostly related to coverage of bulky or extracapsular disease seen on MRI. Freedom from PSA progression at a mean follow-up of 38 months was used as the endpoint. Cox regression analysis showed that only the percentage of positive cores ($P = 0.001$) and failure to have MRI staging ($P = 0.0008$) predicted for failure. This suggests that MRI does improve treatment planning, not only in terms of technical success but also with respect to clinical outcome.

Post-Treatment Follow-Up

The role of MRI and MRSI in post-treatment follow-up of patients with prostate cancer is not well established, largely because it is frequently clinically unclear as to whether patients with a rising PSA after treatment have local or distant recurrence. In our experience, MRI and MRSI are of limited utility after prostatectomy, and only the occasional patient demonstrates an unequivocal locally recurrent tumor. After radiation or hormonal therapy, the prostate becomes shrunken with diffusely low T2 signal intensity and indistinct zonal anatomy.[146,147] These changes greatly limit the role of MRI alone in the detection of local recurrence, and it is possible that MRSI would be helpful in this setting. In a preliminary study of 21 patients with biochemical failure after external beam radiation therapy for prostate cancer in whom subsequent biopsy confirmed locally recurrent prostate cancer in nine hemiprostates of six patients, Teh et al found that the presence of three or more MRSI voxels with isolated (i.e., absent citrate) elevation of choline showed a sensitivity and specificity of 87% and 72%, respectively (Fig. 89-22).[148] In the presence of detectable creatine, choline elevation was defined as a choline-to-creatine ratio greater than 1.5. In the absence of detectable creatine, choline elevation was defined as a choline peak area-to-noise ratio of greater than 5. This study was limited by the small number of patients and the use of sextant biopsy rather than salvage prostatectomy specimens as the standard of reference, but suggests that MRSI may have a role in post-radiation evaluation of prostate cancer. However, it should be noted that the MRSI criteria used to identify prostate cancer after therapy require adjustment due to a time-dependent loss of prostate metabolites following therapy. Published studies have indicated that residual or recurrent prostate cancer can be metabolically discriminated from benign and atrophied/necrotic tissue after cryosurgery and androgen-deprivation therapy based on elevated choline to creatine levels.[48,149-152]

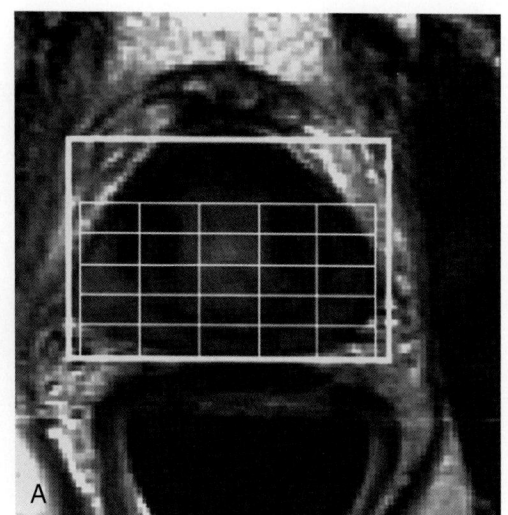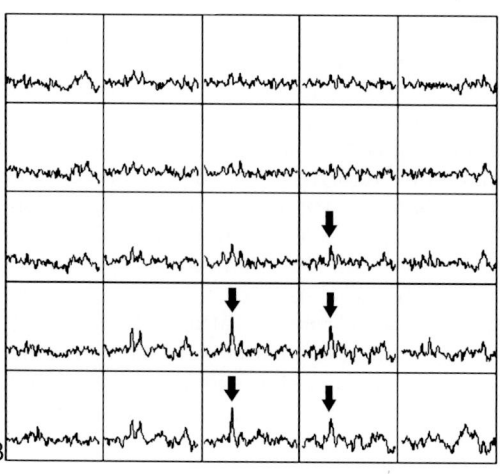

FIGURE 89-22

A, Axial T2-weighted MR image of the prostate in a 60-year-old man with a rising prostatic-specific antigen level 3 years after radiation therapy for prostate cancer. **B,** Proton spectral array corresponds to the grid on **A**. MR spectroscopic imaging demonstrates several suspicious voxels with elevated choline peaks in the left side of the gland. Transrectal ultrasound-guided biopsy confirmed the presence of locally recurrent prostate cancer in the left gland. The detection of local recurrence after radiation treatment of prostate cancer may become one of the primary indications for this modality.

148. Coakley FV, The HS, Qayyum A, et al: Endorectal MR imaging and MR spectroscopic imaging for locally recurrent prostate cancer after external beam radiation therapy: Preliminary experience. Radiology 233:441-448, 2004.

149. Parivar F, Hricak H, Shinohara K, et al: Detection of locally recurrent prostate cancer after cryosurgery: evaluation by transrectal ultrasound, magnetic resonance imaging, and three-dimensional proton magnetic resonance spectroscopy. Urology 48:594-599, 1996.

150. Parivar F, Kurhanewicz J: Detection of recurrent prostate cancer after cryosurgery. Curr Opin Urol 8:83-86, 1998.

151. Mueller-Lisse UG, Vigneron DB, Hricak H, et al: Localized prostate cancer: Effect of hormone deprivation therapy measured by using combined three-dimensional H-1 MR spectroscopy and MR imaging: Clinicopathologic case-controlled study. Radiology 221:380-390, 2001.

152. Mueller-Lisse UG, Swanson MG, Vigneron DB, et al: Time-dependent effects of hormone-deprivation therapy on prostate metabolism as detected by combined magnetic resonance imaging and 3D magnetic resonance spectroscopic imaging. Magn Reson Med 46:49-57, 2001.

153. Chelsky MJ, Schnall MD, Seidmon EJ, Pollack HM: Use of endorectal surface coil magnetic resonance imaging for local staging of prostate cancer. J Urol 150:391-395, 1993.

154. Schnall MD, Imai Y, Tomaszeeoski J, et al: Prostate cancer: local staging with endorectal surface coil MR imaging. Radiology 178:797-802, 1991.

155. White S, Hricak H, Forstner R, et al: Prostate cancer: Effect of post-biopsy hemorrhage on interpretation of MR images. Radiology 195:385-390, 1995.

156. Ramchandani P, Schnall MD: Magnetic resonance imaging of the prostate. Semin Roentgenol 28:74-82, 1993.

157. Ikonen S, Kivisaari L, Vehmas T, et al: Optimal timing of post-biopsy MR imaging of the prostate. Acta Radiol 42:70-73, 2001.

158. Bauer JJ, Zeng J, Zhang W, et al: Lateral biopsies added to the traditional sextant prostate biopsy pattern increases the detection rate of prostate cancer. Prostate Cancer Prostatic Dis 3:43-46, 2000.

159. Qayyum A, Coakley FV, Kurhanewicz J, et al: Relationship between endorectal MR imaging and MR spectroscopic imaging findings in organ-confined prostate cancer and prior transrectal biopsy. Radiology 225(P):628, 2002.

160. Engelhard K, Hollenbach HP, Deimling M, et al: Combination of signal intensity measurements of lesions in the peripheral zone of prostate with MRI and serum PSA level for differentiating benign disease from prostate cancer. Eur Radiol 10:1947-1953, 2000.

161. Van Dorsten FA, Van der Graaf M, De La Rosette J, et al: Differentiation of prostatis from prostate carcinoma using 1H MR spectroscopic imaging and dynamic contrast-enhanced MRI. Proc Int Soc Magn Reson Med 9:632, 2001.

162. Quint LE, Van Erp JS, Bland PH, et al: Carcinoma of the prostate: MR images obtained with body coils do not accurately reflect tumor volume. Am J Roentgenol 156:511-516, 1991.

163. Rifkin MD, McGlynn ET, Choi H: Echogenicity of prostate cancer correlated with histologic grade and stromal fibrosis: endorectal US studies. Radiology 170:549-552, 1989.

164. Tuxhorn JA, Ayala GE, Rowley DR: Reactive stroma in prostate cancer progression. J Urol 166:2472-2483, 2001.

165. McNeal JE, Villers AA, Redwine EA, et al: Histologic differentiation, cancer volume, and pelvic lymph node metastasis in adenocarcinoma of the prostate. Cancer 66:1225-1233, 1990.

166. D'Amico AV, Chang H, Holupka E, et al: Calculated prostate cancer volume: the optimal predictor of actual cancer volume and pathologic stage. Urology 49:385-391, 1997.

167. Carroll PR, Presti JC Jr, Small E, Roach M III: Focal therapy for prostate cancer 1996: maximizing outcome. Urology 49(Suppl 3A):84, 1997.

168. Blute M, Bostwick DG, Bergstralh EJ, et al: Anatomic site-specific positive margins in organ-confined prostate cancer and its impact on outcome after radical prostatectomy. Urology 50:733, 1997.

169. Kooy HM, Cormack RA, Mathiowitz G, et al: A software system for interventional magnetic resonance image-guided prostate brachytherapy. Comput Aided Surg 5:401, 2000.

170. Hata N, Jinzaki M, Kacher D, et al: MR imaging-guided prostate biopsy with surgical navigation software: device validation and feasibility. Radiology 220:263, 2001.

171. Harisinghani MG, Barentsz J, Hahn PF, et al: Noninvasive detection of clinically occult lymph-node metastases in prostate cancer. N Engl J Med 348:2491-2499, 2003.

SCROTUM AND TESTES

Robert F. Mattrey

A variety of imaging techniques have been used to supplement physical examination in the evaluation of scrotal disease. High-resolution ultrasonography is currently the imaging modality of choice. Its contribution has been widely documented.[1-5] The success of ultrasonography is based on its excellent depiction of scrotal anatomy; its display of testicular disease; its low cost, easy accessibility, and speed; and its lack of ionizing radiation. However, high-resolution ultrasonography is limited by its small field of view (FOV), high dependence on technical expertise, and lack of specificity in many disease conditions. Color Doppler imaging has added both anatomic and functional details for evaluation of the testis and its surrounding structures, essentially eliminating the need for nuclear scanning in the setting of acute scrotal pain.[6-12]

MRI provides outstanding contrast resolution and, with the use of high field strengths and surface coils, satisfactory spatial resolution.[13-17] MRI, like ultrasonography, is nonionizing and has, as yet, no known harmful effects. With its wide FOV, MRI is well suited for imaging and evaluation of the scrotum. Since the first reports,[13,14] our experience and that of others has increased.[15-18] The ability of MRI to characterize scrotal disease,[14] has been substantiated with this added experience.[15,16,18] Many disease processes have characteristic appearances to allow their recognition with sufficient specificity. Although the true sensitivity of MRI has not been substantiated, it is likely to equal or may exceed that of ultrasonography.[17] The ability to recognize each intrascrotal structure because of its signal intensity, appearance, and location separate from any other structure, the ability to view the right and left hemiscrotum along with the inguinal region, and the high contrast afforded by MRI make MRI less subjective than ultrasonography. MRI changed the ultrasonographic diagnosis of testicular disease from normal to cancer in 4 of 23 (17%) patients in one study,[17] and from cancer to benign disease in nearly 6% of our cases.[19] The proven efficacy of ultrasonography based on several years of experience, its unlimited access, and its low cost have hindered the advance of this new application of MRI to truly assess its impact on patient care.

This chapter is intended to describe the imaging techniques found to be optimal, to present the normal appearance of the scrotum by MRI, and to demonstrate some common pathologic conditions to provide the reader with the necessary data to obtain and interpret scrotal MR images.

IMAGING TECHNIQUE

Positioning and Preparation of Patients

The patient is positioned supine on the imaging table, feet first, and the scrotum is elevated by means of a support between the thighs to ensure that both testes are in the same horizontal plane for proper coronal imaging. The penis is angled to the side and the whole region is draped. To improve spatial and contrast resolution and signal homogeneity, a 12.5-cm standard equipment circular surface coil is centered over the scrotum and placed horizontally on a 1-cm standoff. The coil is positioned such that the bottom of the coil is over the caudal tip of the scrotal sac. The entire area is then wrapped with the 14-inch table strap to minimize motion. The isocenter is positioned at the middle of the scrotum. In infants, the standard 9-cm circular coil is used in lieu of the 12.5-cm coil.

The air surrounding the scrotum can produce susceptibility artifacts at the edge of the testis. The use of an air-displacing support structure of equal magnetic susceptibility to water, such as the Sat Pad, reduces this artifact.[20]

Pulse Sequence

Multislice imaging begins with a sagittal localizer using a 20-cm FOV. The center of the FOV is shifted anteriorly by 5 cm to ensure that the scrotum is properly centered.

With the advent of the fast spin-echo technique, the standard spin-echo technique has been abandoned. We now obtain four sequences in addition to the sagittal localizer, a heavily T1-weighted (repetition time (TR), 400 ms; echo time (TE), 12 ms; 256×128 acquisition matrix; two excitations) and a fast spin-echo T2-weighted series (TR, 3500 ms; TE, 120 ms, 256×192 matrix, two excitations, 16 echoes) in the coronal and axial planes. Both sequences are obtained with an FOV of 16 cm and a slice thickness of 3 mm with a 1.5-mm interslice gap to ensure proper T2 weighting. The coronal series covers from the posterior aspect of the scrotum to the anterior aspect of the external inguinal ring. The testes must be at the center of the volume for proper prescan optimization; otherwise, the scan will be optimized to tissues other than the testes. The axial series covers from the inferior aspect of the scrotal sac to the top of the symphysis pubis, again ensuring that the testes are at the center of the volume. Note that fat suppression is not necessary because the scrotum contains little fat. Furthermore, because of magnetic field inhomogeneities, water rather than fat could become suppressed, increasing the confusion.

The use of intravenous contrast medium is occasionally needed. In general, however, contrast medium enhancement is reserved for patients with subtle, atypical, or complex findings.

Imaging Planes

The coronal plane is the ideal plane for imaging the scrotum.[13,14] It allows complete visualization of all important anatomic structures and demonstrates the epididymis and spermatic cord optimally. It also allows comparison of the right and left hemiscrotal and inguinal regions. The coronal plane is parallel to the plane of the surface coil, so coronal images are the most pleasing to view because the signal across the field is homogeneous and can be photographed with optimal window and center settings. Although the sagittal plane defines the full anteroposterior dimension of the scrotum and occasionally displays the "bare area" of the testes and cord to better advantage, it offers limited recognition of the epididymis, epididymis-scrotal wall interface, and epididymis-testis interface, and does not allow right and left comparison on the same image. Although the coronal series is sufficient in more than 70% of cases, the axial series clarifies complex findings, allows optimal visualization of the anterior and posterior aspect of the

testis and the body of the epididymis, as well as the epididymis-testis interface, and allows for right and left comparison.

ANATOMY

Embryology

The testis and its efferent duct systems, epididymis, and vas deferens develop from the gonadal ridges and mesonephric duct. The germ cells, which originate from the endodermal cells in the yolk sac, must migrate to and invade the gonadal ridges for the gonads to develop. The primitive sex cords develop in the fifth to sixth week of gestation by the proliferation and penetration of the gonadal ridge into the underlying mesenchyme. Under the influence of the Y chromosome, the primitive sex cords develop into the medullary cords, which split into a network of tiny cell strands that point toward the hilum to give rise to the tubules of the rete testis. During development the medullary cords are separated from the coelomic epithelium by a dense fibrous connective tissue, the tunica albuginea. During the fourth month of development, the testis cords are composed of primitive germ cells and sustentacular cells of Sertoli derived from the surface epithelium gland. The testis cords remain solid until puberty, at which time they form the seminiferous tubules. At puberty they become canalized and join the rete testis tubules, which in turn enter the efferent ductules that are linked to the ductus deferens.[21-23]

The interstitial cells of Leydig are derived from the mesenchyme of the gonadal ridge. The Leydig cells produce testosterone by the eighth week of gestation which effects sexual differentiation of the genital duct and external genitalia. Initially, the embryo has two pairs of genital ducts, the mesonephric duct and the paramesonephric duct. In the male, as the mesonephros regresses, the mesonephric duct persists to form the main genital ducts, the ductus deferens, and the epididymis. As the most cranial portion of the mesonephric duct regresses, it forms the appendix epididymis, and as the paramesonephric duct regresses, it forms the appendix testis. The caudal portion of the regressed mesonephros forms the paradidymis.[23,24]

The primitive testis is found in the posterior abdominal wall until the end of the second month of gestation. As the mesonephros degenerates, ligamentous bands (known as the caudal genital ligament and gubernaculum) descend to the inguinal region from the lower pole of the testes. Each gubernaculum then passes through the abdominal wall and attaches to the scrotal swelling. Independent from the descent of the testis, the peritoneal cavity evaginates, following the course of the gubernaculum into the scrotal swelling to form the vaginal process. The vaginal process exits the fascial layers of the abdominal wall that form the inguinal canal accompanying the gubernaculum. By the 28th week of gestation, the testes descend to the level of the inguinal canal, and by the 32nd week they enter the scrotum. As the testis descends through the inguinal canal, it is covered by and becomes fused with reflected folds of

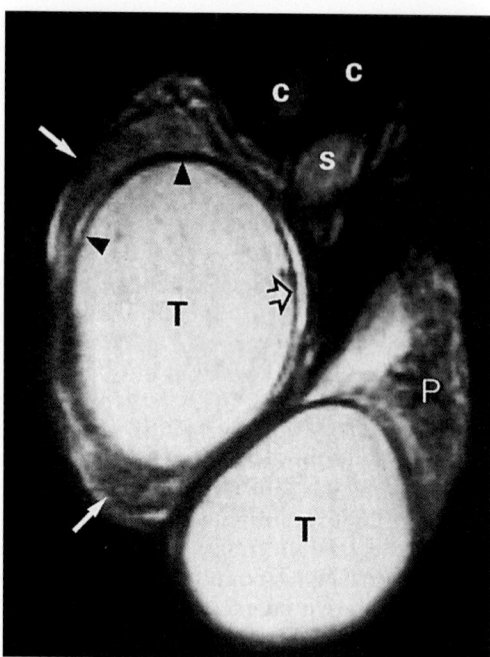

FIGURE 90-1

Normal testes (T), epididymis (*arrows*), and tunica albuginea (*arrowheads*) shown in the coronal plane on a T2-weighted image. A small amount of fluid between the tunical layers, shown best on T2-weighted images, is frequently seen (*open arrow*). The pampiniform plexus (P) can be seen at the base of the scrotum. A cross-section of the penis is seen superior to the scrotum demonstrating the corpora cavernosa (c) and corpora spongiosa (s). The corpora cavernosa is surrounded by a thick dark band, the tunica albuginea of the penis. (*Modified with permission from Baker LL, Hajek PC, Burkhard TK, et al: MR imaging of the scrotum: normal anatomy. Radiology 163:89-92, 1987.*)

the vaginal process to form the tunica vaginalis. Regression of the gubernaculum produces testicular fixation to the scrotum. At birth, 3% of male infants have undescended testes, and this percentage decreases to 0.8% during the first year.[21,23]

The mechanism of descent is not entirely clear. However, it has been shown that outgrowth of the extra-abdominal gubernaculum produces intra-abdominal migration of the testis, and increased intra-abdominal pressure due to growth of intra-abdominal organs promotes the passage of the testis into the inguinal canal. The process of descent is controlled by hormones, which may be androgens and müllerian-inhibiting substances excreted by the Sertoli cells.[21,23]

Normal Anatomy at MRI

The normal testis on MR images is a sharply demarcated oval structure of homogeneous signal intensity brighter than water and darker than fat on T1-weighted images. Testes become slightly darker than water but much brighter than fat on T2-weighted images (Fig. 90-1). The intensity of the testis on T2-weighted images contrasts with the fluid frequently present between the layers of the tunica vaginalis, allowing the assessment of its signal

behavior. The testis is completely surrounded by the tunica albuginea, a thick layer of dense fibrous tissue that is of low signal intensity on T2-weighted images. It can adopt a slightly brighter signal owing to partial volume when the slice plane is near tangential to the testicular surface. The tunica vaginalis, an extension of the peritoneum, is fused to the tunica albuginea except along the bare area of the testis, which becomes highlighted by hydrocele (Fig. 90-2). Along the bare area, the tunica albuginea invaginates the testis to produce the mediastinum testis, through which the testis receives part of its blood supply, and delivers the tubules to the epididymis. The mediastinum is a longitudinal structure 1 to 3 cm in length which is isointense with testis on T1-weighted images and darker than testis on T2-weighted images (see Fig. 90-2). Intrinsic testicular signal, although homogeneous, displays internal texture outlining lobules and rete testes. Intratesticular vessels are infrequently seen in normal testes, but, at times, a major bundle can be seen emanating from the superior mediastinum toward the lateral aspect of the upper pole to reach the tunica (see Fig. 90-23). These vessels have been well described in the literature on ultrasonography.[25]

The epididymis is inhomogeneous with intermediate signal intensity less than that of normal testicular tissue on T2-weighted images. The degree of darkening of the epididymis is variable but when much darker than testis raises the possibility of fibrosis from prior infection. The head, body, and tail of the normal epididymis are easily delineated (see Fig. 90-1). The head of the epididymis, lying lateral to the upper pole of the testis, drapes the tunical signal (see Fig. 90-1). The normal tail, best seen when highlighted by fluid, is smaller than the epididymal head. The body of the epididymis lies in the bare area alongside the mediastinum testis and is therefore extravaginal. It can be easily recognized from testis because it has a darker signal on T2-weighted images and is separated from testicular tissue by the dark band of the tunica albuginea.

The outer parietal and inner visceral layers of the tunica vaginalis are frequently separated by a small amount of fluid (see Fig. 90-1). On T2-weighted images and in the presence of hydrocele, the fluid completely surrounds the testes except posteromedially along the bare area where the testis is attached to the scrotal wall (see Fig. 90-2). The scrotal sac structures, such as fat and dartos muscle, can at times be seen (Fig. 90-3).

The spermatic cord is easily imaged in all cases. Tortuous tubular structures of low signal intensity located at the posterosuperior aspect of the scrotal sac represent the pampiniform plexus (see Fig. 90-1), which can be followed into the inguinal canal (Fig. 90-4). At times, the cremasteric reflex causes foreshortening of the cord, which may give the cord a nodular appearance on a coronal section (see Fig. 90-4). Smooth, undulating tubular structures similar in signal intensity to testis (Fig. 90-5) can at times be seen in the cord or epididymis. They may represent a prominent vas deferens, a serpiginous spermatocele, or a varicocele with stagnant blood. Enhancement with contrast medium would allow the distinction of varicocele from the other two structures.

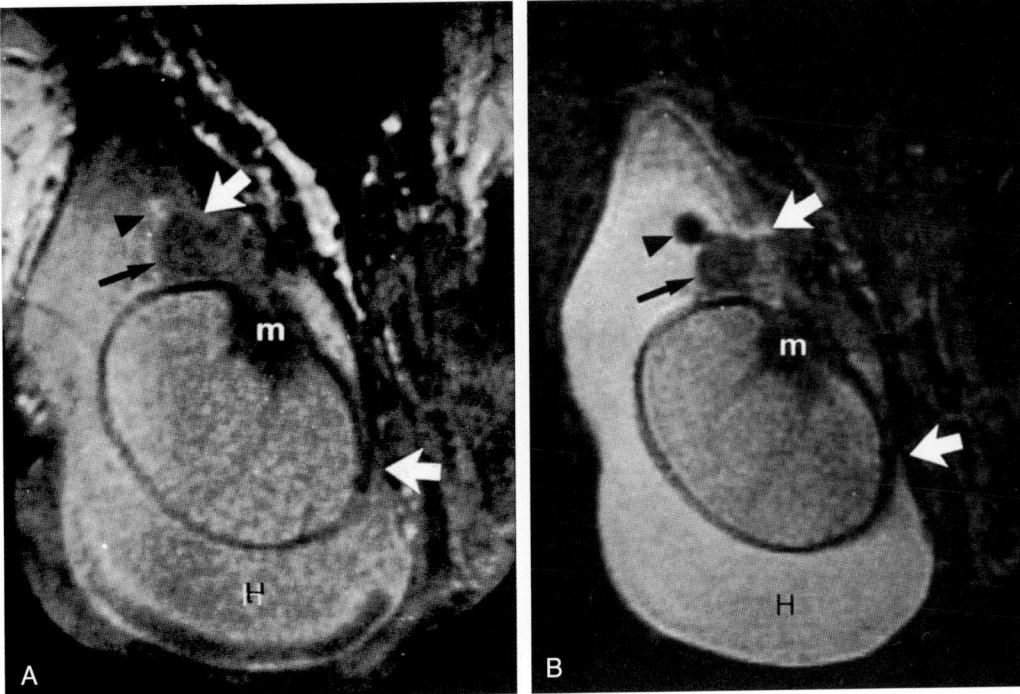

FIGURE 90-2

Acute simple hydrocele is shown on **A,** proton-density–weighted and **B,** T2-weighted images. Note that the signal of hydrocele is consistent with that of water (intermediate with proton-density weighting and bright with T2 weighting). This sympathetic hydrocele is thought to be due to torsion of the epididymal appendix, shown to be hemorrhagic on MR images (*arrowhead*) (slightly bright with proton-density weighting and dark with T2 weighting) and attached to the normal epididymis (*black arrow*). In this example, the lobular septa can be seen with T2 weighting (**B**) emanating from the mediastinum testes (m). Note that the presence of sizable hydrocele demonstrates the "bare area" of the testis, the edges of which are marked by large white arrows. *(Reproduced with permission from Baker LL, Hajek PC, Burkhard TK, et al: MR imaging of the scrotum: Pathologic conditions. Radiology 163:93-98, 1987.)*

FIGURE 90-3

A, Sagittal T2-weighted image shows clear delineation of the tunica albuginea (*arrowheads*), epididymal head and tail (*arrows*), and the various layers of the scrotal wall, including the dartos muscle (*open arrow*). **B,** Cadaveric specimen from a different subject shows similar anatomy. Note that the mediastinum testis (*open arrow*) and the vas deferens (*curved arrow*) can be seen on this section. *(Reproduced with permission from Baker LL, Hajek PC, Burkhard TK, et al: MR imaging of the scrotum: normal anatomy. Radiology 163:89-92, 1987.)*

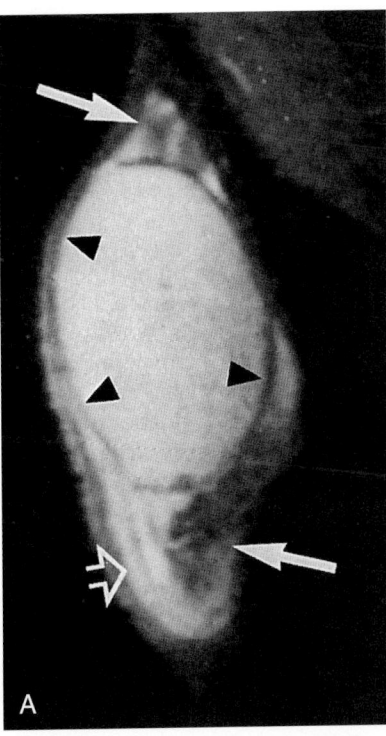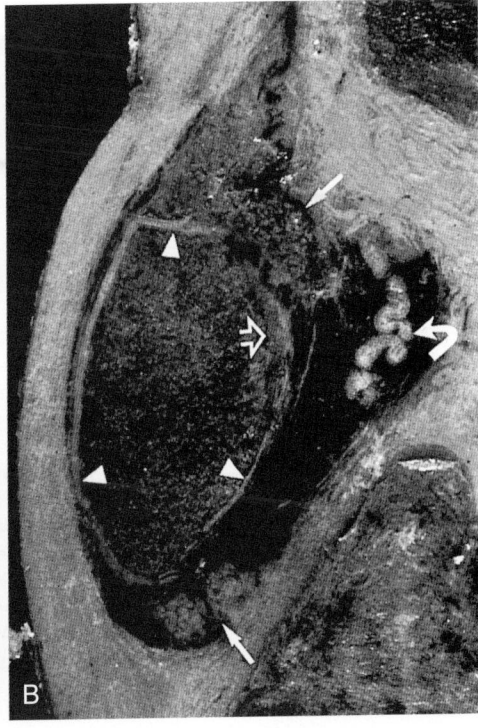

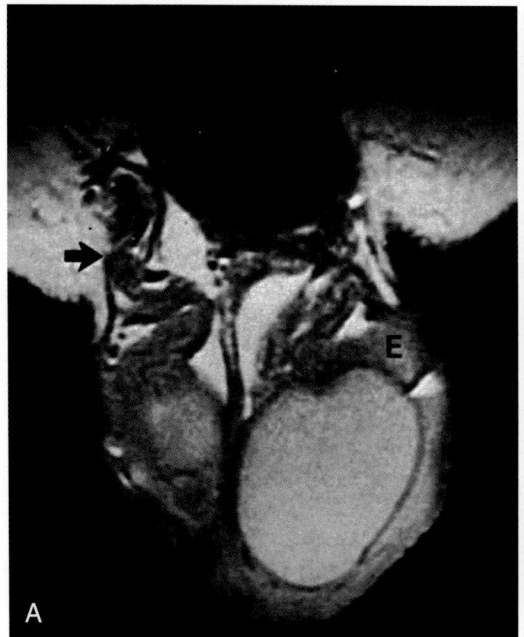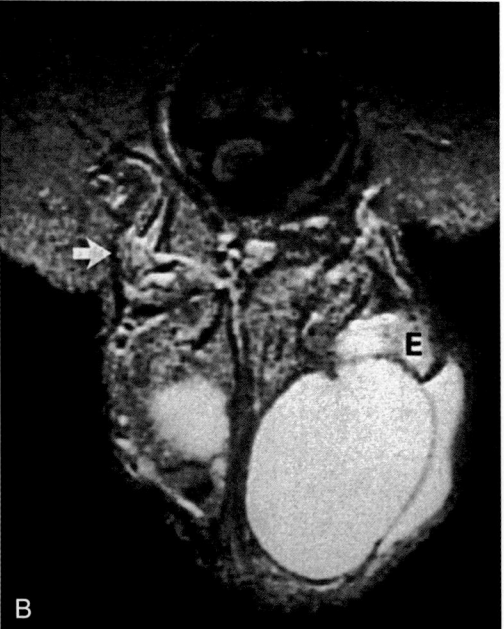

FIGURE 90-4

A, Proton-density–weighted and **B,** T2-weighted images in the coronal plane show the accordion-shaped spermatic cord (*arrow*) entering the base of the right hemiscrotum. Note that the small hydrocele on the left outlines the epididymal head (E). (*Reproduced with permission from Baker LL, Hajek PC, Burkhead TK, et al: MR imaging of the scrotum: normal anatomy. Radiology 163:89-92, 1987.*)

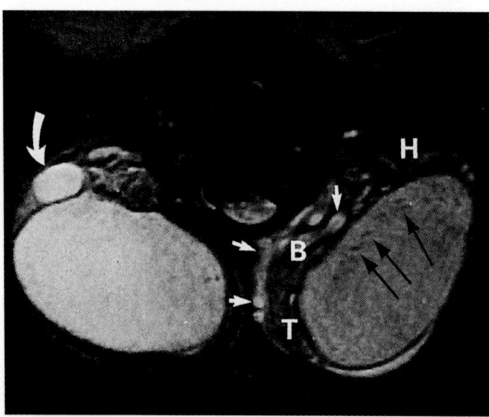

FIGURE 90-5

Coronal T2-weighted image shows a prominent serpentine structure in the body of the epididymis (*white arrows*). Its signal was similar to testis on all sequences (not shown). This is presumed to represent dilated ducts or spermatocele but could also represent a dilated vein or varicocele with stagnant blood. Intravenous contrast medium could allow this distinction. Note that the entire epididymis can be seen: head (H), body (B), and tail (T). Also note the clear delineation of the testis from the epididymis by the dark tunica albuginea. Small linear dark signals (*black arrows*) within the testis are interlobular septa converging toward the mediastinum seen on the next slice (not shown). Also note the presence of an epididymal cyst (*curved arrow*) on the right. Because it was dark with proton-density weighting (not shown), it behaved similarly to water. The difference in the right and left testicular signals is due to the coil position.

PATHOLOGY

The homogeneous high signal intensity of the normal testes on T2-weighted images provides an excellent background for visualizing intratesticular disease. Except for old blood or epidermoid cysts, all intratesticular disease has been less intense than normal testicular tissue on T2-weighted images. The integrity of the tunica albuginea can be assessed; however, partial volume may assign the tunica a brighter signal. If the integrity of the tunica albuginea must be assessed, the slice must be obtained perpendicular to the area of interest.

The majority of pathologic conditions of the scrotum are best visualized on the T2-weighted images. The T1-weighted images allow for tissue characterization. Complete assessment of the scrotum is possible in most cases with coronal sections only. Axial T2-weighted images add confidence, demonstrate to a better advantage the small lesions abutting the anterior or posterior surfaces, and help define complex anatomy.

Neoplasms

Tumors are typically isointense with normal testis on T1-weighted images, becoming inhomogeneous and slightly darker on proton-density–weighted images and moderately darker on T2-weighted images. Their margination and extent, as well as their influence on normal testicular size and shape, are well demonstrated. Extension of mass into extratesticular locations, such as the epididymis or cord, is clearly shown.[14] Local staging of testicular cancer is done histologically. Staging by imaging is reserved for the assessment of regional and retroperitoneal lymph nodes.

Although complete replacement of the testis by cancer has been reported,[17] it is unusual. Cancer typically leaves a rim of normal testicular tissue, even when the mass is large (Fig. 90-6). It is possible in infiltrative disorders (lymphoma or leukemia) for the testis to become totally replaced.[17] In such instances, the signal of the affected testis can be compared with the contralateral testis or surrounding structures and hydrocele. When a fibrous tumor capsule is seen histologically about the tumor, which is typical for nonseminomatous lesions, it is also seen by MRI (see Fig. 90-6).[26] Hemorrhage in lesions is clearly depicted and is assigned signal patterns dependent on its age (see Fig. 90-6).

In one study,[17] although MRI did not miss any lesion seen ultrasonographically and detected all 14 cancers, including the 4 missed by ultrasonography, it was not clear what would be the minimal consistently detectable lesion size. It is possible, given the long imaging time and the continuous contraction of the dartos muscle producing wormian motion of the scrotal wall and constant motion of the testes, that small lesions may be partial volumed with the bright testicular background, significantly decreasing their contrast and detectability.

The smallest lesion detected by MRI prospectively and proven surgically was a 3-mm germ cell tumor (Fig. 90-7). Given that the partial-volume effect is increased by testicular motion, any study aimed at detecting testicular neoplasm and compromised by motion should be repeated if no lesions are found. On the other hand, when clear depiction of the interlobular septa or intratesticular morphology is achieved, it should be regarded as evidence of sufficient quality to negate the presence of disease (see Fig. 90-2). Further clinical experience is, however, required to define the true sensitivity of MRI.

Testicular neoplasms can be primary or metastatic. Primary cancers can originate from any cell type present in normal testes and account for 5000 new cases and 1000 deaths per year in the United States.[27] Testicular neoplasms are most frequent before 10 years of age, between 20 and 40 years, and then after the age 60 years. These neoplasms have their peak occurrence and are the most common solid tumors affecting men between the ages of 20 and 34 years. Primary testicular neoplasms, from the imaging as well as treatment perspective, are grouped into germ cell and stromal tumors. Germ cell tumors account for 90% to 95% of all primary testicular malignancies, whereas non-germ cell or stromal tumors account for 5% to 10%. Germ cell lesions are, in turn, grouped into seminomatous and nonseminomatous lesions. Pure seminomas account for nearly 40% of all primary tumors, whereas nonseminomatous tumors form the remaining 55%. Mixed cellularity, seminomatous, and nonseminomatous elements occur in 10% to 15% of

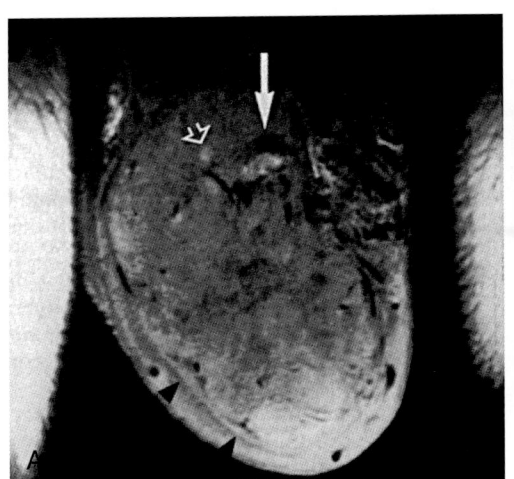
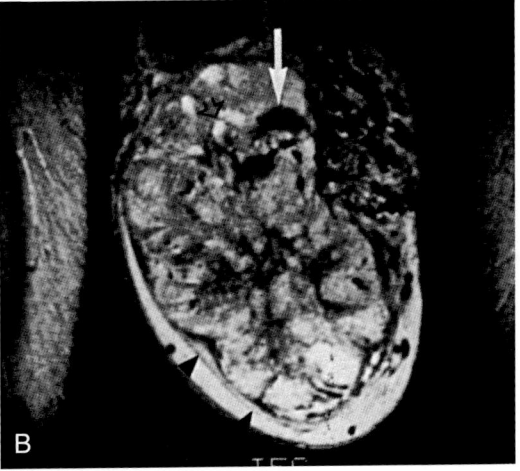

FIGURE 90-6

Coronal **A,** proton-density–weighted and **B,** T2-weighted images of a large (7 × 10 cm) mixed nonseminomatous tumor. The heterogeneous appearance reflects the mixed histology, which includes varied mesenchymal elements and blood. Note that even with this large lesion, a rim of normal testicular tissue is still seen (*arrowheads*) separated from the tumor by a thick fibrous tumor capsule proven pathologically. Note region of high signal intensity density weighting (**A**) that remains high with T2 weighting (**B**) (*open arrow*). Also note the areas of intermediate signal intensity with proton-density weighting (**A**) that become darker with T2 weighting (**B**) (*arrow*). These are areas of hemorrhage characteristic of this tumor type. Note the hypervascularity observed along the scrotal wall and pampiniform plexus. (*Reproduced with permission from Johnson JO, Mattrey RF, Phillipson J: Differentiation of seminomatous from nonseminomatous testicular tumors with MR imaging. Am J Roentgenol 154:539-543, 1990. Reprinted with permission from the American Journal of Roentgenology.*)

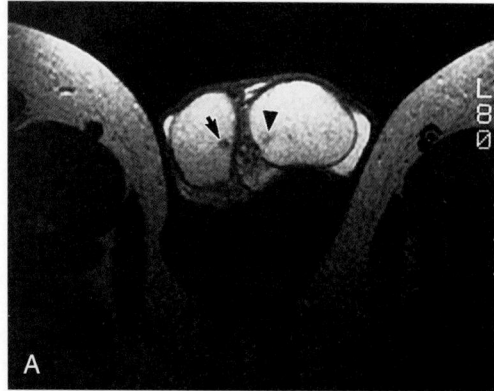

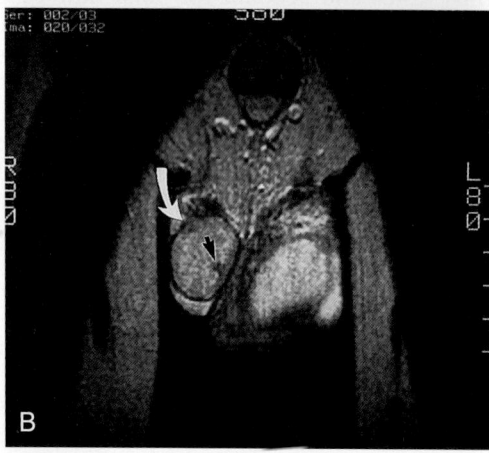

FIGURE 90-7

A, Transaxial and **B,** coronal T2-weighted images show a small 3-mm focus (*black arrows*) in the right testis. This lesion was an embryonal cell tumor with hemorrhage. The left (*arrowhead in* **A**) and right (*curved arrow in* **B**) mediastinum testis can also be seen. This lesion was too small to allow proper characterization. (*Reproduced with permission from Mattrey R: MRI of the male genitalia: testes, seminal vesicles, and urethra. In Goldman SM, Gatewood OMB (eds): Contemporary Issues in Computed Tomography, vol 13, CT and MRI of the Genitourinary Tract. New York: Churchill Livingstone, 1990, pp 245-285.*)

cases. When seminoma is mixed with nonseminomatous elements, the lesion is regarded and treated as a nonseminomatous tumor. Germ cell tumors of yolk sac origin are the predominant lesions of infancy. Testicular lymphoma is the most common neoplasm affecting the testis of men older than 50 years of age.

Testicular tumors are bilateral, either at the time of diagnosis or on follow-up, in 1% to 3% of cases.[28] Therefore, careful examination of the contralateral testis at the time of diagnosis and close follow-up are mandatory.

The differentiation of seminomatous from nonseminomatous lesions is critical in that patients with pure seminomatous lesions are irradiated and those with nonseminomatous lesions undergo retroperitoneal dissection and chemotherapy. These modes of therapy remain controversial,[27] but noninvasive therapy is presently favored. Because seminomatous lesions may harbor small islands of nonseminomatous histology in 10% to 15% of cases,[27] treatment is planned after detailed histologic analysis of the resected testis. This is particu-

larly true when there is elevation of β-human chorionic gonadotropin or α-fetoprotein, findings suggesting the presence of nonseminomatous elements.

In this section, the characteristics of each lesion type are presented. Although the preoperative histologic diagnosis is less critical for treatment, some characteristic findings for seminomatous and nonseminomatous cancers may allow their specific diagnosis.[15-17,26]

Seminomas

Seminoma is rare in patients younger than 10 and older than 60 years but is the most common cell type, accounting for 40% of all testicular neoplasms, and has its peak incidence in the late 30s. Spermatocystic seminoma, a subtype accounting for 10% of all detected seminomas, occurs most frequently after the age of 50 years. Nearly 10% to 15% of seminomatous lesions are not pure seminomas. They have islands of nonseminomatous cells, which changes their classification to a nonseminomatous lesion. Thus, seminomatous lesions mandate a careful pathologic search to ensure their pure cell types and allow for proper treatment planning. Elevation of β-human chorionic gonadotropin or α-fetoprotein levels suggests mixed cellularity. Seminomatous lesions are sheets of cells intermixed with fibrous strands presenting a homogeneous histologic pattern. They rarely bleed or necrose centrally.

The MRI appearance of this tumor type, like its histology, has been consistent. The signal is mildly inhomogeneous. These lesions are rarely visible on T1-weighted and proton-density–weighted images. Their intensity is consistently lower than normal testicular tissue or hydrocele fluid on T2-weighted images. They may contain well-defined regions of low signal intensity (Fig. 90-8) thought to be due to a region with increased condensation of cells and fibrosis.[26] Although atypical, some seminomatous lesions may bleed internally, resulting in a focus of different signal dependent on the age of the hemorrhage. In the setting of hemorrhage, the majority of the lesion will have a signal behavior typical of seminoma. Metastasis to the epididymis and cord is easily demonstrated (see Fig. 90-8) and assumes signal intensities similar to those of the intratesticular mass.[14]

A small rim of normal testicular tissue has been consistently seen to highlight a well-demarcated tumor margin (Fig. 90-9). The appearance of the mass suggests coalescence of multiple nodules (see Fig. 90-8). Indeed, when smaller lesions were imaged, daughter nodules could be detected (not shown). Although seminomatous lesions present a darker signal pattern than testis, similar to infection or infarction, characteristic features allow their distinction (see "Differential Diagnosis").

Nonseminomatous Tumors

Listed in order of occurrence in this category are teratocarcinomas, embryonal cell tumors, teratomas, and choriocarcinomas. Nearly 40% of nonseminomatous lesions are a mixture of two or three elements. They all

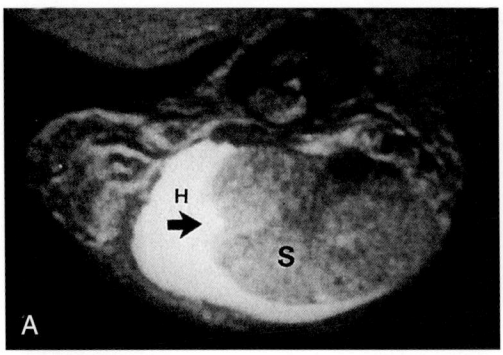 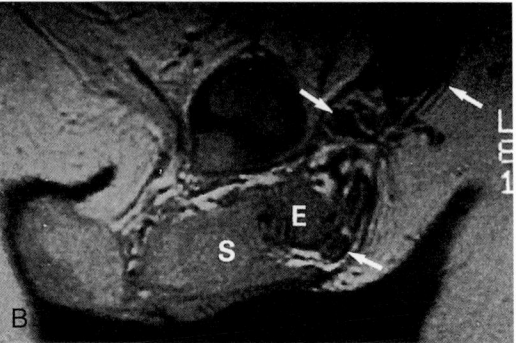

FIGURE 90-8

A, Left testicular seminoma (S) is mildly inhomogeneous on a T2-weighted image and of markedly lower signal intensity than the remaining normal testicular tissue (*arrow*) and hydrocele (H). **B,** Proton-density–weighted image obtained at a different level from **A** demonstrates the upper aspect of testicular tumor (S) along with epididymal (E) and spermatic cord involvement (*arrows*). Extratesticular nodules had a similar signal to intratesticular lesion on both proton-density–weighted (**B**) and T2-weighted images (not shown). *(Reproduced with permission from Baker LL, Hajek PC, Burkhard TK, et al: MR imaging of the scrotum: pathologic conditions. Radiology 163:93-98, 1987.)*

carry similar prognosis and are treated in a similar fashion. Therefore, preoperative distinction of the cell type is not necessary. These lesions account for nearly 50% of all primary testicular neoplasms with a peak incidence in the 20s and early 30s. They therefore afflict slightly younger men than seminomatous lesions do. These lesions present heterogeneous histology, owing to their mixed cellularity, their attempt at tubular formation, and the mixed mesenchymal elements that may be contained in teratomatous lesions (bone, cartilage, muscle, and so on). Furthermore, they have a high propensity to invade vessels, causing internal hemorrhage and necrosis.

These tumors, given their histologic patterns, are markedly inhomogeneous on MR images, which represents their most distinctive feature when compared with seminomatous lesions. Over the background that is typically isointense or slightly brighter than normal testis on T2-weighted images, multiple areas of high and low signal intensities on T1-, proton-density–, and T2-weighted images are seen, representing hemorrhage of various ages or islands of muscle or cartilage within the mass and so characteristic of these lesions (see Fig. 90-6). The degree of heterogeneity and the overall signal intensity are much greater than those seen with seminoma. A band of low signal intensity circumscribing the mass in most cases represents the fibrous tumor capsule, also typical for these lesions. Remaining normal testicular tissue is easily differentiated from tumor by its homogeneous and characteristic intensity, even when the lesion is quite large (see Fig. 90-6). Although some lesions may have a dominant signal lower than that of testis, their heterogeneity and visibility on T1-weighted images distinguish them from seminomatous lesions.

A study assessing the ability of MRI to distinguish seminomatous from nonseminomatous lesions prospectively[26] found that of 12 patients with sizable lesions that could be characterized, MRI allowed the correct

classification of 11 lesions. The remaining lesion (see Fig. 90-7) was too small to characterize. The degree of heterogeneity of signals was the most discriminating factor, with nonseminomatous lesions being more heterogeneous than seminomatous lesions.[26] Hemorrhage may rarely occur in pure seminomas, appearing as a high signal intensity region. It may still be possible to recognize the seminoma by assessing the overall appearance of the lesion. When nonseminomatous islands occur in

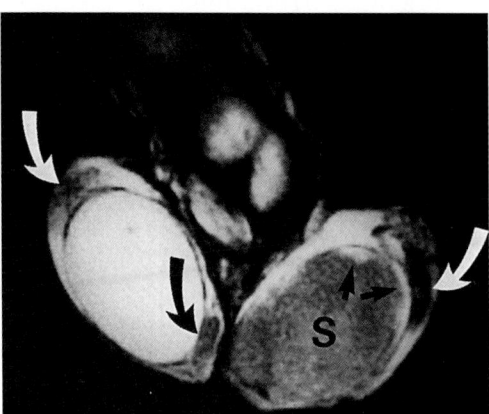

FIGURE 90-9

Left testicular seminoma (S) is of significantly darker signal intensity than normal testis on a T2-weighted image. It was mildly inhomogeneous and of slightly lower signal intensity with proton-density weighting (not shown). Note the well-marginated small rim of normal testicular tissue near the upper pole of testis (*arrows*). Also note the small ipsilateral hydrocele and normal epididymal head (*curved black arrow*). A normal epididymal head and tail are seen on the normal contralateral side (*curved white arrows*). *(Reproduced with permission from Johnson JO, Mattrey RF, Phillipson J: Differentiation of seminomatous from nonseminomatous testicular tumors with MR imaging. Am J Roentgenol 154:539-543, 1990. Reprinted with permission from the American Journal of Roentgenology.)*

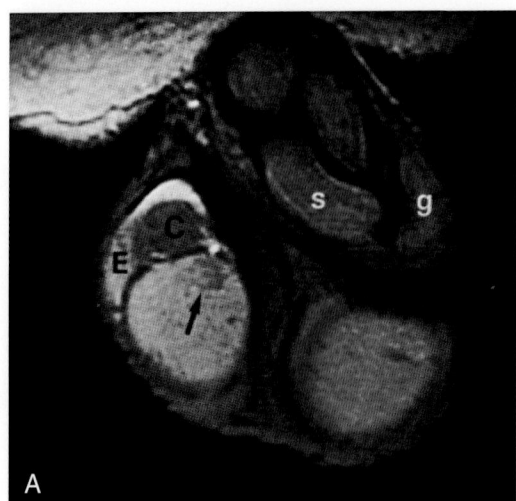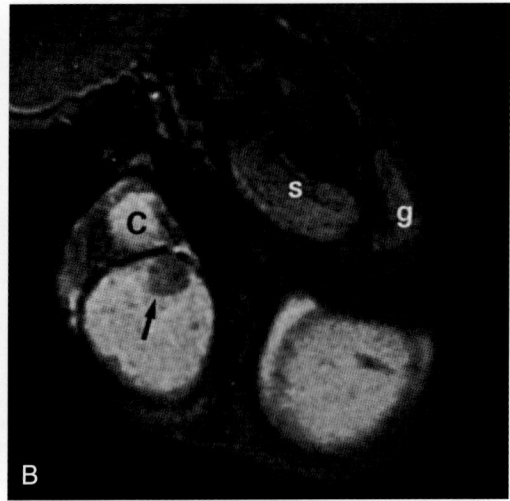

FIGURE 90-10

Mildly inhomogeneous well-marginated testicular tumor (*arrow*), which proved histologically to be a Leydig cell tumor, is better seen on **B,** the T2-weighted image than **A,** the proton-density–weighted image. The epididymal cyst (C) within the normal epididymal head (E) has MRI characteristics similar to those of water. Oblique section through the penis shows the paired corpora cavernosa each surrounded by the dark signal intensity of the tunica albuginea of the penis. Also seen are the brighter corpora spongiosa (s) and glans (g). *(Reproduced with permission from Baker LL, Hajek PC, Burkhard TK, et al: MR imaging of the scrotum: pathologic conditions. Radiology 163:93-98, 1987.)*

seminoma, they are diffusely distributed throughout the lesion rather than occurring as a single large focus. From a review of the literature,[14-17] tumor signal patterns illustrated in figures match the description just given, suggesting that MRI may indeed be able to differentiate these two tumor types. Although ultrasonography demonstrates characteristic echographic findings for seminomatous and nonseminomatous lesions, there is significant overlap in their appearance.[29]

Stromal Tumors

Stromal tumors occur between 20 and 60 years of age and account for nearly 5% of all primary testicular tumors. They are well circumscribed and rarely exhibit hemorrhage or necrosis. Because these lesions generally produce hormones, prepubertal boys can present with precocious puberty and adults with gynecomastia. The cell types include Leydig and Sertoli cells. These lesions are malignant in 10% of cases. Malignancy is suspected histologically when lesions are large, necrotic, or infiltrative or invade blood vessels. Malignancy is clearly established when there are metastases. It could be hypothesized that given their homogeneous histology and lack of hemorrhage and necrosis, their MRI appearance would mimic seminomatous lesions.[14,17] However, when malignant, the hemorrhage and necrosis would change their appearance to mimic nonseminomatous lesions. The experience with these lesions is limited to test this hypothesis.

Two published proven cases of Leydig cell tumor show the mass on T2-weighted images to be of moderately darker signal intensity than normal testis.[14,17] One was small, well circumscribed, and homogeneous, as would be expected from the tumor's histology (Fig. 90-10).[14] The other showed total infiltration of the testis on MR images in a prepubertal boy, and ultrasonography did not show the lesion.[17] It is not yet clear that these lesions can be differentiated from seminomatous lesions.

Other Tumors

Lymphomatous or leukemic infiltration of the testis is common. Lymphoma accounts for nearly 5% of all testicular neoplasms.[27] It may be primary in the testis, the manifestation of occult disease seated elsewhere, or a late manifestation of disseminated disease. Lymphomatous lesions are the most common testicular lesions in men older than 50 years of age.[27] The majority of these lesions are infiltrative and may extend into or originate in the epididymis (Fig. 90-11). The major cell type is histiocytic lymphoma.

The testis is the prime site of relapse of leukemia in children. A blood-testis barrier exists, similar to the blood-brain barrier, which prevents chemotherapeutics from eradicating disease in the testes. Testicular evaluation and biopsy are commonly performed at the end of chemotherapy to exclude testicular involvement. Although ultrasonography can detect leukemic infiltration,[30] it has poor sensitivity.[17] The role of MRI in this setting to determine sensitivity has not been performed, but MRI was more sensitive than ultrasonography in a limited series in which leukemic infiltrates affected the entire testis.[17]

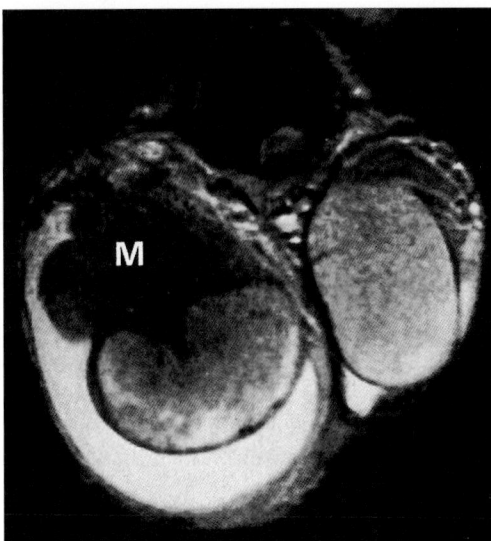

FIGURE 90-11

Scrotal lymphoma involving the right epididymis and testis is shown on a T2-weighted image. Note that the center of the mass (M) is in the epididymis and infiltrates the testis from the hilum. The mass, located along the bare area of the testis, rotated the testis into a horizontal position. Note that the mass within the testis is patchy and its margins with normal testicular tissue are generally poorly defined. Mild hypervascularity and moderate ipsilateral hydrocele are seen.

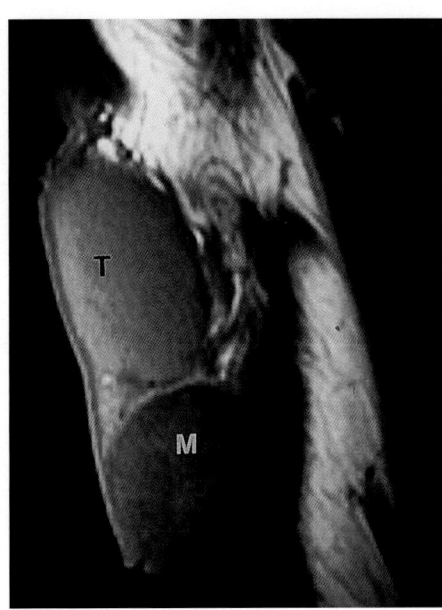

FIGURE 90-12

Sagittal proton-density–weighted image through the hemiscrotum shows a spherical extratesticular mass (M) inferior to the normal testis (T). This mass, which is slightly darker than testis with proton-density weighting, was isointense with testis on T2-weighted images (not shown). It proved to be an epidermoid cyst at surgery.

Benign Testicular Lesions

Teratomas

Benign testicular tumors are relatively uncommon. The most common is benign intratesticular teratoma.[22,31] The ultrasonographic and possibly the MRI appearance of teratoma would be similar to teratocarcinoma from which differentiation may be difficult.

Epidermoid Cyst

Epidermoid inclusion cysts are benign solitary tumors of germ cell origin accounting for approximately 1% of all testicular tumors.[32,33] They are limited by a fibrous capsule with an epithelial lining. The center contains keratin without teratomatous elements. Epidermoid cysts are typically intratesticular but may be extratesticular. These lesions are well defined and homogeneous at ultrasonography. They may be hyper-reflective owing to calcifications. Only a few internal echoes are noted throughout the tumor.[34,35] One reported case imaged by MRI showed a bull's-eye appearance in the testis.[36] We have imaged four cases by MRI, all of which displayed similar findings. The epidermoid cysts were nearly isointense with testis on all pulsing sequences, with a tendency to be slightly darker on T1-weighted images and slightly brighter on T2-weighted images. A low signal intensity wall was observed on the T2-weighted images in all cases caused by the fibrous capsule. The lesions failed to enhance after the infusion of gadolinium

diethylenetriaminepenta-acetic acid (Gd-DTPA), confirming their avascular core (Fig. 90-12). Because normal testicular tissue enhances significantly, the post-contrast images increase not only the conspicuity of these lesions but also their specificity.

Adenomatoid Tumors

Adenomatoid tumors are benign lesions characteristic of the genital tract and consisting of fibrous stroma and epithelial cells. These lesions are benign and usually occur in the epididymis but may rarely occur in the testis. We have imaged two such tumors and one was surgically proved (Fig. 90-13). Dependent on the degree of fibrosis, their signal may vary from being similar to testis to darker than testis. Because the testicular appendix may have a similar appearance, particularly if fibrotic, it might be difficult to differentiate these two entities. This differentiation is not important because neither condition requires surgical intervention.

Cysts

Since the advent of high-resolution ultrasonography, simple intratesticular cysts can be detected on 8% to 10% of ultrasound images.[37-39] Most are 2 to 18 mm and are solitary. They can be intratesticular or tunical. Intratesticular cysts are nonpalpable and incidental.[22,31] They can occur anywhere within the testis and likely originate from the rete testis in that their histology is similar to

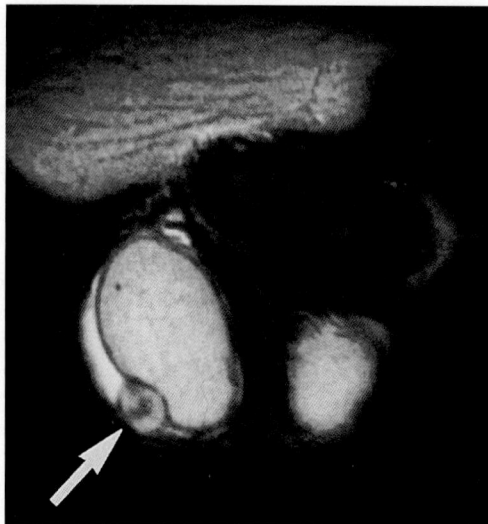

FIGURE 90-13

Adenomatoid tumor (*arrow*) proven surgically has similar signal patterns as testis on a T2-weighted image. Its signal intensity was also similar to that of testis with proton-density weighting (not shown). Note its extratesticular location as it deviates the tunica albuginea medially. Indentation of the testis suggested that the lesion was between the layers of the tunica albuginea and tunica vaginalis, which was where it was at surgery.

that of the rete testes.[40] Another hypothesis is degeneration after trauma or inflammation.[39] Tunical cysts are palpable, small, and usually detected in middle-aged men. The cause of these lesions was considered to be post-traumatic or inflammatory degeneration[41]; however, evidence suggests that they may be from an embryologic remnant of mesothelial rest or from efferent ductules.[42] MRI displays characteristic findings for cysts. Although they are well depicted when they assume water signal (darker with T1 weighting and brighter with T2 weighting than testis), they can be isointense with testis and require use of Gd-DTPA to increase their conspicuity.[43]

Dilated Seminiferous Tubule

The appearance of a dilated intratesticular seminiferous tubule has been recognized and described by both ultrasonography and MRI.[43-45] The findings are somewhat characteristic with ultrasonography, potentially allowing a specific diagnosis to be made to obviate the need for surgery. Among the three publications, 48 patients were reported. Most were older than 50 years and had similar ultrasonographic findings. The intratesticular process was associated with large ipsilateral spermatoceles, was centered at the mediastinum testis, and was contiguous with the body of the epididymis. It appeared hypoechoic with a coarse echotexture due to multitudes of small reflectors caused by the dilated tubules. It may also be associated with mediastinal cysts (Fig. 90-14). It was frequently bilateral and nonpalpable, although the testicular examination was compromised by the associated

large spermatoceles. When this constellation of findings is encountered at ultrasonography, there is no need for further work-up; however, short of that, we recommend the use of MRI to confirm the diagnosis. With MRI, the findings are specific for this entity and distinguishable from those of neoplastic lesions. The mass of ectatic tubules at the mediastinum is homogeneous and of lower signal intensity on T1-weighted and intermediately-weighted images and isointense relative to testis on T2-weighted images; the signal intensity is identical to that of the ipsilateral spermatoceles on all sequences (see Fig. 90-14). The MRI appearance of dilated tubules is different from that of seminomatous tumors in that the latter are typically isointense relative to testis on T1-weighted images and darker than testis on T2-weighted images.[14,26] Nonseminomatous lesions are also different because they are heterogeneous in signal intensity with all pulse sequences, especially on T2-weighted images.[14,26] Because the tubules do not enhance with gadolinium, their conspicuity and tubular pattern become apparent after contrast medium administration (see Fig. 90-14).

The cause of the dilatation of seminiferous tubules is unclear. However, of the 12 testes with tubular ectasia reported, 3 had had an associated ipsilateral hernia repair 3, 10, or 40 years before presentation.[43] Although this could be coincidental, it raises the possibility of an obstructive cause in which surgical scarring or injury to the vas deferens might have occurred. In a series of intratesticular cysts, an inflammatory or traumatic cause was also suspected.[39] In this study, six (46%) of the patients had inflammation of the epididymis shown by histologic examination and two (15%) had prior biopsy.[39]

Intratesticular Varicocele

Intratesticular varicocele, which also occurs in the mediastinum testis, may be indistinguishable from the dilated seminiferous tubule by gray-scale ultrasonography.[46] However, in the two cases reported, the hypoechoic spaces filled with color on Doppler imaging, indicating flow.[46] The intratesticular varicoceles were associated with ipsilateral varicoceles in both patients. MRI should also allow this distinction, although none has been reported, because of the characteristic appearance of flowing blood and because slowly flowing or static blood enhances markedly with intravenous contrast agents, unlike seminiferous tubules.

Microlithiasis

Testicular microlithiasis is caused by tiny (<2 mm) concentric calcifications within the seminiferous tubules throughout both testes. It is typically incidental to the primary cause that brought the patient to medical attention. It is believed that these concretions form from degenerated tubular epithelial cells. Collagenous lamellate form and offer a nidus for dystrophic calcification to occur. Although an exact etiology is not known, diffuse microlithiasis is more frequent in cryptorchidism

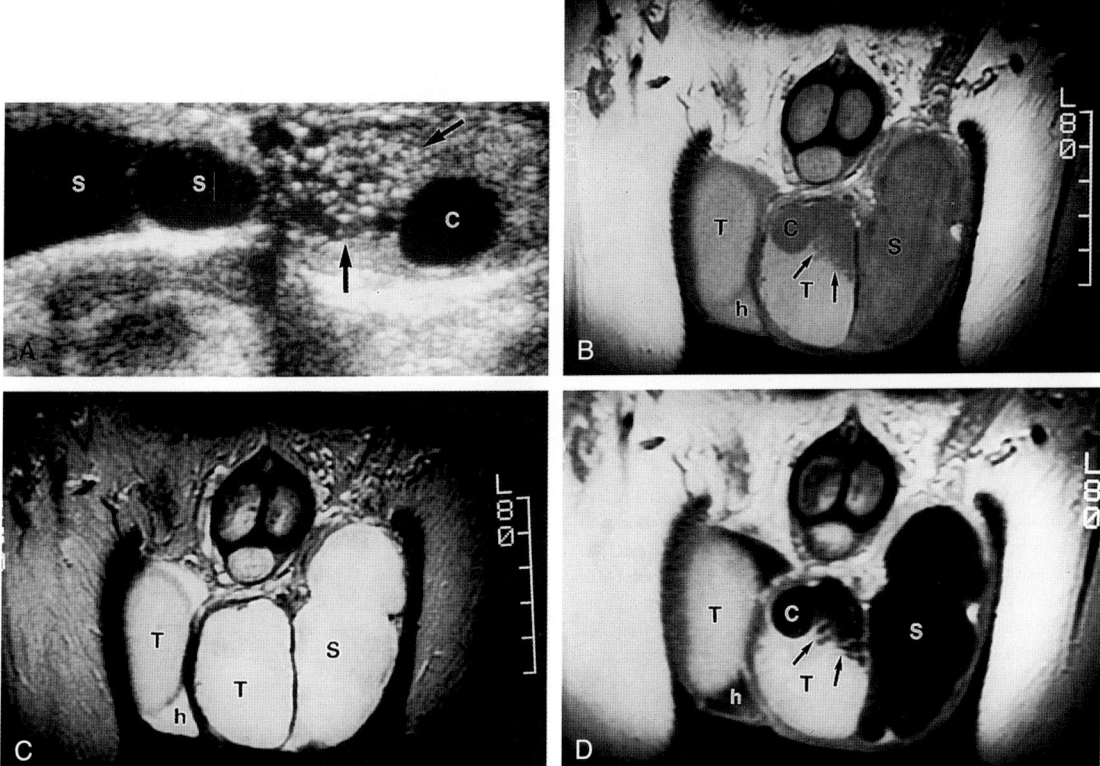

FIGURE 90-14

A 57-year-old man presented with an enlarging, symptomatic left-sided spermatocele and underwent ultrasonography before elective spermatocelectomy. **A,** Longitudinal ultrasound image through the left hemiscrotum shows several locules of a large multilocular spermatocele (S). The mediastinal lesion (*arrow*) has a coarse echotexture, with multiple contiguous tiny cysts and a 1.5-cm diameter intratesticular cyst (C). The mediastinal lesion had no flow on color Doppler imaging (not shown). **B,** Proton-density–weighted and **C,** T2-weighted coronal images show the large spermatocele (S), intratesticular cyst (C), and mediastinal lesion (*arrows*) to be homogeneous and hypointense relative to the testicular parenchyma (T) with proton-density weighting (**B**), becoming isointense relative to and difficult to distinguish from testis on T2 weighting (**C**). Note the small hydrocele (h) in the right hemiscrotum. **D,** After the infusion of 0.1 mmol/kg of Gd-DTPA, the testes (T) enhance markedly, increasing contrast between testes and spermatocele (S), intratesticular cyst (C), mediastinal seminiferous tubule ectasia (*arrows*), and the hydrocele (h). Because of the increased contrast, recognition of tubular structures at the margin between the abnormal mediastinum and testis become more apparent (*arrows*). (*Reproduced with permission from Tartar VM, Trambert MA, Balsara ZN, Mattrey RF: Tubular ectasia of the testicle: sonographic and MR imaging appearance. Am J Roentgenol 160:539-542, 1993. Reprinted with permission from the American Journal of Roentgenology.*)

or delayed testicular descent, and in patients with a variety of genetic conditions, as well as those with pulmonary alveolar microlithiasis. Although cancer and infertility have been associated with this condition, it is believed that the relationship with diffuse bilateral microlithiasis is incidental or may be related to the fact that these conditions also occur in association with cryptorchidism.[47,48]

In our experience, the MRI appearance of the testis with microlithiasis has been diffuse, patchy, poorly demarcated regions of signal loss on T2-weighted images. The tiny calcific regions depicted at ultrasonography could not be seen by MRI. The exact reason for this is unclear. Although it could be a spatial resolution issue, it is more likely due to the presence of mobile protons within these concretions.

Inflammation

Epididymitis

Epididymitis is the most common intrascrotal infection. It may be diffuse or focal and is frequently secondary to prostatitis. Most cases of epididymitis are treated conservatively. Surgery is reserved for complications such as abscess formation. Therefore, diagnostic follow-up in patients with a poor response to therapy may be warranted.

Patients with clinical evidence of acute epididymitis consistently show epididymal enlargement (Fig. 90-15). The epididymis, which is normally of lower signal intensity than testis on T2-weighted images, maintains a higher signal intensity that can be nearly equal to that of testis.

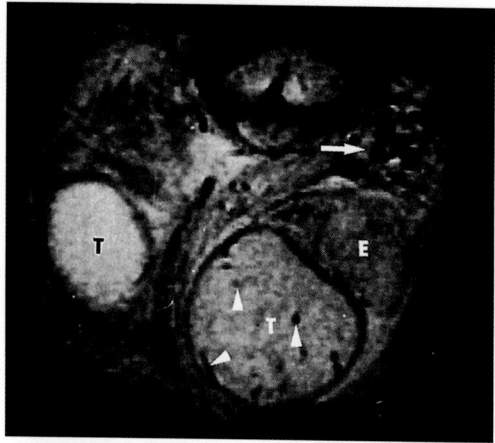

FIGURE 90-15

Acute epididymitis shown on a T2-weighted image in the coronal plane. The testis (T) is of slightly lower signal intensity than the contralateral side and is hypervascular (*arrowheads*). The epididymis (E) is enlarged and assumes a higher signal intensity with T2 weighting than is normally observed. Note the hypervascularity in the pampiniform plexus (*arrow*) and cord (not shown) typical of this condition. (*Reproduced with permission from Trambert MA, Mattrey RF, Levine D, Berthoty D: Subacute scrotal pain: evaluation of torsion versus epididymitis with MR imaging. Radiology 175:53-56, 1990.*)

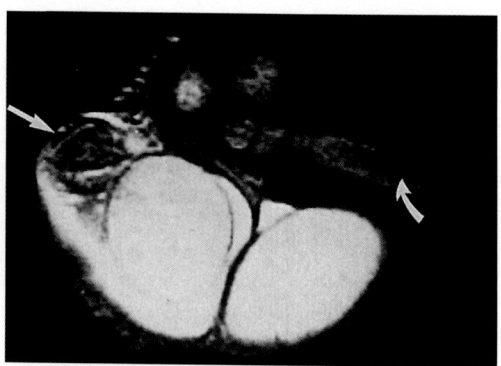

FIGURE 90-16

Focal chronic epididymitis involving the head of the right epididymis shown on a T2-weighted image. Note the enlarged dark epididymis (*arrow*). The patient was known to have chronic epididymitis and now presents with acute exacerbation. There is mild reactive ipsilateral hydrocele. Acute exacerbations may be difficult to diagnose in the setting of chronic changes. The oblique view of the penis shows the urethra (*curved arrow*) within the corpora spongiosa. (*Reproduced with permission from Baker LL, Hajek PC, Burkhard TK: MR imaging of the scrotum: pathologic conditions. Radiology 163:93-98, 1987.*)

In chronic epididymitis, the epididymis is enlarged in a focal (Fig. 90-16) or diffuse (Fig. 90-17) manner and assumes darker signal patterns than normal with T2 weighting, becoming moderately darker than testis. In the setting of chronic epididymitis, acute exacerbation may not affect signal intensity (see Fig. 90-16). Therefore, when the epididymis is enlarged and assumes a dark signal, acute epididymitis cannot be excluded.

Acute epididymitis, particularly when severe, may be associated with hemorrhage within the epididymis (Fig. 90-18). If hemorrhage is present, the MR signal follows its resorptive stages. In acute epididymitis there is hypervascularity, thickening, and swelling of the spermatic cord, increasing its signal on T2-weighted images (Fig. 90-19; see Fig. 90-15). Although the degree of hypervascularity has been variable, it has been consistently present in all patients. Hypervascularity is seen as multiple serpiginous vessels with signal void due to high flow. This is in contradistinction to normal vessels,

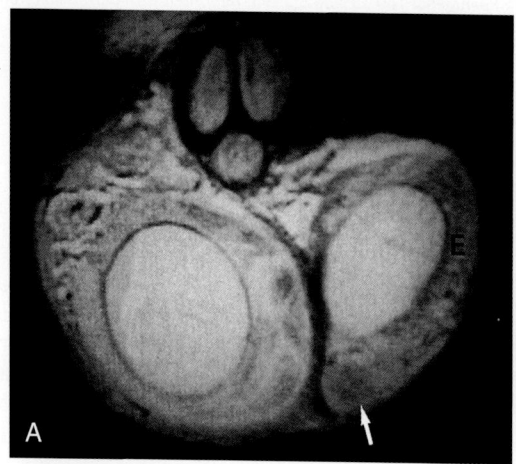
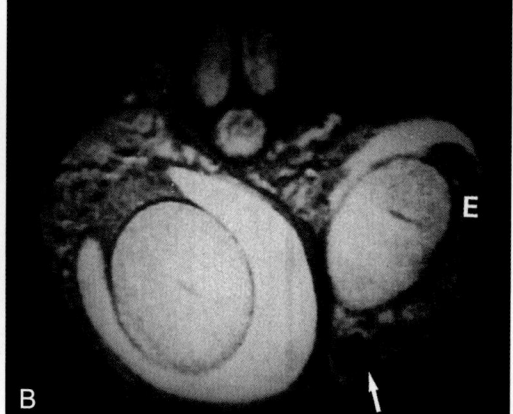

FIGURE 90-17

Diffuse chronic epididymitis involving the entire epididymis on the left and shown in the coronal plane on **A,** proton density–weighted and **B,** T2-weighted images. Note the diffuse enlargement of the entire epididymis (E) with possible hemorrhage in the tail (*arrows*). Mild ipsilateral and moderate contralateral hydroceles are present. The right hydrocele outlines the bare area in its transverse direction (**B**). Note the motion-related signal intensity loss in the right hydrocele better appreciated with proton-density weighting (**A**).

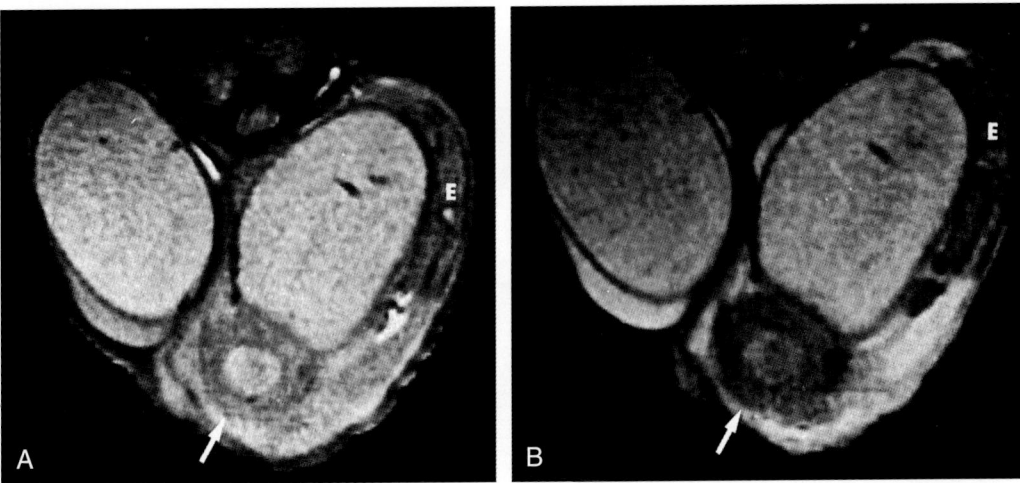

FIGURE 90-18

Focal epididymitis involving the tail shown in the coronal plane on **A,** proton-density–weighted and **B,** T2-weighted images. Note the focal enlargement of the tail (*arrows*) with probable hemorrhage and associated ipsilateral hydrocele. The upper epididymis (E) is darker than normal but is not enlarged.

which are usually thinner, less abundant, and lack the flow void (see Fig. 90-4). Hypervascularity of the testis associated with epididymitis has also been observed in some patients (see Fig. 90-15). Scrotal skin thickening and swelling can easily be seen and are detected in most patients (see Fig. 90-19); however, this finding is not specific to infection. Sympathetic hydrocele is present in most patients and assumes signal patterns identical to those of water (dark on T1-weighted images, isointense on proton-density–weighted images, and brighter than testis on T2-weighted images) (see Fig. 90-17). Extensive inguinal adenopathy is frequent in these patients (see Fig. 90-19). However, it is also frequently found in normal patients or those with a variety of conditions, decreasing the specificity of this finding.

Orchitis

Orchitis is frequently the sequela of epididymitis. Pure orchitis without epididymitis suggests viral etiology. When orchitis accompanies epididymitis, treatment is extended over a longer period owing to the blood-testis barrier. Orchitis, even when appropriately treated, can develop into an abscess requiring surgical intervention (see Fig. 90-19). Therefore, when a focus of orchitis is found, follow-up is necessary to ensure its resolution.

Tuberculous orchitis is usually associated with tuberculous epididymitis and typically occurs in patients with known disease. Epididymal changes at MRI are less severe than those seen with bacterial epididymitis, and the degree of hypervascularity is less prominent. Testicular changes are patchy, poorly marginated areas of slightly lower signal intensity than testis (Fig. 90-20). In one patient with surgically proven diffuse chronic tuberculous orchitis, the testis was diffusely inhomogeneous with low signal intensity on T2-weighted images but without mass effect (Fig. 90-21).

In some patients with fulminant epididymitis, epididymal swelling may be so severe that it can compromise the blood supply to the testis, resulting in infarction.[49] It would be expected, therefore, that such ischemia would result from venous occlusion followed by arterial occlusion, as with spermatic cord torsion. Such infarction would more likely be hemorrhagic and should present different signal patterns than the patchy ill-defined diminished signal of orchitis. This hypothesis requires further clinical evaluation.

Trauma

Surgical intervention in scrotal trauma is generally reserved for patients with testicular fracture or rupture or when the intratesticular hematoma is extensive. MRI is well suited for assessing both the integrity of the tunica albuginea and the degree of intratesticular hematoma. Because the normal tunica is well visualized as a band of low signal intensity surrounding the testes on both proton-density–weighted and T2-weighted images, clear assessment of its integrity is possible. In this setting, multiple imaging planes may be required to ensure that all surfaces are optimally imaged without partial volume. When it is known that multiple planes are required, only T2-weighted sequences need to be performed beyond the T1- and T2-weighted coronal pair.

Overall, the traumatized testes are highly inhomogeneous with regions of high and low signal intensity compared with normal testicular tissue on both T1- and T2-weighted images secondary to intratesticular hemorrhage (Fig. 90-22). Hematocele frequently accompanies trauma and assumes signal patterns commensurate with the age of the hemorrhage (see Fig. 90-22). The classic signals described for hematoma are observed when hematoceles develop, because hemorrhage in this space,

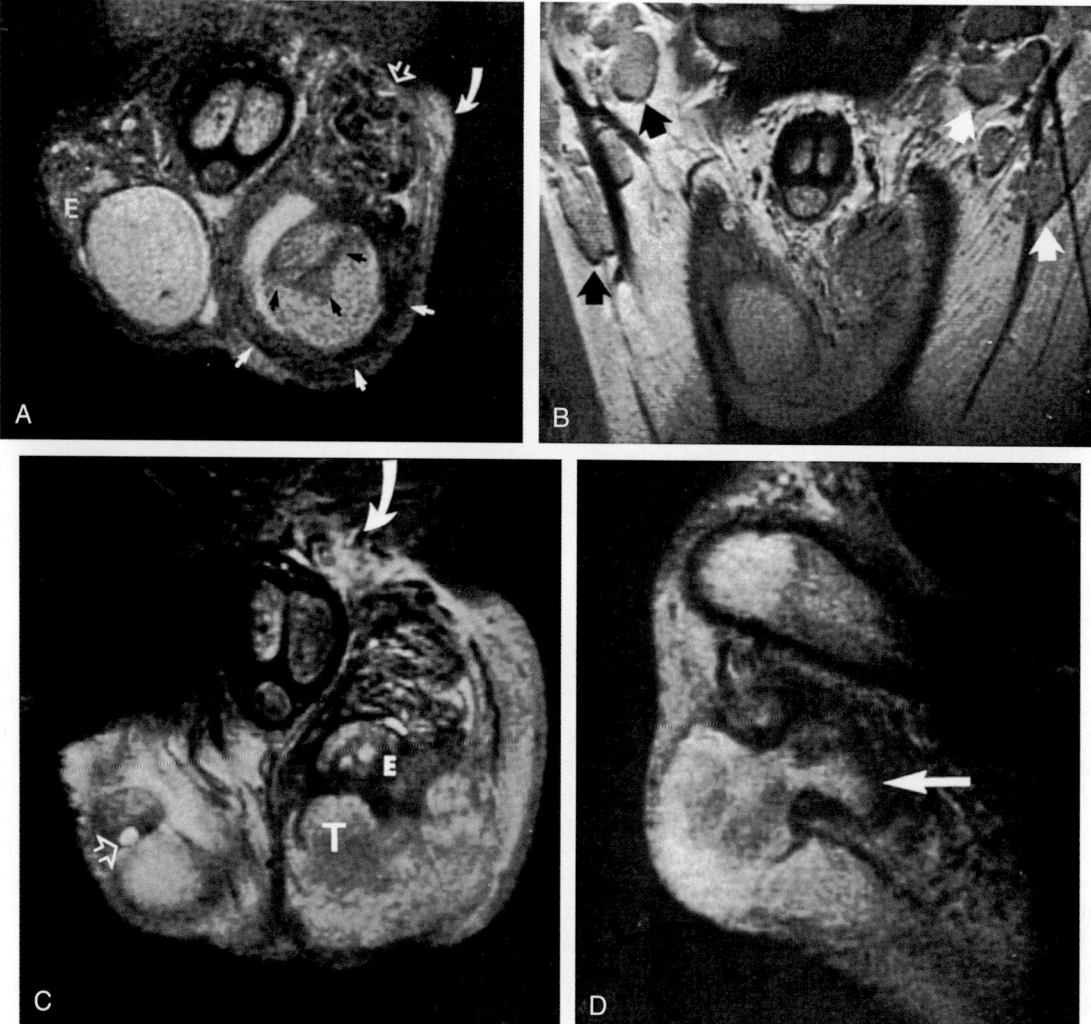

FIGURE 90-19

A, Acute left epididymo-orchitis shown in the coronal plane on a T2-weighted image. Note the diffuse loss of signal intensity of the affected testis, hypervascular cord, and pampiniform plexus (*open arrow*) at the base of the scrotum, associated skin thickening including scrotal septum (*white arrows*), and edema (*curved arrow*). Although the focus of orchitis (*black arrows*) could be confused for tumor at first look, note the associated diffuse loss of testicular signal and the changes in the scrotal wall and cord. These, in conjunction with the clinical history, should eliminate such confusion. Note on **A** the enlarged contralateral darkened epididymis (E), suggesting the occurrence of previous episodes. **B,** Proton-density–weighted image obtained a few levels posterior to **A**. Note the associated bilateral inguinal adenopathy (*arrows*). **C,** T2-weighted image obtained 10 days after **A** at nearly the same level, showing complete destruction of the testis (T) and loss of intrascrotal anatomic detail despite antibiotic therapy. Note the cephalic extension of the scrotal wall involvement and the spread of edema to the base of the penis (*curved arrow*) compared with the image in **A**. There is a small hemorrhagic cyst (*open arrow*) in the right epididymis that was bright with proton-density weighting (not shown). **D,** Changes at this time were due to an epididymal abscess (*arrow*) that involved the testis and pointed along the anterior scrotal wall. (*Reproduced with permission from Baker LL, Hajek PC, Burkhard TK: MR imaging of the scrotum: pathologic conditions. Radiology 163:93-98, 1987.*)

FIGURE 90-20

Acute tuberculous epididymo-orchitis involving the upper pole of the left testis (*arrow*) and epididymal head (*curved arrow*) shown in the coronal plane on a T2-weighted image. Note the patchy involvement of the testis, which was seen only with T2 weighting, and the enlarged epididymis that fails to darken on this T2-weighted image. The mild degree of hypervascularity suggests subacute inflammation.

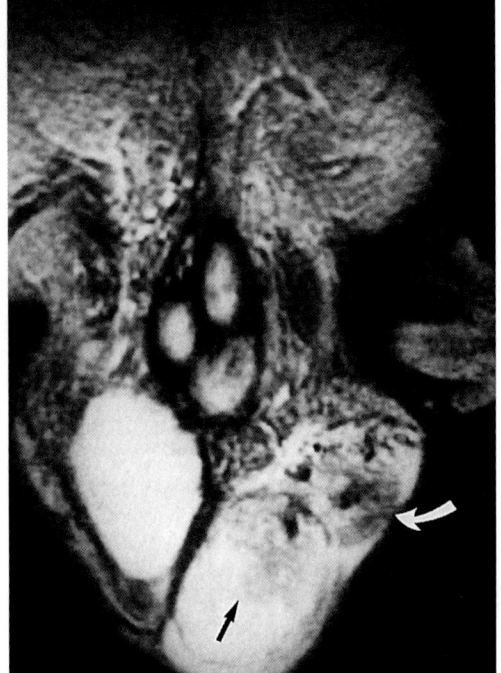

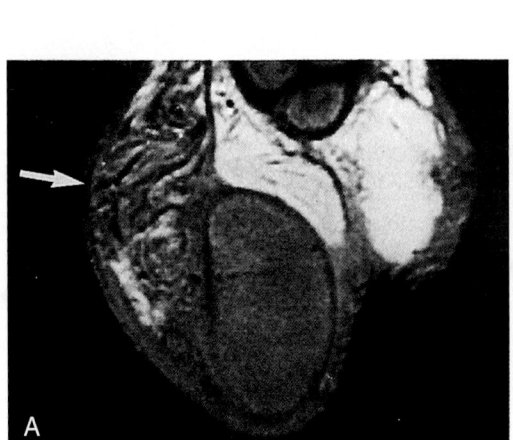 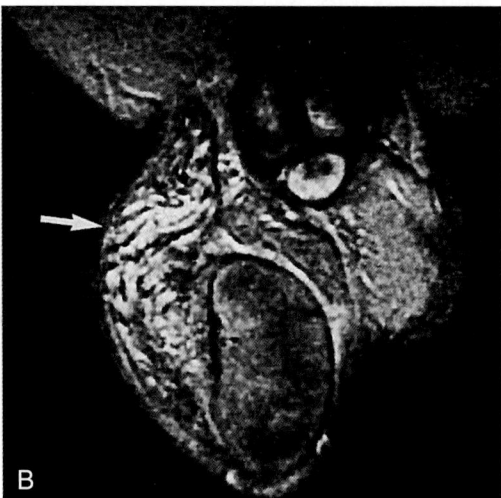

FIGURE 90-21

Chronic tuberculous orchitis shown in the coronal plane on **A,** proton-density–weighted and **B,** T2-weighted images. Note the diffuse, poorly defined process involving the entire testis on **A**. The prominent pampiniform plexus at the base of the scrotum (*arrows*) is compatible with a varicocele. The left testis had been removed because of a tuberculous infection. *(Reproduced with permission from Baker LL, Hajek PC, Burkhard TK, et al: MR imaging of the scrotum: pathologic conditions. Radiology 163:93-98, 1987.)*

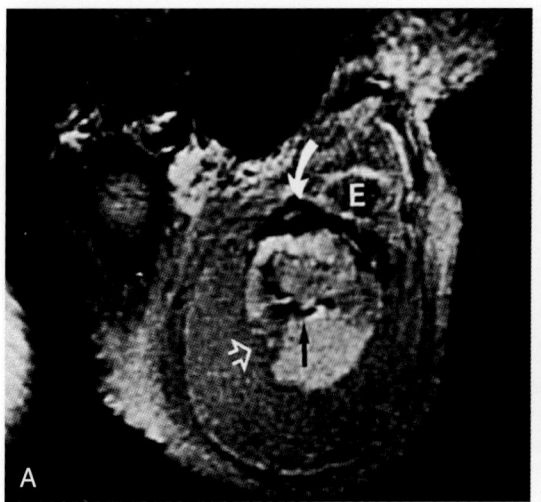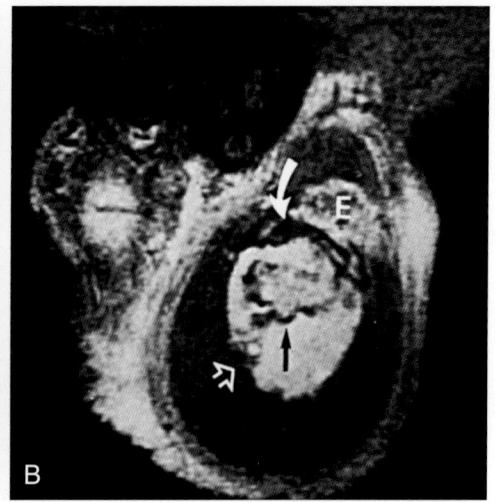

FIGURE 90-22

Three-day-old scrotal trauma is shown in the coronal plane on **A,** proton-density–weighted and **B,** T2-weighted images. Note the hematoma outlining the tunica along the upper pole of the testis is dark (*curved arrow*) and the intratesticular hematoma, although darker than the testis, is brighter than the upper pole collection (*arrow*). The reason for the discrepancy of signals is not clear. The central hemorrhage is incompletely surrounded by a dark band. Given the age of these hematomas (3 days), the dark band cannot represent hemosiderin-filled macrophages. Note that the tunica is interrupted along the medial lower pole (*open arrow*). The tunical fluid, hematocele, has a signal pattern indicating subacute hemorrhage [intermediate with proton-density weighting (**A**) and dark with T2 weighting (**B**)]. Also note that the epididymis (E) is enlarged, swollen, and inhomogeneous. *(Reproduced with permission from Baker LL, Hajek PC, Burkhard TK: MR imaging of the scrotum: pathologic conditions. Radiology 163:93-98, 1987.)*

like in the central nervous system, is reasonably well isolated. Intratesticular trauma causes more linear than spherical changes (Fig. 90-23), reducing its confusion with mass lesions.

Although clinical and scrotal changes with trauma differ from those of tumors, an underlying tumor, particularly a nonseminomatous lesion, could be masked by the intratesticular hemorrhage. Therefore, if the intratesticular change is greater than would be expected for the degree of trauma that occurred, a follow-up evaluation may be warranted to exclude cancer.

Torsion

Intravaginal Spermatic Cord Torsion

The testis, like other abdominal organs, is retroperitoneal. When descended into the scrotum, the testis is accompanied by a peritoneal reflection, the vaginal process that forms the tunica vaginalis. This membrane invests the entire contour of the testis except for a strip that extends from the upper to lower pole. The region of the testis that is left uncovered is called the *bare area* (see Fig. 90-2). The transverse dimension of the bare area is variable but typically extends for at least one third of the perimeter of the testis (see Fig. 90-17). This bare area not only serves as a passage for support structures into and out of the mediastinum testis but also more

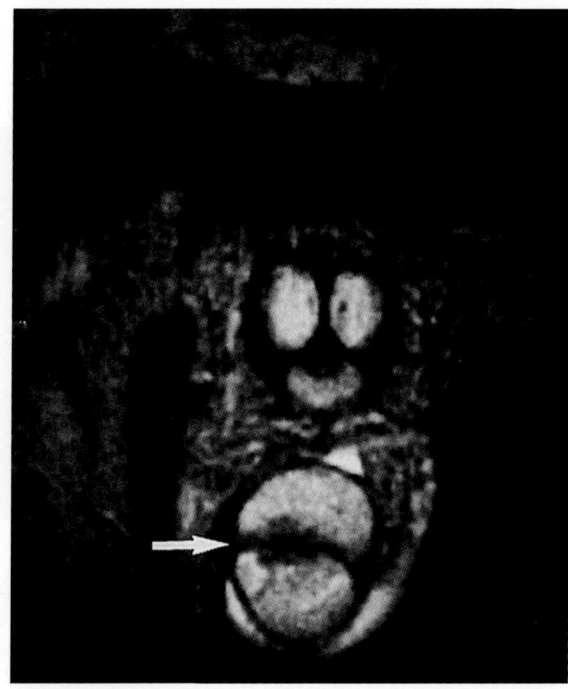

FIGURE 90-23

Seven-day-old trauma that resulted in testicular fracture is shown on a T2-weighted image. Note that the intratesticular abnormality is a linear process that presumably follows the fracture line (*arrow*). Note also the presence of hydrocele rather than hematocele.

importantly anchors the testis to the posteromedial scrotal wall. This broad attachment prevents the testis from twisting. The surface area of this attachment can be variable dependent on the degree the tunica vaginalis invests the testis. The tunica vaginalis can undermine the support structures and epididymis to such a degree that only a thin stalk remains. This anomalous condition, called the "bell clapper" deformity, predisposes the affected testis to twist and strangulate. When the testis rotates on its stalk, the veins become occluded. The intratesticular veins dilate and the testis swells. When intratesticular pressure exceeds arterial pressure, blood flow ceases and the testis undergoes hemorrhagic necrosis. The bell clapper deformity is thought to occur bilaterally in a large percentage of patients who present with torsion, because subsequent contralateral torsion, if the condition is not corrected, has been observed in as many as 40% in one series.[50]

Spermatic cord torsion typically occurs in the teens and 20s and affects 1 in 4000 males younger than 25 years old.[50] The classic presentation is waking up with testicular pain radiating to the abdomen or groin that gradually worsens. Torsion may, however, present with acute onset of pain that can be so severe as to cause nausea and vomiting.[51] The affected hemiscrotum appears indurated, enlarged, and tender, mimicking epididymitis and leading to clinical misdiagnosis in a large percentage of cases. If torsion is suspected, immediate surgery is required, because salvage of testicular function decreases with time. Although nearly all testes can be salvaged if ischemic for 5 hours or less, the salvage rate decreases to 20% if surgery is done at or beyond 12 hours.[52] When patients present in the subacute phase (24 hours or later), surgery is still required to remove the torsed testis and fix the contralateral testis to the scrotum. The torsed testis should be removed to establish the diagnosis, stop the pain, which would otherwise last for 3 to 4 weeks, and prevent the development of infertility in the contralateral testis owing to the possible development of antisperm antibodies, although this latter reason is controversial.[53,54]

Acute torsion can be adequately diagnosed with color Doppler imaging, particularly when the equipment is sensitive to slow flow. Experience with MRI has been limited to subacute torsion (greater than 24 hours) in which several characteristic findings have been observed, three of which are specific, allowing for 100% accuracy.[55]

The first is the appearance of the point of twist itself. The twisted stalk, which contains vessels, lymphatics, tubules, and fat, is usually near the posterosuperior aspect of the scrotum. The point of twist is quite dark, presumably owing to the water being squeezed out of the tissues, similar to the wringing of a wet towel (Figs. 90-24 to 90-26). From this dark point (point of twist) emanates several curvilinear dark lines, presumably representing the spiraling facial planes resembling a whirlpool. To best demonstrate the point of twist, the stalk must be imaged perpendicular to its axis. The "whirlpool" sign was clearly seen in three of six cases with torsion.[55] The absence of this sign in the other three is presumably due to a suboptimal imaging plane. In an experiment conducted in rats with surgically

induced unilateral torsion, the whirlpool sign was the single most accurate finding, allowing the recognition of torsion in all torsed testes from sham control subjects.[56] In the rat study, the whirlpool sign disappeared 2 weeks after torsion owing to necrosis and resorption of tissues.[56] In humans, the whirlpool pattern was seen in a patient in whom the acute episode occurred approximately 3 weeks before imaging.[55]

The second finding is the appearance of the testis and epididymis. In all cases, the epididymis was markedly thickened with areas of swelling and areas of subacute hemorrhage (intermediate signal intensity on proton-density–weighted and darker on T2-weighted images) (see Figs. 90-24 and 90-25). The epididymis was in an abnormal position in most patients (superoanterior and in a transverse orientation rather than posteromedial and longitudinal orientation). The position of the epididymis was, however, not specific, especially because this orientation can be altered by the positioning of the patient. The testis in the subacute phase (more than 5 days) was smaller than the contralateral testis (see Figs. 90-24 to 90-26). Its signal intensity was diminished and inhomogeneous. The inhomogeneity was due to linear bands of slightly diminished signal patterns separated by thin lines of increased signal intensity emanating from the mediastinum testis, possibly representing the affected lobules (see Fig. 90-24). In some cases, branching lines of higher signal intensity than background could be seen, possibly representing thrombosed vessels (see Fig. 90-25). A finding seen in some cases imaged in the subacute setting was thickening of the tunica albuginea, possibly related to the fact that the testis had lost volume. When imaging was performed more than 3 weeks after the acute episode, the loss of testicular volume and the tunical thickening was striking (see Fig. 90-26). Of interest, the testis becomes exceedingly dark on T2-weighted images, probably owing to the hemorrhagic necrosis leaving behind significant accumulation of hemosiderin and fibrosis. The entire testis becomes dark with no residual normal signal pattern, unlike the dark signal pattern of testicular masses leaving residual normal tissue (see Fig. 90-26). The combination of tunical thickening, loss of testicular volume, and loss of signal intensity of the entire testis is characteristic of old torsion.

The third finding is the appearance of the proximal cord, which was thickened in all cases. All cords had absent or diminished vascularity (see Figs. 90-24 to 90-26). This is in contradistinction to the hypervascular cord associated with epididymitis (see Figs. 90-15 and 90-19). If the marked swelling and hemorrhage of the epididymis were due to infection, the infection would have to be severe to account for the epididymal changes. Severe infection should produce marked hypervascularity. It is the discrepancy between epididymal and spermatic cord changes that is so striking in torsion.

Other associated findings that are helpful include a hematocele that may be seen in torsion (see Figs. 90-24 and 90-25) in lieu of a hydrocele that is present in epididymitis. When these fluid collections are large, they may demonstrate the bell clapper deformity (see Fig. 90-24) or the testicular bare area (see Fig. 90-2), ruling in or out testicular torsion.

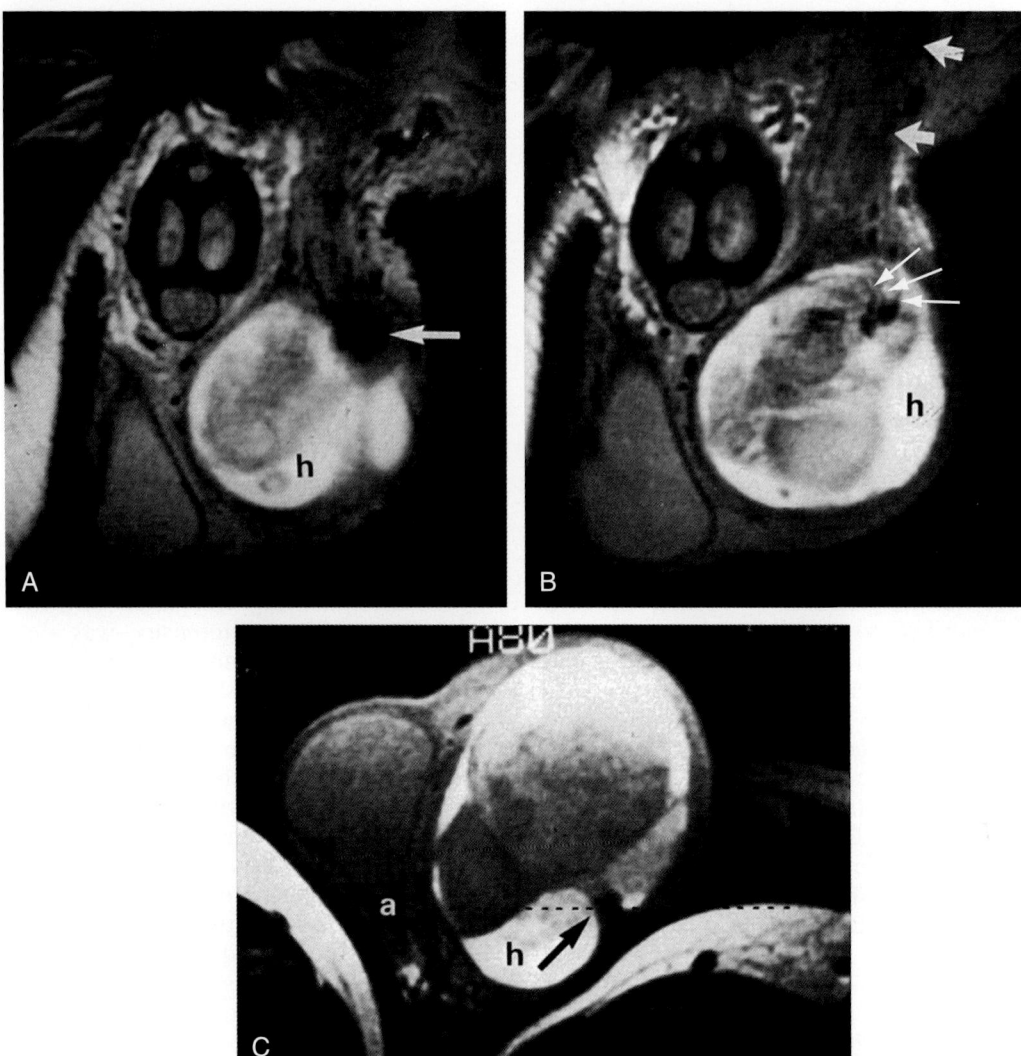

FIGURE 90-24

Five-day-old torsion. **A, B,** and **D** are proton-density–weighted coronal images. **C,** T1-weighted axial image. **E,** T2-weighted coronal image (second echo of **D**). This case demonstrates all the constellation of findings seen in torsion: 1. torsion knot (*arrow* in **A**) is a dark region that represents the point of twist taken at approximately the level shown in **C**; it is thought to be due to the wringing out of water from the cord at the point of twist; 2. whirlpool pattern (*small arrows* in **B**) represents the twisted facial planes of the cord emanating from the point of twist seen just anterior to **A**; 3. the swollen hypovascular cord (*large white arrows* in **B**) when compared with the normal contralateral cord seen on **D** (*arrow*); 4. the bell clapper deformity is seen because the hematocele highlights the stalk (*arrow* on **C**), proven surgically, perpendicular to which images **A** and **B** were obtained (dashed line is level of image in **A**); 5. the hematocele (h) is seen as bright fluid with T1 weighting (**C**), proton-density weighting (**A, B,** and **D**), and T2 weighting (**E**); 6. the enlarged hemorrhagic epididymis (E) shown on coronal images obtained with proton-density weighting (**D**) and T2 weighting (**E**); 7. the superior and transverse position of the epididymis (**D** and **E**); and 8. the testis with overall signal loss (**E**). Note that the intratesticular changes are oriented in the direction of the interlobular septa emanating from the region of the mediastinum (*arrows* on **E**) (*Reproduced with permission from Trambert MA, Mattrey RF, Levine D, Berthoty D: Subacute scrotal pain: evaluation of torsion versus epididymitis with MR imaging. Radiology 175:53-56, 1990.*)

Continued

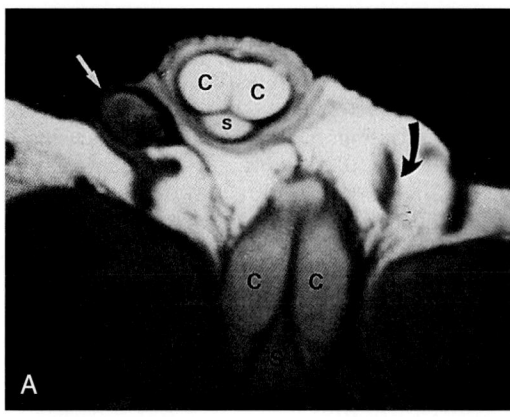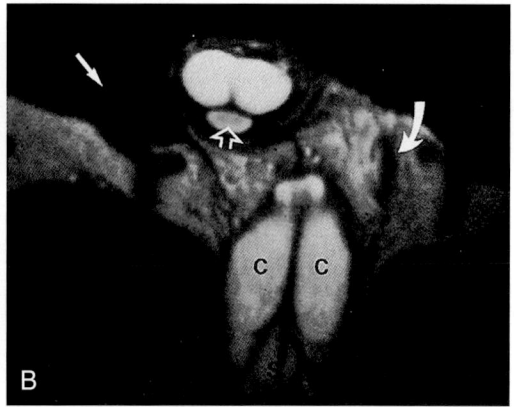

FIGURE 90-27

Axial **A,** proton-density–weighted and **B,** T2-weighted images obtained in a 6-month-old infant with neonatal extravaginal torsion at the level of the affected testis (*arrow*). Note the loss of testicular volume, thickened tunica albuginea, and complete darkening of the testis with no remaining normal testicular tissue similar to the testis seen in Figure 90-23B. Also note that the testis is located in the spermatic canal at the level of the normal contralateral cord (*curved arrow*). Also well seen is the penile anatomy. Corpora cavernosa (C) and spongiosa (S) are bright on both images and are surrounded by the tunica albuginea of the penis. Note that the urethra is better seen on the T2-weighted image (*open arrow*). The lesser signal of the corpora at the base of the penis is due to increased distance from the surface coil.

MRI shows the attached mass containing blood of variable degrees of degradation. Hydrocele is present in two thirds of cases, and associated inflammation of the epididymis is seen in one third. In this setting, MRI can exclude with confidence testicular torsion, infection, or hemorrhage within a tumor, the three clinical conditions that can present with similar signs and symptoms.

In one child with torsion of the appendix proven clinically (Fig. 90-28), the torsed appendix was hemorrhagic and was no longer present at follow-up MRI 6 weeks later. The images were sufficiently characteristic to exclude testicular torsion and allowed for con-servative management. Surgery in this condition is performed to exclude testicular torsion when the diagnosis is unclear.[50] Old torsion of an epididymal appendix is recognized as a spherical mass filled with blood (see Fig. 90-2).

Ischemia and Infarction

Ischemia and partial infarction can result from intermittent torsion, trauma, infection, embolization, or vasculitis. Acute infarction will likely present as hemorrhage or

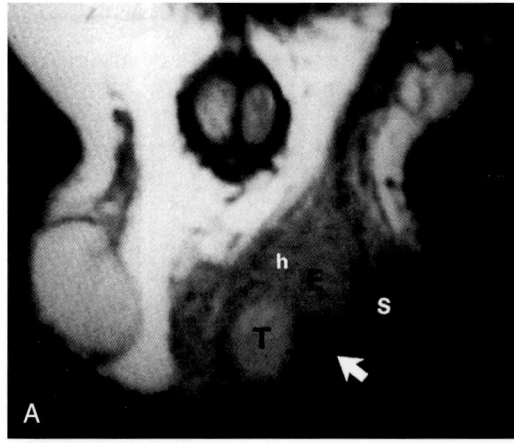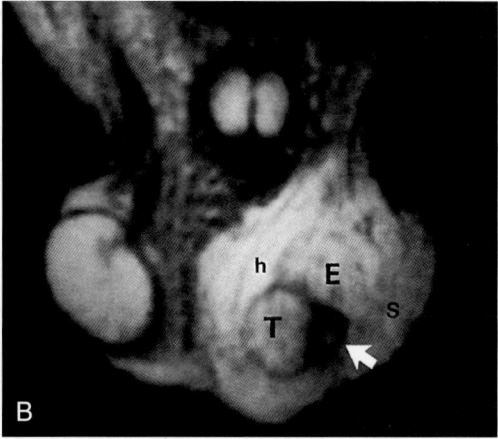

FIGURE 90-28

Torsion of the testicular appendix in a prepubertal boy shown on coronal **A,** proton-density–weighted and **B,** T2-weighted images. Note the darkened testicular appendix (*arrow*) located between the slightly darkened testis (T) and the swollen epididymis (E). Also note the associated hemiscrotal swelling (S) and hydrocele (h). Because of MRI findings, the patient was treated conservatively. A follow-up MR image 6 weeks later was normal (not shown).

focal signal loss with T2 weighting, whereas old infarction will appear as a scar that assumes a dark, sharply demarcated band which typically reaches the tunica and deforms the shape of the testis on T2-weighted sequences. The specific appearance and distribution depend on the cause. Although vasculitis typically produces microinfarcts that are diffusely distributed,[62] trauma and infection may be more focal.

Ischemic change is more difficult to diagnose because no definitive study has addressed this issue where the appearance has been documented histologically. Changes that are presumed to represent ischemic injury have been observed in several patients with testicular pain. Ultrasonography has shown hypoechoic bands alternating with normal testicular echogenicity traversing the testis from the mediastinum to the tunica. At MRI, the testis has appeared patchy on T2-weighted images, at times with alternating bands of low and normal signal intensity that follow the rete testes. When intravenous contrast media were given, interestingly the dark bands enhanced more prominently than the normal bands. This effect is presumed to be due to the disruption of the blood-testis barrier, which leads to excessive gadolinium entrapment analogous to the disruption of the blood-brain barrier.

To test this hypothesis, rats with testicular injury were used. After surgical occlusion of the spermatic cord, rats were reperfused 1 hour ($n = 5$) or 12 hours ($n = 5$) later. A sham group ($n = 2$) or nonreperfused group ($n = 3$) served as negative and positive controls. T1-weighted images were taken every 5 minutes after Gd-DTPA up to 90 minutes immediately after reperfusion and then a week later. Immediately after reperfusion, the normal and 1-hour occlusion groups were indistinguishable. The occluded testes and the testes with 12 hours of occlusion showed delayed wash-in and wash-out. At 1 week, the 1-hour occlusion group enhanced to a greater degree than normal testes. The other two groups again showed delayed wash-in and wash-out. These observations suggest that 12 hours of occlusion, even 1 week later, has a profound effect on testicular flow, whereas 1 hour of occlusion causes some damage that results in leakage and entrapment of Gd-DTPA within the testis.

Extratesticular Lesions

Spermatocele

Spermatoceles are easily identified within the epididymis by MRI. The most frequent site of involvement is the globus major (head). Spermatoceles are round, well-circumscribed structures displaying signal intensity similar to that of hydrocele fluid (see Figs. 90-5 and 90-10). In a minority of cases, the spermatocele may be brighter than water on proton-density–weighted images and remain bright on T2-weighted images (see Fig. 90-19). We are uncertain whether the contents were old blood or high proteinaceous fluid. Indeed, the signal pattern within these lesions does reflect their contents (Fig. 90-29).

Hydrocele

Simple hydrocele has typical fluid characteristics at MRI that are intermediate on proton-density–weighted and high on T2-weighted images relative to fat (see Fig. 90–2). Complicated hydroceles demonstrate signal intensities characteristic of their content (see Figs. 90-24

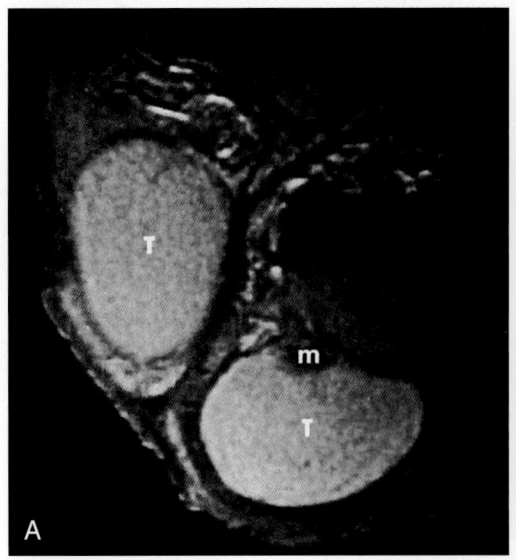 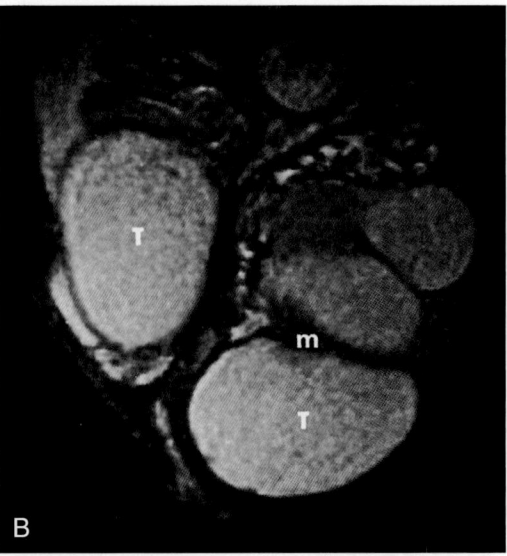

FIGURE 90-29

Septated spermatocele is shown on **A,** proton-density–weighted and **B,** T2-weighted images. Note the rotation of the testis (T) by the multilocular spermatocele in the upper half of the epididymis [spermatocele reaches the mediastinum testis (m)]. Also note the variable signals of each of the locules.

and 90-25). Because fluid is typically present in most subjects, the term hydrocele is reserved for those patients in whom the fluid surrounds the entire equator of the testis or highlights the bare area.

Varicocele

MRI clearly shows the entire spermatic cord from the inguinal ring to the mediastinum testis. Patients with varicocele have widening of the spermatic canal and prominence of the pampiniform plexus (see Fig. 90-21). The plexus is more heterogeneous, with a greater number of serpiginous structures with increased signal intensity on both proton-density– and T2-weighted images. An insufficient number of patients have been studied with this condition to ascertain the role of MRI in this setting. In a prepubertal boy with varicocele, vessels with flow void in the cord as well as prominence of the pampiniform plexus at the base of the scrotum were evident (Fig. 90-30). In one study, abdominal compression, similar to that applied during intravenous urography, exaggerated the appearance of vessels in the cord in patients with varicoceles.[63] The degree of hypervascularity is not prominent, as is seen in epididymitis. Although clinically palpable varicocele are easily depicted by MRI, it is unclear whether MRI will be able to diagnose subclinical varicoceles with sufficient accuracy.

CRYPTORCHIDISM

Cryptorchidism represents the most common disorder of sexual differentiation in humans. It occurs in 2.7% to 6% of full-term male neonates with 0.8% prevalence at 1 year of age. Spontaneous descent is unlikely after the first year.[64-66] Because of a significantly increased risk of malignancy[67,68] and impaired spermatogenic function

in the contralateral descended testis,[69] many techniques have been developed to aid in the diagnosis and treatment of the cryptorchid testis so as to monitor the testis for neoplasia and diminish the incidence of infertility.

An undescended testis may be intra-abdominal, intracanalicular, ectopic, atrophic, or congenitally absent. Undescended testes may be located anywhere from the renal hilum to the superior scrotum. They may also be found in an ectopic location, such as the perineum or superficial abdominal wall. Testes located proximal to the external inguinal ring are usually impalpable, as may be small or atrophic testes located distal to the external inguinal ring.

Surgical treatment consists of orchiopexy of a normal testis in children or orchiectomy in postpubertal patients. The standard surgical treatment of an undescended testis involves division of an associated patent vaginal process and straightening of the cord vessels to achieve sufficient length for the testis to easily reach the caudal extent of the scrotum. An intra-abdominal testis is usually associated with insufficient vessel length to allow for a standard procedure to be performed. These testes are treated by ligating the testicular vessels at a point proximal to their junction with the vas deferens and relying on collateral revascularization from the artery supplying the vas deferens. Testicular autotransplantation is sometimes performed to improve on the 60% to 70% viability rate of the standard procedure. Autotransplantation involves the anastomosis of the distal testicular artery stump to the deep inferior epigastric artery, requiring a microvascular surgical technique and a longer operative procedure.

Neonatal extravaginal torsion results in complete replacement of testicular tissue with scar. If neonatal extravaginal torsion is missed at birth, the patient may present later in life with a nonpalpable undescended testis but possibly a palpable cord. Such a patient requires surgery for diagnosis. If the diagnosis of testicular atrophy

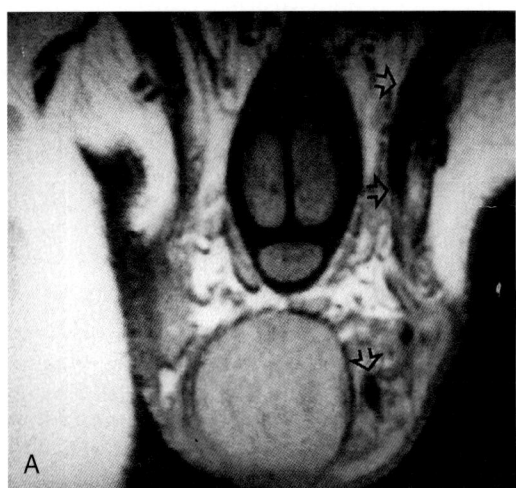 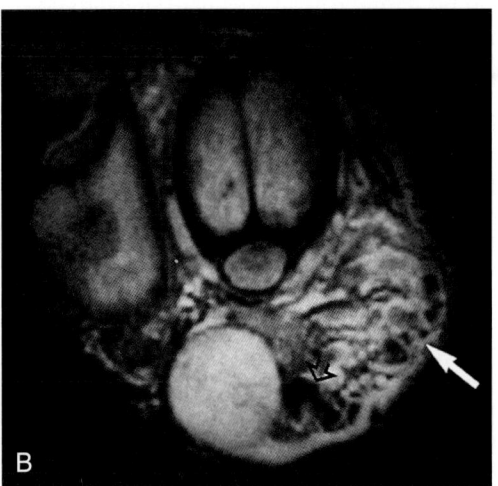

FIGURE 90-30

Left varicocele is seen on coronal **A,** proton-density–weighted and **B,** T2-weighted images obtained at different levels. Note the prominence of the cord and pampiniform plexus at the base of the scrotum (*arrow on* **B**) and the increased flow within their vessels (*open arrows*).

can be reliably made preoperatively, surgery can be avoided or limited to those wanting prosthetic replacement.

Therefore, the adequate preoperative assessment and localization of the undescended testis are useful in guiding clinical management and surgical exploration, making a more limited operative procedure possible.

Various diagnostic modalities, such as ultrasonography,[70,71] computed tomography,[71-73] spermatic venography, and arteriography,[73-75] have been used to localize the cryptorchid testis. These modalities, however, have disadvantages, such as invasiveness, technical difficulties, poor sensitivity and/or specificity, operator dependence, and exposure to ionizing radiation. Laparoscopy was introduced to evaluate the nonpalpable testis before exploration.[76] If testicular vessels and vas deferens end blindly in the abdomen, no exploration is performed. If tissue is present at the end of the vas deferens, exploration follows. However, if the vas deferens enters the internal inguinal ring, exploration of the inguinal canal is required to ensure the absence of testicular tissue. Although laparoscopy is 100% accurate in localizing the potential location of the testis and may obviate surgery in some patients, it is not useful if the cord enters the internal inguinal ring. Laparoscopy does not allow for preoperative planning. It also increases anesthesia and operating room time.

We have studied more than 35 patients with undescended testes. There were 48 total testes with surgical proof available in 27 testes and clinical proof in 5.[77] MRI seems to be the most accurate noninvasive examination. These data are in concordance with other published reports.[78-81] The following discussion details the imaging technique used and presents the capabilities of MRI in this setting.

Imaging Techniques

Although a high-field system is ideal, lower fields can be used if thin slices (3-5 mm) and heavily T2-weighted sequences can be acquired at an adequate signal-to-noise ratio. Patients between 6 months and 6 years of age require sedation. Patients are placed directly in the head coil if they are small enough to fit. A standard 5-inch circular surface coil is centered approximately over the symphysis pubis to ensure that the base of the scrotum and lower pelvis are included in the FOV. The coil is placed on a 1-cm standoff to decrease the high near-field signal. The diaper serves as a standoff in infants and toddlers. A 16-cm FOV, a 256×256 acquisition matrix, and a 3-mm slice thickness are used (voxel size, $0.63 \times 0.63 \times 3$ mm). In small infants, a 3-inch circular surface coil is used and the FOV is reduced to 12 cm while keeping the other parameters constant.

Two series are sufficient in most cases, requiring less than 30 minutes for imaging. Keeping imaging time short is important because most patients require sedation. The first series is T1-weighted (TR/TE, 400/12 ms) and obtained in the transverse plane with 3-, 5-, or 10-mm slice thickness (dependent on the patient's size) and an interslice gap of 50% of the slice thickness. The series should include from the base of the scrotum to

the middle of the bladder to cover the entire course of the spermatic cord. It also serves as a localizer for the subsequent T2-weighted series.

The coronal T1- and T2-weighted series covers the region from the posterior aspect of the scrotum to the anterior abdominal wall. Slice thickness for this series is set at 3 mm in all patients and is obtained with a 50% interslice gap to ensure proper T2 weighting. Alternatively, an interleaved series can be acquired. The sequence is fast spin-echo with a TR of 3500 ms and a TE of 120 ms, 16-cm FOV, 256×192 matrix, two excitations, and an echo train of 16. This series, which can be obtained with fat suppression if magnetic homogeneity is acceptable, allows further assessment of the cord within the spermatic canal and provides testicular tissue characterization. These two series are sufficient if the testes and cord are atrophic and are in the spermatic canal or if the testis is intracanalicular or more distal. This was true in 23 of the 35 patients (63%) we studied. However, if the testes are not seen or are intra-abdominal, a third series is required.

If testes are seen and are intra-abdominal near the internal inguinal ring, a T1-weighted image and a fast spin-echo T2-weighted image are then obtained in the transverse plane over the testis using the surface coil with all parameters unchanged from the coronal series. This series helps to further characterize testicular tissue and locate more precisely the position of the testis relative to the inguinal canal.

If, on the other hand, neither the cryptorchid testis nor its cord structures can be seen on the coronal series, the T1- and T2-weighted fast spin-echo sequences are obtained in the transverse plane from the symphysis pubis to the upper pole of both kidneys using either the head or body coil, dependent on the patient's size, with similar imaging parameters except for a different slice thickness and FOV.

MRI data to be related to the surgeon should describe the testis and the spermatic cord. If the testis is seen, its location, size, and signal behavior should be reported. If the testis is not visualized, visualization of the spermatic cord should be reported, together with the location of its distal end, its thickness, and whether it enters the internal inguinal ring. These data allow the surgeon to assess whether surgery is necessary, to plan the surgical approach and treatment, and to determine if laparoscopy is required.

Role of MRI

High-resolution MRI with surface coils clearly delineates the spermatic cord, inguinal canal, inguinal ring, pubic tubercle, testes, and regional lymph nodes.[13-17,77-80] Both the coronal and axial planes are useful for imaging the spermatic cords. Undescended testes are best seen and recognized on coronal images.[77,78] The axial plane more precisely locates the testis relative to the internal or external inguinal rings and femoral vessels and increases observer confidence. In most patients (23 of 34), two series (transaxial T1- and coronal T1- and T2-weighted sequences) were deemed sufficient for

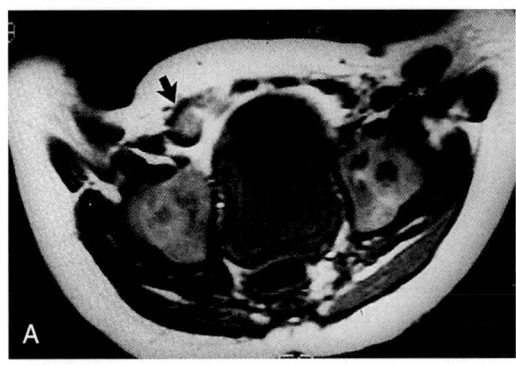
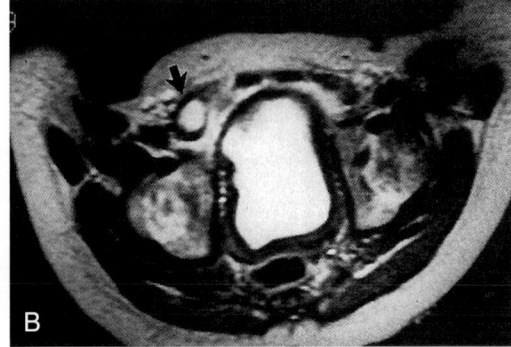

FIGURE 90-31

Right nonpalpable undescended testis located at the internal inguinal ring (*arrows*) shown on **A,** proton-density–weighted and **B,** T2-weighted images. Note the normal testicular signal (intermediate with proton-density weighting and bright with T2 weighting).

complete evaluation, requiring less than 30 minutes of magnet time.[77] The remainder of cases required the additional T1- and T2-weighted transverse series because the testes were intra-abdominal or not visualized.

The undescended testes in our series with surgical or clinical proof were found to be either intra-abdominal (19%), intracanalicular (37%), or atrophic within the spermatic canal (44%). These relationships were similar to the experience of others, but they referred to the group with atrophic testes as absent.[79-81] Four of the six intra-abdominal testes were correctly located. Errors made by others were also related to testes in intra-abdominal locations.[79-81] We believe that these errors should be avoidable with added experience. The overall accuracy of MRI in our prospective series was 93.8% (30 of 32 testes),[77] which is comparable to previously published reports of 94% (15 of 16),[79] 93% (retrospec-

tive data, 13 of 14),[80] and 82% (retrospective data done with body coil). Accuracy was lowest for intra-abdominal testes. Given the intense enhancement of testes with gadolinium, data evaluating undescended testes with fat suppression techniques after administration of intravenous contrast medium are still not available. It would be suspected that accuracy should improve significantly.

Intra-abdominal Testes

Intra-abdominal testes located near or at the internal inguinal ring should be easily evaluated by MRI (Figs. 90-31 and 90-32). However, with lack of experience, we missed two of six testes located near the internal inguinal ring that were easily seen in retrospect (Figs. 90-33 and 90-34). In two published reports, each missed a high intra-abdominal testis.[79,80]

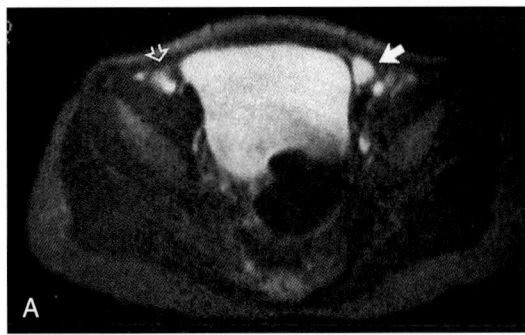
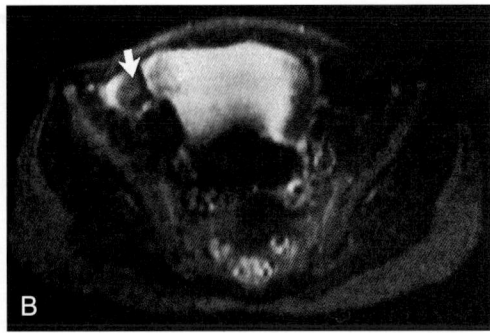

FIGURE 90-32

A and **B,** Bilaterally nonpalpable undescended testes shown on T2-weighted images. The left testis is at the level of the internal inguinal ring (*arrow*). The left testis had normal signal intensity, intermediate to bright with proton-density weighting (not shown), and bright with T2 weighting (**A**). The bright area to the right of the bladder (*open arrow*) is not testis because it was also bright with proton-density weighting (not shown). The right testis is best seen on the next cephalic slice near the level of the internal inguinal ring (*arrow* on **B**). Note that the testicular signal pattern, although it was intermediate with proton-density weighting (not shown), is dark with T2 weighting (**B**). Testicular biopsy showed normal left testis and moderately fibrotic right testis.

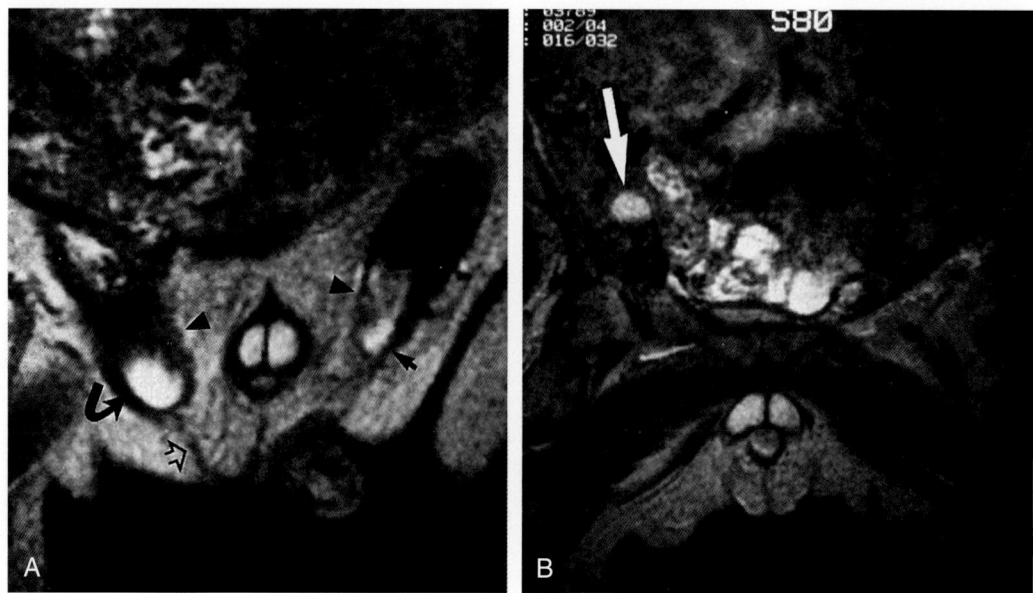

FIGURE 90-33

Newborn with bilateral hernias and bilateral undescended testes. **A,** The right and left hernia sacs shown on a T2-weighted image extend halfway into the spermatic canal (*arrowheads*). Note that the gubernaculum continues into the base of the scrotum better seen on the right (*open arrow*). The right testis was thought to be at the distal end of the hernia sac (*curved arrow*). This proved to be a loop of bowel at surgery. **B,** The right testis was located, in retrospect, three slices posterior to **A** in a typical intra-abdominal location shown on a T2-weighted image (*arrow*). The left testis was small and located at the distal end of its hernia sac (*black arrow on* **A**), proven surgically.

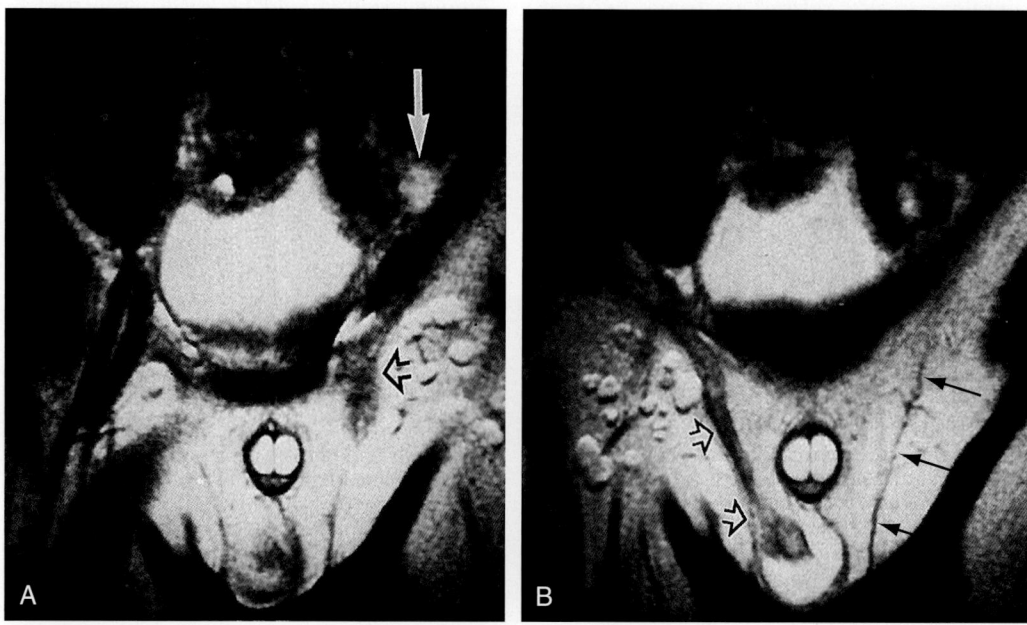

FIGURE 90-34

Left undescended and nonpalpable testis. **A,** T2-weighted image shows a dark band thought to be a flattened end of the cord of an atrophic streak testis at the proximal spermatic canal is shown in a coronal plane (*open arrow*). **B,** T2-weighted image also shows the normal right cord and testis (*open arrows*) and the gubernaculum of the left testis (*small black arrows*) are also shown. At surgery, the normal left undescended testis was intra-abdominal, shown on **A** in a typical intra-abdominal location just superior and lateral to the internal inguinal ring (*arrow*), clearly seen in retrospect. The dark region seen by MRI (*open arrow in* **A**) indicates cord structures preceding the testis. Note the presence of right inguinal adenopathy lateral to the cord in **B**.

The task of locating intra-abdominal testes is the most difficult with MRI. Confusion with lymph nodes and bowel higher in the abdomen becomes possible. With the availability of oral contrast agents and with added experience, this problem could be partially overcome. However, there will always be a certain degree of uncertainty when testes are not clearly depicted. In our series, testes of six patients could not be localized. None of these patients have had surgery to assess the role of MRI when testes are located proximal to the internal inguinal ring. Although it is important to visualize these high intra-abdominal testes,[82] it is our belief that there will always be a certain degree of uncertainty. However, the inability to visualize the high intra-abdominal testis is less critical for management because patients with absent cord and testis will have to undergo surgical exploration that would be preceded by laparoscopy. When the testis and/or cord are well evaluated, laparoscopy is not necessary. MRI in our series could have potentially decreased laparoscopy that was performed in 100% of patients to only 13%.

Assessment of the spermatic cord and testis together is essential for proper diagnosis. An empty spermatic canal is visible by MRI. It appears as a thin line extending from the inguinal canal to the base of the scrotum (Fig. 90-35; see Fig. 90-34), most likely representing the gubernaculum, which is a thin fibrous strand. This thin strand should not be mistaken for an atrophic cord. The latter has significant width but is thinner than the normal contralateral cord (Fig. 90-36). Although an empty canal and an absent cord suggested the possibility of an intra-abdominal testis, the presence of cord structures in the canal does not exclude this possibility (see Fig. 90-34). Cord structures may precede the testis, or the testis

if attached to a long mesentery may flip-flop between an intracanalicular and an intra-abdominal location.

The majority of intra-abdominal testes are found near the internal inguinal ring, where MRI should be reasonably accurate. Therefore, the goal of the imaging schemes should be to maximize the assessment of the internal inguinal ring. The technique described earlier would allow such assessment. The 5-inch surface coil should be centered over the pubic tubercle to place the testis at an optimal position in the field.

Intracanalicular Testes

MRI is extremely accurate in locating these testes. MR image interpretation is simple because these testes are contrasted to fat, are seen in association with intravaginal fluid in many cases, and are seen with their epididymis (see Fig. 90-35). The testis has a normal ovoid shape with clear demonstration of the tunica albuginea. These testes assume three positions: in the subcutaneous space anterior to the external inguinal ring (Fig. 90-37), in the spermatic canal (see Fig. 90-33), or in the inguinal canal (see Fig. 90-35). When testes do not exit the inguinal canal, they frequently proceed laterally and insinuate themselves over the femoral vessels. In this location, they are frequently nonpalpable.

Intracanalicular testes are easily differentiated from lymph nodes because their tunica albuginea can be discerned, they are associated with cord structures or epididymis, they are surrounded by fluid, and they are located in the path of the spermatic cord on axial scans (see Fig. 90-35). Lymph nodes, although of similar signal behavior, present different morphology and are lateral to the cord (see Figs. 90-34 to 90-37).

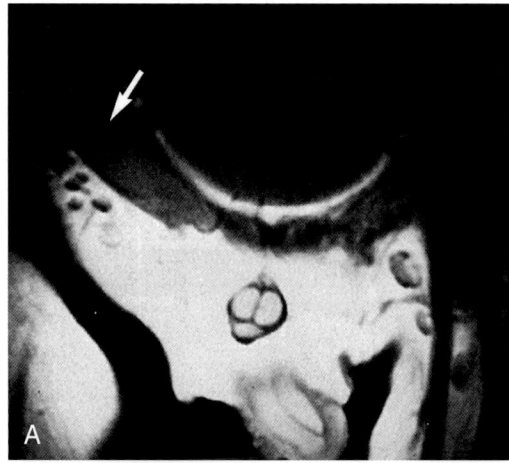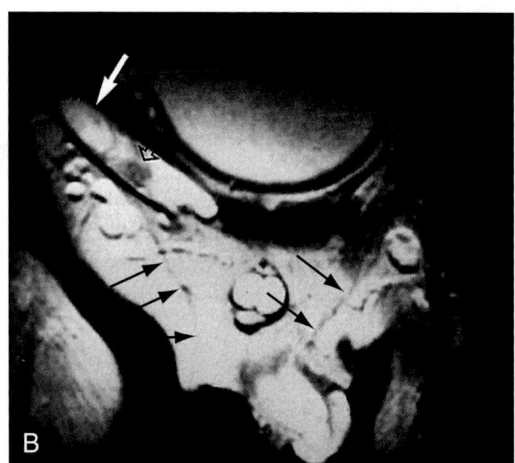

FIGURE 90-35

Undescended nonpalpable right testis in a typical intracanalicular location. Note that the testis has normal signal behavior when seen on **A,** proton-density–weighted and **B,** T2-weighted images (*arrow*) and has an associated normal epididymis (*open arrow*) and ascites. In this location, fluid is technically ascitic because the vaginal process is patent. The other testis was intra-abdominal and is not shown here. Note the gubernaculum best seen on the T2-weighted image bilaterally extending from the external inguinal ring to the base of the scrotum (*small black arrows* on **B**). Note also the presence of inguinal adenopathy lateral to the right and left canals.

REFERENCES

1. Leopold GR, Woo VL, Scheible FW, et al: High resolution ultrasonography of scrotal pathology. Radiology 131:719-722, 1979.
2. Leopold GR: Superficial organs. In Goldberg B (ed): Ultrasound in Cancer. New York, Churchill Livingstone, 1981, pp 123-135.
3. Hricak H, Filly RA: Sonography of the scrotum. Invest Radiol 18:112-121, 1983.
4. Glazer HS, Lee JKT, Melson GL, McClennan BL: Sonographic detection of occult testicular neoplasms. Am J Roentgenol 138:673-675, 1982.
5. Carroll BA, Gross DM: High frequency scrotal sonography. Am J Roentgenol 140:511-515, 1983.
6. Middleton WD, Melson GL: Testicular ischemia: color Doppler sonographic findings in five patients. Am J Roentgenol 152:1237-1239, 1989.
7. Middleton WD, Siegel BA, Melson GL, et al: Acute scrotal disorders: prospective comparison of color Doppler US and testicular scintigraphy. Radiology 177:177-181, 1990.
8. Burks DD, Markey BJ, Burkhard TK, et al: Suspected testicular torsion and ischemia: evaluation with color Doppler sonography. Radiology 175:815-821, 1990.
9. Krieger JN, Wang K, Mack L: Preliminary evaluation of color Doppler imaging for investigation of intrascrotal pathology. J Urol 144:904-907, 1990.
10. Lerner RM, Mevorach RA, Hulbert WC, Rabinowitz R: Color Doppler US in the evaluation of acute scrotal disease. Radiology 176:355-358, 1990.
11. Horstman WG, Middleton WD, Melson GL, Siegel BA: Color Doppler US of the scrotum. RadioGraphics 11:941-957, 1991.
12. Horstman WG, Middleton WD, Melson GL, et al: Scrotal inflammatory disease: color Doppler US findings. Radiology 179:55-59, 1991.
13. Baker LL, Hajek PC, Burkhard TK, et al: Magnetic resonance imaging of the scrotum: normal anatomy. Radiology 163:89-92, 1987.
14. Baker LL, Hajek PC, Burkhard TK, et al: Magnetic resonance imaging of the scrotum: pathologic conditions. Radiology 163:93-98, 1987.
15. Rholl KS, Lee JKT, Ling D, et al: MR imaging of the scrotum with a high resolution surface coil. Radiology 163:99-103, 1987.
16. Seidenwurm D, Smathers RL, Lo RK, et al: Testes and scrotum: MR imaging at 1.5T. Radiology 164:393-398, 1987.
17. Thurnher S, Hricak H, Carroll PR, et al: Imaging the testis: comparison between MR imaging and US. Radiology 167:631-636, 1988.
18. Cramer BM, Schlegel EA, Thueroff JW: MR imaging in the differential diagnosis of scrotal and testicular disease. RadioGraphics 11:9-21, 1991.
19. Semba CP, Trambert MA, Mattrey RF: Specificity of MRI in scrotal disease versus sonography [abstract]. Radiology 177(Suppl):129, 1990.
20. Eilenberg SS, Tartar VM, Mattrey RF: Reducing magnetic susceptibility differences using liquid fluorocarbon pads (Sat Pad): results with spectral presaturation of fat. Artif Cells Blood Substit Immobil Biotechnol 22:1447-1483, 1994.
21. Moore KL: The Developing Human. Clinical Oriented Embryology, 4th ed. Philadelphia: WB Saunders, 1988, pp 246-285.
22. O'Mara EM, Rifkin MD: Scrotum and contents. In Resnick MI, Rifkin MD (eds): Ultrasonography of the Urinary Tract, 3rd ed. Baltimore: Williams & Wilkins, 1991, pp 386-435.
23. Sadler TW: Urogenital system. In Langman's Medical Embryology, 6th ed. Baltimore, Williams & Wilkins, 1990, pp 260-296.
24. Rolnick D, Kowanous S, Szanto P, Bush IM: Anatomical incidence of testicular appendages. J Urol 100:775-766, 1968.
25. Fakhry J, Khoury A, Barakat K: The hypoechoic band: a normal finding on testicular sonography. Am J Roentgenol 153:321-323, 1989.
26. Johnson JO, Mattrey RF, Phillipson J: Differentiation of seminomatous from nonseminomatous testicular tumors with MR imaging. Am J Roentgenol 154:539-543, 1990.
27. Morse MJ, Whitmore WF: Neoplasms of the testes. In Walsh PC, Gittes RF, Permutter AD, Stamey TA (eds): Campbell's Urology. Philadelphia, WB Saunders, 1986, pp 1535-1582.
28. Sokal M, Peckham MJ, Hendry WF: Bilateral germ cell tumours of the testis. Br J Urol 52:158-162, 1980.
29. Schwerk WB, Schwerk WN, Rodeck G: Testicular tumors: prospective analysis of real-time ultrasound patterns and abdominal staging. Radiology 164:369-374, 1987.
30. Lupetin AR, King W III, Rich P, Lederman RB: Ultrasound diagnosis of testicular leukemia. Radiology 146:171-172, 1983.
31. Krone KD, Carroll BA: Scrotal ultrasound. Radiol Clin North Am 23:121-139, 1985.
32. Shah KH, Maxted WC, Chun B: Epidermoid cysts of the testis: a report of three cases and an analysis of 141 cases from the world literature. Cancer 47:577-582, 1981.
33. Berger Y, Srinivas V, Hajdu SI, Herr HW: Epidermoid cysts of the testis: role of conservative surgery. J Urol 134:962-963, 1985.
34. Maxwell AJ, Mamtora H: Sonographic appearance of epidermoid cyst of the testis. J Clin Ultrasound 18:188-190, 1990.
35. Meiches MD, Nurenberg P: Sonographic appearance of a calcified simple epidermoid cyst of the testis. J Clin Ultrasound 19:498-500, 1991.
36. Brenner JS, Cumming WA, Ros PR: Testicular epidermoid cyst: sonographic and MR findings. Am J Roentgenol 152:1344, 1989.
37. Leung ML, Gooding GAW, Williams RD: High-resolution sonography of scrotal contents in asymptomatic subjects. Am J Roentgenol 143:161-164, 1984.
38. Gooding GAW, Leonhardt W, Stein R: Testicular cysts: US findings. Radiology 163:537-538, 1987.
39. Hamm B, Frobbe F, Loy V: Testicular cysts: differentiation with US and clinical findings. Radiology 168:19-23, 1988.
40. Trainer TD: Histology of the normal testis. Am J Surg Pathol 11:797-809, 1987.
41. Arcadia JA: Cysts of the tunica albuginea testis. J Urol 68:631-635, 1952.
42. Mennemeyer RP, Mason JT: Non-neoplastic cystic lesions of the tunica albuginea: an electron microscopic and clinical study of 2 cases. J Urol 121:373-375, 1979.
43. Tartar VM, Trambert MA, Balsara ZN, Mattrey RF: Tubular ectasia of the testicle: sonographic and MR imaging appearance. Am J Roentgenol 160:539-542, 1993.
44. Brown DL, Benson CB, Doherty FJ, et al: Cystic testicular mass caused by dilated rete testis: sonographic findings in 31 cases. Am J Roentgenol 158:1257-1259, 1992.
45. Weingarten BJ, Kellman GM, Middleton WD, Gross ML: Tubular ectasia within the mediastinum testis. J Ultrasound Med 11:349-353, 1992.
46. Weiss AJ, Kellman GM, Middleton WD, Kirkemo A: Intratesticular varicocele: sonographic findings in two patients. Am J Roentgenol 158:1061-1063, 1992.
47. Smith WS, Brammer HM, Henry M, Frazier H: Testicular microlithiasis: sonographic features with pathologic correlation. Am J Roentgenol 157:1003-1004, 1991.
48. Janzen DL, Mathieson JR, Marsh JI, et al: Testicular microlithiasis: sonographic and clinical features. Am J Roentgenol 158:1057-1060, 1992.
49. Bird K, Rosenfield AT: Testicular infarction secondary to acute inflammatory disease: demonstration by B-scan ultrasound. Radiology 152:785-788, 1984.
50. Gullenwater JY, Grayhack JT, Howards SS, Duckett JW: Adult and Pediatric Urology. Chicago, Year Book Medical Publishers, 1987, pp 1955-1962.
51. Finkelstein MS, Rosenberg HK, Snyder HM III, Duckett JW: Ultrasound evaluation of scrotum in pediatrics. Urology 27:1-9, 1986.
52. Hricak H, Jeffrey RB: Sonography of acute scrotal abnormalities. Radiol Clin North Am 21:595-603, 1983.
53. Williamson RCN, Anderson JB: The fate of the human testes following unilateral torsion. Br J Urol 58:698-704, 1986.
54. Ryan PC, Whelan CA, Gaffney EF, Fitzpatrick JM: The effect of unilateral experimental testicular torsion on spermatogenesis and fertility. Br J Urol 62:359-366, 1988.
55. Trambert MA, Mattrey RF, Levine D, Berthoty DP: Subacute scrotal pain: evaluation of torsion versus epididymitis with MR imaging. Radiology 175:53-56, 1990.
56. Landa HM, Gylys-Morin V, Mattrey RF, et al: Detection of testicular torsion by magnetic resonance imaging in a rat model. J Urol 140:1178-1180, 1988.
57. Mueller DL, Amundson GM, Rubin SZ, Wesenberg RL: Acute scrotal abnormalities in children: diagnosis by combined sonography and scintigraphy. Am J Roentgenol 150:643-646, 1988.
58. Bretan PN Jr, Vigneron DB, Hricak H, et al: Assessment of testicular metabolic integrity with P-31 MR spectroscopy. Radiology 162:867-871, 1987.
59. Ben Chaim J, Leibovitch I, Ramon J, et al: Etiology of acute scrotum at surgical exploration in children, adolescents and adults. Eur Urol 21:45-47, 1992.
60. Cohen HL, Shapiro MA, Haller JO, Glassberg K: Torsion of the testicular appendage sonographic diagnosis. J Ultrasound Med 11:81-83, 1992.
61. Atkinson GO Jr, Patrick LE, Ball TI Jr, et al: The normal and abnormal scrotum in children: evaluation with color Doppler sonography. Am J Roentgenol 158:613-617, 1992.
62. Hayward I, Trambert MA, Mattrey RF, et al: Case report: MR imaging of vasculitis of the testis. J Comput Assist Tomogr 15:502-504, 1990.
63. Ziffer JA, Nelson RC, Chezmar JL, et al: Subclinical varicoceles: detection with MRI [abstract]. Magn Reson Imaging 7(Suppl):78, 1989.
64. Scorer CG, Farrington GH: Congenital Deformities of the Testis and Epididymis. New York, Appleton-Century-Crofts, 1972.
65. Cour-Palais IJ: Spontaneous descent of the testicle. Lancet 1:1403-1405, 1966.
66. Hadziselimovic F: Cryptorchidism. Berlin: Springer-Verlag, 1983.
67. Batata MA, Whitmore WF Jr, Hilaris BS, et al: Cryptorchidism and testicular cancer. J Urol 124:382-387, 1980.
68. Pinch L, Aceto T Jr, Meyer-Bahlburg HFL: Cryptorchidism. A pediatric review. Urol Clin North Am 1:573-592, 1974.
69. Rajfer J: The testis and epididymis: cryptorchidism. In Kaufmann JJ (ed): Current Urologic Therapy. Philadelphia, WB Saunders, 1986, pp 422-423.
70. Weiss RM, Carter AR, Rosenfield AT: High resolution real-time ultrasonography in the localization of the undescended testis. J Urol 135:936-938, 1986.
71. Wolverson MK, Houttin E, Heiberh E, et al: Comparison of CT with high resolution ultrasound in the localization of the undescended testis. Radiology 146:133-136, 1983.
72. Lee JKT, McClennan BL, Stanley RJ, Sagel SS: Utility of CT in the localization of the undescended testis. Radiology 135:121-125, 1980.
73. Green JR: Computerized axial tomography vs. spermatic venography in localization of the cryptorchid testis. Urology 26:513-517, 1985.

74. Glickman MF, Weiss RM, Itzchak Y: Testicular venography for undescended testes. Am J Roentgenol 129:67-70, 1977.

75. Diamond AB, Meng CH, Kodroff M, Goldman SM: Testicular venography in the nonpalpable testis. Am J Roentgenol 129:71-75, 1977.

76. Lowe DH, Brock WA, Kaplan GW: Laparoscopy for localization of the nonpalpable testis. J Urol 131:728-729, 1984.

77. Gylys-Morin V, Landa HM, Fitzmorris-Glass R, et al: MR imaging of the cryptorchid testis [abstract]. Radiology 165(P):59, 1987.

78. Landa HM, Gylys-Morin V, Mattrey RF, et al: MRI of the cryptorchid testis. Eur J Pediatr 146(Suppl):S16-S17, 1987.

79. Fritzsche PJ, Hricak H, Kogan BA, et al: Undescended testis: value of MRI. Radiology 164:169-173, 1987.

80. Kier R, McCarthy S, Rosenfield AT, et al: Nonpalpable testes in young boys: evaluation with MR imaging. Radiology 169:429-433, 1988.

81. Tripathi RP, Jena AN, Gulati P, et al: Undescended testis: evaluation by magnetic resonance imaging. Indian Pediatr 29:433-438, 1992.

82. Friedland GW, Chang P: The role of imaging in the management of impalpable undescended testis. Am J Roentgenol 151:1107-1111, 1988.

83. Cho KS, Auh YH, Lee MG, et al: Testicular tumor: conventional MR imaging and Gd-DTPA enhancement. Radiology 181(Suppl):115, 1991.

84. Just M, Melchior S, Grebe P, et al: MR tomography in testicular processes. The significance of Gd-DTPA enhanced sequence in comparison with plain T2-weighted sequences. Rofo Fortschr Geb Rontgenstr Neuen Bildgeb Verfahr 166:527-531, 1992.

CHAPTER **91**

MALIGNANT DISORDERS
OF THE FEMALE PELVIS

Karen Kinkel ● Michele Brown ● Claude B. Sirlin

Magnetic resonance imaging (MRI) of the female pelvis has become one of the primary imaging modalities to diagnose the extent of endometrial or cervical cancer and to characterize the malignant or benign nature of complex adnexal masses or post-treatment changes. Treatment options for gynecological neoplasms vary according to the extent of disease—generally assessed clinically, and often associated with a large percentage of under- or over-staging of the tumor. Magnetic resonance imaging has been shown to be the most accurate imaging tool in defining the extent of cervical cancer, compared with clinical staging, and to define the extent of endometrial cancer, compared with other imaging techniques.[1,2] To avoid under- or over-staging by clinical assessment alone and to allow treatment options to be adapted to tumor volume and location, MRI is increasingly used before planning treatment of malignant disorders of the female pelvis.

From a technical point of view, high-resolution T2-weighted fast spin-echo (FSE) sequences allow adequate assessment of both normal pelvic anatomy and a wide range of benign and malignant pathologies. However, in the diagnosis of tumor extension, T1-weighted contrast-enhanced imaging techniques are often required to increase the diagnostic confidence of deep myometrial invasion of endometrial cancer, to identify morphological signs of malignancy of ovarian cancer, and to diagnose recurrence of female pelvic cancer. A variety of benign uterine diseases can mask or simulate the extension of endometrial or cervical cancer. In this context, dynamic contrast-enhanced T1-weighted sequences can be helpful in clarifying the position of anatomical landmarks, such as the junctional zone, or to visualize isointense small cervical cancers. Normal uterine enhancement is known to change rapidly over time after intravenous injection of contrast media. In the normal uterus, initial slight enhancement of the junction between endometrium and myometrium is followed by strong enhancement of the entire myometrium and little

delayed enhancement of the endometrium.[3,4] Optimal contrast between tumor and normal uterine enhancement requires different timing of sequence acquisition depending on the cervical or endometrial location of the tumor. For endometrial cancer, increased contrast between the delayed enhancement of the tumor and the early enhancement of normal myometrium is identified at approximately 2 minutes after contrast injection.[4] For cervical cancer, the maximum contrast between tumor and normal cervical stroma has been identified at 1 minute after contrast injection.[3] Dynamic contrast-enhanced T1-weighted sequences should, therefore, not last more than 2 minutes for endometrial cancer and 1 minute for cervical cancer. Native T1-weighted sequences with and without fat suppression and contrast-enhanced fat suppressed T1-weighted sequences are important for the diagnosis of complex adnexal masses. MR urography can be added to the examination in the event of suspected urinary obstruction including both non-enhanced heavily T2-weighted spin-echo sequence (TR 8000 ms) and gadolinium-enhanced T1-weighted fast-field-echo sequence.[5-7] As for all MRI of the pelvis, pelvic or torso phased-array surface coils provide high quality images of uterine zonal anatomy. To minimize respiratory artifacts and motion-related phase ghosting, anterior nonselective saturation pulses are positioned over the subcutaneous fat without covering the abdominal wall muscles. Intramuscular or intravenous intestinal movement inhibitors are injected to reduce bowel movement artifacts, provided no medical contraindications are present. Fat suppression is usually not necessary for uterine tumors unless the tumor extends beyond the uterine contour or parametrium. In these circumstances, fat suppressed contrast-enhanced T1-weighted sequences may help diagnose tumor extension into the pelvic sidewall, rectum, or bladder. For the characterization of ovarian masses, fat-suppressed sequences easily differentiate an endometrioma from a mature cystic teratoma of the ovary, and better delineate the anatomical location of pelvic tumor recurrence. Section thickness should not exceed 5 mm, but smaller sections of 3 mm can be helpful in post-menopausal uteri of decreased size. The majority of published studies have been performed at high field strength between 1 and 1.5 T. Studies at low field strength MR (between 0.1 and 0.2 T) reported less adequate results for staging of cervical cancer than those reported for high-field MRI.[8,9]

ENDOMETRIAL CANCER

Cancer of the endometrium is the most common invasive gynecologic malignancy in North America. Most patients with endometrial cancer are post-menopausal and present with uterine bleeding. Transvaginal sonography is the initial imaging technique to identify abnormal thickening of the endometrium. A threshold value above 5 mm helps with patient selection for subsequent endometrial biopsy.[10,11] Once the diagnosis of endometrial cancer has been established at biopsy, local tumor extension defines the treatment options. In 1988, the International Federation of Gynecology and Obstetrics (FIGO) adopted a surgicopathologic system for the staging of endometrial adenocarcinoma (Box 91-1).[12] The rationale behind the change from the clinical to the surgicopathologic staging system was based on the inaccuracy of clinical staging and on the subsequent limitations of treatment planning.[13] The histologic tumor grade and the depth of myometrial invasion in patients with endometrial cancer correlate strongly with the prevalence of lymph node metastasis and with patient survival.[13] Tumor grade is the most commonly used prognostic factor that guides treatment decisions and surgical planning. Because of the higher prevalence of

lymph node metastases in patients with grade 3 carcinomas, these patients are more likely to undergo surgical lymph node assessment than patients with grade 1 endometrial carcinoma. Patients with grade 1 or grade 2 carcinomas represent a clinical challenge and a treatment dilemma: whether or not to perform lymphadenectomy. The removal of pelvic and/or para-aortic lymph nodes requires special surgical training and is usually performed in tertiary care centers. The preoperative assessment of pelvic lymph node invasion by imaging techniques suffers from an insufficient sensitivity for both computed tomography (CT) and MRI.[14] Due to the excellent correlation between deep myometrial invasion and lymph node invasion,[15] pre- or intra-operative assessment of deep myometrial invasion can be used to decide whether lymphadenectomy should be performed at the time of initial hysterectomy. Intra-operative assessment of deep myometrial invasion with frozen section of the myometrium is a valid but time-consuming technique; moreover, if deep myometrial invasion is identified during this intervention, referral of the patient to a tertiary care center for treatment by a specialist in gynecologic oncologic surgery would imply a second intervention. Preoperative imaging techniques that have been proposed for the evaluation of myometrial invasion include transvaginal ultrasound (US), CT, and MRI. Among these imaging modalities, contrast-enhanced MRI has a substantially higher sensitivity and specificity than US or CT.[2] Moreover, MRI is able to diagnose cervical extension of endometrial cancer, another important risk factor of lymph node metastasis.

The diagnosis of myometrial invasion is suspected with T2-weighted MRI when the hypointense junctional zone is interrupted or presents an irregular interface with the endometrium[16] (Fig. 91-1A). A complete, noninterrupted junctional zone without cervical extension is considered to represent stage IA endometrial cancer.[17] Visibility of the endometrial tumor itself can be impaired if the signal is isointense to the normal endometrium (Fig. 91-1A). In most circumstances the endometrial thickness is increased and associated with an enlarged endometrial cavity. This situation can lead to thinning of the myometrial layer without any myometrial invasion.[18] The depth of myometrial invasion is divided into superficial, less than 50% invasion of the total myometrial thickness (stage IB), and deep, more than 50% invasion (stage IC). When the total thickness of the myometrium measures less than 10 mm due to extensive stretching of the myometrium by an enlarged uterine cavity, the distinction between deep and superficial myometrial invasion can be difficult and might require 3-mm sections through the uterus. A common false-negative result of deep myometrial invasion is at the location of the tubal isthmus (uterine cornua), also shown on intra-operative frozen section analysis.[19] Systematic acquisition of T2-weighted images in three planes following the long and short uterine axis with sagittal, oblique coronal, and oblique axial sections through the uterine cavity may be necessary to avoid false-negative results of deep myometrial invasion. Even when the junctional zone and the tumor are easily

---

Box 91-1   FIGO Staging of Endometrial Carcinoma

Stage I   Tumor confined to the corpus
　　IA　Tumor limited to endometrium
　　IB　Invasion of less than 50% of myometrium
　　IC　Invasion of more than 50% of myometrium

Stage II　Involvement of the cervix
　　IIA　Glandular involvement only
　　IIB　Cervical stromal involvement

Stage III　Spread outside of the uterus and confined to pelvis (does not include rectal or bladder involvement)
　　IIIA　Involvement of uterine serosa, adnexae; positive peritoneal cytologic findings
　　IIIB　Spread to vagina
　　IIIC　Metastases to pelvic and/or para-aortic lymph nodes

Stage IV　Spread outside of true pelvis or invasion of bladder or rectal mucosa
　　IVA　Spread to the bladder and/or rectal mucosa
　　IVB　Distant metastasis (includes intra-abdominal or inguinal lymphadenopathy)

identified on T2-weighted images, combined reading with dynamic contrast-enhanced T1-weighted sequences still performs better than interpretation of T2-weighted FSE sequences alone[20] (Fig. 91-1B and C). When the junctional zone remains indistinct from the rest of the myometrium, occurring most often when adenomyosis or polyfibromatosis is associated, dynamic contrast-enhanced T1-weighted images are crucial to distinguish the early enhancing normal myometrium from the delayed enhancement of the tumor[21] (Figs. 91-2 and 91-3). Our endometrial cancer protocol includes one T1-weighted precontrast aquisition and two early post-contrast acquisitions at 1 and 2 minutes after contrast injection. Myometrial invasion corresponds to the non- or poorly enhancing portion of the myometrium in continuation with the endometrial tumor on images acquired at 2 minutes.[16] Fibroids can also demonstrate

reduced myometrial enhancement and should not be misdiagnosed as myometrial invasion (see Fig. 91-3). Comparison with T2-weighted images acquired in identical image sections and orientation helps to avoid this false-positive result. The overall accuracy of contrast-enhanced MRI in predicting deep myometrial invasion has been estimated at 91%.[2]

Cervical invasion is diagnosed when an endometrial tumor extends into the endocervical channel.[16] Widening of the diameter can be the only imaging characteristic of stage IIA endometrial cancer. Stromal invasion of the cervix (stage IIB) corresponds to an interrupted hypointense stromal ring (Fig. 91-4). On dynamic images, early enhancement of the normal endocervical epithelium occurs prior to delayed enhancement of the normal cervical stroma. Stromal invasion shows a hypointense lack of enhancement

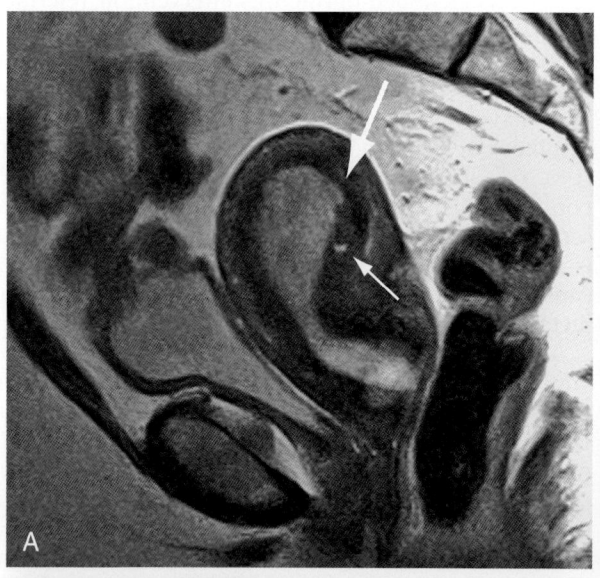

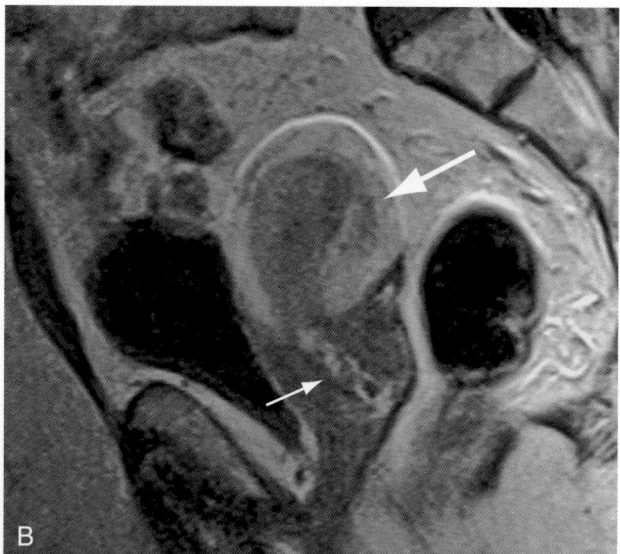

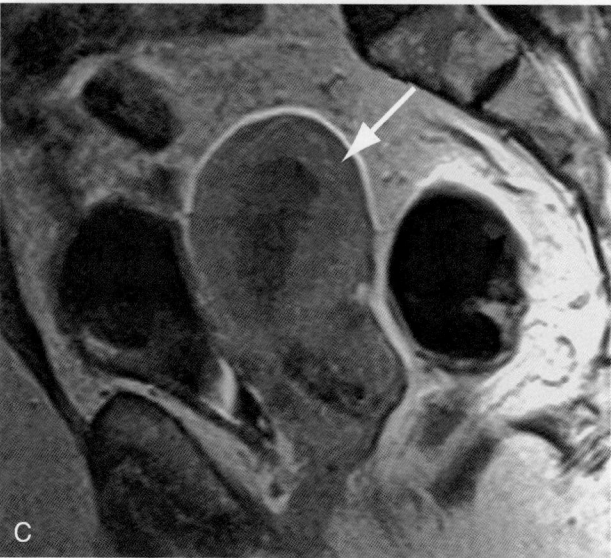

FIGURE 91-1

Post-menopausal woman with vaginal bleeding and intermediate grade adenocarcinoma of the endometrium at endometrial biopsy. **A,** T2-weighted fast spin-echo (FSE) sagittal image through the uterus demonstrating a thickened endometrium associated with a posterior protrusion into the junctional zone (JZ; *large arrow*). The irregular interface between the upper posterior JZ and the endometrium indicate myometrial invasion. The percentage of invasion covers less than 50% of the total thickness of the myometrium suggesting superficial myometrial invasion (stage IB). The hyperintense spot *(small arrow)* and moderate thickening of the JZ suggests associated adenomyosis; stage IB and adenomyosis were confirmed at pathology of the hysterectomy specimen. **B,** Early contrast-enhanced T1-weighted FSE image acquired at 1 minute shows decreased myometrial enhancement of the upper posterior myometrium *(large arrow)* confirming superficial myometrial invasion. Heterogeneous enhancement of the slightly widened mid-endocervical channel *(small arrow)* corresponded to an associated polyp. Differentiation with an endocervical extension of the tumor (stage IIA) is difficult but unlikely due to the preserved upper endocervical os. **C,** Delayed contrast-enhanced T1-weighted image FSE acquired at 5 minutes is less informative than that acquired at an early enhancing phase (**B**) due to a rapid washout phenomena of the normal myometrium that becomes indistinct from the invaded myometrium *(arrow)*.

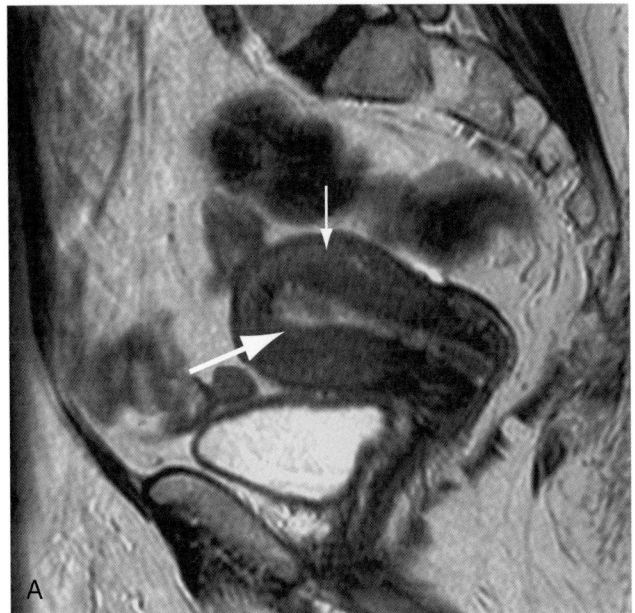

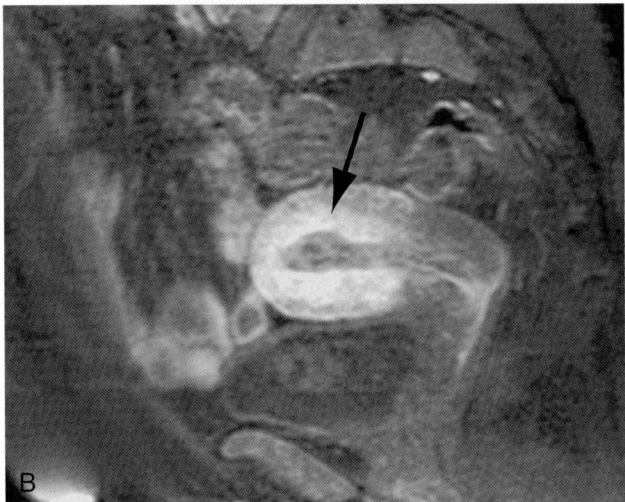

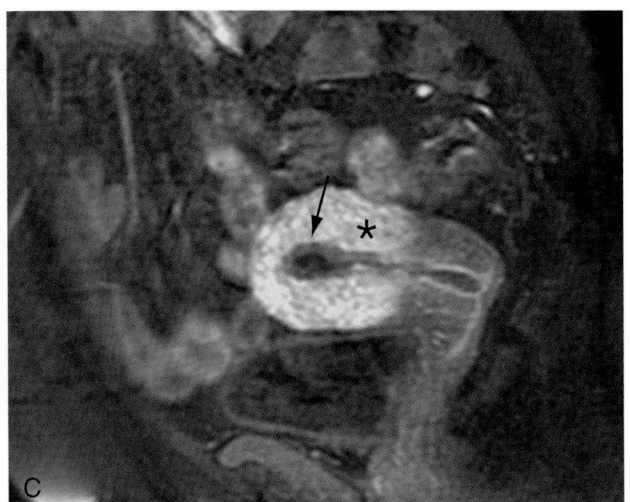

FIGURE 91-2

Low-grade adenocarcinoma of the uterus with superficial myometrial invasion. **A,** Sagittal T2-weighted fast spin-echo (FSE) image shows a heterogeneous signal intensity of the endometrium *(large arrow)* associated with an ill defined junctional zone *(small arrow)*. **B,** Early contrast-enhanced T1-weighted fat-suppressed gradient-echo image at 1 minute shows irregularity of the strongly enhancing junctional zone *(arrow)* indicating myometrial invasion. **C,** Strong enhancement of the entire outer and inner normal myometrium *(asterisk)* at 2 minutes after contrast injection allows differentiation of the less enhancing invaded myometrium *(arrow)*, which accounts for less than 50% of the total myometrial thickness.

extending from the endocervical channel to the stromal ring.[22] The accuracy of MRI in the diagnosis of cervical invasion has been estimated at 92%.[2] Diagnosis of stromal invasion of the cervix is better defined with oblique axial image orientation than with parasagittal image orientation.[23] Due to the different axes of the cervical and endometrial channels, section orientation is crucial and might require careful technician training or the presence of the radiologists during image acquisition. General female pelvic imaging recommendations follow oblique parallel and perpendicular section orientation according to the axis of the endometrial cavity. For the diagnosis of cervical invasion, extra sections may be necessary in a parallel or perpendicular orientation to the cervical channel. Coronal image orientation, parallel to the endocervical channel, is helpful when the cervix exhibits an oblique orientation in the right-left direction (see Fig. 91-4). Parametrial invasion due to endometrial cancer is identified when the tumor signal intensity

invades the cervical stroma with bulging into the parametrial fat. It occurs only in patients with stage IIB disease or greater and has a high rate of recurrence and mortality.[24] Preoperative diagnosis is important due to the need for extended parametrial removal during surgery.[25]

When the tumor demonstrates full-thickness myometrial invasion with uterine contour changes, invasion of the uterine serosa can be suspected, and this corresponds to stage III disease. A suspicious ovarian mass, invasion of the vagina, or pelvic and/or para-aortic lymph nodes are other indications of stage III disease. Stage IV disease is present if the tumor spreads to the bladder or rectal mucosa, or if there are distant metastases including involvement of abdominal or inguinal lymph nodes (Fig. 91-5). The diagnosis of lymphadenopathy is suggested when the short axis of lymph nodes measures more than 10 mm. Due to the excellent soft-tissue contrast between lymph nodes and the surrounding hyperintense fat,

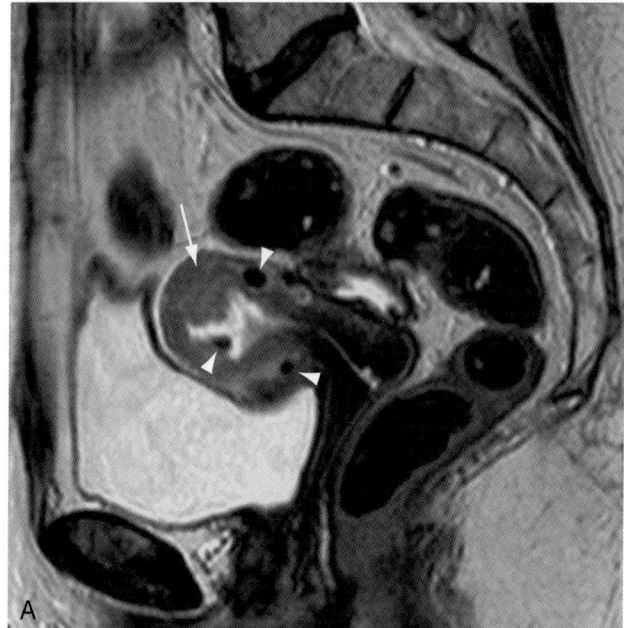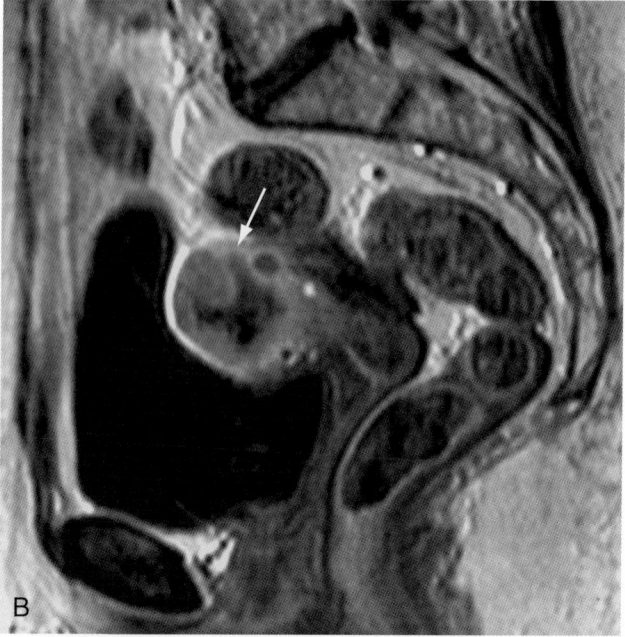

FIGURE 91-3

High-grade endometrioid adenocarcinoma of the uterus with deep myometrial invasion. **A,** Sagittal T2-weighted FSE image of the uterus demonstrates an enlarged uterine cavity with an isointense endometrial mass associated with fluid, an ill-defined junctional zone *(arrow)* and hypointense round myometrial abnormalities *(arrowheads)* suggesting submucosal and interstitial fibroids. **B,** Contrast-enhanced T1-weighted FSE image at 2 minutes shows a lack of enhancement of the endometrial cavity extending to the outer posterior myometrium *(arrow)* suggesting stage IC disease. The associated uterine fibroids demonstrate well-circumscribed reduced myometrial enhancement.

T1-weighted unenhanced sequences detect lymph nodes of increased size quicker than T2-weighted or contrast-enhanced T1-weighted fat-suppressed sequences. However, sensitivity and specificity remain low (see section on cervical cancer) (Fig. 91-6). The use of intravenous superparamagnetic iron oxide contrast media appears to be more helpful in differentiating pelvic metastasis from benign lymph nodes in prostate cancer than in gynecological cancers.[26]

In conclusion, diagnosis of myometrial and cervical invasion by endometrial cancer is a difficult but important step in diagnosing the local extension of endometrial cancer. The mean weighted pretest probabilities of deep myometrial invasion in patients with tumor grades 1, 2, or 3 have been estimated at 13%, 35%, or 54%, respectively.[27] In this Bayesian analysis using contrast-enhanced MRI to determine the utility of MRI according to tumor grade of endometrial carcinoma, post-test probabilities of deep myometrial invasion for grades 1, 2, or 3 increased to 60%, 84%, or 92%, respectively, for positive and decreased to 1%, 5%, or 10%, respectively, for negative MRI findings. Therefore, the use of contrast-enhanced MRI significantly affected the post-test probability of deep myometrial invasion in all patients regardless the grade of endometrial cancer. MRI should be used systematically to select patients for specialist referral. However, careful comparison between T2-weighted and dynamic contrast-enhanced T1-weighted images is required to avoid under- or overstaging due to associated benign disease.

UTERINE SARCOMA

Magnetic resonance imaging reports on uterine sarcoma are rare due to the low incidence of this uterine tumor (2% to 3%). Uterine sarcomas are classified into four subtypes deriving either from stromal cells (malignant mixed mesodermal tumor, endometrial stromal sarcoma, and adenosarcoma) or from smooth muscle cells (leiomyosarcoma). Most of these tumors are diagnosed at hysterectomy due to insufficient tissue sampling during endometrial biopsy. One case report of endometrial stromal sarcoma describes uterine enlargement and complete replacement by neoplastic tissue, with full-thickness myometrial infiltration.[28] Endometrial sarcoma had an isointense signal on T1- and a heterogeneous hyperintense signal on T2-weighted images (Fig. 91-7). Contrast-enhanced dynamic T1-weighted images showed centripetal enhancement. Another study compared dynamic enhancement of 11 endometrial carcinomas with 4 malignant mixed mesodermal tumors.[29] Malignant mixed mesodermal tumors demonstrated areas of early and persistent marked enhancement similar to that of the normal myometrium, mixed with areas of gradual and delayed marked enhancement. The portions showing early and persistent enhancement corresponded histologically to predominantly sarcomatous components with prominent vascularity. Ten of 11 endometrial carcinomas did not show such enhancement, and only one showed a rapid enhancement in the early phase that was diminished in the delayed phase. Although MRI with

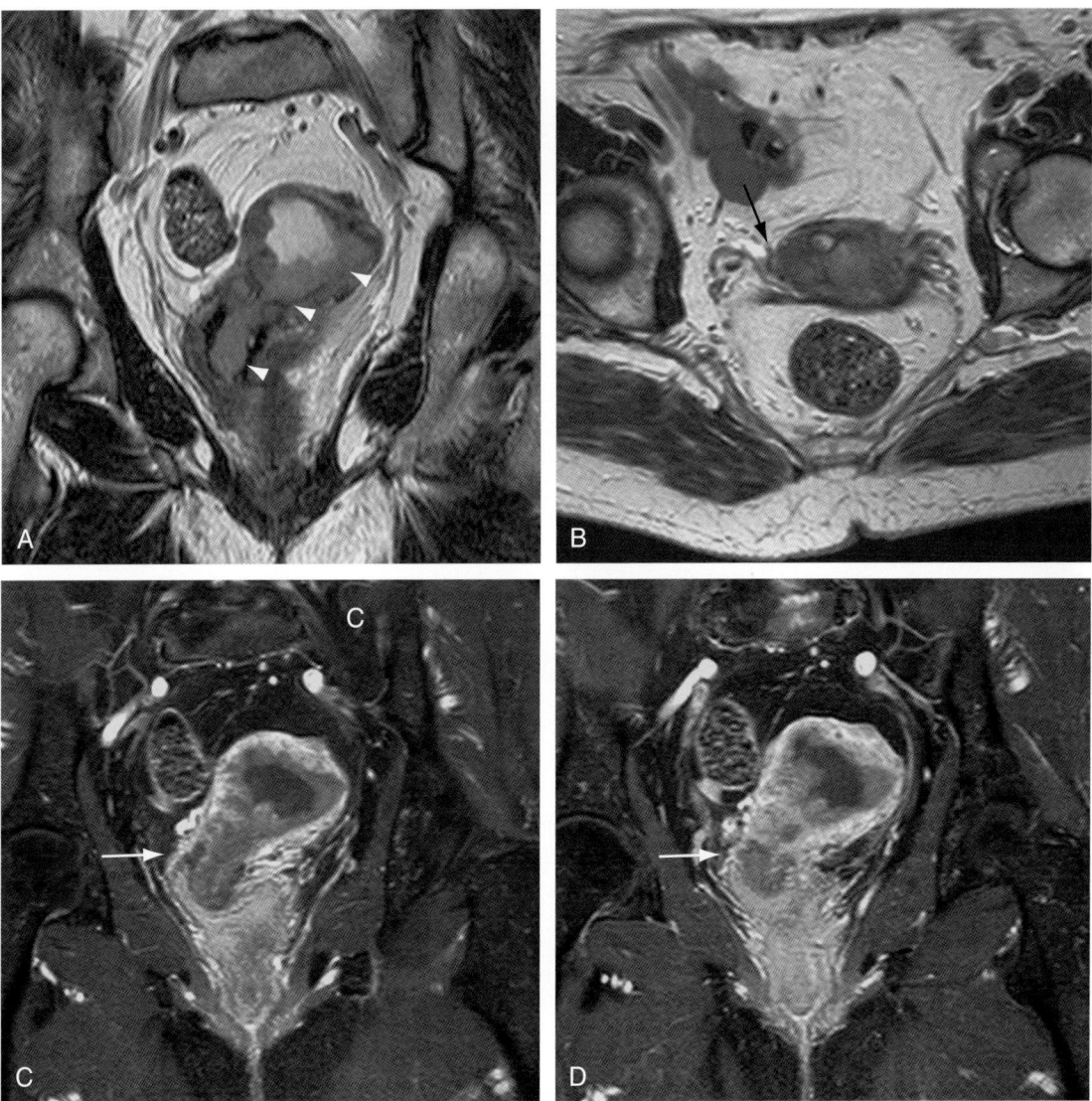

FIGURE 91-4

High-grade adenocarcinoma of the uterus with deep stromal invasion of the cervix. **A,** Oblique coronal T2-weighted image of the uterus shows an isointense endometrial mass extending into the cervical channel and associated with deep myometrial invasion (*arrowheads*). Although most of the hypointense stromal ring is visible, irregularity of the stroma suggests deep stromal invasion. **B,** Oblique axial T2-weighted images confirm interruption of the cervical stroma particularly with suspicion of parametrial invasion at the right side (*arrow*). **C** and **D,** Contiguous delayed fat-suppressed contrast-enhanced T1-weighted images at 4 minutes show tumor extension of the cervical stroma without crossing the outer stromal edge indicating absent parametrial invasion (*arrows*).

a gadolinium-enhanced dynamic study seems to be able to differentiate uterine sarcoma from endometrial carcinoma, the purpose of MRI is not lesion diagnosis but to assess the extent of local tumor invasion. The enhancement characteristics of uterine sarcoma may lead to understaging, because the enhancement may be similar to that of normal myometrium. Careful comparison with T2-weighted images demonstrating a heterogeneous hyperintense myometrial signal may help avoid this pitfall. Most malignant mixed meso-

dermal tumors are identified at advanced stages with invasion of adjacent vessels, pelvic sidewall, or adjacent pelvic organs. Computed tomography of the chest is useful to exclude lung metastasis.

Leiomyosarcoma of the uterus occurs in premenopausal woman with or without preexisting leiomyomas. To date, there have been no imaging characteristics to differentiate leiomyoma from leiomyosarcoma except for increased speed of growth and pelvic sidewall invasion by leiomyosarcoma.

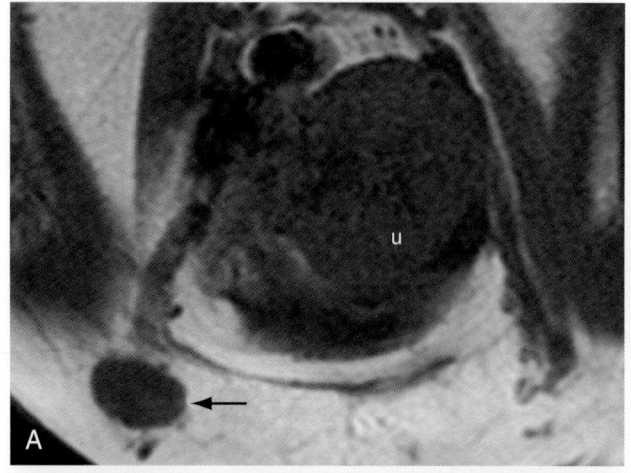

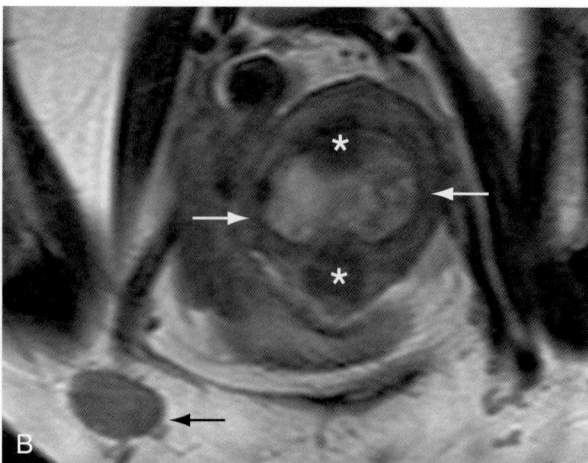

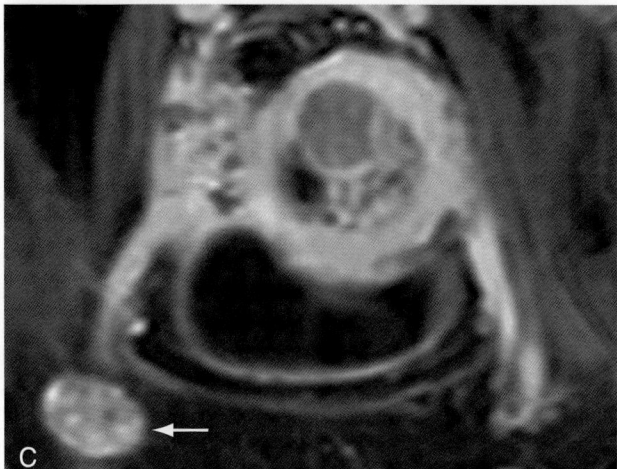

FIGURE 91-5

Stage IV endometrial adenocarcinoma. **A,** Oblique axial T1-weighted image demonstrates an enlarged uterus (u) and an enlarged right inguinal lymph node *(arrow)*. **B,** T2-weighted image shows heterogeneous endometrial thickening *(arrows)*. Two fibroids are also seen *(asterisks)* **C,** Delayed gadolinium-enhanced fat-suppressed T1-weighted image shows enhancement of the endometrium and inguinal lymph node *(arrow)*.

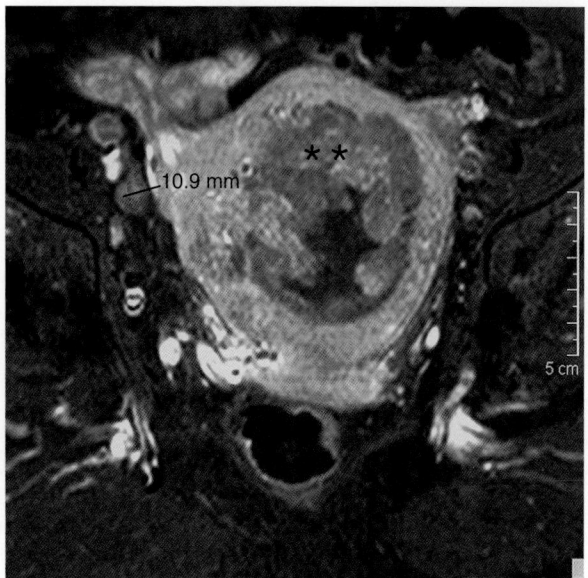

FIGURE 91-6

Adenocarcinoma of the endometrium with deep myometrial invasion and fibroids. Axial fat-suppressed contrast-enhanced T1-weighted image shows an irregular hypoenhancing endometrial mass (**) and an enlarged external iliac lymph node. Subsequent pelvic lymphadenectomy showed absent lymph node invasion and simple lymphatic hyperplasia.

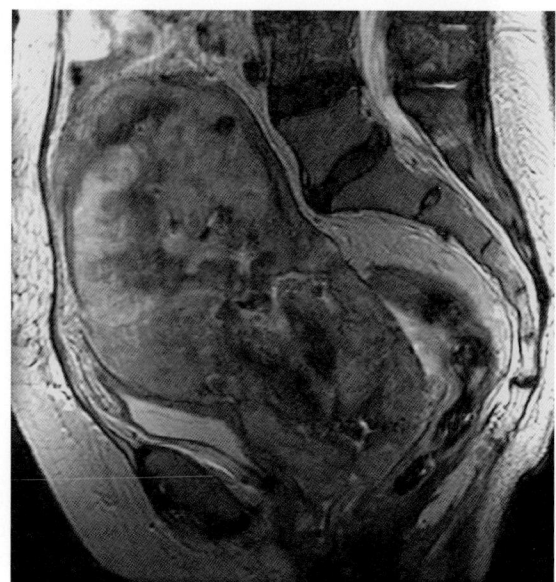

FIGURE 91-7

Endometrial sarcoma of a post-menopausal woman with a pelvic mass. Sagittal T2-weighted image of the uterus demonstrates heterogeneous signal intensity of both the endometrium and myometrium, which are indistinct. *(Courtesy of Dr Corinne Balleyguier, Institut Gustave Roussy, Villejuif, France.)*

CERVICAL CARCINOMA

Early detection of invasive cervical carcinoma with Papanicolaou (Pap) smears led to a significant decrease in mortality and frequency of this tumor during the second half of the last century. The majority of all cervical carcinomas are squamous-cell carcinomas; other tumor types such as adenocarcinomas and adenosquamous carcinomas have increased proportionly during the last 20 years,[30] and now comprise up to one third of cervical carcinomas. Adenocarcinoma of the cervix tends to be located between the external and internal os of the cervical channel rather than at the level of the external os, the typical location of squamous-cell carcinomas. Cervical carcinoma is staged clinically according to the FIGO staging system (Box 91-2) using findings from bimanual pelvic examinations, chest radiography, and intravenous pyelography. In stage IB disease greater than 2 cm or higher stages, MRI has progressively replaced the use of barium enema, cystoscopy, and proctoscopy due to higher cost-effectiveness and better prediction of tumor response, tumor local control, and disease-free survival than FIGO staging alone.[31-34]

Treatment planning for high-stage cervical cancer has evolved during the last 4 years due to greater disease-free survival with combined chemoradiation therapy than with radiation therapy alone.[35] The place of subsequent surgery remains controversial after complete response to chemoradiation. Surgical treatment options in patients with small cervical cancers vary according to tumor stage and size from conization (FIGO stage 0) to simple hysterectomy to radical hysterectomy and possible lymphadenectomy. Stages IB and IIA can be treated with either radical hysterectomy or radiation therapy, depending upon the patient's health and preference.[36] Intracavitary brachytherapy is used as an adjunct to surgery in patients with tumors larger than 2 cm. In patients who desire conserving fertility, trachelectomy and lymphadenectomy is performed for invasive tumors smaller than 2 cm and without parametrial and vaginal extension.[37] In this context, MRI has been shown to be an accurate tool to assess the relationship of the tumor to the internal os and to predict feasibility of the fertility conservative approach.[38]

MRI is the preferred imaging modality for staging cervical cancer. To allow an adequate treatment decision, MRI assesses tumor size, extension to the parametrium, vagina, pelvic sidewall, bladder wall, and rectal wall, as well as lymph node involvement. To reduce respiratory and bowel movement artifacts, technical MRI recommendations include the use of anterior presaturation bands and intramuscular injection of intestinal movement inhibitors, such as glucagon or other antispasmodic agents if not contraindicated. At least axially and sagittally oriented T2-weighted FSE sequences are performed from the symphysis pubis to the renal hilum. The axial orientation for parametrial invasion is oriented perpendicular to the long axis of the cervical canal. High spatial resolution images (512 matrix) of 3-mm axial sections may help differentiate the signal intensity of the tumor from surrounding cervical stroma. The signal intensity of the tumor is usually iso- or hyperintense on T2-weighted images (Fig. 91-8); a visible cervical tumor corresponds to at least stage IB. Dynamic contrast-enhanced T1-weighted images, obtained 30 to 60 seconds after intravenous contrast injection, are useful if the tumor is not identified on T2- or unenhanced T1-weighted images and shows increased early contrast enhancement relative to the cervical stroma. Contrast-enhanced T1-weighted images are necessary to identify bladder or rectal wall invasion or fistulas, and to differentiate fibrosis from tumor recurrence.[39-41] Some have found endocavitary coils to have a higher performance in the diagnosis of parametrial invasion than a body coil[42] or pelvic phased array coil.[43] However, in one study, a pelvic phased array coil did not change the overall staging results in cervical cancer compared with a body coil.[44]

Comparative studies have shown higher staging accuracy of MRI compared with CT for both parametrial invasion (sensitivity of 74% and 55%, respectively) and tumor size assessment. Tumor size measured with MRI demonstrated a correlation coefficient of 0.93 compared with pathological tumor size.[45,46] To diagnose parametrial invasion with MRI, the hypointense cervical stroma serves as an anatomical landmark. Interruption of the stromal ring with tumor bulging into the parametrium is considered the best diagnostic criteria for stage IIB disease (Fig. 91-9). Stage IIA disease with vaginal invasion is implied by the interruption of the hypointense vaginal wall without parametrial invasion (Fig. 91-10). Ureteral obstruction suggests stage III

Box 91-2	FIGO Staging of Cervical Carcinoma

Stage 0   Carcinoma in situ

Stage I   Tumor confined to cervix
  IA   Microinvasion (invasive component <5 mm in depth and <7 mm in horizontal spread)
  IB   Clinically visible or invasive component >5 mm in depth and >7 mm in horizontal spread
    IB1   Tumor size <4 cm
    IB2   Tumor size >4 cm

Stage II   Tumor extends beyond cervix
  IIA   Vaginal invasion not extending to lower third of vagina (no parametrial invasion)
  IIB   Parametrial invasion, but no extension to pelvic sidewall or ureter

Stage III   Tumor extends to lower third of vagina or pelvic sidewall; or ureter obstruction.
  IIIA   Invasion of lower third of vagina (no pelvic sidewall invasion)
  IIIB   Pelvic sidewall extension or ureteral obstruction

Stage IV   Tumor extends outside true pelvis or invades bladder or rectal mucosa
  IVA   Invasion of bladder or rectal mucosa
  IVB   Distant metastases (including para-aortic lymph node invasion)

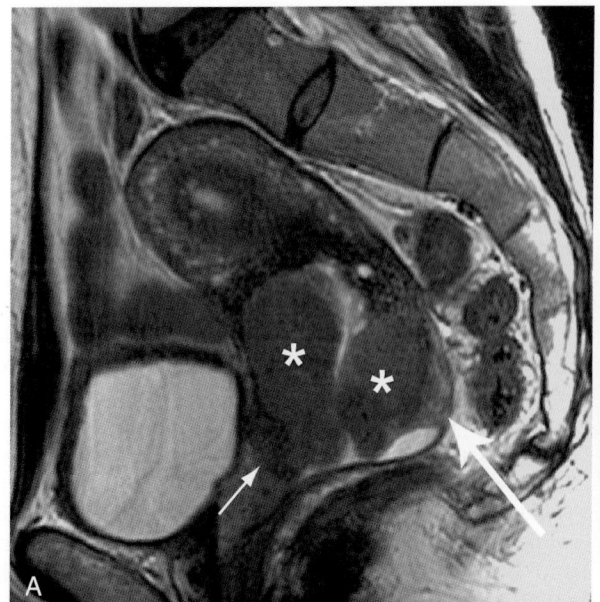

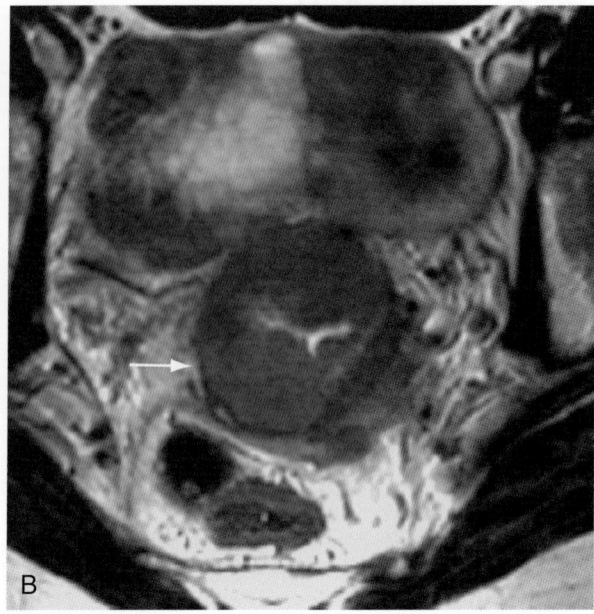

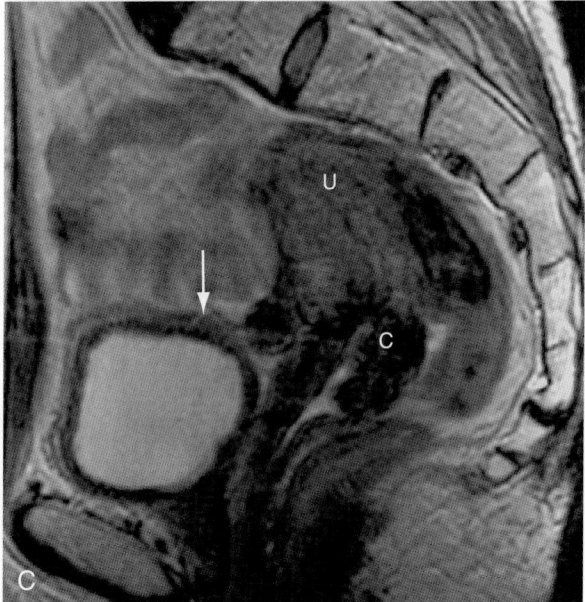

FIGURE 91-8

Adenocarcinoma of the cervix invading the vaginal fornices without parametrial invasion. **A,** Sagittal T2-weighted image of the uterus shows a large endocervical tumor *(asterisks)* with disappearance of the cervical stroma. Tumor size larger than 4 cm suggests at least stage IB2. However, increased signal intensity of the posterior and anterior vaginal fornices *(arrows)* indicates stage IIA. **B,** Axial T2-weighted image demonstrates preservation of the external hypointense cervical stroma *(arrow)* excluding parametrial invasion. **C,** Sagittal T2-weighted image after completion of external radiation therapy, concomitant chemotherapy and complementary brachytherapy shows marked decrease in signal intensity and size of the cervix (c) and uterine body (u) without visibility of any remaining cervical tumor. Thickened bladder wall *(arrow)* and fatty infiltration of the bone marrow correspond to radiation-induced changes of the pelvis. *(Courtesy of Dr Peter Petrow, Geneva University Hospital, Geneva, France.)*

FIGURE 91-9

Squamous carcinoma of the cervix in a 33-year-old patient with bilateral parametrial invasion. Axial T2-weighted image of the cervix shows absence of the hypointense stromal ring indistinct from the cervical tumor bulging into the right parametrium *(thick arrow)*. The left tumor border is irregular *(thin arrows)* suggesting associated left parametrial invasion. *(Courtesy of Dr Peter Petrow, Geneva University Hospital, Geneva, France.)*

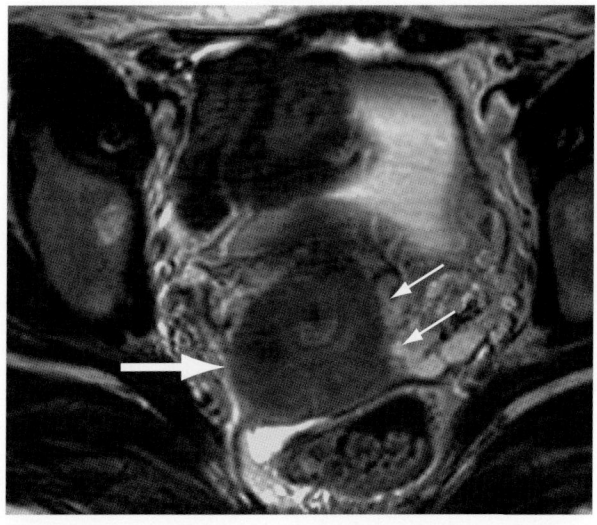

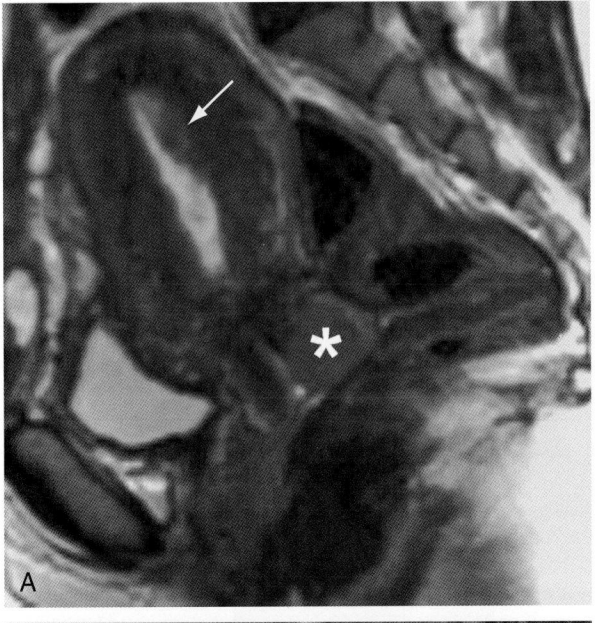
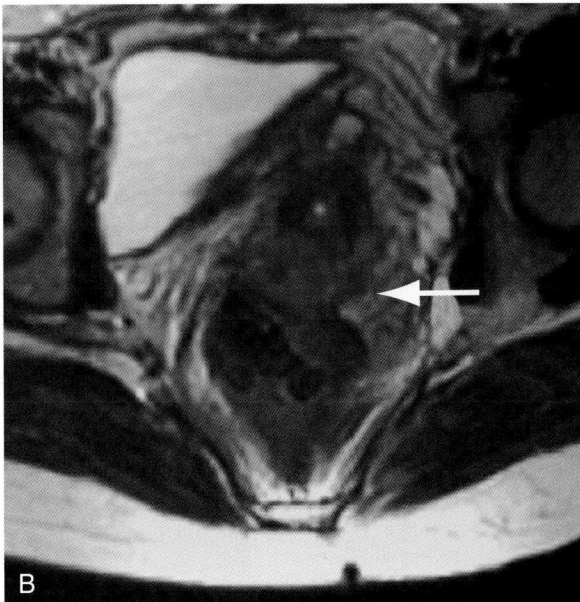
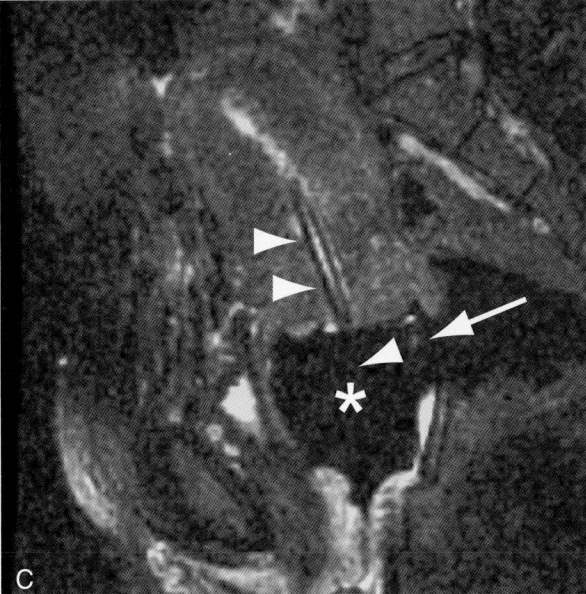

FIGURE 91-10

Squamous carcinoma of the cervix in a 35-year-old patient. **A,** Sagittal T2-weighted image shows the slightly hyperintense tumor of the posterior cervical lip *(asterisk)* with indistinct posterior vaginal fornix. Hypointense signal intensity of the endometrial cavity *(arrow)* corresponded to an associated polyp at hysteroscopy. **B,** Axial T2-weighted image demonstrates interruption of the posterior vaginal wall *(arrow)* indicating stage IIA disease. **C,** Sagittal fat-suppressed T2-weighted image shows a hypointense vaginal applicator *(asterisk)* stretching the vaginal walls. The uterine tube *(arrowheads)* is placed through the applicator into the lower half of the endometrial cavity. The vaginal tumor extension can be seen at the posterior edge of the applicator *(arrow).* *(Courtesy of Dr Peter Petrow, Geneva University Hospital, Geneva, France.)*

disease (Fig. 91-11). After radiochemotherapy, false-positive results of parametrial or vaginal invasion might occur due to similar signal intensities of cervical tumor and surrounding edema or inflammation on T2-weighted images.[47] The role of contrast-enhanced MRI after radiochemotherapy has not yet been assessed.

For bladder invasion, the interruption of the hypointense wall with MRI demonstrated higher sensitivity (75%) and specificity (91%) than CT, but performance was similar for rectal invasion.[46] Contrast-enhanced MRI appeared superior in accuracy (90%) to T2-weighted sequences (69%) for bladder or rectal wall invasion.[39,48]

The assessment of lymph node involvement with receiver operator characteristic analysis showed no significant differences in the overall performance of CT and MRI using a 10 mm small axis cut-off point.[14] One of the major limitations of both cross-sectional imaging methods in detecting lymph node metastasis is the low sensitivity of 60% (95% CI: 52% to 68%) for MRI and 43% (95% CI: 37 to 57%) for CT.[46] Therefore, Bayesian analysis of clinical utility showed only moderate increases in positive post-test probability of lymph node metastasis for all methods.[14] Negative test results had a greater impact and decreased the probability of lymph node metastasis in stage I-IIA from 18.6% to 6% and in stage IIB from 44% to 15%.[14] With a 6% risk of lymph node invasion in patients staged I-IIA and negative lymph node MRI evaluation, lymphadenectomy may not be appropriate considering the risk of retroperitoneal fibrosis and lymphocele formation due to this surgical procedure. Sentinel lymph node mapping, an important development in the surgical management of solid

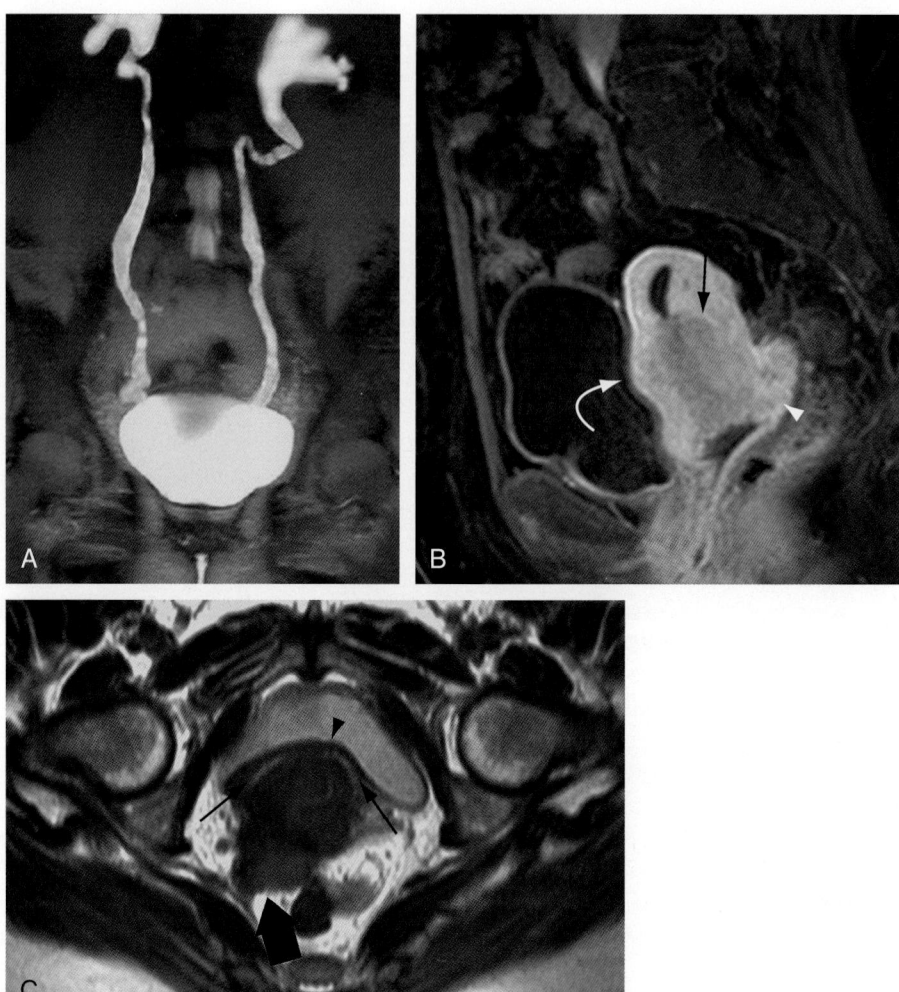

FIGURE 91-11

Stage IIIB cervical carcinoma. **A,** Coronal HASTE maximum-intensity projection shows bilateral hydronephroureter. **B,** Sagittal delayed post-gadolinium fat-suppressed T1-weighted image shows a large hypo-enhancing cervical mass *(arrow)* that protrudes anteriorly, deforming the bladder *(curved arrow)* and posteriorly to involve the vaginal fornix *(arrowhead)*. **C,** Axial T2-weighted image demonstrates parametrial invasion *(thick arrow)* with an intact bladder wall *(arrowhead)* and fat plane *(thin arrows)* suggesting that, although both distal ureters are involved, the bladder is not involved. Bladder involvement would indicate stage IV disease.

tumors, is expected to improve lymph node management in gynecological tumors.[49]

Moreover, T2-weighted and dynamic contrast-enhanced T1-weighted images may have prognostic importance. Mayr et al[50] demonstrated that the percentage of tumor volume regression estimated on T2-weighted images correctly predicted disease-free survival after 40 to 50 Gy of radiation therapy; in patients demonstrating less than 20% of initial tumor volume after 1 month of radiation therapy, the 2-year disease-free survival was 88% versus 45% for patients with more than 20% initial tumor volume.[50] In patients with intermediate tumor volumes, of 40 to 99 cm³, the combined analysis of tumor volume and dynamic enhancement pattern over 120 seconds better predicted local recurrence than volume analysis or dynamic enhancement pattern analysis alone.[51] Low tumor vascularity assessed with pixel analysis of dynamic contrast-enhanced MRI appeared to correlate with a higher incidence of local recurrence in patients treated with radiation therapy alone.[52] The reduced tumor radiosensitivity in patients with decreased tumor microcirculation may be an important factor in deciding between surgery and radiochemotherapy.

In conclusion, MRI of the pelvis is a valuable tool in planning treatment and assessing response to radiochemotherapy in patients with cervical cancer. Treatment trends towards the increased used of combined radiochemotherapy should prompt the development of simple methods of contrast-enhanced MRI to predict treatment response.

ADNEXAL MASSES

Ultrasonography is accepted as the primary imaging modality in the diagnosis of an ovarian mass. The use of US in the detection of a suspected ovarian mass, and in its differentiation from a uterine mass, has been well established. Because US depicts the mass, characterization of the mass is typically performed during the same examination. Thus, de facto, sonography becomes the main triage method prior to treatment.

The majority of ovarian masses are functional cysts. However, when a lesion is suspected of being a neoplasm, surgical intervention must be considered. In most institutions, the type of surgery performed (laparoscopy versus laparotomy) depends on the probability of malignancy. The risk of malignancy depends on the patient's pre- or post-menopausal status. The prevalence of malignancy in surgically removed ovarian masses varies from 7% to 16% in premenopausal women and from 22% to 45% in post-menopausal women.[53-56] For this reason, surgical removal of a suspected ovarian neoplasm is the standard procedure. Because the treatment of ovarian cancer differs considerably from the treatment of a benign ovarian mass, the gynecologist tries to increase the diagnostic confidence of the malignant nature of the mass to allow optimal scheduling of surgical intervention and prior consultation with an oncologist. The purpose of secondary imaging after an initial, indeterminate sonographic result is, therefore, to confirm the indeterminate nature of the mass and to assess the extent of possible malignant disease. Because a combination of sonographic techniques performs better than gray scale (conventional) sonographic assessment alone,[57] the gynecologist most often sends the patient to a specialist in gynecological sonography trained in both conventional and color Doppler imaging. A large prospective study comparing the value of Doppler sonography, CT, and MRI in ovarian lesion characterization and staging demonstrated MRI to have greater accuracy than CT or Doppler sonography in lesion characterization and found no difference in staging performance.[58]

Ovarian tumors are classified according to the origin of the tumor cell, deriving from the surface epithelium (75%, serous, mucinous, endometrioid, and clear cell tumors), germ cells (15%, benign teratoma, dysgerminoma, endodermal sinus tumor, immature teratoma), ovarian stroma or sex cord cells (10%, granulosa and thecal cell tumors) or metastatic cells (5%, most common primary tumors are gastrointestinal, breast, other pelvic cancers, or lymphoma). Serous and mucinous tumor of the ovary can be benign, malignant, or borderline (without invasion); the latter are usually treated as malignant ovarian tumors.

To characterize an adnexal mass, MRI uses primary findings predictive of malignancy, such as papillary projections or solid components in a cystic lesion, necrosis in a solid lesion, and wall or septa thicker than 3 mm. In addition to these primary criteria, the presence of the ancillary findings of ascites or peritoneal metastasis further increases the likelihood of malignancy. A multivariate analysis demonstrated highest odds ratios for malignancy for the following criteria: ascites or peritoneal metastasis (odds ratio 168), necrosis in a solid lesion (odds ratio 107) and vegetation in a cystic lesion (odds ratio 40).[59] Contrast-enhanced T1-weighted sequences better allow identification of solid portions in cystic lesions or necrosis in solid lesions than does non-enhanced MRI, and they are mandatory for the diagnosis of ovarian cancer[59] (Fig. 91-12). A common pitfall of ovarian lesion characterization is the presence of solid portions identified in a cystic teratoma, a benign neoplasm containing fat. Therefore, native T1-weighted non-enhanced sequences with and without fat suppression are important to identify this benign lesion[60] (Fig. 91-13). The diagnosis of specific benign ovarian

tumor types helps to confirm the benign nature of an ovarian mass.[61] Ovarian fibroma, another benign solid lesion type, demonstrates well-defined borders and low signal intensity on both T1- and T2-weighted images.[62] However, the T2-weighted signal intensity of ovarian fibromas increases with the degree of myxomatous change[63] (Fig. 91-14). The diagnosis of endometrioma, frequently suspected in patients with infertility and chronic pain, can be confirmed on MRI due to high signal intensity within the ovarian cyst on fat-suppressed T1-weighted sequences associated with shadowing on T2-weighted sequences[61,64] (Fig. 91-15). T2-hypointense nodules located at the uterosacral ligaments, the posterior portion of the cervix, the vaginal fornices or the rectal wall indicate associated posterior pelvic endometriosis.[65] T2- and T1-hyperintense spots within these nodules correspond to recent blood products. Bladder endometriosis exhibits posterior-wall thickening and has the same predominantly hypointense signal on T2-weighted images as seen in posterior endometriosis.

Mucinous cystadenoma is a common source of false-positive diagnosis of ovarian cancer on US.[57] It is frequently a multilocular tumor with multiple cysts filled with mucin separated by highly vascular septa. On MRI, mucinous cystadenoma demonstrates different signal intensities in each locule[66] (Fig. 91-16). Serous cystadenomas are more typically unilocular. The differentiation of a benign mucinous or serous adenoma from a malignant cystadenocarcinoma on MRI relies on the identification of a thickened septum/wall or the presence of a solid component within the predominantly cystic mass (Fig. 91-17). The specific diagnosis of borderline tumors cannot be made with MRI, but requires a careful histopathologic examination of the specimen. However, a study including 14 borderline tumors reported MRI findings of malignancy in all borderline tumors.[67] Endometrioid carcinoma presents as predominantly solid lesions with necrosis and is often bilateral (25%) or associated with a second primary cancer or hyperplasia of the endometrium (33%). Clear cell cancers are less common. They are invasive, but they typically present with local rather than widely metastatic disease. They are usually unilocular with mural nodules (Fig. 91-18). The malignant germ cell tumors are more common in younger patients and often exhibit rapid growth (Fig. 91-19). Tumors of sex cell stromal origin are most commonly of the granulosa cell type. These tumors are typically solid, with areas of cystic change and hemorrhage (Fig. 91-20). Other primary malignant tumors of the ovary are more rare, but primary ovarian lymphoma and various types of sarcomas have been reported (Fig. 91-21).

False-negative results for the diagnosis of ovarian cancer on MRI can occur for lesions smaller than 2 cm but account for less than 5% of ovarian cancers.[59,68] In addition to imaging techniques, assessment of serum level of cancer antigen 125 (CA-125) is also used for the diagnosis of malignant epithelial ovarian neoplasm. The sensitivity in diagnosing primary epithelial ovarian cancer with increased CA-125 levels is low and depends on tumor stage (50% in stage I disease).[69] False-positive results can occur in patients with endometriosis, uterine

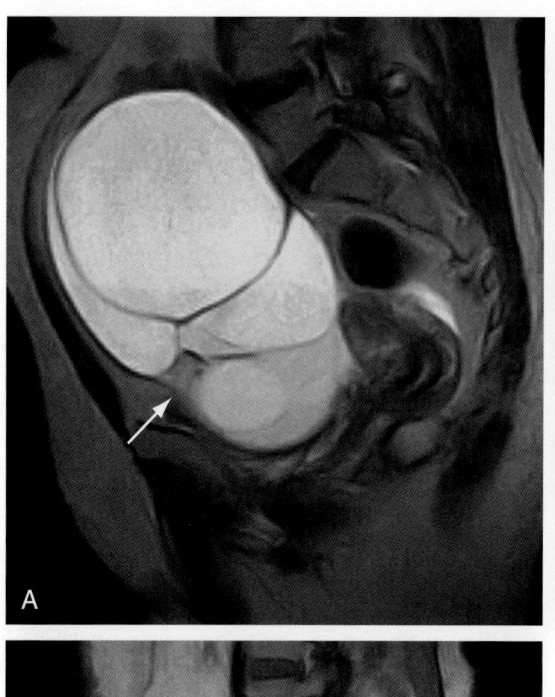

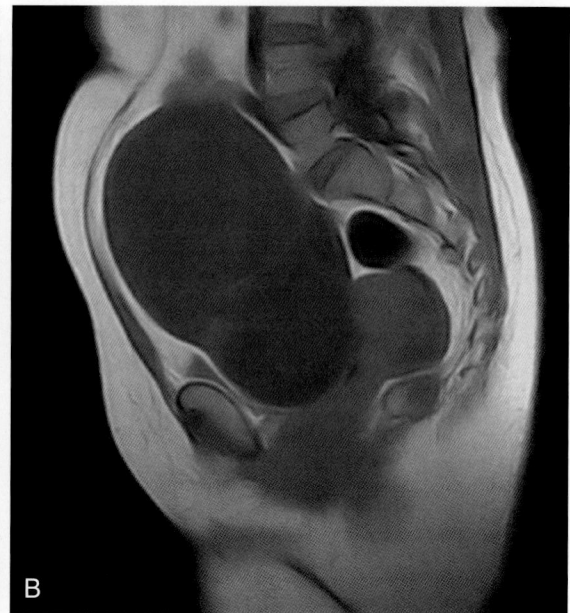

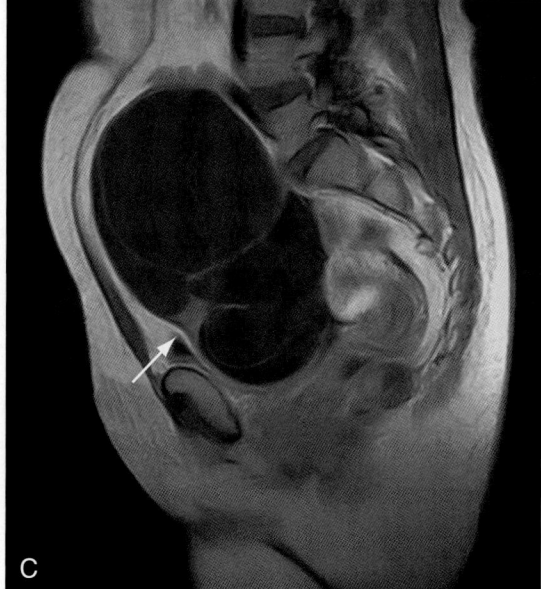

FIGURE 91-12

A 56-year old woman with abdominal swelling and a suspicious mass at sonography. **A,** Sagittal T2-weighted image at 0.23 T demonstrates a multilocular cyst with anterior wall thickening *(arrow)*. **B,** Native sagittal T1-weighted image in the same section as **A** shows the predominantly cystic mass. **C,** After intravenous contrast injection of gadolinium complex, the anterior solid portion enhances *(arrow)* and confirms the suspicion of cancer. Mucinous cystadenocarcinoma was identified at pathology of the specimen.

fibroids, pregnancy, and pelvic inflammatory disease. However, an increasing CA-125 value after completion of surgery indicates possible recurrence and is helpful in the follow-up evaluation of treated patients.[69]

Once the diagnosis of ovarian cancer is suspected at imaging, subsequent staging of the abdomen and pelvis with MRI can help evaluate the feasibility of complete tumor resection. Indeed, ovarian cancer mainly spreads through exfoliation of cells into the peritoneal cavity and may implant anywhere in the peritoneum, such as the pouch of Douglas, subdiaphragmatic regions, paracolic gutters, the omentum (also called "omental cake"), or the mesentery. Tumor locations on the gastrosplenic ligament, gastrohepatic ligament, portal hilus, posterior right subdiaphragmatic region, or the mesentery are considered specific sites that may be unresectable and benefit from chemotherapy prior to debulking surgery. Lymphadenopathy can occur up to the renal hilum due to direct lymphatic spread from the ovaries to the retroperitoneal space. MRI and CT are equivalent techniques in staging ovarian cancer for peritoneal disease and lymphadenopathy.[70] Contrast-enhanced T1-weighted breath-hold fat-suppressed SGE techniques have been shown to demonstrate peritoneal disease better than unenhanced spin-echo techniques.[71] However, peritoneal lesions smaller than 1 cm are often not depicted on MRI. The sensitivity for peritoneal disease in a pelvic location was higher (73% to 83%) than for locations at the greater omentum (38%), or pelvic lymph nodes (28%).[72] Complete staging of ovarian carcinoma is performed at

Text continues on page 2983

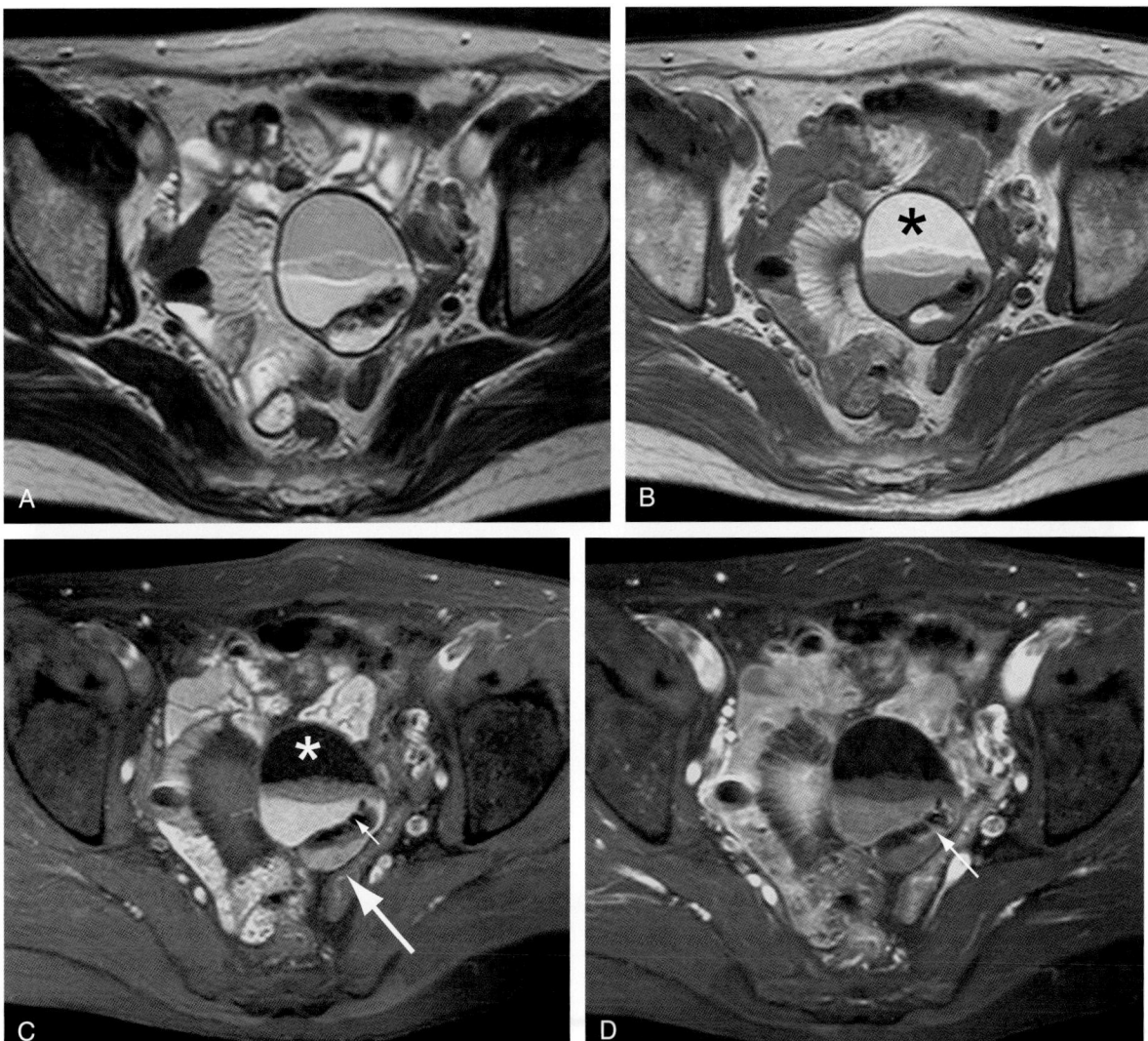

FIGURE 91-13

A 32-year-old woman with an indeterminate mass at sonography. **A,** Axial T2-weighted image shows a heterogeneous mass with multiple layers and posterior wall thickening. **B,** Axial T1-weighted image shows a hyperintense upper layer *(asterisk)* possibly corresponding to blood or fat. **C,** Axial T1-weighted fat-suppressed image of the mass *(thick arrow)* at the same level as **B** proves the fatty content of the upper portion of the lesion *(asterisk)* and the posterior wall thickening *(thin arrow)*, both highly suggestive of mature cystic teratoma of the ovary. **D,** In an axial contrast-enhanced T1-weighted image, enhancement of the posterior portion of the lesion *(arrow)* corresponds to the Rokitansky nodule of the teratoma and should not be mistaken for a vegetation of ovarian cancer. Subsequent surgery confirmed mature cystic teratoma (dermoid cyst).

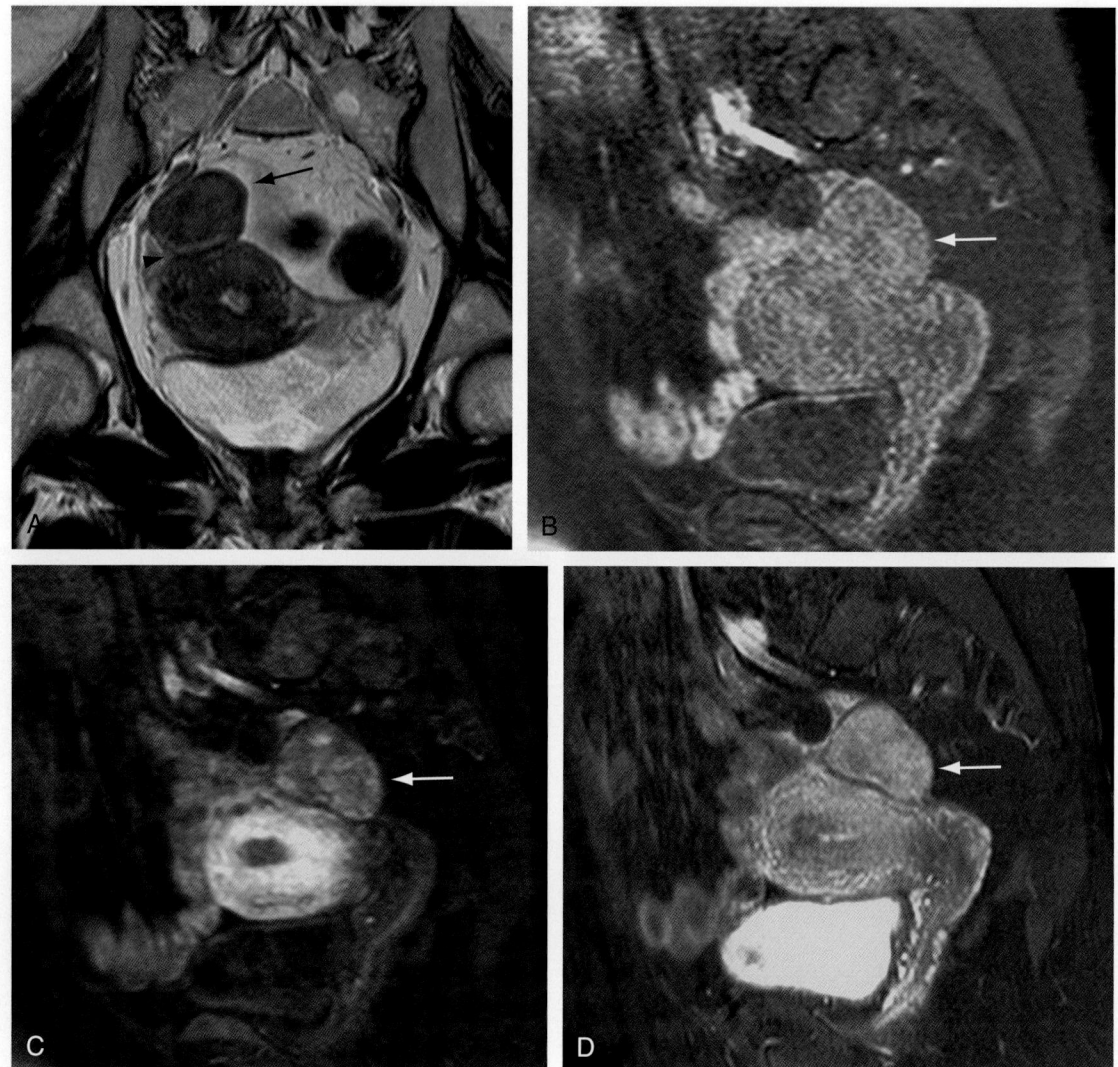

FIGURE 91-14

A patient with low-grade adenocarcinoma of the uterus demonstrates a solid right adnexal mass that could be of ovarian or uterine origin (patient presented in Fig. 91-2). **A,** Coronal T2-weighted image demonstrates a well-circumscribed mass *(arrow)* isointense to the myometrium with a hypointense interface *(arrowhead)* and no visible myometrial stalk excluding the hypothesis of a pedunculated subserosal fibroid. **B,** Native fat-suppressed sagittal T1-weighted image shows a mass *(arrow)* T1-homogeneous and isointense to the myometrium. **C,** Early contrast-enhanced T1-weighted dynamic fat-suppressed sagittal image at 1 minute shows intense contrast uptake by the normal myometrium and less enhancement of the upper solid adnexal mass *(arrow)* corresponding to ovarian fibroma at surgery. **D,** Delayed contrast-enhanced fat-suppressed image shows similar delayed uptake by both normal myometrium and the ovarian fibroma *(arrow)*. The possibility of an ovarian metastasis from endometrial adenocarcinoma has a lower probability due to unilaterality and the homogeneous content of the adnexal mass.

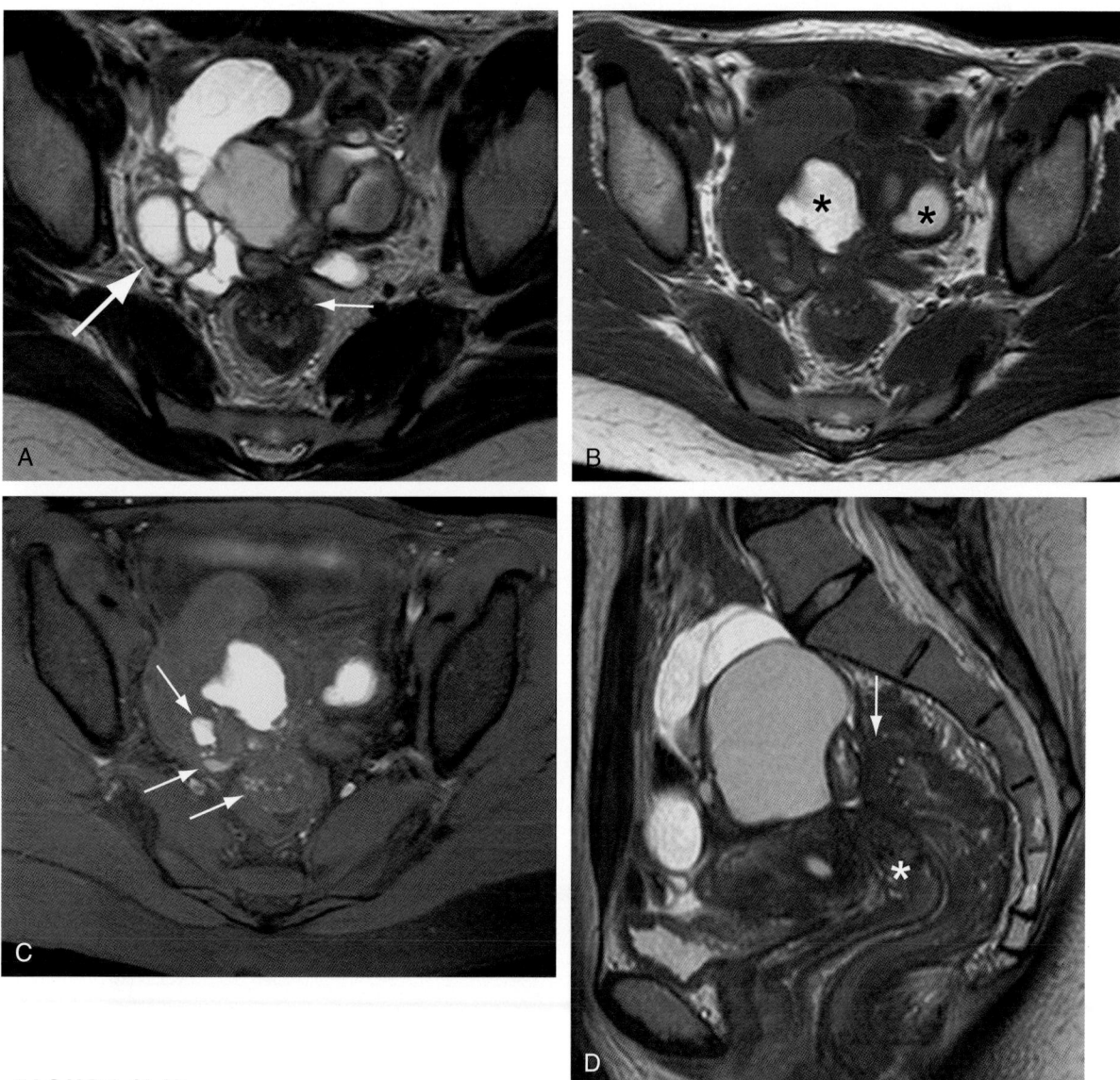

FIGURE 91-15

A 41-year-old woman with chronic pelvic pain and a suspicious multicystic pelvic mass at sonography. **A,** Axial T2-weighted image shows a complex cystic mass associated with normal hyperintense follicles at the right posterior *(thick arrow)* and anterior left side suggesting a bilateral adnexal origin. Shadowing of the left part of the cyst suggests blood products. The anterior rectal wall is abnormally thickened and contains hyperintense spots *(thin arrow)*. **B,** Axial T1-weighted image at the same level as **A** shows hyperintense portions *(asterisks)*. **C,** Fat-suppressed T1-weighted image shows that the hyperintense areas seen in **B** persist, confirming the suspicion of bilateral endometrioma. Multiple smaller high intensity foci are better seen with fat suppression *(arrows)*. **D,** Sagittal T2-weighted image confirms abnormal thickening of the anterior rectal wall posterior to the ovary *(arrow)* and a hypointense nodule in the pouch of Douglas posterior to the cervix *(asterisk)*. Subsequent laparotomy with bilateral oophorectomy and anterior rectal resection confirmed bilateral endometriomas (8 cm rectal and 2 cm peritoneal endometriosis of the pouch of Douglas), associated with functional ovarian cysts.

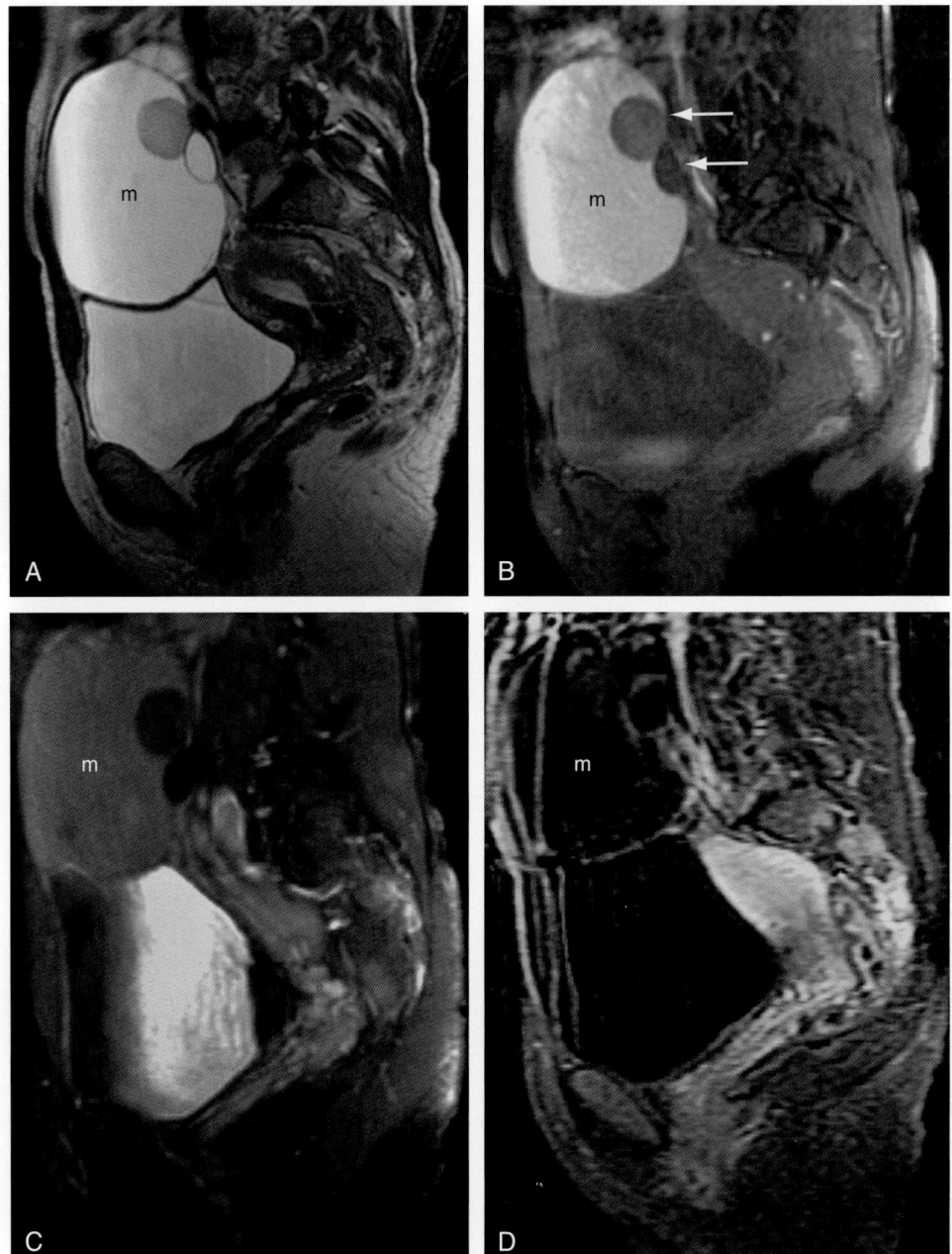

FIGURE 91-16

A 55-year-old woman with a suspicious abdominal mass. **A,** Sagittal T2-weighted image shows a multilocular mass (m) above the normal uterus with different signal intensity in each loculus. **B,** Sagittal fat-suppressed image shows a slightly hyperintense anterior part and two posterior loculi of lower signal intensity *(arrows)*. **C,** After contrast injection, the absence of enhancement of each loculus is difficult to confirm on the standard fat-suppressed T1-weighted image. **D,** Subtraction of image **B** from image **C** provides a subtracted image and confirms the absence of enhancement within the hyperintense loculus except for a thin anterior septation and enhancement of the normal ovarian parenchyma at the upper uterine interface. Benign mucinous cystadenoma was confirmed at pathology. *(Courtesy of Dr Corinne Balleyguier, Institut Gustave Roussy, Villejuif, France.)*

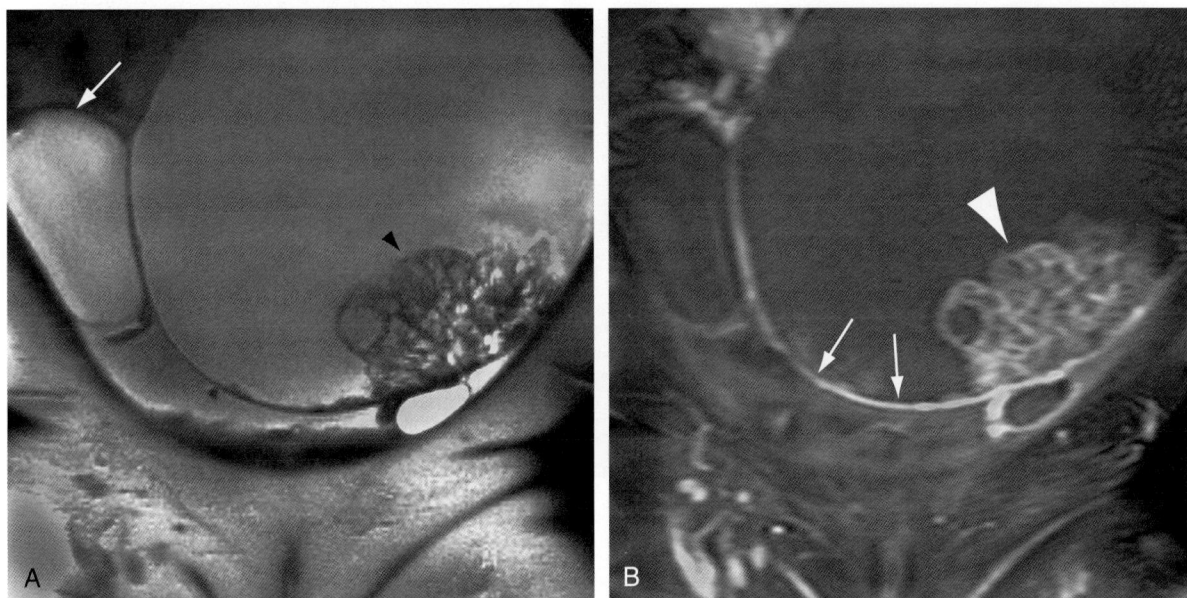

FIGURE 91-17

Serous cyst adenocarcinoma of the ovary. **A,** Coronal T2-weighted image shows a large right ovarian cystic mass with mural vegetation *(arrowhead)* and a smaller left ovarian cystic mass *(arrow)*. **B,** Post-gadolinium fat-suppressed T1-weighted image shows enhancement of the mural projection *(arrowhead)* and the cyst wall *(arrows)*.

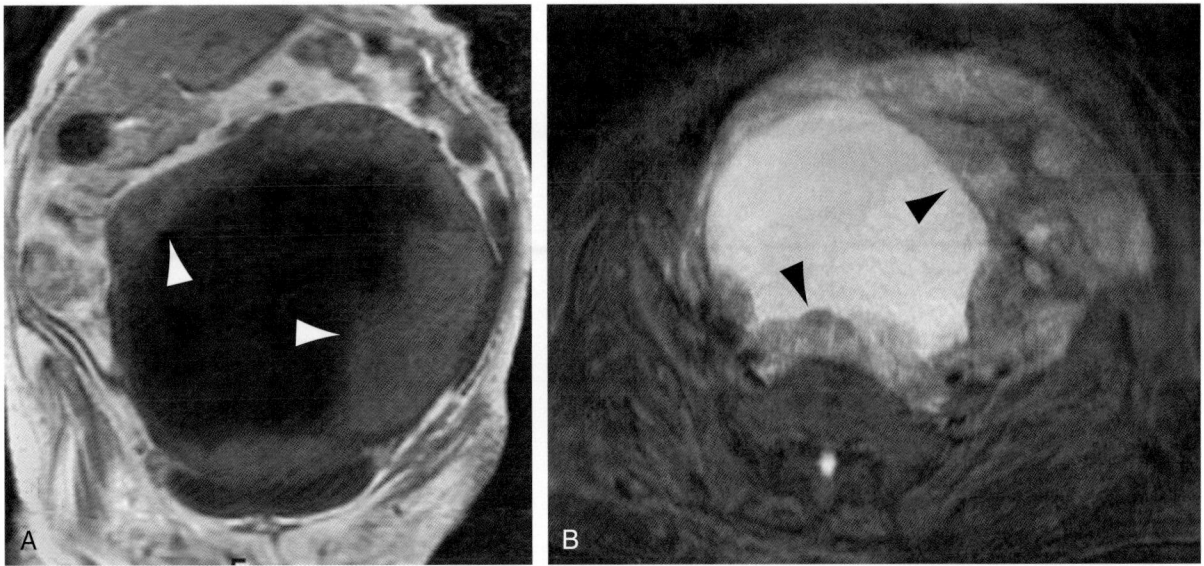

FIGURE 91-18

Clear cell carcinoma of the ovary. **A,** Coronal T1-weighted image shows a large mass arising from the pelvis with central cystic region and a thick irregular wall of intermediate signal *(arrowheads)*. **B,** Axial fat-suppressed T2-weighted image shows heterogenous signal within the soft-tissue component *(arrowheads)*.

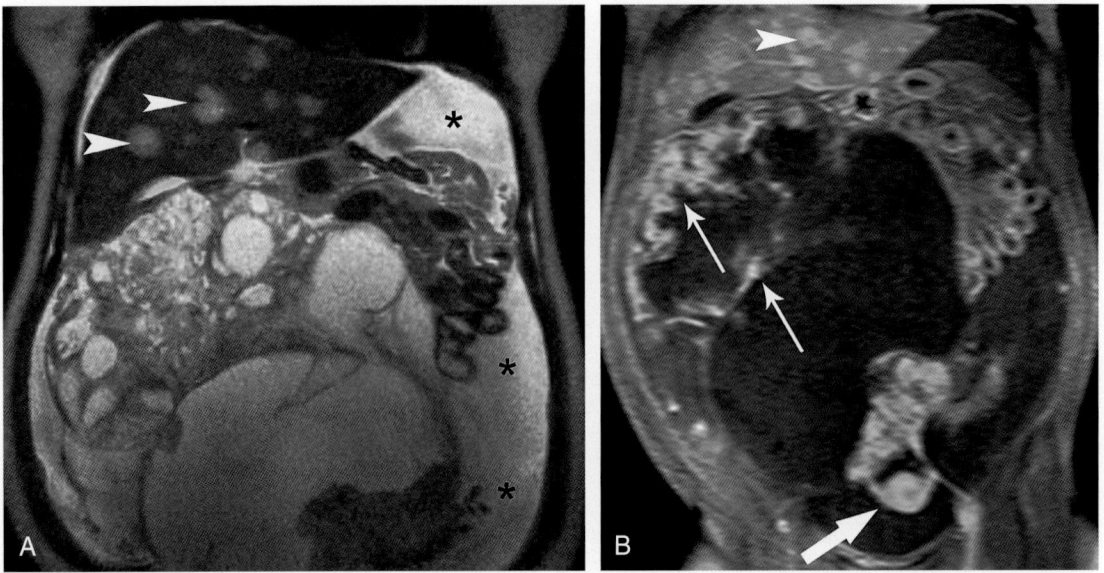

FIGURE 91-19

Endodermal sinus tumor. **A,** Coronal T2-weighted image shows a large heterogeneous ovarian mass with cystic and solid components arising in a 29-year-old woman. Ascites *(asterisks)* is present as well as liver metastases *(arrowheads)*. **B,** Post-gadolinium fat-suppressed T1-weighted image shows enhancement of the solid components *(thin arrows)* and the liver lesions *(arrowhead)*. The normal uterus is also seen *(thick arrow)*.

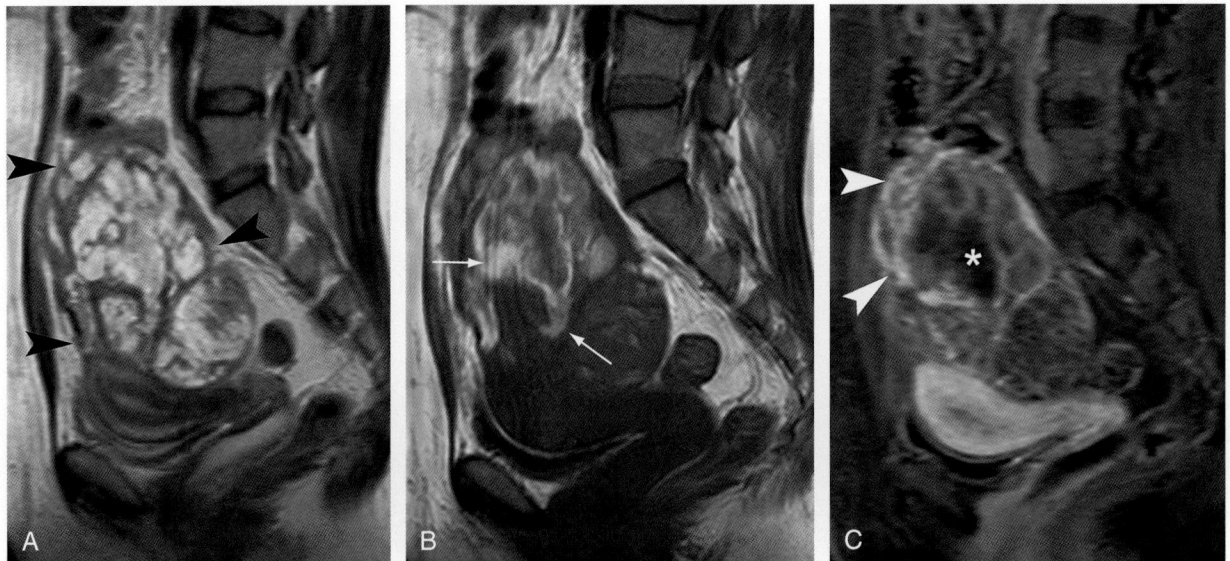

FIGURE 91-20

Granulosa cell tumor. **A,** Sagittal T2-weighted image shows a large heterogeneous mass *(arrowheads)*. **B,** T1-weighted image shows a high-intensity signal within the lesion *(arrows)* indicating intratumoral hemorrhage. **C,** Post-gadolinium fat-suppressed T1-weigthed image shows heterogeneous enhancement *(arrowheads)* with areas of nonenhancing hemorrhage and necrosis *(asterisk)*.

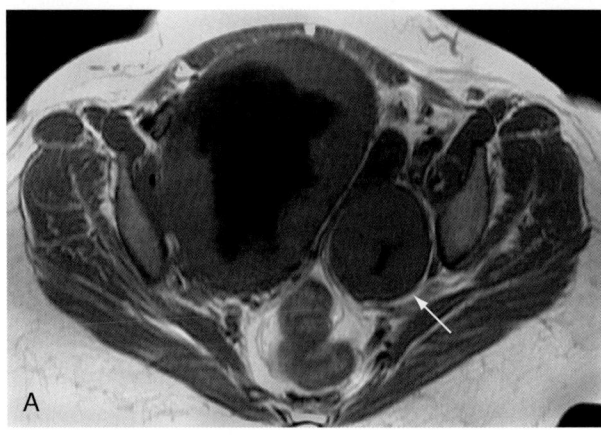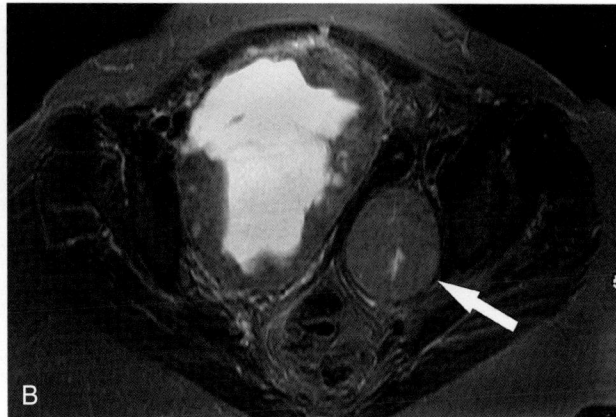

FIGURE 91-21

Ovarian endometrial stromal sarcoma. Axial T1-weighted (**A**) and T2-weighted (**B**) images show a large right ovarian mass with central cystic portion and an irregular soft-tissue rim. There is also a smaller more solid appearing left ovarian mass *(arrows)*.

surgery according to the FIGO guidelines (Box 91-3) and includes total abdominal hysterectomy with bilateral salpingo-oophorectomy, pelvic and para-aortic lymph node sampling, omentectomy, peritoneal washing with cytology, and peritoneal biopsies at various sites. About 75% of ovarian cancers are diagnosed at advances stages (stages III and IV) and have little or no chance of cure. The most important prognostic factors are tumor grade and residual tumor after initial surgery. Patients with residual disease greater than 2 cm are not considered for further surgery. For patients with advanced primary or relapsed ovarian carcinoma, MRI based on contrast-enhanced fat-saturated T1-weighted sequences improves planning of surgical tumor reduction preceding chemotherapy with reported positive and negative predictive values for nonresectable disease of 91% and 97%, respectively.[72,73]

Ovarian metastasis accounts for approximately 5% to 10% of all malignant ovarian neoplasms. Imaging characteristics of secondary compared with primary malignant tumors of the ovary are not different. They most often present as bilateral ovoid solid masses with heterogeneous signal intensities on T2-weighted and at T1-weighted contrast-enhanced images and sharp margins.[74,75] When histologic examination identifies signet ring cells invading an abundant hypercellular ovarian stroma, the metastatic tumor is called Krukenberg's tumor. These tumors can derive from gastrointestinal (90%), breast, or pancreatic primary carcinoma and demonstrate nonspecific imaging features similar to ovarian metastasis without signet ring cells (Fig. 91-22). Low signal intensity on T2-weighted images has been reported to be more suggestive of Krukenberg's tumor than of primary ovarian cancers.[75] Distinction with thecomas, fibrothecomas, or poorly differentiated adenocarcinoma of the ovary might be difficult if the Krukenberg's tumor is unilateral. Ovarian metastases can result from direct extension, peritoneal seeding, or lymphatic or hematogenous spread (Fig. 91-23).

Primary fallopian tube carcinoma is rare, but can be identified during characterization of a suspicious adnexal mass. On MRI, the tumor presents as a lobular or fusiform solid adnexal mass with relatively high signal intensity on T2-weighted images.[76] After contrast injection, the lesion enhances homogeneously. Nearly all patients present with clinical symptoms such as abdominal pain, vaginal bleeding, or discharge. A common reason of missed diagnosis with ultrasound is its similar appearance to uterine leiomyoma because of their adjacent position and fixation to the uterus. Differentiation between leiomyoma and fallopian tube carcinoma is easier on MRI due to the typical low signal intensity or whirled appearance on T2-weighted images. Associated ascites or metastasis to other pelvic organs, peritoneum, or lymph nodes helps to diagnose this rare malignant pelvic neoplasm.

Box 91-3	FIGO Staging of Primary Ovarian Carcinoma

Stage I	Tumor limited to the ovaries
	IA Extension to one ovary
	IB Extension to both ovaries without ascites
	IC Extension to one or both ovaries with ascites or positive peritoneal washing
Stage II	Involvement of the pelvis
	IIA Extension to uterus or fallopian tube
	IIB Extension to other pelvic tissues
Stage III	Tumor with intraperitoneal metastasis outside the pelvis and/or positive retroperitoneal nodes
Stage IV	Distant metastasis or pleural effusion with positive cytology or hepatic metastasis

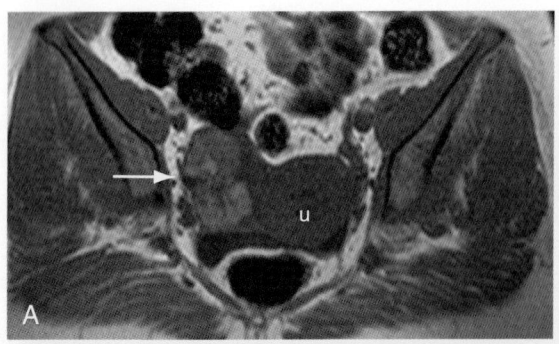

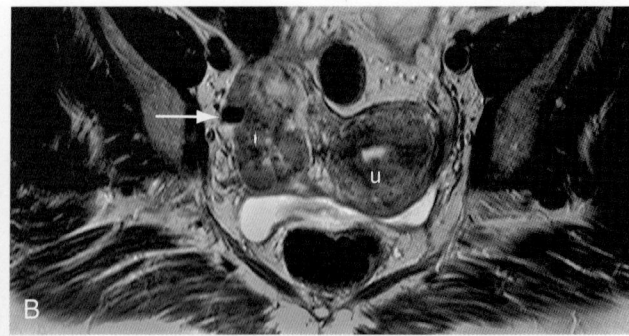

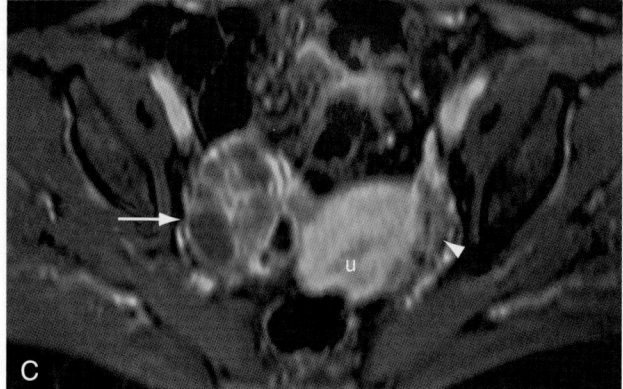

FIGURE 91-22

Krukenberg tumors from colon carcinoma primary. Axial T1-weighted (**A**) T2-weighted (**B**), and post-gadolinium fat-suppressed T1-weighted (**C**) images show a heterogeneous right adnexal mass *(arrow)* adjacent to the uterus (u), which is normal. Post-gadolinium images best demonstrated the smaller left ovarian metastasis *(arrowhead in* **C**).

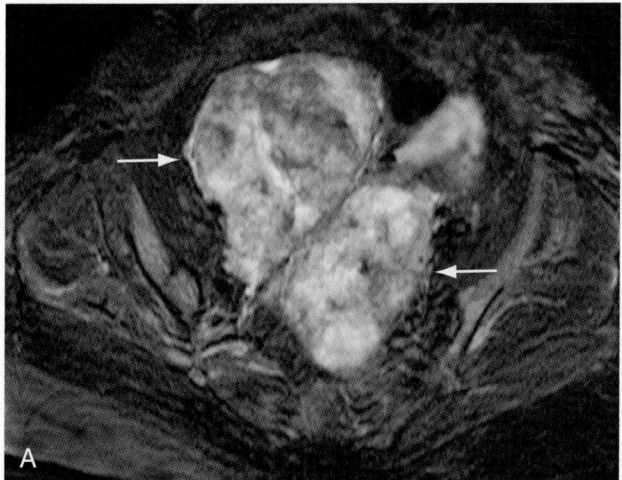

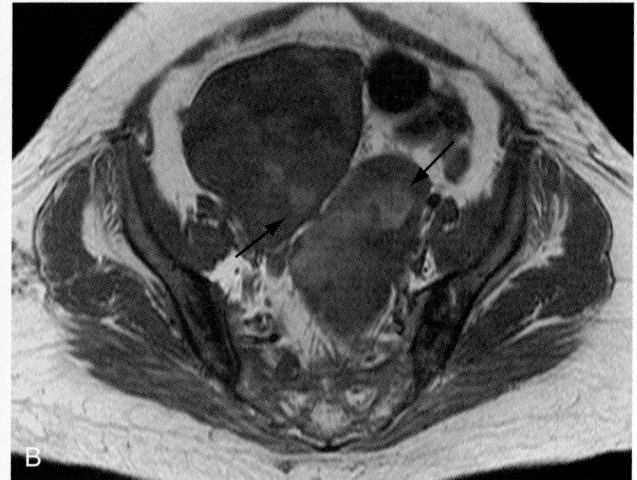

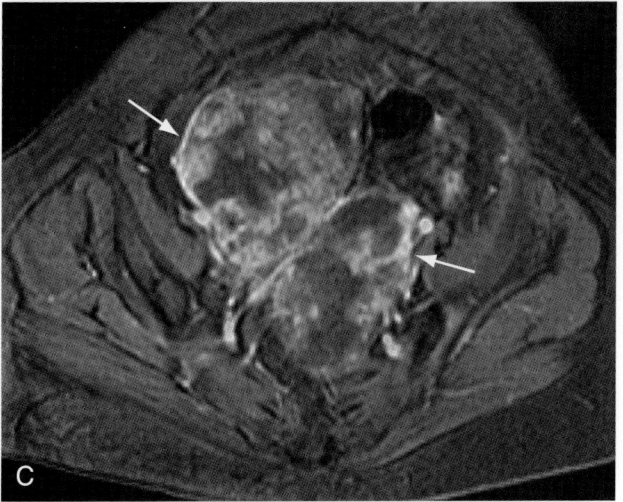

FIGURE 91-23

Hematogenous ovarian metastases due to angiosarcoma. Axial T2-weighted (**A**) T1-weighted (**B**), and post-gadolinium fat-suppressed T1-weighted (**C**) images show bilateral solid ovarian masses *(arrows in* **A**) with heterogeneous signal. High signal intensity on T1-weighted images suggest areas of hemorrhage *(arrows in* **B**). After gadolinium, there is enhancement of the rim and solid components within the metastases *(arrows in* **C**).

menopause. It is divided into the fundus, body, and cervix; the fallopian tubes enter the superolateral corners (cornua), and the fundus lies above this level. The body narrows at the isthmus, which is between the body and the cervix. The mucosal surface of the isthmus is the same as the endometrium of the body of the uterus. The internal os opens into the cervical canal, which ends at the external os, opening into the vagina.

There are three zones of the uterus: the endometrium, myometrium, and subserosa.[8] The endometrium is of variable thickness and composed of endometrial glands, the zona functionale, and the zona basale. These glands interdigitate with the myometrium. The two endometrial leaflets are often in apposition, with a thin layer of fluid, mucus, or blood between them. Beneath the endometrium is the myometrium. Two distinct histologic layers comprise the myometrium: the more superficial subendometrial layer of smooth muscle and the deeper stratum vasculare, where the arcuate vessels course. The outermost uterine zone is the subserosal muscle.

The uterine fundus and body are covered by a layer of visceral peritoneum. Posteriorly, the peritoneum reflects down deeply to the rectum, forming the rectouterine pouch (pouch of Douglas), which extends to the level of the posterior fornix of the vagina; while anteriorly it reflects downward to the bladder to a lesser extent forming the vesicovaginal pouch. The paired round ligaments are muscular bands, 5 to 6 mm in diameter that originate at the level of the fallopian tubes isthmus and traverse the inguinal canal to fuse with the subcutaneous tissue of the labia majora. The broad ligament is a double sheet of peritoneum that reflects off the ventral and dorsal surfaces of the uterus and extends to the pelvic sidewall. The broad ligament contains the parametria which are adjacent to the lateral margins of the uterine corpus and cervix. The lower border of the broad ligament is a coalescence of connective tissue and smooth muscle fibers that form the paired cardinal ligaments. The cardinal ligaments fuse with the paired uterosacral ligaments. Together, the cardinal, uterosacral, and uterovesical ligaments are the main suspensory ligaments of the uterus, whereas the main function of the round ligaments is to prevent retrodisplacement.

The lymphatic drainage of the uterus is by means of three networks from the endometrium, myometrium, and superficial subperitoneal surface. The channels pass out through the broad ligament folds to the pelvic sidewall and then into the iliac chain of nodes. Some of the drainage passes out with the round ligament down to the inguinal nodes, with the lower channels draining into the parametrial nodes lateral to the ureter. A few channels drain posteriorly along the uterosacral ligament to the sacral nodes.

MRI Appearance

Three distinct uterine zones are clearly demarcated on T2-weighted images. These zones, or layers, from the inside out, are the endometrium, junctional zone, and myometrium (Fig. 92-4). These zones are under hormonal stimulation and both the endometrium and myometrium have varying MRI appearances depending on the phase

of the menstrual cycle and menstrual status (i.e., before or after menopause). Hormone status also affects the dynamic contrast-enhancement characteristics of the uterus. In contradistinction, uterine zonal anatomy is indistinguishable on T1-weighted images: the uterus images as a homogeneous intermediate signal intensity structure.

Kinematic studies of uterine peristalsis are now possible using ultrafast sequences (e.g., true fast imaging steady-state free precession).[9] The direction, periodicity, and amplitude of uterine peristalsis are variable and appear to be, in part, a function of the hormonal milieu (Fig. 92-5). Feature analysis of uterine peristalsis may help further our understanding of infertility.

Endometrium

The endometrial cavity has high signal intensity on T2-weighted images, best seen in the sagittal plane. At standard T2-weighted parameters, the signal contributions from blood, fluid in the cavity, and the glandular layer cannot be separated. When assessing endometrial width (bilayer), the measurement should be taken in the sagittal plane in the body of the uterus and excluding the dark junctional zone.

In women of reproductive age, the width of the endometrium varies with the menstrual cycle, ranging from 3 to 13 mm.[10-12] The endometrium is usually thinnest just after menses and thickens progressively toward ovulation and into the secretory phase. The cavity reaches its maximal thickness, up to 13 mm, in the late

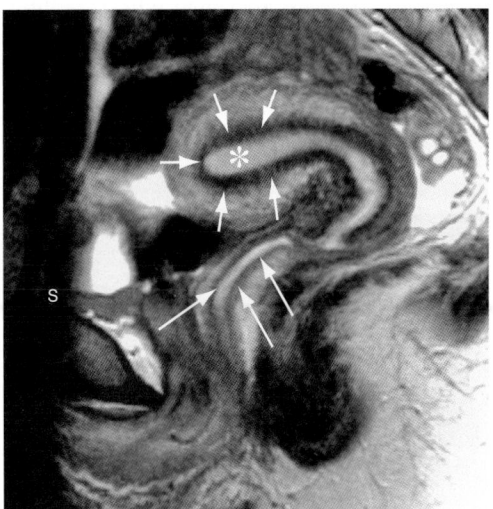

FIGURE 92-4

Normal uterine corpus. Midline sagittal T2-weighted fast spin-echo image shows the major uterine zonal anatomy: high signal intensity endometrium (*), low signal intensity junctional zone (*short arrows*) and intermediate signal intensity myometrium. The uterine serosa, the outermost zone, is not clearly demarcated and blends in with the myometrium. The zonal anatomy of the vagina and cervix are also well demarcated, especially the high signal intensity endovaginal canal and surrounding low signal muscular wall (*long arrows*). Note that the endometrial canal is slightly lower in signal intensity than the endocervical canal due to apposition of the endometrial leaflets. Also note the placement of the anterior saturation band (S) that limits motion artifact in the image.

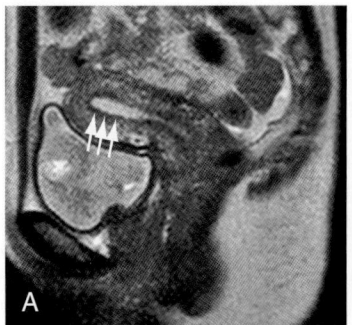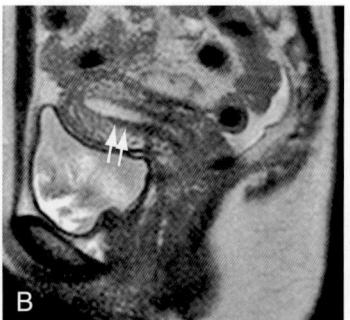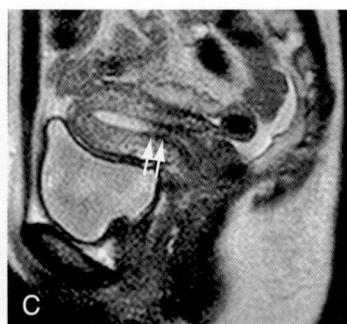

FIGURE 92-5

Uterine peristalsis. **A-C,** Sequential sagittal true fast imaging with steady-state precession (FISP) images show a wave progressive widening of the subedometrial myometrium from the lower uterine segment (*arrows* in **A**), through the mid uterus (*arrows* in **B**), and towards the fundus (*arrows* in **C**). *(Courtesy of Aki Kido, MD and Kaori Togashi, MD, Graduate School of Medicine, Kyoto University, Kyoto, Japan.)*

secretory phase just before menses; whereas it measures up to 6 mm in the follicular phase. In women who are taking birth control pills, the endometrium no longer cycles and remains quite thin (approximately 1-2 mm) throughout the "cycle" (Fig. 92-6). Intrauterine devices image as interrupted linear or curvilinear low signal within the endometrial canal (Fig. 92-7).

In postmenopausal women, the endometrium atrophies and no longer undergoes monthly hormonal stimulation. In a postmenopausal woman who is not taking exogenous hormones, the endometrium should measure no more than 2 to 3 mm (Fig. 92-8).[13] An exception to this is the postmenopausal woman who is being treated with exogenous estrogen. This therapy maintains hormonal stimulation to the uterus resulting in increased signal intensity in the myometrium and increased thick-

ening of the endometrial cavity (up to 1 cm). Similar changes can be seen in postmenopausal women on tamoxifen treatment and/or prophylaxis.[14,15] Therefore, it is important not only to determine the menstrual status but also the exogenous hormonal status of patients prior to interpreting MRI examinations.

Junctional Zone

The middle layer of the uterus, or junctional zone, represents the basal layer of the myometrium. It is composed of longitudinally oriented smooth muscle.[9] It is in fact two layers, the inner compact portion and the outer transitional portion, which blend into the myometrium proper. The muscle in the transitional layer is less compact.[16] The mean thickness of the junctional zone

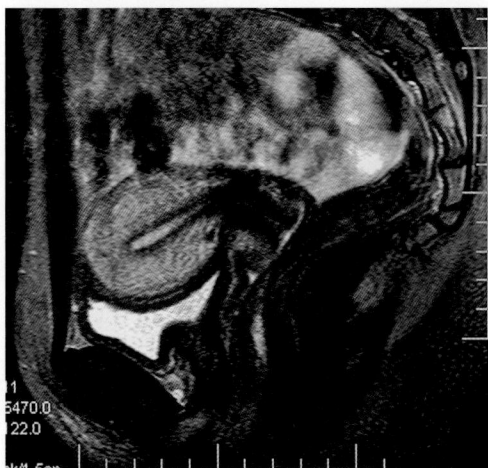

FIGURE 92-6

Normal uterus: oral contraceptives. Sagittal T2-weighted fast spin-echo image shows the typical appearance of the uterus in a woman on oral contraceptives with a thin junctional zone relative to the rest of the myometrium. Similarly, the endometrium is thin. *(Courtesy of Aki Kido, MD and Kaori Togashi, MD, Graduate School of Medicine, Kyoto University, Kyoto, Japan.)*

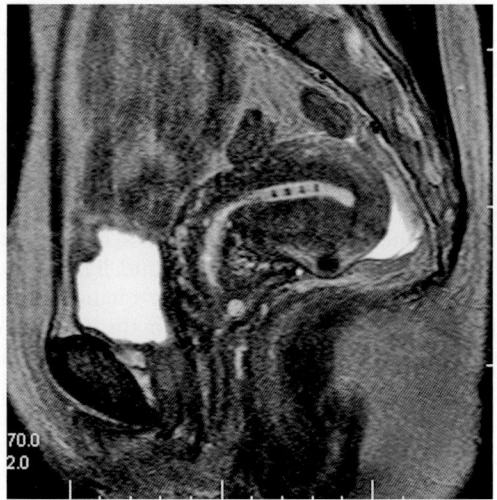

FIGURE 92-7

Normal uterus: intrauterine device (IUD). Sagittal T2-weighted fast spin-echo image shows the typical interrupted linear low signal of an IUD within the endometrial canal. *(Courtesy of Aki Kido, MD and Kaori Togashi, MD, Graduate School of Medicine, Kyoto University, Kyoto, Japan.)*

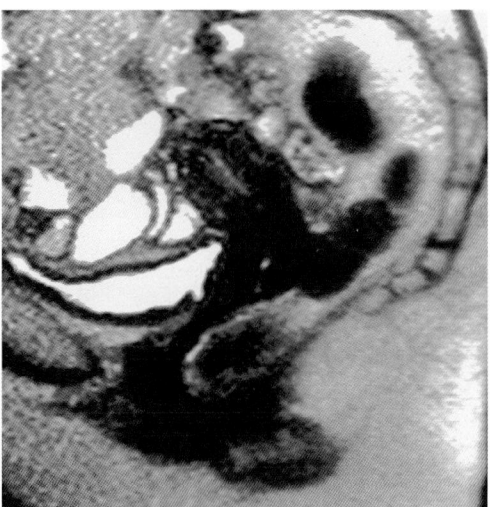

FIGURE 92-8

Normal postmenopausal uterus. Sagittal T2-weighted single-shot fast spin-echo image of a postmenopausal uterus is characterized by a thin endometrium and absent junctional zone. Note that the uterine corpus-to-uterine cervix ratio approaches 1:1, another characteristic of the postmenopausal uterus.

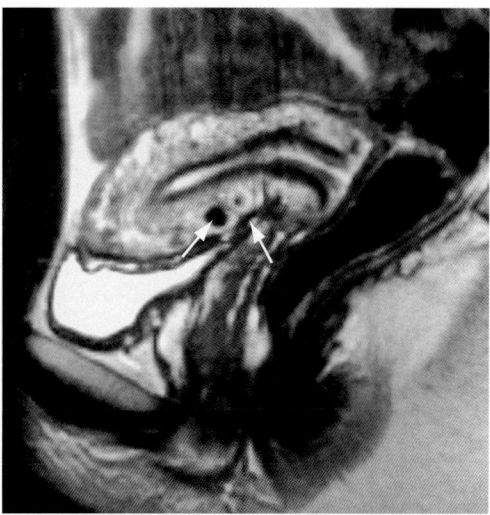

FIGURE 92-9

Normal uterus: arcuate vessels. Sagittal T2-weighted single-shot fast spin-echo image shows the normal arcuate vessels within the myometrium (*arrows*).

ranges from 2 to 8 mm. It images as a low signal intensity band between the endometrium and myometrium on T2-weighted images (see Fig. 92-4). The low signal intensity pattern may be accounted for, in part, by the compact nature of the muscle bundles with little extracellular space. In addition, there is also a difference in the nuclear area (number of cells per unit volume) in the junctional zone. Specifically, the nuclear area of the junctional zone is higher than the nuclear area in the remaining myometrium.[17]

The junctional zone's interface with the endometrium is sharp, but that with the myometrium is less well defined. The uterine arcuate arteries are at the level of this transition from junctional zone to stratum vasculare of the myometrium proper (Fig. 92-9). The junctional zone is routinely visible and is a continuous line in the premenopausal woman. It extends from the endocervical canal up around the uterine body and fundus. This layer does not respond hormonally and thus does not change during the menstrual cycle. In postmenopausal women, the junctional zone is usually absent and if present may be incomplete. That is, with the progressive atrophy and progressive drop in T2-weighted signal intensity of the postmenopausal myometrium, the junctional zone becomes less apparent (see Fig. 92-8).

Myometrium

In the premenopausal woman in the follicular phase of the cycle, the myometrium has diffuse intermediate signal intensity on T2-weighted images (see Fig. 92-4). In the secretory phase of the cycle, the myometrial signal increases, with increasing fluid content and vascular flow. The myometrial morphology and signal may even change during a single examination. That is,

the myometrium may exhibit transient bulges of lower signal intensity over the course of the examination due to myometrial contractions.[18] As the patient ages, the uterus atrophies and decreases in overall size.

Interesting work has been done to correlate the MR signal of the myometrium and its histologic counterpart. Brown et al[16] found that the MR appearance of myometrium is multilayered. The inner one third is the junctional zone. The myometrium proper begins when the junctional zone ends at the level of the arcuate arteries; this layer is known as the stratum vasculare. The third layer is the subserosal layer.

Serosa

Surrounding the smooth muscle of the myometrium is the serosa. It is inconsistently imaged. On high-resolution T2-weighted images the serosa may appear as a discrete thin low signal intensity line. It can be distorted owing to a chemical-shift artifact, which can make one side appear thicker than the other.

Parametrium and Ligaments

The MR appearance of the parametrium and pelvic ligaments reflects their composition: fibrous, muscular, loose connective tissue and/or venous plexuses. That is, the uterosacral ligaments are low in signal intensity on T1-weighted sequences and variable signal intensity on T2-weighted sequences; the round ligaments are low in signal intensity on both T1- and T2-weighted sequences; the cardinal ligaments are intermediate in signal intensity on T1-weighted images and isointense or high in signal intensity on T2-weighted sequences; and the broad ligaments (best seen in patients with ascites) also tend to be low in signal intensity on both T1- and T2-weighted sequences.

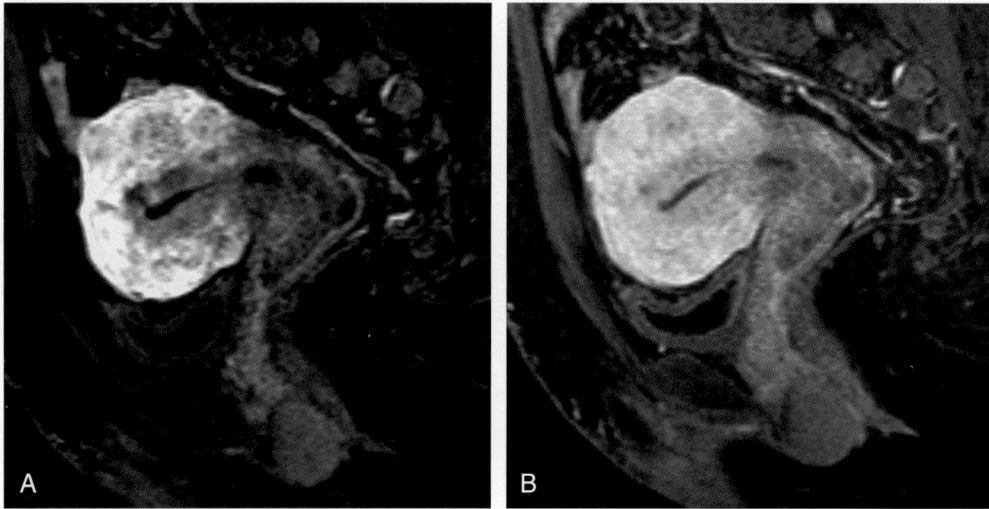

F I G U R E 92-10

Normal dynamic contrast enhancement of the uterus during the secretory phase. **A,** Initial contrast-enhanced sagittal T1-weighted fat-suppressed volume-interpolated breath-hold examination (VIBE) shows relatively greater enhancement of the outer myometrium compared to the junctional zone and cervix. **B,** These differences are less marked on the subsequent sagittal T1 fat-suppressed VIBE.

Contrast-Enhanced Appearance of the Uterus

The contrast enhancement characteristics of the uterus change with the menstrual cycle. During the proliferative phase, there is early enhancement of the thin subendometrium with subsequent enhancement of the remaining myometrium. The junctional zone and inner myometrium exhibit early enhancement during menses whereas early enhancement of the outer myometrium characterizes the secretory phase (Fig. 92-10). Regardless of the cycle phase, the endometrium progressively enhances over time becoming iso- or hyper-intense to myometrium on delayed images (Fig. 92-11). The endometrial enhancement characteristics of a postmenopausal uterus parallel the proliferative-phase endometrium in a woman of reproductive age.

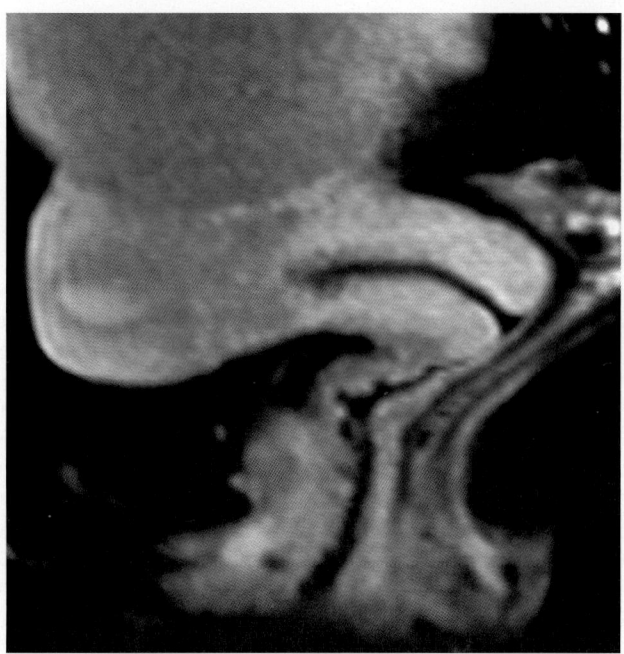

F I G U R E 92-11

Normal uterus: delayed enhancement. Delayed contrast-enhanced sagittal T1-weighted fat-suppressed spoiled gradient-echo image shows relatively greater enhancement of the endometrium compared to the rest of the uterine zones. Note that fluid in the endovaginal and endocervical canals does not enhance. Incidental note is made of a large endometrioma atop the uterus.

TABLE 92-1   Protocol Guidelines

Sequence coil type	Plane	TR/TE (ms)	FOV (mm) appropriate to body habitus	Thickness (mm)	Flip angle (degrees)	Matrix
Scout	Variable	15/6	500	10	30	
T2-weighted SSFSE phased array	Axial pelvis (uterus localizer)	64/4.4	320-380 rec FOV 6/8	6-8	150	128 × 256
T2-weighted SSFSE phased array	Sagittal uterus (long axis)	64/4.4	300-330	6-8	150	128 × 256
T2-weighted SSFSE phased array	Axial uterus (short axis)	64/4.4	300	6-8	150	128 × 256
SSFSE phased array	Coronal uterus*	64/4.4	360-380	6-8	150	128 × 256
T2-weighted SSFSE body	Coronal abdomen/pelvis*	64/4.4	400-450	6-8	150	128 × 256
T1-weighted SGE phased array	Axial pelvis	160/5.3	300 rec FOV 6/8	6-8	80	128 × 256
Fat-suppressed T1-weighted SGE phased array	Axial pelvis	170/2.3	300 rec FOV 6/8	6-8	80	128 × 256
T2 FSE[†] phased array	Variable	4700/132	320	5-7	180	256 × 512
Pre- and 3 dynamic post-contrast fat-suppressed T1 VIBE[‡] phased array	Sagittal	4.5/1.9	330 rec FOV 6/8	3 mm effective	15	80 × 256

FSE, fast spin-echo; SGE, spoiled gradient-echo; SSFSE, single-shot fast spin-echo. VIBE, volume-interpolated breath-hold examination.
Optional: for evaluation of Müllerian duct anomalies. Coronal of uterus to identify uterine fundal contour. Coronal of abdomen and pelvis to identify renal anomalies.
[†] Optional: to clarify or confirm a finding on SSFSE sequences.
[‡] Optional: For evaluation of potential uterine artery embolization (UAE) candidates and to monitor treatment response following uterine artery embolization (UAE).

The 3D data set also allows for multiplanar reconstructions. Occasionally, we perform a delayed fat-suppressed T1-weighted spoiled gradient-echo sequence, especially if we want to obtain more lateral coverage than our 3D sequence.[32]

For evaluating women with known or suspected Müllerian duct anomalies we perform two additional sequences. We acquire a large FOV coronal image using the body coil to assess for urinary tract anomalies, and we also perform a true coronal T2-weighted SSFSE sequence of the uterus to assess the fundal contour. Contrast is not necessary in the evaluation of Müllerian duct anomalies.

CONGENITAL ANOMALIES OF THE UTERUS

Congenital uterine anomalies represent a spectrum of morphologic abnormalities caused by agenesis, hypoplasia, or defects of vertical and lateral fusion of the paramesonephric (Müllerian) ducts early in embryonic development. The incidence of these anomalies has been reported to range from 0.16% to 10%, reflecting selection bias, lack of prospective data, and differences in diagnostic data acquisition. The overall data suggest an incidence of 1% in the general population and 3% in women with recurrent pregnancy loss and poor reproductive outcomes.[35-45] While conception rates in women with congenital anomalies are similar to the general population, spontaneous abortion, premature delivery, fetal malpresentation, and poor reproductive

outcomes is reported to occur in 25% of these women and in 10% of the general population.[35-45] Adverse reproductive outcomes not only reflect the type of anomaly, but also the associated increased incidence of cervical incompetence and endometriosis in these patients.[37,39,46-48] While many of these anomalies are initially suspected or diagnosed by hysterosalpingography and ultrasound, MRI has reported accuracies of up to 100% in the elaboration of these anomalies and is currently the modality of choice in further characterizing the anomaly and diagnosing secondary findings.[49-53] This is especially important given their varying clinical presentations, management regimens, and prognoses for fetal survival.

Patients are optimally evaluated on a 1.5-T magnet with a phased-array surface coil and an empty urinary bladder. Following a localizing series of the uterus in the sagittal plane, a fast spin-echo T2-weighted image series should be performed parallel to the long axis of the uterus, using the endometrial cavity as a guide, to characterize the external uterine contour (Fig. 92-17). Subsequently standard T1-weighted images and multiplanar fast spin-echo T2-weighted images are performed as needed to secure the diagnosis and elaborate secondary findings. Finally, imaging of the retroperitoneum with a gradient-echo or single-shot fast spin-echo T2-weighted series performed in a body coil with a large field of view is recommended to assess the kidneys.

Embryologically, the male and female genital systems are formed by two pairs of symmetric genital ducts: the paramesonephric (Müllerian) ducts and the mesonephric (Wolffian) ducts. In the absence of a factor associated

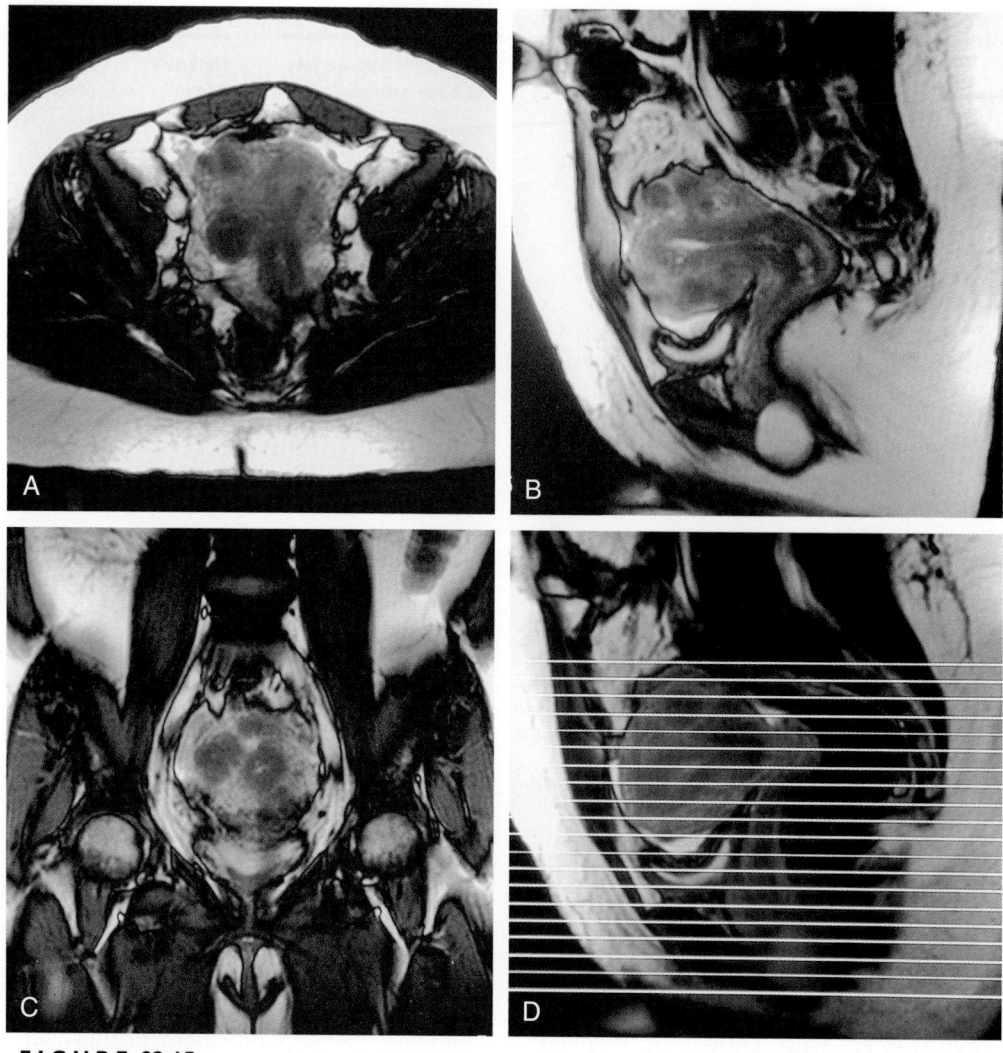

FIGURE 92-15

Normal technique: Scout images. **A,** Axial; **B,** sagittal; and **C,** coronal gradient-echo scout images provide information for acquiring the appropriate imaging planes. **D,** Same image as **B** with slices positioned for obtaining true axial images of the pelvis.

with the Y chromosome at 6 weeks, the mesonephric ducts begin to degenerate and induce the paramesonephric ducts to develop concurrently along the lateral aspects of the gonads. The distal segments of the paramesonephric ducts elongate caudomedially giving rise to the uterine corpus, cervix, and upper two thirds of the vagina, and eventually fuse. The proximal segments remain unfused and form the fallopian tubes. The septum between the fused paramesonephric ducts begins to regress, and at 12 weeks, the normal configuration of the uterus and upper vagina is attained. Synchronously, the sinovaginal bulbs of the urogenital sinus develop into the lower third of the vagina and eventually fuse with the uterovaginal complex.[54]

Development of the ovaries is a separate process, arising from the gonadal ridge, and therefore is not associated with Müllerian duct anomalies. However, the kidneys arise from a ridge of mesoderm in common with the uterovaginal complex which is derived from the mesonephric ducts; hence, abnormal development of the paramesonephric ducts may also disturb embryogenesis of the kidneys and ureters. Renal anomalies are subsequently associated with congenital uterine anomalies.[53-56]

Classification of Müllerian duct anomalies is based on a system proposed by Buttram and Gibbons in 1979, which reflects the degree of failure of normal development, and takes into account similar clinical features, management, and prognosis for fetal survival.[57] In 1988, the classification was modified by the American Fertility Society in 1988 [now the American Society of Reproductive Medicine (ARSM)], and remains the most widely accepted schematization for reporting Müllerian duct anomalies (Fig. 92-18).[58] Anomalies can be categorized by features, which overlap between these classes and should be described by their component parts. Additionally, associated cervical and vaginal malformations, not addressed in the ARSM system, require complete elaboration.

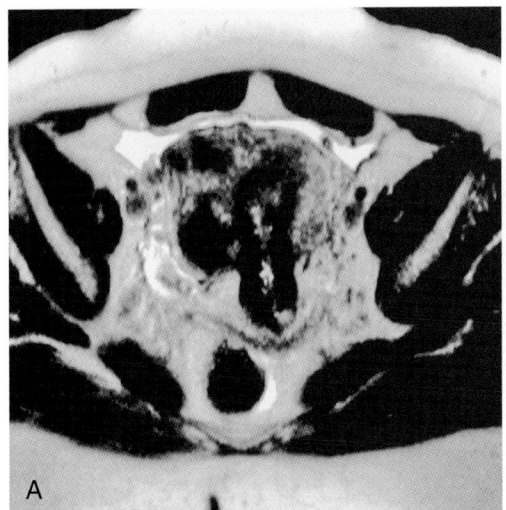

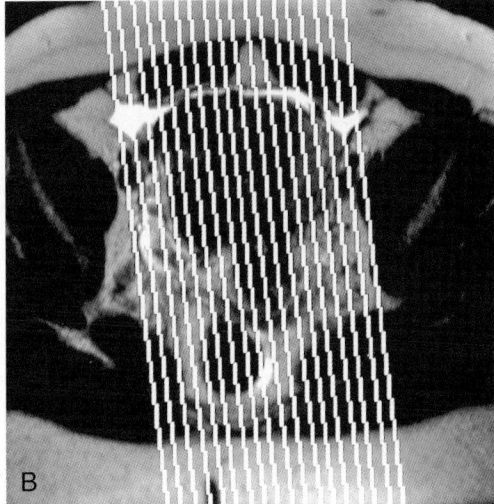

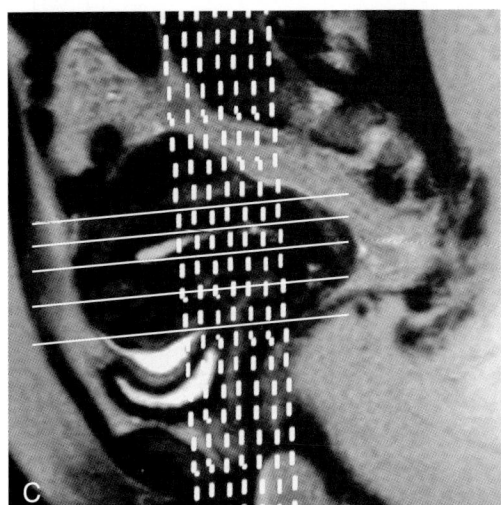

FIGURE 92-16

Normal technique: Orthogonal planes. **A,** T2-weighted single-shot fast spin-echo (SSFSE) true axial image of the pelvis allows a true sagittal image of the uterus to be obtained. **B,** Same image as **A** with angled slices for obtaining a true sagittal image of the uterus. **C,** T2-weighted SSFSE true sagittal image of the uterus prescribed from image **A** with slices positioned for acquiring true short/axial axis (*broken lines*) and true coronal axis (*solid lines*) of the uterus.

FIGURE 92-17

Orientation for acquisition of oblique images (*long arrow*) parallel to the long axis of the uterus using the endometrium (*short arrow*) as the center slice determined from sagittal plane localizing image.

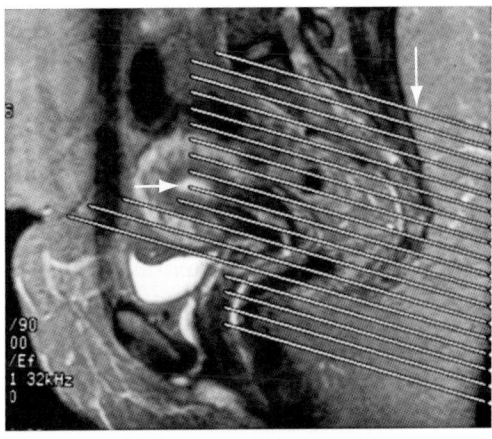

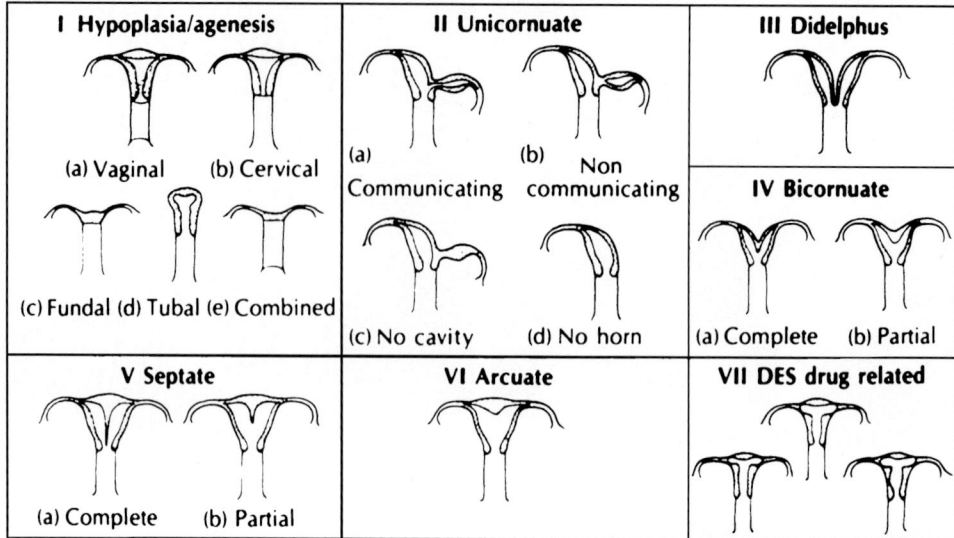

FIGURE 92-18

Classification system of Müllerian duct anomalies modified and adopted by the American Fertility Society. DES, diethylstilbestrol.

Class I: Müllerian Agenesis and Hypoplasia

Early failure to form the Müllerian ducts prior to fusion results in variable degrees of agenesis and hypoplasia, and comprises approximatey 10% of anomalies. Mayer-Rokitansky-Kuster-Hauser syndrome is the most common presentation and reflects complete agenesis of the upper two thirds of the vagina with associated uterine agenesis in 90% of cases. The remaining cases have a small rudimentary uterus, without or with a segment of functioning endometrium.[59] Severe cyclic pelvic pain may reflect a functioning endometrium within an obstructed segment, causing severe hematometria. Ovaries are normal in the majority resulting in the development of secondary sexual characteristics. Vaginal dilatation and reconstruction is performed, especially in patients with an obstructed uterus. Even in patients with functioning endometrial segments within rudimentary uteri, there is little to no potential for a viable pregnancy.[60]

On imaging, a discernible uterus is not visualized with uterine agenesis and is best appreciated in the sagittal plane. If present, the hypoplastic uterus is small, with diminished zonal anatomy and diffuse low signal intensity on T2-weighted images. An endometrial segment may demonstrate increased signal intensity and be expanded, depending on the presence of associated obstruction.[61-63] Vaginal agenesis is best characterized on the axial plane with no normal vaginal zonal anatomy identified between the rectum and urethra (Fig. 92-19).

Class II: Unicornuate Uterus

Unicornuate uteri arise from hypoplasia or agenesis of one Müllerian duct while the other elongates normally, and represent approximately 20% of uterine anomalies. Complete agenesis of a horn occurs in 35% of women, while variable degrees of hypoplasia occur in 65% and result in a rudimentary horn. Uteri with a rudimentary horn are subdivided into rudimentary horns without an associated endometrial segment, designated "noncavitary" (33%), and those with an associated endometrial segment, designated "cavitary" (32%). A cavitary horn is described as "communicating" if the endometrium is in continuity with the endometrium of the contralateral horn (10%), and "noncommunicating" if the endometrium is isolated within the rudimentary horn (22%) and has no connection with the dominant horn. Management reflects the presence of the associated endometrial segment, if present. Unicornuate uteri without rudimentary horns or those with noncavitary rudimentary horns are managed expectantly. Those with rudimentary horns with endometrial segments are usually surgically resected secondary to dysmenorrhea and hematometria, as well as the potential for pregnancy within the hypoplastic horn. The vast majority of pregnancies arising in these rudimentary horns result in uterine rupture.[64,65] Pregnancies that arise in the nonrudimentary horn have a 50% rate of spontaneous abortion, increased rates of premature births, and are at increased risk of fetal malpresentation and intrauterine growth retardation.[66] However, the length of subsequent pregnancies often increases with increasing parity.[64,67-71] Associated renal anomalies are always ipsilateral to the hypoplastic horn and occur in up to 40%, with renal agenesis being the most common abnormality.[42,56,67]

On imaging, the uterus appears elongated and curved, shifted off the midline and with a "banana" shape. Zonal anatomy is maintained, although uterine volume is diminished. For unknown embryologic reasons the preserved horn is most often located on the right. The endometrium may be narrow or may be slightly widened,

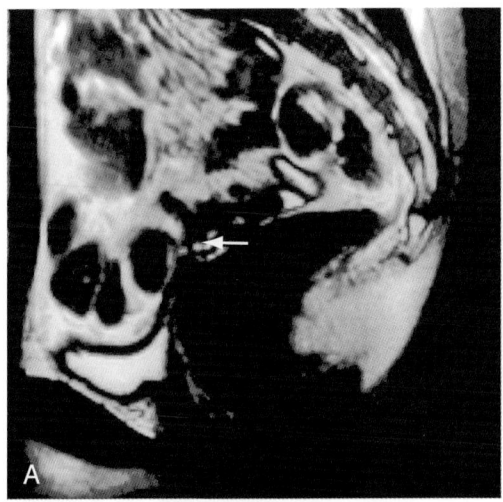
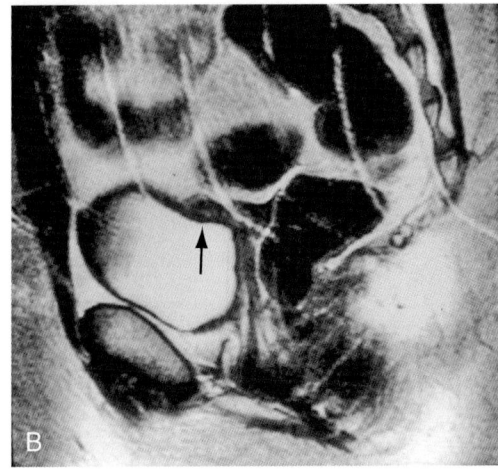
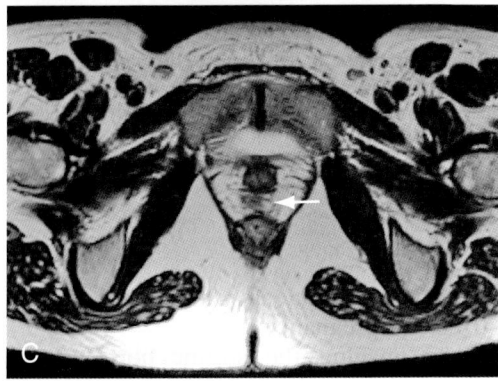

FIGURE 92-19

Uterine agenesis, hypoplasia, and vaginal agenesis. **A** and **B,** Sagittal and **C,** axial T2-weighted fast spin-echo images. **A,** Uterine agenesis. Absence of a normal uterus at the anticipated level of the vaginal apex (*arrow*). **B,** Uterine hypoplasia. Small uterine remnant with loss of normal zonal anatomy (*arrow*). **C,** Vaginal agenesis. Nonspecific rudimentary soft-tissue (*arrow*) insinuated between the urethra and rectum.

tapering at the apex and projecting into a single cornua. The appearance of the rudimentary horn depends on the presence of endometrial tissue. In noncavitary horns, low signal asymmetric soft-tissue thickening is noted on T2-weighted imaging. In cavitary horns, the increased signal intensity of the endometrium is seen, with variable degrees of preserved zonal anatomy (Fig. 92-20).[50,51]

Class III: Uterus Didelphys

Uterus didelphys arises from near complete failure of fusion of the Müllerian ducts, resulting in symmetric duplication of the uterine horns and cervices with no communication between the endometrial cavities, and represent approximately 5% to 7% of uterine anomalies. While the cervices may demonstrate a minor degree of fusion along their medial margins, the horns widely diverge, and an associated vertical vaginal septum is seen in up to 75% of cases. Associated secondary fusion defects may be seen, such as an associated horizontal vaginal septum causing obstruction of the hemiuterus and resulting in hematometrocolpos and dysmenorrhea. The incidence of spontaneous abortion rates approximates 40% and premature birth rates are also increased.[37,68,69] Surgical intervention is usually not indicated, and the length of subsequent gestations often increases with

increasing parity, similar to the unicornuate uterus. The benefits of therapeutic surgical intervention remain unclear, although Strassman metroplasty, in which the medial walls of each horn are resected and the lateral walls reapproximated, has been considered in women with recurrent pregnancy loss.[64,65]

On imaging, two separate uterine horns and cervices are seen demonstrating normal zonal anatomy within each hemiuterus, although the uterine volume of each horn is reduced. While the horns are widely divergent, the cervices often lie in close approximation. A low signal vertical septum may be seen extending to the vagina. A superimposed unilateral horizontal vaginal septum may appear as variable degrees of dilatation of the vaginal segment and endometrium, with differential signal intensity of acute and chronic blood and debris on T2-weighted images (Fig. 92-21).[49,50,53]

Class IV: Bicornuate Uterus

Bicornuate uteri arise from incomplete fusion of the uterine horns and account for approximately 10% of Müllerian duct anomalies. The horns are symmetrical in size with divergence and an intervening cleft of variable length, extending to the internal cervical os in "complete" bicornuate uteri, and to lesser, variable

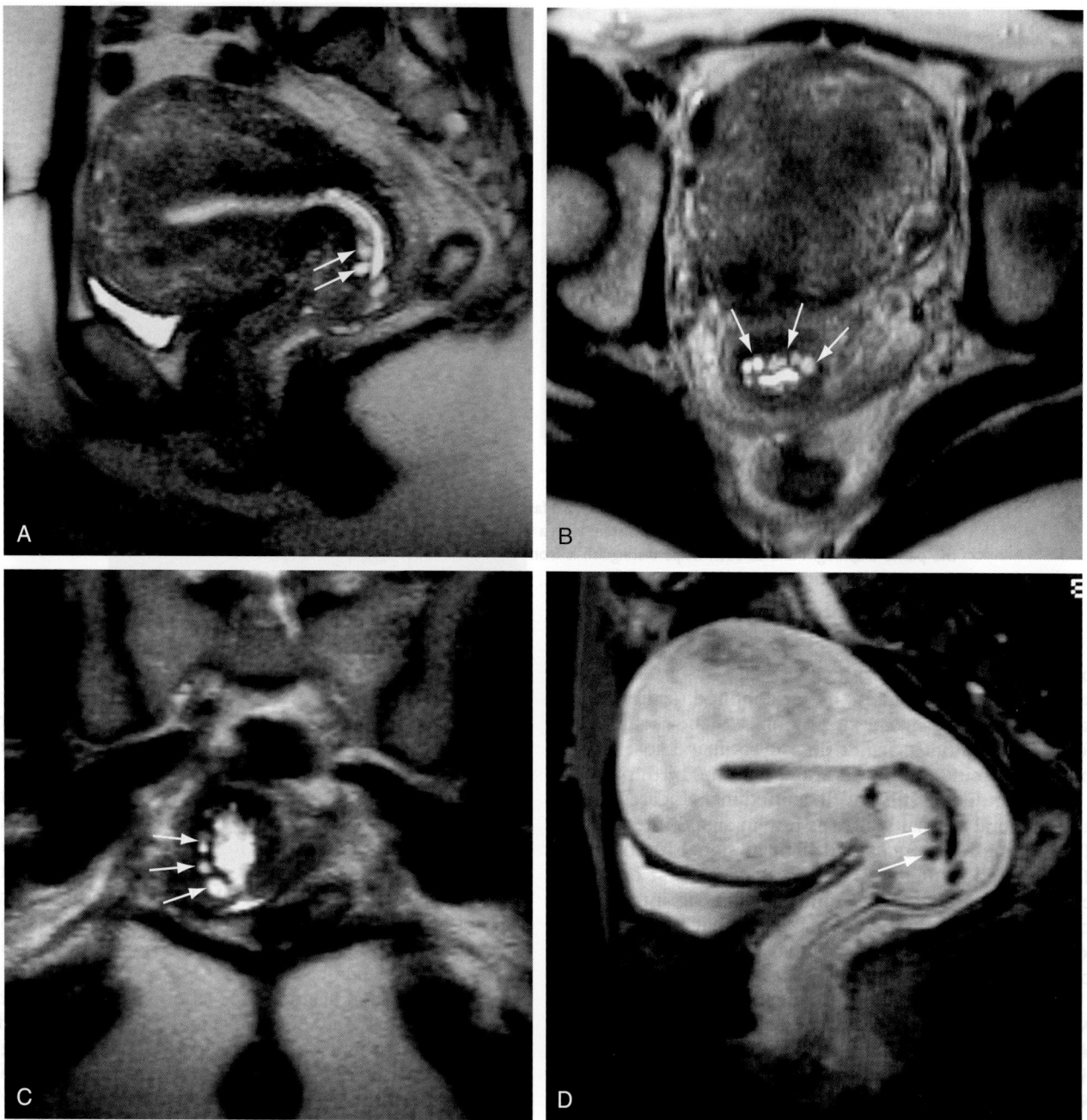

FIGURE 92-31

Nabothian cysts. **A,** Sagittal; **B,** axial; and **C,** coronal T2-weighted single-shot fast spin-echo images of the uterine cervix show multiple high signal intensity nabothian cysts within the cervical tissue *(arrows).* **D,** Sagittal post-contrast T1-weighted fast spin volume-interpolated breath-hold examination highlights the signal void cysts which do not enhance *(arrows).*

uterine distension. Cervical stenosis results from either an organic or iatrogenic etiology. Organic causes include senile atrophy, chronic infection, or tumor. Common iatrogenic causes include radiation therapy, laser therapy, cryosurgery, or cervical endometriosis secondary to combined cervical conization and endometrial curettage.[106] In severe cases of cervical stenosis, egress of endometrial fluids is hampered and retained uterine secretions dilate the uterus causing pelvic pain. In women of reproductive age, narrowing of the cervix

may also cause retrograde menses with resultant endometriosis and hemoperitoneum.

T1- and T2-weighted images are both used when evaluating patients with suspected cervical stenosis. In the absence of mechanical obstruction secondary to a cervical or endometrial tumor, the cervix has normal morphology and signal intensity on T1-weighted sequences. If the uterine corpus is dilated, the contents may be low in signal intensity (i.e., simple fluid) or high in signal intensity (i.e., proteinaceous fluid or blood)

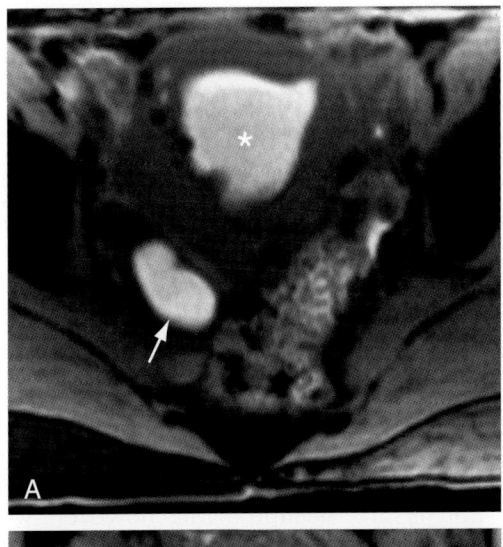
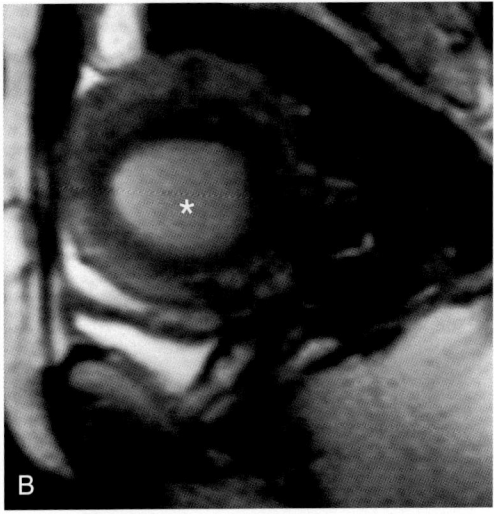
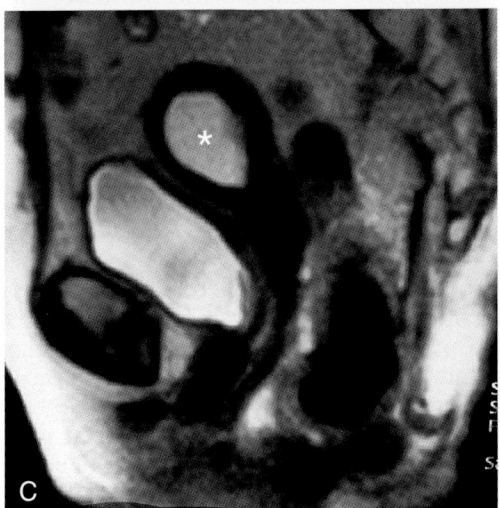

FIGURE 92-32

Cervical stenosis. **A,** Axial T1-weighted fat-suppressed spoiled gradient-echo and **B,** sagittal T2-weighted single-shot fast spin-echo (SSFSE) images show a distended endometrial canal. The contents in the canal are high signal intensity on the T1-weighted fat-suppressed technique (* in **A**) and decrease slightly in signal intensity on the T2-weighted technique (* in **B**), consistent with hematometra secondary to cervical stenosis following myomectomy. Note the susceptibility artifact on the T1-weighted fast spin image from surgery and the right endometrioma from retrograde menses (*arrow* in **A**). **C,** Sagittal T2-weighted SSFSE image in a woman post radiation therapy for colon cancer shows high signal intensity hydrometra (*). Note the loss of normal cervical zonal anatomy that is common in both menopausal women and in women after radiation therapy.

(Fig. 92-32). On T2-weighted sequences the cervical zonal anatomy may be preserved, or there may be loss of the expected zonal architecture. Lack of distinct cervical zones is primarily noted in postmenopausal women (e.g., senile atrophy) and women following radiation therapy to the pelvis (Fig. 92-32).[106] The absence of normal cervical zonal architecture is not diagnostic of cervical stenosis and MR findings need to be interpreted in light of clinical history and reproductive status. If there is concomitant uterine distension, the junctional zone and myometrium may be thinned. The signal intensity of the endometrial cavity reflects the composition of the retained fluid (e.g., hematometra). Both enhanced and nonenhanced sequences are performed to differentiate blood/secretions and/or tumor in the endometrial canal.

The differential diagnosis of cervical stenosis is limited. In women of reproductive age with uterine dilation, uterine didelphys or a complex uterine anomaly with an obstructing transverse vaginal septum should be diagnostic considerations. In most cases, the history (amenorrhea) and duplicated uterus, cervix or vagina will be obvious and the vagina is usually distended out of proportion to the rest of the uterus.

Transvaginal ultrasound (TVS) is often the initial modality to evaluate patients with suspected cervical stenosis and identify the underlying cause. Before ascribing senile atrophy, infection or post-treatment change as the cause of cervical narrowing, malignancy must be excluded. MRI is a useful problem-solving tool in cases of an equivocal or nondiagnostic ultrasound.

The natural history of cervical stenosis depends on the degree of canal narrowing. Some cases resolve spontaneously, in others endometrial fluid egress is not significantly impeded. If the patient is symptomatic, cervical dilation and evacuation of the dilated endometrial canal is performed. In patients with concomitant endometrial thickening, the endometrium is sampled.[107] If long-term drainage is needed, a catheter may be placed.

Cervical Incompetence

Cervical incompetence or insufficiency refers to a short cervix (measured from internal to external os) that predisposes women to recurrent fetal loss. It affects 1%

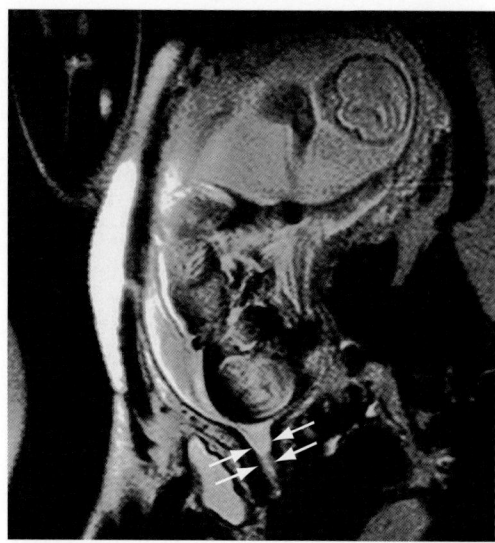

FIGURE 92-33

Cervical incompetence. Sagittal T2 single-shot fast spin-echo image shows a funnel-shaped cervix with a widened internal os (*arrows*) consistent with cervical incompetence in a woman with 19-week-gestation twins. *(Courtesy of Deborah Levine, Beth Israel Deaconess Medical Center, Boston, MA.)*

of pregnant women. Women present with painless cervical dilation followed by fetal expulsion that typically occurs in the second trimester. Patients may also complain of vaginal spotting. Risk factors for cervical incompetence include congenital uterine malformation, in utero DES exposure, and cervical trauma (laceration or iatrogenic, e.g., cone biopsy).[108]

MRI features suggestive of cervical incompetence in a non-gravid woman include one or more of the following: cervical length less than or equal to 3 cm, internal cervical os greater than or equal to 4.3 mm, thinning or increased signal intensity of fibrous stroma, and/or asymmetric irregular widening of the endocervical canal (Fig. 92-33).[109] Assessment is made on sagittal T2-weighted sequences. Of note, in women with cervical incompetence secondary to DES exposure, the endocervical canal is less than 2.5 cm and both cervical stroma signal intensity and internal os width remain normal. Because a full bladder may falsely elongate the cervix, women should void prior to the examination. In a gravid patient a short cervix is not necessarily diagnostic of cervical incompetence. Rather, cervical shortening can be seen with normal cervical effacement at term gestation, placental abruption, and/or subclinical chorioamnionitis.

TVS is the imaging modality of choice for diagnosing cervical incompetence. It has a high degree of consistency for cervical length measurement. In cases that are problematic for ultrasound, MRI is an attractive, noninvasive, nonionizing radiation alternative. Additionally, MR may suggest the diagnosis of cervical incompetence during a pelvic examination performed for another reason.

Cervical cerclage at 12 to 15 mean menstrual weeks is the standard of care for women with cervical incompetence. Bedrest and tocolytics may be prescribed after 24 mean menstrual weeks.[108]

BENIGN CONDITIONS OF THE UTERINE CORPUS

Endometrial Polyp

Endometrial polyps are focal excrescences of endometrial hyperplasia covered by endometrium. There are three type of polyps: hyperplastic (resembling glands of endometrial hyperplasia); atrophic (cystically dilated atrophic glands); and functional (undergo cyclical endometrial changes). They occur most commonly in the fundus and cornua and may be sessile or pedunculated. If pedunculated, polyps may protrude into the endocervical canal. Endometrial polyps are common, being found in 10% of women in autopsy studies. Multiple polyps are found in up to 20% of affected women. Most polyps are asymptomatic; however, when symptomatic they can cause postmenopausal bleeding, intermenopausal bleeding, menorrhagia/menometrorrhagia, mucous discharge, and infertility. There is no direct evidence that there is a continuum between benign and malignant polyps; however, about 0.5% of polyps are malignant and 12% to 34% of women with endometrial cancer have associated polyps.[110]

Women on tamoxifen therapy for breast cancer treatment or prophylaxis have an increased relative risk for developing endometrial polyps. Specifically, while tamoxifen is an estrogen antagonist in breast tissue, it is a weak estrogen agonist in the postmenopausal uterus and a spectrum of endometrial abnormalities has been reported: proliferative changes, hyperplasia, polyps, and cancer. Tamoxifen is also associated with subendometrial cysts, adenomyosis, leiomyomas and intraperitoneal fluid.

The MRI appearance of polyps is variable, especially on T2-weighted sequences.[111] Most often they are slightly lower in signal intensity than adjacent normal endometrium. However, they may be isointense to normal endometrium and present as focal or diffuse widening of the endometrium, or they may be heterogeneous with both cystic and solid areas, and/or they may have a low signal intensity fibrous core or stalk (Fig. 92-34). On T1-weighted sequences, polyps are isointense to endometrium. Polyps enhance following contrast, typically less than normal endometrium but more than normal myometrium. The pattern of contrast enhancement is not specific. The only definitive way to diagnose a cancerous polyp is to detect myometrial invasion.

For patients on tamoxifen therapy, Ascher et al[14] described two distinct MRI patterns. In patients with atrophy or proliferative changes at histopathology, the endometrium is homogeneous and high in signal intensity on T2-weighted images. Following contrast administration, the endometrial-myometrial interface enhances with a persistent signal void lumen. In patients with polyps, the endometrium is heterogenous on T2-weighted sequences (see Fig. 92-21). After contrast administration there is lattice-like enhancement traversing the endometrial cavity. Cystic atrophy is noted in both groups.

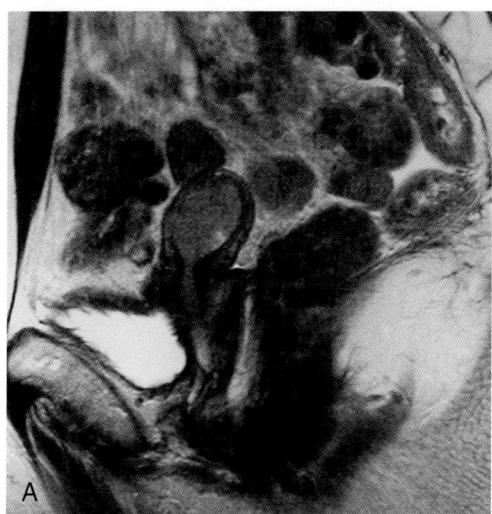 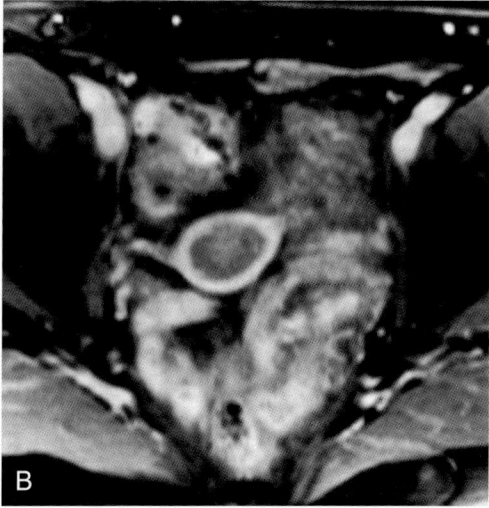

FIGURE 92-34

Endometrial polyp. **A,** Sagittal T2-weightd fast spin-echo image shows the endometrial canal distended by intermediate signal intensity. **B,** Axial contrast-enhanced T1-weighted fat-suppressed T1-weighted spoiled gradient-echo image shows an enhancing mass distending the canal. A benign polyp was diagnosed on histopathology.

Most endometrial polyps can be reliably differentiated from submucosal leiomyomas. The latter are myometrial in origin and are lower in signal intensity than polyps. However, overlap in signal intensity may occur, especially if the submucosal fibroid is degenerated.

The majority of endometrial polyps are asymptomatic, but if symptomatic or incidentally detected, most women undergo hysteroscopic resection. Hysterectomy is reserved for polyps that harbor atypical endometrial hyperplasia or carcinoma. TVS is the modality of choice for the initial investigation of suspected polyps. It is sensitive (56-96%) and specific (82%).[112] Sonohysterography is especially helpful in patients with nonspecific endometrial thickening. However, MRI should be considered in cases where the endometrium cannot be adequately evaluated with ultrasound (equivocal or nondiagnostic studies). For example, morbid obesity, a vertically oriented uterus, multiple or large distorting fibroids, and/or extensive adenomyosis may hamper full ultrasonographic examination. Additionally, MRI is helpful in patients for whom sampling would be difficult (e.g., cervical stenosis).

No definitive screening guidelines for women on tamoxifen therapy have been established, but a combination of TVS and endometrial sampling is most frequently undertaken. As earlier, if the ultrasound or hysteroscopic examinations are equivocal or nondiagnostic, MRI should be considered (Fig. 92-35).

Endometrial Hyperplasia

Endometrial hyperplasia is excessive proliferation of the endometrial glands. Specifically, the endometrial-gland-to-stroma ratio is increased and the glands may be cystically dilated. It may be focal or diffuse. Endometrial hyperplasia is most often the result of unopposed estrogen stimulation (e.g., chronic anovulatory states, unopposed exogenous estrogen use, tamoxifen therapy, obesity, estrogen-producing ovarian tumors). The condition is subdivided into two broad categories: endometrial hyperplasia with cellular atypia and endometrial hyperplasia without cellular atypia. Twenty-five percent of women with hyperplasia and atypia either harbor foci of endometrial carcinoma or will develop endometrial carcinoma in the future. In contradistinction, the risk of endometrial cancer is much smaller, less than 2% for women with endometrial hyperplasia without atypia. Women with endometrial hyperplasia usually present with postmenopausal bleeding: endometrial hyperplasia accounts for up to 8% of cases of postmenopausal bleeding.[113]

Endometrial hyperplasia usually images as diffuse widening of the endometrium on T2-weighted images. The signal intensity of the hyperplastic endometrium is either iso- or hypo-intense relative to normal endometrium (Fig. 92-36). Small, high signal intensity, cystically dilated glands, may be embedded in the thickened endometrium. Following dynamic contrast administration, endometrial hyperplasia enhances less than adjacent myometrium. With time, it enhances either in a similar fashion or more than myometrium. If there are cystically dilated glands, the lumina do not enhance after contrast.[114] The cut-off value for normal versus abnormal endometrial width is controversial, but is a function of the patient's hormone status [e.g., premenopausal, postmenopausal with and without hormone replacement therapy (HRT)]. Data from ultrasound series suggest that for symptomatic postmenopausal women (irrespective of HRT status), a bilayer endometrial width greater than 5 mm is abnormal. In asymptomatic, postmenopausal women on HRT, cut-off values range

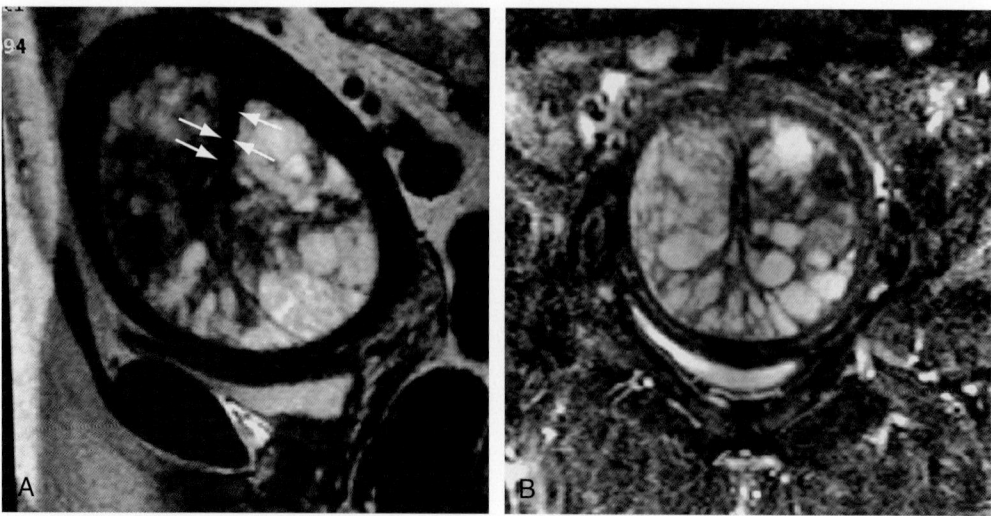

FIGURE 92-35

Tamoxifen-induced polyp. **A,** Sagittal and **B,** coronal T2-weighted fast spin-echo images show a large heterogeneous tamoxifen-induced polyp distending the endometrial cavity. Note the low signal intensity stalk posteriorly (*arrows* on **A**). The polyp was benign at histopathology.

between less than 5 to greater than 8 mm. For premenopausal women, a bilayer endometrial width greater than 8 mm during the proliferative and greater than 16 mm during the secretory phase is considered abnormal.[115]

The MRI appearance of endometrial hyperplasia is nonspecific. Secretory endometria, endometrial polyps, and noninvasive (stage IA) endometrial carcinomas may image similarly. If the diagnosis of endometrial hyperplasia is raised in a premenopausal woman, correlation with the patient's menstrual cycle is important for deciding if a normal secretory endometrium is responsible for apparent endometrial widening. Endometrial polyps are usually more focal and masslike, but may mimic focal endometrial hyperplasia. Identification of a stalk, when present, distinguishes an endometrial polyp from hyperplasia. Endometrial carcinoma is usually lower in signal intensity to normal endometrium on T2-weighted images and enhances less than myometrium following contrast. If there is evidence of myometrial invasion, the diagnosis of carcinoma can be made with confidence.

Ultrasound, both TVS and sonohysterography, are the first line modalities for screening for endometrial pathology. If diffuse or focal endometrial widening is identified, patients undergo office pipelle biopsy or hysteroscopic biopsy/resection, respectively. MRI may be reserved for patients with an inconclusive ultrasound and/or those who have cervical stenosis precluding biopsy. Once the diagnosis of endometrial hyperplasia is made, treatment depends on the type of hyperplasia. For women without atypia, a trial of progesterone therapy followed by TVS and endometrial biopsy is undertaken. For women with atypia, the risk of coexistant and/or future carcinoma is high enough that hysterectomy is recommended.[113]

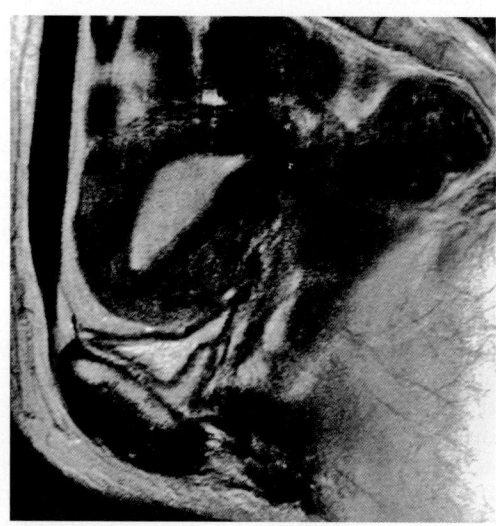

FIGURE 92-36

Endometrial hyperplasia. Sagittal T2-weighted fast spin-echo image shows the endometrial canal to be widened with intermediate signal intensity. These findings are nonspecific as endometrial hyperplasia, endometrial polyps, and stage IA endometrial cancer all image similarly.

Endometrial Synechiae

Endometrial synechiae are bridging myometrial adhesions that form in response to trauma (e.g., post curettage), infection, and/or inflammation. Predisposing factors for developing synechiae are a gravid uterus, infection, and/or missed abortion. When severe, Asherman's syndrome with complete or near complete obliteration

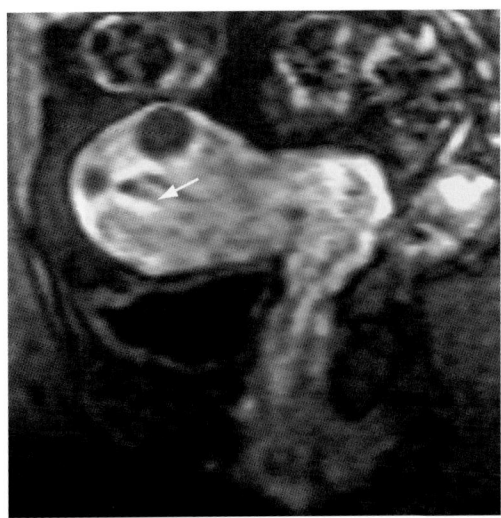

FIGURE 92-37

Endometrial synechia. Sagittal contrast-enhanced T1-weighted fat-suppressed volume-interpolated breath-hold examination demonstrates an enhancing linear adhesion traversing the endometrial cavity (*arrow*) consistent with an endometrial synechia.

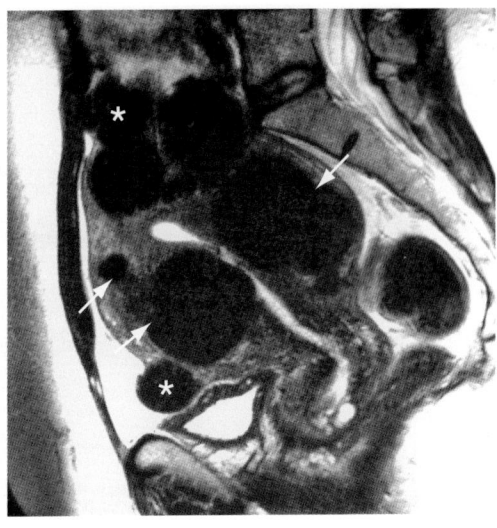

FIGURE 92-38

Subserosal and intramural fibroids. Sagittal T2-weighted fast spin-echo image shows multiple, low signal intensity, well circumscribed fibroids in both subserosal (*) and intramural (*arrows*) locations.

of the of the uterine cavity results. Infertility, recurrent pregnancy loss, and amenorrhea characterize this syndrome.[116]

Endometrial synechiae image as low signal intensity bands that traverse the endometrial cavity on T2-weighted images and enhance after administration of contrast, especially in the early phase (Fig. 92-37).

Hysterosalpingography followed by hysteroscopy are the primary modalities to diagnose and treat synechiae, respectively. MRI is complementary; it provides information on the etiology of synechiae.[117] Additionally, MRI provides a global image of the uterus and offers information on the uterine cavity above the adhesions; this area is a blind spot for hysteroscopy. Specifically, MRI can detect the presence of endometrial remnants above the adhesions which has both therapeutic and prognostic significance.[118]

Leiomyomas

Leiomyomas, or fibroids, are benign neoplasms and are the most common tumor of the female genital tract, occurring in up to 25% of the female population older than 35 years. They are composed of smooth muscle cells arranged in a whorl-like pattern with a variable amount of collagen, extracellular matrix, and fibrous tissue. Leiomyomas are well demarcated by a pseudocapsule of areolar tissue.[119,120] Risk factors for the presence of leiomyomas are younger age at menarche, higher education, obesity as well as race (African-American women having a two-fold relative risk). Lower risk has been suggested with increasing parity, tobacco abuse and, in some studies, oral contraceptive use.[121-124] Leiomyomas are classified according to their location within the

uterine corpus: intramural (the most common), submucosal (the most symptomatic), or subserosal. They may also occur, albeit less frequently, in the uterine cervix, broad ligament, or completely detached from the genital tract where they parasitize pelvic and/or abdominal vasculature (e.g., the omentum).[125] Estrogen stimulates and progesterone inhibits their growth and therefore leiomyomas decrease in size after menopause, but may increase in size during pregnancy.[126,127] As leiomyomas enlarge, they may outgrow their blood supply and degenerate. Types of degeneration include hemorrhagic or carneous, hyaline, fatty, cystic or much less likely, sarcomatous. Rarely, leiomyomas undergo sarcomatous degeneration (<2%) and while this is a rare event, it bears keeping in mind for women who fail conservative therapies for symptomatic fibroids. Leiomyomas may also calcify, especially in older women

The symptoms associated with leiomyomas may be protean, though most women are generally asymptomatic. The most common symptom is bleeding; however, pressure effects, infertility, fetal wastage, dystocia, and a palpable mass do occur. Rarely, leiomyomas may torse or become infected. Acute pain is usually a manifestation of acute degeneration that may result from torsion of a pedunculated subserosal leiomyoma, infarction of a leiomyoma during pregnancy, or prolapse of a submucosal leiomyoma.[119]

Leiomyomas are most conspicuous on T2-weighted images and appear as sharply marginated, low signal intensity masses relative to the myometrium (lesions as small as 0.5 cm are routinely imaged).[128] Orthogonal images allow for accurate localization of leiomyomas as submucosal, intramural, or subserosal (Fig. 92-38). MRI is even able to reliably identify the stalk in a prolapsed submucosal leiomyoma (Fig. 92-39). This is important

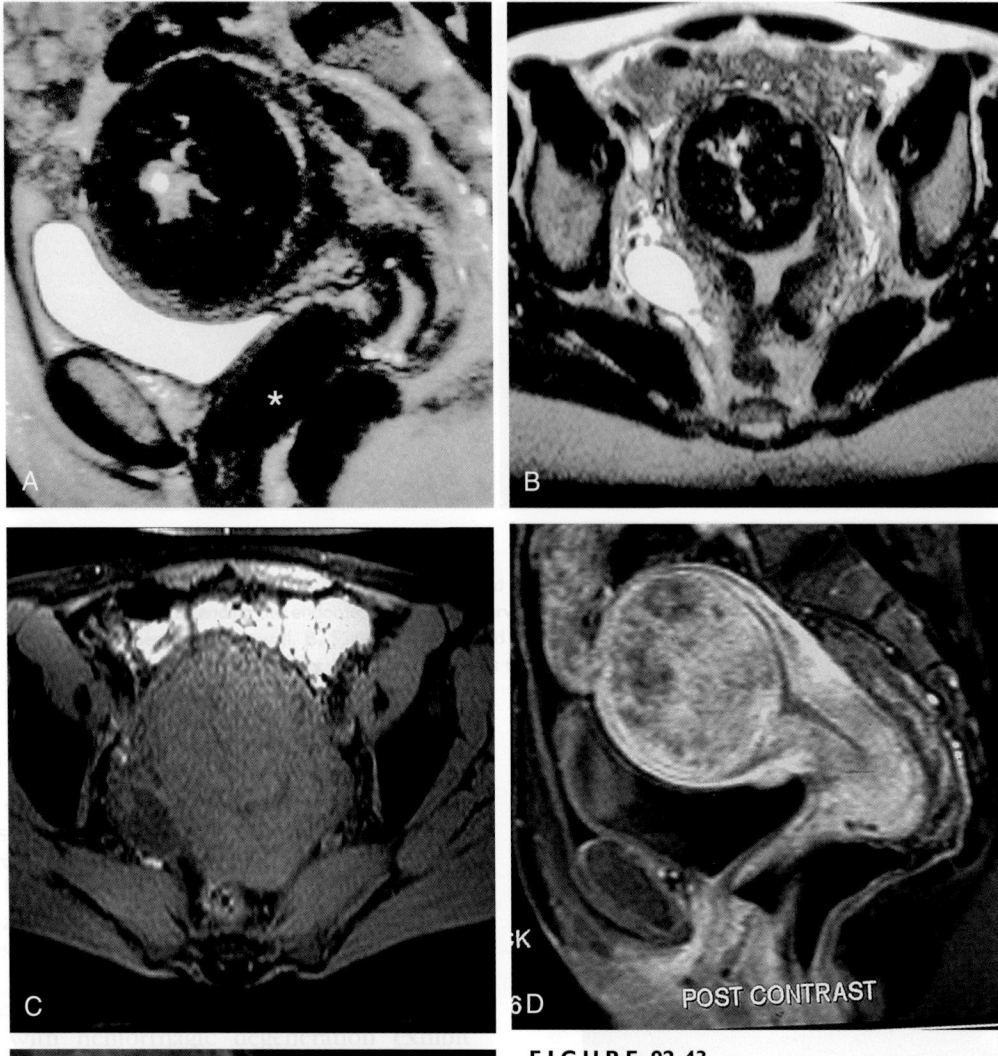

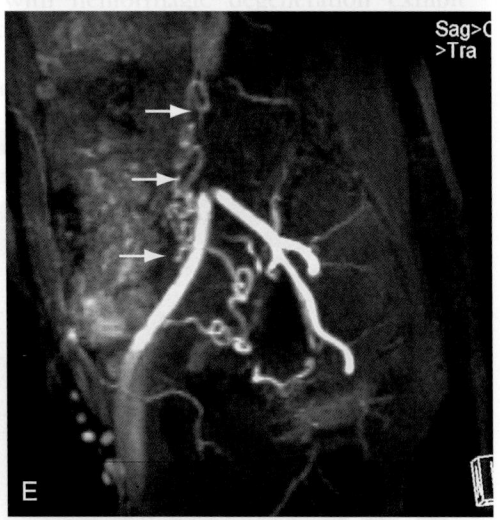

FIGURE 92-43

Fibroid, pre-uterine artery embolization (UAE) evaluation. **A,** Sagittal and **B,** axial T2-weighted single-shot fast spin-echo; **C,** axial T1-weighted fat-suppressed spoiled gradient-echo; **D,** sagittal contrast-enhanced T1-weighted fat-suppressed volume-interpolated breath-hold examination; and **E,** Sagittal maximum intensity projection (MIP) MR angiography images in a candidate for UAE. There is a single, large intramural fibroid with a submucosal component. The fibroid is heterogeneous on T2 images suggesting some form of degeneration. That the fibroid is isointense to myometrium on the T1 image, excludes hemorrhagic degeneration. The fibroid enhances post contrast. Note the unilateral ovarian artery seen on the MR angiogram (*arrows* in **E**). The patient should be counseled that despite a technical success, she may not achieve a complete clinical success, may not have a durable response, and/or may risk embolization of her ovary on that side. Incidental note is made of a tampon in the endovaginal canal (* in **A**)

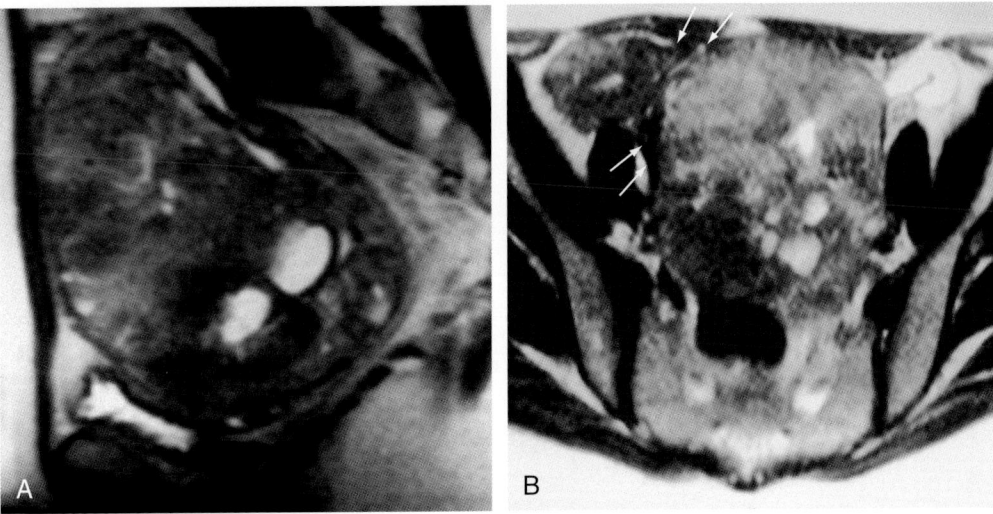

FIGURE 92-44

Subserosal fibroid. **A,** Sagittal T2-weighted single-shot fast spin-echo (SSFSE) image shows a large heterogeneous pelvic mass, but its location is difficult to ascertain. **B,** Axial T2-weighted SSFSE image shows the mass originates from the left uterine corpus as evidenced by a claw of myometrium along its anterior and right aspects (*arrows*). This constellation of findings is consistent with a degenerated subserosal fibroid.

nondiagnostic or equivocal ultrasound.[133] Specifically, an intermediate signal intensity mass on T1-weighted images that is low in signal intensity on T2-weighted images and splays the uterine serosa or myometrium allows the diagnosis of leiomyoma to be made with confidence (Fig. 92-44). The presence of feeding vessels originating in the myometrium further supports the uterine origin of the mass. However, if a mass is adjacent to the uterus and is of intermediate or high signal intensity relative to the myometrium on T2-weighted images, the differential diagnosis includes both degenerated leiomyoma and extrauterine tumors (benign and malignant). In these patients, the diagnosis of leiomyoma should be reserved only for cases where the uterine origin of the mass is firmly established. Occasionally, it may be difficult to distinguish a pedunculated subserosal leiomyoma from an ovarian fibroma. This distinction is likely not significant as the latter is rarely malignant.[120,128] Submucosal leiomyomas are usually distinguished from endometrial polyps by identifying their myometrial origin and low signal intensity on T2-weighted images. Submucosal leiomyomas must also be distinguished from adenomyomas. This topic will be covered in the following section on adenomyosis. Finally, myometrial contractions may mimic both submucosal leiomyomas and adenomyomas. Contractions image as low signal intensity within the myometrium that deform the endometrium while sparing the outer uterine contour.[18,134] Their low signal intensity may be a function of regional decrease in perfusion. Myometrial contractions are distinguished from leiomyomas by noting the transient and changing appearance on subsequent T2-weighted sequences after the initial T2-weighted sequence.[18,134]

Malignant degeneration of a leiomyoma is a rare occurrence. Unfortunately, signal characteristics do not reliably distinguish a benign leiomyoma from a leiomyomosarcoma. However, if a leiomyoma suddenly enlarges, especially after the menopause, and/or has a shaggy or indistinct border, the possibility of sarcomatous transformation should be raised.

In patients with suspected leiomyomas, imaging is used to detect, localize, and characterize the tumors. TVS continues to be the initial imaging modality in evaluating these patients[135,136] however, there are instances where a more thorough analysis is warranted and MRI is the most accurate modality to diagnose leiomyomas. Specifically, a more sophisticated analysis of their number, size, location, and vascularity may be needed to help identify appropriate patients for uterine-conserving alternatives to hysterectomy: myomectomy (hysteroscopic approach versus laparoscopic approach for pedunculated submucosal and subserosal leiomyomas, respectively), UAE, and hormonal manipulation. Additionally, TVS can be hampered by its limited FOV, patient's body habitus, and/or distorted anatomy secondary to large and/or multiple leiomyomas.[137,138] While TVS has superior spatial resolution compared to transabdominal ultrasound, leiomyomas of less than 2 cm may not be routinely identified, even when symptomatic.[139] Finally, there are cases where ultrasound is equivocal or non-diagnostic for either identifying comorbid conditions such as adenomyosis which may cause or contribute to the patient's symptoms, and/or determining the origin of a pelvic mass (pedunculated subserosal leiomyoma versus solid ovarian mass).[133,140] Therefore, MRI is indicated in cases where a more complete evaluation of suspected leiomyomas is needed and as a problem-solving tool in cases with inconclusive ultrasound results.[129,133,137,141]

UAE is gaining momentum as an alternative to hysterectomy. It is attractive because not only is the

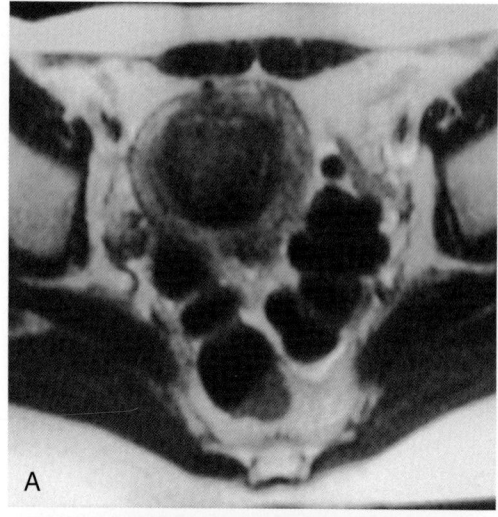

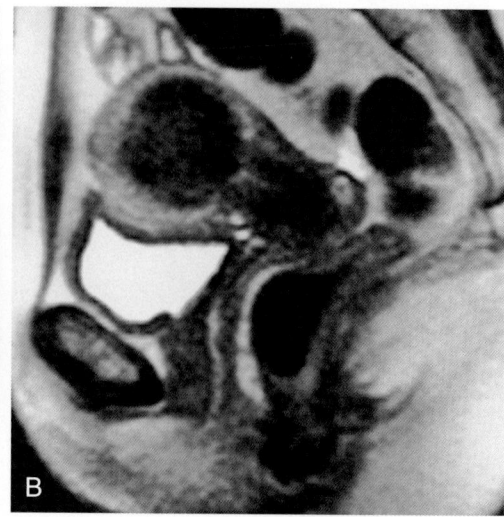

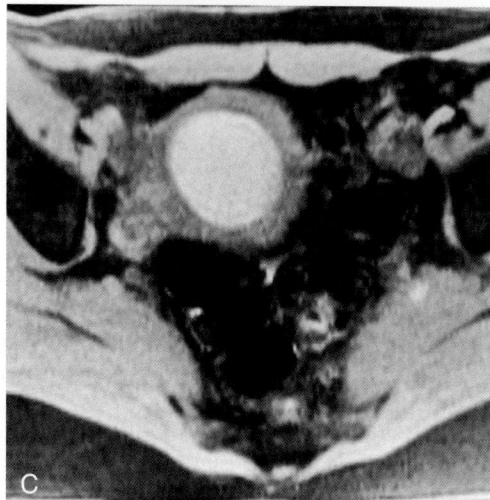

FIGURE 92-45

Cellular fibroid post uterine artery embolization (UAE). **A,** Axial and **B,** sagittal images of a cellular fibroid following UAE show the fibroid to be smaller with homogenous low signal intensity in contrast to its high signal intensity before embolization (see Fig. 92-42). **C,** Axial T1-weighted fat-suppressed spoiled gradient-echo image shows the fibroid to have high signal intensity. This constellation of imaging findings is compatible with hemorrhagic infarction.

uterus preserved while the fibroid undergoes hemorrhagic infarction, but the time to return to full activity post UAE is significantly shorter than with hysterectomy (8 versus 42 days) (Fig. 92-45).[142,143] To date, more than 25,000 procedures have been performed worldwide.[144] Studies of women post UAE have reported a significant decrease in both uterine and dominant-fibroid volumes as well as a concomitant decrease in bleeding and bulk-related symptoms (Fig. 92-46).[142,145-151] In one of the largest studies of 200 consecutive women who underwent UAE, Spies et al[142] reported improvement of bleeding and bulk symptoms in 90% and 91% of patients, respectively, at 1 year after therapy. Another study by the same team of investigators documented a 33.5% reduction in uterine volume and a 40.4% reduction in leiomyoma volume post UAE.[148] These changes appear to be durable in the majority of patients to at least 2 years, with smaller studies reporting longer durability after therapy. It is important to note that while the embolized leiomyomas undergo hemorrhagic infarction, myometrial perfusion is maintained despite a transient decrease immediately after UAE.[152,153] Similarly, ovarian function is overwhelmingly preserved in the majority of patients.[142]

While complications are rare, minor ones that require little or no intervention include hematoma, transient recurrent pain, leiomyoma passage, and phlebitis. More significant complications such as endometritis necessitating hysterectomy, tubo-ovarian abscess, pulmonary embolism, and deep venous thrombosis have also been reported (Fig. 92-47).[145,149,150] A cost-effectiveness study of UAE and hysterectomy for fibroids found that UAE is a cost-effective alternative across a wide range of assumptions about the costs and effectiveness of the two procedures, though the study test results were sensitive to changes in quality-of-life values.[154]

Most practices consider a desire to get pregnant a contraindication to UAE, however; Ravina et al[155] published a series of 12 pregnancies in 9 patients after UAE. Seven of these pregnancies were carried to term and five ended in miscarriage. Our own experience includes several patients who had term pregnancies following UAE. Although Ravina et al's small study coupled with ours and other investigators' anecdotal experiences is encouraging, myomectomy remains the standard of care for women with symptomatic leiomyomas who desire to become pregnant.

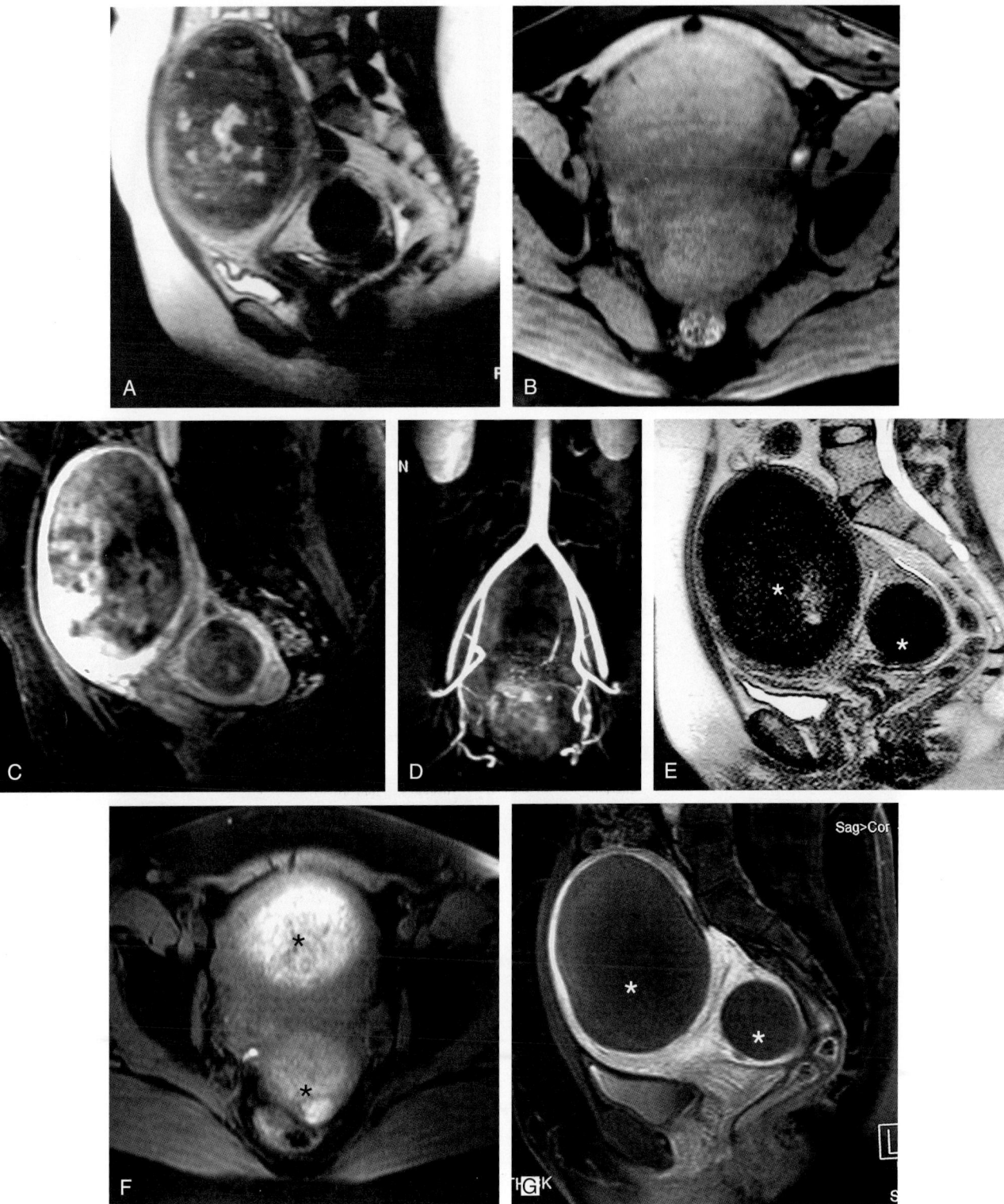

FIGURE 92-46

Fibroids pre and post uterine artery embolization (UAE). **A,** Sagittal T2-weighted single-shot fast spin-echo (SSFSE); **B,** axial T1-weighted fat-suppressed spoiled gradient-echo (SGE); **C,** sagittal contrast-enhanced T1-weighted fat-suppressed volume-interpolated breath-hold examination (VIBE); and **D,** coronal maximum intensity projection (MIP) MR angiography before UAE show two intramural fibroids. The fibroids enhance following contrast and there is no significant ovarian arterial supply to the uterus. **E,** Sagittal T2-weighted SSFSE; **F,** axial T1-weighted fat-suppressed SGE; and **G,** sagittal contrast-enhanced T1-weighted fat-suppressed VIBE after UAE show interval decrease in fibroid size, interval increase in signal intensity on T1-weighted fat-suppressed technique, and interval devascularization consistent with hemorrhagic infarction (* in **E-G**).

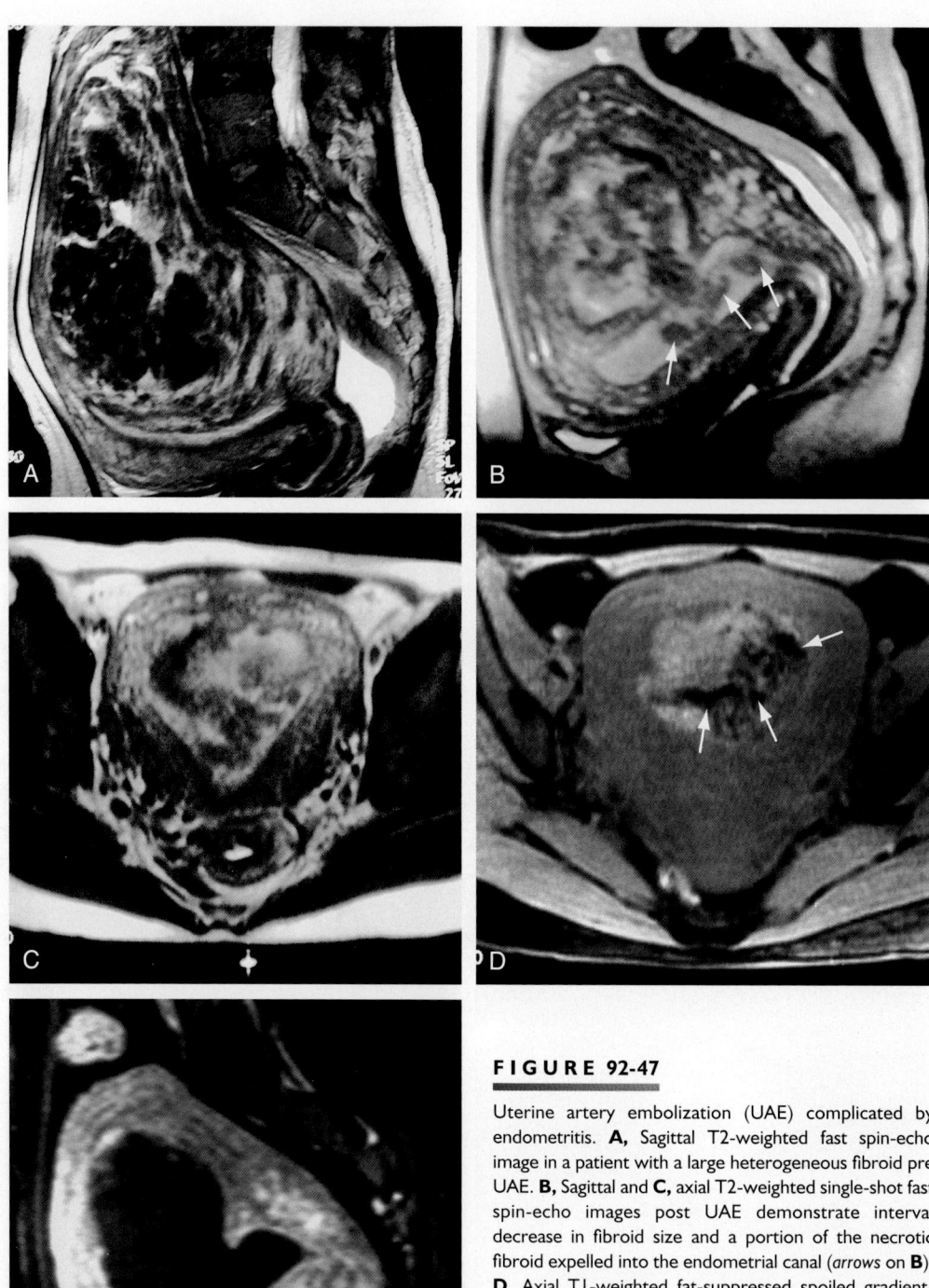

FIGURE 92-47

Uterine artery embolization (UAE) complicated by endometritis. **A,** Sagittal T2-weighted fast spin-echo image in a patient with a large heterogeneous fibroid pre UAE. **B,** Sagittal and **C,** axial T2-weighted single-shot fast spin-echo images post UAE demonstrate interval decrease in fibroid size and a portion of the necrotic fibroid expelled into the endometrial canal (*arrows* on **B**). **D,** Axial T1-weighted fat-suppressed spoiled gradient-echo image shows mixed signal within the endometrial canal—high signal of blood products and susceptibility artifact (*arrows*) from gas associated with an acute super-infection and endometritis. **E,** Sagittal contrast-enhanced T1-weighted fat-suppressed volume-interpolated breath-hold examination image confirms hemorrhagic infarction as evidenced by absent enhancement of the fibroid.

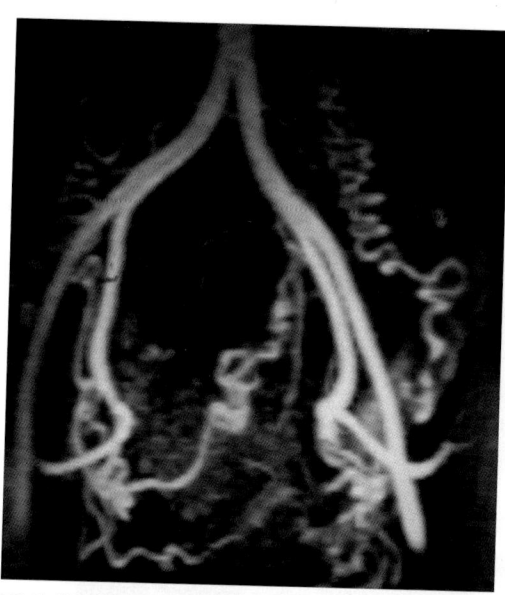

FIGURE 92-48

Bilateral ovarian arterial supply to the uterus. Coronal maximum intensity projection (MIP) MR angiogram highlights bilateral ovarian arteries supplying the uterus. This feature may result in uterine artery embolization failure or a nondurable result.

mi
on
Ni
wa
sig
zo
92
ar
ac
a
ai
U
U
w
fc
t
a
f
t
v

Leiomyoma hypervascularity correlates with a good response post UAE.[148] In contradistinction, leiomyomas with negligible enhancement and high signal intensity on T1-weighted sequences do not respond to UAE. These imaging features suggest that these leiomyomas have already undergone hemorrhagic infarction and as such, patients derive no further benefit from embolizing an already infarcted leiomyoma. In addition to information regarding leiomyoma vascularity, 3D contrast-enhanced images provide angiographic information. Specifically, pre-UAE MR angiograms are helpful for identifying patients with leiomyomas supplied by parasitized ovarian arteries (Fig. 92-48). These patients may not respond to UAE and/or do not have durable results as evidenced by revascularization and regrowth of their tumor; such patients may benefit from retreatment or alternative treatments (Fig. 92-49).[156-158]

Adenomyosis

Adenomyosis is the presence of ectopic endometrial glands and stroma embedded within the myometrium. The ectopic glands and stroma are often accompanied by myometrial hyperplasia. Morphologically adenomyosis exists in two forms: diffuse and focal.[159,160] The presence of adenomyosis in hysterectomy specimens varies between 19% and 62%.[159] This wide range likely relates to differences in pathologic criteria for determining what constitutes an ectopic endometrial gland. That is, clinicians and pathologists distinguish between superficial and deep adenomyosis.[161,162] Superficial

adenomyosis is defined as islands of ectopic glands and stroma that reside within several millimeters of the zona basalis of the endometrium; in fact, this may be a normal finding as women with this condition are usually asymptomatic. In contrast, the ectopic endometrial glands and stroma of deep adenomyosis are flagrant histologically and correlate with patients' symptoms and uterine enlargement. The adenomyotic endometrial glands do not typically undergo cyclical bleeding. This reflects the predominance of endometrial zona basale in adenomyosis—zona basale is relatively refractive to the cyclic hormonal milieu. Cystic adenomyosis is a subcategory of either focal or diffuse disease. In these instances, there is extensive hemorrhage within ectopic endometrial glands.

Adenomyosis is a common gynecologic disorder that affects women during their reproductive and perimenopausal years, in the fifth and sixth decades. Symptoms include pelvic pain, menorrhagia, and dysmenorrhea of increasing severity.[159,160] The etiology is unknown, though one report suggests a hereditary component.[163] The uterus in women with adenomyosis is frequently enlarged and globular. Women with cystic adenomyosis may present with a palpable mass. While the signs and symptoms of adenomyosis mimic other conditions, such as leiomyomas, endometriosis, and dysfunctional uterine bleeding, the importance of making the correct preoperative diagnosis is not trivial. Whereas leiomyomas are amenable to minimally invasive therapies, hysterectomy is curative for symptomatic women and is the mainstay of treatment. GnRH analog, endometrial ablation, and even UAE are currently under investigation for the treatment of adenomyosis.[159,160,164]

T2-weighted sequences that highlight uterine zonal anatomy are used to diagnose adenomyosis. The diagnostic criteria include: 1. focal or diffuse widening of the low signal intensity junctional zone; or 2. an ill-defined low signal intensity myometrial mass.[165-167] Cut-off values for junctional zone width to distinguish patients with from patients without adenomyosis vary between 6 and 12 mm (Fig. 92-50). Based on a retrospective receiver operating characteristic curve (ROC) analysis, Reinhold et al[168] reported that the optimal junctional zone value for the diagnosis of adenomyosis is greater than or equal to 12 mm. A junctional zone width of less than or equal to 8 mm reliably excludes the disease, whereas a junctional zone width of 9 to 11 mm is equivocal. In the latter instance, ancillary findings may aid diagnosis. Ancillary findings in adenomyosis include: 1. poorly defined margins; 2. high signal intensity foci on T1- or T2-weighted sequences; and 3. linear high signal intensity striations radiating out from the endometrial surface. These striations are thought to represent direct invasion of the endometrial zona basale into the underlying myometrium (Fig. 99-51). That adenomyosis images as low signal intensity on T2-weighted images is not surprising; the low signal intensity is a function of the associated smooth muscle hyperplasia. The hypertrophied smooth muscle is so densely packed that it resembles the innermost portion of the myometrium, the histopathologic correlate of the junctional zone.[166] The high signal

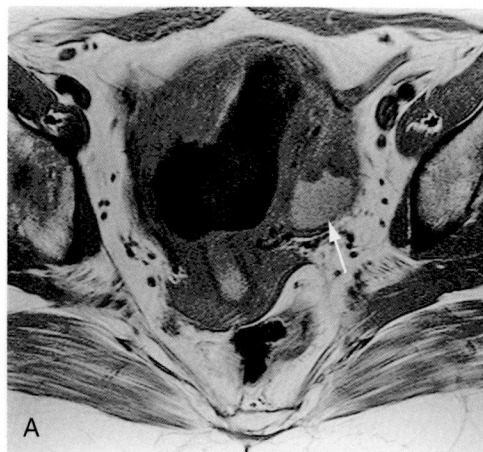
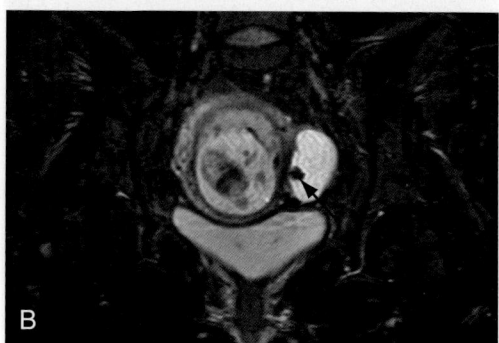

FIGURE 92-56

Hemorrhagic corpus luteum cyst. **A,** Axial T1 SE image demonstrates hyperintense cyst contents in the dependent portion of a left adnexal cyst (arrow) which may be secondary to hemorrhagic products or proteinaceous fluid. **B,** Coronal STIR image demonstrates low signal intensity debris (arrow) within the corpus luteum cyst. The cyst had resolved completely on follow-up ultrasound. (Courtesy of Deborah Levine, MD, Beth Israel Deaconess Medical Center, Boston.)

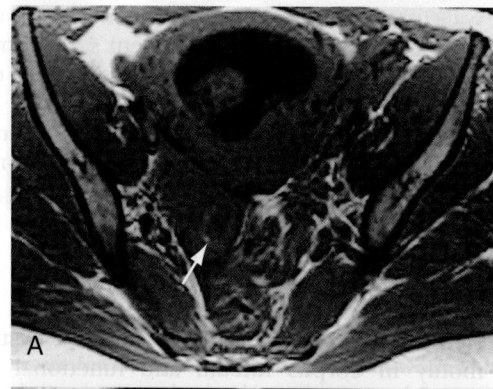
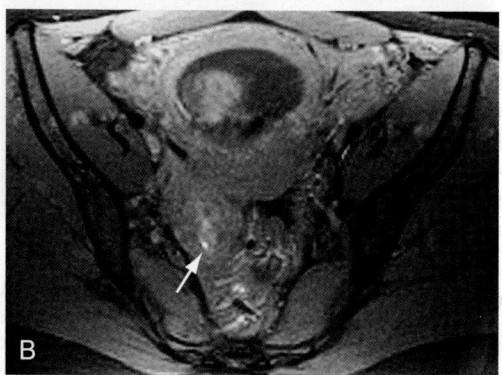
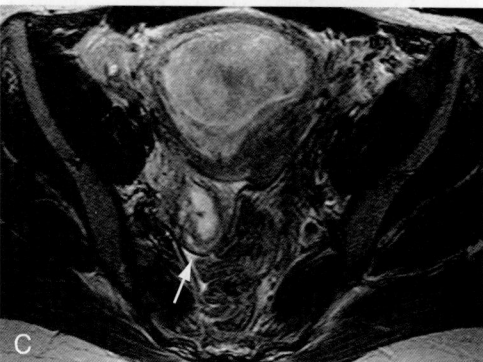

FIGURE 92-57

Hemorrhagic corpus luteum cyst presenting as a complex adnexal mass. **A,** Axial T1-weighted spin-echo image demonstrates a complex right adnexal mass with heterogeneous signal intensity (arrow). **B,** On axial T1-weighted spoiled gradient-echo image with fat saturation high signal intensity foci persist (arrow), confirming hemorrhage into the lesion. **C,** On axial T2-weighted turbo spin-echo the mass appears as heterogeneous signal intensity (arrow). Follow-up ultrasound demonstrated resolution of the mass consistent with corpus luteum of pregnancy. (Courtesy of Deborah Levine, MD, Beth Israel Deaconess Medical Center, Boston.)

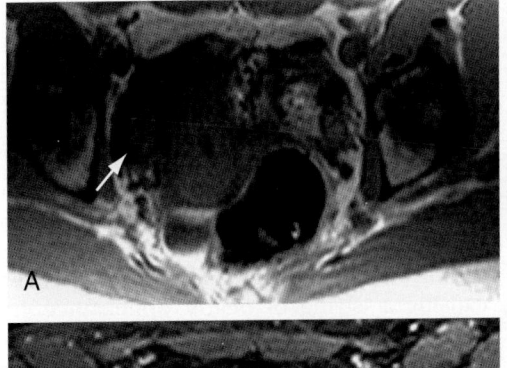
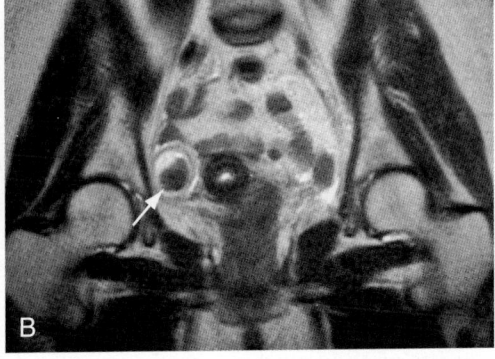
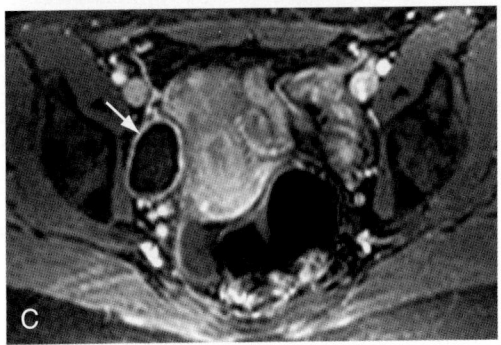

FIGURE 92-58

Hemorrhagic cyst. **A,** Axial T1-weighted spin-echo image demonstrates a mass of heterogeneous signal intensity in the right ovary with areas of high signal intensity (*arrow*) consistent with hemorrhagic products or proteinaceous fluid, as the high signal intensity foci persisted on T1-weighted fast spin-echo images (not shown). **B,** On coronal T2-weighted turbo spin-echo imaging an eccentric focus of low signal intensity is seen within the lesion consistent with a retracted clot (*arrow*)

C, Axial contrast-enhanced 3D fast spin T1-weighted gradient-recalled echo image confirms the absence of internal enhancement within the cyst. Note the thin enhancing wall (*arrow*) with no solid enhancing nodules.

Hemorrhagic cysts are treated conservatively if no underlying mass is noted on MRI or if no other underlying condition, such as ovarian torsion or rupture, that may require surgical intervention is diagnosed in a clinically unstable patient. Follow-up ultrasound is performed 6 weeks following the initial examination preferably in the first week after menstruation to allow time for resolution of the cyst and to avoid confusion with new physiologic cysts.[179]

Hyperreactio Luteinalis

Hyperreactio luteinalis represents ovarian enlargement due to multiple luteinized follicle cysts. This results from abnormal human chorionic gonadotropin (hCG) stimulation. It is believed to be due either to hypersensitivity of the ovary to normal circulating amounts of hCG or to elevated hCG. The latter include gestational trophoblastic disease, multiple gestations, fetal hydrops, and otherwise normal pregnancy with hyperstimulation syndrome.[190] Clinical presentation includes abdominal pain and distention, abnormal liver function tests, shortness of breath, as well as hirsutism, but is generally much milder than that seen in ovarian hyperstimulation syndrome. Severe fluid depletion from ascites and pleural effusion are, in contrast to ovarian hyperstimulation syndrome, not part of the disease process. Patients are usually asymptomatic and lesions are discovered incidentally on imaging studies or during surgery. Abdominal pain occurs with hemorrhage into one of the cysts.

Hyperreactio luteinalis resolves spontaneously after delivery. In an otherwise normal pregnancy, the differential diagnosis for an enlarged ovary with multiple cysts

(Fig. 92-59) includes neoplastic processes such as multiloculated cystic neoplasia or struma ovarii.[191] The clinical history, rapid growth of the ovaries, and bilaterality of the process in hyperstimulation syndrome and hyperreactio luteinalis usually avoid confusion with these entities. In addition, the cysts in multilocular cystic neoplasia are of variable size and shape,[192] in contrast to a uniform

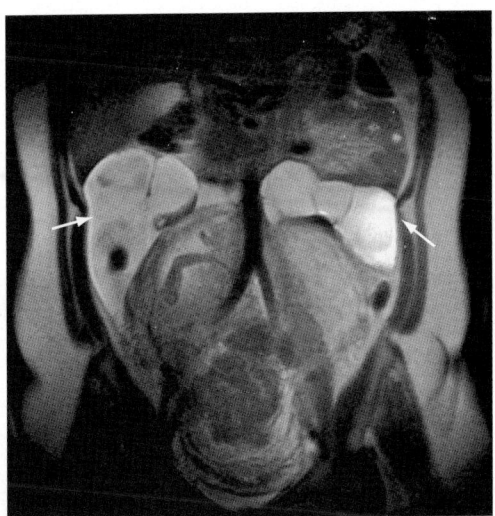

FIGURE 92-59

Hyperreactio luteinalis in a patient with an otherwise normal pregnancy. On this coronal T2-weighted HASTE image, bilateral enlarged ovaries with multiple cysts of uniform size are noted (*arrows*). (*Courtesy of Deborah Levine, MD, Beth Israel Deaconess Medical Center, Boston.*)

appearance in the benign entities. MRI can be used to exclude ancillary signs of malignancy such as peritoneal implants or lymphadenopathy.

Ovarian Hyperstimulation Syndrome

Hyperstimulated ovaries occur as a complication of ovulation induction. The ovaries are enlarged and contain multiple cysts. While a mild version of the syndrome has been demonstrated in up to 65% of patients undergoing ovulation induction,[175] only 0.2% to 0.3% of patients develop a severe form requiring hospitalization. Clinical presentation consists of abdominal pain and distention, nausea and vomiting or diarrhea. Exudation of fluid can cause ascites and pleural effusions with hemoconcentration, impaired renal function, and coagulation disorders.

The ovaries are diffusely enlarged and demonstrate multiple large cysts of uniform size varying from 1 to 3 cm with low signal intensity on T1-weighted images and high signal intensity on T2-weighted images (Fig. 92-60). Cysts have a thin wall that can enhance. Signal intensity of the cysts can vary due to internal hemorrhage.[193] Ascites or intraperitoneal hemorrhage can occur from fluid secreted by the ovaries.

Treatment is conservative as about 90% of hyperstimulated ovaries resolve spontaneously later in pregnancy or following delivery. If ascites is present, ultrasound-guided paracentesis may be beneficial. However, the syndrome can be complicated by ovarian hemorrhage, torsion or rupture, which may require surgical intervention.

Polycystic Ovarian Syndrome

Polycystic ovarian disease or Stein-Leventhal syndrome is a clinical diagnosis consisting of oligomenorrhea or amenorrhea and infertility in conjunction with bilaterally enlarged ovaries on physical examination. Obesity and hirsutism are commonly associated with the disease but are not a prerequisite for making the diagnosis. While follicle-stimulating hormone and estrogen levels are normal, luteinizing hormone is elevated with no luteinizing hormone surge. The syndrome is seen in up to 50% of patients in infertility clinics and involves approximately 3.5% to 7% of the female population.

Classic sonographic and MRI features are bilateral ovarian enlargement with multiple (10 or more) small peripheral follicles of uniform size, measuring 2 to 18 mm in diameter. Two patterns of cyst distribution have been described.[194,195] In the peripheral cystic pattern, the cysts are present beneath the ovarian capsule causing a "string of pearls" appearance. In the general cystic pattern, the cysts can be seen in both the subcapsular and stromal parts of the ovary and can vary in size. The cysts are uniformly of high signal intensity on T2-weighted images. Abundant medullary stroma is depicted as broad central areas of low T1 and T2 signal intensity. However, less than 50% of patients with the disease exhibit these distinctive findings on MRI. In approximately 30% of patients, the ovaries are normal in size.

The diagnosis is typically made by clinical features and laboratory analysis. The diagnosis can be confirmed with ultrasound when bilaterally enlarged ovaries with small peripheral follicles are visualized. While MRI has been shown to be superior to ultrasound in demonstrating the typical appearance of this disease,[196] it has played no role in the evaluation of patients suspected of polycystic ovarian syndrome. However, the ovarian findings may be seen incidentally on MRI. Caution is necessary in the interpretation of these findings out of clinical context, as MRI findings typical of polycystic ovarian syndrome have been noted in asymptomatic women.[197]

Benign Ovarian Neoplasms

Ovarian tumors are classified by the cell type of origin, such as surface epithelial, germ cell, or stromal tumors. Approximately 80% of ovarian tumors are benign. The

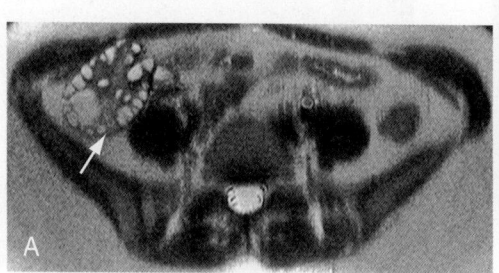
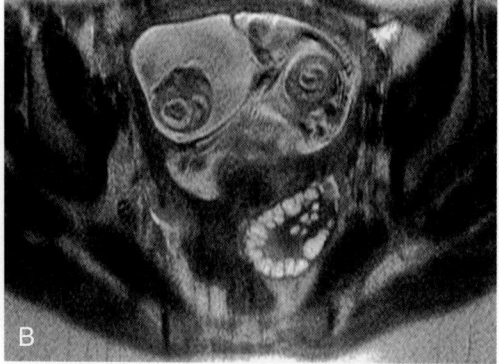

FIGURE 92-60

Ovarian hyperstimulation syndrome in a patient who underwent ovulation induction. **A,** Axial HASTE image at the level of the iliac crest demonstrates an enlarged right ovary with multiple cysts of uniform size (*arrow*). **B,** Axial HASTE image at the level of the uterus demonstrates a similar appearance of the left ovary. (*Courtesy of Deborah Levine, MD, Beth Israel Deaconess Medical Center, Boston.*)

clinical presentation is nonspecific and is due to a mass effect of enlarging tumors. Urinary frequency, constipation, or pelvic pressure may be present. Larger lesions can cause abdominal pain or swelling, abnormal uterine bleeding, nausea and vomiting or weight loss. If the lesions are complicated by torsion, hemorrhage or rupture, they can present with acute abdominal pain.[20]

Surface Epithelial Tumors

Serous and mucinous tumors are the most common surface epithelial tumors and account for 45% to 50% of all benign ovarian neoplasms. While 50% to 70% of all serous neoplasms are benign, the percentage is even higher in mucinous tumors where 75% to 85% are benign. Bilateral tumors are noted in 20% of serous and 2% to 3% of mucinous tumors. Calcifications can be present. In the postmenopausal population, serous cystadenomas represent 80% of benign lesions.[179]

Serous cystadenomas are most commonly unilocular and fluid filled with a thin wall. They can be multilocular, in which case the depicted septations are thin (Fig. 92-61). Tumor size can reach 30 cm with a mean diameter of 10 cm. Usually the cysts contain simple fluid with low signal intensity on T1- and high signal intensity on T2-weighted images. However, signal intensities may vary as the tumors are rarely entirely solid, or the cyst contents can be complex due to high protein content or hemorrhage. On T1-weighted images after the administration of gadolinium, the cyst wall and septa enhance. However, no enhancing solid component is identified.

In contrast, mucinous cystadenomas are multilocular containing many small daughter cysts. Occasionally, they may appear as a unilocular cyst difficult to differentiate from a functional cyst. They can be larger than serous cystadenomas reaching 50 cm in size. The cyst content contains thick, mucinous material with high signal intensity on T1- and low signal intensity on T2-weighted images. The loculations in these cysts vary in signal intensity, giving a "stained glass" appearance.[198]

In ovarian cystadenofibromas, multiloculated cystic ovarian masses, cyst formation, and edema can be noted. Cysts may be central or peripheral and can be distinguished from necrosis by their thin wall and smooth appearance. These areas are identified on T2-weighted images as foci of high signal intensity.[199] The fibrous part of the tumor can vary in size from 2 mm to 4 cm and can be present in the form of a rim, plaque, or nodule.

An interesting feature still under investigation is the variation in apparent diffusion coefficients in the cystic components of ovarian lesions. While some investigators have demonstrated ovarian cysts and serous cystadenomas to exhibit higher apparent diffusion coefficients than malignant cystic ovarian lesions,[200] others could not establish a difference between benign and malignant lesions.[201,202]

The diagnosis of cystadenoma is usually made by ultrasound. MRI is helpful for the evaluation of indeterminate adnexal masses noted on ultrasound due to its superior tissue characterization and evaluation of possible malignant features of an adnexal mass.[203,204] MRI is also helpful in determining the origin of a lesion as intra- or extra-ovarian with an accuracy of 94%, as opposed to 81% by ultrasound.[205]

Diagnosis of a benign ovarian neoplasm should only be made if the lesion is truly simple and none of the following findings concerning for malignancy is present: wall or septa thickness greater than 3 mm and soft-tissue nodules or vegetations. Papillary projections are specific features of epithelial neoplasms.[206] On T2-weighted images they appear as high signal intensity edematous tissue surrounding a fibrous stalk of low signal intensity. The two components are best identified in larger papillary projections; in smaller lesions it may be impossible to discern them. Contrast-enhanced T1-weighted sequences allow distinction of the enhancing papillary projections from nonenhancing debris or intracystic clot. As papillary projections are absent in benign lesions, their presence suggests a malignancy. Ancillary findings raising concern for malignancy are adenopathy, ascites, peritoneal, omental, or mesenteric implants, and involvement of the pelvic side wall.[207,208]

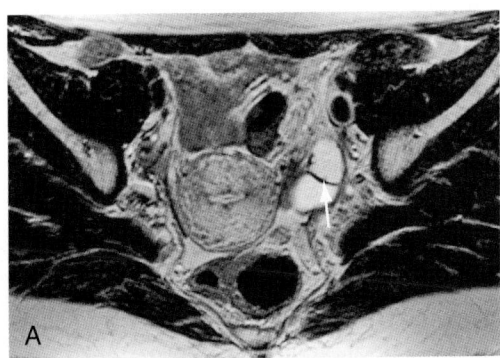
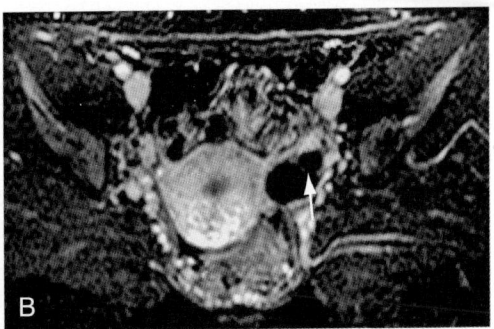

FIGURE 92-61

Serous cystadenoma. **A,** Axial T2-weighted turbo spin-echo image demonstrates a high signal intensity left ovarian mass with a thin septation (*arrow*). **B,** On axial T1 contrast-enhanced volume-interpolated breath-hold examination image there is enhancement of the cyst wall and the thin septation (*arrow*). No enhancing nodules are noted.

Dermoid Tumor

Dermoid cysts are also referred to as mature cystic teratomas and comprise 99% of germ cell tumors and 10% to 15% of ovarian neoplasms. They are the most common tumors in children and young adults but can appear at any age. They are bilateral in 10% to 15% of cases. Dermoid cysts contain all three germ layers; however, the ectodermal layer predominates. On gross pathology, a unilocular cyst filled with sebaceous material is noted. Additional contents of the mass can include fat, hemorrhage, hair, bones, and teeth. These tissues can be scattered diffusely, but demonstrate an orderly organoid arrangement into cutaneous, gastrointestinal, and bronchial tissues. Lesions vary from 0.5 cm to more than 40 cm in size. Malignant conversion to squamous cell carcinoma occurs in 2%[209] and has been described in lesions larger than 10 cm and in postmenopausal women.

Most tumors are discovered incidentally on physical examination, imaging studies, or surgery. If clinical symptoms are present they are often nonspecific and include pelvic pain or pressure, abdominal swelling or mass, and abnormal uterine bleeding. However, dermoid cysts can present with acute abdominal pain when complications are present. The most common complication is ovarian torsion, seen in 16% of cases. Rupture-inducing chemical peritonitis and infection are less frequent.[210]

Classic signal characteristics of dermoid cysts are high signal intensity on T1- and T2-weighted images due to the presence of sebaceous fluid (Fig. 92-62). Occasionally, fluid-fluid and fat-fluid levels can be present. Macroscopic fat is less commonly present. Several sequences can be utilized to document the presence of fat within the lesion and one of these sequences should be performed to differentiate a lesion that is of high signal intensity on non–fat-suppressed T1-weighted images from hemorrhagic cysts or endometriomas.[211-213] T1-weighted images can be obtained with and without proton-selective fat- or water-saturation pulse. Dermoid cysts are of low signal intensity on T1-weighted images with selective fat-saturation pulses (Fig. 92-62)[208,214] and maintain high signal intensity on T1-weighted images obtained with water saturation. Occasionally, a dermoid cyst may not contain fat within the cyst cavity; however, fat may be present in a Rokitansky nodule or the cyst wall or intracellular lipid may be present. In this setting gradient-echo opposed-phase imaging may be helpful in demonstrating focal chemical shift artifacts within the

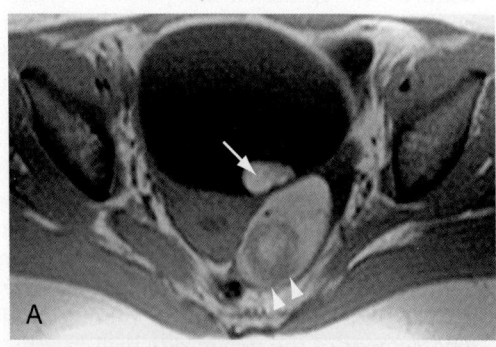
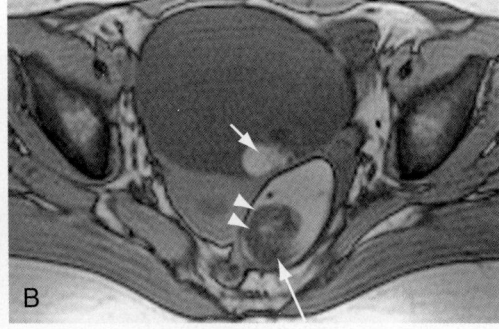
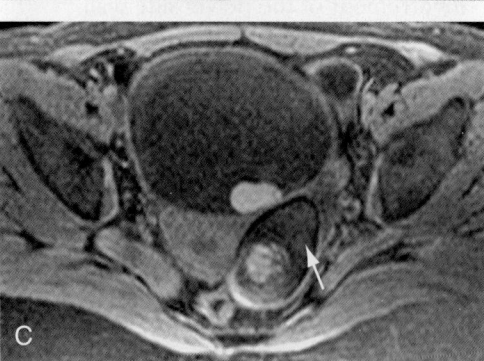

FIGURE 92-62

Bilateral dermoid tumors. **A,** Axial T1-weighted gradient-recalled echo in-phase image demonstrates bilateral adnexal masses. A large low signal intensity mass arising from the right ovary is seen anterior to the uterus and contains a small nodule of high signal intensity (*arrow*). A mass in the left adnexa is predominantly of high signal intensity with a focus of intermediate signal intensity posteriorly (*arrowheads*). **B,** Axial T1-weighted gradient-recalled echo out-of-phase image shows decreased signal intensity in the posterior component of the left ovarian mass (*long arrow*) due to the intravoxel coexistence of fat and water. Note the India-ink effect at the interface between the fatty component of the mass and the uterus and left ovarian tissue (*arrowheads*). The hyperintense focus in the right ovarian mass anterior to the uterus demonstrates no drop of signal or India-ink effect at its interface with the rest of the mass (*short arrow*); these findings suggest hemorrhagic contents but no fat within this focus. **C,** Axial 3D frequency-selective fat-saturated T1-weighted gradient-recalled (volume-interpolated breath-hold examination) image. Note the suppression of the signal in those areas with high signal intensity seen on **A** within the left adnexal mass (*arrow*) confirming the presence of macroscopic fat in the lesion. Again, a focus of high signal intensity is noted in the right ovarian mass and is most likely consistent with hemorrhagic products. (*Courtesy of Ivan Pedrosa, MD, Beth Israel Deaconess Medical Center, Boston.*)

cyst wall or nodule.[215] Misregistration in the frequency-encoding direction on spin-echo images can be seen at fat-fluid interfaces. Visualization of this artifact has been demonstrated to be as equally effective as standard fat-saturation techniques for demonstrating fat in dermoids.[216] While short tau inversion recovery (STIR) sequences have been used for fat suppression, the use of this technique is problematic in this setting as other substances with T1 values similar to fat will be equally suppressed. Unfortunately, the hemorrhagic lesions from which dermoids must be distinguished can have T1 values similar to fat and thus lose signal on STIR images.

Frequently, a solid nodular component is identified (on non–contrast-enhanced T1-weighted images) projecting from the cyst wall. These are known as dermoid plugs or Rokitansky nodules and represent solid fat, hair, and/or teeth. On contrast-enhanced T1-weighted images, there is no enhancement within these nodules, which enables differentiation from ovarian carcinoma (see Fig. 92-62).

Dermoid cysts are usually diagnosed with sonography. However, occasionally the high echogenicity of the lesion is difficult to differentiate from normal pelvic fat; or in case of a large lesion, the full extent may be difficult to appreciate on ultrasound. In these cases, MRI is able to establish the presence and dimensions of a dermoid cyst. The size is important to determine the operative approach (laparoscopy versus mini-laparotomy versus laparotomy).

Treatment of dermoid tumors consists of laparoscopic excision (if the lesion is small enough to allow for this approach). Conservation of part of the ovary is attempted if technically feasible. Therefore, it is useful to try to establish the benign nature of the mass with MRI prior to surgery if ultrasound is inconclusive. However, due to the variable content of dermoid cysts, the MRI appearance can be atypical and an accurate MRI diagnosis may not be possible if the lesion does not contain fat. For example, huge dermoid cysts in the younger age groups can be filled with simple fluid and contain scant fatty tissue.[215] Differentiation from immature teratomas may be impossible in this setting and correlation with tumor markers can be helpful. While elevated serum levels of CA 19-9 can be seen in all germ cell tumors, including dermoids, elevated α-fetoprotein is concerning for an immature teratoma.

Brenner Tumor

A Brenner tumor is a benign tumor consisting of transitional cells in prominent fibrous connective tissue. About 20% are associated with epithelial neoplasms, typically mucinous cystadenoma in the ipsilateral or contralateral ovary. Most Brenner tumors are smaller than 2 cm in diameter and rarely exceed 10 cm. Usually the Brenner tumor is discovered as an incidental lesion at pathology.[21]

The solid nodule in a Brenner tumor is isointense to uterine muscle on T1-weighted images and low on T2-weighted images.[209] Following injection of gadolinium mild patchy enhancement is seen within the nodule.

Extensive calcification may be noted. Cystic areas usually represent a coexistent cystadenoma.

The Brenner tumor is the exception to the rule that an enhancing soft-tissue nodule in a cystic mass indicates malignancy. MR signal characteristics may help make the preoperative diagnosis of this tumor.

Fibrous Tumors

Fibromas, fibrothecomas, and thecomas account for more than 50% of sex cord stromal tumors and represent approximately 4% of ovarian tumors. Their common histologic features are varying degrees of fibrosis and edema. Fibromas are composed of spindle cells that produce a variable amount of collagen and are not hormonally active. Fibromas can be complicated by ascites and pleural effusions, known as Meigs' syndrome, which occurs in 1% of cases. Ascites and pleural effusions resolve spontaneously after removal of the tumor. In large fibromas measuring over 10 cm, ascites is seen in 10% to 15% of cases.[217] These tumors most commonly occur in middle age. Fibrothecomas contain fibrous tissue and theca cells and often are hormonally active. These can be associated with a thickened endometrial stripe, representing endometrial hyperplasia from hormonal stimulation. Calcifications can occasionally be seen.

Fibromas and fibrothecomas have the same signal characteristics as leiomyomas (Fig. 92-63). They are of intermediate signal intensity on T1-weighted and low signal intensity on T2-weighted images[199,218] due to dense fibrotic tissue within the lesion. However, intratumoral edema may be present, particularly in larger lesions, and can explain the high signal intensity on T2-weighted images. On contrast-enhanced T1-weighted images, these may demonstrate mild enhancement. If calcifications are present, they are usually difficult to identify as foci of low signal intensity on both T1- and T2-weighted images.

Sclerosing stromal tumors occur in the second or third decade of life. The tumors have characteristic imaging features, including striking enhancement, brighter than the uterus on post-contrast T1-weighted images. On T2-weighted images, pseudolobulation is noted with low signal intensity nodules against a high signal intensity background.[219,220] Sclerosing stromal tumors are benign lesions, but can be mistaken for a Krukenberg tumor on histology. The imaging diagnosis is therefore critical.

Diagnosis of fibrous ovarian lesions is usually made by ultrasound if classic sonographic features of a hypoechoic, attenuating mass separate from the uterus with a nonvisualized ovary are present. MRI is used if sonographic appearance is nonspecific or if the ovarian origin of the lesion is questionable. Treatment is removal of the affected ovary when the lesion is large. Preoperative diagnosis of these solid but benign ovarian lesions may modify the surgical approach to a less invasive, laparoscopic procedure compared to an open laparotomy for cases where malignancy is suspected.

Differential diagnosis includes a fibroid of the broad ligament (see Fig. 92-63) and Krukenberg tumors. The former is easy to differentiate with MRI due to its location separate from the ovary and uterus. Low signal intensity

location. In addition, MRI can be used for staging the disease, differentiating endometriomas from other adnexal masses, and evaluating response to treatment.

MRI can be used in staging the disease when relaxation times are measured,[245,256] thus enabling differentiation of new from old lesions. This can be helpful in surgical planning.[245]

Differential diagnosis for lesions with high signal intensity on T1-weighted images includes fat-containing lesions, such as dermoid tumors, and other hemorrhagic lesions, such as hemorrhagic or corpus luteum cysts. A T1-weighted sequence with fat suppression is important in the distinction between endometriomas and dermoid cysts and establishes the presence of blood products within the cyst should high signal intensity persist within the lesion. The differentiation of endometriomas from other hemorrhagic lesions may be difficult and sometimes impossible based on imaging criteria alone, particularly when a solitary lesion is present. While this is a hallmark of hemorrhagic and corpus luteum cysts, endometriomas can on occasion be solitary as well. Multiplicity of adnexal lesions, lesions in the cul-de-sac, or a dilated fallopian tube with high signal intensity on T1-weighted images support a diagnosis of endometriosis.[239,241] Hemorrhagic cysts have a thin wall, with corpus luteum cysts demonstrating a slightly thicker, convoluted appearing wall. As there is no repeated hemorrhage into these lesions, marked loss of signal intensity on T2-weighted images i.e., "shading" is generally not observed.

Medical treatment of endometriosis is aimed at suppression of cyclic hemorrhage with danazol and GnRH analogues.[242] MRI can be used to triage patients for medical therapy and to monitor response to treatment.[252] Larger endometriomas with pronounced T2 shading have been reported to benefit less from medical treatment.[256] This may relate to the more concentrated blood products in older endometriomas, with obliterated glandular tissue due to increased internal pressure. A low signal intensity rim, multiplicity of lesions, and irregularity of the lesions were also noted more commonly in the nonresponder group. A reduction in T2 signal intensity following treatment with GnRH may reflect a good response.[257]

Peritoneal Inclusion Cysts

These cysts can develop as a complication of prior surgery, PID, trauma, or endometriosis. While the normal peritoneum absorbs fluid produced by the ovaries, this ability can be lost following inflammation or adhesion formation. Fluid-filled cysts of variable size up to 20 cm with multiple septations can thus develop adherent to pelvic organs. Peritoneal inclusion cysts can rarely be seen in the upper abdomen, retroperitoneum, or hernia sacs. While they can present with lower abdominal pain and/or as a palpable mass, some are noted incidentally on imaging studies or during surgery.

Peritoneal inclusion cysts have a characteristic appearance on MRI bordered by pelvic side wall (Fig. 92-71), pelvic organs, and bowel loops without a distinct

wall.[258] Usually there is no mass effect on adjacent structures, although this can be seen in large lesions. Signal intensity is variable depending on the nature of the fluid content. Typically, they are of low signal intensity on T1- and high signal intensity on T2-weighted images. If protein content in the lesion is high or hemorrhage into the cyst has occurred the signal intensity on T1-weighted images may be intermediate to hyperintense. They usually contain thin septations, however, occasionally thick septations may be seen. The ovary and fallopian tubes can be located inside the inclusion cyst, surrounded by septations and fluid, or be seen inside the wall of the inclusion cyst. Thus, they can mimic a mural mass or papillary projections.

An accurate diagnosis can usually be made on MRI, thus averting multiple surgeries that may result from suspicion of a cystic ovarian neoplasm. Treatment for this condition is conservative as inclusion cysts recur after extensive surgery in 30% to 50%.[259-261] Ovarian suppression with oral contraceptive agents can be considered.[262] Image-guided percutaneous or transvaginal aspiration and drainage, possibly with instillation of a sclerosing agent, can be performed[263] if the patient is symptomatic. If surgery is warranted, more conservative procedures, such as adhesiotomy and marsupialization of the cyst, are feasible.

Ectopic Pregnancy

Ectopic pregnancy occurs in 1 in 7000 pregnancies, but the incidence is higher in patients undergoing infertility treatment with ovulation induction or in vitro fertilization. The extrauterine gestational sac is most commonly located along the course of the fallopian tube in the ampulla or isthmus (95-97%). Rarely is it seen at

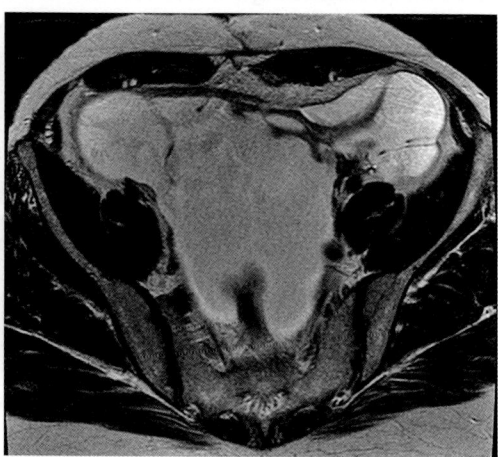

FIGURE 92-71

Peritoneal inclusion cyst. Axial T2-weighted fast spin-echo image demonstrates a cystic mass with thin septations and no distinct wall bordered by the pelvic side wall. The mass fills the peritoneal space without causing significant mass effect upon the pelvic structures. (*Courtesy of Ivan Pedrosa, MD, Beth Israel Deaconess Medical Center, Boston.*)

the cornua (2-5%) (Fig. 92-72). The ovary itself (0.5-1%) and the uterine cervix are other uncommon locations. The classic clinical presentation consists of acute abdominal pain and bleeding in a patient with positive β-human chorionic gonadotropin. Because many ectopic pregnancies are now diagnosed earlier, in an nonruptured condition, the majority of patients present with minimal or no symptoms.

Ectopic pregnancy appears as a complex cystic or solid adnexal mass representing the ectopic gestational sac and hematoma, usually separate from the ovary. The gestational sac can be visualized as a cystic structure surrounded by a thick enhancing rim. Hemosalpinx and hemorrhagic ascites may be present. Acute hemorrhage is seen as intermediate signal intensity on T1-weighted and low signal intensity on T2-weighted images, representing deoxyhemoglobin.[264]

Surgery remains the treatment of choice for ruptured ectopic pregnancy. However, recent approaches to management of nonruptured ectopic pregnancies include medical therapy with methotrexate or expectant management. Sonography is the imaging modality of choice for making the diagnosis; however, if sonographic findings are inconclusive, MRI may help to make a more confident diagnosis of ectopic pregnancy by demonstrating blood products. This may be particularly useful when conservative management is considered. While the differentiation between a hemorrhagic ovarian lesion and ectopic pregnancy may be difficult based on imaging criteria alone, the demonstration of a hemorrhagic adnexal mass distinct from the ovary is suggestive, as ectopic pregnancy commonly occurs in the fallopian tube. In addition, MRI is helpful in assessing unusual locations such as intra-abdominal presentations.

CONCLUSION

MRI is synonymous with comprehensive gynecologic imaging in the 21st century. It provides the most detailed anatomic images of the uterus and ovary to date (form), coupled with advances in fast imaging techniques that provide information on motion (function). To be sure, ultrasound, especially transvaginal ultrasound, is the initial imaging modality in evaluating gynecologic conditions, but in instances where a more thorough or sophisticated analysis is warranted, or in cases where the ultrasound is inconclusive, MRI should be routinely performed.

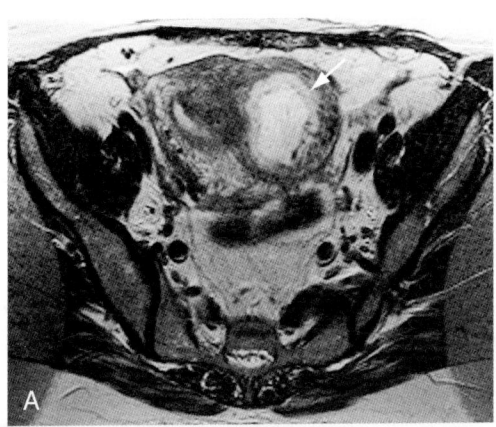
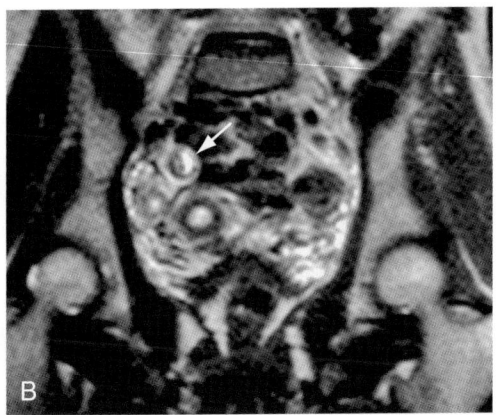
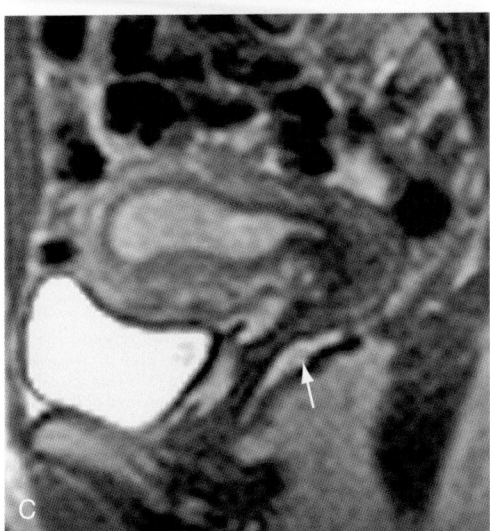

FIGURE 92-72

Ectopic pregnancy. **A,** Axial T2-weighted fast spin-echo (FSE) image demonstrates an ectopic gestational sac in the left cornu (*arrow*). **B,** Coronal T2-weighted FSE in a different patient demonstrates a dilated fallopian tube containing layering blood products (*arrow*) adjacent to the normal ovary. **C,** Sagittal T2-weighted fast spin-echo image shows free fluid in the cul-de-sac (*arrow*). The endometrium is thickened although no gestational sac is visualized within the endometrial cavity. (*Courtesy of Ivan Pedrosa, MD, Beth Israel Deaconess Medical Center, Boston.*)

REFERENCES

1. Sedlis A, Robboy SJ: Disease of the vagina. In Kurman R (ed): Blaustein's Pathology of the Female Genital Tract, 3rd ed. New York, Springer-Verlag, 1987, pp 98-101.
2. Llewellyn-Jones D: Anatomy of the female genital tract. In Fundamentals of Obstetrics and Gynecology, vol II. London, Faber & Faber, 1969, pp 24-36.
3. Hricak H, Chang YC, Thurnher S: Vagina: Evaluation with MR imaging. Part I. Normal anatomy and congenital anomalies. Radiology 169:169-174, 1998.
4. Ferenczy A, Winkler B: Anatomy and histology of the cervix. In Kurman R (ed): Blaustein's Pathology of the Female Genital Tract, 3rd ed. New York, Springer-Verlag, 1987, pp 141-145.
5. Hricak H, Alpers C, Crooks LE, Sheldon PE: Magnetic resonance of the female pelvis: initial experience. Am J Roentgenol 141:1119-1128, 1983.
6. Scoutt LM, McCauley TR, Flynn SD, et al: Zonal anatomy of the cervix: correlation of MR imaging and histological examination of hysterectomy specimens. Radiology 186:159-162, 1993.
7. Smith RC, Reinhold CR, McCauley TR, et al: Multicoil high resolution fast spin-echo MR imaging of the female pelvis. Radiology 184:671-676, 1992.
8. Schwalm H, Dubrauszky V: The structure of the musculature of the human uterus—muscles and connective tissue. Am J Obstet Gynecol 94:391-404, 1966.
9. Nakai A, Togashi K, Fujiwara T, et al: Uterine peristalsis shown on cine MR imaging using ultra sequence. J Magn Reson Imaging 18:726-733, 2003.
10. McCarthy S, Taubert C, Gore J: Female pelvic anatomy: MR assessment of variations during the menstrual cycle and with use of oral contraceptives. Radiology 160:111-123, 1986.
11. Kubik-Huch R, Reinhold C, Semelka RC, et al: Uterus and cervix. In Semelka RC (ed): Abdominal-Pelvic MRI. New York, Wiley-Liss, 2002, pp 1049-1122.
12. Chaudhry S, Reinhold C, Guermazi A, et al: Benign and malignant diseases of the endometrium. Top Magn Reson Imaging 14:339-358, 2003.
13. Demas BE, Hricak H, Jaffe RB: Uterine MR imaging: Effects of hormonal stimulation. Radiology 159:123-126, 1986.
14. Ascher SM, Johnson JC, Barnes W, et al: Spin echo and dynamic contrast-enhanced gradient echo imaging of the uterus with histopathologic correlation in postmenopausal women receiving tamoxifen therapy. Radiology 200:105-110, 1996.
15. Ascher SM, Imaoka I, Lage J: Tamoxifen-induced uterine abnormalities: The role of imaging. Radiology 214:29-38, 2000.
16. Brown HK, Stoll BS, Nicosia SV, et al: Uterine junctional zone: correlation between histological findings and MR imaging. Radiology 179:409-413, 1991.
17. Scoutt LM, Flynn SD, Luthringer DJ, et al: Junctional zone of the uterus: correlation of MR imaging and histological examination of hysterectomy specimens. Radiology 179:403-407, 1991.
18. Togashi K, Kawakami S, Kimura I, et al: Uterine contractions: possible diagnostic pitfall at MR imaging. J Magn Reson Imaging 3:889-893, 1993.
19. Williams PL, Bannister LH, Berry MM, et al: The female genital organs. In Gray's Anatomy, 38th ed. Edinburgh, Churchill Livingstone, 1995.
20. Cohen HL, Tice HM, Mandel FS: Ovarian volumes measured by US: bigger than we think. Radiology 177:189-190, 1990.
21. Kurman RF (ed): Blaustein's Pathology of the Female Genital Tract, 4th ed. New York, Springer-Verlag, 1994.
22. Outwater EK, Talerman A, Dunton C: Normal adnexa uteri specimens: Anatomic basis of MR imaging features. Radiology 201:751-755, 1996.
23. Outwater EK, Mitchell DG: Normal ovaries and functional cysts: MR appearance. Radiology 198:397-402, 1996.
24. Mattrey RF, Trambert MA, Brown JJ, et al: Oral contrast agents of magnetic resonance imaging, result of phase III trials with Imagent® GI as an oral magnetic resonance contrast agent. Invest Radiol 26:S65-S66, 1991.
25. Brown JJ, Duncan JR, Heiken JP, et al: Perfluoroctylbromide as a gastrointestinal contrast agent for MR imaging: use with and without glucagon. Radiology 181:455-460, 1991.
26. Ros PR, Steinman RM, Torres GM, et al: The value of barium as a gastrointestinal contrast agent in MR imaging: a comparison study in normal volunteers. Am J Roentgenol 157:761-767, 1991.
27. Hricak H: Current trends in MR imaging of the female pelvis. RadioGraphics 13:913-919, 1993.
28. Baudouin CJ, Soutter WP, Gilderdale DJ, Coutts GA: Magnetic resonance imaging of the uterine cervix using an intravaginal coil. Magn Reson Med 24:196-203, 1993.
29. Moulopoulos LA, Varma DG, Charnsangavej C, et al: Magnetic resonance imaging and computed tomography appearance of asymptomatic para-vaginal cysts. Clin Imaging 17:126-132, 1993.
30. Ascher SM: Gartner's duct cyst. In Hricak H, Reinhold C, Ascher SM (eds): PocketRadiologist: Gynecology—Top 100 Diagnoses. Salt Lake City, Amirsys™, 2004, pp 195-197.
31. Ascher SM, Agrawal R, Bis KG, et al: Endometriosis: Appearance and detection with conventional, fat suppressed, and contrast-enhanced fat suppressed, spin echo techniques. J Magn Reson Imaging 5:251-257, 1995.
32. Outwater EK, Ascher SM: Bartholin's gland cyst. In Hricak H, Reinhold C, Ascher SM (eds): PocketRadiologist: Gynecology—Top 100 Diagnoses. Salt Lake City, Amirsys™, 2004, pp 265-267.
33. Siegelman ES, Outwater EK, Banner MP, et al: High-resolution MR imaging of the vagina. RadioGraphics 17:1183-1203, 1997.
34. Llauger J, Palmer J, Roson N, et al: The normal and pathologic ischiorectal fossa at CT and MR imaging. RadioGraphics 18:61-82, 1998.
35. Ashton D, Amin HK, Richart RM, Neuwirth RS: The incidence of asymptomatic uterine anomalies in women undergoing transcervical tubal sterilization. Obstet Gynecol 72:28-30, 1988.
36. Byrne J, Nussbaum-Blask A, Rubin A, et al: Prevalence of mullerian duct anomalies detected at ultrasound. Am J Med Genet 94:9-12, 2000.
37. Heinonen PK, Saarikoski S, Pystynen P: Reproductive performance of women with uterine anomalies. An evaluation of 182 cases. Acta Obstet Gynecol Scand 61:224-236, 1982.
38. Maneschi F, Zupi E, Marconi D, et al: Hysteroscopically detected asymptomatic mullerian anomalies: Prevalence and reproductive implications. J Reprod Med 40: 684-688, 1995.
39. Simon C, Martinez L, Pardo F, et al: Mullerian defects in women with normal reproductive outcome. Fertil Steril 56:1192-1193, 1991.
40. Sorenson S: Estimated prevalence of mullerian duct anomalies. Acta Obstet Gynecol Scand 67:441, 1988.
41. Stray-Pedersen B, Stray-Pedersen S: Etiologic factors and subsequent reproductive performance in 195 couples with a prior history of habitual abortion. Am J Obstet Gynecol 148:140-146, 1984.
42. Rock JA, Schlaff WD: The obstetric consequences of uterovaginal anomalies. Fertil Steril 43:681, 1985.
43. Green LK, Harris RE: Uterine anomalies: Frequency of diagnosis and obstetric complications. Obstet Gynecol 47:427, 1976.
44. Homer HA, Li TC, Cooke ID: The septate uterus: A review of management and reproductive outcome. Fertil Steril 73:1-14, 2000.
45. Raga F, Bauset C, Remohi J, et al: Reproductive impact of congenital mullerian anomalies. Hum Reprod 12:2277-2281, 1997.
46. Wajntraub A, Milwidsky A, Weiss D: Prevention of premature delivery in a unicornuate uterus by cervical cerclage. Acta Obstet Gynecol Scand 54:497-498, 1975.
47. Olive DL, Henderson DY: Endometriosis and mullerian anomalies. Obstet Gynecol 69:412-415, 1987.
48. Ugur M, Turan C, Mungan T, et al: Endometriosis in association with mullerian anomalies. Gynecol Obstet Invest 40:261-264, 1995.
49. Carrington BM, Hricak H, Nuruddin RN, et al: Mullerian duct anomalies: MR imaging evaluation. Radiology 176:715-720, 1990.
50. Pellerito JS, McCarthy SM, Doyle MB, et al: Diagnosis of uterine anomalies: Relative accuracy of MR imaging, endovaginal ultrasound, and hysterosalpingography. Radiology 183:795-800, 1992.
51. Doyle MB: Magnetic resonance imaging in mullerian fusion defects. J Reprod Med 37:33-38, 1992.
52. Fielding JR: MR imaging of mullerian anomalies: Impact on therapy. Am J Roentgenol 167:1491-1495, 1996.
53. Fedele L, Dorta M, Brioschi D, et al: Magnetic resonance evaluation of double uteri. Obstet Gynecol 74:844-847, 1989.
54. Larsen WJ: Development of the urogenital system. In Human Embryology. New York, Churchill Livingstone, 1993, pp 235-279.
55. Daly DC, Witten CA, Soto-Albors CE, Riddick DH: Hysteroscopic metroplasty: surgical technique and obstetric outcome. Fertil Steril 39:623-628, 1983.
56. Fedele L, Bianchi S, Agnoli B, et al: Urinary tract anomalies associated with unicornuate uterus. J Urol 155:847-848, 1996.
57. Buttram VC, Gibbons WE: Mullerian anomalies: A proposed classification (an analysis of 144 cases). Fertil Steril 32:40-46, 1979.
58. The American Fertility Society. The American Fertility Society Classifications of Adnexal Adhesions, Distal Tubal Obstruction, Tubal Occlusion Secondary to Tubal Ligation, Tubal Pregnancies, Mullerian Anomalies and Intrauterine Adhesions. Fertil Steril 49:944-955, 1988.
59. Murray JM, Gambrell RD: Complete and partial vaginal agenesis. J Reprod Med 22:101, 1979.
60. Lindenman E, Shepard MK, Pescovitz OH: Mullerian agenesis: An update. Obstet Gynecol 90:307-312, 1997.
61. Fedele L, Dorta M, Brioschi D, et al: Magnetic resonance imaging in Mayer-Rokitansky-Kuster-Hauser syndrome. Obstet Gynecol 76:593-596, 1990.
62. Togashi K, Nishimura K, Itoh K, et al: Vaginal agenesis: Classification by MR imaging. Radiology 162:675-677, 1987.
63. Vainright JR, Fulp CJ, Schiebler ML: MR imaging of vaginal agenesis with hematocolpos. J Comput Assist Tomogr 12:891-893, 1988.
64. Fedele L, Zamberletti D, Vercellini P, et al: Reproductive performance of women with unicornuate uterus. Fertil Steril 47:416-419, 1987.
65. Rolen AC, Choquette AJ, Semmens JP: Rudimentary uterine horn: Obstetric and gynecologic implications. Gynecol Obstset 27: 806-813, 1966.
66. Andrews MC, Jones HW: Impaired reproductive performance of the unicornuate uterus: intrauterine growth retardation, infertility, and recurrent abortion in five cases. Am J Obstet Gynecol 144:173-176, 1982.
67. Patton PE, Novy MJ: Reproductive potential of the anomalous uterus. Semin Reprod Endocrinol 6:217-233, 1988.
68. Propst AM, Hill JA: Anatomic factors associated with recurrent pregnancy loss. Semin Reprod Med 18:341-350, 2000.
69. Buttram VC: Mullerian anomalies and their management. Fertil Steril 40:159-163, 1983.

70. Heinonen PK: Unicornuate uterus and rudimentary horn. Fertil Steril 68:224-230, 1997.

71. Brody JM, Koelliker SL, Frishman GN: Unicornuate uterus: Imaging appearance, associated anomalies, and clinical applications. Am J Roentgenol 171:1341-1347, 1988.

72. Rock JA, Jones HW: The clinical management of the double uterus. Fertil Steril 28: 798-806, 1977.

73. Raziel A, Arieli S, Bukovsky I, et al: Investigation of the uterine cavity in recurrent aborters. Fertil Steril 62:1080-1082, 1994.

74. Clifford K, Rai R, Watson H, Regan L: An informative protocol for the investigation of recurrent miscarriage: preliminary experience of 500 consecutive cases. Hum Reprod 9:1328-1332, 1994.

75. Harger JH, Archer DF, Marchese SG, et al: Etiology of recurrent pregnancy losses and outcome of subsequent pregnancies. Obstet Gynecol 62:574, 1983.

76. Kupesic S, Kurjak A: Septate uterus: Detection and prediction of obstetrical complications by different forms of ultrasonography. J Ultrasound Med 17:631-636, 1998.

77. Fedele L, Bianchi S, Marchini M, et al: Residual uterine septum of less than 1 cm after hysteroscopic metroplasty does not impair reproductive outcome. Human Reprod 11:727-729, 1996.

78. Fedele L, Bianchi S: Hysteroscopic metroplasty for septate uterus. Obstet Gynecol Clin North Am 22:473-489, 1995.

79. Fayez JA: Comparison between abdominal and hysteroscopic metroplasty. Obstet Gynecol 68:399-403, 1986.

80. Dabirashrafi H, Bahodori M, Mohammad K, et al: Septate uterus: New idea on the histologic features of the septum in the abnormal uterus. Am J Obstet Gynecol 172:105-107, 1995.

81. Candiani GB, Federle L, Zamberletti D, et al: Endometrial patterns in malformed uteri. Acta Europ Fertil 14:311-318, 1983.

82. Fedele L, Bianchi S, Marchini M, et al: Ultrastructural aspects of endometrium in infertile women with septate uterus. Fertil Steril 65:750-752, 1996.

83. Valle RF: Hysteroscopic treatment of partial and complete uterine septum. Int J Fertil Menopausal Stud 41:310-315, 1996.

84. DeCherney AH, Russell JB, Graebe RA, Polan ML: Resectoscopic management of Mullerian fusion defects. Fertil Steril 45:726-728, 1986.

85. Gray SE, Roberts DK, Franklin RR: Fertility after metroplasty of the uterus. J Reprod Med 29:185-188, 1984.

86. Zreik TG, Troiano RN, Ghoussoub RAD, et al: Myometrial tissue in uterine septa. J Am Assoc Gynecol Laparoscopists 5:155-160, 1998.

87. Tulandi T, Arronet GH, McInnes RA: Arcuate and bicornuate uterine anomalies and infertility. Fertil Steril 34:362-664, 1980.

88. Musich JR, Behrman SJ: Obstetric outcome after metroplasty in women with uterine anomalies. Obstet Gynecol 52:1, 1978.

89. Sorenson SS: Fundal contour of the uterine cavity in the new syndrome of minor mullerian duct anomalies and oligomenorrhea: a prospective controlled study. Am J Obstet Gynecol 145:659-667, 1983.

90. Herbst AL, Senekjian EK, Frey KW: Abortion and pregnancy loss among diethylstilbestrol-exposed women. Semin Endocrinol 7:124-129, 1989.

91. Herbst AL, Ulfelder H, Poskanzer DC: Adenocarcinoma of the vagina. Association of maternal stilbesterol therapy with tumor appearance in young women. N Engl J Med 284:878-881, 1971.

92. Goldberg JM, Falcone T: Effect of diethylstilbestrol on reproductive function. Fertil Steril 72:1-7, 1999.

93. Kaufman RH, Adam E, Binder GL, Gerthoffer E: Upper genital tract changes and pregnancy outcome in offspring exposed in utero to diethylstilbestrol. Am J Obstet Gynecol 137:299-308, 1980.

94. Winfield AC, Wentz AC: Diethylstilbestrol exposure in utero. In Winfield AC, Wentz AC (eds): Diagnostic Imaging of Infertlity, 2nd ed. Baltimore, Williams and Wilkins, 1992, pp 85-95.

95. van Gils AP, Than RT, Falke TH, Peters AA: Abnormalities of the uterus and cervix after diethylstilbestrol exposure: Correlation of findings on MR and hysterosalpingography. Am J Roentgenol 153:1235-1238, 1989.

96. DeCherney AH, Cholst I, Naftolin F: Structure and function of the fallopian tubes following exposure to diethylstilbestrol (DES) during gestation. Fertil Steril 36:741-745, 1981.

97. Kaufman RH, Adam E, Hatch EE, et al: Continued follow-up of pregnancy outcomes in diethylstilbestrol-exposed offspring. Obstet Gynecol 96:483-489, 2000.

98. Rennell CL: T-shaped uterus in diethylstilbestrol (DES) exposure. Am J Roentgenol 132:979-980, 1979.

99. Kipersztok S, Javitt M, Hill MC, Stillman RJ: Comparison of magnetic resonance imaging and transvaginal sonography with hysterosonography in the evaluation of women exposed to diethylstilbestrol. J Reprod Med 41:347-351, 1996.

100. Nussbaum-Blask AR, Sanders RC, Rock JA: Obstructed uterovaginal anomalies: Demonstration with sonography. Part II. Teenagers. Radiology 179:84-88, 1991.

101. Rock JA: Anomalous development of the vagina. Semin Reprod Endocrinol 4:13-31, 1986.

102. Arnold BW, Gilfeather M, Woodward PJ: Mullerian duct anomalies complicated by obstruction. Evaluation with pelvic magnetic resonance imaging. J Women Imaging 3:146-152, 2001.

103. Outwater E, Ascher SM: Nabothian cyst. In Hricak H, Reinhold C, Ascher SM (eds): PocketRadiologist: Gynecology—Top 100 Diagnoses. Salt Lake City, Amirsys™, 2004, pp 235-237.

104. Li H, Sugimura K, Okizuka H, et al: Markedly high-signal intensity lesions in the uterine cervix on T2-weighted imaging: Differentiation between mucin-producing carcinomas and nabothian cysts. Radiation Med 17:137-143, 1999.

105. Daya D, Young RH: Florid deep glands of the uterine cervix: Another mimic of adnoma malignum. Am J Clin Pathol 103:614-617, 1995.

106. Ascher SM, Allison S: Cervical stenosis. In Hricak H, Reinhold C, Ascher SM (eds): PocketRadiologist: Gynecology—Top 100 Diagnoses. Salt Lake City: Amirsys™, 2004, pp 218-220.

107. Zalel Y, Tepper R, Altaras M, Beyth Y, et al: Clinical significance of endometrial fluid collections in asymptomatic postmenopausal women. J Ultrasound Med 15:515-515, 1996.

108. Allison S, Ascher SM: Cervical incompetence. In Hricak H, Reinhold C, Ascher SM, eds. PocketRadiologist: Gynecology—Top 100 Diagnoses. Salt Lake City: Amirsys™, 2004, pp 238-240.

109. Hricak H: Cervical incompetence: Preliminary evaluation with MR imaging. Radiology 174:821-826, 1990.

110. Atri M, Reinhold C: Endometrial polyp. In Hricak H, Reinhold C, Ascher SM (eds): PocketRadiologist: Gynecology—Top 100 Diagnoses. Salt Lake City: Amirsys™, 2004, pp 3-5.

111. Grasel RP, Outwater EK, Siegelman ES, et al: Endometrial polyps: MR imaging features and distinction from endometrial carcinoma. Radiology 214:47-52, 2000.

112. Atri M, Nazarnia S, Aldis AE, et al: Transvaginal ultrasound appearance of endometrial abnormalities. RadioGraphics 14:483-492, 1994.

113. Reinhold C, Atri M: Endometrial hyperplasia. In Hricak H, Reinhold C, Ascher SM (eds): PocketRadiologist: Gynecology—Top 100 Diagnoses. Salt Lake City: Amirsys™, 2004, pp 8-10.

114. Reinhold C, Khalili I: Postmenopausal bleeding: Value of imaging. Radiol Clin North Am 40:527-562, 2002.

115. Smith-Bindman R, Kerlikowske K, Feldstein VA, et al: Endovaginal ultrasound to exclude endometrial cancer and other endometrial abnormalities. JAMA 280:1510-1617, 1998.

116. Schenker JG: Etiology of and therapeutic approach to synechia uteri. Europ J Obstet Gynecol Reprod Biol 65:109-113, 1996.

117. Letterie GS, Haggerty MF: Magnetic resonance imaging of intrauterine synechiae. Gynecol Obstet Invest 37:66-68, 1994.

118. Bacelar AC, Wilcock D, Powell M, et al: The value of MRI in the assessment of traumatic intra-uterine adhesions (Asherman's syndrome). Clin Radiol 50:80-83, 1995.

119. Ascher SM, Jha RC, Reinhold C: Benign myometrial conditions: Leiomyomas and adenomyosis. Top Magn Reson Imaging 14:281-304, 2003.

120. Jones HW, Jones GS (eds): Gynecology, 3rd ed. Baltimore: Williams & Wilkins, 1982, pp 245-253.

121. Ross PK, Pike MC, Vessey MP, et al: Risk factors for uterine fibroids: Reduced risk associated with oral contraceptives. BMJ 293:59, 1986.

122. Parazzini F, Vecchia CL, Negri E, et al: Epidemiologic characteristics of women with uterine fibroids: a case-control study. Obstet Gynecol 72:853-857, 1988.

123. Kjerulff KH, Guzinski GM, Langenberg PW, et al: Hysterectomy and race. Obstet Gynecol 82:757, 1991.

124. Ratner H: Risk factors for uterine fibroids: reduced risk associated with oral contraceptives. BMJ 293:1027, 1986.

125. Rader JS, Binette SP, Brandt TD, et al: Ileal hemorrhage caused by a parasitic uterine leiomyoma. Obstet Gynecol 76: 531-534, 1990.

126. Friedman AJ, Iobel SM, Rein MS, et al: Efficacy and safety considerations in women with leiomyomas treated with gonadotropin-releasing hormone agonists: The estrogen threshold hypothesis. Am J Obstet Gynecol 163:1114-1119, 1990.

127. Buttram VC Jr: Uterine leiomyomata—etiology, symptomatology, and management. Prog Clin Biol Res 293:59, 1986.

128. Hricak H, Tscholakoff D, Heinrichs L, et al: Uterine leiomyomas: Correlation of MR histopathologic findings and symptoms. Radiology 158:385-391, 1986.

129. Mittl RL, Yeh I, Kressel HY: High-signal-intensity rim surrounding uterine leiomyomas on MR images: Pathologic correlation. Radiology 180:81-83, 1991.

130. Yamashita Y, Torashima M, Takahashi M: Hyperintense uterine leiomyoma at T2-weighted MR imaging: Differentiation with dynamic enhanced MR imaging and clinical implications. Radiology 189:721-725, 1993.

131. Horie Y, Ikawa S, Kadowaki K, et al: Lipoadenofibroma of the uterine corpus: Report of a new variant of adenofibroma (benign mullerian mixed tumor). Arch Pathol Lab Med 119:274-276, 1996.

132. Hricak H, Finck S, Honda G, Goeranson H: MR imaging in the evaluation of benign uterine masses: Value of gadopentatate dimeglumine-enhanced T1-weighted images. Am J Roentgenol 158:1043-1050, 1992.

133. Weinreb JC, Barkoff ND, Megibow A, et al: The value of MR imaging in distinguishing leiomyomas form other solid pelvis masses when sonography is indeterminate. Am J Roentgenol 154:295-299, 1990.

134. Togashi K, Kawakami S, Kimura I, et al: Sustained uterine contractions: A cause of hypointense myometrial bulging. Radiology 187:707-710, 1993.

135. Gross BH, Silver TM, Jaffe MH: Sonographic features of uterine leiomyomas: Analysis of 41 proven cases. J Ultrasound Med 2:401-406, 1983.

136. Karasick S, Lev-Toaff AS, Toaff ME: Imaging of uterine leiomyomas. Am J Roentgenol 158:799-805, 1992.

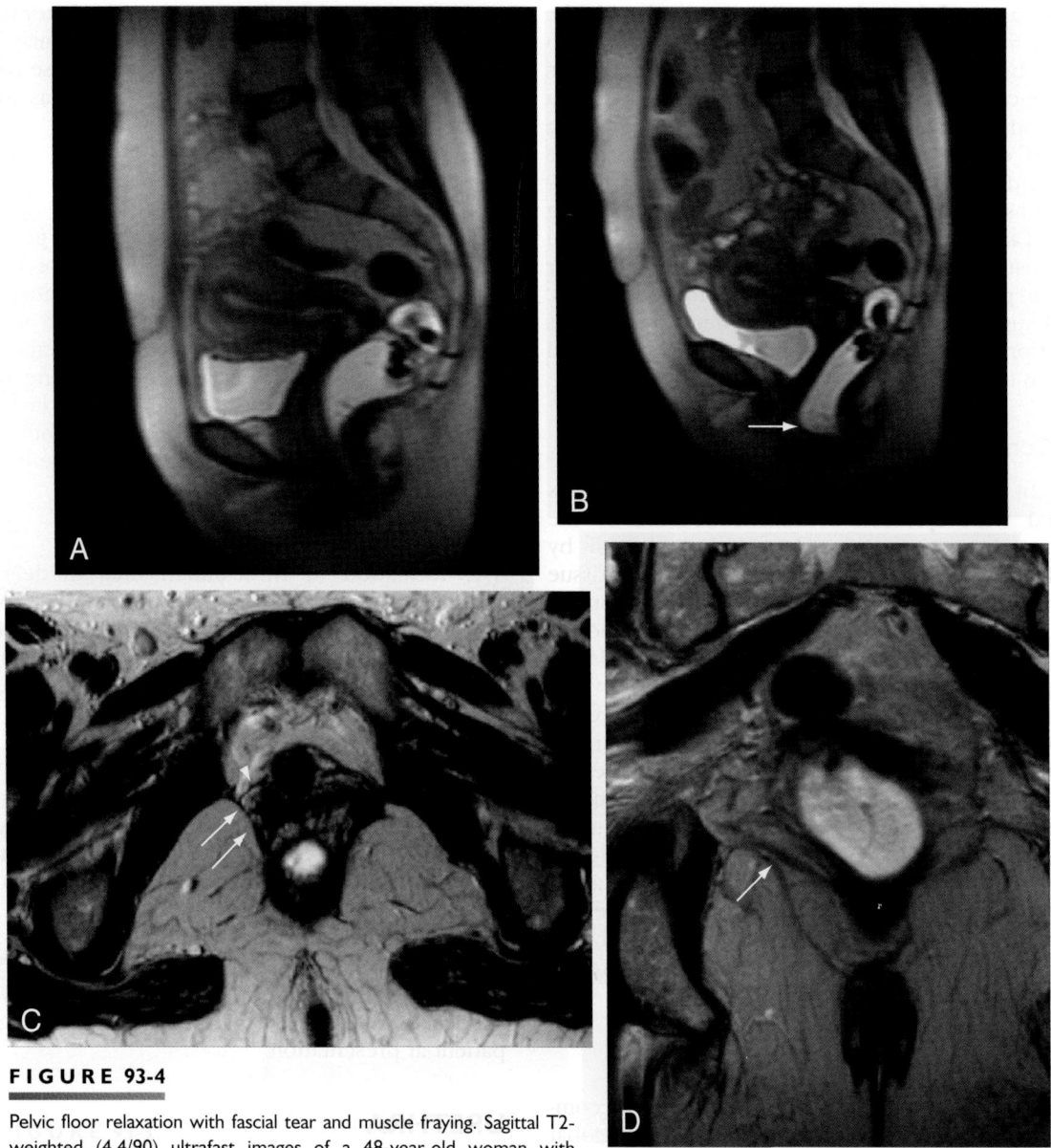

FIGURE 93-4

Pelvic floor relaxation with fascial tear and muscle fraying. Sagittal T2-weighted (4.4/90) ultrafast images of a 48-year-old woman with occasional episodes of urinary and fecal incontinence at rest (**A**) and at strain (**B**) show increased descent of the posterior compartment with formation of a small anterior rectocele (*arrow*). **C,** Axial T2-weighted (5000/132) image shows thinning of the right aspect of the puborectalis (*arrows*), asymmetry of the vagina within the sling, and tear of the right lateral pubovesical ligaments (*arrowheads*). **D,** Coronal T2-weighted (5000/132) image at rest shows fraying of the right iliococcygeus with some fibers displaced inferiorly (*arrow*).

The walls of the urethra are filled with glands, the greatest number posteriorly. Skene's glands arise from the lower urethra but drain on the vestibular surface on either side of the urethral meatus. Obstruction presents as a fluctuant mass extending inferiorly from the perineum. The obstruction of the smaller, secretory glands leads to the formation of a diverticulum. These outpouchings may be sacular, bilobed, or circumferential. Presentation is that of recurrent urinary dribbling or infection, and physical exam reveals a labial mass. It is important to identify the neck of the diverticulum with as great a degree of accuracy as possible because surgery is often technically difficult.

Multiple imaging tests can be used to diagnose urethral diverticula, the simplest being a voiding cystourethrogram. When this fails, transperineal ultrasound and MRI should be considered. On ultrasound examination, the diverticulum appears as a hypo- or anechoic fluid collection arising lateral to the urethra.[27,28] MRI should be performed using a multicoil array wrapped low around the pelvis. T2-weighted images centered on the bladder neck and employing fast or turbo spin-echo pulse sequences in the axial, sagittal, and coronal plane will usually suffice. Ultrafast T2-weighted pulse sequences, such as SSFSE or HASTE, usually do not provide adequate resolution. Good general scanning parameters include

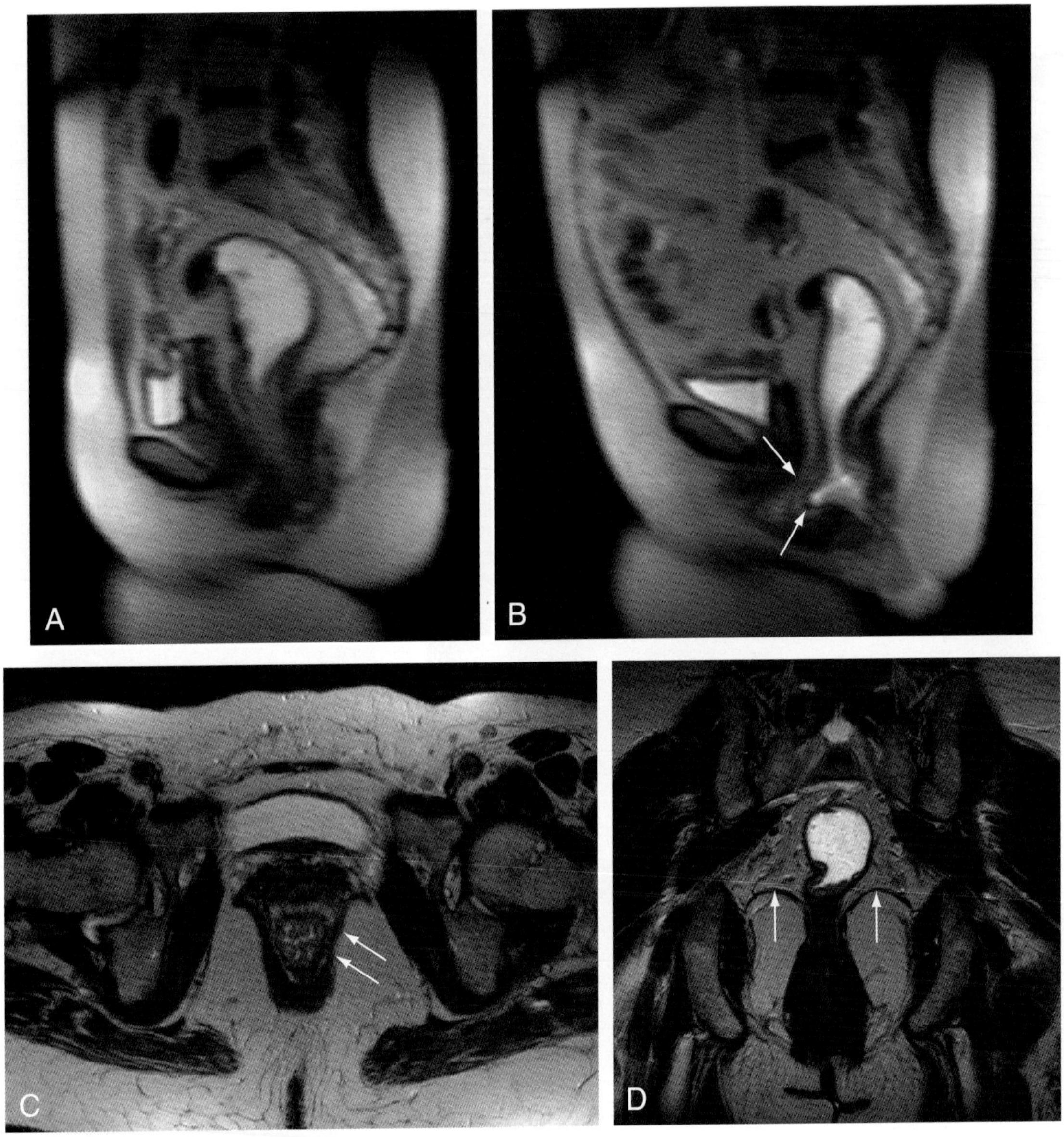

FIGURE 93-5

Anterior rectocele. Sagittal T2-weighted (4.4/90) ultrafast images of a 56-year-old woman with incomplete defecation at rest (**A**) and at strain (**B**) show formation of an anterior rectocele and adjacent herniation of the pelvic floor fat *(arrows)*. **C,** Axial T2-weighted (5000/132) image shows some thinning of the left aspect of the puborectalis muscle *(arrows)* but is otherwise unremarkable. **D,** Coronal T2-weighted (5000/132) image shows normal-appearing iliococcygeus muscles that remain bowed superiorly even during strain *(arrows)*.

a 16 to 20 cm field of view, 3 mm contiguous slices obtained using interpolation, 4000 msec TR, 130 msec effective TE, 256 phase encodes, and 2 acquisitions. Fat saturation is optional. No intravenous contrast agents are required when clinical findings strongly suggest the presence of a diverticulum. Gadolinium diethylenetriaminepentaacetic acid (Gd-DTPA) should be administered and axial, dynamic images obtained using a gradient-echo based pulse sequence, such as fast multiplanar spoiled gradient recall (FMPSGR) or fast low-angle shot (FLASH) when a rare urethral tumor is considered in the differential.

A diverticulum will appear as a bright focus with well-defined border on the T2-weighted images.[29,30] Debris may be identified in the dependent portion of the diverticulum (Fig. 93-6). In addition to locating the neck of the diverticulum, it is important to search for other diverticula arising from the urethra.

Tumor arising within a urethral diverticulum is a rare occurrence. Unfortunately, because no muscle layer separates the diverticulum from adjacent tissues, tumor extension beyond the confines of the urethra is usually rapid (Fig. 93-7). Lymphatic drainage may involve the inguinal nodes as well as the pelvic sidewall chains knowledgeable in fetal anatomy and the clinical question to be answered present during the study. This typically means that a radiologist should be present to oversee the examination. Since the fetus is in nearly constant motion, decisions regarding choice of image plane and whether the anatomy has been sufficiently evaluated need to be made relatively quickly.

Software advances now allow for parallel imaging, where fewer phase-encoding steps are needed to obtain images.[36-38] This allows for less blur with RARE imaging. Although there is a lower SNR overall, the images are obtained much faster, and some of this time can be used to either increase SNR, or increase resolution. One problem with parallel imaging is the increase in aliasing artifacts. We are currently testing various imaging strategies to determine if these are worthwhile in fetal imaging (Fig. 94-5).

Real-time imaging of the fetus is another relatively new development that allows for interactive optimization of imaging parameters such as slice thickness, FOV, echo spacing, and slice orientation.[39,40] This commonly results in images of superior diagnostic quality to standard single shot fast spin-echo imaging (Fig. 94-6).

T1-Weighted Imaging

T1-weighted imaging (Fig. 94-7) is more difficult than T2-weighted imaging of the fetus since there is less inherent soft-tissue contrast. In addition, since most T1-weighted sequences are not single shot, the images are degraded by motion that occurs during the breath-hold. We currently employ spoiled gradient-echo technique in and out of phase with the following parameters: TR = 180; TE = 2.2 and 4.5; flip angle = 80°; 5 mm slice thickness; FOV = 36 cm; matrix = 160 × 256; scan time = 17 seconds (breath-hold). T1-weighted imaging is used to assess for hemorrhage or fat in a lesion, and to assess the liver position in cases of congenital diaphragmatic hernia.

NORMAL FETAL ANATOMY

Central Nervous System

Sulcal development is a marker of cortical maturation and is used as an indicator of fetal maturity. Studies have shown that MR evaluation of CNS development[41-43] often lags behind neuroanatomic landmarks described in the pathology literature.[44] Earliest to form is the interhemispheric fissure present in all normal fetuses examined at 14 weeks. The Sylvian fissure begins as a shallow depression at 14 weeks and becomes grooved by 16 weeks. Major occipital gyri are present by weeks 18 to 19. Appearance of the cingulate gyrus is variable and generally present by the 26th week. Further progression of sulcation occurs after the 26th week and continues through the end of gestation. Coronal views of the varying appearance of the brain during development are shown in Figure 94-8. The corpus callosum is fully formed by 20 weeks, although it may be difficult to visualize on MR images until 24 weeks gestational age (Fig. 94-9). Midline views are particularly helpful in assessing the normal appearance of the corpus callosum and cerebellar vermis (see Fig. 94-9). The cavum septum pellucidum is seen in all normal fetuses. Occasionally, it may appear slightly dilated and more prominent; this finding is of unclear significance (Fig. 94-10).

The ventricular-to-brain diameter ratio decreases progressively throughout gestation: from >0.5 before 20 weeks,[45] it decreases rapidly to <0.5 after 20 weeks, with more gradual decreases thereafter to near childhood proportions, with a ratio approaching 0.35 to 0.4 beginning at around 30 weeks.[46]

Distinction of the spinal cord from the cerebrospinal fluid (CSF) can be made beginning early in the second trimester.[47] The conus medullaris, when visualized, terminates at the level of the fetal kidneys (Fig. 94-11).[35]

Face

Amniotic fluid is of high signal intensity in T2-weighted images and allows for sharp contrast for the external contour of the fetus, allowing for excellent visualization of the fetal profile in the sagittal plane (see Figs. 94-5 and 94-9). As the fetus swallows fluid, the contrast afforded by the amniotic fluid allows visualization of the oropharynx, soft palate, and tongue (see Figs. 94-5 and 94-9). The orbits are best evaluated in the fetal coronal and axial planes (Fig. 94-12).

Thorax

The fetal lungs fill with secretions as they develop. While they appear of slightly lower signal intensity than the surrounding amniotic fluid during the first and early second trimester (Fig. 94-13), with time, they become of high signal intensity, only slightly lower than that of amniotic fluid in the third trimester.[48] This signal intensity analysis has the potential to serve as a guide to fetal lung maturity, although further research is needed to determine the accuracy of this indirect evaluation of lung maturation. Pulmonary vessels are seen as hypointense linear structures.

Cardiac evaluation remains limited due to inherent motion. Fetal motion, rapid fetal heart rate, and variability of fetal heart rate make gated sequences impractical in the fetus. Occasionally, the interventricular septum and atrioventricular valves can be visualized, but a satisfactory four-chamber view, as can be obtained with sonography, is not routinely visualized.

When filled with amniotic fluid, the esophagus is visible as a posterior thoracic structure with a tubular shape and a hyperintense signal (see Fig. 94-13D). The trachea may also be seen medial to the major bronchi as a high-signal-intensity tubular structure (see Fig. 94-13E). The diaphragm is clearly visible as a thin hypointense band separating the abdomen from the thorax on coronal and sagittal images (see Fig. 94-13C). The thymus may be prominent in the third trimester (see Fig. 94-13F).

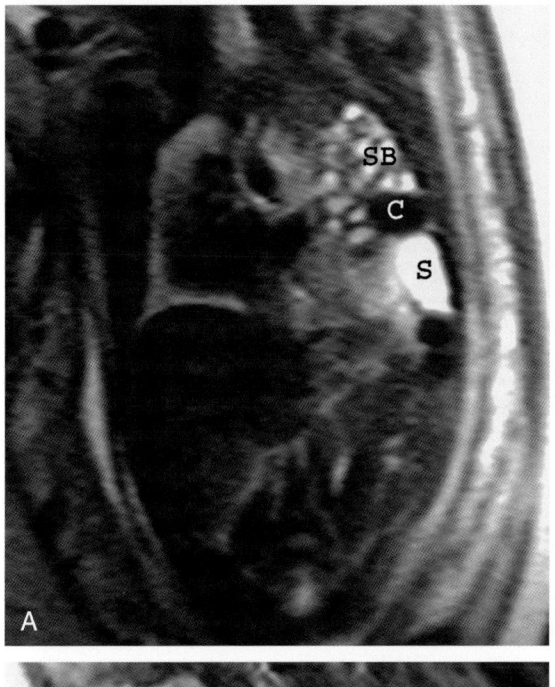

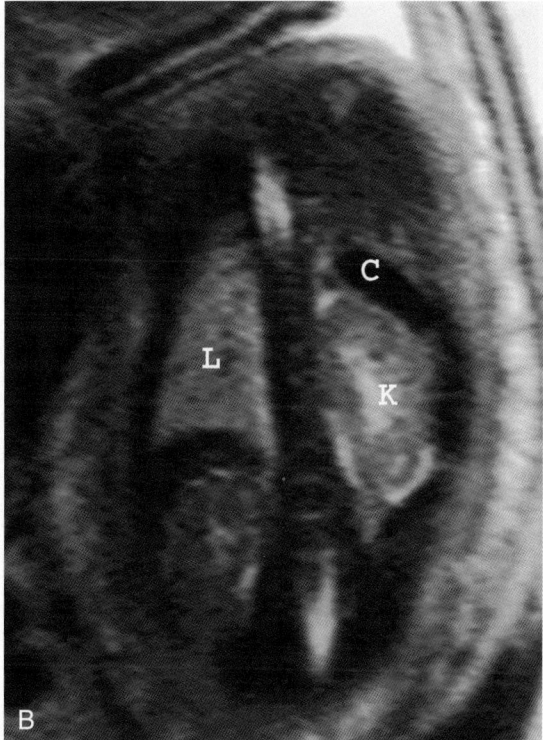

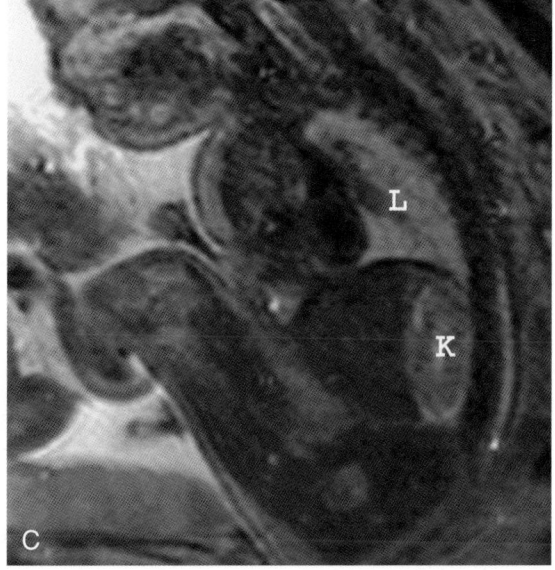

FIGURE 94-21

Images of fetus with congenital diaphragmatic hernia at 31 weeks gestational age. The stomach, colon, small bowel, and kidney are in the chest. **C,** Note the normal appearance to the right hemidiaphragm and right lung. (C, colon; K, kidney; L, lung; S, stomach; SB, small bowel.)

with ultrasound, but MRI can clearly demonstrate the region of the cleft soft palate in both normal (see Fig. 94-8) and abnormal fetuses (Fig. 94-22). This has important implications in patient counseling, since clefts in the soft palate are associated with speech and hearing difficulties.

The Fetal Surgery Patient

A rapidly expanding area for MRI is the evaluation of fetuses that potentially will undergo in-utero surgery and in fetuses being assessed for potential ex-utero intrapartum treatment (EXIT) procedure. In this procedure, while still attached to umbilical blood circulation, the appropriate diagnostic and therapeutic maneuvers

are undertaken to either provide ventilation or put the fetus on extra corporeal membrane oxygenation prior to clamping the umbilical cord. Assessment of airway obstruction is, therefore, an important indication for prenatal MRI. This is typically undertaken to define the extent of neck masses such as a cervical teratoma or lymphatic malformation.[86-88] It is increasingly common for fetuses with proven or suspected airway obstruction to undergo the EXIT procedure.[88,89] In patients being evaluated for EXIT procedure, MRI is helpful for visualizing potential airway obstruction, and in planning for intervention at the time of delivery (Fig. 94-23).[76,90]

For all fetal surgery patients, MRI is very helpful to ensure that unexpected anomalies are not present prior to undertaking the risk of fetal surgery.[91,92] In patients undergoing surgery for neural tube defects, MRI is

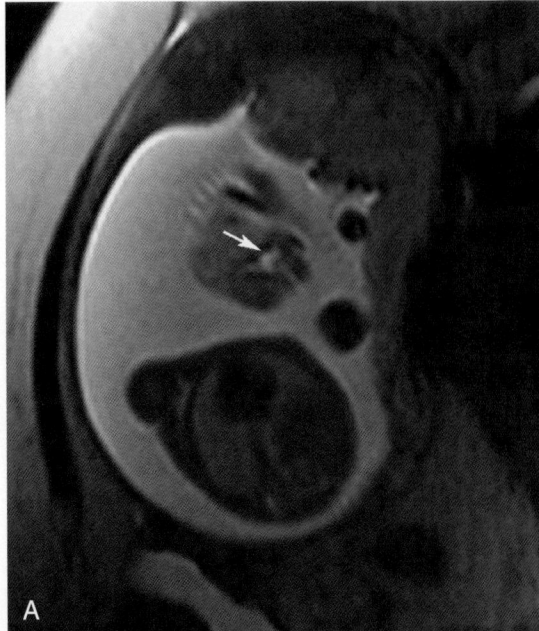

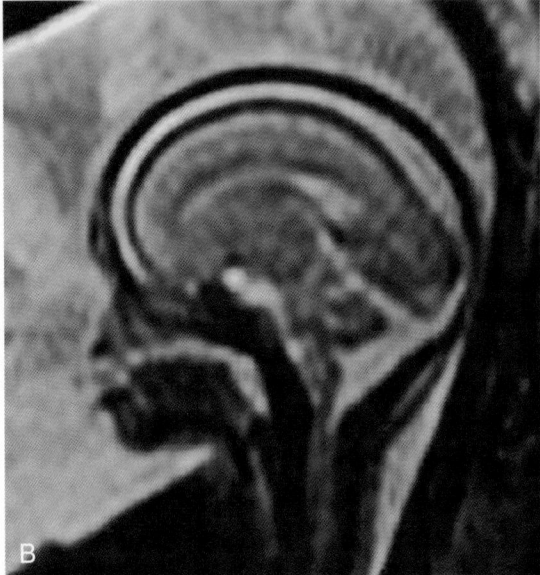

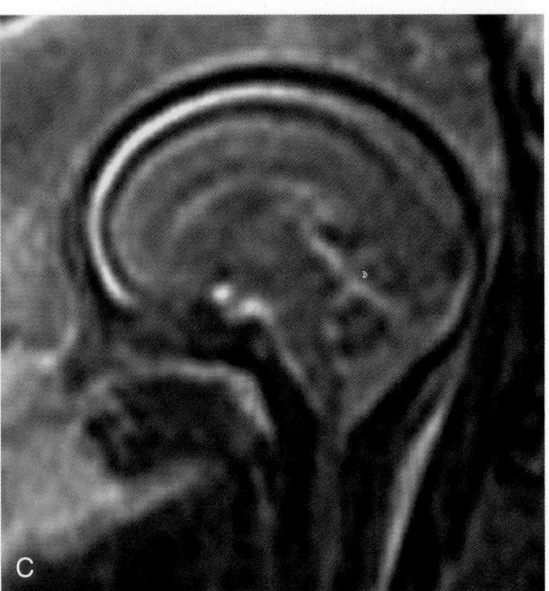

FIGURE 94-22

Cleft palate. Coronal (**A**) and Sagittal (**B** and **C**) views of fetus with cleft lip *(arrow)* and cleft palate. Note that despite amniotic fluid filling the oropharynx the dark band of the soft palate (see Fig. 94-6C) is not visualized.

helpful in characterizing the Chiari malformation, since the amount of cerebellar herniation is easily followed on serial MR examinations.

MAGNETIC RESONANCE VOLUMETRY

The data obtained from fast scan techniques can be used to assess the volume of the fetus and supporting structures. The expectation is that fetal weight estimates based on fetal volume determinations will be more accurate than those obtained with ultrasound. While sonographic estimates of fetal weight are reasonably accurate for the majority of the fetal population, at the extremes of weight, in the intrauterine growth-restricted (IUGR) and in the macrosomic fetus, where accuracy is most important, sonographic biometry frequently is limited. MRI has the promise of being less affected by patient body habitus (unless the patient cannot fit into the magnet bore), and instead of two-dimensional measurements being used for estimation of weight, a true fetal mass can be assessed.[93] A number of different methods have been described for obtaining the data upon which fetal volumetry can be performed.[94-99]

MR measurements of liver show that a single fetal liver volume measurement, performed several weeks before delivery, can distinguish fetuses subsequently diagnosed as being growth restricted with greater accuracy than ultrasound.[100,101]

Oligohydramnios is another finding in the IUGR fetus. Variations in technique for assessing amniotic fluid volume, typically by use of the amniotic fluid index

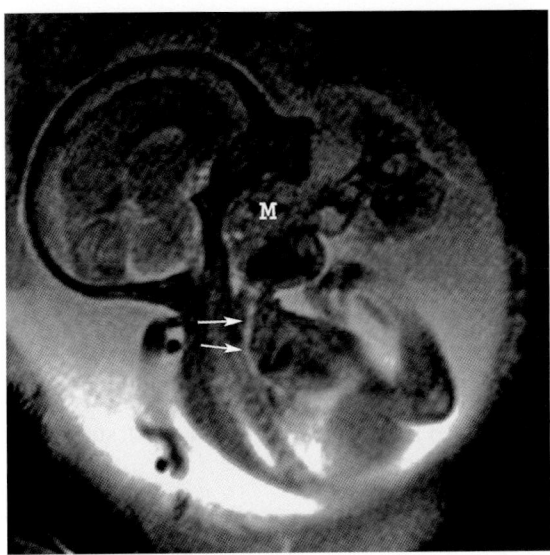

FIGURE 94-23

Oropharyngeal teratoma. Sagittal view of the fetus shows a large mass (M) distending the oropharynx. However, the trachea *(arrows)* appears distended with fluid. This information allowed for planning delivery by ex utero intrapartum treatment procedure with plan for tracheostomy placement, if needed, while the fetus was still on umbilical cord circulation, prior to cutting the umbilical cord.

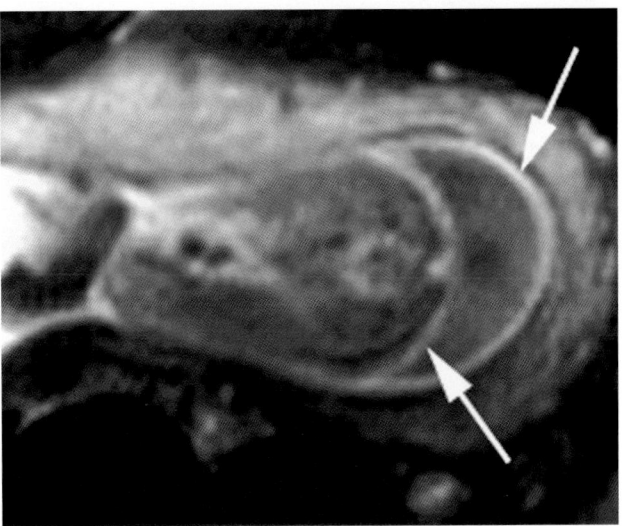

FIGURE 94-24

Fluid motion around a fetus at 20 weeks gestation. At times, fluid motion will be visualized as low signal in the amniotic fluid rimmed by a bright "layer" *(arrows)*. This brightness is generally due to a lack of motion at the periphery of the fluid space, however, the high signal intensity may also be due to subcutaneous fat (adjacent to the fetus) or fluid in the subamniotic space. *(Reproduced with permission from Levine D, Stroustrup Smith A, McKenzie C: Tips and Tricks of Fetal MRI. Rad Clin N Am 41:729-746, 2003.)*

(AFI), hamper our ability to standardize assessment of oligohydramnios. It is possible that MRI will allow for a more reliable means of assessing amniotic fluid volume. Information regarding fetal fat,[102] functional evaluation of the placenta,[103,104] and placental volume assessments will likely be used in combination with other data to better distinguish between the constitutionally small but appropriately grown fetus and the fetus at risk due to placental insufficiency.

Similarly, additional information about the macrosomic fetus will be available with MRI including pelvimetry,[105] fetal shoulder width,[105] and fetal fat.[102] The incremental benefit of MRI beyond that of ultrasound in the assessment of fetuses at the extremes of fetal growth remains to be determined in clinical practice.

ARTIFACTS

Motion Artifact

Motion affects all fetal MR examinations due to the combination of maternal breathing or whole body motion, maternal bowel peristalsis and arterial pulsations, and fetal motion. Since images are obtained with a single shot sequence, it is typical that we can obtain diagnostic quality imaging despite motion, since only the slice that was obtained during the motion will be affected. In general, breath-holding is not needed during sub-second imaging sequences, but if the patient is moving during imaging, a breath-hold could be helpful. If the fetus moves during the sequence, and the move-

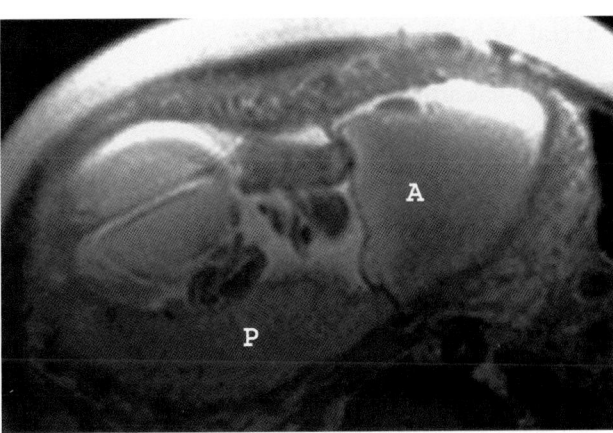

FIGURE 94-25

Abruption at 26 weeks gestational age. Note the low signal intensity fluid of the blood products (A) adjacent to the placenta (P).

ment is in plane with imaging, it is possible that a portion of the anatomy will be seen more than once. More commonly, an extremity will move out of the image plane during sequence acquisition and will not be visualized.[106]

Fluid motion artifact is characterized by a signal void occurring in fluid such as amniotic fluid (Fig. 94-24), cerebrospinal fluid, and fetal urine. A pitfall in the assumption that dark fluid on RARE imaging is due to motion is shown in Figure 94-25, where the low signal is due to blood products.

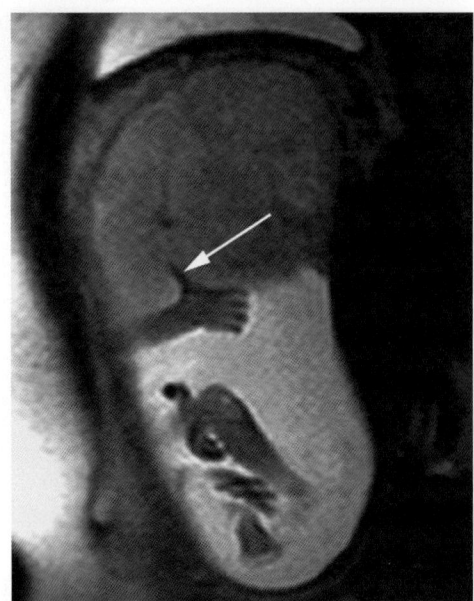

FIGURE 94-26

Partial volume artifact in a fetus at 19 weeks gestation. This image shows the fetal hand adjacent to the placenta. A prominent vein *(arrow)* in the placenta looks like a hyperextended thumb. *(Reproduced with permission from Levine D, Stroustrup Smith A, McKenzie C: Tips and Tricks of Fetal MRI. Rad Clin N Am 41:729-746, 2003.)*

Partial Volume Artifact

Partial volume artifact can complicate fetal imaging. As in all tomographic imaging, if only a portion of an anatomic region is in the slice, partial volume artifact can occur. What is different in obstetric imaging, is that this artifact can include structures outside of the fetus, for example,

in the placenta (Fig. 94-26). Because of SNR limitations, small fetal structures may be difficult to identify and evaluate. Thin structures surrounded by fluid can be difficult to visualize due to partial volume averaging occurring over the thickness of the slice. Examples include the membranous sac of a neural tube defect, the wall of an arachnoid cyst, and the forming corpus callosum in the second trimester.

Due to partial volume averaging, some pathologies have a slightly unexpected appearance on MRI. For example, in some cases of nuchal thickening (Fig. 94-27), the more complex cystic and solid appearance on ultrasound corresponds to a simple cystic appearance on MRI. Additionally, there are areas of pathology that are better assessed by ultrasound than by MRI, such as small calcifications (Fig. 94-28).[106]

FUTURE DEVELOPMENTS

In the future it is possible that use of MRI in fetuses with mild ventriculomegaly can improve our ability to counsel patients. It may be possible to use MRI to assess for other indices besides ventricular volume (e.g., cortical maturation, cortical volume, and ventricular morphology) that will allow us to stratify patients into those in whom a normal outcome can be expected as opposed to those at risk for developmental delay.

Functional imaging is also on the horizon, with diffusion-weighted brain imaging and brain spectroscopy. These tools may allow for earlier identification of brain damage or hypoxia.

Three-dimentional volumetry is easily performed on fetal MRI. In addition to fetal lung volumes in cases of chest masses, it may be that 3D volumetry allows for a better assessment of fetal weight, such as in diabetics

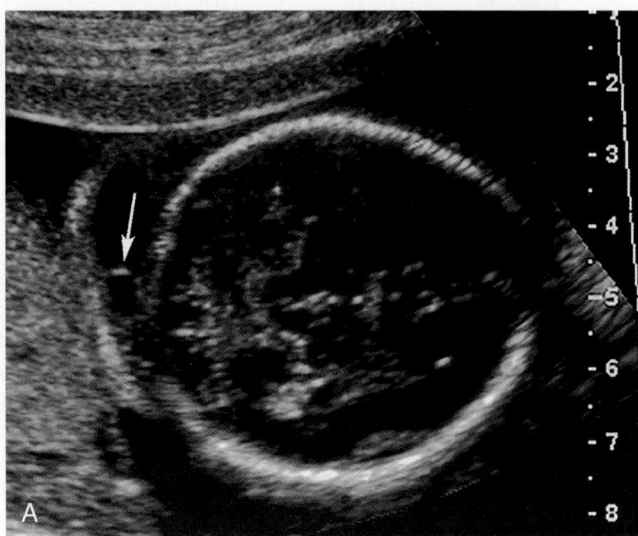
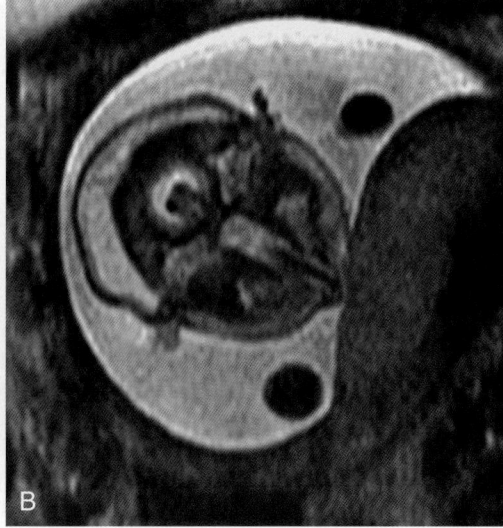

FIGURE 94-27

Nuchal thickening. Sonogram (**A**) and MR image (**B**) in fetus at 21 weeks gestational age with nuchal thickening. The septation in the nuchal region *(arrow)* is better seen on the sonogram than the MR image.

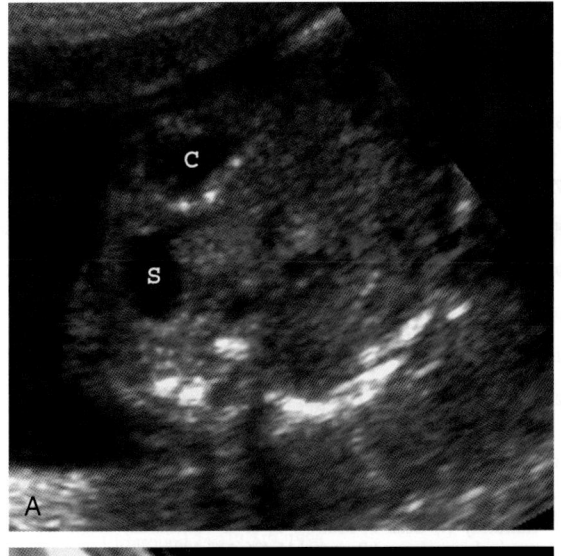

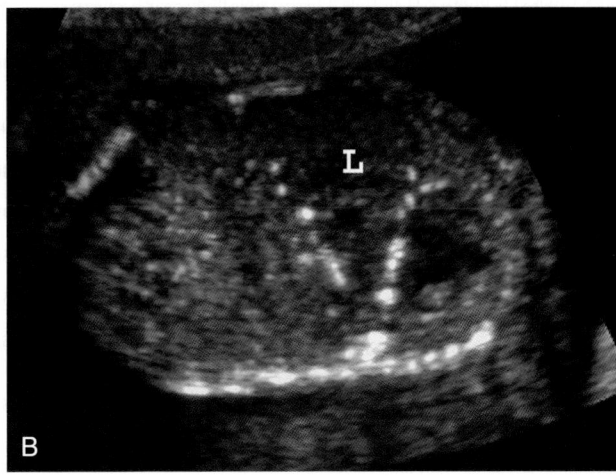

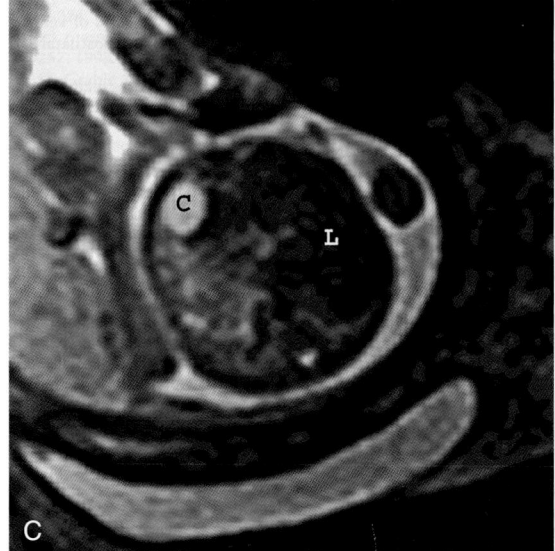

FIGURE 94-28

Meconium peritonitis. **A** and **B,** Transverse and sagittal sonograms on the abdomen demonstrate a cyst (C) with calcifications along the wall of the cyst and around the edge of the liver (L) consistent with meconium peritonitis. **C,** MR image demonstrates the cyst, but not the calcifications. (S, stomach.)

with macrosomia, potentially allowing for a decreased cesarean section rate or, for example, in differentiating between the growth restricted fetus from the normal but small-for-gestational-age fetus.

CONCLUSION

Ultrasound continues to be the screening modality of choice in the evaluation of the fetus due to its relatively low cost and real-time capability. However, there are many cases in which alternative imaging is useful as an adjunct to ultrasound. Fast MR techniques allow for superb imaging of fetal anatomy. In the future, faster imaging, 3D volumetry, and functional imaging will add to our ability to better assess the fetus, and optimize patient care. As our experience with fast MR techniques increases, we will continue to identify patients in whom MRI contributes to patient evaluation.

REFERENCES

1. Weinreb JC, Lowe T, Cohen JM, Kutler M: Human fetal anatomy: MR imaging. Radiology 157:715-720, 1985.
2. Antuaco TL, Shah HR, Mattison DR, Quirk JG Jr: MR imaging in high-risk obstetric patients: a valuable complement to US. Radiographics 12:91-109, 1992.
3. Powell MC, Worthington BS, Buckley JM, Symonds EM: Magnetic resonance imaging (MRI) in obstetrics. II. Fetal anatomy. Br J Obstet Gynaecol 95:38-46, 1988.
4. Williamson RA, Weiner CP, Yuh WT, Abu-Yousef MM: Magnetic resonance imaging of anomalous fetuses. Obstet Gynecol 73:952-956, 1989.
5. Stark DD, McCarthy SM, Filly RA, et al: Intrauterine growth retardation: evaluation by magnetic resonance. Work in progress. Radiology 155:425-427, 1985.
6. Lenke RR, Persutte WH, Nemes JM: Use of pancuronium bromide to inhibit fetal movement during magnetic resonance imaging. A case report. J Reprod Med 34:315-317, 1989.
7. Horvath L, Seeds JW: Temporary arrest of fetal movement with pancuronium bromide to enable antenatal magnetic resonance imaging of holoprosencephaly. Am J Perinatol 6:418-420, 1989.
8. Mansfield P, Stehling MK, Ordidge RJ, et al: Echo planar imaging of the human fetus in utero at 0.5 T. Br J Radiol 63:833-841, 1990.
9. Edelman RR, Wielopolski PA: Fast MRI, 2nd ed. Philadelphia: Saunders, 1996, pp302-352.

PEDIATRIC BODY APPLICATIONS OF MRI

Marilyn J. Siegel ● Fredric A. Hoffer

INTRODUCTION

Imaging of pediatric diseases has been revolutionized with the development of MRI. MRI is increasingly utilized as the primary study to evaluate soft-tissue and paraspinal masses as well as joint abnormalities, and it is employed as a secondary test to assess abnormalities observed on sonography or CT scans. This chapter will highlight the diagnostic applications of MRI in a wide variety of disease processes of the pediatric chest, abdomen, and pelvis.

TECHNICAL CONSIDERATIONS

Receiver Coil Selection

The smallest coil that fits tightly around the body part of interest should be used to improve the signal-to-noise ratio and spatial resolution.[1,2] A head coil or phased-array coil can usually be used to study infants and small children, while a phased-array or whole-body coil is required for imaging larger children and adolescents. The phased-array coils are preferred over the body coils for imaging the pelvis because they provide better anatomic resolution. A perineal coil may improve resolution in patients who have tumors localized to the perineum. Intrarectal coils are rarely needed in the pediatric population. In addition, their use in very young children usually requires parenteral sedation. Surface coils, which can be useful in the evaluation of superficial structures such as the spine, have limited value in the evaluation of deeper abdominal structures because of the drop off in signal strength with increasing distance from the center of the coil.

Image-Specific Parameters

Images of the pelvis are typically acquired in two or three orthogonal planes: coronal, sagittal, and/or axial. Slice thickness varies with patient size and area of interest. Thicker slices (4-8 mm) are usually adequate for a general survey of the chest, abdomen, or pelvis and larger lesions. Thinner slices (3-4 mm) are used in evaluating small lesions and areas of maximum interest. Most MR examinations in children are performed with a 128 or 192 matrix and one or two signal acquisitions to shorten imaging time. A 286×286 matrix may be needed in areas where more anatomic detail is desired.

A square shape is used when the body part being examined fills the field of view. An asymmetric field of view is ideal for body parts that are narrow in one direction, such as the abdomen or pelvis in a thin patient. A large field of view is preferred over a smaller one to achieve a better signal-to-noise ratio. Decreasing the field of view improves spatial resolution, but it decreases the pixel size, which increases noise.

Pulse Sequences and Image Contrast

Spin-Echo Sequences

T1- and T2-weighted spin-echo sequences are obtained in virtually all patients. T1-weighted sequences [short repetition time (TR), short time to echo (TE)] provide excellent contrast between soft-tissue structures and fat and thus, they help in tissue characterization (i.e., fluid, fat, or blood). T2-weighted images, usually acquired by fast (turbo) spin-echo techniques to shorten imaging time, provide excellent contrast between tumor and adjacent soft-tissues. The fast spin-echo techniques, however, may result in some loss of contrast between fat and similar intense fluid, and thus, they should be used in combination with fat-suppression techniques. When a lesion of high signal intensity is noted on routine T1-weighted images, fat-saturated images are useful to differentiate hemorrhagic from fat-containing lesions.

Two basic methods of fat suppression are widely available: short tau inversion recovery (STIR) and radio-frequency presaturation of the lipid peak (fat saturation). Signal from fat is nulled on STIR and fat-saturated images, while most pathologic lesions, with increased free water and prolonged T1 and T2 values, are bright on the fat-suppressed sequences.

Contrast Provided by Other Pulse Sequences

Gradient-Echo Images

The gradient-recalled echo (GRE) technique is used to evaluate the patency of vascular structures and to differentiate between vessels and lymph nodes.[3] GRE sequences result in high signal in flowing blood. By comparison, flowing blood appears as areas of flow void or decreased signal within the vessel lumen on spin-echo sequences. Images acquired with large flip angles (>45 degrees) are T1 weighted, while those acquired with small flip angles (<30 degrees) are T2 weighted. The relatively short acquisition time required to obtain GRE images also allows serial dynamic imaging immediately following intravenous administration of gadolinium chelate agents. Arterial and venous phases can be acquired and reformatted in a three-dimensional (3D) display.[4-6]

Gadolinium-enhanced T1-weighted images can help in lesion characterization by depicting the presence of areas of vascularized tumor, necrosis, and cyst formation. They also may improve contrast between tumor and normal tissues, thus contributing to the determination of extent of disease.

Single-shot fast spin-echo imaging uses extremely long echo-train lengths and half-Fourier imaging to provide fast images. It is the sequence of choice for MR cholangiopancreatography[7] and MR urography.[8] There are two basic approaches for abdominal single-shot fast spin-echo imaging. One technique is to image a 30 to 40-mm thick slab of tissue. This has the advantage of displaying convoluted structures, such as the ureter, in one image. The thick slabs are prescribed in conjunction with very long echo times; resulting in heavy T2-weighted images, which eliminates the signal from structures that are not fluid filled. The second approach uses thin, continuous images that are less T2 weighted. These can be reviewed individually or as a maximal intensity projection.

In general, most lesions have a low signal intensity on T1-weighted images and a high signal intensity on T2-weighted images. Blood, proteinaceous fluid, and cartilage can increase the T1 signal. Administration of gadolinium chelates also results in a high T1 signal intensity. A low T2 signal intensity is seen with mineralization, hemosiderin and other blood products, iron oxide, and fibrosis.

Optimizing Image Quality

Motion artifacts, including voluntary motion and physiologic motion due to respiration and bowel peristalsis, can be a problem because of the relatively long time period required to obtain images. Methods for suppressing motion artifacts include conscious sedation, cardiac gating, and fast MR imaging sequences.

Conscious Sedation

Voluntary motion can be minimized or eliminated by the use of conscious sedation. The American Academy of Pediatrics guidelines are recommended for administering and monitoring the sedation of pediatric patients.[9]

Children over 6 years of age will usually cooperate for the MR examination after an explanation of the procedure and reassurance. It also helps to assure that the patient is comfortable, free of pain, and has an empty bladder. Conscious sedation is essential when imaging children younger than 6 years of age. The drugs most frequently used for sedation are oral chloral hydrate and intravenous pentobarbital sodium.[10] Oral chloral hydrate is the most common sedative in children younger than 18 months. The dose of this sedative drug is 50 to 100 mg/kg, with a maximum dosage not to exceed 2000 mg. In children aged 18 months to 6 years, intravenous pentobarbital sodium is the drug of choice. Initially, 2.5 mg/kg is given as a slow bolus over 1 to 2 minutes. Sedation will be successful at this dose in most patients. If adequate sedation is not obtained, an additional 1.25 mg/kg is given. This dose can be repeated 1 to 2 minutes later if necessary, up to a maximum dose of 6 mg/kg or 200 mg (whichever is smaller). Patients who are to receive parenteral sedation should have no liquids by mouth for 3 hours and no solid foods for 6 hours prior to their examination. Propofol, because it has a short half-life, has been used in some centers. However, its use usually requires the assistance of an anesthesiologist.

Fast MR Imaging Techniques

Respiratory motion can produce ghosting and blurring artifacts. These artifacts can be reduced or eliminated by the use of faster imaging sequences. These fast techniques (gradient-echo, fast spin-echo, single-shot fast spin-echo) were discussed earlier.

Cardiac Gating

Electrocardiographic (ECG)-cardiac gating reduces motion unsharpness and is used in MR examinations of the thorax. This technique entails an increase in scan time, but it markedly improves the image quality. MRI-compatible electrodes are placed on either the patient's ventral or dorsal surface. Triggering is commonly performed to the R-wave of the ECG. In general, image acquisition is during systole.

CHEST

The common clinical indications for MRI of the pediatric chest are: 1. evaluation of mediastinal masses; 2. characterization of vascular anomalies; and 3. evaluation of congenital heart diseases. The role of MRI in imaging mediastinal masses is discussed below. MRI features of vascular and cardiac lesions are described elsewhere in this textbook.

Mediastinal Masses

CT remains the study of choice to evaluate most mediastinal masses. The major application of MRI has been as a problem-solving tool in patients in whom the CT examination is indeterminate, often because there is a contraindication to the use of iodinated contrast material. MRI has been most helpful in two specific clinical scenarios: the evaluation of complex mediastinal cysts and the determination of intraspinal extension of neurogenic tumors.[11]

Congenital Mediastinal Cysts

Congenital mediastinal cysts include foregut (bronchogenic, enteric, and neurenteric), thymic, and pericardial cysts. Bronchogenic cysts are usually located in the subcarinal or right paratracheal regions, while enteric cysts usually are located close to or within the esophageal wall. Neurenteric cysts are posterior mediastinal lesions that are connected to the meninges through a midline defect in one or more vertebral bodies and are easily recognized by the associated vertebral body anomalies. Pericardial cysts are most frequently seen in the right cardiophrenic angle. Thymic cysts are located in the anterior mediastinum.

On MRI, most foregut cysts appear as well-marginated, round or oval, nonenhancing masses. The cyst contents are usually homogeneous and have a low signal intensity on T1-weighted images and a high signal intensity on T2-weighted images, reflecting their serous nature. On occasion, foregut cysts may have a signal intensity equal to that of muscle or soft-tissue on T1-weighted images because of viscid mucoid or hemorrhagic contents or calcium (Fig. 95-1). They may contain air or air-fluid levels when they communicate with the bronchial tree or gastrointestinal tract, usually due to superimposed infection or perforation.

Neurogenic Tumors

Posterior mediastinal masses are of neural origin in approximately 95% of cases and may arise from sympathetic ganglion cells (neuroblastoma, ganglioneuroblastoma, or ganglioneuroma) or from nerve sheaths (neurofibroma or schwannoma). Rarer causes of posterior mediastinal masses in children include neurenteric cyst, lateral meningocele, and extramedullary hematopoiesis. MRI is particularly well suited for

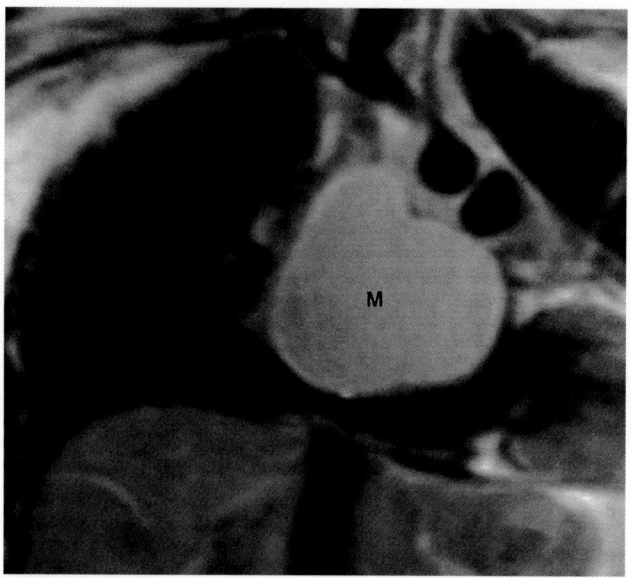

FIGURE 95-1

Mediastinal cyst. T1-weighted coronal MR image shows a homogenous intermediate mass (M). The signal intensity reflects the high protein content of the cyst fluid.

identifying intraspinal extension, which is an important clinical question in patients with neurogenic tumors.[12] Recognition of intraspinal invasion is critical because such involvement usually requires radiation therapy or a laminectomy prior to tumor debulking.

Ganglion cell tumors tend to have an elongated configuration and parallel the spinal column, in contradistinction to nerve sheath tumors, which have a rounder shape. On T1-weighted images, most neurogenic tumors have a low to intermediate signal intensity. On T2-weighted images, the tumors have a high signal intensity. Areas of low signal intensity, corresponding to calcification or collagenous fibrous tissue, may be noted on T2-weighted images. Because of their origin from neural tissue, neurogenic tumors have a tendency to invade the spinal canal. Intraspinal extension is extradural in location, displacing and occasionally compressing the cord (Fig. 95-2).

ABDOMEN

The most common indication for MRI of the pediatric abdomen is determination of the site of origin, extent, and character of an abdominal mass. Less often, MRI is used to evaluate parenchymal diseases of the liver and abnormalities of the major abdominal vessels.

Abdominal Masses

Abdominal masses in the pediatric population are predominantly retroperitoneal in location, with the kidney being the site of origin in over one half of cases. Generally in neonates and infants younger than 2 months

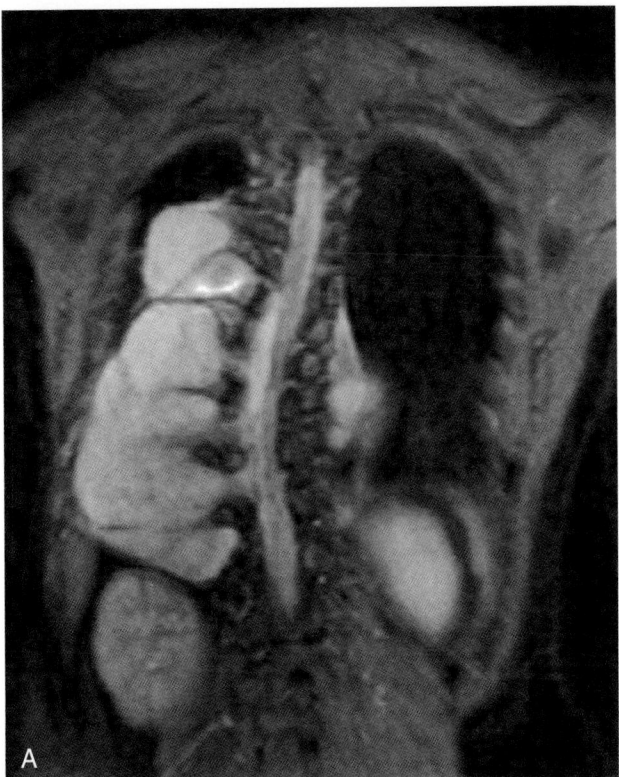

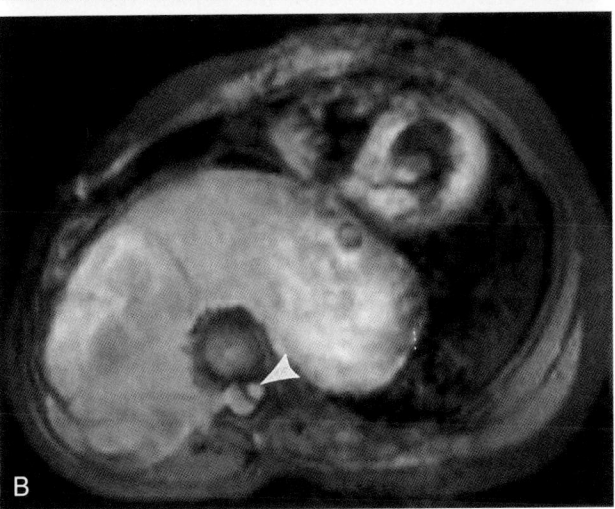

FIGURE 95-2

Mediastinal ganglioneuroblastoma, 7-year–old girl. **A,** Short tau inversion recovery (STIR) coronal image (TR/TE 3500/18, flip angle 140 degrees) shows a large right posterior mediastinal mass entering the spinal canal through multiple neural foramen. **B,** Axial T1-weighted gadolinium-enhanced and fat-suppressed image (TR/TE 804/15) demonstrates the tumor entering the right neural foramen and displacing the spinal cord (*arrowhead*) to the left. The intraspinal component was removed 3 years later and had matured to a ganglioneuroma.

of age, most abdominal masses are benign and have an excellent prognosis, while with increasing age the frequency of malignant neoplasms increases.[13]

The choice of examination for evaluation of a suspected abdominal mass varies with the age of the patient, the expertise at a given institution, and the

relative advantages and disadvantages of each imaging method. Ultrasonography is considered the screening technique of choice for identification of a pediatric abdominal mass. If the sonogram is normal, additional radiographic evaluation generally is not required. If sonography cannot provide adequate information or if more information is needed about the character or extent of a neoplasm, either CT or MRI can be performed.[14] In general, CT, because of its ready availability and established accuracy, is more widely used than MRI. However, MRI is a reliable alternative to CT.[14] MRI can provide important diagnostic information about location and tumor extent, particularly in the older infant and child with solid masses.

Kidneys

Normal Anatomy

T1-weighted coronal images are best to demonstrate the two major zones of the kidney—cortex and medulla. The renal cortex has a relatively high signal intensity in contrast to the medulla, which has a lower intensity. On T2-weighted images, the signal intensity of the renal medulla increases relative to the renal cortex, and they become isointense to each other. The renal artery and vein, the ureter, and the pelvicalyceal system are imaged as tubular areas of low signal intensity on T1-weighted images and high signal intensity on T2-weighted sequences. The medullary pyramids are better defined on T1- than on T2-weighted images. They are relatively more prominent in neonates and young children than in older children and adolescents. In young children, adipose tissue, characterized by high signal intensity, is not easily identified on either sequence in the renal hili. Renal sinus fat increases with age, and by adolescence it is clearly seen on T1-weighted images.

Wilms' Tumor

Wilms' tumor is the most common primary malignant renal tumor of childhood, accounting for 7% of all childhood cancers.[15-17] The mean patient age at diagnosis is 3.5 years. Wilms' tumors are rare in children younger than 6 months of age and older than 6 years of age. Affected children usually present with a palpable abdominal mass, and on occasion with abdominal pain, fever, and hematuria. Other clinical findings include hypertension, polycythemia, fever, malaise, and left-sided varicoceles due to tumor compressing the left renal vein.[15]

At gross examination, Wilms' tumors are typically solitary intrarenal masses that contain areas of hemorrhage, necrosis, and cyst formation. Histologically, there is undifferentiated renal tissue as well as skeletal muscle, cartilage, and squamous epithelium. Metastases are seen in about 10% of children at diagnosis. These are most often to the lungs and less often to the lymph nodes and liver.[17]

Wilms' tumor usually develops sporadically, but approximately 20% of children have a family history.[18]

TABLE 95-1 Wilms' Tumor Staging by the National Wilms' Tumor Study Group

Stage	Definition
1	Tumor limited to kidney and completely excised. The renal capsule has an intact outer surface. No evidence of tumor at or beyond the margins of resection
2	Tumor extends beyond the kidney, but is completely excised. May have regional extension (i.e., penetration of renal capsule or invasion of renal sinus). No evidence of tumor at or beyond the margins of resection
3	Residual nonhematogenous tumor present and confined to the abdomen
4	Hematogenous metastases (lung, liver, bone, brain, etc.) or lymph node metastases outside the abdominopelvic region
5	Bilateral renal involvement is present at diagnosis

From Green DM: Paediatric oncology update: Wilms' tumour. Eur J Cancer 33:409-418, 1997.

In these patients, the tumor is inherited as an autosomal dominant trait. Other risk factors for development of Wilms' tumor include aniridia, the overgrowth syndromes (hemihypertrophy, Beckwith-Weidemann, Simpson-Golabi-Behmel, Sotos), Drash syndrome, and neurofibromatosis.[16,17]

Clinical Staging

The National Wilms' Tumor Staging System is shown in Table 95-1.[17] The staging of Wilms' tumor is based on surgical and preoperative imaging findings. Two-year survival rates after treatment are approximately 96% for stage I, 90% for stage II, 90% for stage III, 80% for stage IV, and 85% for stage IV.[17]

Diagnostic Imaging

Imaging is performed to confirm the intrarenal origin of the tumor, to evaluate the potential for resectability by identifying local invasion and vascular extension, and to detect bilateral or metastatic disease.

Wilms' tumor usually appears as a large, spherical, at least partially intrarenal mass, which is often associated with dilatation and distortion of the renal pelvis and calyces. Tumors may be homogeneous, but are more often heterogeneous (Fig. 95-3) with a predominantly intermediate signal intensity on T1-weighted sequences and a high signal intensity on T2-weighted sequences.[16,20-23] Most enhance after the administration of gadolinium chelate compounds.

Local spread of tumor may take the form of extension through the capsule into the perinephric space, retroperitoneal lymphadenopathy, or renal vein or inferior vena caval thrombosis.[17] Perinephric extension, which occurs in about 20% of patients with Wilms' tumor, produces a thickened renal capsule or perirenal soft-tissue stranding.

Spread to regional lymph nodes also occurs in about 20% of patients. The diagnosis of nodal metastases is based on demonstration of lymph node enlargement. In contrast to adults, lymph nodes, even small ones, are not common findings in the retroperitoneum of young children. Thus, the demonstration of hilar, periaortic, paracaval, or other retroperitoneal nodes, regardless of size, should be considered abnormal and suspicious for tumor metastases. Lymph nodes have medium

signal intensity on T1-weighted image (Fig. 95-4) and high signal intensity on T2-weighted and gadolinium-enhanced images.

Vascular invasion occurs in up to 10% of cases. It does not adversely affect prognosis if the thrombus is resected, but the presence of caval invasion is a determinant of the surgical approach. Removal of tumor thrombus extending to or above the confluence of the hepatic veins may require a thoracoabdominal approach to prevent tumor embolization to the pulmonary arteries. An abdominal approach alone is satisfactory for intravascular thrombus below the hepatic veins. Tumor thrombus is hyperintense to flowing blood on spin-echo sequences and is hypointense to flowing blood on gradient-echo images (Fig. 95-5).[4]

Several pitfalls in the interpretation of vascular extension need to be recognized. Flow entry artifacts related to slowly flowing blood can cause increased intravascular signal on axial spin-echo images and loss of intravascular signal on gradient-echo images, mimicking tumor thrombus. Turbulent flow, as a result of the

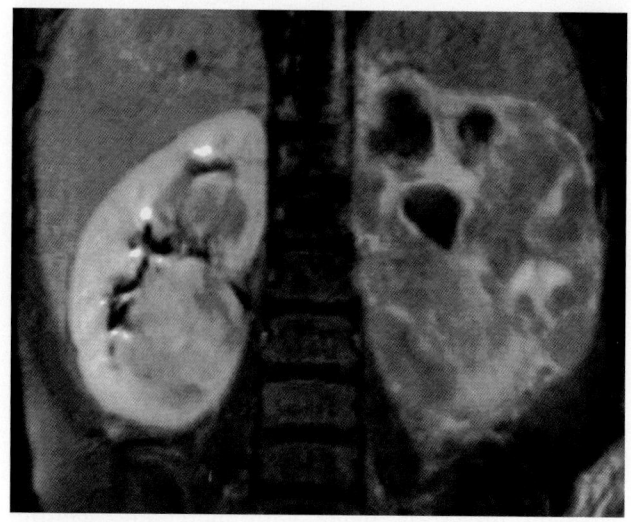

FIGURE 95-3

Bilateral Wilms' tumors, 2-year–old girl. T1-weighted gadolinium contrast-enhanced coronal MR image shows large intermediate signal intensity masses in both kidneys.

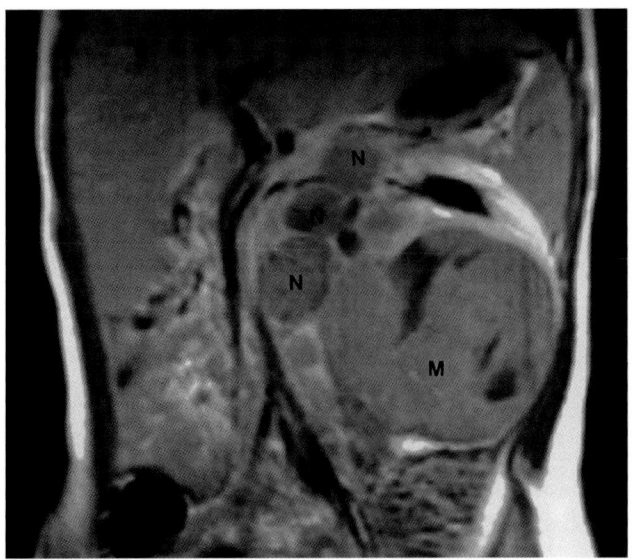

FIGURE 95-4

Wilms' tumor with retroperitoneal adenopathy, 3-year–old boy. T1-weighted (TR/TE 450/15) coronal image shows a large mass (M) arising within the left kidney and enlarged retroperitoneal lymph nodes (N).

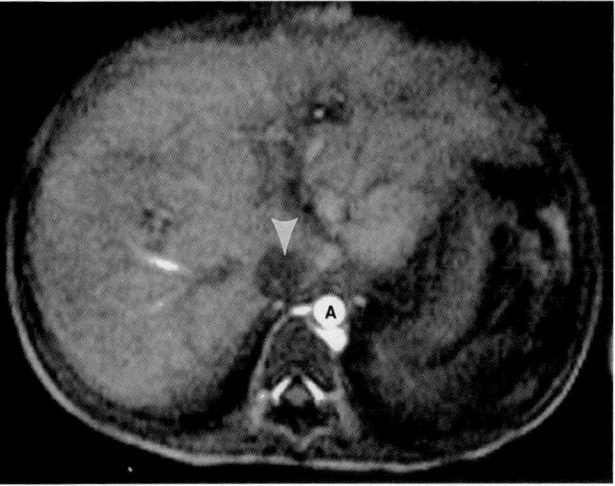

FIGURE 95-5

Wilms' tumor with intracaval extension, 3-year–old girl. Axial gradient-echo MR image (TR/TE 50/8, flip angle 50 degrees) shows flow in the aorta (A), but absence of flow in the inferior vena cava (*arrowhead*). This patient had a large Wilms' tumor in the right kidney which invaded the renal vein and propagated into the inferior vena cava and hepatic veins. The patient presented with findings of a Budd-Chiari syndrome.

multiplicity of flow velocities and phase shifts, also can decrease intravascular signal on gradient-echo images. Reviewing the combination of spin-echo and gradient-echo images can eliminate errors in diagnosis.

Bilateral tumors, present in as many as 10% of patients, also may be identified by MRI (see Fig. 95-3). These are usually synchronous and present at the time of initial diagnosis. Liver metastases are easily evaluated by MRI at the same time that the primary tumor is imaged. CT is the method of choice to detect pulmonary metastases.

Patients with incomplete resection of tumor, lymph node involvement, and vascular invasion have the highest risk for postoperative recurrence. Features that suggest localized recurrence are a soft-tissue mass in the empty renal fossa and ipsilateral psoas muscle enlargement.

Nephroblastomatosis

Nephroblastomatosis is an abnormality of nephrogenesis and is characterized by the persistence of nephrogenic rests (i.e., persistent fetal renal blastema) beyond 36 weeks of intrauterine gestation. Nephroblastomatosis itself is not a malignant condition, but it is a precursor to Wilms' tumor.[21,24-27] There are two basic types of nephrogenic rests: perilobar, which is found at the periphery of a renal lobe, and intralobar, which may be found anywhere within a renal lobe. Perilobar rests are much more common than intralobar rests.[21] The risk of Wilms' tumor is approximately 1% to 2% in patients with perilobar rests and 4% to 5% in those with intralobar rests.[21] Nephrogenic rests may be further subdivided into sclerosing, hyperplastic, or neoplastic types.

Nephrogenic rests are usually hypointense relative to normal renal tissue on gadolinium-enhanced T1-weighted MR images and hypo-, iso- or slightly hyper-intense to renal parenchyma on T2-weighted images (Fig. 95-6).[20,21] Hyperplastic and neoplastic nephrogenic rests are more likely to appear iso- or hyper-intense on T2-weighted images than are sclerotic or inactive rests, which often appear as hypointense foci.[20] The overall sensitivity and specificity of MRI for depicting foci of nephroblastomatosis is about 55% and 100%, respectively. Nephrogenic rests are best seen on gadolinium-enhanced sequences.[20]

Mesoblastic Nephroma

Mesoblastic nephroma, also termed fetal renal hamartoma, is a benign neoplasm, and it is the most common solid renal tumor of neonates and infants younger than 6 months of age. This tumor occurs in two forms; a typical form that is benign and most often seen in young infants, and an atypical form that is potentially malignant and usually seen in older children, but may also occur in infants.[28-30] On MRI, the tumor has a signal intensity similar to renal parenchyma on T1- and T2-weighted sequences. The MR appearance is nonspecific and overlaps with that of Wilms' tumor, but the diagnosis should be considered in infants with solid renal masses.

Clear-Cell Sarcoma and Rhabdoid Tumor

Clear-cell sarcomas and rhabdoid tumors account for about 4% and 2% of pediatric renal tumors, respectively. Both typically affect children under 2 years of age.

TABLE 95-2 International Neuroblastoma Staging System for Neuroblastoma

Stage	Definition
1	Localized tumor with complete resection, with or without microscopic residual disease; representative ipsilateral lymph nodes negative for tumor microscopically (nodes attached to and removed with the primary tumor may be positive)
2A	Localized tumor with incomplete gross excision; representative ipsilateral nonadherent lymph nodes negative for tumor microscopically
2B	Localized tumor with or without complete gross excision, with representative ipsilateral nonadherent lymph nodes positive for tumor. Enlarged contralateral lymph nodes must be negative microscopically
3	Unresectable unilateral tumor infiltrating across the midline, with or without regional lymph node involvement; or localized unilateral tumor with contralateral regional lymph node involvement; or midline tumor with bilateral extension by infiltration (unresectable) or by lymph node involvement
4	Any primary tumor with dissemination to distant lymph nodes, bone, bone marrow, liver, skin and/or other organs (except as defined for stage 4S)
4S	Localized primary tumor (as defined for stages 1, 2A, or 2B), with dissemination limited to skin, liver, and/or bone marrow. Bone marrow involvement should be minimal (<10% of total nucleated cells identified as malignant on bone marrow biopsy or on marrow aspirate). Limited to infants younger than 1 year of age

From Brodeur GM, Pritchard J, Berthold F, et al: Revision of the international criteria for neuroblastoma diagnosis, staging, and response to treatment. J Clin Oncol 11:1466-1477, 1993.

Neonatal neuroblastoma can be hemorrhagic and thus, have an appearance similar to that of benign hemorrhage. Differentiating between these two conditions is possible when there are hepatic metastases or when serum vanillylmandelic acid (VMA) levels are elevated. Serial imaging also can help to differentiate between these lesions. A hematoma decreases in size over 1 to 2 weeks, while neuroblastoma will either remain the same size or enlarge.

Neuroblastoma

Neuroblastoma is one of the small, blue, round cell tumors and accounts for 8% to 10% of all abdominal tumors.[13] Neuroblastoma can arise anywhere along the sympathetic chain from the neck through the pelvis. However, more than half of all neuroblastomas originate in the abdomen, and two thirds of these arise in the adrenal gland, with another 30% occurring in the pelvic or visceral ganglia, paraganglia or the organ of Zuckerkandl, and 15% to 20% arising in the neck or chest.[37]

Patients with neuroblastoma usually are between 1 and 5 years of age; mean patient age at diagnosis is 2 years. Most children with neuroblastoma are symptomatic. Common clinical complaints include skeletal pain; neurologic abnormalities such as nystagmus, ataxia, opsoclonus, and paraplegia; ophthalmic signs such as proptosis and periorbital ecchymosis; and diarrhea.[37] These findings are the result of metastatic spread of tumor or the production of catecholamines or vasoactive intestinal polypeptides. The most common clinical finding is a palpable abdominal or pelvic mass. Metastases are present in approximately 70% of children with neuroblastoma at the time of diagnosis.

Neuroblastoma is part of a spectrum of tumors, which includes ganglioneuroblastoma and ganglioneuroma. Neuroblastoma is the most undifferentiated tumor in the spectrum. Histologically, neuroblastomas are characterized by small, blue, round cells with hyperchromic or densely speckled nuclei arranged in rosettes. Ganglio-neuroblastoma is characterized by the presence of these neuroblasts as well as ganglion cells. Ganglioneuroma is the most differentiated tumor of sympathetic origin, consisting of well-differentiated ganglion cells that lack metastatic potential. Imaging findings of these tumors are similar.

Clinical Staging

The most recent staging system for neuroblastoma is the International Neuroblastoma Staging System (INSS) (Table 95-2).[38] This classification takes into account radiologic findings, surgical resectability, and lymph node and bone marrow involvement.[38]

Patient survival is affected by stage of disease, patient age at diagnosis, site of primary tumor, tumor histology, and biologic markers. Two-year survival rates for infants younger than 1 year of age with early-stage tumors are 85% to 90% versus 15% to 30% for older children with advanced-stage disease. Given the same stage of disease, survival rates are better for infants than for older children. Patients with extra-abdominal primaries or well-differentiated histology have better prognoses than those with adrenal primaries or those with poorly differentiated histology. Biological predictors of unfavorable outcome are elevated lactate dehydrogenase and blood ferritin levels, "diploid" (decreased DNA) karyotype, N-myc amplification, and allelic loss of chromosome 1p.[39]

Diagnostic Imaging

The role of imaging is to establish the diagnosis, define the resectability of the primary tumor, and ascertain the presence or absence of metastatic disease.

Neuroblastoma appears as an irregular, lobulated, extrarenal mass, which has intermediate signal intensity on T1-weighted images and high signal intensity on T2-weighted images. Most enhance after the administration of intravenous gadolinium chelate compounds. Heterogeneity is common because of the presence of

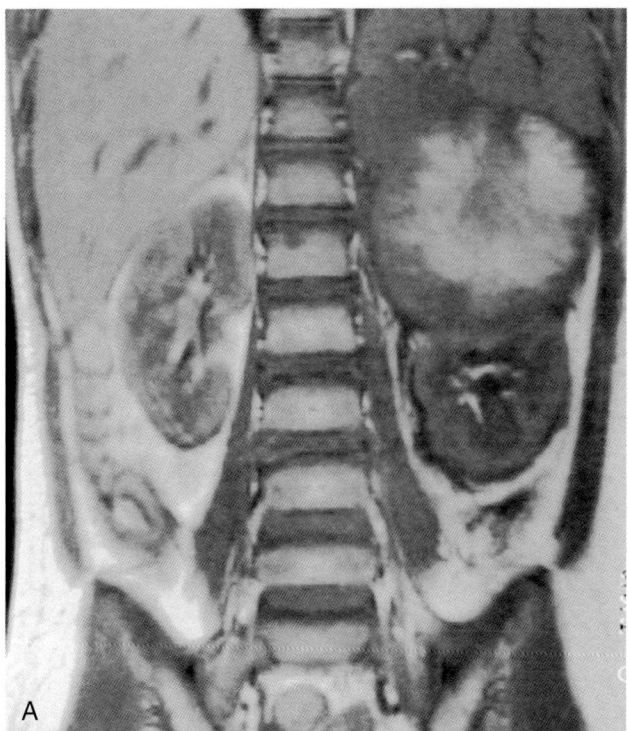

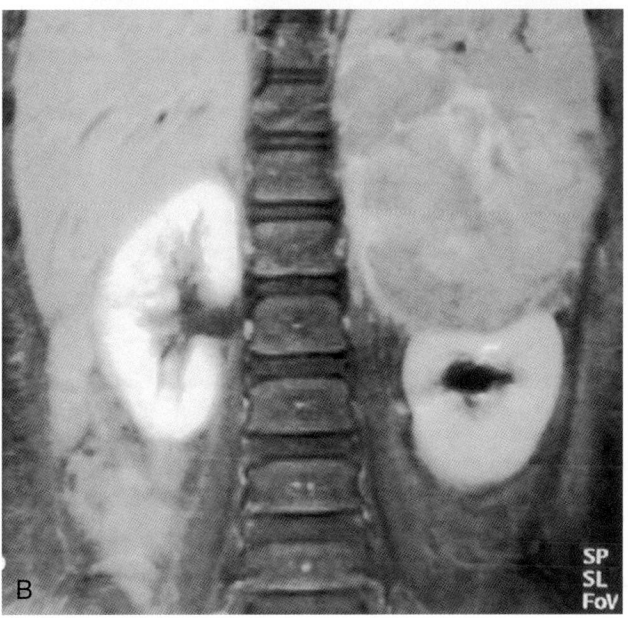

FIGURE 95-10

Neuroblastoma, 2-year–old boy. **A,** T1-weighted image (TR/TE 450/15) shows a large left suprarenal mass. Central high signal intensity represents hemorrhage. **B,** On a T1-weighted gadolinium-enhanced and fat-suppressed image, the tumor shows heterogeneous enhancement.

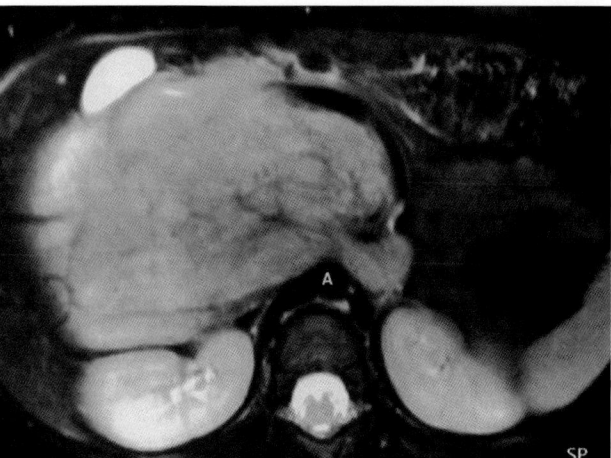

FIGURE 95-11

Neuroblastoma, 6-month–old girl. T2-weighted image (TR/TE 3000/119) demonstrates a large suprarenal mass with high signal intensity arising in the right side of the abdomen. The tumor crosses the midline anterior to the aorta (A).

Local spread of tumor may take the form of midline extension, vessel encasement, intraspinal invasion, and/or regional lymph node involvement (Figs. 95-11 and 95-12).[13-15] Midline extension and lymph node enlargement are important because they change tumor stage. Vessel encasement is often a contraindication to complete surgical resection. Detection of intraspinal extension is important because it may require a decompressive laminectomy or radiation treatment prior to debulking of the main tumor.

Neuroblastoma metastasizes to skin, liver, distant nodes, cortical bone, and bone marrow. Skin metastases occur in 20% to 25% of tumors, almost always in association with stage 4S disease. Hepatic metastases occur in 5% to 10% of children with neuroblastoma, usually in stage 4S disease and rarely in stage 4 disease. Hepatic metastases (Fig. 95-13) have a varying appearance depending on patient age. In patients older than 1 year of age, the lesions tend to be well defined and may be single or multiple. In patients younger than 1 year of age, metastases are more often diffuse, replacing most of the liver, and are also ill defined.[15] The most common site of distant nodal spread is the left supraclavicular location.[45]

Skeletal involvement, which may be to cortex or marrow, occurs in 50% to 60% of patients. Bone and bone marrow metastases may be either focal or diffuse. In long bones, metastases are typically asymmetrical and metaphyseal in location. On T1-weighted sequences, marrow metastases have signal intensity equal to or slightly greater than that of skeletal muscle. On fat-saturated sequences, the signal intensity of the tumor is close to that of fat (Fig. 95-14).[44,46-48] Focal lesions may increase in signal intensity on gadolinium-enhanced sequences. In neonates and infants, care must be taken to avoid confusing the diffuse low signal intensity of normal hematopoietic marrow on T1-weighted sequences for metastatic disease.

hemorrhage, necrosis, or calcification (Fig. 95-10). Hemorrhage results in variable signal intensity, dependent on the age of the blood. Necrotic foci are usually hypointense on T1-weighted images and hyperintense on T2-weighted images, and do not enhance following gadolinium administration. Tumor calcification has low signal intensity on all imaging sequences.[40-44]

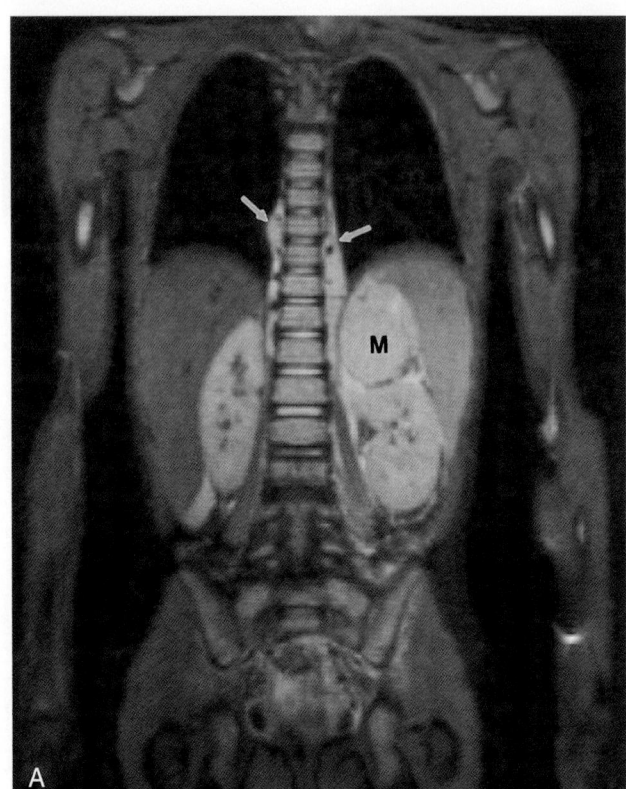

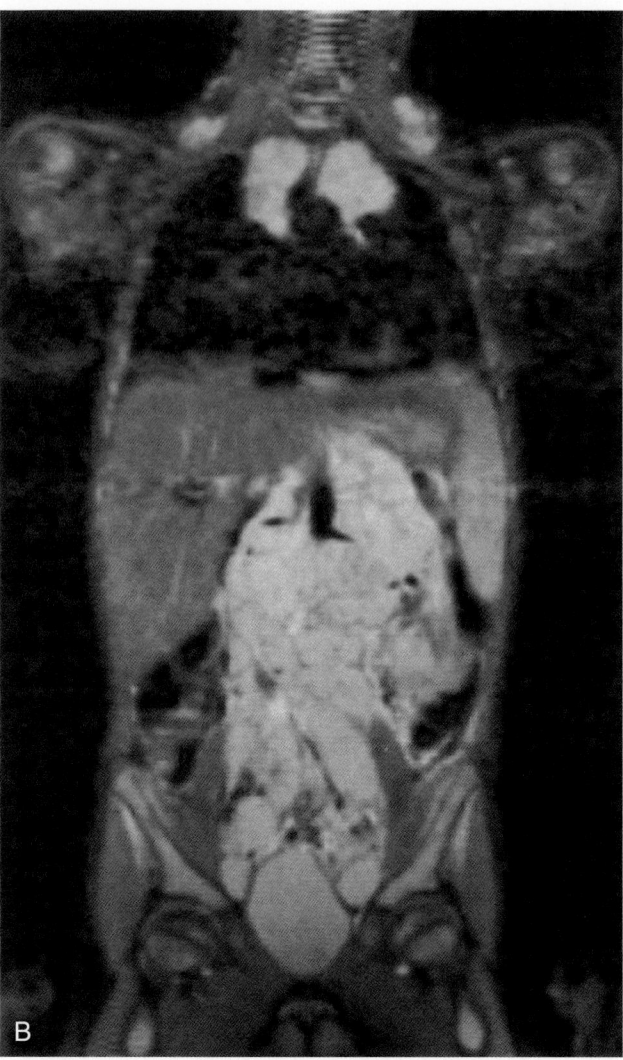

FIGURE 95-12

Neuroblastoma, 5-year–old girl. **A,** Short tau inversion recovery (STIR) image (TR/TE 3390/18, flip angle 140 degrees) shows a left adrenal mass (M) displacing the kidney inferiorly. Also noted is extensive retrocrural adenopathy (*arrows*) extending into the posterior mediastinum. The high signal intensity marrow in the vertebral bodies indicates marrow metastases. In a patient of this age, the marrow should be hypointense on STIR images. **B,** A more anterior section demonstrates extensive retroperitoneal adenopathy extending from the upper abdomen to the lower pelvis. Also "sentinel" supraclavicular and retroclavicular adenopathy is noted in the neck and superior mediastinum.

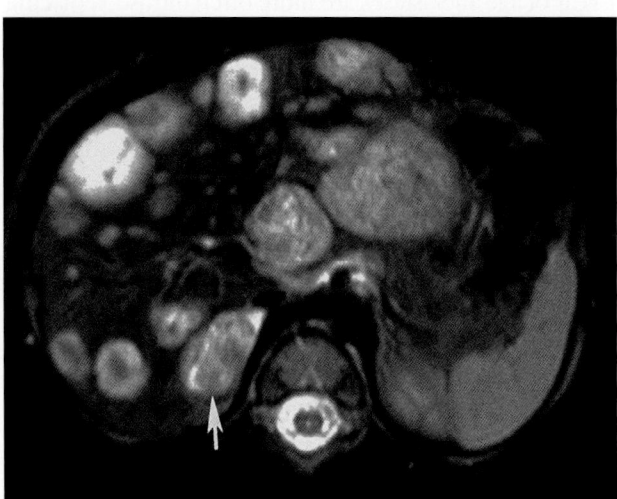

FIGURE 95-13

Neuroblastoma. Hepatic metastases, 7-month–old boy with a right adrenal primary. Axial T2-weighted fat-suppressed MR image shows multiple high signal intensity liver metastases and a right adrenal primary (*arrow*).

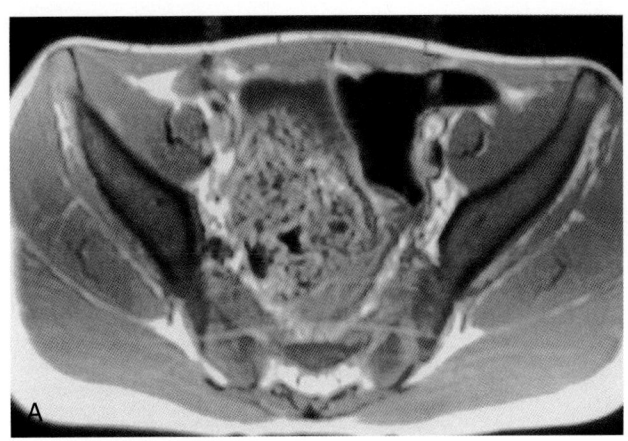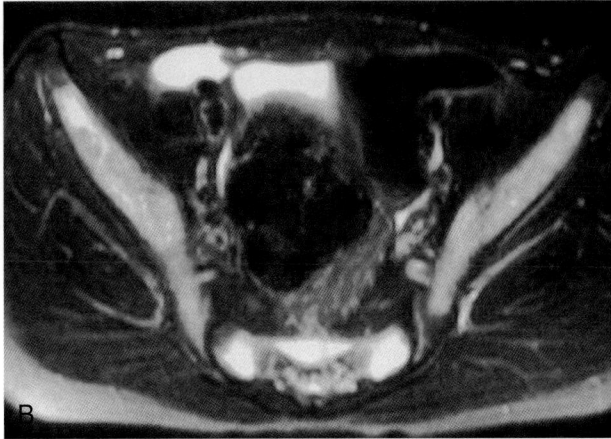

FIGURE 95-14

Neuroblastoma. Bone marrow metastases, 3-year–old boy. **A,** Axial T1-weighted image of both femora shows diffusely low signal intensity marrow in both iliac crests and the sacrum. **B,** Axial fat-saturated T1-weighted image (TR/TE 2500/18, flip angle 140 degrees). The signal intensity is higher than that of muscle indicating diffuse marrow replacement by tumor.

Comparative Imaging

The results of a multi-institutional study of 95 children, aged 9 days to 12.4 years, with newly diagnosed neuroblastoma have shown that MRI is more sensitive than CT for diagnosis of stage 4 disease.[44] For the diagnosis of stage 4 disease, MRI and CT had a sensitivity of 82% and 43%, respectively ($P < 0.0001$) and areas under the receive operating characteristic (ROC) curve of 0.85 and 0.81, respectively. When combined with bone scintigraphy, CT and MRI had similar areas under the ROC curves (0.90 and 0.88, respectively). For the diagnosis of bone/bone marrow metastases, the accuracy of MRI (ROC area 0.86) and scintigraphy (0.85) was significantly higher than that of CT (0.59). These results suggest that MRI can be used as a single study to replace the combination of CT and bone scintigraphy in staging neuroblastoma.

Post-Treatment Evaluation

Following therapy, MRI can be used to monitor tumor regression and detect recurrence. Demonstration of a residual mass with low signal intensity on both T1- and T2-weighted images suggests the diagnosis of fibrosis, while high signal on the T2-weighted sequence may be seen with either residual tumor or fibrosis with an inflammatory component.

Other Adrenal Neoplasms

Adrenal carcinomas account for less than 1% of all adrenal neoplasms in children. The mean age of affected children is 6 years.[49] Most carcinomas are hormonally active, producing virilization in girls and pseudoprecocious puberty in boys. Less often, these tumors produce excess glucocorticoids, estrogens, or aldosterone. Adrenal carcinomas are large masses, usually greater than 5 cm in diameter, and have an MRI appearance similar to that of neuroblastoma (Fig. 95-15).[15,49] Local invasion

occurs in 50% of cases. Adrenal adenomas and aldosteronomas are very rare in childhood.

Pheochromocytomas are catecholamine-producing tumors. Clinical manifestations include paroxysmal hypertension, headache, sweating, palpitations, tremor, and micturation syncope. Most pheochromocytomas in children are sporadic; however, they may be associated with multiple endocrine neoplastic (MEN) syndromes and the phakomatoses, including neurofibromatosis, tuberous sclerosis, von Hippel-Lindau disease, and Sturge-Weber disease.[50] Approximately 85% arise in the adrenal medulla; the remainder are in the sympathetic ganglia adjacent to the vena cava or aorta, near the organ of Zuckerkandl, or in the wall of the urinary bladder.[50] As many as one third of tumors are bilateral and about 5% to 10% are malignant. Pheochromocytomas are usually greater than 2 cm in diameter and have a low signal intensity similar to that of liver on T1-weighted sequences and a high signal intensity similar to that of fat on T2-weighted sequences (Fig. 95-16).[51] They show intense enhancement after gadolinium administration.

Retroperitoneal Soft-Tissue Masses

Although rare, both benign and malignant primary tumors occur in the retroperitoneal soft-tissues. Benign tumors include teratoma, lymphangioma, neurofibroma, lipomatosis, and desmoid tumors. Teratomas appear as well-defined, fluid-filled masses with a variable amount of fat or calcium. Lymphangiomas are well-circumscribed, multiloculated, fluid-filled masses. Neurofibromas are usually well-defined, cylindrical, soft-tissue lesions with a characteristic location in the neurovascular bundle. Lipomatosis appears as a diffuse, infiltrative mass with a signal intensity equal to fat; it grows along fascial planes and may invade muscle. Desmoid tumor (aggressive fibromatosis) contains areas of high and low signal intensity (Fig. 95-17).

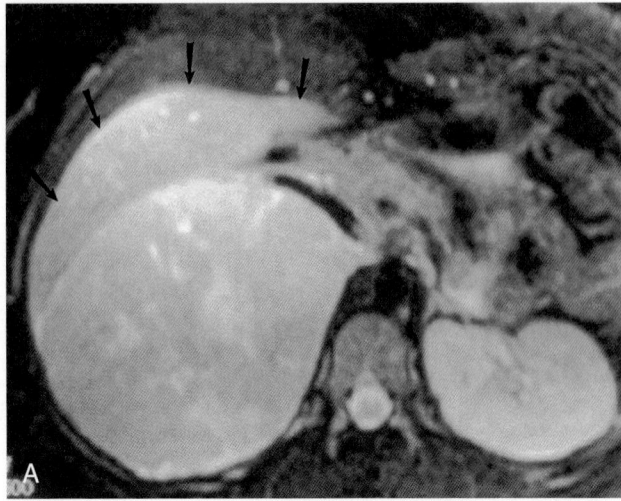

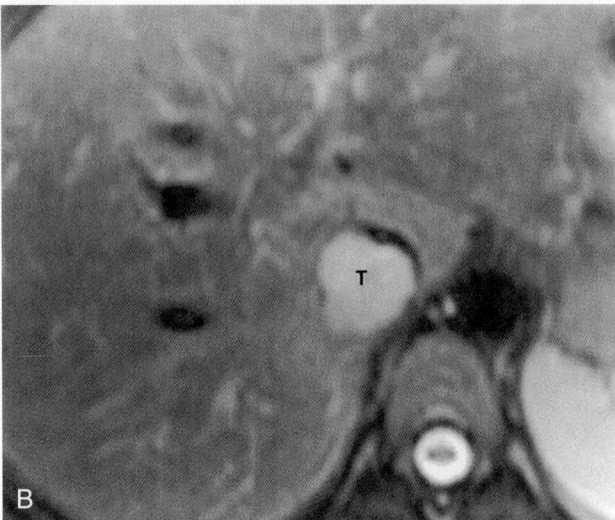

FIGURE 95-15

Adrenocortical carcinoma, 14-year–old boy. **A,** T2-weighted axial fat-suppressed MR image (TR/TE 2500/90, flip angle 140 degrees) shows a bilobed right adrenal tumor (*arrows*). **B,** T2-weighted axial fat-saturated MR image at a higher level shows a large tumor thrombus (T) in the inferior vena cava.

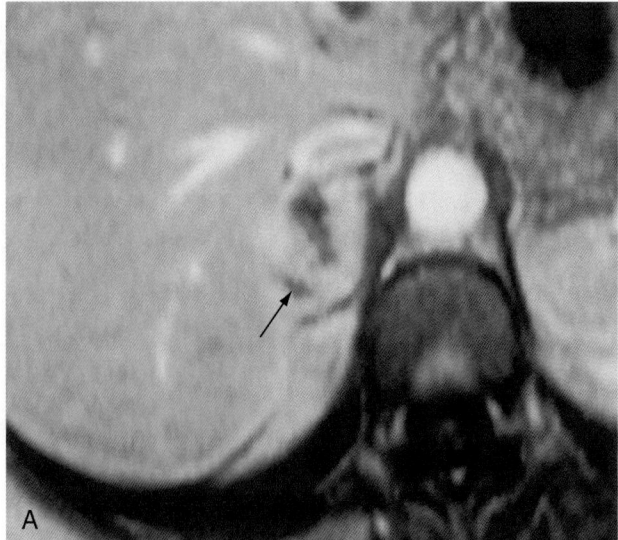

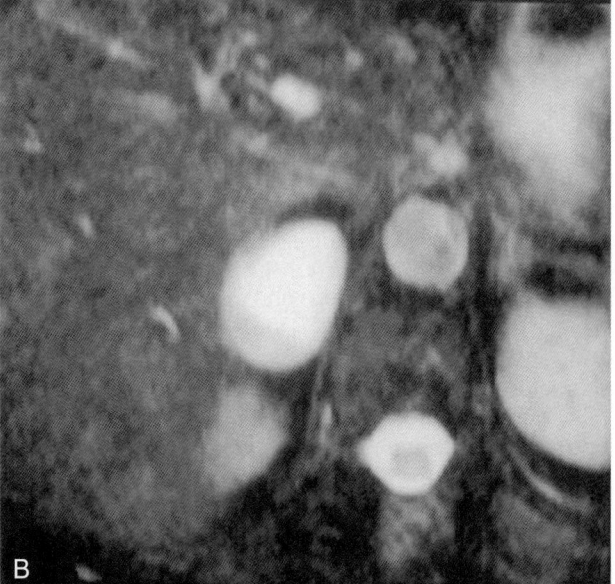

FIGURE 95-16

Adrenal pheochromocytoma. **A,** Axial T1-weighted gradient-echo gadolinium-enhanced and fat-suppressed image demonstrates a small heterogeneously enhancing mass in the right adrenal gland (*arrow*). **B,** T2-weighted turbo spin-echo sequence. The mass has become hyperintense to adjacent liver.

Rhabdomyosarcoma is the most common malignant tumor of the retroperitoneum, followed by neurofibrosarcoma, fibrosarcoma, and extragonadal germ cell tumors. These tumors appear as bulky, soft-tissue masses. On T1-weighted MR images, they appear either hypo- or iso-intense to liver, kidney, and muscle. On T2-weighted images, they have a signal intensity equal to or greater than that of fat. Vessel displacement or encasement sometimes occurs and can be seen easily with gradient-echo imaging.

Hepatic Masses

Primary hepatic tumors account for approximately 0.5% to 2% of pediatric tumors and are the third most frequent neoplasm after Wilms' tumor and neuroblastoma.[52-55]

Malignant hepatic tumors are twice as frequent as benign tumors, and most of these are hepatoblastomas and hepatocellular carcinomas.

Hepatoblastoma and Hepatocellular Carcinoma

Hepatoblastoma typically affects infants and young children; median patient age at diagnosis is 1 year. Conditions associated with an increased risk of hepatoblastoma include Beckwith-Wiedemann syndrome, hemihypertrophy, fetal alcohol syndrome, familial polyposis coli, and Gardner's syndrome.[54] There is no association with cirrhosis. Hepatoblastoma most often

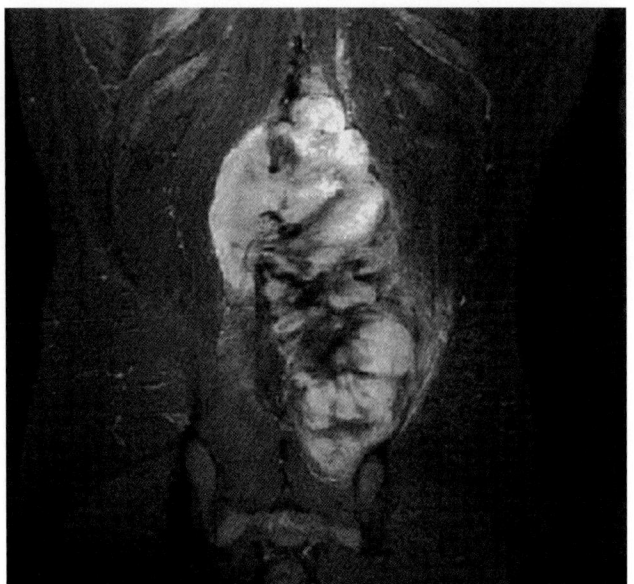

FIGURE 95-17

Aggressive fibromatosis, 20-year–old man with Gardner's syndrome. Short tau inversion recovery (STIR) coronal image shows a large paraspinal mass with a combination of high and low signal intensity areas, typical of desmoid tumor (aggressive fibromatosis). The bright areas represent active fibroblastic disease and the dark areas inactive fibrosis, biopsy proven.

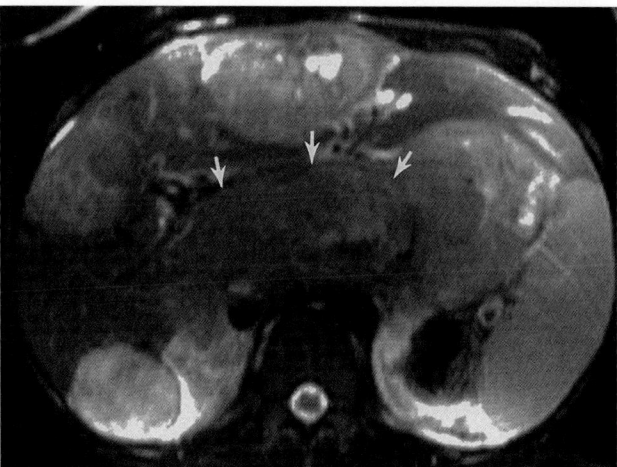

FIGURE 95-18

Hepatocellular carcinoma, 17-year–old man. Axial T2-weighted, fat-suppressed, breath-hold MR image shows multiple high signal intensity hepatic masses. Note the extensive retroperitoneal lymphadenopathy (*arrows*) splaying the inferior vena cava away from the aorta.

presents as an asymptomatic mass. Other features include abdominal pain, anorexia, weight loss, jaundice, and precocious puberty related to the secretion of chorionic gonadotropins. Serum α-fetoprotein levels are elevated in 80% to 90% of patients.[53,54,56] Metastases occur in 10% to 20% of patients and are chiefly to the lungs and less commonly to the brain and skeleton.

The median age of children with hepatocellular carcinoma is 12 years, with a range of 5 to 15 years. The tumor is relatively rare in patients under 5 years of age.[53,54] Pre-existing liver disease, such as hepatitis B infection, type I glycogen storage disease, tyrosinemia, familial cholestatic cirrhosis, hemochromatosis or α1-antitrypsin deficiency, is present in approximately one half of cases. Abdominal distention and right upper quadrant mass are the most common presenting features. Serum α-fetoprotein levels are elevated in up to 50% of cases.

Pathology

Pathologic differentiation of hepatoblastoma and hepatocellular carcinoma is based on cellular maturity. Hepatoblastoma contains small, primitive epithelial cells, resembling fetal liver, while hepatocellular carcinoma contains large, pleomorphic multinucleated cells with variable degrees of differentiation.[53,57,58] Invasion of the portal or hepatic veins is frequent in both tumors.

Staging

The staging system used most widely in the United States is that of the Children's Cancer Study Group and the

Southwest Oncology Group (Table 95-3).[53,54] The treatment of hepatoblastoma and hepatocellular carcinoma is chemotherapy followed by surgical resection.

MR Imaging

The role of imaging is to determine the extent of the primary tumor, particularly the presence of tumor in surgically critical areas such as the porta hepatis, portal vein, and inferior vena cava, and the presence of regional extrahepatic spread and distant metastases.

Hepatoblastoma and hepatocellular carcinoma have similar imaging features. Both usually appear as a solitary mass confined to a single lobe, with the right lobe involved twice as often as the left lobe. Less frequently, they are multifocal or diffusely replace hepatic parenchyma. Malignant hepatic lesions are predominantly hypo- or iso-intense relative to normal hepatic parenchyma on T1-weighted images and hyperintense on T2-weighted images (Fig. 95-18).[59-62] High signal intensity foci due to areas of steatosis, hemorrhage, or excessive glycogen deposition can be seen in some cases on T1-weighted images. Some enhancement is typical after administration of intravenous gadolinium chelates (Fig. 95-19). Tumor margins generally are well defined

TABLE 95-3   Clinical Grouping of Malignant Hepatic Tumors

Group I	Complete resection as initial treatment
Group IIA	Complete resection following initial irradiation or chemotherapy
Group IIB	Residual disease in one lobe
Group IIIA	Residual disease in both lobes of the liver
Group IIIB	Regional node involvement
Group IV	Distant metastases

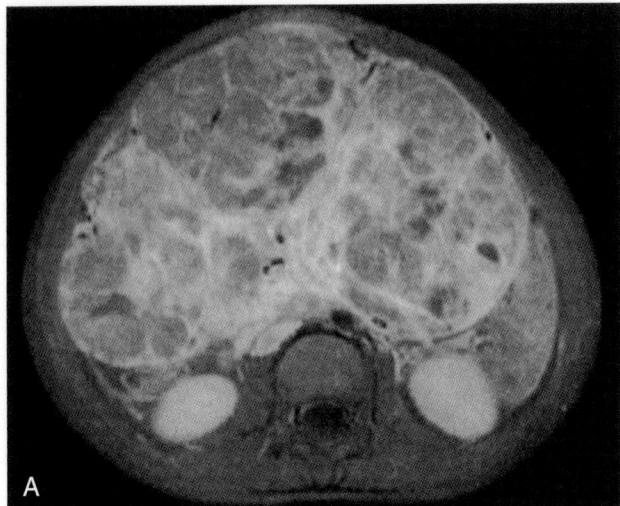

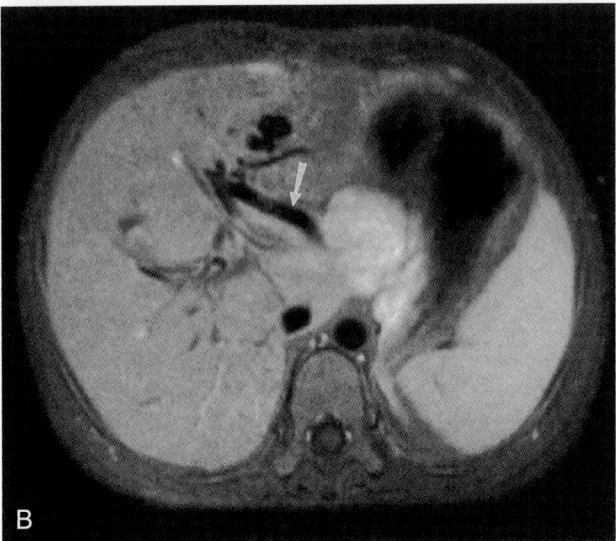

FIGURE 95-19

Hepatoblastoma, 7-year–old boy. **A,** T1-weighted axial gadolinium-enhanced and fat-suppressed MR image shows a large, heterogeneously enhancing tumor replacing most of the upper abdomen. **B,** A more superior T1-weighted contrast-enhanced MR section shows the enhancing regional lymphadenopathy next to the large hepatic artery (*arrow*).

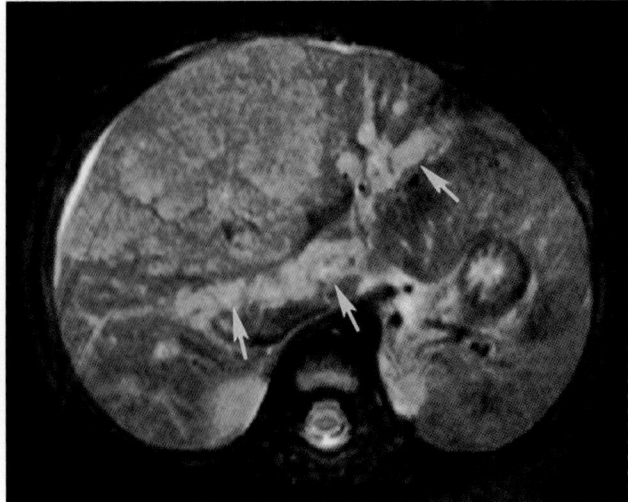

FIGURE 95-20

Hepatoblastoma, 2-yearold girl. Axial T2-weighted, fat-suppressed image (TR/TE: 4090/100, flip angle 140 degrees) shows a large tumor in the medial segment of the left lobe and anterior segment of the right lobe of the liver. High signal intensity in the portal vein represents tumor thrombus (*arrows*).

and, in cases of hepatocellular carcinoma, there may be a low attenuation or low signal intensity rim, corresponding to a fibrous capsule.[63] Tumor thrombus appears as a focus of increased signal within a normally echo-free vessel on spin-echo sequences or as a low intensity area on gradient-echo imaging (Fig. 95-20).

Hepatic malignancies usually metastasize to portal lymph nodes and lung. Portal lymph nodes are easily evaluated by MRI at the same time that the primary tumor is imaged. CT scanning is the best imaging examination for detecting pulmonary metastases.

Other Rare Malignant Hepatic Neoplasms

Fibrolamellar hepatocellular carcinoma is a histologic subtype of hepatocellular carcinoma that occurs predominantly in adolescent and younger adults. Histologically, it contains eosinophilic-laden hepatocytes separated by thin, fibrous bands arranged in a lamellar pattern, hence, the term "fibrolamellar." A central scar and calcifications are common. Serum α-fetoprotein levels are usually normal.[64-66] Fibrolamellar carcinoma is less aggressive than the typical variety of hepatocellular carcinoma and patients have a more favorable prognosis.

Fibrolamellar carcinoma is hypointense to liver on T1-weighted MR images and hyperintense on T2-weighted images. The central scar is hypointense on both sequences.[65,67,68] The tumor parenchyma, but not the central scar, enhances after administration of gadolinium chelates. Central calcifications are common (68% of cases). Associated findings include intrahepatic biliary obstruction, portal or hepatic vein invasion, and lymphadenopathy.

Undifferentiated embryonal sarcoma, also known as mesenchymal sarcoma, embryonal sarcoma, and malignant mesenchymoma, affects older children and adolescents, usually between 6 and 10 years of age, and 90% occur by 15 years of age.[67,69-71] Clinical manifestations include a palpable mass, fever, and normal levels of α-fetoprotein.[67] Prognosis is poor, with a median survival of approximately 1 year. At gross examination, the tumor contains cystic spaces, representing necrosis and hemorrhage, and cellular areas. Histologically, it contains undifferentiated sarcomatous tissue in a myxoid matrix.

At MRI, embryonal sarcoma usually has a low signal intensity on T1-weighted images and a high signal intensity on T2-weighted and gadolinium-enhanced images. Signal intensity on T1-weighted images can be increased if the contents are hemorrhagic (Fig. 95-21). Septations are also an occasional finding. The septa are

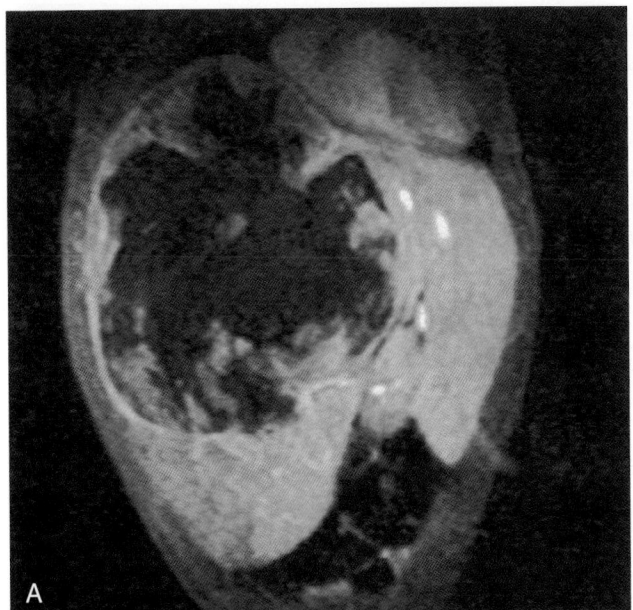

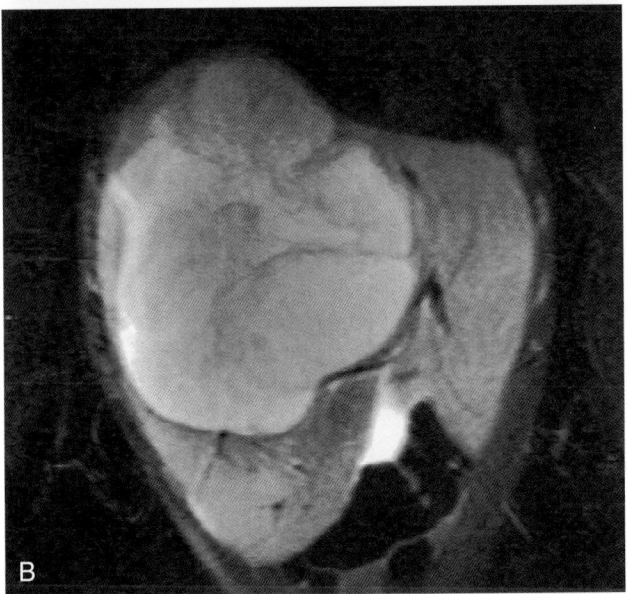

FIGURE 95-21

Embryonal sarcoma, 12-year–old boy with a large abdominal mass. **A,** Breath-hold coronal short tau inversion recovery (STIR) image (TR/TE 4000/76, flip angle 130 degrees) demonstrates a large, predominantly low signal intensity hepatic mass with areas of high signal intensity representing hemorrhage. **B,** Coronal source images from contrast-enhanced MR angiogram (TR/TE 5/2, flip angle 25 degrees) shows a predominantly intermediate signal intensity mass with some low signal intensity septations. At surgery, only the periphery of this tumor was viable.

hypointense on both pulse sequences. After gadolinium administration, the solid areas enhance, whereas the cystic spaces remain hypointense. Metastases are to lung and bone.

Rhabdomyosarcoma usually arises in the biliary tract and tends to affect children under 5 years of age.[72,73] Obstructive jaundice, hepatomegaly, and abdominal distention are common clinical findings. Extension into the liver parenchyma is common. The imaging findings are those of intra- and extra-hepatic ductal dilatation and a mass, which usually is in the porta hepatis. Similar to other hepatic malignancies, the tumor is hypointense on T1-weighted images and hyperintense on T2-weighted images. Sites of metastatic disease are the liver, lungs, peritoneal surfaces, lymph nodes, and bone.

Hemangioendothelioma and Cavernous Hemangioma

Hemangioendothelioma is the most common benign hepatic neoplasm in childhood. Most affected patients are diagnosed in the first 6 months of life and present with hepatomegaly or congestive heart failure due to high output overcirculation.[59,62,67,74] Occasionally, affected patients present with bleeding diathesis secondary to platelet sequestration (Kasabach-Merritt syndrome) or hemoperitoneum due to spontaneous tumor rupture. MRI can establish the diagnosis of hemangioendothelioma and differentiate it from malignant hepatic tumors. Most hemangioendotheliomas are solitary, but multicentricity can occur.

Cavernous hemangioma is the most common benign tumor of the liver in adults. Although it can occur in children, it is a rare lesion. It is usually asymptomatic and detected as an incidental finding on sonography, CT, or MRI.

Pathology

Histologically, hemangioendothelioma is composed of a network of vascular channels lined by plump endothelial cells that are supported by reticular fibers. Areas of fibrosis, calcification, hemorrhage, and cystic degeneration are common in larger lesions. Cavernous hemangioma is composed of multiple blood-filled spaces that are lined by a single layer of flat endothelial cells supported by fibrous septa.

MR Imaging

Hemangioendothelioma and cavernous hemangioma tend to be well-circumscribed lesions. Characteristically, they are hypointense to normal liver on T1-weighted images and markedly hyperintense on T2-weighted images (Fig. 95-22).[59,67,74-76] Signal intensity in larger lesions can be heterogeneous due to the presence of hemorrhage, necrosis, or fibrosis. Internal heterogeneity is especially common in larger lesions.

Dynamic imaging with gadolinium chelate agents may show three patterns of enhancement. The characteristic appearance is peripheral nodular enhancement progressing centripetally to complete central enhancement (Fig. 95-23). However, small lesions may show complete early enhancement, while very large lesions may demonstrate peripheral nodular enhancement with a persistent central hypointense area, reflecting the presence of fibrosis, thrombus, or degeneration. A secondary finding in neonates with multiple hemangioendotheliomas is a small infrahepatic aorta distal to the level of the celiac artery. This is related to shunting of

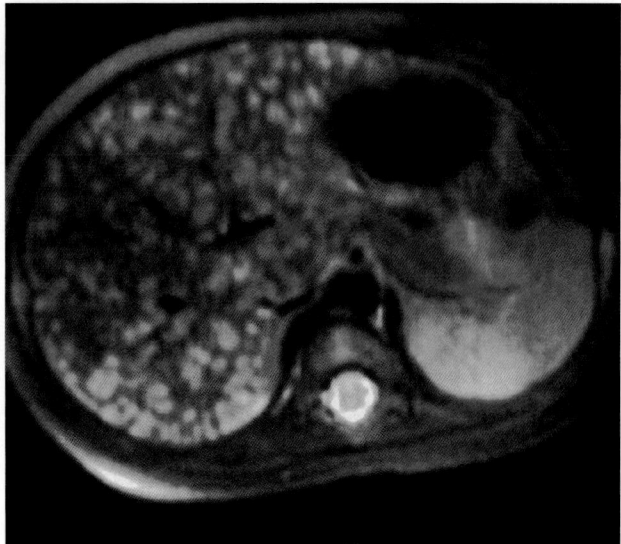

FIGURE 95-22

Multiple hemangioendotheliomas in a newborn girl. Axial T2-weighed spin-echo fat-suppressed image shows multiple lesions that are hyperintense to the normal liver parenchyma. *(Courtesy of Sudha Anupindi, MD.)*

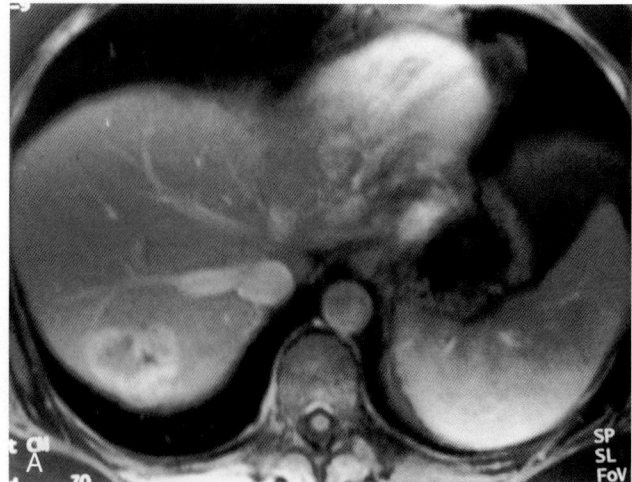

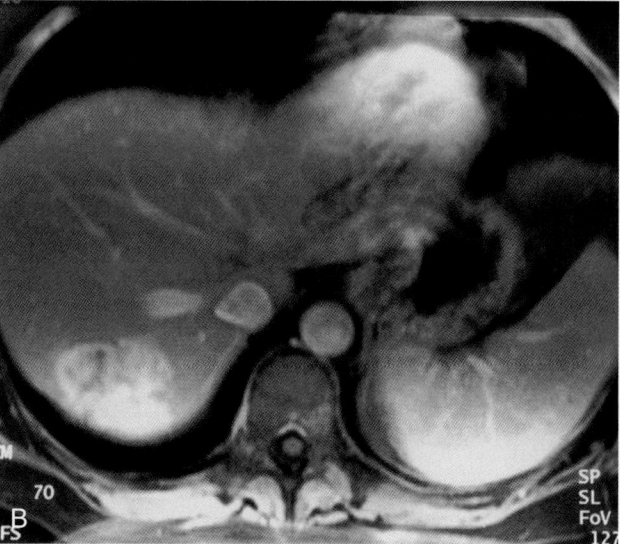

FIGURE 95-23

Cavernous hemangioma. **A,** Early-contrast gradient-echo fat-suppressed image (TR/TE 200/6, flip angle 70 degrees) shows peripheral enhancement in a lesion in the right lobe posteriorly. **B,** An image 2 minutes later shows nearly complete enhancement of the mass.

blood into the tumor via the celiac artery. If the typical findings of centripetal enhancement and filling-in are present, the diagnosis of a vascular lesion can be made with certainty. Biopsy is not necessary.

Other Benign Hepatic Tumors

Mesenchymal hamartoma is a benign lesion composed of varying sized cysts and fibrous septations.[67,77] Most affected children are under 2 years of age and present with a palpable mass or painless abdominal enlargement. Boys are affected twice as often as girls. MRI findings are a well-circumscribed multicystic lesion. The fluid-filled locules have a low signal intensity on T1-weighted images and high signal intensity on T2-weighted images, and are separated by low signal intensity septa (Fig. 95-24).[67,77] Higher signal intensity may be seen on T1-weighted images if the tumor contains large amounts of protein or debris. The septal components, but not the cystic spaces, usually enhance after the administration of gadolinium chelate agents.

Focal nodular hyperplasia and hepatic adenomas are uncommon lesions in childhood, accounting for less than 5% of hepatic tumors.[78] Focal nodular hyperplasia has no strong association with preexisting abnormalities.[79] Histologically, it is composed of normal hepatocytes, bile ducts, blood vessels, and Kupffer cells, and often contains a central fibrous scar. Internal hemorrhage and necrosis are usually absent. The lesion is most often an incidental finding on imaging examinations, but patients with large lesions may present with hepatomegaly or right upper quadrant discomfort. Typically, focal nodular hyperplasia, including the central scar, is iso- or hypo-intense on T1-weighted images and iso- or slightly hyper-intense to normal hepatic parenchyma

on T2-weighted images (Fig. 95-25).[78-80] Most lesions show intense enhancement during the hepatic arterial phase and rapid washout during the portal venous phase. The central scar, however, may show delayed enhancement. By comparison, the central scar in fibrolamellar hepatocellular carcinoma has low signal intensity on both arterial and portal venous phases of enhancement.

Hepatic adenoma in childhood has been associated with type I glycogen storage disease (von Gierke's disease), Fanconi's anemia, and galactosemia. Histologically, it is composed of hepatocytes, which often contain fat and glycogen; bile ducts and portal tracts are absent. Patients may be asymptomatic or they may present with hepatomegaly or abdominal pain secondary to tumor infarction, hemorrhage, or rupture. On T1-weighted images, hepatic adenomas are often heterogenous,

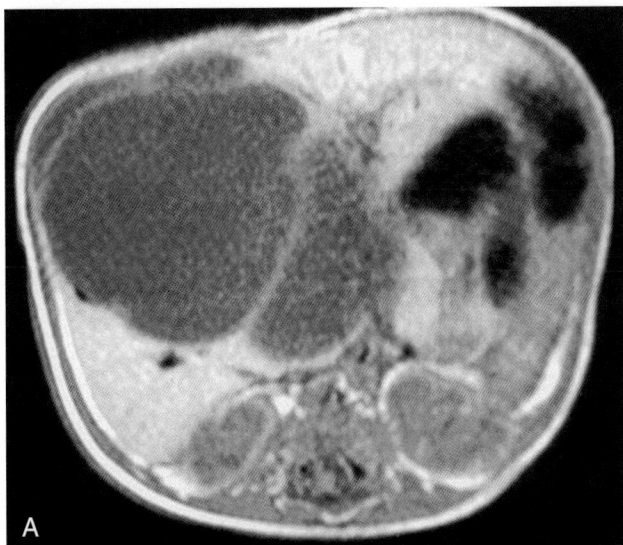

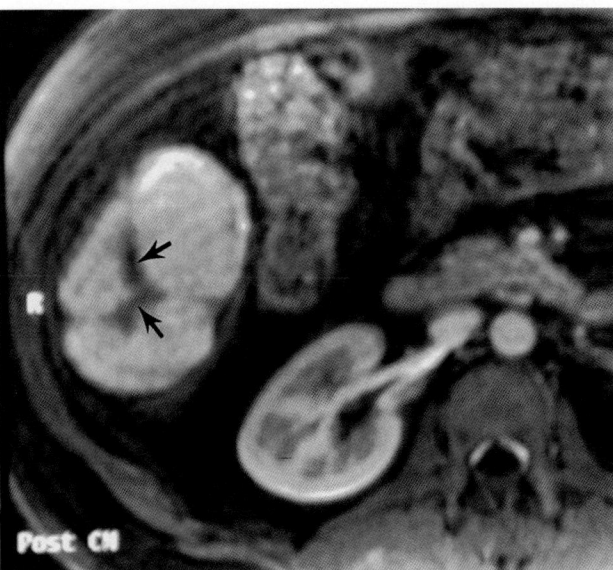

FIGURE 95-25

Focal nodular hyperplasia. Gradient-echo image soon after the administration of gadolinium chelate agent. A well-circumscribed hyperintense
lesion is present in the tip of the right hepatic lobe. The central scar
(*arrows*) is hypointense.

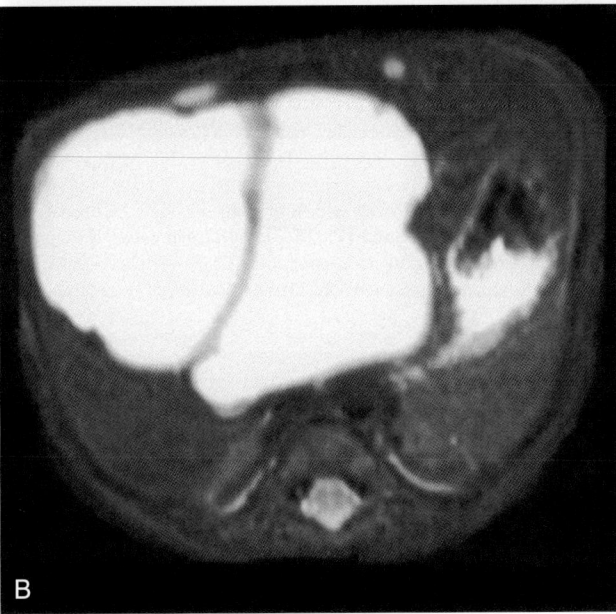

FIGURE 95-24

Mesenchymal hamartoma, 3-week–old infant. **A,** T1-weighted image shows
a low signal intensity mass in the right hepatic lobe. **B,** T2-weighted (TR/TE
3500/85) image. The lesion has become hyperintense to adjacent parenchyma.
Several septations can be noted. (*Courtesy of Lane Donnelly.*)

containing hyperintense areas due to the presence of
hemorrhage, glycogen or fat, and hypointense areas
resulting from necrosis.[77,78] On T2-weighted images,
they appear hyper- or iso-intense to normal parenchyma.
On contrast-enhanced images, most adenomas show
intense enhancement during the arterial phase and
rapid washout during the portal venous phase of
enhancement.

Hepatic Metastases

The malignant tumors of childhood that most frequently
metastasize to the liver are Wilms' tumor, neuroblastoma,

rhabdomyosarcoma, and lymphoma. Neuroblastoma
may affect the liver in either stage IV or IV-S disease.
Stage IV disease is characterized by the presence of a
retroperitoneal mass and distant metastases to skeleton,
liver, or nodes. Stage IV-S neuroblastoma occurs in
patients younger than 1 year of age, who have small
ipsilateral tumors (not crossing the midline) and metastases to the liver, skin and bone marrow, but not to
cortical bone. Patients with hepatic metastases present
with hepatomegaly, jaundice, abdominal pain or mass, or
abnormal hepatic function tests.

Hepatic metastases typically appear as multiple, well-
circumscribed lesions. They usually are hypointense on
T1-weighted MR images and hyperintense on T2-
weighted images (see Fig. 95-13). Other findings include
mass effect with displacement of vessels and vessel
invasion or amputation. Most metastases are hypovascular and do not enhance following the administration of
gadolinium agents. However, some will show peripheral
(ring) enhancement during the hepatic arterial phase.

Hepatic Cysts

Hepatic cysts may be congenital or acquired in origin.
The former arise from intrahepatic biliary ducts, which
fail to involute, while the latter are the result of
inflammation, trauma, or parasitic disease. Most hepatic
cysts are detected incidentally on examinations performed for other clinical indications. Large cysts,
however, may present as abdominal masses or hepatomegaly or they may produce abdominal pain secondary
to mass effect. On MRI, cysts are sharply circumscribed,
homogenous masses that are hypointense on T1-weighted

images and hyperintense on T2-weighted images. They characteristically show no enhancement on contrast-enhanced dynamic MRI studies.

Biliary Masses

Choledochal cyst is the most common mass arising in the biliary ductal tree. Classically, patients present with jaundice, pain, and a palpable abdominal mass, though the complete triad is present in only about one third of patients.[81]

Ultrasonography is the preliminary imaging procedure to detect intrahepatic ductal dilatation associated with obstruction. This can be supplemented by radionuclide studies using hepatobiliary imaging agents or CT.[82] MR cholangiography has proven to be a useful, noninvasive alternative to endoscopic retrograde pancreatography to delineate the anatomy of the biliary system when the results of other studies are indeterminate or additional information is needed for surgical planning. Images are acquired in the coronal and axial plane with two-dimensional, fat-suppressed, fast T2-weighted spin-echo sequences. In neonates in whom non–breath-hold techniques are required, the signal acquisitions are increased to increase the signal-to-noise ratio and to compensate for motion. MR images are acquired with a breath-hold in cooperative children. Source images are post-processed using a maximum intensity projection algorithm to produce reconstructed 3D models.

Choledochal cysts can be classified into five types.[83] The type 1 cysts (80% to 90% of cases) is characterized by dilatation of the common bile duct. The type 2 cyst is a true diverticulum arising from the common duct. The type 3 cyst is a choledochocele, involving only the intraduodenal portion of the duct. The type 4 cyst is characterized by multiple extrahepatic cysts; the intrahepatic ducts may or may not be dilated. The type 5 cyst, or Caroli's disease, is characterized by multiple intrahepatic cysts. Choledochal cysts in neonates and young infants may coexist with biliary atresia. The dilated common and intrahepatic bile ducts are easily shown by MR cholangiography (Fig. 95-26).[84-87]

Mesenteric Masses

Lymphangiomatous malformations, also termed mesenteric cysts, account for most benign mesenteric masses. Mesenteric cysts have a signal intensity equal to or slightly less than that of muscle on T1-weighted MR images, though the signal intensity may be higher if the lesions contain blood or proteinaceous material. On T2-weighted images, the signal intensity is greater than that of fat.

Lymphadenopathy due to lymphoma and occasionally to leukemia is another cause of a mesenteric mass. The appearance varies from mildly enlarged nodes in a single area to large conglomerate masses in multiple regions. Typically, the enlarged nodes have well-defined margins and a signal intensity greater or equal to that of muscle

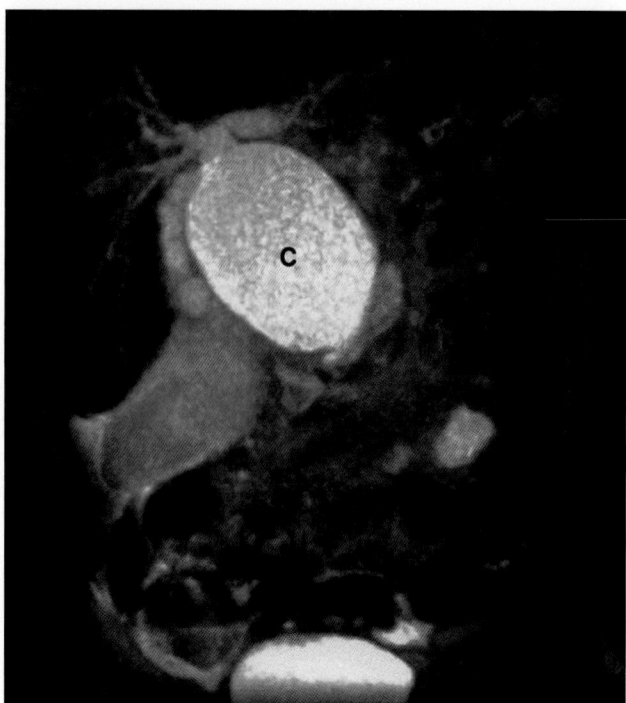

FIGURE 95-26

Choledochal cyst in a 2-year–old boy with jaundice. Coronal fat-suppressed turbo T2-weighted (TR/TE 3157/189, flip angle 90 degrees) image demonstrates a high signal intensity cyst (C) in the porta hepatis. The right and left hepatic ducts are mildly dilated. (Courtesy of Peter Strouse.)

on T1-weighted images and close to that of fat on T2-weighted and fat-suppressed images (Fig. 95-27). They show little enhancement after the administration of gadolinium agents.

PELVIS

Normal Anatomy

Ovaries

The ovaries descend from the upper abdomen into the pelvis during gestation, and at birth they usually lie within the superior margin of the broad ligaments. In some individuals, descent is incomplete, and the ovaries remain high in the pelvis, lying dorsal or cephalad to the uterus. With activation of the hypothalamic-pituitary-ovarian axis at the time of puberty, the ovaries move deeper into the pelvis, reaching their adult position posterolateral to the body of the uterus, though not necessarily at the same horizontal level. If ligamentous attachments are lax, the ovaries may be seen posterior to the uterus. Adult or post-menarchal ovaries measure between 3.0 × 1.5 × 0.6 cm and 5.0 × 3.0 × 2.5 cm.[88,89]

Histologically, the ovaries are composed of an outer cortex and inner medulla. Both layers contain follicles. Primordial or unstimulated follicles, which have a

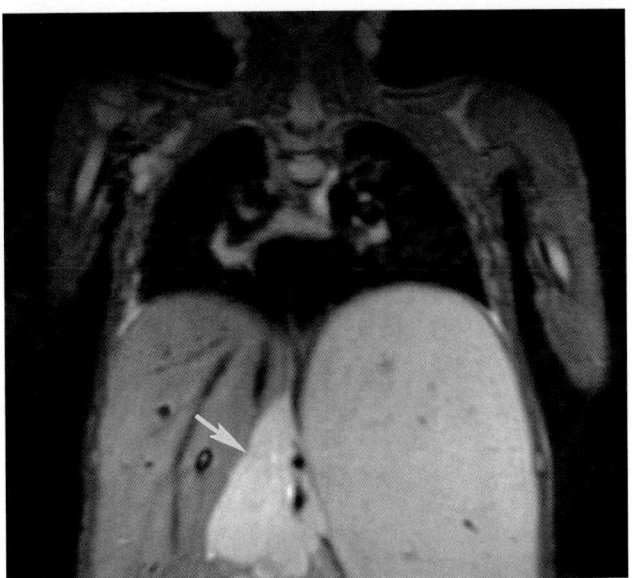

FIGURE 95-27

Mesenteric adenopathy, 4-year–old boy with juvenile myelomonocytic leukemia. Coronal short tau inversion recovery (STIR) (TR/TE 4845/30, flip angle 140 degrees) image shows massive splenomegaly and celiac and mesenteric adenopathy (*arrow*). In addition the patient has axillary, cervical and pulmonary hilar adenopathy and generalized marrow disease, shown as high signal intensity areas in the humeri.

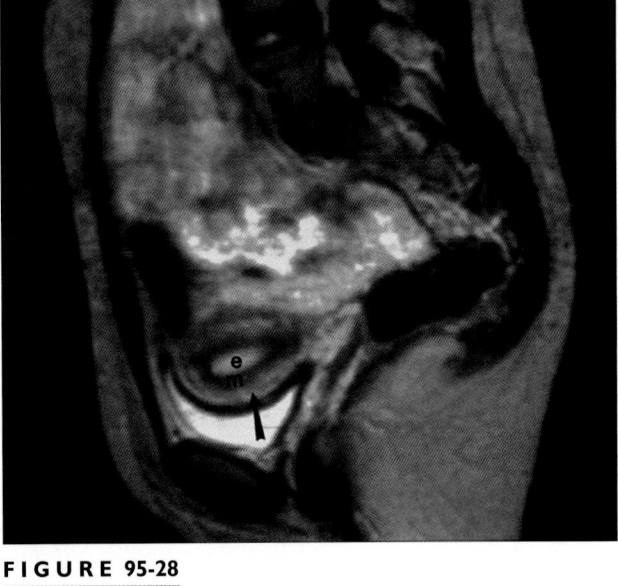

FIGURE 95-28

Normal post-menarchal female pelvis. T2-weighted fat-saturated (TR/TE 3500/98) MR image of a 14-year–old girl demonstrates normal zonal anatomy of the uterus: (e) high signal intensity endometrial canal (e), low signal inner myometrium (m), and intermediate signal intensity outer myometrium (*arrow*).

diameter of less than 9 mm, are typical of the premenarcheal ovary. Primordial and stimulated follicles, either graafian or corpus luteum follicles, are typical of the menarcheal ovary.[90] Graafian or corpus luteum follicles range between 9 mm and 3 cm in diameter. A cystic mass greater than 3 cm in diameter is considered pathologic and usually represents a stimulated follicle that failed to involute.

Normal ovarian parenchyma has a homogeneous signal intensity that is isointense to myometrium on T1-weighted images. A high signal intensity outer cortex and a lower signal intensity central medulla can be seen on T2-weighted images. The outer zone contains the hormonally unstimulated (primordial) follicles and the stimulated graafian or corpus luteum follicles. The ovaries enhance following the injection of gadolinium chelate compounds. The walls of the follicles are typically thin or imperceptible. Most follicles have a low signal intensity on T1-weighted images and a high signal intensity on T2-weighted images. Some mature follicles will have a high signal intensity on T1-weighted images due to the presence of blood.

Uterus and Vagina

The mean uterine volumes range between 0.5 and 1.3 cm³ in girls under 8 years of age and between 4.1 and 37.3 cm³ in older girls.[88,89] In post-pubertal girls, the uterus has a homogeneous medium signal intensity on T1-weighted images. Three distinct zones can be seen

within the fundus on T2-weighted images (Fig. 95-28).[91] The high signal intensity central zone represents endometrium; the low intensity middle layer corresponds to inner myometrium; and the medium signal intensity outer layer corresponds to the outer myometrium. Endometrial width varies during the menstrual cycle. It is thinnest immediately after menses and is thickest at midcycle. The endometrium and myometrium enhance, while the junctional zone continues to show a low signal intensity.

The normal cervix has a homogenous low-to-intermediate signal intensity on T1-weighted images. Two zones can be seen on T2-weighted images: a central area of high signal intensity representing endocervical glands and a lower signal intensity wall. The vagina also has a low-to-medium signal intensity on T1-weighted images and shows two distinct zones on T2-weighted images: the central high signal intensity canal and the intermediate signal intensity wall.[91]

Male Pelvis

The prostate gland and seminal vesicles are usually too small to be appreciated on routine pelvic MRI studies in infants and young boys. As these structures increase in size at the time of puberty, they are easier to recognize. If the prostate and seminal vesicles are seen in prepubertal boys, they appear as homogeneous intermediate signal intensity structures on both T1- and T2-weighted sequences. Zonal anatomy can be seen on

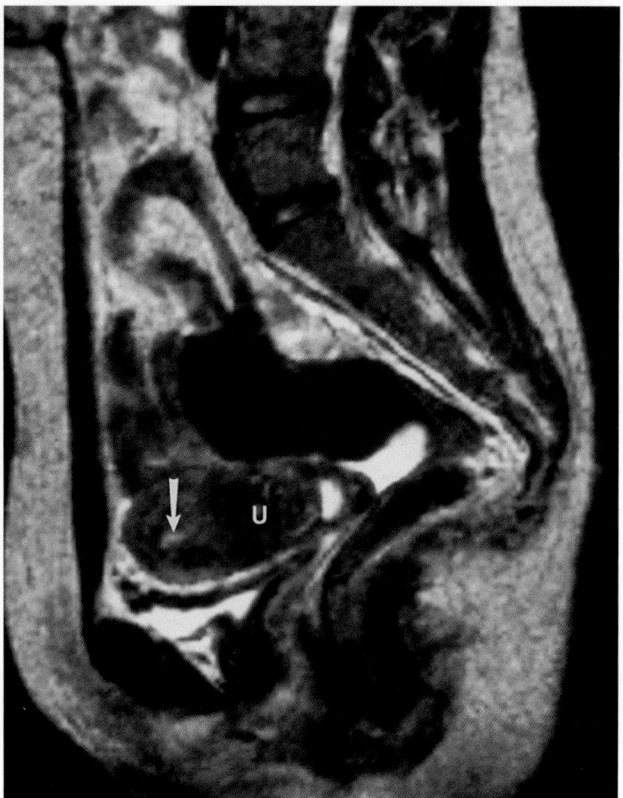

FIGURE 95-29

Uterine hypoplasia in a 16-year-old girl with Mayer-Rokitansky-Kuster-Hauser syndrome, who presents with amenorrhea. Sagittal T2-weighted image (TR/TE 4400/99) shows absence of the vaginal canal and a hypoplastic uterus (U). A small portion of the endometrial canal (arrow) is seen in the fundus. Otherwise there is no zonal differentiation. This patient had normal ovaries and no associated renal anomalies.

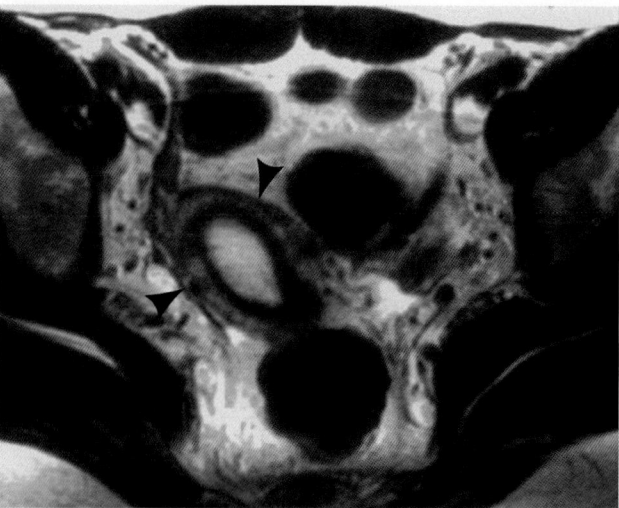

FIGURE 95-30

Unicornuate uterus with a noncommunicating rudimentary horn. Axial T2-weighted image (TR/TE 3500/90) shows a single fusiform uterine cavity (arrowheads) which is deviated to the right.

T2-weighted images after puberty. The peripheral zone of the prostate has a high signal intensity similar to that of adjacent fat. The central zone has an intermediate signal intensity and is hypointense relative to the peripheral zone. The seminal vesicles have a low-to-medium signal intensity on T1-weighted images and a high signal intensity on T2-weighted images. The outer walls of the tubules have a low signal intensity.[92]

Urinary Bladder

The urinary bladder is a midline structure with varying size and configuration depending on the degree of distention. The bladder wall has a signal intensity equal to that of soft-tissue, whereas the urine has a signal intensity near that of water.

Congenital Anomalies

Ultrasonography, especially transvaginal sonography, is probably the best initial examination in the evaluation of patients with suspected uterine anomalies. If the results

of sonography are indeterminate or if additional information is needed to characterize an anomaly seen on sonography, then MRI is indicated.[93-98] The features of the more common lesions seen in the pediatric population are briefly described in the following sections.

Uterine Anomalies

Uterine Agenesis and Hypoplasia

Uterine agenesis and hypoplasia are the result of non-development or arrested development of the Müllerian ducts bilaterally. This can be an isolated finding or occur in association with the Mayer-Rokitansky-Kuster-Hauser syndrome. Patients most commonly present with primary amenorrhea.[99,100] The Mayer-Rokitansky-Kuster-Hauser syndrome is characterized by vaginal atresia and a spectrum of uterine anomalies, including absence, hypoplasia, and duplication.[99,100] External genitalia, secondary sexual development, ovaries, and fallopian tubes are normal. Renal anomalies, usually agenesis and rarely ectopia or hydronephrosis, occur in about 50% of patients and skeletal anomalies in about 15% of patients.

In agenesis, there is no recognizable uterine tissue. In uterine hypoplasia, the uterus is small and exhibits poorly differentiated zonal anatomy and reduced endometrial and myometrial width (Fig. 95-29).[95] The myometrial signal intensity also is reduced.

Unicornuate Uterus

The unicornuate uterus results from failure or incomplete development of one of the two Müllerian ducts. The classic banana-shaped uterus (single fusiform uterine cavity with lateral deviation) results when there is development of only one of the Müllerian ducts

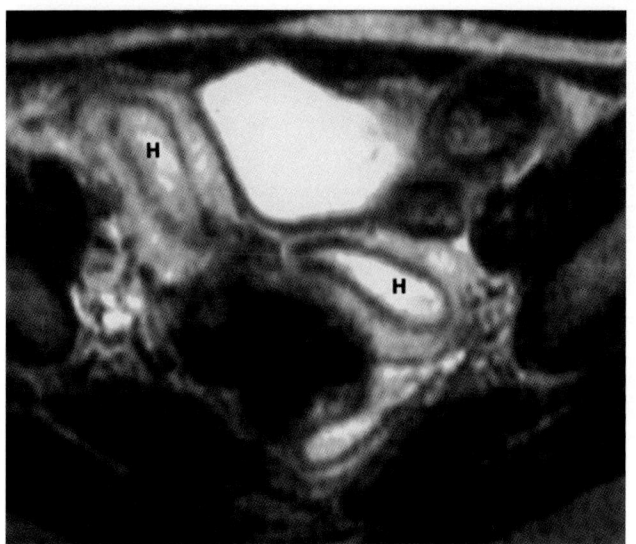

FIGURE 95-31

Uterus didelphys. Axial T2-weighted (TR/TE 3500/90) MR image demonstrates two uterine horns (H) with a widened intercornual distance. Two cervices and two vaginas were seen at a more caudal level.

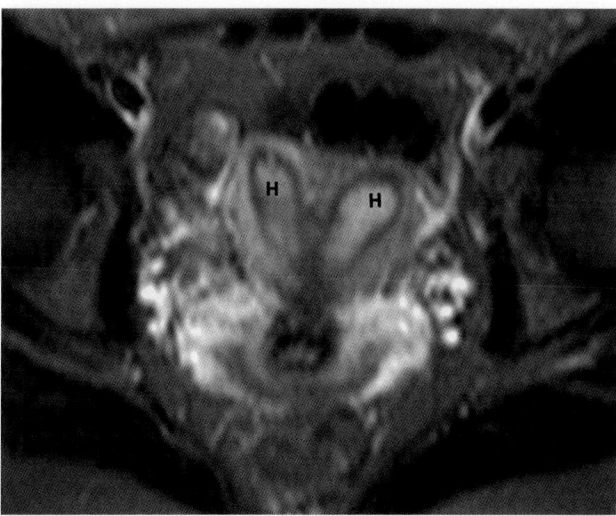

FIGURE 95-32

Septate uterus, 18-year-old woman. Axial gradient-echo image (TR/TE 2500/18, flip angle 140 degrees) shows two uterine horns (H) with normal zonal anatomy. A continuous band of myometrium surrounds the horns. The fundal contour is normal.

(Fig. 95-30). A rudimentary contralateral horn, which may or may not communicate with the main uterine body, may be seen when there is partial development of the second Müllerian duct. Renal anomalies occur in about 25% of cases.[95,101]

Double Uteri: Didelphys and Bicornuate Uteri

Double uteri result from nonfusion of the Müllerian ducts. Uterus didelphys is characterized by two uterine horns and two cervices. Bicornuate uterus is characterized by two uterine horns and a single cervix. In both anomalies, the fundal contour is concave and there is a deep cleft (>1 cm) between the two uterine horns which are widely divergent (Fig. 95-31).[95,102-105] Each horn has a fusiform shape, convex lateral margins, and a central endometrial cavity surrounded by a junctional zone. The tissue between the two horns is composed of myometrium and has an intermediate signal intensity on T1-weighted images and a higher signal intensity on T2-weighted images.

Septate Uterus

The septate uterus is the result of failure of resorption of the fibrous septum between the two Müllerian ducts. There is a single uterus, cervix, and vagina with a septum dividing the uterus into two cavities. The fundal contour is normal (convex) or shows a minimal (<1 cm) concavity.[95] The signal intensity of the septum depends on the relative amounts of fibrous tissue or myometrium. A fibrous septum has a relatively low signal intensity on both T1- and T2-weighted sequences, whereas myometrium has a bright signal on T2-weighted images (Fig. 95-32).

Ovarian Masses

Neonatal genital masses are usually the result of vaginal obstruction or ovarian cysts, whereas in older children almost all genital masses are of ovarian origin and either benign simple cysts or germ cell tumors. Sonography is the initial examination of choice to confirm the pelvic origin of the mass and its internal contents.[93,94,106] However, if sonography is nondiagnostic or if the mass appears malignant, MRI can be useful for further evaluation. Gynecologic masses may be discovered incidentally on imaging examinations or they may present as lower abdominal or pelvic pain secondary to mass effect, hemorrhage, or torsion.

Ovarian Cysts

Follicular and corpus luteum cysts account for the majority of ovarian masses in children. Follicular cysts result when a follicle continues to grow after failed ovulation, while corpus luteum cysts arise when the follicle fails to collapse after ovulation occurs. The cysts vary in size from 3 to 20 cm, but most are usually between 3 and 5 cm.[88,90,107,108]

Ovarian cysts typically appear as well-circumscribed, round, masses with a low signal intensity on T1-weighted images and a high signal intensity on T2-weighted images.[108] Follicular and corpus luteal cysts cannot be differentiated on the basis of the MR findings alone.

If blood vessels within the cyst rupture, a hemorrhagic cyst develops. Acute hemorrhagic cysts contain intact blood cells and have an intermediate or high signal intensity on T1-weighted images and a low signal intensity on T2-weighted images. Subacute hemorrhage will be bright on both T1- and T2-weighted images, related to the formation of methemoglobin.[90,106]

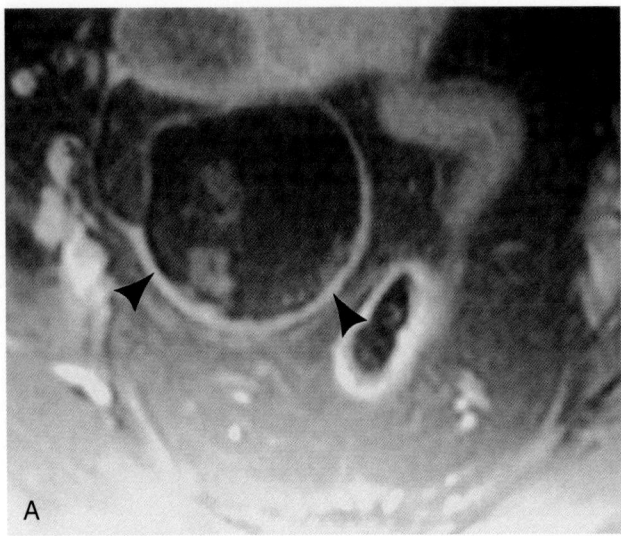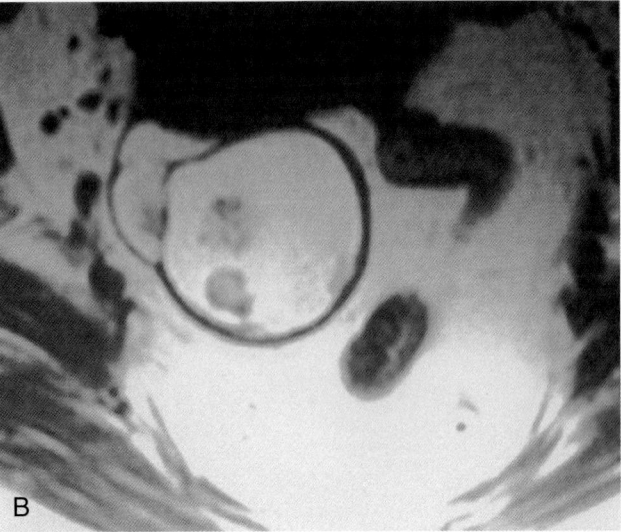

FIGURE 95-33

Benign ovarian teratoma in a young woman with a palpable pelvic mass. **A,** Axial T1-weighted image (TR/TE 672/12) shows a right adnexal mass (*arrowheads*). The mass has areas of low and high signal intensity related to fluid and fat, respectively. **B,** T2-weighted image (TR/TE 6000/119). The signal intensity of the fluid components has increased and is equal to that of subcutaneous fat. The signal intensity of fat has slightly decreased, but still remains brighter than muscle. *(Courtesy of Jeffrey Brown, MD.)*

Cystic Teratoma

Approximately 65% of ovarian tumors are benign,[109-111] and the majority of these are teratomas with cystadenomas occurring less frequently. Ovarian teratomas (also known as cystic teratomas and dermoid cysts) are congenital lesions, containing tissue derivatives from all three germ cell layers (endoderm, ectoderm, and mesoderm). On pathologic examination, teratomas are subdivided into mature, immature (containing embryonic neural elements), and malignant types.[109,112] The first subtype accounts for greater than 90% of ovarian germ cell tumors. Ovarian teratomas usually range in diameter from 5 to 10 cm and are bilateral in 25% of cases. Most cystic teratomas are composed of a cystic cavity filled with sebum, which is liquid at body temperature, or serous fluid. A protuberance, termed a dermoid plug or Rokitansky nodule, typically projects into the cavity. This protuberance contains an admixture of tissues, including bone, teeth, fat, and hair.

Signal characteristics vary depending on the amount of sebum, serous fluid, calcification, hair, and fibrous tissue present.[106,113,114] Serous contents and liquid sebum demonstrate low signal intensity on T1-weighted images and high signal intensity on T2-weighted images. Fat has high signal intensity on T1-weighted images and intermediate or high signal intensity on T2-weighted sequences (Fig. 95-33). Calcifications, bone, hair, and fibrous tissue demonstrate low signal intensity on both pulse sequences. Fat is the most characteristic feature of a teratoma and gradient-echo and fat-suppression techniques are the best sequences to confirm the presence of lipid contents.[115] Other diagnostic features include gravity-dependent layering or floating debris, peripheral nodules (dermoid plugs), intracystic fat balls, and fat-

fluid levels.[116] The cyst wall, Rokitansky nodule, and soft-tissue elements enhance after the administration of gadolinium chelate compounds; the intracystic fluid does not enhance.

Cystadenoma

Cystadenomas account for less than 5% of benign ovarian neoplasms in the pediatric population. Serous forms are more common than mucinous forms. On MRI, cystadenomas are usually cystic, unilocular masses with thin, smooth walls. They typically have a low signal intensity on T1-weighted images and a high signal intensity on T2-weighted images (Fig. 95-34), reflecting their serous fluid. When the cyst contents contain thick mucin or hemorrhage, the signal intensity on T1-weighted images may increase. The cyst wall and papillary projections often enhance after the administration of gadolinium chelates.

Malignant Ovarian Neoplasms

Malignant ovarian neoplasms account for 2% to 3% of childhood cancers and are usually germ cell tumors (dysgerminoma, immature teratoma, endodermal sinus tumor, embryonal carcinoma, and choriocarcinoma) rather than stromal tumors (Sertoli-Leydig, granulosa theca, undifferentiated neoplasm) or epithelial carcinomas.[109,110-112]

By comparison with benign cystic teratomas, the malignant neoplasms have a predominance of soft-tissue elements and therefore, appear as large heterogeneous pelvic and/or abdominal masses with intermediate signal intensity on T1-weighted images and intermediate or high signal intensity on T2-weighted images.[117] Other

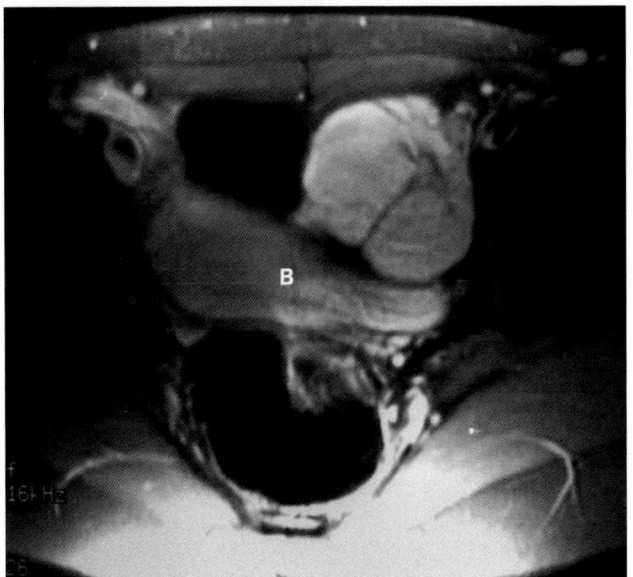

FIGURE 95-34

Cystadenoma. T2-weighted MR image (TR/TE 5000/16) in a 16-year–old girl shows a high signal intensity mass with septations in the left adnexal region. B, bladder. *(Courtesy of Philipp Silberberg, MD.)*

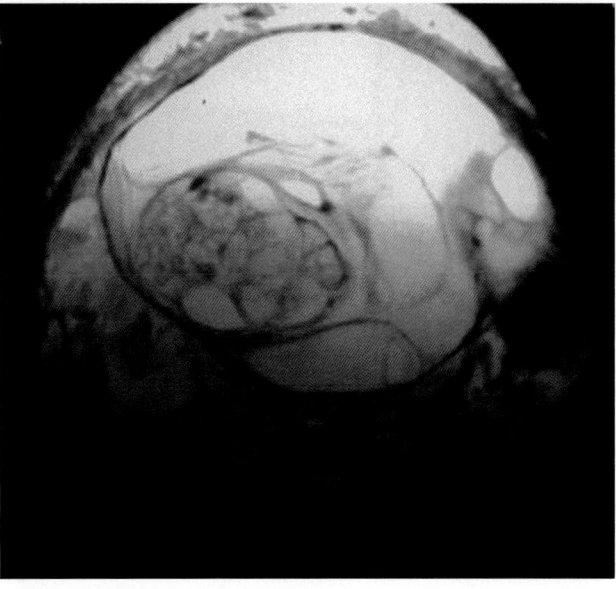

FIGURE 95-35

Malignant ovarian germ cell tumors. Axial fat-suppressed T2-weighted images (TR/TE 4000/54, flip angle 130 degrees) shows a large mass with septations and nodules, filling most of the abdomen.

frequent findings include calcifications, thick septa, and papillary projections (Fig. 95-35). Secondary findings include ascites, lymph node enlargement, and hepatic metastases. Peritoneal and omental implants are not typical features of the malignant germ cell tumors, but they can be seen with ovarian carcinoma. Peritoneal tumor implants appear as nodules on the lateral peritoneal surfaces or in the ligaments and mesenteries of the abdomen. Omental implants appear as discrete nodules or as conglomerate soft-tissue masses ("omental cake") beneath the anterior abdominal wall. Both have a medium signal intensity on MRI. Peritoneal and omental implants may enhance after intravenous contrast administration.

Vaginal Obstruction

Vaginal obstruction is a cause of a pelvic or lower abdominal mass in neonates. This condition has also been referred to as hydrocolpos when the dilated vagina contains serous fluid, hydrometrocolpos when both the vagina and uterus contain serous fluid, hematocolpos when the vagina is dilated by blood, and hematocolpos when both the vagina and uterus contain blood. Causes of vaginal obstruction include vaginal atresia or stenosis and an imperforate membrane. These conditions result in the accumulation of fluid in the vaginal canal and sometimes in the uterus. The end result is a pelvic or lower abdominal mass. Almost all patients with vaginal or cervical atresia or stenosis have associated anomalies, including bicornuate uterus,

urogenital sinus, imperforate anus, esophageal or duodenal atresia, and congenital heart disease.[118]

MR findings of vaginal obstruction are a tubular, fluid-filled, midline mass, representing the dilated vagina and uterus. The vagina typically is larger than the uterus. The distended vagina has a thin, almost imperceptible wall, while the uterus has a thicker muscular wall. The appearance of the internal contents is variable depending on the nature of the fluid. Serous fluid has a low signal intensity on T1-weighted images and high signal intensity on T2-weighted images (Fig. 95-36). The signal intensity increases on T1-weighted images if the contents are hemorrhagic.[119] Additional findings on MRI include hydro- or hemato-salpinx, ureterectasis, and hydronephrosis.

Vaginal and Uterine Tumors

Rhabdomyosarcoma is the most common tumor of the vagina/uterus in the first two decades of life.[120-122] It ranks fourth after central nervous system neoplasms, neuroblastoma, and Wilms' tumor. The tumor has a bimodal age distribution. The first peak occurs between 2 and 6 years of age and the second between 14 and 18 years of age. The common histologic subtype of rhabdomyosarcoma of the genitourinary tract is the embryonic or botryoid subtype. The botryoid rhabdomyosarcoma is a subtype of embryonal rhabdomyosarcoma and shows a polypoid growth pattern. The margins of the tumor may be infiltrative or well defined by a compressive pseudocapsule. Metastatic disease is

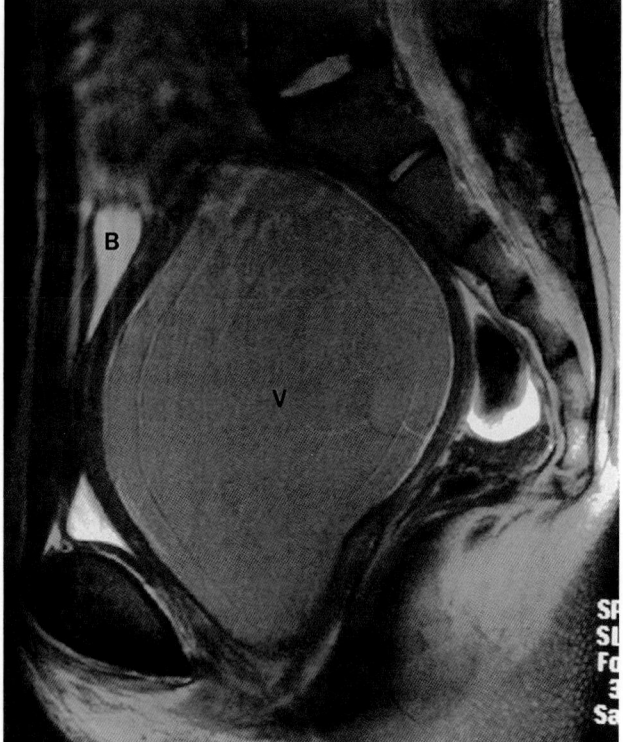

FIGURE 95-36

Vaginal obstruction, hematometrocolpos in a 14-year-old girl with pelvic pain and a palpable pelvic mass. Sagittal T2-weighted image (TR/TE 5000/120) shows a markedly dilated vaginal canal (V) posterior to the bladder (B). The intermediate signal intensity reflects the presence of blood products.

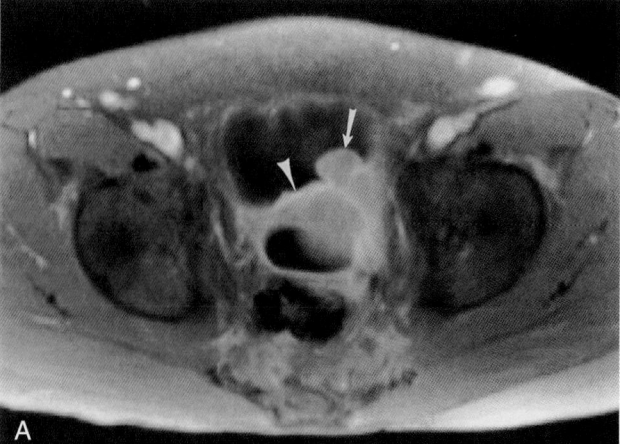

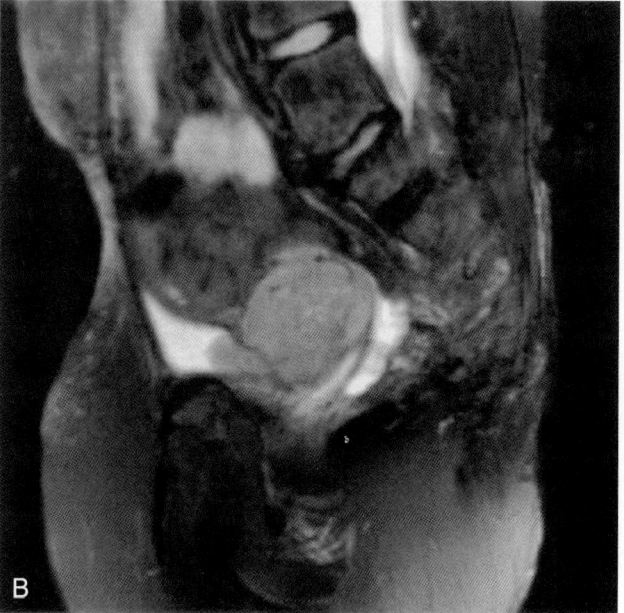

FIGURE 95-37

Epithelioid leiomyosarcoma involving the uterus and bladder. This 19-year-old woman had a sacrococcygeal teratoma at age 2 years treated with surgery, chemotherapy, and radiotherapy. Now she presents with a secondary tumor, shown to be a leiomyosarcoma at biopsy. **A,** Axial T1-weighted contrast-enhanced and fat-suppressed MR image (TR/TE 86/4.1, flip angle 60 degrees) demonstrates an enhancing uterine mass (*arrow*) invading the left posterior wall of the bladder (*arrowhead*). **B,** Sagittal fat-saturated T2-weighted image (TR/TE 4550/99, flip angle 180 degrees) image again shows the intermediate signal uterine mass invading the bladder.

most commonly to para-aortic lymph nodes, lungs, bone, bone marrow, and liver. Between 10% and 20% of all patients with rhabdomyosarcoma will have metastases at the time of diagnosis.[120-122] Most patients with vaginal or uterine tumors present with vaginal bleeding or a vaginal, perineal, or vulvar mass.

Malignant gynecologic tumors result in a soft-tissue mass enlarging the vaginal and/or uterine lumen (Fig. 95-37). These tumors demonstrate intermediate signal intensity on T1-weighted images and high signal intensity on T2-weighed and gadolinium-enhanced images.[120,123] If the tumor is hemorrhagic, the signal intensity on T1-weighted images may be close to that of fat. Tumor heterogeneity secondary to necrosis and calcification are common.

Signs of regional spread include lymph node enlargement and invasion of the adjacent soft-tissues. Lymphadenopathy has a spectrum of appearances ranging from small discrete nodules to large conglomerate masses. Regional tumor invasion is seen as stranding of the soft-tissue or an eccentric mass extending into the soft-tissues from the primary tumor. Enhanced T1-weighted images with fat suppression are best for depicting lymphadenopathy and invasion of perivesical fat, whereas T2-weighted images with fat-suppression are best for demonstrating invasion of adjacent soft-tissues or muscle. Vaginal tumors also may invade the bladder base or obstruct the ureters, leading to hydronephrosis.

Prostate and Bladder Neoplasms

Malignant tumors of the prostate and bladder in children are nearly always rhabdomyosarcomas. The pathology, epidemiology, and sites of distant spread are similar

21. Lonergan GJ, Martinez-Leon MI, Agrons GA, et al: Nephrogenic rests, nephroblastomatosis, and associated lesions of the kidney. Radiographics 18: 947-968, 1998.
22. Morello FP, Donaldson JS: Nephroblastomatosis. In Siegel BA, Proto AV (eds): Pediatric Disease (Fourth Series) Test and Syllabus. Reston, VA, American College of Radiology, 1993, pp 584-615.
23. Siegel MJ: MRI of the pediatric abdomen. MRI Clin North Am 3:161-182, 1995.
24. Beckwith JB, Kiviat NB, Bonadio JF: Nephrogenic rests, nephroblastomatosis, and the pathogenesis of Wilm tumor. Pediatr Pathol 10:1-36, 1990.
25. Bove KE, McAdams AJ: The nephroblastomatosis complex and its relationship to Wilm tumor: a clinicopathologic treatise. Perspect Pediatr Pathol 3:185-223, 1976.
26. Fernbach DJ, Hawkins EP, Pokorny WJ: Nephroblastoma and other renal tumors. In Fernbach DJ, Vietti TJ (eds): Clinical Pediatric Oncology, 4th ed. St Louis, Mosby Year Book, 1991, pp 465-489.
27. Rohrschneider WK, Weirich A, Rieden K, et al: US, CT and MR imaging characteristics of nephroblastomatosis. Pediatr Radiol 28:435-443, 1998.
28. Broecker B: Non-Wilms' renal tumors in children. Urol Clin North Am 27:463-469, 2000.
29. Rieumont MJ, Whitman GJ: Mesoblastic nephroma. Am J Roentgenol 162:76, 1994.
30. Wootton SL, Rowen SJ, Griscom NT: Pediatric case of the day. Radiographics 11:719-721, 1991.
31. Hugosson C, Nyman R, Jacobsson B, et al: Imaging of solid kidney tumours in children. Acta Radiol 36:254-260, 1995.
32. Argons GA, Kingsman KD, Wagner BJ, Sotelo-Avila C: Rhabdoid tumor of the kidney in children: a comparison of 21 cases. Am J Radiol 168:447-451, 1997.
33. Eftekhari F, Erly WK, Jaffe N: Malignant rhabdoid tumor of the kidney: imaging features in two cases. Pediatr Radiol 21:39-42, 1990.
34. Han TI, Kim M-J, Yoon H-K, et al: Rhabdoid tumour of the kidney: Imaging findings. Pediatr Radiol 31:233-237, 2001.
35. Sisler CL, Siegel MJ: Malignant rhabdoid tumor of the kidney: radiologic features. Radiology 172:211-212, 1989.
36. Westra SJ, Zaninovic AC, Hall TR, et al: Imaging of the adrenal gland in children. RadioGraphics 14:1323-1340, 1994.
37. Brodeur GM, Castleberry RP: Neuroblastoma. In Pizzo PA, Poplack DG (eds): Principles and Practice of Pediatric Oncology. Philadelphia: Lippincott-Raven, 1997, pp 761-797.
38. Brodeur GM, Pritchard J, Berthold F, et al: Revisions of the international criteria for neuroblastoma diagnosis, staging, and response to treatment. J Clin Oncol 11:1466, 1993.
39. Caron H, van Sluis P, de Kraker J, et al: Allelic loss of chromosome 1p as a predictor of unfavorable outcome in patients with neuroblastoma. N Engl J Med 334:225-230, 1996.
40. Borrello JA, Mirowitz SA, Siegel MJ: Neuroblastoma. In Siegel BA, Proto AV (eds): Pediatric Disease (Fourth Series) Test and Syllabus. Reston, VA, American College of Radiology, 1993, pp 640-665.
41. Dietrich RB, Kangarloo H, Lenarsky C, et al: Neuroblastoma: the role of MR imaging. Am J Roentgenol 148:937-942, 1987.
42. Fletcher BD, Kopiwoda SY, Strandjord SE, et al: Abdominal neuroblastoma: magnetic resonance imaging and tissue characterization. Radiology 155:699-703, 1985.
43. Siegel MJ: MRI of the pediatric abdomen. MRI Clin North Am 3:161-182, 1995.
44. Siegel MJ, Ishwaran H, Fletcher BD, et al: Staging of neuroblastoma at imaging: report of the Radiology Diagnostic Oncology Group. Radiology 223:168-175, 2002.
45. Abramson SJ, Berdon W, Stolar C, et al: Stage IV N neuroblastoma: MRI diagnosis of left supraclavicular "Virchow's" nodal spread. Pediatr Radiol 26:717-719, 1996.
46. Ruzal-Shapiro C, Berdon WE, Cohen MD, Abramson SJ: MR imaging of diffuse bone marrow replacement in pediatric patients with cancer. Radiology 181:587-589, 1991.
47. Siegel MJ, Luker GD: Bone marrow imaging in children. MRI Clin North Am 4:771-796, 1996.
48. Sofka CM, Semelka RC, Kelekis NL, et al: Magnetic resonance imaging of neuroblastoma using current techniques. Magn Reson Imaging 17:193-198, 1999.
49. Daneman A: Adrenal neoplasms in children. Semin Roentgenol 23:205-215, 1988.
50. Stratakis CA, Chrousos GP: Endocrine tumors. In Pizzo PA, Poplack DG (eds): Principles and Practice of Pediatric Oncology. Philadelphia, Lippincott-Raven, 1997, pp 947-976.
51. Van Gils AP, Falke THM, van Erkel AR, et al: MR imaging and MIBG scintigraphy of pheochromocytomas and extraadrenal functioning paragangliomas. Radiographics 11:37-57, 1991.
52. Chandra RS, Stocker JT, Dehner LP: Liver, gallbladder, and biliary tract. In Stocker JT, Dehner LP (eds): Pediatric Pathology. Philadelphia, JB Lippincott, 1992, pp 703-789.
53. Greenberg M, Filler RM: Hepatic tumors. In Pizzo PA, Poplack DC (eds): Principles and Practice of Pediatric Oncology. Philadelphia, Lippincott-Raven, 1997, pp 717-732.

54. Pizzo PA, Poplack DG, Horowitz ME, et al: Solid tumors of childhood. In DeVita VT, Hellman S, Rosenberg SA (eds): Cancer: Principles and Practice of Oncology, 4th ed. Philadelphia: JB Lippincott, 1993, pp 1738-1791.
55. Weinberg AG, Finegold MJ: Primary hepatic tumors of childhood. Human Pathol 14: 512-537, 1983.
56. Davey MS, Cohen MD: Imaging of gastrointestinal malignancy in childhood. Radiol Clin North Am 34:717-742, 1996.
57. Finegold MJ: Tumors of the liver. Semin Liver Dis 14:270-281, 1994.
58. Ni Y-H, Chang M-H, Hsu H-Y, et al: Hepatocellular carcinoma in childhood: clinical manifestations and prognosis. Cancer 68:1737-1741, 1991.
59. Pobeil RS, Bisset GS: Pictorial essay: imaging of liver tumors in the infant and child. Pediatr Radiol 25:495-506, 1995.
60. Boechat MI, Kangarloo H, Ortega J, et al: Primary liver tumors in children: comparison of CT and MR imaging. Radiology 169:727-732, 1988.
61. Finn JP, Hall-Craggs MA, Dicks-Mireaux C, et al: Primary malignant liver tumors in childhood: assessment of resectability with high-field MR and comparison with CT. Pediatr Radiol 21:34-38, 1990.
62. Siegel MJ, Luker GD: MR imaging of the liver in children. MRI Clin North Am 4:637-656, 1996.
63. Kelekis NL, Semelka RC, Worawattanakul S, et al: Hepatocellular carcinoma in North America: a multi-institutional study of appearance on T1-weighted, T2-weighted, and serial gadolinium-enhanced gradient-echo images. Am J Roentgenol 170:1005-1013, 1988.
64. Brandt DJ, Johnson CD, Stephens DH, Weiland LH: Imaging of fibrolamellar hepatocellular carcinoma. Am J Roentgenol 151:295-299, 1988.
65. McLarney JK, Rucker PT, Bender GN, et al: Fibrolamellar carcinoma of the liver: radiologic-pathologic correlation. RadioGraphics 19:453-471, 1999.
66. Stevens WR, Johnson CD, Stephens DH, Nogorney DM: Fibrolamellar hepatocellular carcinomas: stage at presentation and results of aggressive surgical management. Am J Roentgenol 164:1153-1158, 1995.
67. Powers C, Ross PR, Stoupis C, et al: Primary liver neoplasms: MR imaging with pathologic correlation. RadioGraphics 14:459-482, 1994.
68. Ichikawa T, Federle MP, Grazioli L, et al: Fibrolamellar hepatocellular carcinoma: imaging and pathologic findings in 31 recent cases. Radiology 213:352-361, 1999.
69. Newman KD, Schisgall R, Rearman G, Guzzetta PC: Malignant mesenchymoma of the liver in children. J Pediatr Surg 24:781-783, 1989.
70. Buetow PC, Buck JL, Pantongrag-Brown L, et al: Undifferentiated (embryonal) sarcoma of the liver: pathologic basis of imaging findings in 28 cases. Radiology 203:779-783, 1997.
71. Ros PR, Olmsted WW, Dahman AH, et al: Undifferentiated (embryonal) sarcoma of the liver: radiologic-pathologic correlation. Radiology 160:141-145, 1986.
72. Roebuck DJ, Yang WT, Lam WWM, Stanely P: Hepatobiliary rhabdomyosarcoma in children: diagnostic radiology. Pediatr Radiol 28:101-108, 1998.
73. Sanz N, Florez ML de F, Rollan V: Rhabdomyosarcoma of the biliary tree. Pediatr Surg Int 12:200-201, 1997.
74. Kesslar PJ, Buck JL, Selby DM: Infantile hemangioendothelioma of the liver revisited. RadioGraphics 13:657-670, 1993.
75. Mortele K, Mergo PJ, Urrutia M, Ros PR: Dynamic gadolinium-enhanced MR findings in infantile hepatic hemangioendothelioma. J Comput Assist Tomogr 22:714-717, 1998.
76. Semelka RC, Sofka CM: Hepatic hemangiomas. Magn Reson Imaging Clin North Am 5:241-253, 1997.
77. Ros PR, Goodman AD, Ishak KG, et al: Mesenchymal hamartoma of the liver: radiologic-pathologic correlation. Radiology 158:619-624, 1986.
78. Horton KM, Bluemke DA, Hruban RH, et al: CT and MR imaging of benign hepatic and biliary tumors. RadioGraphics 19:431-451, 1999.
79. Toma P, Taccone A, Martinoli C: MRI of hepatic focal nodular hyperplasia: a report of two new cases in the pediatric age group. Pediatr Radiol 20:267-269, 1990.
80. Buetow PC, Pantongrag-Brown L, Buck JL, et al: Focal nodular hyperplasia of the liver: radiologic-pathologic correlation. RadioGraphics 16:369-388, 1996.
81. Gubernick JA, Rosenberg HK, Ilaslan H, Kessler A: US approach to jaundice in infants and children. Radiographics 20:173-195, 2000.
82. Kim OH, Chung HJ, Choi BG: Imaging of the choledochal cyst. RadioGraphics 15:69-88, 1995.
83. Savader SJ, Benenati JF, Venbrux AC, et al: Choledochal cysts: classification and cholangiographic appearance. Am J Roentgenol 156:327-331, 1991.
84. Irie H, Honda J, Jimi M, et al: Value of MR cholangiopancreatography in evaluating choledochal cysts. Am J Roentgenol 171:1381-1385, 1988.
85. Jaw T-S, Kuo Y-T, Liu G-C, et al: MR cholangiography in the evaluation of neonatal cholestasis. Radiology 212:249-256, 1999.
86. Matos C, Nicaise N, Deviere J, et al: Choledochal cysts: comparison of findings at MR cholangiopancreatography and endoscopic retrograde cholangiopancreatography in eight patients. Radiology 209:4443-448, 1998.
87. Miyazaki T, Yamashita Y, Tang Y, et al: Single-shot MR cholangiopancreatography of neonates, infants, and young children. Am J Roentgenol 170:33-37, 1998.
88. Siegel MJ: Female pelvis. In Siegel MJ, ed. Pediatric Sonography, 3rd ed. Philadelphia: Lippincott, Williams & Wilkins, 2002, pp 529-577.
89. Siegel MJ: Pelvic organs and soft tissues. In Siegel MJ, ed: Pediatric Body CT. Philadelphia, Lippincott, Williams and Wilkins, 1999.

90. Yu KK, Hricak H: The adnexa. In Higgins CB, Hricak H, Helms CA (eds): Magnetic Resonance Imaging of the Body, 3rd ed. Philadelphia, Lippincott-Raven, 1997, pp 815-844.

91. McCarthy S, Hricak H: The uterus and vagina. In Higgins CB, Hricak H, Helms CA (eds): Magnetic Resonance Imaging of the Body, 3rd ed. Philadelphia, Lippincott-Raven, 1997, pp 761-814.

92. Chernoff DM, Hricak H: The male pelvis: prostate and seminal vesicles. In Higgins CB, Hricak H, Helms CA (eds): Magnetic Reonance Imaging of the Body, 3rd ed. Philadelphia: Lippincott-Raven, 1997, pp 875-927.

93. Siegel MJ: Pediatric and adolescent pelvis. In Haaga J, Lanzieri CF, Gilkerson RC (eds): CT and MRI of the Whole Body, 4th ed. St. Louis, Mosby, 2003, pp 2075-2094.

94. Boechat IN: MR imaging of the pediatric pelvis. MRI Clin North Am 4:679-697, 1996.

95. Carrington BM, Hricak H, Nuruddin RN, et al: Mullerian duct anomalies: MR imaging evaluation. Radiology 176:715-720, 1990.

96. Fielding JR: MR imaging of Mullerian anomalies: impact on therapy. Am J Roentgenol 167:1491-1495, 1996.

97. Golan A, Langer R, Bukovsky I, Caspi E: Congenital anomalies of the Mullerian system. Fertil Steril 51:747-755, 1989.

98. Javitt MC: Magnetic resonance imaging in the diagnosis of congenital uterine anomalies. In Fleischer AC, Javitt MC, Jeffrey RB, Jones HW III (eds): Clinical Gynecologic Imaging. Philadelphia: Lippincott-Raven, 1997, pp 299-310.

99. Fedele L, Dorta M, Brioschi D, et al: Magnetic resonance imaging in Mayer-Rokitansky-Küster-Hauser syndrome. Obstet Gynecol 76:593-596, 1990.

100. Reinhold C, Hricak J, Forstner B, et al: Primary amenorrhea: evaluation with MR imaging. Radiology 203:383-390, 1997.

101. Fedele L, Dorta M, Brioschi D: Magnetic resonance imaging of unicornuate uterus. Acta Obstet Gynecol Scand 69:511-513, 1990.

102. Fedele L, Dorta M, Brioschi D, et al: Magnetic resonance evaluation of double uteri. Obstet Gynecol 74:844-847, 1989.

103. Hamlin DJ, Pettersson H, Ramey SL, Moazam F: Magnetic resonance imaging of bicornuate uterus with unilateral hematometrosalpinx and ipsilateral renal agenesis. Urol Radiol 8:52-55, 1986.

104. Mintz MC, Grumbach K: Imaging of congenial uterine anomalies. Semin US CT MRI 9:167-174, 1988.

105. Mintz MC, Thickman DI, Gussman D, Kressel HY: MR evaluation of uterine anomalies. Am J Roentgenol 148:287-290, 1987.

106. Mitchell DG, Outwater EK: Benign gynecologic disease: applications of magnetic resonance imaging. Top Magn Reson Imaging 7:26-43, 1995.

107. Clement PB: Nonneoplastic lesions of the ovary. In Kurman RJ, ed: Blaustein's Pathology of the Female Genital Tract. New York, Springer-Verlag, 1994, pp 606-616.

108. Outwater EK, Mitchell DG: Normal ovaries and functional cysts: MR appearance. Radiology 198:397-402, 1996.

109. Breen JL, Bonamo JF, Maxson WS: Genital tract tumors in children. Pediatr Clin North Am 28:355-367, 1981.

110. Castleberry RP, Cushing B, Perlman E, Hawkins EP: Germ cell tumors. In Pizzo PA, Poplack DG (eds): Principles and Practice of Pediatric Oncology. Philadelphia: Lippincott Raven, 1997, pp 921-945.

111. Ehren IM, Mahour GH, Isaacs H: Benign and malignant ovarian tumors in children and adolescents. Am J Surg 147:339-344, 1984.

112. Pizzo PA, Poplack DG, Horowitz ME, et al: Solid tumors of childhood. In DeVita VT, Hellman S, Rosenberg SA (eds): Cancer: Principles and Practice of Oncology, 4th ed. Philadelphia: JB Lippincott, 1993, pp 1738-1791.

113. Togashi K, Nishimura I, Itoh K, et al: Ovarian cystic teratomas: MR imaging. Radiology 162:669-673, 1987.

114. Yamashita Y, Hatanka Y, Torashima M, et al: Mature cystic teratomas of the ovary without fat in the cystic cavity: MR features in 12 cases. Am J Roentgenol 163:613-616, 1994.

115. Stevens SK, Hricak H, Campos Z: Teratomas versus cystic hemorrhagic adnexal lesions: differentiation with proton-selective fat-saturation MR imaging. Radiology 186:481-488, 1993.

116. Muramatsu Y, Moriyama N, Takayasu K, et al: CT and MR imaging of cystic ovarian teratoma with intracystic fat balls. J Comput Assist Tomogr 15:528-529, 1991.

117. Brammer HM, Buck JL, Hayes WS, et al: Malignant germ cell tumors of the ovary: radiologic-pathologic correlation. RadioGraphics 10:715-724, 1990.

118. Gambino J, Caldwell B, Dietrich R, et al: Congenital disorders of sexual differentiation: MR findings. Am J Radiol 158:363-367, 1992.

119. Hricak H, Chang YCF, Thurnher S: Vagina: evaluation with MR imaging. Part I. Normal anatomy and congenital anomalies. Radiology 169:169-174, 1988.

120. Argons GA, Wagner BJ, Lonergan GJ, et al: Genitourinary rhabdomyosarcoma in children: radiologic-pathologic correlation. RadioGraphics 17:919-937, 1997.

121. Maurer HM, Ragab A: Rhabdomyosarcoma. In Fernbach DJ, Vietti TJ (eds): Clinical Pediatric Oncology, 4th ed. St Louis, Mosby-Year Book, 1991, pp 491-515.

122. Wexler LH, Helman LJ: Rhabdomyosarcoma and the undifferentiated sarcomas. In Pizzo PA, Poplack DG (eds): Principles and Practice of Pediatric Oncology. Philadelphia, Lippincott Raven, 1997, pp 799-829.

123. Fletcher BD, Kaste SC: Magnetic resonance imaging for diagnosis and follow-up of genitourinary, pelvic, and perineal rhabdomyosarcoma. Urol Radiol 14:262-272, 1992.

124. Bartolozzi C, Selli C, Olmastroni M, et al: Rhabdomyosarcoma of the prostate: MR findings. Am J Roentgenol 150:1333-1334, 1988.

125. Castleberry RP, Cushing B, Perlman E, Hawkins EP: Germ cell tumors. In Pizzo PA, Poplack DG (eds): Principles and Practice of Pediatric Oncology. Philadelphia, Lippincott Raven, 1997, pp 921-945.

126. Kesslar PJ, Buck JL, Suarez ES: Germ cell tumors of the sacrococcygeal region: radiologic-pathologic correlation. RadioGraphics 14:607-620, 1994.

127. Wells RG, Sty JR: Imaging of sacrococcygeal germ cell tumors. RadioGraphics 10:701-713, 1990.

128. Kaste SC, Bridges JO, Marina NM: Sacrococcygeal yolk sac carcinoma: imaging findings during treatment. Pediatr Radiol 26:212-219, 1996.

129. Berdon WE, Stylianos S, Ruzal-Shapiro C, et al: Neuroblastoma arising from the organ of Zuckerkandl: an unusual site with a favorable biologic outcome. Pediatr Radiol 29:497-502, 1999.

130. Macpherson RI: Gastrointestinal tract duplications: clinical, pathologic, etiologic, and radiologic considerations. RadioGraphics 13:1063-1080, 1993.

131. Siegel MJ: Pelvic tumors. Radiol Clin North Am 35:1455-147, 1997.

132. Siegel MJ, Hoffer FA: Magnetic resonance imaging of nongynecologic pelvic masses in children. Magn Reson Imaging Clin N Am 10:325-344, 2002.

133. Bhargava R, Parham DM, Lasater OE, et al: MR imaging differentiation of benign and malignant peripheral nerve sheath tumors: use of the target sign. Pediatr Radiol 27:124-129, 1997.

134. Suh JS, Abenoza P, Galloway HR, et al: Peripheral (extracranial) nerve tumors: correlation of MR imaging and histologic findings. Radiology 183:341-346, 1992.

135. Johnson JO, Mattrey RF, Phillipson J: Differentiation of seminomatous from nonseminomatous testicular tumors with MR imaging. Am J Roentgenol 154:539-543, 1990.

136. Hricak H: MRI for evaluating abnormalities of the testes. Contemp Urol 2:13-22,1990.

137. Schultz-Lampel D, Bogaert G, Thüroff JW, et al: MRI for evaluaion of scrotal pathology. Urol Res 19:289-292, 1991.

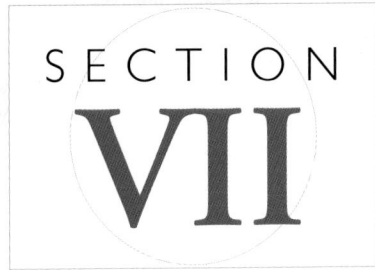

MUSCULOSKELETAL SYSTEM

CHAPTER **96**

Musculoskeletal MRI Techniques

John V. Crues III ● Michael B. Zlatkin ● Scott A. Mirowitz

After its introduction in the mid-1980s, magnetic resonance imaging (MRI) rapidly became the imaging modality of choice for evaluating the majority of bone and joint derangements, and a plethora of ongoing technical advances continues to improve its ability to evaluate these problems. This article reviews basic principles in patient setup, radiofrequency (RF) coil design, and optimization of advanced pulse sequences. We also emphasize the necessity for appropriate clinical information, including operative reports, to be available to the radiologist as the imaging protocol is being determined and while interpreting the study. The goal of this chapter is not to provide imaging recommendations of specific anatomic locations or clinical scenarios, since these are discussed in other chapters; rather its intention is to discuss general approaches for optimizing musculoskeletal MR imaging adaptable to a variety of clinical circumstances.

OBJECTIVES FOR OPTIMIZATION OF MUSCULOSKELETAL PROTOCOLS

Whereas there are many options for performing musculoskeletal MRI, several objectives form the basis for optimization of imaging protocols. These include signal-to-noise ratio (SNR), spatial resolution, anatomic depiction, tissue contrast, artifact control, and imaging time. Adequate SNR is essential for producing diagnostic MR images, as low SNR images appear grainy with poor contrast, compromising visualization of anatomic and pathologic features. Major factors contributing to increased SNR include long repetition time (TR), short echo time (TE), increased number of excitations (NEX), narrow receiver bandwidth, large voxel sizes, high-field-strength systems,[1] and use of a local coil, features discussed in greater detail in the physics chapters of this book (2-5, 7, 8, 13, 18, 22 and 24).

Adequate spatial resolution is critical to depiction of small structures, for detection of injuries to the internal components of the joints, and for characterizing pathologic changes. Spatial resolution improves (i.e., pixel diameters decrease in size) directly with increasing matrix size (i.e., number of phase and frequency encoding steps) and inversely with slice thickness (voxel depth), interslice gap, and field-of-view (FOV). Improved spatial resolution is associated with smaller voxel volumes, but smaller voxel volumes include fewer hydrogen nuclei, leading to less signal and poorer SNR.[2] Therefore, in acquiring diagnostic-quality, high-resolution images, the use of high-field-strength systems, local coils, and increased NEX is often essential. Optimization of anatomic depiction requires proper patient positioning, selection of imaging planes, and coverage of the region of interest, factors dependent on the anatomy being evaluated and the type of pathology suspected. Consequently, the details of imaging of each joint will be described in specified chapters, including functional, dynamic, and kinematic information.

Tissue contrast refers to the ability of any imaging modality to provide differing intensities between tissues that allow characterization of normal and abnormal tissues, such as distinguishing synovial fluid from hyaline cartilage or infiltrating tumor from surrounding normal bone marrow. A major advantage of MRI over other competing imaging technologies is that contrast varies according to the type of pulse sequence used (i.e., spin-echo versus gradient-echo) and imaging parameters (i.e., choice of TR, TE, and flip angle). As the number and types of pulse sequences continue to expand, MRI is increasingly robust in its ability to characterize internal structure. Suppression of background signal intensity (e.g., fat) or use of exogenous contrast agents may also be employed to improve the inherent tissue contrast. With increased complexity of pulse sequences and exogenously infused contrast agents come a variety of potential artifacts that may obscure or simulate pathology in the musculoskeletal system, including motion-induced phase-encoding errors, chemical shift misregistration, aliasing, inhomogeneity of fat suppression, and many others, which are discussed in greater detail in chapters specific to body regions.[3-6]

Finally, it is desirable to keep image acquisition time to a minimum in order to improve patient tolerance, reduce motion artifacts, increase efficiency for utilization of the MR system, and to accommodate special techniques requiring short acquisition times, such as three-dimensional Fourier transform imaging, kinematic imaging, and dynamic contrast-enhanced imaging.

PATIENT SETUP

Patient Positioning

The area of interest should be positioned as close to the isocenter of the magnet as possible, where homogeneity of the main magnetic field is greatest and where images are most likely to yield optimal SNR and uniform intensity. Signal inhomogeneity at the periphery of the magnetic field (shading artifacts) may be encountered that can reduce the ability to detect subtle abnormalities or simulate abnormalities that are not present. For example, artifactually reduced signal intensity in the marrow space due to shading or magnetic field inhomogeneity can simulate marrow replacement on T1-weighted images or fat-suppressed images (Fig. 96-1). Positioning can also have a significant impact on patient comfort.

Because many patients experience some anxiety or claustrophobia within the MR scanner, it is preferable to allow as much of the patient's head and upper torso to remain outside of the magnet bore as is feasible. Contact of the patient with the sides of the magnet should be avoided, as this can also contribute to shading artifacts and may predispose to patient injury.[7] Patients should be instructed to keep their arms and legs toward the center of the magnet bore; sponges and other positioning devices may help decrease patient fatigue, especially for larger patients. Although patients are usually positioned supine for MR examinations, the prone position may be optimal: for example, some claustrophobic patients better tolerate imaging in the prone position, since this allows them to see outside the bore of the magnet, and the sternum may be better imaged prone to minimize breathing motion artifact. One should also consider prone positioning for patients with suspected soft-tissue abnormalities involving posterior structures, such as the gluteal region or the superficial back, since pressure exerted on these regions with the patient supine can flatten or deform the soft-tissues. In some circumstances, oblique or other nontraditional positions may be considered, depending on the anatomic region being evaluated and the type of suspected pathology. For example, slight external rotation of the leg may be advantageous for routine knee imaging, since it improves alignment of the anterior cruciate ligament along the sagittal plane,[8] although this may not be necessary if thinner sections are obtained. For evaluation of the fibrocartilaginous glenoid labrum, some centers place the arm in slight internal or external rotation, depending on the portion of the labrum most likely to be injured.

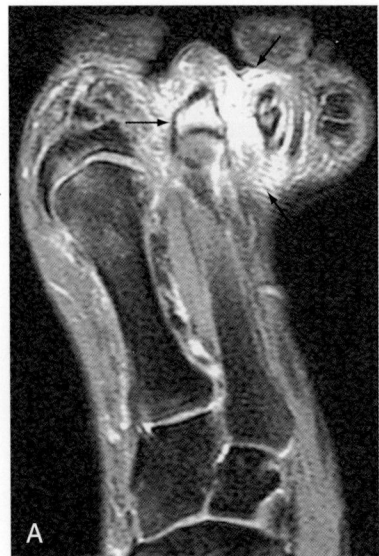
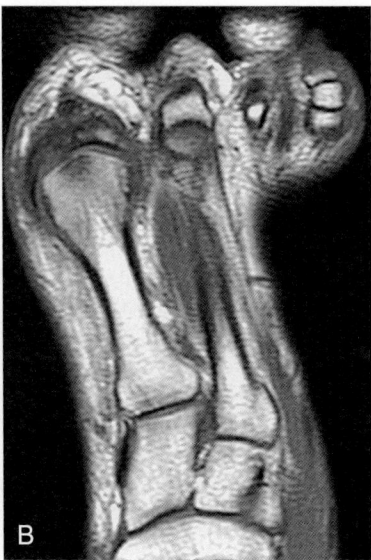
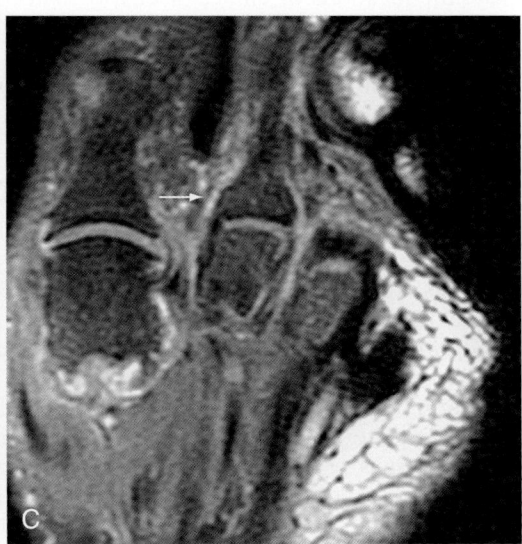

FIGURE 96-1

Inhomogeneous fat suppression. **A,** This fat-suppressed proton density (FSPD) image obtained through the foot shows high signal intensity within the proximal phalanx of the second toe and within the surrounding soft-tissues *(arrows)*. This was initially interpreted as osteomyelitis. **B,** The T1-weighted image is normal. The patient had no symptoms to suggest infection, and the signal abnormality on the FSPD was due to failure of fat suppression from magnetic field inhomogeneity. **C,** Re-scanning using a STIR technique showed normal marrow signal without evidence of marrow edema *(arrow)*.

Patient Comfort

As mentioned above, many patients experience anxiety or claustrophobia during MR imaging. Surveys indicate that in up to 10% of patients this may interfere with performance of the examination. Attempts to avert claustrophobia or discomfort at the outset of the examination will allow many patients to undergo MR imaging who would not otherwise be able to do so, will improve patient acceptability in many others, and will assist with improving examination quality by minimizing motion-related artifacts. A thorough explanation of the examination, including the reason it is being performed, its estimated duration, and the physical setup of the scanner, is helpful in allaying patient apprehension. Ample opportunity for answering patient questions should be permitted, and it may be helpful to allow anxious patients to visualize the scan room directly or to view a videotape about the procedure prior to being placed in the magnet. Patients should be informed that they will be able to communicate with the technologist throughout the examination. Many centers have the capability for patients to listen to music or watch videos during the examination, which can be helpful in diverting their attention. Other alternatives for improving patient cooperation include the use of prism glasses that allow patients to see outside of the magnet bore, or use of gauze pads or other materials to cover the patient's eyes. Magnets with shorter and wider bore sizes are also now available, and may be useful for alleviating claustrophobia. Because many patients are evaluated for painful conditions, simple steps for ensuring patient comfort should always be considered. For example, in patients with back or leg pain the use of a foam wedge beneath their legs can help make them more comfortable. When the above steps are not successful in relieving patient anxiety or discomfort, it may be necessary to use sedation or analgesia. The specific protocols for inpatient and outpatient sedation vary widely at different centers, and should involve consideration of the patient's age and medical history. In addition, adequate monitoring of sedated patients should be provided both during and after the imaging examination.[9-12]

Clinical Information

It is important to obtain an adequate patient history prior to beginning the examination. Most critically, every person entering the magnet room must be screened for potential metallic and ferromagnetic articles, such as aneurysm clips and pacemakers, as such devices may produce injuries in the presence of a large magnetic field.[11-21] Most insurance companies and government agencies in the United States require documentation in the MRI report justifying the medical indications for the procedure, making obtaining clinical information from the referring physician essential for all MRI studies. It is also helpful to have clinical information from the patient. This may be acquired through a written survey asking directed questions of the patient regarding symptoms, including the site, duration, and other features

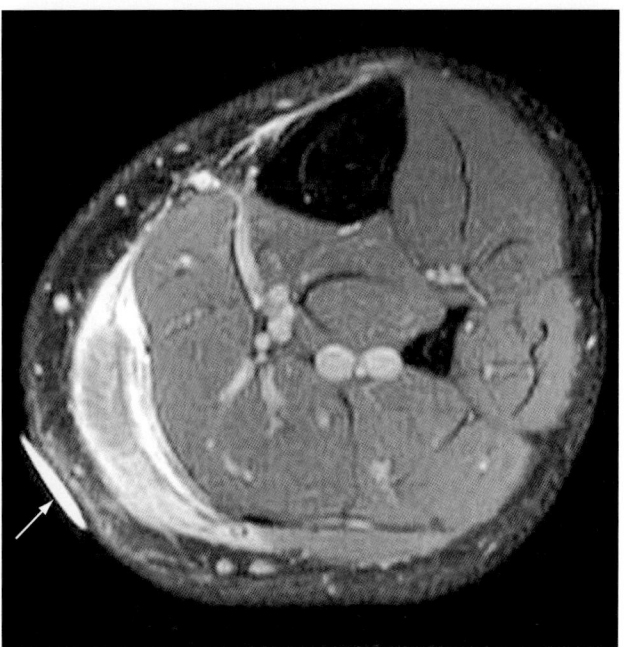

FIGURE 96-2

Vitamin E marker. A vitamin E capsule is placed over a region of suspected muscle tear *(arrow)* displayed on an FSPD axial image.

of any discomfort the patient may be experiencing, as well as any precipitating factors which he or she can identify. Patients should also be questioned as to previous diagnostic or surgical procedures they may have undergone, as this may be important in determining the appropriate imaging protocol and in interpreting the study. Operative reports of prior surgery can be valuable to proper interpretation of the examinations, as well as previous relevant radiologic images and reports. Placement of a marker over any site of localized pain, tenderness, or palpable mass so that this region is easily identified on the MR images is also very useful. Markers help direct the interpreter's eye to the relevant anatomy, and they ensure that the appropriate body location has been included in the images. Many items can be used as surface markers: perhaps the most widely available is a vitamin E capsule taped to the skin surface (Fig. 96-2). This will appear moderately intense on T1-weighted and proton density–weighted (PD) images. It is important to tape such markers rather loosely to the skin surface, in order to avoid distortion of the soft-tissues.

LOCAL COILS

A local coil is a radiofrequency receiver coil placed adjacent to the area to be imaged. Such a coil may surround the tissue to be imaged (commonly known as a volume or whole volume coil) or may be placed on the skin without surrounding the area of interest (commonly known as a surface coil). Coils that partially surround the tissue of interest are known as partial volume coils. Local receiver coils are critical to joint MR imaging

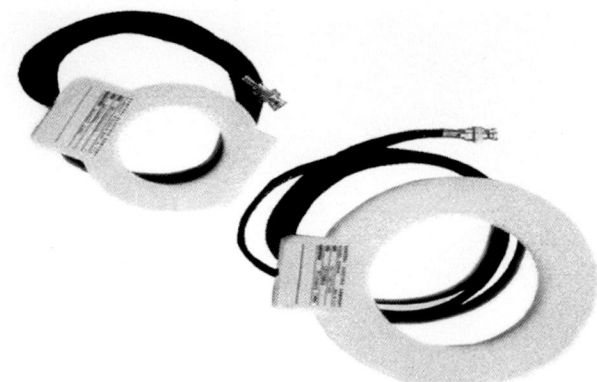

FIGURE 96-3

Single loop coils. These are two linear surface coils of different sizes. When the coils are placed on the skin, tissue near the center of the coils can be imaged with good SNR.

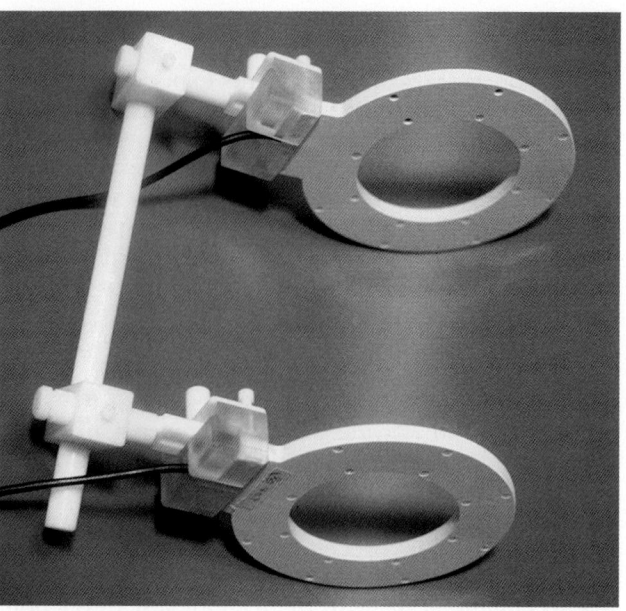

FIGURE 96-4

Helmholtz coils. The Helmholtz arrangement is two linear coils spaced apart, allowing for a larger region of near homogeneous signal acquisition than a single linear surface coil.

as they provide greater diagnostic capability from an increase in SNR.[22-29] Since noise is inherent in the tissue being imaged, it is important that RF coils adequately cover the area of interest but include as little unwanted tissue as possible. In general, larger coils have lower SNR; therefore the aim is to use as small a coil as feasible for the area of interest.

Coil Placement

The geometry of the coil and body part to be imaged restricts coil placement. For a coil to work optimally, the B_1 field of the coil (located in the direction at right angles to the plane of the coil) must lie in a plane perpendicular to the main magnetic field, B_0. For example, if the loop coil is placed such that its B_1 axis is parallel or coincident with the B_0 field of the magnet, there will be minimal radiofrequency voltage induced in the coil, and hence minimal RF signal received by the MR system. Closed MR magnets have a B_0 field that is horizontal and oriented down the axis of the body coil, so a coil loop around the body in the axial plane would be very inefficient. Instead, planar coils in the sagittal, oblique sagittal, or coronal plane must be used. Open MR magnets typically have a vertical B_0 field, hence coils looped around the body are commonly used for body and spine imaging. A planar coil in the coronal plane would not work.

Linear coils are the most basic coils currently in use, often consisting of a single loop (Fig. 96-3). A single loop is an effective coil, if the anatomy of interest lies in the center of the loop. The homogeneity of the image and the SNR degrade sharply away from the center of the loop, often producing suboptimal image quality in adjacent anatomic structures of interest. Other types of linear coil designs, including butterfly coils and rectangular coils, can improve the volume of uniform signal acquisition.

More complex coils using more than one loop can increase the anatomic coverage imaged with uniform

signal acquisition and allow more advanced imaging, such as quadrature, phased-array, and coil-sensitivity imaging.[28,30,31] Helmholtz coils (Fig. 96-4) consist of two parallel loops connected electrically in parallel with a single channel output to the MR system. With the anatomy of interest sandwiched between the coils, the SNR performance is somewhat lower than at the center of a loop, but this configuration has the benefit of reducing the fall-off in signal intensity with distance from the coil; this is helpful in imaging deeper structures and generally improves the uniformity of the resulting image over linear coils. In the shoulder, one coil element is typically positioned under the posterior aspect of the joint, while the other coil element is positioned above the anterior aspect of the joint. This approach also has some limitations. As the separation of the anterior loop and posterior loop changes due to patient size, the coil frequency also changes, resulting in degraded SNR performance unless automatic or manual retuning restores the Helmholtz coil to optimal performance levels. Since proper positioning is always important, MRI manufacturers and practitioners have developed various coil-positioning aids, similar to chemistry laboratory ring stands, to help in coil placement. Although commonly used in the past to image the shoulder,[29] wrist,[32] and other joints, their use has diminished as more efficient quadrature and array coils have become available.

Flexible coils are used very commonly at present (Fig. 96-5). Because many anatomic regions in the extremities are difficult to cover with a good filling factor using rigid coils, they have been difficult to image using standard surface coils. Flexible coils can fit closer to the tissue of interest, thus obtaining a better SNR and patient comfort. Applications include the elbow and long bones, but they

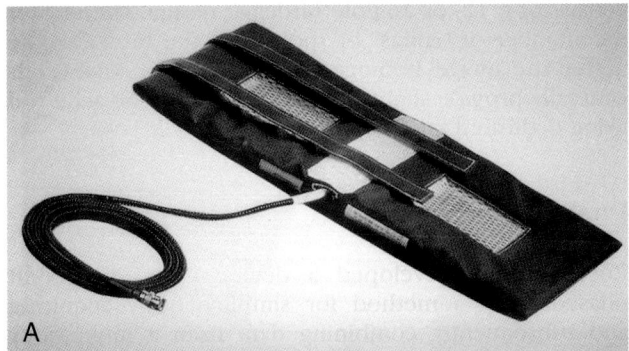

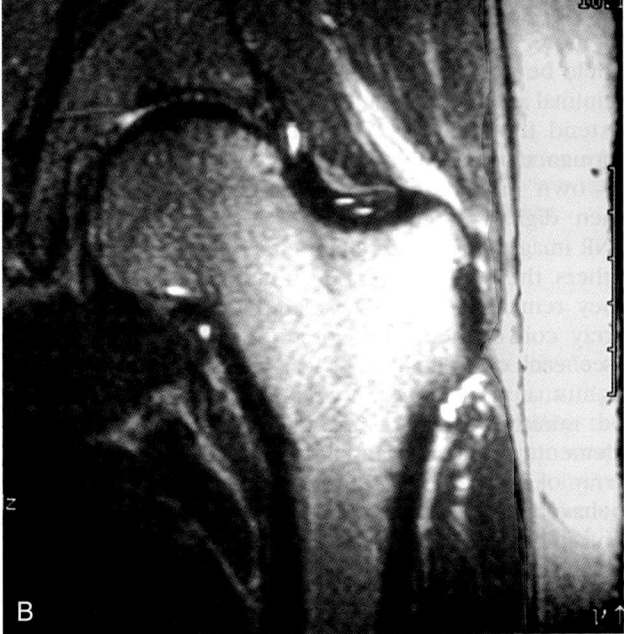

FIGURE 96-5

Linear flexible coil. **A,** Flexible coils are more malleable to the skin surface than rigid coils but suffer from similar signal drop-off. **B,** T1-weighted coronal image of the hip obtained with a flexible surface coil shows characteristic signal drop-off away from the center of the coil.

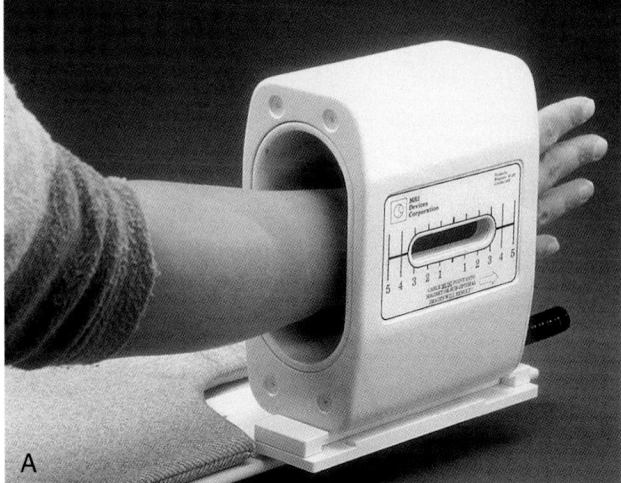

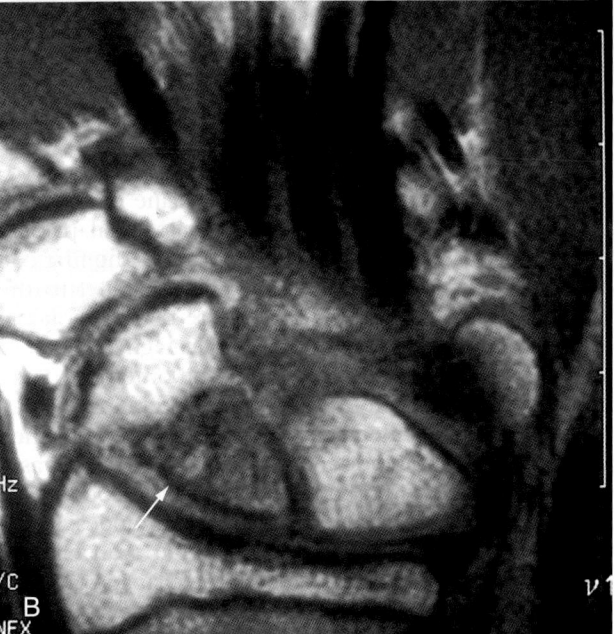

FIGURE 96-6

Quadrature coils. **A,** A typical quadrature-designed volume coil for the wrist. **B,** The high SNR obtainable with quadrature coils allows excellent display of avascular necrosis of the proximal aspect of the scaphoid (arrow).

are also used in the shoulder, hip, wrist, knee, foot, and ankle. Presently these coils consist of one or more linear loops that wrap (once) around the area of interest, but quadrature flexible coils are also becoming widely available with improved SNR. Since flexible coils can be closely coupled to the anatomy, coil loading is fairly constant, resulting in a good impedance match through a range of geometric distortion of the coil. While flexible coils offer good patient comfort and reasonable diagnostic capability for a variety of uses, rigid quadrature or array coils designed for a specific joint generally surpass flexible coils in SNR.

Linear coils detect linearly polarized RF signal from the patient. By designing coils to detect circularly polarized signals, several improvements can be exploited. First, the RF power deposition into the patient can be cut in half and a square-root-of-two improvement in SNR can be obtained over linear polarization. Consequently, RF coil design for joint imaging progressed from linear

designs to quadrature designs in the 1990s (Fig. 96-6).[33,34] Quadrature requires two orthogonal elements feeding into a quadrature combiner, which shifts the phase of the two signals by 90° and adds the signals from the coils in an analog fashion, yielding a single channel output to the MRI system.[35,36] Quadrature design coils are also known as circularly polarized (CP) coils. CP coils have a polarity; if they are placed backwards with respect to the B_0 field of the MR magnet, the signals from the two elements will subtract from each other, rather than add, resulting in poor image quality. The earliest work, by Hyde[26] in 1986, described a quadrature detection system containing two surface coils. One of the two coils was a device called a counter-rotating coil, a two-turn coplanar surface coil with the turns wound in series to create a mode with a

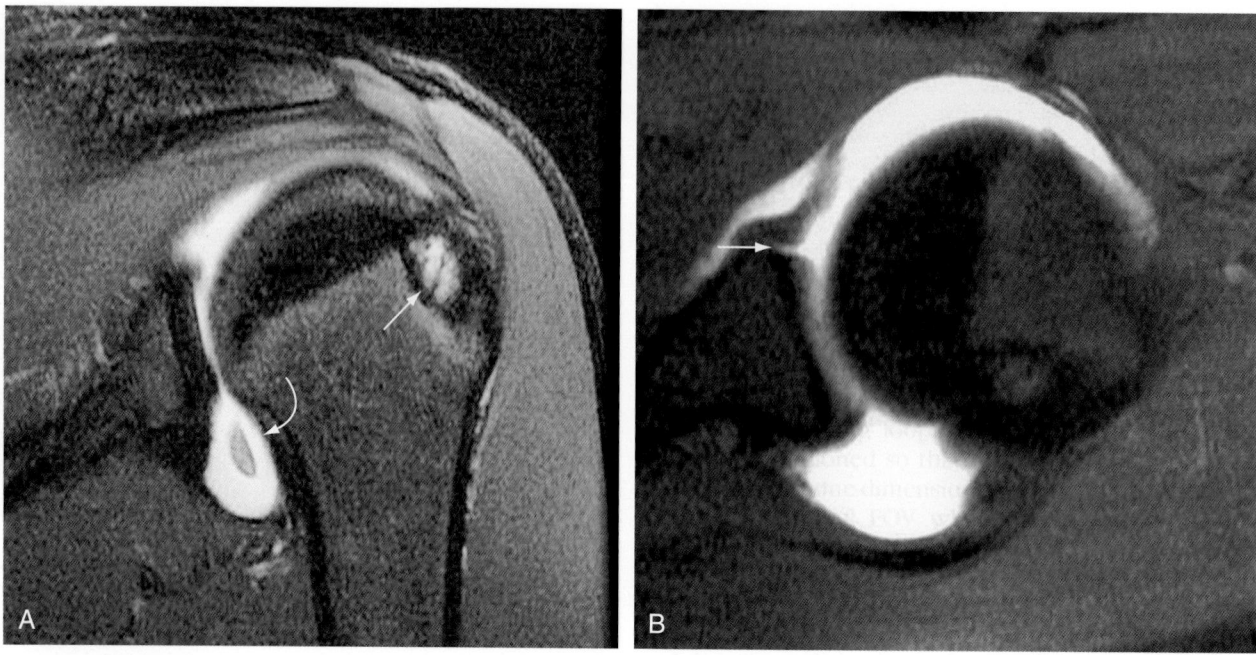

FIGURE 96-9

Fat-suppressed T1-weighted images used in arthrography. **A,** This coronal FS T1-weighted image after dilute gadolinium-DTPA was introduced into the shoulder joint shows both the Hill-Sachs injury *(arrow)* and loose body *(curved arrow)*. **B,** The anterior labral tear *(arrow)* is well seen on this axial FS T1-weighted image with the humerus placed in the abducted, externally rotated position (ABER view).

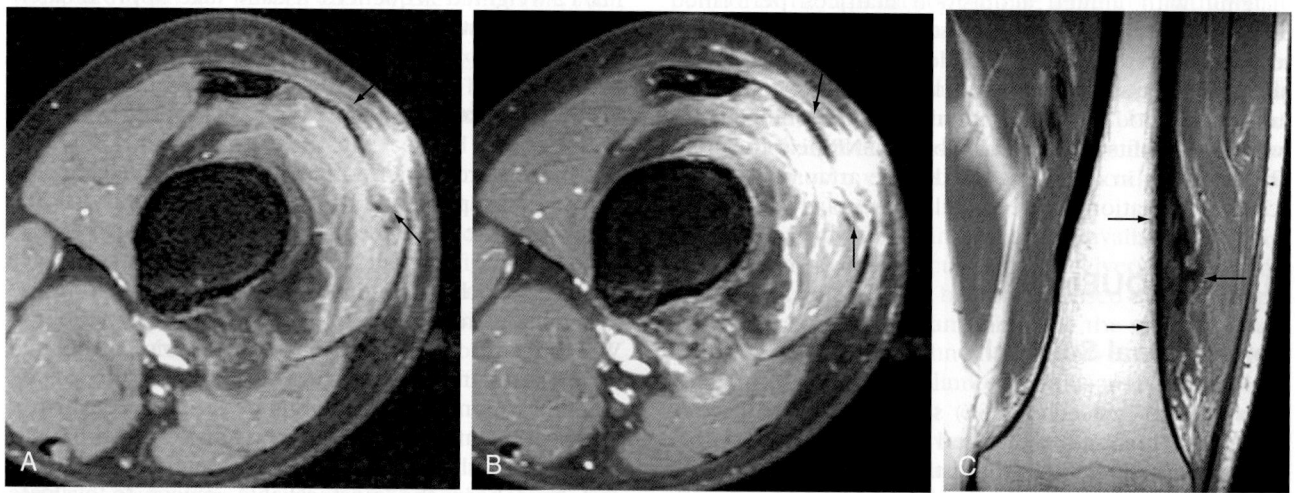

FIGURE 96-10

T1-weighted spectral fat-suppressed images before and after IV gadolinium. **A,** Abnormal signal intensity is seen on this T1-weighted fat-suppressed axial image before gadolinium infusion *(arrows)*. **B,** Marked enhancement is seen after infusion *(arrows)*. **C,** The periosteal osteosarcoma is also seen on this coronal T1-weighted image without fat suppression *(arrows)*.

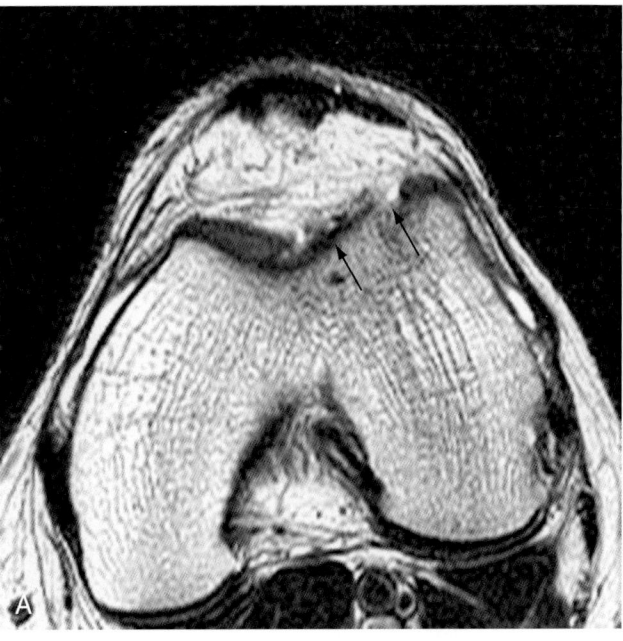
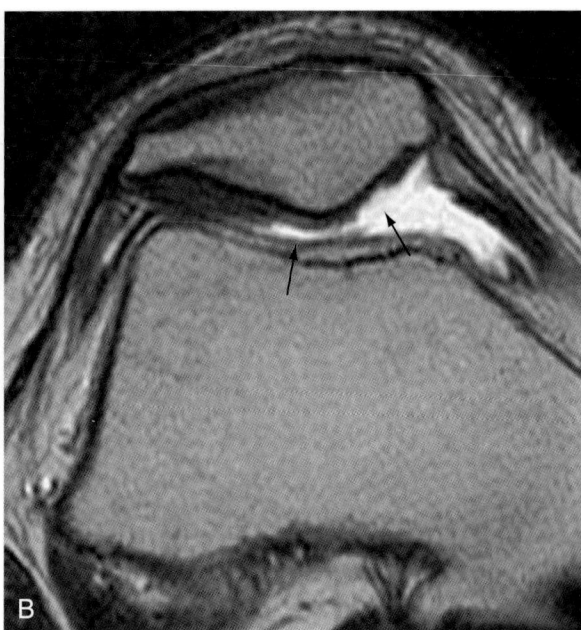

FIGURE 96-18

Articular cartilage injury on T2-weighted images. **A,** Articular cartilage defect of the trochlea on a T2-weighted axial image *(arrows)*. **B,** Patellar articular cartilage injury (grade IV chondromalacia) on a T2-weighted FSE image *(arrows)*.

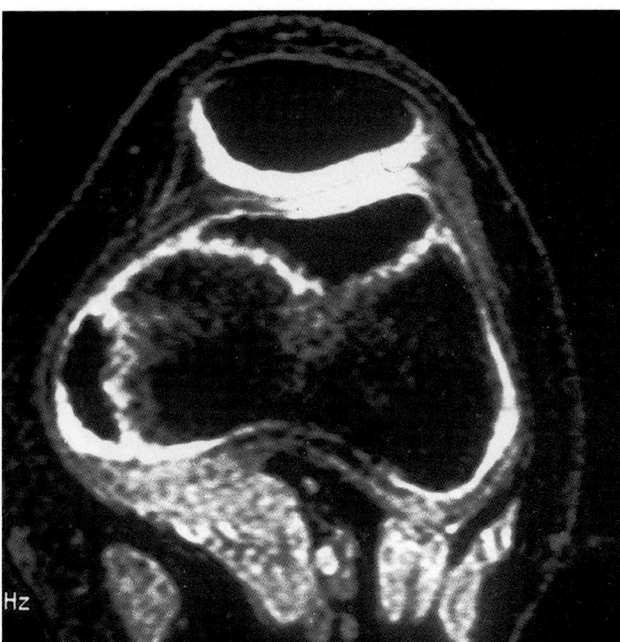

FIGURE 96-19

Short spoiled GRASS (SPGR). Axial 3D spoiled gradient-echo image shows high contrast for the articular cartilage.

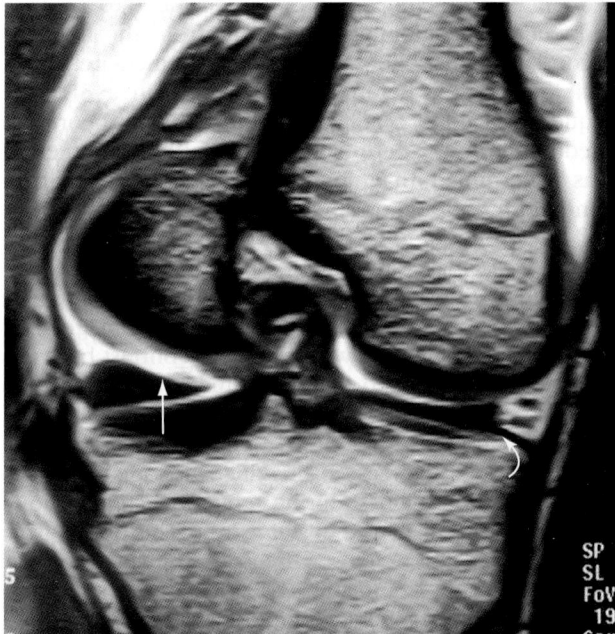

FIGURE 96-20

T2* gradient-echo. This T2* GRASS image shows a full-thickness articular defect *(arrow)* and a meniscal tear *(curved arrow)*.

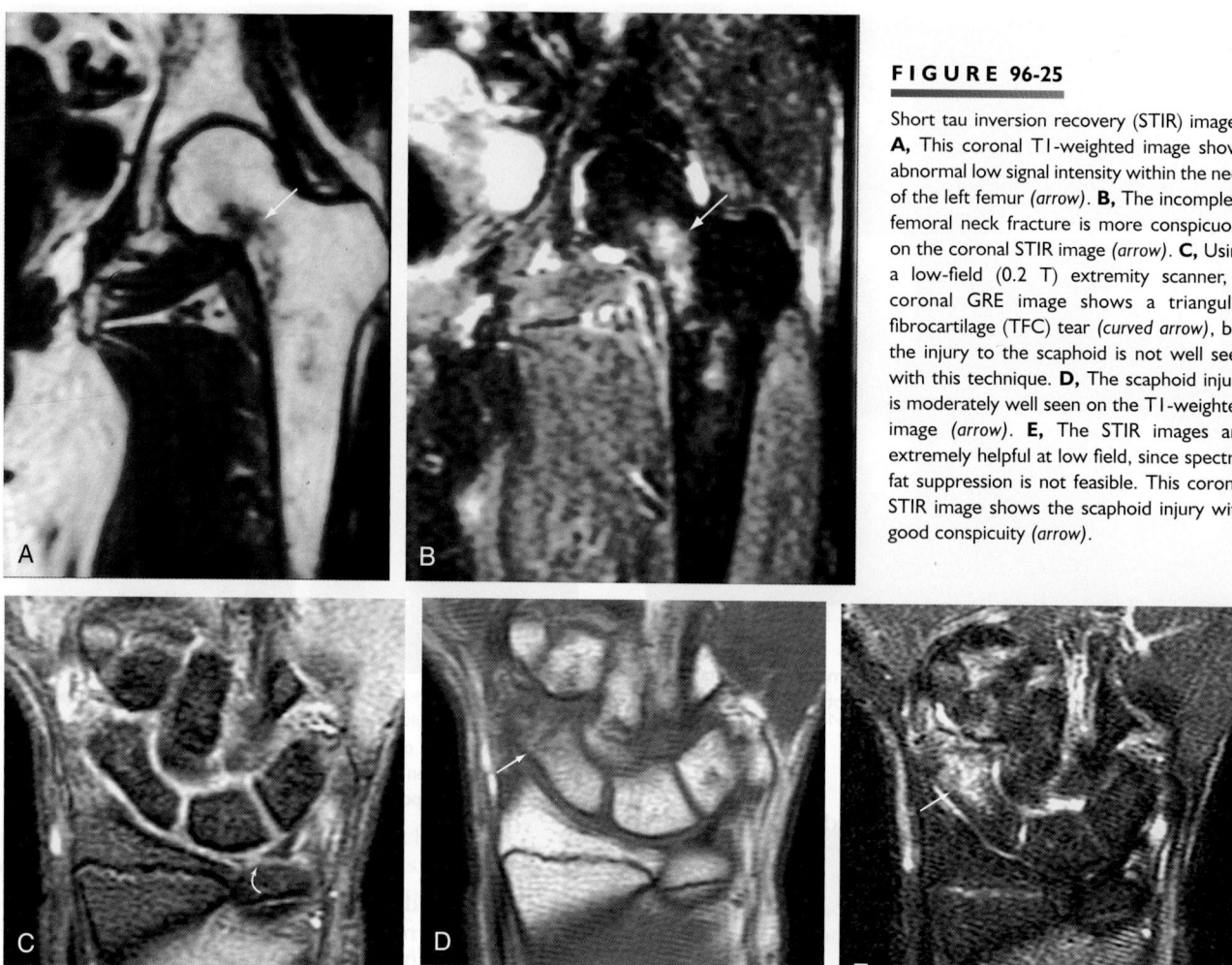

FIGURE 96-25

Short tau inversion recovery (STIR) images. **A,** This coronal T1-weighted image shows abnormal low signal intensity within the neck of the left femur (*arrow*). **B,** The incomplete femoral neck fracture is more conspicuous on the coronal STIR image (*arrow*). **C,** Using a low-field (0.2 T) extremity scanner, a coronal GRE image shows a triangular fibrocartilage (TFC) tear (*curved arrow*), but the injury to the scaphoid is not well seen with this technique. **D,** The scaphoid injury is moderately well seen on the T1-weighted image (*arrow*). **E,** The STIR images are extremely helpful at low field, since spectral fat suppression is not feasible. This coronal STIR image shows the scaphoid injury with good conspicuity (*arrow*).

increased signal intensity in STIR images is not specific for tissue characterization.[124] The advent of FSE inversion recovery has ameliorated the problems of long imaging time, limited slices, motion artifacts, and poor SNR that plagued conventional STIR imaging. Because tissues with short T1 times on the order of fat will also be suppressed on STIR images, nonspecific unwanted signal suppression is possible. In practice, this is a clinical concern only with contrast enhancement, as gadolinium-type contrast agents are effective by shortening tissue T1 relaxation times (Fig. 96-26), either with intravenous infusion or intra-articular injection. Overall, the contrast in STIR images is very similar to tissue contrast in FSPD images, but fat suppression on STIR images is not as affected by minor inhomogeneities in the magnetic field (see Fig. 96-1) and is an excellent technique at low magnetic fields where spectral fat suppression is not feasible (see Fig. 96-25).[50,69,80,122,125] At high field strengths, FSPD FSE imaging provides images with higher SNR than STIR imaging with a shorter acquisition time.

Spectral fat saturation uses a chemical-shift selective radiofrequency presaturation pulse applied at the resonant frequency of fat, followed by a gradient pulse designed to spoil any residual fat signal intensity.[3,126,127] Fat saturation can be used with SE, FSE, and GRE sequences but is more robust in high-field-strength systems because the separation of the fat and water peaks increases linearly with field strength, allowing the presaturation pulse to be more selective. It is also more effective with highly uniform magnetic fields, which may be affected by imperfections in the magnet, poor shimming, or the presence of air or ferromagnetic objects.[49,50] Consequently, we prefer to use STIR imaging to evaluate joints after surgery to minimize artifact from retained metal (Fig. 96-27). Fat saturation is also less effective when used with a large field-of-view due to nonuniformity of the magnetic field across large areas. Another disadvantage of fat suppression is that it results in reduced SNR, since fat is a major source of signal in the musculoskeletal system, making fat suppression difficult to apply in situations requiring high spatial resolution, such as imaging the ligaments of the wrist.

Fat-suppression techniques are used to evaluate many disorders of the musculoskeletal system. As discussed above, marrow abnormalities such as bone marrow contusions, occult fractures or stress fractures, and other

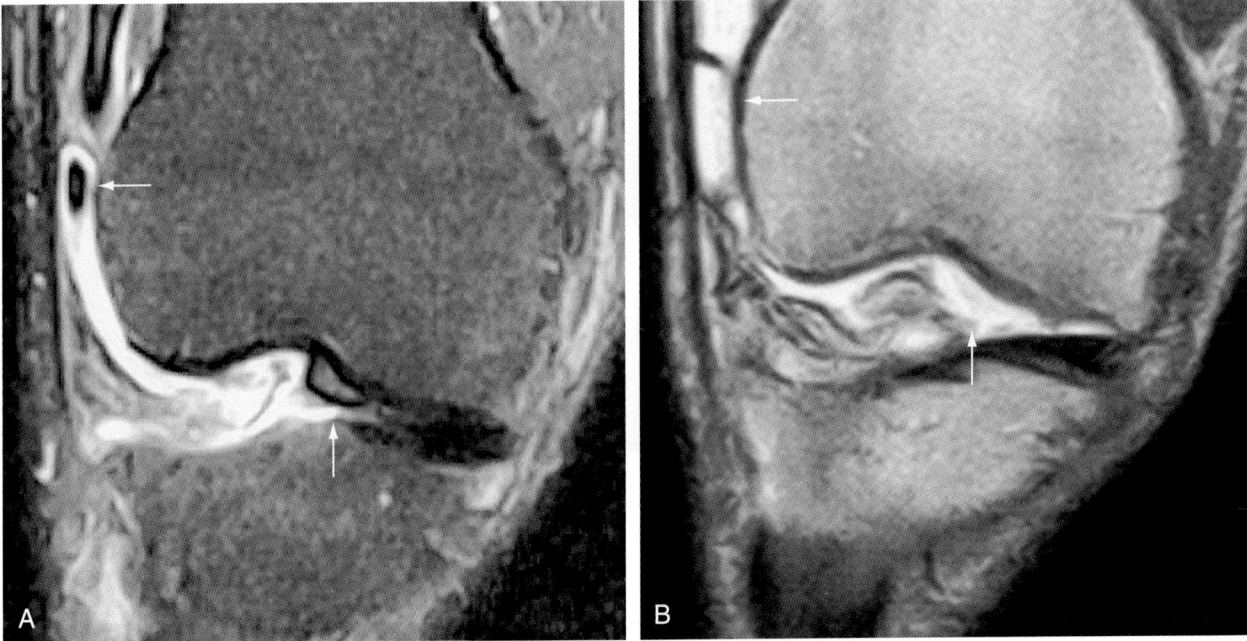

FIGURE 96-26

Artifact using STIR with gadolinium. **A,** This coronal STIR image obtained during an MR arthrogram was initially interpreted as showing two loose bodies within the joint space *(arrows)*. **B,** The corresponding T1-weighted coronal image obtained without fat suppression shows no loose bodies *(arrows)*. The "loose bodies" were regions within the dilute contrast where the T1 time was similar to fat, and thus suppressed with the STIR technique.

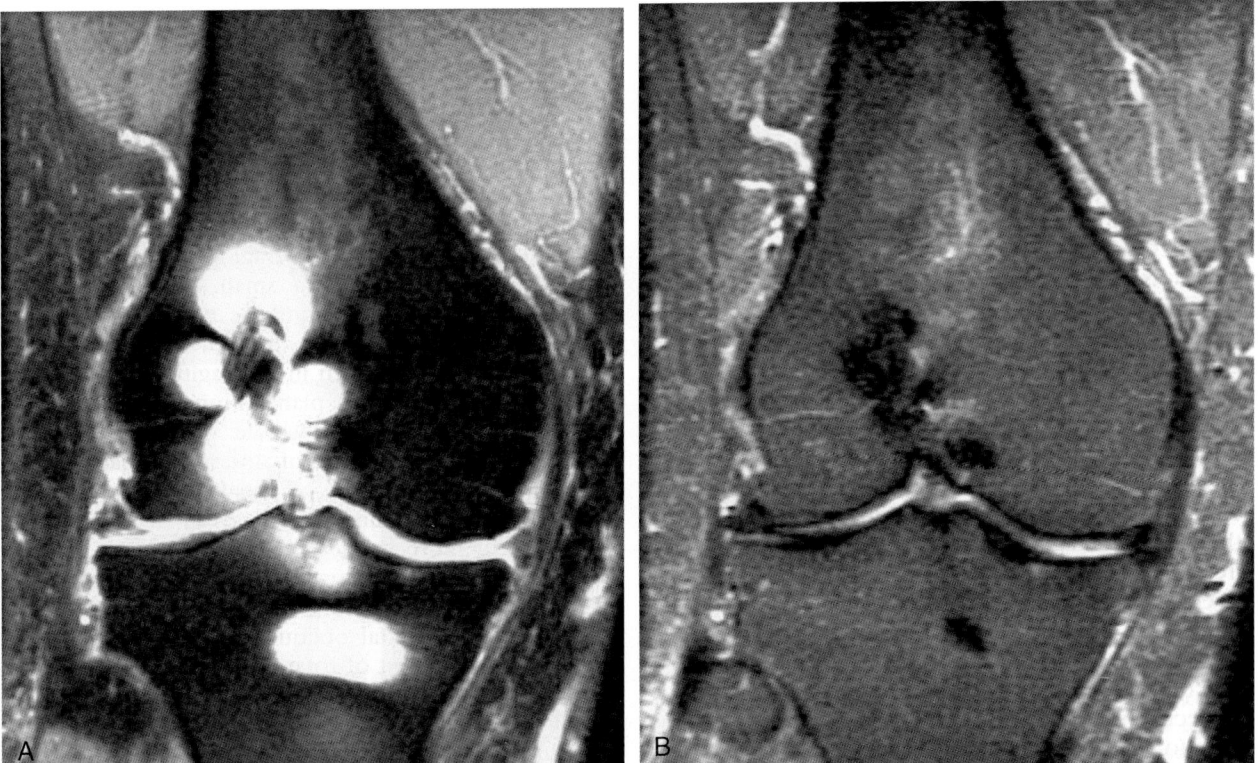

FIGURE 96-27

Ferromagnetic artifacts on fat-suppressed images. **A,** Artifact from ferromagnetic remnants is present in this postoperative patient on this FSPD coronal image. **B,** Markedly less artifact is present on the corresponding STIR image. We routinely replace FSPD sequences in our standard protocols if patients have undergone prior surgery, as pathology can be obscured by susceptibility artifact on FSPD images.

Choosing an appropriate imaging matrix is usually related to finding a balance between the need for high spatial resolution and the cost in terms of the scan time and poor SNR.[49,50] Joint images are usually acquired with a matrix of 256 frequency-encoded steps and 192 or 256 phase-encoded steps are applied, the larger may be preferable with FSE imaging to decrease blurring. The ability to image with even larger matrices is now available on many scanners, with systems capable of performing 512×512 matrices or even 1024×1024 matrices. These large matrices place demands on the performance of computer and gradient systems, but newer systems routinely include faster, more robust gradient amplifiers and computers than older systems. Fast imaging techniques at high-field strengths need to be used with these techniques to keep imaging time reasonable for improved visualization of subtle abnormalities of the menisci, the labrum, and rotator cuff, and small ligaments of the wrist and TFCC, especially when used in conjunction with MR arthrography (see Fig. 96-21).[145,146]

The acquisition FOV is another important parameter to consider in obtaining appropriate spatial resolution for accurate diagnostic interpretations, as FOV is inversely related to spatial resolution.[49] When evaluating small structures and subtle abnormalities, such as small articular cartilage defects or subtle injuries to the labrum or TFCC, it is important to use the smallest FOV that includes the anatomy of interest.[24,146,147] Fields of view as small as 4 to 6 cm are routinely available on current scanners; however, the use of both large matrices and small FOV is limited by available SNR. With the development of better local coils, changes in scan protocols (such as increases in the number of excitations and longer repetition time), and new hardware, some of the loss in SNR at high resolution can be ameliorated. Narrowing the receiver bandwidth can increase the SNR with associated worsening of chemical-shift artifacts, especially annoying in the joints without fat suppression as it interferes with imaging articular cartilage. When a small FOV is used, aliasing (wrap-around) artifacts can become a problem. Oversampling techniques, such as no phase wrap or no frequency wrap, are techniques available on most scanners that minimize these artifacts. More recent scanners with receiver arrays can use coil sensitivity encoding to correct for aliasing.[30,31] Local coils also can help diminish aliasing artifacts because of their inherent drop-off in sensitivity of signal detection from tissues distant from the coil. With recent improvements in magnet homogeneity and the ability to shim actively away from the magnet center (auto-shimming), off-center field-of-view imaging is now more easily applied. Small joints away from the magnet center such as the shoulder, wrist, and elbow can now be more easily imaged with the patient's arm by his or her side. This is much more desirable than placing the arm overhead for the wrist or elbow, where patients usually tire quickly and are more likely to move. One of the drivers stimulating interest in 3.0 T imaging in the musculoskeletal system is the need for greater SNR in high-resolution imaging.

The slice thickness has an important effect on spatial resolution. As when choosing the FOV and imaging matrix, a balance between the spatial resolution needed clinically and the resultant SNR loss must be considered. Thinner slices improve spatial resolution in the direction orthogonal to the slice plane, but thinner images with a constant interslice gap means more slices are required to cover the same anatomic volume, leading to a potential penalty in scan time, as a longer TR may be needed on 2D imaging sequences and a larger slab needed on 3D acquisitions to cover the area of interest. Slice thicknesses of 2 mm or less on 2D spin-echo and gradient-echo sequences and thicknesses of 1 mm or less on 3DFT images are available routinely on many scanners. Cross-excitation (crosstalk) is minimized on 2D contiguous slices with square RF profiles. A major advantage of 3D is the acquisition of adjacent cuts without degradation from crosstalk, minimizing partial volume averaging effects.[95,96,98] Thin sections are needed when evaluating the knee meniscus, the glenoid labrum, the TFCC and wrist ligaments, and subtle injuries of articular cartilage.[32,102,104,134,146]

MR ARTHROGRAPHY

MR arthrography is discussed in more detail in Chapter 97. The term refers to MR imaging of joints after fluid has been injected into the joint to improve contrast.[51,116,142,143] In X-ray arthrography both gas and liquid are commonly injected as contrast agents; in MR imaging air produces excessive susceptibility artifacts, so either saline or dilute gadolinium-DTPA is used. Although saline can be effective,[143] most people prefer gadolinium as its signal characteristics are distinct from those of normal joint fluid (Fig. 96-31). Due to the T1 shortening effects of gadolinium it does not require T2-weighted images to be visualized, as would be the case with saline injection. This shortens the imaging time and decreases degradation of the images from patient motion. After a test injection of iodinated contrast to confirm intra-articular location, a saline/gadopentetate dimeglumine mixture (1.0 mL of gadopentetate dimeglumine/250 mL of saline) is injected, the amount depending on the capacity of the joint—typically 35 mL for the knee, 12 to 15 mL for the shoulder, and 3 to 4 mL for each compartment of the wrist. In certain circumstances it may be desirable to obtain a conventional arthrogram concurrently, such as in the knee and wrist. In this circumstance the gadolinium can be diluted in a combination of saline and iodinated contrast and the appropriate conventional arthrographic images taken prior to MRI. When using dilute gadolinium, fat-suppressed T1-weighted images are usually obtained in at least two orthogonal planes (many practitioners obtain them in all three planes), but it is essential that a true T2-weighted image be obtained in at least one plane (Fig. 96-32). We routinely image the patient after contrast is injected and do not perform pre-injection MR images. By distending the joint, intra-articular gadolinium often improves visualization of a broad spectrum of joint injuries.[51,116,142,148]

MR arthrography is possible in any joint in which standard arthrography is performed, especially in the assessment of complex anatomic structures and intra-articular

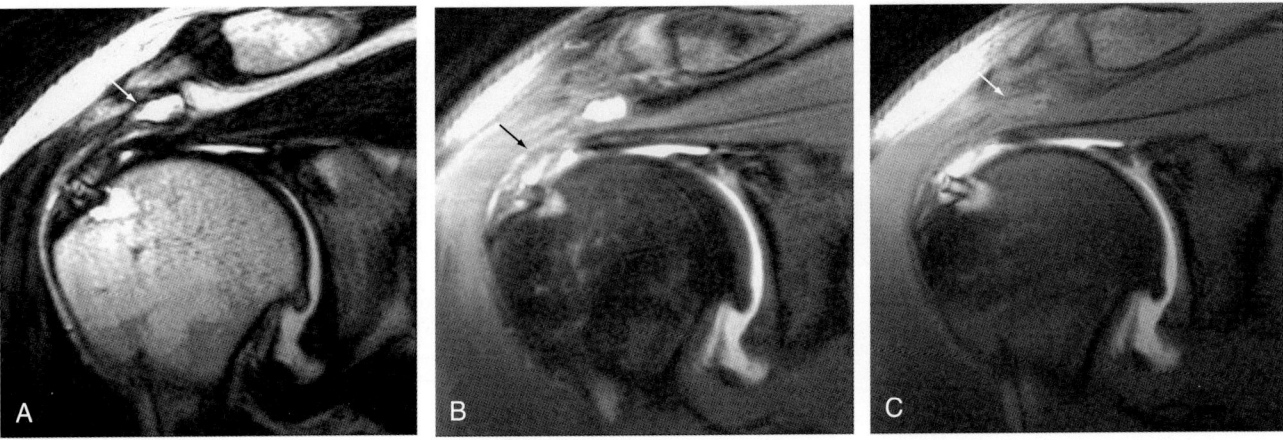

F I G U R E 96-31

Value of dilute gadolinium over normal saline in MR arthrography. **A,** This T2-weighted oblique coronal image performed in a patient with shoulder pain after a previous supraspinatus tendon repair shows fluid in the subacromial bursae, consistent with communication with the glenohumeral joint and a recurrent tear *(arrow)*. **B,** The FSPD sequence also suggests recurrent tear *(arrow)*. **C,** The FS T1-weighted image, however, shows that the fluid collection in the subacromial bursae does not display signal characteristics of contrast (bright) but rather characteristics of bursal fluid, which is not communicating with the glenohumeral joint (low signal intensity, *arrow*). The supraspinatus tendon was not re-torn.

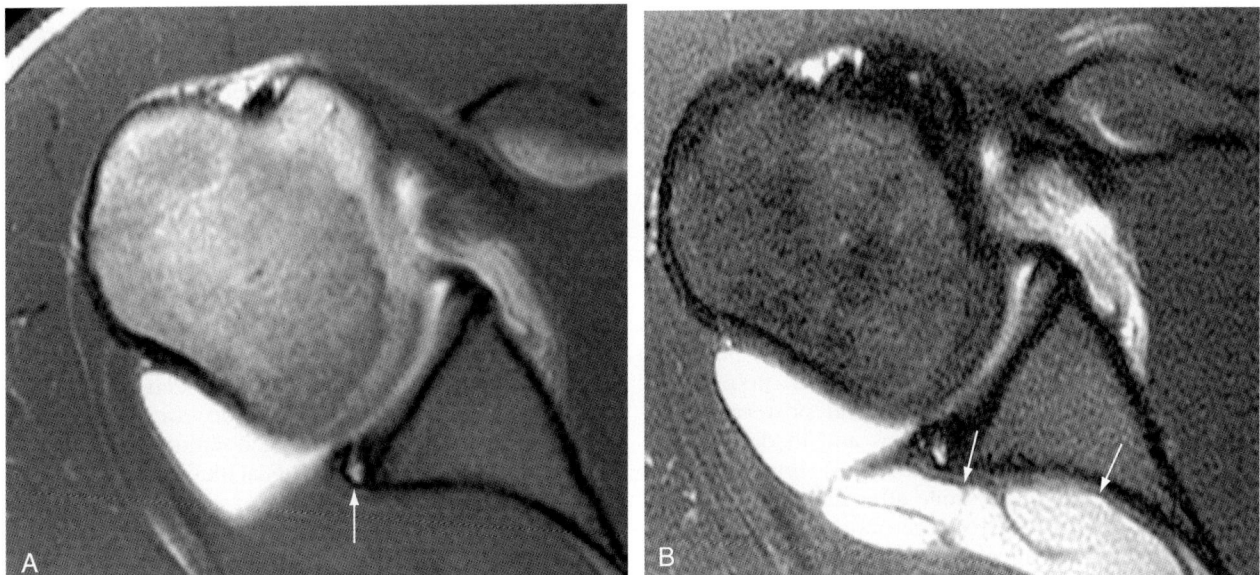

F I G U R E 96-32

The necessity to obtain T2-weighted images in MR arthrography. **A,** This T1-weighted axial image obtained after dilute gadolinium was injected into the glenohumeral joint shows a posterior labral tear *(arrow)*. **B,** Since the large paralabral cyst did not communicate with the glenohumeral joint during or after the injection, its presence might have been missed without the T2-weighted images *(arrows)*.

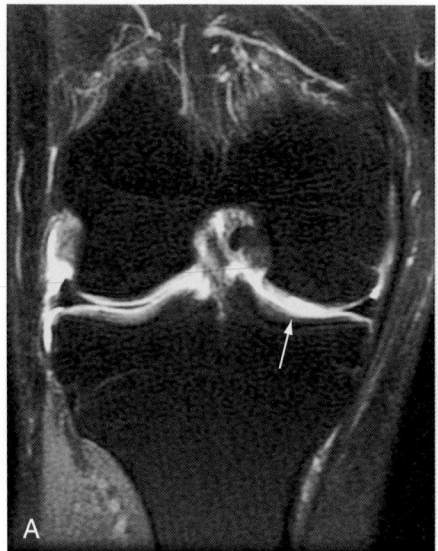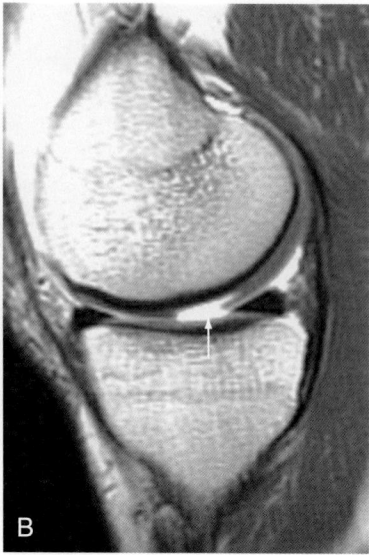

FIGURE 96-33

Arthrography in osteochondral injuries. **A,** This coronal FSPD image obtained with dilute gadolinium-DTPA in the knee joint shows an acute cartilaginous injury *(arrow).* **B,** The sagittal non–fat-suppressed PD image shows the defect *(arrow).*

abnormalities that are difficult to visualize on conventional MR images.[148,149] Current applications of MR arthrography are in the shoulder, knee, wrist, elbow, ankle, and hip.[51,150] In the shoulder it is utilized to assess the rotator cuff undersurface, to identify partial cuff tears or undersurface fraying, to distinguish high-grade partial tears from complete tears, and if used in the setting of complete tears, can help determine cuff tear size and the status of the torn tendon edges (see Figs. 96-9 and 96-30 to 96-32).[140,142,151,152] In patients with suspected glenohumeral instability, especially when there is no native effusion, it is of value to assess the integrity of the labrum, glenohumeral ligaments, and capsule, as well as the biceps labral complex on the superior glenoid margin. It is of critical value in evaluating the post-operative shoulder for recurrent cuff tears (see Fig. 96-31).[140] Imaging of patients in an abducted and externally rotated position (ABER) has become popular at some centers and may be particularly helpful in assessing anterior labral pathology and posterior cuff partial defects in throwing athletes and in diagnosing postero-superior subglenoid (internal) impingement (see Fig. 96-9).[152,153] In the knee after meniscectomy or meniscal repair it may better determine the presence of residual or recurrent meniscal tears and determine the presence of meniscal healing.[130,149,154-156] It assesses the articular cartilage surfaces in osteochondral injuries (Fig. 96-33) and for chondromalacia,[99] helps diagnose unstable lesions in osteochondritis dissecans and assists in the search for loose bodies.[157] In the wrist it may be the most efficacious method of diagnosing ligament injuries, both intrinsic and extrinsic (Fig. 96-34).[53,146,158-161] It can also assess early articular cartilage degeneration at the radioscaphoid articulation in patients with scapholunate instability, a prognostic sign important in deciding on ligament reconstruction.[146] In the elbow it can be useful in evaluating lateral collateral ligament injuries, particularly in high-profile throwing athletes (Fig. 96-35),[162,163] in assessing the status of the articular cartilage in osteochondral injuries, and in delineating loose bodies.

In the ankle it has been used to confirm injuries of the lateral collateral ligament complex, evaluate and stage osteochondral injuries, and detect impinging lesions.[154,164] In the hip it has been found useful to confirm tears of the acetabular labrum.[165-167]

Disadvantages of MR arthrography are that it requires an injection into the joint, making the study semi-invasive. Fluoroscopy is often required for injection, increasing the total examination time, although most knee injections can be done without the use of fluoroscopy, and it may be logistically difficult to perform if the scanner is remote from the fluoroscopic unit. We have performed MRI-guided arthrography in cadaver models, particularly in the wrist.[146] Others have used direct injections into the wrist or shoulder in patients using known anatomic guidelines,[168] ultrasound guidance,[169] MR guidance with specially designed MR interventional units,[170] or CT guidance. Gadolinium had been approved by the FDA for intravenous injections, but has not been approved for intra-articular use, though no toxic effects are known from the intra-articular use of gadolinium-DTPA.[171]

Indirect MR arthrography is achieved by injection of paramagnetic MR contrast media intravenously instead of intra-articular injection as in direct MR arthrography.[154,172-174] In some uses, exercising the joint results in considerable signal intensity increase within the joint cavity where fat-saturated MR sequences yield arthrographic images (Fig. 96-36).[175] The method is less invasive than direct MR arthrography and initial results claim comparable sensitivities and specificities for rotator cuff and glenoid labrum pathology (Fig. 96-37).[176] Other areas where it has been found to be of value include recurrent tears of the menisci, articular cartilage (Fig. 96-38), and in the classification of osteochondritis dissecans. More recent work, however, suggests that indirect arthrography is limited in diagnostic value in the large joints, but possibly superior to direct arthrography in small joints, where intra-articular contrast can be excellent with the indirect technique and surrounding soft-tissues are enhanced from the intravenous injection.[154]

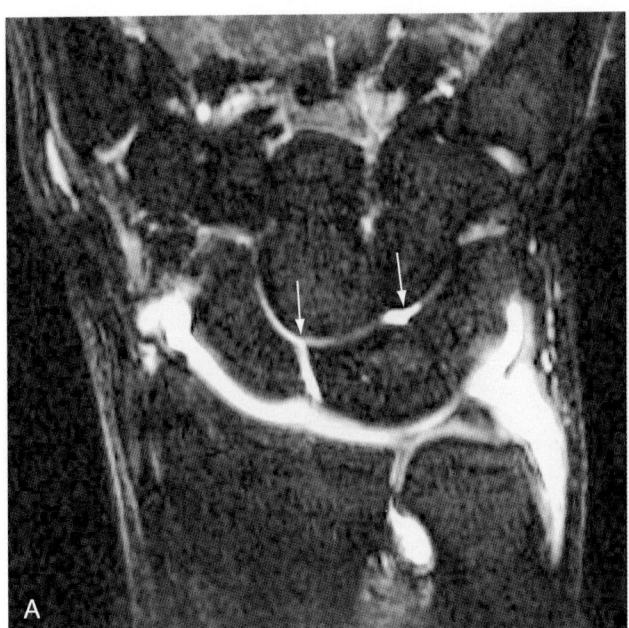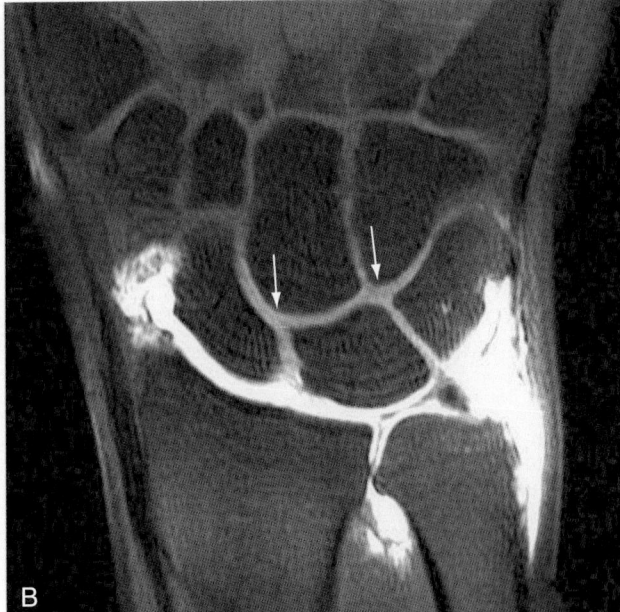

FIGURE 96-34

MR arthrography of the wrist. **A,** This coronal STIR image from an arthrogram through the wrist shows fluid within the scapholunate ligament and the middle compartment, suggestive of a ligament tear *(arrows)*. **B,** The FS T1-weighted coronal image shows that the fluid within the middle compartment does not display signal characteristics of gadolinium and does not communicate with the proximal compartment. A scapholunate ligament tear was not present.

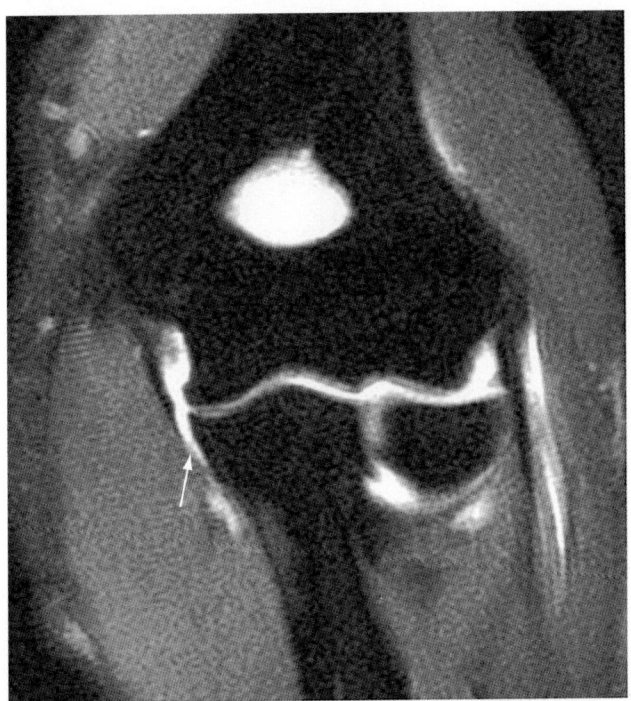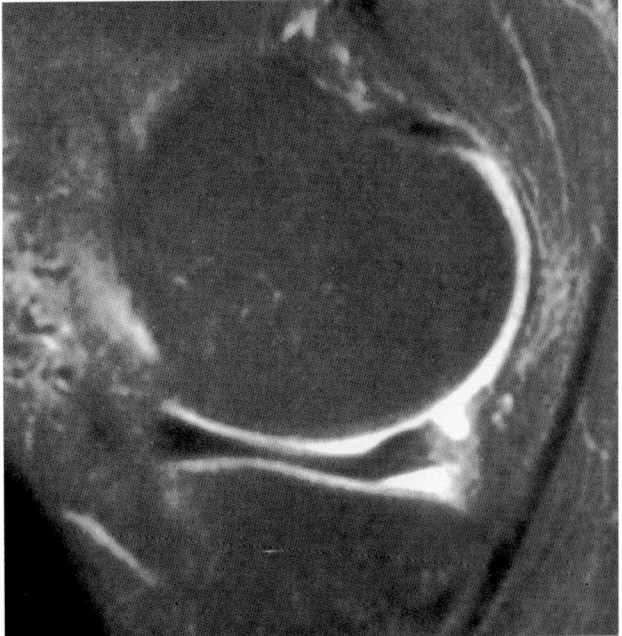

FIGURE 96-35

Ulnar collateral ligament tear. This FS T1-weighted coronal arthrogram image shows a tear of the distal attachment of the ulnar collateral ligament in this professional baseball pitcher *(arrow)*.

FIGURE 96-36

IV arthrogram of the knee. This FS T1-weighted sagittal image shows excellent contrast in the joint after IV gadolinium injection.

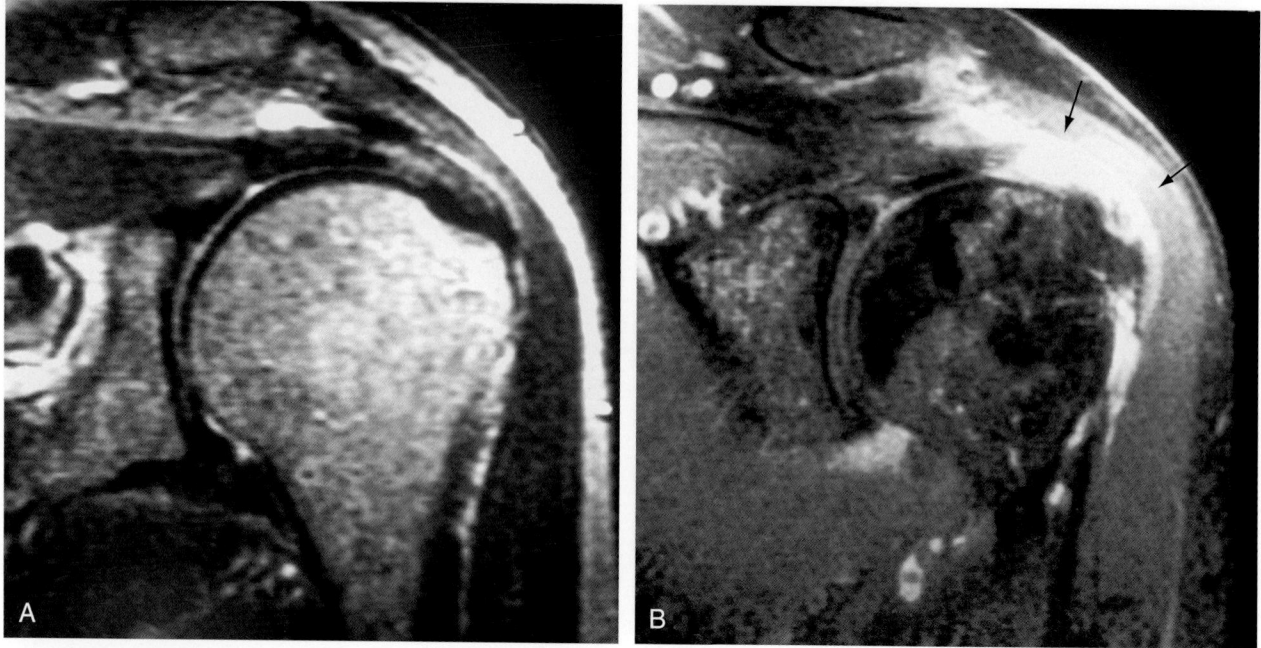

FIGURE 96-37

IV arthrogram of the shoulder. **A,** Precontrast T2-weighted oblique coronal view of the shoulder. **B,** Prominent cuff enhancement *(arrows)* is seen after IV contrast administration.

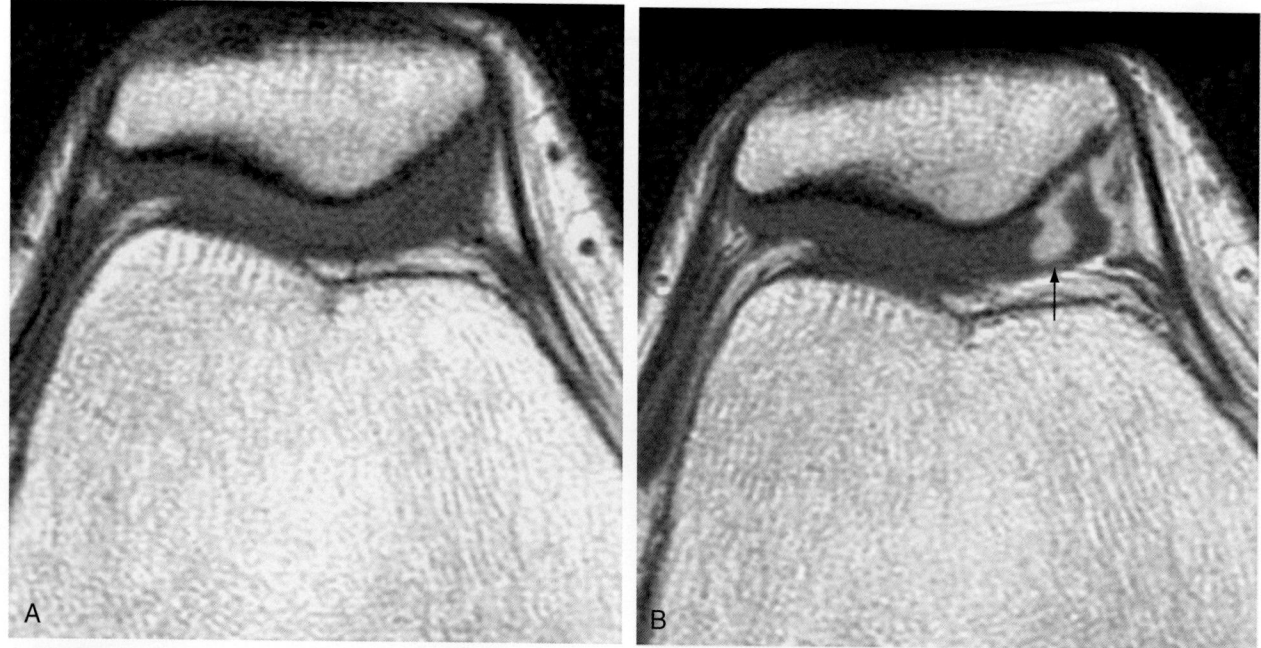

FIGURE 96-38

IV gadolinium enhancement of articular cartilage injury. **A,** T1-weighted images are known to be insensitive for articular cartilage injuries. This axial T1-weighted image is unremarkable. **B,** After IV gadolinium infusion, the cartilage abnormality (region of glycosaminoglycan loss) is well seen *(arrow)*. See Chapter 109.

REFERENCES

1. Fischer SP, Fox JM, Del Pizzo W, et al: Accuracy of diagnoses from magnetic resonance imaging of the knee. J Bone Joint Surg 73:2-10, 1991.
2. Bradley WG, Kortman KE, Crues JV: Central nervous system high-resolution magnetic resonance imaging: Effect of increasing spatial resolution on resolving power. Radiology 156:93-98, 1985.
3. Axel L, Kolman L, Charafeddine K, et al: Origin of a signal intensity loss artifact in fat-saturation MR imaging. Radiology 217:911-915, 2000.
4. Frank LR, Brossman J, Buxton RB, et al: MR imaging truncation artifacts can create a false laminar appearance in cartilage. Am J Roentgenol 168:547-554, 1997.
5. Peh WCG, Chan JHM: Artifacts in musculoskeletal magnetic resonance imaging: Identification and correction. Skeletal Radiol 30:179-191, 2001.
6. Suh J, Jeong EK, Shin KH, et al: Minimizing artifacts caused by metallic implants at MR imaging: Experimental and clinical studies. Am J Roentgenol 171:1207-1213, 1998.
7. Shellock FG: Radiofrequency energy-induced heating during MR procedures: A review. J Magn Reson Imaging, 12:30-36, 2000.
8. Reicher MA, Bassett LW, Gold RH: High-resolution magnetic resonance imaging of the knee joint: Pathologic correlations. Am J Roentgenol 145:903-909, 1985.
9. Berlin L: Sedation and analgesia in MR imaging. Am J Roentgenol 177:293-299, 2001.
10. Bluemke DA, Breiter SN: Sedation procedures in MR imaging: Safety, effectiveness, and nursing effect on examinations. Radiology 216:645-652, 2000.
11. Kanal E, Borgstede JP, Barkovich AJ, et al: American College of Radiology white paper on MR safety. Am J Roentgenol 178:1335-1347, 2002.
12. Shellock FG, Crues JV: MR safety and the American College of Radiology white paper. Am J Roentgenol 178:1349-1352, 2002.
13. Chaljub G, Kramer LA, Johnson RF 3rd, et al: Projectile cylinder accidents resulting from the presence of ferromagnetic nitrous oxide or oxygen tanks in the MR suite. Am J Roentgenol 177:27-30, 2001.
14. Dempsey MF, Condon B, Hadley DM: Investigation of the factors responsible for burns during MRI. J Magn Reson Imaging 13:627-631, 2001.
15. Edwards M, Ordidge RJ, Thomas DL, et al: Translational and rotational forces on heart valve prostheses subjected ex vivo to a 4.7-T MR system. J Magn Reson Imaging 16:653-659, 2002.
16. Shellock FG, Tkach JA, Ruggieri PM, et al: Cardiac pacemakers, ICDs, and loop recorder: Evaluation of translational attraction using conventional ("long-bore") 1.5- and 3.0-Tesla MR systems. J Cardiovasc Magn Reson 5:387-397, 2003.
17. Ho HS: Safety of metallic implants in magnetic resonance imaging. J Magn Reson Imaging 14:472-477, 2001.
18. Seidenwurm DJ, McDonnell CH 3rd, Raghavan N, et al: Cost utility analysis of radiographic screening for an orbital foreign body before MR imaging. Am J Neuroradiol 21:426-433, 2000.
19. Shellock FG: Metallic neurosurgical implants: Evaluation of magnetic field interactions, heating, and artifacts at 1.5-Tesla. J Magn Reson Imaging 14:295-299, 2001.
20. Shellock FG: Magnetic resonance safety update 2002: Implants and devices. J Magn Reson Imaging 16:485-496, 2002.
21. Shellock FG: Biomechanical implants and devices: Assessment of magnetic field interactions with a 3.0-Tesla MR system. J Magn Reson Imaging 16:721-732, 2002.
22. Alley M, Grist T, Swan J: Development of a phased-array coil for the lower extremities. Magn Reson Med 34:260, 1995.
23. Axel L: Surface coil magnetic resonance imaging. J Comput Assist Tomogr 8:381, 1984.
24. Foo TK, Shellock FG, Hayes CE, et al: High-resolution MR imaging of the wrist and eye with short TR, short TE, and partial-echo acquisition. Radiology 183:277-281, 1992.
25. Hayes CE, Tsuruda JS, Mathis CM, et al: Brachial plexus: MR imaging with a dedicated phased array of surface coils. Radiology 203:286, 1997.
26. Kneeland JB, Carrera GF, Middleton WD, et al: Rotator cuff tears: preliminary application of high-resolution MR imaging with counter rotating current loop-gap resonators. Radiology 160:695-699, 1986.
27. Niitsu M, Mishima H, Miyakawa S, et al: High resolution MR imaging of the bilateral hips with dual phased-array coil. J Magn Reson Imaging 6:950, 1996.
28. Roemer PB, Edelstein WA, Hayes CE, et al: The NMR phased array. Magn Reson Med 16:192-225, 1990.
29. Zlatkin MB, Iannotti JP, Roberts MC, et al: Rotator cuff tears: Diagnostic performance of MR imaging. Radiology 172:223-229, 1989.
30. Pruessmann KP, Weiger M, Boesinger P: Sensitivity-encoded MRI. Medica Mundi, 44(2):10-17, 2000.
31. Kurihara Y, Yakushijii YK, Tam I, et al: Coil sensitivity encoding in MR imaging: Advantages and disadvantages in clinical practice. Am J Roentgenol 178:1087-1091, 2002.
32. Zlatkin MB, Chao PL, Osterman AL, et al: Chronic wrist pain: Evaluation with high-resolution MR imaging. Radiology 173:723-729, 1989.
33. Hyde JS, Jesmanowicz A: A quadrature detection surface coil. U.S. Patent #4,721,913, 1988.
34. Mehdizadeh M, Molyneaux D, Morich M: Quadrature surface coils for magnetic resonance. U.S. Patent # 4,918,388, 1990.
35. Mehdizadeh M, Molyneaux D, Morich M: Quadrature planar surface coil. In SMRM. 1998, p 271.
36. Hyde JS, Jesmanowicz A: Quadrature detection surface coil. Magn Reson Med 4(2):179-184, 1987.
37. Beltran J, Noto AM, Mosure JC, et al: Ankle: surface coil MR imaging at 1.5 T. Radiology 161:203-205, 1986.
38. Crues JV, Fareed DO: Magnetic resonance imaging of shoulder impingement. Top Magn Reson Imaging 3:39-49, 1991.
39. Crues JV, Mink J, Levy TL, et al: Meniscal tears of the knee: Accuracy of magnetic resonance imaging. Radiology 164:445-448, 1987.
40. Herzog R: Magnetic resonance imaging of the elbow. Magn Reson Quart 9:188-210, 1993.
41. Iannotti JP, Zlatkin MB, Esterhai JL, et al: Magnetic resonance imaging of the shoulder: Sensitivity, specificity and predictive value. J Bone Joint Surg Am 73:17-29, 1991.
42. Mink JH, Levy T, Crues JV: Tears of the anterior cruciate ligament and menisci of the knee: MR imaging evaluation. Radiology 167:769-774, 1988.
43. Mitchell D, Kundel HL, Steinberg ME, et al: Avascular necrosis of the hip: Comparison of MR, CT, and scintigraphy. Am J Roentgenol 147:67-71, 1986.
44. Needell S, Zlatkin MB, Sher JS, et al: Imaging of the rotator cuff: Peritendinous and bony abnormalities in an asymptomatic population. Am J Roentgenol 166:863-867, 1996.
45. Sperling J, Potter HG, Craig EV, et al: Magnetic resonance imaging of painful shoulder arthroplasty. J Shoulder Elbow Surg 11:315-321, 2002.
46. Umans H, Wimpfheimer O, Haramati N, et al: Diagnosis of partial tears of the anterior cruciate ligament of the knee: Value of MR imaging. Am J Roentgenol 165:893-897, 1995.
47. Zlatkin M: Techniques in MR imaging of joints in sports medicine. Magn Reson Imaging Clin N Am 7:1-21, 1999.
48. Crues JVI: Technical considerations. In Mink JH, et al (eds): MRI of the Knee. New York: Raven Press, 1993, pp 1-23.
49. Buxton R: Technical considerations. In Resnick D, Kang H (eds): Internal Derangement of Joints. Philadelphia: WB Saunders, 1997, pp 3-25.
50. Mirowitz S: Musculoskeletal MRI techniques. In Hesselink J, Edelman R, Zlatkin M (eds): Clinical MRI. Philadelphia: WB Saunders, 1996, pp 1797-1817.
51. Steinbach LS, Palmer WE, Schweitzer ME: MR arthrography. Radiographics 22:1223-1246, 2002.
52. Legan JM, Burkhard TK, Goff WB, et al: Tears of the glenoid labrum: MR imaging of 88 arthroscopically confirmed cases. Radiology 179:241-246, 1991.
53. Schweitzer ME, Brahme SK, Hodler J, et al: Chronic wrist pain: Spin-echo and short tau inversion recovery MR imaging and conventional and MR arthrography. Radiology 182:205-211, 1992.
54. Falchook FS, Zlatkin MB, Erbacher GE, et al: Rupture of the distal biceps tendon: Evaluation with MR imaging. Radiology 190:659-663, 1994.
55. Quinn SF, Murray WT, Clark RA, et al: Achilles tendon: MR imaging at 1.5T. Radiology 164:767-770, 1987.
56. Rosenberg R: Chronic rupture of the posterior tibial tendon. Magn Reson Imaging Clin N Am 2:79-87, 1994.
57. Listerud J, Einstein S, Outwater E, et al: First principles of fast spin echo. Magn Reson Quart 8:199-224, 1992.
58. Henkelman RM, Hardy PA, Bishop JE, et al: Why fat is bright in RARE and fast spin-echo imaging. J Magn Reson Imaging 2:533-540, 1992.
59. Constable RT, Anderson AW, Zhong J, et al: Factors influencing contrast in fast spin-echo MR imaging. Magn Reson Imaging 10:497-511, 1992.
60. Henning J, Naureth A, Friedburg H: RARE imaging: A fast imaging method for clinical MR. Magn Reson Med 3:823-833, 1986.
61. Zhou X, Liang ZP, Cofer GP, et al: Reduction of ringing and blurring artifacts in fast spin-echo imaging. J Magn Reson Imaging 3:803-807, 1993.
62. Kowalchuk RM, Kneeland JB, Dalinka MK, et al: MRI of the knee: Value of short echo time fast spin-echo using high performance gradients versus conventional spin-echo imaging for the detection of meniscal rears. Skeletal Radiol 29:520-524, 2000.
63. Helms CA: The meniscus: Recent advances in MR imaging of the knee. Am J Roentgenol 179:1115-1122, 2002.
64. Sonin AH, Pensy RA, Mulligan ME, et al: Grading articular cartilage of the knee using fast spin-echo proton density-weighted MR imaging without fat suppression. Am J Roentgenol 179:1159-1166, 2002.
65. Cheung L, Li KC, Hollett MD, et al: Meniscal tears of the knee: Accuracy of detection with fast MR imaging and arthroscopic correlation in 293 patients. Radiology 203:508-512, 1997.
66. Anderson M, Raghavan N, Seidenwurm D: Evaluation of meniscal tears: Fast spin-echo versus conventional spin-echo magnetic resonance imaging. Acad Radiol 2:209, 1995.
67. Escobedo EM, Hunter JC, Zinc-Brody GC, et al: Usefulness of turbo spin-echo MR imaging in the evaluation of meniscal tears: Comparison with a conventional spin-echo sequence. Am J Roentgenol 167:1223-1227, 1996.
68. Gusmer PB, Potter HG, Schatz JA, et al: Labral injuries: Accuracy of detection with unenhanced MR imaging of the shoulder. Radiology 200:519-524, 1996.
69. Needel S, Zlatkin M: Comparison of fat-saturation fast spin echo versus conventional spin echo MRI in the detection of rotator cuff pathology. J Magn Reson Imaging 7:674, 1996.
70. Sofka C, Potter HG, Figgie M, et al: Magnetic resonance imaging of total knee arthroplasty. Clin Orthop 406:129-135, 2003.

71. Tuite MJ, Shinners TJ, Hollister MC, et al: Fat-suppressed fast spin-echo mid-TE (TE[effective]=34) MR images: Comparison with fast spin-echo T2-weighted images for the diagnosis of tears and anatomic variants of the glenoid labrum. Skeletal Radiol 28:685-690, 1999.

72. Constable R, Smith R, Gore J: Signal-to-noise and contrast in fast spin echo (FSE) and inversion recovery FSE imaging. J Comput Assist Tomogr 16:41-47, 1992.

73. Arndt WF, Truax AL, Barnett FM, et al: MR diagnosis of bone contusions of the knee: Comparison of coronal T2-weighted fast spin-echo with fat saturation and fast spin-echo STIR images with conventional STIR images. Am J Roentgenol 166:119-124, 1996.

74. Chrysikopoulos H, Pappas J, Papanikolaou N, et al: Bone marrow lesions: evaluation with fat-suppression turbo spin echo MR imaging at 0.5 T. Eur Radiol 6:895, 1996.

75. Kapelov SR, Teresi LM, Bradley WG, et al: Bone contusions of the knee: Increased lesion detection with fast spin-echo MR imaging with spectroscopic fat saturation. Radiology 189:901-904, 1993.

76. Li KCP, Hiette P: Contrast-enhanced fat saturation magnetic resonance imaging for studying the pathophysiology of osteonecrosis of the hips. Skeletal Radiol 21:375-379, 1992.

77. Quinn SF, Sheley RC, Demlow TA, et al: Rotator cuff tendon tears: Evaluation with fat-suppressed MR imaging with arthroscopic correlation in 100 patients. Radiology 195:497-501, 1995.

78. Carrino J, McCauley TR, Katz LD, et al: Rotator cuff: evaluation with fast spin-echo versus conventional spin-echo MR imaging. Radiology 202:533-539, 1997.

79. Singson R, Hoang T, Dan S, et al: MR evaluation of rotator cuff pathology using T2-weighted fast spin-echo technique with and without fat suppression. Am J Roentgenol 166:1061-1065, 1996.

80. Sahin-Akyar G, Miller TT, Staron RB, et al: Gradient-echo versus fat-suppressed fast spin-echo MR imaging of rotator cuff tears. Am J Roentgenol 171:223-227, 1998.

81. Rubin DA, Kneeland JB, Listerud J, et al: MR diagnosis of meniscal tears of the knee: Value of fast spin-echo vs conventional spin-echo pulse sequences. Am J Roentgenol 162:1131-1135, 1994.

82. Ha TP, Li KC, Beaulieu CF, et al: Anterior cruciate ligament injury: Fast spin-echo MR imaging with arthroscopic correlation in 217 examinations. Am J Roentgenol 170:1215-1219, 1998.

83. Munk P, Lee MJ, Poon PY, et al: Diagnostic equivalence of conventional and fast spin echo magnetic resonance imaging of the anterior cruciate ligament of the knee. Australas Radiol 41:238-242, 1997.

84. Mulkern RV, Wong ST, Winalski C, et al: Contrast manipulation and artifact assessment of 2D and 3D RARE sequences. Magn Reson Imaging 8:557-566, 1990.

85. Oshio K, Melki PS, Jolesz FA: Multislab 3D RARE: A fast T2 weighted 3D acquisition. In The Ninth Annual Meeting of the Society for Magnetic Resonance Imaging. 1991. Chicago: JMRI.

86. Smith HE, Mosher TJ, Dardzinski BJ, et al: Spatial variation in cartilage T2 of the knee. J Magn Reson Imaging 14:50-55, 2001.

87. Potter HG, Linklater JM, Allen AA, et al: Magnetic resonance imaging of articular cartilage in the knee. An evaluation with use of fast-spin-echo imaging. J Bone Joint Surg Am 80:1276-1284, 1998.

88. Burstein D, Gray M: New MRI techniques for imaging cartilage. J Bone Joint Surg Am 85:70-77, 2003.

89. Haacke EM: A guide to understanding key aspects of fast gradient-echo imaging. J Magn Reson Imaging 1:621-624, 1991.

90. McCauley TR, Pope CF, Jokl P: Normal and abnormal glenoid labrum: Assessment with multiplanar gradient-echo MR imaging. Radiology 183:35-37, 1992.

91. Tuite MJ, DeSmet AA, Norris M, et al: Anteroinferior tears of the glenoid labrum: fat-suppressed fast spin-echo T2 versus gradient-recalled echo MR images. Skeletal Radiol 26:293-297, 1997.

92. Tuite MJ, DeSmet AA, Norris M, et al: MR diagnosis of labral tears of the shoulder: Value of T2*-weighted gradient-recalled echo images made in external rotation. Am J Roentgenol 164:941-944, 1995.

93. Buckwalter K, Pennes D-R: Anterior cruciate ligament: oblique sagittal MR imaging. Radiology 175:276-277, 1990.

94. Piplani MA, Disler DG, McCauley TR, et al: Articular cartilage volume in the knee: Semiautomated determination from three-dimensional reformations of MR images. Radiology 198:855-859, 1996.

95. Haggar AM, Froelich JW, Hearshen DO, et al: Meniscal abnormalities of the knee: 3DFT fast-scan GRASS MR imaging. Am J Roentgenol 150:1341-1344, 1988.

96. Reeder JD, Malz SO, Becker L, et al: MR imaging of the knee in the sagittal projection: comparison of three-dimensional gradient-echo and spin-echo sequences. Am J Roentgenol 153:537-540, 1989.

97. Reiser MF, Bongartz G, Erlemann R, et al: Magnetic resonance in cartilaginous lesions of the knee joint with three-dimensional gradient-echo imaging. Skeletal Radiol 17:465-471, 1988.

98. Heron CW, Calvert PT: Three-dimensional gradient-echo MR imaging of the knee: comparison with arthroscopy in 100 patients. Radiology 183:839-844, 1992.

99. Chandnani V, Ho C, Chu P, et al: Knee hyaline cartilage evaluated with MR imaging: a cadaveric study involving multiple imaging sequences and intra-articular injection of gadolinium and saline solution. Radiology 178:557-561, 1991.

100. Disler DG: Fat-suppressed three-dimensional spoiled gradient-recalled MR imaging: assessment of articular and physeal hyaline cartilage. Am J Roentgenol 169:1117, 1997.

101. Disler DG, McCauley TR, Kelman CG, et al: Fat-suppressed three-dimensional spoiled gradient-echo MR imaging of hyaline cartilage defects in the knee: Comparison with standard MR imaging and arthroscopy. Am J Roentgenol 167:127-132, 1996.

102. Recht MP, Piraino DW, Paletta GA, et al: Accuracy of fat-suppressed three-dimensional spoiled gradient-echo FLASH MR imaging in the detection of patellofemoral articular cartilage abnormalities. Radiology 198:209-212, 1996.

103. Stoller D, et al: Three dimensional rendering and classification of meniscal tears disarticulated from 3-D FT images. Society of Magnetic Resonance in Medicine, Abstracts 1:346, 1990.

104. Smith DK: Volar carpal ligaments of the wrist: Normal appearance on multiplanar reconstructions of three-dimensional Fourier transform MR imaging. Am J Roentgenol 161:353-357, 1993.

105. Loehr S, Pope TL Jr, Martin DF, et al: Three-dimensional MRI of the glenoid labrum. Skeletal Radiol 24:117, 1995.

106. Hardy P, Recht MP, Piraino D, et al: Optimization of a dual echo in the steady state (DESS) free-precession sequence for imaging cartilage. J Magn Reson Imaging 6:329-335, 1996.

107. Brossmann J, Muhle C, Bull CC, et al: Evaluation of patellar tracking in patients with suspected patellar malalignment: cine MR imaging vs arthroscopy. Am J Roentgenol 162:361-367, 1994.

108. Shellock FG, Mink JH, Deutsch AL, et al: Patellar tracking abnormalities: clinical experience with kinematic MR imaging in 130 patients. Radiology 172:799-804, 1989.

109. Shellock FG, Foo TK, Deutsch AL, et al: Patellofemoral joint: Evaluation during active flexion with ultrafast spoiled Grass MR imaging. Radiology 180:581-585, 1991.

110. Shellock FG, Mink JH, Deutsch AL, et al: Kinematic magnetic resonance imaging of the joints: techniques and clinical applications. Magn Reson Q 7:104-135, 1991.

111. Shellock FG, Mink JH, Deutsch AL, et al: Kinematic MR imaging of the patellofemoral joint: Comparison of passive positioning and active movement techniques. Radiology 184:574-577, 1992.

112. Brown S, Rosenbach D, Zlatkin M: Kinematic MR imaging of joints. In Hesselink J, Edelman R, Zlatkin M (eds): Clinical MRI. Philadelphia: WB Saunders, 1996.

113. Cardinal E, Buckwalter K, Braunstein E: Kinematic magnetic resonance imaging of the normal shoulder: assessment of the labrum and capsule. Can Assoc Radiol J 47:44-50, 1996.

114. Boden B, Hanks G, Chesnick R: Diagnosis of biceps tendon dislocation by kinematic magnetic resonance imaging. Am J Orthop 25:709-711, 1996.

115. Shellock F, Feske W, Frey C: Peroneal tendons: use of kinematic MR imaging of the ankle to determine subluxation. J Magn Reson Imaging 7:451-454, 1997.

116. Beltran J, Chandnani V, McGhee RA, et al: Gadopentetate dimeglumine-enhanced MR imaging of the musculoskeletal system. Am J Roentgenol 156:457-466, 1991.

117. Nakahara N, Uetani M, Hayoshi K, et al: Gadolinium-enhanced MR imaging of the wrist in rheumatoid arthritis: value of fat suppression pulse sequences. Skeletal Radiol 25:639, 1996.

118. Balaban RS, Ceckler TL: Magnetization transfer contrast in magnetic resonance imaging. Magn Reson Quart 8:116-137, 1992.

119. Yao L, Thomasson D: Magnetization transfer contrast in rapid three-dimensional MR imaging using segmented radiofrequency prepulses. Am J Roentgenol 179:863-865, 2002.

120. Mansfield P: Real-time echo-planar imaging by NMR. Br Med Bull 40:187-190, 1984.

121. Karantanas A, Zibis A, Papanikolaou N: Comparison of echo planar imaging, gradient echo and fast spin echo MR scans of knee menisci. Comput Med Imaging Graph 24:309-316, 2000.

122. Mirowitz SA: Normal rotator cuff: MR imaging with conventional and fat-suppression techniques. Radiology 180:735-740, 1991.

123. Bydder GM, Pennock JM, Steiner RE, et al: The short TI inversion recovery sequence—an approach to MR imaging of the abdomen. Magn Reson Imaging 3:251-254, 1985.

124. Krinsky G, Rofsky N, Weinreb J: Nonspecificity of short inversion time inversion recovery (STIR) as a technique of fat suppression: pitfalls in image interpretation. Am J Roentgenol 166:523, 1996.

125. Rubin DA, Harner CD, Costello JM: Treatable chondral injuries of the knee: Frequency of associated focal subchondral edema. Am J Roentgenol 174:1099-1106, 2000.

126. Helms CA: The use of fat suppression in gadolinium-enhanced MR imaging of the musculoskeletal system: A potential source of error. Am J Roentgenol 173:234-236, 1999.

127. Delfaut EM, Beltran J, Johnson G, et al: Fat suppression in MR imaging: Techniques and pitfalls. Radiographics 19:373-382, 1999.
128. Mirowitz S, Shu H: MR imaging evaluation of knee collateral ligament and related injuries: Comparison of T1 weighted, T2 weighted and fat saturation T2 weighted sequences—correlation with clinical findings. J Magn Reson Imaging 4:725, 1994.
129. Singson RD, Feldman F, Staron R, et al: MR imaging of displaced bucket-handle tear of the medial meniscus. Am J Roentgenol 156:121-124, 1991.
130. Broderick L, Turner DA, Renfrew DL, et al: Severity of articular cartilage abnormality in patients with osteoarthritis: evaluation with fast spin-echo MR vs arthroscopy. Am J Roentgenol 162:99-103, 1994.
131. Hodler J, Trudell D, Pathria MN, et al: Width of the articular cartilage of the hip: quantification by using fat-suppression spin-echo MR imaging in cadavers. Am J Roentgenol 159:351-355, 1992.
132. Rose PM, Demlow TA, Szumowski J, et al: Chondromalacia patellae: Fat-suppressed MR imaging. Radiology 193:437-440, 1994.
133. Hauger O, Dumont E, Chateil JF, et al: Water excitation as an alternative to fat saturation in MR imaging: Preliminary results in musculoskeletal imaging. Radiology 224:657-663, 2002.
134. Resnick D: Magnetic resonance imaging: Typical protocols. In Resnick D, Kang H (eds): Internal Derangement of Joints. Philadelphia: WB Saunders, 1997, pp 22-45.
135. Reicher MA, Hartzman S, Duckwiler GR, et al: Meniscal injuries: Detection using MR imaging. Radiology 159:753-757, 1986.
136. Crues JV, Stoller DW: The menisci. In Mink JH, Reicher MA, Crues JV (eds): Magnetic Resonance Imaging of the Knee. New York: Raven Press, 1987, pp 55-92.
137. Wright D, De Smet A, Norris M: Bucket-handle tears of the medial and lateral menisci of the knee: Value of MR imaging in detecting displaced fragments. Am J Roentgenol 165:621-624, 1995.
138. Roychowdhury S, Fitzgerald SW, Sonin AH, et al: Using MR imaging to diagnose partial tears of the anterior cruciate ligament: Value of axial images. Am J Roentgenol 168:1487-1491, 1997.
139. Crues JV, Stoller DW, Ryu RKN: Shoulder. In Stark DD, Bradley WG (eds): Magnetic Resonance Imaging. Mosby: St. Louis, 1999, pp 691-732.
140. Zlatkin M: Shoulder. In Hesselink J, Edelman R, Zlatkin M (eds): Clinical Magnetic Resonance Imaging. Philadelphia: WB Saunders, 1996, pp 1819-1875.
141. Cartland JP, Crues JV 3rd, Stauffer A, et al: MR imaging in the evaluation of SLAP injuries of the shoulder: Findings in 10 patients. Am J Roentgenol 159:787-792, 1992.
142. Tirman PF, Applegate GR, Flannigan BD, et al: MR arthrography of the shoulder. Magn Reson Imaging Clin N Am 1:125-142, 1993.
143. Tirman PF, Stauffer AE, Crues JV 3rd, et al: Saline magnetic resonance arthrography in the evaluation of glenohumeral instability. Arthroscopy 9:550-559, 1993.
144. Tirman PF, Bost FW, Garvin GJ, et al: Posterosuperior glenoid impingement of the shoulder: Findings at MR imaging and MR arthrography with arthroscopic correlation. Radiology 193:431-436, 1994.
145. Potter H, Asnis-Emberg L, Weiland AJ, et al: The utility of high-resolution magnetic resonance imaging in the evaluation of the triangular fibrocartilage complex of the wrist. J Bone Joint Surg Am 79:1675-1684, 1997.
146. Zlatkin M, Ouellette E, Needell S: High resolution MRI and MR arthrography of wrist ligament anatomy. Proceedings of the ISMRM. Fourth Scientific Meeting, 1996. 1: p 213.
147. Erickson S: High-resolution imaging of the musculoskeletal system. Radiology 205:593, 1997.
148. Palmer W: MR arthrography: is it worthwhile? Top Magn Reson Imaging 8:24-43, 1996.
149. Schulte-Altedorneburg G, Gebhard M, Wohlgemuth WA, et al: MR arthrography: Pharmacology, efficacy and safety in clinical trials. Skeletal Radiol 32:1-12, 2003.
150. Zlatkin M, Chambers T, Uribe J, et al: MRI arthrography of meniscal repairs. Florida Orthopedic Society meeting, 1997.
151. Palmer W: MR arthrography of the rotator cuff and labral-ligamentous complex. Semin Ultrasound CT MR 18:278, 1997.

152. Tirman PF, Bost FW, Steinbach LS, et al: MR arthrographic depiction of tears of the rotator cuff: Benefit of abduction and external rotation of the arm. Radiology 192:851-856, 1994.
153. Cvitanic O, Tirman PF, Feller JF, et al: Using abduction and external rotation of the shoulder to increase the sensitivity of MR arthrography in revealing tears of the anterior glenoid labrum. Am J Roentgenol 169:837, 1997.
154. Bergin D, Schweitzer ME: Indirect magnetic resonance arthrography. Skeletal Radiol 32:551-558, 2003.
155. Magee T, Shapiro M, Rodriguez J, et al: MR arthrography of postoperative knee: For which patients is it useful? Radiology 229:159-163, 2003.
156. Crues JV, Ryu R, Morgan FW: Meniscal pathology: The expanding role of magnetic resonance imaging. Clin Orthop 252:80-87, 1990.
157. Brossmann J, Preidler KW, Daenen B, et al: Imaging of osseous and cartilaginous intraarticular bodies in the knee: Comparison of MR imaging and MR arthrography with CT and CT arthrography in cadavers. Radiology 200:509-517, 1996.
158. Kovanlikaya I, Camli D: Diagnostic value of MR arthrography in detection of intrinsic carpal ligament lesions: use of cine-MR arthrography as a new approach. Eur Radiol 7:1441-1445, 1997.
159. Scheck R, Kubitzek C, Hiemer R, et al: The scapholunate interosseous ligament in MR arthrography of the wrist: correlation with non-enhanced MRI and wrist arthroscopy. Skeletal Radiol 26:263-271, 1997.
160. Zanetti M, Bram J, Hodler J: Triangular fibrocartilage and intercarpal ligaments of the wrist: Does MR arthrography improve standard MRI? J Magn Reson Imaging 7:590-594, 1997.
161. Zlatkin M: The wrist. In Hesselink J, Edelman R, Zlatkin M (eds): Clinical Magnetic Resonance Imaging. Philadelphia: WB Saunders, 1996.
162. Schwartz M, al-Zahrani S, Morwessel RM, et al: Ulnar collateral ligament injury in the throwing athlete: evaluation with saline-enhanced MR arthrography. Radiology 197:297, 1995.
163. Cotten A, Jacobson J, Brossmann J, et al: Collateral ligaments of the elbow: conventional MR imaging and MR arthrography with coronal oblique plane and elbow flexion. Radiology 204:806, 1997.
164. Cerezal L, Abascal F, Canga A, et al: MR imaging of ankle impingement syndromes. Am J Roentgenol 181:551-559, 2003.
165. Czerny C, Hoffman S, Neuhold A, et al: Lesions of the acetabular labrum: accuracy of MR imaging and MR arthrography in detection and staging. Radiology 200:225, 1996.
166. Hodler J, Yu JS, Goodwin D, et al: MR arthrography of the hip: improved imaging of the acetabular labrum with histologic correlation in cadavers. Am J Roentgenol 165:887, 1995.
167. Petersilge CA: Current concepts of MR arthrography of the hip. Semin Ultrasound CT MR 8:291, 1997.
168. DeMouy E, Menedez CJ, Bodin C: Palpation directed saline enhanced MR arthrography of the shoulder. Am J Roentgenol 169:229, 1997.
169. Valls R, Melloni P: Sonographic guidance of needle position for MR arthrography of joints. Am J Roentgenol 169:845-847, 1997.
170. Beaulieu C, Ladd A: MR arthrography of the wrist: scanning-room injection of the radiocarpal joint based on clinical landmarks. Am J Roentgenol 170:606-608, 1998.
171. Hajek P, Sartoris DJ, Gylys-Morin V, et al: The effect of intrarticular gadolinium-DTPA on synovial membrane and cartilage. Invest Radiol 25:179, 1990.
172. Vahlensieck M, et al: Indirect MR arthrography: techniques and applications. Semin Ultrasound CT MR 18:302-306, 1997.
173. Vahlensieck M, Peterfy CG, Wischer T, et al: Indirect MR arthrography: Optimization and clinical applications. Radiology 200:249-254, 1996.
174. Weishaupt D, Schweitzer ME, Rawool NM, et al: Indirect MR arthrography of the knee: effects of low-intensity ultrasound on the diffusion rate of intravenously administered Gd-DTPA in healthy volunteers. Invest Radiol 36:493-499, 2001.
175. Schweitzer ME, Natale P, Winalski CS, et al: Indirect wrist MT arthrography: The effects of passive motion versus active exercise. Skeletal Radiol 29:10-14, 2000.
176. Allmann K, Schafer O, Hauer M, et al: Indirect MR arthrography of the unexercised glenohumeral joint in patients with rotator cuff tears. Invest Radiol 34:435-440, 1999.

CHAPTER 97

MR Arthrography

Oliver A. Cvitanic

DEFINITIONS

"Direct" magnetic resonance (MR) arthrography is defined as MR imaging following the injection of either dilute gadolinium or saline directly into a joint space and is implied throughout this chapter unless otherwise stated. "Indirect" MR arthrography is defined as MR imaging following passive diffusion of intravenously injected gadolinium into the joint and is discussed in the final section of this chapter.

INTRODUCTION

In MR arthrography, dilute solutions of gadolinium are generally preferred over saline as contrast media for the slightly superior anatomic detail revealed on T1-weighted imaging compared to T2-weighted imaging, as well as the added ability to determine if any extra-articular fluid collection communicates with the joint. For maximum effectiveness, gadolinium MR arthrography relies upon the combination of four imaging techniques: joint distension, short echo times (TE), dilute solutions of gadolinium, and fat suppression (Fig. 97-1). Distension of the joint is advantageous for separating capsular and ligamentous structures and opening physiologically closed tears. Short echo times (TE) raise the sensitivity for tears by increasing the signal-to-noise ratio, and the use of fat suppression further increases tear conspicuity

by narrowing the window. The choice of a dilute solution of gadolinium to distend the joint provides an arthrographic effect that is compatible with the use of a short TE and may even modestly facilitate tear penetration since gadolinium has a lower viscosity than joint fluid. T2-weighted imaging is routinely added to MR arthrography protocols to highlight fluid-containing extra-articular structures. Table 97-1 illustrates one simple method of weighing the clinical and imaging considerations involved in deciding whether an MR arthrogram is indicated.

PREPARATION OF THE DILUTE SOLUTION OF GADOLINIUM FOR INJECTION

The greatest T1 shortening of joint fluid is achieved using gadolinium at a concentration of 2 mmol/L or 1:250, which approximates the concentration of gadolinium in the blood following IV administration.[1] However, any concentration between 0.5 and 2.5 mmol/L is effective for use in any joint in the body.[2,3] A 2 mmol/L concentration can be obtained by injecting 0.4 mL of gadolinium dimeglumine (Magnevist: Berlex Laboratories, Wynne, NJ) in a concentration of 467.01 mg/mL (from the vial without dilution) into a 100 mL bag of normal saline. Alternatively, 1 mL can be injected into a 250 mL bag of

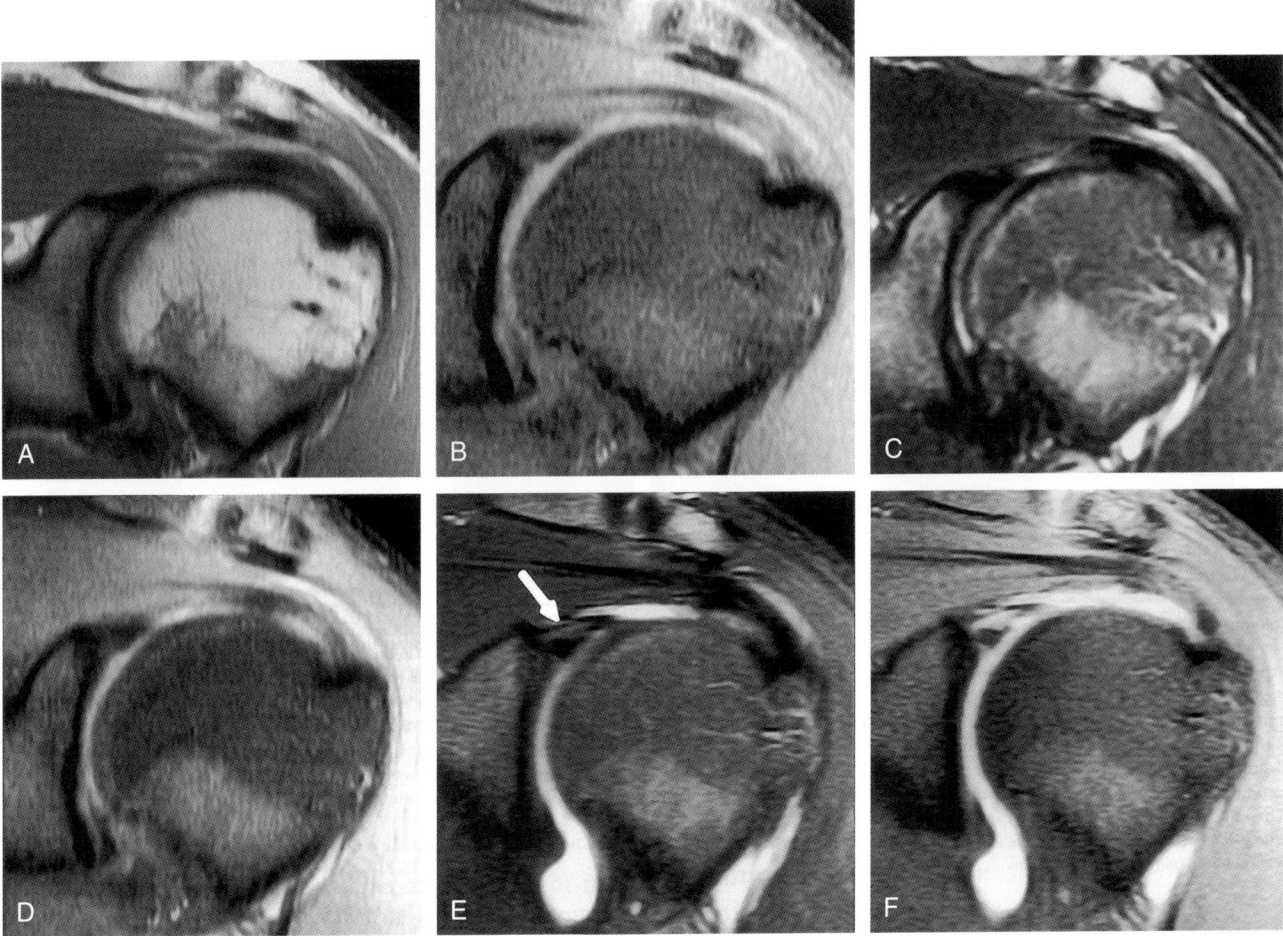

FIGURE 97-1

Relative value of joint distension, fat suppression, dilute gadolinium solutions, and echo times (TE) in the ability of MR arthrography to reveal a surgically confirmed detached superior labral tear (SLAP IV) at the 12 o'clock position. **A** to **D,** Proton density–weighted (**A**), fat-suppressed T1 (**B**), fat-suppressed T2 (**C**), and fat-suppressed proton density–weighted (**D**) coronal MR images obtained through the superior labrum at 12 o'clock prior to the intra-articular administration of contrast material. Neither the use of a short TE, fat suppression, nor the combination of the two was effective in revealing the labral tear. **E,** Fat-suppressed T2-weighted sagittal MR arthrogram in the same patient as **A** through **D** following distension of the joint with dilute gadolinium reveals intermediate signal intensity within the labrum *(arrow),* suggestive of a tear. Joint distension has improved the sensitivity for tear (compare with **C** above). **F,** Fat-suppressed T1-weighted coronal MR arthrogram in the same patient as **A** through **D** following joint distension with dilute gadolinium reveals hyperintense contrast material penetrating deeply into the superior labrum. This image shows the advantage of combining joint distension, fat suppression, a short TE, and dilute solutions of gadolinium in maximizing sensitivity for labral tears.

normal saline, or, for a single patient, 0.1 mL into a 20 mL bottle of saline. The small amount of gadolinium needed for preparing the solution is usually borrowed from the vial of a patient undergoing intravenous injection of gadolinium instead of opening a new vial.[4] If a conventional arthrogram is desired in conjunction with the MR arthrogram, iodinated contrast material can be safely added to the injecting syringe.[5] In this case, the desired mixture is obtained by drawing up the dilute gadolinium solution into a 20 mL syringe which has been prefilled with 10 mL of iodinated contrast material. If a short-acting local anesthetic is also desired, the syringe is prefilled with a combination of 5 mL of 1% lidocaine and 5 mL of iodinated contrast material.

Saline MR arthrograms are most often relegated to low-field-strength MR scanners since spectral fat suppression is not available and the relaxivity of gadolinium starts to decline below 0.4 T.[6,7] If a saline arthrogram is desired, simply substitute normal saline for the dilute gadolinium solution.

Since both dilute gadolinium and saline solutions are gradually absorbed through the synovial lining of the joint, MR imaging should ideally be initiated within one hour of the injection so that scanning can be performed while the joint remains distended. Some investigators have advocated adding 0.3 mL of 1:1000 epinephrine into the 20 mL syringe containing the dilute gadolinium mix to slow absorption of the injected solution, but the

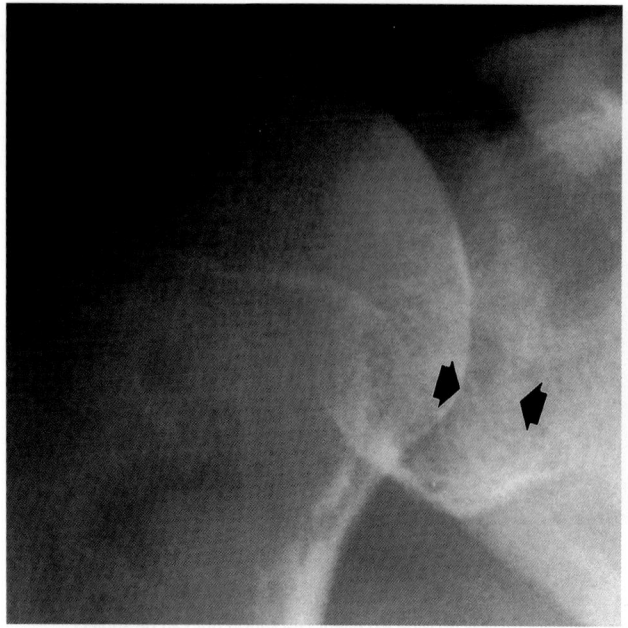

FIGURE 97-3

An AP radiograph with standard supine shoulder positioning shows an oblique glenohumeral joint with limited accessibility using the standard anterior approach which targets the inferior third of the joint (arrows).

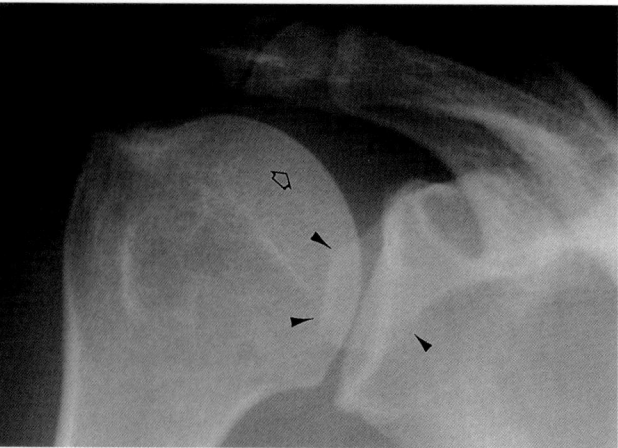

FIGURE 97-4

An AP radiograph reveals a long coracoid process (arrowheads) which partially obstructs access to the glenohumeral joint using the standard anterior approach. Targeting the rotator interval (open arrow) avoids the coracoid process.

placing the anterior labrum in the path of the needle.[10] In our experience, however, slow advancement of the needle along the medial margin of the humeral head with frequent test injections of lidocaine to indicate capsular penetration avoids labral injury.

Another modification of anterior approach shoulder arthrography which can overcome an oblique glenohumeral joint is to target the rotator interval instead of the inferior third of the glenohumeral joint.[11] In this technique, which is also performed with the patient supine, the needle is aimed at the superomedial aspect of the humeral head and advanced until bone is encountered. Once bone is struck, the needle may need to be withdrawn between 1 and 3 mm and twisted slightly while gently depressing the plunger of the lidocaine syringe to confirm that the tip is intra-articular. Since mild resistance to injection is common in this technique even with appropriate placement, needle position should be reconfirmed with iodinated contrast material prior to injecting the gadolinium solution to make sure the tip is not embedded in a cuff muscle.

Another common anatomic variant that can frustrate anterior access to the glenohumeral joint using the standard anterior approach is the long coracoid process (Fig. 97-4). Although easily recognized on conventional radiographs, long coracoid processes can occasionally be missed on fluoroscopy, particularly when the study is performed using a C-arm. Since the Grashey position tends to shift the coracoid process to the front of the glenohumeral joint, it is not recommended in patients

with long coracoid processes (Fig. 97-5). Joint access in the presence of a long coracoid process is easily achieved by directing the needle above or below the coracoid using either the standard anterior or the rotator interval targeting approaches.

Another potential source of frustration in attempting to access the joint using the standard anterior approach is the presence of degenerative joint disease. This common condition, which is associated with thinning of the articular cartilage, osteophyte formation, and adhesive capsulitis, can severely impede access. Both the Grashey and the rotator interval targeting approaches are effective in patients with degenerative joint disease.

There are several advantages to using the rotator interval targeting technique: avoidance of the anterior glenoid labrum, simplification of patient positioning, reduction in the necessary depth of needle penetration, near-total elimination of muscle spasm, and decreased skin exposure. Overall, the rotator interval targeting approach is regarded as safe, rapid, and better tolerated than any other approach[11]; however, the technique is not without risk. The tendency to rely on single-look fluoroscopy, a common way of saving time in the rotator interval targeting technique, does increase the chances of inadvertently infiltrating the subscapularis and supraspinatus muscles or of impaling the long biceps tendon, the coracohumeral ligament, or superior glenohumeral ligament. Local infiltrations of muscle with dilute contrast material are not associated with any adverse clinical consequences but can mimic undersurface cuff tears on MR arthrography. The incidence and significance of perforations involving the long biceps tendon or a ligament are less well known since such injuries can be difficult to identify on MR arthrography and may initially be asymptomatic (Fig. 97-6).

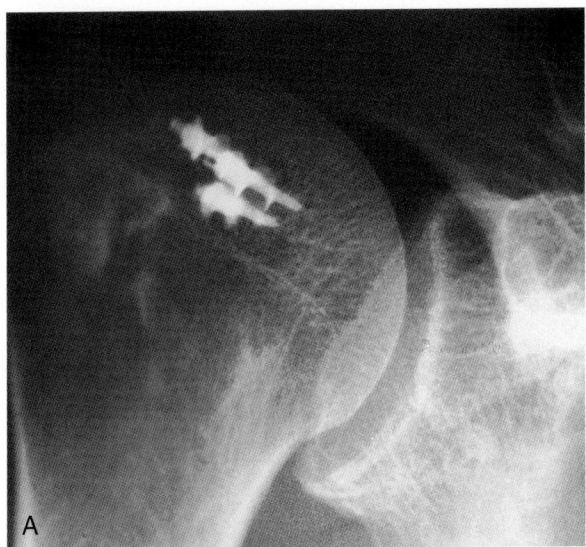

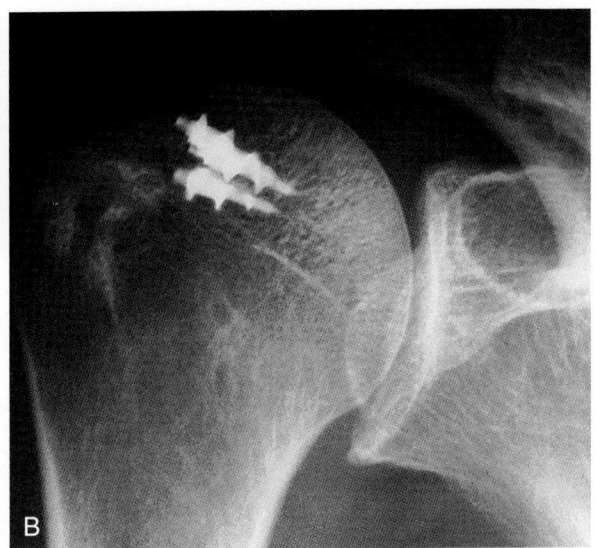

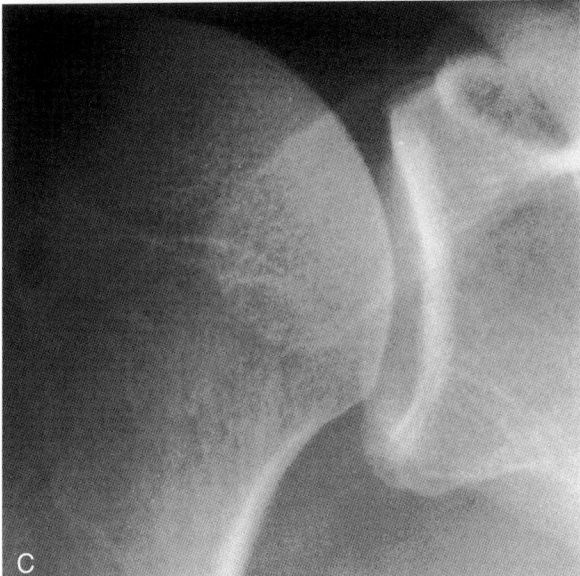

FIGURE 97-5

Effect of shoulder position on anterior joint access. **A,** AP radiograph with standard supine positioning reveals an oblique glenohumeral joint, which limits access in a standard anterior approach. **B,** AP radiograph with Grashey positioning in the same patient as **A** shows the glenohumeral joint now in profile but the standard anterior approach has become almost completely obstructed by the coracoid process. **C,** AP radiograph with Grashey positioning in a different patient than **A** and **B** reveals a long coracoid process that partially covers the target zone for rotator interval targeting approach.

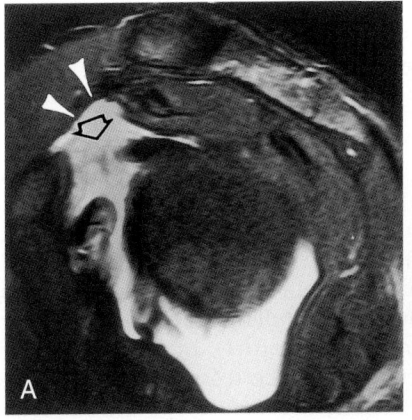

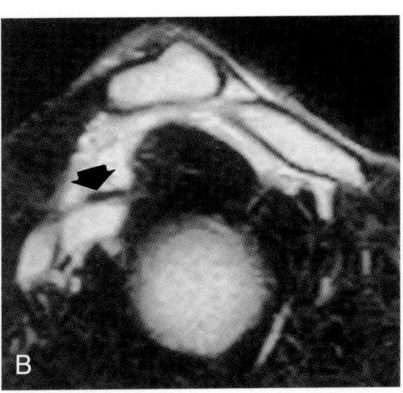

FIGURE 97-6

Acute coracohumeral ligament disruption. **A,** Fat-suppressed T1-weighted sagittal MR arthrogram obtained following multiple blind adjustments of needle position during the rotator interval targeting technique reveals the wispy remains of the torn coracohumeral ligament *(open arrow)* in the presence of an intact capsule *(arrowheads)*. **B,** Conventional T2-weighted sagittal MR image in the same patient as **A** 9 months earlier reveals an intact coracohumeral ligament *(arrow)*.

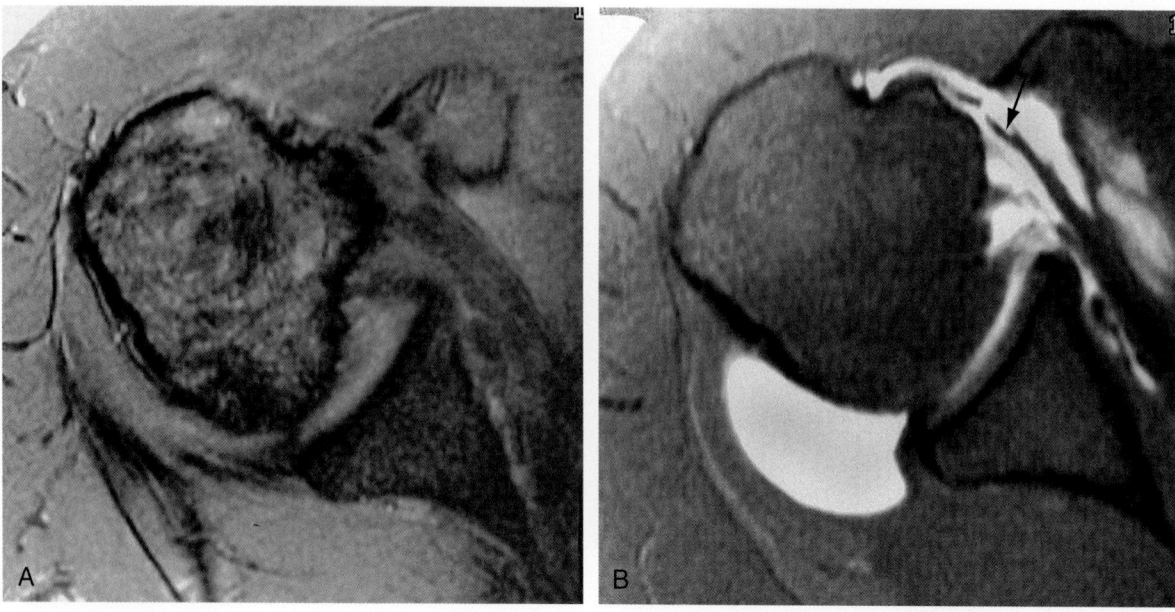

FIGURE 97-7

Superior sensitivity of MR arthrography in the diagnosis of subscapularis tendon tears. **A,** T2* axial MR image reveals a normal-appearing subscapularis tendon. **B,** Fat-suppressed T1-weighted axial MR arthrogram in the same patient as **A** reveals complete avulsion of the subscapularis tendon *(arrow)* from the lesser tuberosity of the humerus.

Recent work has proposed using a posterior approach to shoulder arthrography when the anterior labrum is a focal point for the evaluation in order to eliminate the possibility of damaging that structure with the needle while entering the joint.[12] However, for the reasons described above, the rotator interval targeting approach is currently favored for all patients. The recommended volume of injection in shoulder arthrography is between 6 and 15 mL.[8]

Applications

Full-Thickness Tears of the Rotator Cuff

Perhaps the most obvious finding on conventional MRI in full-thickness rotator cuff tears is an accumulation of fluid in the subacromial-subdeltoid bursa. However, fluid alone cannot be used to diagnose a full-thickness tear since subacromial bursitis may accompany partial-thickness bursal surface tears or occur in isolation. The lack of specificity regarding subacromial fluid accumulations is also a key drawback of saline MR arthrography. Conversely, the appearance of contrast material in the subacromial-subdeltoid bursa on an MR arthrogram is considered a reliable sign of a full-thickness tear provided the test injection of iodinated contrast material has confirmed intra-articular needle placement. Failure to find a tear on coronal images despite the presence of contrast material in the subacromial-subdeltoid bursa should prompt close scrutiny of the sagittal images for a vertical cuff tear. Vertical or "longitudinal" cuff tears are difficult to diagnose on coronal images because they are

not associated with tendon retraction. This type of tear most commonly occurs at the junction between the supraspinatus and infraspinatus tendons. Regarding the subscapularis tendon, MR arthrography has also proved superior to conventional MRI in the depiction and characterization of full-thickness tears even though such tears do not always result in communication with the subacromial-subdeltoid bursa (Fig. 97-7).[13] Accumulations of contrast material in the subcoracoid bursa also correlate with full-thickness tears of the rotator cuff.[14] Overall, the addition of intra-articular contrast material prior to MRI improves the sensitivity for full-thickness rotator cuff tears from 77% to 99%.[15] As focal full-thickness tears enlarge and the tendon begins to retract, there is a corresponding decline in the advantage of MR arthrography over conventional MRI in their diagnosis.

Partial-Thickness Articular Surface Injuries of the Rotator Cuff

Conventional MRI is less effective in diagnosing partial-thickness articular surface tears than full-thickness tears. The difficulties are manifold: the potential for small tears to be effaced by the humeral head with the arm in adduction; the potential for partial tears to be mistaken for tendinosis; and the potential for high-grade partial tears occurring in conjunction with subacromial bursitis to be mistaken for small full-thickness tears. Intra-articular contrast material improves the sensitivity for partial-thickness articular surface tears by mildly elevating the cuff and penetrating defects in the articular surface (Fig. 97-8).[16] Abduction external rotation (ABER) positioning is a useful supplement to conventional

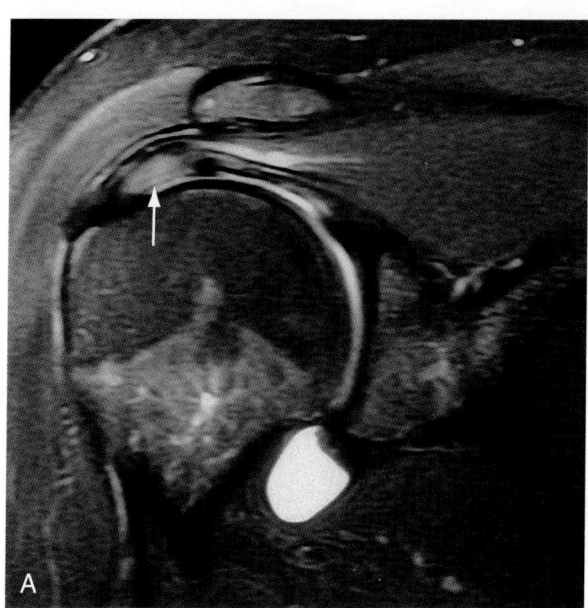
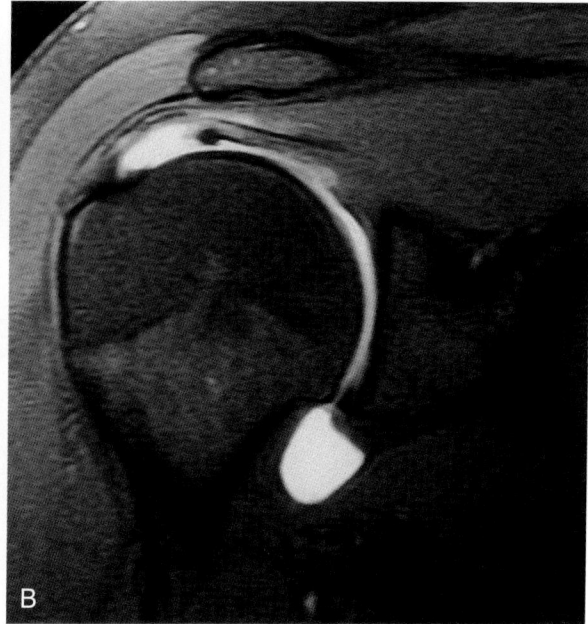

FIGURE 97-8

Superior specificity of MR arthrography obtained with fat-suppressed T1 weighting in diagnosing partial-thickness articular surface tears of the rotator cuff in the shoulder. **A,** Fat-suppressed proton density–weighted coronal MR image obtained following joint distension reveals an area of intermediate signal intensity involving the substance and undersurface of the anterior aspect of the infraspinatus tendon *(arrow)*. **B,** Fat-suppressed T1-weighted MR arthrogram in the same shoulder as **A** reveals contrast material outlining a 1.3 cm defect with 60% tendon penetration in the same area shown in **A**.

positioning in MR arthrography since this position introduces laxity into the infraspinatus tendon which allows laminar and flap tears to better fill with contrast material (Fig. 97-9).[17,18] In general, the smaller the tendon tear, the greater the diagnostic advantage of MR arthrography compared to conventional MRI.

Articular Surface–Sparing Injuries of the Rotator Cuff

Tendinosis, interstitial tears, post-traumatic inflammation, and partial-thickness bursal surface tears of the rotator cuff can have similar appearances on MR arthrography since none involves a defect in the articular surface of the tendon. MR arthrography remains useful in confirming the absence of articular surface defects, but diagnosis of these various conditions depends on subtle differences in the appearance of the tendon on T2-weighted pulse sequences. Fat suppression is routinely added to counter the fat-brightening effect of fast spin-echo techniques.[19]

Injuries of the Rotator Interval including the Reflection Pulley

The rotator interval refers to the capsule-covered gap between the supraspinatus and subscapularis tendons which is traversed and thickened by the coracohumeral ligament.[20] Tears of the rotator interval are important to recognize on MR arthrography because they can allow communication between the glenohumeral joint and the subacromial-subdeltoid bursa in the absence of a cuff tear. Rotator interval tears are more readily diagnosed with MR arthrography than with conventional MRI (Fig. 97-10).[21]

The "reflection pulley" is considered to be a part of the rotator interval.[22-24] Anatomically, the reflection pulley refers to the sling formed by the common attachment of the coracohumeral and superior glenohumeral ligaments to the lesser tuberosity of the humerus through which the long biceps tendon passes immediately prior to its descent into the intertubercular groove. Reflection pulley injuries occur when tension in the long biceps tendon from a sudden deceleration is transmitted to these ligaments.[21] This tension can avulse the coracohumeral and superior glenohumeral ligaments from the lesser tuberosity as well as from their secondary attachments to the superior margin of the subscapularis and the anterior margin of the supraspinatus tendons (Fig. 97-11). Such avulsions can tear these tendons, particularly the superior fibers of the subscapularis tendon, and can also lead to medial subluxation of the biceps tendon. The reflection pulley mechanism of injury may help explain the known association between injuries of the biceps tendon and those of the anterior superior portion of the rotator cuff.[25] Reflection pulley injuries have been described as "the hidden lesions of the rotator cuff" because the ligament disruptions are not visible arthroscopically (but only on open surgery), and the clinical findings are nonspecific.

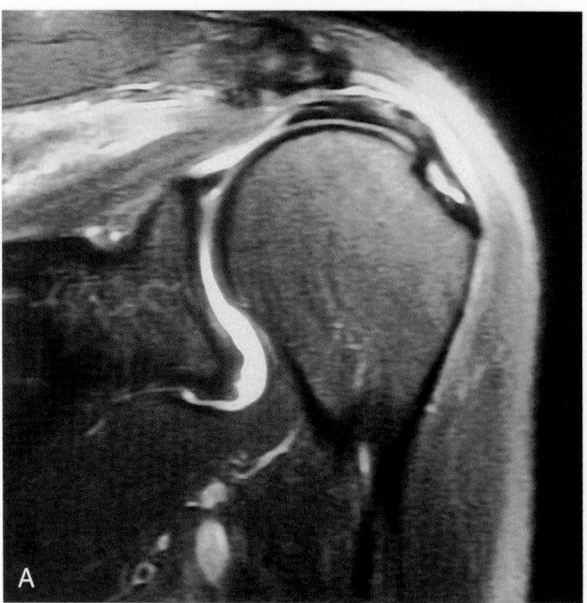
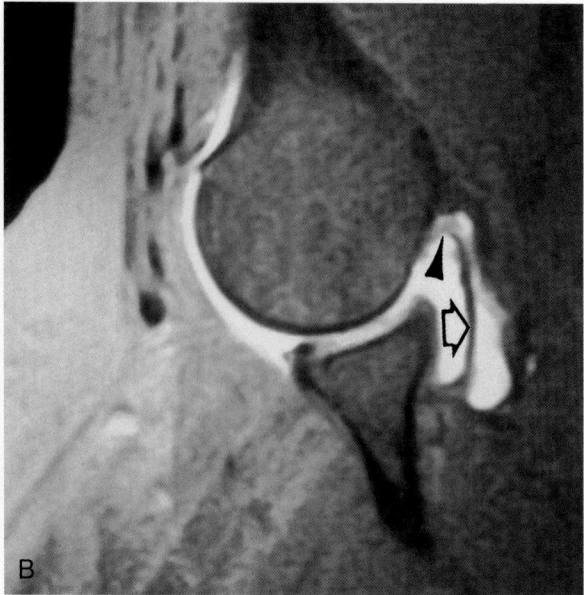

FIGURE 97-9

Superior specificity of abduction and external rotation (ABER) positioning in assessing the infraspinatus tendon using MR arthrography. **A,** Fat-suppressed proton density–weighted coronal MR image obtained following distension of the joint with dilute gadolinium reveals a circumscribed area of high signal intensity within the substance of the anterior aspect of the infraspinatus tendon. **B,** Fat-suppressed T1-weighted ABER MR arthrogram of the same shoulder as **A** reveals contrast material entering a plane of dissection deep to the articular surface *(open arrow)* of the infraspinatus tendon through a small perforation *(arrowhead)*.

Acromioclavicular Joint Cysts

Superior migration of the humeral head in relation to the bony glenoid often accompanies endstage rotator cuff disease. Such migration can result in undersurface impingement of the acromioclavicular joint leading to possible perforation of the inferior capsular ligament of the joint and secondary communication between the glenohumeral and acromioclavicular joints. The appearance of contrast material extravasating superiorly into the acromioclavicular joint on a conventional shoulder arthrogram has been referred to as a "geyser sign,"[26] and can also be seen on MR arthrography (Fig. 97-12). In certain patients and for reasons not fully understood, communication between the glenohumeral and acromioclavicular joints can eventually lead to the development of an acromioclavicular joint cyst.[27] The propensity of these cysts to recur following aspiration and local resection makes their accurate diagnosis a priority. Conventional MRI is adequate to make the diagnosis.

Surgical Treatment and Reporting of Rotator Cuff Tears

Due to the evolving nature of treatment recommendations, it is important to provide detailed descriptions of rotator cuff tears. At the time of this writing, arthroscopic repair is considered feasible for partial tears of the supraspinatus and infraspinatus tendons involving up to 67% of tendon thickness, while those involving greater than 67% of tendon thickness require open surgery.[28] Regarding focal full-thickness tears, arthroscopic repair is

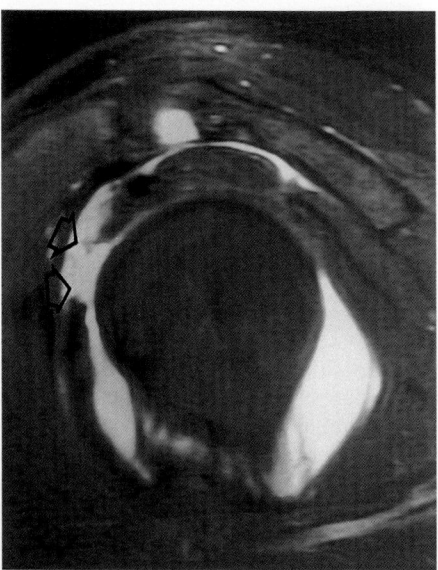

FIGURE 97-10

Rotator interval tear. Fat-suppressed T1-weighted sagittal MR arthrogram reveals discontinuity of the joint capsule in the rotator interval *(open arrows)*.

possible for those up to 1.0 cm in diameter while those over 1.0 cm require open surgery. Such precise surgical criteria demand the most accurate preoperative assessment possible and argue in favor of using MR arthrography. Findings which should be reported routinely on

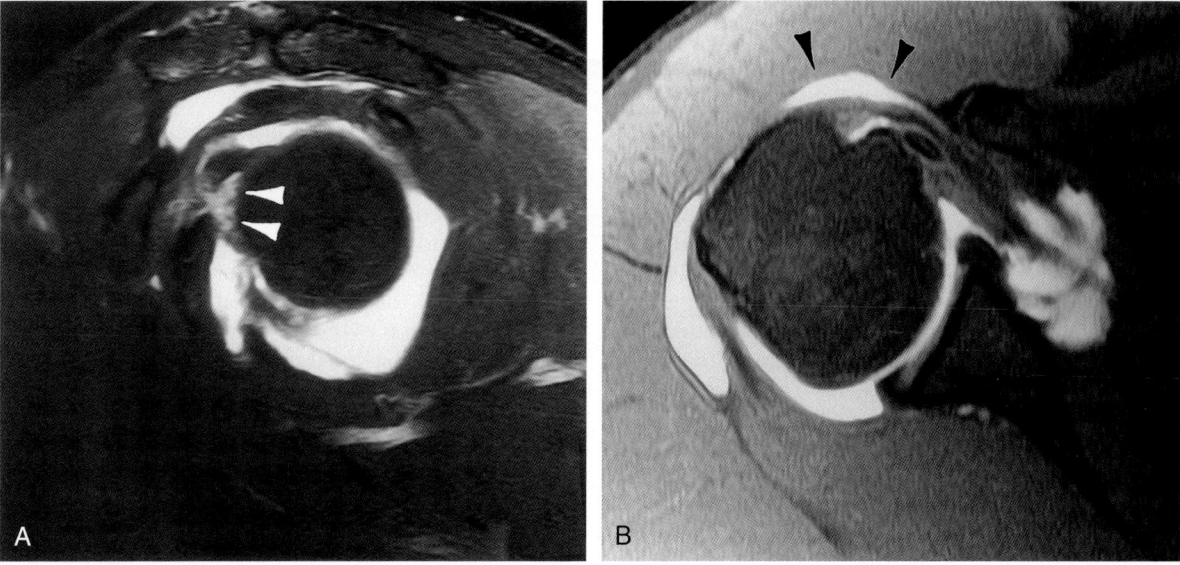

FIGURE 97-11

Reflection pulley injury. **A,** Fat-suppressed T1-weighted sagittal MR arthrogram reveals contrast material undermining the humeral insertion of the superior glenohumeral ligament *(arrowheads)*. **B,** Fat-suppressed T1-weighted axial MR arthrogram reveals medial subluxation of the long biceps tendon. The presence of contrast material superficial to the biceps and subscapularis tendons *(arrowheads)* has been referred to as the "pulley sign."

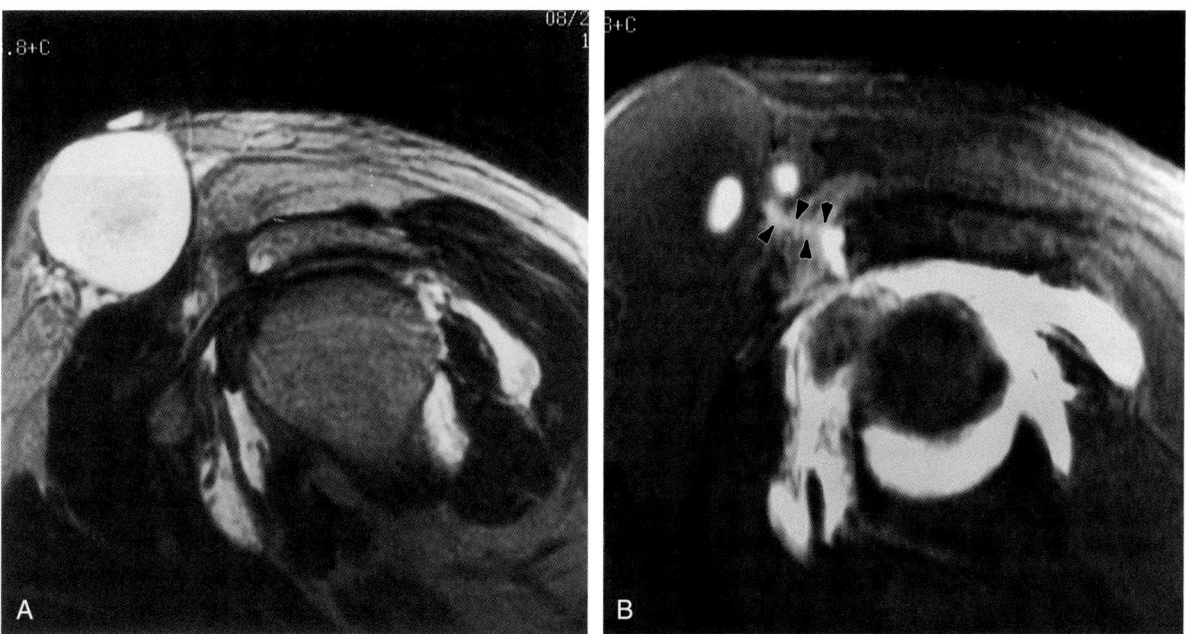

FIGURE 97-12

Acromioclavicular joint cyst on MR arthrography. **A,** T2-weighted sagittal MR image reveals a 3.0 cm subcutaneous cyst in the anterior superior shoulder. **B,** Fat-suppressed T1-weighted sagittal MR arthrogram in the same shoulder as **A** reveals a slender but uninterrupted column of contrast material *(arrowheads)* between the glenohumeral joint, acromioclavicular joint, and cyst.

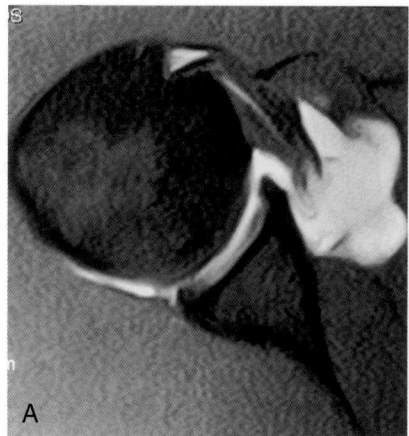

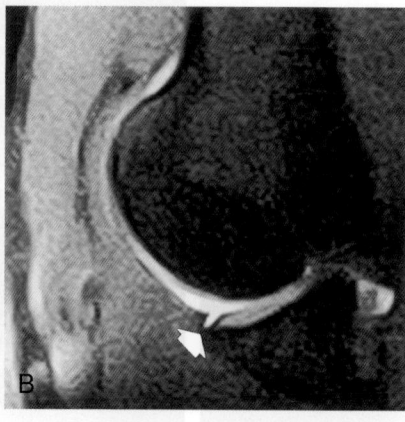

FIGURE 97-17

Superior sensitivity of ABER arm positioning compared to conventional arm positioning (adduction) in detecting tears of the anterior glenoid labrum using MR arthrography. **A,** Fat-suppressed T1-weighted axial MR arthrogram with the arm in adduction fails to reveal a tear of the anterior glenoid labrum. **B,** Fat-suppressed T1-weighted ABER MR arthrogram in the same patient as **A** reveals contrast material in a cleft which opened up at the base of the labrum (*arrow*). A partially detached tear involving the anterior inferior labrum was found at surgery.

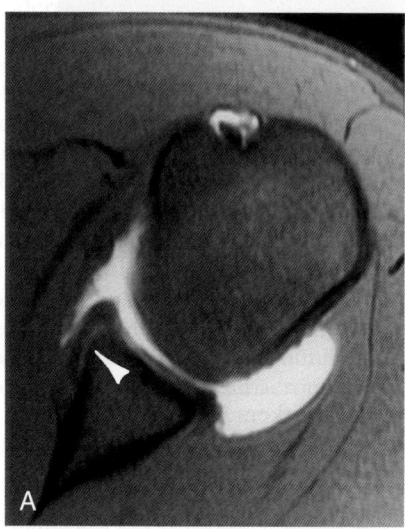

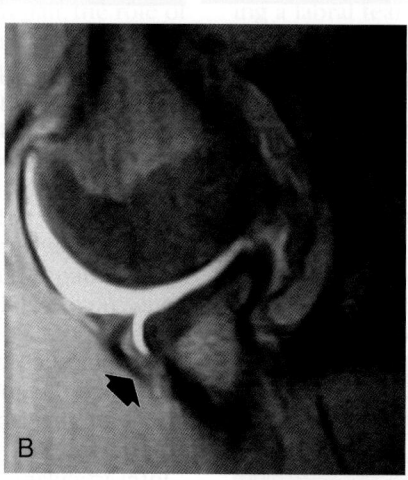

FIGURE 97-18

Superior specificity of ABER positioning compared to conventional arm positioning (adduction) in the diagnosis of a Perthes lesion (Bankart variant) using MR arthrography. **A,** Fat-suppressed T1-weighted axial MR arthrogram with the arm in adduction hints at the presence of contrast material (*arrowhead*) between the bony glenoid and the anterior labrum. **B,** Fat-suppressed T1-weighted ABER MR arthrogram in the same patient as **A** reveals contrast material displacing the torn anterior glenoid labrum which has remained tethered to the glenoid by the intact anterior scapular periosteum (*arrow*).

The greatest challenge in diagnosing SLAP lesions with MRI stems from overlap between the appearance of normal sublabral recesses and the most common form of SLAP lesion: type II (Figs. 97-19 and 97-20).[43] The identification of a paralabral cyst facilitates the diagnosis of a superior labral tear on MRI.[44] These cysts are thought to occur when synovial fluid is expressed slowly through a tear in the labrum and distends the overlying capsule. Paralabral cysts often expand into the spinoglenoid notch and can occasionally impinge upon a branch of the suprascapular nerve causing denervation atrophy of the infraspinatus muscle. The gelatinous consistency of the fluid in paralabral cysts discourages filling on MR arthrography (Fig. 97-21). Tears in the superior glenoid labrum are diagnosed with up to 94% accuracy using MR arthrography.[45,46]

Tears of the Posterior Glenoid Labrum

Posterior labral tears are nearly as common as anterior labral tears but less prone to cause clinically significant instability and more difficult to visualize arthroscopically. Posterior labral tears resemble superior labral tears in their association with paralabral cysts. Additional findings that can be seen in association with posterior labral tears include posterior scapulohumeral imbalance, diagnosed when there is posterior displacement of the humeral head in relation to the main axis of the scapula on an axial image, and erosion of the articular cartilage in the posterior aspect of the glenoid fossa.[47] Displaced tears of the posterior labrum which remain attached to the scapular periosteum have been termed posterior labrum periosteal sleeve avulsion (POLPSA) lesions (Fig. 97-22).[48] The accuracy of MR arthrography in diagnosing posterior labral tears is approximately 90%.[8,33,47]

Biceps Tendinopathy

The long biceps tendon is a dynamic stabilizer of the shoulder that most often tears in concert with massive rotator cuff disruptions in elderly individuals but can also tear in young adults engaged in heavy lifting. Ruptures of the proximal tendon usually occur within 2.0 cm of its origin on the supraglenoid tubercle (Fig. 97-23).

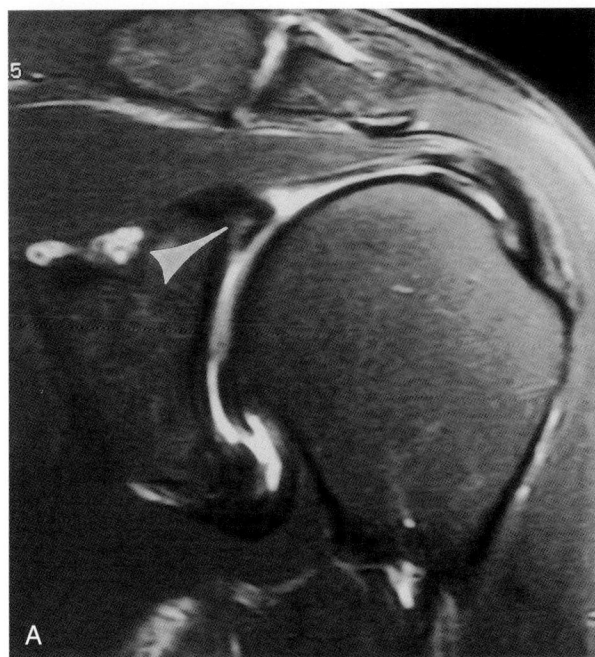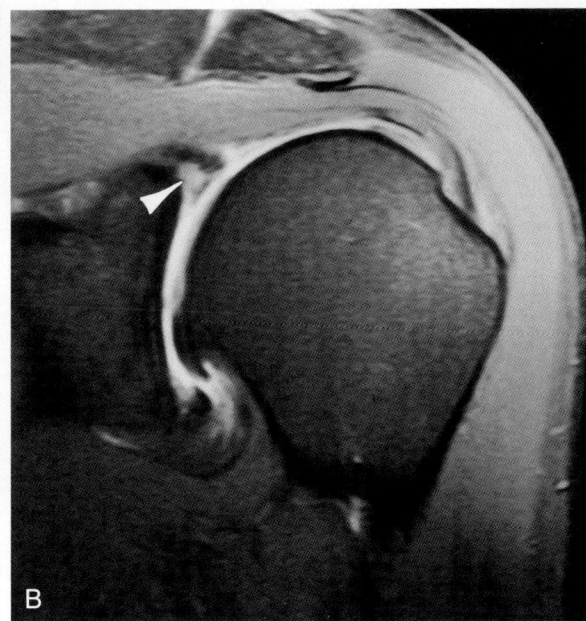

FIGURE 97-19

Superior specificity of fat suppression and T1 weighting over fat suppression and proton density weighting for diagnosing superior labrum anterior posterior (SLAP) lesions in MR arthrography. **A,** Fat-suppressed proton density–weighted coronal MR image following joint distension reveals mildly increased signal intensity at the base of the superior labrum *(arrowhead)*. **B,** Fat-suppressed T1-weighted coronal MR arthrogram in the same patient as **A** reveals contrast material penetrating superolaterally into the labrum *(arrowhead)*. This appearance indicates labral detachment and is classified as a type II SLAP lesion.

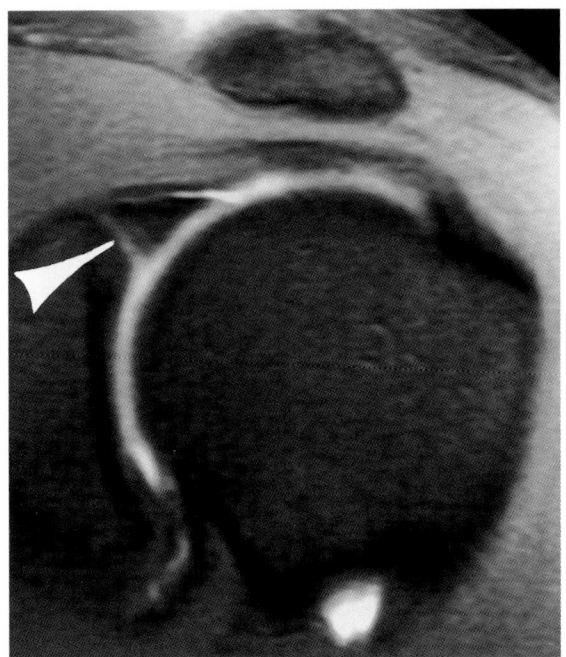

FIGURE 97-20

"Pseudo" SLAP lesion. Fat-suppressed T1-weighted coronal MR arthrogram reveals a slender contrast material–filled cleft *(arrowhead)* extending superomedially along the margin of the bone. The presence of a normal sublabral recess was confirmed at arthroscopy.

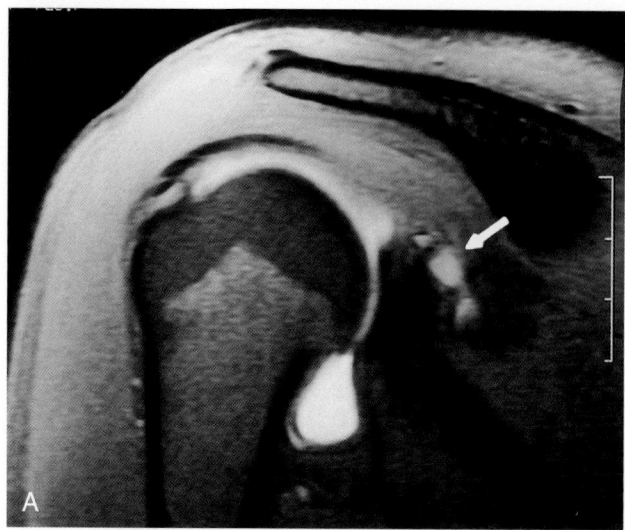

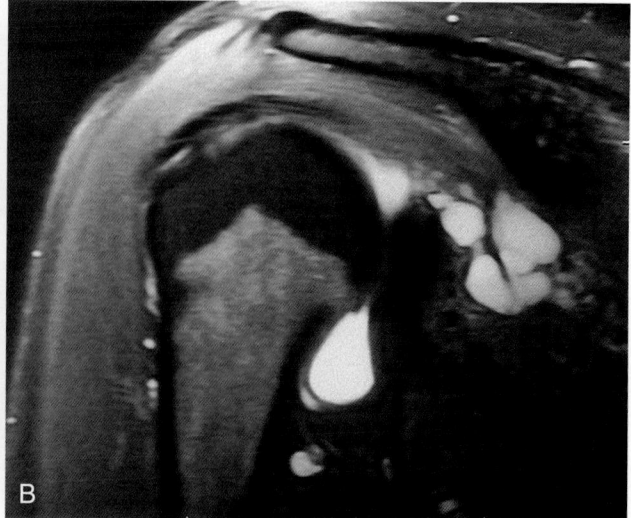

FIGURE 97-21

Superior sensitivity of fat-suppressed proton density–weighted MRI following joint distension over a fat-suppressed T1-weighted MR arthrography in the diagnosis of paralabral cysts in the shoulder. **A,** Fat-suppressed T1-weighted coronal MR arthrogram reveals a small amount of contrast material *(arrow)* entering a cyst in the suprascapular notch. **B,** Fat-suppressed proton density–weighted coronal MR image in the same shoulder as **A** (following joint distension) confirms a 2.5 cm multilocular cyst. Paralabral cysts are associated with tears in the adjacent labrum.

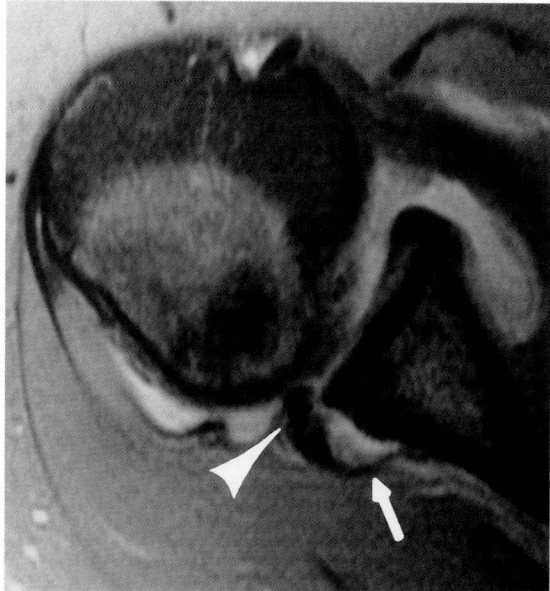

FIGURE 97-22

The posterior labrum periosteal sleeve avulsion (POLPSA) lesion. Fat-suppressed T1-weighted coronal MR arthrogram reveals the torn and displaced posterior glenoid labrum *(large arrowhead)*, which remains attached to the intact posterior scapular periosteum *(arrow)*.

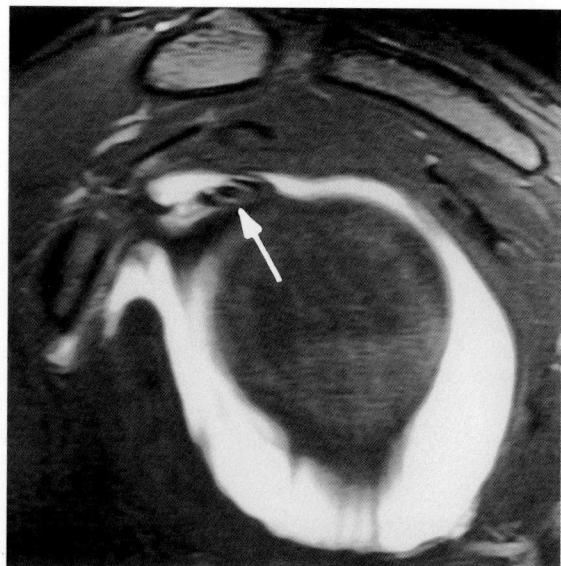

FIGURE 97-23

Biceps tendon in a type IV SLAP lesion. Fat-suppressed T1-weighted sagittal MR arthrogram reveals longitudinal splitting of the proximal long biceps tendon into three separate bands *(arrow)*.

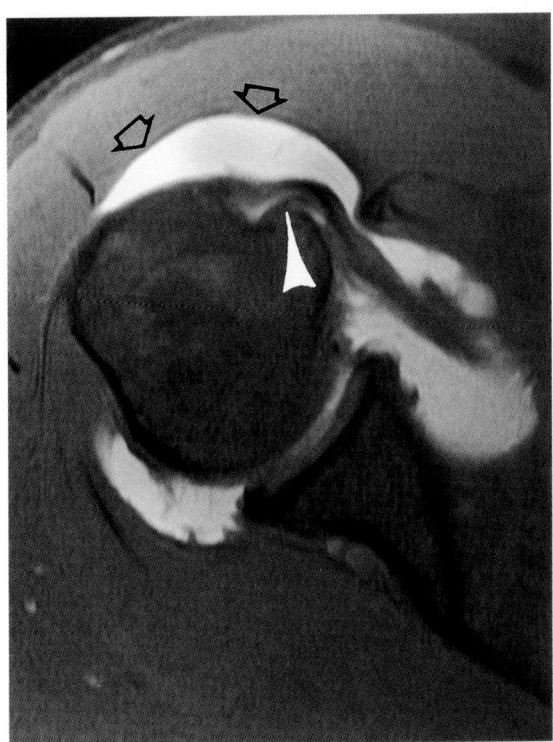

FIGURE 97-24

The "perched" biceps tendon. Fat-suppressed T1-weighted axial MR arthrogram reveals a flattened biceps tendon *(large arrowhead)* draped over the lesser tuberosity in the presence of a normally configured bicipital groove. The presence of contrast material in the subacromial-subdeltoid bursa *(open arrowheads)* indicates a co-existing full-thickness tear of the rotator cuff.

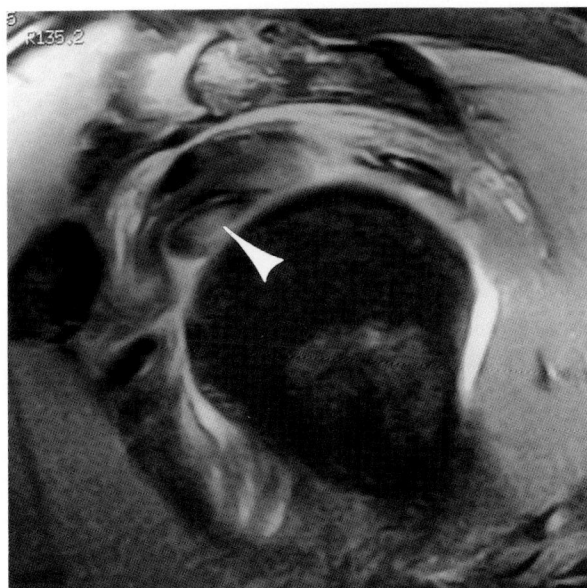

FIGURE 97-25

Biceps tendinosis. Fat-suppressed T2-weighted coronal MR image following joint distension reveals marked thickening and internally increased signal intensity in the proximal biceps tendon *(arrowhead)*.

The long biceps tendon can also dislocate medially[49] or sublux ("perch") onto the lesser tuberosity of the humerus, a condition requiring open surgery for confirmation and correction (Fig. 97-24).[50] Conventional MRI is highly sensitive for detecting tendon ruptures and dislocations, but intra-articular contrast material enhances the sensitivity of MRI for tendinosis and partial tears (Figs. 97-23 and 97-25). The intracapsular biceps tendon is one rare anomaly in which MR arthrography is more effective in diagnosis than either arthroscopy or conventional MRI.[51]

Chondral Lesions

The articular cartilage of both the humeral head and glenoid fossa is less than 2 mm in average thickness.[52] Chondral lesions in the shoulder correlate with tears of the glenoid labrum and also with cuff tendinopathy.[53] In anterior humeral instability, the most common sites of chondral injury are the anterior inferior quadrant of the glenoid fossa and the posterior superior aspect of the humeral head. In posterior instability, on the other hand, chondral lesions tend to involve the posterior aspect of the glenoid fossa and the anterior medial aspect of the humeral head (Fig. 97-26). Chondral lesions occurring adjacent to anterior labral tears have been termed glenoid

labrum articular disruption (GLAD) lesions.[54] Superior migration of the humeral head in endstage rotator cuff disease is associated with chondral lesions in the superior aspect of the glenoid fossa and the superior medial aspect of the humeral head. The humeral changes in endstage cuff disease can, if severe enough, resemble avascular necrosis which also tends to occur in the superior medial aspect of the humeral head.[55] Patterns of chondral injury which do not conform with clinical assessments may reflect undiagnosed multidirectional instability. The accuracy of MR arthrography in identifying defects in the articular cartilage of the glenoid fossa or humeral head is between 65% and 70%.[56]

THE WRIST

Applications

The wrist contains three spaces that can be injected for the purpose of arthrography: the radiocarpal, midcarpal, and distal radioulnar compartments. The major indications for MR arthrography of the wrist are to assess the triangular fibrocartilage complex and intrinsic ligaments of the wrist.[57] Minor indications include the confirmation of nonunion following scaphoid fractures and the evaluation of the dorsal extrinsic ligaments. MR scanning is usually performed following injection of the radiocarpal compartment but can also be performed following injection of the midcarpal or distal radioulnar compartments depending on the provisional diagnosis.[58] The remaining wrist compartments are then usually studied using conventional arthrography.

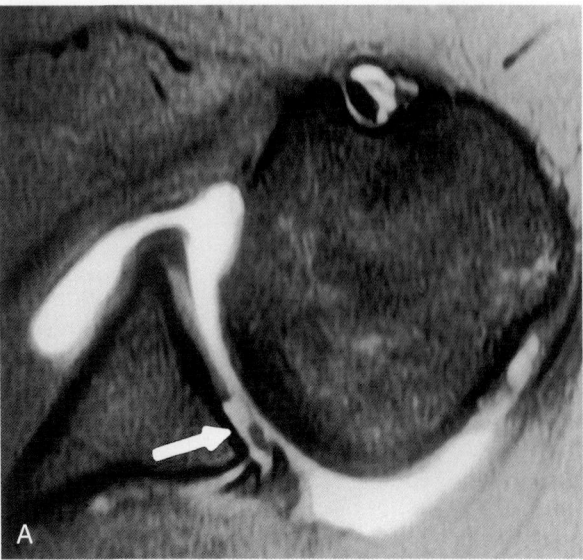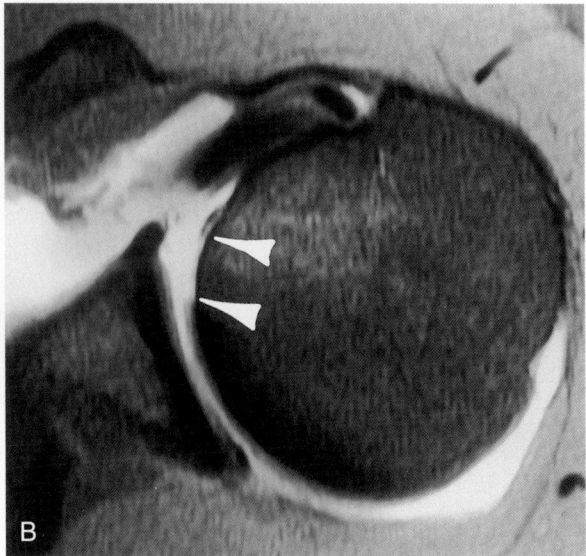

FIGURE 97-26

Chondral defects in posterior shoulder instability. **A,** Fat-suppressed T1-weighted axial MR arthrogram reveals an 8-mm chondral defect *(arrow)* in the posterior aspect of the glenoid fossa adjacent to a detached tear of the posterior labrum. **B,** Fat-suppressed T1-weighted axial MR arthrogram in the same patient as **A** reveals a 7-mm chondral defect in the anteromedial aspect of the humeral head *(arrowheads)*.

Technique for Wrist Arthrography

(Box 97-2)

Injection of the radiocarpal compartment is performed using a dorsal approach with a 25-gauge butterfly needle oriented in a slightly volar direction while aiming at the scaphoid side of the radioscaphoid articulation (Fig. 97-27). The injection is usually performed using fluoroscopic guidance, but the radioscaphoid articulation can also be palpated using bony landmarks.[59] The radiocarpal compartment is typically filled with 4 mL of contrast material. The wrist is observed fluoroscopically or videotaped during the injection so that the initial passage of contrast material through either the scapholunate or lunotriquetral ligaments or the triangular fibrocartilage can be observed. Once the contrast material has been injected, fluoroscopic spot radiographs are obtained with the wrist in radial and ulnar deviation to mildly stress the ligaments and raise the sensitivity for tears. After 1 minute of exercise, MRI scanning is performed.

The rationale for performing a midcarpal arthrogram following the radiocarpal arthrogram is to raise the sensitivity for intrinsic ligament perforations by identifying those perforations that permit only unidirectional passage of contrast material from the midcarpal to the radiocarpal compartment. Injection of the midcarpal compartment should only be performed after all the contrast material from the earlier radiocarpal injection has been absorbed, a process that usually requires 2 hours but occasionally takes longer. This delay affords patients a 1-hour rest between the MRI and the midcarpal arthrogram. It is our policy to allow patients to temporarily leave the imaging facility during this time. If the contrast material has not been absorbed from the

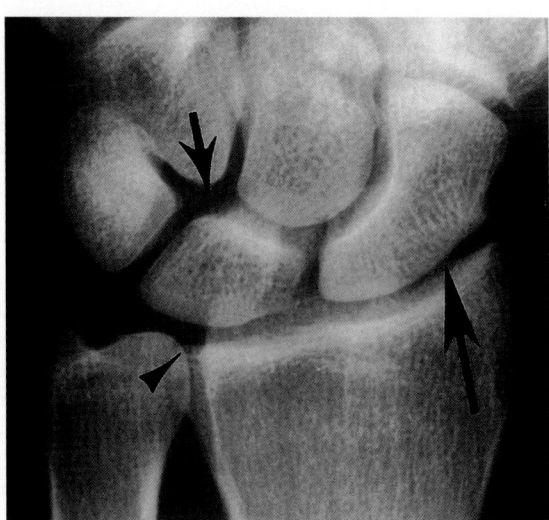

FIGURE 97-27

An AP radiograph of a hand. The *long arrow* indicates the target site for injecting the radiocarpal compartment. The *short arrow* identifies the target site for injecting the midcarpal compartment. The *arrowhead* indicates the target site for injecting the distal radioulnar compartment.

Box 97-2	Sample Scanning Protocol for MR Arthrography of the Wrist

T1-weighted coronal
Fat-suppressed T1-weighted coronal
Fat-suppressed T2-weighted coronal
T2* coronal
T1-weighted sagittal
T2* axial

radiocarpal compartment after 2 hours, the patient is given the option to reschedule the midcarpal and distal radioulnar joint injections.

To perform the midcarpal arthrogram, a 25-gauge butterfly needle is aimed at the space between the capitate, lunate, and triquetrum under fluoroscopy. Unless MR scanning is to be performed following injection of the midcarpal compartment, undiluted iodinated contrast material is used. The midcarpal compartment is filled by 1.0 to 4.0 mL of contrast material. A 3 mL syringe is recommended for the injection in order to maximize sensitivity to minor changes in resistance as the plunger is being depressed. Once moderate resistance is encountered, the needle is withdrawn, and fluoroscopic spot radiographs are obtained with the wrist in ulnar and radial deviation.

The rationale behind performing arthrography of the distal radioulnar joint (DRUJ) is to improve the sensitivity for noncommunicating tears of the triangular fibrocartilage complex (TFCC). If contrast material has not passed into the radiocarpal compartment during the midcarpal arthrogram, the DRUJ arthrogram can be undertaken immediately following the midcarpal arthrogram. If contrast material has passed into the radiocarpal compartment, the DRUJ arthrogram should be delayed until the radiocarpal compartment is fluoroscopically clear. If the contrast material has not cleared from the radiocarpal compartment after 2 hours, we give the patient the option to reschedule the DRUJ injection.

Injection of the DRUJ is performed with a 25-gauge butterfly needle aimed at the radial margin of the distal ulna. This is the most technically challenging of all three wrist injections and use of the 3 mL syringe is strongly recommended. Successful needle placement is characterized by a palpable decrease in resistance to injection associated with rapid outline of the DRUJ. The DRUJ is filled by 0.5 to 1.0 mL of contrast material. Unless MR scanning is to be performed following injection of the DRUJ, undiluted iodinated contrast material is used. Fluoroscopic spot radiographs are obtained with the wrist in the anteroposterior and bilateral oblique projections to improve sensitivity for noncommunicating defects in the TFCC.

Triangular Fibrocartilage Complex

Anatomy

The TFCC is composed of a central relatively avascular fibrocartilaginous disk (the triangular fibrocartilage or "TFC proper") and its surrounding ligamentous reinforcements. The TFCC serves to cushion the ulnocarpal articulation and stabilize the distal radioulnar joint while facilitating a wide range of motion in the wrist. The triangular fibrocartilage inserts on the sigmoid notch of the distal radius and on the base of the styloid process of the ulna. On its volar surface, the triangular fibrocartilage is supported by the ulnolunate, ulnotriquetral, and volar radioulnar ligaments. On its dorsal surface, the triangular fibrocartilage is supported by the dorsal radioulnar ligament.

Injuries of the Triangular Fibrocartilage Complex

The most common abnormality of the TFCC is central perforation, with a prevalence of over 50% in the cadaveric wrists of subjects over 50 years of age.[60] Perforations of the articular disk of the triangular fibrocartilage which are central in location are generally considered to be degenerative in origin while defects occurring in the radial and ulnar aspects of the TFCC are regarded as traumatic. In ulnolunate impaction syndrome, a long ulna (positive ulnar variance) predisposes to compressive forces leading to degeneration and perforation of the TFC proper.[61,62] In the more advanced stages, chondromalacia can develop in the proximal poles of the lunate and triquetrum. In ulnoradial impingement syndrome, a short ulna predisposes to mechanical irritation at the distal radioulnar articulation leading to synovitis and fluid accumulation in the DRUJ without perforation of the TFC proper.

Conventional MRI has 72% to 100% sensitivity for central communicating perforations of the TFCC,[62-64] and 17% to 50% sensitivity for ulnar-sided tears of the TFCC.[61,65,66] MR arthrography also has 80% to 100% sensitivity for central communicating perforations of the TFCC (Fig. 97-28),[63,66] but is considered more sensitive than conventional MRI for ulnar-sided tears and noncommunicating defects of the TFCC (Palmer Class 1B lesions).[58] Since ulnar-sided and noncommunicating defects of the TFCC correlate better with wrist pain than do central communicating defects, there is a greater incentive to use MR arthrography to detect them.[58]

Ligaments

The scapholunate and lunotriquetral or "intrinsic" ligaments of the proximal carpal row in the wrist are crucial to carpal stability. Each ligament is triangular in shape from the anteroposterior perspective and contains three zones: dorsal, volar, and intermediate. The dorsal and volar zones are strong static stabilizers of the proximal carpal row while the intermediate zone is comparatively thin and weakly attached. Developmental and degenerative perforations occur in the intermediate zone and tend to be asymptomatic with little functional significance. Tears of the dorsal and volar zones, on the other hand, are more likely to be traumatic in origin and symptomatic. From an anteroposterior perspective, tears of the dorsal and volar zones can occur in the midline or in the periphery.

Early studies using conventional MRI to identify complete tears of the scapholunate and lunotriquetral ligaments described 50% sensitivity for each ligament.[63,67,68] More recent work has reported 56% sensitivity using conventional MRI to diagnose partial tears of these ligaments.[69] Complete tears of the intrinsic ligaments are diagnosed on MR arthrography if, and only if, contrast material passes completely through the ligament. The sensitivity of MR arthrography for complete tears of the intrinsic ligaments of the wrist is between 83% and 90% (Figs. 97-29 to 97-31).[63,67] Some investigators have advocated performing arthrography in the contralateral

20 mL. If iodinated contrast material has been included in the injectant, anteroposterior and lateral radiographs may be obtained to complete the conventional arthrogram. In one potential pitfall of MR arthrography, intra-articular contrast material normally distributes into the sheaths of the flexor hallucis longus and flexor digitorum longus tendons as well as the subtalar joints in up to 25% of individuals.[81,82]

Ligament Tears on MR Arthrography

The anterior talofibular ligament is a focal capsular thickening that originates on the anterior aspect of the distal fibula and inserts on the neck of the talus (Fig. 97-32). The extravasation of intra-articular contrast material through the ligament into the anterior soft-tissues of the ankle indicates a complete tear (Fig. 97-33). The calcaneofibular ligament, also a capsular thickening, originates on the posterior aspect of the lateral malleolus and passes posteriorly and inferiorly to insert on the superior aspect of the calcaneus. Extravasation of intra-articular contrast material laterally through that ligament, often to surround the peroneal tendons, indicates a complete tear (Fig. 97-34). The posterior talofibular ligament originates on the posteromedial aspect of the fibula and inserts on the posterior aspect of the talus. Extravasation of intra-articular contrast material posteriorly through that ligament indicates a complete tear. Secondary signs of ligament disruption, including laxity and discontinuity, can be used to diagnose a tear in the absence of contrast material extravasation.[76]

Treatment

As previously described, treatment of torn anterior talofibular ligaments is initially conservative. All presumptive tears are immobilized to allow healing by scar formation. If instability persists, the lateral ligament complex can be surgically reinforced using either the joint capsule (Broström repair) or rerouted peroneal tendons (Evans, Watson-Jones, or Chrisman-Snook procedures).[77]

Impingement Syndromes in the Ankle

Anterolateral impingement syndrome (AIS) is a clinical diagnosis characterized by localized tenderness, swelling, and pain in the anterolateral ankle on certain maneuvers such as single leg squatting and dorsiflexion/eversion of the foot. The pathophysiology involves repetitive microtrauma from forced plantar flexion and supination resulting in synovitis, hemorrhage, and fibrosis in the anterolateral recess of the ankle. There is no correlation with acute trauma, mechanical instability, or degenerative joint disease. AIS can be excluded on arthroscopy if there is no evidence of synovitis in the anterolateral recess of the ankle. The converse, however, is not true. Specifically, arthroscopic evidence of synovitis in the anterolateral recess is not sufficient for diagnosing AIS in the absence of the appropriate clinical symptoms and signs.

MR arthrography can support the diagnosis of AIS by facilitating the identification of a nodular soft-tissue build-up in the anterolateral recess, a space bounded by the fibula laterally, the tibia posteromedially, and the anterior talofibular ligament anteriorly. For example, a

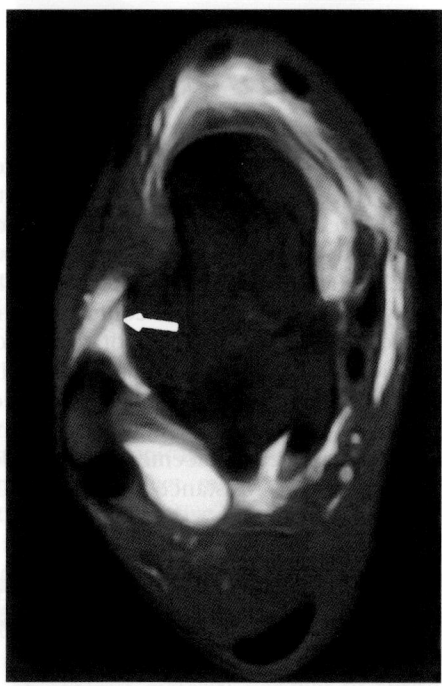

FIGURE 97-32

Normal anterior talofibular ligament of the ankle on MR arthrography. Fat-suppressed T1-weighted axial MR arthrogram reveals an intact anterior talofibular ligament (*arrow*) saddle-bagged by the distended joint capsule.

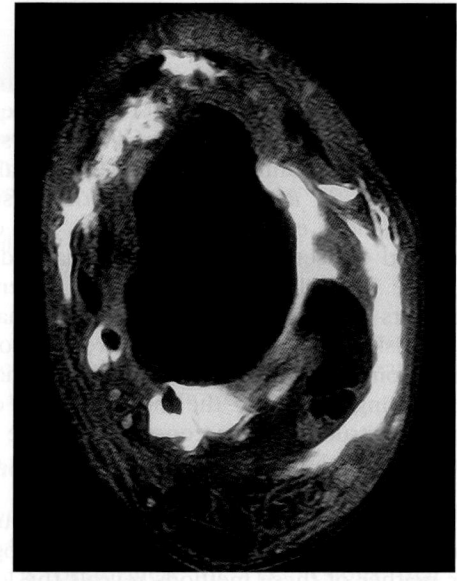

FIGURE 97-33

Disruption of anterior talofibular ligament of the ankle. Fat-suppressed T1-weighted axial MR arthrogram reveals contrast material extravasating through the anterior talofibular ligament into the anterior (and lateral) soft-tissues.

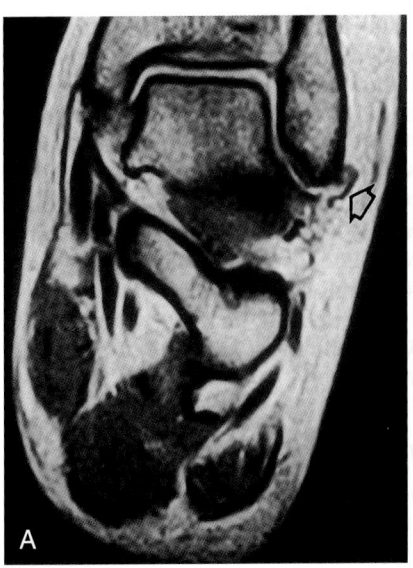 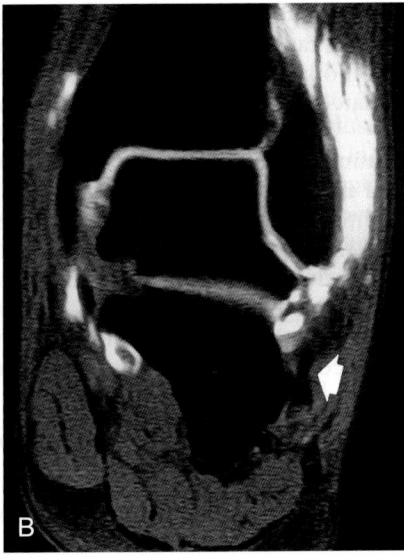

FIGURE 97-34

Disruption of the calcaneofibular ligament of the ankle. **A,** Proton density–weighted coronal MR image reveals discontinuity of the calcaneofibular ligament (*open arrowhead*). **B,** Fat-suppressed T1-weighted coronal MR arthrogram of the same patient as **A** reveals the extravasation of contrast material through the calcaneofibular ligament into the lateral soft-tissues. The peroneal tendons (*arrow*) remain isolated from the tear.

recent study using MR arthrography accurately identified abnormal soft-tissue in the anterolateral recesses of all 13 ankles clinically diagnosed with anterolateral impingement syndrome. Unfortunately, similar findings were also identified on the MR arthrograms of 11 of 19 asymptomatic "control" subjects.[83] Thus, in attempting to diagnose AIS using MR arthrography, correlation with clinical signs is imperative.

Impingement syndromes have also been described in the anteromedial and posterior aspects of the ankle joint. These syndromes are thought to arise from inversion and forced plantar flexion type injuries, respectively. Anteromedial impingement is associated with synovial hypertrophy in the anteromedial recess of the ankle joint, injuries of the deltoid ligament complex, and the development of tibial and talar osteophytes (Fig. 97-35).[84] Posterior impingement is associated with contusion of the lateral talar tubercle and os trigonum as well as synovitis in the posterior recesses of the tibiotalar and subtalar joints.[85,86]

Intra-articular Loose Bodies

Conventional MRI and MR arthrography are equally effective in the identification of loose bodies when a joint effusion is present. Loose bodies can usually be differentiated from air bubbles by their irregular configurations and dependent locations. However, loose bodies that are embedded in the synovium can be difficult to differentiate from osteophytes.

THE ELBOW

Introduction

Considering the popular appeal of throwing sports, it is not surprising that overuse injuries of the elbow are second only to those of the shoulder in terms of frequency. Any activity in which an individual grips an object, such as a ball or club, and then thrusts it forcefully away from the body, including baseball, tennis, and golf, will subject the elbow to some degree of valgus or varus stress. Valgus stress creates medial tension and lateral compression in the elbow. Injuries associated with medial tension include sprains and tears or tear of the ulnar collateral ligament (UCL), flexor tendinopathy, ulnar traction spurs, and ulnar neuropathy. Injuries associated with lateral compression include osteochondritis dissecans of the capitellum and radial head as well as degenerative joint disease and the formation of loose bodies. Varus stress creates lateral tension and medial

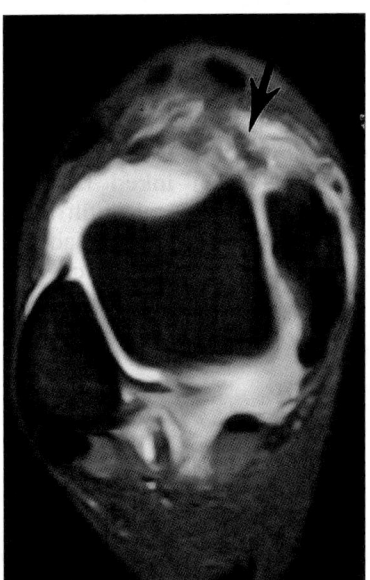

FIGURE 97-35

Anteromedial impingement syndrome. A 19-year-old ballerina complaining of pain and popping in the anterior aspect of the ankle. Fat-suppressed T1-weighted axial MR arthrogram through the ankle joint reveals synovitis (*arrow*) and mild capsular thickening in the anteromedial recess.

Indications

Chronic hip pain is a common cause of disability with important socioeconomic ramifications.[102] Hips with clicking, locking, snapping, or sudden weakness are termed functionally unstable. Radiographic findings in the functionally unstable but non-dysplastic hip are typically nil.[103] While there may be some risk for developing degenerative joint disease, osseous changes tend to be late manifestations of instability. In most cases, the primary underlying etiology for functional instability in the hip is thought to be a labral tear, and this is the primary indication for MR arthrography. Minor indications for MR arthrography in the hip include the identification of capsular tears, chondral defects, and loose bodies.

Single-contrast hip arthrograms have not proven effective for revealing labral tears.[104] Double-contrast CT arthrography has shown more promise but no large series has yet been published. Conventional MRI is currently the most popular imaging study for evaluating the acetabular labrum. In most cases, however, insufficient joint distension and the use of large fields of view make it difficult to separate labrum, capsule, cartilage, and bone. In one published series, the accuracy of conventional MRI for acetabular labral tears was only 36%.[105] By contrast, MR arthrography is approximately 90% accurate for diagnosing acetabular labral tears.[105-108]

Technique for Hip Arthrography
(Box 97-6)

With the patient supine on the fluoroscopy table, the hips are fixed into internal rotation by taping the feet together. A bolster may be placed under the knees for comfort. The common femoral artery is then localized by palpation. Following this, the skin is marked at a point that is lateral to the femoral artery, inferior to the inguinal ligament, and over the mid femoral neck on fluoroscopy. A 20-gauge spinal needle is then advanced directly downward until bone is encountered. The needle tip may need to be withdrawn 1 to 3 mm and twisted while gently depressing the plunger of a 10 mL syringe containing 1% lidocaine to confirm that the tip is intra-articular. After positive resistance testing using a lidocaine syringe, the location of the needle tip is reconfirmed using a few drops of iodinated contrast material. Once successful needle placement has been confirmed, dilute gadolinium may be instilled until resistance is encountered, usually between 6 and 12 mL. Intra-articular lidocaine can be

used to help confirm internal derangement as the cause for hip pain.

MR imaging of the hip is performed using any type of surface coil that is capable of acquiring a small field of view for optimal resolution. Phased-array flex coils, phased-array PA shoulder coils (for small hips only), and anterior neck coils have been employed with success. In MR arthrography, fat-suppressed T1-weighted images are acquired in all three planes, but oblique axials are usually substituted for orthogonal axials since the oblique slices are more perpendicular to the anterior superior labrum. The oblique axial cuts are prescribed perpendicular to the long axis of the femoral neck on a coronal localizer. Lastly, STIR or fat-suppressed proton density–weighted coronals and axials are performed to facilitate the identification of paralabral cysts, subchondral cysts, and bursitis.

Tears of the Acetabular Labrum

The acetabular labrum is a fibrocartilaginous rim, which is triangular in cross-section and attaches directly to the osseous rim of the acetabulum to deepen the hip joint. The labrum is thickest posterosuperiorly and thinnest anteroinferiorly including the acetabular notch where the labrum becomes the transverse acetabular ligament. The capsule of the hip joint also attaches directly to the osseous rim of the acetabulum, resulting in the creation of a small paralabral recess between the labrum and capsule. Closure of this recess has been associated with labral pathology as well as prior hip surgery which can scar and shrink the joint capsule.[99] In assessing the acetabular labrum, it is important to bear in mind that most morphologic changes represent normal variations, analogous to the glenoid labrum. Normal variations include shape (rounding or flattening), size (hypertrophy), the presence of sulci (in the anterior superior quadrant), and signal intensity (intermediate signal intensity due to fibrovascular structure, magic angle effect, or degeneration).

The diagnosis of an acetabular labral tear on MR arthrography requires the depiction of contrast material either completely undermining the labrum in a detached tear or penetrating the labrum in a nondetached tear (Figs. 97-37 and 97-38). The majority of traumatic tears are detached, and the most common location is in the anterior superior quadrant.[105] In one pitfall, normal undercutting of the labrum by articular cartilage can be mistaken for a detached tear. Tear location has been found to correlate with the cause of the injury and the age of the patient. For example, sports-related labral tears most often occur in the anterior superior quadrant while those associated with hip dysplasia tend to be lateral.[100,103,107,108] In children and adolescents, labral tears are often posterior in location (Fig. 97-39).[109,110] Childhood Legg-Calvé-Perthes disease is associated with an increased incidence of acetabular labral tears. Paralabral cysts are also known to occur adjacent to tears of the acetabular labrum and may be the only sign of an underlying labral tear on MRI.[111,112] Since paralabral cysts do not tend to fill with contrast material, their diagnosis depends on T2-weighted imaging (Fig. 97-40).

Box 97-6	Sample Protocol for Unilateral MR Arthrography of the Hip

T1-weighted coronal
Fat-suppressed T1-weighted coronal
Fat-suppressed T1-weighted sagittal
Fat-suppressed T1-weighted oblique axial
STIR coronal

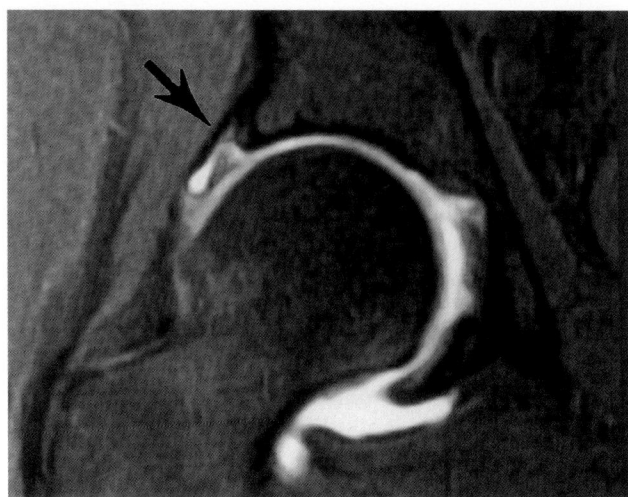

F I G U R E 97-37

Detached tear of the lateral acetabular labrum. Fat-suppressed T1-weighted coronal MR arthrogram reveals contrast material completely undermining the lateral aspect of the acetabular labrum *(arrow)*.

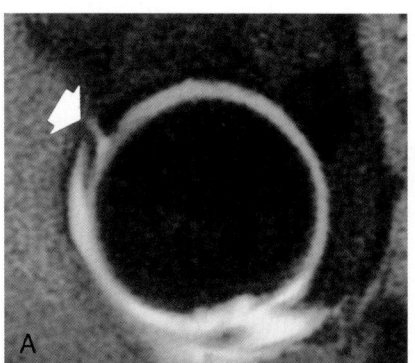 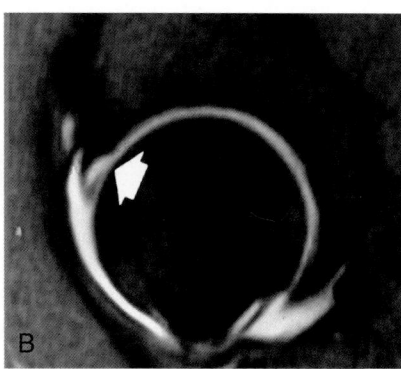

F I G U R E 97-38

Detached and nondetached tears of the anterior acetabular labrum. **A,** Fat-suppressed T1-weighted sagittal MR arthrogram reveals contrast material *(arrow)* completely undermining the anterior labrum. **B,** Fat-suppressed T1-weighted sagittal MR arthrogram reveals contrast material deeply penetrating the anterior labrum *(arrow)* without detachment.

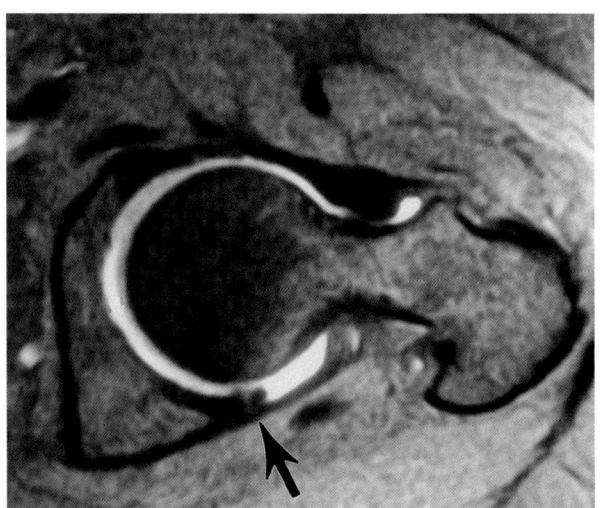

F I G U R E 97-39

Nondetached tear of the posterior acetabular labrum. Fat-suppressed T1-weighted oblique axial MR arthrogram reveals subtle penetration of contrast material into the posterior aspect of the acetabular labrum *(arrow)*.

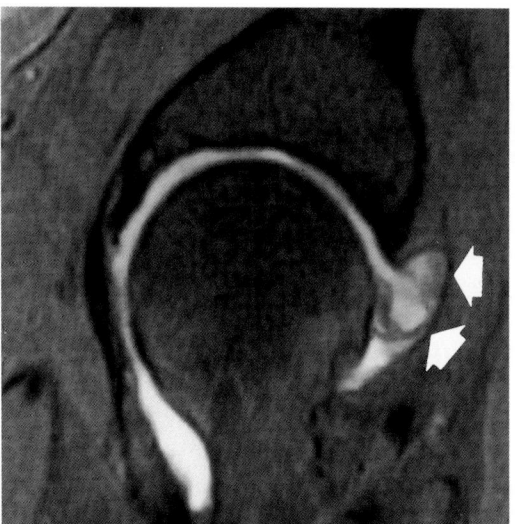

F I G U R E 97-40

Fat-suppressed T2-weighted sagittal MR image following joint distension reveals a 1.0 cm posterior paralabral cyst *(arrows)*.

Capsular Tears in the Hip

Capsular tears in the hip are rare, but any extravasation of contrast material on an MR arthrogram is suggestive of the diagnosis. Capsular tears in the hip are most often medial or superior in location. Medial tears may be associated with injuries of the obturator externus muscle. In one pitfall, the iliopsoas bursa communicates with the hip joint in up to 15% of normal individuals.[113]

Chondral Defects

The articular cartilage of the acetabulum is horseshoe-shaped and very thin, measuring as little as 2.0 mm anterosuperiorly and 1.0 mm posteroinferiorly.[114] Chondral defects are more commonly found in the acetabulum than in the femoral head, and an association exists between chondral defects in the acetabulum and labral tears.[115] It has been postulated that impingement of the femur on the acetabular rim, thought to occur when the hip is flexed, adducted, and internally rotated, may account for the high proportion of chondral injuries identified in the anterior superior quadrant of the acetabulum. Femoral dysplasia predisposes to femoro-acetabular impingement.

Conventional MRI identifies chondral tears in the hip indirectly based upon secondary signs such as joint space narrowing, subchondral sclerosis, subchondral cysts, and osteophytes. MR arthrography, should, in theory, be more sensitive than conventional MRI for chondral tears and erosion since such injuries are directly outlined by contrast material. However, recent work evaluating the efficacy of MR arthrography using two independent observers yielded sensitivities of (only) 50% and 79% and specificities of 77% and 84% with poor interobserver agreement.[116] The authors postulated that the lower than anticipated levels of sensitivity accuracy and agreement were due to volume averaging between bone, cartilage, and the enhanced joint fluid.

Loose Bodies

Loose bodies are relatively rare in the hip. As in other joints, the sensitivity of conventional MRI for loose bodies correlates with the amount of fluid in the joint. The main advantage of MR arthrography is joint distension. The propensity for loose bodies to lodge in the acetabular fossa of the hip joint has recently been recognized.

THE KNEE

Introduction

Thousands of arthroscopic meniscal resections and repairs are performed on a daily basis in the United States, and the trend shows no sign of slowing. The proportion of MRI exams evaluating postoperative knees for recurrent meniscal tears has risen in kind. However, while the accuracy of conventional MRI for diagnosing meniscal tears in non-operated knees is well established

at between 90% and 100%, the accuracy of conventional MRI for recurrent meniscal tears languishes between 38% and 82%.[117,118] This reduction in accuracy stems from two problems associated with partial meniscal resection: the tendency for pre-existing linear intrameniscal signal to come to the surface following surgery, and the tendency for suture lines and scar tissue to create linear intermediate signal intensity on short TE sequences which can intersect a meniscal surface and be indistinguishable from an acute tear. The first problem may be alleviated if a preoperative MRI is available at the time of interpretation. The second problem is more difficult to resolve, prompting several investigators to advocate revising the criteria for diagnosing recurrent tears on conventional MRI.[118-120] In one such proposal, if less than 25% of the meniscus has been resected, the standard tear criterion of surfacing linear hyperintensity on proton density–weighted imaging still applies. However, if greater than or equal to 25% of the meniscus has been resected, only surfacing linear hyperintensity on T2-weighted imaging qualifies for a tear. The rationale for this modification is to improve specificity by excluding intrameniscal scar tissue, which can mimic a recurrent tear on proton density–weighted imaging. Using these modified criteria, the accuracy of conventional MRI for recurrent meniscal tear reportedly rises to between 77% and 80%.[119,120]

Indications

The best-recognized indication for performing MR arthrography in the knee is in the evaluation of the postoperative meniscus. Other conditions whose evaluation is facilitated by MR arthrography include anterior cruciate ligament grafts, OCD, loose bodies, chondral defects, and synovial plica. However, since each of these conditions can be diagnosed reasonably accurately on conventional MRI, they are considered minor indications for the procedure.

Technique for Knee Arthrography

(Box 97-7)

Fluoroscopy is not necessary to perform knee arthrography. The patient is placed on a table in the supine position with the knee fully extended. Using sterile technique and 1% lidocaine for local anesthesia, a puncture is made either medial or lateral to the patella using a 3.8 cm 22-gauge needle attached to a lidocaine syringe. The needle is then gingerly advanced between the patella and trochlea, avoiding the articular surfaces of

Box 97-7	Sample Protocol for MR Arthrography of the Knee

Fat-suppressed T1-weighted sagittal
Fat-suppressed proton density–weighted sagittal
Fat-suppressed T1-weighted coronal
Fat-suppressed proton density–weighted coronal
Fat-suppressed proton density–weighted axial

the patella and trochlea, which can be tender. While the needle is being advanced, the plunger is intermittently depressed to check resistance. Once the lidocaine passes into the joint with little or no resistance, the needle tip is presumed to be intra-articular. There is generally no need to reconfirm with iodinated contrast material. After attempting to aspirate the joint, 20 to 40 mL of dilute gadolinium solution is injected. MR imaging is preceded by a short period of mild exercise.

Postoperative Meniscus

Both direct and indirect techniques of MR arthrography outperform conventional MRI in the evaluation of the postoperative meniscus.[119-121] In each technique, meniscal tears are diagnosed if and only if contrast material directly penetrates a meniscal surface (Fig. 97-41).[121] In repaired menisci, the absence of penetrating contrast material is interpreted as a healed tear while the penetration of contrast material a short distance into a known suture line is interpreted as a partially healed tear. Deep penetration of contrast material into a known suture line is interpreted as a failed repair. In 1994, Applegate et al reported that direct MR arthrography had a 72% accuracy for recurrent meniscal tears in cases in which at least 25% of the meniscus had been previously resected.[118] However, more recent studies on the same topic have yielded conflicting data regarding the need for MR arthrography in evaluating postoperative menisci.[119,120] Nevertheless, many musculoskeletal radiologists and orthopedists continue to favor MR arthrography for this purpose.

Anterior Cruciate Ligament Grafts

Conventional MRI has had mixed success in evaluating anterior cruciate ligament (ACL) grafts with accuracy rates ranging from 50% to 100%.[122-124] Radiologists have traditionally recommended MR imaging with intravenous gadolinium in the evaluation of anterior cruciate ligament grafts because of the known tendency of the intact grafts to develop a richly vascularized soft-tissue envelope within a month of the surgery.[125,126] Unfortunately, graft impingement can induce a similar hypervascular response. By contrast, direct MR arthrography enables assessment of the graft itself rather than the periligamentous envelope. Recent work investigating the ability of direct MR arthrography to evaluate ACL grafts has yielded accuracy rates of 93% and 100%.[127]

Osteochondritis Dissecans

Osteochondritis dissecans (OCD), defined as a focal lesion of bone and overlying articular cartilage characterized by fragmentation and possible separation, is more commonly found in the knee than any other joint in the body. The condition is particularly prevalent among adolescents where the most common location is in the lateral aspect of the medial femoral condyle. Preventing an acceleration of degenerative joint disease depends initially on accurate staging.[78] As in other joints, MR arthrography is preferred over conventional MRI for staging OCD because of the slightly superior conspicuity of gadolinium on fat-suppressed T1-weighted images compared to nonenhanced joint fluid on fat-suppressed T2-weighted images.

Loose Bodies

The knee develops more loose bodies than any other joint in the body, and many do not contain bone. Since radiography and CT have limited abilities to detect nonossific loose bodies, MRI is often requested for this purpose. Conventional MRI has a sensitivity of 86% in detecting loose bodies in the knee, but the greater joint

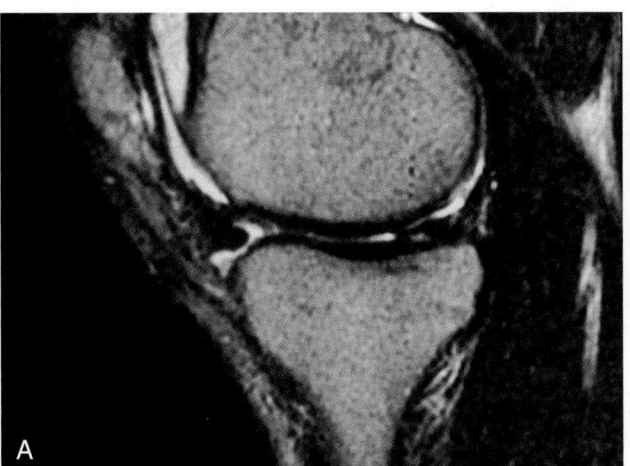
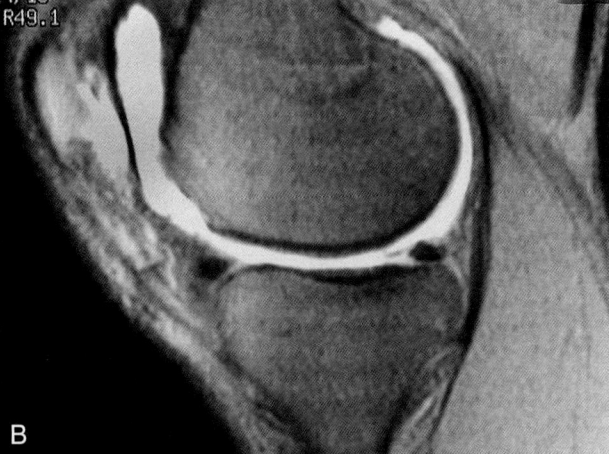

FIGURE 97-41

Superior specificity of direct MR arthrography over T2-weighted imaging in diagnosing recurrent meniscal tears in the knee. **A,** T2-weighted sagittal MR image of the medial meniscus shows 35% previous meniscal resection and obliquely oriented linear intermediate signal intensity intersecting the undersurface of the remnant of the posterior horn. **B,** Fat-suppressed T1-weighted sagittal MR arthrogram in the same patient as **A** reveals a recurrent vertical tear in the remnant of the posterior horn.

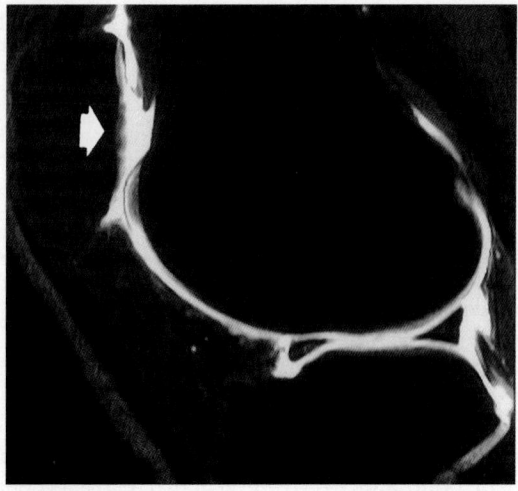

FIGURE 97-42

Grade 2 chondromalacia patellae. Fat-suppressed T1-weighted sagittal MR arthrogram reveals contrast material outlining numerous superficial fissures in the patellar cartilage (arrow).

distension afforded by MR arthrography may give it a minor advantage in this regard.[128] In one common pitfall, an ossific structure that appears separate from the tibia or femur in one imaging plane but cannot be separated from those bones in the other imaging planes may be an osteophyte rather than a loose body.

Chondral Lesions

Chondral defects are commonly found on all weight-bearing articular surfaces in the knee as well as in the patella and trochlea. Arthroscopists grade chondromalacia from 1 to 4 based primarily on the depth of chondral tears, fissures, and erosions. Grades 3 and 4 changes are easily recognized on radiography, CT, and conventional MRI based upon secondary findings such as joint space narrowing, subchondral sclerosis, subchondral cyst formation, and periarticular spurring. Various pulse sequences have been proposed to improve the sensitivity of conventional MRI for early (grades 1 and 2) chondromalacia with mixed results.[129-131] MR arthrography achieves 90% and 100% accuracy for chondromalacia in the knee by delivering contrast material directly into the pits and fissures found in grade 2 chondromalacia as well as the cavities found in more advanced stages (Fig. 97-42).[78,132-134]

Synovial Plica

Of the three synovial plicae in the knee, the medial is the most likely to undergo pathologic thickening. "Plica syndrome," which is characterized by pain and locking on the medial aspect of the knee, can mimic a medial meniscal tear clinically.[135] On conventional MRI, medial plicae are best identified in the presence of a joint effusion but can also be recognized against a background of adipose tissue in the absence of an effusion.[136] MR arthrography improves the characterization of plicae

including size, thickness, and position but these anatomic details have yet to be shown to correlate with symptoms and may have limited clinical relevance.[135-137]

INDIRECT MR ARTHROGRAPHY

Introduction

Indirect MR arthrography is a technique that exploits the tendency of intravenously injected gadolinium to diffuse into joint fluid. Since blood vessels in the synovium lack a basement membrane, gadolinium quickly passes from blood plasma into joint fluid to establish an equilibrium.[138] The primary objective of indirect MR arthrography is to achieve an arthrographic effect less invasively and without the need for a radiologist to perform the injection. Indirect MR arthrography also provides physiologic information not available using direct MR arthrography by enhancing hyperemic and inflamed structures.

Comparison with Direct MR Arthrography

Indirect MR arthrography has clear-cut advantages over direct MR arthrography in terms of logistics, convenience, and patient tolerance. Indirect MR arthrography is also more sensitive than direct MR arthrography for inflammation involving tendons, bursae, muscles, and synovium. By contrast, however, indirect MR arthrography is generally considered less sensitive than direct MR arthrography for detecting small tears involving the labrum, ligaments, and articular cartilage.[8] The reduced sensitivity of indirect MR arthrography reflects the difficulty in attaining high enough concentrations of contrast material and sufficient joint distension in large joints to achieve an adequate arthrographic effect.[139] In well-vascularized areas, indirect MR arthrography is also considered less specific than direct MR arthrography. For example, following IV contrast administration, there is normally intense enhancement in the meniscocapsular junction of the knee and the ulnar aspect of the TFCC—two areas that are vulnerable to injury.[138,139] In the shoulder, isolated subacromial bursitis and small full-thickness tears of the rotator cuff may be difficult to distinguish on indirect MR arthrography.[139] In terms of economics, direct and indirect MR arthrography are reimbursed similarly at present.

Techniques of Indirect MR Arthrography

Two techniques are available for performing indirect MR arthrography. The first is the so-called "biphasic technique," which involves obtaining an immediate post-contrast "vascular phase" T1-weighted pulse sequence and then T2-weighted imaging in the same plane, followed by T1-weighted imaging with fat suppression in all three orthogonal planes (Fig. 97-43). The second technique involves only delayed postexercise imaging.

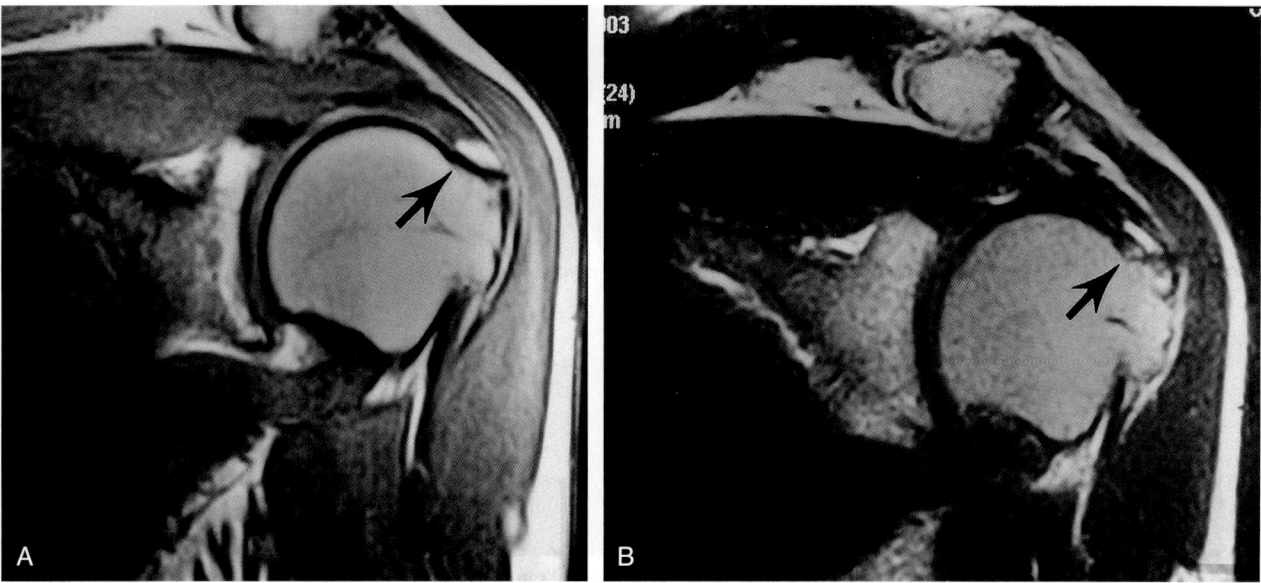

FIGURE 97-43

Comparison of T2-weighted imaging and indirect MR arthrography in diagnosing intrasubstance tears of the rotator cuff. **A,** Vascular phase T1-weighted coronal indirect MR arthrogram reveals a focal area of intense contrast enhancement in the interstitium of the distal tendon *(arrow)*. **B,** T2-weighted coronal MR image in the same patient as **A** confirms a small area of hyperintensity in the distal supraspinatus tendon *(arrow)* which does not involve either the articular or bursal surfaces.

Using this technique, contrast material is administrated intravenously in the waiting room followed by a period of passive exercise prior to scanning. The length of the period of exercise is directly proportional to the size of the joint in question. In small to medium-sized joints such as the wrist, elbow, and ankle, no more than 5 or 10 minutes of passive exercise is required. For the shoulder or hip, 15 minutes is recommended. In the knee, however, 30 minutes is optimal (Fig. 97-44).[138,140] These times may be lengthened in the presence of a hemarthrosis or large native joint effusion since these conditions raise intra-articular pressures and slow the rate of diffusion into the joint. Conversely, times may be reduced if hyperemia or synovitis is present. The scanning protocols used in delayed postexercise indirect MR arthrography are identical to those used in direct MR arthrography.

Indications

Certain niche applications for indirect MR arthrography have been reported.[141] In the wrist, enhancement around the flexor tendons is considered a relatively specific sign of carpal tunnel syndrome while the degree of intraosseous enhancement in the proximal fragment of a fractured scaphoid corresponds to healing potential.[142] In the elbow, focal enhancement of the common flexor or extensor tendons has been described as diagnostic for epicondylitis while perineural enhancement in the cubital tunnel is suggestive of ulnar neuritis. In the ankle, enhancement of fluid in tendon sheaths helps differentiate tenosynovitis from passive fluid accumulation, while localized synovial enhancement has been associated with tarsal tunnel syndrome, sinus tarsi

syndrome, and the various ankle impingement syndromes. In the shoulder, synovial enhancement in the rotator interval on indirect MR arthrography is reportedly a more sensitive marker for adhesive capsulitis than any finding on direct MR arthrography.[143] In the knee, indirect arthrography has been described as having equal effectiveness with direct MR arthrography in the diagnosis of recurrent meniscal tears.[120,144] Indirect MR arthrography can also help differentiate inflammatory arthritis from simple reactive joint effusions in large joints (Fig. 97-45).

CONCLUSION

Since its inception in 1990, MR arthrography has fostered the understanding of joint derangements and lengthened the roster of pathologic conditions that can be reliably diagnosed on imaging. However, despite the increased accuracy and expanded applications being realized with MR arthrography, we estimate that less than 5% of patients sent for MR imaging of a medium-sized or large joint currently receive an intra-articular injection of dilute gadolinium prior to scanning. Logistic issues are partly to blame but in many cases the opportunity to perform an MR arthrogram is missed because the radiologist is reluctant to convert a noninvasive procedure into a minimally invasive one, or because he or she feels that the small additional reimbursement for the arthrogram falls short of justifying the extra work. Technologists may also have objections to MR arthrography because of the extra time required in preparing the syringes, fluoroscopy suite, and consent form. While the probability of obtaining additional information must always be weighed against concerns for invasiveness

74. Helgason JW, Chandnani VP: Magnetic resonance imaging arthrography of the ankle. Top Magn Reson Imaging 9:286-294, 1998.

75. Oloff LM, Sullivan BT, Heard GS, et al: Magnetic resonance imaging of traumatized ligaments of the ankle. J Am Podiatr Med Assoc 82:25-32, 1992.

76. Chandnani VP, Harper MT, Ficke JR, et al: Chronic ankle instability: evaluation with MR arthrography, MR imaging, and stress radiography. Radiology 192:189-194, 1994.

77. Canale S: Ankle injuries. In Canale S (ed): Campbell's Operative Orthopedics. St. Louis: Mosby, 1998.

78. Kramer J, Stiglbauer R, Engel A, et al: MR contrast arthrography (MRA) in osteochondrosis dissecans. J Comput Assist Tomogr 16:254-260, 1992.

79. Mintz DN, Tashjian GS, Connell DA, et al: Osteochondral lesions of the talus: a new magnetic resonance grading system with arthroscopic correlation. Arthroscopy 19:353-359, 2003.

80. Schmid MR, Pfirrmann CWA, Hodler J, et al: Cartilage lesions in the ankle joint: comparison of MR arthrography and CT arthrography. Skeletal Radiol 32:259-265, 2003.

81. Boruta PM, Bishop JO, Braly WG, et al: Acute lateral ankle ligament injuries: a literature review. Foot Ankle Int 11:107-113, 1990.

82. Haller J, Resnick D, Sartoris D, et al: Arthrography, tenography, and bursography of the ankle and foot. Clin Podiatr Med Surg 5:839-909, 1988.

83. Robinson P, White LM, Salonen DC, et al: Anterolateral ankle impingement: MR arthrographic assessment of the anterolateral recess. Radiology 221:186-190, 2001.

84. Robinson P, White LM, Salonen D, et al: Anteromedial impingement of the ankle: Using MR arthrography to assess the anteromedial recess. Am J Roentgenol 178:601-604, 2002.

85. Bureau NJ, Cardinal E, Hobden R, et al: Posterior ankle impingement syndrome: MR imaging findings in seven patients. Radiology 215:497-503, 2000.

86. Karasick D, Schweitzer ME: The os trigonum syndrome: imaging features. Am J Roentgenol 166:125-129, 1996.

87. Rijke AM, Goitz HT, McCue FC, et al: Stress radiography of the medial elbow ligaments. Radiology 191:213-216, 1994.

88. Hill NB, Bucchieri JS, Shon F, et al: Magnetic resonance imaging of injury to the medial collateral ligament of the elbow: a cadaver model. J Shoulder Elbow Surg 9:418-422, 2000.

89. Mirowitz SA, London SL: Ulnar collateral ligament injury in baseball pitchers: MR imaging evaluation. Radiology 185:573-576, 1992.

90. Timmerman LA, Schwartz ML, Andrews JA: Preoperative evaluation of the ulnar collateral ligament by magnetic resonance imaging and computed tomography arthrography. Evaluation of 25 baseball players with surgical confirmation. Am J Sports Med 22:26-31, 1994.

91. Carrino JA, Morrison WB, Zou KH, et al: Noncontrast MR imaging and MR arthrography of the ulnar collateral ligament of the elbow: prospective evaluation of two dimensional pulse sequences for detection of complete tears. Skeletal Radiol 30:625-632, 2001.

92. Schwartz ML, Al-Zahrani S, Morwessel RM, et al: Ulnar collateral ligament injury in the throwing athlete: evaluation with saline-enhanced MR arthrography. Radiology 197:297-299, 1995.

93. Nakanishi K, Masatomi T, Ochi T, et al: MR arthrography of the elbow: evaluation of the ulnar collateral ligament of the elbow. Skeletal Radiol 25:269-634, 1996.

94. Munshi M, Pretterklieber ML, Chung C, et al: Anterior bundle of ulnar collateral ligament: evaluation of anatomic relationships by using MR imaging, MR arthrography, and gross anatomic and histologic analysis. Radiology 231:797-803, 2004.

95. O'Driscoll SW, Bell DF, Morrey BG: Posterolateral rotary instability of the elbow. J Bone Joint Surg Am 73:440-446, 1991.

96. Potter HG, Weiland AJ, Schatz JA, et al: Posterolateral rotatory instability of the elbow: usefulness of MR imaging in the diagnosis. Radiology 204:185-189, 1994.

97. Cotton A, Jacobson J, Brossman J, et al: MR arthrography of the elbow: normal anatomy and diagnostic pitfalls. J Comput Assist Tomogr 21:516-522, 1997.

98. Fitzgerald RH: Acetabular labrum tears: diagnosis and treatment. Clin Orthop 311:60-68, 1995.

99. Czerny C, Hofmann S, Urban M, et al: MR arthrography of the adult acetabular capsular-labral complex: correlation with surgery and anatomy. Am J Roentgenol 173:345-349, 1999.

100. Konrath GA, Hamel AJ, Olson SA, et al: The role of the acetabular labrum and the transverse acetabular ligament in load transmission in the hip. J Bone Joint Surg Am 80:1781-1788, 1998.

101. Klaue K, Durnian CW, Ganz R: The acetabular rim syndrome: a clinical presentation of dysplasia of the hip. J Bone Joint Surg Br 73:423-429, 1991.

102. Doherty M: Common regional pain syndromes I. Practitioner 233:1380, 1989.

103. Petersilge CA: Chronic adult hip pain: MR arthrography of the hip. Radiographics 20:S43-S52, 2000.

104. Ikeda T, Awaya G, Suzuki S: Torn acetabular labrum in young patients. Arthroscopic diagnosis and management. J Bone Joint Surg Br 70:13-16, 1988.

105. Czerny C, Hofmann S, Nuhold A, et al: Lesions of the acetabular labrum: accuracy of MR imaging and MR arthrography in detection and staging. Radiology 200:225-230, 1996.

106. Petersilge CA, Haque MA, Petersilge WJ, et al: Acetabular labral tears: evaluation with MR arthrography. Radiology 200:231-235, 1996.

107. Leunig M, Werlen S, Ungersbock A, et al: Evaluation of the acetabular labrum by MR arthrography. J Bone Joint Surg Br 79:230-234, 1997.

108. Santori N, Villar RN: Acetabular labrum tears: result of arthroscopic partial limbectomy. Arthroscopy 16:11-15, 2000.

109. Altenberg AR: Acetabular labrum tears: a cause of hip pain and degenerative arthritis. South Med J 70:174-175, 1977.

110. Hase T, Ueo T: Acetabular labral tear: arthroscopic diagnosis and treatment. Arthroscopy 15:138-141, 1999.

111. Edwards DJ, Lomas D, Villar RH: Diagnosis of the painful hip by magnetic resonance imaging and arthrography. J Bone Joint Surg Br 77:374-376, 1995.

112. Haller J, Resnick D, Greenway G, et al: Juxtaacetabular ganglionic (or synovial) cysts: CT and MR features. J Comput Assist Tomogr 13:976-983, 1989.

113. Williams PL, Warwick R (eds): Arthrology: the joints of the lower limb: the hip (coxal) joint. In: Gray's Anatomy, 36th ed. Philadelphia: WB Saunders, 1980.

114. Hodler J, Trudell D, Pathria MN, et al: Width of the articular cartilage of the hip: quantification by using fat-suppression spin-echo MR imaging in cadavers. Am J Roentgenol 159:351-355,1992.

115. Ito K, Minka MA II, Leunig M, et al: Femoroacetabular impingement and the cam-effect: A MRI based quantitative anatomical study of the femoral neck offset. J Bone Joint Surg Br 83:171-176, 2001.

116. Schmid MR, Notzli HP, Zanetti M: Cartilage lesions in the hip: diagnostic effectiveness of MR arthrography. Radiology 226:382-386, 2003.

117. Totty WG, Matava MJ: Imaging the postoperative meniscus. Magn Reson Imaging Clin N Am 8:271-283, 2000.

118. Applegate GR, Flannigan BD, Tolin BS, et al: MR diagnosis of recurrent tears in the knee: value of intraarticular contrast material. Am J Roentgenol 161:821-825, 1993.

119. Sciulli RL, Boutin RD, Brown RR, et al: Evaluation of the postoperative meniscus of the knee: a study comparing conventional arthrography, conventional MR imaging, MR arthrography with iodinated contrast material, and MR arthrography with gadolinium-based contrast material. Skeletal Radiol 28:508-514, 1999.

120. White LM, Schweitzer ME, Weishaupt D, et al: Diagnosis of recurrent meniscal tears: prospective evaluation of conventional MR imaging, indirect MR arthrography, and direct MR arthrography. Radiology 222:421-429, 2002.

121. Magee T, Shapiro M, Rodriguez J, et al: MR arthrography of postoperative knee: for which patients is it useful? Radiology 229:159-163, 2003.

122. Moeser P, Bechtold RE, Clark T, et al: MR imaging of anterior cruciate ligament repair. J Comput Assist Tomogr 13:105-109, 1989.

123. Horton LK, Jacobson JA, Lin J, et al: MR imaging of anterior cruciate ligament reconstruction graft. Am J Roentgenol 175:1091-1097, 2000.

124. Rak KM, Gillogly SD, Schaefer RA, et al: Anterior cruciate ligament reconstruction: evaluation with MR imaging. Radiology 178:553-556, 1991.

125. Jansson KA, Karjalainen PT, Harilainen A, et al: MRI of anterior cruciate ligament repair with patellar and hamstring tendon autografts. Skeletal Radiol 30:8-14, 2001.

126. Howell SM, Knox KE, Farley TE, et al: Revascularization of a human anterior cruciate ligament graft during the first two years of implantation. Am J Sports Med 23:42-49, 1995.

127. McCauley TR, Elfar A, Moore A, et al: MR arthrography of anterior cruciate ligament reconstruction grafts. Am J Roentgenol 181:1217-1223, 2003.

128. Brossmann J, Priedler KW, Daenen B: Imaging of osseous and cartilaginous intra-articular bodies in the knee: comparison of MR imaging and MR arthrography with CT and CT arthrography in cadavers. Radiology 200:509-517, 1996.

129. Disler D, McCauley TR, Wirth CR, et al: Detection of knee hyaline cartilage defects using fat-suppressed 3D spoiled gradient-echo MR imaging: comparison with standard MR imaging and correlation with arthroscopy. Am J Roentgenol 165:377-382, 1995.

130. Peterfy CG, Majumdar S, Lang P, et al: MR imaging of the arthritic knee: improved discrimination of cartilage, synovium, and effusion with pulsed saturation transfer and fat-suppressed T1-weighted sequences. Radiology 191:413-419, 1994.

131. Recht MP, Piraino D, Paletta GA, et al: Accuracy of fat-suppressed 3D spoiled gradient-echo FLASH MR imaging in the detection of patellofemoral articular cartilage abnormalities. Radiology 198:209-212, 1996.

132. Gagliardi JA, Chung EM, Chandnani VP: Detection and staging of chondromalacia patellae: relative efficacies of conventional MR imaging, MR arthrography and CT arthrography. Am J Roentgenol 163:629-636, 1994.

133. Kramer J, Recht MP, Imhoff, et al: Post-contrast MR arthrography in assessment of cartilage lesions. J Comput Assist Tomogr 18:218-224, 1994.

134. Chandnani VP, Ho C, Chu P, et al: Knee hyaline cartilage evaluated with MRI imaging: a cadaveric study involving multiple imaging sequences and intra-articular injection of gadolinium and saline solution. Radiology 178:557-561, 1991.

135. Boles CA, Butler J, Lee JA, et al: Magnetic resonance characteristics of medial plica of the knee. Correlation with arthroscopic resection. J Comput Assist Tomogr 28:397-401, 2004.
136. Garcia-Valtuille R, Abascal F, Cerezal L, et al: Anatomy and MRI imaging appearances of synovial plicae of the knee. Radiographics 22:775-784, 2002.
137. Kobayashi Y, Murakami R, Tajima H: Direct MR arthrography of plica synovialis mediopatellaris. Acta Radiol 42:286-290, 2001.
138. Schweitzer ME, Natale P, Winalski CS, et al: Indirect wrist arthrography: the effects of passive motion versus active exercise. Skeletal Radiol 29:10-14, 2000.
139. Winalski CS, Aliabadi P, Wright RJ, et al: Enhancement of joint fluid with intravenously administered gadopentetate dimeglumine: technique, rationale, and implications. Radiology 187:179-185, 1993.
140. Matsuzaki S, Yoneda M, Kobayashi Y, et al: Dynamic enhanced MRI of the subacromial bursa: correlation with arthroscopic and histologic findings. Skeletal Radiol 32:510-520, 2003.
141. Bergin D, Schweitzer ME: Indirect magnetic resonance arthrography. Skeletal Radiol 32:551-558, 2003.
142. Cerezal L, Abascal S, Canga A, et al: Usefulness of gadolinium-enhanced MR imaging in the evaluation of the vascularity of scaphoid nonunions. Am J Roentgenol 174:141-149, 2000.
143. Manton GL, Schweitzer ME, Weishaupt D, et al: Utility of MR arthrography in adhesive capsulitis. Skeletal Radiol 30:326-330, 2001.
144. Vives MJ, Homesley D, Ciccotti MG, et al: Evaluation of recurring meniscal tears with gadolinium enhanced magnetic resonance imaging. A randomized, prospective study. Am J Sports Med 31:868-873, 2003.

FUNCTIONAL ASSESSMENT OF THE JOINTS USING KINEMATIC MAGNETIC RESONANCE IMAGING*

Frank G. Shellock

INTRODUCTION

"Kinematics" is the branch of mechanics dealing with the study of motion of a body without specific reference to force or mass.[1] While traditional kinematic analyses (i.e., motion analysis systems that utilize external markers) form the cornerstone to the biomechanical assessment of joint function, interpretation of such data is limited with respect to identifying the internal factors contributing to abnormal joint motion (pathokinematics) and dysfunction. On the other hand, kinematic magnetic resonance imaging (MRI) provides a means by which the intricacies of joint function can be evaluated for both diagnostic and research purposes.[2] The fact that images can also be obtained during active motion, that is "dynamically", provides the ability to thoroughly evaluate the interactions of osseous structures and the contribution of muscle action and other soft-tissues to joint function.

Kinematic MRI techniques were developed in recognition of the fact that certain pathologic conditions that affect the joints are position dependent and/or associated with stressed or "loaded" conditions.[2-4] Information obtained using kinematic MRI procedures often serves to definitively identify and characterize the underlying abnormality or to supplement the findings acquired with standard MRI techniques. Combining kinematic MRI with routine MRI views of the joint provides a means of conducting a more thorough examination and can improve the diagnostic yield of the imaging procedure.[2-4]

To date, kinematic MRI methods have been applied to evaluate virtually every articulation.[2-70] A comprehensive description of functional anatomy, kinesiology, and clinical applications of kinematic MRI techniques has been published.[2] Because of the prevalence of pathology and abnormal conditions, this chapter presents information for kinematic MRI applications applied to the temporomandibular and patellofemoral joints, with a discussion of the normal kinematics and pathokinematics. In addition, other kinematic MRI procedures applied to the ankle, wrist, cervical spine, shoulder and lumbar spine will be discussed briefly.

[*Portions of this chapter were excerpted with permission from Shellock FG, Powers CM: Kinematic MRI of the Joints: Functional Anatomy, Kinesiology, and Clinical Applications. Boca Raton, FL: CRC Press, 2001. © FG Shellock, 2001.]

GENERAL ASPECTS OF KINEMATIC MAGNETIC RESONANCE IMAGING

Magnetic Resonance System

Most types of commercially available MR systems have been utilized for kinematic MRI examinations of the joints, including high-field, long-bore, and short-bore MR systems; high-field and mid-field, "open" MR systems; low-field, C-shaped magnet MR systems; and low-field, dedicated extremity MR systems.[2] Obviously, MR systems with open configurations offer the potential advantages of being able to accomplish greater incremental movements for certain body parts (e.g., the shoulder) and are inherently more comfortable for patients undergoing kinematic MRI procedures.

Techniques

Kinematic MRI protocols have utilized a variety of pulse sequences and joint positioning strategies. In general, kinematic MRI methods are divided into four primary types:

1. incremental, passive positioning
2. cine-cyclic
3. active-movement or dynamic
4. active-movement, against-resistance.[2,4,24-26,43]

The incremental, passive positioning technique involves the gradual movement and sequential imaging of the joint through a specific range of motion.[2] T1-weighted, spin-echo or gradient-echo pulse sequences are typically used to acquire MR images during kinematic MRI procedures that utilize the incremental, passive positioning technique.

The cine-cyclic method (also referred to as "motion-triggered" MR imaging) is similar to gated MR imaging used for cardiac- or respiratory-gated studies.[26] During this type of kinematic MRI procedure, the active, physical motion of the joint is repeated throughout the imaging acquisition cycle, which may last for several minutes.[26] MR imaging is performed using the cine-cyclic method with a spin-echo pulse sequence. Because of the inherent time and repeated movements that are required, this type of protocol is not considered to be advantageous for the evaluation of joints, especially in patients who are symptomatic during movement.

The active-movement technique is performed using fast gradient-echo pulse sequences or echo-planar imaging to permit imaging of the joint during dynamic motion.[2,24] A temporal resolution of approximately one image per second or less is believed to be optimal for this type of kinematic MRI examination.

The active-movement, against-resistance method is similar to the active-movement technique with respect to the MR imaging parameter requirements.[2,25] This type of kinematic MRI procedure involves application of a resistive load to stress the joint during dynamic motion.

Positioning Devices

Positioning devices are an important requirement for the performance of kinematic MRI examinations.[2-4] Positioning devices are used to guide the joint in a specific plane of imaging and through a specific range of motion. Obviously, these devices must be constructed of components or materials that are compatible with the electromagnetic fields used for MR imaging.

The positioning devices also need to be designed with a thorough understanding of the biomechanical aspects of the particular joint that is undergoing evaluation. For example, positioning devices designed for the patellofemoral joint should permit unrestricted rotational movements of the lower extremity, while the joint moves from approximately 45° of flexion to extension (i.e., the critical range of motion for the patellar articulation with the femoral trochlear groove that is necessary to accurately visualize patellar tracking abnormalities).[2,4] This movement of the patellofemoral joint can only be accomplished appropriately with the patient in a prone or supine position. Placement of the patient on his or her side in a lateral position for kinematic MRI of the patellofemoral joint prevents rotational movements of the lower extremity and will adversely influence patellofemoral joint kinematics.[2] Accordingly, the diagnostic capability of the kinematic MRI examination is impaired.

Positioning devices may incorporate surface radiofrequency (RF) coils to facilitate imaging of the joints and may be used to apply a resistance or to load the joint during kinematic MRI. Resistance or load is imposed using various types of mechanisms including elastic bands, vacuum or pneumatic techniques, and friction methods. Interestingly, there are now devices designed to impose axial loading on supine patients undergoing MRI to obtain a functional assessment of the spine. Several commercially available positioning devices have been developed for kinematic MRI in consideration of the above-mentioned important factors including those from Chamco (Cocoa, FL), Captain Plastic (Seattle, WA), Medrad (Pittsburgh, PA), General Electric Medical Systems (Milwaukee, WI), and Portal Inc (North Logan, UT).

Assessment of Kinematic Magnetic Resonance Imaging Examinations

MR images obtained using kinematic MRI techniques may be visualized as individual, static images or displayed as a cine-loop.[2-4] Visualization of the MR images as a cine-loop involves using the basic software provided with the MR system to produce a forward-and-backward "paging" format of the multiple images obtained at a single section location for a given range of motion. Display of the images acquired for the kinematic MRI procedure in this manner facilitates the rapid viewing of multiple images that are usually obtained at the different section locations of the joint that is being evaluated.[2-4]

Compared with viewing individual static images of the kinematic MRI study, the cine-loop display is considered to provide the best diagnostic information regarding the joint with respect to the various patterns of normal or abnormal motions that may exist.[2-4] This is particularly important for cases where the kinematic-related abnormality may be subtle. Furthermore, making recordings (i.e., using video tapes, CDs, DVD or MPEG files) of the kinematic MRI cine-loops enables the examinations to be easily maintained as permanent records for the imaging facility and to be sent to the referring physicians so that they can view the studies and share the findings with their patients.

The kinematic MRI examination is usually evaluated using qualitative criteria developed and applied in consideration of the specific biomechanical aspects of the joint with regard to the interactions between soft-tissue structures and osseous anatomy that occur during a given range of motion.[2-4] This information will be further discussed below for the various joints.

TEMPOROMANDIBULAR JOINT

Internal derangement of the temporomandibular joint (TMJ) occurs in a high percentage of the adult population and is associated with marked pain and functional abnormalities.[71-73] Thus, identification and characterization of TMJ disorders are of great interest, particularly since objective documentation of internal derangement is often required by third-party payers before long-term therapy or surgical intervention is approved. Compared to other radiographic techniques, MRI is unsurpassed for depicting the important soft-tissue and osseous components of the TMJ including the disk, mandibular condyle, glenoid fossa, articular eminence, hyaline cartilage, marrow, and associated muscular structures.[9,10,71-73]

Initially, the inability to obtain a functional assessment of jaw biomechanics and disk-condyle complex co-ordination was considered to be a limitation of MRI. Fortunately, Burnett et al[8] developed a kinematic MRI technique to examine the function of the TMJ. With further refinements of kinematic MRI methodology,[9,10,72] this imaging application emerged as a routine method of determining the functional aspects of this joint.

A comprehensive diagnostic imaging evaluation of the patient with TMJ dysfunction is currently accomplished using static view and kinematic MRI procedures to obtain both anatomic and functional information. This has proven to be extremely valuable in the examination and characterization of TMJ abnormalities.[9,10,72,74]

Protocol

Most kinematic MRI investigations of the TMJ have been accomplished using the incremental, passive positioning technique. Various types of positioning devices may be used for this kinematic MRI procedure, whereby the goal is to open the mouth in specific, predetermined increments.[2-4,9,10] Dental wedges, bite blocks, a patient-activated incrementing device, and a hydraulic jaw opener have all been utilized for this purpose.[2]

The most widely used, commercially available apparatus for kinematic MRI is the Burnett TMJ Positioning Device (Medrad, Pittsburgh, PA).[8] This plastic device has a ratchet and gearing mechanism that allows 1 mm incremental opening or closing of its "jaws" when the handle is depressed (Fig. 98-1). The Burnett TMJ Positioning Device was designed to be operated by the patient while inside the MR system.[8]

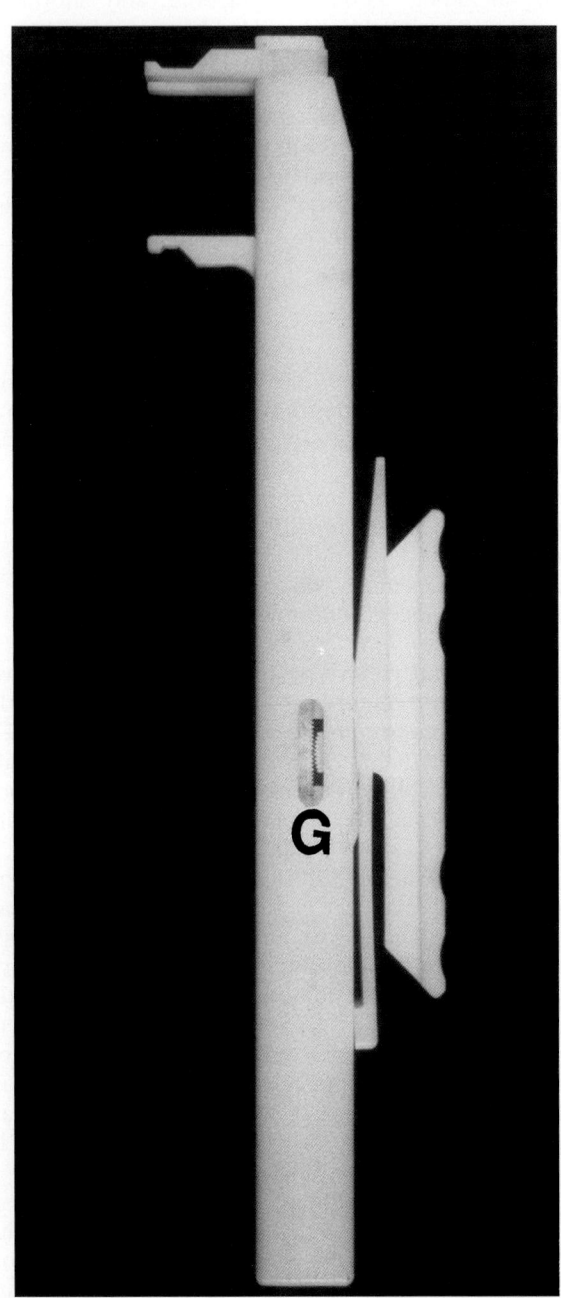

FIGURE 98-1

Positioning device used to perform kinematic MRI examination of the TMJ using the incremental, passive positioning technique (Burnett TMJ Positioning Device, Medrad Inc, Pittsburgh, PA). Movement of the device is controlled by the patient using the handle mechanism. A gauge (G) indicates the relative extent of mouth opening. This device has disposable mouthpieces. *(Reprinted with permission from Shellock FG, Powers CM: Kinematic MRI of the Joints: Functional Anatomy, Kinesiology, and Clinical Applications. Boca Raton, FL: CRC Press, 2001. © FG Shellock, 2001.)*

Because the degree of mouth opening is different for each patient, the range of motion must be determined using the Burnett TMJ Positioning Device prior to the kinematic MRI examination. The fully closed device (i.e., the "start" position) is placed into the patient's mouth and then opened incrementally until the fully opened mouth position is reached. This is done without forcing the joint or causing pain. The millimeter incrementing gauge on the positioning device indicates the extent of the range of motion for the patient. Information pertaining to the patient's range of motion is used to guide the kinematic MRI examination.

Obtaining high-resolution detail of the anatomy of the TMJ is crucial for an optimal evaluation.[2,10,71-74] Acquisition of MR images with a high signal-to-noise ratio is accomplished using a surface or local RF coil. Obviously, the position of the TMJ is ideally suited for surface RF coil imaging because the anatomy of interest is located close to the skin in a confined area.

For static view or kinematic MRI examinations of the TMJ, a 3-inch circular or loop surface RF coil is typically used, centering the coil slightly anterior to the external auditory canal. Alternatively, since the TMJ is easily palpated, an open-configured surface coil may be centered on the anatomic region of interest, making this a technically simple procedure to perform.[72]

Since there is a bilateral articulation with the cranium, the right and left TMJ articulations must function together. Therefore, it is not surprising that there is a high incidence of bilateral abnormalities in patients with TMJ disorders.[72] Even though the patient may only present with unilateral symptoms, each TMJ is affected by the contralateral side. Thus, a thorough assessment of the patient for TMJ dysfunction requires MR imaging of both joints.

From an examination time consideration, it is advisable to perform MRI on both joints simultaneously. Furthermore, for the kinematic MRI examination, simultaneous imaging of bilateral TMJs permits MR images to be obtained for a direct comparison between the joints at the same relative degree of mouth opening. Side-to-side differences in translation or asymmetrical motion of the TMJ may be optimally visualized utilizing this technique.[2,4,9,10]

Simultaneous, bilateral MR imaging of the TMJ can be accomplished easily using various types of coil configurations including:

1. dual 3-inch, circular surface coils
2. phased-array coils
3. a quadrature head coil.

Because unwanted patient motion during MRI is problematic from an image quality consideration, a variety of commercially available coil holders and patient stabilization systems have been developed and are recommended for use during static view and kinematic MRI procedures.

The TMJ consists of tissues with mostly short T2 times.[71,72] Therefore, it is best to use pulse sequences with short echo times (short TEs) when imaging the TMJ to properly visualize anatomic details. The repetition time (TR) is not as critical insofar as MR images obtained using either T1-weighted (i.e., short TE, short TR) or proton density-weighted (i.e., short TE, long TR) sequences will provide acceptable tissue contrast characteristics for proper assessment of this joint.[2,4,9,10,71,72]

For the kinematic MRI study, images are typically obtained using a T1-weighted, spin-echo pulse sequence to best depict the disk-condyle complex through the range of motion of this joint. Partial flip angle or gradient-echo pulse sequences have also been used for kinematic MRI but these techniques have intrinsically poor contrast and are more susceptible to artifacts when metallic implants or dental appliances are present. Furthermore, since the kinematic MRI examination is routinely performed using an incremental, passive positioning technique, there is no justification for using a gradient-echo pulse sequence over a T1-weighted, spin-echo sequence when one considers the relative small amount of time that is "saved".

The kinematic MRI procedure begins by acquiring images in the axial plane that are used to show the relative orientation of the mandibular condyles. The mandibular condyles are generally positioned at oblique angles in both the sagittal and coronal planes. Investigations have demonstrated that the best orientation for images of the TMJ is with reference to the long axis of the condylar head because a significant number of both normal individuals and patients have abnormally configured condyles. Therefore, section locations used for kinematic MRI of the TMJ should be selected perpendicular (i.e., oblique sagittals) to the long axis of the condylar head, as viewed on the axial plane localizer scan (Fig. 98-2). This permits

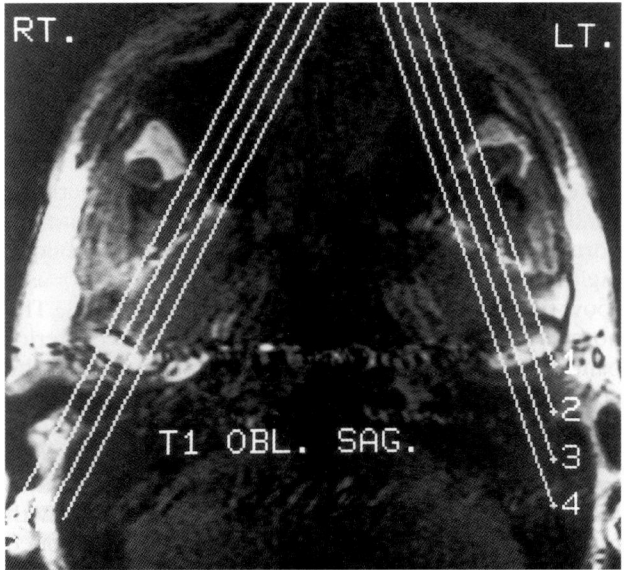

FIGURE 98-2

T1-weighted spin-echo, axial plane localizer (TR/TE, 400/20 ms; slice thickness, 5 mm) used to obtain section locations oriented perpendicular to the condylar heads to obtain oblique sagittal plane images. Note the areas of lateral high signal intensity resulting from the dual 3" surface coils used for this examination. *(Reprinted with permission from Shellock FG, Powers CM: Kinematic MRI of the Joints: Functional Anatomy, Kinesiology, and Clinical Applications. Boca Raton, FL: CRC Press, 2001. © FG Shellock, 2001.)*

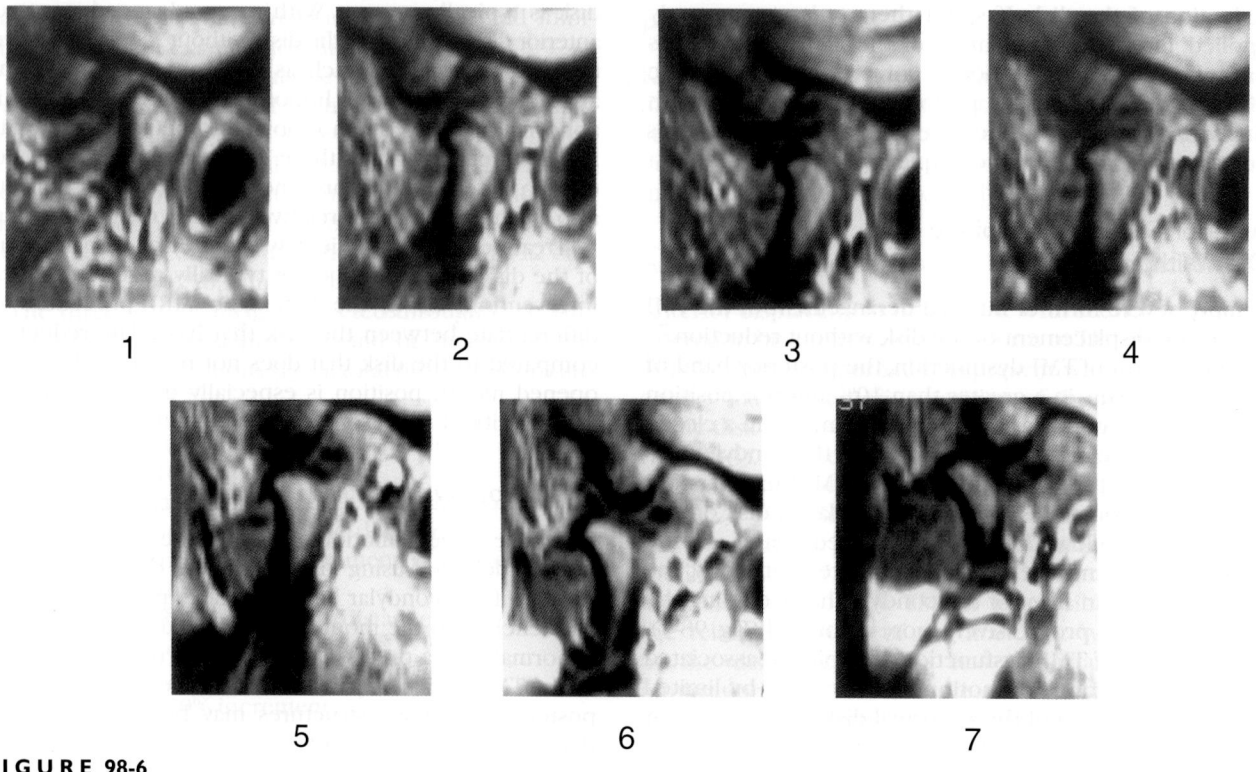

FIGURE 98-6

Hypermobile TMJ and anterior displacement of the disk with reduction. MR images obtained in oblique sagittal plane using a T1-weighted, spin-echo pulse sequence. This kinematic MRI examination shows anterior displacement of the disk relative to the condylar head in the closed-mouth view (1). The disk is recaptured early (2, the condylar head moves onto the intermediate zone), as the mouth incrementally opens and the condyle translates anteriorly (2-7). Notably, the condylar head translates beyond the articular eminence (7, fully opened mouth view), indicating a hypermobile TMJ. This condition predisposes to internal derangement. *(Reprinted with permission from Shellock FG, Powers CM: Kinematic MRI of the Joints: Functional Anatomy, Kinesiology, and Clinical Applications. Boca Raton, FL: CRC Press, 2001. © FG Shellock, 2001.)*

Asymmetric Motion

Because the mandible has a bilateral articulation with the cranium, both TMJs should function synchronously. As the mouth opens, both condylar heads should initially rotate then translate anteriorly. Thus, this movement pattern should occur for both TMJs, simultaneously. Any disordered, asynchronous movement comparing the right TMJ to the left TMJ is regarded as an abnormality. Asymmetric motion may be associated with lateral deviation of the mandible as the mouth opens or other more unusual or complex movements.[2-4] For example, there may be progressive anterior translation of one condyle as the mouth opens, while the other condyle remains in a fixed position or moves in a retrograde manner. To identify and characterize asymmetric motion, it is necessary to perform kinematic MRI using the simultaneous, bilateral imaging technique.

PATELLOFEMORAL JOINT

Abnormalities of the patellofemoral joint are a primary cause of pain and functional instability.[77-82] Imperfect congruence between the patella and femoral trochlear groove is the main causative mechanism responsible for patellofemoral pain. Patellar malalignment and abnor-

mal tracking are believed to produce significant shearing forces and excessive contact stress that cause degeneration of the articular cartilage.[78,79] Chronic patellar displacement also may change the load distribution in the patellofemoral joint, producing pain in the absence of a detectable cartilage defect.

The detection and characterization of patellofemoral joint abnormalities by physical examination are often difficult because the associated symptoms may mimic internal derangement of the knee and co-existing pathologic conditions are common. Patients with persistent symptoms following patellar realignment surgery present a particular challenge. Because identification of abnormal patellofemoral relationships is known to be crucial for proper treatment decisions, diagnostic imaging has played an important role in the evaluation of patients with patellofemoral pain.[2-7]

Abnormal patellar alignment and tracking typically exist during the earliest portion of the range of motion (e.g., <20°), as the patella enters and begins to articulate with the femoral trochlear groove.[77] As flexion increases, the patella moves deeper into the femoral trochlear groove. Within this anatomic area, patellar displacement is less likely to occur because the osseous anatomy of the trochlear groove functions to buttress and stabilize the patella.[2-7,77]

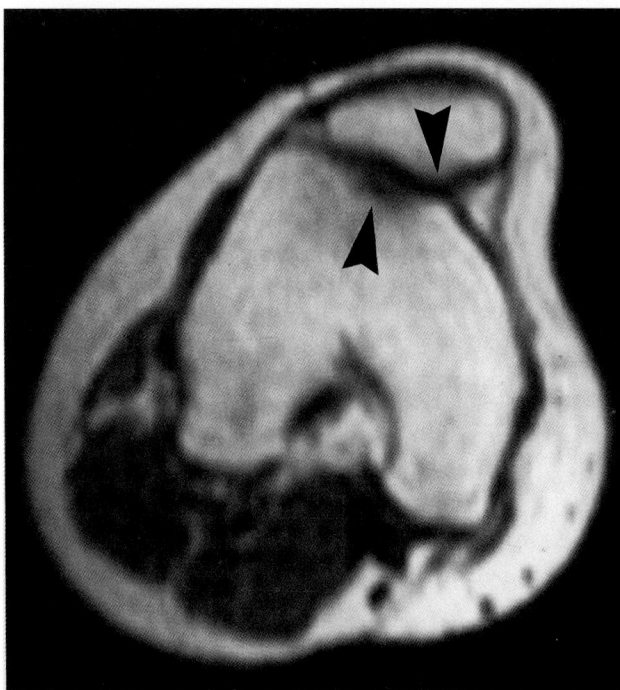

FIGURE 98-10

MR image acquired during kinematic MRI examination using the incremental, passive positioning technique (axial plane; T1-weighted, spin-echo) showing example of medial subluxation of the patella. Note the substantial medial displacement of the patellar median ridge relative to the femoral trochlear groove (arrowheads). (Reprinted with permission from Shellock FG, Powers CM: Kinematic MRI of the Joints: Functional Anatomy, Kinesiology, and Clinical Applications. Boca Raton, FL: CRC Press, 2001. © FG Shellock, 2001.)

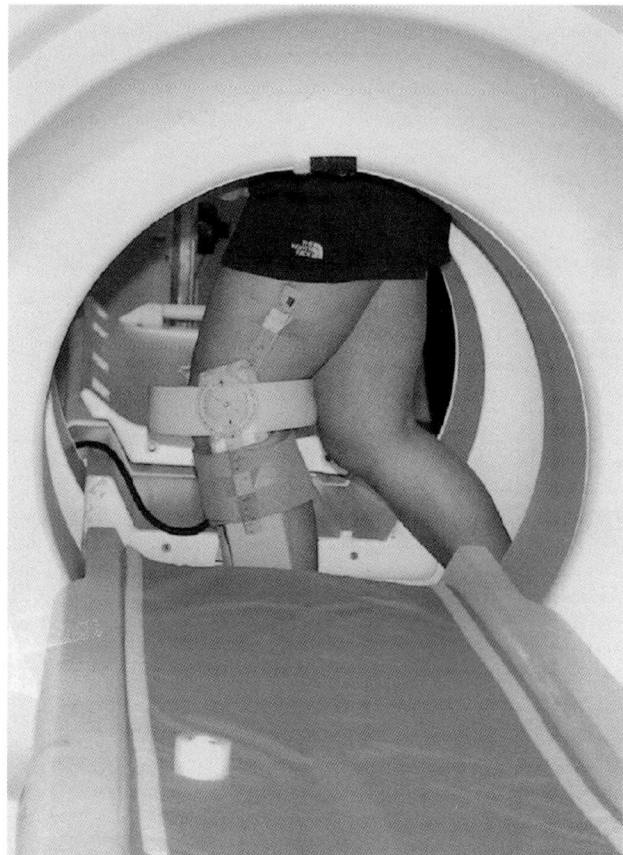

FIGURE 98-11

Use of the vertically opened MR system (0.5 tesla, Signa SP, General Electric Medical Systems, Milwaukee, WI) for upright, loaded kinematic MRI examination, showing the flexible transmit-receive RF coil used for this procedure. (Reprinted with permission from Shellock FG, Powers CM: Kinematic MRI of the Joints: Functional Anatomy, Kinesiology, and Clinical Applications. Boca Raton, FL: CRC Press, 2001. © FG Shellock, 2001.)

Besides being used in the initial diagnostic evaluation of the patellofemoral joint, kinematic MRI has been applied to assess the effect of conservative treatments and surgical interventions on patellofemoral relationships. Additionally, for patients with persistent symptoms following surgery, this diagnostic imaging technique has been reported to be beneficial for assessment of problematic cases. For example, symptomatic patients following lateral retinacular release were found to have unresolved patellar malalignment as demonstrated by kinematic MRI.[2,12]

When a conservative treatment like bracing or taping is used, it is advantageous to immediately determine if there has been improvement in patellar displacement. Otherwise, valuable time may be wasted or, more importantly, unwanted cartilage contact stress may be induced that creates another problem for the patient (e.g., if bracing or taping moves the patella in an unacceptable manner). Theoretically, the function of bracing is to reduce the displaced patella, with secondary functions that include providing warmth to the tissues, changing tension of soft-tissue structures, and reducing sensations of joint instability. Various investigations have used kinematic MRI to examine the effect of bracing on patellofemoral relationships.[21,50,33,34,40] Kinematic MRI may be used effectively in a timely manner to obtain objective findings regarding whether or not bracing is successful in treating subluxation of the patella.

Assessment During Closed-Chain Weight Bearing

Recently, an investigation designed to assess the patellofemoral joint during open-chain (i.e., with the foot off the ground, the tibia moving "freely") and closed-chain (i.e., with the foot on the ground, the tibia "fixed" during weight-bearing movement) activities was conducted.[2] To accomplish this, a vertically opened MR system (0.5 tesla, Signa SP, General Electric Medical Systems, Milwaukee, WI) was used that permits the patient to undergo dynamic MR imaging (i.e., using a fast spoiled gradient-echo pulse sequence) in upright (closed-chain activity) and seated (open-chain activity) positions (Fig. 98-11). Results indicated that patellar tracking is qualitatively different, with abnormalities demonstrated in a more profound manner by the open-chain activity.

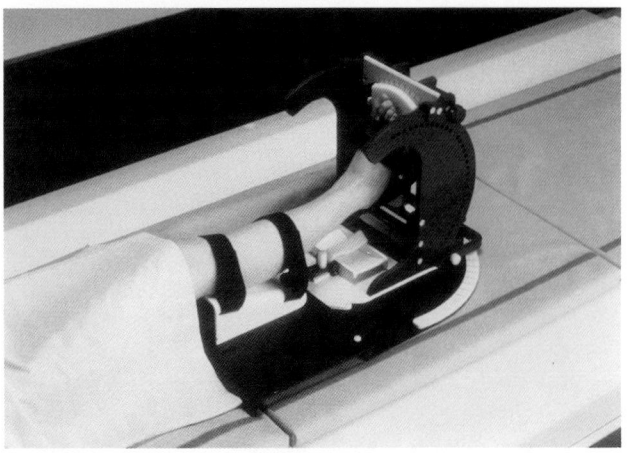

FIGURE 98-12

Positioning device designed to allow single or combined incremental positions of the ankle (General Electric Medical Systems, Milwaukee, WI). This positioning device is typically used with a circumferential, receive-only surface coil. *(Reprinted with permission from Shellock FG, Powers CM: Kinematic MRI of the Joints: Functional Anatomy, Kinesiology, and Clinical Applications. Boca Raton, FL: CRC Press, 2001. © FG Shellock, 2001.)*

ANKLE

Despite the initial description in 1990 by Shellock and Mandelbaum,[3] kinematic MRI of the ankle has not become a common part of the diagnostic imager's armamentarium of clinical studies. This is surprising, since the ankle is prone to a variety of derangements that might best be evaluated by such a unique diagnostic method. Reports suggest that kinematic MR imaging helps provide a more thorough examination of the ankle, particularly in cases of functional abnormalities associated with bony subluxations or soft-tissue impingement.[2,4,42-44] A recent review by Terk[44] described the important aspects of kinematic MRI techniques applied to the ankle.

Protocol

A variety of positioning devices have been developed for kinematic MRI of the ankle.[2] In general, they all allow a reproducible range of motion and control the movement of the ankle (Fig. 98-12). The small size and complex anatomy of the ankle make high-resolution kinematic MR views essential for optimal examination of this joint. Therefore, the positioning apparatus must be able to incorporate a RF coil to permit the signal-to-noise ratio necessary for MR imaging of the ankle. RF coils shown to be useful for kinematic MRI of the ankle include dual 5-inch, flexible, circular (circumferential), and dedicated-extremity RF coils. The positioning device should also permit acquisition of both static high-resolution MRI views and kinematic MRI studies without the need for an equipment change.

T1-weighted or proton density-weighted images provide good anatomic visualization of the anatomic features of the ankle and may be acquired in a relatively rapid manner if some compromises are made to resolution and/or signal to noise. With the reduction of inter-echo spacing, T1-weighted, fast spin-echo images have become practical with substantial reductions in acquisition time or increases in resolution. Gradient-echo, spoiled gradient-echo, and "fast" versions of these pulse sequences may also be used if greater speed is desired or required.

The appropriate plane for kinematic MRI of the ankle may be selected based on the anatomic structure or the pathologic feature being evaluated. For example, the axial plane should be selected for investigation of peroneal tendon subluxation, while the sagittal plane better demonstrates anterior impingement or osseous syndromes with plantarflexion and dorsiflexion of the ankle.[2,44] Alternatively, if inversion and eversion are to be studied (e.g., for assessment of subtalar instability or assessment of lateral and medial soft-tissues), the coronal plane of imaging tends to be most suitable.

Clinical Applications

While many abnormal ankle conditions can be effectively demonstrated by static-view MR imaging,[2-4,42-44] it is evident that abnormalities that are position dependent or that may only be detected transiently (e.g., peroneal tendon subluxation, impingement syndromes, subtalar instability, etc.), lend themselves to evaluation by kinematic MRI.

Peroneal Tendon Subluxation

In the case of peroneal tendon subluxation, the positional abnormality may be transient and not observable with static imaging techniques. There are two main anatomic abnormalities that predispose these tendons to subluxation: a deficiency of the peroneal retinaculum and a convex or shallow posterior surface of the fibula forming the peroneal groove.[44] While these abnormalities are, at times, detectable with static imaging, they are frequently difficult to image or, if present, may not be related to symptomatic subluxation. It is the very transient nature of peroneal subluxation that makes kinematic MRI of the ankle a useful examination in the detection of this condition (Fig. 98-13).[2,44]

The presence of peroneal tendon subluxation may have associated serious sequelae. If this abnormality is not repaired or treated in the early stages following injury, there is a poor long-term prognosis. Therefore, a rapid and accurate diagnosis of this condition is critical for appropriate patient management.

Repaired Achilles Tendon

Kinematic MRI of the ankle has been used to assess the Achilles tendon after surgical repair.[2] Imaging is typically performed in the mid-sagittal plane, with the ankle dorsiflexed to apply "stress" to this tendon.

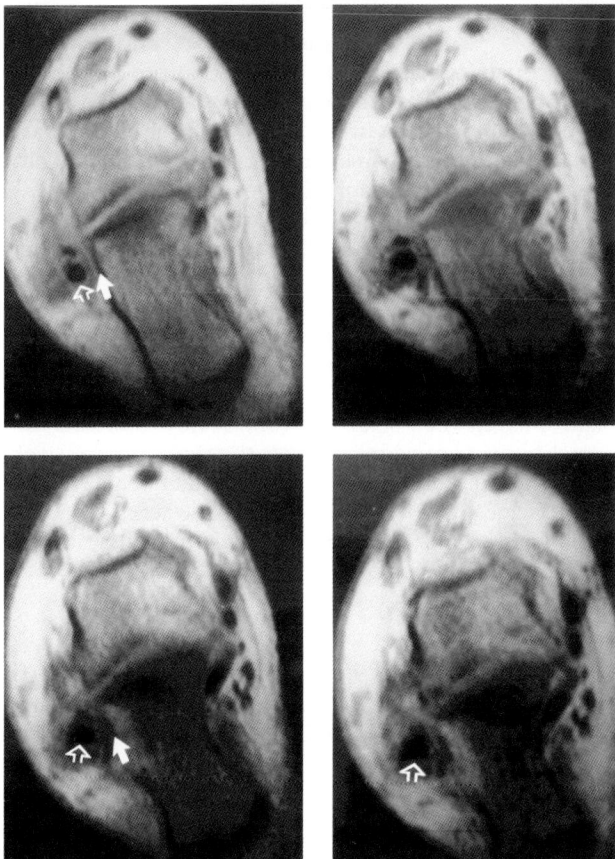

FIGURE 98-13

Kinematic MRI examination of the ankle in dorsiflexion *(left, upper image)*, neutral *(right, upper image)*, partial plantarflexion *(left, bottom image)*, and full plantarflexion *(right, bottom image)* positions using incremental, passive positioning technique (axial plane, fast spoiled gradient-echo). Lateral subluxation of the abnormally enlarged peroneus longus *(open arrow)* relative to the lateral border of the calcaneus can be seen on the successive, incremental images. *(Reprinted with permission from Shellock FG, Powers CM: Kinematic MRI of the Joints: Functional Anatomy, Kinesiology, and Clinical Applications. Boca Raton, FL: CRC Press, 2001. © FG Shellock, 2001.)*

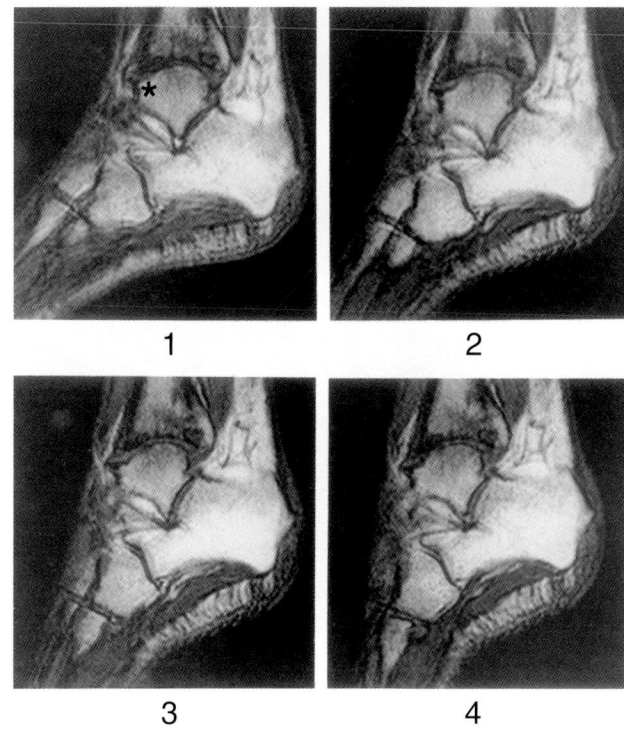

FIGURE 98-14

Kinematic MRI examination of the ankle in dorsiflexion (1), neutral (2), partial plantarflexion (3), and full plantarflexion (4) (sagittal plane, fast spoiled gradient-echo pulse sequence). There is osseous impingement resulting from the presence of an osteophyte (1, *asterisk*) that prevents proper movement into the dorsiflexion position. This disorder would go undetected using routine MRI of the ankle because it is position dependent. *(Reprinted with permission from Shellock FG, Powers CM: Kinematic MRI of the Joints: Functional Anatomy, Kinesiology, and Clinical Applications. Boca Raton, FL: CRC Press, 2001. © FG Shellock, 2001.)*

Impingement Syndromes

Previously, it was believed that impingement syndromes of the ankle were caused primarily by osseous structures, such as an osteophyte on the anterior aspect of the tibia impacting with the talus during dorsiflexion. However, soft-tissue impingement syndromes associated with plantarflexion-inversion injuries of the ankle also have been described. These abnormalities frequently result in a loss in range of motion.[2] The ability to view the process of impingement syndromes using kinematic MRI offers hope for a better understanding of these clinical entities (Fig. 98-14).

Osteochondral Defects and Loose Bodies

Osteochondral defects of the talus are thought to result from impaction of the talus on the tibia during transient instability of the ankle. With osteochondral injuries, there may be a situation where a fragment is either loose within the donor site or moves freely within the joint space. This diagnosis can be made using kinematic MRI of the ankle.[2,43]

WRIST

The combination of static-view MR imaging with kinematic MRI of the wrist offers an extremely effective diagnostic means of evaluating this joint. Kinematic MRI has been applied in a variety of ways to examine the function of the wrist.[2,3,7,45-48] Reeder[47] recently provided a thorough review of this topic. To date, these kinematic examination procedures have been reported to be useful for detection of subtle abnormalities of carpal motion, instability patterns, transitory subluxation, and other conditions that are not seen using routine static-view MR imaging.[2,3,7,45-48] Thus, to improve the diagnostic yield of MRI of the wrist, a kinematic MRI procedure should be utilized to assist in identifying additional conditions that affect this joint.

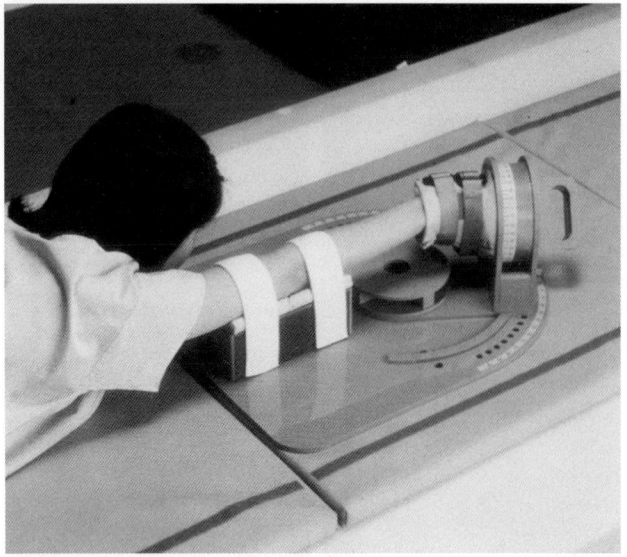

FIGURE 98-15

Positioning device designed for incremental positions of the wrist (General Electric Medical Systems, Milwaukee, WI). This device supports and stabilizes the upper extremity and permits progressive movements of the wrist through single or multiple ranges of motions. A circumferential receive-only surface coil is typically used with this positioning device. (Reprinted with permission from Shellock FG, Powers CM: Kinematic MRI of the Joints: Functional Anatomy, Kinesiology, and Clinical Applications. Boca Raton, FL: CRC Press, 2001. © FG Shellock, 2001.)

Protocol

The use of an MR-compatible positioning device is crucial for standardized, repeatable kinematic MRI examinations of the wrist. Several different types of commercially available positioning devices have been developed for this kinematic MRI application (Fig. 98-15). The small size of the wrist makes it necessary to use a RF coil to obtain adequate signal-to-noise ratio for the small field of view and high-resolution images necessary for the kinematic MRI examination. RF coils used for kinematic MRI studies include single or dual 3- or 5-inch receive-only, circular surface coils, flexible, wrap-around coils or transmit/receive extremity coils.[2,3,7] Furthermore, it is advantageous to employ the same RF coil equipment to obtain high-resolution MR images, thus combining static-view and kinematic MRI examinations to acquire a comprehensive view of the wrist.

Since it is currently not possible to rapidly obtain MR images using imaging parameters that provide the high signal-to-noise ratio required to assess the wrist dynamically, an incremental, passive positioning kinematic MRI technique is typically used to examine this joint.[2,3,7] In general, using this technique, the wrist is incrementally moved using the positioning device at specific intervals through a specified range of motion, in a given plane of interest.

A variety of pulse sequences are acceptable for the incremental, passive positioning kinematic MRI technique, including conventional T1-weighted or T2-weighted spin-echo, T1-weighted or T2-weighted fast spin-echo, gradient-echo or fast gradient-echo pulse sequences.[2,3,7,45-48] Obviously, the selection of the specific imaging parameters used to evaluate the wrist is highly dependent on the suspected or known pathology or abnormality that is present. A small section thickness (e.g., 2 to 4 mm) and small field of view (e.g., 8 to 10 cm) are also a requirement for this procedure.

With regard to the plane of imaging, adjustments need to be made based on the anatomy and abnormality that is being assessed. For example, to evaluate distal radioulnar joint instability, axial plane images of the distal radioulnar joint are acquired with the wrist incrementally placed into pronation and supination. To examine carpal instability or impingement syndromes, coronal plane images (i.e., selected from a view showing the carpal bones) are acquired with the wrist progressively moved in radial and ulnar deviation. Additionally, sagittal plane images may be obtained with the wrist placed in flexion and extension and in radial and ulnar deviation to identify instability patterns.

Clinical Applications

Distal Radioulnar Joint Instability

The kinematic MRI application for assessment of the distal radioulnar joint instability has been described by Reeder.[47] A tear of the volar distal radioulnar ligament, typically a result of hyperpronation, results in dorsal dislocation of the ulna relative to the distal radius. Distal radioulnar joint injuries may also involve the extensor carpi ulnaris tendon located within the dorsal groove of the distal ulna.

To evaluate distal radioulnar relationships using kinematic MRI, axial plane images are obtained during progressive rotation of the wrist at specific intervals from pronation to supination.[47] Although static-view MR imaging may adequately allow detection and characterization of tears and tenosynovitis of the extensor carpi ulnaris tendon, the kinematic MRI examination improves the sensitivity of identifying tendon subluxation because this finding is frequently dependent upon the rotational position of the wrist.

Carpal Instability

Carpal instability patterns have been classified as either static or dynamic.[2,45,47] Static instabilities are typically recognizable on conventional radiographs because of fixed carpal malalignment. Assessment of dynamic instabilities may require a particular stress or movement to produce symptoms associated with abnormal carpal orientation. Kinematic MRI techniques can be applied to the evaluation of both static and dynamic carpal instabilities, with imaging performed during the relevant wrist movements in the coronal and/or sagittal plane.

Scapholunate and Lunotriquetral Ligament Tears

A tear of the scapholunate ligament is frequently associated with both static and dynamic carpal instability.

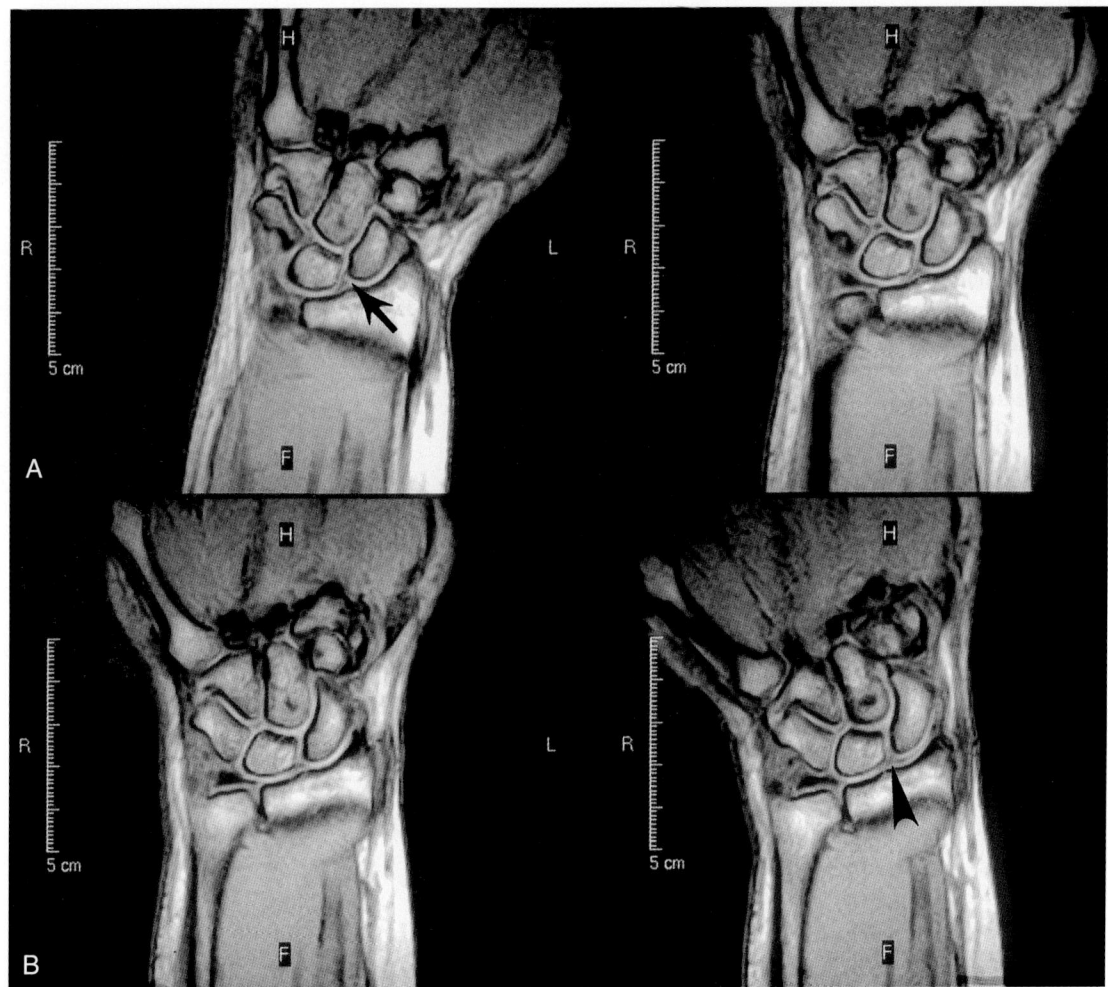

FIGURE 98-16

Kinematic MRI of the wrist performed using coronal plane imaging (gradient-echo pulse sequence) with passive, incremental movements. This example shows a scapholunate ligament tear. With the wrist in radial deviation, the scapholunate distance appears normal (**A,** *upper left image, arrow*). As the wrist moves towards ulnar deviation, the scapholunate joint widens (**B,** *lower right image, arrowhead*), indicating a tear of the scapholunate ligament and resultant scapholunate instability. *(Reprinted with permission from Shellock FG, Powers CM: Kinematic MRI of the Joints: Functional Anatomy, Kinesiology, and Clinical Applications. Boca Raton, FL: CRC Press, 2001. © FG Shellock, 2001.)*

In the absence of a fixed rotational subluxation of the scaphoid, conventional radiographs remain normal. High-resolution, small field-of-view, MR imaging techniques have improved the detection of scapholunate ligament tears but kinematic MRI improves sensitivity by imaging during the application of a tensile stress applied to the ligament.[45-47]

Coronal plane kinematic MRI is performed at the level of the scapholunate joint while moving from progressive radial to ulnar deviation. Normally, the scaphoid and lunate bones move together, with the intercarpal distance remaining constant. In the presence of a scapholunate ligament tear or pathologic ligamentous laxity, a dynamic scapholunate diastasis develops as tensile stress increases during ulnar deviation (Fig. 98-16). Radial deviation of the wrist applies tensile stress to the lunotriquetral ligament, thereby improving the probability of detect-

ing lunotriquetral ligament tears and laxity with kinematic MRI.[46,47]

Additionally, close attention to intercarpal spacing on coronal plane images with the wrist positioned from radial to ulnar deviation may provide evidence of an abnormality. Spacing should be evenly distributed between the carpal bones, without any significant or uneven intercarpal widening, proximal or distal movement, or anterior or posterior displacement of the carpal bones.

Ulnolunate Impaction Syndrome

Coronal plane images obtained using kinematic MRI techniques during examination of radial and ulnar deviation of the wrist also contribute to the evaluation of ulnolunate impaction syndrome.[47] Ulnolunate impaction syndrome is typically associated with positive ulnar variance and patients present with a history of pain involving the ulnar aspect of the wrist. Abnormal compressive forces transmitted from the distal ulna to the lunate and triquetrum result in the development of secondary osteoarthritis and chondromalacia.

Furthermore, coronal plane kinematic MR images acquired during radial and ulnar deviation permit detection of abnormal ulnocarpal abutment prior to the development of the irreversible structural findings that are evident on static MRI views. Documenting the resolution of an abnormal dynamic ulnocarpal relationship following ulnar-shortening osteotomy or ulnar head resection is an additional application for kinematic MRI of the wrist.[47]

CERVICAL SPINE

According to the recent comprehensive review by Karju and Koskinen,[57] a valuable functional assessment of the cervical spine may be conducted using kinematic MRI techniques. Since there may be a significant change in spinal canal and cord compression during flexion and extension of the cervical spine, kinematic MRI is especially useful for further assessment of the cervical spine during these movements.[49-58] Importantly, common abnormalities that may affect this anatomic region may go undetected using routine static-view MR imaging. The primary reason for this is because the cervical spine is typically imaged with the patient's neck in a comfortable, neutral position; however, certain disorders are position dependent. Thus, to improve the diagnostic yield of MRI, it may be necessary to assess the cervical spine using a kinematic MRI procedure.[49-56,58] Kinematic MRI is capable of showing the relationship between the odontoid, foramen magnum, spinal cord, and other related anatomic structures as the patient's cervical spine is moved through a given range of motion.[49-58]

Protocol

Various positioning devices are available for kinematic MRI of the cervical spine that permit studies to be accomplished during flexion and extension, side-bending, rotation, or a combination of movements (Fig. 98-17).[49-58] The complex anatomy of the cervical spine requires that the kinematic MRI examination be performed using a RF surface coil to obtain adequate signal-to-noise ratio for imaging. A variety of RF coil configurations have been used for kinematic MRI studies, including dual 5-inch receive-only circular surface coils, flexible wrap-around coils, and posterior neck coils. Furthermore, since high-resolution MR of images of the cervical spine are frequently needed in addition to the kinematic MRI examination, it is advantageous to use the same positioning device and RF coil equipment to eliminate the need to reposition the patient and unnecessarily lengthen the overall imaging procedure.

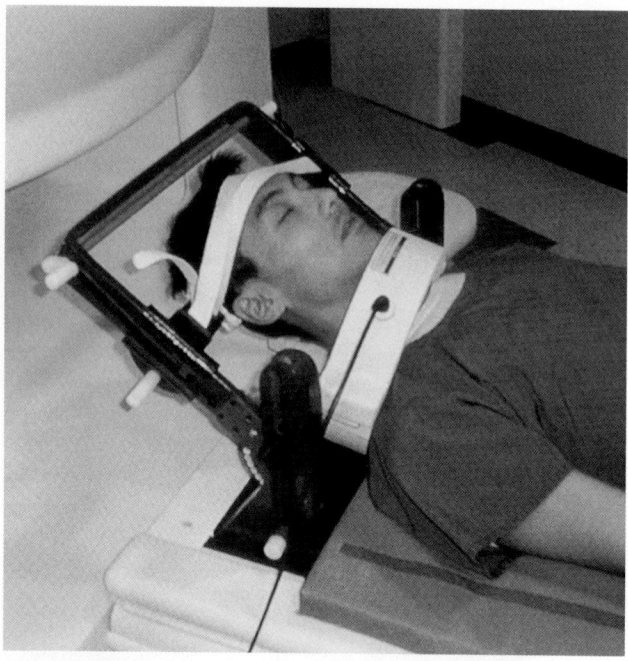

FIGURE 98-17

Positioning device designed for kinematic MRI of the cervical spine (General Electric Medical Systems, Milwaukee, WI). This device supports and stabilizes the subject's head and neck during the kinematic MRI examination. *(Reprinted with permission from Shellock FG, Powers CM: Kinematic MRI of the Joints: Functional Anatomy, Kinesiology, and Clinical Applications. Boca Raton, FL: CRC Press, 2001. © FG Shellock, 2001.)*

A variety of pulse sequences and protocols have been used for kinematic MRI of the cervical spine.[49-58] For example, T1-weighted, T2-weighted spin-echo, T2-weighted fast spin-echo, gradient-echo, fast gradient-echo, and echo-planar imaging parameters have been reportedly used for this procedure. However, T2-weighted, fast spin-echo imaging parameters selected to produce a "myelographic effect" are considered to be optimal for most kinematic MRI examinations.

The selection of specific imaging parameters for kinematic MRI is based on the desired image contrast and resolution necessary to assess the suspected cervical spine abnormality or disorder. Additionally, the temporal resolution of the imaging parameters must be considered with respect to the type of kinematic MRI procedure that is used. Kinematic MRI may be conducted using either an incremental, passive positioning or an active-movement (i.e., dynamic) technique.[57]

The major movements of the cervical spine that have been assessed using kinematic MRI techniques are flexion and extension (sagittal plane), side-bending (frontal or coronal plane), and rotation (axial plane).[49-58] If an abnormality is seen on a mid-sagittal plane image, obliqued axial plane images may be obtained through the area of affected anatomy, in the coronal plane during side-bending and in the axial plane during rotation. In general, the imaging plane used for the kinematic MRI procedure must be selected in consideration of the suspected pathology or condition that is present.

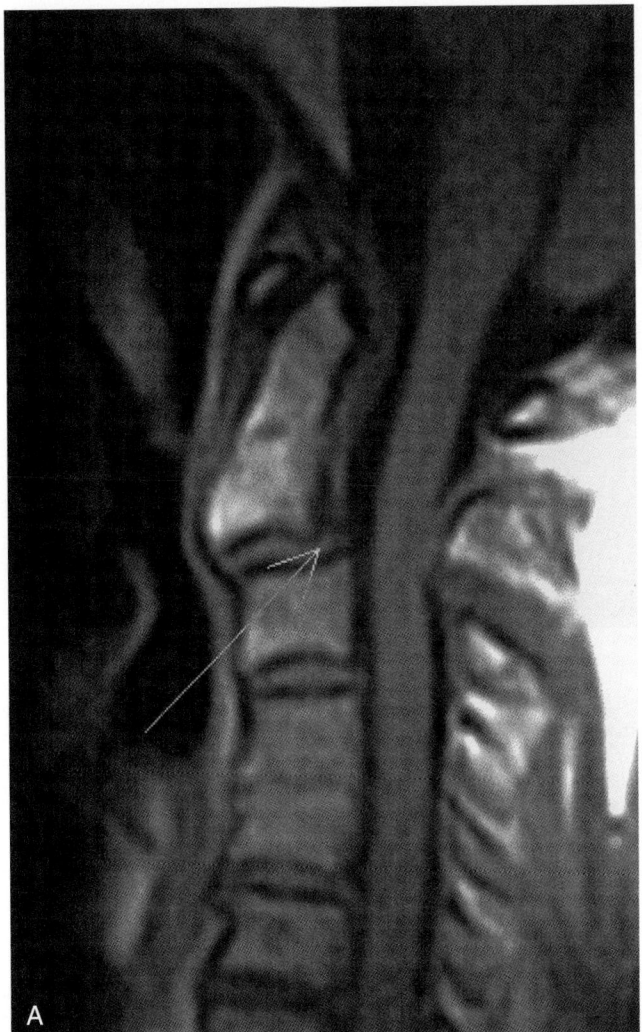
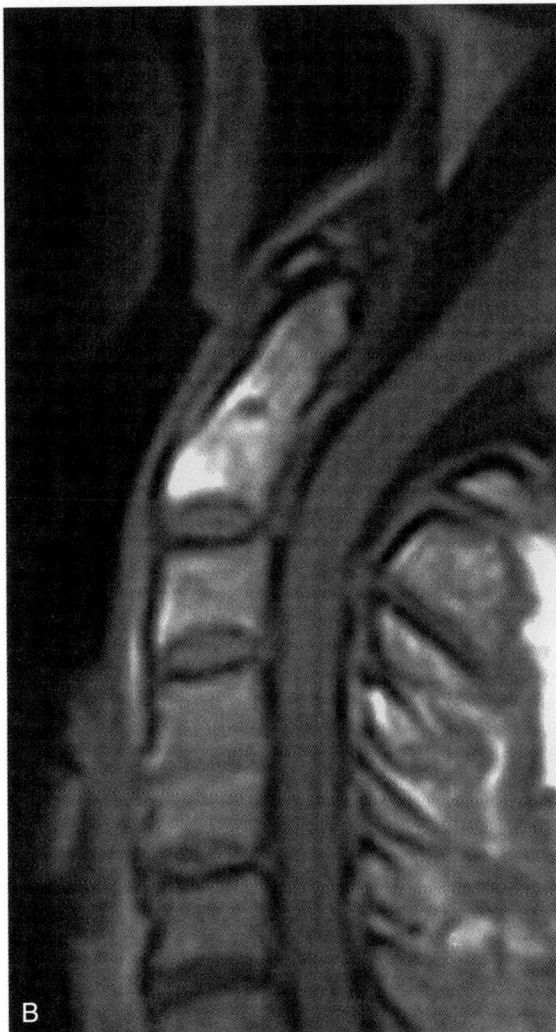

FIGURE 98-18

Kinematic MRI of the cervical spine performed in a patient with systemic lupus erythematosus and subaxial instability of the segment C2-C3. Subluxation of C2 *(arrow)* is evident in flexion (**A**), but not in extension (**B**). *(Reprinted with permission from Shellock FG, Powers CM: Kinematic MRI of the Joints: Functional Anatomy, Kinesiology, and Clinical Applications. Boca Raton, FL: CRC Press, 2001. © FG Shellock, 2001.)*

Clinical Applications

Knowledge of normal cervical spine anatomy, motion patterns, and ranges of motion forms the basis for interpreting kinematic MRI examinations of the cervical spine.[49-58] In general, kinematic MRI studies are usually analyzed qualitatively because quantitative parameters may have only limited diagnostic value.

Pathokinematics

The use of kinematic MRI contributes to a more thorough evaluation of the cervical spine in patients with abnormalities secondary to trauma, cervical spondylotic disease, and rheumatoid arthritis, as well as with other conditions.[49-58] Furthermore, kinematic MRI may provide critical information for staging disorders and planning conservative or surgical treatments of the cervical spine.[57]

Kinematic MRI of the cervical spine has been used to evaluate patients with cervical instabilities, rheumatoid arthritis, and cervical spondylotic disease as well as other abnormalities and disorders.[49-58] Kinematic MRI has also been applied to evaluate a patient diagnosed with os odontoideum. This is the most common form of odontoid anomaly and is associated with atlantoaxial instability. Additionally, instability due to post-traumatic pseudoarthrosis of the odontoid can be evaluated using kinematic MRI of the cervical spine.

Degenerative changes of the cervical spine, including loss of disk height, disk protrusion or herniation, foraminal stenosis, osteophytic formation, hypertrophy and buckling of the ligamentum flavum, and spondylolisthesis with possible segmental instability, may result in radicular compression or cervical myelopathy (Fig. 98-18).

Functional disorders of the cervical spine are often present in patients with rheumatoid arthritis. Kinematic

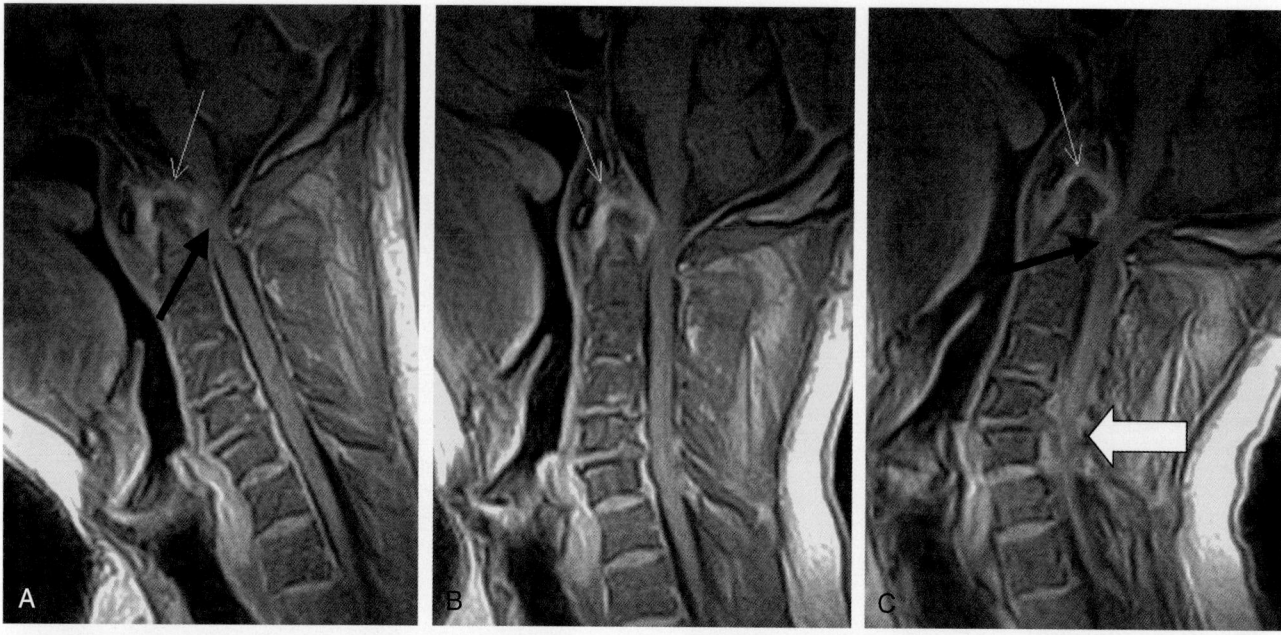

FIGURE 98-19

Kinematic MRI of the cervical spine obtained in a patient with rheumatoid arthritis using the contrast-enhanced technique. Enhancement of the inflammatory pannus tissue is seen around the dens *(white arrow)*. **A,** Flexion: the cord compression *(black arrow)* is caused by the pannus and atlantoaxial subluxation. **B,** Neutral position. **C,** Extension: the compression and distortion of the cord *(black arrow)* are even more evident than in flexion. There is also subaxial spinal stenosis at the C5-C6 level *(white block arrow)*. *(Reprinted with permission from Shellock FG, Powers CM: Kinematic MRI of the Joints: Functional Anatomy, Kinesiology, and Clinical Applications. Boca Raton, FL: CRC Press, 2001. © FG Shellock, 2001.)*

MRI is well suited to diagnose and stage the severity of these abnormalities. In patients with rheumatoid arthritis or other inflammatory diseases, the kinematic MRI study should optimally be performed using gadolinium enhancement (Fig. 98-19).

Evaluation of Treatment

Kinematic MRI of the cervical spine can influence the therapeutic or intraoperative management of patients with spondylotic myelopathy and radiculopathy associated with spinal stenosis.[57] Furthermore, this diagnostic procedure is considered to be particularly useful in the planning of stabilization and decompressive operations of the rheumatoid upper cervical spine.[57]

SHOULDER

The shoulder or glenohumeral (GH) joint permits a high degree of upper limb mobility, which is necessary to move the hand through space. Unfortunately, this aspect of the shoulder articulation sacrifices stability. As a result, the shoulder requires substantial muscle activity and ligamentous support to maintain its integrity and to move against resistance. The combination of a high degree of mobility, limited bony stability, and high muscular demand places the shoulder at risk for various injuries and joint pathology.

While static-view MR imaging is considered to be the noninvasive procedure of choice to evaluate abnormal shoulder conditions, especially with regard to identifying lesions of the rotator cuff and glenoid labrum, various abnormalities that are movement related are not optimally demonstrated using routine MR examinations. As such, kinematic MRI procedures have been developed to study the shoulder.[2,59-64]

Protocol

Kinematic MRI of the shoulder has been conducted using low-field, mid-field, high-field and, most recently, the 0.5 tesla, vertically opened MR system[2,59-64] (Figs. 98-20 and 98-21). Unfortunately, conventional "tunnel-configured" MR systems have limitations with regard to shoulder movements and, thus, kinematic MRI of the shoulder may only be used to examine internal and external rotation. By comparison, open-configured MR systems allow additional critical shoulder movements to be assessed, including abduction and adduction. However, these studies must be performed with the patient in a lying position, which may not be optimal with regard to evaluating physiologic loading of this joint. Importantly, the utilization of the vertically opened MR system to conduct kinematic MRI of the shoulder with the patient in an upright, seated position is believed to lead to a better understanding of the biomechanics of the shoulder.[62-64]

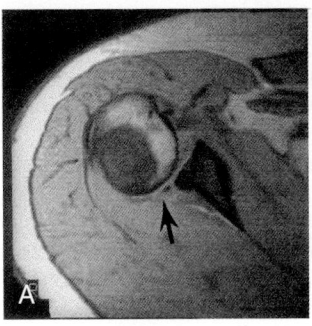
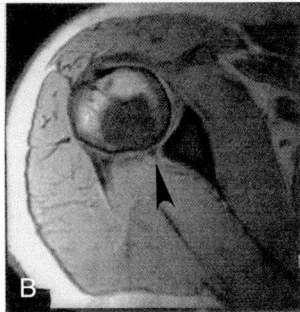

FIGURE 98-20

Glenohumeral instability demonstrated by kinematic MRI of the shoulder. This study was done using a conventional open MR system. Axial plane MR images were obtained using kinematic MRI in a patient who demonstrated posterior subluxation *(arrow)* of the humeral head relative to the glenoid in internal rotation (**A**) with reduction of the malalignment *(arrowhead)* occurring during external rotation. (**B**) By placing rotational demands on the capsular mechanism of the shoulder, the use of the kinematic MRI technique improves the sensitivity of MRI in the detection of glenohumeral instability. *(Reprinted with permission from Shellock FG, Powers CM: Kinematic MRI of the Joints: Functional Anatomy, Kinesiology, and Clinical Applications. Boca Raton, FL: CRC Press, 2001. © FG Shellock, 2001.)*

Kinematic MRI examinations of the shoulder have involved the use of several different positioning devices, including those designed to permit examination of internal and external rotation, abduction and adduction, and a combination of other movements.[2,59-64] At least one positioning device (Chamco, Cocoa Beach, FL) has been designed to assess virtually all shoulder movements for patients undergoing kinematic MRI using an open-configured MR system. A dedicated shoulder coil or flex-coil is typically used to acquire MR images for this procedure.

Kinematic MRI studies of the shoulder have been accomplished using various techniques. For the incremental passive positioning technique, a series of images are obtained at different positions through a specific range of motion of the joint. For the active-movement technique, the patient freely moves the joint limb and a rapid MR imaging technique is used to acquire images for the kinematic MRI examination. Finally, for the active-movement, against-resistance technique, stress is applied to load or resist the joint while the patient freely moves the joint and/or limb and a rapid imaging technique is used to acquire MR images. Interestingly, MR-guided physical examinations of the shoulder have also been conducted, whereby the examiner is able to actually perform provocative maneuvers to assess the joint.[62-64]

A variety of pulse sequences and positioning strategies have been used for this diagnostic procedure.[2,59-65] As with other kinematic applications, the selection of the plane of imaging and the pulse sequence that is used is based on the suspected pathology under evaluation during kinematic MRI of the shoulder. In general, the techniques that have been applied may be categorized with respect to the position of the patient during the kinematic examination. That is, during a lying position versus an upright, seated position.

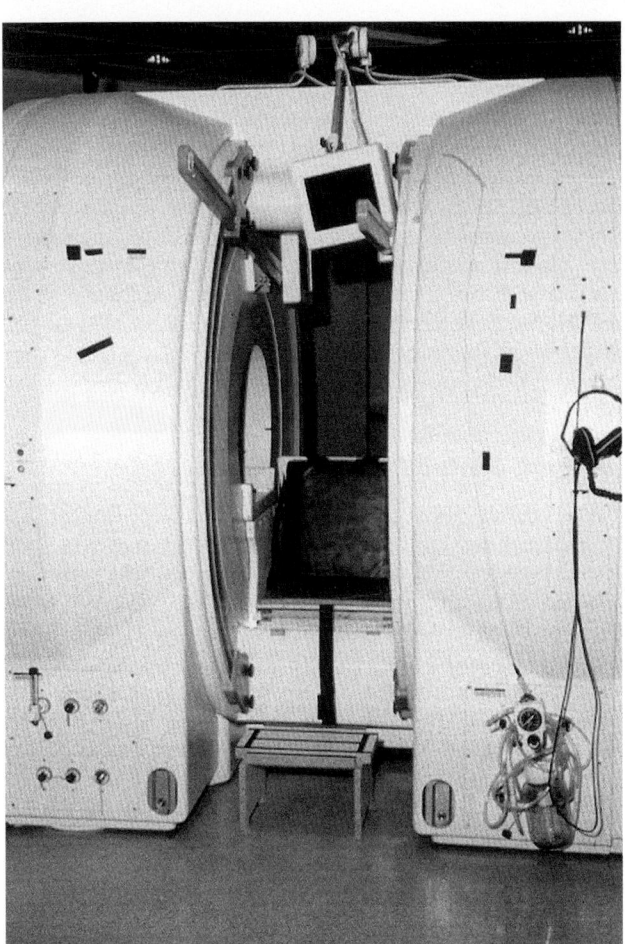

FIGURE 98-21

The vertically opened MR system (0.5 tesla, Signa SP, General Electric Medical Systems, Milwaukee, WI). This unique scanner permits kinematic MRI of the shoulder to be performed during physical examinations. *(Reprinted with permission from Shellock FG, Powers CM: Kinematic MRI of the Joints: Functional Anatomy, Kinesiology, and Clinical Applications. Boca Raton, FL: CRC Press, 2001. © FG Shellock, 2001.)*

Clinical Applications

Lying Position

In the lying position, internal and external rotation has been assessed in patients using tunnel-shaped or open MR systems. For example, using this technique, Bonutti et al[59] reported that there was good visualization of the anterior glenoid labrum (AGL) and demonstrated the role of the AGL in stabilizing the glenohumeral joint anteriorly, in conjunction with the capsular ligaments. Avulsions of the AGL may be better characterized using kinematic MRI of the shoulder during internal and external rotation compared to static-view MR imaging.[59]

A study conducted by Allmann et al[60] assessed shoulder lesions in a variety of positions utilizing an open 0.2 T MR system and a conventional 1.0 T MR system with kinematic MRI examinations in the axial and oblique coronal planes. These investigators reported that normal variations of the glenohumeral joint were easy to recognize. With regard to pathologic conditions, subluxation of the humeral head and rupture of the labrum were well demonstrated, along with abnormal distances between osseous structures during dynamic movements.[60] Accordingly, Allmann et al[60] concluded that kinematic MRI studies of the shoulder appear to be useful in visualizing the capsular ligament complex of the glenohumeral joint associated with impingement and instability syndromes (see Fig. 98-20).[60] With additional experience, the role of kinematic MRI of the shoulder of the patient in a lying position will be further refined.

Upright, Seated Position

Investigators have stated that there are limitations in performing kinematic MRI studies in patients in a lying position.[61-64] Therefore, kinematic MRI physical examinations of the shoulder with the patient in an upright, seated position have been described by Beaulieu and Gold[63] and Dufour et al.[64] These kinematic applications require the use of an MR system designed for interventional or MR-guided procedures (Signa SP, General Electric Medical Systems, Milwaukee, WI, USA) (see Fig. 98-21).

Specialized hardware and software are necessary for performing the kinematic MRI examination of the shoulder with the patient in an upright, seated position. The MR Tracking System (General Electric Medical Systems, Milwaukee, WI) is utilized to actively localize the anatomy of interest.[63,64] Basically, this device performs as a miniature untuned RF-receiving coil sensitive to only those hydrogen spins immediately surrounding it.[63,64] The spatially limited sensitivity of the miniature coil leads to a direct relationship between its position within a magnetic field gradient and the frequency spectrum of its received MR signal.[63,64] A transmit/receive flexible RF surface coil is used to facilitate imaging for the kinematic procedure. By interactively adjusting the location of the tracker coil on the patient, the scan location is also modified. Thus, image acquisition may be accomplished in a "near real-time" manner using fast gradient-echo or other similar pulse sequence.[63,64]

Shoulder Impingement Syndrome

Dufour et al[64] developed the upright, seated kinematic MRI technique to permit measurements of the acromiohumeral distance at controlled angles of flexion and abduction. The comprehensive experience of this group's efforts have been recently described[64] with respect to findings in healthy volunteer subjects and patients with shoulder pathology.

A high percentage of shoulder pain and dysfunction is attributed to "shoulder impingement syndrome", which is believed to result from irritation of the structures contained within the subacromial space. The etiology of this syndrome involves narrowing of the subacromial space during elevation of the arm against gravity, which reflects painful compression of the supraspinatus tendon, the subacromial-subdeltoid bursa, and the long head of the biceps tendon between the humeral head and the acromion. Importantly, the clinical signs and symptoms of shoulder impingement syndrome are only manifested during free motions or at arm angles at approximately 90° of elevation.

According to Dufour et al,[64] shoulder impingement syndrome may best be evaluated using kinematic MRI to examine the shoulder during active, unrestricted motions, with this diagnostic imaging procedure reproducing the conditions in which impingement is more likely to occur. In fact, Dufour et al[64] reported the feasibility of using the upright, seated kinematic MRI technique to monitor active movement-related changes of acromiohumeral distance in healthy subjects as well as in patients diagnosed with impingement syndrome. This procedure provides an outcome measure to discriminate between shoulders with and without impingement.[64]

Glenohumeral Instability

Whereas there is considerable literature on the appearance of the glenohumeral joint with static-view MR imaging and MR arthrography, there are no systematic reports of kinematic MRI of the shoulder in patients with instability. Beaulieu and Gold[62,63] and Hodge et al[61] used the vertically opened MR system to study glenohumeral relationships. Each shoulder was studied through a range of abduction/adduction and internal/external rotation to quantify translation of the humeral head in relation to the glenoid. Additionally, an examiner performed MR-guided stress testing on each shoulder. In these investigations, pathologic motion patterns and anatomic derangements were identified in many instability patients using kinematic MRI of the shoulder. Importantly, there was a relatively good correlation between kinematic MRI stress testing and clinical instability grade, suggesting that relevant information was being derived from this examination. Beaulieu and Gold[63] reported that while the overall patient numbers remain small, the results obtained to date for kinematic MRI examinations of the shoulder are generally encouraging.

LUMBAR SPINE

The lumbar spine is a highly dynamic structure composed of numerous functional spinal units. It is well documented that changes associated with load and position result in alterations in the space of the spinal canal. Importantly, clinical data indicate that a change in body position or certain physical activities may significantly alter symptoms in patients with low back pain. These effects may relate to axial loading of the spine as it occurs during standing upright, with or without carrying weight, or in a seated position. Notably, in studying patients with low back pain, there is often a discrepancy between symptoms reported by the patient and findings as documented by MR imaging. Therefore, in order to optimally visualize findings related to "loading", a special kinematic MRI technique was developed to examine the

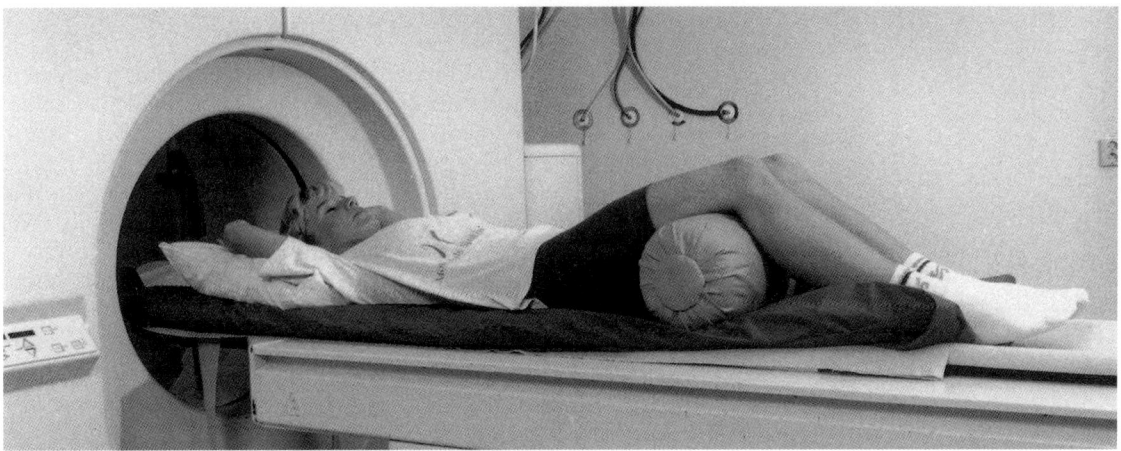

FIGURE 98-22

Subject prepared for a kinematic MRI examination using the axial compression technique. The patient is placed on a low friction mat on top of the examination table. The patient harness is connected to a compression device using straps and the axial load is measured by a balance mechanism in the compression device (DynaMed AB, Stockholm, Sweden). *(Reprinted with permission from Shellock FG, Powers CM: Kinematic MRI of the Joints: Functional Anatomy, Kinesiology, and Clinical Applications. Boca Raton, FL: CRC Press, 2001. © FG Shellock, 2001.)*

lumbar spine with the patient in an axial loaded, supine position with the goal of obtaining improved diagnostic information to assess this anatomic region.[65,67,68,70] This topic has been reviewed by Willen et al.[65]

Additionally, considerable work has been reported on the performance of a kinematic MRI procedure that involves obtaining flexion and extension views of the lumbar spine with the patient in an upright-seated position.[66,69,70] This procedure requires the use of a vertically opened MR system designed for interventional MR imaging (0.5 tesla, Signa SP, General Electric Medical Systems, Milwaukee, WI). Currently, there are less than 20 of these MR systems in existence worldwide. Therefore, this topic will not be covered here but interested readers are referred to the compelling review by Weishaupt et al.[69]

Protocol

Axial Loading of the Supine Patient

In 1994, a specially designed compression device was developed to perform axial loaded examinations of the supine patient in a conventional MR system. This device consists of a plastic compression device and a neoprene/nylon harness (DynaMed AB, Stockholm, Sweden) (Fig. 98-22). The harness is attached to the compression device using nylon straps, which are tightened to provide axial loading of the lumbar spine with the subject in a supine position. The harness is constructed to ensure that the pressure is evenly distributed across the lower part of the chest rather than the shoulders. This positioning device enables the examination of patients in a supine position, with straightened legs, thus simulating the axial load on the lumbar spine in an upright position (i.e., the posture associated with most

symptoms of sciatica and spinal stenosis).[65] More recently another device, the Portal Gravity System (Portal Inc, North Logan, UT), was developed to allow "weight-bearing" studies in patients undergoing MR imaging and computed tomography examinations.

The kinematic MRI procedure involves the use of a flat or flexible RF surface coil along with imaging sequences similar to those commonly used to obtain routine static-view MR images, such as sagittal and axial plane, T1- and T2-weighted, spin-echo or fast (or turbo) spin-echo (FSE) pulse sequences.

If it is intended to perform this procedure in a patient, it is crucial to *first* begin with a routine MR imaging study to avoid loading a spine with a malignant disease or other similar significant pathologic condition that would constitute a contraindication for the axial loaded, supine kinematic MRI examination.

To ensure that the images chosen for assessment are comparable in every position, it is important to compare nerve roots, other soft-tissues, and bony structures such as facet joints and the lamina. Furthermore, it is essential to look for signs of narrowing of the lateral recess and compression or flattening of the nerve roots in any level, especially from L3 to S1. Any deformation of the dural sac should be noted as well as a suspicion of a disk herniation, narrowing of an intervertebral foramen, ligamentum flavum thickening or a synovial cyst adjacent to a facet joint.

Clinical Applications

Kinematic MRI of the lumbar spine permits new diagnostic possibilities for the evaluation of structural position-dependent changes in patients with chronic low back pain, with and without sciatica, or suspected segmental instability. Based on their extensive experience

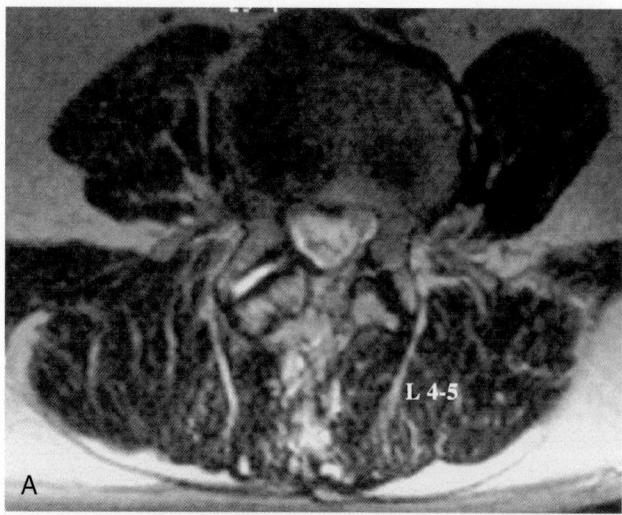

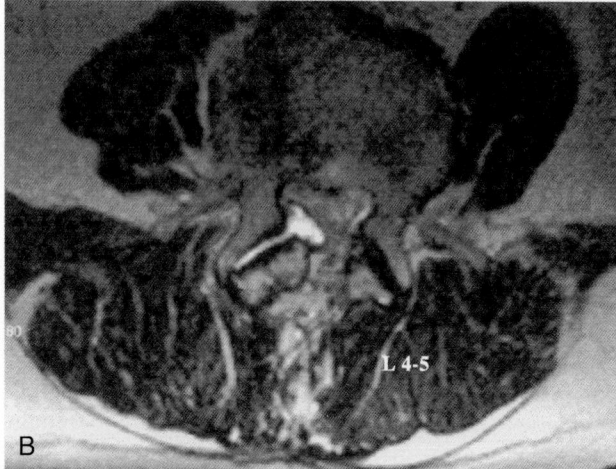

FIGURE 98-23

Kinematic MRI examination performed in an elderly male patient. This patient had a previous surgical procedure for spinal stenosis at the L3-L5 disk level with a good result. After 2 years, he experienced a severe L4 rhizopathy at the ventral part of his right thigh. Examination in a relaxed position (**A**) did not reveal any pathology but during axial loading (**B**), a large synovial cyst appeared to bulge from the right facet joint into the spinal canal, explaining the origin of the patient's painful symptoms. *(Reprinted with permission from Shellock FG, Powers CM: Kinematic MRI of the Joints: Functional Anatomy, Kinesiology, and Clinical Applications. Boca Raton, FL: CRC Press, 2001. © FG Shellock, 2001.)*

with this procedure, Willen et al[65] recommend using the axial loaded, kinematic MRI examination of the lumbar spine in the patient with:

1. neurogenic claudication
2. sciatica
3. suspected disk herniation, narrow lateral recess or foraminal stenosis
4. suspected synovial cyst (Fig. 98-23).

Combining this kinematic procedure with routine, static-view MR images is considered to improve the diagnostic yield of MR examinations of the lumbar spine.[65,68]

Acknowledgments

The following individuals are acknowledged for their important contributions to the field of kinematic MRI and, thus, to the content of this chapter: Christopher M Powers, Susan Mais Requejo, Michael Terk, Kornelia Kulig, Jari O Karhu, Seppo K Koskinen, Jan Willen, Nils Schönström, Barbro Danielson, Dominik Weishaupt, Simon Wildermuth, Marius Schmid, Juerg Hodler, Gretchen B Salsich, Samuel Ward, Christopher Beaulieu, Garry Gold, Marie Dufour, Hélène Moffet, Luc J Hébert, Christian Moisan, Sally Ho, Elizabeth F Souza, John Reeder, W M W Gedroyc, and A Williams.

REFERENCES

1. Nordin M, Frankel VH: Basic Biomechanics of the Musculoskeletal System, 2nd ed. Philadelphia: Lea & Febiger, 1989.
2. Shellock FG, Powers CM: Kinematic MRI of the Joints: Functional Anatomy, Kinesiology, and Clinical Applications. Boca Raton, FL: CRC Press, 2001.
3. Shellock FG, Mandelbaum B: Kinematic MR imaging of the joints. In Mink JH, Deutsch A (eds): MRI of the Musculoskeletal System: A Teaching File. New York: Raven Press, 1990.
4. Shellock FG, Mink JH, Deutsch A, Pressman B: Kinematic MRI of the joints: techniques and clinical applications. Magn Reson Q 7:104-135, 1991.
5. Deutsch AL, Shellock FG: The patellofemoral joint and extensor mechanism. In Mink J, Reicher MA, Crues JV, Deutsch AL (eds): Magnetic Resonance Imaging of the Knee, 2nd ed. New York: Raven Press, 1992.
6. Deutsch AD, Shellock FG, Mink JH: Imaging of the patellofemoral joint: emphasis on advanced techniques. In Fox J, Del Pizzo W (eds): The Patellofemoral Joint. New York: McGraw-Hill, 1993.
7. Shellock FG: Kinematic magnetic resonance imaging. In Stoller DW (ed): Magnetic Resonance Imaging in Orthopaedics and Sports Medicine, 2nd ed. Philadelphia: Lippincott-Raven, 1997.
8. Burnett KR, Davis CL, Read J: Dynamic display of the temporomandibular joint meniscus by using "fast-scan" MR imaging. Am J Roentgenol 149:959-962, 1987.
9. Shellock FG, Pressman BD: Dual-surface-coil MR imaging of bilateral temporomandibular joint: improvements in the imaging protocol. Am J Neuroradiol 10:595-598, 1989.
10. Pressman BD, Shellock FG: The temporomandibular joint. In Mink JH, Deutsch AL (eds): MRI of the Musculoskeletal System: A Teaching File. New York: Raven Press, 1990.
11. Shellock FG, Mink JH, Deutsch A, Fox JM: Patellar tracking abnormalities: clinical experience with kinematic MR imaging in 130 patients. Radiology 172:799-804, 1989.
12. Shellock FG, Mink JH, Deutsch A, Fox JM, Ferkel RD: Evaluation of patients with persistent symptoms following lateral retinacular release by kinematic MRI of the patellofemoral joint. Arthroscopy 6:226-234, 1990.
13. Shellock FG, Mink JH, Fox JM: Patellofemoral joint: kinematic MR imaging to assess tracking abnormalities. Radiology 68:551-553, 1988.
14. Shellock FG, Mink JH, Deutsch A, Fox JM: Kinematic magnetic resonance imaging for evaluation of patellar tracking: a case report. Physician Sportsmed 17:99-108, 1989.
15. Kujala UM, Osterman K, Kormano M, Komu M, Schlenzka D: Patellar motion analyzed by magnetic resonance imaging. Acta Orthop Scand 60:13-16, 1989.
16. Kujala UM, Osterman K, Kormano M, Nelimarkka O, Hurme M, Taimela S: Patellofemoral relationships in recurrent patellar dislocation. J Bone Joint Surg [Br] 71B:788-792, 1989.
17. Koskinen SK, Hurme M, Kujala UM, Kormano M: Effect of lateral release on patellar motion in chondromalacia: an MRI study of 11 knees. Acta Orthop Scand 61: 311-312, 1990.
18. Shellock FG, Mink JH, Fox JM: Identification of medial subluxation of the patella in a dancer using kinematic MRI of the patellofemoral joint: a case report. Kinesiol Med Dance 13:1-9, 1991.
19. Shellock FG: Patellofemoral joint abnormalities in athletes: evaluation by kinematic MRI. Top Magn Reson Imaging 3:1-30, 1991.
20. Shellock FG, Foo TKF, Deutsch A, Mink JH: Patellofemoral joint: evaluation during active flexion with ultrafast spoiled GRASS MR imaging. Radiology 180:581-585, 1991.
21. Koskinen SP, Kujala UM: Effect of patellar brace on patellofemoral relationships. Scand J Med Sci Sports 1:119-122, 1991.
22. Koskinen SK, Hurme M, Kujala UM: Restoration of patellofemoral congruity by combined lateral release and tibial tuberosity transposition as assessed by MRI analysis. Int Orthopedics 15:363-366, 1991.
23. Koskinen SK, Kujala UM: Patellofemoral relationships and distal insertion of the vastus medialis muscle: a magnetic resonance imaging study in nonsymptomatic subjects and in patients with patellar dislocation. Arthroscopy 8:865-868, 1992.

24. Shellock FG, Mink JH, Deutsch AL, Foo TKF: Kinematic MR imaging of the patellofemoral joint: comparison between passive positioning and active movement techniques. Radiology 184:574-577, 1992.

25. Shellock FG, Mink JH, Deutsch AL, Foo TKF, Sullenberger P: Patellofemoral joint: identification of abnormalities using active movement, "unloaded" vs "loaded" kinematic MR imaging techniques. Radiology 88:575-578, 1993.

26. Brossman J, Muhle C, Schroder C, Melchert UH, Spielmann RP, Heller M: Motion-triggered cine MR imaging: evaluation of patellar tracking patterns during active and passive knee extension. Radiology 187:205-212, 1993.

27. Brossman J, Muhle C, Bull CC, et al: Evaluation of patellar tracking in patients with suspected patellar malalignment: cine MR imaging vs. arthroscopy. Am J Roentgenol 62:361-367, 1993.

28. Brossman J, Muhle C, Bull CC, et al: Evaluation of patellar tracking in patients with suspected patellar malalignment: cine MR imaging vs arthroscopy. Am J Roentgenol 162:361-367, 1994.

29. Shellock FG, Mink JH, Deutsch AL, Fox J, Molnar T, Kvitne R: Effect of a patellar realignment brace on patellofemoral relationships: evaluation using kinematic MR imaging. J Magn Reson Imaging 4:590-594, 1994.

30. Worrell TW, Ingersoll CD, Farr J: Effect of patellar taping and bracing on patellar position. An MRI study. J Sports Rehabil 3:146-153, 1994.

31. Brown SM, Bradley WG: Kinematic magnetic resonance imaging of the knee. MRI Clin North Am 2:441-449, 1994.

32. Brossman J, Muhle C, Bull CC, et al: Cine MR imaging before and after realignment surgery for patellar tracking: comparison with axial radiographs. Skelet Radiol 24:191-196, 1995.

33. Shellock FG, Mink JH, Deutsch DL, Molnar T: Effect of a newly-designed patellar realignment brace on patellofemoral relationships: a case report. Med Sci Sports Exercise 27:469-472, 1995.

34. Worrell T, Ingersoll CD, Brockrath-Pugliese K, Minis P: Effect of patellar taping and bracing on patellar position as determined by MRI in patients with patellofemoral pain. J Athletic Training 33:16-20, 1998.

35. Powers CM, Pfaff M, Shellock FG: Active movement, loaded kinematic MRI of the patellofemoral joint: reliability of quantitative measurements. J Magn Reson Imaging 8:724-732, 1998.

36. Witonski D, Goraj B: Pateller motion analyzed by kinematic and dynamic axial magnetic resonance imaging in patients with anterior knee pain syndrome. Arch Orthop Trauma Surg 119:46-49, 1999.

37. Muhle C, Brossman J, Heller M: Kinematic CT and MR imaging of the patello-femoral joint. Eur Radiol 9:508-518, 1999.

38. Shellock FG, Stone KR, Crues JV: Development and clinical application of kinematic MRI of the patellofemoral joint using an extremity MR system. Med Sci Sports Exercise 31:788-791, 1999.

39. Powers CM, Shellock FG, Beering TV, Garrido DE, Goldbach RM, Molnar T: Effect of bracing on patellar kinematics in patients with patellofemoral joint pain. Med Sci Sports Exercise 31:1714-1720, 1999.

40. Shellock FG: The effect of a patellar stabilizing brace on lateral subluxation of the patella: assessment using kinematic MRI. Am J Knee Surg 3:137-142, 2000.

41. Ward SR, Shellock FG, Terk MR, Salsich GB, Powers CM: Assessment of patellofemoral relationships using kinematic MRI: comparison between qualitative and quantitative methods. J Magn Reson Imaging 16:69-74, 2002.

42. Shellock FG, Feske W, Frey C, Terk M: Peroneal tendons: use of kinematic MR imaging to determine subluxation. J Magn Reson Imaging 7:451-454, 1997.

43. Muhle C, Brinkmann G, Brossman J, Wesner F, Heller M: Kinematic MR imaging of the ankle: initial results with ultra-fast imaging. Acta Radiol 38:885-889, 1997.

44. Terk M: Kinematic MRI of the ankle. In Shellock FG, Powers CM (eds): Kinematic MRI of the Joints: Functional Anatomy, Kinesiology, and Clinical Applications. Boca Raton, FL: CRC Press, 2001.

45. Reicher MA, Kellerhouse LE: Normal wrist anatomy, biomechanics, basic imaging protocol, and normal multiplanar MRI of the wrist. In Reicher MA, Kellerhouse LE (eds): MRI of the Hand and Wrist. New York: Raven Press, 1990.

46. Ton ER, Pattynama PM, Bloem JL, Obermann WR: Interosseous ligaments: device for applying stress in wrist MR imaging. Radiology 196:863-864, 1995.

47. Reeder J: Kinematic MRI of the wrist. In Shellock FG, Powers CM (eds): Kinematic MRI of the Joints: Functional Anatomy, Kinesiology, and Clinical Applications. Boca Raton, FL: CRC Press, 2001.

48. Miller RJ: Wrist MRI and carpal instability: what the surgeon needs to know, and the case for dynamic imaging. Semin Musculoskelet Radiol 5:235-240, 2001.

49. Bell GR, Stearns KL: Flexion-extension MRI of the upper rheumatoid cervical spine. Orthopedics 14:969-973, 1991.

50. Shellock FG, Sullenberger P, Mink JH, et al: MRI of the cervical spine during flexion and extension: development and implementation of a new technique. J Magn Reson Imaging WIP:S21, 1994.

51. Muhle C, Weinert D, Falliner A, et al: Dynamic changes of the cervical spinal canal in patients with cervical spondylosis at flexion and extension using magnetic resonance imaging. Invest Radiol 33:444-449, 1998.

52. Muhle C, Wiskirchen J, Weinert D, et al: Biomechanical aspects of the subarachnoid space and cervical cord in healthy individuals examined with kinematic magnetic resonance imaging. Spine 23:556-567, 1998.

53. Muhle C, Bischoff L, Weinert D, et al: Exacerbated pain in cervical radiculopathy at axial rotation, flexion, extension, and coupled motions of the cervical spine: evaluation by kinematic magnetic resonance imaging. Invest Radiol 33:279-288, 1998.

54. Muhle C, Metzner J, Weinert D, et al: Classification system based on kinematic MR imaging in cervical spondylitic myelopathy. Am J Neuroradiol 19:1763-1771, 1998.

55. Muhle C, Metzner J, Weinert D, et al: Kinematic MR imaging in surgical management of cervical spine disk disease, spondylois, and spondylotic myelopathy. Acta Radiol 40:146-153, 1998.

56. Allmann KH, Schafer O, Uhl M, et al: Kinematic versus static MRI study of the cervical spine in patients with rheumatoid arthritis. Rofo Fortscher Geb Rontgenstr Neuen Bildgeb Verfahr 170:22-27, 1999.

57. Karhu JO, Koskinen SK: Kinematic MRI of the cervical spine, In Shellock FG, Powers CM (eds): Kinematic MRI of the Joints: Functional Anatomy, Kinesiology, and Clinical Applications. Boca Raton, FL: CRC Press, 2001.

58. Muhle C, Resnick D, Ahn JM, Sudmeyer M, Heller M: In vivo changes in the neuroforaminal size at flexion-extension and axial rotation of the cervical spine in healthy persons examined using kinematic magnetic resonance imaging. Spine 26:E287-293, 2001.

59. Bonutti PM, Norfray JF, Friedman RJ, Genez BM: Kinematic MRI of the shoulder. J Comput Assist Tomogr 17:666-669, 1993.

60. Allmann KH, Uhl M, Gufler H, et al: Cine-MR imaging of the shoulder. Acta Radiol 38:1043-1046, 1997.

61. Hodge DK, Beaulieu CF, Tabit GH, et al: Dynamic MR imaging and stress testing in glenuhumeral instability: comparison with normal shoulders and clinical/surgical findings. J Magn Reson Imaging 13:748-756, 2001.

62. Beaulieu CF, Hodge DK, Bergman AG, et al: Glenohumeral relationships during physiologic shoulder motion and stress testing: initial experience with open MR imaging and active imaging-plane registration. Radiology 212:699-705, 1999.

63. Beaulieu C, Gold G: Kinematic MRI of the shoulder: stress testing and MR-guided physical examination. In Shellock FG, Powers CM (eds): Kinematic MRI of the Joints: Functional Anatomy, Kinesiology, and Clinical Applications. Boca Raton, FL: CRC Press, 2001.

64. Dufour M, Moffet H, Herbert LJ, Moisan C: Kinematic MRI of the shoulder in the upright, seated position. In Shellock FG, Powers CM (eds): Kinematic MRI of the Joints: Functional Anatomy, Kinesiology, and Clinical Applications. Boca Raton, FL: CRC Press, 2001.

65. Willen J, Danielson B, Gaulitz A, Niklason T, Schonstrom N, Hansson T: Dynamic effects on the lumbar spinal canal. Spine 22:2968-2976, 1997.

66. Wildermuth S, Zanetti M, Duewell S, et al: Lumbar spine: quantitative and qualitative assessment of positional (upright flexion and extension) MR imaging and myelography. Radiology 207:391-398, 1998.

67. Danielson BI, Willen J, Gaulitz A, Niklason T, Hansson TH: Axial loading of the spine during CT and MR in patients with suspected lumbar spinal stenosis. Acta Radiol 40: 604-611, 1998.

68. Willen J, Schönström J, Danielson B: Kinematic MRI of the lumbar spine: assessment in the axial loaded, supine position. In Shellock FG, Powers CM (eds): Kinematic MRI of the Joints: Functional Anatomy, Kinesiology, and Clinical Applications. Boca Raton, FL: CRC Press, 2001.

69. Weishaupt D, Wildermuth S, Schmid M, Hodler J: Kinematic MRI of the lumbar spine: assessment in the upright, seated position. In Shellock FG, Powers CM (eds): Kinematic MRI of the Joints: Functional Anatomy, Kinesiology, and Clinical Applications. Boca Raton, FL: CRC Press, 2001.

70. Wisleder D, Smith MB, Mosher TJ, Zatsiorsky V: Lumbar spine mechanical response to axial compression load in vivo. Spine 26:E403-409, 2001.

71. Helms CA, Richardson ML, Moon KL, Ware WH: Nuclear magnetic resonance imaging of the temporomandibular joint: preliminary observations. J Craniomand Pract 2:219, 1984.

72. Harms SE: Temporomandibular joint. In Stark DD, Bradley WG Jr (eds): Magnetic Resonance Imaging, Vol. II, 3rd ed. New York: Mosby, 1999.

73. Schellhas KP, Piper MA, Omlie MR: Facial skeletal remodeling due to temporomandibular joint degeneration: an imaging study of 100 patients. Am J Neuroradiol 11:541, 1990.

74. Drace JE, Enzmann DR: Defining the normal temporomandibular joint: closed-, partially open-, and open mouth MR imaging of asymptomatic subjects. Radiology 177:67, 1990.

75. Manzione JV, Tallents RF, Katzberg RW, Oster C, Miller TL: Arthrographically guided therapy for recapturing the temporomandibular joint meniscus. Oral Surg Oral Med Oral Pathol 57:235, 1984.

76. Tallents RH, Katzberg RW, Miller TL, Manzione JV, Oster C: Arthrographically assisted splint therapy. J Prosthet Dent 53:235, 1985.

77. Fulkerson JP, Hungerford DS: Disorders of the Patellofemoral Joint, 2nd ed. Baltimore: Williams and Wilkins, 1990.

78. Moller BN, Krebs B, Jurik AG: Patellofemoral incongruence in chondromalacia and instability of the patella. Acta Orthop Scand 57:232-234, 1986.

79. Moller BN, Moller-Larsen F, Frich LH: Chondromalacia induced by patellar subluxation in the rabbit. Acta Orthop Scand 60:188-191, 1989.

80. Eppley RA: Medial patellar subluxation. In Fox J, Del Pizzo W (eds): The Patellofemoral Joint. New York: McGraw-Hill, 1993.

81. Hughston JC, Deese M: Medial subluxation of the patella as a complication of lateral release. Am J Sports Med 16:383, 1988.

82. Molnar TJ: Patellar rehabilitation. In Fox J, Del Pizzo W (eds): The Patellofemoral Joint. New York: McGraw-Hill, 1993.

SHOULDER

Michael B. Zlatkin

INTRODUCTION

The shoulder is a joint capable of great freedom and motion. It is therefore both inherently unstable and subject to injury. Shoulder pain is thus a common clinical problem. It has a number of different etiologies, including subacromial and other forms of impingement leading to rotator cuff tendon failure, and various forms of glenohumeral joint instability. These diseases may be misdiagnosed clinically or dismissed with nonspecific diagnoses, including bursitis or synovitis. In the absence of a precise diagnosis, treatment may fail to relieve the symptoms, resulting in chronic limitation of motion, atrophy, and persistent pain.

MRI is accepted as the imaging modality of choice in patients with shoulder pain. It is a useful and accurate technique in noninvasively diagnosing many shoulder disorders, particularly those due to rotator cuff disease and shoulder instability. This chapter will review current experience with this modality and discuss relevant technical, anatomic, and pathologic issues.

TECHNICAL FACTORS

Local Coils

Local radiofrequency coils are critical to MRI of joints,[1] including the shoulder, as they provide greater diagnostic capability through an increase in signal-to-noise ratio (SNR). Since noise is inherent in the tissue being imaged, it is important that a radiofrequency coil adequately covers the area of interest, but covers as little unwanted tissue as possible. In general, larger coils have lower SNR; therefore, it is important to use the smallest coil feasible to adequately encompass the area of interest. Linear coils which consist of a single loop are limited as the homogeneity of the image and SNR degrade sharply away from the center of the loop, producing suboptimal image quality for diagnosis of deeper structures such as the labrum. Helmholtz coils, consisting of two parallel loops with the anatomy of interest sandwiched between them, provide better homogeneity than a linear loop coil. The SNR performance is somewhat less than at the center of a loop. Flexible coils are used commonly by some manufacturers. They consist of one or more linear loops that wrap (once) around the area of interest. While flexible coils offer good patient comfort and reasonable diagnostic capability, their performance is easily surpassed by quadrature or array coils designed specifically for imaging the shoulder. Quadrature (circularly polarized, CP) coils provide significant improvements in image quality over linear loop coils, with good SNR and homogeneity available over the entire joint. Some flexible coils may have a quadrature design. Flexible quadrature coils have the "flexible" positioning options of flex coils, but with superior SNR performance.

A multicoil (also known as phased) array consists of two or more resonating loops. The output signal of each loop is fed into an independent channel of the MRI system. Since each channel is independent from the others, the coil receivers do not share noise as long as

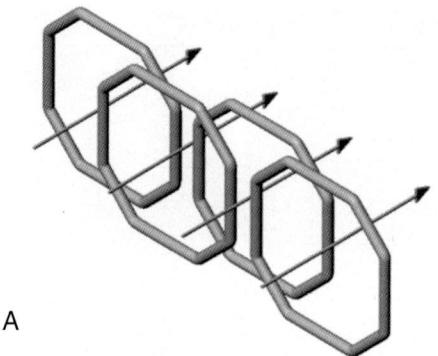
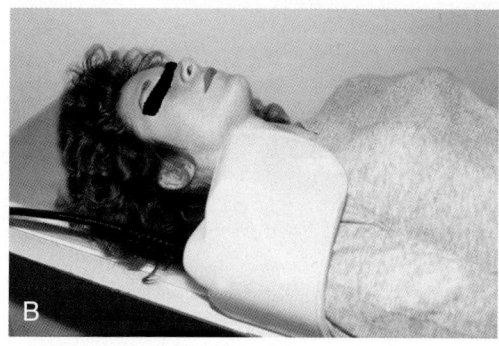

A

B

FIGURE 99-1

Technique. **A,** Four-channel array coil consisting of four linear coils arranged in a strip. The arrows represent the B1 field of each coil in the array. **B,** Four-channel array shoulder coil positioned on a normal volunteer. Patients are imaged in a supine position, with their arm by the side in the neutral rotation. *(Courtesy of Tom Schubert, MRI Devices Corporation, Waukesha, WI.)*

they remain electrically isolated from each other. Although MRI scanners can handle as many as 8 or 16 multicoil array channels, currently most shoulder array coils are four-channel arrays (Fig. 99-1). Shoulder multicoil arrays will permit imaging with high resolution, small fields of view, and thin sections.

Pulse Sequences and Parameters

Conventional spin-echo sequences have for the most part been replaced in MRI by fast spin-echo imaging sequences. Short repetition time (TR)/time to echo (TE) images are still, however, helpful to demonstrate anatomic details and are most often used in MR arthrography.

The tissue contrast is similar in fast spin-echo imaging sequences to that seen with conventional spin echo; however, fat is more intense on T2-weighted fast spin-echo images, and therefore differentiating fat from fluid signal can sometimes be difficult. Blurring of anatomic structures is another problem, especially on short TE sequences. Comparative studies have established the efficacy of fast spin-echo techniques.[2-6] Since marrow fat is brighter, marrow edema can be obscured and fluid in tears or in effusions may be more difficult to identify. Thus most commonly, fat-suppression techniques are added.

Gradient-echo sequences[2,5,7-9] may be applied in imaging the shoulder. These techniques can be used for kinematic imaging[10-15] and are also used to evaluate the glenoid labrum. Problems with the gradient-echo technique include the vacuum phenomenon,[16] which may simulate loose bodies or calcification, and increased magnetic-susceptibility artifact.

Fat suppression is useful in shoulder MRI as it can increase the conspicuity of an abnormality. This effect is most prominent on T2-weighted sequences. Detection of abnormal enhancement after contrast injection is improved on T1-weighted images by using fat sup-

pression. TR and TE can also be reduced on T2-weighted fast spin-echo sequences without loss of tissue contrast, and imaging sequences with TEs in the 35 to 45 ms range are often used with fat saturation in place of imaging sequences with longer TEs and poorer SNR. Fat suppression also reduces phase-encoding and chemical shift artifacts. The two most common types of fat suppression are short tau inversion recovery (STIR) imaging and fat saturation. STIR images exhibit combined T1 and T2 contrast, which enhance sensitivity but diminish specificity. Fat saturation uses a radiofrequency pre-saturation pulse applied at the resonant frequency of lipid protons, followed by a gradient pulse designed to spoil any residual signal intensity of fat. This technique is better with high field-strength systems and a highly uniform magnetic field.[6,17] Methods such as STIR and fat-saturation T2 can improve visualization of rotator cuff tendon injuries (Fig. 99-2) and hyaline cartilage lesions, and are also used to evaluate marrow abnormalities, and inflammatory and post-traumatic processes. They may also be useful to evaluate labral tears.

Performance of high-resolution imaging using large matrices has recently become available, with systems capable of performing 512×512 matrices. Using parallel imaging, 3-T magnets, and appropriate coils even higher matrices may be employed (Fig. 99-3). These techniques may improve visualization of subtle abnormalities involving the labrum and rotator cuff. Smaller fields of view[18] are also helpful in the evaluation of the shoulder. Large matrix and/or small field of view imaging is made possible by higher field strength, improvements in scanner hardware, better local coils, or such standard factors as increased excitations and longer repetition time. A narrow receiver bandwidth also improves SNR.

The slice thickness is also an important determinant of spatial resolution. Slice thicknesses of 2 mm on two-dimensional (2D) spin- and gradient-echo sequences and thicknesses of 1 mm or less on 3D Fourier transform (FT) images are available on most scanners for routine usage. These are also very useful for evaluating such

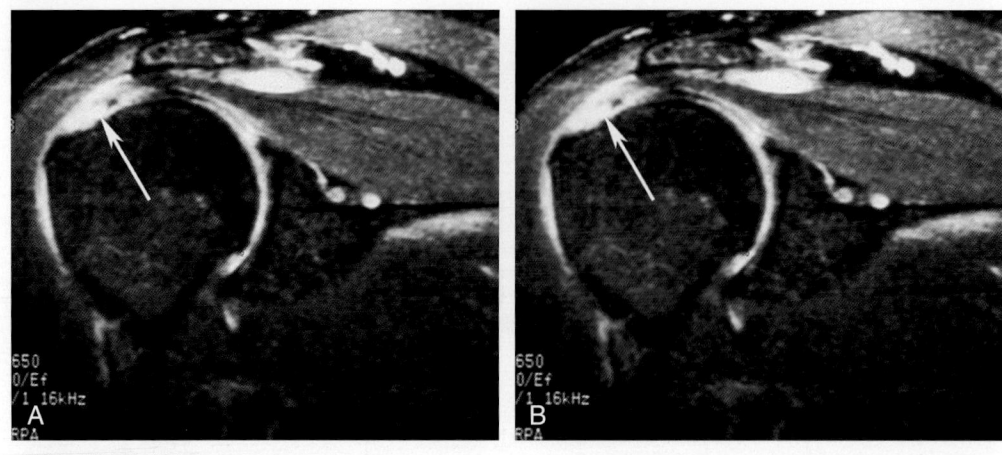

FIGURE 99-2

Fat suppression. **A,** Conventional spin-echo T2-weighted image. **B,** T2-weighted fast spin-echo (FSE) image with fat saturation. Fat saturation increases the conspicuity of the tendon disruption (*arrows* in **A** and **B**).

structures as the glenoid labrum and subtle injuries of articular cartilage. Contiguous thin slices ensure that the relevant anatomy is adequately covered and also reduce partial volume averaging.

MRI Arthrography

In the absence of a native effusion MRI can be performed after the injection of saline or a gadopentate dimeglumine/saline mixture for MR arthrography.[19-35] A saline/gadopentate dimeglumine mixture (1.0 mL of gadopentate dimeglumine/200 mL of saline) is injected. This can be achieved by diluting 0.1 mL of gadolinium in 20 mL of saline. The amount depends on the capacity of the joint, but is typically 12 to 15 mL, which is somewhat greater than for conventional arthrography. The patient is then taken to the MRI scanner and the appropriate image sequences are obtained. As mentioned earlier, fat-saturation techniques are often utilized in conjunction to increase the conspicuity of the contrast.[32,34,36] Intra-articular gadolinium distends the joint and potentially can more directly identify abnormalities (Fig. 99-4). In the shoulder, it is utilized to assess the rotator cuff undersurface and to improve assessment of torn tendon edges in complete cuff tears. It is very helpful in evaluating the postoperative shoulder and in assessing patients with glenohumeral instability and SLAP tears, when findings are uncertain, or when there is no native effusion.[1] Positioning patients in abduction and external rotation (ABER)[37-39] may help visualize posterior under-surface lesions in posterosuperior subglenoid impingement and help to visualize labroligamentous abnormalities in complex instability cases, including Bankart lesion variants. MR arthrography may help locate loose bodies but may not be as effective as CT air arthrography for this application.

Disadvantages of gadolinium injection are that it requires an injection into the joint, making the study

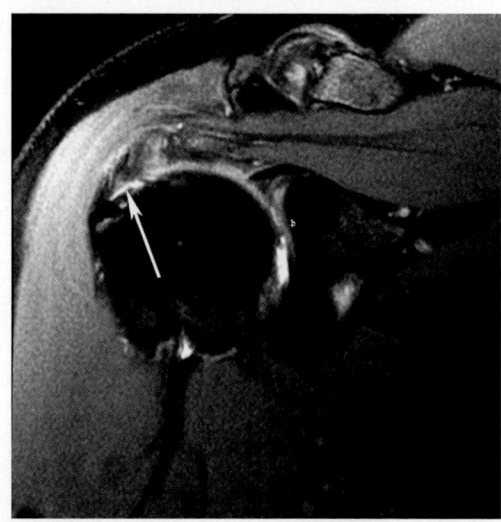

FIGURE 99-3

Image of the shoulder obtained with a four-channel phased-array coil at 3 T. Note the severe tendinosis and small undersurface anterodistal partial tear (*arrow*). (*Courtesy of Larry Tannenbaum MD, Edison, NJ.*)

semi-invasive. Fluoroscopy is required for injection and therefore the total examination time is increased. Our patients are injected under C arm fluoroscopic guidance. In addition, imaging may be logistically difficult to perform if the scanner is remote from the fluoroscopic unit. Although no toxic effects are known, the intra-articular use of gadolinium[21] has not yet been approved by the Food and Drug Administration (FDA).

Indirect MR arthrography is achieved by injection of paramagnetic MR contrast media intravenously instead of as an intra-articular injection as in direct MR arthrography.[40-43] In some cases, exercising the joint results in considerable signal intensity increase within

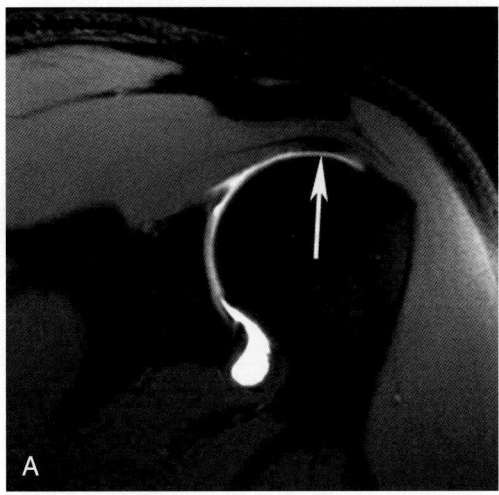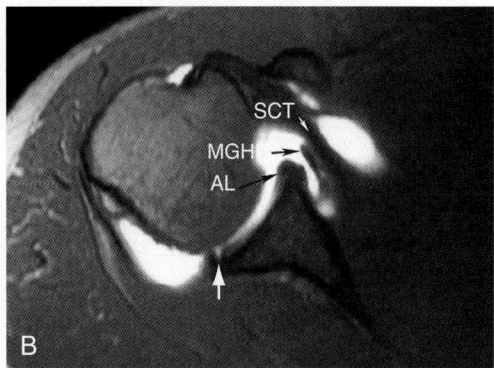

FIGURE 99-4

MR arthrography. T1-weighted images with fat saturation obtained after intra-articular gadolinium injection (1/200 dilution of gadolinium in saline). **A,** Coronal oblique image. Note the high signal obtained from gadolinium outlining the cuff undersurface (*arrow*). **B,** Axial image shows the excellent delineation of the anterior labrum (AL), middle glenohumeral ligament (MGHL), and subscapularis tendon (SCT) when the joint is distended with contrast. A small posterior labral tear is seen (*arrow*).

the joint cavity where fat-saturated MR sequences yield arthrographic images.[44] The method is less invasive than direct MR arthrography and initial results claim comparable sensitivities and specificities for rotator cuff and glenoid labrum pathology.[45-47]

Imaging Protocols

In shoulder imaging, patients are typically positioned supine, with the arm at the side in a neutral rotation (see Fig. 99-1B). With the arm in external rotation the capsule is generally taut; with the arm in internal rotation it may appear more redundant. External rotation is generally avoided except under special circumstances, as this is uncomfortable and may result in motion artifact. The arm should not be placed on the chest or abdomen to avoid transmitted respiratory motion.

In the routine shoulder protocol an axial dual-echo proton-density and T2-weighted fast spin-echo pulse sequence is obtained first with fat saturation. Some examiners perform this sequence as an intermediate-echo fast spin-echo sequence (TE 35-45 ms) with fat saturation. Especially in patients with shoulder instability this is followed by a sliced interleaved gradient-echo (MPGR) T2* gradient-echo sequence, also in the axial plane. The oblique coronal images are performed next and are oriented from the axial images perpendicular to the glenoid margin. Others orient these parallel to the course of the supraspinatus tendon on axial images. This sequence best evaluates the rotator cuff. A fast spin-echo proton-density–weighted sequence is carried out, without fat suppression, followed by a T2-weighted fast spin-echo sequence with fat saturation. Sagittal oblique

images can be obtained with an intermediate-echo fast spin-echo sequence with fat saturation.

MRI arthrography is performed in selected cases as discussed earlier (see Fig. 99-4). Twelve to 15 mL of contrast is injected. T1-weighted images with fat saturation in the axial, coronal oblique, and sagittal oblique planes are obtained. This is then followed by a T2-weighted fast spin-echo sequence, typically in the axial and coronal oblique planes.

The field of view is 12 to 14 cm and the slice thickness is 3 to 4 mm. The matrix size is 256×192 or 256×256 for the T1 and gradient-echo sequences. For fast spin-echo imaging, a 384×256 matrix is employed with an echo train of three to four for the proton-density–weighted images and seven to eight for the T2-weighted images.

General Shoulder Anatomy

The shoulder enjoys a greater range of motion than any other joint in the body. In fact it is not a single joint, but the synergistic action of four separate articulations: glenohumeral, acromioclavicular, sternoclavicular, and scapulothoracic joints.

Glenohumeral Joint

The glenohumeral joint is a multiaxial ball and socket joint lying between the roughly hemispheric humeral head and the shallow glenoid fossa of the scapula.[48] The glenoid fossa is essentially a pear-shaped cavity with dimensions approximately a quarter the size of the humeral head.[49] The glenoid is covered by articular

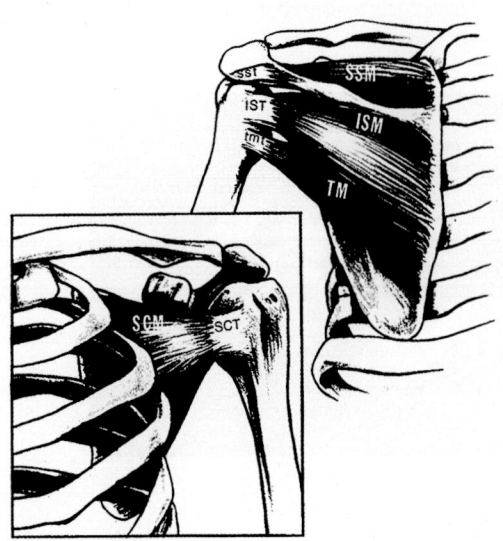

FIGURE 99-5

Rotator cuff muscles and tendons. Note the supraspinatus tendon inserts more superiorly and anteriorly on the greater tuberosity, and the infraspinatus and teres minor more posteriorly and inferiorly. The subscapularis is anterior and inserts broadly in a fanlike fashion on the lesser tuberosity. ISM, infraspinatus muscle; IST, infraspinatus tendon; SSM, supraspinatus muscle; SST, supraspinatus tendon; SCM, subscapularis muscle; SCT, subscapularis tendon; TM, teres minor muscle; TMT, teres minor tendon. *(Reproduced with permission from Zlatkin MB: MRI of the Shoulder, 2nd ed. Philadelphia, Lippincott, Williams and Wilkins, 2003.)*

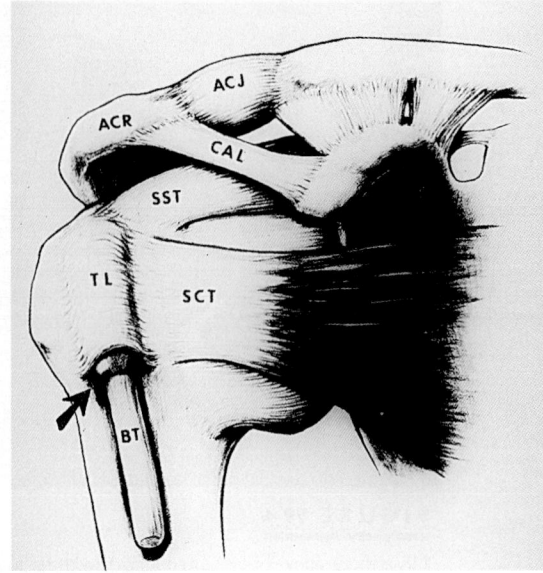

FIGURE 99-6

Coracoacromial arch and surrounding structures. Note the relationship of the supraspinatus tendon to the anterior acromion, acromioclavicular joint, and coracoacromial ligament. The long head of the biceps tendon is also an important relation of this arch. ACJ, acromioclavicular ligament; ACR, acromion; BT, biceps tendon; CAL, coracoacromial ligament; SCT subscapularis tendon; SST, supraspinatus tendon; TL, transverse humeral ligament. *Arrow*, biceps tendon sheath. *(Reproduced with permission from Zlatkin MB: MRI of the Shoulder, 2nd ed. Philadelphia, Lippincott, Williams and Wilkins, 2003.)*

cartilage that is thinner centrally. The humeral head is also covered with articular cartilage which thins slightly at the periphery to accentuate glenohumeral joint congruity.[50] This anatomy permits a wider range of motion than is possible at any other joint. The shoulder is capable of flexion-extension, abduction-adduction, circumduction, and medial and lateral rotation.[48] This anatomy provides mobility, but renders the joint unstable and prone to subluxation and dislocation. This is due to the small size of the glenoid fossa compared to the humeral head and the relative laxity of the joint capsule. These movements and the associated inherent instability of the glenohumeral joint may also be important in the development of internal impingement in the overhead throwing athlete.[51]

The proximal end of the humerus consists of the head and greater and lesser tuberosities. The humeral head is normally retroverted approximately 30 degrees with the arm in the anatomic position. The articular surface is directed superiorly, medially, and posteriorly with an axis angled 130 to 150 degrees relative to the humeral shaft.[50] The anatomic neck of the humerus lies at the base of the articular surface at the proximal end of the bone. The neck is the site of attachment of the inferior aspect of the joint capsule. The greater tuberosity is located on the lateral aspect of the proximal humerus and is the site of insertion of the supraspinatus, infraspinatus, and teres minor tendons (Fig. 99-5). The supraspinatus tendon

inserts on the highest point of the greater tuberosity (Fig. 99-5). The infraspinatus and teres minor tendons localize, respectively, to the middle and lower thirds of the greater tuberosity and lie somewhat more posteriorly than the supraspinatus tendon insertion. The lesser tuberosity is situated on the anterior portion of the proximal humerus, medial to the greater tuberosity. The subscapularis tendon inserts here in a broad band (Fig. 99-5).

The intertubercular (bicipital) groove is located between the greater and lesser tuberosities. The transverse humeral ligament stretches between the two tuberosities, forming the roof of the intertubercular groove. The tendon of the long head of the biceps brachii muscle passes through here, surrounded by a synovial sheath (Fig. 99-6). The width of the groove can vary and if shallow this may predispose it to impingement. Below the greater and lessor tuberosities, the humerus tapers to the surgical neck. The intertubercular groove at this level normally then becomes shallower, and its medial lip provides the insertion site for the latissimus dorsi and teres major tendons; its lateral lip provides the insertion site for the pectoralis major.[50] The deltoid inserts along the deltoid tuberosity, a smooth broad bony prominence on the midportion of the diaphysis. The coracobrachialis also inserts at this level along the medial border of the humerus. The long head of the triceps muscle attaches to the infraglenoid tubercle, which is a

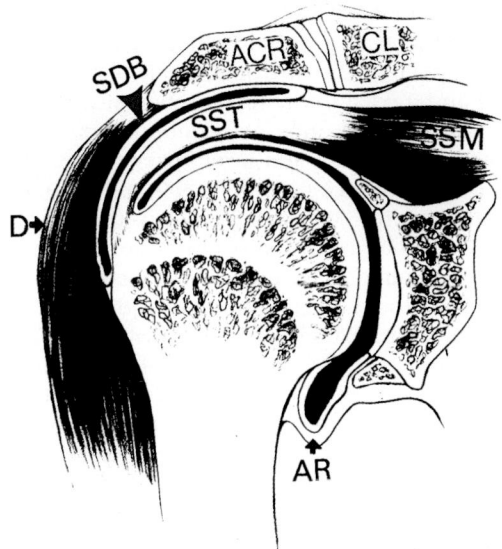

FIGURE 99-7

Cross-sectional diagram illustrating important structures and relations of the shoulder. ACR, acromion; AR, axillary recess; CL, clavicle; D, deltoid muscle; SDB, subacromial-subdeltoid bursa; SSM, supraspinatus muscle; SST, supraspinatus tendon. (*Reproduced with permission from Zlatkin MB: MRI of the Shoulder, 2nd ed. Philadelphia, Lippincott, Williams and Wilkins, 2003.*)

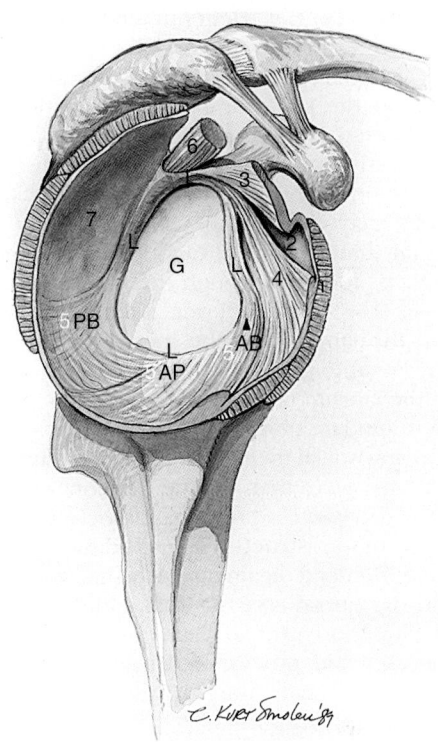

FIGURE 99-8

Capsular mechanism and surrounding structures. The capsule and glenohumeral ligaments are seen. The superior labrum, superior glenohumeral ligament, and biceps tendon converge superiorly. The convergence of the superior labrum and biceps tendon superiorly is known as the biceps labral anchor. There is an opening into the subscapularis bursa between the middle and superior glenohumeral ligaments. The inferior glenohumeral ligament merges with the labrum inferiorly. It is divided into an anterior band, axillary pouch, and posterior band. 1, subscapularis muscle; 2, anterior capsule; 3, superior glenohumeral ligament; 4, middle glenohumeral ligament; 5, inferior glenohumeral ligament; AB, anterior band; AP, axillary pouch; PB, posterior band; 6, biceps tendon, long head; 7, posterior capsule; 8, posterior rotator cuff; L, glenoid labrum; G, glenoid. (*Reproduced with permission from Zlatkin MB, Bjorkengren AG, Gylys-Morin V, et al: Cross-sectional imaging of the capsular mechanism of the glenohumeral joint. Am J Roentgenol 150:151-158, 1988. Reprinted with permission from the American Journal of Roentgenology.*)

triangular surface where the inferior glenoid rim joins the lateral scapular border.[50]

Hyaline articular cartilage lines the surfaces of the humeral head. The cartilage on the humeral head is thickest at its center. The blood supply to the humeral head is via the anterior humeral circumflex artery. There is a normal "sulcus" located posteriorly on the humeral head.[52] This represents an area of "bare bone" between the insertion of the posterior capsule and overlying synovial membrane and the edge of the articular surface of the humeral head. The appearance of this sulcus on cross-sectional images has sometimes been confused with a Hill-Sachs lesion.

The glenoid fossa is situated on the superolateral aspect of the scapula (Figs. 99-7 and 99-8). The superior portion of the fossa is narrow and the inferior portion is broad. In man there is greater anterior tilt to the glenoid fossa and therefore greater anterior instability.[53,54] The glenoid fossa is lined by articular cartilage, thinner in the center. The glenoid labrum rims the glenoid cavity, and provides inherent stability to the glenohumeral joint, restricting anterior and posterior excursion of the humerus (Figs. 99-7 and 99-8).[49] The labrum consists of hyaline cartilage, fibrocartilage, and fibrous tissue. Fibrocartilage is present in the labrum only in a small transition zone at the attachment to the osseous glenoid rim. The blood supply of the labrum is mainly to the outermost portion of the labrum. The inner portion is without vessels.

The glenoid labrum is variable in size and thickness. In young patients the labrum is closely attached at its base to the glenoid, blending with the fibrils of hyaline articular cartilage. In later years especially the superior portion of the labrum may rest free on the edge of the glenoid. This may arise as a result of pull by the superior glenohumeral ligament and biceps tendon and may be distinguished from a labral tear by its smooth borders. In young athletes superior quadrant labral tears may result from traction by these same two structures in overhead throwing.[55]

The fibrous glenoid labrum deepens and enlarges the shallow glenoid fossa. The glenoid is also deepened by the thin cartilaginous lining in the center of this structure. The labrum is also important as a site for ligamentous attachment (see Fig. 99-8).[56] It is believed that the strong intertwining between the collagen fibers of the glenohumeral ligaments and the labrum is more resistant to injury than the glenolabral junction/union. There appears to be a strong pathophysiologic relationship between the locations of labral lesions and the attachment sites of the glenohumeral ligaments and proximal biceps tendon (see Fig. 99-8).[57,58] The inferior portion of the labral-ligamentous complex is more important than the superior portion in stabilizing the glenohumeral joint. It is this portion of the labrum that is more commonly injured in patients with anterior glenohumeral instability. Nonethelesss, the superior labrum does play some role in the stability of the glenohumeral joint where it functions in conjunction with the biceps tendon, through the biceps labral complex (see Fig. 99-8). The superior and anterior superior portions of the labrum are the more variable in their attachment to the glenoid, while the more inferior portion of the labrum is typically fixed.

A loose, redundant fibrous capsule envelops the joint. It is lined by a synovial membrane, and has a surface area approximately twice that of the humeral head (see Figs. 99-7 and 99-8).[50] It encompasses all the intra-capsular soft-tissue structures, including the biceps tendon, glenohumeral ligaments, labrum, and synovial recesses. In the bursal recesses this membrane may be redundant. Superiorly, the capsule encroaches on the root of the coracoid process and inserts in the supra-glenoid region. Laterally the capsule inserts into the anatomic neck of the humerus and inferiorly into the periosteum of the humeral shaft. With the arm at the side the lower part of the capsule is lax, forming the axillary recess (see Figs. 99-7 and 99-8). Posteriorly and inferiorly, the capsule is continuous with the capsular border of the labrum and the adjacent bone. Medially, the anterior capsular insertion may be variable[59] based on its relationship to the glenoid labrum. It may insert directly into the labrum.[60] In a smaller percentage of cases it may insert progressively more medially along the scapular neck, which has been considered to be less stable. Investigation with MRI and MR arthography has called into question the correlation between the type of capsular insertion and glenohumeral instability.[61]

The fibrous capsule is strengthened in several areas. The coracohumeral ligament is a strong fibrous band extending from the coracoid process over the humerus to attach to the greater tuberosity. It has a more important function in shoulder stability than previously thought.[62-65] It also supports the long head of the biceps tendon in the intertubercular groove, and it is disruption of this structure rather than the subscapularis tendon, or its extension into the transverse humeral ligament, that appears to be the main cause of intra-articular subluxation of the biceps tendon. Anteriorly, the capsule may thicken to form the superior (SGHL), middle (MGHL), and inferior glenohumeral ligaments (IGHL) (Figs. 99-8 and 99-9).[66-68] These ligaments reinforce the anterior portion of the capsule and act as a check to external rotation of the humeral head.[66,69] They extend from adjacent to the lesser tuberosity to the anterior border of the glenoid fossa.

The superior glenohumeral ligament, together with the coracohumeral ligament, stabilizes the shoulder joint when the arm is in the adducted dependent position. The ligament consists of two proximal attachments; one to the superoanterior aspect of the labrum conjoined with the biceps tendon, and the other to the base of the

coracoid process (Figs. 99-8, 99-9, and 99-10). This ligament projects in a lateral fashion to insert along the anterior aspect of the anatomic neck of the humerus, superior and medial to the lesser tuberosity.[49,52]

The middle and inferior glenohumeral ligaments blend with the labrum at a level lower than that of the superior ligament (see Figs. 99-8, 99-9, and 99-10). These ligaments and the recesses between them are quite variable.[66,69] The greatest variation is in relation to the middle glenohumeral ligament. This ligament provides stabilization to the glenohumeral joint when the shoulder is abducted 45 degrees. It originates from just beneath the superior glenohumeral ligament along the anterior border of the glenoid to the junctions of the middle and inferior third of the glenoid rim. It blends with the anteroinferior aspect of the capsule, and inserts along the anterior aspect of the surgical neck of the humerus, anterior and inferior to the lesser tuberosity.[49,52]

The inferior glenohumeral ligament has a complex configuration (see Figs. 99-8, 99-9, and 99-10).[70,71] It may be identified as a distinct structure or as just a diffuse thickening of the capsule. It is the thickest portion of the capsule. It consists of three portions: anterior band, posterior band, and axillary pouch/recess of the capsule. It stabilizes the glenohumeral joint when the arm is abducted to approximately 90 degrees (see Figs. 99-8, 99-9, and 99-10).[22,72] The ligament has a triangular configuration with its origin from the anteroinferior and posterior margin of the glenoid rim below its epiphyseal line and its origin is inseparable from the base of the labrum. The inferior glenohumeral ligament inserts along the inferior aspect of the surgical neck of the humerus.

The capsule is reinforced by the tendons of the rotator cuff muscles: the supraspinatus, infraspinatus, teres minor, and subscapularis muscles. These tendons all blend with the fibrous capsule to form the musculo-tendinous cuff (see Fig. 99-5). The primary function of the supraspinatus muscle and tendon complex is to abduct the humerus, but it also has a role in humeral rotation, and also functions as a counterbalance to the deltoid by depressing the humeral head.[50] The innervation of the supraspinatus muscle is by the supra-scapular nerve (C5 and C6 roots), which passes through the suprascapular notch. The suprapinatus tendon may consist of two distinct portions. The ventral portion originates from the anterior supraspinatus fossa inserting anteriorly onto the greater tuberosity. This ventral portion of the supraspinatus tendon may additionally have a site of insertion onto the lesser tuberosity and there may function as an internal rotator of the arm. The second portion of the supraspinatus is located more posteriorly, in a "straplike" configuration. It has several small tendon slips which coalesce into a broad fibrous attachment inserting more posteriorly onto the greater tuberosity. This portion acts primarily as a shoulder abductor.[73] In addition, medially originating fibers from both muscle portions merge in a bipennate fashion to form a strong tendon eccentrically located within the muscle.

The main function of the infraspinatus muscle-tendon unit is external rotation. It also functions to depress the

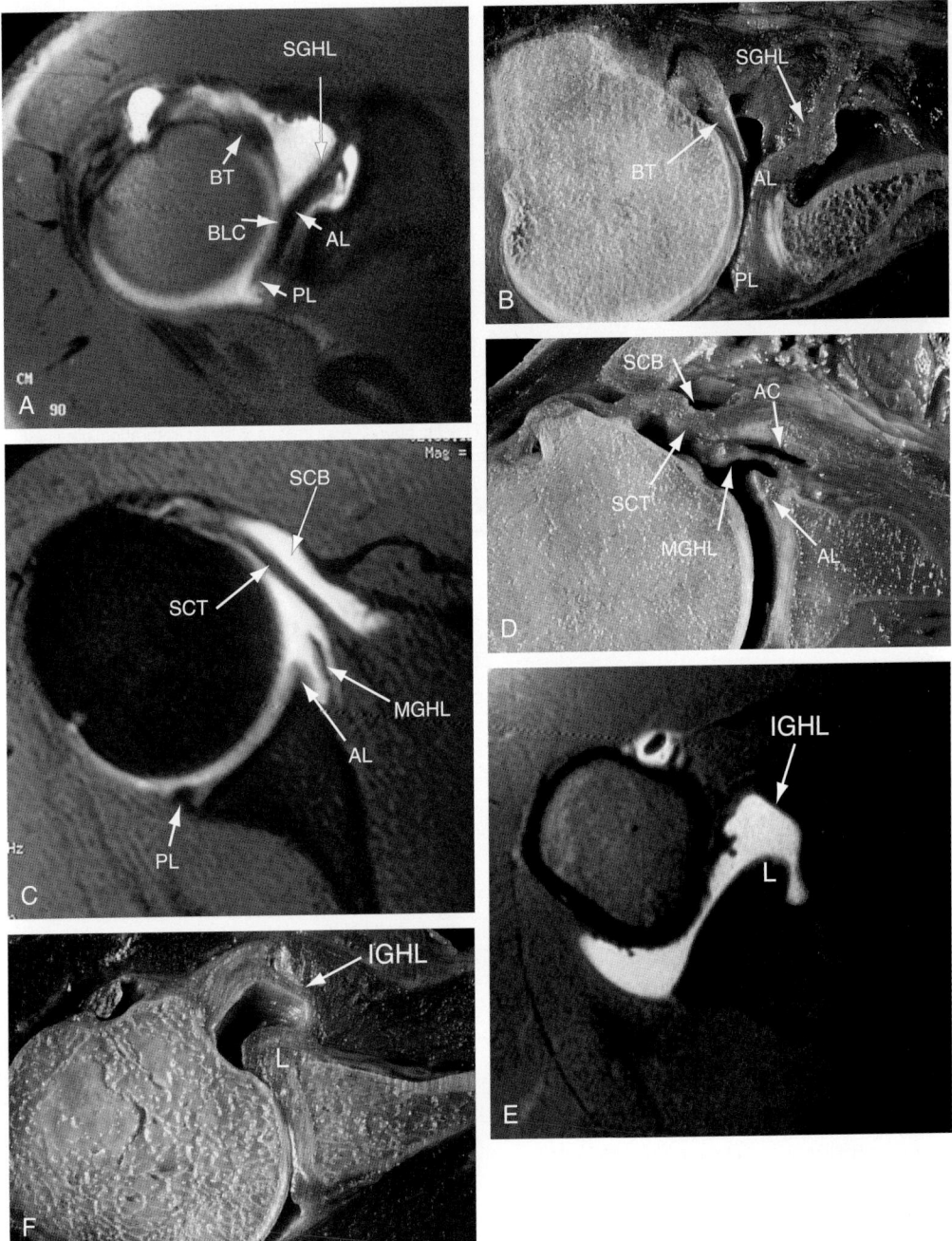

FIGURE 99-9

Cross-sectional anatomy of the glenohumeral ligaments and surrounding structures (axial plane). MR images (TR/TE 800/20 ms) with fat saturation obtained after intra-articular gadolinium injection, and corresponding cadaver sections. **A** and **B,** Superior attachments of the superior glenohumeral ligament are seen with the biceps tendon into the superior glenoid, with the superior labrum, and more anteriorly along the coracoid. The confluence of the biceps tendon long head and superior labrum forming the biceps-labral anchor is also seen. AL, anterior superior labrum; BLC, biceps-labral complex; BT, biceps tendon long head; PL, posterior superior labrum; SGHL, superior gleno-humeral ligament. **C** and **D,** Midglenoid level shows the relationship of the anterior labrum (AL) to the middle glenohumeral ligament (MGHL), anterior capsule (AC), and subscapularis tendon (SCT). The subscapularis bursa is continuous with the joint and extends anterior to the subscapularis tendon (SCB). **E** and **F,** Anterior inferior glenoid level. Here the anterior band of the inferior glenohumeral ligament (IGHL) and subjacent capsule is thick and forms a complex with the labrum (L), which is usually also round and thick at this level.

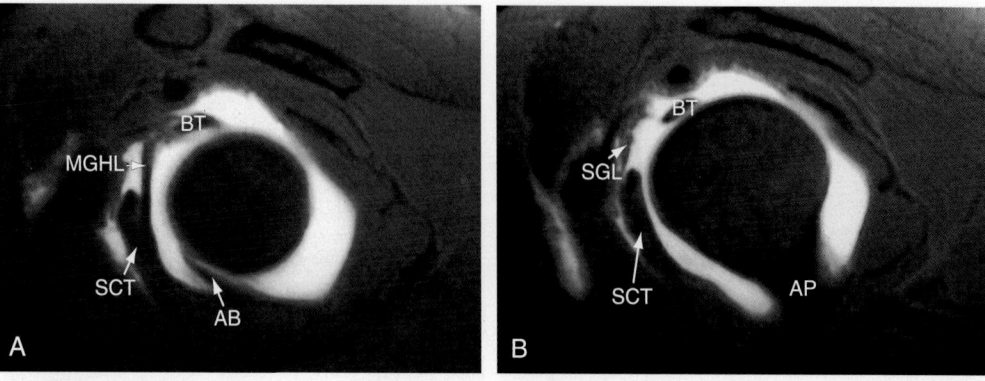

FIGURE 99-10

Glenohumeral ligaments. **A** and **B**, Sagittal oblique MR (TR/TE 600/20 ms) images with fat saturation obtained after intra-articular gadolinium injection. The anterior band (AB) (**A**) and axillary pouch portions (AP) (**B**) of the inferior glenohumeral ligament can be well seen in this plane when contrast is present. The oblique course of the middle glenohumeral ligament is noted (MGL) (**A**). A small portion of the superior glenohumeral ligament (SGL) is visible (**B**). BT, biceps tendon; SCT, subscapularis tendon.

humeral head, and as a static stabilizer of the gleno-humeral joint, resists posterior subluxation.[50] The infraspinatus muscle is innervated by the distal fibers of the suprascapular nerve. The infraspinatus tendon is posterior to the supraspinatus tendon and inserts on the middle facet of the greater tuberosity, inferior and posterior to the supraspinatus tendon.

The teres minor is posteroinferior to the infraspinatus (see Fig. 99-5). It is a powerful external rotator of the humerus. It also helps resist subluxation of the humeral head.[50] The teres minor muscle is innervated by branches of the axillary nerve. It also forms part of the border of the quadrilateral space as well as the triangular space.

The subscapularis is the largest and most powerful muscle of the rotator cuff with a broad-based belly that originates from the anterior scapula (see Fig. 99-5). It has four to six strong tendon slips that arise medially deep within the muscle. These slips converge to form a main tendon that inserts along the superior aspect of the lesser tuberosity.[74] Additional tendon fibers from the subscapularis merge with the transverse humeral ligament and extend across the floor of the bicipital groove, fusing with those of the supraspinatus tendon into a sheath that encompasses the biceps tendon.[75] The subscapularis muscle is supplied by the upper and lower subscapular nerve.[50] In addition to the subscapularis' primary role in active internal rotation, it also functions in adduction, depression, flexion, and extension. The subscapularis tendon also reinforces the anterior joint capsule. It is separated from the rest of the rotator cuff tendons by the rotator cuff interval.

The rotator cuff tendons fuse along their distal attachments to the greater and lesser tuberosities to provide a continuous water-tight unit.[76] Prior to their

fusion, the anatomic space between the supraspinatus and subscapularis along the anterosuperior aspect of the shoulder is the rotator interval (Fig. 99-11). It is a complex region and can be conceptualized in layers.[68,77,78] The outermost layer consists of fibrofatty tissue and beneath this is the coracohumeral ligament, the rotator interval capsule, and then the superior glenohumeral ligament. The coracohumeral ligament courses from the coracoid process into the interval, fusing with the interval capsule. This capsule/ligament complex extends superiorly merging and fusing with the anterior margin and superficial/deep fascial fibers of the supraspinatus anteriorly. The interval capsule and ligament also extend inferiorly to the superior margin of the subscapularis, and project laterally to insert on the greater and lesser tuberosities. The superior glenohumeral ligament also is a contributor to this complex of structures, originating from the supraglenoid tubercle contiguous to the attachment of the long head of the biceps tendon (LHB), and then coursing laterally to insert at the lesser tuberosity, where it fuses with the coracohumeral ligament.[76] This fused rotator interval capsule and coracohumeral ligament are important stabilizers and anterosuperior supporting structures for shoulder function, and can be conceptualized as a roof over the intra-articular course of the biceps tendon, which is the deepest structure in the interval. When the interval capsule and coracohumeral ligament are disrupted, the shoulder may be susceptible to posterior inferior subluxation and instability.[76]

The biceps brachii functions primarily as a supinator of the forearm and a flexor of the elbow joint. There are two tendinous origins of the biceps muscle. Its role is in stabilizing the humeral head in the glenoid during abduction of the shoulder.[79] The intra-articular portion of

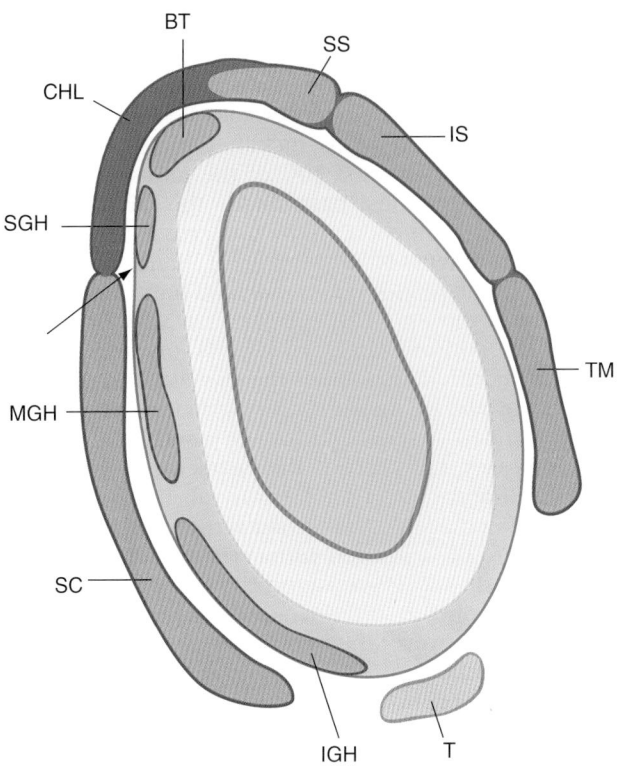

FIGURE 99-11

Rotator interval structures. Sagittal diagram through the left shoulder showing structures of the anterior interval. The first layer of the interval includes the subscapularis (SC) and supraspinatus (SS) tendons, and the coracohumeral ligament (CHL). Deep to this is the articular capsule (*arrow*) followed by the superior glenohumeral ligament (SGH) and the biceps tendon (BT) and its sheath. Also shown is the infraspinatus (IS), teres minor (TM), middle glenohumeral ligament (MGH), inferior glenohumeral ligament (IGH), and triceps long head (T).

the LHB arises from the supraglenoid tubercle (see Figs. 99-8, 99-9, 99-10, and 99-12) and the posterosuperior glenoid labrum. It runs across the superomedial aspect of the humeral head and enters the intertubercular sulcus which is formed by the greater tuberosity, lesser tuberosity, and soft-tissues, including the insertion of the subscapularis tendon and coracohumeral ligament.[79] It penetrates the rotator cuff between the supraspinatus and subscapularis at the rotator interval. The biceps tendon is surrounded by a synovial sheath, which is continuous with the synovial sheath of the shoulder joint (see Fig. 99-6). The anterior relationships of the proximal long head of the biceps include the coracohumeral ligament, the superior glenohumeral ligament, the anterior supraspinatus tendon, and the subscapularis tendon. These are the stabilizers of this portion of the tendon. The tendon is secured within the groove by the transverse humeral ligament, which passes between the tuberosities, over the synovial sheath of the tendon. The transverse humeral ligament is formed by a few fibers of the capsule, or as a continuation of the subscapularis tendon. The biceps tendon mainly functions through its distal insertion at the elbow, but also has some function at the shoulder where it acts as a stabilizer, as well as a humeral head depressor. It is closely associated functionally with the rotator cuff. The short head of the biceps arises from the tip of the coracoid process. The conjoined tendon of the coracobrachialis muscle and the short head of the biceps brachii muscle join on the tip of the coracoid process.

There are a number of bursae about the glenohumeral joint. The subdeltoid bursa is the largest bursa in the human body (see Fig. 99-7). It is comprised primarily of a subacromial and subdeltoid portion which communicate. The size and configuration of the subdeltoid bursa varies. The bursa is firmly adherent to the periosteum

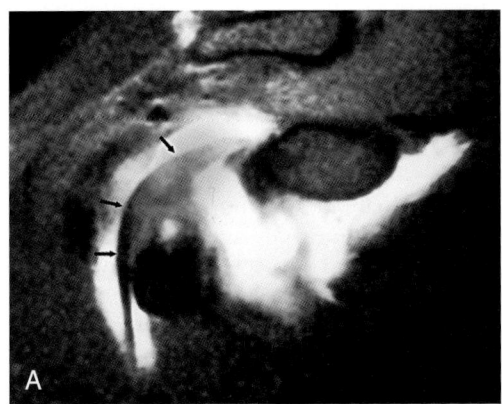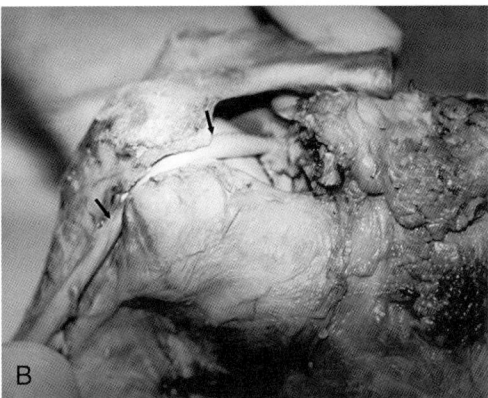

FIGURE 99-12

Biceps tendon. **A,** Coronal oblique MR images (TR/TE 600/20 ms) with fat saturation obtained after intra-articular gadolinium injection. **B,** Corresponding anatomic section. The long head of the biceps tendon is seen extending from the supraglenoid region into the intertubercular groove (*arrows* in **A** and **B**).

of the undersurface of the acromion, coracoacromial ligament, and superior surface of the rotator cuff. Its lateral extent projects deep to the deltoid muscle approximately 3 cm along the outer margin of the greater tuberosity. Medially, the bursa exhibits considerable variability extending as far as 2 cm medial to the acromioclavicular joint. Anteriorly, the bursa covers the superior aspect of the bicipital groove; posteriorly, the bursa extends between the deltoid muscle and rotator cuff musculature. There is continuity between the subdeltoid and subacromial components. The bursa is a synovial-lined potential space within a fine layer of mature areolar/adipose tissue that lubricates motion between the rotator cuff and the acromion and acromioclavicular joint; hence it is often inflamed in patients with impingement and rotator cuff disease. It only communicates with the joint if a full-thickness tear of the rotator cuff opens through the joint capsule into the floor of the bursa.

The subcoracoid bursa resides between the subscapularis tendon and the combined tendon of the coracobrachialis and the short head of the biceps tendon. It is identified in nearly 97% of gross specimens, and communicates with the subdeltoid bursa in 11% of anatomic specimens.[80] The subcoracoid bursa should not communicate with the glenohumeral joint. Subcoracoid bursitis may be a rare cause of nonspecific anterior shoulder discomfort.

The subscapularis bursa is found in up to 90% of the population (see Figs. 99-8 and 99-9). It is really an outpouching of the glenohumeral joint protruding between the superior and middle glenohumeral ligaments and residing between the posterior aspect of the subscapularis muscle/tendon and the anterior surface of the scapula. The opening into the bursa between these two ligaments is known as the foramen of Weitbrecht. The subscapularis bursa communicates with the joint cavity and protects the subscapularis tendon as it passes under the coracoid, or over the neck of the scapula. The subscapularis recess may extend anterior to the subscapularis tendon and acts as a gliding mechanism for it (see Fig. 99-9).

Acromioclavicular Joint

The acromioclavicular joint is a small, immobile synovial articulation between the medial aspect of the acromion and the lateral portion of the clavicle (see Figs. 99-6 and 99-7). The articular surfaces of the acromion and clavicle are covered with fibrocartilage. In the central portion of the joint there is an articular disk which is fibrocartilaginous. A synovium-lined articular capsule surrounds the joint. It is reinforced by the superior and inferior acromioclavicular ligaments. The inferior portion of the joint is also reinforced by fibers of the coracoacromial ligament.[50] The coracoclavicular ligament is more important to stability and forms a fanshaped ligament complex that connects the base of the coracoid process to the overlying clavicle. This ligament has two components, the posteromedial conoid and anterolateral trapezoid ligaments.

The coracoacromial arch (see Fig. 99-6) is a strong bony and ligamentous arch that protects the humeral head and rotator cuff tendons from direct trauma.[59] It consists of the acromion, acromioclavicular joint, coracoid process, and coracoacromial ligament. Portions of the rotator cuff tendons, including the supraspinatus tendon and the superior 20% of the infraspinatus and subscapularis tendons, pass under this arch as they extend to their insertion on the humerus.[50] The coracoacromial ligament is unyielding. It limits the space available to the rotator cuff, subdeltoid bursa, and biceps in overhead motion. The ligament can vary in appearance.[81] In approximately two-thirds of subjects the ligament morphology follows the classical description; a strong, fibrous, triangular-shaped structure comprising two conjoined or closely adjacent bands. In the other third of cases, the base of the ligamentous triangle is broadened and extends posteriorly all the way to the base of the coracoid. This broad acromial insertion site is thought to be worsened with certain acromial shapes, thickening of the coracoacromial ligament, and bony osteophytes on the anterior acromion or acromioclavicular joint. This may then contribute to the process of chronic impingement.

Acromial morphology has been categorized utilizing plain radiographic analysis: type I flat, type II curved, and type III hooked (Fig. 99-13).[82-84] This configuration can be assessed with sagittal MR images, though this has met with variability and poor reliability among investigators.[85,86] The J- or hook-shaped type III morphology has the highest association with impingement syndrome and rotator cuff abnormalities.[87]

The coracohumeral ligament originates from the lateral margin of the base of the coracoid process, blends with the supraspinatus tendon, and attaches to both the greater and lesser tuberosities, creating a tunnel for the biceps tendon. This ligament stabilizes the long head of the biceps tendon and also projects within the rotator interval (see Fig. 99-11).[88,89]

The suprascapular notch lies just lateral to the base of the coracoid process. The superior transverse scapular ligament converts the notch to a foramen through which the suprascapular nerve passes. The suprascapular vessels project superior to this ligament.[50]

MRI Anatomy (Figs. 99-14 to 99-16)

The normal MR appearance of the shoulder in the axial, coronal oblique and sagittal oblique planes is illustrated in Figures 99-14 to 99-16. In the normal state, subcutaneous fat, intermuscular fat planes, and bone marrow normally have the highest signal on short TR/TE or long TR short TE images, due to their relatively short T1. On long TR/TE images, they are of intermediate signal intensity. Muscles and hyaline cartilage have an intermediate-to-high signal intensity on all spin-echo pulse sequences, and on gradient-echo sequences articular cartilage tends to have high signal intensity. Due to a relative lack of mobile protons, a long T1, and a short T2, certain structures should have essentially a very

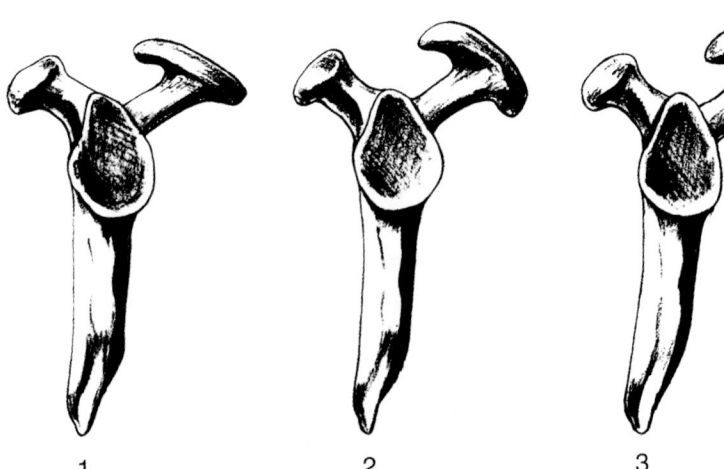

FIGURE 99-13

Acromion shape. Three types of anterior acromion: type 1, flat; type 2, curved; type 3, hook shaped. *(Reproduced with permission from Zlatkin MB: MRI of the Shoulder, 2nd ed. Philadelphia, Lippincott, Williams and Wilkins, 2003.)*

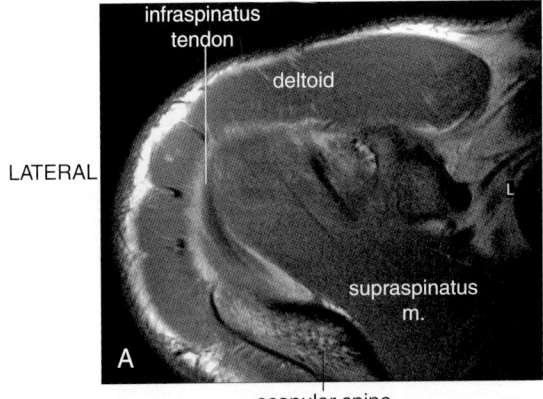

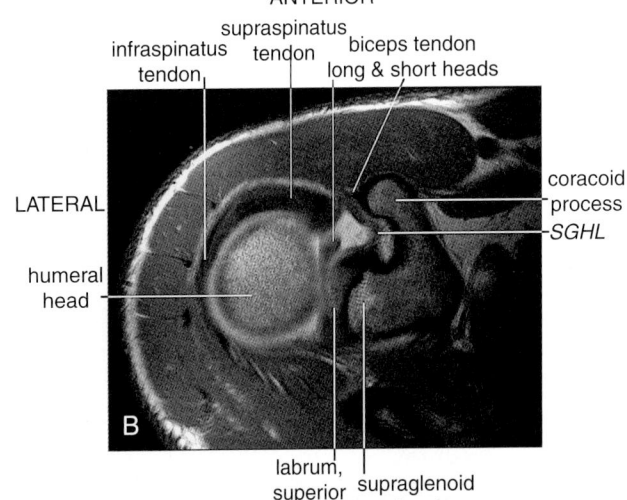

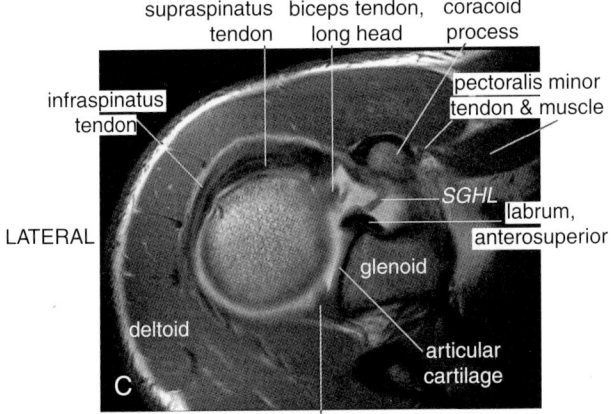

FIGURE 99-14

A-C, Axial MRI and MR arthrographic anatomy. Superior to inferior. Short TR/TE images (800/20 ms). IGHL, inferior glenohumeral ligament; MGHL, middle glenohumeral ligament; SGHL, superior glenohumeral ligament; a., artery; m., muscle; n., nerve; t., tendon. *(Prepared by Steven Needell, MD; reproduced with permission from Zlatkin MB: MRI of the Shoulder, 2nd ed. Philadelphia, Lippincott, Williams and Wilkins, 2003.)*

Continued

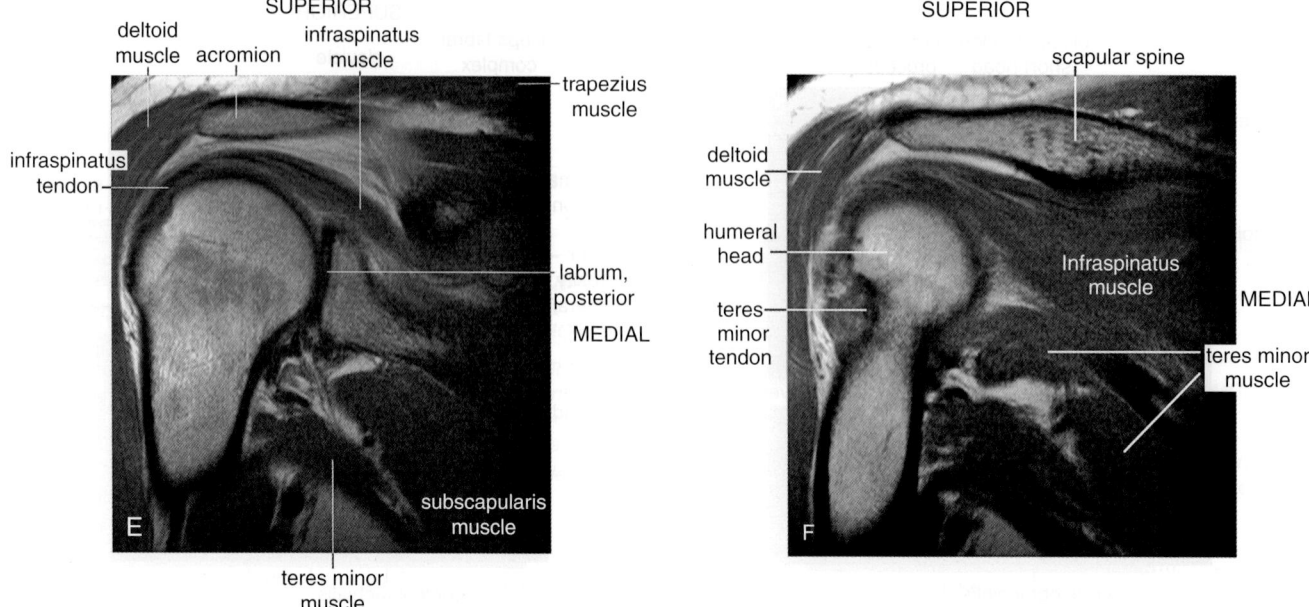

FIGURE 99-15, cont'd

E and **F,** Coronal oblique MRI and MR arthrographic anatomy. Anterior to posterior. Short TR/TE images (800/20 ms). IGHL, inferior glenohumeral ligament MGHL; middle glenohumeral ligament; SGHL, superior glenohumeral ligament; subscap, subscapularis; pect., pectoralis; m., muscle; t., tendon. *(Prepared by Steven Needell, MD; reproduced with permission from Zlatkin MB: MRI of the Shoulder, 2nd ed. Philadelphia, Lippincott, Williams and Wilkins, 2003.)*

low or no MR signal. These structures include cortical bone, glenoid labrum, fibrous capsule, glenohumeral and other ligaments and tendons, such as the tendinous insertions of the rotator cuff musculature, and long head of biceps tendon, as it courses in the bicipital groove.[90,91] Numerous studies have shown that signal may be present in the ligaments, tendons, and fibrocartilage of asymptomatic people due to age-related degeneration, subclinical pathology, partial volume averaging of normal tissues, or artifacts including magic angle effects.[92-99]

Axial images (Fig. 99-14) demonstrate the relationship between the humeral head and glenoid fossa. Articular cartilage and the glenoid labrum are well depicted. The superior and middle portions of the anterior glenoid labrum are usually triangular in this plane, whereas the more anterior inferior labrum may be round. The anterior labrum can be variable in appearance and size, may be rounded or cleaved, or may even rarely be absent (Fig. 99-17).[100] The posterior labrum is also said typically to be triangular, but may be rounded, flat or absent.[101] The normal bright signal of hyaline cartilage at the base of the labrum should not be mistaken for a tear or detachment (Fig. 99-17).[102] Linear or globular foci of increased signal can be observed near the base of the labrum in normal subjects.[103] Magic angle phenomenon can cause areas of increased signal in the postero-superior/anteroinferior labrum on proton-density– and T1-weighted images. This signal should not approach that of fluid on T2-weighted images.[103-105] On MRI, labral

shape may vary with humeral rotation. Cleaved or notched[101] configurations are normal variants and should not be mistaken for tears. Labral size, shape, and appearance are also not necessarily bilateral and symmetric. Partial imaging of the glenohumeral ligaments (see Figs. 99-9 and 99-14)[106] may also simulate cleavage planes or notches in the labrum, or even tears or avulsed fragments. A similar problem may also occur with partial imaging of the subscapularis tendon. This may be most notable in the absence of an effusion when the glenohumeral ligaments and subscapularis tendons are closely applied to the anterior labrum. Superiorly, fluid may be seen in a sublabral recess or foramen (Fig. 99-18).[89,107-109] Fluid or contrast beneath the labrum at the level of the coracoid or below (below the equator or epiphyseal line) is considered pathologic and indicative of a tear or detachment. The vacuum phenomenon[16] is where low signal intensity gas is seen intra-articularly on gradient-recalled echo (GRE) images and should not be mistaken for a labral tear or cartilage lesion. It is accentuated with the arm in external rotation and is located superiorly.

The subscapularis muscle and tendon are also well visualized in the axial plane (Figs. 99-9 and 99-14). The subscapularis recess or bursa is identified in the presence of synovial fluid. This bursa can extend anterior to the subscapularis tendon, as well as between the capsule and posterior surface of the tendon (Figs. 99-9 and 99-14). The anterior capsule and its insertion into

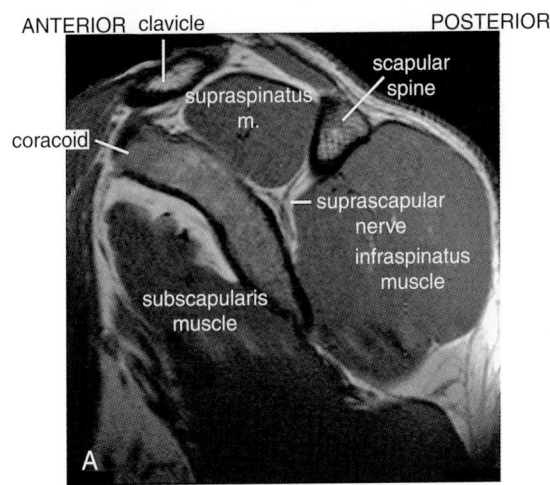

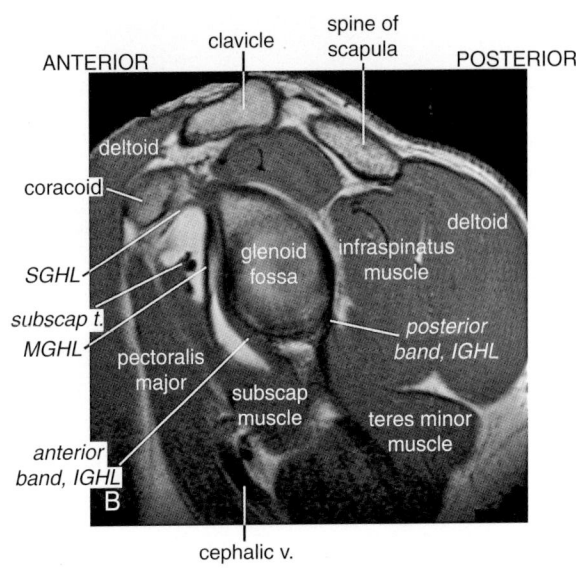

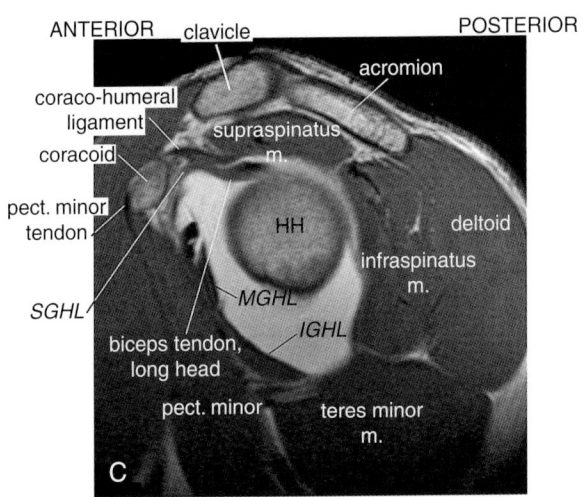

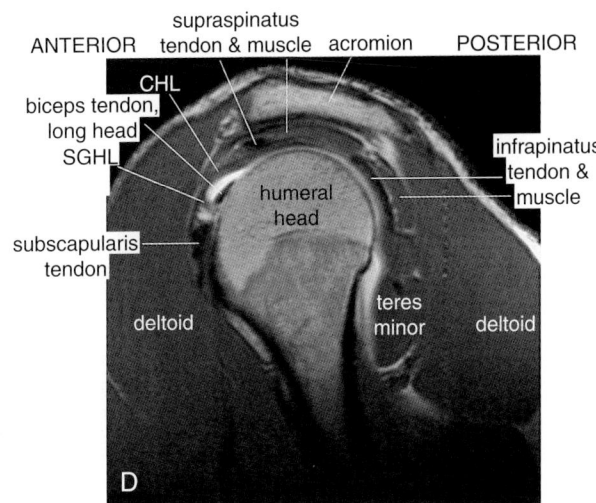

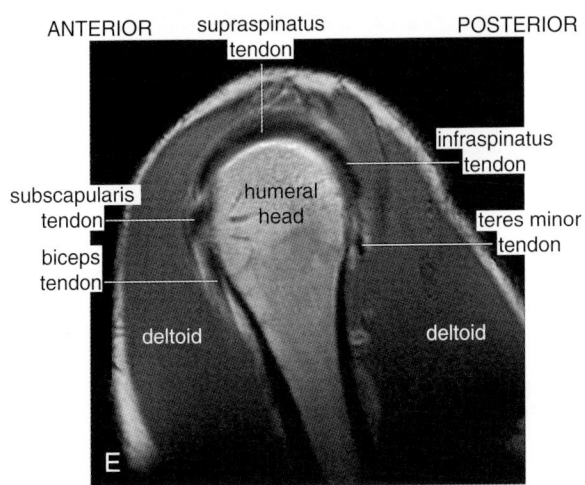

FIGURE 99-16

A-E, Sagittal oblique MRI and MR arthrographic anatomy. Medial to lateral. Short TR/TE images (800/20 ms). IGHL, inferior glenohumeral ligament; MGHL, middle glenohumeral ligament; SGHL, superior glenohumeral ligament; subscap, subscapularis; pect., pectoralis; m., muscle; t., tendon. *(Prepared by Steven Needell, MD; reproduced with permission from Zlatkin MB: MRI of the Shoulder, 2nd ed. Philadelphia, Lippincott, Williams and Wilkins, 2003.)*

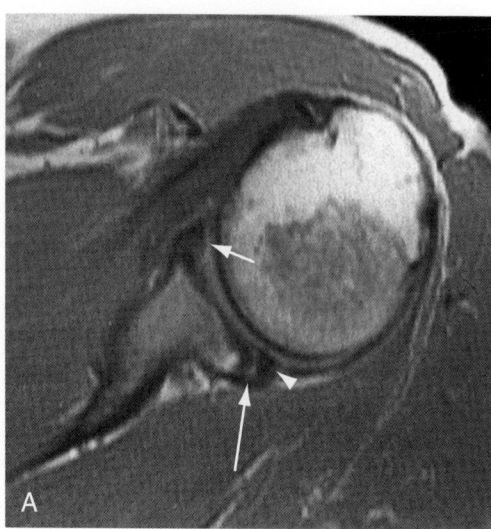 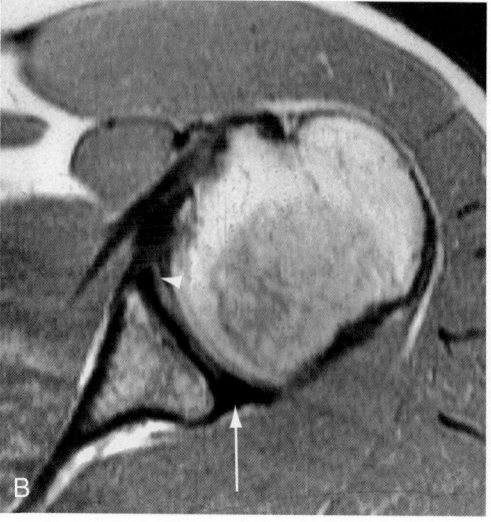

FIGURE 99-17

Labral shape and variation. Axial short TR/TE (800/20 ms) images. **A,** Triangular appearance of the anterior labrum (*short arrow*) and the smaller more round appearance of the posterior labrum (*arrowhead*). The hyaline articular cartilage undercutting the posterior labrum is also seen (*long arrow*). **B,** Image reveals the small near absent anterior labrum (*arrowhead*) and the posterior labrum (*arrow*) to be larger and more triangular. *(Prepared by Steven Needell, MD; reproduced with permission from Zlatkin MB: MRI of the Shoulder, 2nd ed. Philadelphia, Lippincott, Williams and Wilkins, 2003.)*

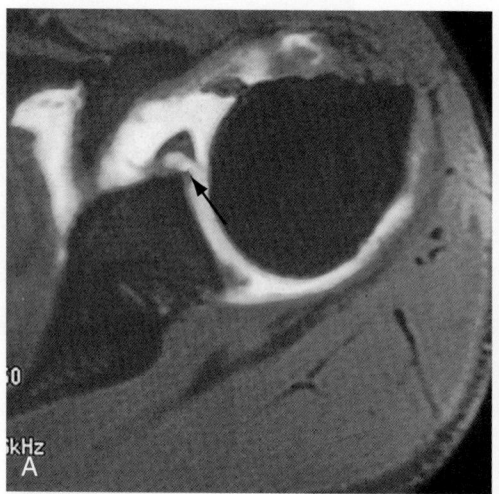 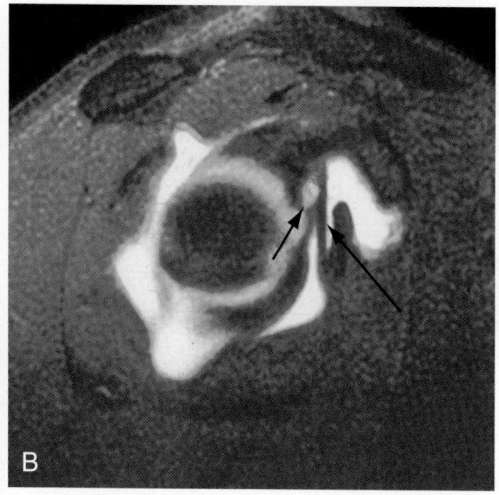

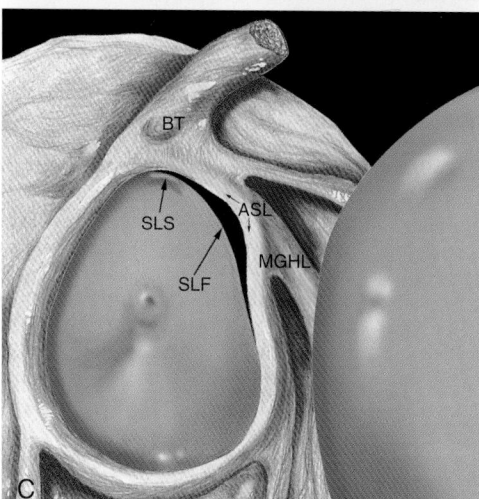

FIGURE 99-18

Sublabral foramen. **A,** Axial spoiled gradient-echo image and **B,** sagittal oblique MR arthrogram with short TR/TE image (800/20 ms) and fat suppression. High signal contrast outlines a smooth appearing sublabral foramen (*short arrow* in **A** and **B**). A thick middle glenohumeral attaches anterosuperiorly (*long arrow* in **B**). Note there is no sublabral sulcus more superiorly. **C,** Lateral view illustrates the sublabral foramen. It is anterior and inferior to the sublabral sulcus. ASL, anterior superior labrum; BT, long head of the biceps tendon; MGHL, middle glenohumeral ligament; SLF, sublabral foramen; SLS, sublabral sulcus. *(Drawn by Salvador Beltran; reproduced with permission from Zlatkin MB: MRI of the Shoulder, 2nd ed. Philadelphia, Lippincott, Williams and Wilkins, 2003.)*

the glenoid margin can be identified on axial images. It is best seen on long TR/TE images in the presence of joint fluid, with gradient-echo imaging, or with MR arthrography. The glenohumeral ligaments may not be easily separated from the subscapularis tendon on routine spin-echo axial images but are more easily identified when an effusion is present. They may also be better seen with MRI arthrography (Figs. 99-9 and 99-14 to 99-16). On superior sections, the superior glenohumeral ligament and superior capsule may be seen inserting into the supraglenoid region, where the superior labrum and biceps tendon may be identified. At the midglenoid level the middle glenohumeral ligament is best identified posterior to the subscapularis tendon and the capsule. At the inferior portion of the glenoid cavity the inferior glenohumeral ligament inserts as a thick complex with the inferior capsule into the labrum. When an effusion is present or with MR arthrography the three bands of the inferior glenohumeral ligament may be identified separately and of particular importance in the setting of anterior instability is visualization of the anterior band as it forms part of the anterior inferior labral-ligamentous complex (Figs. 99-9 and 99-14 to 99-16).

The biceps brachii functions as a supinator of the forearm and a flexor of the elbow joint. It is also believed to be a flexor of the shoulder joint. The long head of the biceps tendon is seen arising from the supraglenoid region (see Fig. 99-12). At the level of the superior pole of the glenoid, four separate attachments of the biceps tendon may be observed. These include the supraglenoid tubercle, the posterior superior labrum, the anterior superior labrum, and an extra-articular attachment to the lateral edge of the base of the coracoid process. The biceps labral complex corresponds to the superior one third of the glenoid. Stoller has described variability in the pattern of insertion of the long head into the supraglenoid region as it forms part of the biceps labral anchor complex.[110] As it exits the supraglenoid region the tendon courses obliquely and anteriorly over the humeral head. Proximally it may be best seen on coronal and sagittal oblique images (see Figs. 99-15 and 99-16). It then courses inferiorly into the intertubercular groove, where it is well seen on axial sections and appears as a round signal void (see Fig. 99-14). Its synovial sheath is seen as a ring of moderate signal intensity,[110] which often contains a small amount of fluid as a normal finding.[111]

The tendons of the rotator cuff complex are well seen on serial coronal oblique images, since this plane courses parallel to the supraspinatus muscle and tendon (see Fig. 99-15). The infraspinatus and teres minor tendons are also well delineated in this orientation. The subscapularis tendon is identified on more anterior coronal oblique images but is better evaluated on axial images (Fig. 99-14 and 99-15). It may also be delineated on sagittal oblique images (Fig. 99-16). The subdeltoid bursa is a potential space and therefore is not visualized as a separate structure, unless filled with fluid, though on occasion a thin rim of fluid signal may be seen on fat-suppressed images in this region.[17,74] The subdeltoid peribursal fat plane[112] is seen on short TR/TE and proton-density–weighted sequences, as a high signal intensity line separating the rotator cuff tendons from the acromioclavicular joint, acromion, and overlying deltoid muscle.

On anterior coronal oblique images, the coracoclavicular (coronoid and trapezoid) and acromioclavicular ligaments, as well as the acromioclavicular joint, may be identified. The anterior acromion can be seen. The coracoacromial ligament may also be delineated, though less constantly identified. The anterior edge of the supraspinatus tendon can be depicted, along with the long head of the biceps tendon and the subscapularis muscle and tendon. The rotator interval may be seen on these sections as well (see Fig. 99-15). The superior and inferior labrum can be identified in this plane as can the axillary recess.

The sagittal oblique plane demonstrates the rotator cuff muscles and tendons in cross section (see Fig. 99-16). The anteroposterior extent of the rotator cuff tendons can be visualized. The relationship of the acromion process, the acromioclavicular joint, and the coracoacromial ligament to the supraspinatus and other cuff tendons is best depicted. The shape of the anterior acromion can be discerned on sagittal oblique images. With fluid in the joint or with MRI arthrography (see Figs. 99-10 and 99-16), the labrum, capsule, and glenohumeral ligaments can be depicted, and in particular the three limbs of the inferior glenohumeral ligament are well seen.

The rotator interval may be well evaluated on oblique sagittal images (see Fig. 99-16). The coracohumeral ligament is an important landmark on sagittal images, coursing from the coracoid process into the interval to blend with the interval capsule. The most proximal portion of the biceps can be found immediately inferior and deep to the posterior aspect of the coracohumeral ligament and interval capsule at the level of the superior biceps labral anchor complex. The fused coracohumeral ligament and capsule may be followed posterosuperiorly to the level of the anterior margin and leading edge of the supraspinatus.[76] The long head of the biceps tendon should be demonstrated as a smooth low signal intensity structure which on sequential sagittal images (see Fig. 99-18) can be followed within the rotator interval from medial to lateral to the bicipital groove, after which axial images are best for following the tendon from the proximal bicipital groove (see Fig. 99-14) more distally along the humeral shaft.[76]

Although a detailed discussion of anatomic pitfalls about the glenohumeral joint is beyond the scope of this chapter, those about the anterosuperior labrum are so common and give rise to so many difficulties in interpretation that they warrant separate discussion. The anterosuperior labrum is the most common site of normal anatomic variations, with specific variations described in up to 13.5% of those studied.[27,107,109] These variations in labral attachment occur above the equator of the glenoid, which occurs at the 3 o'clock position on the glenoid margin. Below the equator the labrum should be firmly attached. The anterosuperior labrum is not attached to the bony glenoid in 8% to 12% of the population, referred to as a sublabral foramen, also

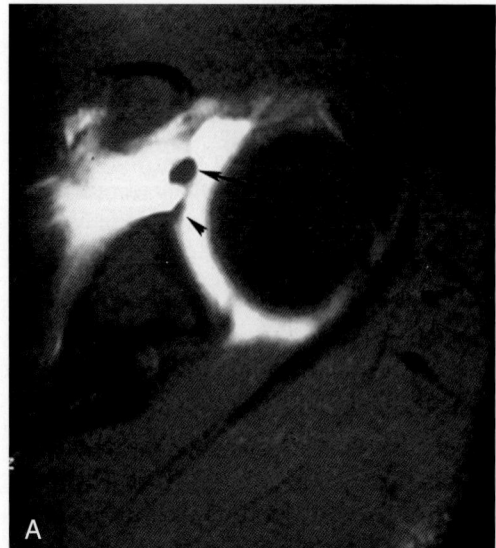

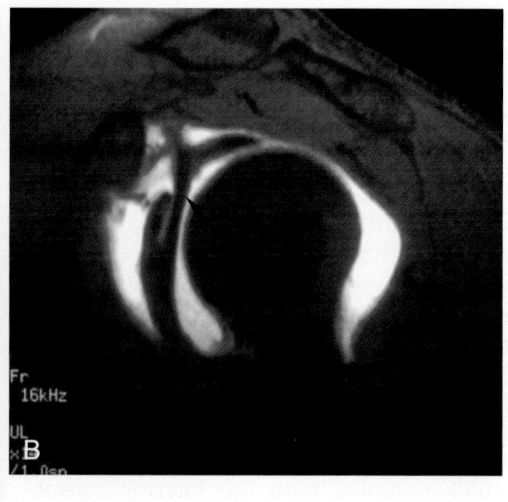

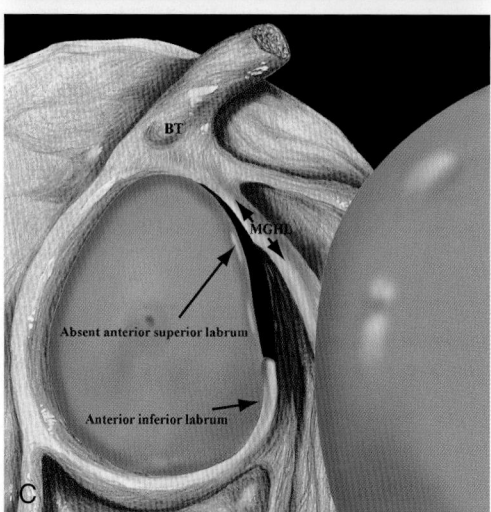

FIGURE 99-19

Buford complex. **A,** Axial and **B,** sagittal oblique MR arthrograms. Short TR/TE images (800/20 ms) with fat suppression. The labrum is nearly absent antero-superiorly (*arrowhead* on **A**). The thick cordlike middle glenohumeral ligament is identified partially in **A** and continuously in **B**, attaching to the superior labrum directly (*arrow*). **C,** Lateral view of the Buford complex. Note the absent anterior superior labrum and the thick, cordlike, middle glenohumeral ligament which is attaching anterosuperiorly. BT, long head of the biceps tendon; MGHL, middle glenohumeral ligament. (*Drawn by Salvador Beltran; reproduced with permission from Zlatkin MB: MRI of the Shoulder, 2nd ed. Philadelphia, Lippincott, Williams and Wilkins, 2003.*)

known as a sublabral hole (see Fig. 99-18).[113] This finding is located anterior to the biceps-labral complex.[114] A sublabral recess, also referred to as a sublabral sulcus, is a recess/synovial reflection between the biceps-labral complex and the superior margin of the glenoid.[113] On occasion, a sublabral recess can be continuous with a sublabral foramen.[114] In cadaver studies, a sublabral recess has been demonstrated in up to 73% of shoulders.[115] The anterosuperior labrum can also be focally absent, usually associated with a thickened, cordlike middle glenohumeral ligament. This entity is referred to as the Buford complex, believed to be present in approximately 1.5% of patients (Fig. 99-19).[114] Pathologic lesions occurring or originating in, or extending into, the antero-superior labral quadrant can also be distinguished from normal anatomic variations if they extend below the level of the coracoid process tip (which helps mark the equator) towards or into the anteroinferior labrum, or posteriorly into the posterosuperior quadrant (beyond the biceps labral anchor).[103] Therefore, a Buford complex should be suspected if the contiguous anteroinferior

and superior labrum appear normal.[116] Morphologic alterations help to distinguish pathologic lesions as well. MR arthrography will delineate this anatomy to better advantage and help distinguish variant anatomy from pathologic lesions.

ROTATOR CUFF DISEASE

Pathophysiology

A variety of different factors are considered to be important in the etiology of rotator cuff disease and ultimately rotator cuff tears. The most discussed mechanisms include rotator cuff impingement beneath the coracoacromial arch (extrinsic impingement), and primary degeneration of the cuff. Trauma, overuse related to occupational and athletic activities, and glenohumeral joint instability also play a role. Acute and chronic inflammation such as seen in rheumatoid arthritis is a less common cause.

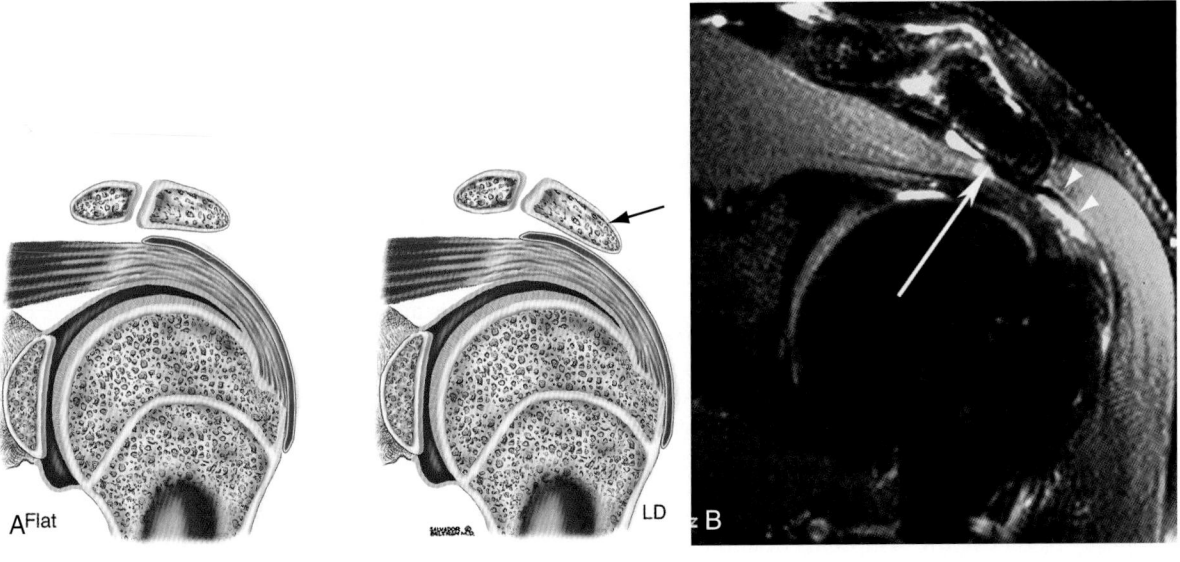

FIGURE 99-20

A, Lateral downsloping (LD) of the anterior acromion as seen on coronal section (*arrow*). **B,** Coronal T2-weighted MRI with fat suppression revealing LD (*arrow*). Note the corresponding alterations on the bursal surface of the rotator cuff and the thickened subdeltoid bursa filled with fluid (*arrowheads*). *(Drawn by Salvador Beltran; reproduced with permission from Zlatkin MB: MRI of the Shoulder, 2nd ed. Philadelphia, Lippincott, Williams and Wilkins, 2003.)*

Impingement

Rotator cuff impingement may be divided into primary extrinsic impingement, secondary extrinsic impingement (secondary to instability), internal impingement (posterosubglenoid), and subscoracoid impingement.

Primary Extrinsic Impingement

Neer[117-120] is most responsible for popularizing this concept and using this as an aid in clinical management of patients. Neer[119,120] showed that when the shoulder elevates in its functional arc the rotator cuff and surrounding soft-tissue structures impinge in the space beneath the coracoacromial arch. Neer[119,120] stated that 95% of rotator cuff tears occur as a result of chronic impingement beneath this arch. The space below this arch is defined by the acromion superiorly, the coracoacromial ligament superomedially, and the coracoid process anteriorly. Known sites of impingement in this arch include the anteroinferior edge of the acromion, the coracoacromial ligament, and, occasionally, the undersurface of the acromioclavicular joint.[121]

Variation in anterior acromion shape also correlates with cuff tears (see Fig. 99-13).[83,122-124] Three types of acromion have been described, based on their shape. A type 1 acromion has a flat surface, type 2 has a curved undersurface, and type 3 has a hooked undersurface. A fourth type of acromion shape (type 4) has also been recently described. This has a convex inferior surface.[124] As yet no statistical correlation has been found between this type of acromion and impingement.

The hook-shaped acromion (type 3) has been shown to have the most significance (see Fig. 99-13).[83,122] It has the highest correlation with rotator cuff pathology and particularly rotator cuff tears. Correlation with surgical and arthrographic results revealed a 70% to 80% association of rotator cuff tears with type 3 acromions.[83]

Lateral or anterior downward sloping of the acromion, relative to the distal clavicle may also contribute to impingement and narrowing of the suprapinatus outlet (Fig. 99-20).[125] A low lying acromial position, relative to the distal clavicle, may decrease the space between the acromion and the humerus and may predispose certain individuals to shoulder impingement.

Osteophytes arising from the acromioclavicular joint and extending inferiorly may play some role in the impingement process as well. A study by Petersson et al[121] revealed an association between the acromioclavicular joint osteophytes and supraspinatus tendon pathology. Kessel and Watson[126] found these changes in one third of their patients with a "painful arc syndrome" and lesions of the supraspinatus tendon. In this study these osteophytes were found to be more common than anterior subacromial spurs, though they frequently occur together. Osteoarthritis of the acromioclavicular joint, however, may be identified on MRI examination in a large percentage of asymptomatic individuals.[111]

Spurs on the anterior and inferior aspect of the acromion are also important.[119] These spurs extend from the anteroinferior surface of the acromion in a medial and slightly inferior direction toward the coracoid process. They arise at the acromial attachment of the coracoacromial ligament. The presence of these spurs is considered presumptive evidence of shoulder impingement. Spur size may be strongly associated with the incidence of a rotator cuff tear.[127] Subacromial spurs are considered to be a more correlative marker of impingement changes and rotator cuff disease[128] than acromioclavicular joint osteophytes. Variation in size and thickness of the coracoacromial ligament, especially the wide portion inferior to the acromion, may be an additional factor in narrowing the subacromial space and thus causing attritional changes of the rotator cuff.[129]

An unfused apophysis of the anterior acromion, known as the os acromiale, may contribute to shoulder impingement.[130-132] These normally fuse by 25 years of age. Fusion failure may occur in 8% of the population and thus form an os acromiale.[133] The os acromiale may cause impingement because, if it is unstable, it may be pulled inferiorly during abduction by the deltoid, which attaches here. In addition, hypertrophy and spurring may develop at the junction of the os acromiale and the more posterior aspect of the acromion along its undersurface, and may contribute to impingement and subsequent rotator cuff tears in this manner.[134]

The clinical syndrome of impingement was outlined by Neer.[119] He described the technique of anterior acromioplasty to relieve the symptoms of impingement. Three progressive stages of impingement lesions were described. This was based on the age of the patient, the type of activity that presumably led to the injury, and the pathologic findings. Stage 1 typically results from excessive overhead use such as in sports. It usually occurs in patients younger than 25 years of age, but may occur at any age. Histologically, edema and hemorrhage are said to be present in the rotator cuff tendons at this stage. If treated conservatively, this phase of the disease is usually reversible and these patients may return to normal function.

Stage 2 disease consists of fibrosis and thickening of the rotator cuff tendons as well as the subacromial-subdeltoid bursa. It occurs in patients between 25 to 40 years of age and is less common than stage 1. The shoulder will usually become symptomatic after vigorous overhead use such as in throwing sports. Traditionally, surgery is considered in these patients when a conservative approach to therapy has failed. The procedure at this stage is removal of the thickened subacromial bursa and dividing the coracoacromial ligament. According to Neer,[119,120] anterior acromioplasty in this group of patients who are younger than 40 years old should not be performed unless overhang and prominence of the undersurface of the anterior acromion is present.

Stage 3 results from further impingement wear. At this stage incomplete (3A) or complete tears (3B) of the rotator cuff are present. These lesions are most common in patients older than 40 years of age. Lesions of the biceps tendon are usually present, though true tears of the biceps tendon are much less common than the associated cuff tears. Secondary bone changes are very common. Acromioplasty and cuff repair are often required.

Secondary Extrinsic Impingement (Impingement Associated with Instability)

Fu et al[134] subdivided impingement syndromes into two major categories: primary extrinsic impingement which occurs in nonathletic persons and is related to alterations in the coracoaromial arch as discussed earlier;

and secondary impingement occurring mainly in athletes involved in sports requiring overhead motion of the arm and which has a relationship to glenohumeral joint instability.[135,136] These patients may develop symptoms without any abnormality of the bony anatomy of the coracoacromial arch. These patients usually have less advanced rotator cuff pathology, including tendinosis or partial or very small rotator cuff tears.[136] This distinction is important, since therapy should be directed to the underlying instability. Conservative treatment is aimed at strengthening the rotator cuff and scapular rotators. Throwing athletes with glenohumeral instability and secondary impingement that do not respond to conservative treatment may be treated with an anterior capsular labral reconstruction. In the less common situation where alterations of the bony coracoacromial arch may also be identified (mixed pathology), then subacromial decompression may be necessary in addition to anterior stabilization.

Posterosubglenoid (Internal) Impingement

This is impingement of the rotator cuff on the posterosuperior portion of the glenoid in throwing athletes.[38,137-144] This is also known as internal impingement. This particular type of impingement occurs during the late cocking phase of throwing with abnormal contact between the posterosuperior portion of the glenoid rim and the undersurface of the rotator cuff, and is thought to occur at the extremes of abduction and external rotation. It has also been recognized in nonathletes who frequently rotate the shoulder into the extremes of abduction and external rotation.[139,145]

A triad of findings will be present including injury to the rotator cuff undersurface at the junction of the infraspinatus and supraspinatus tendons, degenerative tearing of the posterosuperior glenoid labrum, as well as subcortical cysts and chondral lesions in the postero-superior glenoid and humerus due to repetitive impaction. There may in addition be an injury to the inferior glenohumeral ligament and anterior inferior labrum.

Subcoracoid Impingement

Impingement beneath the coracoid process relates to encroachment of the subscapularis tendon insertion on the lesser tuberosity,[146-148] secondary to narrowing of this space between the coracoid process and the humeral head. Developmental enlargement of the coracoid process that projects more laterally may be the underlying cause.

Subcoracoid impingement may occur when the distance between the coracoid and lesser tuberosity measures less than 11 mm, with the arm positioned in maximal internal rotation.[15]

Other Causes

These may include such entities as supraspinatus muscle hypertrophy in athletes who perform repetitive overhead activity, such as swimmers. In these patients, the enlarged supraspinatus muscle belly may seem to be deformed beneath the acromioclavicular joint on coronal oblique MR images.[149] Impingement may also occur related to prominent healed callus from a greater tuberosity fracture.

Primary Rotator Cuff Degeneration (Intrinsic Causes)

There are other theories on the etiology of rotator cuff tears and many who disagree with the predominant or exclusive role of impingement in the development of cuff tears. Codman[150,151] suggested that degenerative changes within the cuff itself lead to tears. This may have a vascular or ischemic basis. Codman[150,151] described a critical portion in the rotator cuff at the distal supraspinatus tendon approximately 1 cm medial to its insertion into the greater tuberosity. Codman[150-152] described the pattern of degenerative cuff failure as a "rim rent" in which the deep surface of the cuff is torn at its attachment to the tuberosity. He stated that these tears tend to begin on the deep surface and then extend outward until they become full-thickness defects. He pointed out that it would be hard to explain this on the basis of erosion from contact with the acromion process.

Uthoff et al[153-155] found that most rotator cuff tears begin from the articular side. They indicated that if rotator cuff tears arose primarily from extrinsic impingement, then the majority of rotator cuff tears should begin from the bursal side. On the basis of this they considered that rotator cuff tears are therefore degenerative in origin and nature and that extrinsic causes therefore play a secondary role. Ozaki et al[156] have shown in cadavers that the majority of pathologic changes of the undersurface of the acromion occurred in specimens in which the cuff tear was incomplete and on the bursal side of the cuff.

The critical portion in the rotator cuff has been described as "the critical zone." This region is said to be a watershed area, occurring between osseous and tendinous vessels supplying the rotator cuff tendons.[153,157]

The histologic pattern of age-related degeneration in the tendon reveals changes in cell arrangement, calcium deposition, fibrinoid thickening, fatty degeneration, necrosis, and rents. There is an alteration in the pattern of collagen fibers in such patients, with transformation from type II to fibrovascular-containing type III collagen.[158,159]

In contrast, intraoperative laser Doppler flowmetry has also been used to assess the rotator cuff tendon vascularity in symptomatic patients.[160] These studies were considered to support impingement as a mechanism of rotator cuff pathology. Particularly in patients with intact tendons and tendinosis but also in patients with partial and complete tears, increased vascularity was found in the region of the critical zone. Brooks et al[161] also carried out perfusion studies which they considered did not support an ischemic zone in the distal anterior supraspinatus tendon. They concluded that factors other than vascularity are important in the pathogenesis of supraspinatus rupture.

Budoff et al[162] argued that most patients with rotator cuff abnormalities have as their primary underlying etiology intrinsic, rather than extrinsic, impingement, which they believe occurs secondary to rotator cuff failure. They stated that the suprapinatus, since it is a small and relatively weak muscle, is in a key position and is therefore susceptible to overuse and injury. When eccentric tensile overload occurs at a rate greater than the ability of the cuff to repair itself, injury occurs, resulting in weakness of the musculotendinous rotator cuff unit. Trauma to the shoulder may initiate the process as well, and a weak, fatigued or injured rotator cuff is unable to oppose the superior pull of the deltoid effectively, which is then unable to keep the humeral head centered on the glenoid during elevation of the arm, causing it to elevate, which then functionally narrows the subacromial space. Continued dysfunction of the rotator cuff and further superior migration of the humeral head cause the greater tuberosity and rotator cuff to abut against the undersurface of the acromion and the coracoacromial ligament, leading to signs of secondary extrinsic impingement. These authors believe that changes to the coracoacromial ligament and the undersurface of the anterior acromion are secondary processes, and since they do not occur in many patients, these structures should be preserved if their anatomy is not altered. They believe that these structures play an important role as passive stabilizers against superior migration of the humeral head, and therefore should not be sacrificed. These authors therefore recommend debridement of the degenerated cuff tissue arthroscopically, and resection only of clearly identified excrescences. They do not perform a complete acromioplasty and do not remove the coracoacromial ligament.

Trauma

Trauma is considered to play a secondary role in the etiology of rotator cuff tears.[119,120] Little force may be needed to tear a tendon that is already degenerated by long-standing impingement wear, perhaps related to underlying tendinosis and repeated episodes of peritendinous inflammation. The trauma from a fall or dislocation may, therefore, complete or enlarge a preexistent small or incomplete tear, or tear an already degenerated tendon.

Notwithstanding the above, a tear may occur following an anterior dislocation of the shoulder, usually in an older patient in whom a cuff rupture occurs rather than an injury to the glenoid labrum and/or shoulder capsule. Studies show that a cuff tear may occur in 14% to 63% of patients with acute anterior dislocations. The incidence will be higher in older patients.[163-166] The supraspinatus tendon may tear with variable degrees of infraspinatus involvement.

Traumatic tears of the subscapularis tendon may occur due to traumatic hyperextension or external rotation of the abducted arm.[167] Concomitant biceps tendon pathologic conditions include subluxation, dislocation, or rupture. Isolated ruptures of the subscapularis may also occur with anterior dislocations, again predominantly in male patients older than 40.[164,168]

Avulsive fractures of the lesser tuberosity at the site of insertion of the subscapularis may occur in elderly women and men. With a posterior dislocation there may be disruption of the infraspinatus or teres minor tendons.[169] Superior dislocations of the humeral head may also result in cuff rupture as the humeral head is driven upward acutely through the cuff.

A cuff tear may also arise following a dislocation when the greater tuberosity is fractured. It may also develop following an avulsion fracture of the greater tuberosity. Posterior dislocations may also result in a fracture of the lesser tuberosity, in which case a tear of the subscapularis tendon may result. Although a non-displaced greater tuberosity fracture may result in injury to the cuff, recent evidence with MRI[170,171] indicates that this may more often result in a tendon contusion or intact cuff, rather than a tear, and the pain may more commonly be related to the bony injury.

Classification, Location, and Incidence of Rotator Cuff Tears

A full-thickness rotator cuff tear extends from the articular surface to the bursal surface of the cuff. A complete tear is one in which the whole thickness of the rotator cuff and capsule are torn, resulting in direct communication between the subdeltoid bursa and the joint cavity.[172] In contrast, partial-thickness tears (Fig. 99-21) involve only one surface of the cuff, either the inferior or superficial surface, or only the midsubstance of the cuff. Tears of the inferior surface are also referred to as deep or articular surface tears, those of the midsubstance as intrasubstance tears, and those of the superficial surface as superior or bursal surface tears. Retraction of tendinous fibers from the greater tuberosity may also be considered a partial tear.[96]

Partial tears have been classified by Ellman[173] as follows: grade 1 (low grade) are less than 3 mm deep and only the capsule or superficial fibers are involved; grade 2 (intermediate) are 3 to 6 mm deep and less than 50% of the cuff thickness is involved; and grade 3 (high grade or deep) greater than 6 mm, in which more than 50% of the cuff thickness is involved.

Complete cuff tears can be classified by size. Small tears are less than 1 cm, medium tears are less than 3 cm, large tears are 3 to 5 cm, and massive tears are greater than 5 cm.[174] Ellman[175] proposed that the area of a tear be measured in square centimeters using the base of the tear along the former insertion site times the depth of the muscle retraction. The size of the rotator cuff tear in both anterior posterior and mediolateral dimensions is a very important prognostic factor in determining surgical outcome.[176]

Most partial and small full-thickness rotator cuff tears are centered in the anterior half of the supraspinatus.[177] Supraspinatus tears begin on the deep surface anteriorly and distally at the greater tuberosity insertion, near the biceps tendon, and then extend outward until they become full-thickness defects. Once in the supraspinatus the defects then propagate posteriorly and medially through the remaining portions of the supraspinatus and then into the infraspinatus. This then puts progressive stress on the biceps tendon. Changes in the biceps tendon may initially be of a less severe degree, and may only consist of tendinosis, but it may eventually rupture, especially in chronic defects. The defect may then propagate across the bicipital groove to involve the subscapularis tendon, starting at the top of the lesser tuberosity and extending inferiorly.

Involvement of the subscapularis tendon may occur with larger tears and anterior tears. In this case it may often involve the superior articular surface fibers and the rotator interval capsule. It may also be involved in subcoracoid impingement. Acute ruptures of the subscapularis can occur with severe trauma, or in elderly patients with recurrent anterior dislocations. As the lesions propagate anteriorly into the subscapularis they may result in medial dislocation of the biceps tendon.[75,167,168,178-182]

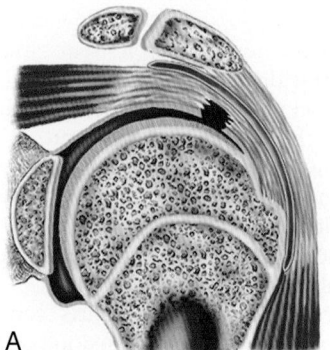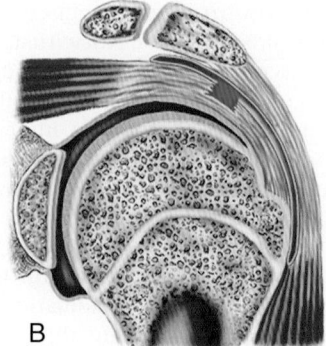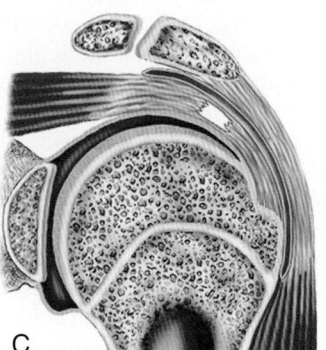

A   B   C

FIGURE 99-21

Classification of partial tears by location. **A,** Articular surface partial tear; **B,** bursal surface partial tear; and **C,** intrasubstance (interstitial) partial tear. *(Drawn by Salvador Beltran; reproduced with permission from Zlatkin MB: MRI of the Shoulder, 2nd ed. Philadelphia, Lippincott, Williams and Wilkins, 2003.)*

Isolated infraspinatus full-thickness tears are uncommon. They can occur in the spectrum of posterior superior (internal) subglenoid impingement or with severe trauma with posterior dislocation. Partial tears occurring at the junction of the posterior supraspinatus and anterior infraspinatus can occur in overhead throwing athletes in association with posterior superior (internal) subglenoid impingement.[141] Tears of the teres minor tendon are distinctly rare, even in the setting of massive tears, though partial tears of the superior aspect of the teres minor have been reported in a series of massive, irreparable, rotator cuff tears.[183] They may occur with trauma, in association with posterior capsular rupture as well as infraspinatus tendon tears, or in the setting of a posterior dislocation. In this situation, teres minor muscle and capsular injuries may occur without the typical reverse Bankart lesion.[184]

With progressive disruption of the rotator cuff tendons, the humeral head can then rise under the pull of the deltoid muscle. This then leads to abrasion of the humeral head articular cartilage against the coraco-acromial arch, causing subacromial impingement that in time erodes the anterior portion of the acromion and the acromioclavicular joint. There are also nutritional factors related to the rotator cuff tear that cause atrophy of the glenohumeral articular cartilage and osteoporosis of the subchondral bone of the humeral head. Eventually, the soft, atrophic head collapses, producing the complete syndrome of rotator cuff tear arthropathy.[185,186]

One other factor that is important when evaluating rotator cuff tears is the assessment of the status of the torn rotator cuff tendon edges. On imaging examinations as well as at surgery the appearance of the torn edges may be classified as good, fair or poor.[187,188] The status of the rotator cuff musculature with regard to the degree of atrophy, as well as fatty infiltration, can be also be quantified in a relative manner as mild, moderate, or severe.[187,188] Another system classifies both atrophy and fatty infiltration. Goutallier et al[189,190] graded muscular fatty degeneration into five stages in patients with rotator cuff tears.

Magnetic Resonance Imaging

Bone Changes Associated with Extrinsic Impingement

The most common secondary bone changes that have been described in association with extrinsic impingement include acromioclavicular joint osteophytes, subacromial spur formation, and cysts and sclerosis in the greater tuberosity.

Subacromial spurs are less common but are more correlative of rotator cuff disease than acromioclavicular osteoarthrosis (Fig. 99-22).[111] They are the most specific finding on MR examination for shoulder impingement.[191] Small subacromial spurs may appear on MRI examination as a signal void that projects from the acromion tip in a medial and inferior direction, and may be surrounded by a rim of signal void representing cortical bone,[192] and must be distinguished from the insertion of

the coracoacromial ligament or the deltoid insertion.[99] The inferior tendon slip of the deltoid inserts on the inferolateral acromion, coracoacromial ligament, and inferomedial acromion.[99] Larger spurs frequently contain marrow and thus have brighter signal.[193] The anterior and inferior location of the spurs are often best shown on sagittal oblique images. Larger spurs may be evident on coronal oblique images.

Degenerative osteophytes of the acromioclavicular joint have similar appearances. They may be inferiorly projecting. These osteophytes of the acromioclavicular joint may precede the presence of anterior acromial spurs. Hypertrophy and callus formation of the acromioclavicular joint capsule may also be visualized, which appears as a rounded mass of medium signal intensity surrounding the joint, which often projects inferiorly[194-196] and may encroach on the bursal surface of the musculotendinous junction of the supraspinatus. The relationship of the acromioclavicular joint arthrosis to the subacromial space and bursal surface of the cuff are best seen on the sagittal oblique and coronal oblique sequences (see Figs. 99-15 to 99-18). Fluid may be seen in the acromioclavicular joint, especially on fat-saturated images, and there may also be increased signal on these fat-saturated images in the bony margins of this joint. The significance of fluid within the acromioclavicular joint has also been debated, however.[195,197,198] It is speculated that marginal edema in the bones about the acromio-clavicular joint may be a marker of this joint as a site or source of pain in patients with this finding. Edema in the distal clavicle alone may be stress related and may be particularly common in athletes such as weight lifters, throwers, and swimmers (Fig. 99-23). Low signal intensity sclerosis, erosions, and subchondral cysts are also identified on MR images in patients with acromio-clavicular joint arthrosis.

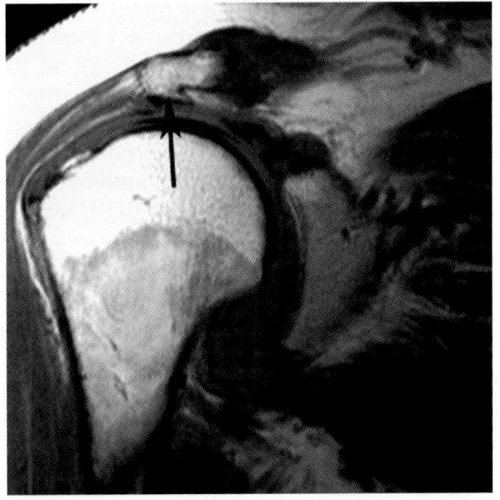

FIGURE 99-22

Sub-acromial spur. Coronal oblique T1-weighted image. Note the mature appearing subacromial spur (*arrow*).

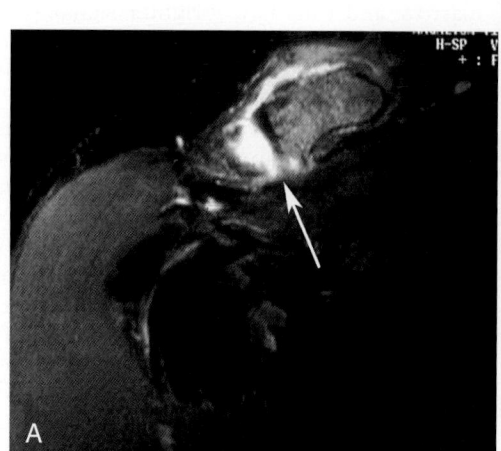
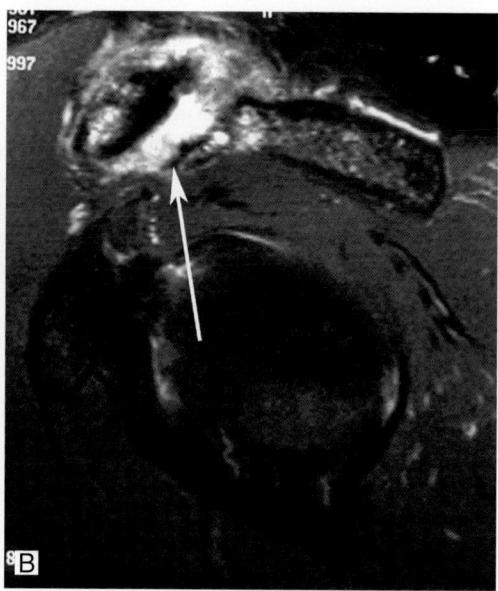

FIGURE 99-23

Acromioclavicular joint osteoarthritis. **A,** Coronal oblique and **B,** sagittal oblique fast spin-echo T2-weighted MR images with fat suppression. The acromioclavicular joint shows advanced degenerative changes with inferiorly projecting spurs, capsular hypertrophy, and marginal edema (*arrows*).

The three types of acromion shape described for plain radiographic examination can be adapted for MRI (Figs. 99-13 and 99-24). Type 1 has a flat or straight inferior surface. Type 2 demonstrates a smooth curved inferior surface that approximately parallels the superior humeral head in the sagittal oblique plane. Type 3 has an inferiorly curved or hook shape on sagittal images (Fig. 99-24). Type 3 acromions are statistically associated with an increased incidence of rotator cuff tears. Studies that have used sagittal oblique MRI to determine the presence of hook-shaped anterior acromions have also found an association with clinical impingement and rotator cuff tears.[199] A type 4 acromion can be appreciated on MR examination when the acromion appears convex near its distal end.[124] Peh et al[85] found that the apparent acromial shape is sensitive to the minor changes in the MR section viewed. More medial sections closer to the acromioclavicular joint may falsely produce the appearance of a hooked anterior acromion, which has a flat appearance on more peripheral sagittal oblique images.

Lateral or anterior downward sloping of the acromion, or a low lying acromion, relative to the distal clavicle may contribute to impingement and narrowing of the supraspinatus outlet, and can be discerned on MRI images. Impingement related to lateral downsloping of the anterior acromion may cause impingement of the mid portion of the supraspinatus tendon. It may cause impingement on the superior aspect of the subscapularis tendon.[125,200] This type of acromial position may also be associated with lateral supraspinatus injury near the greater tuberosity insertion, especially in patients who perform forceful abduction of the shoulder.[196] Anterior

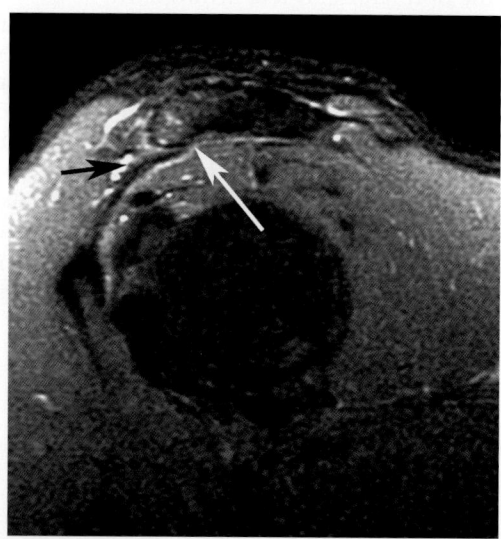

FIGURE 99-24

Type 3 acromion. Sagittal oblique fast-spin echo T2-weighted MR image with fat suppression. Note the hook-shaped, type 3 acromion (*white arrow*). A thickened coracoacromial ligament is also present (*black arrow*).

downsloping is best seen on sagittal MR images and lateral downsloping on coronal MR images. Anterior downsloping of the acromion is present when the anterior inferior cortex of the acromion is more inferiorly located relative to the posterior cortex on sagittal oblique images. Lateral downsloping is identified when the inferior surface of the distal acromion is inferior or

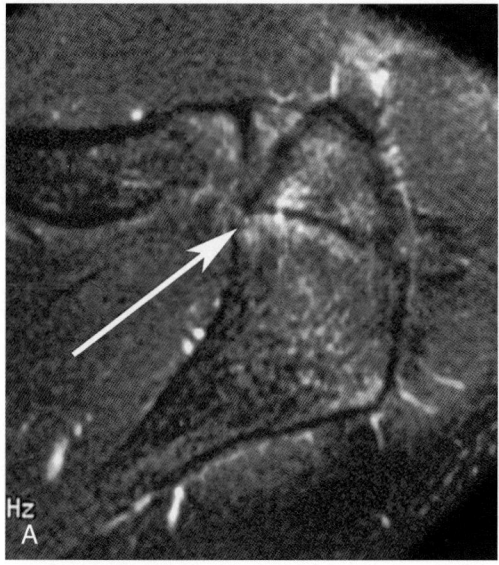
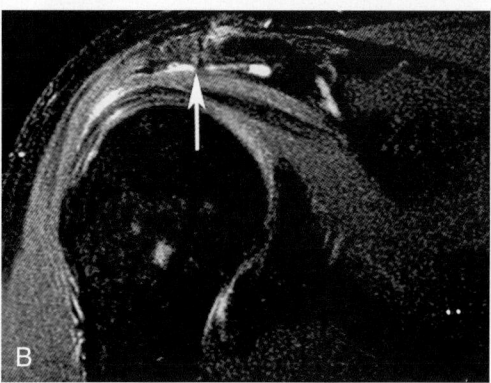

FIGURE 99-25

Os acromiale. **A,** On this superior axial section the os acromiale is well seen (*arrow*). Marginal edema is present. **B,** Posterior coronal oblique images may also identify the presence of the os acromiale (*arrow*). Note the pseudo acromioclavicular joint, more posterior in location.

caudally located, relative to the inferior surface of the more proximal aspect of the acromion, adjacent to the acromioclavicular joint (see Fig. 99-20).

Thickening of the coracoacoromial ligament may contribute to narrowing of the supraspinatus outlet and is best seen on sagittal oblique images (see Fig. 99-24). This includes assessment of its size and whether the thickening is smooth or irregular.[129,192,201-203]

The os acromiale is identified best on superior axial sections that demonstrate the entire acromion (Fig. 99-25A). The synchondrosis should not be mistaken for the subjacent acromioclavicular joint. When superior axial sections are not available this pattern of mimicking the acromioclavicular joint on sagittal and coronal oblique images may also be used to help identify the presence of the os acromiale (Fig. 99-25B).[130,131,204-206] Increased signal on either side of the fusion defect may be seen on both STIR and fat-suppressed T2-weighted fast spin-echo sequences (Fig. 99-25A). This hyperintensity may correlate with degenerative changes or instability of the os acromiale. It is important to identify the os acromiale because removal of the acromion distal to the synchrondrosis at the time of acromioplasty may further destabilize the synchondrosis and allow for even greater mobility of the os acromiale after surgery and worsening of the impingment.[204]

Hypertrophic changes or flattening and sclerosis may occur in the region of the greater tuberosity in patients with impingement. This is likely as noted above to be due to traumatization of the greater tuberosity on the undersurface of the acromion during abduction. These may be appreciated on MR examination as areas of cortical thickening or prominent low signal in the region of the greater tuberosity.[149]

Humeral head or greater tuberosity cysts have been associated with shoulder impingement. This is a very common finding on MR examination. More recently these cysts, which can become quite large, have been considered to be nonspecific and are as well correlated with increasing age as they are with alterations in the rotator cuff, reflective of impingement.[111] These cysts are often posteriorly located at the greater tuberosity or at its junction with the humeral head near the capsular insertion. Cysts may also occur more superiorly or anteriorly as well.[149]

Tendon Lesions

Tendinosis

A variety of terms may be used to describe the injured tendon in the absence of a tendon defect. The term most commonly used in the past was tendonitis. Most authors prefer the term tendinosis or tendinopathy as the pathologic changes found within such tendons most often do not include inflammation,[207-209] except in the peritendinous tissues. The MRI findings of tendinosis (Fig. 99-26) are moderate increase in signal intensity within the tendon on short TR/TE and proton-density images, oriented along the long axis of the tendon, which may be homogeneous (focal, diffuse or bandlike)[96] or inhomogeneous, and which fades or is absent on long TR/TE (T2-weighted images) whether obtained with conventional[96,187,188,210] or fast spin-echo imaging sequences without fat suppression. Fat-suppressed conventional or fast spin-echo T2-weighted sequences, or STIR imaging sequences, may make this signal more

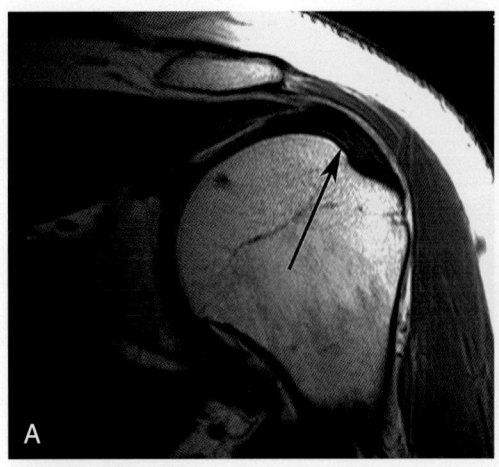
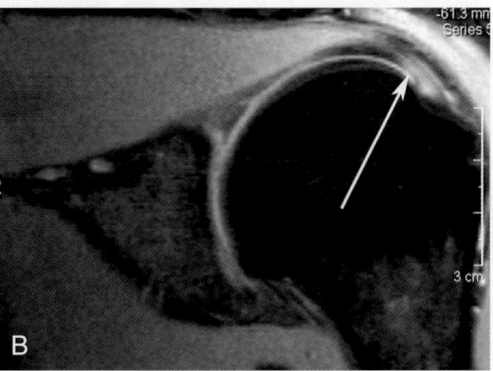

FIGURE 99-26

Tendinosis. **A,** Coronal oblique T1-weighted image. Diffuse increased signal in the supraspinatus tendon is present (*arrow*). The articular and bursal surfaces of the tendon are intact. **B,** Coronal oblique fast spin-echo proton-density–weighted sequence with fat suppression. Note the relative increase in tendon signal, which can be seen when fat suppression is present but does not approach fluid signal (*arrow*).

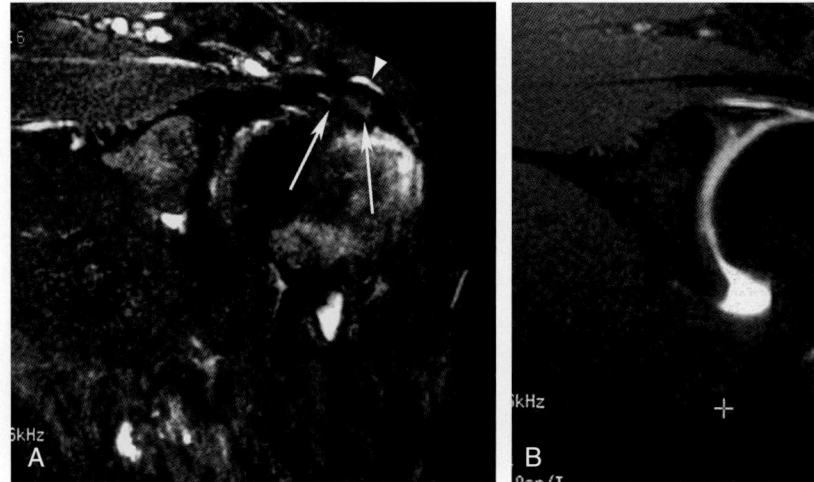

FIGURE 99-27

Tendinosis. Articular surface fraying/fibrillation. MR arthrography. **A,** Coronal oblique fast spin-echo T2-weighted sequence with fat suppression. Moderate tendinosis is seen in the supraspinatus tendon and there is undersurface fraying and irregularity (*arrows*). A small amount of fluid is seen in the subdeltoid bursa, likely reflective of bursal inflammation (*arrowhead*). **B,** Coronal oblique T1-weighted MR arthrogram with fat suppression outlines the undersurface fraying and irregularity (*arrows*), but no focal tendon defect is seen.

conspicuous and should be distinguished from true fluid signal as seen in a rotator cuff tear (see Fig. 99-26).[188] Tendon thickening may be present, and increased and more diffuse thickening may be associated with more advanced tendinosis. It is proposed that persistence of increased signal within the tendon on images with T2 weighting, but less intense than fluid signal, may indicate more advanced tendinosis, related to a greater degree of collagen breakdown in the tendon.[211]

Fat-saturated T2-weighted fast spin-echo images are more sensitive to the presence of fluid in the subdeltoid bursa (Figs. 99-27 and 99-28). With the use of these sequences, identifying fluid in the subdeltoid bursa region is a more common correlate of disease at this stage than previously thought.[187,188] When evident, fluid is considered to be indicative of associated subdeltoid bursal inflammation. Persistent low signal intensity in a thickened subacromial subdeltoid bursa on imaging sequences with both T1 and T2 contrast has also been described[96] and is said to indicate proliferative chronic subdeltoid bursitis, but this appearance is more difficult to discern on MRI studies.

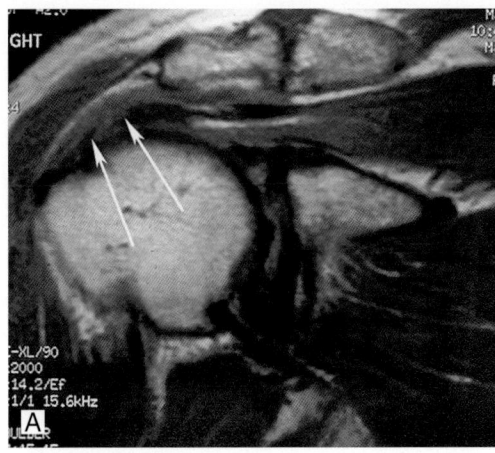
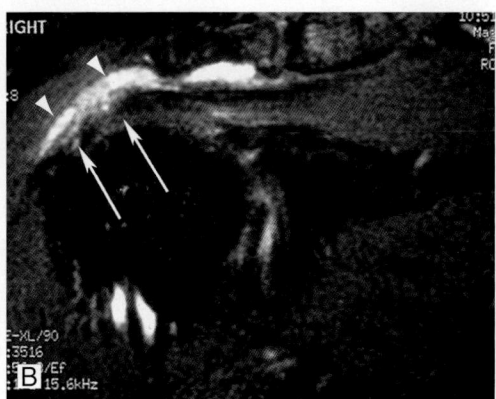

FIGURE 99-28

Tendinosis. Bursal surface fraying/fibrillation. **A,** Coronal oblique fast spin-echo proton-density–weighted image and **B,** fast spin-echo T2-weighted sequence with fat suppression. Moderate/severe tendinosis is seen in the supraspinatus tendon and there is bursal surface fraying and irregularity (*arrows*). A moderate amount of fluid is seen in the subdeltoid bursa (*arrowheads*), reflective of bursal inflammation.

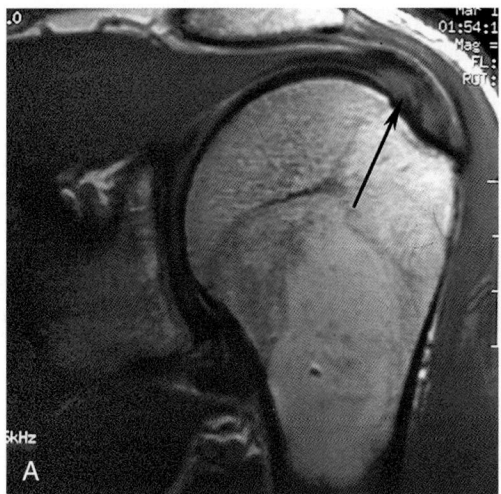
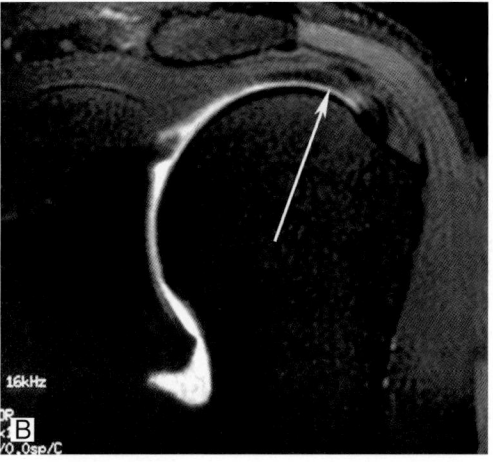

FIGURE 99-29

Tendinosis. MR arthrography. **A,** Coronal oblique fast spin-echo proton-density–weighted image. Diffuse increased signal in the supraspinatus tendon is noted (*arrow*). The articular and bursal surfaces of the tendon are smooth. **B,** Coronal oblique T1-weighted MR arthrogram with fat suppression. No contrast-filled tendon defect is seen (*arrow*).

The arthroscopic findings in patients with these MRI findings are hyperemia of the tendon surface and bursal scarring and inflammation.[187] Biopsy of the tendon in patients with MRI findings consistent with tendinosis has been carried out in a small number of patients and has shown mucoid degenerative changes and some inflammation.[212] Histologic sectioning in cadavers with similar MRI findings revealed eosinophilic, mucoid, and fibrillary degeneration.[94]

MR arthrography (Fig. 99-29) may confirm the integrity of the articular surface of the cuff. In patients with tendinosis the articular surface should be linear in contour and low in signal intensity.[29]

Anzilotti et al[213] described a subset of young patients (<35 years) with acute, post-traumatic insults to the rotator cuff which mimic the signal intensity changes of tendinosis. Patients had signal intensity that was similar to tendinosis, but was localized more in atypical locations of the supraspinatus tendon and was associated with bone bruise, suggesting the possibility of post-traumatic strain.

Tendons with a similar MRI appearance to tendinosis have been detected in asymptomatic individuals.[97,214,215] They should be distinguished from advanced rotator disease and rotator cuff tears as they are not associated with morphologic alterations and do not brighten like fluid on long TR/TE images.

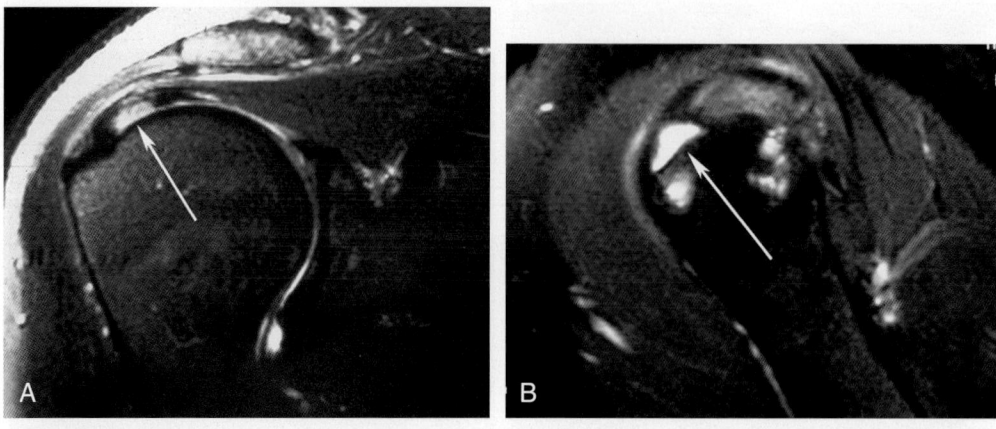

FIGURE 99-30

Articular surface partial tears. **A,** Coronal oblique T2-weighted image. A high-grade partial tear of the supraspinatus tendon undersurface is seen. Note the focal tendon defect outlined by the fluid signal (*arrow*). **B,** Sagittal oblique fast spin-echo T2-weighted image with fat suppression in another patient. A deep articular surface defect is again identified. The addition of fat suppression increases the conspicuity of the lesion (*arrow*).

Other MRI changes beyond tendinosis, not indicative of either a partial or complete tear but considered abnormal, include tendon thinning or irregularity of the tendon surface (see Figs. 99.27 and 99.28). MR arthrography will outline those findings that occur on the articular side (see Fig. 99-27B). Such irregularities in contour and signal intensity indicate fraying of the superficial fibers of the tendon. At arthroscopy the tendon surface is described as showing "fraying, roughening or degeneration."[158,187] On the bursal side of the tendon, T2-weighted images, especially with fat suppression, will show some fluid in the subdeltoid bursa that likely reflects bursal and peribursal inflammation. These findings may be reflective of the wear and tear of impingement. The distinction between this stage of disease and early partial-thickness tears may be difficult to define both by MRI and at arthroscopy, though by definition[173] in order to describe a partial tear a discrete tendon defect should be seen.

Partial Tears

Using MRI the diagnosis of partial tears is less sensitive and accurate than for complete tears.[3,6,8,96,187,188,216-220] A partial tear can be diagnosed when there is a defect that extends to one surface only, either the articular surface (Fig. 99-30), which is more common, or the bursal surface (Fig. 99-31), or is within the tendon substance (intrasubstance or interstitial), and that shows increased signal on long TR/TE images, or on other imaging sequences with T2 contrast. When the increased signal is that of fluid the diagnosis can be made with confidence. Tears of the bursal surface and of the undersurface will be perpendicular to the long axis of the tendon on coronal oblique imaging sequences, whereas those in the tendon substance are parallel to the long axis of the tendon (Fig. 99-32).

Some partial tears may be partially healed or quite small and, therefore, the signal increase may not be as strong. In such situations they may be difficult to distinguish from tendinosis. Fat saturation or STIR images may help (see Figs. 99-30 and 99-32).[3,6,210,217,221] T2-weighted fast spin-echo techniques with fat saturation can obtain this type of contrast in a more efficient manner. STIR imaging has also been suggested to increase diagnostic performance as well. Partial tears may less commonly be manifested by significant loss of tendon thickness. T1-weighted images with fat saturation after the intra-articular injection of gadolinium diethylenetriamine pentetate (Gd-DTPA) are of value in the diagnosis of partial tears of the articular surface of the tendon (Fig. 99-33).[19,23,26,32,35,39,222] In this situation MR arthrography maximizes anatomic resolution and diagnostic confidence. Partial-thickness tears occur and begin commonly along the undersurface of the antero-distal insertion of the cuff near the "critical zone," and therefore evaluating this region of the cuff undersurface with MR arthrography is of considerable importance in the differentiation of a normal cuff and cuff tendinosis from one with a partial tear. On MR arthrography a partial-thickness tear is diagnosed when contrast extends in a focal manner into a tendon defect, but does not extend into the subacromial subdeltoid bursa. MR arthrography is also very effective at depicting the extent of morphologic alterations and their depth of involvement by showing contrast imbibition and the depth of loss of tendon thickness (Fig. 99.33). This is again helpful in distinguishing these alterations from those associated with tendinosis and tendon surface degeneration.

Partial tears associated with posterosuperior subglenoid impingement (Fig. 99-34) may have areas of delamination of the rotator cuff undersurface and loose flaps of cuff tissue may be seen on the cuff undersurface. These partial tears which commonly occur posteriorly at the junction of the suprapsinatus and infraspinatus are

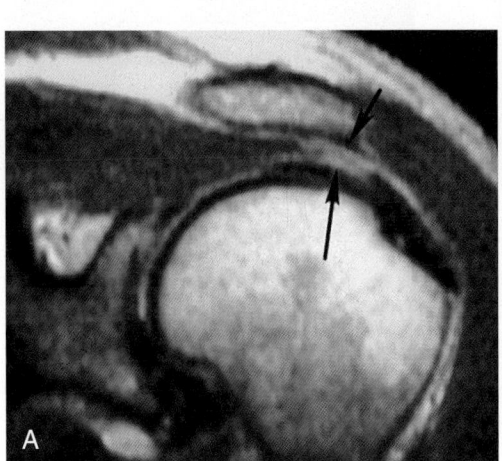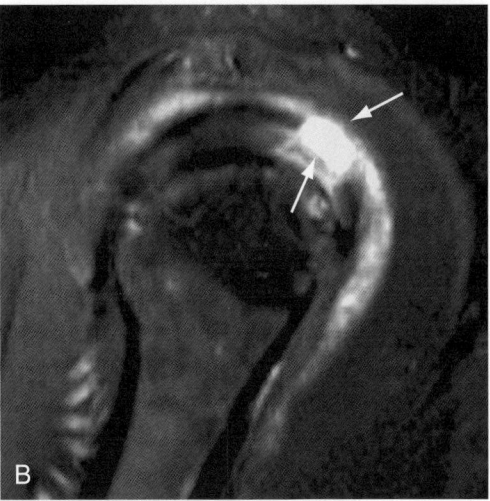

FIGURE 99-31

Bursal surface partial tears. **A,** Coronal oblique T2-weighted image. An intermediate-grade partial tear of the supraspinatus tendon superior surface is seen. A focal tendon defect outlined by fluid signal is seen (outlined by *short* and *long arrows*). **B,** Sagittal oblique fast spin-echo T2-weighted image with fat suppression. Note the fluid signal outlining a high-grade bursal surface partial tear of the supraspinatus tendon (*arrows*).

sometimes referred to as posterior interval tears.[141,143,223] MR arthrography and the arm placed in ABER position[39,141,223] may be useful in such patients. This position also allows better depiction of the other lesions in the spectrum of this process, including the osteochondral compression fracture of the posterosuperior humeral head, degenerative fraying or tear of the posterosuperior glenoid labrum and alterations of the subjacent glenoid, and the less common involvement of the inferior glenohumeral ligament and anterior inferior labrum.

Intrasubstance partial tears are difficult to confirm with either surgery or arthroscopy, unless the tendon is incised. This diagnosis is considered on MR images when fluid signal is present on long TR/TE images in the substance of the tendon, i.e., parallel to the long axis of the tendon, and not extending to either the bursal or articular surface (see Fig. 99-32). Acute tendonitis or tendon contusions after trauma can theoretically have a similar pattern of increased signal as well. Combinations of partial tears may also be seen.

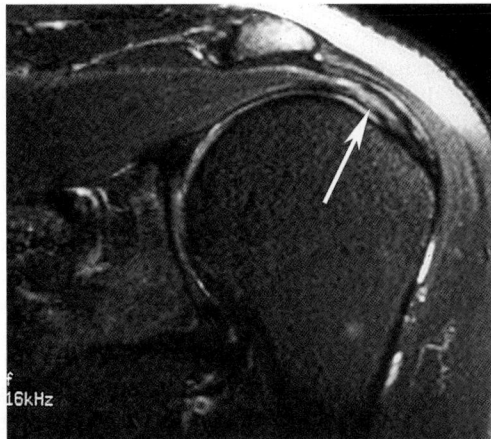

FIGURE 99-32

Intrasubstance partial tears. Coronal oblique fast spin-echo T2-weighted image with fat saturation. Longitudinal increased signal in the tendon substance approaching that of fluid is seen (*arrow*). The signal is oriented parallel to the tendon.

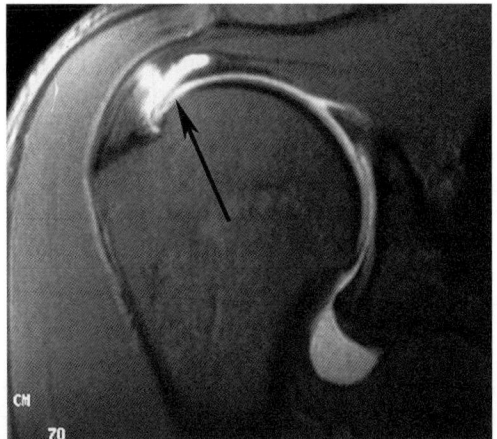

FIGURE 99-33

Partial tears. Coronal oblique T1-weighted MR arthrogram with fat saturation. A high-grade articular surface partial-thickness tear of the supraspinatus tendon is seen (*arrow*). MR arthrography clearly outlines the extent and depth of the tendon defect.

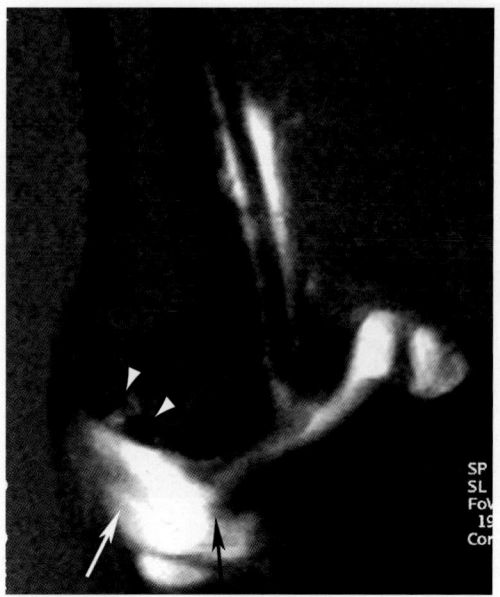

FIGURE 99-34

Subglenoid impingement. Axial oblique T1-weighted MR arthrogram with fat saturation performed with the patient in the abduction and external rotation (ABER) position. Note the flaplike areas of undersurface partial tearing of the supraspinatus tendon (*white arrow*). There is fraying of the posterosuperior labrum (*black arrow*). Note the cystic areas of the posterosuperior humeral head (*arrowheads*).

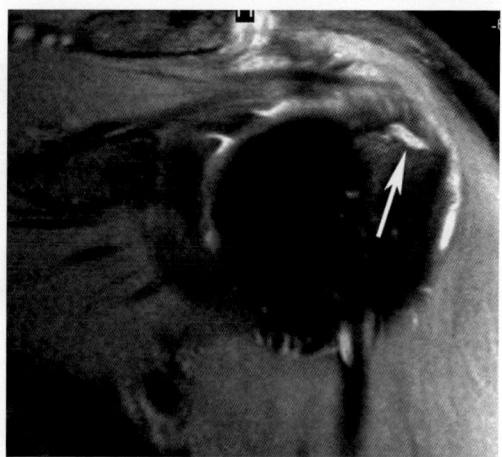

FIGURE 99-35

Insertional partial tear. Coronal oblique fast spin-echo proton-density–weighted image with fat saturation. A fluid-filled insertional defect is seen at the supraspinatus tendon insertion into the greater tuberosity (*arrow*).

Fluid in the subdeltoid bursa may commonly be identified in bursal-side partial-thickness tears and may make it easier to assess the size and depth of these tears.[82] Bursal-side partial tears cannot be identified with MR arthrography from the articular side. Preliminary work with MR bursography has the potential to improve the accuracy for diagnosis of bursal-side partial tears, but as yet has not been used very often in clinical practice.

Retraction of tendinous fibers from the distal insertion into the greater tuberosity may also be considered a partial tear (Fig. 99-35). This may occur in the throwing athlete, specifically baseball players.[224] These lesions appear as small regions of high signal intensity on long TR/TE images in this location, with associated bony defects on the greater tuberosity. Partial tears of differing size and nature may coexist in different portions of the rotator cuff or at the posterior margin of a larger tear.

Full-Thickness Tears

This diagnosis is made with the visualization of a complete defect in the tendon, extending from the articular to the bursal surface of the tendon, most commonly involving the supraspinatus tendon.[3,4,6,82,96,187,188,217,220,225-229] The defects in the rotator cuff are filled with fluid, granulation tissue, or hypertrophied synovium, and therefore in the majority of cases (80% or greater) with a cuff defect, fluid-like signal is present within the defect on long TR/TE images,[229] which can be

made more conspicuous with the use of fast spin-echo sequences with fat suppression or fast inversion recovery sequences (STIR). The presence of a tendon defect filled with fluid is the most direct and definite sign of a rotator cuff tear.

In the presence of a full-thickness tear, especially larger tears, tendon retraction may be present and the supraspinatus may take on a more globular configuration (Fig. 99-36).[229] The location of the musculotendinous junction can vary even in asymptomatic individuals and depends on the position of the arm during the MR examination. Therefore, the use of retraction of the musculotendinous junction alone as a direct sign of a rotator cuff tear in the absence of a clear tendon defect is not recommended. In large to massive tears the tendon may retract as far as the medial glenoid margin (Fig. 99-37).

MR arthrography is most helpful in distinguishing small from partial tears and tendinosis, and in assessing the reparability of the cuff and the postoperative prognosis in larger cuff tears. MR arthrography is helpful in determining the size and location of cuff tears and in assessing the status of the torn tendon edges (Fig. 99-38). The diagnosis of a full-thickness rotator cuff tear on MR arthrography is made when contrast extends through a defect in the tendon from the cuff undersurface into the subacromial-subdeltoid bursa. The retracted tendon margins may be thickened in response to healing or attenuated in more chronic tears. The uninvolved areas of tendon adjacent to the tear site may demonstrate changes of degeneration or partial-thickness tear. The quality of the retracted tendon edges can be assessed on conventional MRI by assessing their appearance and describing them according to the classification scheme discussed earlier (good, fair or poor),[187] and at MR arthrography by evaluating for the presence of contrast imbibition.[23,32,57,230]

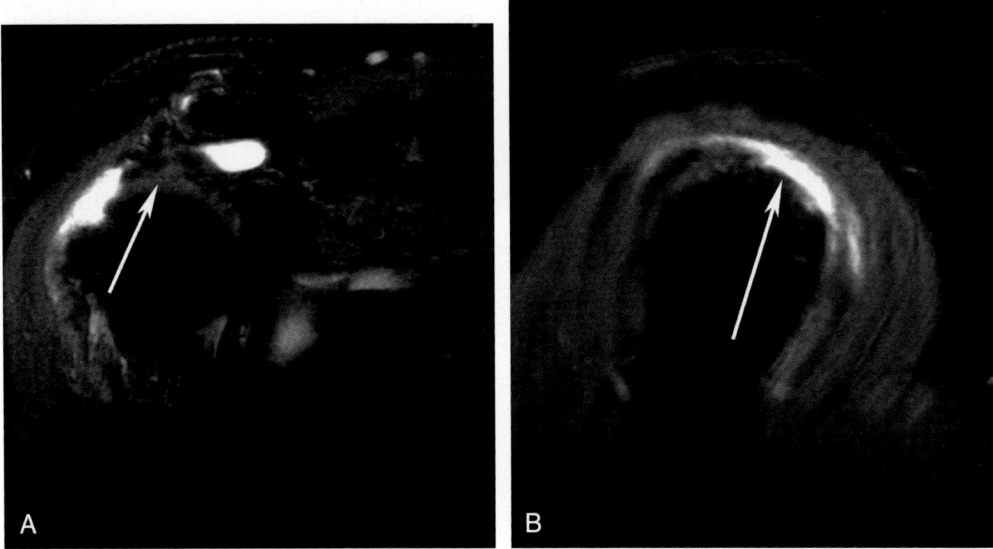

FIGURE 99-36

Moderate complete tear. **A,** Coronal oblique and **B,** sagittal oblique fast spin-echo T2-weighted images with fat saturation. There is a complete tear of the supraspinatus tendon, retracted to the mid humeral head, involving the central to anterior aspect. There is degeneration of the medial tendon edges (*arrows*).

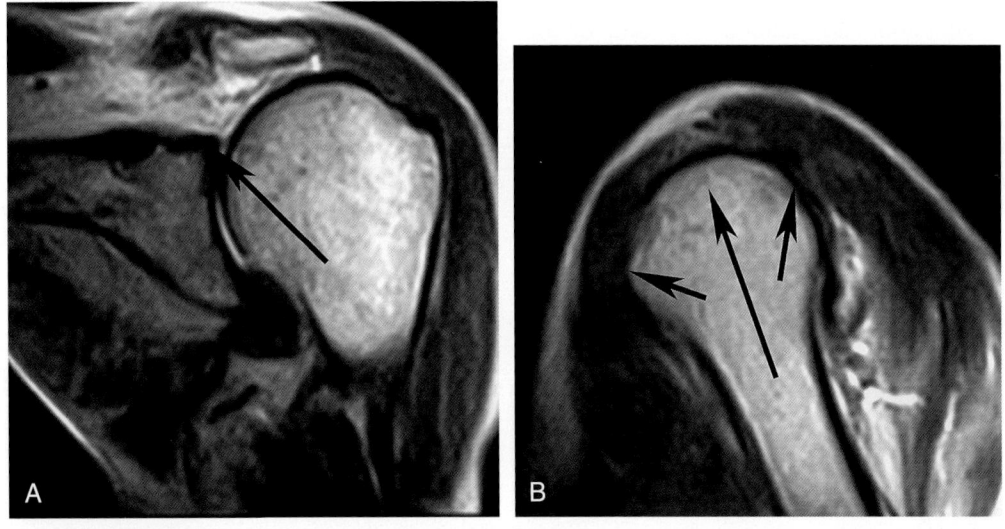

FIGURE 99-37

Massive tear. **A,** Coronal oblique T2-weighted image. The supraspinatus tendon is retracted to the medial glenoid margin (*arrow*). There is severe atrophy. **B,** Sagittal oblique T2-weighted image. Note the "bald humeral head." The tear extends from the subscapularis to the infraspinatus tendon (*arrows*).

Secondary signs[188,229] of rotator cuff tears are utilized less commonly, with increased experience, and with better depiction of the primary tendon defects. These secondary signs include diffuse loss of the peribursal fat plane and the presence of fluid in the subdeltoid bursa. Loss of the peribursal fat plane in association with a rotator cuff tear is most likely related to the presence of

bursal fluid and/or inflammatory change, granulation or scar tissue.[112,231] A large amount of fluid in the subdeltoid bursa is believed to represent extension of joint fluid through the capsule and tendon defect into the bursa. It has been considered a more specific finding of a complete cuff tear, particularly if a large volume of liquid signal is present.[229] Nonetheless, smaller amounts of

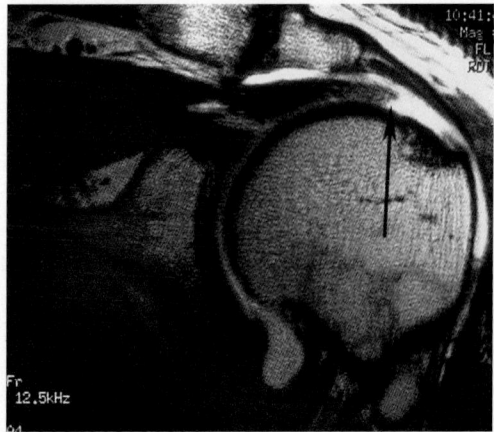

FIGURE 99-38

Moderate size full-thickness tear. Coronal oblique T1-weighted MR arthrogram with fat saturation. High signal contrast outlines a defect in the supraspinatus tendon. The tendon edges are mildly frayed (*arrow*).

fluid in the subdeltoid bursa can be identified quite commonly in patients without a tendon defect, especially on fat-suppressed images, and may be indicative of bursal inflammation (see Figs. 99-20, 99-27, and 99-28). Fluid in the subdeltoid bursa may also be seen in patients with partial tears, especially those on the bursal surface. Although less common, large amounts of fluid in the subdeltoid bursa may also be identified with primary subdeltoid bursitis in patients with calcium hydroxyapatite deposition disease (HADD) (see later) and other inflammatory causes.[96]

Muscle atrophy is a secondary sign seen especially in association with large tears and chronic tears (Figs. 99-37, 99-39, and 99-40).[187,232-237] It is best identified on

T1- and proton-density–weighted images, particularly in the sagittal oblique plane, and is not easily seen on fat-suppressed imaging sequences. Atrophy may, however, be seen in association with neurologic compromise, adhesive capsulitis, and other conditions in which shoulder movement is restricted or absent, and therefore in and of itself is not diagnostic of tendon disruption.[238-240]

Other findings associated with large or chronic rotator cuff tears include a decrease in the acromial-humeral distance to less than 7 mm and the presence of acromioclavicular joint cysts (Fig. 99-41). The former can be seen on plain radiographs as well, but if associated with a tear, MRI can be helpful to assess the extent of the defect. Acromioclavicular joint cysts are associated with full-thickness tears, usually large to massive, and occur when a high riding humeral head impacts on the overlying acromioclavicular joint. This leads to wear on the inferior aspect of the acromioclavicular joint capsule, with resultant tear. Fluid from the joint can then extend through the tear and subdeltoid bursa, into the acromioclavicular joint. Removal of the cyst alone must be avoided because the condition tends to recur if the cuff tear is not repaired. The rotator cuff should be repaired and the cyst excised.[241-243] Large joint effusions may also accompany rotator cuff tears. This is a nonspecific finding. A recent study revealed the relationship between intramuscular cysts of the rotator cuff and tears of the rotator cuff[244]: intramuscular cysts of the rotator cuff are associated with small, full-thickness tears or partial undersurface tears of the rotator cuff (Fig. 99-42). These cysts are best identified on imaging sequences with T2-weighted contrast.

In more chronic tears a discrete tendon defect can be more difficult to discern due to partial or complete obliteration of the tear due to scarring. Severe morphologic changes, a decrease in the acromial-humeral distance, atrophy, and peribursal and bursal changes can

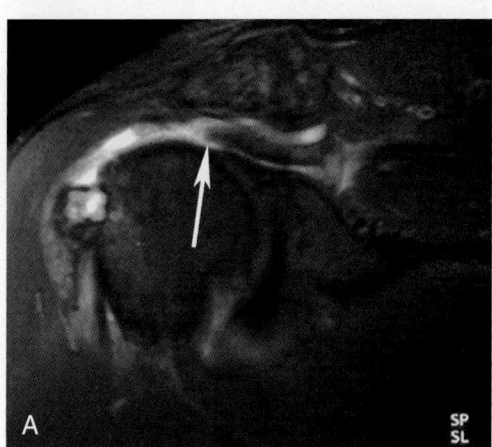
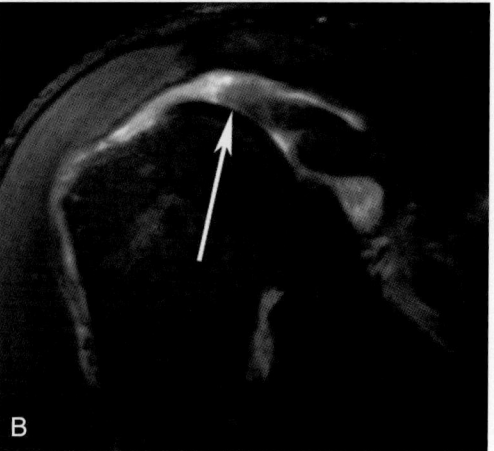

FIGURE 99-39

Posterior extension of large full-thickness tear. **A** and **B,** Coronal oblique fast spin-echo inversion-recovery–weighted images. The tendon defect is retracted to the medial one third of the humeral head (*arrow* in **A**). In **B** the posterior extension of the tear into the infraspinatus tendon is seen (*arrow*). The retracted tendon edges are globular and degenerated.

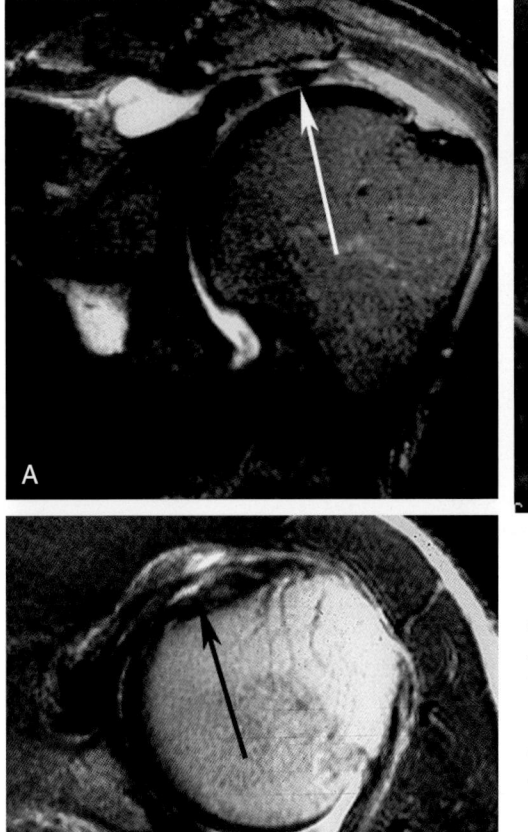
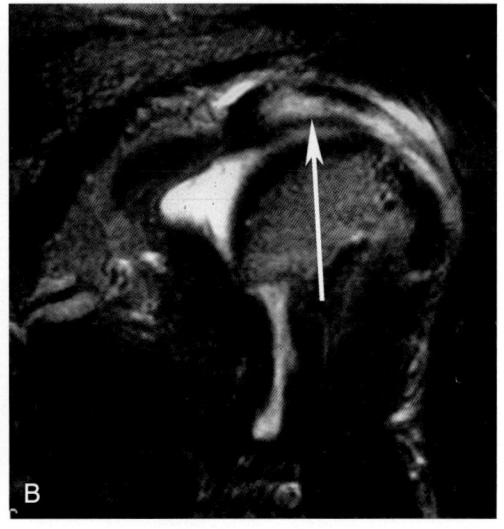

FIGURE 99-40

Anterior and posterior extension of large full-thickness tear. **A,** Coronal oblique T2-weighted image. The supraspinatus tendon is retracted to the medial one third of the humeral head (*arrow*). The tendon edges are thin. There is moderate muscle atrophy. **B,** Coronal oblique T2-weighted image, more posteriorly. The defect extends posteriorly to the infraspinatus tendon in a fluid filled longitudinal cleavage plane (*arrow*). **C,** Axial T2-weighted image. The tendon lesion extends anteriorly across the rotator interval to involve the superodistal subscapularis tendon (*arrow*).

help in the recognition of these lesions on conventional MR images.[96] MR arthrography may be helpful in such cases if doubt remains about the presence and extent of such tears and surgery is contemplated.

MRI can also accurately determine the size of the tendon defects,[187,188,245-247] including the amount of medial retraction, the anteroposterior extent of the defect, as well as the overall cross-sectional area. As noted earlier the cross-sectional area of the tendon defect may be the most important factor in surgical planning. Sagittal and coronal oblique sequences can assess the medial and anteroposterior extent of cuff tears. In conjunction with axial views they can also determine the number of tendons involved, including supraspinatus, infraspinatus, and subscapularis tendons, as well as the location of the tendon defect (see Figs. 99-39 and 99-40).

The site of rotator cuff tears can also be determined with MRI.[82,177,179,187,188,234,248,249] Small full-thickness tears are often found in the anterior portion of the distal supraspinatus tendon, near its insertion into the greater tuberosity at the junction with the biceps and subscapularis tendon (near the rotator interval). They

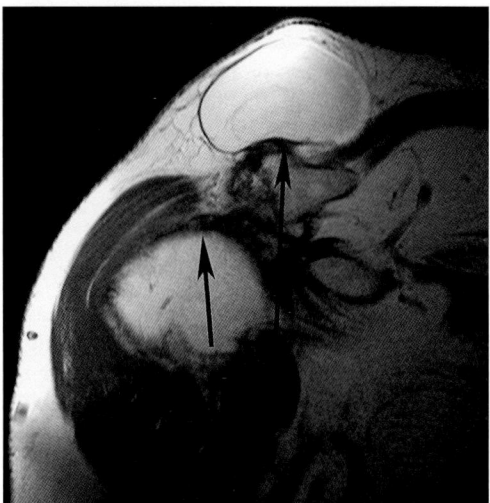

FIGURE 99-41

Acromioclavicular joint cyst. Coronal oblique fast spin-echo T2-weighted image. A large acromioclavicular joint cyst is seen (*long arrow*), associated with a retracted full-thickness rotator cuff tear (*short arrow*).

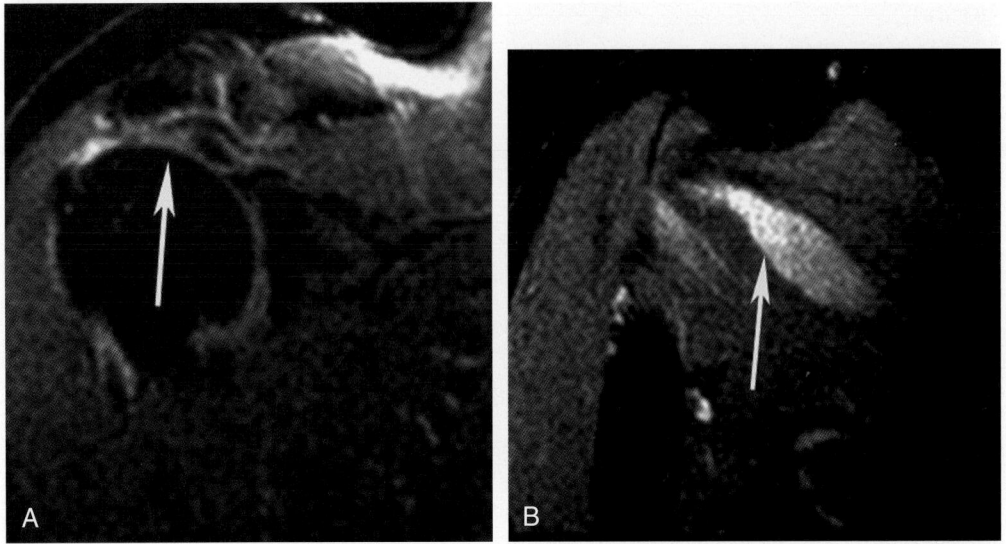

FIGURE 99-42

Intramuscular cyst. **A** and **B,** Coronal oblique STIR images. Note the full-thickness tear in **A** (*arrow*) and the associated intramuscular cyst in **B** (*arrow*).

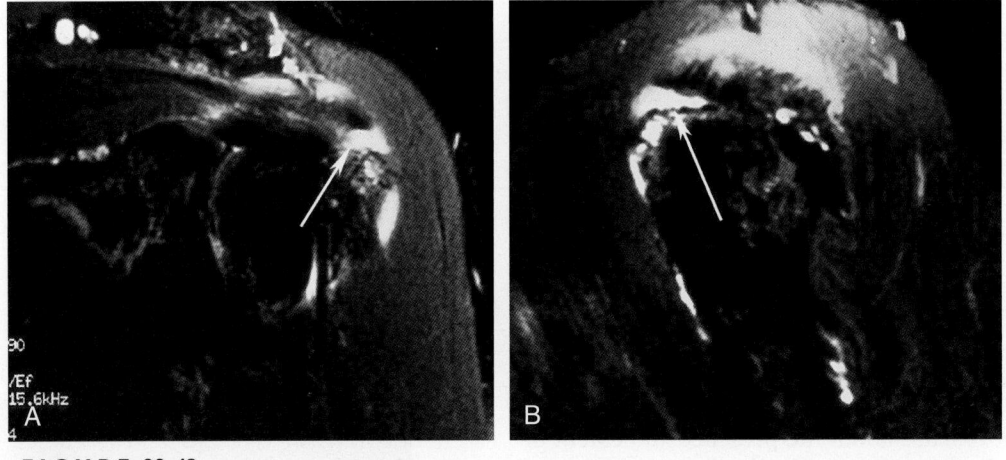

FIGURE 99-43

Small complete tear. **A,** Coronal oblique and **B,** sagittal oblique fast spin-echo T2-weighted images with fat saturation. Note the small rotator cuff tear outlined by fluid signal (*arrows*). Small tears tend to begin and occur at the anterior distal supraspinatus tendon near its insertion.

are therefore best seen on far anterior coronal oblique images or on lateral sagittal oblique images (Fig. 99-43). Partial-thickness tears show a predilection for this area as well. When larger, the tears extend to involve the infraspinatus tendon from anterior to posterior aspect (see Figs. 99-37, 99-39, and 99-40). The component of the tear involving the infraspinatus is seen on the more posterior coronal oblique images or on sagittal oblique images. Anterior tears and larger tears may extend to involve the rotator interval capsule and the subscapularis tendon and there may be an associated lesion of the biceps tendon (Figs. 99-40 and 99-44). The biceps tendon is often implicated in these situations since it lies beneath the anterior aspect of the supraspinatus tendon, which then subjects it to even further impingement between the humeral head and acromion when the supraspinatus tendon is torn. Subscapularis and infraspinatus tears may also be visualized in the sagittal oblique and axial plane images in addition to the coronal oblique plane where the supraspinatus tendon defects are best seen. In larger tears and anterior tears of the supraspinatus tendon, axial images superior to the glenohumeral joint may also demonstrate the fluid-filled tendinous gap.

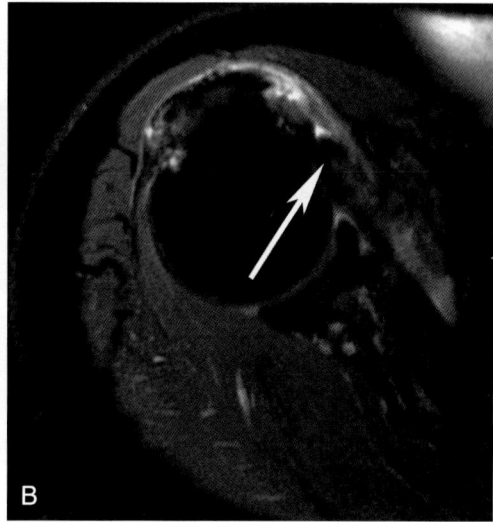

FIGURE 99-44

Rotator interval anterior tear. Biceps lesion. **A,** Coronal oblique fast spin-echo T2-weighted image with fat saturation. Note the tear in the anterior supraspinatus tendon. The torn tendon fibers are markedly thickened and show degeneration of the edges (*arrow*). **B,** Axial fast spin-echo T2-weighted image with fat saturation. The tear extends anteriorly, likely disrupting the rotator interval, and the superodistal aspect of the subscapularis tendon, leading to instability of the proximal aspect of the long head of the biceps tendon which migrates medially ("hidden lesion") (*arrow*).

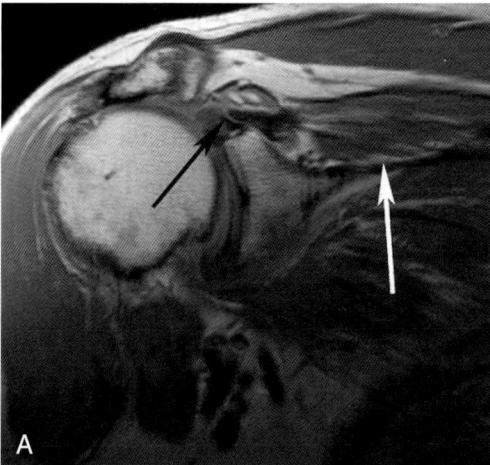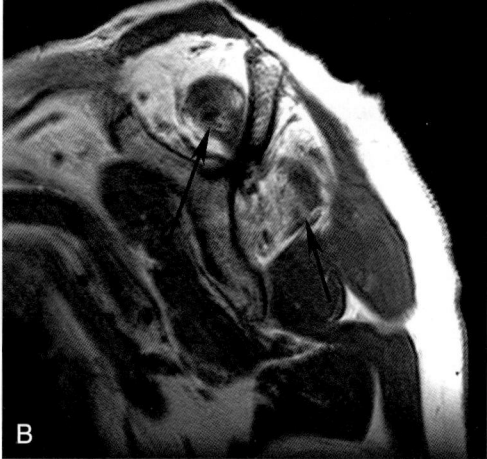

FIGURE 99-45

Muscle atrophy. **A,** Coronal oblique proton-density–weighted image. Note the retracted supraspinatus (*black arrow*). The supraspinatus muscle reveals muscle atrophy manifested by a decrease in bulk and infiltration by fat (*white arrow*). **B,** Sagittal oblique T1-weighted image. Note the presence of atrophy in both the supraspinatus and infraspinatus muscle bellies (*arrows*).

The presence of muscle atrophy[187,232,234-237,250,251] is, as noted earlier, a secondary sign associated with a rotator cuff tear, and the degree and presence of muscle atrophy is highly correlative with the size of the tear. Muscle atrophy has importance in determining surgical outcome with regard to return of muscle strength. Atrophy is identified as a decrease in muscle bulk and size. There will be an increase in fat signal within the muscle belly, often appearing as linear bands of high signal on T1- and proton-density–weighted images, though other patterns may be seen (Fig. 99-45). This may be separately described as fatty infiltration (degeneration).[190,235,251] Images with fat suppression only are less helpful in evaluating muscle atrophy except for visualization of a decrease in muscle bulk. The degree of muscle atrophy and fatty infiltration is most commonly graded as mild,

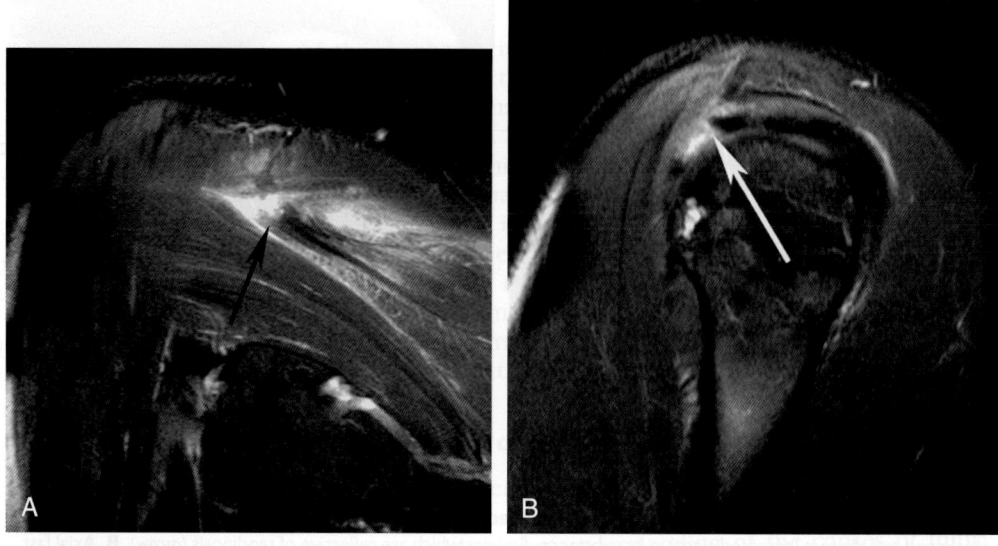

FIGURE 99-48

Infraspinatus tear. **A,** Coronal and **B,** sagittal fast spin-echo T2-weighted images with fat saturation. Note the isolated tear of the infraspinatus tendon (*arrows*).

The rotator interval is defined as the space between the superior border of the subscapularis muscle and tendon below and the supraspinatus muscle and tendon above[77,78,268] (Fig. 99-11). It is a complex region and can be conceptualized in layers.[68,269] The outermost layer consists of fibrofatty tissue and beneath this is the coracohumeral ligament, the joint capsule, and then the superior glenohumeral ligament. The deepest structure in the anterior interval is the long head of the biceps tendon. Surgeons may enter the joint through this region for an arthrotomy. It is through this interval that the long head of the biceps tendon enters the shoulder joint from the proximal bicipital groove to extend to the superior labral-biceps anchor and the supraglenoid tubercle attachment. The interval is bridged by the rotator interval capsule.[270] The fused rotator interval capsule and the coracohumeral ligament may be seen as a roof over the biceps tendon, and are important anterior supporting structures for shoulder function.

It is believed that injury or deficiency of the rotator interval capsule and coracohumeral ligament may lead to posterior inferior laxity and instability.[270] Lesions of the rotator interval may also be seen in association with shoulder subluxations and dislocations, where this region may be an area of relative weakness susceptible to injury and therefore during which time this region may be torn or enlarged. As such many surgeons believe this area should be repaired or reinforced during stabilization procedures for instability.

Injuries to this interval may also occur in individuals without a history of instability.[268] In this circumstance there may be an anterior tear of the supraspinatus tendon as well as a tear of the superior subscapularis tendon, in association with the tear of the interval. Isolated lesions of the rotator interval appear thin and longitudinal, and are not associated with muscle retraction.[267] Tears of the rotator interval may cause communication with the subdeltoid bursa, and fluid or contrast may be seen in this region on conventional MRI and MR arthrography. This may be identified along with altered signal in the region of the interval involving structures such as the coracohumeral ligament and the long head of the biceps tendon, without necessarily involving the supraspinatus tendon. This may be confusing if this anatomy and lesion are not understood. Lesions of the rotator interval may often be best discerned on sagittal oblique T2-weighted imaging sequences with fat suppression, or with MR arthrography.

The structures that contribute to the functional anatomy of this region, or may be injured in association with them, include the anterior margin of the supraspinatus tendon, distal superior margin of the subscapularis tendon, coracohumeral ligament, rotator interval capsule, superior glenohumeral ligament, and long head of the biceps tendon. Injuries to the superior labrum and biceps labral anchor may also occur, as well as the ligamentous reflection pulley for the long head of the biceps tendon formed by these structures at the lateral margin of the rotator interval, extending to the lesser tuberosity and proximal bicipital groove. It also includes the transverse humeral ligament.

The lesions may be acute as after a dislocation, or chronic as in overuse injuries. If acute, the alterations may be identified as areas of edema, fluid signal, and synovitis, and have high signal on T2-weighted images, or if chronic, show areas of thickening and scarring, revealed as areas of low-to-intermediate signal in the region of the interval, including the coracohumeral ligament and capsule (Fig. 99-49). Other associated injuries may occur to the biceps tendon, including inflammation and tear, or with disruption of the transverse humeral ligament, or tear of the subscapularis tendon at

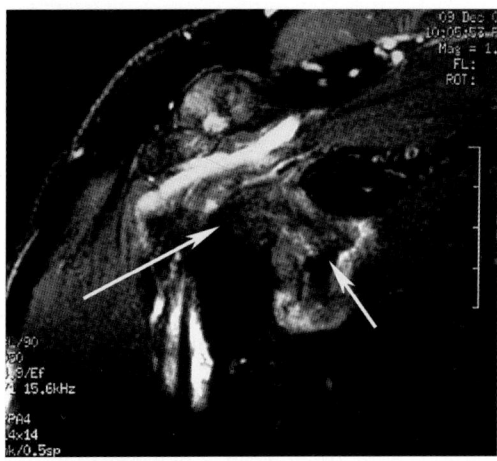

FIGURE 99-49

Rotator interval injury. Coronal oblique T2-weighted fast spin-echo sequences with fat saturation. Fluid signal due to edema and synovitis, as well as areas of thickening and scarring, revealed as areas of low-to-intermediate signal in the region of the rotator interval, are noted (*arrows*). Fluid is also present in the anterior aspect of the subdeltoid bursa.

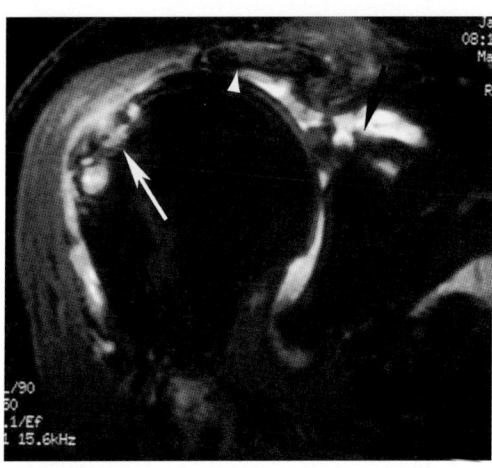

FIGURE 99-50

Rotator cuff arthropathy. Coronal oblique fast spin-echo T2-weighted image with fat saturation. There is a large retracted full-thickness tear (*black arrow*). Changes of rotator cuff arthropathy are seen. Note the decrease in the acromiohumeral distance, the scalloping and resorption of the undersurface of the anterior acromion (*arrowhead*), and the fraying and thinning of the articular cartilage of the humeral head, along with cystic change (*white arrow*).

its attachment to the lesser tuberosity, biceps instability including medial dislocation. With interval disruption tearing of the distal anterior supraspinatus tendon at its insertion into the greater tuberosity, "the anterior or leading edge" at the lateral rotator interval may also occur. Owing to the course of the long head of the biceps through the interval to the superior labrum, SLAP lesions may also occur.[76]

These lesions are often better recognized on sagittal oblique sections or axial sections, acquired as either T2-weighted fast spin-echo imaging with fat suppression or with MR arthrography. When any one of the spectrum of these associated injuries is suspected or found all other possible associated injuries should be searched for on MR examination.[76]

Rotator Cuff Tear Arthropathy

Rotator cuff tear arthropathy[186,271,272] occurs in the setting of large-to-massive tears (Fig. 99-50). In addition to the presence of the advanced disruption of the cuff there is abrasion of the humeral head articular cartilage against the coracoacromial arch, causing subacromial impingement that in time erodes the anterior portion of the acromion and the acromioclavicular joint. There may be collapse of the soft, atrophic humeral head,[186] with eventual erosion of the glenoid and coracoid. While many of these findings may be visible on plain radiographs,[185] MRI can help assess the full extent of bone and soft-tissue involvement. This process should be recognized and described at the time of MRI evaluation, as the best treatment for this may be total shoulder replacement, if possible with rotator-cuff reconstruction.[186]

Biceps Tendon

The biceps tendon may also become involved in patients with impingement and rotator cuff tears.[79,89,223,273-281] In general the extent of disease in the biceps is less severe than that in the cuff, but follows the progression seen in the rotator cuff. A small amount of fluid may be observed in the biceps tendon sheath even in asymptomatic individuals.[111] Since the tendon sheath communicates with the joint it may fill with fluid when a shoulder joint effusion is present from some other cause; therefore, this is a nonspecific finding. Tenosynovitis can be diagnosed when the amount of fluid in the tendon sheath is out of proportion to that in the joint.

Tendinosis of the biceps tendon may manifest by an increase in tendon size and increased signal in its substance on T1- and proton-density–weighted images (Fig. 99-51). With T2-weighted fast spin-echo imaging with fat suppression or fast spin-echo STIR the increased signal may persist or mildly increase.

In shoulders with tears of the rotator cuff the biceps also becomes an active depressor of the head of the humerus.[282] On MRI examination the biceps may enlarge as a response to this increased workload. This is sometimes termed "tendonization."

Partial-thickness tears may be more easily discerned when there is alteration in morphology, such as thinning, irregularity, or splitting of the tendon. Biceps tendon ruptures may be seen with anterior tears of the rotator cuff (Fig. 99-52). Up to 7% of large rotator cuff tears are also accompanied by biceps tendon rupture. After a tear, the intracapsular portion of the tendon lies free in the joint cavity while the extra-articular portion is pulled distally. With MRI the tendon is absent from the groove which is filled with fluid. Distal retraction of the muscle

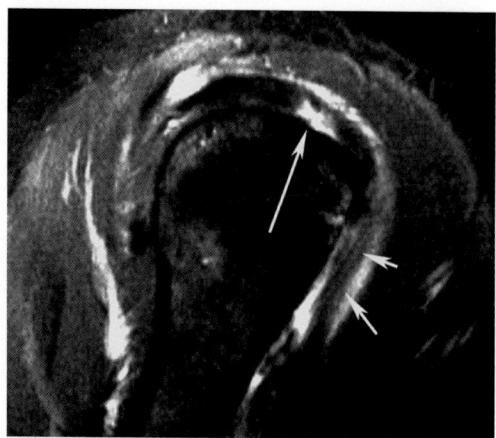

FIGURE 99-51

Biceps tendinosis. Sagittal oblique T2-weighted image with fat saturation. Note the high-grade partial tear in the supraspinatus tendon (*long arrow*). The biceps tendon is thickened and shows increased signal in its substance reflective of tendinosis (*short arrows*).

and tendon may be seen, best identified in longitudinal planes of section. Occasionally the intertubercular groove may fill with scar tissue of low signal and may lead to a false-negative diagnosis.

Medial dislocation of the biceps tendon may also result from chronic impingement, associated with a large anterior cuff tear.[13,179,273,277-279] There is tearing of the secondary biceps stabilizers, including the anterior supraspinatus and subscapularis tendons, and the coracohumeral ligament. The low signal tendon is displaced medially outside the intertubercular groove (see Figs. 99-44 and 99-47). This is best seen on axial

views. There may be an extra-articular tendon dislocation with an intact subscapularis. With rupture of the subscapularis tendon either post trauma or with a large or massive cuff tear the biceps tendon may also dislocate intra-articularly. The biceps tendon may then extend into and be entrapped in the joint.

Calcium Hydroxyapatite Deposition Disease

The shoulder is the most common site of involvement with calcium hydroxyapatite crystal deposition disease (HADD). Patients may often be asymptomatic, but clinical symptoms occur in 30% to 45% of patients in whom calcifications are present. The disorder occurs in both males and females, usually between the ages of 40 and 70 years. The pathogenesis of hydroxyapatite crystal deposition is unknown, though trauma, ischemia, or other systemic factors may induce abnormalities in the connective tissue, leading to crystal deposition.[283-285] Crystal deposition most commonly occurs in the tendinous and bursal structures about the shoulder, particularly the supraspinatus tendon (see Fig. 99-53) (52%). It may become bilateral in up to 50% of patients.[283] In the supraspinatus tendon it may target the critical zone, as this may be an area of both altered vascularity and mechanical pressure, which therefore may predispose it to hydroxyapatite crystal deposition. It may also occur in the other tendons of the rotator cuff, or in the biceps tendon. Bursal calcification is most common in the subacromial-subdeltoid bursa. These crystals incite a synovitis, tendinitis or bursitis and periarticular inflammation. The calcification alone may not be the inciting agent, but symptoms may occur with the dissolution of the calcium. With rupture of a calcific deposit, hydroxyapatite crystals are spilled into the surrounding soft-tissue space or bursa, setting off an

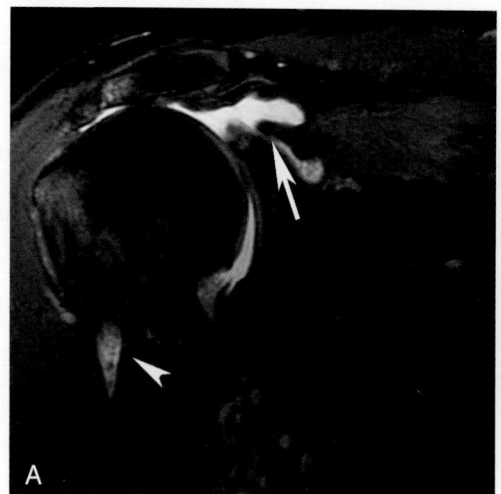
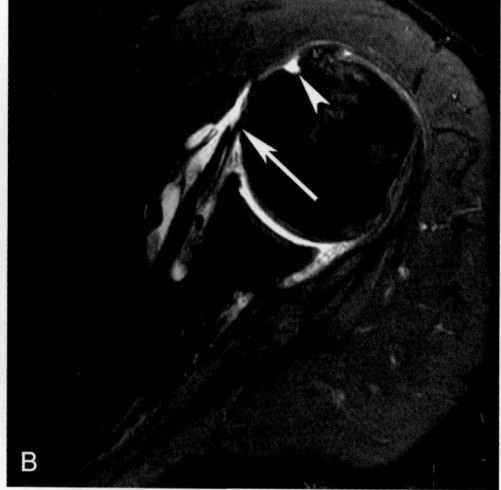

FIGURE 99-52

Biceps tendon rupture. **A,** Coronal oblique and **B,** axial T2-weighted images with fat saturation reveal the torn rotator cuff involving the supraspinatus tendon in **A** and subscapularis tendon in **B** (*arrows*). The biceps tendon is ruptured and retracted to the region just below the humeral neck (*arrowheads*). Note the empty, fluid-filled groove in **B**.

acute inflammatory response. Milwaukee shoulder consists of a destructive arthropathy, hydroxyapatite deposits, high collagenase activity in the synovial fluid, and rotator cuff tears.[271,286]

The nodular calcific deposits in HADD can usually be easily seen with plain radiographs and the combination of radiographs and the characteristic history is usually sufficient for diagnosis and subsequent therapy. When MRI is obtained in these patients the calcific densities, usually of low signal intensity, may be difficult to see, especially when small, due to the lack of contrast with the low signal of the tendons (Fig. 99-53). They are difficult to differentiate from a thickened tendon without calcification.[287] It may be difficult to distinguish a calcified tendon from a thickened tendon without calcification. They may be more easily identified when they are large, or if there is subjacent high signal on images with T2-type contrast, related to peritendinous edema and inflammation. T2*–gradient-echo images may also enhance visualization by providing a blooming effect. Although areas of high signal intensity may be observed about foci of calcification in tendons and bursae on T2-weighted spin-echo MR images and after injection of gadolinium intravenously, the correlation of such findings to calcific tendinitis and bursitis has not been proved.[191,288]

When the calcifications are seen, MRI can localize the specific tendons or bursa involved and document associated changes such as tendinitis, or the less common tears. Tears of the rotator cuff can occur in association with calcific tendonitis, though the mechanism is not yet clear.[289] It may relate to localized hyperemia in the tendon, which may lead to impingement.

The presence of effusions in the subacromial-subdeltoid bursa can be identified, particularly after extrusion of the calcifications into the bursa. MRI may also be helpful in these patients to exclude other causes of shoulder pain. In patients with Milwaukee shoulder the extent of joint destruction may be determined and the presence of a rotator cuff tear, as well as its extent, can be documented.

Bone Injuries

Nondisplaced fractures and bone contusions about the humeral head (Fig. 99-54) and greater tuberosity may result in pain and associated contusion-like injuries of the rotator cuff that may mimic pain due to rotator cuff tears. Anzilloti et al[213] found that this tended to occur in younger patients and in atypical locations of the supraspinatus tendon. This post-traumatic strain of the rotator cuff was typically associated with a bone bruise in this study.[213]

SHOULDER INSTABILITY

General Features

The shoulder is considered the most unstable joint in the human body. A simple definition of instability indicates that the humeral head slips out of its socket during activities. In the past it was considered to be present only if a previous dislocation had occurred. Now more subtle degrees of instability are well recognized, including

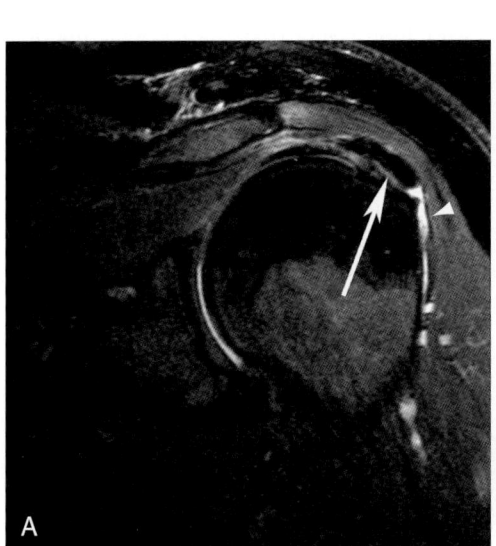
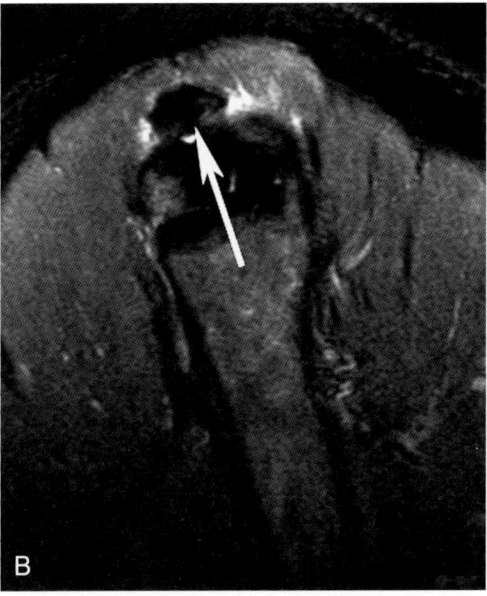

FIGURE 99-53

Calcium hydroxyapatite crystal deposition disease (HADD). **A,** Coronal and **B,** sagittal oblique fast spin-echo T2-weighted images with fat saturation. There is a nodular focus of low signal consistent with calcium in the central aspect of the supraspinatus tendon (*arrows*). Fluid is also seen in the subdeltoid bursa (*arrowhead*).

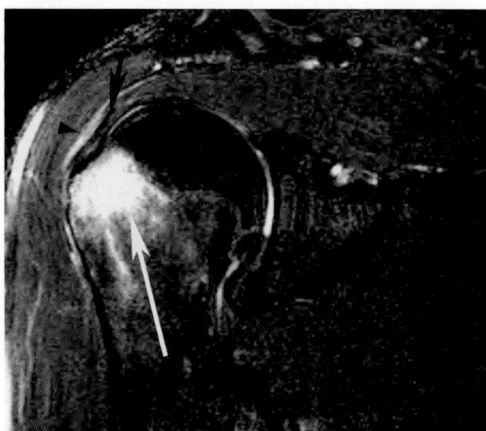

FIGURE 99-54

Greater tuberosity contusion. Coronal inversion-recovery–weighted image reveals a greater tuberosity contusion (*long arrow*). Also note there is mildly increased signal in the supraspinatus tendon which could reflect post-traumatic strain or contusion (*short arrow*). The small amount of fluid in the subdeltoid bursa may indicate some post-traumatic bursitis (*arrowhead*).

subluxation and instability that results from microtrauma.[70,290] Although the humeral head may translate a small amount during daily activities, these more subtle types of instability may result in pain from spasm or capsular stretching. The traditional forms of instability should be differentiated from glenohumeral joint laxity, in which asymptomatic passive translation of the humeral head on the glenoid fossa is observed. Glenohumeral joint laxity and instability may however coexist.

Instability may be classified according to frequency (acute, recurrent, or chronic), degree (subluxation or dislocation), etiology, and direction.[291,292] With regard to etiology, instability may result from one specific traumatic episode (termed traumatic instability), from repetitive microtrauma in activities such as swimming or throwing, or without any history of trauma (termed atraumatic instability). In the latter cases there is often a coexistent history of congenital ligamentous laxity. Shoulder instability can also be described by direction as anterior, posterior, or inferior to the glenoid, or multidirectional.[291,292] Anterior instability is by far the most common type of instability. Functional instability is another term used to describe instability and it indicates that derangement of the shoulder is caused by damage that may be confined to the glenoid labrum.[293,294] The shoulder may catch, slip, or lock and may not exhibit subluxation or dislocation. Another term in current use to define different types of minor instability is microinstability. This is said to occur in some 5% of patients. It is a spectrum of disorders involving the upper half of the shoulder joint, as opposed to more traditional instability which involves the lower third to half. Involved in the etiology of this process are entities such as a lax rotator interval and there may also be a history of overuse in these patients.[295,296]

Anterior Instability

Clinical Features

Recurrent subluxation or dislocation (shoulder instability) is the most frequent complication of acute traumatic dislocation. When the initial event occurs between the ages of 15 and 35 years the dislocations usually become recurrent or habitual. Once a second dislocation has occurred the patient becomes a "recurrent dislocator." The recurrence rate in the younger age group of patients is very high and may be as high as 80% to 90%.[297,298] Recurrences usually occur in the first 2 years. The damage to the shoulder seems to occur at the time of the original trauma, though each redislocation may cause further damage. The incidence of recurrence seems to be inversely related to the severity of the initial trauma.[293,299-301] There does not appear to be a relationship between the length and type of immobilization and the development of redislocation,[293,294,302-304] though many surgeons still immobilize the shoulders of younger patients for up 6 weeks in the hope of allowing the damaged tissues to heal. Recurrences are more common in men.

Over the age of 40 years the recurrence rate typically drops to 15% or less.[166] In older patients the spectrum of lesions is different and there is more often a tear of the rotator cuff or fracture of the greater tuberosity.

Pathologic Lesions

Patients with recurrent subluxations and dislocations incur lesions to the capsular mechanism. The essential lesion of instability described by Bankart is detachment of the glenoid labrum and capsule from the anterior glenoid margin.[305] Others believe the most important abnormality is a Hill Sachs defect.[306-309] Fractures of the inferior glenoid margin, insufficiency, stretching, or avulsion of the subscapularis muscle and tendon, and stretching rather than actual detachment of the anterior capsule may also be important. Other factors include aplasia or hypoplasia of the glenoid, variations in contour of the glenoid fossa, excessive anteversion of the glenoid, increased anteversion of the humeral head, and muscle imbalances.[54,310]

True Bankart lesions are more commonly found in patients with a history of complete traumatic dislocation. In patient with a history of a subluxating shoulder there may just be laxity or redundancy of the capsule, though labral lesions, fractures of the glenoid rim, and articular defects of the posterolateral humeral head may also be seen. Damage to the glenoid rim and Hill-Sachs lesions are more frequently found in complete traumatic dislocation.[310-314]

Bone Abnormalities

The two most common bone abnormalities are Hill-Sachs lesions and fractures of the inferior glenoid margin. A Hill-Sachs lesion is a specific indicator of a prior anterior glenohumeral joint dislocation. It is a posterolateral notch defect in the humeral head that is

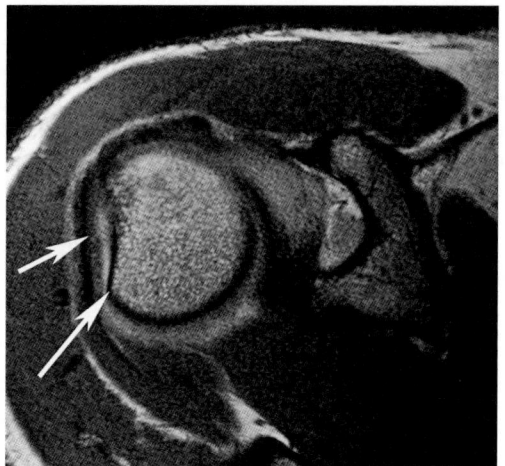

FIGURE 99-55

Hill-Sachs lesions. Axial T1-weighted image (TR/TE 800/17 ms) at the level of the coracoid process. A wedge-like defect is seen at the posterior superior lateral aspect of the humeral head (*arrows*).

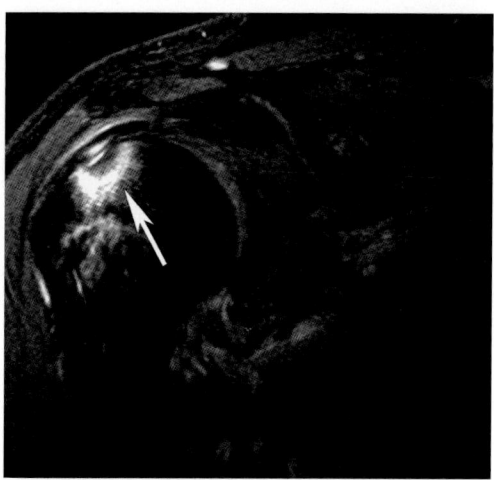

FIGURE 99-56

Hill-Sachs lesion. Coronal oblique fast spin-echo T2-weighted image (TR/TE 3916/54 ms) with fat suppression. A Hill-Sachs lesion with associated marrow edema is seen along the posterior superior aspect of the humeral head (*arrow*).

created by impingement of the articular surface of this portion of the humerus against the anteroinferior rim of the glenoid fossa. It is most common in patients with recurrent anterior subluxation and dislocation,[315] and uncommon in patients with anterior subluxation alone,[292] multidirectional instability, or labral pathology not associated with recurrent subluxations or dislocations.

On MRI, Hill-Sachs lesions appear as wedgelike defects on the posterolateral aspect of the humeral head (Fig. 99-55). They are identified above the level of the coracoid process.[315-318] They are best seen on axial images, but may also be apparent on coronal and sagittal oblique images (Fig. 99-56). Both the larger, more traditional Hill-Sachs lesions and the minor impaction injuries of the humeral articular cartilage and subchondral plates that may be more easily appreciated with arthroscopy can be seen. Hill-Sachs lesions should not be confused with the normal posterolateral flattening seen in the inferior aspect of the humeral head and which is typically present below the level of the coracoid.[318] Depending on their age, Hill-Sachs lesions may be associated with marrow edema (see Fig. 99-56) or trabecular sclerosis. MRI imaging was found to have a sensitivity of 97%, a specificity of 91%, and an accuracy of 94% in the detection of a Hill-Sachs lesion.[315]

The osseous Bankart lesion (Figs. 99-57 and 99-58) is a defect in the anterior inferior margin of the glenoid rim.[319] Cross-sectional imaging with either CT or MRI with or without intra-articular contrast injection can be helpful in depicting these lesions[273,320-322] and determining their size and location. It is generally thought that a large defect should be treated with bone-grafting, but there is a lack of consensus with regard to how large a defect must be in order to necessitate this procedure. Some investigators have proposed that a defect must

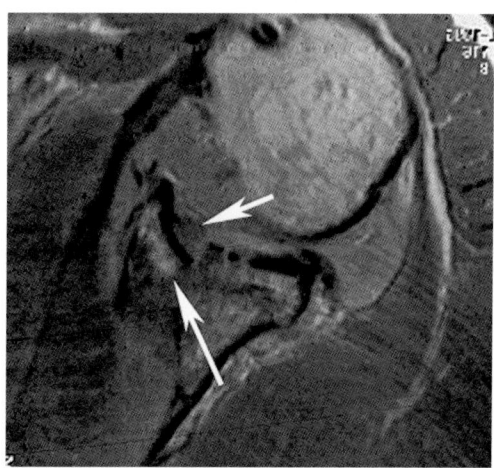

FIGURE 99-57

Bony glenoid margin lesions ("bony Bankart"). Axial proton-density–weighted image. A large fracture fragment from the mid to anterior inferior glenoid is seen in this patient after anterior dislocation (*arrows*).

involve at least one third of the glenoid surface in order to necessitate bone grafting.[319,323] When large, bony Bankart lesions may lead to reversal of the normal pear shape of the glenoid surface, a situation that promotes recurrent dislocations. The bony glenoid rim lesions may be easier to interpret with CT, especially fractures and ectopic ossification, although lesions in the subchondral bone and marrow are more easily identified with MRI. On MRI cystic change and sclerosis may be seen. STIR images and/or intermediate or T2-weighted MRI images with fat suppression in the sagittal oblique plane may depict particularly well bone and marrow alterations

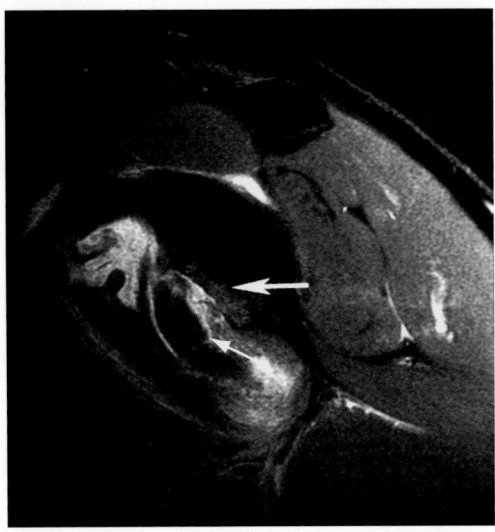

FIGURE 99-58

Bony glenoid margin lesions ("bony Bankart"). Sagittal oblique T2-weighted fast spin-echo image with fat suppression. A bone defect with marrow edema of the anterior more inferior glenoid (*large arrow*) parallels the labroligamentous avulsion. Note the anteriorly displaced, low signal bone fragment (*small arrow*).

associated with Bankart lesions (Fig. 99-58). CT with reformatted images with 3D reconstruction may aid in determining the size of the defect and the need for bone grafting to prevent recurrence after surgery.[323-325]

Labral, Capsular, and Ligamentous Lesions

General Features

The soft-tissue lesions associated with recurrent anterior subluxation and dislocation include damage to the anterior glenoid labrum, associated glenohumeral ligaments (labroligamentous complex), and anterior capsule.[292,293,305,326-329] Specifically the "cartilaginous" lesion as originally described by Bankart has been considered to be an avulsion or tear of the glenoid labrum and/or stripping of the joint capsule. The damage to the anterior labrum that is seen at surgery, however, may vary from detachment of the labrum from the glenoid rim, to tears of the substance of the labrum, to a completely destroyed or absent labrum.[293]

Injury to the labroligamentous complex typically will involve the region of the anterior band of the inferior glenohumeral ligament. Failure of this complex may occur at its glenoid insertion site (70-75% of cases). The labrum tears as it is avulsed by the glenohumeral ligaments at the time of injury. Failure of this complex may also occur at its humeral insertion site (5-10% of cases), or in its substance (15-20%), whereby there will be capsular failure due to tear or laxity. Those associated with glenoid-sided failure include the Bankart lesion described earlier and its less common variants, the Perthes lesion and the anterior labroligamentous peri-

osteal sleeve avulsion (ALPSA) lesion. Lesions associated with humeral failure include humeral avulsion of the glenohumeral ligament (HAGL) and its bone counterpart (BHAGL) lesion. Failure of this ligament at both its glenoid and humeral insertion destabilizes both ends of the anterior band of the inferior glenohumeral ligament [floating avulsion of the inferior glenohumeral ligament (AIGHL)].

A typical Bankart lesion would be an avulsion of the labroligamentous complex from the anteroinferior portion of the glenoid.[329-331] The periosteum of the scapula is lifted and disrupted. It occurs at the 3 to 6 o'clock position, but may extend upward. The soft-tissue lesion may be avulsed together with a piece of bone, the "bony" Bankart lesion, along the anteroinferior aspect of the glenoid rim.[307]

Labral Lesions

The labrum has been divided into six quadrants: I, superior; II, anterior superior; III, anterior inferior; IV, inferior; V, posterior inferior; and VI, posterior superior. Lesions of the glenoid labrum are considered to be a reliable sign of instability. Normal variation occurs in the superior and anterior superior portion from the 11 to 3 o'clock position, including the sublabral foramen and the Buford complex. Pathology in the labrum associated with anterior instability typically occurs in the anterior inferior portion from the 3 to 6 o'clock position. Intermediate signal occurs in the sublabral zone between the articular cartilage of the glenoid.[105] Another cause of difficulty is the occurrence of magic angle phenomenon in the labrum on short TE sequences.

The criteria used to diagnose an abnormality of the glenoid labrum include alterations in its morphology and/or signal intensity. Increased signal within the labrum not extending to the surface reflects internal labral degeneration.[187] A torn labrum has moderate or intense signal on short TR/TE, density-weighted or gradient-echo images, extending to the surface of the labrum, and brightens on T2-weighted or fat-suppressed proton-density images (Fig. 99-59A) or imbibes contrast into the defect at MR arthrography (Fig. 99-59B).[105,187,273,332-334] Abnormal labra may also be blunted, eroded, or frayed and irregular.

The diagnostic performance of MRI and MR arthrography in the evaluation of labral tears has been evaluated. One study of conventional MRI found a sensitivity of 93% and a specificity 87%.[187] A larger study found a sensitivity of 89% and a specificity of 97%.[5] MRI was found to be most sensitive in the evaluation of anterior labral tears and least sensitive in superior and posterior tears. MRI arthrography reveals a diagnostic performance similar to or better than conventional MRI and better reveals labral separation/detachment.[33,56,273,335-338]

Capsular Lesions

In patients with shoulder instability after one or repeated dislocations and or subluxations there may be traumatic avulsion of the capsule from its glenoid

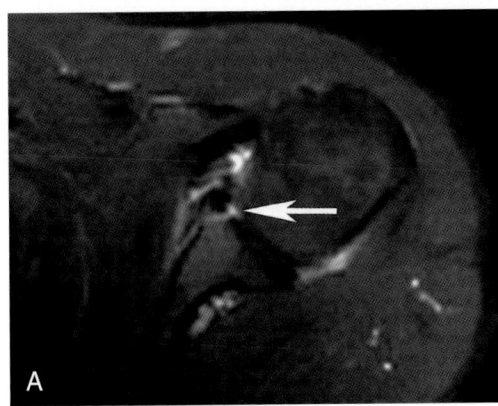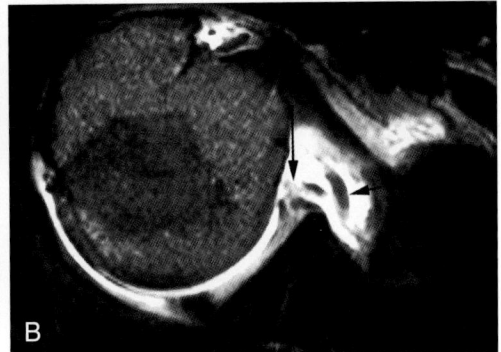

FIGURE 99-59

Labral lesion. **A,** Anterior labral separation outlined by fluid signal on an axial fast spin-echo T2-weighted image with fat suppression (*arrow*). The anterior labrum is also blunted and attenuated. **B,** Axial T1-weighted MR arthrogram (TR/TE 800/20 ms) in another patient. Contrast outlines and imbibes into a complex tear in the anterior labrum (*long arrow*). Note the attenuated glenohumeral ligament (*middle*) anterior to this (*short arrow*).

insertion. In the latter circumstance the capsule would be peeled back to the neck of the scapula with the first and subsequent dislocation. This is described as capsular stripping or shearing.

The anterior inferior capsule and associated glenohumeral ligaments (especially the anterior band of the inferior glenohumeral ligament) can often best be seen on arthrographic MR examination on fast spin-echo proton-density, intermediate, or T2-weighted images with fat suppression, or with T2*-weighted 2D gradient-echo techniques, particularly when there is a significant effusion. In the absence of an effusion MR arthrography is very useful, especially to clearly identify the anterior inferior labrum and inferior glenohumeral ligament. With injury to this region fluid or contrast may also be seen to extend beneath the soft-tissue mantle. In a typical Bankart lesion the labrum will be torn or detached with the capsular structures and fluid signal or contrast may extend within or beneath the labrum as well (Figs. 99-60, 99-61, and 99-62). The assessment of the capsule should be at the midglenoid or below, since on the more superior images a distended subscapularis bursa or medial capsular insertion may mimic capsular stripping.[339] Evaluation of capsular stripping may then better reflect disruption of the anterior inferior labral ligamentous complex.[223,340]

Bankart Lesion Variants

The earlier discussion focuses on the typical lesion of anterior instability—the Bankart lesion, which is an avulsion of the anterior inferior labrum, capsule, and inferior glenohumeral ligament complex, with an associated disruption of the scapular periosteum (see Fig. 60-62). There are however a number of variants of this typical lesion.

Perthes Lesion

This lesion[341] is a labral ligamentous avulsion in which the scapular periosteum remains intact but is stripped medially. The periosteum may then become redundant, and recurrent instability may occur as the humeral head moves forward into this region of acquired laxity (pseudojoint). The labrum may then lay back down into a relatively normal position on the glenoid and resynovialize (heal back). It may then be very difficult to diagnose as the detachment may not be easily identified on conventional MRI or even on MR arthrography (Fig. 99-63) (or at arthroscopy), unless specialized imaging positions such as ABER are employed (Fig. 99-63).[29,39,341] With distension from MR arthrography and when needed with ABER positioning, only subtle displacement of the labral tissue may be seen (see Fig. 99-63).

Anterior Labroligamentous Periosteal Sleeve Avulsion

The ALPSA lesion[342,343] is anterior labroligamentous sleeve avulsion. In these cases the scapular periosteum does not rupture, resulting in a medial displacement and inferior rotation of the labroligamentous structures as they are stripped down to the scapular neck. The ALPSA lesion may then heal in this displaced position. This has also been termed a medialized Bankart lesion. A small cleft or separation can then be seen between the glenoid margin and the labrum. With a chronic ALPSA lesion fibrous tissue is deposited on the medially displaced labral ligamentous complex and the entire lesion then resynovializes along the articular surface. This may leave a deformed and redundant labrum. This lesion may require a different repair from the typical Bankart lesion

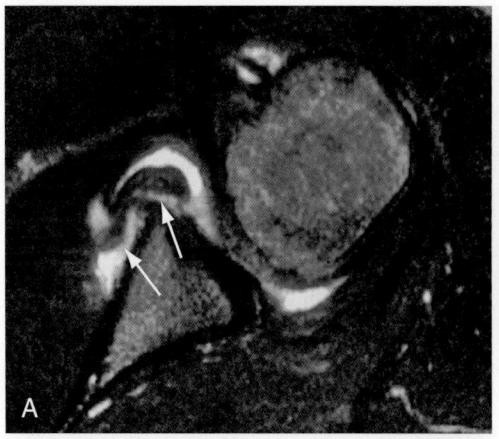

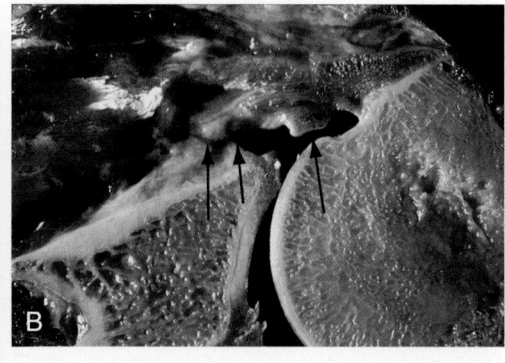

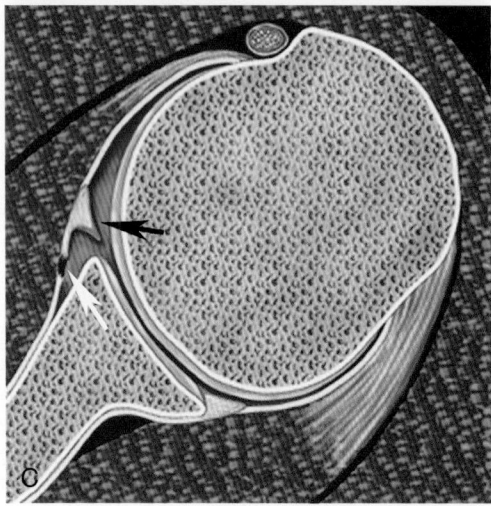

FIGURE 99-60

Bankart lesion. **A,** Axial fast spin-echo T2-weighted image with fat suppression. There is evidence of detachment of the anterior inferior labroligamentous complex from the glenoid margin (*arrows*). **B,** Axial cadaver section from a specimen subjected to simulated dislocations in the laboratory. Tear and detachment of the anterior labrum is seen with disruption of the capsule and scapular periosteum (*black arrows*). **C,** Bankart lesion showing the anterior labroligamentous tear and detachment (*black arrow*) with disruption of the scapular periosteum (*white arrow*). (*Reproduced with permission from Zlatkin MB. MRI of the Shoulder, 2nd ed. Philadelphia, Lippincott, Williams and Wilkins, 2003. Drawn by Salvador Beltran.*)

and therefore it is important to recognize it.[343-345] In the absence of an effusion the ALPSA lesion may be missed on conventional MRI if the lesion does not extend to the mid anterior labrum, as the fibrous medialized resynovialized mass may not be well seen on MRI imaging (Fig. 99-64) in a patient with a paucity of joint fluid and magic angle artifact.[29] MR arthrography, including the ABER position, may be valuable in revealing these lesion (Fig. 99-64).

Humeral Avulsion of the Glenohumeral Ligament

The HAGL lesion refers to humeral avulsion of the glenohumeral ligament.[346-349] This lesion more typically occurs in individuals older than 30 years.[349] It may be seen in conjunction with a tear of the rotator cuff or fracture of the greater tuberosity of the humerus. It is not uncommonly associated with a tear of the subscapularis tendon. This lesion can be seen on conventional MRI as well as with MR arthrography (Fig. 99-65).[346,347] On MRI examination the torn glenohumeral ligament may appear thick, wavy and irregular, with increased signal intensity.[346] MR arthrography may also show contrast material extravasating from the joint through the capsular disruption at its humeral insertion. It may be feasible to repair this lesion athroscopically via reattach-

ment to the humerus via sutures. Recently, the HAGL lesion was also seen after successful Bankart repair.[350]

The bony humeral avulsion of the glenohumeral ligaments (BHAGL)[351,352] is a rare lesion that may occur after anterior dislocation of the shoulder. The bone fragment may appear similar to a bony glenoid avulsion. CT or MRI can show that the bone is attached to the glenohumeral ligaments and does not originate from the glenoid but rather from the bone at the site of humeral attachment of the inferior glenohumeral ligament.

Posterior Instability

Posterior instability of the shoulder is not as well understood as anterior stability, in part because it is uncommon but also because of the confusion in terminology differentiating posterior subluxations and dislocations.[291,353-355]

Isolated posterior instability is uncommon and accounts for only 5% of instability. Acute posterior dislocations of the glenohumeral joint are rare (approximately 2% to 4% of all dislocations of the shoulder).[356,357] They may occur following trauma but are commonly associated with electric shocks or seizures. Recurrence is not common.

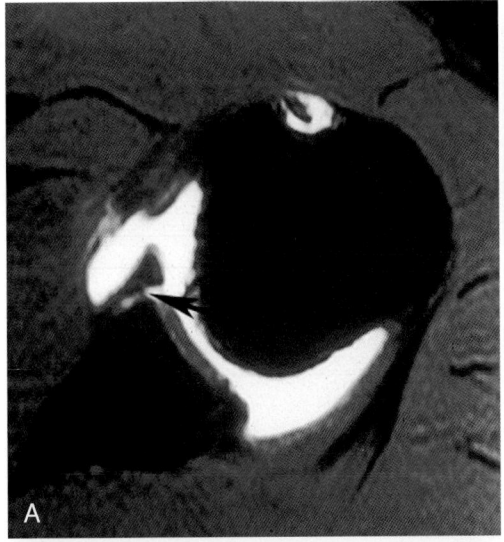
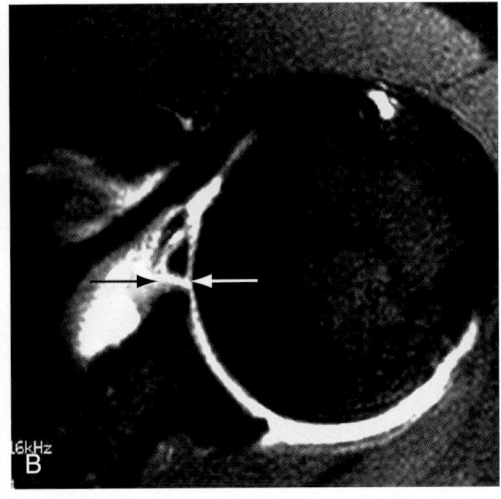
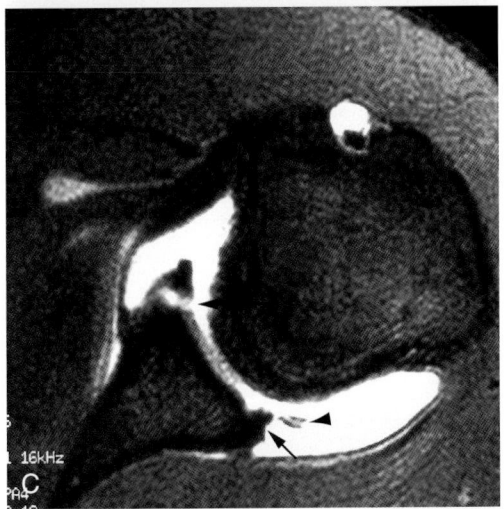

FIGURE 99-61

Bankart lesion. **A,** Axial T1-weighted MR arthrogram with fat suppression. There is evidence of detachment of the anterior inferior labroligamentous complex from the glenoid margin (true "Bankart" lesion) (*arrow*). **B** and **C,** Axial T1-weighted MR arthrograms with fat suppression. Similar findings of a labroligamentous tear and detachment are seen (*white* and *black arrows* in **B**, *large arrow* in **C**). Note the small defect in the posterior labrum (*small arrow* in **C**) and subjacent fragment (*arrowhead*).

Recurrence is very common with atraumatic posterior dislocations and in patients with a history of a traumatic dislocation when large bony defects of the humerus and glenoid occur. Recurrent posterior subluxation rather than dislocation is however the more common lesion. Overuse as in athletics is usually involved. Abduction, flexion, and internal rotation are the mechanisms involved (swimming, throwing, and punching), reflective of repeated microtrauma. These patients, who are often young athletes, may present with pain rather than signs of instability. There may be some association with posterior laxity.[353-355,358-364]

The posterior band of the inferior glenohumeral ligament is a primary static stabilizer of the glenohumeral joint with respect to translation posteriorly of the humeral head. Injury sufficient to cause posterior instability, however, requires injury to the posterior inferior labroligamentous complex as well as the posterior capsule. Pathologic findings in patients with prior posterior dislocations and resultant instability may be the reverse of those for recurrent anterior

dislocations and include posterior labral and capsular detachments and tears, as well as posterior capsular laxity.[365] An impaction type defect on the anteromedial aspect of the humeral head is known as a reverse Hill-Sachs lesion (notch sign or trough lesion). Fractures of the posterior glenoid margin and of the lesser tuberosity may also occur. The subscapularis tendon may be stretched or detached, and tears of the teres minor tendon may occur. Posterior labrocapsular periosteal sleeve avulsion (POLPSA) has also been described.[366,367]

The MR and MR arthrographic findings associated with patients with posterior instability mirror those described for anterior instability except they involve the posterior capsule and labrum.[339,361,368] The reverse Hill-Sachs lesion is well seen on MR images (Fig. 99-66). MRI and MR arthrography may be used to identify the presence and extent of a tear and detachment of the posterior labroligamentous complex (Fig. 99-66). Although the posterior capsule is injured, the capsular abnormalities may be less prominent than in anterior instability.[339] MR-evident abnormalities that involve

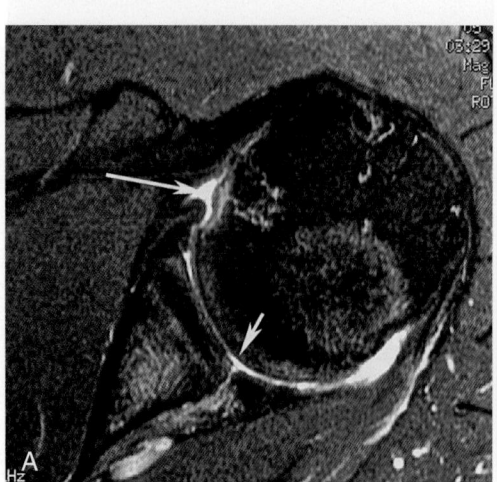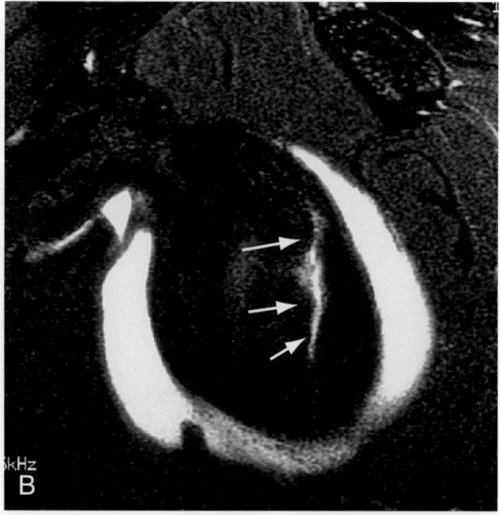

FIGURE 99-66

Posterior instability. **A,** Axial T2-weighted (TR/TE 3100/47 ms) fast spin-echo image with fat suppression. The posterior glenoid labrum and capsule are torn along the posterior glenoid margin (*short arrow*). There is a bony defect on the anteromedial aspect of the humeral head consistent with a "reverse Hill-Sachs deformity." It is associated with marrow edema (*long arrow*). **B,** Sagittal oblique T2-weighted fast spin-echo image with fat suppression, carried out after intra-articular fluid injection. The superior inferior extent of the labral tear/detachment is seen best in this projection, outlined by the fluid signal and joint distension (*arrows*).

the bony glenoid include fractures or defects, although findings of marrow edema or sclerosis and cystic lesions may also be identified. In patients with atraumatic recurrent posterior subluxation, joint laxity with redundancy of the posterior capsule may be the most prominent finding and a posterior labral tear may not be found.[354] This may also be associated with inferior redundancy[353,369] in which case multidirectional instability may result. MR arthrography may be the only means of imaging able to reveal this laxity.

Isolated Labral Tears

The labrum can tear in the absence of subluxation or dislocation. The tears that have been described in this circumstance include flap or bucket-handle tears and these lesions may be present in the anterior superior portion of the labrum. They may respond to arthroscopic excision. Isolated glenoid labrum lesions may occur in the throwing athlete as fraying or separation in the superior quadrant of the labrum adjacent to the origin of the long head of the biceps. These patients present with a painful catching or snapping sensation during throwing. This is related to overloading of the biceps tendon and subsequent avulsion of the superior part of the labrum during the follow through. These lesions in the labrum may be associated with pathology in the rotator cuff. Injuries seen in the rotator cuff are often partial tears of the rotator cuff undersurface more posteriorly. MR arthrography may reveal these lesions best, as contrast will leak into the labral tears, imbibe into areas of labral fraying, detect areas of labral separation or detachment, and leak or imbibe into undersurface rotator cuff injuries.

Posterosuperior subglenoid impingement (see earlier) occurs during the late cocking phase of throwing with abnormal contact between the posterosuperior portion of the glenoid rim and the undersurface of the rotator cuff, and is thought to occur at the extremes of abduction and external rotation. A triad of findings has been described in association with this lesion (Figs. 99-34 and 99-67): injury to the rotator cuff undersurface at the junction of the infraspinatus and supraspinatus tendons; degenerative tearing of the posterosuperior glenoid labrum; and subcortical cysts and chondral lesions in the posterosuperior glenoid and humerus due to repetitive impaction. There may in addition be an injury to the inferior glenohumeral ligament because it limits abduction in external rotation of the glenohumeral joint and is therefore under tension in this position.

SLAP Lesions

Snyder et al[370-372] introduced this term to define injuries to the superior portion of the labrum and adjacent biceps tendon. A superior quadrant labral tear with anterior and posterior components of the tear is labeled a SLAP lesion (superior labrum anterior posterior). The lesion may be acute or chronic and when acute they may result from a fall onto the outstretched arm with the shoulder in abduction and forward flexion. It also may occur in athletes repetitively overusing the arm,[295,373-375] including baseball, tennis, or volleyball players. The injury to the superior portion of the glenoid labrum may result from sudden forced abduction of the arm, i.e., excessive traction related to a sudden pull from the long head of the biceps tendon. The lesion may typically begin posteriorly and then extend anteriorly and terminate at

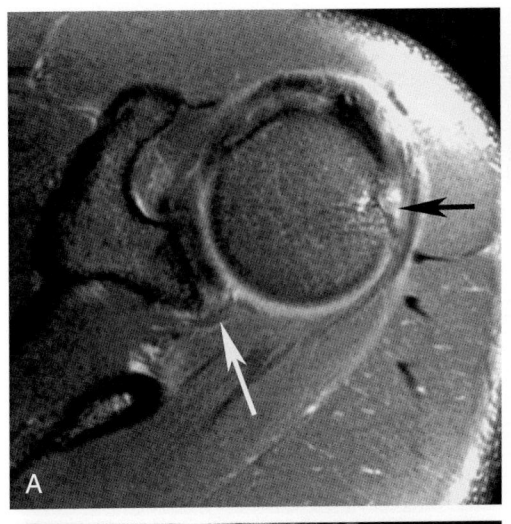

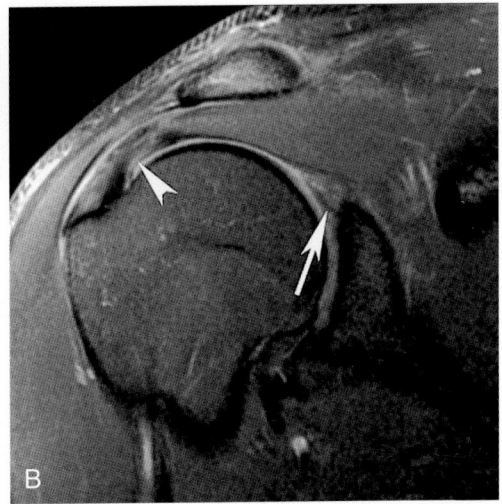

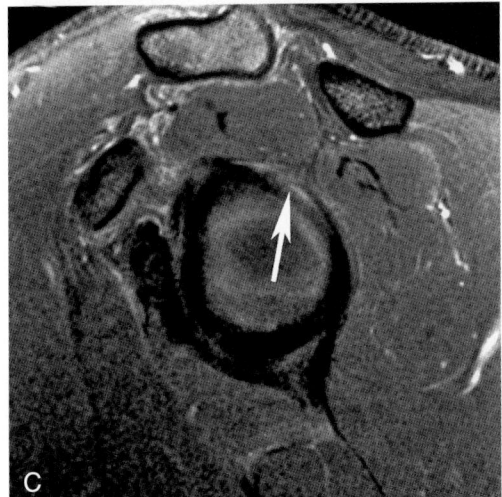

FIGURE 99-67

A, Axial; **B,** coronal; and **C,** sagittal oblique T1-weighted images after intravenous gadolinium injection for intravenous MR arthrography. The rotator cuff shows tendinosis more posteriorly (*arrowhead* in **B**). There is cystic change in the humeral head posterosuperiorly (*black arrow* in **A**). The labrum imbibes contrast, reflective of degenerative-type tearing (*white arrows*). Findings are consistent with posterosuperior glenoid impingement.

or before the midglenoid notch. It includes the biceps labral anchor.

SLAP tears were categorized into four basic types by Snyder et al.[372] Type 1 (10% of SLAP lesions) reveals superior labral roughening and degeneration. The labrum remains firmly attached to the glenoid. This lesion may represent a degenerative tear of the labrum. Type 2 is the most common lesion (40%) and is a detachment of this roughened superior portion of the labrum and its biceps tendon anchor. Burkhart et al[295,374] described three distinct categories of type 2 SLAP lesions: anterior, posterior, and combined anteroposterior. Type 3 (30%) is a bucket-handle tear of the superior portion of the labrum. It does not involve the biceps labral anchor. Type 4 (15%) has in addition to the bucket handle tear a split tear of the biceps tendon.

Additional types of SLAP lesions have been described.[273,373,376,377] Type 5 is a Bankart lesion of the anterior inferior labrum that then extends superiorly to include separation of the biceps tendon anchor. Type 6 lesions are unstable radial or flap tears that also involve separation of the biceps anchor. A type 7 lesion consists of anterior extension of the SLAP lesion to involve the middle glenohumeral ligament. Type 8 lesions extend posteroinferiorly with extensive detachment of the posterior labrum. A type 9 lesion is a complete concentric avulsion of the labrum circumferentially around the entire glenoid rim.[375]

MRI and MR arthrography may be used in the detection of SLAP lesions (Figs. 99-68, 99-69, 99-70, and 99-71).[273,376,378-383] In the study by Cartland et al[384] on MRI examination, type 1 lesions exhibited irregularity of the labral contour with mildly increased signal intensity. Type 2 lesions may have revealed a globular region of increased signal interposed between the superior labrum and glenoid margin. Type 3 showed typical linear increased signal extending to the labral surface. Type 4 lesions showed high signal within the superior labrum and extending into the proximal biceps tendon. SLAP lesions may be difficult to detect on conventional MR imaging. The more superior portions of the tear can be difficult to visualize on axial images. External rotation, as well as coronal oblique images, help define these lesions.[382] MR arthrography can be very helpful in

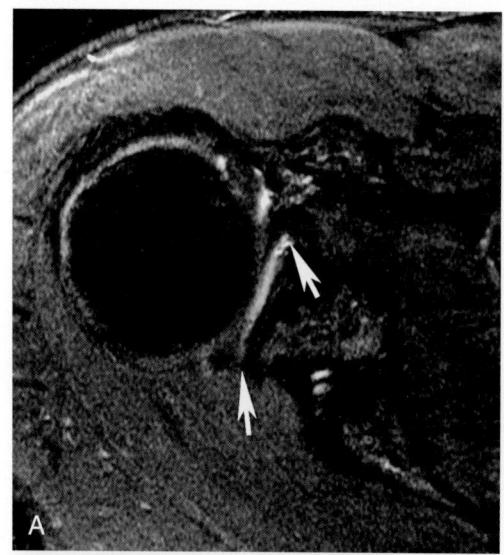

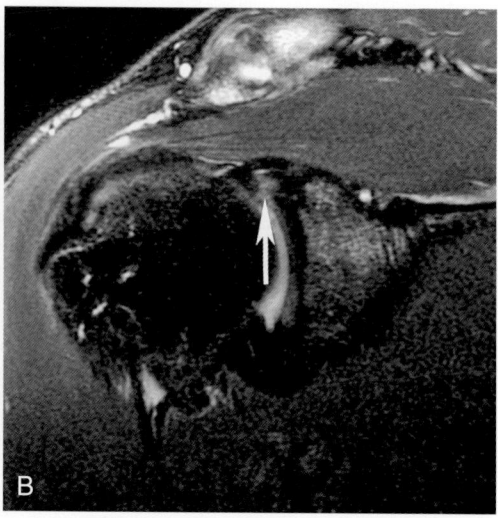

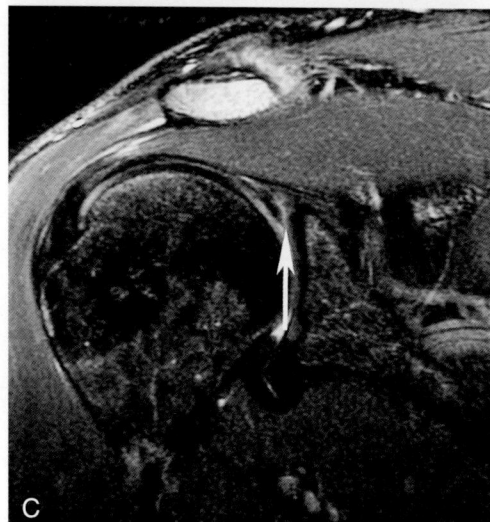

FIGURE 99-68

Superior labrum anterior posterior (SLAP) lesion. **A,** Axial, and **B** and **C,** coronal oblique fast spin-echo images (**B,** anterior; **C,** more posterior) with fat suppression. A continuous tear and detachment is identified in the superior labrum, anterior and posterior (SLAP type 2) (*white arrows* in **A-C**).

FIGURE 99-69

Superior labrum anterior posterior (SLAP) lesion. Type 3 lesion. Coronal oblique T1-weighted MR arthrogram. Contrast extension reveals detachment and mild displacement of the superior labrum from the glenoid rim (*arrow*). The biceps tendon insertion remains intact (*arrowhead*). (*Courtesy of Javier Beltran MD, New York.*)

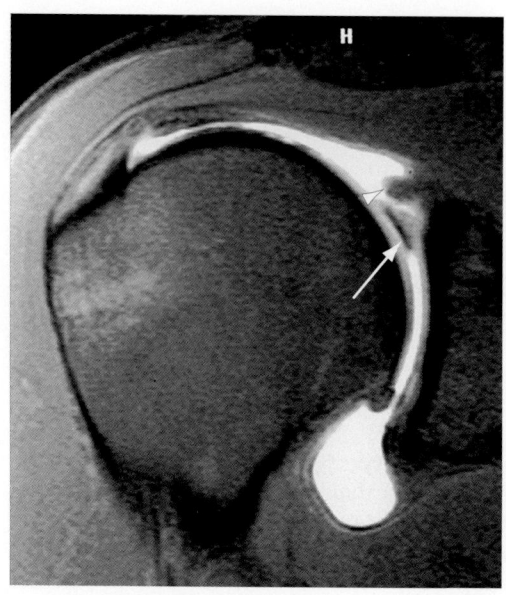

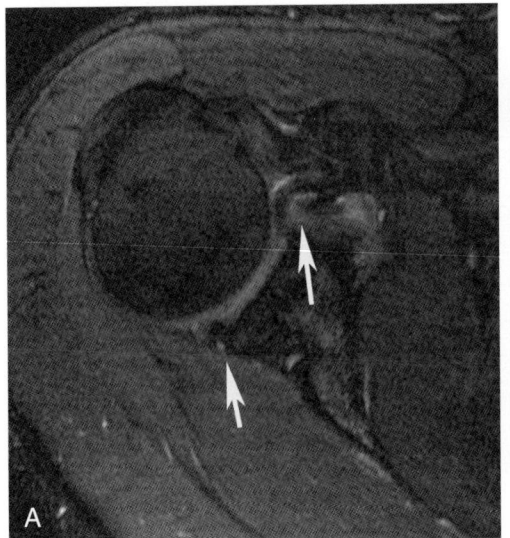 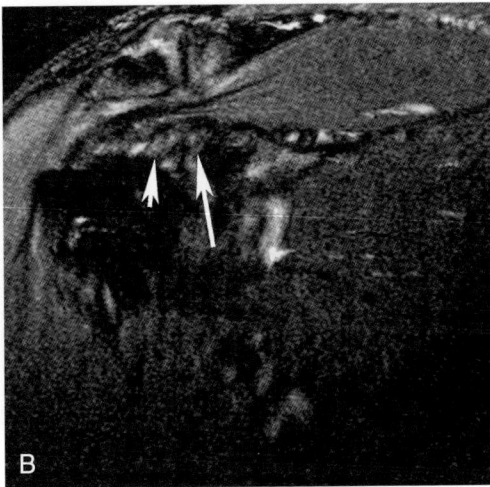

FIGURE 99-70

Superior labrum anterior posterior (SLAP) lesion. Type 4 lesion. **A,** Axial and **B,** coronal oblique fast spin-echo images with fat suppression. A tear is identified in the superior labrum, anterior and posterior (*long arrows*) extending into the proximal biceps tendon (*short arrow* in **B**).

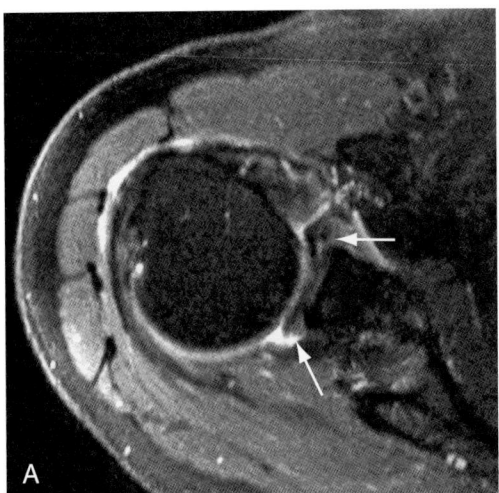 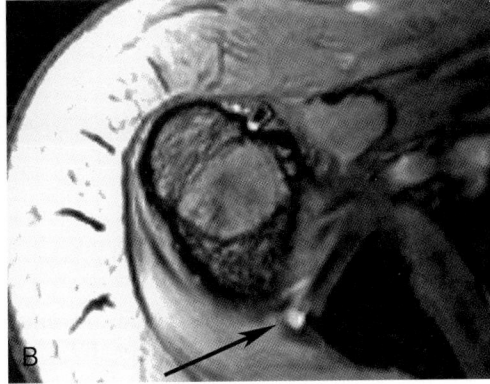

FIGURE 99-71

Superior labrum anterior posterior (SLAP) lesion. Type 8 lesion. **A,** Axial fast spin-echo T2-weighted image (TR/TE 3000/55) with fat suppression. **B,** 2D gradient-echo image (TR/TE 400/22 ms, flip angle 25 degrees). There is a tear of the superior labrum which extends posteroinferiorly (*arrows*).

detecting SLAP lesions, including the use of traction in some select situations.[385] It will distend out buckle-handle type tears, outline morphologic alterations, and imbibe into areas of degeneration and fraying of the labrum and biceps tendon. MR arthrography demonstrates the following signs in SLAP lesions[386]: 1. contrast material may extend superiorly into the glenoid attachment of the long head of the biceps tendon (LHBT) on oblique coronal images; 2. irregularity of the insertion of the LHBT on oblique coronal and sagittal images; 3. accumulation of contrast material between the labrum and glenoid fossa on axial images; 4. detachment and displacement of the superior labrum on oblique sagittal and coronal images; and 5. a fragment of the labrum displayed inferiorly between the glenoid fossa and the humeral head. In addition, as noted later, a paralabral cyst

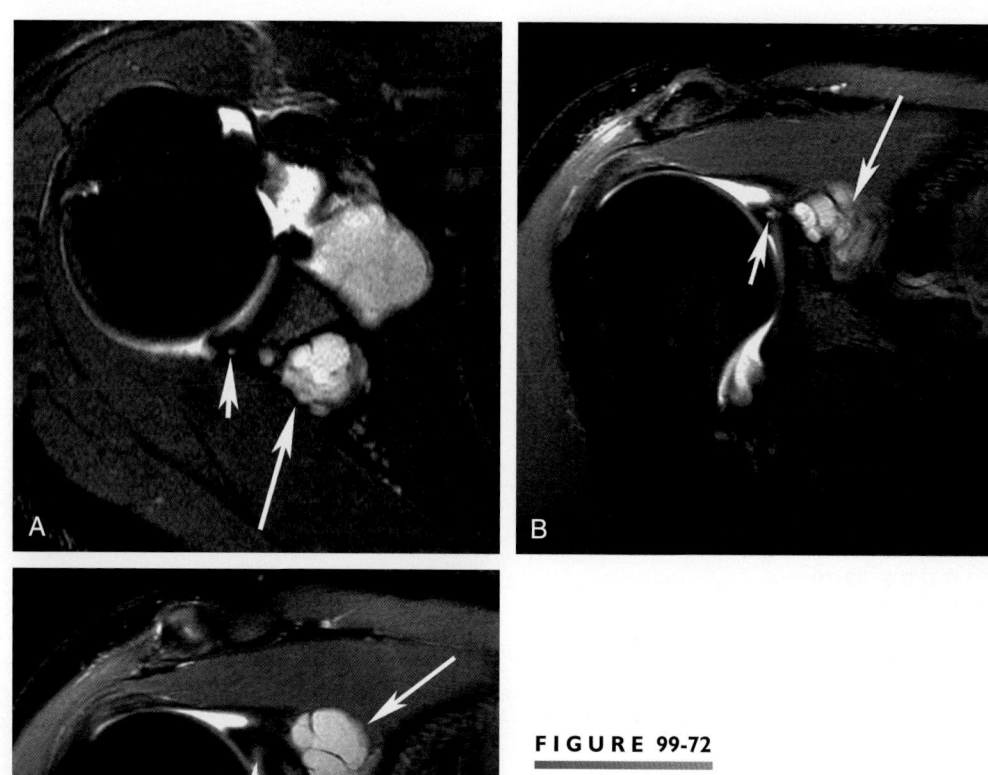

FIGURE 99-72

Paralabral cyst. **A,** Axial; and **B** and **C,** (both posterior) coronal oblique fast spin-echo T2-weighted sequences with fat suppression. A large paralabral cyst is identified (*long arrows*) arising in relation to a posterosuperior labral tear (*short arrows*) and extending into the spinoglenoid notch region.

may be frequently associated with these lesions. In one study MR arthrography had a sensitivity of 89%, a specificity of 91%, and an accuracy of 90%.[376]

Tears of the superior portion of the labrum must be distinguished from the normal variants of the labrum and its attachments in this region. Among the criteria for distinguishing these lesions from SLAP tears are that these lesions do not extend to involve the superior or posterior labrum beyond the level of the biceps labral anchor and there should be no associated morphologic alterations. In addition they should not extend below the level of the equator of the glenoid which may be marked by the coracoid process. Increased distance between the labrum and the glenoid, an irregular appearance of the labral margin, or lateral extension of the separation may suggest a SLAP lesion rather than a normal anatomic variant.[380] As with other tears of the superior labrum, SLAP lesions are frequently associated with rotator cuff lesions, particularly partial tears. One study found such lesions in 42% of cases.[376]

Paralabral Ganglion Cysts

These are ganglion cysts arising adjacent to the glenoid labrum[387-389] and most commonly associated with a labral tear (see Figs. 99-72 and 99-73). This labral tear is often a SLAP lesion and the paralabral cyst most commonly arises in relation to the posterosuperior component (Fig. 99-72). It may, however, occur anywhere in the glenohumeral joint. Pathophysiologically they may be similar to cysts of this nature elsewhere in the body, such as meniscal cysts or cysts associated with tears of the acetabular labrum. In this situation fluid arising from the joint extends through the labral tear into the surrounding soft-tissues and leads to ganglion cyst formation. Paralabral cysts may be difficult to identify on MR arthrography unless some form of T2-weighted sequence is performed as direct communication between a cyst and the joint space rarely occurs (see Fig. 99-46). A posterior or inferior cyst may cause compression neuropathy of the suprascapular or axillary nerve, respectively. Compression of the suprascapular nerve is

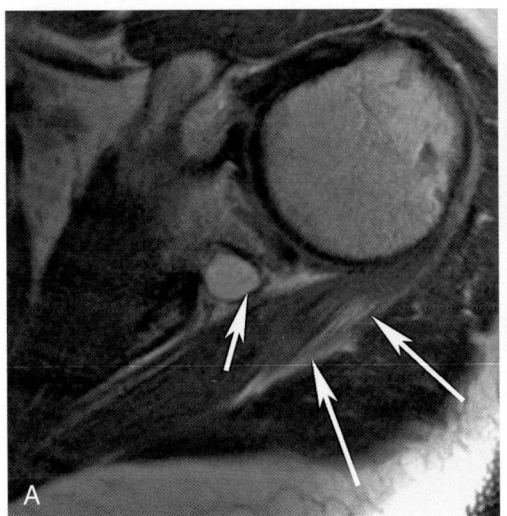
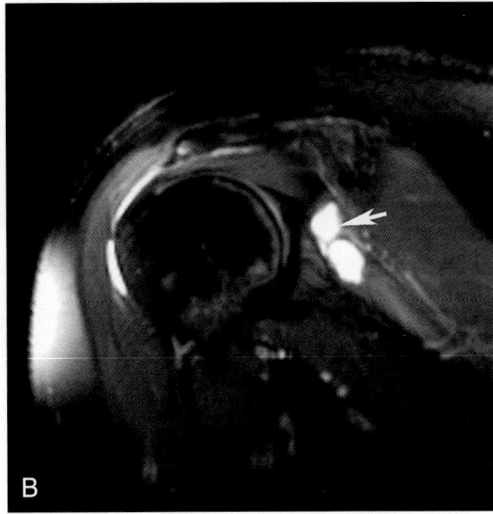

FIGURE 99-73

Paralabral cyst. Infraspinatus atrophy. **A,** Axial fast spin-echo T2-weighted sequence and **B,** coronal oblique fast spin-echo T2-weighted sequence with fat suppression. A paralabral cyst is identified (*short arrows*) which extends into the spinoglenoid notch region. Note the atrophy of the infraspinatus muscle (*long arrows* in **A**).

usually with extension of the posterior cyst into the spinoglenoid notch. Cysts that cause nerve compression are usually large (mean size 3.1 cm). Infraspinatus muscle atrophy may be seen (Fig. 99-73). Compression of the axillary nerve may be an unusual cause of quadrilateral space syndrome.[390] Atrophy of the teres minor muscle may also be seen.

Glenoid Labrum Articular Disruption

Another recently described lesion occurs in athletes and has been described at arthroscopy.[391] The GLAD lesion (glenoid labrum articular disruption) is a tear of the superficial anterior inferior labrum and also involves articular cartilage (Fig. 99-74). It results from a forced adduction across the chest from an abducted and externally rotated position. The labral tear is an inferior flap-type tear. It is not associated with glenohumeral instability. In addition, there is fibrillation and erosion of the articular cartilage in the anteroinferior quadrant of the glenoid fossa. These lesions may be visible on MRI and MR arthrography may improve the sensitivity to these lesions.[392,393]

Glenohumeral Internal Rotation Deficit in Abduction

This refers to the concept proposed by Burkart and Morgan[295,374,394] that reflects the fact that many of the problems associated with shoulder disability in older throwing athletes is due to contracture and thickening of the posterior inferior capsule, which results in a glenohumeral internal rotation deficit in abduction

(GIRD). This is associated with secondary hyperexternal rotation. Other associated lesions include the posterior peel back lesion of the glenoid labrum from the biceps tendon insertion to the posterior superior labrum,[324,394,395] SLAP type 2 lesions, and dead arm syndrome.[374] Shear and torsional forces result in injury to the posterosuperior aspect of the rotator cuff. Although lesions similar to those described in posterior superior glenoid impingement are seen, the posterior inferior capsular lesion rather than the act of subglenoid impingement is considered to be the underlying cause. The anterior capsular stretching, often seen in older throwing athletes, is also considered to be secondary to the posterior capsular contracture. These lesions, including the presence of posterior capsular thickening, may be best outlined with MRI arthrography (Fig. 99-75).

POSTOPERATIVE SHOULDER

Imaging the postoperative shoulder is challenging both from an imaging point of view and a technical point of view.[396-405] Certain technical factors must be taken into consideration. Postoperative artifact is problematic in imaging the postoperative patient. This includes ferromagnetic screws or staples. Small metal shavings from the use of a burr during acromioplasty may yield considerable artifact. The use of gradient-echo sequences should be minimized and fast spin-echo imaging is useful to minimize the degree of magnetic susceptibility artifact. Additionally, fat saturation may be incomplete and fast spin-echo inversion recovery sequences may be more useful. MR arthrography can be a useful tool to help image postoperative patients more successfully.

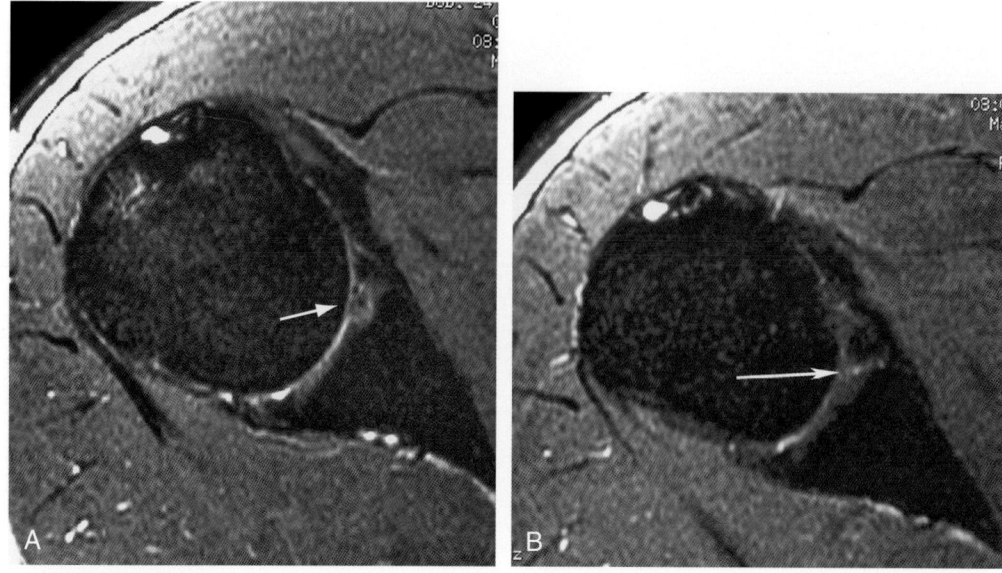

FIGURE 99-74

Glenoid labrum articular disruption (GLAD) lesion. **A** and **B,** Axial 2D gradient-echo images. There is a tear of the anterior inferior labrum (*arrow* in **B**). It is associated with an osteochondral-like lesion of the inferior anterior margin of the glenoid articular surface (*arrow* in **A**). The capsuloligamentous structures are intact.

Impingement and Rotator Cuff Disease

Subacromial Decompression without Rotator Cuff Repair

Surgical Technique

The first category of postoperative patients is those who have had a prior acromioplasty for impingement with an intact rotator cuff and no rotator cuff repair. This procedure may be done open, via an anterolateral deltoid splitting incision, or via arthroscopy. The anteroinferior acromion is removed, from the acromioclavicular joint to the deltoid insertion, removing that portion anterior to the clavicle. Most often the subdeltoid bursa is also resected as well as a variable part of the coracoacromial ligament. The acromioclavicular joint and the distal 2.5 cm of the clavicle may also be removed.

MRI Findings

MRI findings associated with acromioplasty include a flattened acromial undersurface, nonvisualization of the anterior one third of the acromion, and decreased marrow signal in the remaining distal acromion due to marrow fibrosis. Low signal due to artifacts from small metal fragments are often present, related to burring of the acromion. Removal of the subacromial bursa and subdeltoid fat pad results in the absence of these structures on postoperative studies, and most often a small amount of fluid signal on images with T2 contrast. If the acromioclavicular joint has been excised, scar tissue may be the most prominent finding (Fig. 99-76).[397,400,403,405]

Causes of persistent pain after subacromial decompression include inadequate acromioplasty and residual osteoarthrosis of the acromioclavicular joint (Fig. 99-77). Sagittal oblique MR images evaluate the adequacy of the decompression and any persistent impingement due to insufficient acromion resection or the persistence of a large subacromial spur. Large osteophytes projecting from the acromioclavicular joint may be seen on coronal and sagittal images. After acromioplasty, there may be progression of rotator cuff disease, including the interval development of a rotator cuff tear, partial or complete (Fig. 99-77). Unrecognized partial tears or small complete tears may extend. Progression may occur if the acromioplasty and decompression are inadequate, with persistent subacromial roughening.[397,400,403,405]

In the setting of interval development of a cuff tear or extension and/or progression of existing cuff pathology, such as tendinosis, the integrity of the cuff is more difficult to determine in the postoperative situation. MRI remains sensitive but less specific than MRI without prior surgery. Criteria include a definite region of discontinuity in the cuff, accompanied by fluid signal on images with T2 contrast, STIR or T2*-weighted gradient-echo sequences, or when contrast extravasation is seen through the cuff defect at MR arthrography (see Fig. 99-77).[397,400,403,405]

Rotator Cuff Repair or Debridement

Surgical Technique

The second category involves patients who have had a prior rotator cuff repair. In patients with partial-thickness tears, treatment depends on the area, depth, and severity

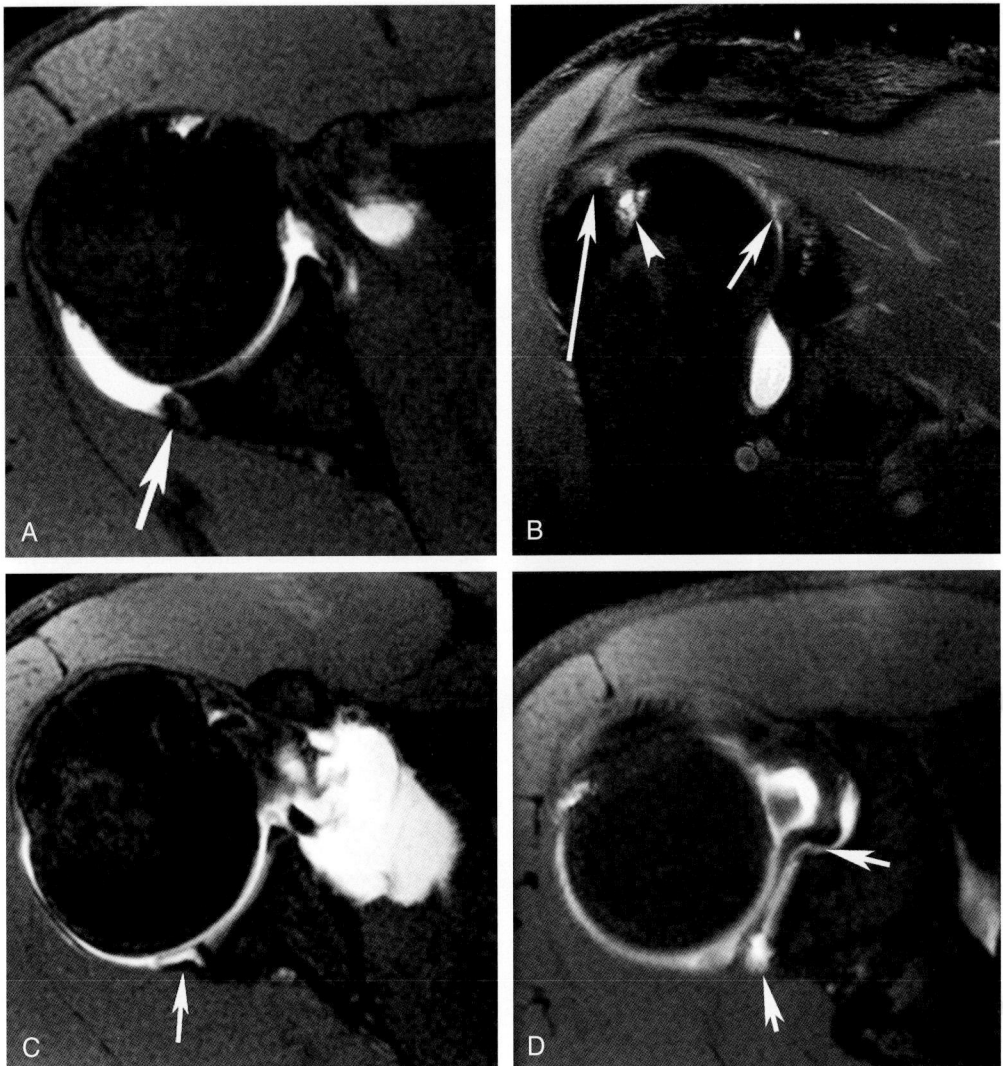

FIGURE 99-75

Glenohumeral internal rotation deficit (GIRD). **A,** Axial T1-weighted MR arthrogram. Note the thickened posterior capsule at the site of insertion into the glenoid (*arrow*). **B,** Coronal oblique T1-weighted MR arthrogram in the same patient as in **A**. Note the alterations in the posterior rotator cuff (*long arrow*), the degenerative-type tear of the posterior superior labrum (*short arrow*), and the cystic changes in the humeral head (*arrowhead*). **C,** Axial T1-weighted MR arthrogram in a different patient. Note the thickened posterior capsule, similar to that in **A** (*arrow*). **D,** Axial T1-weighted MR arthrogram in the same patient as in **C**. Note the superior labrum anterior posterior (SLAP) type 2 tear of the superior labrum (*arrows*).

of tendon involvement. Treatment may vary from debridement of frayed tissue in more superficial partial tears, to completely excising the area of the partial defect and repairing the defect as if it were a small full-thickness defect. Repairs of high-grade partial- or full-thickness tears are either a side-to-side or tendon-to-bone repair and may be accompanied by decompression. This may be done arthroscopically, open, or with a combined approach.

MRI Findings

MRI findings following cuff repair (Fig. 99-78) include distortion of the soft-tissues adjacent to the cuff and nonvisualization of the subdeltoid fat/bursa and fluid in the region of the subdeltoid bursa. Soft-tissue metal or suture artifacts occur due to nonabsorbable sutures and suture anchors, especially if ferromagnetic suture anchors are used. Granulation tissue surrounding sutures may result in intermediate or high signal on images with T2 contrast in the peritendinous tissues. A surgical trough in the humeral head is present with tendon-to-bone repairs. Intermediate signal within the rotator cuff substance may be present due to granulation tissue. Mild superior subluxation of the humeral head may occur due to capsular tightening, scarring, cuff atrophy, or bursectomy. Mild marrow edema in the humeral head may be seen.[397,400,403,405]

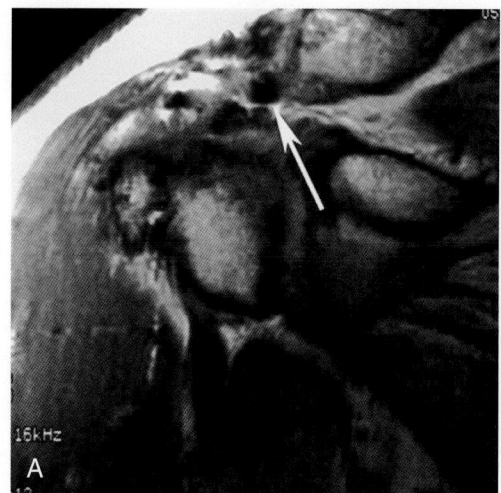

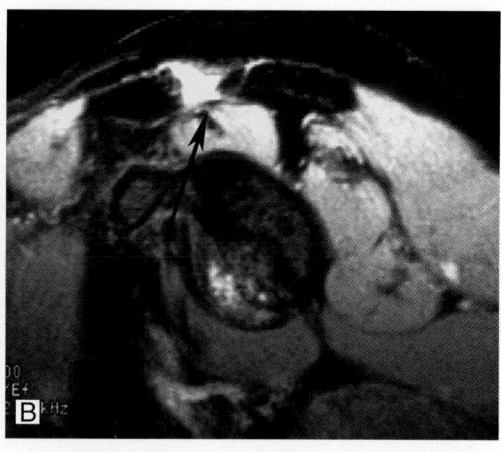

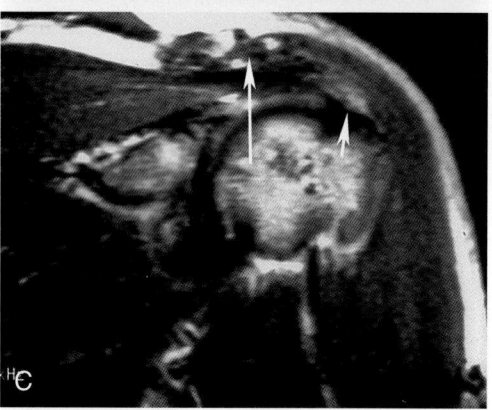

FIGURE 99-76

Status post acromioplasty, distal clavicle excision. **A,** Coronal oblique proton-density–weighted image. The anterior portion of the acromion has been removed (*arrow*). Also note the low signal post-surgical artifact. **B,** Sagittal oblique proton-density–weighted image. The extent of the decompression is often best seen in this position. The anterior acromion, acromioclavicular joint, and distal clavicle have been excised (*arrow*). **C,** Coronal T2-weighted image. Increased signal or fluid is often identified in the subdeltoid bursal region post decompression, due to accompanying resection or debridement of the bursa. The bursal surface of the tendon is thin, likely post debridement (*short arrow*). There has been an acromioplasty and distal clavicle excision (*long arrow*).

Fluid signal on T2-weighted images seen within a recurrent rotator cuff tendon defect or nonvisualization of a portion of the cuff are the more reliable indicators of full-thickness tears in the postoperative patient, with complete absence of the tendon the most specific finding. In the postoperative situation there may be a higher incidence of low signal tears due to chronic granulation tissue. Secondary signs such as muscle atrophy and tendon retraction may be helpful (Fig. 99-79). MR arthrography can document leakage of contrast through a cuff defect directly, and the cuff tissues and tendon edges may be better delineated with this technique (Fig. 99-80). The location of the musculotendinous junction is not a reliable sign after surgery because its position may change if the cuff is mobilized during surgery.[397,400,403,405]

The criteria for a recurrent partial tear is fluid signal on images with T2-weighted contrast replacing a portion of the tendon. Small recurrent full-thickness tears may be underestimated as partial tears. MR arthrography may help to resolve these difficulties.[397,400,403,405]

Deltoid Detachment

Postoperative detachment of the deltoid from its insertion to the acromion may occur. On MRI images, the presence of deltoid detachment can be identified by retraction of the deltoid from the acromion with fluid filling the defect.[397,406,407] If the detachment is chronic, atrophy will be present.

Biceps Tendon Rupture

MRI is accurate in the diagnosis of biceps tendon rupture in patients after surgery. This is diagnosed by lack of visualization of the biceps tendon in the intertubercular groove.

Shoulder Instability

Surgical Approach

The surgical treatment of patients with anterior instability has involved different approaches. Most commonly a direct repair of the labral and capsular lesions is done, usually a Bankart-type repair, or less commonly staple capsulorraphy. Other types of repair are those that tighten the capsule indirectly, usually through manipulation of the subscapularis, most commonly the Putti Platt or Magnusson-Stack procedure, and those that involve movement of the coracoid process, most commonly the Bristow procedure.

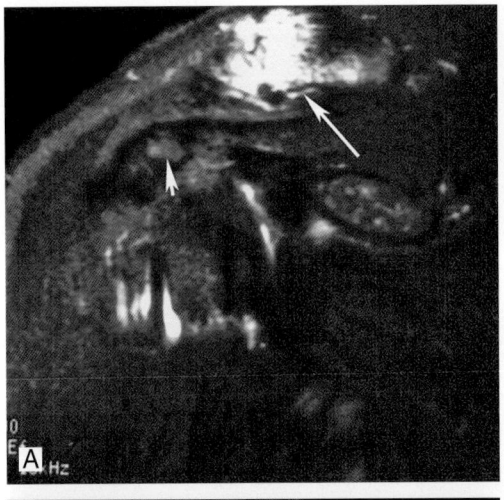
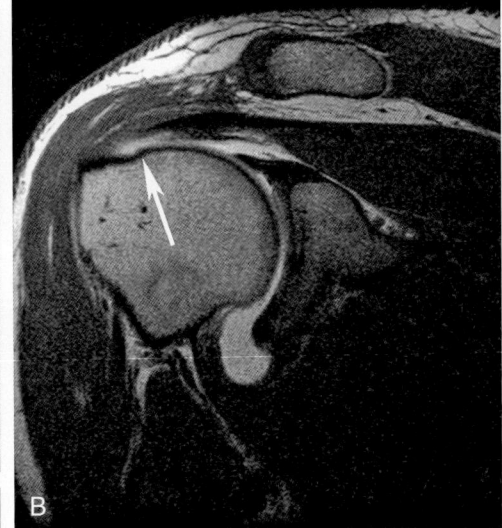
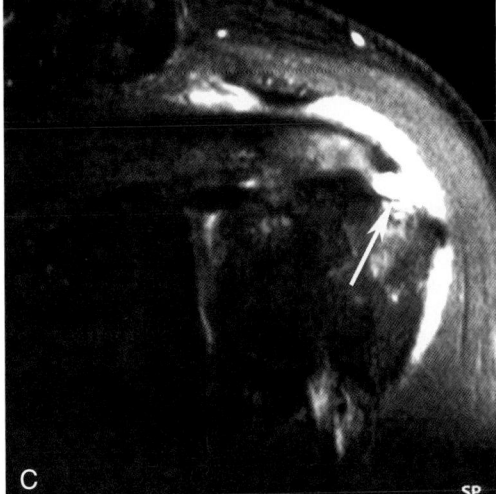

FIGURE 99-77

Postacromioplasty pain. **A,** Coronal oblique T2-weighted fast spin-echo sequence with fat saturation. There is persistent acromioclavicular joint arthritis with marginal edema (*long arrow*). A small undersurface partial tear is also seen (*short arrow*). **B,** Coronal oblique T1-weighted MR arthrogram. The patient has had an acromioplasty. There is an intermediate-grade undersurface partial thickness tear (*arrow*). **C,** Coronal oblique, fast inversion-recovery sequence in another patient. The patient has had an anterior acromioplasty. There has been interval development of a full-thickness tear of the supraspinatus tendon, anterodistally (*arrow*).

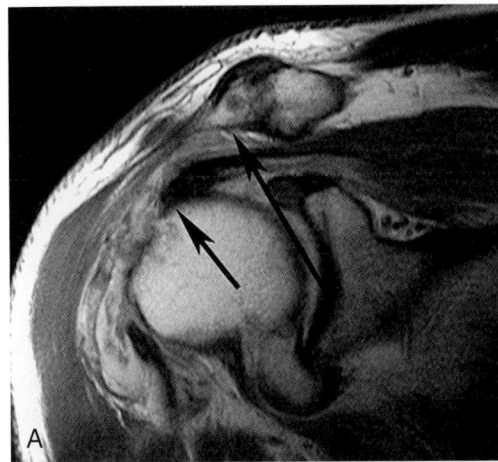
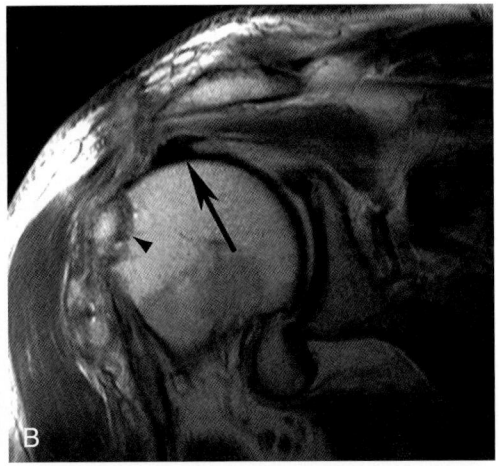

FIGURE 99-78

Postoperative shoulder. Rotator cuff repair. **A** and **B,** Coronal oblique proton-density–weighted images. There has been a tendon-to-bone repair (*short arrows*). Note the bone trough for the sutures (*arrowhead* in **B**). There has been an acromioplasty (*long arrow* in **A**).

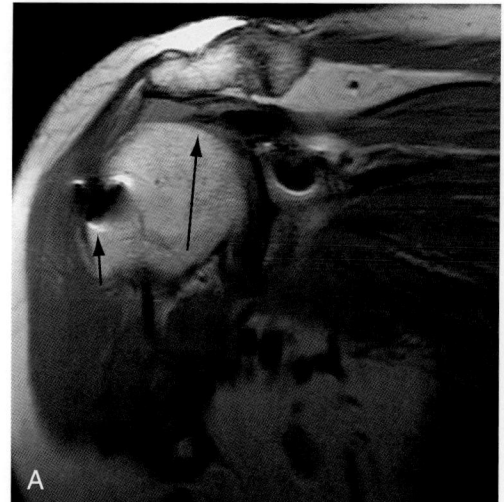

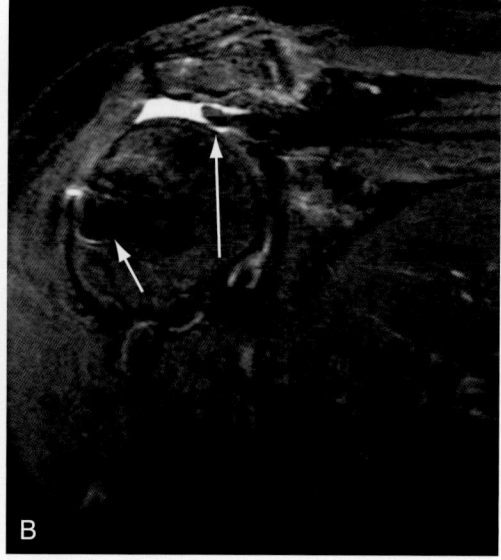

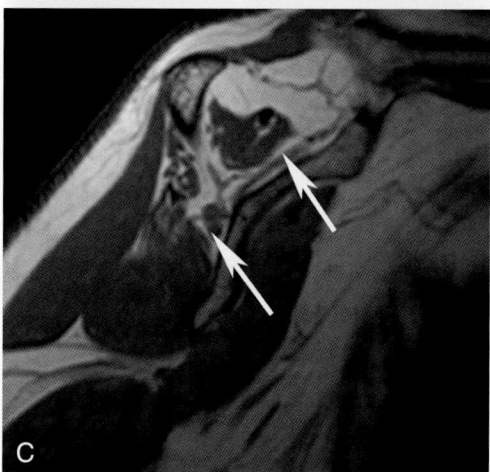

FIGURE 99-79

Recurrent rotator cuff tear. Coronal oblique **A,** proton-density– and **B,** T2-weighted fast spin-echo sequence with fat saturation. There is a recurrent full-thickness tear (*long arrows*). The tendon is retracted medially with thin edges. Note the site of repair (*short arrows*). There is persistent subacromial spur formation and acromoclavicular joint osteoarthritis. **C,** Sagittal oblique T1-weighted images. Note the muscle atrophy and fat infiltration (*arrows*).

FIGURE 99-80

Coronal oblique T1-weighted MR arthrogram. A moderate size recurrent tear of the supraspinatus tendon is identified (*arrow*). Depiction of the tear size and status of the tendon edges is aided by MR arthrography.

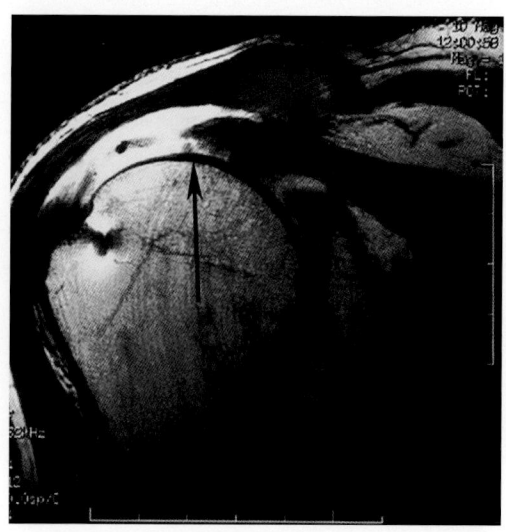

Normal Postoperative MRI Findings

The artifacts from surgery impair visualization, including metal and suture artifacts, especially screw fixation of the coracoid in the Bristow procedure, or the placement of suture anchors, staples, or tacks. Scarring from the incisions as well as suture repair may impair visualization. In Bankart repairs (Fig. 99-81) even nonferromagnetic suture anchors may be apparent within the glenoid neck. If transglenoid sutures are placed, channels will be seen traversing the glenoid neck and scapula. In addition the suture knot placed posteriorly, i.e., tied over fascia, may show some surrounding intermediate or high signal on images with T2-type contrast due to hyperemic granulation tissue. In patients with anatomic repairs, such as the Bankart repair, there should be an anatomic position and morphology of the labrum and capsule post repair. In procedures that do not directly repair the labral and capsular lesions, as noted earlier, the abnormality from these lesions remains.[396,397,408]

Recurrent Lesions

Causes of recurrent instability (Fig. 99-82) include inadequate or incorrect procedures and the uncovering of missed anterior or posterior instability with isolated treatment of one. An overtight repair can lead either to degenerative change or may precipitate instability in the other direction. This may be more common in procedures such as the Putti Platt or Magnusson-Stack, which may also result in loss of external rotation. Inferior

capsular shifts or other types of capsular plications can also be overtightened. Signs of an overtightened inferior capsular shift include loss of the axillary pouch and subtle posterior subluxation of the humeral head relative to the glenoid. Degenerative arthritis may also occur if there is persistent instability from inadequate repair. Misplaced or detached staples, tacks or anchors (Fig. 99-83) from labral and capsular repairs or misplaced screws or coracoid nonunion in a Bristow procedure may also cause joint derangement. If left unrecognized it may lead to degenerative changes as well.

In patients after repair of the labrum and capsule the postoperative labrum may be thickened and irregular due to scar tissue or suture material, but should not be detached. Signal alterations may be present post-operatively and high signal on images with T2 contrast may be present in the earlier postoperative periods due to hyperemic granulation tissue.[399] As such, outlining the labrum and capsule with intra-articular contrast is the best means of discerning recurrent tears and detachments, by outlining any surface irregularities and revealing any contrast extension into or beneath the labrum.[401,409] Failed Bankart repairs may show persistence or recurrence of the detached labrum and capsule. This may occur due to breakdown of the fixation from suture breakage, anchor device pullout, or failure of the reapproximated labral and capsular tissues. The repaired labrum may also become blunted, attenuated, or fragmented.

Postoperatively the joint capsule may appear thickened and nodular. Measurements of capsular thickening have been described for adhesive capsulitis,[410] and can be measured best in the axillary recess on MR

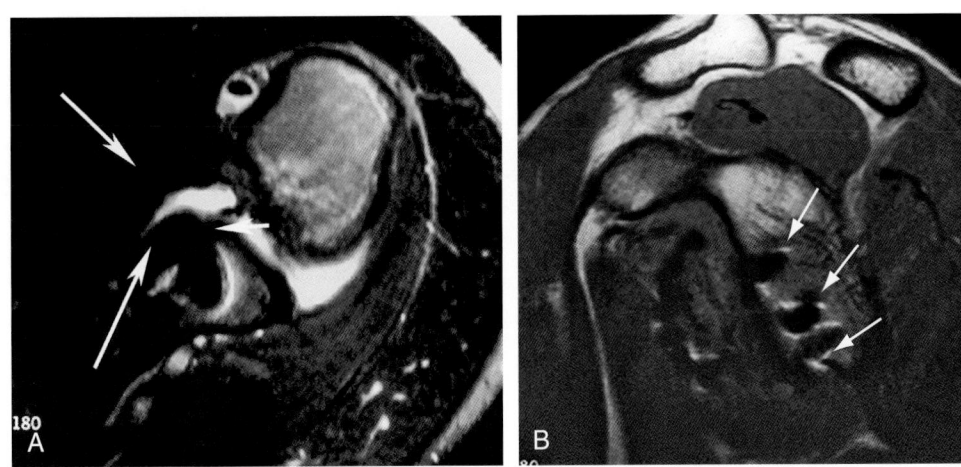

FIGURE 99-81

Post Bankart repair. **A,** Axial turbo spin-echo T2-weighted image. Note the artifact from the suture anchor in the anterior inferior glenoid (*short arrow*). Low signal from scarring of the labroligamentous tissue is noted after surgery (*long arrows*). **B,** Sagittal oblique fast spin-echo proton-density–weighted image in another patient. Post-surgical artifact outlines the sites of fixation in the anterior glenoid (*arrows*).

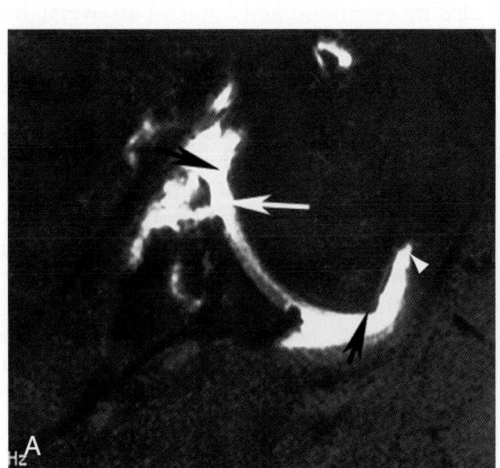 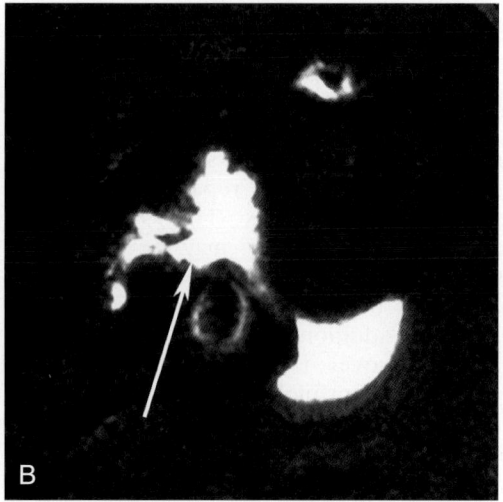

FIGURE 99-82

Post Bankart repair. Recurrent lesion. **A** and **B,** MR arthrogram. Axial T1-weighted images with fat suppression (**B** is inferior to **A**). The anterior inferior labrum is detached (*white arrow* in **A**). Note is also made of early glenohumeral joint degenerative change. Note the small osteophytes projecting from the humeral head in **A** (*black arrows*). There is bone loss along the inferior glenoid (*arrow* in **B**). A Hill-Sachs lesion is present (*arrowhead* in **A**).

arthrography as a band of low signal adjacent to the hyperintense signal of contrast medially, and the hyperintense signal of the fat stripe laterally on T1-weighted images. A measurement of 4 mm indicates adhesive capsulitis and one of 2 to 4 mm is considered consistent with the thickening expected after Bankart repair. The glenohumeral ligaments may also appear thickened and nodular post repair. In patients with recurrent instability the repaired capsule may become stretched and redundant. These changes are best identified by MR arthrography. Rand[401] indicates that an anterior capsular width/posterior capsular width ratio of less than 1 on MR arthrography may predict a good outcome post surgery, particularly if a capsulorraphy, open or arthroscopic, has been done. The glenohumeral ligaments, if abnormal, may appear thin, elongated, irregular, and discontinuous.

OTHER DISORDERS

Occult Fractures

Occult fractures of the proximal humerus often involve the greater tuberosity and occur as a result of injuries such as seizures, glenohumeral dislocations, and forced abduction. Mason et al[170] described the MRI findings of occult greater tuberosity fractures in 12 patients in whom plain films failed to demonstrate minimally displaced fractures. All patients had partial tears or tendinosis of the rotator cuff, but none had full thickness tears. These authors postulate that the presence of a fracture precludes a full-thickness tear of the cuff. Conversely, Zanneti et al[411] found nondisplaced greater tuberosity fractures in 9 of 24 patients following acute

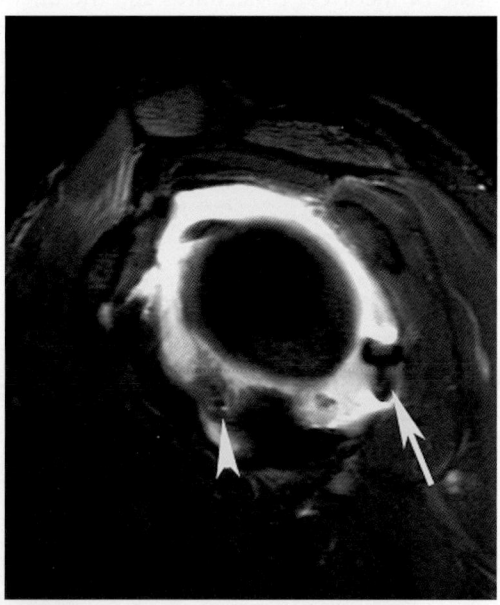

FIGURE 99-83

Displaced anchor. Sagittal oblique T1-weighted MR arthrogram with fat suppression. Note the displaced suture anchor (*arrow*) from a prior Bankart repair (*arrowhead*) in the posterior inferior joint recess.

substantial trauma to the shoulder associated with complete tears of the supraspinatus, infraspinatus, and subscapularis tendons.[411]

MRI demonstrates the fracture line as a low signal irregular area surrounded by bone marrow edema (Fig. 99-84). Clinically, these patients present with symptoms that simulate rotator cuff tears.

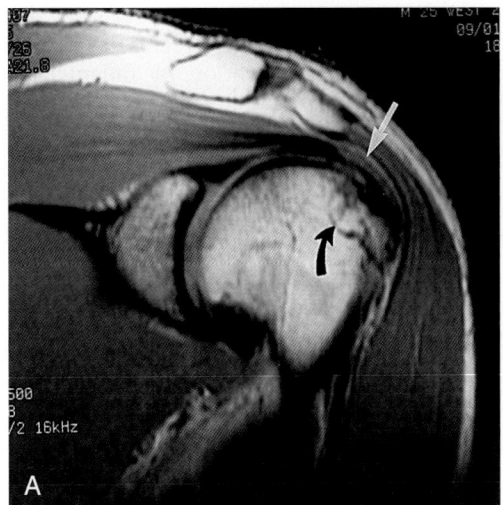
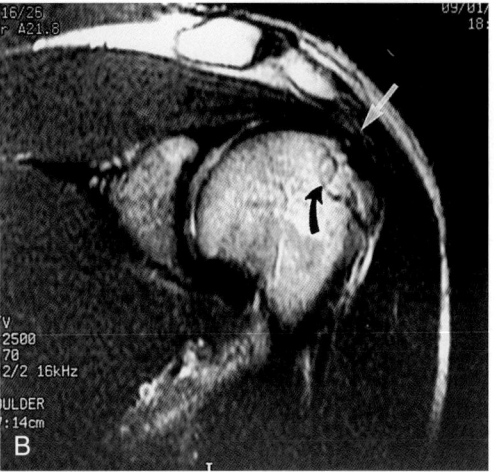

FIGURE 99-84

Occult greater tuberosity fracture. **A,** Coronal oblique proton-density image and **B,** T2-weighted image. A linear region of low signal represents the fracture line (*curved black arrows*). There is adjacent marrow edema. There is evidence of injury (strain or contusion) to the cuff and fluid in the bursa (*white arrows*), but no cuff tear.

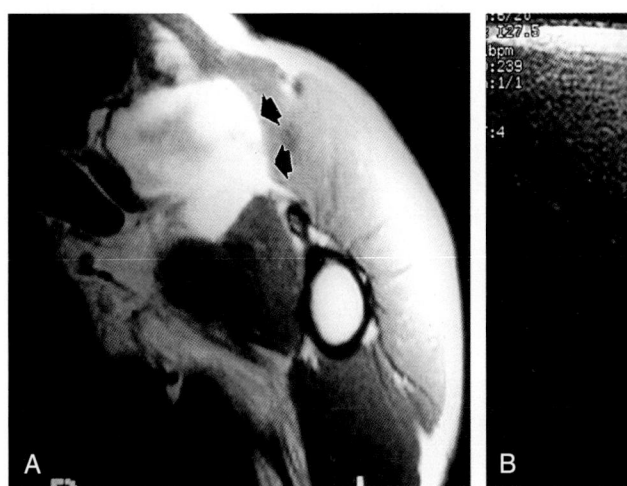
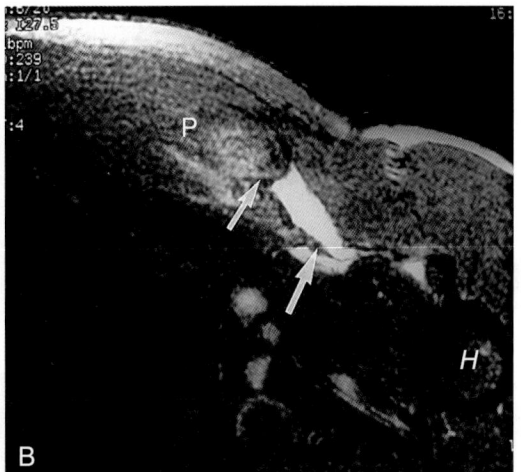

FIGURE 99-85

Pectoralis major rupture. **A,** Axial T1-weighted image. In the acute phase the muscle rupture is manifested by and obscured by a focal hematoma. Note the high signal mass (*arrows*). **B,** Axial T2-weighted fast spin-echo image with fat saturation. The retracted torn pectoralis muscle and tendon are now evident (*arrows*). H, humerus; P, pectoralis major muscle.

Muscle Injuries

Muscle contusions, hematomas, and ruptures may involve the muscles of the shoulder girdle, not only the rotator cuff muscles such as the subscapularis, but also the surrounding musculature such as the deltoid, trapezius, or pectoralis muscles.[412-414] Muscle hematomas may have high signal intensity on both T1- and T2-weighted images (Fig. 99-85). Complete rupture of the muscles of the shoulder girdle such as the deltoid, pectoralis, or triceps are relatively uncommon lesions.

Evaluation of pectoralis major ruptures with MRI (Fig. 99-85) has been described.[415-418] This occurs most commonly in weightlifters. Fat-saturated T2-weighted fast spin-echo sequences in the axial plane with surface coils are the most useful in diagnosing this lesion and its extent. Surgical repair of these lesions is difficult but it is likely that MRI can be very helpful if surgery is contemplated, to assess the extent, type, and pattern of rupture, and determine the status of the torn muscle and tendon edges.

Inflammatory and Degenerative Joint Processes

Many forms of inflammatory and degenerative joint processes involve the shoulder. These include rheumatoid arthritis, ankylosing spondylitis, other seronegative spondyloarthropathies, and degenerative arthritis.[419-423] Involvement of the shoulder is not uncommon in rheumatoid arthritis and its variants, particularly in long-standing disease. Osseous erosions occur predominantly on the humeral side of the joint. The acromioclavicular joint is also often involved.[197] Inflammatory arthritis may also affect the surrounding bursae, muscles, and rotator cuff tendons.[388,424,425] Although loss of articular cartilage and osseous erosions may be observed with conventional radiography, they may be visualized at an earlier stage with MRI and their extent may be better assessed. Soft-tissue changes, including rotator cuff atrophy and tears, inflammation of the subacromial bursa, ruptures of the biceps tendon, and synovial cysts can also be identified with MRI.[419,421,425,426] MRI can be used to follow patients to assess the response to medical therapy. Intravenous gadolinium injection is useful in differentiating a joint effusion from acutely inflamed synovium (Fig. 99-86).[426]

In septic arthritis MRI may be particularly useful in establishing an early diagnosis and determining the extent of the disease. This is important as septic arthritis in the shoulder in adults rarely responds well to treatment. Early joint aspiration still needs to be performed for definitive diagnosis and to obtain fluid for culture. Tears of the rotator cuff may be associated with septic

arthritis of the shoulder and can be documented on MR images. This is likely related to erosion of the inferior aspect of the tendon by inflamed synovium. The presence of a cuff tear may be more responsible for a poor functional result after treatment than damage to the articular cartilage. MRI may also be helpful in documenting extra-articular spread of infection, such as cavities that may communicate with the joint space. When osteomyelitis develops, MRI[407] will show marrow edema on short TR/TE, fast spin-echo T2-weighted images with fat suppression, or STIR images.

Degenerative arthritis in the absence of prior trauma, or an underlying systemic disorder, is uncommon in the shoulder (see Fig. 99-86). Changes observed include joint space narrowing, sclerosis of the subchondral bone and cyst formation that involves the glenoid and humeral head. Osteophytes may be seen at the circumference of the glenoid fossa, along the inferior aspect of the humeral head and adjacent to the bicipital groove. MRI is rarely required to assess patients for this clinical problem alone, but may on occasion be found on imaging patients with shoulder pain suspected of other disorders. Degenerative joint disease of the acromioclavicular joint is very common, particularly in older patients. It may contribute to rotator cuff disease and shoulder impingement, but may also be a source of shoulder pain. Ganglion cysts may develop in relation to this joint.

Other synovial processes, such as pigmented villonodular synovitis (PVNS) or synovial osteochondromatosis, may be visualized with MRI. The shoulder is the fourth most common site of involvement of PVNS, but is still a rare site of involvement.[427,428] On MRI, nodules and villous projections of synovium which

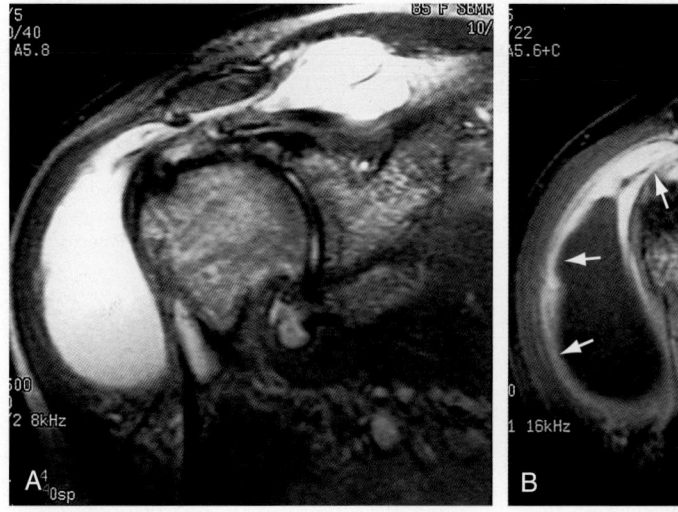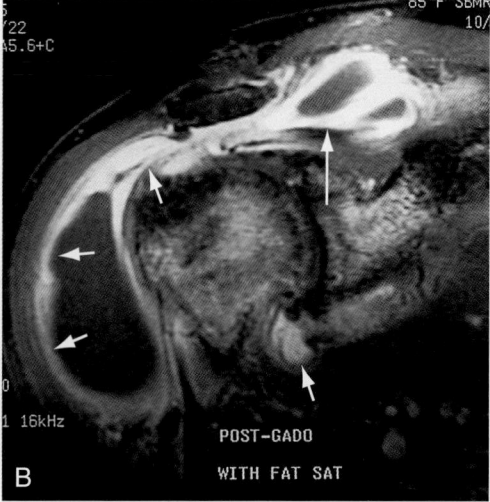

FIGURE 99-86

Osteoarthritis. Intravenous gadolinium, synovitis. **A,** Coronal oblique T2-weighted image. Severe joint space narrowing, subchondral sclerosis, and osteophytes are present. There is a massive subdeltoid bursal effusion. **B,** Coronal oblique T1-weighted image after intravenous gadolinium injection with fat saturation. Areas of enhancement in the joint and bursa represent acutely inflamed synovium superimposed on the degenerative process (*arrows*).

contain hemosiderin are seen as areas of intermediate signal intensity on all pulse sequences. There is usually a large joint effusion and periarticular cysts may develop. Cystic erosions may be evident as well-defined areas of low signal intensity on short TR/TE images and increased signal intensity on long TR/TE images. Hemosiderin deposition is more apparent on gradient-echo sequences because of increased susceptibility effects.

Idiopathic synovial osteochondromatosis (SOC) is a chronic, progressive, monoarticular disorder caused by metaplasia of the synovial membrane, with the formation of numerous cartilaginous intra-articular nodules. Shoulder involvement is less common than that of the hip and knee.[429] MRI can be helpful in verifying the diagnosis and can demonstrate the nodules, even if these are not calcified.[430-432] Calcified nodules appear as areas of low intensity on short TR/TE, proton-density–weighted, and long TR/TE images (Fig. 99-87). Nodules that do not calcify should have a high signal on long TR/TE images due to the abundant water content of hyaline cartilage, with interspersed areas of low signal due to fibrous tissue between the cartilage nodules. The surrounding tissue may include areas of inflamed and/or hyperplastic synovium and reactive fluid.

Osteocartilaginous loose bodies are usually fragments of bone and cartilage that may be sheared off the glenoid or humeral head, often secondary to osteochondral fractures. Other causes of loose bodies include osteo-arthritis and neuropathic disease. Osteocartilaginous loose bodies may occur in the joint of patients with recurrent shoulder dislocations. These may result from Hill-Sachs lesions or may be fragments from fractures of the glenoid rim. Clinically, they may cause recurrent effusions, a locking or grating sensation, as well as a decreased range of motion. More commonly, they fall into the inferior capsular recess and do not produce any

significant problem. In general, MRI is not the procedure of choice to identify loose bodies. When encountered, densely calcified loose bodies on MRI appear as low signal intensity structures. When ossified they may be of high-to-intermediate signal with a low signal intensity rim due to the presence of mature marrow elements within. MRI arthrography may be helpful to outline some of these lesions by distending the joint and by improving overall contrast resolution.

Osteochondral Lesions

Osteochondral lesions of the shoulder are rare. Different names and descriptions have been used by different authors to describe a group of lesions that involve the articular surface of the glenoid fossa, including osteo-chondritis dissecans (OCD),[433] subchondral avascular necrosis,[434] juxta-articular bone cyst or post-traumatic subchondral cyst,[435] and glenoid articular rim divot (GARD).[370,371,436] These lesions may be related to acute trauma and are often associated with glenohumeral instability, labral tears, and intra-articular loose bodies (Fig. 99-88).[433] Cystic changes in the subchondral bone of the glenoid fossa are the most frequent feature. Occasionally, loose bodies are found. Careful attention to the articular surface of the glenoid may reveal the presence of a chondral or osteochondral defect.

The glenoid articular rim divot (GARD) has been described based on arthroscopic findings.[370,371] MRI examination in these patients may reveal the chondral defect as well as a cartilaginous loose fragment in a joint recess. A similar entity was reported by Chan et al[437] in which multiloculated subchondral cysts are present in the posterior superior quadrant of the glenoid fossa. These authors used the same acronym, GARD, to indicate

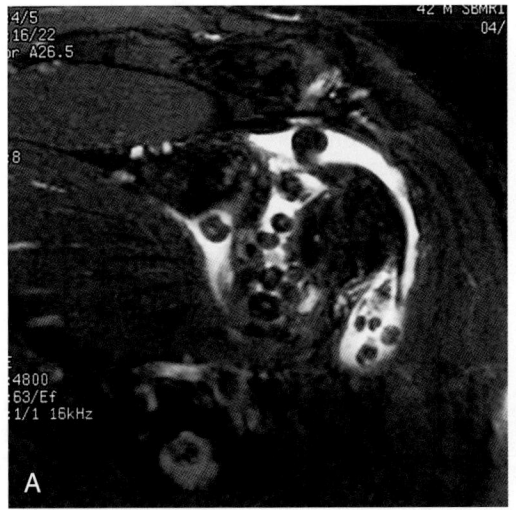
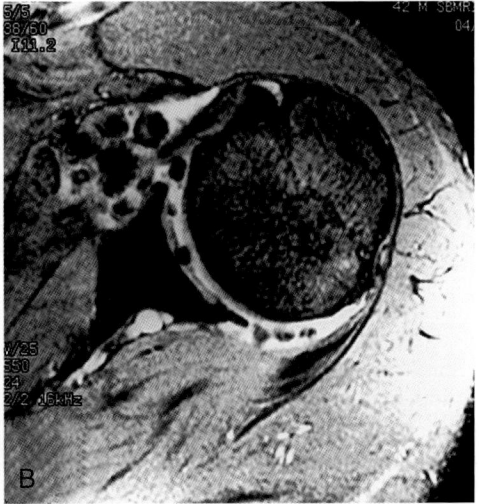

FIGURE 99-87

Synovial osteochondromatosis. **A,** Coronal oblique T2-weighted fast spin-echo image with fat saturation and **B,** axial gradient-echo image. Numerous small and large calcified nodules appear as areas of low signal intensity.

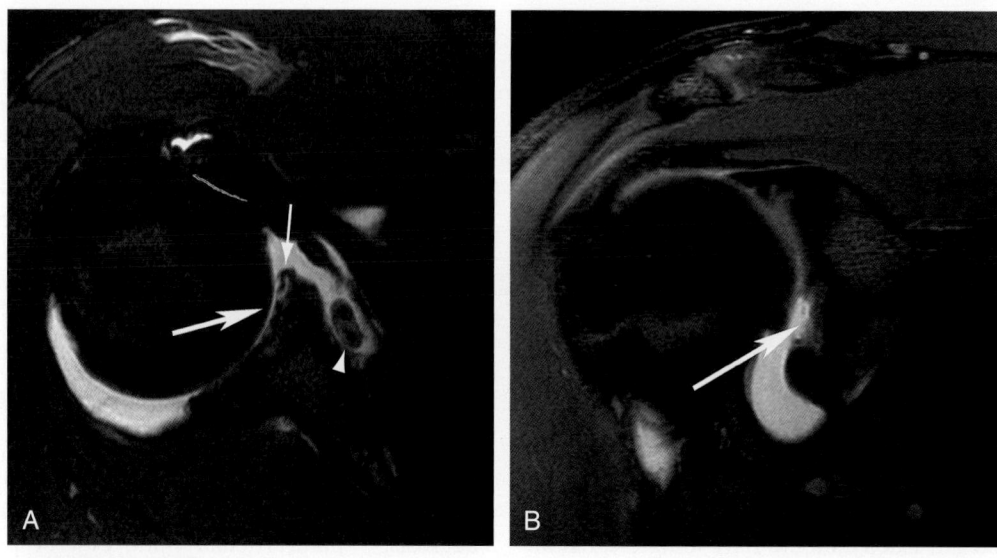

FIGURE 99-88

Osteochondral lesion (OCD). **A,** Axial and **B,** coronal oblique T2-weighted fast spin-echo MR arthrogram with fat saturation. Note the osteochondral lesion in the anterior inferior glenoid (*arrows*). There is a loose body in the subscapularis bursa (*arrowhead* in **A**). The labrum is blunted and torn (*thin white arrow* in **A**).

glenoid articular rim disruption. The specific location of these lesions is thought to be related to a developmentally weak area of the glenoid fossa at an area of junction between the ossification centers of the glenoid. These osteochondral lesions are often detected in the throwing athlete.

Avascular Necrosis

This entity results from a significant decrease or loss of the blood supply to the affected region. The most common cause is trauma. Other causes such as steroid use may be implicated. Avascular necrosis may occur in patients receiving high doses of corticosteroids, though it is only one third as common as femoral head avascular necrosis.[438,439] The vessels that supply the humeral head pierce the bony cortex just distal to the anatomic neck. Fractures proximal to this level, most commonly involving the anatomic neck, may result in ischemic necrosis of the humeral head (Fig. 99-89). The MRI findings in osteonecrosis of the shoulder appear as focal subarticular regions of decreased signal intensity (79%) or as a dark signal intensity band surrounding more normal marrow fat (21%).[440] A double line sign, similar to what has been described in the femoral head, may be seen (Fig. 99-89). Chronic osteonecrosis demonstrates an increase in dark fibrosis-like marrow signal, often complicated by fragmentation and collapse of the articular surface. Areas of infarction in the diaphyseal and metadiaphyseal are completely surrounded by a reactive interface and may have a more geographic or doughnut appearance.[440] There are central regions of

high signal intensity representing regions of isolated marrow fat, surrounded by bands of low signal intensity representing fibrosis and or calcification in subacute or chronic infarcts, or a subjacent band of high signal intensity representing reactive granulation tissue in more acute infarcts.

Quadrilateral Space Syndrome

Another entity whose diagnosis on MRI has been recently described is the quadrilateral space syndrome. This refers to impingement of the axillary nerve in the quadrilateral space. This is a space bounded by the teres minor muscle superiorly, the long head of triceps medially, the teres major inferiorly, and the surgical neck of the humerus laterally. The posterior humeral circumflex artery and axillary nerve course here and may be entrapped by fibrous bands in this region.

Proximal humeral and scapular fractures or axillary mass lesions can result in damage or compression of the axillary nerve. Injury to the nerve may also occur after anterior dislocation. Entrapment of this nerve can also be produced by extreme abduction of the arm during sleep, hypertrophy of the teres minor muscle in paraplegic patients, or by a fibrous band within the quadrilateral space.[441,442] In advanced cases, atrophy of the deltoid and teres minor muscles can occur. A paralabral cyst has been noted as a rare cause of quadrilateral space syndrome.[390]

The axillary nerve can be visualized on sagittal oblique MR images. Osseous lesions involving the axillary nerve may be better seen with plain film radiography or CT.

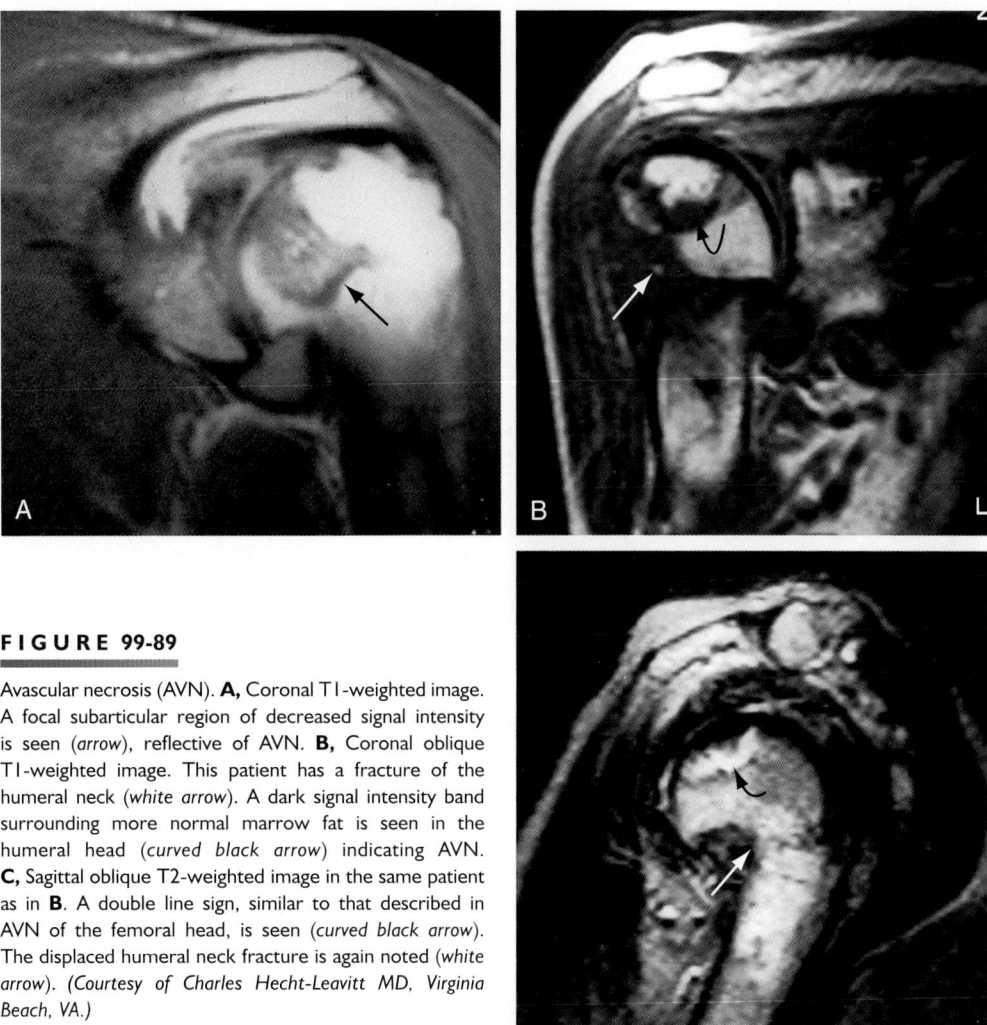

FIGURE 99-89

Avascular necrosis (AVN). **A,** Coronal T1-weighted image. A focal subarticular region of decreased signal intensity is seen (*arrow*), reflective of AVN. **B,** Coronal oblique T1-weighted image. This patient has a fracture of the humeral neck (*white arrow*). A dark signal intensity band surrounding more normal marrow fat is seen in the humeral head (*curved black arrow*) indicating AVN. **C,** Sagittal oblique T2-weighted image in the same patient as in **B**. A double line sign, similar to that described in AVN of the femoral head, is seen (*curved black arrow*). The displaced humeral neck fracture is again noted (*white arrow*). (*Courtesy of Charles Hecht-Leavitt MD, Virginia Beach, VA.*)

Soft-tissue lesions can be detected with MRI. Selective atrophy or edema of the teres minor muscle and less commonly the deltoid caused by axillary nerve compression may be identified (Fig. 99-90).[443,444]

Parsonage-Turner Syndrome

Parsonage-Turner syndrome, also referred to as acute brachial neuritis, is characterized by the sudden onset of severe atraumatic pain in the shoulder girdle.[445] The pain typically decreases spontaneously in 1 to 3 weeks and is followed by weakness of at least one of the muscles about the shoulder. The exact etiology has not been established but viral and immunologic causes have been considered.

Originally the long thoracic nerve was thought to be most frequently compromised, but suprascapular nerve disease may be more common. The axillary, radial,

and phrenic nerves may also be affected as well as the entire brachial plexus. Bilateral involvement may be present.

MRI findings in the acute stage include diffuse increased signal intensity on T2-weighted images consistent with interstitial muscle edema associated with denervation (Fig. 99-91). The most commonly affected muscles are those innervated by the suprascapular nerve, including the supraspinatus and infraspinatus. The deltoid muscle can also be compromised in cases of axillary nerve involvement. Later in the course of the disease, muscle atrophy manifested by decreased muscle bulk may be visualized.[239,446]

This disorder can resemble a variety of other clinical diagnoses, but the most confusing differential diagnosis is compressive neuropathy of the suprascapular nerve.[447] MRI can exclude suprascapular nerve entrapment related to paralabral ganglions or other impinging mass lesions.[239,446,448] Rotator cuff pathology can also be readily excluded using MRI.

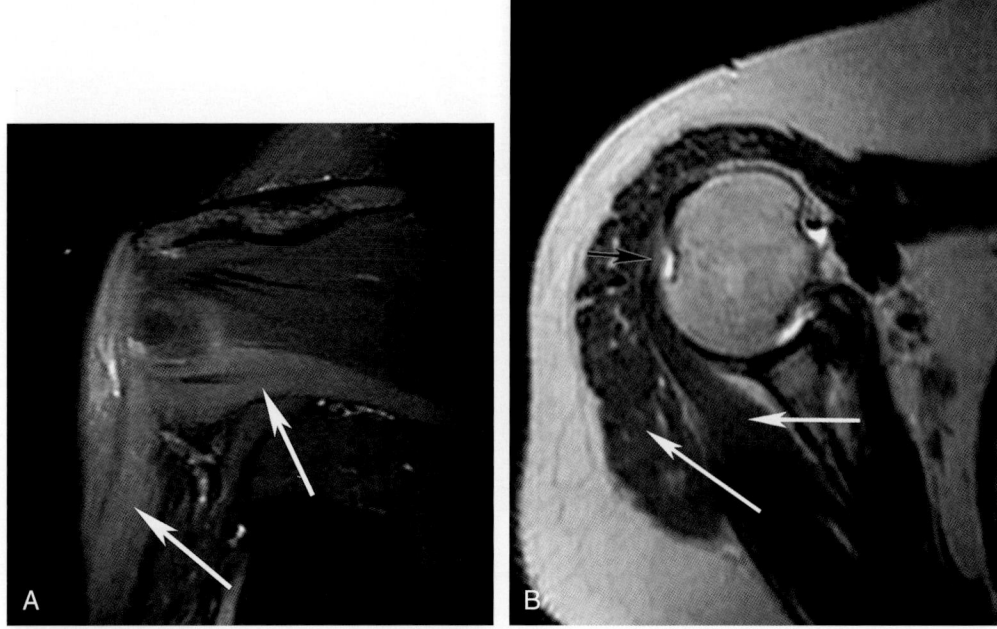

FIGURE 99-90

Quadrilateral space syndrome. **A,** Coronal short tau inversion recovery (STIR) and **B,** axial T2-weighted fast spin-echo images. Patient sustained an anterior dislocation. Note the Hill-Sachs lesion in **B** (*black arrow*). There is denervation edema in the deltoid and teres minor muscles (*white arrows*).

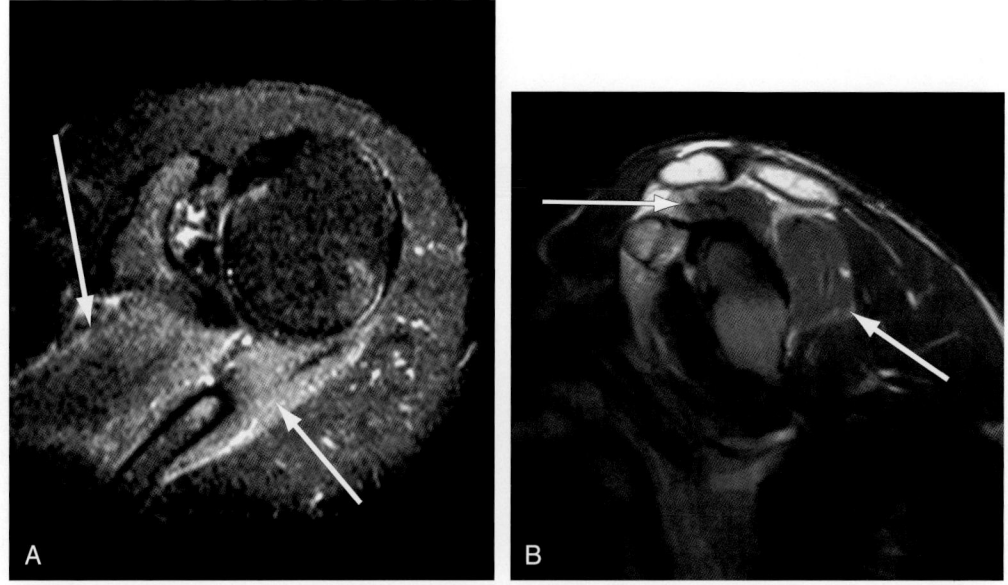

FIGURE 99-91

Parsonage Turner syndrome. **A,** Axial short tau inversion recovery (STIR) and **B,** sagittal oblique T2-weighted images. Increased signal intensity consistent with interstitial muscle edema associated with denervation is seen in the supraspinatus and infraspinatus muscles (*arrows*).

REFERENCES

1. Zlatkin MB: Techniques for MR imaging of joints in sports medicine. Magn Reson Imaging Clin North Am 7:1-21, vii, 1999.
2. Sahin-Akyar G, Miller TT, Staron RB, et al: Gradient-echo versus fat-suppressed fast spin-echo MR imaging of rotator cuff tears. Am J Roentgenol 171:223-227, 1998.
3. Needell SD, Zlatkin MB: Comparison of fat-saturation fast spin echo versus conventional spin-echo MRI in the detection of rotator cuff pathology. J Magn Reson Imaging 7:674-677, 1997.
4. Carrino JA, McCauley TR, Katz LD, et al: Rotator cuff: evaluation with fast spin-echo versus conventional spin-echo MR imaging. Radiology 202:533-539, 1997.
5. Gusmer PB, Potter HG, Schatz JA, et al: Labral injuries: accuracy of detection with unenhanced MR imaging of the shoulder. Radiology 200:519-524, 1996.
6. Singson RD, Hoang T, Dan S, Friedman M: MR evaluation of rotator cuff pathology using T2-weighted fast spin-echo technique with and without fat suppression. Am J Roentgenol 166:1061-1065, 1996.
7. Parsa M, Tuite M, Norris M, Orwin J: MR imaging of rotator cuff tendon tears: comparison of T2*-weighted gradient-echo and conventional dual-echo sequences. Am J Roentgenol 168:1519-1524, 1997.
8. Tuite MJ, Yandow DR, DeSmet AA, et al: Diagnosis of partial and complete rotator cuff tears using combined gradient echo and spin-echo imaging. Skeletal Radiol 23:541-545, 1994.
9. Resendes M, Helms CA, Eddy R, Knox K: Double-echo MPGR imaging of the rotator cuff. J Comput Assist Tomogr 15:1077-1079, 1991.
10. Shellock FG: Functional assessment of the joints using kinematic magnetic resonance imaging. Semin Musculoskelet Radiol 7:249-276, 2003.
11. Tokuda O, Kunihiro Y, Matsunaga N: Kinematic MRI of the normal shoulder using a specially designed positioning device. J Comput Assist Tomogr 26:849-854, 2002.
12. Sans N, Richardi G, Railhac JJ, et al: Kinematic MR imaging of the shoulder: normal patterns. Am J Roentgenol 167:1517-1522, 1996.
13. Boden BP, Hanks GA, Chesnick RM: Diagnosis of biceps tendon dislocation by kinematic magnetic resonance imaging. J Am Orthop 25:709-711, 1996.
14. Cardinal E, Buckwalter KA, Braunstein EM: Kinematic magnetic resonance imaging of the normal shoulder: assessment of the labrum and capsule. Can Assoc Radiol J 47:44-50, 1996.
15. Bonutti PM, Norfray JF, Friedman RJ, Genez BM: Kinematic MRI of the shoulder. J Comput Assist Tomogr 17:666-669, 1993.
16. Patten RM: Vacuum phenomenon: a potential pitfall in the interpretation of gradient-recalled-echo MR images of the shoulder. Am J Roentgenol 162:1383-1386, 1994.
17. Mirowitz SA: Normal rotator cuff: MR imaging with conventional and fat-suppression techniques. Radiology 180:735-740, 1991.
18. Foo TK, Shellock FG, Hayes CE, et al: High-resolution MR imaging of the wrist and eye with short TR, short TE, and partial-echo acquisition. Radiology 183:277-281, 1992.
19. Meister K, Thesing J, Montgomery WJ, et al: MR arthrography of partial thickness tears of the undersurface of the rotator cuff: an arthroscopic correlation. Skeletal Radiol 33:136-141, 2004.
20. Kreitner KF, Loew R, Runkel M, et al: Low-field MR arthrography of the shoulder joint: technique, indications, and clinical results. Eur Radiol 13:320-329, 2003.
21. Schulte-Altedorneburg G, Gebhard M, Wohlgemuth WA, et al. MR arthrography: pharmacology, efficacy and safety in clinical trials. Skeletal Radiol 32:1-12, 2003.
22. Parmar H, Jhankaria B, Maheshwari M, et al: Magnetic resonance arthrography in recurrent anterior shoulder instability as compared to arthroscopy: a prospective comparative study. J Postgrad Med 48:270-273, discussion 273-274, 2002.
23. Steinbach LS, Palmer WE, Schweitzer ME: Special focus session. MR arthrography. RadioGraphics 22:1223-1246, 2002.
24. Loew R, Kreitner KF, Runkel M, et al: MR arthrography of the shoulder: comparison of low-field (0.2 T) vs high-field (1.5 T) imaging. Eur Radiol 10:989-996, 2000.
25. Zanetti M, Jost B, Lustenberger A, Hodler J: Clinical impact of MR arthrography of the shoulder. Acta Radiol 40:296-302, 1999.
26. Shuman WP: Gadolinium MR arthrography of the rotator cuff. Semin Musculoskelet Radiol 2:377-384, 1998.
27. Beltran J, Bencardino J, Mellado J, et al: MR arthrography of the shoulder: variants and pitfalls. RadioGraphics 17:1403-1412, discussion 1412-1405, 1997.
28. Petersilge CA, Lewin JS, Duerk JL, Hatem SF: MR arthrography of the shoulder: rethinking traditional imaging procedures to meet the technical requirements of MR imaging guidance. Am J Roentgenol 169:1453-1457, 1997.
29. Tirman PF, Palmer WE, Feller JF: MR arthrography of the shoulder. Magn Reson Imaging Clin North Am 5:811-839, 1997.
30. Palmer WE: MR arthrography: is it worthwhile? Top Magn Reson Imaging 8:24-43, 1996.
31. Kopka L, Funke M, Fischer U, et al: MR arthrography of the shoulder with gadopentetate dimeglumine: influence of concentration, iodinated contrast material, and time on signal intensity. Am J Roentgenol 163:621-623, 1994.
32. Palmer WE, Brown JH, Rosenthal DI: Rotator cuff: evaluation with fat-suppressed MR arthrography. Radiology 188:683-687, 1993.
33. Tirman PF, Stauffer AE, Crues JV, 3rd, et al: Saline magnetic resonance arthrography in the evaluation of glenohumeral instability. Arthroscopy 9:550-559, 1993.
34. Fritz RC, Stoller DW: Fat-suppression MR arthrography of the shoulder. Radiology 185:614-615, 1992.
35. Flannigan B, Kursunoglu-Brahme S, Snyder S, et al: MR arthrography of the shoulder: comparison with conventional MR imaging. Am J Roentgenol 155:829-832, 1990.
36. Funke M, Kopka L, Vosshenrich R, et al: MR arthrography in the diagnosis of rotator cuff tears. Standard spin-echo alone or with fat suppression? Acta Radiol 37:627-632, 1996.
37. Lee SY, Lee JK: Horizontal component of partial-thickness tears of rotator cuff: imaging characteristics and comparison of ABER view with oblique coronal view at MR arthrography initial results. Radiology 224:470-476, 2002.
38. Halbrecht JL, Tirman P, Atkin D: Internal impingement of the shoulder: comparison of findings between the throwing and nonthrowing shoulders of college baseball players. Arthroscopy 15:253-258, 1999.
39. Tirman PF, Bost FW, Steinbach LS, et al: MR arthrographic depiction of tears of the rotator cuff: benefit of abduction and external rotation of the arm. Radiology 192:851-856, 1994.
40. Bergin D, Schweitzer ME: Indirect magnetic resonance arthrography. Skeletal Radiol 32:551-558, 2003.
41. Vahlensieck M, Lang P, Sommer T, et al: Indirect MR arthrography: techniques and applications. Semin US CT MR 18:302-306, 1997.
42. Vahlensieck M, Peterfy CG, Wischer T, et al: Indirect MR arthrography: Optimization and clinical applications. Radiology 200:249-254, 1996.
43. Weishaupt D, Schweitzer M, Rawool N, et al: Indirect MR arthrography of the knee: effects of low-intensity ultrasound on the diffusion rate of intravenously administered Gd-DTPA in healthy volunteers. Invest Radiol 36:493-499, 2001.
44. Schweitzer ME, Natale P, Winalski CS, Culp R: Indirect wrist MT arthrography: The effects of passive motion versus active exercise. Skeletal Radiol 29:10-14, 2000.
45. Allmann K, Schafer O, Hauer M, et al: Indirect MR arthrography of the unexercised glenohumeral joint in patients with rotator cuff tears. Invest Radiol 34:435-440, 1999.
46. Wagner SC, Schweitzer ME, Morrison WB, et al: Shoulder instability: accuracy of MR imaging performed after surgery in depicting recurrent injury—initial findings. Radiology 222:196-203, 2002.
47. Yagci B, Manisali M, Yilmaz E, et al: Indirect MR arthrography of the shoulder in detection of rotator cuff ruptures. Eur Radiol 11:258-262, 2001.
48. Warwick RWP: Arthrology. In Gray's Anatomy, 35th ed. London, Churchill Livingstone, 1973, pp 424-429.
49. Carson WG, Jr: Arthroscopy of the shoulder: anatomy and technique. Orthop Rev 21:143-153, 1992.
50. Petersilge CA, Witte DH, Sewell BO, et al: Normal regional anatomy of the shoulder. Magn Reson Imaging Clin North Am 5:667-681, 1997.
51. Davidson PA, Elattrache NS, Jobe CM, Jobe FW: Rotator cuff and posterior-superior glenoid labrum injury associated with increased glenohumeral motion: a new site of impingement. J Shoulder Elbow Surg 4:384-390, 1995.
52. Matthews LS, Terry G, Vetter WL: Shoulder anatomy for the arthroscopist. Arthroscopy 1:83-91, 1985.
53. Hill JA, Tkach L, Hendrix RW: A study of glenohumeral orientation in patients with anterior recurrent shoulder dislocations using computerized axial tomography. Orthop Rev 18:84-91, 1989.
54. Saha AK: Dynamic stability of the glenohumeral joint. Acta Orthop Scand 42:491-505, 1971.
55. Andrews JR, Carson WG, Jr, McLeod WD: Glenoid labrum tears related to the long head of the biceps. Am J Sports Med 13:337-341, 1985.
56. Beltran J, Rosenberg ZS, Chandnani VP, et al: Glenohumeral instability: evaluation with MR arthrography. RadioGraphics 17:657-673, 1997.
57. Palmer WE: MR arthrography of the rotator cuff and labral-ligamentous complex. Semin Ultrasound CT MR 18:278-290, 1997.
58. Palmer WE, Caslowitz PL, Chew FS: MR arthrography of the shoulder: normal intraarticular structures and common abnormalities. Am J Roentgenol 164:141-146, 1995.
59. Rothman RH, Marvel JP, Jr, Heppenstall RB: Anatomic considerations in glenohumeral joint. Orthop Clin North Am 6:341-352, 1975.
60. Uhthoff HK, Piscopo M: Anterior capsular redundancy of the shoulder: congenital or traumatic? An embryological study. J Bone Joint Surg Br 67:363-366, 1985.
61. Palmer WE, Caslowitz PL: Anterior shoulder instability: diagnostic criteria determined from prospective analysis of 121 MR arthrograms. Radiology 197:819-825, 1995.
62. Ferrari FS, Governi S, Burresi F, et al: Supraspinatus tendon tears: comparison of US and MR arthrography with surgical correlation. Eur Radiol 12:1211-1217, 2002.
63. Coumas JM, Waite RJ, Goss TP, et al: CT and MR evaluation of the labral capsular ligamentous complex of the shoulder. Am J Roentgenol 158:591-597, 1992.
64. Ferrari DA: Capsular ligaments of the shoulder. Anatomical and functional study of the anterior superior capsule. Am J Sports Med 18:20-24, 1990.

65. Neer CS, 2nd, Satterlee CC, Dalsey RM, Flatow EL: The anatomy and potential effects of contracture of the coracohumeral ligament. Clin Orthop 182-185, 1992.

66. Steinbeck J, Liljenqvist U, Jerosch J: The anatomy of the glenohumeral ligamentous complex and its contribution to anterior shoulder stability. J Shoulder Elbow Surg 7:122-126, 1998.

67. Cooper DE, O'Brien SJ, Warren RF: Supporting layers of the glenohumeral joint. An anatomic study. Clin Orthop 144-155, 1993.

68. Clark JM, Harryman DT, 2nd: Tendons, ligaments, and capsule of the rotator cuff. Gross and microscopic anatomy. J Bone Joint Surg Am 74:713-725, 1992.

69. Depalma A: Surgery of the Shoulder. Philadelphia, Lippincott, 1983.

70. O'Brien SJ, Neves MC, Arnoczky SP, et al: The anatomy and histology of the inferior glenohumeral ligament complex of the shoulder. Am J Sports Med 18:449-456, 1990.

71. O'Brien SJ, Schwartz RS, Warren RF, Torzilli PA: Capsular restraints to anterior-posterior motion of the abducted shoulder: a biomechanical study. J Shoulder Elbow Surg 4:298-308, 1995.

72. Bencardino JT, Beltran J: MR imaging of the glenohumeral ligaments. Magn Reson Imaging Clin North Am 12:11-24, v, 2004.

73. Vahlensieck M, van Haack K, Schmidt HM: Two portions of the supraspinatus muscle: a new finding about the muscles macroscopy by dissection and magnetic resonance imaging. Surg Radiol Anat 16:101-104, 1994.

74. Totterman SM, Miller RJ, Meyers SP: Basic anatomy of the shoulder by magnetic resonance imaging. Top Magn Reson Imaging 6:86-93, 1994.

75. Patten RM: Tears of the anterior portion of the rotator cuff (the subscapularis tendon): MR imaging findings. Am J Roentgenol 162:351-354, 1994.

76. Ho CP: MR imaging of rotator interval, long biceps, and associated injuries in the overhead-throwing athlete. Magn Reson Imaging Clin North Am 7:23-37, 1999.

77. Cole BJ, Rodeo SA, O'Brien SJ, et al: The anatomy and histology of the rotator interval capsule of the shoulder. Clin Orthop Sep:129-137, 2001.

78. Chung CB, Dwek JR, Cho GJ, et al: Rotator cuff interval: evaluation with MR imaging and MR arthrography of the shoulder in 32 cadavers. J Comput Assist Tomogr 24:738-743, 2000.

79. Sakurai G, Ozaki J, Tomita Y, et al: Morphologic changes in long head of biceps brachii in rotator cuff dysfunction. J Orthop Sci 3:137-142, 1998.

80. Major NM: Imaging of the subcoracoid bursa. Am J Roentgenol 176:812-813, 2001.

81. Holt EM, Allibone RO: Anatomic variants of the coracoacromial ligament. J Shoulder Elbow Surg 4:370-375, 1995.

82. Fritz RC, Stoller DW: MR imaging of the rotator cuff. Magn Reson Imaging Clin North Am 5:735-754, 1997.

83. Bigliani LU, Levine WN: Subacromial impingement syndrome. J Bone Joint Surg Am 79:1854-1868, 1997.

84. Bigliani LU, Ticker JB, Flatow EL, et al: The relationship of acromial architecture to rotator cuff disease. Clin Sports Med 10:823-838, 1991.

85. Peh WC, Farmer TH, Totty WG: Acromial arch shape: assessment with MR imaging. Radiology 195:501-505, 1995.

86. Haygood TM, Langlotz CP, Kneeland JB, et al: Categorization of acromial shape: interobserver variability with MR imaging and conventional radiography. Am J Roentgenol 162:1377-1382, 1994.

87. Gohlke F, Barthel T, Gandorfer A: The influence of variations of the coracoacromial arch on the development of rotator cuff tears. Arch Orthop Trauma Surg 113:28-32, 1993.

88. Jost B, Koch PP, Gerber C: Anatomy and functional aspects of the rotator interval. J Shoulder Elbow Surg 9:336-341, 2000.

89. Erickson SJ, Fitzgerald SW, Quinn SF, et al: Long bicipital tendon of the shoulder: normal anatomy and pathologic findings on MR imaging. Am J Roentgenol 158:1091-1096, 1992.

90. Kieft GJ, Bloem JL, Obermann WR, et al: Normal shoulder: MR imaging. Radiology 159:741-745, 1986.

91. Seeger LL, Ruszkowski JT, Bassett LW, et al: MR imaging of the normal shoulder: anatomic correlation. Am J Roentgenol 148:83-91, 1987.

92. Neumann CH, Holt RG, Steinbach LS, et al: MR imaging of the shoulder: appearance of the supraspinatus tendon in asymptomatic volunteers. Am J Roentgenol 158:1281-1287, 1992.

93. Chandnani V, Ho C, Gerharter J, et al: MR findings in asymptomatic shoulders: a blind analysis using symptomatic shoulders as controls. Clin Imaging 16:25-30, 1992.

94. Kjellin I, Ho CP, Cervilla V, et al: Alterations in the supraspinatus tendon at MR imaging: correlation with histopathologic findings in cadavers. Radiology 181:837-841, 1991.

95. Davis SJ, Teresi LM, Bradley WG, et al: Effect of arm rotation on MR imaging of the rotator cuff. Radiology 181:265-268, 1991.

96. Rafii M, Firooznia H, Sherman O, et al: Rotator cuff lesions: signal patterns at MR imaging. Radiology 177:817-823, 1990.

97. Sher JS, Uribe JW, Posada A, et al: Abnormal findings on magnetic resonance images of asymptomatic shoulders. J Bone Joint Surg Am 77:10-15, 1995.

98. Erickson SJ, Cox IH, Hyde JS, et al: Effect of tendon orientation on MR imaging signal intensity: a manifestation of the "magic angle" phenomenon. Radiology 181:389-392, 1991.

99. Kaplan PA, Bryans KC, Davick JP, et al: MR imaging of the normal shoulder: variants and pitfalls. Radiology 184:519-524, 1992.

100. McNiesh LM, Callaghan JJ: CT arthrography of the shoulder: variations of the glenoid labrum. Am J Roentgenol 149:963-966, 1987.

101. Neumann CH, Petersen SA, Jahnke AH: MR imaging of the labral-capsular complex: normal variations. Am J Roentgenol 157:1015-1021, 1991.

102. Tsai JC, Zlatkin MB: Magnetic resonance imaging of the shoulder. Radiol Clin North Am 28:279-291, 1990.

103. Tsao LY, Mirowitz SA: MR imaging of the shoulder. Imaging techniques, diagnostic pitfalls, and normal variants. Magn Reson Imaging Clin North 5:683-704, 1997.

104. Longo C, Loredo R, Yu J, et al: Pictorial essay. MRI of the glenoid labrum with gross anatomic correlation. J Comput Assist Tomogr 20:487-495, 1996.

105. Loredo R, Longo C, Salonen D, et al: Glenoid labrum: MR imaging with histologic correlation. Radiology 196:33-41, 1995.

106. Zlatkin MB, Bjorkengren AG, Gylys-Morin V, et al: Cross-sectional imaging of the capsular mechanism of the glenohumeral joint. Am J Roentgenol 150:151-158, 1988.

107. Tuite MJ, Blankenbaker DG, Seifert M, et al: Sublabral foramen and Buford complex: inferior extent of the unattached or absent labrum in 50 patients. Radiology 223:137-142, 2002.

108. Yeh L, Kwak S, Kim YS, et al: Anterior labroligamentous structures of the glenohumeral joint: correlation of MR arthrography and anatomic dissection in cadavers. Am J Roentgenol 171:1229-1236, 1998.

109. Tuite MJ, Orwin JF: Anterosuperior labral variants of the shoulder: appearance on gradient-recalled-echo and fast spin-echo MR images. Radiology 199:537-540, 1996.

110. Stoller DWE: The shoulder. In Stoller DWE (ed): Magnetic Resonance Imaging in Orthopedics and Sports Medicine, 2nd edn. Philadelphia: Lippincott, Williams and Wilkins, 1997, pp 511-633.

111. Needell SD, Zlatkin MB, Sher JS, et al: MR imaging of the rotator cuff: peritendinous and bone abnormalities in an asymptomatic population. Am J Roentgenol 166:863-867, 1996.

112. Mitchell MJ, Causey G, Berthoty DP, et al: Peribursal fat plane of the shoulder: anatomic study and clinical experience. Radiology 168:699-704, 1988.

113. Kwak SM, Brown RR, Resnick D, et al: Anatomy, anatomic variations, and pathology of the 11- to 3-o'clock position of the glenoid labrum: findings on MR arthrography and anatomic sections. Am J Roentgenol 171:235-238, 1998.

114. Stoller DW: MR arthrography of the glenohumeral joint. Radiol Clin North Am 35:97-116, 1997.

115. Smith DK, Chopp TM, Aufdemorte TB, et al: Sublabral recess of the superior glenoid labrum: study of cadavers with conventional nonenhanced MR imaging, MR arthrography, anatomic dissection, and limited histologic examination. Radiology 201:251-256, 1996.

116. Tirman PF, Feller JF, Palmer WE, et al: The Buford complex—a variation of normal shoulder anatomy: MR arthrographic imaging features. Am J Roentgenol 166:869-873, 1996.

117. Rockwood CA, Lyons FR: Shoulder impingement syndrome: diagnosis, radiographic evaluation, and treatment with a modified Neer acromioplasty. J Bone Joint Surg Am 75:409-424, 1993.

118. Bjorkenheim JM, Paavolainen P, Ahovuo J, Slatis P: Subacromial impingement decompressed with anterior acromioplasty. Clin Orthop 150-155, 1990.

119. Neer CS, 2nd: Impingement lesions. Clin Orthop 70-77, 1983.

120. Neer CS, 2nd: Anterior acromioplasty for the chronic impingement syndrome in the shoulder: a preliminary report. J Bone Joint Surg Am 54:41-50, 1972.

121. Petersson CJ, Gentz CF: Ruptures of the supraspinatus tendon. The significance of distally pointing acromioclavicular osteophytes. Clin Orthop 143-148, 1983.

122. Hyvonen P, Paivansalo M, Lehtiniemi H, et al: Supraspinatus outlet view in the diagnosis of stages II and III impingement syndrome. Acta Radiol 42:441-446, 2001.

123. Park TS, Park DW, Kim SI, Kweon TH: Roentgenographic assessment of acromial morphology using supraspinatus outlet radiographs. Arthroscopy 17:496-501, 2001.

124. Vanarthos WJ, Monu JU: Type 4 acromion: a new classification. Contemp Orthop 30:227-229, 1995.

125. Yao L, Lee HY, Gentili A, Shapiro MM: Lateral down-sloping of the acromion: a useful MR sign? Clin Radiol 1996; 51:869-872.

126. Kessel L, Watson M: The painful arc syndrome. Clinical classification as a guide to management. J Bone Joint Surg Br 59:166-172, 1977.

127. Jim YF, Chang CY, Wu JJ, Chang T: Shoulder impingement syndrome: impingement view and arthrography study based on 100 cases. Skeletal Radiol 21:449-451, 1992.

128. Burns WC, 2nd, Whipple TL: Anatomic relationships in the shoulder impingement syndrome. Clin Orthop 96-102, 1993.

129. Gallino M, Battiston B, Annaratone G, Terragnoli F: Coracoacromial ligament: a comparative arthroscopic and anatomic study. Arthroscopy 11:564-567, 1995.

130. Boehm TD, Matzer M, Brazda D, Gohlke FE: Os acromiale associated with tear of the rotator cuff treated operatively. Review of 33 patients. J Bone Joint Surg Br 85:545-549, 2003.

131. Sammarco VJ: Os acromiale: frequency, anatomy, and clinical implications. J Bone Joint Surg Am 82:394-400, 2000.

132. Swain RA, Wilson FD, Harsha DM: The os acromiale: another cause of impingement. Med Sci Sports Exerc 28:1459-1462, 1996.

133. Gold RH, Seeger LL, Yao L: Imaging shoulder impingement. Skeletal Radiol 22:555-561, 1993.
134. Fu FH, Harner CD, Klein AH: Shoulder impingement syndrome. A critical review. Clin Orthop 162-173, 1991.
135. Jobe FW, Kvitne RS, Giangarra CE: Shoulder pain in the overhand or throwing athlete. The relationship of anterior instability and rotator cuff impingement. Orthop Rev 18:963-975, 1989.
136. Jobe FW. Impingement problems in the athlete. Instr Course Lect 38:205-209, 1989.
137. Sonnery-Cottet B, Edwards TB, Noel E, Walch G: Results of arthroscopic treatment of posterosuperior glenoid impingement in tennis players. Am J Sports Med 30:227-232, 2002.
138. Paley KJ, Jobe FW, Pink MM, et al: Arthroscopic findings in the overhand throwing athlete: evidence for posterior internal impingement of the rotator cuff. Arthroscopy 16:35-40, 2000.
139. McFarland EG, Hsu CY, Neira C, O'Neil O: Internal impingement of the shoulder: a clinical and arthroscopic analysis. J Shoulder Elbow Surg 8:458-460, 1999.
140. Giombini A, Rossi F, Pettrone FA, Dragoni S: Posterosuperior glenoid rim impingement as a cause of shoulder pain in top level waterpolo players. J Sports Med Phys Fitness 37:273-278, 1997.
141. Tirman PF, Bost FW, Garvin GJ, et al: Posterosuperior glenoid impingement of the shoulder: findings at MR imaging and MR arthrography with arthroscopic correlation. Radiology 193:431-436, 1994.
142. Walch G, Liotard JP, Boileau P, Noel E: Postero-superior glenoid impingement. Another shoulder impingement [French]. Rev Chir Orthop Reparatrice Appar Mot 77:571-574, 1991.
143. Meister K: Internal impingement in the shoulder of the overhand athlete: pathophysiology, diagnosis, and treatment. Am J Orthop 29:433-438, 2000.
144. Edelson G, Teitz C: Internal impingement in the shoulder. J Shoulder Elbow Surg 9:308-315, 2000.
145. Walch G, Liotard JP, Boileau P, Noel E: Postero-superior glenoid impingement. Another impingement of the shoulder. J Radiol 74:47-50, 1993.
146. Lo IK, Parten PM, Burkhart SS: Combined subcoracoid and subacromial impingement in association with anterosuperior rotator cuff tears: An arthroscopic approach. Arthroscopy 19:1068-1078, 2003.
147. Gerber C, Terrier F, Ganz R: The role of the coracoid process in the chronic impingement syndrome. J Bone Joint Surg Br 67:703-708, 1985.
148. Dines DM, Warren RF, Inglis AE, Pavlov H: The coracoid impingement syndrome. J Bone Joint Surg Br 72:314-316, 1990.
149. Bergman AG: Rotator cuff impingement. Pathogenesis, MR imaging characteristics, and early dynamic MR results. Magn Reson Imaging Clin North Am 5:705-719, 1997.
150. Codman EA: Rupture of the supraspinatus tendon. Clin Orthop 254:3-26, 1990.
151. Codman EA: The Shoulder, Rupture of the Supraspinatus Tendon and Other Lesions in or About the Subacromial Bursa. Boston: Thomas Todd, 1934.
152. Wolfgang GL: Rupture of the musculotendinous cuff of the shoulder. Clin Orthop 134:230-243, 1978.
153. Lohr JF, Uhthoff HK: The microvascular pattern of the supraspinatus tendon. Clin Orthop 35-38, 1990.
154. Uhthoff HK, Sarkar K: Periarticular soft tissue conditions causing pain in the shoulder. Curr Opin Rheumatol 4:241-246, 1992.
155. Uhthoff HK, Sarkar K: Classification and definition of tendinopathies. Clin Sports Med 10:707-720, 1991.
156. Ozaki J, Fujimoto S, Nakagawa Y, et al: Tears of the rotator cuff of the shoulder associated with pathological changes in the acromion. A study in cadavera. J Bone Joint Surg Am 70:1224-1230, 1988.
157. Ling SC, Chen CF, Wan RX: A study on the vascular supply of the supraspinatus tendon. Surg Radiol Anat 32:161-165, 1990.
158. Williams GR, Jr, Iannotti JP, Rosenthal A, et al: Anatomic, histologic, and magnetic resonance imaging abnormalities of the shoulder. Clin Orthop 66-74, 1996.
159. Kumagai J, Sarkar K, Uhthoff HK: The collagen types in the attachment zone of rotator cuff tendons in the elderly: an immunohistochemical study. J Rheumatol 21:2096-2100, 1994.
160. Chansky HA, Iannotti JP: The vascularity of the rotator cuff. Clin Sports Med 10:807-822, 1991.
161. Brooks CH, Revell WJ, Heatley FW: A quantitative histological study of the vascularity of the rotator cuff tendon. J Bone Joint Surg Br 74:151-153, 1992.
162. Budoff JE, Nirschl RP, Guidi EJ: Debridement of partial-thickness tears of the rotator cuff without acromioplasty. Long-term follow-up and review of the literature. J Bone Joint Surg Am 80:733-748, 1998.
163. Neviaser RJ, Neviaser TJ, Neviaser JS: Anterior dislocation of the shoulder and rotator cuff rupture. Clin Orthop 103-106, 1993.
164. Neviaser RJ, Neviaser TJ, Neviaser JS: Concurrent rupture of the rotator cuff and anterior dislocation of the shoulder in the older patient. J Bone Joint Surg Am 70:1308-1311, 1988.
165. Neviaser RJ: Ruptures of the rotator cuff. Orthop Clin North Am 18:387-394, 1987.
166. Pevny T, Hunter RE, Freeman JR: Primary traumatic anterior shoulder dislocation in patients 40 years of age and older. Arthroscopy 14:289-294, 1998.
167. Deutsch A, Altchek DW, Veltri DM, et al: Traumatic tears of the subscapularis tendon. Clinical diagnosis, magnetic resonance imaging findings, and operative treatment. Am J Sports Med 25:13-22, 1997.
168. Gerber C, Krushell RJ: Isolated rupture of the tendon of the subscapularis muscle. Clinical features in 16 cases. J Bone Joint Surg Br 73:389-394, 1991.
169. Itoi E, Tabata S: Rotator cuff tears in anterior dislocation of the shoulder. Int Orthop 16:240-244, 1992.
170. Mason BJ, Kier R, Bindleglass DF: Occult fractures of the greater tuberosity of the humerus: radiographic and MR imaging findings. Am J Roentgenol 172:469-473, 1999.
171. Reinus WR, Hatem SF: Fractures of the greater tuberosity presenting as rotator cuff abnormality: magnetic resonance demonstration. J Trauma 44:670-675, 1998.
172. Matsen FA, Lippitt SB: Rotator cuff. In Rockwood CE (ed): The Shoulder. Philadelphia: WB Saunders, 1998, pp 755-795.
173. Ellman H: Diagnosis and treatment of incomplete rotator cuff tears. Clin Orthop May:64-74, 1990.
174. Ciepiela MD: Classification of rotator cuff tears. In Burkhead WZ Jr (ed): Rotator Cuff Disorders. Baltimore: William and Wilkins, 1996, pp 100-110.
175. Ellman H, Kay SP, Wirth M: Arthroscopic treatment of full-thickness rotator cuff tears: 2- to 7-year follow-up study. Arthroscopy 9:195-200, 1993.
176. Iannotti JP, Bernot MP, Kuhlman JR, et al: Postoperative assessment of shoulder function: a prospective study of full-thickness rotator cuff tears. J Shoulder Elbow Surg 5:449-457, 1996.
177. Tuite MJ, Turnbull JR, Orwin JF: Anterior versus posterior, and rim-rent rotator cuff tears: prevalence and MR sensitivity. Skeletal Radiol 27:237-243, 1998.
178. Clark RJ, Marchessault J, Sizer PS, Jr, Slauterbeck J: Isolated traumatic rupture of the subscapularis tendon. J Am Board Fam Pract 15:304-308, 2002.
179. Tung GA, Yoo DC, Levine SM, et al: Subscapularis tendon tear: primary and associated signs on MRI. J Comput Assist Tomogr 25:417-424, 2001.
180. Pfirrmann CW, Zanetti M, Weishaupt D, et al: Subscapularis tendon tears: detection and grading at MR arthrography. Radiology 213:709-714, 1999.
181. Li XX, Schweitzer ME, Bifano JA, et al: MR evaluation of subscapularis tears. J Comput Assist Tomogr 23:713-717, 1999.
182. Gerber C, Lambert SM: Allograft reconstruction of segmental defects of the humeral head for the treatment of chronic locked posterior dislocation of the shoulder. J Bone Joint Surg Am 78:376-382, 1996.
183. Gartsman GM: Massive, irreparable tears of the rotator cuff. Results of operative debridement and subacromial decompression. J Bone Joint Surg Am 79:715-721, 1997.
184. Hottya GA, Tirman PF, Bost FW, et al: Tear of the posterior shoulder stabilizers after posterior dislocation: MR imaging and MR arthrographic findings with arthroscopic correlation. Am J Roentgenol 171:763-768, 1998.
185. Buirski G: Magnetic resonance imaging in acute and chronic rotator cuff tears. Skeletal Radiol 19:109-111, 1990.
186. Neer CS, 2nd, Craig EV, Fukuda H: Cuff-tear arthropathy. J Bone Joint Surg Am 65:1232-1244, 1983.
187. Iannotti JP, Zlatkin MB, Esterhai JL, et al: Magnetic resonance imaging of the shoulder. Sensitivity, specificity, and predictive value. J Bone Joint Surg Am 73:17-29, 1991.
188. Zlatkin MB, Iannotti JP, Roberts MC, et al: Rotator cuff tears: diagnostic performance of MR imaging. Radiology 172:223-229, 1989.
189. Goutallier D, Postel JM, Gleyze P, et al: Influence of cuff muscle fatty degeneration on anatomic and functional outcomes after simple suture of full-thickness tears. J Shoulder Elbow Surg 12:550-554, 2003.
190. Goutallier D, Postel JM, Bernageau J, et al: Fatty muscle degeneration in cuff ruptures. Pre- and postoperative evaluation by CT scan. Clin Orthop 78-83, 1994.
191. Resnick DKH: Shoulder. In Resnick DKH (ed): Internal Derangement of Joints. Philadelphia, WB Saunders, 1997, pp 163-334.
192. Farley TE, Neumann CH, Steinbach LS, Petersen SA: The coracoacromial arch: MR evaluation and correlation with rotator cuff pathology. Skeletal Radiol 23:641-645, 1994.
193. Seeger LL, Gold RH, Bassett LW, Ellman H: Shoulder impingement syndrome: MR findings in 53 shoulders. Am J Roentgenol 150:343-347, 1988.
194. Seeger LL: Magnetic resonance imaging of the shoulder. Clin Orthop 48-59, 1989.
195. Jordan LK, Kenter K, Griffiths HL: Relationship between MRI and clinical findings in the acromioclavicular joint. Skeletal Radiol 31:516-521, 2002.
196. Crues JV, 3rd, Fareed DO: Magnetic resonance imaging of shoulder impingement. Top Magn Reson Imaging 3:39-49, 1991.
197. Gordon BH, Chew FS: Isolated acromioclavicular joint pathology in the symptomatic shoulder on magnetic resonance imaging: a pictorial essay. J Comput Assist Tomogr 2004; 28:215-222, 1997.
198. Schweitzer ME, Magbalon MJ, Frieman BG, et al: Acromioclavicular joint fluid: determination of clinical significance with MR imaging. Radiology 192:205-207, 1994.
199. Epstein RE, Schweitzer ME, Frieman BG, et al: Hooked acromion: prevalence on MR images of painful shoulders. Radiology 187:479-481, 1993.
200. MacGillivray JD, Fealy S, Potter HG, O'Brien SJ: Multiplanar analysis of acromion morphology. Am J Sports Med 26:836-840, 1998.
201. Fremerey R, Bastian L, Siebert WE: The coracoacromial ligament: anatomical and biomechanical properties with respect to age and rotator cuff disease. Knee Surg Sports Traumatol Arthrosc 8:309-313, 2000.

202. Reichmister JP, Reeder JD, McCarthy E: Ossification of the coracoacromial ligament: association with rotator cuff pathology of the shoulder. Maryland Med J 45:849-852, 1996.

203. Gagey N, Ravaud E, Lassau JP: Anatomy of the acromial arch: correlation of anatomy and magnetic resonance imaging. Surg Radiol Anat 15:63-70, 1993.

204. Uri DS, Kneeland JB, Herzog R: Os acromiale: evaluation of markers for identification on sagittal and coronal oblique MR images. Skeletal Radiol 26:31-34, 1997.

205. Park JG, Lee JK, Phelps CT: Os acromiale associated with rotator cuff impingement: MR imaging of the shoulder. Radiology 193:255-257, 1994.

206. McClure JG, Raney RB: Anomalies of the scapula. Clin Orthop 22-31, 1975.

207. Khan K, Cook J: The painful nonruptured tendon: clinical aspects. Clin Sports Med 22:711-725, 2003.

208. Khan KM, Cook JL, Bonar F, et al: Histopathology of common tendinopathies. Update and implications for clinical management. Sports Med 27:393-408, 1999.

209. Wolf WB, 3rd: Shoulder tendinoses. Clin Sports Med 11:871-890, 1992.

210. Zlatkin MB, Hoffman C, Shellock FG: Assessment of the rotator cuff and glenoid labrum using an extremity MR system: MR results compared to surgical findings from a multi-center study. J Magn Reson Imaging 19:623-631, 2004.

211. Tyson LL, Crues JV, 3rd: Pathogenesis of rotator cuff disorders. Magnetic resonance imaging characteristics. Magn Reson Imaging Clin North Am 1:37-46, 1993.

212. Kieft GJ, Bloem JL, Rozing PM, Obermann WR: Rotator cuff impingement syndrome: MR imaging. Radiology 166:211-214, 1988.

213. Anzilotti KF, Jr, Schweitzer ME, Oliveri M, Marone PJ: Rotator cuff strain: a post-traumatic mimicker of tendonitis on MRI. Skeletal Radiol 25:555-558, 1996.

214. Miniaci A, Mascia AT, Salonen DC, Becker EJ: Magnetic resonance imaging of the shoulder in asymptomatic professional baseball pitchers. Am J Sports Med 30:66-73, 2002.

215. Miniaci A, Dowdy PA, Willits KR, Vellet AD: Magnetic resonance imaging evaluation of the rotator cuff tendons in the asymptomatic shoulder. Am J Sports Med 23:142-145, 1995.

216. Yamakawa S, Hashizume H, Ichikawa N, et al: Comparative studies of MRI and operative findings in rotator cuff tear. Acta Med Okayama 55:261-268, 2001.

217. Reinus WR, Shady KL, Mirowitz SA, Totty WG: MR diagnosis of rotator cuff tears of the shoulder: value of using T2-weighted fat-saturated images. Am J Roentgenol 164:1451-1455, 1995.

218. Quinn SF, Sheley RC, Demlow TA, Szumowski J: Rotator cuff tendon tears: evaluation with fat-suppressed MR imaging with arthroscopic correlation in 100 patients. Radiology 195:497-500, 1995.

219. Traughber PD, Goodwin TE: Shoulder MRI: arthroscopic correlation with emphasis on partial tears. J Comput Assist Tomogr 16:129-133, 1992.

220. Evancho AM, Stiles RG, Fajman WA, et al: MR imaging diagnosis of rotator cuff tears. Am J Roentgenol 151:751-754, 1988.

221. Shellock FG, Bert JM, Fritts HM, et al: Evaluation of the rotator cuff and glenoid labrum using a 0.2-Tesla extremity magnetic resonance (MR) system: MR results compared to surgical findings. J Magn Reson Imaging 14:763-770, 2001.

222. Bradley YC, Chandnani VP, Gagliardi JA, Reeves TQ: Partial thickness supraspinatus tears: diagnosis by magnetic resonance arthrography. Australas Radiol 39:124-127, 1995.

223. Tirman PF, Smith ED, Stoller DW, Fritz RC: Shoulder imaging in athletes. Semin Musculoskelet Radiol 8:29-40, 2004.

224. Burk DL, Jr, Torres JL, Marone PJ, et al: MR imaging of shoulder injuries in professional baseball players. J Magn Reson Imaging 1:385-389, 1991.

225. Uri DS: MR imaging of shoulder impingement and rotator cuff disease. Radiol Clin North Am 35:77-96, 1997.

226. Stoller DW, Fritz RC: Magnetic resonance imaging of impingement and rotator cuff tears. Magn Reson Imaging Clin North Am 1:47-63, 1993.

227. Farley TE, Neumann CH, Steinbach LS, et al: Full-thickness tears of the rotator cuff of the shoulder: diagnosis with MR imaging. Am J Roentgenol 158:347-351, 1992.

228. Burk DL, Jr, Karasick D, Kurtz AB, et al: Rotator cuff tears: prospective comparison of MR imaging with arthrography, sonography, and surgery. Am J Roentgenol 153:87-92, 1989.

229. Zlatkin MB, Reicher MA, Kellerhouse LE, et al: The painful shoulder: MR imaging of the glenohumeral joint. J Comput Assist Tomogr 12:995-1001, 1998.

230. Lehtinen JT, Tingart MJ, Apreleva M, et al: Practical assessment of rotator cuff muscle volumes using shoulder MRI. Acta Orthop Scand 74:722-729, 2003.

231. Vahlensieck M, Resendes M, Lang P, Genant H: Shoulder MRI: the subacromial/subdeltoid bursa fat stripe in healthy and pathologic conditions. Eur J Radiol 14:223-227, 1992.

232. Tingart MJ, Apreleva M, Lehtinen JT, et al: Magnetic resonance imaging in quantitative analysis of rotator cuff muscle volume. Clin Orthop 104-110, 2003.

233. Yao L, Mehta U: Infraspinatus muscle atrophy: implications? Radiology 226:161-164, 2003.

234. Shimizu T, Itoi E, Minagawa H, et al: Atrophy of the rotator cuff muscles and site of cuff tears. Acta Orthop Scand 73:40-43, 2002.

235. Fuchs B, Weishaupt D, Zanetti M, et al: Fatty degeneration of the muscles of the rotator cuff: assessment by computed tomography versus magnetic resonance imaging. J Shoulder Elbow Surg 8:599-605, 1999.

236. Zanetti M, Gerber C, Hodler J: Quantitative assessment of the muscles of the rotator cuff with magnetic resonance imaging. Invest Radiol 33:163-170, 1998.

237. Thomazeau H, Rolland Y, Lucas C, et al: Atrophy of the supraspinatus belly. Assessment by MRI in 55 patients with rotator cuff pathology. Acta Orthop Scand 67:264-268, 1996.

238. Vad VB, Southern D, Warren RF, et al: Prevalence of peripheral neurologic injuries in rotator cuff tears with atrophy. J Shoulder Elbow Surg 12:333-36, 2003.

239. Bredella MA, Tirman PF, Fritz RC, et al: Denervation syndromes of the shoulder girdle: MR imaging with electrophysiologic correlation. Skeletal Radiol 28:567-572, 1999.

240. Goldstein B, Young J, Escobedo EM: Rotator cuff repairs in individuals with paraplegia. Am J Phys Med Rehabil 76:316-322, 1997.

241. Selvi E, Falsetti P, Manganelli S, et al: Acromioclavicular joint cyst: a presenting feature of full thickness rotator cuff tear. J Rheumatol 27:2045-2046, 2000.

242. Marino AJ, Tyrrell PN, el-Houdiri YA, Kelly CP: Acromioclavicular joint cyst and rotator cuff tear. J Shoulder Elbow Surg 7:435-437, 1998.

243. Postacchini F, Perugia D, Gumina S: Acromioclavicular joint cyst associated with rotator cuff tear. A report of three cases. Clin Orthop 111-113, 1993.

244. Sanders TG, Tirman PF, Feller JF, Genant HK: Association of intramuscular cysts of the rotator cuff with tears of the rotator cuff: magnetic resonance imaging findings and clinical significance. Arthroscopy 16:230-235, 2000.

245. Green A: Chronic massive rotator cuff tears: evaluation and management. J Am Acad Orthop Surg 11:321-331, 2003.

246. Bryant L, Shnier R, Bryant C, Murrell GA: A comparison of clinical estimation, ultrasonography, magnetic resonance imaging, and arthroscopy in determining the size of rotator cuff tears. J Shoulder Elbow Surg 11:219-224, 2002.

247. Iannotti JP: Full-thickness rotator cuff tears: Factors affecting surgical outcome. J Am Acad Orthop Surg 2:87-95, 1994.

248. Fritz RC: Magnetic resonance imaging of sports-related injuries to the shoulder: impingement and rotator cuff. Radiol Clin North Am 40:217-234, vi, 2002.

249. Patten RM, Spear RP, Richardson ML: Diagnostic performance of magnetic resonance imaging for the diagnosis of rotator cuff tears using supplemental images in the oblique sagittal plane. Invest Radiol 29:87-93, 1994.

250. Schaefer O, Winterer J, Lohrmann C, et al: Magnetic resonance imaging for supraspinatus muscle atrophy after cuff repair. Clin Orthop 93-99, 2002.

251. Nakagaki K, Ozaki J, Tomita Y, Tamai S: Fatty degeneration in the supraspinatus muscle after rotator cuff tear. J Shoulder Elbow Surg 5:194-200, 1996.

252. Sashi R, Kobayashi M, Hashimoto M, et al: Comparison of fast spin-echo and conventional spin-echo sequences in the MR diagnosis of rotator cuff tears. Radiat Med 15:75-78, 1997.

253. Hodler J, Kursunoglu-Brahme S, Snyder SJ, et al: Rotator cuff disease: assessment with MR arthrography versus standard MR imaging in 36 patients with arthroscopic confirmation. Radiology 182:431-436, 1992.

254. Vahlensieck M, Sommer T, Textor J, et al: Indirect MR arthrography: techniques and applications. Eur Radiol 8:232-235, 1998.

255. Sakurai G, Ozaki J, Tomita Y, et al: Incomplete tears of the subscapularis tendon associated with tears of the supraspinatus tendon: cadaveric and clinical studies. J Shoulder Elbow Surg 7:510-515, 1998.

256. Lo IK, Burkhart SS: The etiology and assessment of subscapularis tendon tears: a case for subcoracoid impingement, the roller-wringer effect, and TUFF lesions of the subscapularis. Arthroscopy 19:1142-1150, 2003.

257. Tan V, Moore RS, Jr, Omarini L, et al: Magnetic resonance imaging analysis of coracoid morphology and its relation to rotator cuff tears. Am J Orthop 31:329-333, 2002.

258. Rossi F: Shoulder impingement syndromes. Eur J Radiol 27(Suppl 1):S42-48, 1998.

259. Friedman RJ, Bonutti PM, Genez B: Cine magnetic resonance imaging of the subcoracoid region. Orthopedics 21:545-548, 1998.

260. Russo R, Togo F: The subcoracoid impingement syndrome: clinical, semeiologic and therapeutic considerations. Ital J Orthop Traumatol 17:351-358, 1991.

261. Grainger AJ, Tirman PF, Elliott JM, et al: MR anatomy of the subcoracoid bursa and the association of subcoracoid effusion with tears of the anterior rotator cuff and the rotator interval. Am J Roentgenol 174:1377-1380, 2000.

262. Gerber C, Hersche O, Farron A: Isolated rupture of the subscapularis tendon. J Bone Joint Surg Am 78:1015-1023, 1996.

263. Neviaser RJ, Neviaser TJ: Recurrent instability of the shoulder after age 40. J Shoulder Elbow Surg 4:416-418, 1995.

264. Walch G, Nove-Josserand L, Boileau P, Levigne C: Subluxations and dislocations of the tendon of the long head of the biceps. J Shoulder Elbow Surg 7:100-108, 1998.

265. Nove-Josserand L, Levigne C, Noel E, Walch G: Isolated lesions of the subscapularis muscle. Apropos of 21 cases [French]. Rev Chir Orthop Reparatrice Appar Mot 80:595-601, 1994.

266. Othman AY, Taylor GJ: Traumatic avulsion of the bony insertion of infraspinatus tendon. J Trauma 50:575-577, 2001.
267. Seeger LL, Lubowitz J, Thomas BJ: Case report 815: Tear of the rotator interval. Skeletal Radiol 22:615-617, 1993.
268. Nobuhara K, Ikeda H: Rotator interval lesion. Clin Orthop 44-50, 1987.
269. Clark J, Sidles JA, Matsen FA: The relationship of the glenohumeral joint capsule to the rotator cuff. Clin Orthop 29-34, 1990.
270. Harryman DT, 2nd, Sidles JA, Clark JM, et al: Translation of the humeral head on the glenoid with passive glenohumeral motion. J Bone Joint Surg Am 72:1334-1343, 1990.
271. Antoniou J, Tsai A, Baker D, et al: Milwaukee shoulder: correlating possible etiologic variables. Clin Orthop 79-85, 2003.
272. Sjoden GO, Movin T, Sperber A, et al: Cuff tear arthropathy with hemarthrosis. A report on 3 elderly patients. Acta Orthop Scand 67:571-574, 1996.
273. Beltran J, Jbara M, Maimon R: Shoulder: labrum and bicipital tendon. Top Magn Reson Imaging 14:35-49, 2003.
274. Spritzer CE, Collins AJ, Cooperman A, Speer KP: Assessment of instability of the long head of the biceps tendon by MRI. Skeletal Radiol 30:199-207, 2001.
275. Murthi AM, Vosburgh CL, Neviaser TJ: The incidence of pathologic changes of the long head of the biceps tendon. J Shoulder Elbow Surg 9:382-385, 2000.
276. Sethi N, Wright R, Yamaguchi K: Disorders of the long head of the biceps tendon. J Shoulder Elbow Surg 8:644-654, 1999.
277. Rokito AS, Bilgen OF, Zuckerman JD, Cuomo F: Medial dislocation of the long head of the biceps tendon. Magnetic resonance imaging evaluation. Am J Orthop 25:314, 318-323, 1996.
278. Tuckman GA: Abnormalities of the long head of the biceps tendon of the shoulder: MR imaging findings. Am J Roentgenol 163:1183-1188, 1994.
279. Cervilla V, Schweitzer ME, Ho C, et al: Medial dislocation of the biceps brachii tendon: appearance at MR imaging. Radiology 180:523-526, 1991.
280. Neviaser TJ: The role of the biceps tendon in the impingement syndrome. Orthop Clin North Am 18:383-386, 1987.
281. Postacchini F: Rupture of the rotator cuff of the shoulder associated with rupture of the tendon of the long head of the biceps. Ital J Orthop Traumatol 12:137-149, 1986.
282. Kido T, Itoi E, Konno N, et al: The depressor function of biceps on the head of the humerus in shoulders with tears of the rotator cuff. J Bone Joint Surg Br 82:416-419, 2000.
283. Hurt G, Baker CL, Jr: Calcific tendinitis of the shoulder. Orthop Clin North Am 34:567-575, 2003.
284. Speed CA, Hazleman BL: Calcific tendinitis of the shoulder. N Engl J Med 340:1582-1584, 1999.
285. Uhthoff HK: Calcifying tendinitis. Ann Chir Gynaecol 85:111-115, 1996.
286. Halverson PB: Crystal deposition disease of the shoulder (including calcific tendonitis and milwaukee shoulder syndrome). Curr Rheumatol Rep 5:244-247, 2003.
287. Burk DL, Jr, Karasick D, Mitchell DG, Rifkin MD: MR imaging of the shoulder: correlation with plain radiography. Am J Roentgenol 154:549-553, 1990.
288. Garcia GM, McCord GC, Kumar R: Hydroxyapatite crystal deposition disease. Semin Musculoskelet Radiol 7:187-193, 2003.
289. Jim YF, Hsu HC, Chang CY, et al: Coexistence of calcific tendinitis and rotator cuff tear: an arthrographic study. Skeletal Radiol 22:183-185, 1993.
290. Wall MS, O'Brien SJ: Arthroscopic evaluation of the unstable shoulder. Clin Sports Med 14:817-839, 1995.
291. Schwartz E, Warren RF, O'Brien SJ, Fronek J: Posterior shoulder instability. Orthop Clin North Am 18:409-419, 1987.
292. O'Brien SJ, Warren RF, Schwartz E: Anterior shoulder instability. Orthop Clin North Am 18:395-408, 1987.
293. Zarins B, McMahon MS, Rowe CR: Diagnosis and treatment of traumatic anterior instability of the shoulder. Clin Orthop 75-84, 1993.
294. Zarins B, Rowe CR: Current concepts in the diagnosis and treatment of shoulder instability in athletes. Med Sci Sports Exerc 16:444-448, 1984.
295. Burkhart SS, Morgan CD, Kibler WB: The disabled throwing shoulder: spectrum of pathology Part I: pathoanatomy and biomechanics. Arthroscopy 19:404-420, 2003.
296. Sperling JW, Anderson K, McCarty EC, Warren RF: Complications of thermal capsulorrhaphy. Instr Course Lect 50:37-41, 2001.
297. Hovelius L: The natural history of primary anterior dislocation of the shoulder in the young. J Orthop Sci 4:307-317, 1999.
298. Hovelius L, Augustini BG, Fredin H, et al: Primary anterior dislocation of the shoulder in young patients. A ten-year prospective study. J Bone Joint Surg Am 78:1677-1684, 1996.
299. Goga IE: Chronic shoulder dislocations. J Shoulder Elbow Surg 12:446-450, 2003.
300. Cai TD, Guo BF: Recurrent anterior dislocation of shoulder joint. Chin Med J (Engl) 103:604-605, 1990.
301. Rowe CR: Acute and recurrent anterior dislocations of the shoulder. Orthop Clin North Am 11:253-270, 1980.
302. Buscayret F, Edwards TB, Szabo I, et al: Glenohumeral arthrosis in anterior instability before and after surgical treatment: incidence and contributing factors. Am J Sports Med 32:1165-1172, 2004.
303. te Slaa RL, Wijffels MP, Brand R, Marti RK: The prognosis following acute primary glenohumeral dislocation. J Bone Joint Surg Br 86:58-64, 2004.
304. Hovelius L, Lind B, Thorling J: Primary dislocation of the shoulder. Factors affecting the two-year prognosis. Clin Orthop 181-185, 1983.
305. Rowe CR, Patel D, Southmayd WW: The Bankart procedure: a long-term end-result study. J Bone Joint Surg Am 60:1-16, 1978.
306. Knight D, Patel V: Use of allograft for the large Hill-Sachs lesion associated with anterior shoulder dislocation. Injury 35:96; author reply 96, 2004.
307. Edelson JG: Bony changes of the glenoid as a consequence of shoulder instability. J Shoulder Elbow Surg 5:293-298, 1996.
308. Calandra JJ, Baker CL, Uribe J: The incidence of Hill-Sachs lesions in initial anterior shoulder dislocations. Arthroscopy 5:254-257, 1989.
309. Danzig LA, Greenway G, Resnick D: The Hill-Sachs lesion. An experimental study. Am J Sports Med 8:328-332, 1980.
310. Morton KS: The unstable shoulder: recurring subluxation. Injury 10:304-306, 1979.
311. Werner CM, Jacob HA, Dumont CE, Gerber C: Static anterior glenohumeral subluxation following coracoid bone block in combination with pectoralis major transfer: a case report and biomechanical considerations [French]. Rev Chir Orthop Reparatrice Appar Mot 90:156-160, 2004.
312. Postacchini F, Mancini A: Anterior instability of the shoulder due to capsular laxity. Ital J Orthop Traumatol 14:175-185, 1988.
313. Rowe CR: Recurrent anterior transient subluxation of the shoulder. The "dead arm" syndrome. Orthop Clin North Am 19:767-772, 1988.
314. Rowe CR, Zarins B: Recurrent transient subluxation of the shoulder. J Bone Joint Surg Am 63:863-872, 1981.
315. Workman TL, Burkhard TK, Resnick D, et al: Hill-Sachs lesion: comparison of detection with MR imaging, radiography, and arthroscopy. Radiology 185:847-852, 1992.
316. Imhoff AB, Hodler J: Correlation of MR imaging, CT arthrography, and arthroscopy of the shoulder. Bull Hosp Joint Dis 54:146-152, 1996.
317. Wintzell G, Haglund-Akerlind Y, Tengvar M, et al: MRI examination of the glenohumeral joint after traumatic primary anterior dislocation. A descriptive evaluation of the acute lesion and at 6-month follow-up. Knee Surg Sports Traumatol Arthrosc 4:232-236, 1996.
318. Richards RD, Sartoris DJ, Pathria MN, Resnick D: Hill-Sachs lesion and normal humeral groove: MR imaging features allowing their differentiation. Radiology 190:665-668, 1994.
319. Itoi E, Lee SB, Berglund LJ, et al: The effect of a glenoid defect on antero-inferior stability of the shoulder after Bankart repair: a cadaveric study. J Bone Joint Surg Am 82:35-46, 2000.
320. Wilson AJ: Computed arthrotomography of glenohumeral instability. Top Magn Reson Imaging 6:139-146, 1994.
321. Calvisi V, Collodel M, Nasi M, et al: CT arthrography and arthroscopy in chronic glenohumeral joint instability. Ital J Orthop Traumatol 18:303-310, 1992.
322. Stevens KJ, Preston BJ, Wallace WA, Kerslake RW: CT imaging and three-dimensional reconstructions of shoulders with anterior glenohumeral instability. Clin Anat 12:326-336, 1999.
323. Burkhart SS, De Beer JF: Traumatic glenohumeral bone defects and their relationship to failure of arthroscopic Bankart repairs: significance of the inverted-pear glenoid and the humeral engaging Hill-Sachs lesion. Arthroscopy 16:677-694, 2000.
324. Lo IK, Parten PM, Burkhart SS: The inverted pear glenoid: an indicator of significant glenoid bone loss. Arthroscopy 20:169-174, 2004.
325. Burkhart SS, Debeer JF, Tehrany AM, Parten PM: Quantifying glenoid bone loss arthroscopically in shoulder instability. Arthroscopy 18:488-491, 2002.
326. Gartsman GM, Roddey TS, Hammerman SM: Arthroscopic treatment of anterior-inferior glenohumeral instability. Two to five-year follow-up. J Bone Joint Surg Am 82-A:991-1003, 2000.
327. Taylor DC, Arciero RA: Pathologic changes associated with shoulder dislocations. Arthroscopic and physical examination findings in first-time, traumatic anterior dislocations. Am J Sports Med 25:306-311, 1997.
328. Walch G. Chronic anterior glenohumeral instability. J Bone Joint Surg Br 78:670-677, 1996.
329. Massengill AD, Seeger LL, Yao L, et al: Labrocapsular ligamentous complex of the shoulder: normal anatomy, anatomic variation, and pitfalls of MR imaging and MR arthrography. RadioGraphics 14:1211-1223, 1994.
330. O'Neill DB: Arthroscopic Bankart repair of anterior detachments of the glenoid labrum. A prospective study. J Bone Joint Surg Am 81:1357-1366, 1999.
331. Cole BJ, L'Insalata J, Irrgang J, Warner JJ: Comparison of arthroscopic and open anterior shoulder stabilization. A two to six-year follow-up study. J Bone Joint Surg Am 82-A:1108-1114, 2000.
332. Tuite MJ, De Smet AA, Norris MA, Orwin JF: Anteroinferior tears of the glenoid labrum: fat-suppressed fast spin-echo T2 versus gradient-recalled echo MR images. Skeletal Radiol 26:293-297, 1997.
333. Suder PA, Frich LH, Hougaard K, et al: Magnetic resonance imaging evaluation of capsulolabral tears after traumatic primary anterior shoulder dislocation. A prospective comparison with arthroscopy of 25 cases. J Shoulder Elbow Surg 4:419-428, 1995.
334. Chandnani VP, Yeager TD, DeBerardino T, et al: Glenoid labral tears: prospective evaluation with MRI imaging, MR arthrography, and CT arthrography. Am J Roentgenol 161:1229-1235, 1993.
335. McCauley TR: MR imaging of the glenoid labrum. Magn Reson Imaging Clin North Am 12:97-109, vi-vii, 2004.

336. Tuite MJ, Rubin D: CT and MR Arthrography of the Glenoid Labroligamentous Complex. Semin Musculoskelet Radiol 2:363-376, 1998.

337. Chandnani VP, Gagliardi JA, Murnane TG, et al: Glenohumeral ligaments and shoulder capsular mechanism: evaluation with MR arthrography. Radiology 196:27-32, 1995.

338. Habibian A, Stauffer A, Resnick D, et al: Comparison of conventional and computed arthrotomography with MR imaging in the evaluation of the shoulder. J Comput Assist Tomogr 13:968-975, 1989.

339. Rafii M, Firooznia H, Golimbu C: MR imaging of glenohumeral instability. Magn Reson Imaging Clin North Am 5:787-809, 1997.

340. Grigorian M, Genant HK, Tirman PF: Magnetic resonance imaging of the glenoid labrum. Semin Roentgenol 35:277-285, 2000.

341. Wischer TK, Bredella MA, Genant HK, et al: Perthes lesion (a variant of the Bankart lesion): MR imaging and MR arthrographic findings with surgical correlation. Am J Roentgenol 178:233-237, 2002.

342. Connell DA, Potter HG: Magnetic resonance evaluation of the labral capsular ligamentous complex: a pictorial review. Australas Radiol 43:419-426, 1999.

343. Neviaser TJ: The anterior labroligamentous periosteal sleeve avulsion lesion: a cause of anterior instability of the shoulder. Arthroscopy 9:17-21, 1993.

344. Sailer J, Imhof H: Shoulder instability [French]. Radiologe 44:578-590, 2004.

345. Yoneda M. Neviaser's contribution to the treatment of ALPSA lesions. J Bone Joint Surg Am 83-A:621-622, 2001.

346. Tirman PF, Steinbach LS, Feller JF, Stauffer AE: Humeral avulsion of the anterior shoulder stabilizing structures after anterior shoulder dislocation: demonstration by MRI and MR arthrography. Skeletal Radiol 25:743-748, 1996.

347. Bui-Mansfield LT, Taylor DC, Uhorchak JM, Tenuta JJ: Humeral avulsions of the glenohumeral ligament: imaging features and a review of the literature. Am J Roentgenol 179:649-655, 2002.

348. Wolf EM, Cheng JC, Dickson K: Humeral avulsion of glenohumeral ligaments as a cause of anterior shoulder instability. Arthroscopy 11:600-607, 1995.

349. Bokor DJ, Conboy VB, Olson C: Anterior instability of the glenohumeral joint with humeral avulsion of the glenohumeral ligament. A review of 41 cases. J Bone Joint Surg Br 81:93-96, 1999.

350. Schippinger G, Vasiu PS, Fankhauser F, Clement HG: HAGL lesion occurring after successful arthroscopic Bankart repair. Arthroscopy 17:206-208, 2001.

351. Coates MH, Breidahl W: Humeral avulsion of the anterior band of the inferior glenohumeral ligament with associated subscapularis bony avulsion in skeletally immature patients. Skeletal Radiol 30:661-666, 2001.

352. Oberlander MA, Morgan BE, Visotsky JL: The BHAGL lesion: a new variant of anterior shoulder instability. Arthroscopy 12:627-633, 1996.

353. Hawkins RJ, Janda DH: Posterior instability of the glenohumeral joint. A technique of repair. Am J Sports Med 24:275-278, 1996.

354. Tibone JE, Bradley JP: The treatment of posterior subluxation in athletes. Clin Orthop 124-137, 1993.

355. Hawkins RJ, Belle RM: Posterior instability of the shoulder. Instr Course Lect 38:211-215, 1989.

356. Pavlov H, Warren RF, Weiss CB, Jr, Dines DM: The roentgenographic evaluation of anterior shoulder instability. Clin Orthop 153-158, 1985.

357. Pavlov H, Freiberger RH: Fractures and dislocations about the shoulder. Semin Roentgenol 13:85-96, 1978.

358. Tuite MJ: MR imaging of sports injuries to the rotator cuff. Magn Reson Imaging Clin North Am 11:207-219, v, 2003.

359. Abrams JS: Arthroscopic repair of posterior instability and reverse humeral glenohumeral ligament avulsion lesions. Orthop Clin North Am 34:475-483, 2003.

360. Kim SH, Ha KI, Park JH, et al: Arthroscopic posterior labral repair and capsular shift for traumatic unidirectional recurrent posterior subluxation of the shoulder. J Bone Joint Surg Am 85-A:479-1487, 2003.

361. Tung GA, Hou DD: MR arthrography of the posterior labrocapsular complex: relationship with glenohumeral joint alignment and clinical posterior instability. Am J Roentgenol 180:369-375, 2003.

362. Hovis WD, Dean MT, Mallon WJ, Hawkins RJ: Posterior instability of the shoulder with secondary impingement in elite golfers. Am J Sports Med 30:886-890, 2002.

363. Misamore GW, Facibene WA: Posterior capsulorrhaphy for the treatment of traumatic recurrent posterior subluxations of the shoulder in athletes. J Shoulder Elbow Surg 9:403-408, 2000.

364. Weinberg J, McFarland EG: Posterior capsular avulsion in a college football player. Am J Sports Med 27:235-237, 1999.

365. Petersen SA: Posterior shoulder instability. Orthop Clin North Am 31:263-274, 2000.

366. Yu JS, Ashman CJ, Jones G: The POLPSA lesion: MR imaging findings with arthroscopic correlation in patients with posterior instability. Skeletal Radiol 31:396-399, 2002.

367. Simons P, Joekes E, Nelissen RG, Bloem JL: Posterior labrocapsular periosteal sleeve avulsion complicating locked posterior shoulder dislocation. Skeletal Radiol 27:588-590, 1998.

368. Jerosch J, Castro WH, Assheuer J: Nuclear magnetic resonance tomography diagnosis of changes in the glenoid process in patients with unstable shoulder joints [German]. Sportverletz Sportschaden 6:106-112, 1992.

369. Hawkins RJ, McCormack RG: Posterior shoulder instability. Orthopedics 11:101-107, 1988.

370. Snyder SJ, Banas MP, Belzer JP: Arthroscopic evaluation and treatment of injuries to the superior glenoid labrum. Instr Course Lect 45:65-70, 1996.

371. Snyder SJ, Banas MP, Karzel RP: An analysis of 140 injuries to the superior glenoid labrum. J Shoulder Elbow Surg 4:243-248, 1995.

372. Snyder SJ, Karzel RP, Del Pizzo W, et al: SLAP lesions of the shoulder. Arthroscopy 6:274-279, 1990.

373. Kim TK, Queale WS, Cosgarea AJ, McFarland EG: Clinical features of the different types of SLAP lesions: an analysis of one hundred and thirty-nine cases. Superior labrum anterior posterior. J Bone Joint Surg Am 85-A:66-71, 2003.

374. Burkhart SS, Morgan CD, Kibler WB: Shoulder injuries in overhead athletes. The "dead arm" revisited. Clin Sports Med 19:125-158, 2000.

375. Mileski RA, Snyder SJ: Superior labral lesions in the shoulder: pathoanatomy and surgical management. J Am Acad Orthop Surg 6:121-131, 1998.

376. Bencardino JT, Beltran J, Rosenberg ZS, et al: Superior labrum anterior-posterior lesions: diagnosis with MR arthrography of the shoulder. Radiology 214:267-271, 2000.

377. Maffet MW, Gartsman GM, Moseley B: Superior labrum-biceps tendon complex lesions of the shoulder. Am J Sports Med 23:93-98, 1995.

378. Waldt S, Burkart A, Lange P, et al: Diagnostic performance of MR arthrography in the assessment of superior labral anteroposterior lesions of the shoulder. Am J Roentgenol 182:1271-1278, 2004.

379. Jee WH, McCauley TR, Katz LD, et al: Superior labral anterior posterior (SLAP) lesions of the glenoid labrum: reliability and accuracy of MR arthrography for diagnosis. Radiology 218:127-132, 2001.

380. De Maeseneer M, Van Roy F, Lenchik L, et al: CT and MR arthrography of the normal and pathologic anterosuperior labrum and labral-bicipital complex. RadioGraphics 20(Spec No):S67-81, 2000.

381. Tung GA, Entzian D, Green A, Brody JM: High-field and low-field MR imaging of superior glenoid labral tears and associated tendon injuries. Am J Roentgenol 174:1107-1114, 2000.

382. Monu JU, Pope TL, Jr, Chabon SJ, Vanarthos WJ: MR diagnosis of superior labral anterior posterior (SLAP) injuries of the glenoid labrum: value of routine imaging without intraarticular injection of contrast material. Am J Roentgenol 163:1425-1429, 1994.

383. Smith AM, McCauley TR, Jokl P: SLAP lesions of the glenoid labrum diagnosed with MR imaging. Skeletal Radiol 22:507-510, 1993.

384. Cartland JP, Crues JV, 3rd, Stauffer A, et al: MR imaging in the evaluation of SLAP injuries of the shoulder: findings in 10 patients. Am J Roentgenol 159:787-792, 1992.

385. Chan KK, Muldoon KA, Yeh L, et al: Superior labral anteroposterior lesions: MR arthrography with arm traction. Am J Roentgenol 1999; 173:1117-1122.

386. Shankman S, Bencardino J, Beltran J: Glenohumeral instability: evaluation using MR arthrography of the shoulder. Skeletal Radiol 28:365-382, 1999.

387. Sherman PM, Sanders TG, De Lone DR: A benign soft tissue mass simulating a glenoid labral cyst on unenhanced magnetic resonance imaging. Mil Med 169:376-378, 2004.

388. Mellado JM, Salvado E, Camins A, et al: Fluid collections and juxta-articular cystic lesions of the shoulder: spectrum of MRI findings. Eur Radiol 12:650-659, 2002.

389. Tung GA, Entzian D, Stern JB, Green A: MR imaging and MR arthrography of paraglenoid labral cysts. Am J Roentgenol 174:1707-1715, 2000.

390. Sanders TG, Tirman PF: Paralabral cyst: an unusual cause of quadrilateral space syndrome. Arthroscopy 15:632-637, 1999.

391. Neviaser TJ: The GLAD lesion: another cause of anterior shoulder pain. Arthroscopy 9:22-23, 1993.

392. Amrami KK, Sperling JW, Bartholmai BJ, Sundaram M: Radiologic case study. Glenolabral articular disruption (GLAD) lesion. Orthopedics 25:95-96, 2002.

393. Sanders TG, Tirman PF, Linares R, et al: The glenolabral articular disruption lesion: MR arthrography with arthroscopic correlation. Am J Roentgenol 172:171-175, 1999.

394. Burkhart SS, Morgan CD: The peel-back mechanism: its role in producing and extending posterior type II SLAP lesions and its effect on SLAP repair rehabilitation. Arthroscopy 14:637-640, 1998.

395. Morgan CD, Burkhart SS, Palmeri M, Gillespie M: Type II SLAP lesions: three subtypes and their relationships to superior instability and rotator cuff tears. Arthroscopy 14:553-565, 1998.

396. Vahlensieck M, Lang P, Wagner U, et al: Shoulder MRI after surgical treatment of instability. Eur J Radiol 30:2-4, 1999.

397. Zlatkin MB. MRI of the postoperative shoulder. Skeletal Radiol 31:63-80, 2002.

398. Zanetti M, Hodler J: MR imaging of the shoulder after surgery. Magn Reson Imaging Clin North Am 12:169-183, viii, 2004.

399. Rand T, Trattnig S, Breitenseher M, et al: The postoperative shoulder. Top Magn Reson Imaging 10:203-213, 1999.

400. Spielmann AL, Forster BB, Kokan P, et al: Shoulder after rotator cuff repair: MR imaging findings in asymptomatic individuals—initial experience. Radiology 213:705-708, 1999.

401. Rand T, Freilinger W, Breitenseher M, et al: Magnetic resonance arthrography (MRA) in the postoperative shoulder. Magn Reson Imaging 17:843-850, 1999.

402. Longobardi RS, Rafii M, Minkoff J: MR imaging of the postoperative shoulder. Magn Reson Imaging Clin North Am 5:841-859, 1997.

403. Gusmer PB, Potter HG, Donovan WD, O'Brien SJ: MR imaging of the shoulder after rotator cuff repair. Am J Roentgenol 168:559-563, 1997.
404. Haygood TM, Oxner KG, Kneeland JB, Dalinka MK: Magnetic resonance imaging of the postoperative shoulder. Magn Reson Imaging Clin North Am 1:143-155, 1993.
405. Owen RS, Iannotti JP, Kneeland JB, et al: Shoulder after surgery: MR imaging with surgical validation. Radiology 186:443-447, 1993.
406. Allen AA, Drakos MC: Partial detachment of the deltoid muscle. A case report. Am J Sports Med 30:133-134, 2002.
407. Oxner KG: Magnetic resonance imaging of the musculoskeletal system. Part 6. The shoulder. Clin Orthop 354-373, 1997.
408. Mohana-Borges AV, Chung CB, Resnick D: MR imaging and MR arthrography of the postoperative shoulder: spectrum of normal and abnormal findings. RadioGraphics 24:69-85, 2004.
409. Rand T, Trattnig S, Breitenseher, et al: MR arthrography of the shoulder joint in a postoperative patient sample [French]. Radiologie 36:966-970, 1996.
410. Emig EW, Schweitzer ME, Karasick D, Lubowitz J: Adhesive capsulitis of the shoulder: MR diagnosis. Am J Roentgenol 164:1457-1459, 1995.
411. Zanetti M, Weishaupt D, Jost B, et al: MR imaging for traumatic tears of the rotator cuff: high prevalence of greater tuberosity fractures and subscapularis tendon tears. Am J Roentgenol 172:463-467, 1999.
412. Donnelly LF, Helms CA, Bisset GS, 3rd: Chronic avulsive injury of the deltoid insertion in adolescents: imaging findings in three cases. Radiology 211:233-236, 1999.
413. Gaffney KM: Avulsion injury of the serratus anterior: a case history. Clin J Sport Med 7:134-136, 1997.
414. Kono M, Johnson EE: Pectoralis major tendon avulsion in association with a proximal humerus fracture. J Orthop Trauma 10:508-510, 1996.
415. Dodds SD, Wolfe SW: Injuries to the pectoralis major. Sports Med 32:945-952, 2002.
416. Carrino JA, Chandnanni VP, Mitchell DB, et al: Pectoralis major muscle and tendon tears: diagnosis and grading using magnetic resonance imaging. Skeletal Radiol 29:305-313, 2000.
417. Ohashi K, El-Khoury GY, Albright JP, Tearse DS: MRI of complete rupture of the pectoralis major muscle. Skeletal Radiol 25:625-628, 1996.
418. Miller MD, Johnson DL, Fu FH, et al: Rupture of the pectoralis major muscle in a collegiate football player. Use of magnetic resonance imaging in early diagnosis. Am J Sports Med 21:475-477, 1993.
419. Hermann KG, Backhaus M, Schneider U, et al: Rheumatoid arthritis of the shoulder joint: comparison of conventional radiography, ultrasound, and dynamic contrast-enhanced magnetic resonance imaging. Arthritis Rheum 48:3338-3349, 2003.
420. Woodward TW, Best TM: The painful shoulder: part II. Acute and chronic disorders. Am Fam Physician 61:3291-3300, 2000.
421. Alasaarela E, Suramo I, Tervonen O, et al: Evaluation of humeral head erosions in rheumatoid arthritis: a comparison of ultrasonography, magnetic resonance imaging, computed tomography and plain radiography. Br J Rheumatol 37:1152-1156, 1998.
422. Alasaarela E, Takalo R, Tervonen O, et al: Sonography and MRI in the evaluation of painful arthritic shoulder. Br J Rheumatol 36:996-1000, 1997.
423. Kieft GJ, Sartoris DJ, Bloem JL, et al: Magnetic resonance imaging of glenohumeral joint diseases. Skeletal Radiol 16:285-290, 1987.
424. Kataria RK, Chaiamnuay S, Jacobson LD, Brent LH: Subacromial bursitis with rice bodies as the presenting manifestation of rheumatoid arthritis. J Rheumatol 30:1354-1355, 2003.
425. Kieft GJ, Dijkmans BA, Bloem JL, Kroon HM: Magnetic resonance imaging of the shoulder in patients with rheumatoid arthritis. Ann Rheum Dis 49:7-11, 1990.
426. Munk PL, Vellet AD, Levin MF, et al: Intravenous administration of gadolinium in the evaluation of rheumatoid arthritis of the shoulder. Can Assoc Radiol J 44:99-106, 1993.
427. Tong KM, Hsu KC, Lee TS, Chang SM: Diffuse pigmented villonodular synovitis of the shoulder: a case report. Zhonghua Yi Xue Za Zhi (Taipei) 53:188-192, 1994.
428. Muller LP, Bitzer M, Degreif J, Rommens PM: Pigmented villonodular synovitis of the shoulder: review and case report. Knee Surg Sports Traumatol Arthrosc 7:249-256, 1999.
429. Buess E, Friedrich B: Synovial chondromatosis of the glenohumeral joint: a rare condition. Arch Orthop Trauma Surg 121:109-111, 2001.
430. Ferraro FA, Winalski CS, Weissman BN: Magnetic resonance imaging of arthritides affecting the shoulder. Magn Reson Imaging Clin North Am 1:157-170, 1993.
431. Tuckman G, Wirth CZ: Synovial osteochondromatosis of the shoulder: MR findings. J Comput Assist Tomogr 13:360-361, 1989.
432. Burnstein MI, Fisher DR, Yandow DR, et al: Case report 502: Intra-articular synovial chondromatosis of shoulder with extra-articular extension. Skeletal Radiol 17:458-461, 1988.
433. Yu JS, Greenway G, Resnick D: Osteochondral defect of the glenoid fossa: cross-sectional imaging features. Radiology 206:35-40, 1988.
434. Shanley DJ, Mulligan ME: Osteochondrosis dissecans of the glenoid. Skeletal Radiol 19:419-421, 1990.
435. Greenan TJ, Zlatkin MB, Dalinka MK, Esterhai JL: Posttraumatic changes in the posterior glenoid and labrum in a handball player. Am J Sports Med 21:153-156, 1993.
436. Barber FA, Snyder SJ, Abrams JS, et al: Arthroscopic Bankart reconstruction with a bioabsorbable anchor. J Shoulder Elbow Surg 12:535-538, 2003.
437. Chan K, Skaf A, Roger B, Resnick DL: Glenoid articular rim disruption (GARD) and its relationship to osteochondritis dissecans: Routine radiography, standard arthrography, CT arthrography, and MR arthrography in eighteen patients. In Radiologic Society of North America Annual Meeting, Chicago, 1998, p 236.
438. Blacksin MF, Kloser PC, Simon J: Avascular necrosis of bone in human immunodeficiency virus infected patients. Clin Imaging 23:314-318, 1999.
439. Wing PC, Nance P, Connell DG, Gagnon F: Risk of avascular necrosis following short term megadose methylprednisolone treatment. Spinal Cord 36:633-636, 1998.
440. Patten RM, Shibata D, Reicher MA: Avascular necrosis of the humeral head. MR characteristics. In Society of Magnetic Resonance in Medicine, Book of Abstracts of Annual Society Meeting, 1990, p 192.
441. Chautems RC, Glauser T, Waeber-Fey MC, et al: Quadrilateral space syndrome: case report and review of the literature. Ann Vasc Surg 14:673-676, 2000.
442. Cormier PJ, Matalon TA, Wolin PM: Quadrilateral space syndrome: a rare cause of shoulder pain. Radiology 167:797-798, 1988.
443. Sofka CM, Lin J, Feinberg J, Potter HG: Teres minor denervation on routine magnetic resonance imaging of the shoulder. Skeletal Radiol 33:514-518, 2004.
444. Linker CS, Helms CA, Fritz RC: Quadrilateral space syndrome: findings at MR imaging. Radiology 188:675-676, 1993.
445. Turner JW, Parsonage MJ: Neuralgic amyotrophy (paralytic brachial neuritis); with special reference to prognosis. Lancet 273:209-212, 1957.
446. Helms CA, Martinez S, Speer KP: Acute brachial neuritis (Parsonage-Turner syndrome): MR imaging appearance—report of three cases. Radiology 207:255-259, 1998.
447. Misamore GW, Lehman DE: Parsonage-Turner syndrome (acute brachial neuritis). J Bone Joint Surg Am 78:1405-1408, 1996.
448. Helms CA: The impact of MR imaging in sports medicine. Radiology 224:631-635, 2002.

CHAPTER 100

MAGNETIC RESONANCE IMAGING OF THE ELBOW

Russell C. Fritz

INTRODUCTION

Magnetic resonance imaging provides clinically useful information in assessing the elbow joint. Superior depiction of muscles, ligaments, and tendons as well as the ability to directly visualize nerves, bone marrow, and hyaline cartilage are advantages of MR imaging relative to other imaging techniques. These features of MR imaging may help establish the cause of elbow pain and dysfunction by accurately depicting the presence and extent of bone and soft-tissue pathology.

Recent clinical experience has shown the utility of MR imaging in detecting and characterizing disorders of the elbow in a noninvasive fashion.[1-7] Direct visualization of the bone marrow makes MR imaging useful and accurate for evaluating osteomyelitis, tumor extension, radiographically occult fractures, and stress-related bony remodeling. Direct visualization of unossified cartilage makes MR imaging useful for evaluating fractures of the growth plate and epiphysis in children.[3,8] MR imaging is also the imaging procedure of choice for evaluating soft-tissue masses and nerve entrapment about the elbow.

IMAGING TECHNIQUES

The elbow may be scanned with the patient in a supine position and the arm at the side or with the patient prone and arm overhead (Fig. 100-1). The patient should be scanned in a comfortable position to avoid motion artifact. A surface coil is essential for obtaining high-quality images regardless of the field strength of the MR imaging system. Ongoing improvements in surface coil design have resulted in higher quality MR images of the elbow that can be obtained more rapidly.

We routinely perform fast spin-echo proton density images as well as fat-suppressed fast spin-echo T2-weighted images in the axial, sagittal, and coronal planes on high-field strength systems. We use short TI inversion recovery (STIR) instead of fat-suppressed T2-weighted images on lower field strength systems. We also use STIR when there is hardware present that distorts the images and results in heterogeneous fat suppression. The images without and with fat suppression are obtained in the exact same locations to facilitate analysis of the anatomy. Anatomic structures are identified on the proton density images and evaluated for their relative water content on the fat-suppressed T2-weighted images. It is essential to have properly displayed and photographed fat-suppressed T2-weighted images that allow differentiation between tissue and fluid. We have found that having control of the grayscale used for image display is quite useful when reading MR scans, therefore we typically interpret the images on computer workstations rather than using the hard-copy film for diagnosis.

We occasionally use intravenous gadolinium or intra-articular injections of dilute gadolinium or saline for problem solving. T1-weighted images with fat suppression are useful whenever gadolinium is administered, either intravenously or directly, into the elbow joint. Intravenous gadolinium may be useful when evaluating tumors and synovial processes about the elbow. MR arthrography may be useful for determination of osteochondral fragment stability in patients with osteochondritis dissecans and may also help to detect small undersurface tears of the medial collateral ligament.[9]

ELBOW ANATOMY

A thorough understanding of the anatomy and function of the elbow is essential for interpretation of the MR images. The anatomic structures of the elbow are reliably depicted with MR imaging. Knowledge of the relative

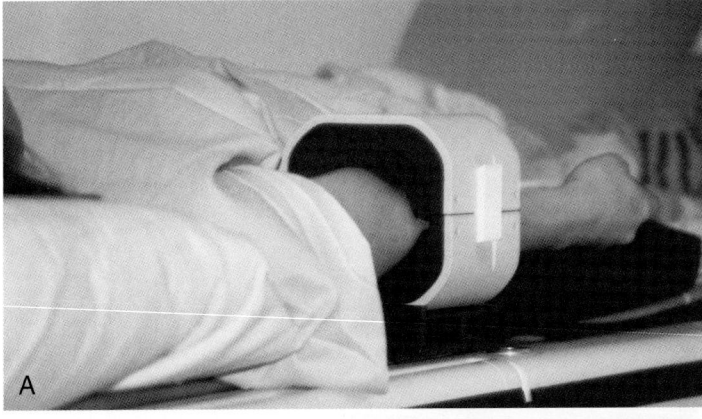

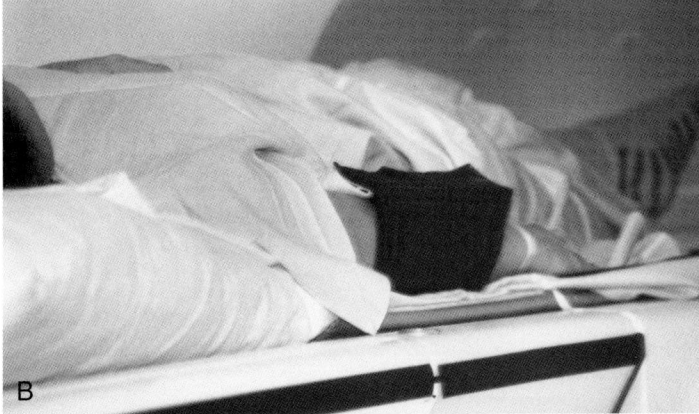

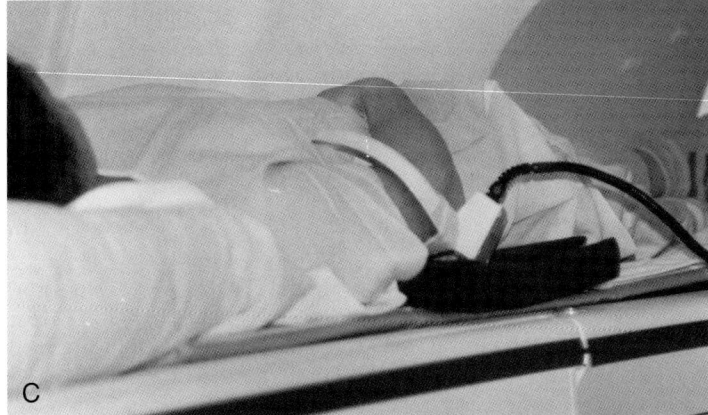

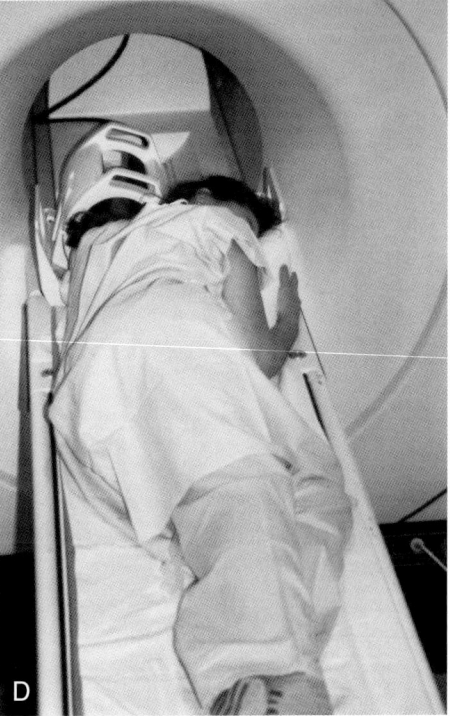

FIGURE 100-1

Surface coil options. **A,** This wrist coil produces excellent elbow images in children and relatively small adults. **B,** This flexible coil is similar to a blood pressure cuff. Even large patients can be scanned in a supine position with this "low profile" coil design. **C,** We have used this shoulder coil when patients cannot fit into smaller coils because of inability to fully extend the elbow. **D,** Larger patients may have to be scanned with the arm overhead in high-field small-bore magnets. This position can be quite uncomfortable, requiring rapid scanning.

functional significance of these structures allows assessment of the clinically important anatomy. Focusing on the relevant anatomic structures leads to more meaningful interpretation of the images and facilitates clinical problem solving.

The elbow is composed of three articulations contained within a common joint cavity. The radial head rotates within the radial notch of the ulna, allowing supination and pronation distally. The radial head is surrounded by the annular ligament that is best seen on the axial images. Disruption of the annular ligament results in proximal radioulnar joint instability. The radius articulates with the capitellum and the ulna articulates with the trochlea in a hinge fashion. The anterior and posterior portions of the joint capsule are relatively thin,

whereas the medial and lateral portions are thickened to form the collateral ligaments.

The medial collateral ligament complex (MCL) consists of anterior and posterior bundles as well as an oblique band also known as the transverse ligament. The transverse ligament and posterior bundle are well seen along the floor of the cubital tunnel on MR imaging. The anterior bundle provides the primary restraint to valgus stress and is commonly damaged in throwing athletes.[10] The functionally important anterior bundle of the MCL extends from the medial epicondyle to the medial aspect of the coronoid process (Fig. 100-2). The anterior fibers of the anterior bundle are taut in extension whereas the posterior fibers of the anterior bundle are taut in flexion, reciprocally tightening and loosening during flexion and

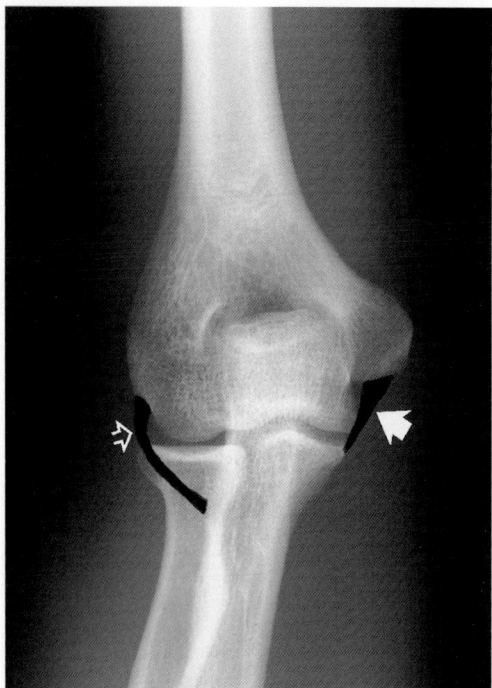

FIGURE 100-2

Primary ligamentous stabilizers of the elbow. The anterior bundle of the medial collateral ligament *(solid arrow)*, which extends from the medial epicondyle to the sublime tubercle of the ulna, provides the primary constraint to valgus stress. The lateral ulnar collateral ligament *(open arrow)*, which extends from the lateral epicondyle to the supinator crest along the lateral margin of the ulna, provides the primary constraint to varus stress.

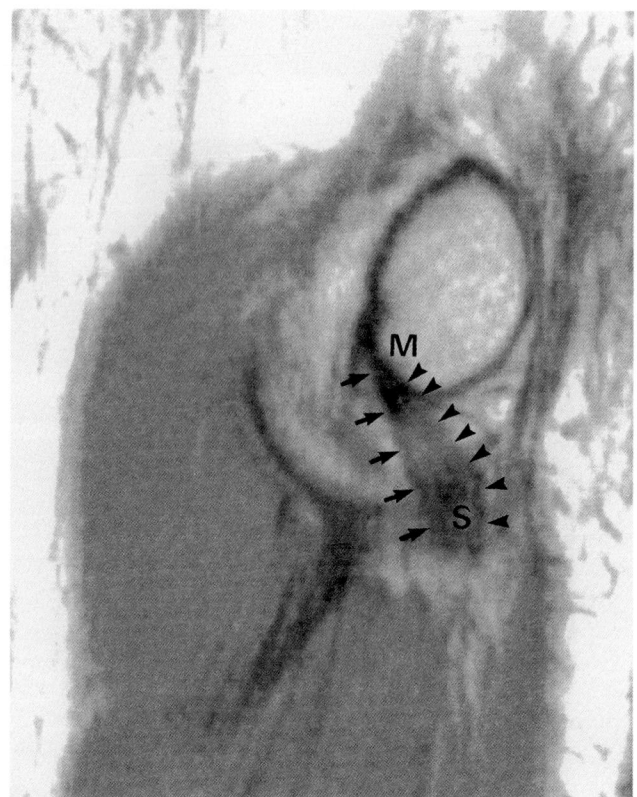

FIGURE 100-3

Normal anterior bundle of the medial collateral ligament (MCL). The anterior bundle of the MCL is well seen on this proton density sagittal image. The ligament extends from the anterior inferior aspect of the medial epicondyle (M) to the sublime tubercle of the ulna (S). The central fibers within the anterior bundle are isometric, remaining taut throughout the arc of flexion and extension. The anterior fibers *(arrows)* are taut in extension whereas the posterior fibers *(arrowheads)* are taut in flexion, undergoing reciprocal tightening and loosening.

extension.[11] The anterior bundle of the MCL arises from the anterior inferior aspect of the medial epicondyle and extends to the sublime tubercle of the ulna further distally. The ligament runs from anterior to posterior when the elbow is imaged in extension, and rotates anteriorly along with the ulna during flexion. This orientation of the anterior bundle of the MCL is well seen on sagittal images (Fig. 100-3). The ligament extends posteriorly towards the sublime tubercle whereas the components of the common flexor tendon extend anteriorly. This relationship is key to differentiating the ligament from the adjacent deep components of the common flexor tendon on axial images.

The lateral collateral ligament complex (LCL) can also be divided into separate components that can be evaluated with MR imaging.[7] The radial collateral ligament proper arises from the lateral epicondyle anteriorly and blends with the fibers of the annular ligament which surrounds the radial head. The annular ligament is the primary stabilizer of the proximal radioulnar joint and is best evaluated on axial images. A more posterior bundle, known as the lateral ulnar collateral ligament (LUCL), arises from the inferior aspect of the lateral epicondyle and extends along the posterior aspect of the radius to insert on the supinator crest of the ulna, adjacent to the most proximal fibers of the supinator muscle. The LUCL acts as a sling or guy-wire that provides the primary ligamentous restraint to varus

stress.[12] Disruption of the LUCL also results in a pivot shift phenomenon and posterolateral rotatory instability of the elbow.[13] Both the radial collateral ligament proper and the lateral ulnar collateral ligament are well seen progressing from anterior to posterior on the coronal images and should be considered separately because of the difference in functional significance of these structures.

The muscles of the elbow can be divided into anterior, posterior, medial, and lateral groups. The anterior group contains the biceps and brachialis muscles that are best evaluated on sagittal and axial images. The brachialis extends along the anterior joint capsule and inserts on the ulnar tuberosity. The biceps lies superficial to the brachialis and inserts on the radial tuberosity. The posterior group contains the triceps and anconeus muscles that are best evaluated on sagittal and axial images. The triceps inserts on the proximal aspect of the olecranon. The anconeus arises from the posterior aspect of the lateral epicondyle and inserts more distally on the olecranon. The anconeus provides dynamic support to the lateral collateral ligament in resisting varus stress. The medial and lateral muscles are best seen on coronal and

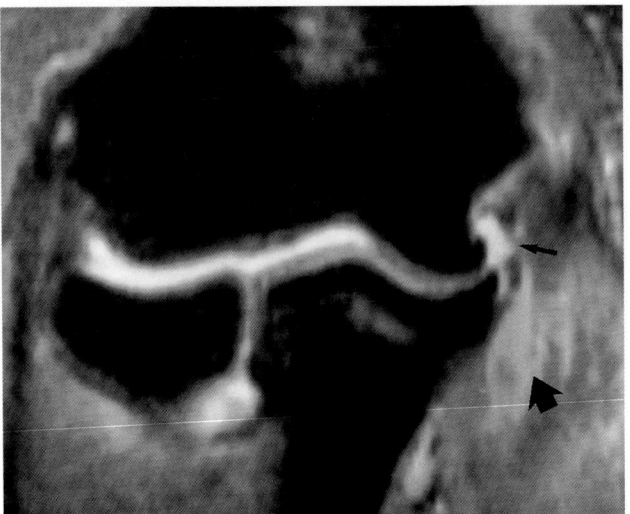

FIGURE 100-4

Muscle strain and partial tear of the medial collateral ligament (MCL). Rupture of the deep capsular fibers of the anterior bundle of the MCL is seen at its distal attachment to the ulna (*small arrow*). A strain of the adjacent flexor digitorum superficialis muscle is also noted (*large arrow*) on this T2*-weighted coronal image.

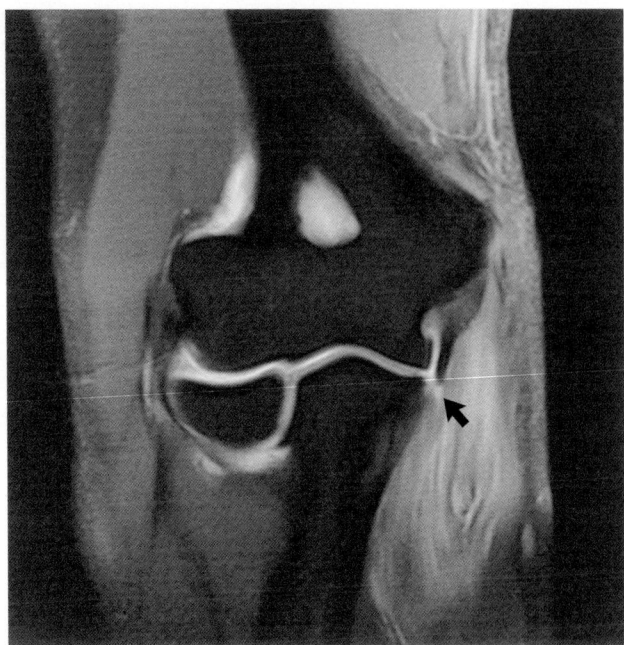

FIGURE 100-5

MR arthrogram of a complete avulsion of the medial collateral ligament (MCL). The anterior bundle of the MCL is torn from its distal attachment to the ulna (*arrow*). There is gadolinium contrast leaking from the elbow joint into the adjacent flexor digitorum superficialis muscle on this fat-suppressed T1-weighted coronal image.

axial images. The medial structures include the pronator teres and the flexors of the hand that arise from the medial epicondyle as the common flexor tendon. The common flexor tendon provides dynamic support to the MCL in resisting valgus stress. The lateral structures include the supinator, the brachioradialis, and the extensors of the hand that arise from the lateral epicondyle as the common extensor tendon.

The ulnar, median, and radial nerves are subject to entrapment in the elbow region. These nerves are normally surrounded by fat and are best seen on the axial images.

ELBOW PATHOLOGY

Valgus Stress Injury

Valgus stress injury in the elbow may occur secondary to chronic repetitive microtrauma or acute macrotrauma. A number of different conditions may occur secondary to the repeated valgus stress to the elbow that occurs with throwing. Medial tension overload typically produces extra-articular injury such as flexor/pronator strain, ulnar collateral ligament sprain, ulnar traction spurring, and ulnar neuropathy. Lateral compression overload typically produces intra-articular injury such as osteochondritis dissecans of the capitellum or radial head, degenerative arthritis, and loose body formation. MR imaging can detect and characterize each of these pathologic processes associated with repeated valgus stress. The information provided by MR imaging can be quite helpful in formulating a logical treatment plan, especially when surgery is being considered.

Medial Collateral Ligament Injury

Degeneration and tearing of the MCL with or without concomitant injury of the common flexor tendon commonly occurs in baseball pitchers and other throwers. Acute injury of the MCL can be detected, localized, and graded with MR imaging. The status of the functionally important anterior bundle of the MCL complex may be determined by assessing the axial and coronal images. Partial detachment of the deep undersurface fibers of the anterior bundle may occur in pitchers with medial elbow pain (Fig. 100-4). These partial tears of the MCL characteristically spare the superficial fibers of the anterior bundle and are therefore not visible from an open surgical approach unless the ligament is incised to inspect the torn capsular fibers.[14,15] As a result, MR imaging is important to localize these partial tears that may require ligament reconstruction. Detection of these undersurface partial tears may be improved when intra-articular contrast is administered and CT or MR arthrography is performed.[16] The capsular fibers of the anterior bundle of the MCL normally insert on the medial margin of the coronoid process. Undersurface partial tears of the anterior bundle are characterized by distal extension of fluid or contrast along the medial margin of the coronoid.[9]

Midsubstance MCL ruptures can be differentiated from proximal or distal avulsions (Fig. 100-5). Midsubstance ruptures of the MCL accounted for 87%, whereas distal and proximal avulsions were found in 10% and 3%, respectively, in a large series of surgically treated throwing

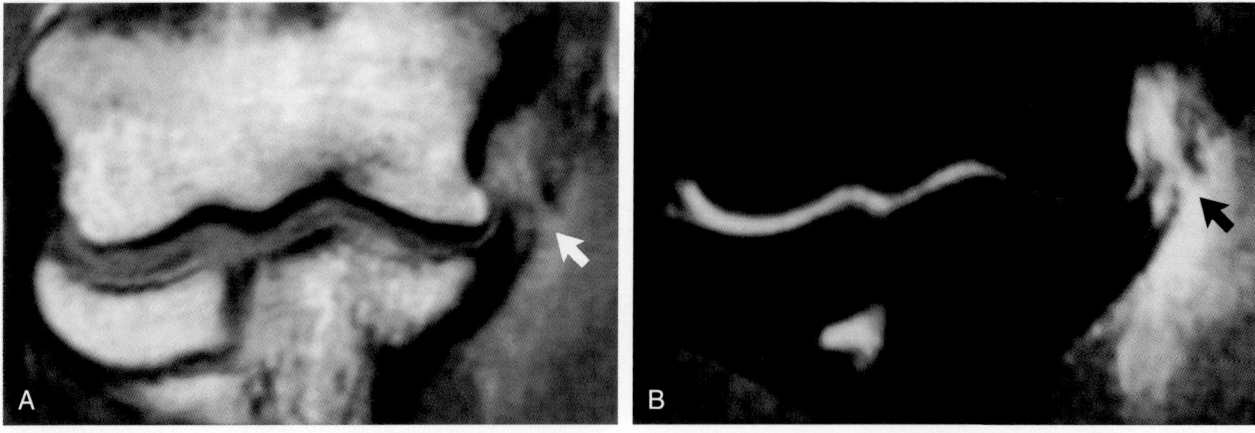

FIGURE 100-6

Medial collateral ligament (MCL) rupture in a 25-year-old baseball pitcher. T1-weighted (**A**) and STIR (**B**) coronal images reveal a midsubstance rupture of the anterior bundle of the MCL (arrows).

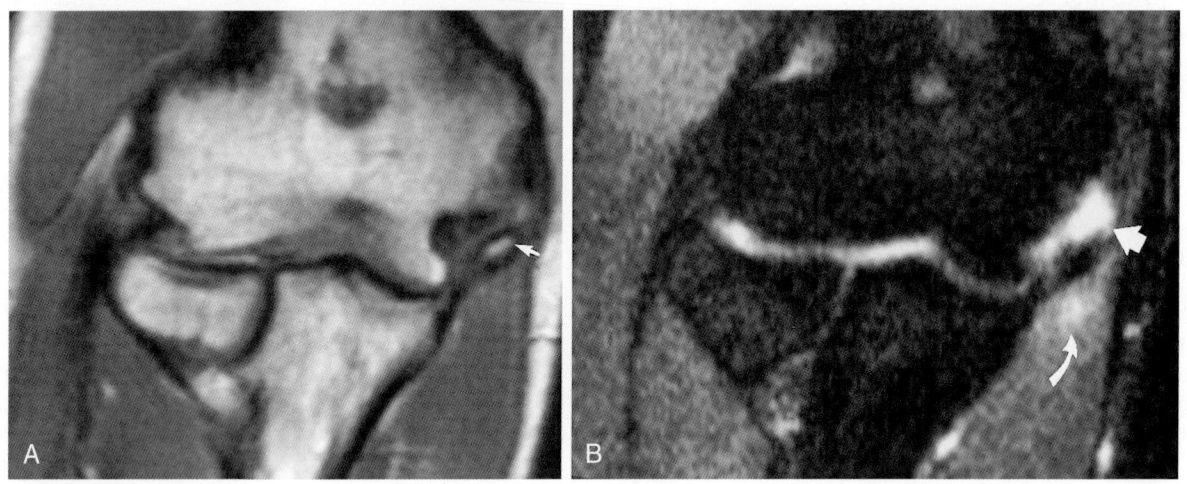

FIGURE 100-7

Chronic detachment of the MCL and acute muscle strain in a 16-year-old baseball player. T1-weighted (**A**) and STIR (**B**) coronal images reveal a small focus of heterotopic ossification (small arrow) versus an old apophyseal avulsion fracture which separates the anterior bundle of the MCL from the epicondyle (large arrow). A strain of the adjacent flexor digitorum superficialis muscle (curved arrow) as well as cubitus valgus is also noted.

athletes.[10] Others have found a lesser percentage of midsubstance ruptures.[17] The fibers of the flexor digitorum superficialis muscle blend with the anterior bundle of the MCL.[15] A strain of the flexor digitorum superficialis muscle is commonly seen when the MCL is injured (Fig. 100-6). Ulnar traction spurs are commonly seen at the insertion of the MCL on the coronoid process due to repetitive valgus stress, occurring in 75% of professional baseball pitchers.[18] Chronic degeneration of the MCL is characterized by thickening of the ligament secondary to scarring which often contains foci of calcification or heterotopic bone (Fig. 100-7).[19] The findings are similar to those seen after healing of medial collateral ligament sprains in the knee, in which the development of heterotopic ossification has been termed the Pellegrini-Stieda phenomenon. Patients with symptomatic MCL insufficiency are usually treated with recon-

struction using a palmaris tendon graft. Graft failure is unusual but may also be evaluated with MR imaging (Fig. 100-8). Lateral compartment bone contusions are occasionally seen in association with acute MCL tears and may provide useful confirmation of recent lateral compartment impaction secondary to valgus instability (see Fig. 100-8).

Medial Epicondylitis

Medial epicondylitis, also known as golfer's elbow, pitcher's elbow or "medial tennis elbow", is less common than lateral epicondylitis.[20] This condition is caused by degeneration of the common flexor tendon secondary to overload of the flexor/pronator muscle group which arises from the medial epicondyle.[21] The spectrum of

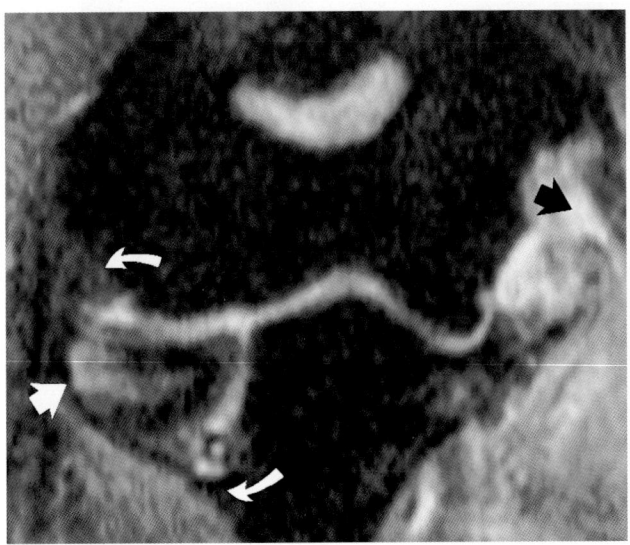

FIGURE 100-8

MCL graft rupture and contusion of the radial head in a professional baseball player. A STIR coronal image reveals increased signal at the site of a ruptured MCL graft *(black arrow)*. Increased signal is also seen within the lateral portion of the radial head secondary to impaction from valgus insufficiency *(white arrow)*. The normal LUCL is also well seen *(curved white arrows)*.

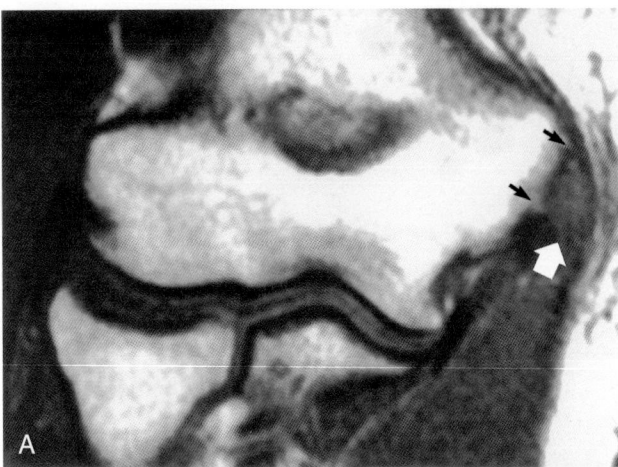

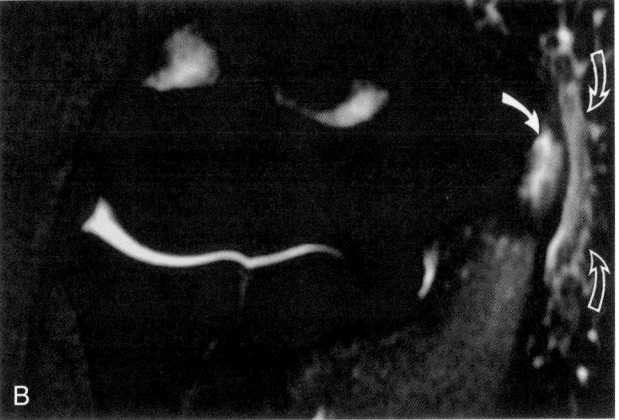

FIGURE 100-9

Medial epicondylitis in a 42-year-old golfer. **A,** A T1-weighted coronal image reveals increased signal in the common flexor tendon *(large arrow)* and spurring of the medial epicondyle *(small arrows)*. **B,** A STIR coronal image reveals a fluid-filled intrasubstance partial tear within the tendon *(solid curved arrow)* as well as edema in the overlying subcutaneous fat compatible with surrounding inflammation *(open curved arrows)*.

damage to the muscle-tendon unit that may be characterized with MR imaging includes muscle strain injury, tendon degeneration (tendinosis), and macroscopic tendon disruption.

MR imaging is useful for detecting and characterizing acute muscle injury as well as following its resolution. The STIR sequence is the most sensitive for detecting muscle pathology. The common flexor tendon and MCL should be carefully evaluated for associated tearing when there is evidence of muscle strain injury on MR imaging. Alternatively, increased signal intensity on STIR and T2-weighted sequences may be seen following an intramuscular injection and persist for as long as one month. Abnormal signal intensity within a muscle may simply be due to the effect of a therapeutic injection for epicondylitis rather than an indication of muscle strain. Inquiring if and when a steroid injection was performed may be useful in recognizing this phenomenon; this information may be easily obtained from the patient questionnaire at the time of MR imaging.

A normal muscle-tendon unit will tear at the myotendinous junction. Tendon degeneration (tendinosis) is quite common about the elbow as patients age so that failure of an overloaded muscle-tendon unit may occur through this weakened tendon tissue.[22] The degree of tendon degeneration and injury can be characterized with MR imaging (Fig. 100-9). Medial and lateral epicondylitis may occur concurrently secondary to flexor and extensor tendinosis (Fig. 100-10). MR imaging can determine if there is tendinosis secondary to degeneration versus macroscopic partial tearing or complete rupture.

The coronal, sagittal, and axial sequences are all useful for assessing the degree of tendon injury (Fig. 100-11).

MR imaging facilitates surgical planning by delineating and grading tears of the common flexor tendon as well as evaluating the underlying MCL and adjacent ulnar nerve (Fig. 100-12). The increased preoperative diagnostic information may lessen the need for extensive surgical exploration in cases in which the MCL is clearly intact on MR imaging. In addition, MR imaging may be useful for problem solving in patients who develop recurrent symptoms after surgery for medial or lateral epicondylitis (Fig. 100-13).

In skeletally immature individuals, the flexor muscle-tendon unit may fail at the unfused apophysis of the medial epicondyle. Stress fracture, avulsion or delayed closure of the medial epicondylar apophysis may occur in young baseball players secondary to overuse (Little Leaguer's elbow). MR imaging may detect these injuries prior to complete avulsion and displacement by revealing soft-tissue or marrow edema about the medial epicondylar apophysis on fat-suppressed T2-weighted or STIR images.[23]

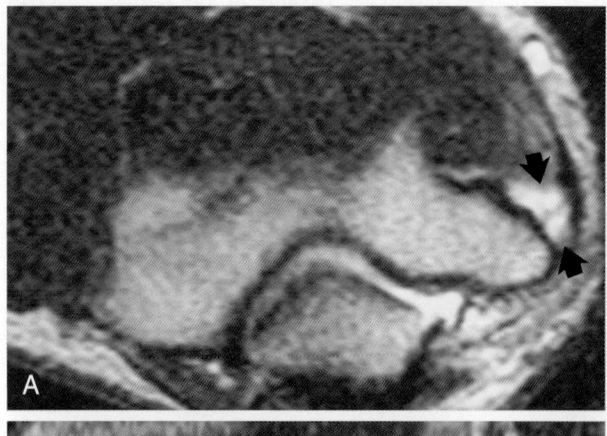
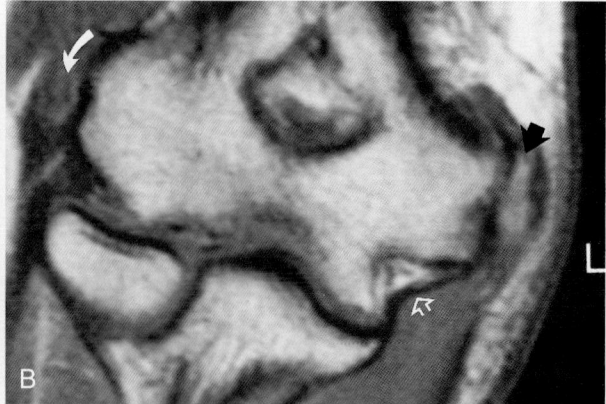
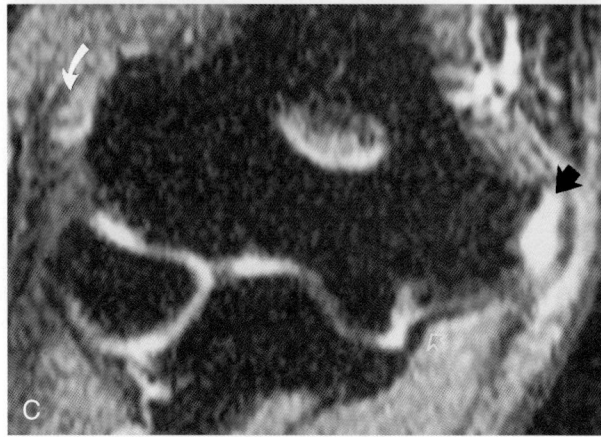

FIGURE 100-10

Severe medial epicondylitis and mild lateral epicondylitis in a 63-year-old golfer. T2-weighted axial (arrows) (**A**) as well as T1-weighted (**B**) and STIR (**C**) coronal images reveal increased signal and poor definition of the common flexor tendon adjacent to the medial epicondyle (black arrows) compatible with a complete tear. Mild thickening and increased signal of the common extensor tendon are seen (curved white arrows) compatible with mild tendinosis. A normal anterior bundle of the medial collateral ligament (open arrows) is also well seen on the coronal images.

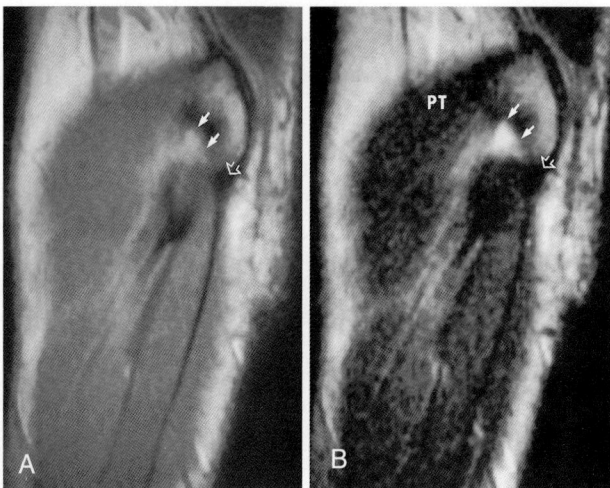

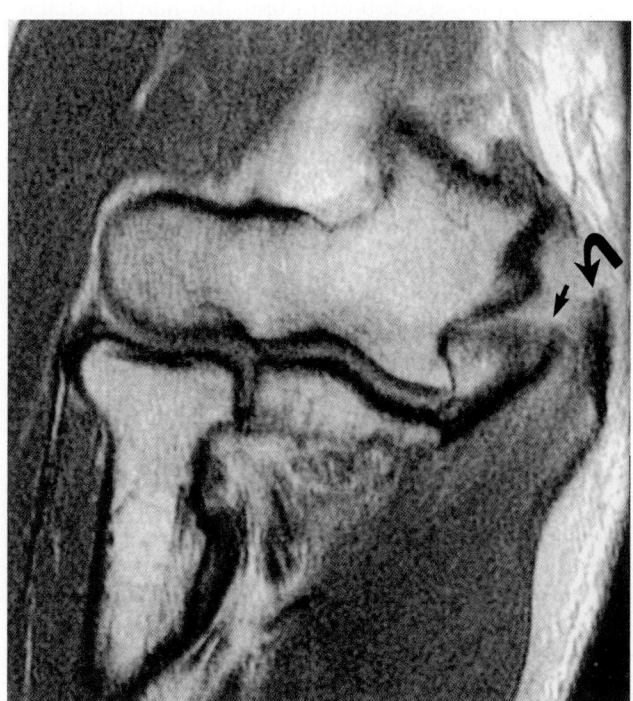

FIGURE 100-11

High-grade tear of the common flexor tendon in a professional quarterback. Proton density (**A**) and T2-weighted (**B**) sagittal images reveal fluid separating the anterior fibers of the common flexor tendon from the medial epicondyle (white arrows). The flexor carpi ulnaris portion of the tendon remains attached posteriorly (open arrow). PT, pronator teres muscle.

FIGURE 100-12

Acute rupture of the common flexor tendon and the medial collateral ligament while arm wrestling. A proton density coronal image reveals detachment of the common flexor tendon (curved arrow) and the underlying anterior bundle of the medial collateral ligament (straight arrow) from the medial epicondyle. There were two successive popping sounds when the ligament and then the tendon gave way as this patient lost the arm-wrestling match.

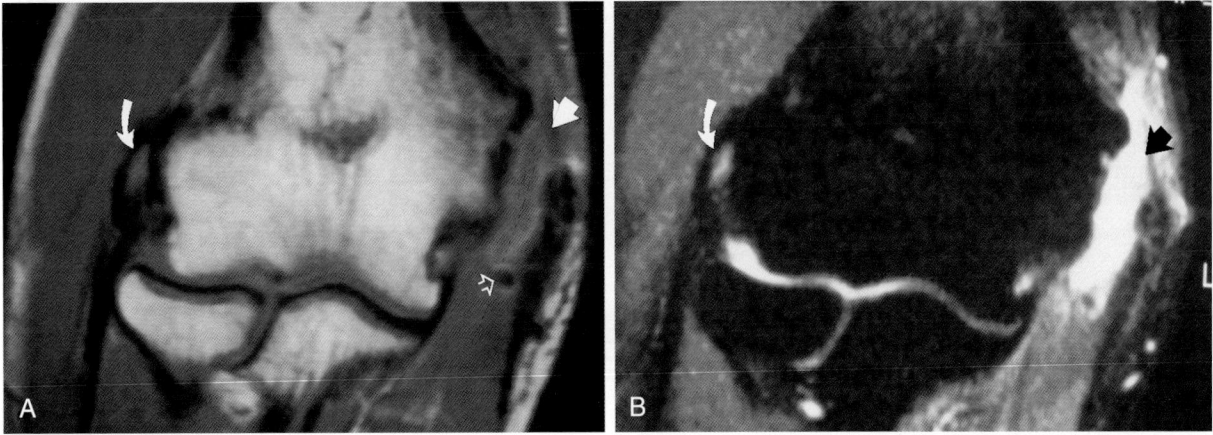

FIGURE 100-13

Reruptured common flexor tendon. T1-weighted (**A**) and STIR (**B**) coronal images reveal complete rupture of a previously repaired common flexor tendon from the medial epicondyle *(large arrows)*. Postoperative micrometallic artifact is seen adjacent to the distally retracted tendon *(open arrow)*. A small partial tear of the common extensor noted is also noted *(curved arrows)*.

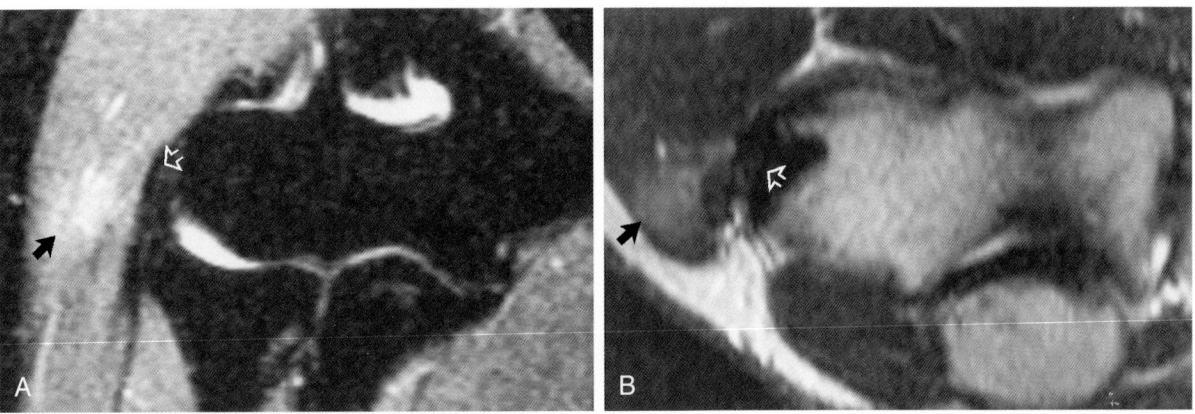

FIGURE 100-14

Clinically suspected tennis elbow in a patient who did not respond to a local steroid injection. A STIR coronal image (**A**) and a T2-weighted axial image (**B**) reveal a completely normal common extensor tendon *(open arrows)* as well as increased signal within the adjacent extensor carpi radialis longus muscle *(solid arrows)* secondary to a recent steroid injection. Abnormal signal may persist for weeks after an injection and be mistaken for primary muscle pathology on MR imaging.

Lateral Epicondylitis

Lateral epicondylitis, also referred to as tennis elbow, is caused by degeneration and tearing of the common extensor tendon.[20] This condition often occurs as a result of repetitive sports-related trauma to the tendon, although it is seen far more commonly in nonathletes. In the typical case, the degenerated extensor carpi radialis brevis tendon is partially avulsed from the lateral epicondyle. Scar tissue forms in response to this partial avulsion, which is then susceptible to further tearing with repeated trauma. Histologic studies have clearly demonstrated angiofibroblastic tendinosis with a lack of inflammation in the surgical specimens of patients with lateral epicondylitis;[20,24] indeed, the abnormal signal seen on MR images is secondary to tendon degeneration and repair rather than tendinitis. Local steroid injections are commonly used to treat lateral epicondylitis and may increase the risk of tendon rupture. Signal alteration in the region of a local steroid injection should not be confused with primary muscle pathology on MR imaging (Fig. 100-14).

Overall, 4% to 10% of cases of lateral epicondylitis are resistant to conservative therapy[20,25]; MR imaging is useful in assessing the degree of tendon damage in such cases. Tendon degeneration (tendinosis) is manifested by normal to increased tendon thickness with increased signal intensity on short TE images that remains less than the signal intensity of fluid on T2-weighted images (Fig. 100-15). Partial tears are characterized by thinning of the tendon that is outlined by adjacent fluid on the T2-weighted images (Fig. 100-16). Tendinosis and tearing

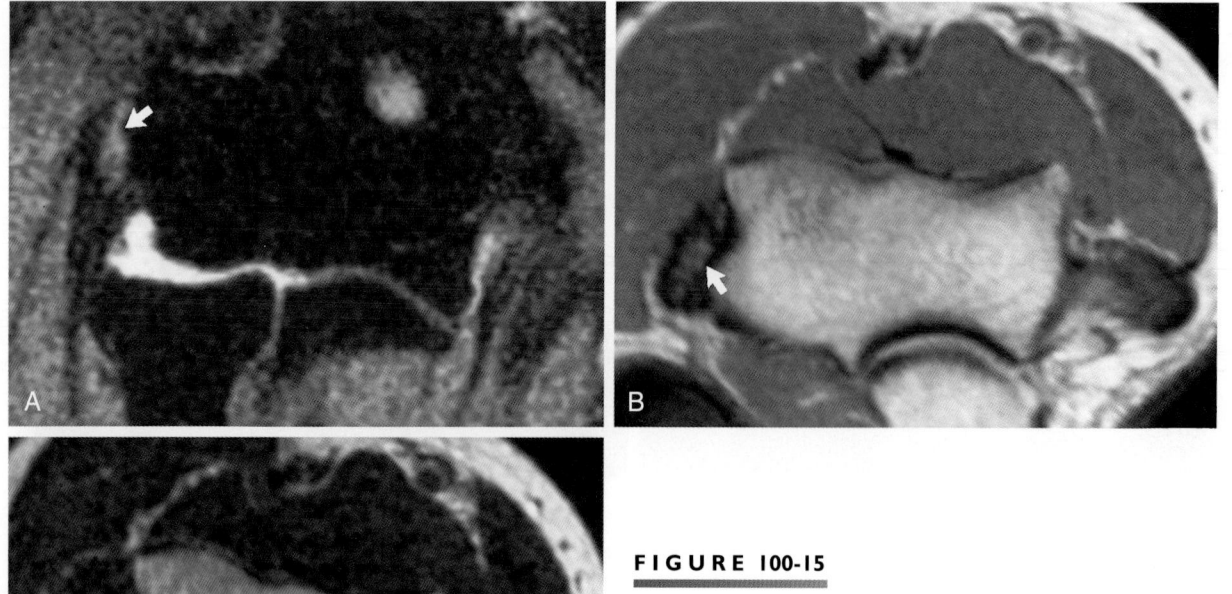

FIGURE 100-15

Tennis elbow secondary to mild tendinosis. A STIR coronal image (**A**) as well as proton density (**B**) and T2-weighted (**C**) axial images reveal faint increased signal within the fibers of the common extensor tendon *(arrows)*. The abnormal signal is much less intense than joint fluid and is compatible with tendinosis.

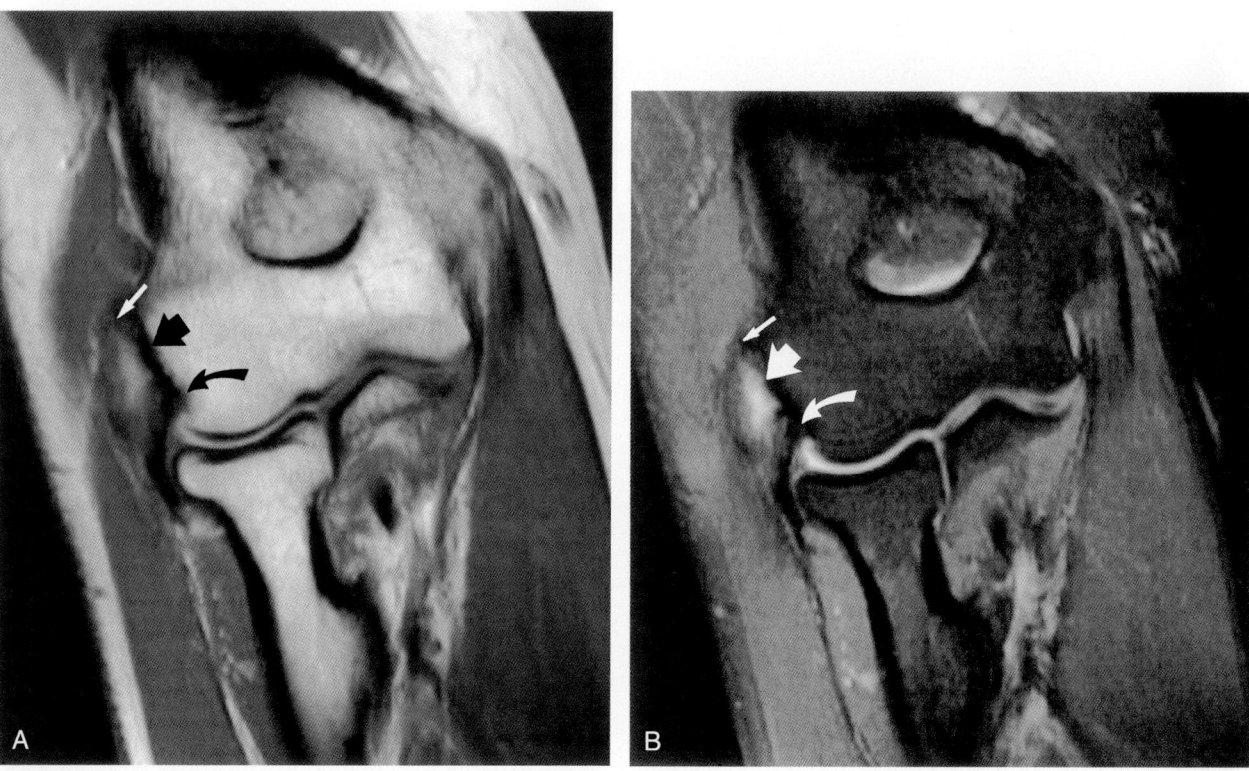

FIGURE 100-16

Forty-year-old tennis player with lateral elbow pain and a high-grade partial tear of the common extensor tendon. Proton density (**A**) and fat-suppressed T2-weighted (**B**) coronal images reveal a fluid-filled defect in the common extensor tendon *(large straight arrows)*. The majority of the tendon is torn, however, the most superficial tendon fibers remain attached to the proximal aspect of the lateral epicondyle *(small straight arrows)*. The underlying lateral collateral ligament *(curved arrows)* is intact.

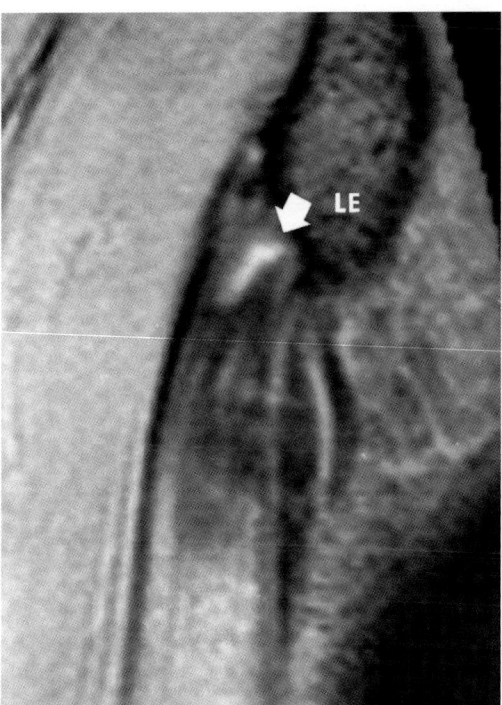

FIGURE 100-17

Partial tear of the extensor carpi radialis brevis. A T2*-weighted sagittal image reveals a small tear *(arrow)* involving the anterior attachment of the common extensor tendon to the lateral epicondyle (LE).

typically involve the extensor carpi radialis brevis portion of the common extensor tendon anteriorly (Fig. 100-17). Complete tears may be diagnosed on MR imaging by identifying a fluid-filled gap separating the tendon from its adjacent bony attachment site.

At surgery for lateral epicondylitis, 97% of the tendons appear scarred and edematous and 35% have macroscopic tears.[20] MR imaging is useful in identifying high-grade partial tears and complete tears which are unlikely to improve with rest and repeated steroid injections. In addition to determining the degree of tendon damage, MR imaging also provides a more global assessment of the elbow and is therefore able to detect additional pathologic conditions that may explain the lack of a therapeutic response. For example, unsuspected ruptures of the lateral collateral ligament complex may occur in association with tears of the common extensor tendon (Fig. 100-18). Morrey has reported a series of 13 patients who underwent reoperation for failed lateral epicondylitis surgery; stabilization procedures were required in four patients with either iatrogenic or unrecognized lateral ligament insufficiency.[26] Iatrogenic tears of the LUCL may occur secondary to overaggressive release of the common extensor tendon (Fig. 100-19). MR imaging can reveal concurrent tears of the LUCL and common extensor tendon in patients with lateral epicondylitis as well as isolated LUCL tears in patients with posterolateral rotatory instability.[1] Moreover, the lack of a significant abnormality involving the common extensor tendon on MR imaging may prompt consideration of an alternative diagnosis such as radial nerve entrapment that may mimic or accompany lateral epicondylitis.[27,28]

Bone Injury

Radiographically occult or equivocal fractures may be assessed with MR imaging, which can be performed with the patient in a cast with only minor degradation of the image quality. A large cast may require using a larger surface coil such as the head coil. In general, the findings of bone injury may be subtle on proton density, T2-weighted, and T2*-weighted sequences and are more conspicuous on T1-weighted, fat-suppressed, T2-weighted or STIR sequences.

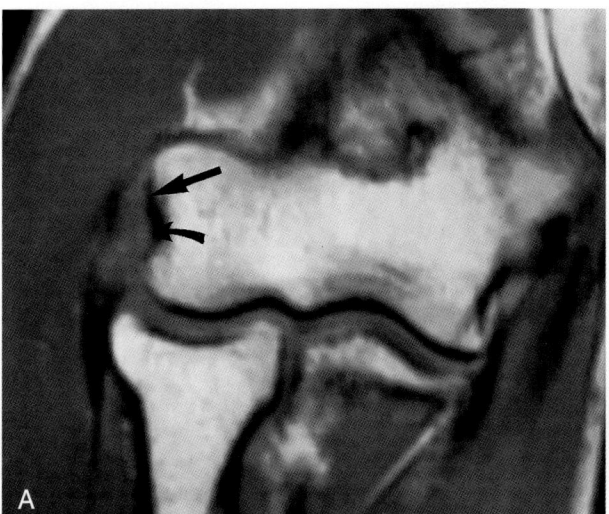
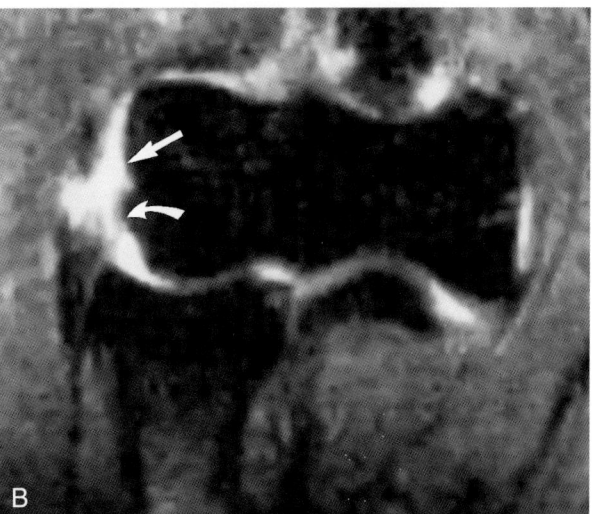

FIGURE 100-18

Lateral epicondylitis in a 40-year-old golfer. T1-weighted (**A**) and STIR (**B**) coronal images reveal a complete tear of the common extensor tendon *(straight arrows)* and a tear of the underlying lateral collateral ligament *(curved arrows)*.

An anterior coronoid process fracture or bone contusion may be seen after posterior elbow dislocation or subluxation that may occur as a consequence of hyperextension injury or a fall on the outstretched arm (Fig. 100-20). These fractures may be subtle on standard radiographs and may predispose to recurrent posterior instability if large and associated with ligament injury.[12,29] Coronoid process fractures occur as a result of direct shear injury by the trochlea during posterior subluxation or dislocation injury and can be seen in association with radial head fractures (Fig. 100-21). Anterior capsular injury and strain of the adjacent brachialis muscle as well as medial and lateral collateral ligament injury are also commonly seen with MR imaging after posterior elbow dislocation.

Chronic lateral impaction may lead to osteochondritis dissecans of the capitellum or radial head in adolescent pitchers or gymnasts. Repeated valgus stress and a relatively tenuous blood supply within the capitellum has been proposed to explain the frequent occurrence of osteochondritis dissecans in this location. Stable osteochondral lesions are usually treated with rest and splinting whereas unstable lesions are either pinned or excised.[30] MR imaging can reliably detect and stage these lesions. Unstable lesions are characterized by fluid encircling the osteochondral fragment on fat-suppressed T2-weighted images. Loose in situ lesions may also be diagnosed by identifying a cyst-like lesion beneath the osteochondral fragment. These apparent "cysts" typically contain loose granulation tissue at surgery rather than fluid, explaining why they may enhance after IV administration of gadolinium.[31]

Osteochondritis dissecans should be distinguished from osteochondrosis of the capitellum which is known as Panner's disease. Osteochondritis dissecans is typically seen in the 13-16 year age range whereas Panner's disease is typically seen in the 5-10 year range. Loose body formation and significant residual deformity of the capitellum are concerns in osteochondritis dissecans but are usually not seen in Panner's disease. Panner's disease is characterized by fragmentation and abnormally decreased signal intensity within the ossifying capitellar epiphysis on short TE images similar in appearance to Legg-Calve-Perthes disease in the hip; subsequent scans reveal normalization of these changes with little or no residual deformity of the capitellar articular surface.

Unstable osteochondral lesions may fragment and migrate throughout the joint as loose bodies. These loose bodies may attach to the synovial lining of the joint and undergo laminar growth with variably thick hyaline cartilage. Loose bodies may become quite large and result in mechanical symptoms such as locking and limitation of motion. Loose bodies are usually arthroscopically removed when detected as they may lead to premature degenerative arthritis in addition to their effects on joint function.

Laxity of the MCL in throwing athletes may lead to incongruity between the medial olecranon and the medial aspect of the olecranon fossa, resulting in loose body formation.[32] These posterior compartment loose bodies frequently occur in baseball pitchers and may be well seen when joint fluid is present (Fig. 100-22). Small loose bodies may be difficult to exclude with conventional MR imaging in the absence of an effusion. Direct intra-articular administration of saline or dilute gadolinium

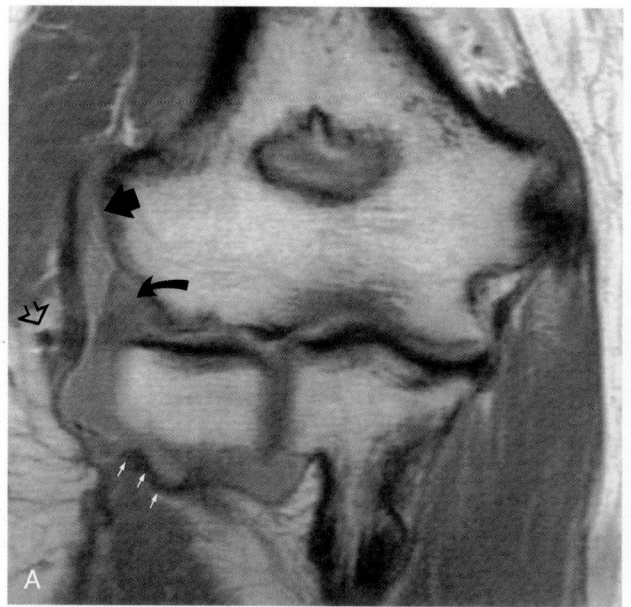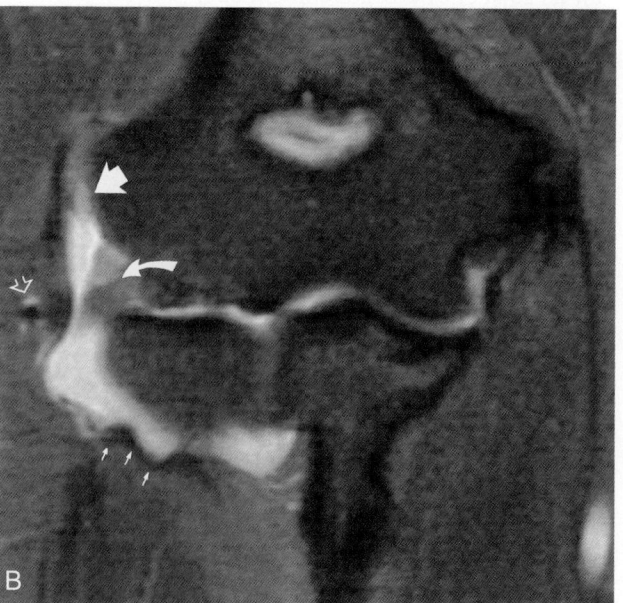

FIGURE 100-19

Torn lateral ulnar collateral ligament (LUCL) in a patient who developed posterolateral rotatory instability after extensor tendon release. Proton density (**A**) and fat-suppressed T2-weighted (**B**) coronal images reveal a fluid-filled defect in the common extensor tendon (*large straight arrows*). A frayed, thickened stump of the underlying lateral collateral ligament (*curved arrows*) remains attached to the inferior aspect of the lateral epicondyle. The distal fibers of the ligament (*small arrows*) are retracted and appear lax. Micrometallic artifact is noted from prior surgical release (*open arrows*).

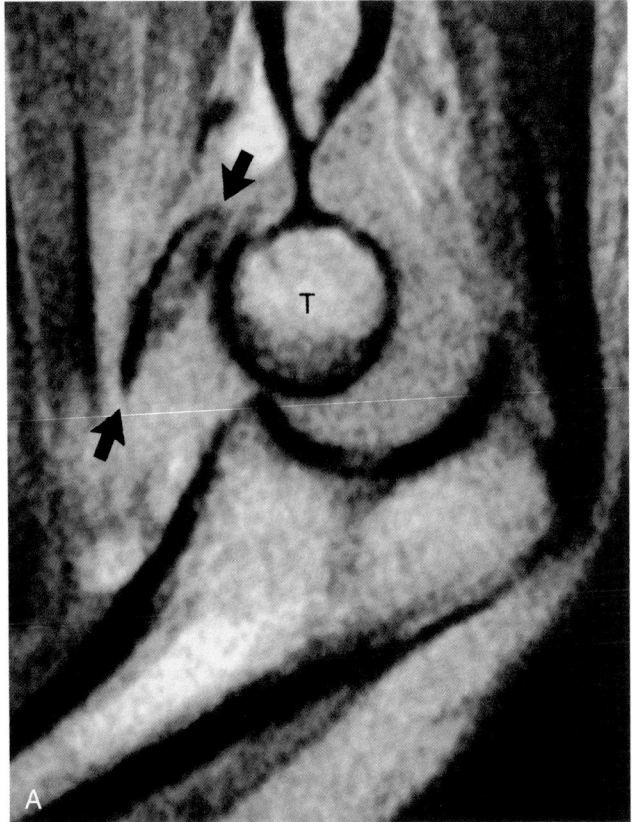

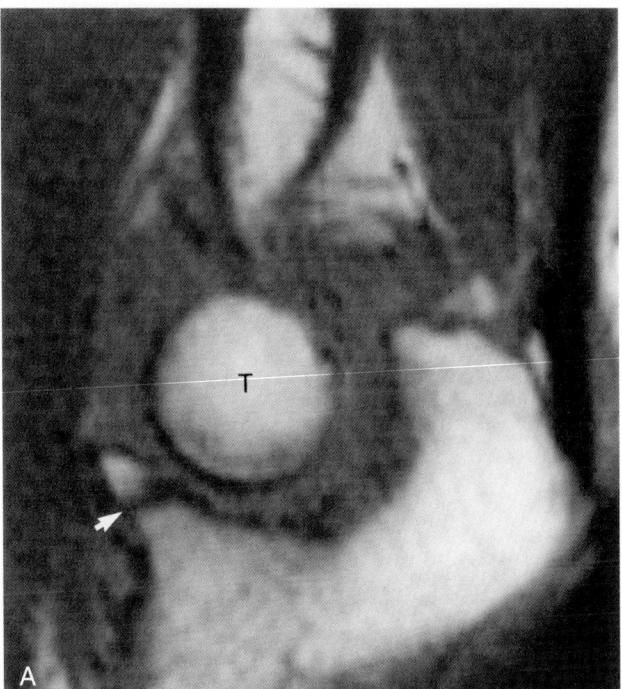

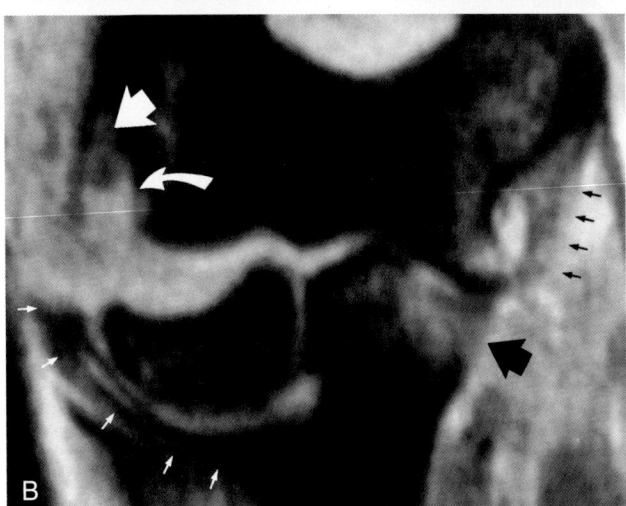

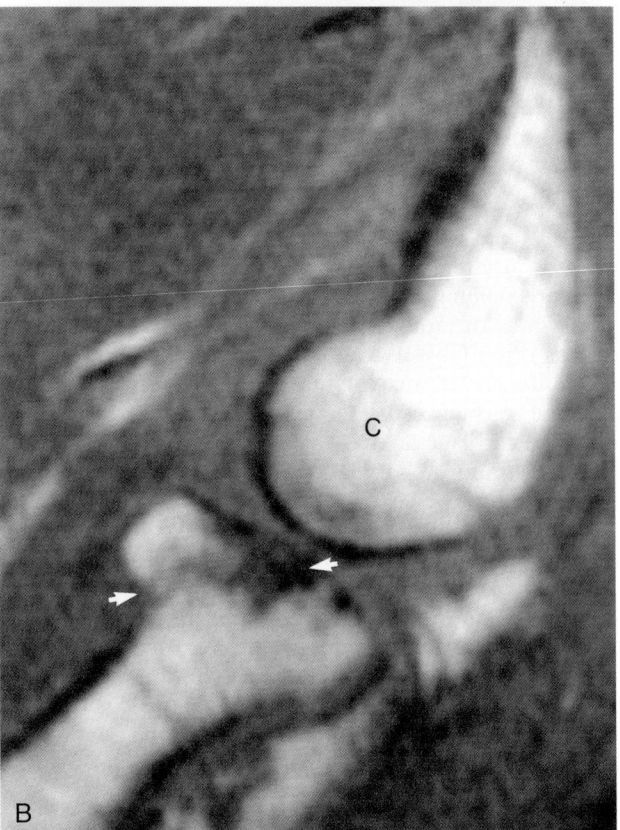

FIGURE 100-20

Rupture of the collateral ligaments and common extensor tendon as well as a coronoid process fracture. This patient had persistent instability after a posterior dislocation of the elbow. **A,** A proton density sagittal image reveals posterior subluxation of the ulna and a large fracture of the coronoid process *(arrows)* that is superiorly displaced. T, trochlea. **B,** A fat-suppressed STIR coronal image reveals a complete tear of the common extensor tendon *(large white arrow)* and the underlying lateral collateral ligament *(curved white arrow)* from the lateral epicondyle. The distal ligament fibers *(small white arrows)* can be seen extending to the supinator crest of the ulna. The anterior bundle of the medial collateral ligament is torn from the sublime tubercle of the ulna *(large black arrow)*. The proximal ligament fibers *(small black arrows)* can be seen extending to the medial epicondyle.

FIGURE 100-21

Radiograpically occult fractures secondary to a fall while skiing. A T1-weighted sagittal image (**A**) reveals a nondisplaced fracture of the tip of the coronoid process of the ulna *(arrow)*. T, trochlea. A T1-weighted sagittal image (**B**) reveals a nondisplaced fracture of the radial head *(arrows)*. C, capitellum.

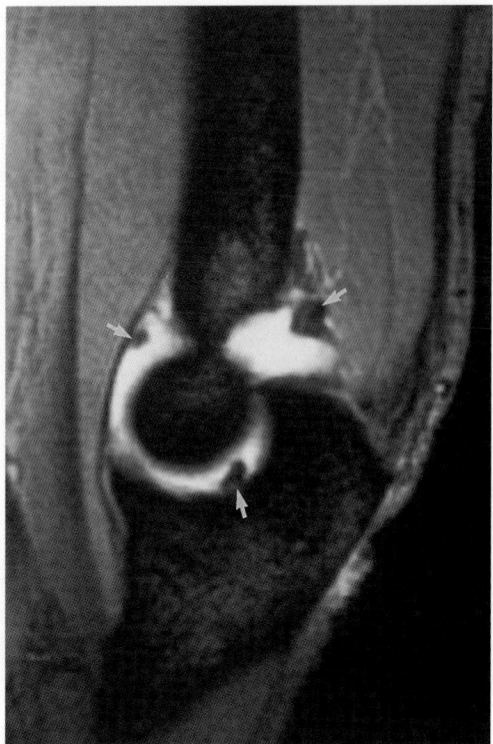

FIGURE 100-22

Multiple loose bodies in a pitcher with intermittent locking of the elbow. A T2*-weighted sagittal image reveals a large joint effusion which increases the conspicuity of multiple loose bodies *(arrows)*.

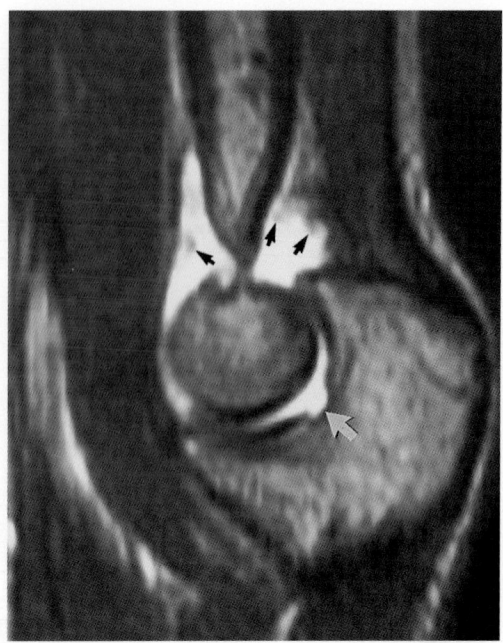

FIGURE 100-23

Saline MR arthrography. A T2-weighted sagittal image obtained after intra-articular saline injection reveals irregular synovial thickening *(black arrows)* compatible with synovitis. A normal, variably sized depression in the trochlear notch of the ulna is noted *(white arrow)* that should not be mistaken for an osteochondral defect. Small loose bodies may lodge in this trough that has been termed the *bare area* of the ulna.

may be useful for identifying small loose bodies and synovitis when there is no evidence of a joint effusion on exam or with radiographs (Fig. 100-23). Chondral loose bodies often have a geographic appearance with a thin black line on MR imaging representing either the surface layer of cartilage (the lamina splendens) or the deep calcified cartilage layer.

Detection of a chondral defect should lead to a careful search for a corresponding loose body (Fig. 100-24). Conversely, the articular cartilage should be inspected carefully on MR imaging when a loose body is detected. An unstable flap of articular cartilage may result in mechanical symptoms such as intermittent locking of the elbow joint. Subarticular bone marrow edema may be an important clue to a deep fissure, chondral flap lesion or chondral defect on MR imaging (Fig. 100-25). A fluid-filled fissure that is parallel to the surface of the articular cartilage may be a clue to a nondisplaced chondral flap lesion on MR imaging (Fig. 100-26). An unstable flap of articular cartilage may ultimately break off and result in a loose body. Unstable chondral flap lesions are typically treated with arthroscopic debridement.

Loss of motion may be due to loose bodies or capsular scarring and contracture that can be detected with MR imaging.[33] Patients with osteoarthritis may develop osteophytes in the olecranon fossa posteriorly that limit full extension as well as osteophytes in the radial fossa or coronoid fossa anteriorly that limit full flexion of the elbow (Fig. 100-27).

Stress fractures of the middle third of the olecranon may occur in throwing athletes as a consequence of overload by the triceps mechanism (Fig. 100-28). These fractures have the potential to displace and are usually treated surgically.[34,35] Similar chronic extension overload in adolescent baseball pitchers leads to nonunion of the olecranon physeal plate that may also require surgery. MR imaging can detect these lesions that may be difficult to diagnose clinically and radiographically.

While MR imaging is quite sensitive to abnormalities of the marrow space, the appearance is often non-specific and close clinical correlation is essential. For example, the appearance of a bone contusion secondary to acute macrotrauma may resemble a stress reaction or stress response secondary to repetitive microtrauma and overuse (Fig. 100-29). An infiltrative neoplasm or early osteomyelitis could also be confused with these traumatic processes (Fig. 100-30).

MR imaging may identify or exclude radial head fractures in adults as well as supracondylar and lateral condylar fractures in children when radiographic evidence of a joint effusion is present and a fracture is not visualized (Fig. 100-31). Injury to the physis as well as the unossified epiphyseal cartilage may be assessed with MR imaging in difficult pediatric cases when the plain film findings are equivocal.[3,36,37] Early diagnosis and proper treatment of these injuries are essential to avoid complications such as nonunion and deformity of the elbow (Fig. 100-32).

Text continues on page 3297

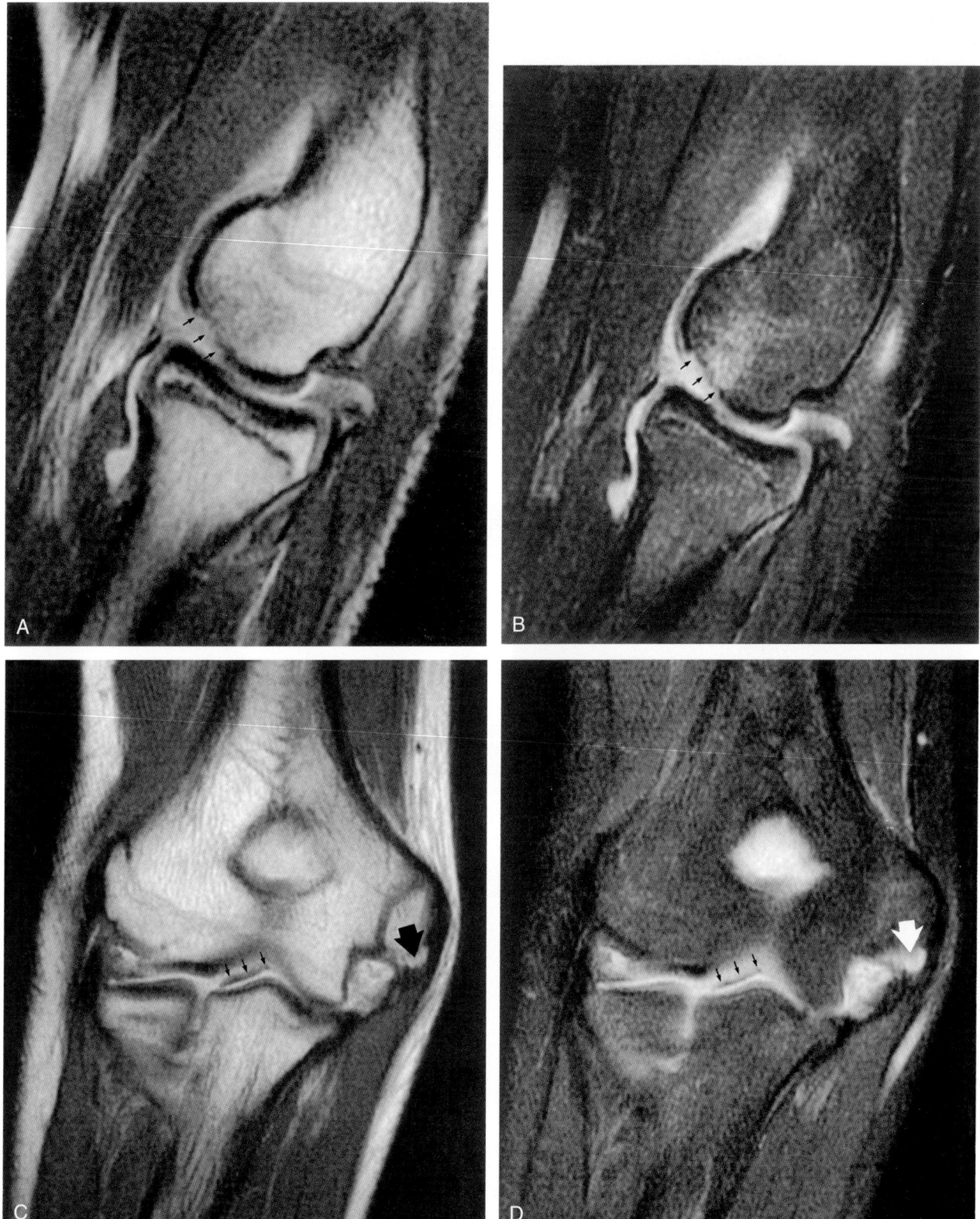

F I G U R E 100-24

Sixteen-year-old baseball pitcher with pain and mechanical symptoms. Proton density (**A**) and fat-suppressed T2-weighted (**B**) sagittal images reveal an osteochondral defect *(arrows)* of the capitellum with underlying bone marrow edema. Proton density (**C**) and fat-suppressed (**D**) coronal images reveal a thin loose body *(arrows)* between the humerus and the ulna. There is a fluid-filled detachment of the anterior bundle of the medial collateral ligament *(large arrows)* from the medial epicondyle.

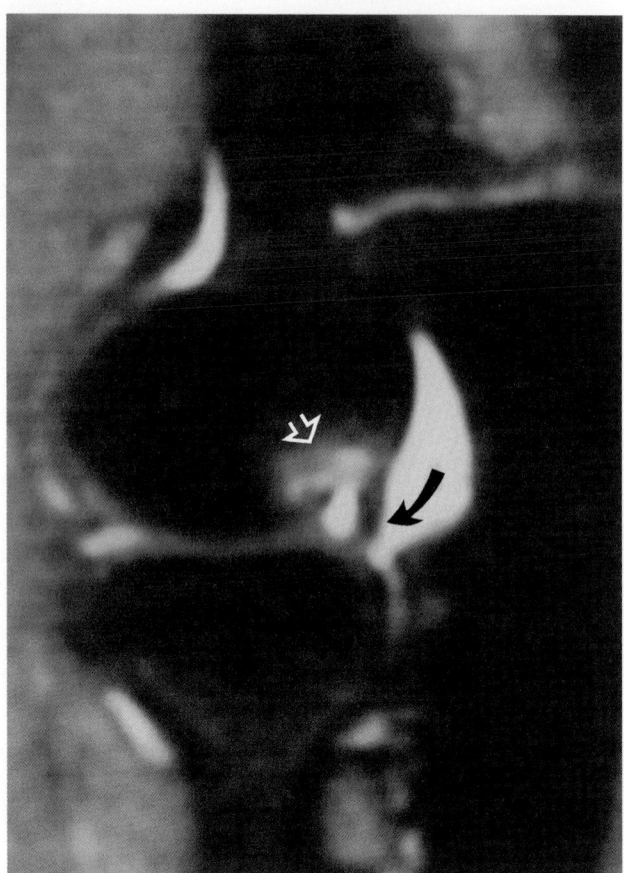

FIGURE 100-25

Displaced osteochondral flap lesion in a 16-year-old gymnast with intermittent locking and pain. A STIR sagittal image reveals bone marrow edema *(open arrow)* adjacent to a flap lesion arising from the posteromedial aspect of the capitellum *(curved arrow)*.

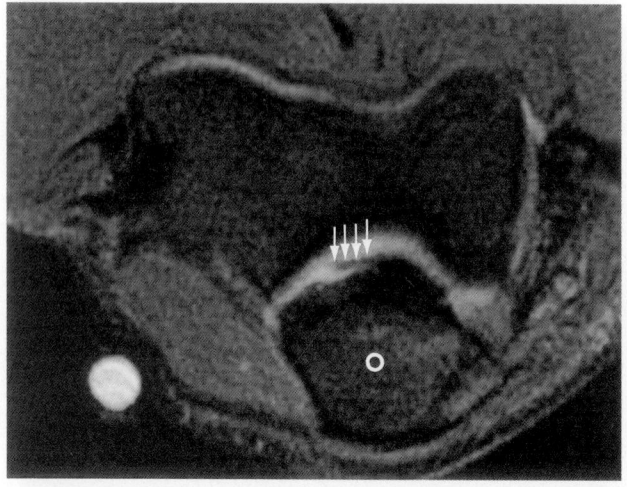

FIGURE 100-26

Nondisplaced chondral flap lesion in a 25-year-old baseball player. A fat-suppressed T2-weighted axial image reveals a fluid-filled fissure extending beneath a strip of articular cartilage *(arrows)* in the central aspect of the olecranon (O), subsequently proved at arthroscopy.

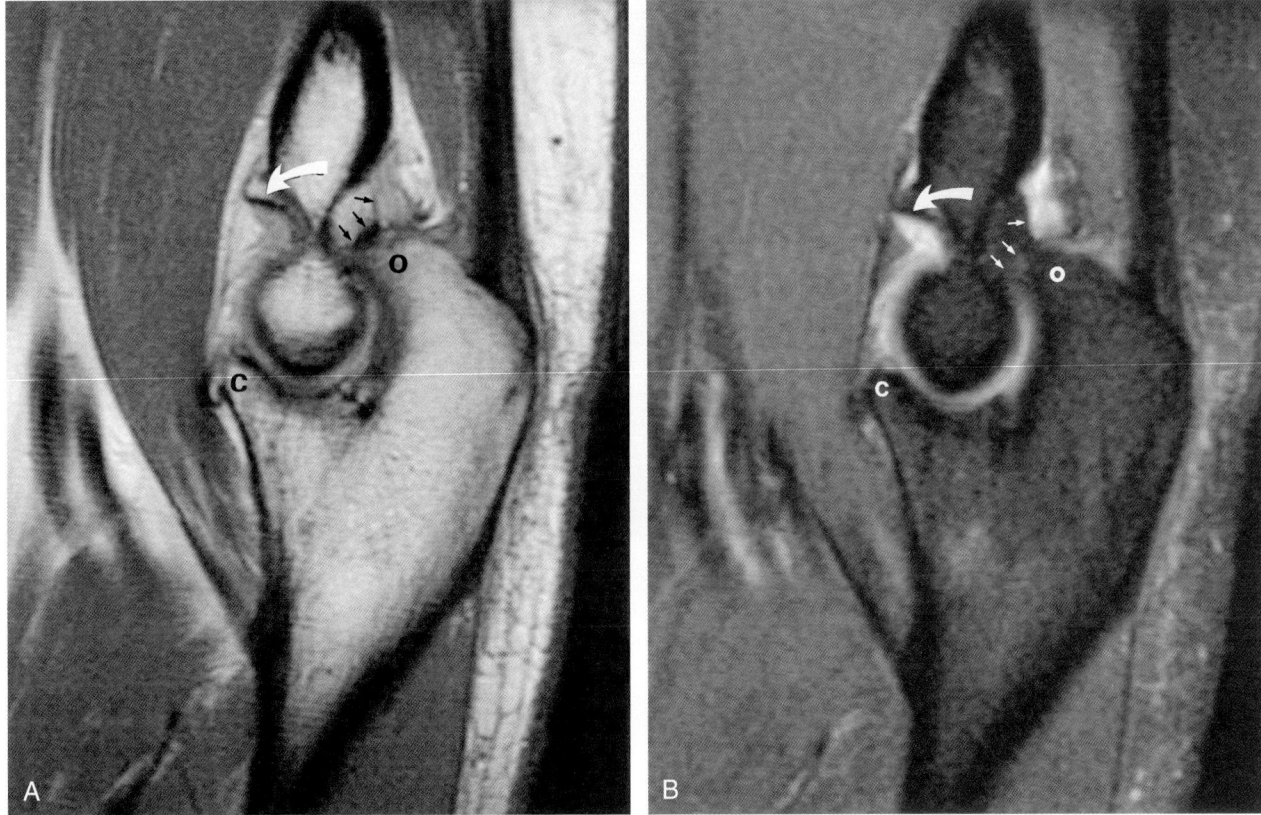

FIGURE 100-27

Osteoarthritis in a 50-year-old man with gradual loss of flexion and extension. Proton density (**A**) and fat-suppressed T2-weighted (**B**) sagittal images reveal impingement of the olecranon (O) against a prominent ridge of hypertrophic bone that fills the olecranon fossa (*small arrows*) and limits full extension of the elbow. Loss of flexion is explained by similar spurring that fills the superior aspect of the coronoid fossa (*curved arrows*). C, coronoid process.

FIGURE 100-28

Olecranon stress fracture in a 25-year-old professional pitcher. T1-weighted (**A**) and STIR (**B**) coronal images reveal a linear fracture line (*arrows*) which is surrounded by low signal intensity sclerosis. Valgus deformity of the elbow is apparent with the fracture oriented perpendicular to the pull of the triceps (tr).

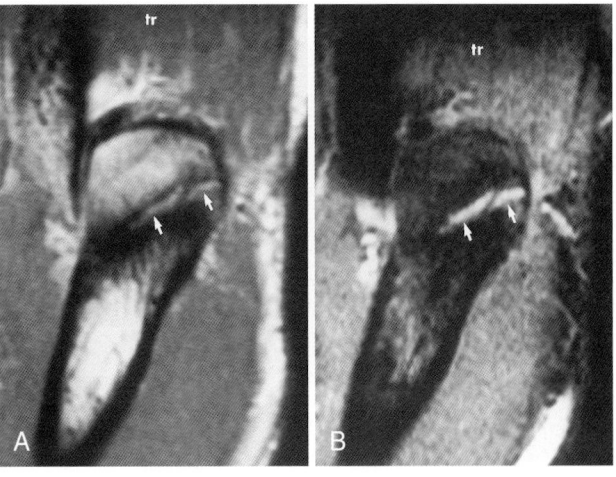

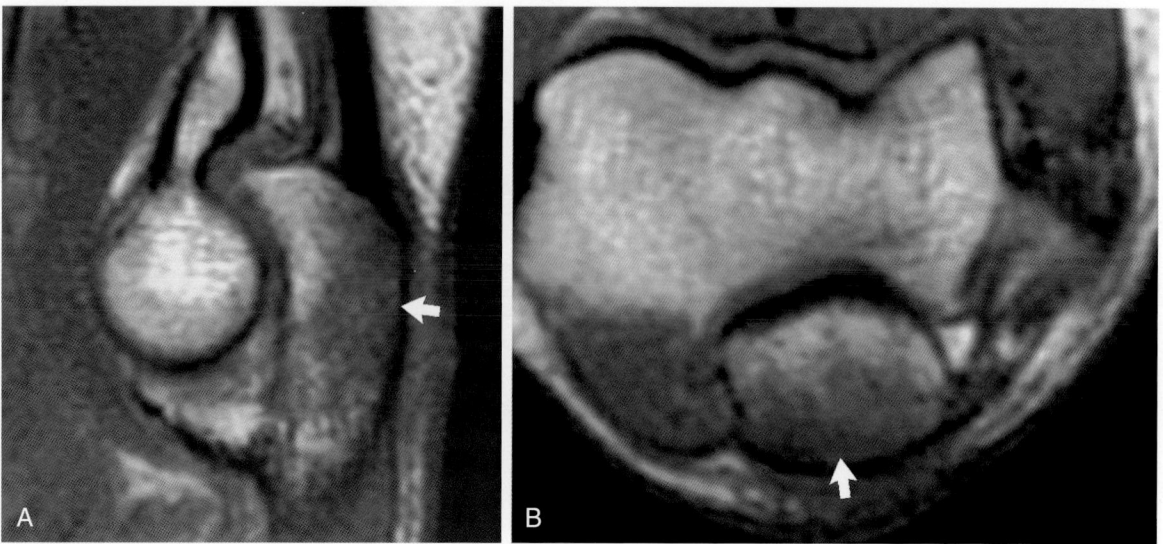

FIGURE 100-29

Olecranon bone contusion sustained during a fall 6 weeks before this scan. T1-weighted sagittal (**A**) and axial (**B**) images reveal decreased signal throughout the posterior aspect of the olecranon *(arrows)* in a tennis player who complained of persistant pain with extension.

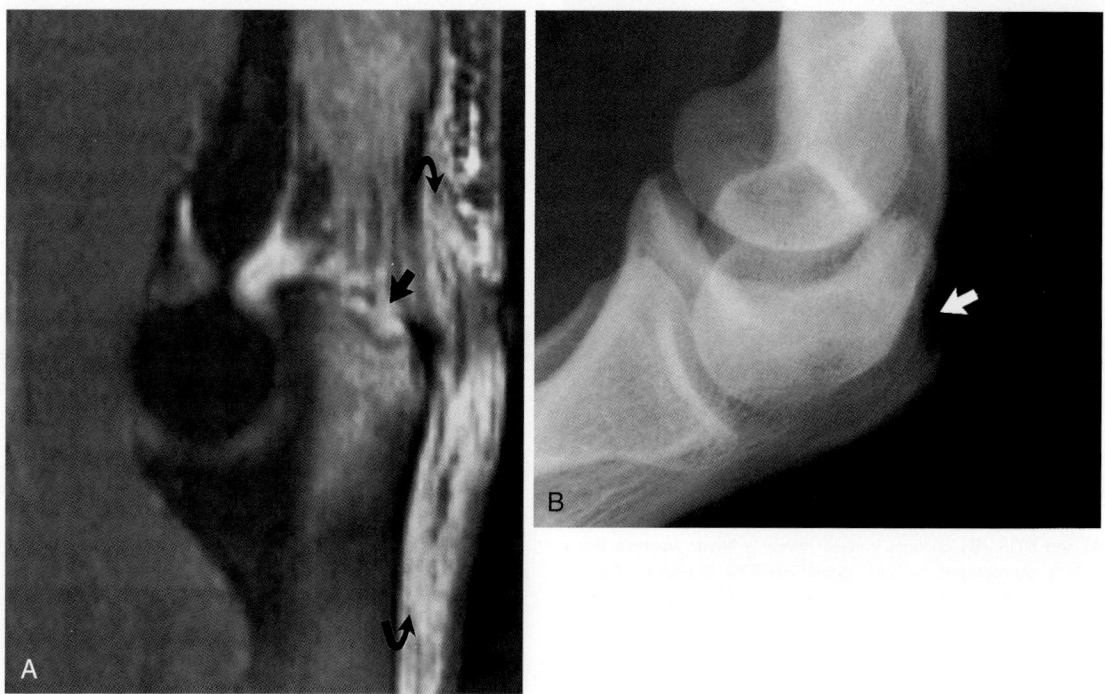

FIGURE 100-30

Osteomyelitis of the olecranon. **A,** STIR sagittal image reveals a cortical defect *(arrow)* with underlying marrow signal alteration. Prominent abnormal signal is also noted in the olecranon bursa and adjacent subcutaneous fat *(curved arrows).* **B,** A subsequent lateral radiograph reveals bony destruction *(arrow)* compatible with osteomyelitis.

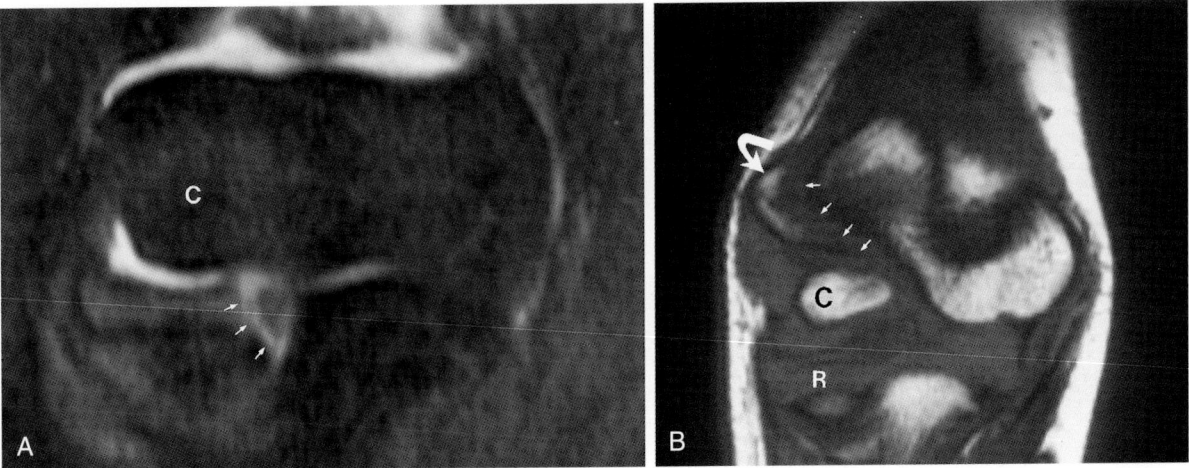

FIGURE 100-31

Radiographically subtle fractures about the elbow. **A,** STIR coronal image reveals a Salter-Harris Type IV fracture *(arrows)* of the medial margin of the radial head in a 14-year-old child with near complete physeal closure. **B,** T1-weighted coronal image reveals a Salter-Harris Type II fracture *(arrows)* with mild lateral displacement of the lateral humeral condyle *(curved arrow)* in a 5-year-old child. C, capitellum; R, unossified radial head cartilage.

Biceps Tendon Injury

Rupture of the distal biceps tendon is a relatively uncommon injury which accounts for 3% to 10% of all biceps tendon tears. The vast majority of distal biceps ruptures occur in men, with the injury involving the dominant arm in 80%. The mechanism of injury is usually contraction of the biceps against resistance, typically in weightlifters or manual laborers who lift heavy objects. Clinical diagnosis can be difficult as the bicipital aponeurosis (lacertus fibrosis) may remain intact with minimal retraction of the muscle. Flexion power at the elbow may be preserved if the lacertus fibrosis remains intact; however, supination of the forearm is usually weakened due to the biceps tendon detachment. Complete tears of the distal biceps are thought to be more common than partial tears.[2] MR imaging is useful in evaluating these injuries as tendinosis, partial tears, and complete ruptures may be distinguished (Fig. 100-33). Early diagnosis and treatment are important as primary repair of the distal biceps becomes increasingly difficult with increasing retraction of the tendon. Delayed diagnosis of this injury may require reconstruction rather than simple repair.

Distal biceps tendinosis is common and has been shown to precede spontaneous tendon rupture.[22,38] Tendinosis of the distal biceps is probably a multifactorial process which involves repetitive mechanical impingement of a poorly vascularized distal segment of the tendon (Fig. 100-34). Irregularity of the radial tuberosity and chronic inflammation of the adjacent radial bicipital bursa may also be contributory. A zone of relatively poor blood supply exists within the distal biceps tendon approximately 1 cm from its insertion on the radial tuberosity.[39] In addition, this hypovascular zone may be trapped between the radius and the ulna during pronation. The space between the radius and ulna progressively narrows with increasing degrees of

pronation, with measurements of 8.5 mm in supination, 6.3 mm in neutral position, and 4.3 mm in pronation recorded in normal volunteers with CT and MR imaging.[39]

The distal biceps tendon is an extrasynovial paratenon-covered tendon which is separated from the radial tuberosity distally by the bicipital radial bursa.[40] Inflammation of this cubital bursa may accompany tendinosis and tearing of the distal biceps (Fig. 100-35). Cubital bursitis, tendinosis, and partial tendon rupture may be impossible to distinguish clinically. Cubital bursitis may present as an antecubital fossa mass or and may also present with entrapment of the adjacent radial nerve.[41,42]

The T2-weighted axial images are most useful for determining the degree of tearing. The axial images must extend from the musculotendinous junction to the insertion of the tendon on the radial tuberosity. The axial images are also useful for evaluating the lacertus fibrosis (Fig. 100-36). The status of the lacertus on MR imaging is not a critical assessment as this structure is usually not repaired during the surgical repair of a biceps tendon rupture. However, surgical repair of a symptomatic lacertus fibrosis rupture has been reported along with repair of a partial tear of the biceps tendon.[43]

MR imaging provides useful information regarding the degree of tearing, the size of the gap, and the location of the tear for preoperative planning. The tendon typically tears from its attachment on the radial tuberosity as a result of forced elbow extension during maximal eccentric contraction of the biceps muscle.

Triceps Tendon Injury

Injuries of the triceps tendon are well seen with MR imaging (Fig. 100-37). The normal triceps tendon often appears lax and redundant when the elbow is imaged in

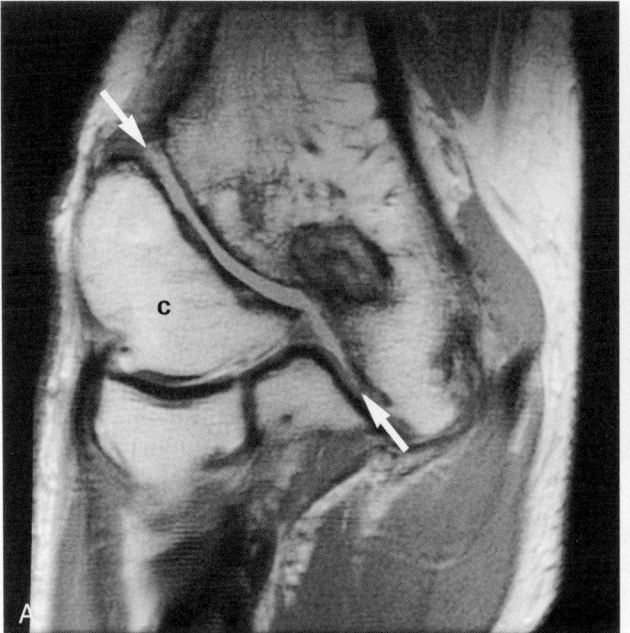

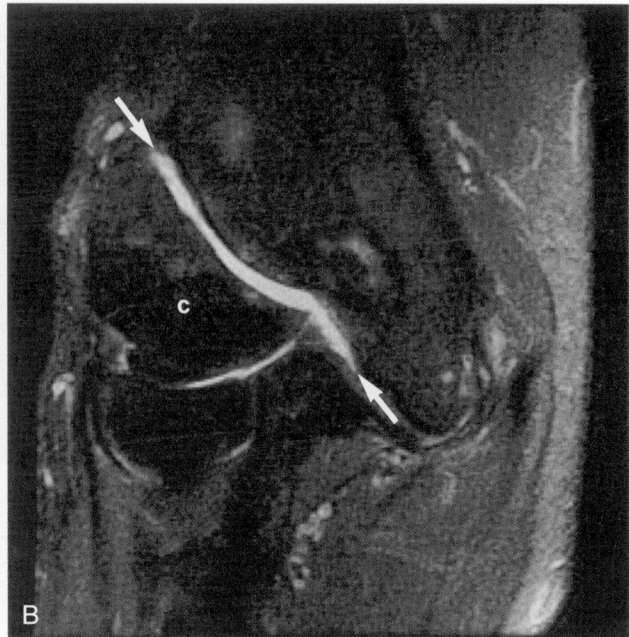

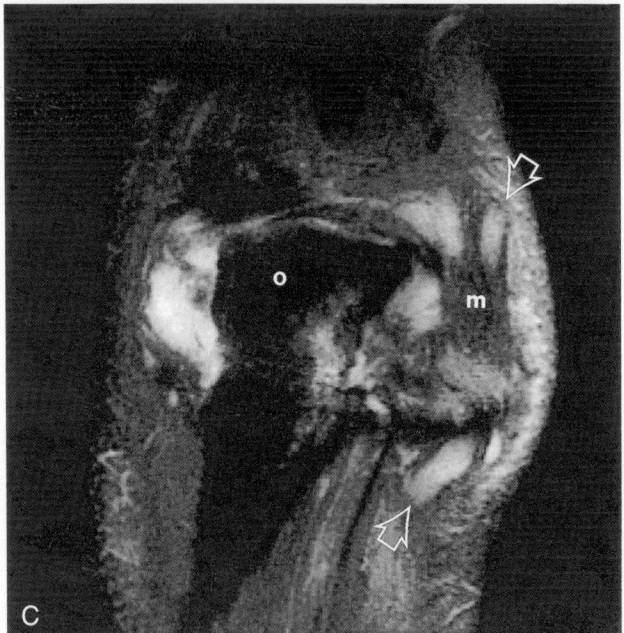

FIGURE 100-32

Nonunion of a Salter-Harris Type IV fracture of the lateral humeral condyle in a 20-year-old man presenting with symptoms of ulnar neuritis. This fracture was not recognized on X-rays at the time of the original injury 13 years before this scan. Proton density (**A**) and fat-suppressed T2-weighted (**B**) coronal images reveal a fluid-filled fracture nonunion (*arrows*). A more posterior fat-suppressed T2-weighted (**C**) coronal image reveals increased signal and enlargement of the ulnar nerve (*open arrows*) extending proximal and distal to the medial epicondyle (m). C, capitellum; o, olecranon.

full extension. This appearance resolves when the elbow is imaged in mild degrees of flexion. Complete avulsion of the distal triceps has been considered one of the least common tendon injuries in the literature. Partial tears have been considered even less common than complete ruptures. Triceps tendon injury has recently been reported with increasing frequency in professional football players and has not been uncommon in our MR imaging practice.[44] Both anabolic steroid abuse and local steroid injections have been implicated in rupture of the triceps tendon.[45]

The tendon typically avulses from its attachment on the olecranon (Fig. 100-38). The usual mechanisms of injury include a direct blow to the tendon, a fall on an outstreched arm or a decelerating counterforce during active extension. Olecranon bursitis may mimic or accompany partial triceps tendon tears.[46]

Entrapment Neuropathies

The ulnar nerve is well seen on axial MR images as it passes through the cubital tunnel.[47] The roof of the cubital tunnel is formed by the flexor carpi ulnaris aponeurosis distally and the cubital tunnel retinaculum proximally (Fig. 100-39). Anatomic variations of the cubital tunnel retinaculum may possibly contribute to ulnar neuropathy.[48] These variations in the cubital tunnel

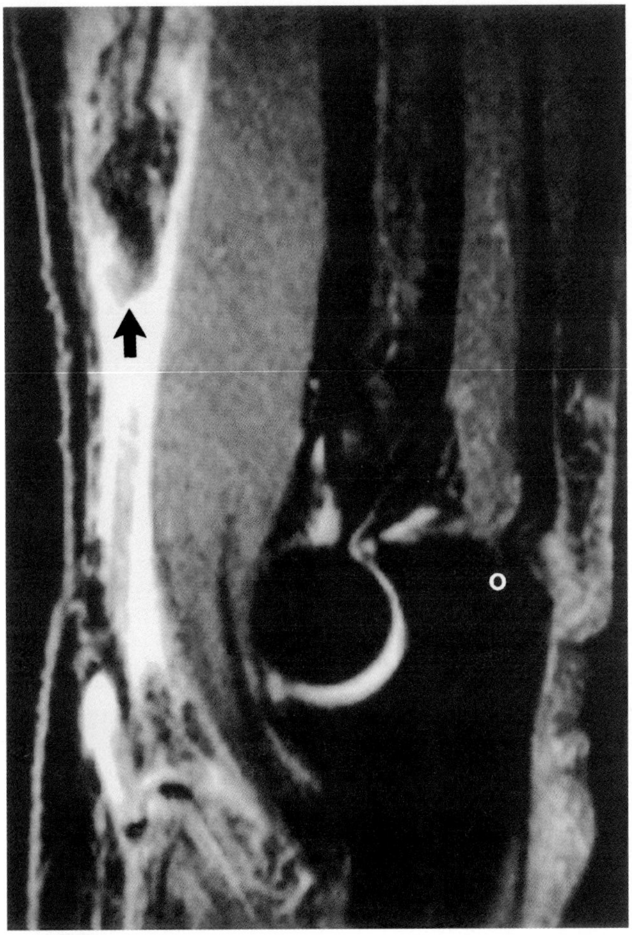

FIGURE 100-33

Subacute distal biceps tendon rupture. A STIR sagittal image reveals prominent proximal retraction of the biceps tendon *(arrow)* with surrounding edema. This patient presented for imaging 3 weeks after injuring his arm. O, olecranon.

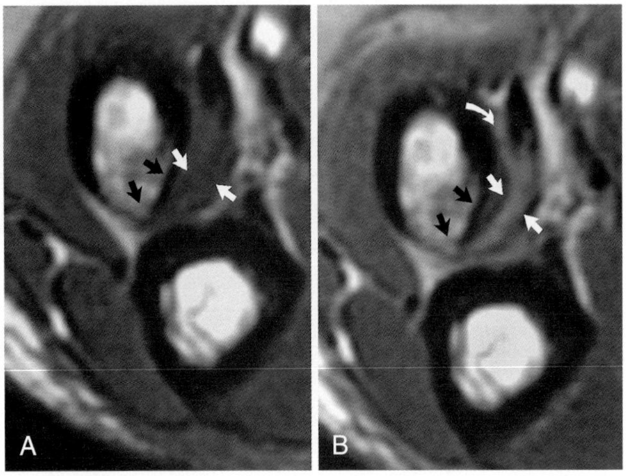

FIGURE 100-34

Distal biceps impingement syndrome. T1-weighted axial images before (**A**) and after (**B**) IV administration of gadolinium reveal prominence of the radial tuberosity *(black arrows)* on images performed with the arm not fully pronated. Further pronation causes impingement of the biceps tendon between the radial tuberosity and the ulna. Abnormal signal is noted in the biceps tendon which enhances with gadolinium consistent with tendinosis *(straight white arrows)*. The synovium within the bicipital radial bursa also mildly enhances with contrast *(curved arrow)*.

retinaculum as well as the appearance of the ulnar nerve itself can be identified with MR imaging.The retinaculum may be thickened in 22% of elbows, resulting in dynamic compression of the ulnar nerve during elbow flexion (Fig. 100-40). The retinaculum may be replaced by an anomalous muscle, the anconeus epitrochlearis, in 11%, possibly resulting in static compression of the ulnar nerve (Fig. 100-41). Alternatively, this muscle could be an adaptive variation that may cushion and protect the ulnar nerve from direct injury. An abnormal ulnar nerve typically demonstrates increased signal intensity on T2-weighted images and may also be enlarged, compressed or flattened (Fig. 100-42).The cubital tunnel retinaculum may be absent in 10% of elbows, allowing anterior dislocation of the nerve over the medial epicondyle during flexion, with subsequent friction neuritis (Fig. 100-43).[48] This anterior displacement of the ulnar nerve may be well seen with MR imaging by scanning the elbow in full flexion.[49] Alternatively, the ulnar nerve can be dynamically evaluated with ultrasound during flexion and extension.[50]

The floor of the cubital tunnel is formed by the capsule of the elbow and the posterior and transverse portions of the MCL.Thickening of the MCL and medial bony spurring may undermine the floor of the cubital tunnel, resulting in ulnar neuropathy.[51] Heterotopic ossification in the MCL, tumors, ganglion cysts or displaced fracture fragments may also result in ulnar nerve entrapment. Synovitis from the elbow joint may undermine the cubital tunnel and compress the ulnar nerve (Fig. 100-44).

Surgical procedures for ulnar nerve entrapment include medial epicondylectomy, decompression of the nerve, and translocation of the nerve.[52] Translocation or transfer of the nerve may be subcutaneous, intramuscular or submuscular. Low signal intensity scarring may be seen along the margins of the surgically translocated ulnar nerve; this finding has also been observed in patients with ulnar nerve subluxation and friction neuritis.

Entrapment of the radial nerve and median nerve may also be evaluated with MR imaging (Fig. 100-45). Median nerve entrapment may be due to a variety of uncommon anatomic variations about the elbow, including the supracondyloid process with a ligament of Struthers, anomalous muscles, an accessory bicipital aponeurosis, and hypertrophy of the ulnar head of the pronator teres. These anatomic variants, as well as pathologic mass lesions, may entrap the median nerve and may be identified with MR imaging. Radial nerve entrapment may occur due to thickening of the arcade of Frohse along the proximal edge of the supinator muscle. Ganglion cysts may arise from the anterior margin of the elbow joint and compress the radial nerve. The radial nerve and its branches may also be entrapped by an enlarged radial bicipital bursa.[41]

Text continues on page 3307

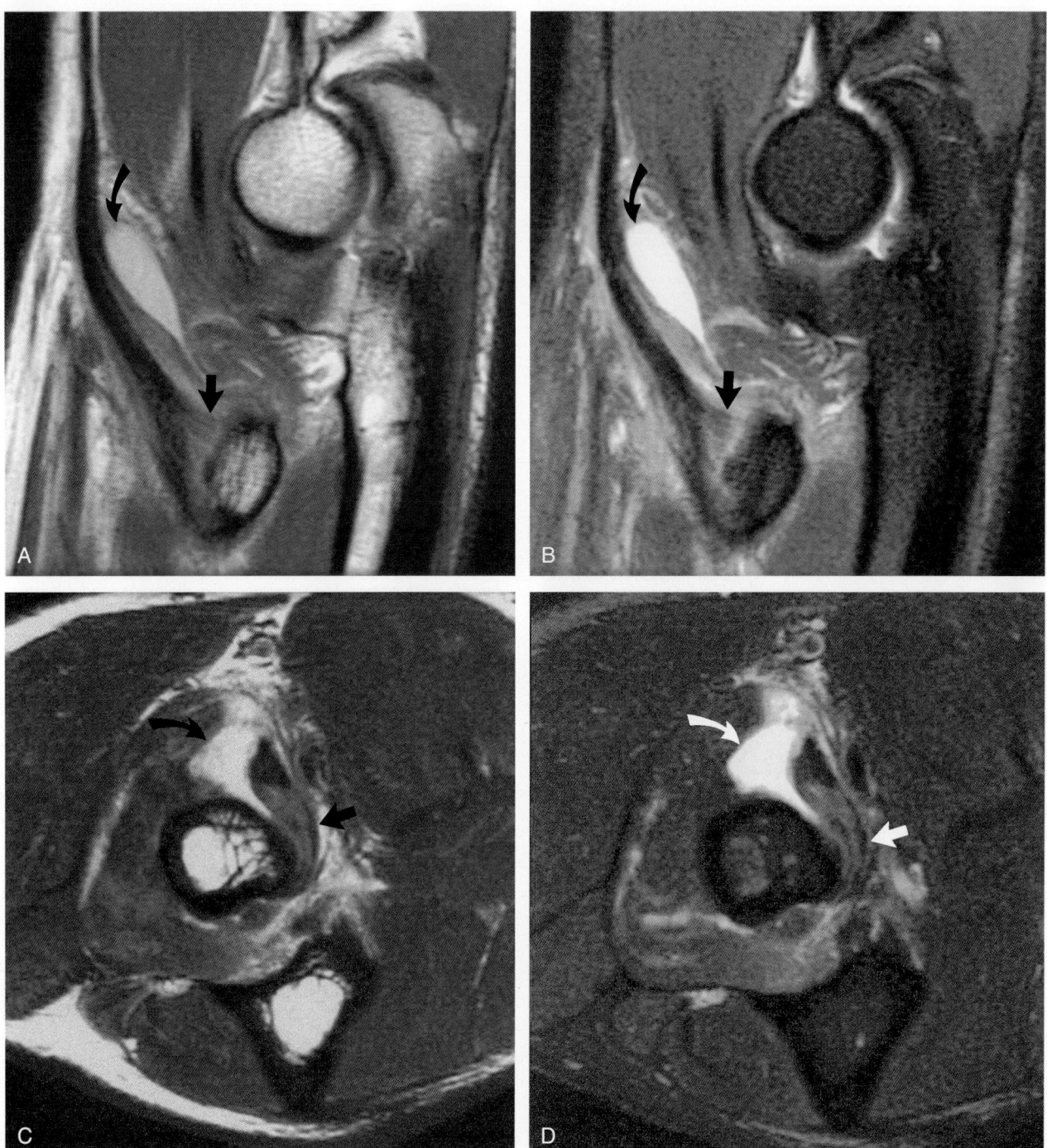

FIGURE 100-35

Cubital bursitis and moderately severe distal biceps tendinosis in a 30-year-old football player. Proton density (**A**) and fat-suppressed T2-weighted (**B**) sagittal images as well as proton density (**C**) and fat-suppressed T2-weighted (**D**) axial images reveal increased signal within the biceps tendon *(straight arrows)* and fluid distending the bicipital radial bursa *(curved arrows)*. The bursa separates the biceps tendon from the radial tuberosity. The scan was performed with the arm partially supinated. Images in pronation can demonstrate distal biceps impingement between the radial tuberosity and the ulna.

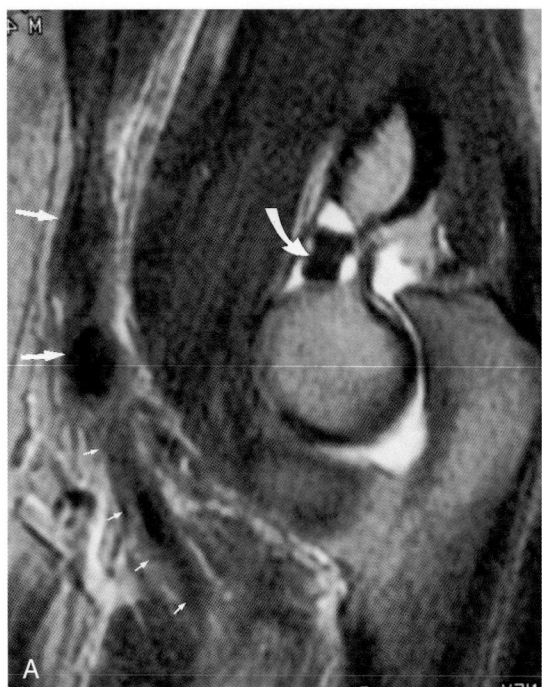

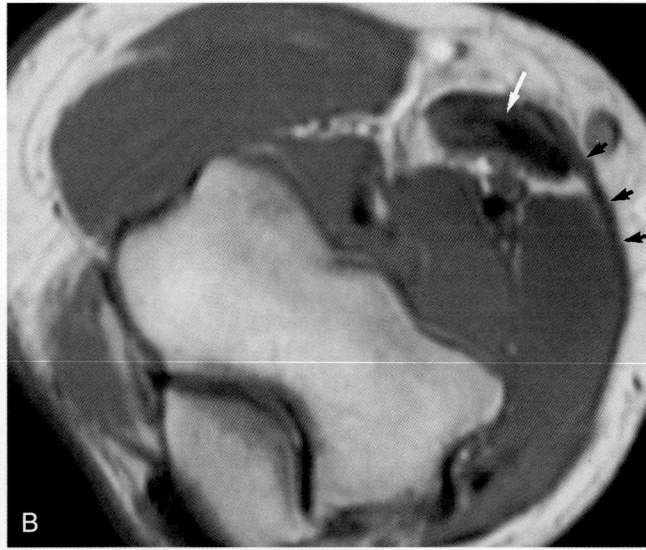

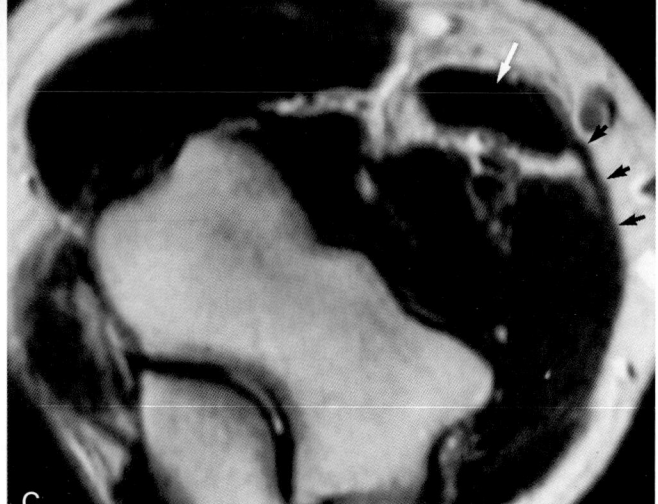

FIGURE 100-36

Chronic partial biceps tendon rupture in a 42-year-old man with painful limitation of elbow flexion. **A,** T2-weighted sagittal image reveals a large loose body *(curved arrow)* in the coronoid which prevented full flexion. The proximal biceps is thickened *(large arrows)* whereas the distal tendon is abnormally thin *(small arrows)* but remains attached to the radial tuberosity. Proton density (**B**) and T2-weighted (**C**) axial images at the level of the distal humerus reveal increased signal and thickening of the biceps tendon *(white arrows)* as well as thickening of the lacertus fibrosus *(small black arrows)*.

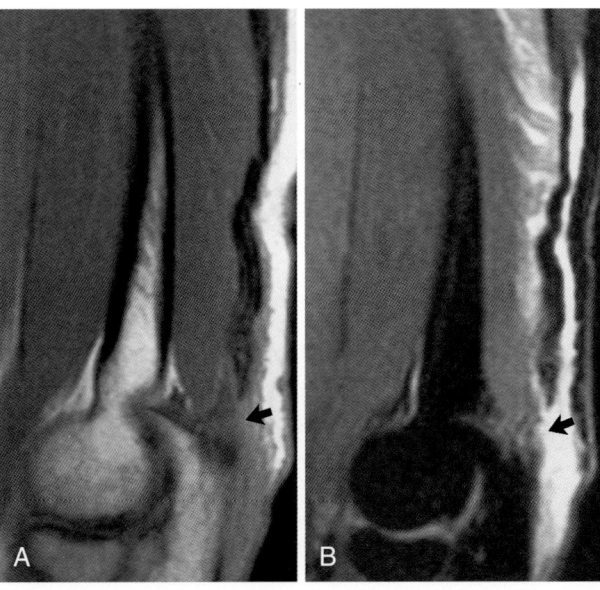

FIGURE 100-37

Acute triceps tendon rupture in a professional football player. T1-weighted (**A**) and STIR (**B**) sagittal images reveal a fluid-filled gap *(arrows)* that separates the distal triceps tendon from the olecranon.

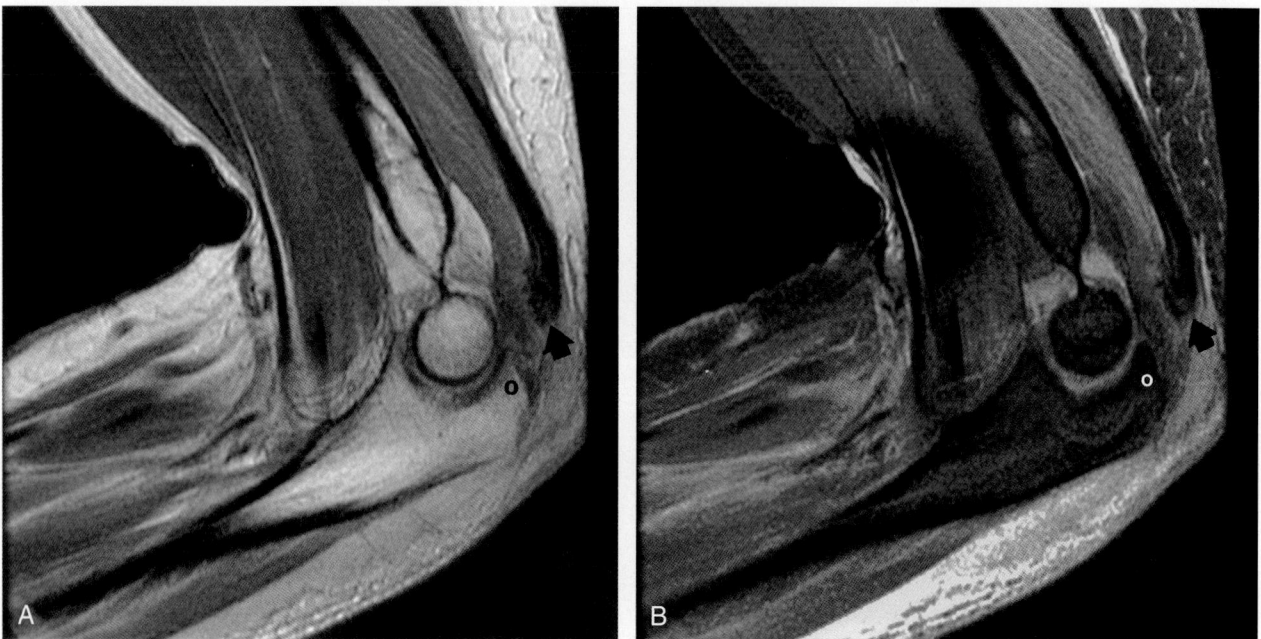

FIGURE 100-38

Triceps tendon rupture imaged in flexion. This patient was unable to extend the elbow due to discomfort. The images were performed on a high-field scanner with the patient prone and the arm flexed overhead. Proton density (**A**) and fat-suppressed T2-weighted (**B**) coronal images reveal a fluid-filled tear of the distal triceps tendon *(arrow)* from the olecranon (O).

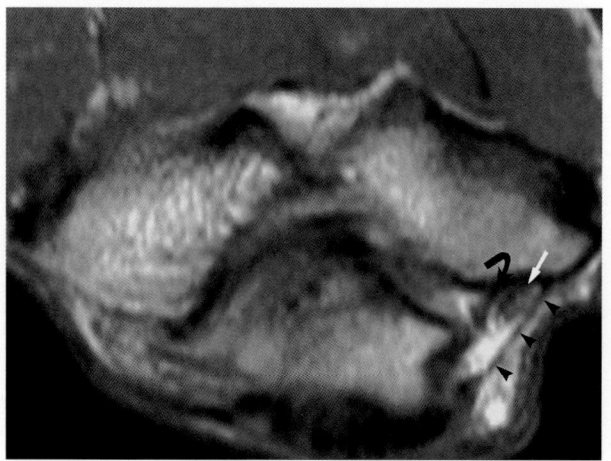

FIGURE 100-39

Anatomy of the cubital tunnel. A proton density axial image reveals the ulnar nerve *(white arrow)* deep to a normal, thin cubital tunnel retinaculum *(arrowheads)* and superficial to the posterior bundle of the medial collateral ligament *(curved arrow)*.

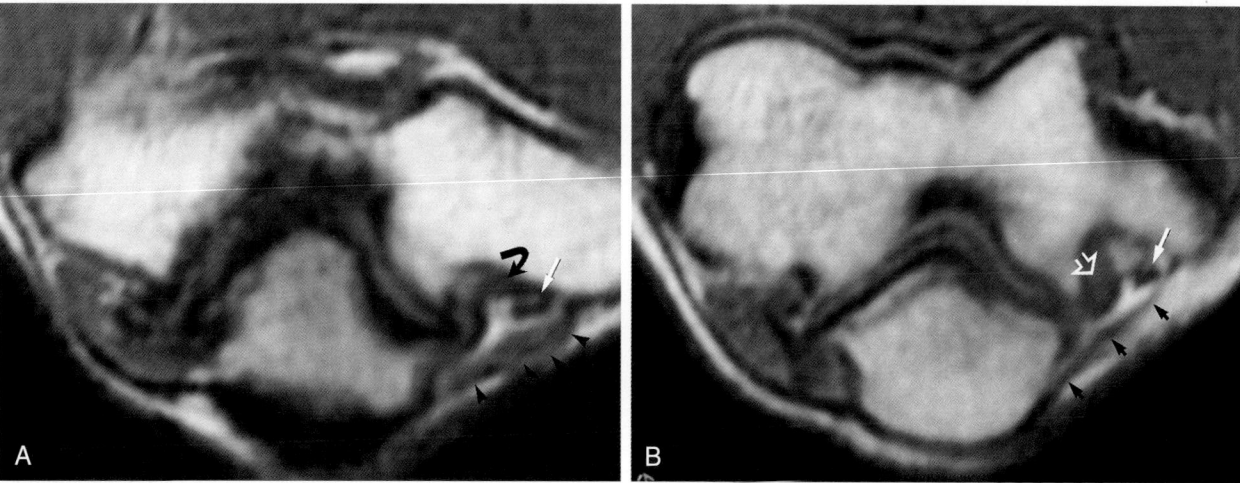

FIGURE 100-40

Thickening of the cubital tunnel retinaculum. **A,** T1-weighted axial image reveals the ulnar nerve *(white arrow)* deep to a thickened cubital tunnel retinaculum *(arrowheads)* and superficial to the posterior bundle of the medial collateral ligament *(curved arrow)*. **B,** An axial image further distally in the same patient reveals the ulnar nerve *(white arrow)* deep to a normal, thin aponeurosis of the flexor carpi ulnaris *(small black arrows)* and superficial to a mildly thickened medial joint capsule *(open arrow)*.

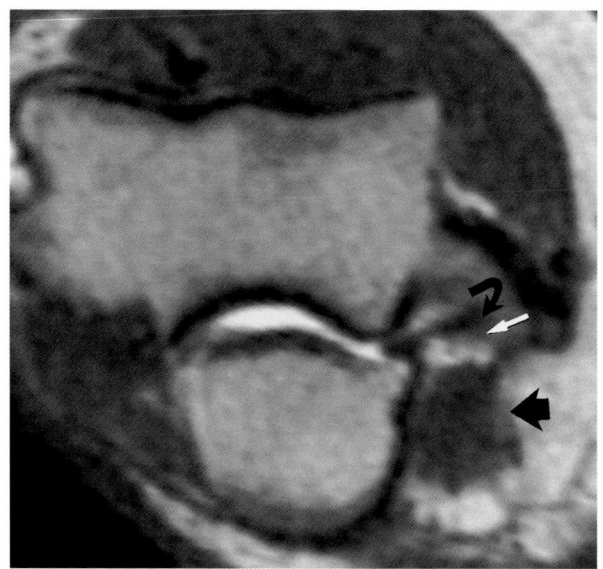

FIGURE 100-41

Anconeus epitrochlearis muscle replacing the cubital tunnel retinaculum. A T2-weighted axial image reveals the ulnar nerve *(white arrow)* deep to an anomalous anconeus epitrochlearis muscle *(black arrow)* and superficial to the posterior bundle of the medial collateral ligament *(curved arrow)*.

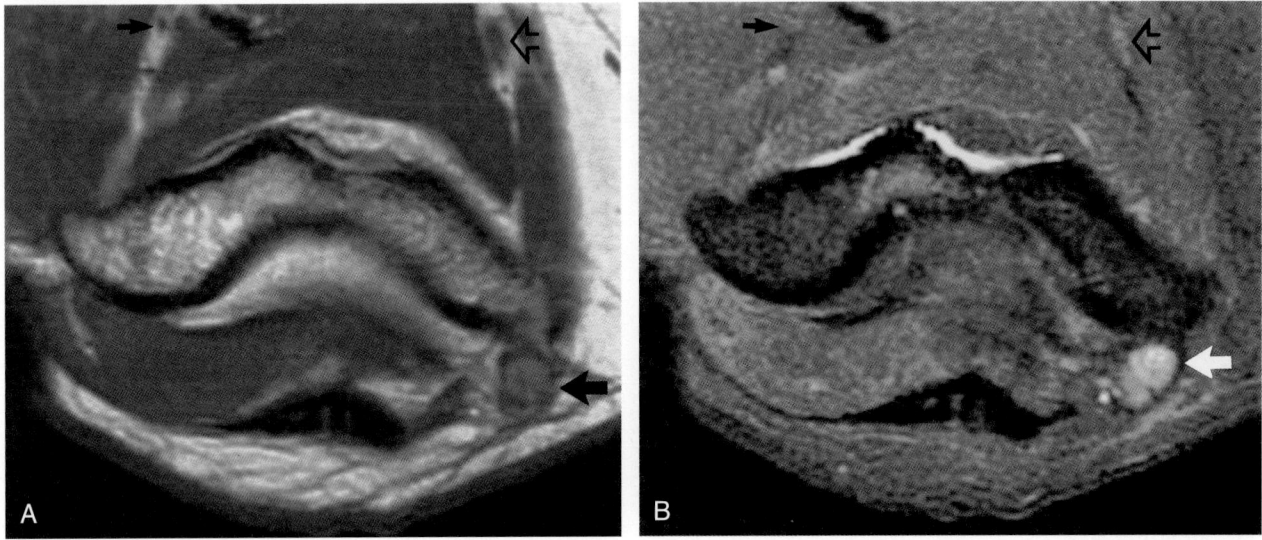

FIGURE 100-42

Severe ulnar neuritis in a 35-year-old golfer. Proton density (**A**) and fat-suppressed T2-weighted (**B**) axial images reveal enlargement and increased signal intensity of the ulnar nerve *(large arrows)* due to edema and neuritis. The signal intensity of the nerve on the fat-suppressed image (**B**) is relatively increased when compared to the signal intensity of normal muscles and nerves. The normal median nerve *(open arrows)* and the normal deep branch of the radial nerve *(small arrows)* can also be identified on the proton density image (**A**).

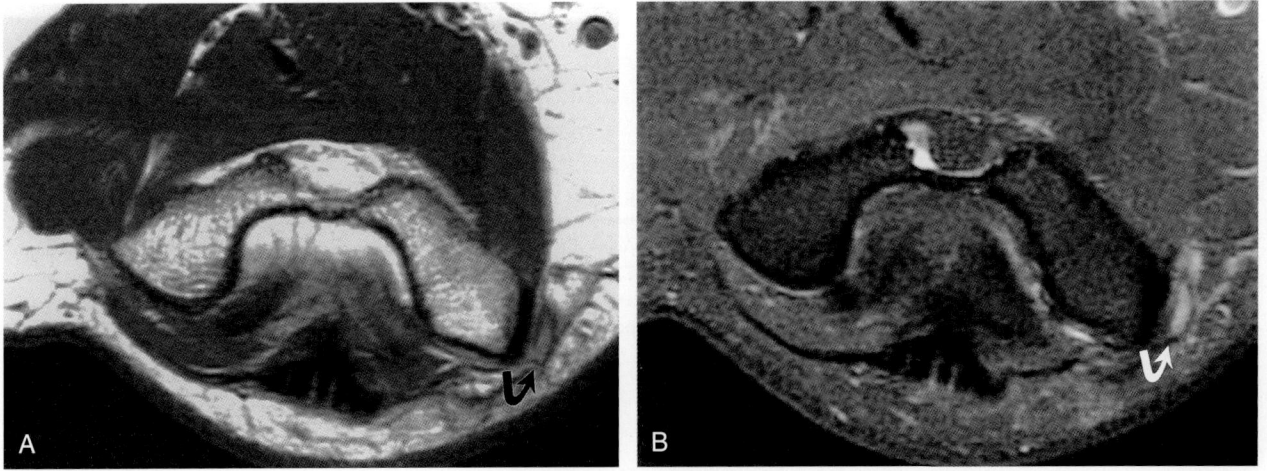

FIGURE 100-43

Ulnar neuritis and subluxation. Proton density (**A**) and fat-suppressed T2-weighted (**B**) axial images reveal flattening and increased signal intensity of the ulnar nerve *(arrows)* due to edema and neuritis. The nerve is anteromedially subluxed from the cubital tunnel due to insufficiency of the overlying cubital tunnel retinaculum.

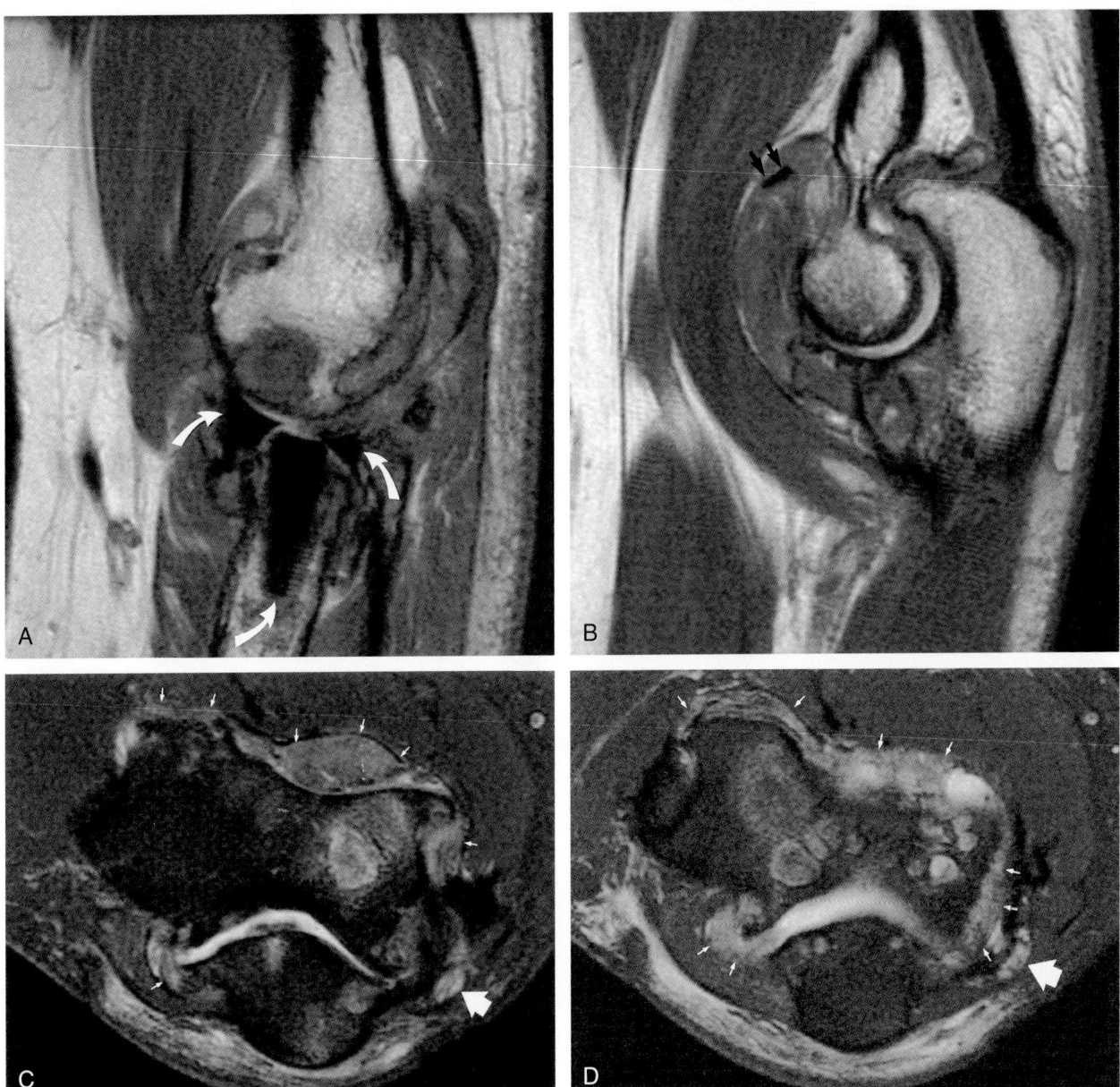

FIGURE 100-44

Silicone synovitis complicated by ulnar neuritis. This patient had previously had a Silastic implant inserted for a comminuted radial head fracture. **A,** A proton density sagittal image reveals a fracture of the low signal intensity implant *(curved arrows)*. The stem of the implant is impacted into a defect in the head. **B,** A proton density sagittal image reveals a fragment of Silastic *(small black arrows)* surrounded by prominent synovitis distending the anterior joint capsule and extending into erosions in the coronoid process. **C,** A fat-suppressed T2-weighted axial image reveals synovitis throughout the joint *(small arrows)* and edema within the fascicles of the ulnar nerve *(large arrow)*. **D,** A fat-suppressed T2-weighted axial image reveals synovitis diffusely *(small arrows)*. There is medial synovitis distending the medial joint capsule, resulting in compression and flattening of the ulnar nerve *(large arrow)*.

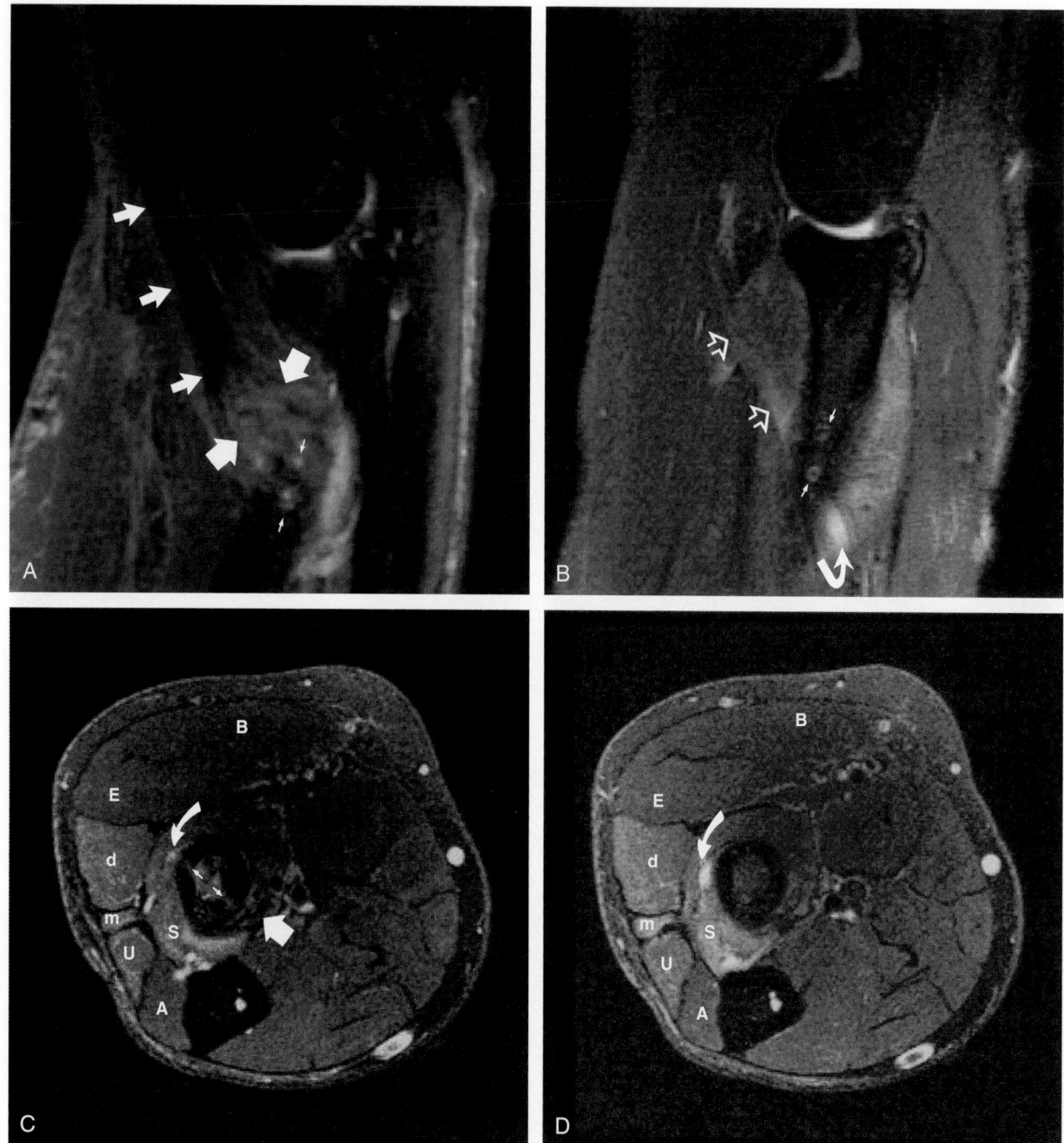

FIGURE 100-45

Biceps tendon repair complicated by radial nerve injury. **A,** A fat-suppressed T2-weighted sagittal image along the medial aspect of the radius reveals the biceps tendon *(arrows)* repaired to the radial tuberosity through two adjacent drill holes *(small arrows)*. There is increased signal within the distal tendon repair secondary to developing scar tissue *(large arrows)*. **B,** A fat-suppressed T2-weighted sagittal image along the lateral aspect of the radius reveals increased signal in the deep branch of the radial nerve *(curved arrow)* once the nerve passes the drill holes *(small arrows)*. The nerve is normal *(open arrows)* proximal to the drill holes. **C,** A fat-suppressed T2-weighted axial image at the level of the distal drill hole *(small arrows)* and biceps tendon *(large arrow)* reveals slight increased signal in the radial nerve. There is increased signal in the posterior aspect of the supinator muscle (S) secondary to subacute denervation. There is also denervation of the extensor carpi ulnaris (u), the extensor digiti minimi (m), and the extensor digitorum (d). The anconeus (A), extensor carpi radialis longus (E), and brachioradialis (B) muscles are normal, having been innervated by more proximal branches of the radial nerve. **D,** A fat-suppressed T2-weighted axial image just distal to the most distal drill hole reveals prominent increased signal in the radial nerve as well as subacute muscle denervation.

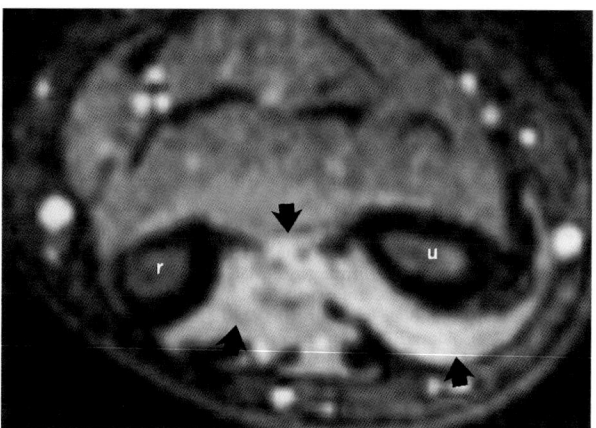

FIGURE 100-46

Muscle denervation due to entrapment of the radial nerve at the level of the elbow. There is abnormal increased signal throughout the extensor musculature of the forearm (arrows) in the distribution of the radial nerve on this STIR axial image. The findings are compatible with subacute denervation. r, radius; u, ulna.

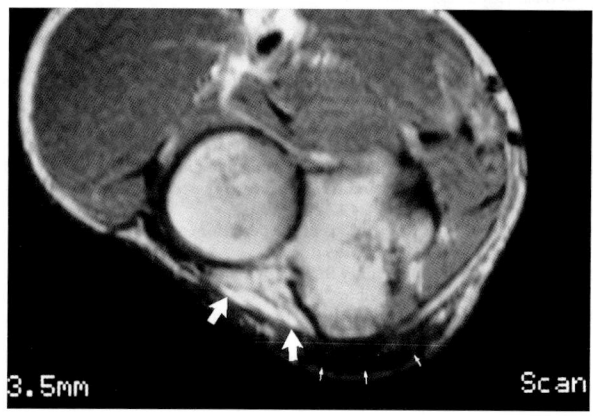

FIGURE 100-47

Fatty infiltration and atrophy of the anconeus muscle secondary to chronic denervation. There is prominent fatty replacement of the anconeus muscle (large arrows) on this T1-weighted axial image. Low signal intensity scarring (small arrows) is noted at the site of a prior olecranon bursectomy that was complicated by damage to the innervation of the anconeus muscle.

MR imaging may be complementary to EMG and nerve conduction studies in cases of nerve entrapment about the elbow.[53] In subacute denervation the affected muscles have prolongation of T1 and T2 relaxation times secondary to muscle fiber shrinkage and associated increases in extracellular water.[54] Entrapment of a nerve about the elbow may therefore cause increased signal within the muscles innervated by that nerve on T2-weighted or STIR images (Fig. 100-46). These changes may be followed to resolution or progressive atrophy and fatty infiltration (Fig. 100-47). Moreover, the site and cause of entrapment may be discovered with MR imaging by following the nerve implicated from the distribution of abnormal muscles on MR imaging.[55]

CONCLUSION

MR imaging currently provides clinically useful information in patients with a variety of traumatic and degenerative disorders that result in elbow pain. MR imaging is perhaps most useful when patients have not responded to conservative therapy and therefore surgery as well as additional diagnoses are being considered.

REFERENCES

1. Bredella MA, Tirman PF, Fritz RC, et al: MR imaging findings of lateral ulnar collateral ligament abnormalities in patients with lateral epicondylitis. Am J Roentgenol 173:1379-1382, 1999.
2. Williams BD, Schweitzer ME, Weishaupt D, et al: Partial tears of the distal biceps tendon: MR appearance and associated clinical findings. Skeletal Radiol 30:560-564, 2001.
3. Horn BD, Herman MJ, Crisci K, et al: Fractures of the lateral humeral condyle: role of the cartilage hinge in fracture stability. J Pediatr Orthop 22:8-11, 2002.
4. Chen AL, Youm T, Ong BC, et al: Imaging of the elbow in the overhead throwing athlete. Am J Sports Med 31:466-473, 2003.
5. Mackay D, Rangan A, Hide G, et al: The objective diagnosis of early tennis elbow by magnetic resonance imaging. Occup Med (Lond) 53:309-312, 2003.
6. Fritz RC: MR imaging of sports injuries of the elbow. Magn Reson Imaging Clin North Am 7:51-72, 1999.
7. Potter HG, Weiland AJ, Schatz JA, et al: Posterolateral rotatory instability of the elbow: usefulness of MR imaging in diagnosis. Radiology 204:185-189, 1997.
8. Beltran J, Rosenberg ZS, Kawelblum M, et al: Pediatric elbow fractures: MRI evaluation. Skeletal Radiol 23:277-281, 1994.
9. Schwartz ML, al-Zahrani S, Morwessel RM, Andrews JR: Ulnar collateral ligament injury in the throwing athlete: evaluation with saline-enhanced MR arthrography. Radiology 197:297-299, 1995.
10. Conway JE, Jobe FW, Glousman RE, Pink M: Medial instability of the elbow in throwing athletes. Treatment by repair or reconstruction of the ulnar collateral ligament. J Bone Joint Surg (Am) 74:67-83, 1992.
11. Callaway GH, Field LD, Deng XH, et al: Biomechanical evaluation of the medial collateral ligament of the elbow. J Bone Joint Surg (Am) 79:1223-1231, 1997.
12. O'Driscoll SW: Classification and evaluation of recurrent instability of the elbow. Clin Orthop 370: 34-43, 2000.
13. Smith JP 3rd, Savoie FH 3rd, Field LD: Posterolateral rotatory instability of the elbow. Clin Sports Med 20:47-58, 2001.
14. Timmerman LA, Andrews JR: Undersurface tear of the ulnar collateral ligament in baseball players. A newly recognized lesion. Am J Sports Med 22:33-36, 1994.
15. Timmerman LA, Andrews JR: Histology and arthroscopic anatomy of the ulnar collateral ligament of the elbow. Am J Sports Med 22:667-673, 1994.
16. Timmerman LA, Schwartz ML, Andrews JR: Preoperative evaluation of the ulnar collateral ligament by magnetic resonance imaging and computed tomography arthrography: evaluation in 25 baseball players with surgical confirmation. Am J Sports Med 22:26-32, 1994.
17. Bennett JB, Green MS, Tullos HS: Surgical management of chronic medial elbow instability. Clin Orthop 278:62-68, 1992.
18. Gore RM, Rogers LF, Bowerman J, et al: Osseous manifestations of elbow stress associated with sports activites. Am J Roentgenol 134:971-977, 1980.
19. Mulligan SA, Schwartz ML, Broussard MF, Andrews JR: Heterotopic calcification and tears of the ulnar collateral ligament: radiographic and MR imaging findings. Am J Roentgenol 175:1099-1102, 2000.
20. Nirschl RP: Elbow tendinosis/tennis elbow. Clin Sports Med 11:851-870, 1992.
21. Vangsness CT, Jobe FW: Surgical treatment of medial epicondylitis. J Bone Joint Surg (Br) 73:409-411, 1992.
22. Kannus P, Jozsa L: Histopathological changes preceding spontaneous rupture of a tendon. A controlled study of 891 patients. J Bone Joint Surg (Am) 73:1507-1525, 1991.
23. Case SL, Hennrikus WL: Surgical treatment of displaced medial epicondyle fractures in adolescent athletes. Am J Sports Med 25:682-686, 1997.
24. Regan W, Wold LE, Coonrad R, Morrey BF: Microscopic histopathology of chronic refractory lateral epicondylitis. Am J Sports Med 20:746-749, 1992.
25. Coonrad RW, Hooper WR: Tennis elbow, its course, natural history, conservative and surgical management. J Bone Joint Surg (Am) 55:1177-1182, 1973.
26. Morrey BF: Reoperation for failed surgical treatment of refractory lateral epicondylitis. J Shoulder Elbow Surg 1:47-55, 1992.

evaluating patients with chronic wrist pain when a wrist coil was not used. Quadrature or phased-array coils are preferred. Recent advances in hardware and software have enabled the use of phased-array coils with multiple channels. Current coils generally utilize four channels or less, but coils with six to eight channels are under development (Fig. 101-1B).

A comprehensive wrist examination for TFCC and intercarpal ligament problems includes sagittal short TR/TE and coronal long TR/short and long TE spin-echo (SE) images. Scout axial views for orientation of the coronal and axial images to obtain true orthogonal images are recommended. A slice-interleaved dual-echo gradient-echo (GRE) sequence in the coronal plane (MPGR) is also employed. 3D volume gradient-echo sequences allow slice thickness of less than 1 mm and reformatted images and are employed as a primary imaging sequence by some. Coronal SE sequences are obtained with contiguous 2 to 3 mm sections. Sagittal and axial images have a section thickness of 3 mm. The field of view (FOV) is 6 to 8 cm. The matrix size is 250×160 for the long TR/TE sequences and 256×192 or 256 for the other sequences. Fast spin-echo sequences (FSE) are now commonly employed in place of conventional spin-echo sequences especially on high-field scanners with higher gradient strength and with newer pulse sequence profiles with shorter interecho spacing, with or without fat saturation.[2a] They allow for T2-weighted imaging with shorter imaging times, or with higher matrices with similar imaging times but with improved spatial resolution. The use of fat suppression, either with fat saturation or with FSE inversion recovery (IR), also improves lesion conspicuity. These sequences may be employed in the coronal or axial plane. On systems with faster gradients (20 mT/m or above) in conjunction with high matrix imaging (384×256 or greater) and FSE sequences with intermediate level TE (30 to 49) and fat suppression the image quality in many cases is of sufficient quality and resolution to replace conventional spin-echo sequences or gradient-echo sequences for evaluating the ligaments and TFCC. These sequences are also of significant benefit in the assessment of occult fractures and other bone and marrow abnormalities, especially when employed with fat suppression. This is true as well for fast spin-echo inversion recovery (FSE-IR/STIR) sequences.

For MR arthrography[3] a saline/gadopentetate dimeglumine (gadolinium) mixture (1.0 mL of gadopentetate dimeglumine/250 mL of saline) is injected. This can be accomplished by diluting 0.05 mL of gadolinium in 10 mL of saline in a 10 mL syringe. If a conventional arthrogram is also desired, then the gadolinium can be diluted in a saline/iodinated contrast mixture (we utilize Isovue 400). Injection and arthrographic filming is done under C-arm fluoroscopic guidance. Injection under MRI guidance has been described.[4] Three to 4 mL of contrast material are injected into the radiocarpal wrist compartment. Intra-articular gadolinium distends the joint and may be the most efficacious method of diagnosing ligament injuries. Fat-saturated T1-weighted images (Fig. 101-2A) can be obtained in all three imaging planes. These are typically done with 3 mm sections, $256 \times 192 \times 256$ matrix, and 8 cm FOV. High-resolution (512×512 matrix, 1 to 2 mm section, 6 cm FOV) 2D and 3D imaging can also be employed, usually without fat suppression (Fig. 101-2B). In general, at least one additional sequence with T2 weighting, usually in the coronal plane with FSE with fat saturation (FS), is also carried out.

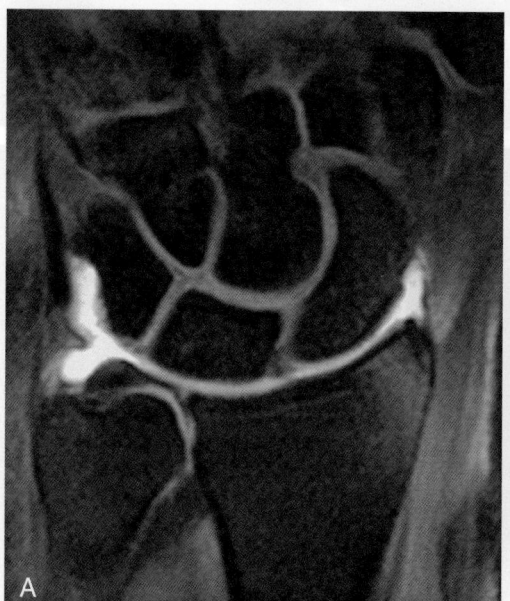
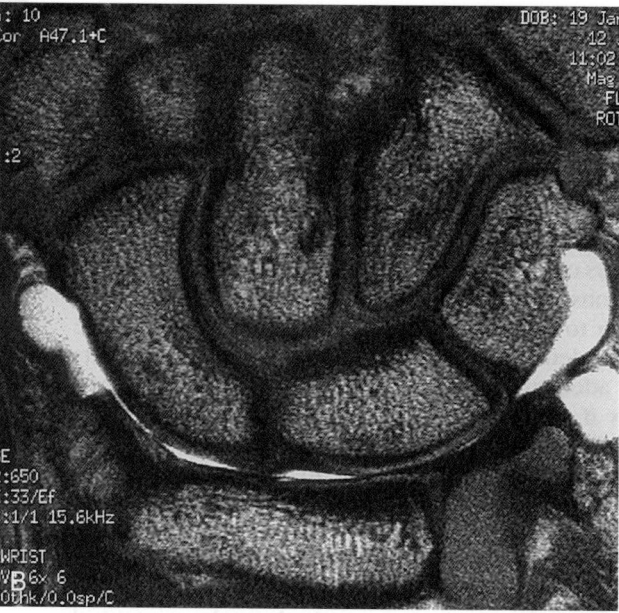

FIGURE 101-2

MR arthrograms. **A,** Coronal T1-weighted image with fat suppression. **B,** Coronal T1-weighted image without fat suppression (6 cm field of view, 2 mm sections, 512×512 matrix).

Intravenous MR arthrography[5-7] has been utilized by some (see Chapter 97). A standard dose of gadolinium is injected. Passive or active motion can be undertaken to exercise the patient to create a joint effusion and to obtain an arthrographic effect, with imaging done 15 minutes after injection. Another technique used to obtain an arthrographic effect is to create a joint effusion with therapeutic ultrasound.[8] Immediate imaging rather than delayed imaging has also been employed to enhance vascularized or inflamed tissue and improve contrast resolution in that manner. This technique can be used when direct techniques are inconvenient or are not logistically feasible. Indirect MR arthrography has been shown to improve sensitivity in the evaluation of scapholunate ligament tears versus unenhanced MRI.[9]

Axial images are necessary in patients with carpal tunnel syndrome (CTS) and masses. Coronal and sagittal T2-weighted imaging sequences are necessary in soft-tissue masses. We obtain one conventional spin-echo sequence, in the axial plane, but the additional imaging sequences can be acquired as FSE sequences. Care should be taken when evaluating the median nerve with fast spin-echo T2-weighted sequences with fat suppression or with FSE-IR images as they may falsely show increased signal in the median nerve in patients without symptoms of CTS. Intravenous gadolinium injection is utilized in patients with wrist synovitis, occasionally with wrist masses, and in evaluating the vascularity of the scaphoid or lunate in avascular necrosis (AVN). Fat-saturated short TR/TE or spoiled gradient-echo sequences (SPGR) are employed. As mentioned above, occult fractures and AVN may be best evaluated with sagittal and coronal T1-weighted, or T2-weighted FSE sequences with fat saturation or FSE-IR sequences. In evaluating scaphoid fractures and nonunion, T2-weighted coronal oblique FSE sequences, with fat suppression, oriented to the plane of the scaphoid may be helpful.

ANATOMY

Osseous Anatomy

The distal radius has on its lateral aspect the radial styloid process, which extends further distally than the rest of the bone. The radial collateral ligament arises from this region. The articular surface of the radius is divided into an ulnar and a radial portion. The radial portion articulates with the scaphoid and the ulnar portion with the lunate. The distal radius articulates with the distal ulna and its medial aspect in the region of the concave ulnar notch. On the volar radial aspect of the radius arise the volar radial carpal ligaments. On the dorsal surface is a prominent ridge, known as the dorsal tubercle. The distal ulna contains a small round head and a styloid process. The ulnar collateral ligament arises from the styloid process. The triangular fibrocartilage attaches to an area between the styloid process and the inferior articular surface. There is a dorsal groove for the extensor carpi ulnaris tendon and tendon sheath.

The carpus is arranged in proximal and distal rows. The proximal row consists of the lunate, triquetrum, and pisiform. The distal row consists of the trapezium, trapezoid, capitate, and hamate. The scaphoid traverses both rows. The dorsal surface of the carpus is convex, and the palmar surface forms a deep concavity, termed the carpal groove or canal.

The distal row of carpal bones articulates with the five metacarpals. The trapezium has a saddle-shaped articulation for the first metacarpal. The trapezoid fits into a deep notch in the second metacarpal. The capitate primarily aligns with the third metacarpal. The hamate articulates with the fourth and fifth metacarpals.

The wrist contains three main compartments: the distal radioulnar, radiocarpal, and midcarpal compartments. Other compartments include the pisiform triquetral compartment, the common carpometacarpal compartment, the first carpometacarpal compartment, and the intermetacarpal compartments. The distal radioulnar compartment is an L-shaped articulation whose proximal border is the cartilage-covered head of the ulna and ulnar notch of the radius. The radiocarpal compartment is formed proximally by the distal surface of the radius and the triangular fibrocartilage (TFC), and distally by the proximal row of carpal bones, exclusive of the pisiform. Its limit is the TFC. The midcarpal compartment extends between the proximal and distal carpal rows.

Ligamentous Anatomy

The carpal ligaments may be classified as either extrinsic or intrinsic. The extrinsic ligaments link the carpal bones to the radius and ulna. The intrinsic or intercarpal ligaments connect the individual carpal bones.

Volar Ligaments

The most functionally significant of the extrinsic ligaments are the volar radiocarpal ligaments.[10] There is considerable variation in the anatomic description of these ligaments.[10-14] These ligaments are the most important stabilizers of wrist motion. They originate from the volar aspect of the styloid process of the radius. Specifically, the radioscaphocapitate ligament (RSC; radiocapitate) connects the radius to the distal carpal row and plays an important role in preventing rotary subluxation of the scaphoid. The second and strongest, the radiolunotriquetral (RLT; radiotriquetral) ligament, connects the radius to the proximal carpal row (Fig. 101-3).

The volar extrinsic ligaments display low signal on MR images (Fig. 101-3), although on 3D images they may have a striated appearance.[15,16] On coronal sequences, the volar radiocarpal ligaments are bands of low signal intensity traversing obliquely from the radius to the carpal bones.[17,18] They can also be seen on sagittal images and this is the preferred plane of review of these ligaments by some.[15,16] The radioscaphocapitate ligament is the most radial of the major volar ligaments. It originates at the radial styloid, crosses the waist of the scaphoid, and attaches to the head of the capitate. Some fibers of the radioscaphocapitate ligament may extend to the triquetrum. The radiolunotriquetral ligament arises on

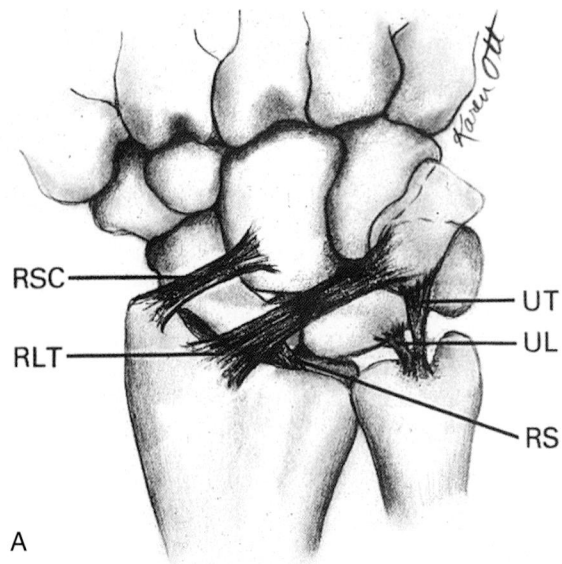

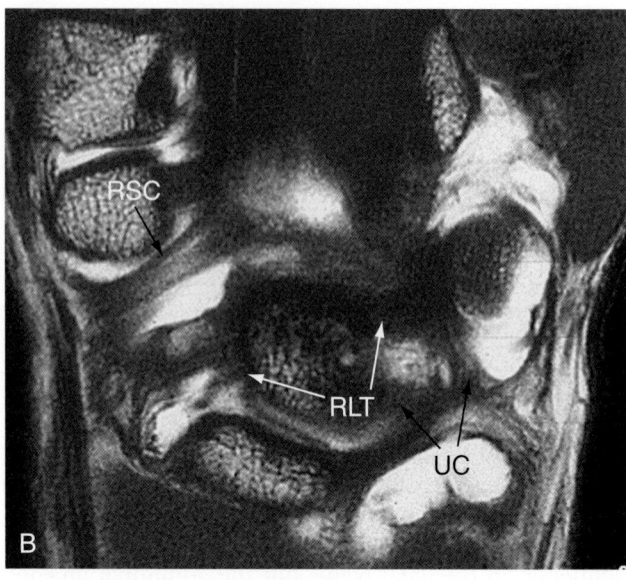

FIGURE 101-3

Anatomy of the volar ligaments. **A,** Diagram illustrating the volar radiocarpal and ulnocarpal ligaments. **B,** Correlative coronal MR arthrogram image. RLT, radiolunotriquetral ligament; RS, radioscaphoid (radioscapholunate) ligament; RSC, radioscaphocapitate ligament; UC, ulnocarpal ligaments; UL, ulnolunate ligament; UT, ulnotriquetral ligament. **(A,** From Greenan TJ, Zlatkin MB: Magnetic resonance imaging of the wrist. Semin Ultrasound CT MR 11:267-287, 1990).

the radial styloid process adjacent to the radioscaphocapitate ligament.[17,19-21] It courses distally and ulnarward to attach to the volar aspect of the triquetrum. It may be visualized in two portions, the radiolunate portion and the lunotriquetral portion. As such it has also been referred to as separate long radiolunate and volar lunotriquetral ligaments. This ligament serves as a volar sling for the lunate.

Of the small ligaments that attach to the palmar aspect of the scaphoid, lunate and scapholunate interosseous ligament, the ligament that attaches to the scapholunate interosseous ligament is most often identified, and it originates more dorsal and medial. It is best seen on coronal images. It has a higher signal intensity than the other extrinsic ligaments. It is best described as the radioscapholunate ligament. It arises from the volar aspect of the distal portion of the radius and inserts into the proximal and volar surfaces of the scapholunate interval.[13,22-24] Others believe that this structure may in fact not be a ligament at all. Rather it is thought to be a neurovascular bundle, with components derived from the anterior interosseous and radial arteries and the anterior interosseous nerve.[24]

The volar ulnocarpal ligaments[10,25] arise from the ulnar styloid process and the anterior margin of the TFCC (Fig. 101-3). The ulnocarpal ligaments can be best seen on coronal sequences, but may also be identified on sagittal sequences.[15,16] They extend distally and laterally to the lunate and triquetral bones respectively. That which inserts on the lunate is the ulnolunate ligament. The band that inserts on the triquetrum is the ulnotriquetral ligament. There is also a distal portion of the ulnotriquetral ligament that extends on to the volar aspect of the capitate and lunate.

The deltoid ligament has a V shape (Fig. 101-4). It is an intrinsic ligament. There is a capitotriquetral (ulnar) and a capitoscaphoid (radial) arm. Disruption of the ulnar arm of the deltoid ligament may lead to dynamic midcarpal instability. The space of Poirier is an area of normal weakness in the volar aspect of the capsule, just proximal to the deltoid ligament. It is through this site of weakness that volar dislocation of the lunate occurs.[26] The deltoid ligament may be difficult to observe on conventional spin-echo images, however Totterman[21] describes good visualization on thin-section 3DFT images. MR arthrography may also aid in its visualization.[4,20,27,28]

Dorsal Ligaments

The dorsal radiocarpal ligament extends from the dorsal aspect of the radial styloid to terminate on the triquetrum[29-31] and in its course traverses the lunate to which it is also attached[25] (Fig. 101-5). It actually represents a thickening of the joint capsule. This structure may be viewed as a single structure or as several separate structures with a multitude of different names. The most consistent of these structures appears to be the radiotriquetral ligament. These ligaments are generally regarded as functionally less important than the volar radiocarpal ligaments.

Of the other dorsal carpal ligaments the most prominent is the dorsal intercarpal ligament (Fig. 101-5). This is an intrinsic ligament. It may have a common proximal origin from the triquetrum with a proximal limb to the scaphoid (triquetroscaphoid) and a distal limb to the trapezium (triquetrotrapezium).[31]

The dorsal ligaments provide stability to wrist motion and are frequently injured in a fall on the outstretched

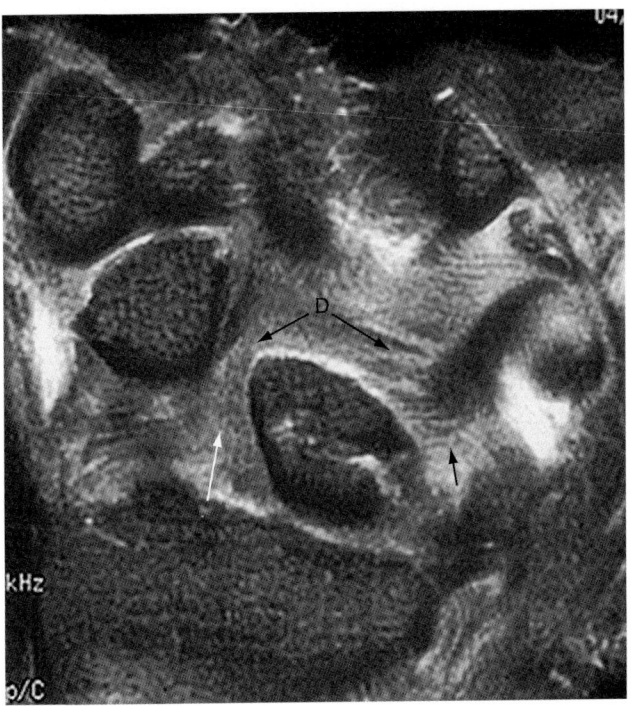

FIGURE 101-4

Coronal MR image. The V-shaped deltoid ligament is shown (D). The volar aspects of the scapholunate *(long white arrow)* and lunotriquetral *(shorter dark arrow)* ligaments are also shown.

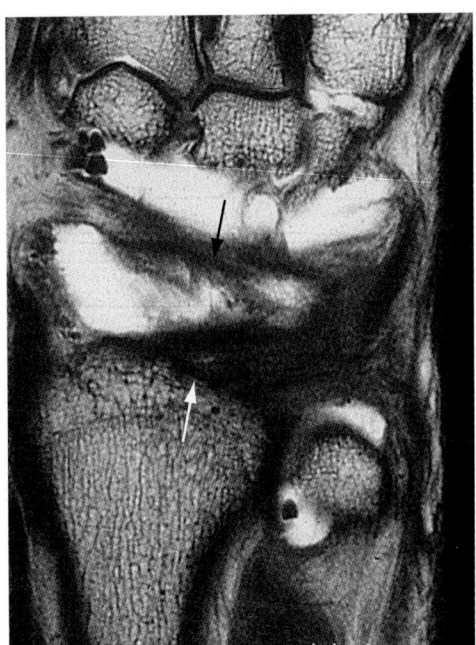

FIGURE 101-5

Dorsal ligaments. Coronal MR arthrogram. The dorsal radiocarpal ligament *(white arrow)* is seen. More distally the dorsal intercarpal ligament is identified *(black arrow)*.

hand, producing a "dorsal wrist sprain." The dorsal ligaments can be seen on sagittal images but are best depicted on dorsal coronal images (Fig. 101-5).[15,29,30,32] Smith[15,29] has described consistent visualization of these ligaments with 3DFT imaging with multiplanar reconstruction. High-resolution MR arthrography depicts these structures better than conventional MRI.[27,28]

Collateral Ligaments

The collateral ligaments are thickenings of the fibrous capsule and are functionally less important than collateral ligaments in other joints such as the knee. The ulnar collateral ligament is a poorly developed capsular thickening that arises from the ulnar styloid and inserts into the triquetrum. It has an extension more proximally to the TFCC. The radial collateral ligament is more volar than lateral and runs from the radial styloid process to the tuberosity of the scaphoid and the flexor carpi radialis tendon. The radial and ulnar collateral ligaments are seen as bands of low signal intensity on coronal sections.[33]

Interosseous Ligaments

The interosseous (intercarpal) ligaments are intrinsic ligaments that connect the adjacent carpal bones and separate the intercarpal compartments. The most important of these ligaments from a clinical and imaging point of view are the proximal interosseous ligaments:

the scapholunate (SL) and lunotriquetral (LT) ligaments (Fig. 101-6). These ligaments bridge the dorsal, proximal, and volar (palmar) aspects of their respective joints, leaving the distal aspect of each joint open to communicate with the midcarpal joint. Both of these ligaments have histologic characteristics that justify their division into dorsal, proximal, and volar (palmar) regions.[34] Both ligaments are deep in the joint. These ligaments have volar and dorsal portions with thinner membranous portions in between.[13,28,35] They separate the radiocarpal from the midcarpal compartments. They provide the flexible linkage for the proximal carpal row to function properly. The lunotriquetral ligament is more taut than the scapholunate ligament, thus there is a more solid relationship between these bones than that between the scaphoid and lunate. The distal carpal row has three intercarpal ligaments that unite the trapezium with the trapezoid, the trapezoid with the capitate, and the capitate with the hamate. The ligament between the capitate and hamate is the strongest. These distal interosseous ligaments do not extend from the volar to the dorsal portions of the wrist capsule, explaining the communication of the midcarpal and common carpometacarpal compartments of the wrist.[36]

The scapholunate and lunotriquetral interosseous ligaments are identified on MR images as bands of low signal intensity traversing the inferior aspect of these bones (Fig. 101-6). The scapholunate ligament is described as having either a linear or triangular configuration.[37] The triangular configuration is the most common. Most ligaments have homogeneous low signal intensity, but central or linear vertical intermediate signal intensity

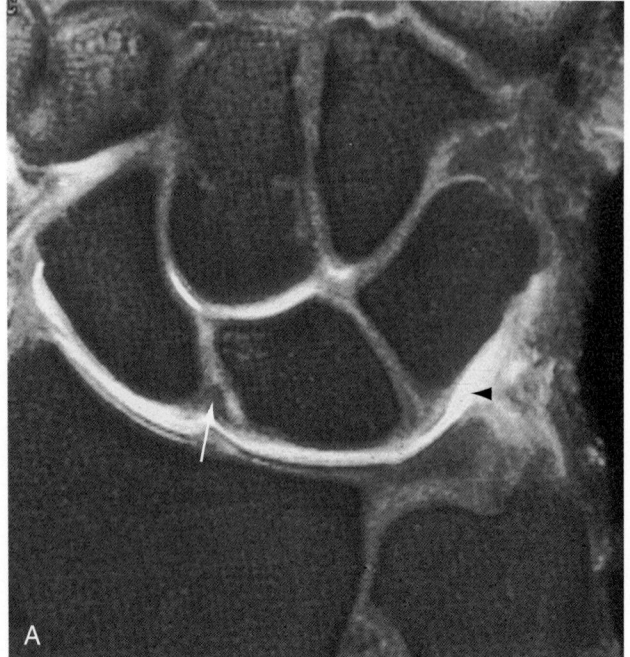

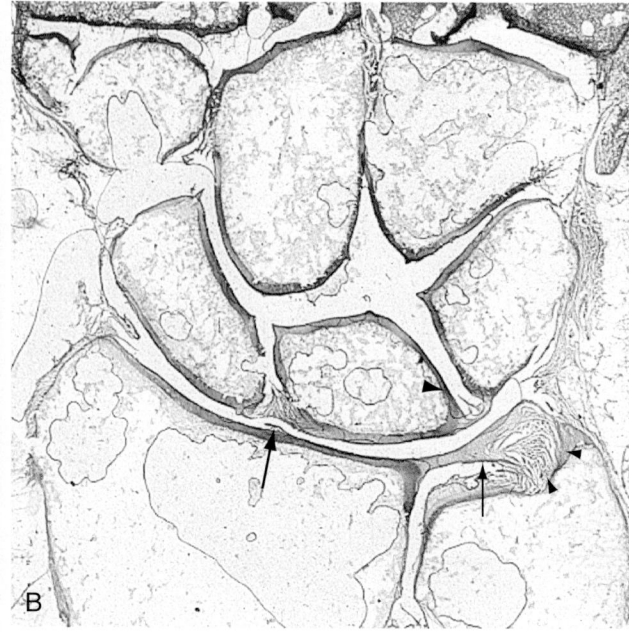

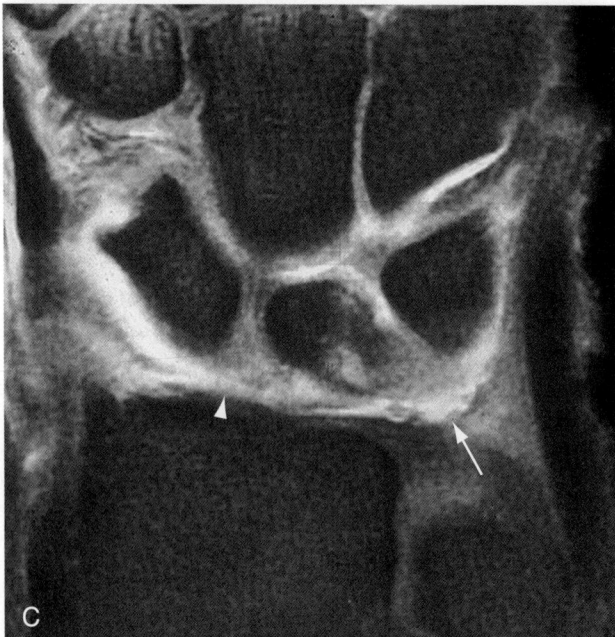

FIGURE 101-6

Normal intercarpal ligaments. **A** and **B,** Central portion. The central portions of the intercarpal ligaments are thinner. They course along the more inferior aspect of the corresponding carpal bones as seen on the coronal MR image in **A** and corresponding thin coronal histologic section in **B**. Note the scapholunate ligament (*white arrow* in **A**, *black arrow* in **B**), and the lunotriquetral (*arrowhead*). The scapholunate ligament may appear triangular in this central region. Also, note on the histologic section the differing characteristics of the TFCC, with the more fibrocartilage-like articular disk (*small black arrow*) and the more ligament-like peripheral ulnar attaching portion (*smaller arrowheads* in **B**), see later discussion. **C,** Dorsal portion of the ligaments. The ligaments in this portion thicken and extend more vertically, especially the scapholunate ligament. Scapholunate ligament (*arrowhead*), lunotriquetral ligament (*white arrow*).

may be seen within the scapholunate ligament.[37] Hyaline cartilage signal intensity may be present at the interface of this ligament with the scaphoid, lunate, or both, but primarily at the central weakest portion. The lunotriquetral ligament is more difficult to visualize because of its smaller size. It may have a linear, delta shape, or amorphous configuration. The delta shape is most common.[38] Although most LT ligaments also have homogeneously low signal intensity, there may also be linear intermediate signal intensity within the ligament and at its interface with the lunate, triquetrum, or both. This intermediate signal intensity seen in both the SL and LT ligaments and

at their bone interfaces should not be mistaken for tears unless fluid signal is seen traversing the ligament or its interface. Due to the convex adjacent surfaces of the scaphoid and lunate bones the scapholunate interosseous interval may appear wider along the far volar and dorsal aspects of the wrist.[39] This should not be mistaken for pathologic widening.[39]

The appearance of the intercarpal ligaments varies from the volar to dorsal aspect and this can be observed on MRI examination (Figs. 101-4, 101-6, and 101-7).[13,28,35] The volar region of the lunotriquetral ligament is a true ligament and is the thickest region of the ligament: it is

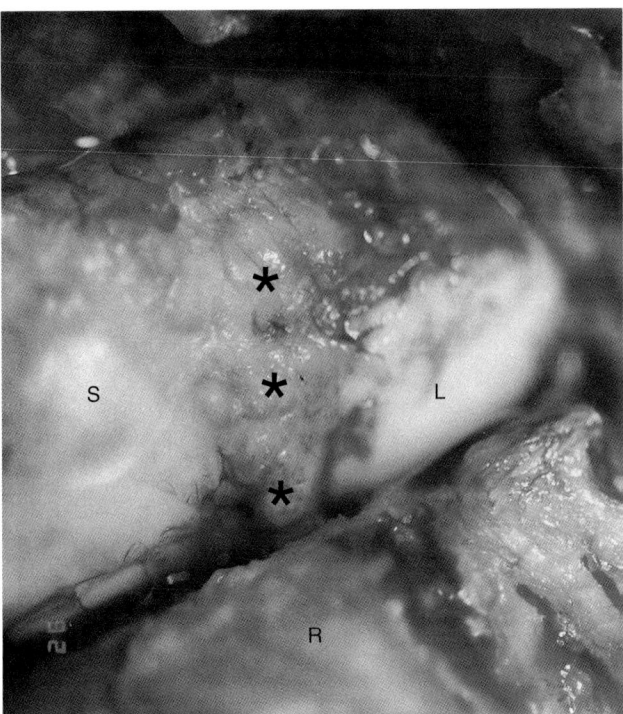

FIGURE 101-7

Normal scapholunate ligament *(asterisks)*. Intraoperative photograph, viewed from below. Note the volar to dorsal extent of the ligament. L, lunate; S, scaphoid; R, radius.

composed of transversely oriented collagen fascicles (see Fig. 101-4). Volarly, on MRI examination the LT ligament may appear to attach to, and be difficult to separate from, fibers of the TFCC, to which it may attach. The volar aspect of the scapholunate ligament is thinner than the dorsal aspect and oriented obliquely from palmar to dorsal, progressing from the scaphoid to the lunate (see Fig. 101-4).[34] It can appear thicker inferiorly and more posteriorly, just anterior to the central portion where the radioscapholunate ligament attaches. Both have a more linear mid portion, which on MRI may appear sling-like, attaching at the inferior margin of the carpal bones (see Fig. 101-6A). This central portion of the ligament may be fibrocartilaginous histologically.[34] Both ligaments thicken again dorsally, and have a broader proximal to distal attachment than at the mid portion, although in general the SL ligament is said to be thicker in the proximal to distal dimension than the LT ligament (see Fig. 101-6B).[21,40] In fact, the dorsal region of the scapholunate interosseous ligament is its thickest region, and is also a true ligament composed of transversely oriented collagen fascicles. The dorsal portion of the SL ligament is considered to be the most important portion for wrist stability. The appearance of these ligaments from volar to dorsal can also be characterized as hammock-like. The volar and dorsal portions extend not only linearly from medial to lateral as in the thinner central portion, but also have a more vertical course

from superior to inferior along the more volar (see Fig. 101-4) and especially along the more dorsal (see Fig. 101-6) aspects of the ligaments.

Triangular Fibrocartilage Complex

The structures that make up the triangular fibrocartilage complex (TFCC) are not universally agreed upon. In most descriptions, however, the TFCC is composed of the triangular fibrocartilage (TFC), the meniscus homologue, the ulnar collateral ligament, the dorsal and volar radioulnar ligaments, and the sheath of the extensor carpi ulnaris tendon[41] (Fig. 101-8). The ulnolunate and ulnotriquetral ligaments may also be considered as part of the TFCC.[42] These structures are a complex unit that functions as a stabilizing element in the pivot movement of the radius and ulna and limits the lateral deviation of the carpus. The distal radioulnar joint is primarily stabilized by the TFCC. The TFC functions as a cushion between the ulnar head and carpal bones.[11] Many of the structures that make up the complex are connected by fibrous bands. Proximally, the TFCC arises from the ulnar aspect of the lunate fossa of the radius, courses toward the ulna, and inserts in the fovea at the base of the ulnar styloid process. Benjamin et al,[43] in a histologic study, describe two ulnar attachments: a proximal one attaching to the base of the ulnar styloid, and a distal one, extending beyond the ulna and blending with the fibrous connective tissue of the extensor carpi ulnaris tendon sheath. The insertion of the disk may occasionally extend up the entire length of the styloid process[44] to its distal tip. Totterman et al also describe two ulnar styloid attachments, one at the ulnar base and one at the distal tip.[45,46] Palmer also describes an insertion along the ulnar head.[47] Distally, the TFCC inserts onto the hamate, triquetrum, and base of the fifth metacarpal.[47] As it extends distally, it is joined by fibers of the ulnar collateral ligament. The TFCC is firmly attached volarly to the triquetrum (ulnotriquetral ligament) and the lunotriquetral interosseous ligament, and less strongly to the lunate (ulnolunate ligament). It is strongly attached dorsally where it incorporates the sheath of the extensor carpi ulnaris tendon.[47] Just distal to the ulnar styloid is the prestyloid recess, which is a site of communication between the TFCC and the radiocarpal joint. The prestyloid recess is a fluid-filled space. It is located between the TFC and the meniscus homologue. It protrudes inferiorly to the apex of the TFC, and variably interfaces with the ulnar styloid process. The TFC separates the radiocarpal compartment from the distal radioulnar joint and acts as a cushion on the ulnar aspect of these joints. It is the most typical site of injury. It is fibrocartilaginous and is thicker at its margins than at the center. It may be fenestrated centrally, especially in older individuals. The thickness of the TFC is inversely proportional to ulnar length, thus a thinner TFC in patients with ulnar positive variance may predispose to TFC tears.[48,49] The thick and strong marginal portions of the TFC which are composed of lamellar collagen are often referred to as the dorsal and volar radioulnar ligaments. These are stabilizers of the distal radioulnar joint in radioulnar rotation. These

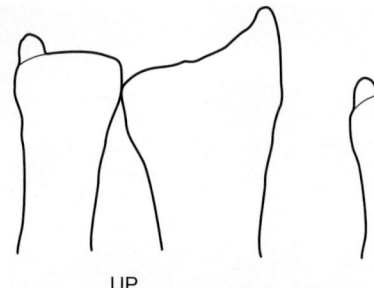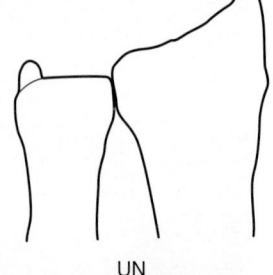

A

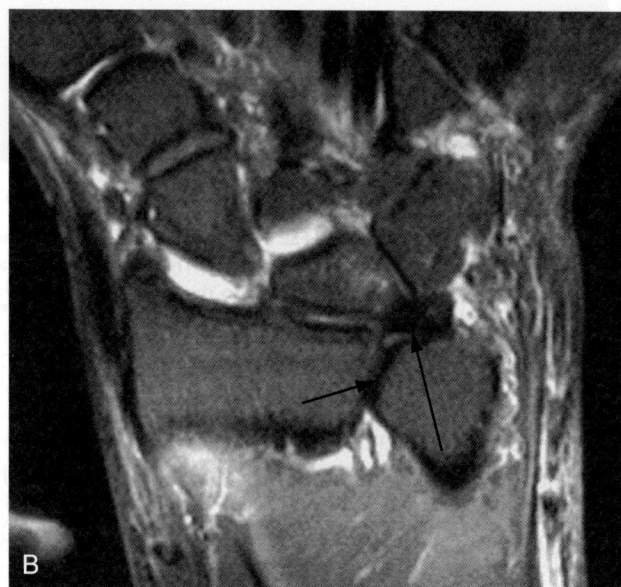

B

FIGURE 101-11

Ulnar variance. **A,** Diagrammatic representation of positive (UP), and negative (UN) variance. **B,** Coronal T2 FSE image. There is negative ulnar variance *(short arrow)*. Note the thickened TFC *(longer arrow)*. **C,** Coronal proton density–weighted FSE image. There is positive ulnar variance *(long arrow)*. There is a large central defect of the TFC *(short arrow)*. The lunotriquetral ligament is also disrupted *(arrowhead)*.

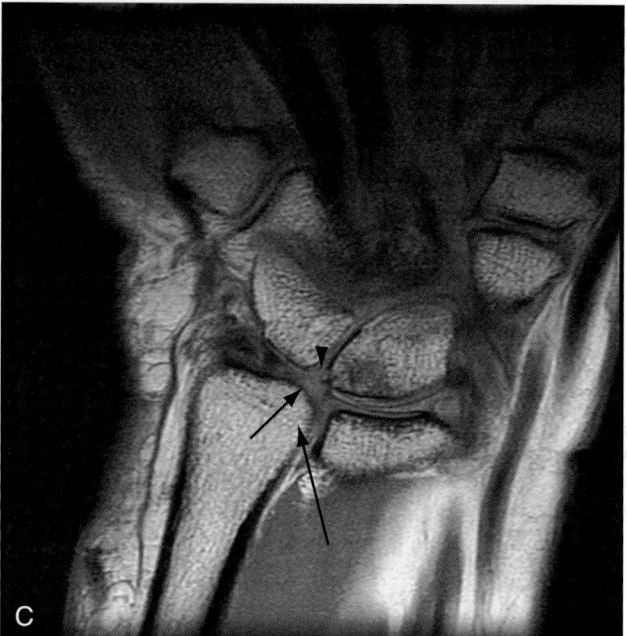

C

Axial MR images depict the distal ulna articulating with the distal radius (Fig. 101-10). The volar and dorsal radioulnar ligaments are also delineated as low signal intensity structures on MR images. Normal congruence of the DRUJ is present when the ulnar head is articulated within the sigmoid notch of the radius and does not project above a line drawn through the dorsal ulnar and radial borders of the radius or below a line drawn through the volar ulnar and radial borders of the radius.[33,57]

Variations of the length of the ulna relative to the radius are referred to as ulnar variance.[48,49,58,59] This can significantly alter the forces borne by the distal radius and ulna. Ulnar variance is measured from the center of the distal articular surfaces of the radius and ulna. It should be measured without any pronation or supination of the forearm, which can change the relative lengths of the distal radius and ulna. If the radius and ulna are of equal length then this is considered neutral: most of the axial loading forces are then transmitted from the ulna to the radius. If the ulna is long relative to the radius this is considered positive or plus, and if the ulna is short relative to the radius then this is considered negative or minus (Fig. 101-11).

As will be discussed in the section on Wrist Abnormalities, ulnar minus leads to a relative decreased load on the distal portion of the ulna, and is seen in association with Kienböck's disease. With such variance the TFCC is thicker (Fig. 101-11) and abnormalities of the TFCC are said to be less common.[48] In an ulnar positive situation there is an increase in the force borne by the distal portion of the ulna. The TFC portion is also thinner in such cases. This is seen in association with the ulnocarpal impaction/abutment syndrome. Ulnocarpal impaction syndrome may be associated with tears of the TFC and of the lunotriquetral interosseous ligament.[42,58,60-63]

Carpal Tunnel

The carpal tunnel is an oval-shaped space bounded ventrally by a ligamentous band, the flexor retinaculum, and dorsally by the volar surfaces of the carpal bones[64] (Fig. 101-12). The flexor retinaculum is composed of a band of transverse fibers attached to the pisiform and hook of the hamate medially and the scaphoid and trapezium laterally. The lunate and capitate form the floor of the carpal tunnel, the tubercle of the trapezium forms the lateral wall, the hook of the hamate the medial wall, and the flexor retinaculum the roof. Ten major structures reside within the carpal tunnel. Specifically these are the

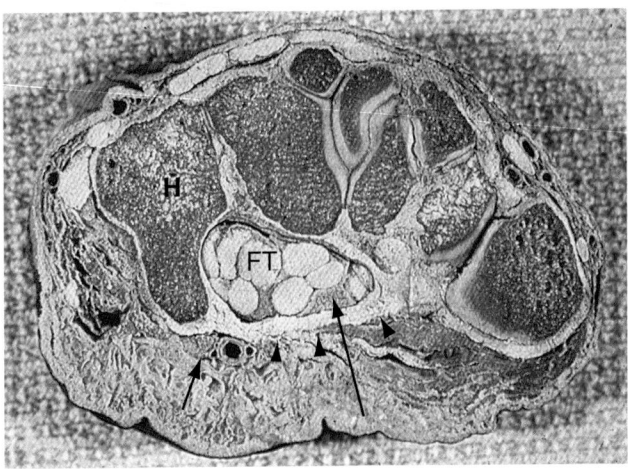

FIGURE 101-12

Carpal tunnel. Axial section at the level of the hamate hook (H). Note the flexor retinaculum (*arrowheads*), median nerve (*arrow*), and flexor tendons (FT). The ulnar nerve (*short arrow*) is outside the confines of the flexor retinaculum.

Guyon's Canal

The ulnar nerve at the wrist passes through a fibro-osseous tunnel known as Guyon's canal or the distal ulnar tunnel[66] (see Fig. 101-12) located at the antero-medial aspect of the wrist.[67] This is a triangular semirigid tunnel that extends from the flexor retinaculum at the proximal edge of the pisiform to the origin of the hypothenar muscles at the level of the hamate hook. It is bounded on the ulnar side by the pisiform and the flexor carpi ulnaris, dorsally by the flexor retinaculum, radially by the hamate hook, and on the flexor side by the volar carpal ligaments. The ulnar artery, occasionally some communicating veins, and fat are located within this canal. Within the canal, the nerve is medial to the artery. These structures within Guyon's canal, similar to the carpal tunnel and its contents, may be best seen on axial images[67] (Fig. 101-13).

Tendons

Extensor Tendons

The synovial sheaths of the extensor tendons are located on the dorsum of the wrist, beneath the dorsal carpal ligament. There are six compartments from medial to lateral. They contain the extensor tendons and their synovial sheaths. The most medial compartment (sixth compartment) contains the extensor carpi ulnaris tendon and its sheath, located at the dorsomedial aspect of the distal ulna. The extensor digiti quinti courses in the fifth compartment, and the fourth compartment contains the tendons of the extensor digitorum communis and the extensor indicis proprius. The third compartment contains the extensor pollicis longus. This tendon may rupture as the result of a Colles fracture, rheumatoid arthritis, or overuse, as it angulates around the dorsal radial (Lister's) tubercle. The second compartment contains the extensor carpi radialis brevis and longus. In the first compartment course the abductor pollicis longus and extensor pollicis brevis tendons, which are involved in De Quervain's tenosynovitis.[68,69]

Flexor Tendons

The long flexor tendons of the fingers and thumb are beneath the flexor retinaculum within the carpal tunnel in the wrist. The four flexor digitorum sublimis tendons are arranged in two rows, with the tendons to the middle and ring finger above the tendons for the index and little finger. The four flexor digitorum profundus tendons are deep to the sublimis. In the finger they are enveloped by digital sheaths. These sheaths usually terminate just proximal to the metacarpophalangeal joint, but the tendon sheaths of the thumb and little finger may communicate with the palmar synovial sacs in the wrist, the radial and ulnar bursae, which envelop the flexor tendons in the wrist and thumb (flexor pollicis longus) and may also communicate with each other through an intermediate bursa.[70] In the finger, these tendons partially decussate and in fact the sublimis tendons pass deep to

tendons of the flexor digitorum superficialis (four), the flexor digitorum profundus (four), and the flexor pollicis longus. The most important structure is the median nerve. It is located in the radial aspect of the tunnel deep to the flexor retinaculum and palmaris longus tendon. It usually lies between the flexor pollicis longus and flexor digitorum superficialis tendons but occasionally may be found more deeply.[65] Occasionally, a persistent median artery is also present.

MR imaging of the carpal tunnel (Fig. 101-13) is best performed in the axial plane. The majority of the space within the carpal tunnel is occupied by the flexor tendons, which appear as low signal intensity tubular structures. Each tendon is invested by an intermediate signal synovial sheath, which enables identification of the individual tendons as separate structures. The walls of the carpal tunnel include the palmar carpal ligaments deeply and the flexor retinaculum superficially. The flexor retinaculum is a volarly situated low signal intensity band. The flexor retinaculum can be oriented horizontally or may be slightly volarly bowed.[39] A small margin of fat is normally seen between the flexor tendons and the volar carpal ligaments and carpal bones. The median nerve is of intermediate signal intensity and remains isointense to muscle on long TR/TE images. On images with fat suppression such as T2 FSE with fat saturation or with STIR images the median nerve may increase in signal. The median nerve can be traced through the carpal tunnel and into the hand. Mesgarzadeh et al[65] describe evaluating the median nerve at six different levels including the distal radioulnar joint, the proximal carpal tunnel, the intermediate carpal tunnel, the distal carpal tunnel, the metacarpal base, and the metacarpal shaft. The normal median nerve in axial cross-section is round or oval in shape at the level of the distal radius, becoming more elliptical distally at the level of the hamate.[39]

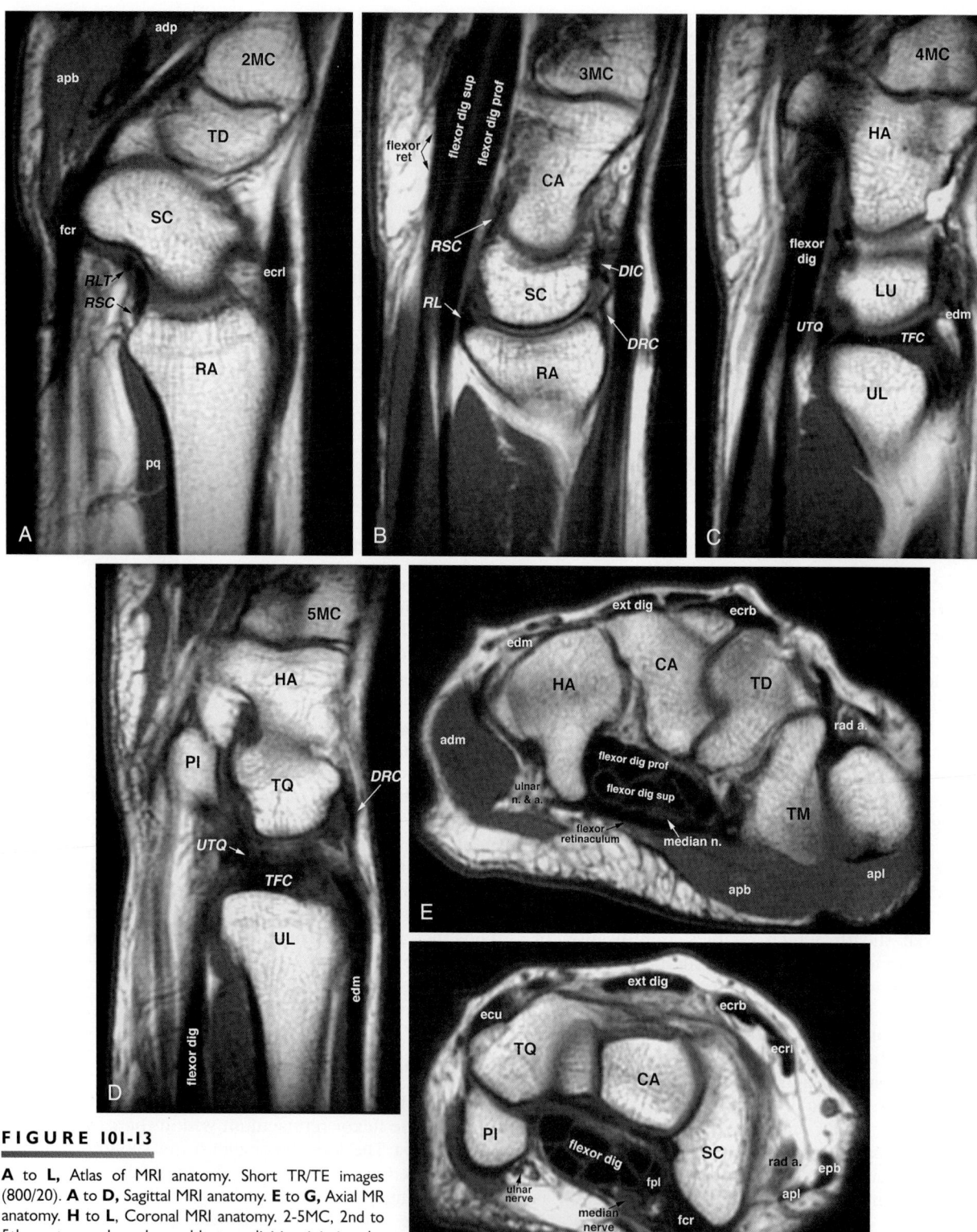

FIGURE 101-13

A to L, Atlas of MRI anatomy. Short TR/TE images (800/20). A to D, Sagittal MRI anatomy. E to G, Axial MR anatomy. H to L, Coronal MRI anatomy. 2-5MC, 2nd to 5th metacarpals; adm, adductor digiti minimi; adp, adductor pollicis; apb, abductor pollicis brevis; apl, abductor pollicis longus; CA, capitate; DIC, dorsal intercarpal ligament; DRC, dorsal radiocarpal ligaments; DRUL, dorsal radioulnar ligament; ecrb, extensor carpi radialis brevis; ecrl, extensor carpi radialis longus; ecu, extensor carpi ulnaris; edm, extensor digiti minimi; epb, extensor pollicis brevis; epl, extensor pollicis longus; ext dig, extensor digitorum; ext ten, extensor tendons; fcr, flexor carpi radialis; fcu, flexor carpi ulnaris; fdp / flexor dig prof, flexor digitorum profundus tendons; fds / flexor dig sup, flexor digitorum superficialis; flexor ret, flexor retinaculum; fpl, flexor pollicis longus; HA, hamate; HH, hh, hamate hook; LTB, Lister (dorsal radial) tubercle; LT, lunotriquetral interosseous ligament; LU, lunate; PH, pisiform-hamate ligament; PI, pisiform; pq, pronator quadratus; RA, radius; rad a., radial artery; RC, radial collateral ligament; RL, radiolunate portion of radio-scapholunate ligament; RLT, radiolunotriquetral ligament; RSC, radioscaphocapitate ligament; SC, scaphoid; SL, scapholunate interosseous ligament; TD, trapezoid; TFC, triangular fibrocartilage; TM, trapezium; TQ, triquetrum; UCL, ulnar collateral ligament; UL, ulna; UTQ, ulnotriquetral ligament; VRUL, volar radioulnar ligament. (J and K, 3 T images courtesy of Paul Clifford MD, University of Miami).   Continued

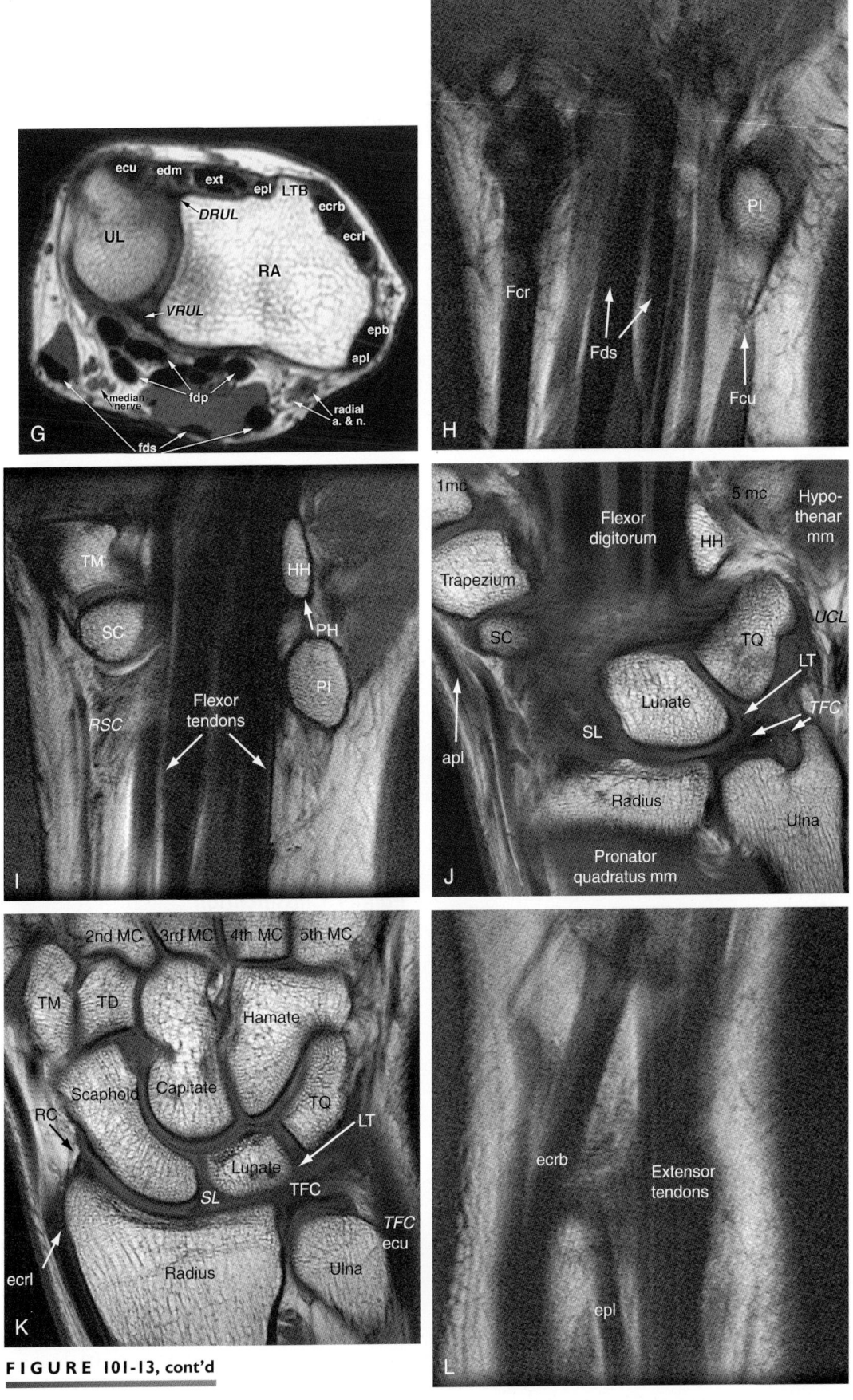

FIGURE 101-13, cont'd

the profundus tendons and attach to the sides of the middle phalanx. The tendons of the profundus attach distally to the base of the terminal phalanx and in fact change from a deep to a superficial location at the level of the middle phalanx.

The tendons should appear as tubular structures of homogeneously low signal intensity on MR images within the intermediate signal synovial sheaths (Fig. 101-13). Fluid within the tendon sheaths may be detected as high signal intensity on long TR/TE images.[69,71]

WRIST ABNORMALITIES

Triangular Fibrocartilage Complex Tears

General Features

Lesions of the TFCC may be variable in their extent of involvement. They may be confined to the horizontal or flat portion of the TFCC, referred to as the TFC or articular disk, or involve one or more components of the TFCC. Such injuries also can involve instability of the DRUJ. Tears of the TFC should be suspected in patients with ulnar-sided wrist pain and tenderness, although some degenerative tears or defects may not be symptomatic. A palpable or audible click or pain may be present with rotation of the forearm. Both degenerative and traumatic tears of the TFC may occur.

Degenerative perforations tend to occur in the central region of the disk where it is thinnest.[47] The incidence of central degenerative tears is age related. According to Mikic,[52] degeneration begins in the third decade and progressively increases in frequency and severity in subsequent decades. The changes comprise reduced cellularity, loss of elastic fibers, mucoid degeneration of the ground substance, exposure of collagen fibers, fibrillation, erosion, ulceration, abnormal thinning, and, ultimately, disk perforation. The changes are more frequent and more intense on the ulnar surface, and they are always situated in the central part of the disk. In Mikic's cadaveric study of 180 wrists, there were no perforations in the first two decades of life, in the third there were 7.6%, in the fourth 18.1%, in the fifth 40.0%, in the sixth 42.8%, and in cadavers of those older than 60 the incidence was 53.1%. There was an associated pattern of degenerative changes in the wrist joint as a whole. The structures adjacent to the articular disk (discal surface of the ulnar head, discal part of the lunate) were much more often involved, and the changes were much more advanced than on non-discal surfaces. As degenerative perforations may be so common in older patients, who may be asymptomatic, Gilula and Palmer[72] have objected to the use of the term "tear" or "perforation" for these lesions and prefer the term "defect."

Longer ulnae are associated with perforations of the triangular fibrocartilage complex (TFCC). Positive ulnar variance may lead to increased ulnar carpal loading with resultant ulnolunate impaction syndrome.[47,58,60,62,73-75] This chronic abutment leads to erosive changes in the cartilage of the ulnar head and lunate, degenerative perforation of the disk, and attrition and eventually a tear of

the lunotriquetral ligament. These associated abnormalities of the lunotriquetral interosseous ligament have been described in up to 70% of patients with degenerative perforation of the TFC.[47] In spite of the stated association of ulnar positive variance with TFC tears and ulnocarpal abutment, Manaster,[76] in a study utilizing plain films and arthrography, was unable to find a significant correlation between ulnar positive variance and TFC tears. This may have been due to the young age of the patients in the study, as the majority were younger than 35 years.[76] Tomaino also has indicated that although the ulnar impaction syndrome occurs most commonly in the ulnar positive wrist, it can also occur in wrists with either ulnar negative or neutral variance.[74]

In patients with negative ulnar variance, TFC tears may more likely be traumatic. Many post-traumatic tears of the TFC occur closer to the radial insertion (within 2 to 3 mm) than the central degenerative tears where the thick collagen bundles connect the avascular portion of the TFC to the radius.[77] Traumatic tears may also be more common in younger patients. Avulsions of the TFC may also occur from the ulnar attachments.[63,78-80] This is typically a less common lesion, although in a study by Golimbu[75] most of the tears that were observed were felt to occur closer to the ulnar insertion site.[63,79,80] Ulnar detachments may be associated with an ulnar styloid fracture.[81,82] This may be associated with instability of the distal radioulnar joint Palmer type 1B (see below).[83] Ulnar styloid fracture associated with an avulsion of the ulnar attachment of the TFC can result in nonunion (type 2).[82] The ununited fracture can cause chondromalacia along the undersurface of the triquetrum.[58] Studies of the microvascular anatomy of the TFC indicate that tears that occur on the ulnar side of the TFC have the ability to heal, whereas those that are centrally or radially located do not.[50,77]

Palmer Classification

The Palmer classification of TFCC tears divides them into traumatic (class IA to D) and degenerative (class IIA to D) (Box 101-1). Palmer indicated that the traumatic type (class I) were relatively uncommon. The traumatic types include central perforation, ulnar avulsion with and without distal ulnar fracture, distal avulsion, and radial avulsion, with and without sigmoid notch fracture. Class IA, the central perforation, represents a tear or perforation of the horizontal portion of the TFCC, usually occurring as a 1 to 2 mm slit, located 2 to 3 mm medial to the radial attachment of the TFCC. The ulnar avulsion, or class 1B, represents a traumatic avulsion of the TFCC from its insertion site into the distal portion of the ulna, sometimes with an associated fracture of the base of the styloid process of the ulna. This is considered to be an unstable lesion. Class IC represents distal avulsion of the TFCC at its site of attachment to the lunate or triquetrum, reflecting a tear of the ulnolunate and/or ulnotriquetral ligaments. A class ID lesion represents avulsion of the TFCC from its attachment to the radius at the distal aspect of the sigmoid notch, which may be associated with an avulsion fracture of this region.[84]

Box 101-1	Palmer Classification of Triangular Fibrocartilage Injuries[41]

Class I (Traumatic Injury)
A   Central perforation
B   Ulnar avulsion ± distal ulnar fracture
C   Distal avulsion at carpal attachment
D   Radial avulsion ± sigmoid notch fracture

Class II (Degenerative Injury)
A   TFCC wear
B   TFCC wear, lunate or ulnar chondromalacia
C   TFCC perforation, lunate or ulnar chondromalacia
D   TFCC perforation, lunate or ulnar chondromalacia, lunotriquetral ligament perforation
E   TFCC perforation, lunate or ulnar chondromalacia, lunotriquetral ligament perforation, ulnocarpal osteoarthritis

The degenerative type is reflected by progressive stages of ulnocarpal impaction. Five types of degenerative lesions were detailed. Class IIA is TFC wear from the undersurface, occurring in the central horizontal portion, without perforation. Class IIB is TFC wear as denoted above, with ulnolunate malacia. The cartilage changes occur on the inferomedial aspect of the lunate, or on the more radial portion of the head of the ulna. Class C is TFC perforation, with ulnolunate malacia. The perforation is in the central, horizontal portion of the TFCC and occurs in a more ulnar location than that seen with the traumatic injury that occurs in this region (class IA). Class D is a TFC perforation in the central horizontal portion, associated with ulnolunate malacia as denoted in IIC, and lunotriquetral ligament perforation. Class E is all of the above with ulnolunate/ulnocarpal arthritis, and there may be degenerative arthritis about the distal radioulnar joint as well.

MRI Findings

Degenerative defects are more common than traumatic defects. The imaging characteristics however may be similar; location, age, and clinical history as discussed above may often be needed to differentiate their origin. Either type of lesion may result in full-thickness defects of the TFCC, and these can be visualized on MRI examination or at MR arthrography.

A radial tear of the TFC appears as a linear band of increased signal intensity on short TR/TE and proton density–weighted SE or GRE images.[33,53] With complete tears the signal extends to both proximal and distal articular surfaces. In partial tears, considered to be less important from a clinical perspective, the signal will only extend to one articular surface, usually the proximal surface (DRUJ), as the proximal surface tends to be subject to greater stresses, particularly in situations of positive ulnar variance. The signal will increase on long TR/TE images, SE images, or T2*-weighted GRE images or T2-weighted FSE sequences with fat suppression (see

Fig. 101-14), consistent with synovial fluid trapped in the defect. Fluid collecting in the DRUJ is an important secondary sign,[85] but the presence of fluid signal intensity alone is not indicative of a tear of the TFC. MR arthrography, either with a radiocarpal or DRUJ injection, will reveal contrast extending through and outlining the TFC defect (Fig. 101-14).

There are no specific differentiating features on MRI examination to separate a traumatically induced tear of the TFC from one due to degeneration. The appearance of these lesions may also be similar in both symptomatic and asymptomatic individuals, therefore it may be difficult to determine the clinical relevance of these lesions and their correlation with the patient's symptoms (i.e., radial- or ulnar-sided wrist pain).[86] As noted above, the age of the patient, the site of the tear, and associated lesions may help in this regard.

Ulnar-sided tears should be differentiated from central tears because of the different therapeutic strategies. As indicated above, peripheral tears have a good vascular supply and are thus repaired, whereas central lesions are avascular and are treated with debridement. Ulnar-sided tears and avulsions can, however, be more difficult to diagnose,[53,87] especially if a large amount of fluid on the ulnar aspect of the wrist is present. Differentiating this joint fluid from focal synovitis related to a peripheral TFCC injury may be difficult. Oneson et al, in their large study of TFCC tears, found only a small number of ulnar-sided tears. They had a poor sensitivity to these lesions. This was attributed to the presence of the striated fascicles at the periphery of the TFCC, which were considered to be difficult to evaluate by MR imaging.[88]

Findings that correlate with these types of tears include altered morphology of the ulnar attachments of the TFC, excessive fluid localizing to this region, especially if it extends below the expected location of the prestyloid recess, and linear fluid signal intensity in the ulnar TFC itself extending to its surface (Fig. 101-15). High signal intensity at the ulnar insertion of the triangular fibrocartilage complex as the only marker for a tear of the ulnar TFCC may be insensitive: in the study of Haims and co-workers[87] this finding revealed a sensitivity of only 42%, a specificity of 63%, and an accuracy of 55%. Use of axial and sagittal imaging may be helpful in assessing these patients. Greater attention to the findings of focal synovitis may also improve sensitivity.[87] Additionally, unenhanced and enhanced MRI may be helpful in differentiating joint fluid from focal synovitis.[87] MR arthrography may also help outline such tears by revealing contrast extending directly into the defect. The results of indirect MR arthrography in this regard are still under investigation and further study is needed in determining its efficacy.[6,9] Not uncommonly, fluid signal and thickening may be present along the ulnar aspect of the TFCC (Fig. 101-16). This appearance may be due to degenerative and/or inflammatory change or the result of an old healed peripheral TFC injury with scarring and chronic synovitis. This may be difficult to differentiate from an acute peripheral TFC injury. Correlation with the patient's clinical history is very helpful in this regard. Nonetheless such findings may often be associated with significant ulnar-sided wrist pain.

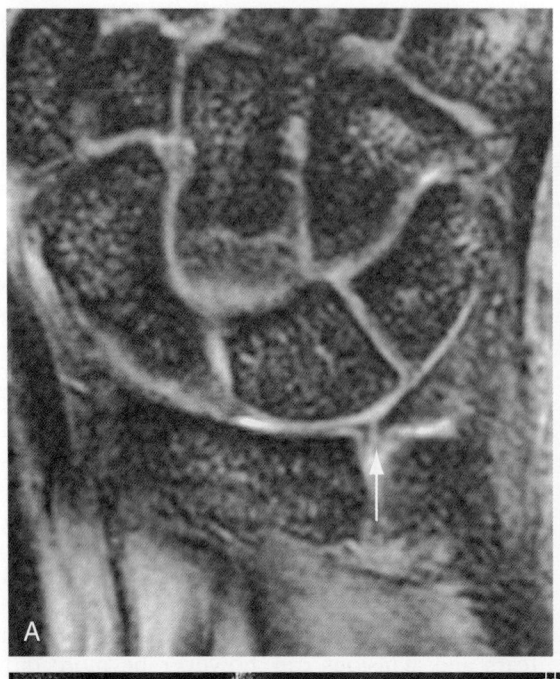

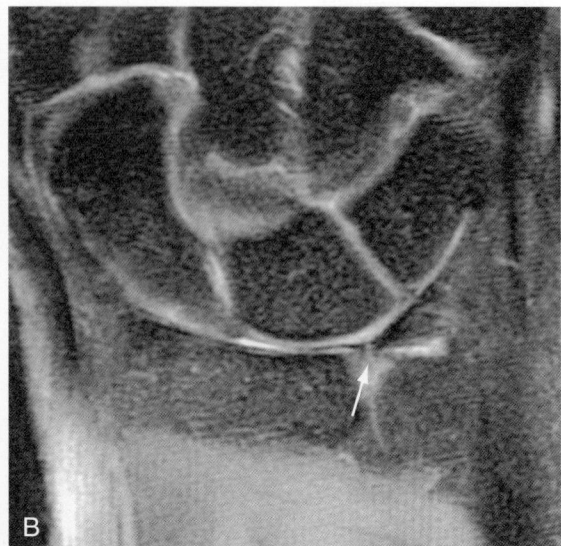

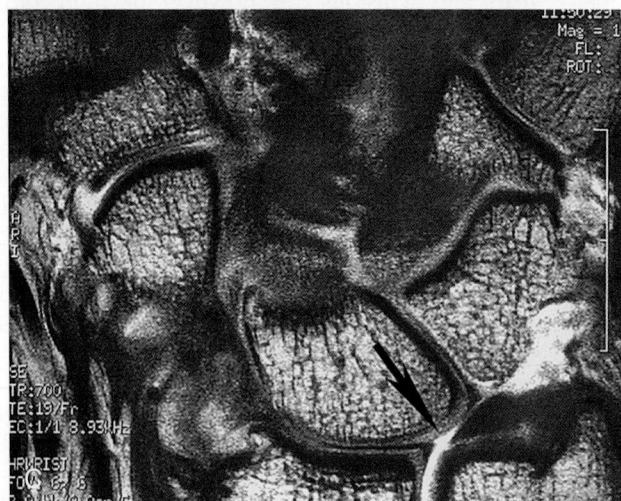

FIGURE 101-14

Radial-sided triangular fibrocartilage (TFC) tears. Coronal 2D T2* gradient-echo image (**A**) and T2 FSE image with fat saturation (**B**) demonstrate fluid signal intensity in the radial aspect of the TFC (*arrow*) which extends to both the radiocarpal and the distal radioulnar joint (DRUJ) articular surfaces. Fluid is seen in the DRUJ. **C,** Coronal high-resolution T1 FSE image after intra-articular contrast injection into the radiocarpal joint in another patient illustrates high-signal-intensity contrast extending through a TFC defect into the DRUJ (*arrow*).

Ulnocarpal Impaction (Abutment)

Ulnocarpal impaction syndrome (Figs. 101-11C, 101-17, and 101-18) is considered a degenerative condition and is characterized by ulnar-sided wrist pain, swelling, and limitation of motion related to excessive load-bearing across the ulnar aspect of the wrist.[58,60,62] There is typically a pattern of ulnar positive variance or a distal ulna prominent enough to allow transfer of excessive compressive force from the ulna and triquetrum and lunate via the TFCC. It is distinguished from ulnar impingement, which consists of a short ulna impinging on the distal portion of the radius and causing a disabling painful pseudoarthrosis. Ulnocarpal abutment can also occur in a secondary manner, via acquired ulnar positive anatomy, after malunited distal radius fractures.[73]

In patients with ulnocarpal abutment (impaction), foci of low signal intensity may be seen within the articular cartilage of the ulnar head and/or lunate, reflecting

the presence of chondromalacia.[51] There may be thinning of the articular cartilage surface. This may be best seen on T2 FSE sequences with fat saturation, or on MR arthrography, if performed. The perforations in these lesions are more centrally located. Degenerative changes in the subchondral marrow of the lunate, including marrow edema and subchondral cystic change, may develop as well (see Fig. 101-17). These may be difficult to distinguish from intraosseous ganglia; however, MRI can document the presence of the central tears of the TFC and lunotriquetral interosseous ligament.

Ulnocarpal abutment cannot be treated via simple partial debridement of the TFC. More extensive procedures, such as ulnar shortening or resection of the ulnar head, must be carried out in order to treat these patients. After such procedures, improvement in some of the articular cartilage and bone marrow alterations discussed above may be identified.[75] In the study by Imaeda

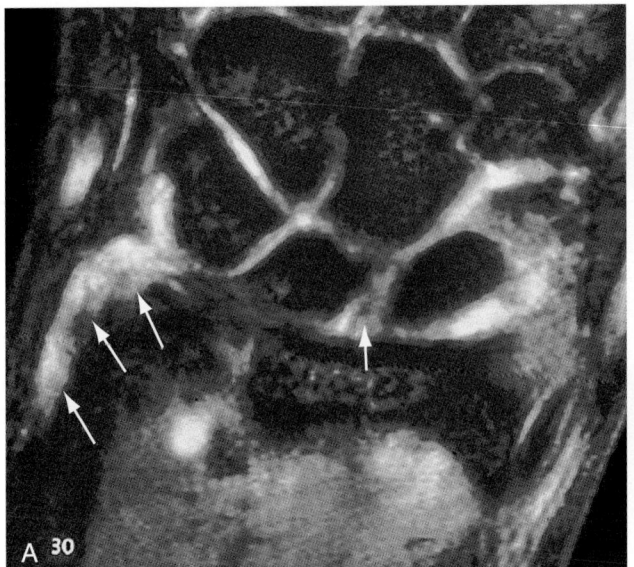

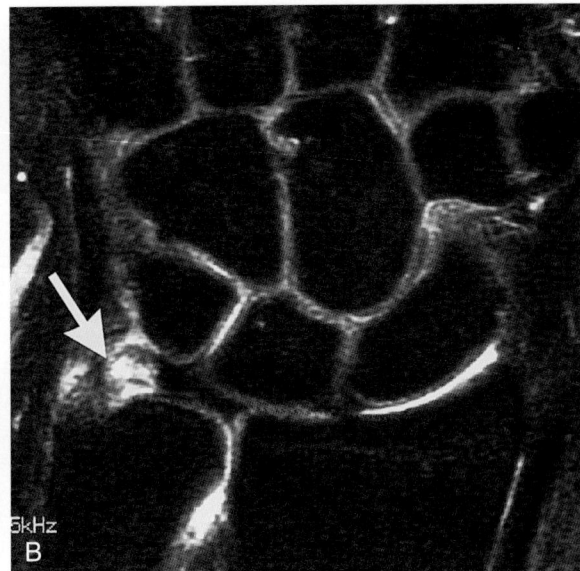

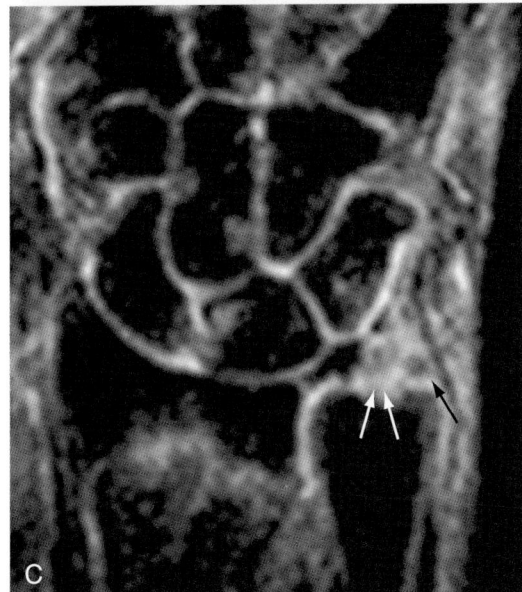

FIGURE 101-15

Ulnar-sided triangular fibrocartilage (TFC) tears. **A,** Coronal 2D T2* gradient-echo image. A large amount of fluid signal is seen replacing the ulnar attachment of the TFC, extending beyond the ulnar capsule, along the extensor carpi ulnaris tendon sheath more proximally *(arrows)*. A tear of the scapholunate ligament is also present *(short arrow)*. **B,** Coronal T2 FSE image with fat saturation reveals fluid signal and altered morphology indicating disruption of the ulnar attachment *(arrow)* of the TFC. **C,** Coronal STIR image. The ulnar aspect of the TFC is torn and detached *(white arrows)*. There is a fracture of the ulnar styloid tip *(black arrow)*.

FIGURE 101-16

Chronic peripheral triangular fibrocartilage complex (TFCC) synovitis. Coronal T2-weighted MR image. Marked thickening and fluid signal is seen along the ulnar attachments and ulnar aspect of the TFCC *(arrows)*.

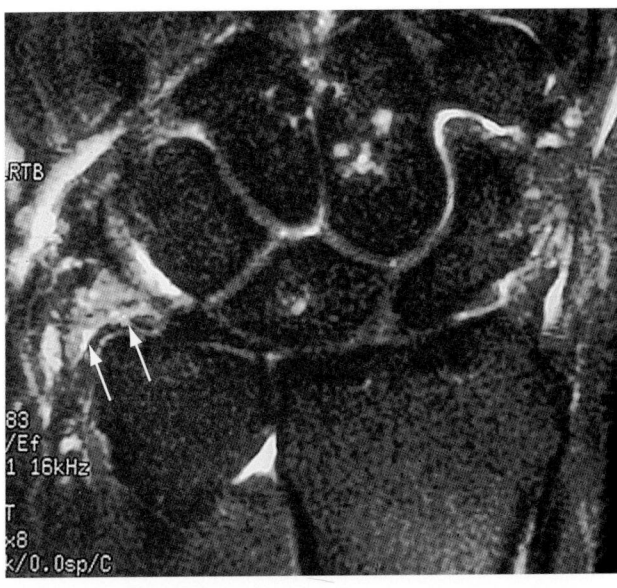

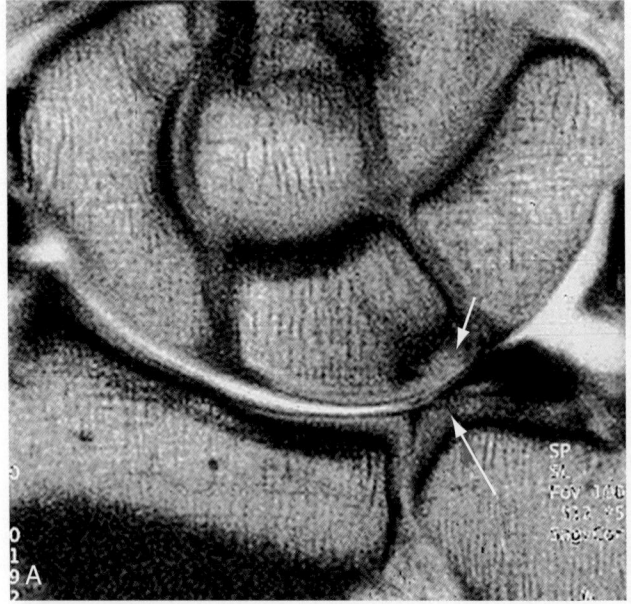

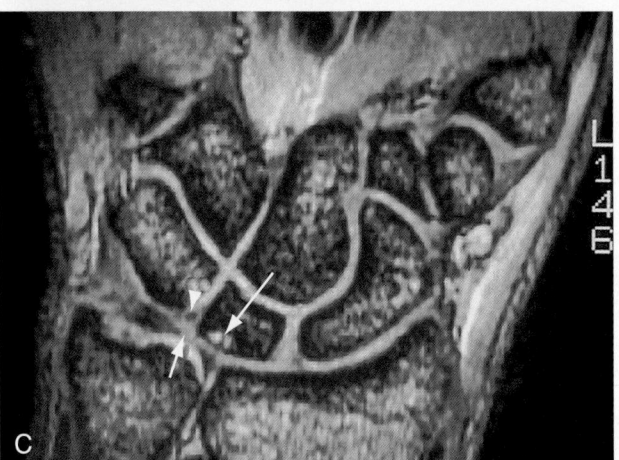

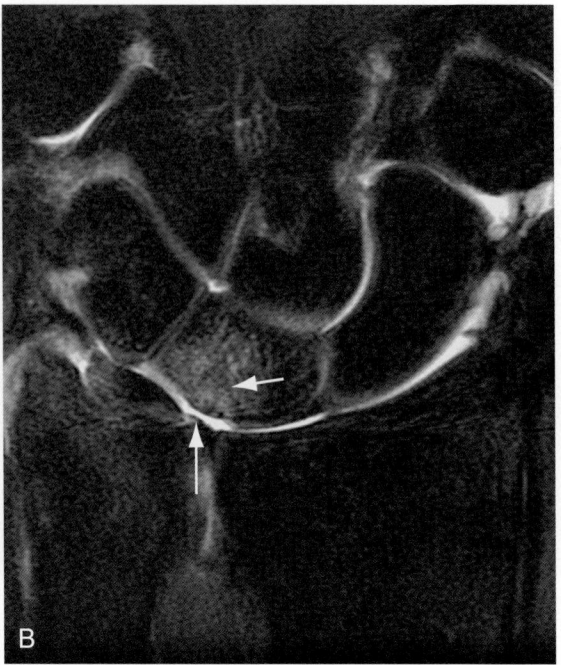

FIGURE 101-17

Ulnocarpal impaction syndrome. **A,** Early stage (stage 2B). High-resolution T1-weighted MR arthrogram reveals prominent thinning of the triangular fibrocartilage (TFC) undersurface *(long arrow),* with corresponding marrow alterations of the inferior medial aspect of the lunate *(short arrow).* **B,** Later stage 2C. Coronal T2-weighted FSE image with fat saturation. A large central TFC defect is seen *(arrow).* There is marked chondro-malacia of the inferomedial lunate with associated marrow edema *(short arrow).* **C,** Late stage (stage 2D). Note the wide central TFC defect *(short arrow),* cystic change in the inferomedial lunate *(long arrow),* and disrupted lunotriquetral ligament *(arrowhead).*

et al[75] there was focal abnormal signal intensity of the ulnar aspect of the lunate in 87% of wrists, of the radial aspects of the triquetrum in 43%, and of the radial aspects of the ulnar head in 10% before surgery. The signal intensity of the abnormalities was decreased on T1-weighted images and decreased or increased on T2-weighted images. After surgery, the signal intensity of the lunate shifted from low through slightly low to normal on T1-weighted images and from low through high to normal on T2-weighted images.

Ulnar Styloid Impaction

Ulnar-sided wrist pain can also be caused by impaction between an excessively long ulnar styloid process and the triquetral bone.[58,89] Onetime or repetitive impaction between the tip of the ulnar styloid process and the triquetral bone results in contusion, which leads to chondromalacia of the opposing articular surfaces, synovitis, and pain. If a single-event trauma is forceful enough, fracture of the dorsal triquetral bone may occur.

Impaction over a long period of time can lead to lunotriquetral instability. The diagnosis of this condition is made on the basis of radiographic evidence of an excessively long ulnar styloid process in combination with positive findings on a provocative clinical test. MR imaging may reveal the prominent ulnar styloid process, chondromalacia of the ulnar styloid process and proximal triquetral bone, associated marrow edema, and a lunotriquetral tear if present (Fig. 101-19). Resection of all but the two most proximal millimeters of the styloid process (so as not to interfere with the TFC complex insertion) is the treatment of choice.

Degenerative Lesions of the Triangular Fibrocartilage Complex

High signal intensity within the TFC may be encountered commonly on T1-weighted and proton density–weighted MR images.[51,86] This signal can be mistaken for a tear. If such a high signal intensity change does not communicate with the inferior or superior surface of the TFC

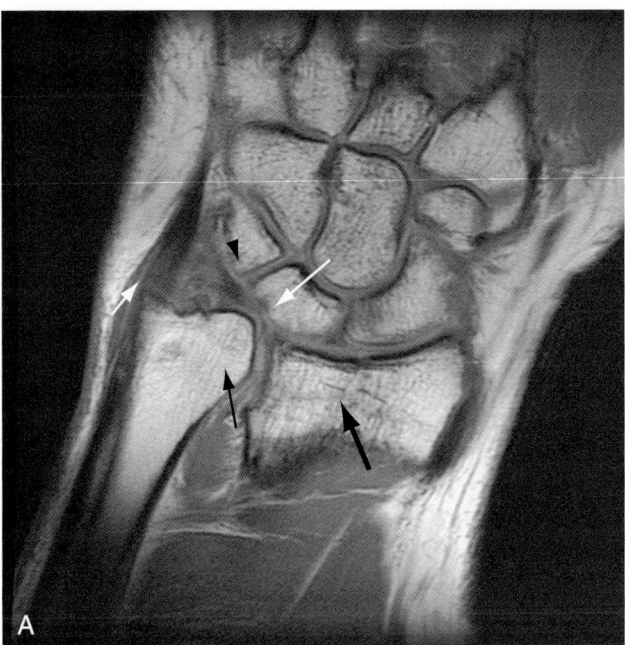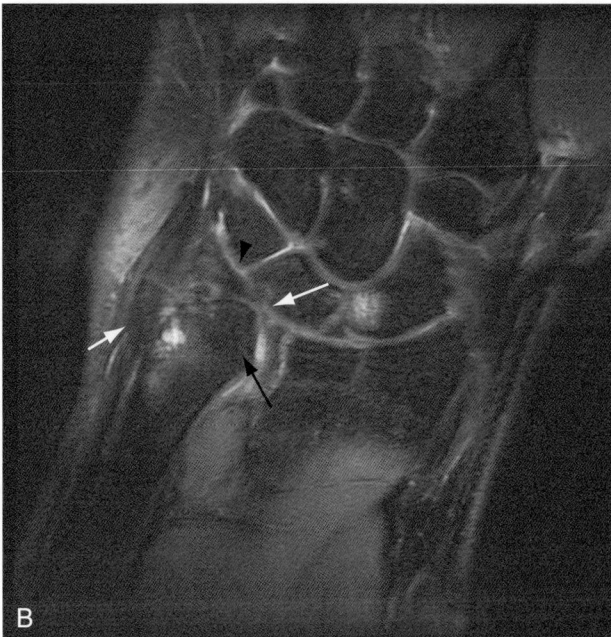

FIGURE 101-18

Secondary ulnocarpal abutment. **A,** Coronal FSE proton density–weighted image; **B,** T2-weighted image with fat saturation. The ulna is positive *(black arrow)* owing to shortening from a prior distal radius fracture *(thick black arrow in **A**)*. There is secondary ulnocarpal abutment. Note the triangular fibrocartilage tear *(long white arrow)*, marrow change in the lunate, and lunotriquetral ligament tear *(black arrowhead)*. Additionally noted is tendinosis of the extensor carpi ulnaris *(short white arrow)*.

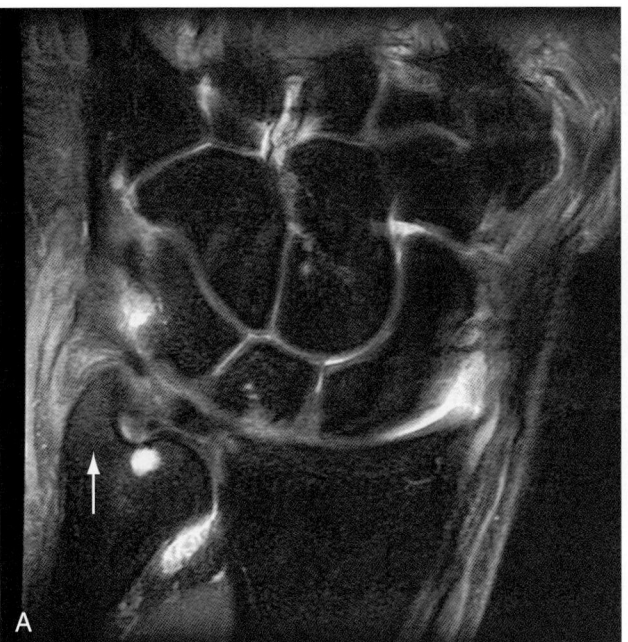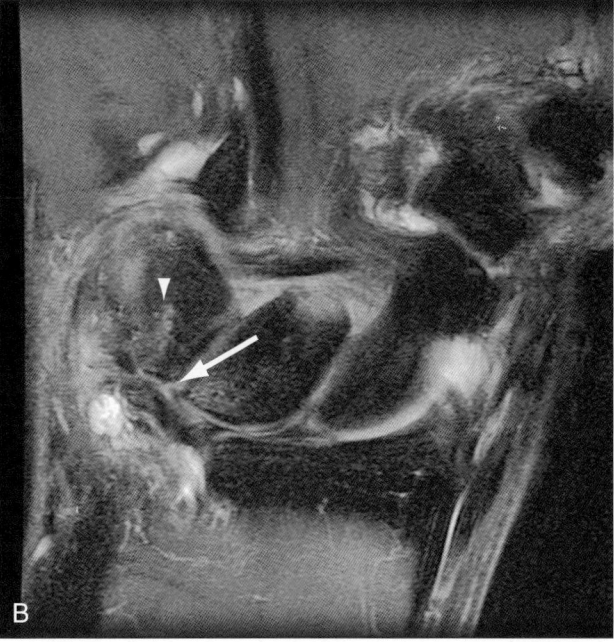

FIGURE 101-19

Ulnar styloid impingement. **A** and **B,** Coronal T2 FSE images with fat saturation. The ulnar styloid is prominent in **A** *(arrow)*. Note the edema in the triquetrum *(arrowhead)*, and the lunotriquetral ligament tear *(long white arrow)*. Abnormalities are also present in the triangular fibrocartilage complex undersurface and peripheral aspect.

and if it does not get bright on images with T2 contrast it is not considered indicative of a tear. In fact, such high signal intensity may diminish on images with T2 contrast, particularly if fat suppression is not applied. This high signal intensity pattern was studied in cadavers[51,86] and was considered to be attributable to degeneration, both mucinous and myxoid in character, and to the age of the person, increasing in frequency with age. Such alterations in high signal intensity and their differentiation are similar to those problems that arise from degenerative-type high signal intensity that occurs in the glenoid labrum of the shoulder and in the meniscus of the knee.

Degenerative change on the surface of the TFC may also be seen in asymptomatic individuals on MRI examination.[51] It is typically more evident on the proximal aspect of the TFC and in its more central portion. It occurs centrally, as this is the thinner portion of the TFC, and also more proximally due to the greater biomechanical stresses on this surface of the TFC. These alterations on the ulnar surface of the TFC may be similar to those changes seen in patients with ulnocarpal abutment and may be accompanied by similar alterations in the distal portion of the ulna and of the inferior surface of the lunate.[51]

Diagnostic Performance

MRI studies of the tears of the TFC when compared to arthrography and arthroscopy, have revealed a sensitivity of 92%, specificity of 89%, and accuracy of 98%.[52,88] Potter et al[90] assessed the diagnostic performance of MRI using thin-section 3D volume gradient-echo sequences. MRI was found to be sensitive and specific in the diagnosis and location of TFC tears when correlated with arthroscopy. The sensitivity of MRI for tears was 100% and the specificity was 90%. In a study by Oneson et al[88] of 56 patients who underwent arthroscopic evaluation of the TFC, using the Palmer classification for TFC pathology, the sensitivity for detecting central degenerative perforations was 91%. The sensitivity for detecting radial slitlike tears was 100% and 86% for observers I and II. The sensitivity for detecting ulnar-sided avulsions was 25% and 50% for observers I and II, indicating at least in this study that ulnar-sided avulsions can be more difficult to detect. In a British study by Johnstone and co-workers,[91] however, results were less favorable when compared to arthroscopy. The sensitivity and specificity of MRI compared with arthroscopy were 80% and 70% for TFCC pathology. Another study utilizing cadavers found that low-field-strength extremity-only magnets may allow visualization of the TFC and allowed accurate assessment of a small number of complete tears. Observer experience may play a role in the accuracy of interpretation and predicting the location of the lesions.

A recent study by Haims et al,[87] also discussed above, found MR imaging not to be sensitive in revealing injuries of the peripheral attachment of the TFCC. High signal intensity at the ulnar insertion of the TFCC as a marker for tear only showed a sensitivity of 42%, a specificity of 63%, and an accuracy of 55%. The authors, however, indicated that all of the peripheral tears in this study were associated with synovitis at arthroscopy. It is possible that the finding of a focal synovitis at the ulnar attachment could be used as a marker for peripheral tear. The authors felt that this focal synovitis could potentially be differentiated from fluid with the use of unenhanced and enhanced imaging.[87]

MR arthrography may be of value in evaluating TFCC lesions, particularly in identifying defects on the ulnar aspect where the anatomy is more complex and more ligamentous in nature. It may also help to outline partial tears of the undersurface. If MR arthrography is carried out, injection of the DRUJ may best outline such partial-thickness defects. Schweitzer and colleagues[6] reported good initial results with indirect MR arthrography in evaluation of the TFCC, although a more recent study by this group revealed less promising results.[9] Herold and co-workers[92] evaluated indirect MR arthrography in detecting TFCC tears. The sensitivity and specificity in the detection of TFCC lesions were calculated as 100% and 77%. The accuracy was 93%. Small degenerative changes of the TFC fibers were most common (Palmer type IIA). In trauma the tears occurred near the insertion of the TFCC at the ulna (Palmer type IB). No deficiency in the evaluation of ulnar-sided lesions was detected in this study.

Treatment

Treatment of TFC tears often can be carried out arthroscopically. Unstable central fragments can be excised or debrided.[93,94] Peripheral separations may be treated with suture repair, due to the more vascular nature of this region.[95,96] Tears associated with a positive ulnar variance can be treated with ulnar shortening–type procedures as described in the discussion of ulnocarpal impaction.[97]

Other Causes of Ulnar-sided Wrist Pain

Other causes of ulnar-sided wrist pain that may mimic TFCC tears include pisiform-triquetral osteoarthritis, fractures of the hamate, DRUJ instability, radioulnar degenerative change (Fig. 101-20), disorders of the extensor carpi ulnaris tendon (ECU; Fig. 101-20), and calcific tendonitis of the flexor carpi ulnaris tendon.[98] Recent assessment of MR imaging and/or MR arthrography for the pisotriquetral joint determined that it allows visualization of all anatomic structures of the pisotriquetral joint.[99] Cartilaginous lesions and osteophytes were easily identified and were detected more often in the pisiform bone than in the triquetral bone. Communication of the pisotriquetral joint with the radiocarpal joint was noted in 82% of wrists. MR arthrography improved the visualization of findings of osteoarthritis. Hamatolunate impingement is a less common cause of ulnar-sided wrist pain.[100] Hamatolunate impingement occurs secondary to an anatomic variant in which the lunate has a separate articulation with the hamate. This is referred to as a type II lunate. In this configuration there is a second lunate facet, medially for articulation with the hamate, in addition to the normal articulation with the capitate. Impingement is felt to occur with repetitive ulnar deviation. As a consequence,

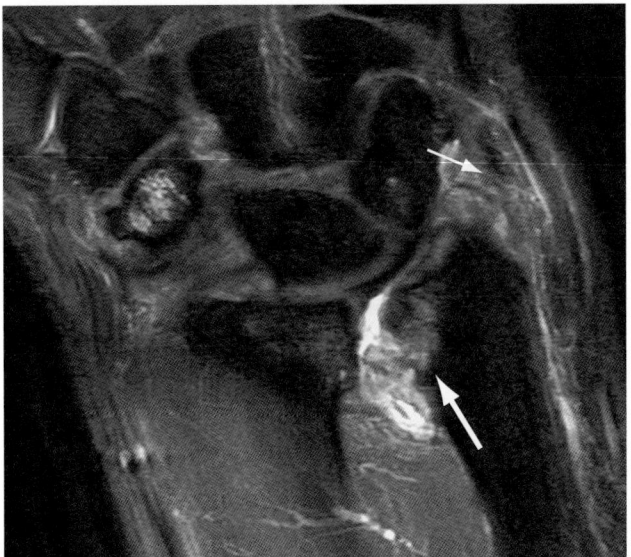

FIGURE 101-20

Distal radioulnar joint arthritis. Marginal cystic change, loss of cartilage, and bony productive change are seen *(larger arrow)*. Also note the severe extensor carpi ulnaris tendinosis, with thickening and increased signal intensity *(smaller arrow)*.

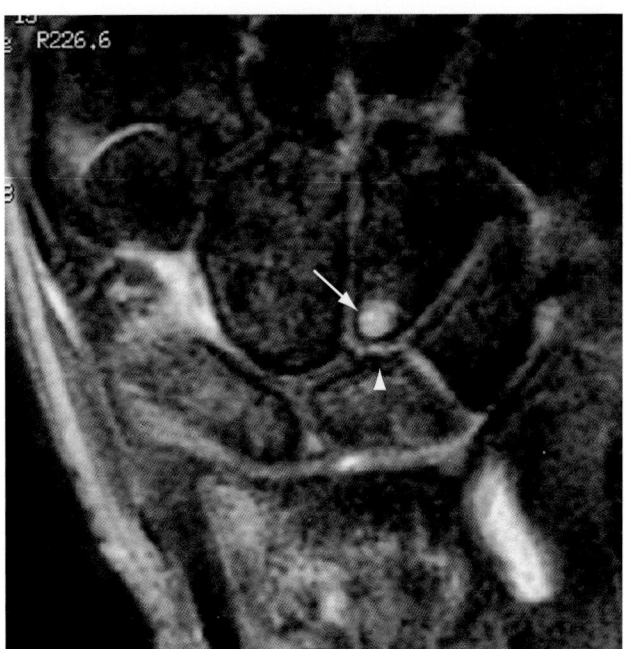

FIGURE 101-21

Hamatolunate abutment. The lunate has a separate medial articulation with the hamate (type II lunate; *arrowhead*). Note the subchondral cysts on the inferior hamate *(arrow)*. The marrow edema in the radius and proximal carpal row is due to unrelated trauma.

there is a propensity for chondromalacia of the base of the hamate. On MRI examination (Fig. 101-21) there may be chondral erosions along the medial lunate facet and the proximal pole of the hamate. Subchondral cysts and sclerosis and marrow edema may be seen, usually on the hamate side. In addition there may be some additional capitate-lunate arthrosis. Arthroscopy with burring of the hamate is the current treatment option.

Instability of the Distal Radioulnar Joint

Nathan and Schneider[101] emphasized the theory that instability of the DRUJ is caused by a deficiency or disruption of various components of the TFCC. Instability of the DRUJ may arise in relation to injury,[102] may be part of a process associated with a fracture of the distal radius or of the styloid process of the ulna, or may accompany such inflammatory processes such as rheumatoid arthritis. The clinical manifestations of DRUJ instability include pain, weakness, loss of forearm rotation, and snapping. Dorsal instability predominates over volar instability. On physical examination a dorsal prominence of the ulnar head may be appreciated, especially in the position of forearm pronation.

The diagnosis, if not evident by clinical examination, can usually be made on the lateral radiograph with the wrist in neutral position.[103] However, if the distal radius is deformed by fracture, or proper positioning is precluded by intractable pain or a plaster cast, then axial imaging will provide a more accurate assessment of the congruity of the DRUJ.[103] Examinations that employ cross-sectional imaging, including CT and MRI, are advantageous over plain radiographic examination in the diagnosis of DRUJ instability.

Although CT[103-105] is generally considered the procedure of choice to make this diagnosis as it is more rapidly obtained and may be less expensive than MRI, the advantage of utilizing MRI instead of CT for this purpose is that associated abnormalities such as tears of the TFC can be evaluated as well. Also, the dorsal and volar radioulnar ligaments can be directly visualized, especially on axial images.[33,106] It is also possible to assess adjacent structures such as the extensor carpi ulnaris tendon and other components of the TFCC that can be affected. Volar radioulnar ligament tears may be associated with dorsal instability.

Short TR/TE axial images through the DRUJ can be obtained rapidly and are satisfactory to demonstrate subluxation and dislocation (Fig. 101-22). It should be remembered that in pronation the distal ulna might rotate slightly dorsally and in supination slightly volarly. When imaging for DRUJ incongruity, scans are routinely obtained in pronation, supination, and neutral positions. Comparison views of the opposite side are helpful to diagnose minor degrees of instability.

Ligamentous Injuries

General Features and Pathophysiology

The ligaments of the wrist, both intrinsic and extrinsic, play an important role in wrist stability. Although the extrinsic volar radiocarpal ligaments are felt to be important factors in carpal stability, injuries to the intrinsic

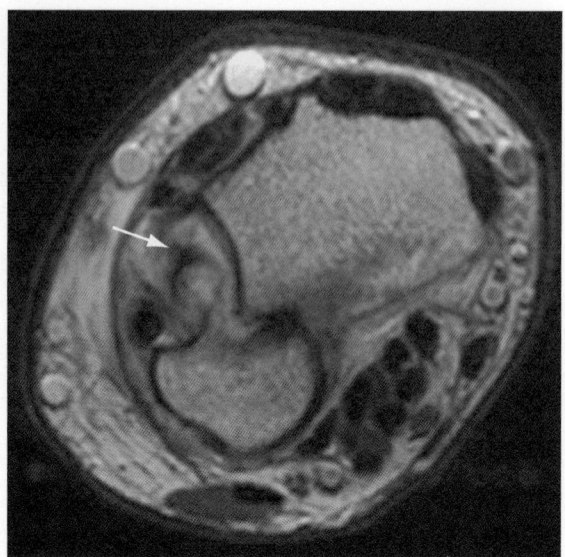

FIGURE 101-22

Distal radioulnar joint (DRUJ) subluxation. Axial MR image. Note volar subluxation of the DRUJ. The dorsal radioulnar ligament is stretched, irregular and attenuated (arrow).

interosseous ligaments of the wrist have been better documented with imaging techniques and may often be a cause of pain and dysfunction in patients. Although MRI demonstrates the anatomy of the extrinsic ligaments,[16,17,27] pathologic lesions of the intrinsic interosseous ligaments are more readily visualized.[9,15,33,37,53,107-111]

The wrist may be injured by a fall on the outstretched arm. In such a situation it can undergo hyperextension, ulnar deviation, and internal supination. When there is ligamentous injury to the wrist, a spectrum of severity[10,112,113] may result. The most common ligamentous injuries occur on the radial side of the wrist. Mayfield,[10,112,113] describes a pattern of progressively severe ligamentous injury as four stages of perilunar instability. According to Mayfield, stage I consists of tearing the volar extrinsic radioscaphoid ligament with elongation or partial tearing of the scapholunate interosseous ligament. With continued loading, total ligamentous failure occurs at the scapholunate joint, followed by failure of the radioscaphoid capitate ligament or an avulsion fracture of the radial styloid (stage II). If loading about the radial aspect of the wrist persists, then ligamentous disruption will occur at the lunate-triquetral joint with radiolunotriquetral ligament and dorsal radiocarpal ligament disruption (stage III). Finally, in stage IV, with a large load of prolonged duration, there occurs the ultimate failure of the dorsal radiocarpal ligament, which renders the lunate free to rotate volarly on its remaining volar ligamentous attachments.

Different schemas exist for classifying wrist instability. The carpus is considered unstable if it exhibits symptomatic malalignment.[26] Some authors have divided carpal instability into carpal instability dissociative (CID) and nondissociative forms (CIND).[114,115] Nondissociative instability represents abnormalities of alignment or relationship of the carpal bones with intact interosseous ligaments, although there may be some attenuation of the palmar and dorsal radiocarpal and ulnocarpal ligaments. These are less common than dissociative instabilities, which include trans-scaphoid fractures and tears of the scapholunate and lunotriquetral interosseous ligaments. These may occur also in association with injuries to the palmar and dorsal extrinsic ligaments. Instabilities may also be classified as static or dynamic.[116-119] Static instabilities are based on the presence of radiographically detectable carpal abnormalities. With dynamic instability, the carpal alignment may be altered from normal to abnormal with certain movements of the wrist or with manipulation of the wrist during clinical examination. If these instabilities are classified anatomically, there are three types of carpal instability[118,119]: lateral between the scaphoid and lunate; medial between the triquetrum and lunate and triquetrum and hamate (less common); and proximal when there is instability related to injury of the radius and/or massive radiocarpal disruption. Instabilities involving the scapholunate articulation may also produce a dorsal intercalated segmental instability pattern (DISI) and those between the lunate and triquetrum a volar segmental instability pattern (VISI). Static patterns of wrist instability such as scapholunate dissociation and lunate-triquetral dissociation with or without DISI or VISI, scapholunate advanced collapse (SLAC), and ulnar translocation may often be identified on plain radiographic examination alone. Stress views and fluoroscopy may help identify some more subtle forms of static instability and some dynamic instabilities.

MR Imaging

MRI and MR arthrography can be helpful to identify some of the ligamentous and soft-tissue injuries that occur in the circumstance of wrist instability. They have been found to be useful in the detection of injuries to the interosseous ligaments, particularly the scapholunate ligament and, to a lesser degree, the lunotriquetral ligament.[18,27,53,85,111,120] Variable success has also been achieved with both techniques in evaluating injuries to the volar and dorsal radiocarpal ligaments.[16,17,27,53,121]

Scapholunate instability

Scapholunate instability presents with pain, swelling, and tenderness over the dorsoradial aspect of the wrist. Tears of this ligament may be partial or complete. On MRI examination[33,53,85] complete tears (Figs. 101-23 and 101-24) appear as distinct areas of discontinuity within the ligament with increased signal intensity on images with T2 type contrast, or complete absence. Severe distortion of the morphology of the ligament (fraying, thinning, or irregularity) may also reflect ligamentous injury. Coursing of the central portion of the ligament in a direction other than horizontal may also be considered abnormal. MR arthrography may aid in revealing contrast extravasation through a complete defect (Fig. 101-25), or help to outline the aforementioned morphologic alterations. Fluid in the midcarpal joint is a sensitive but

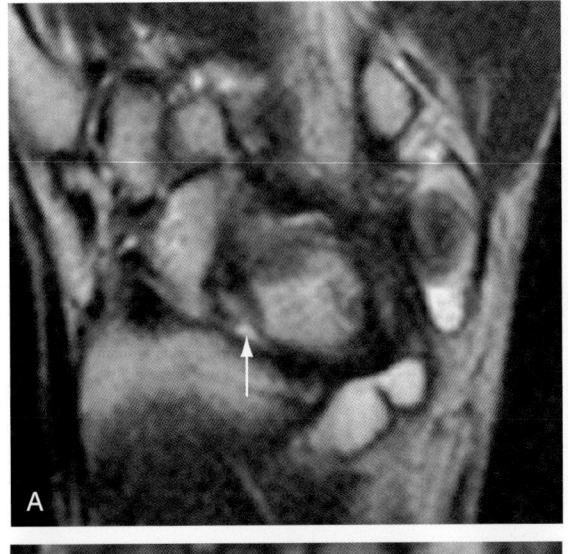

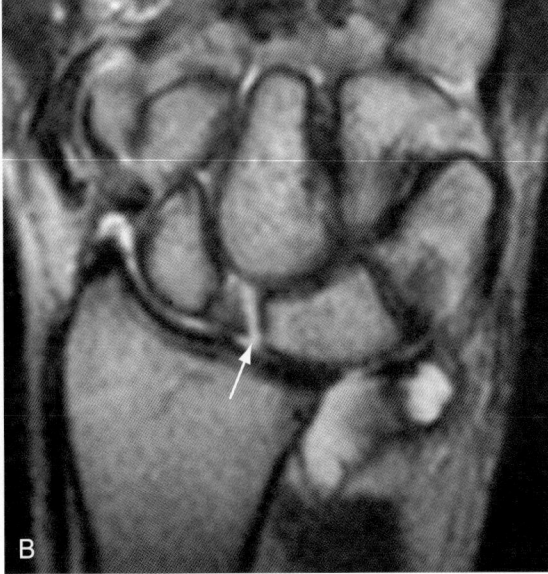

FIGURE 101-23

Scapholunate tear. **A** to **C,** Coronal T2-weighted images reveal widening of the scapholunate interval with an associated fluid-filled tear. The ligament is torn in the volar (**A**), central (**B**), and dorsal portions (**C**) *(arrows).*

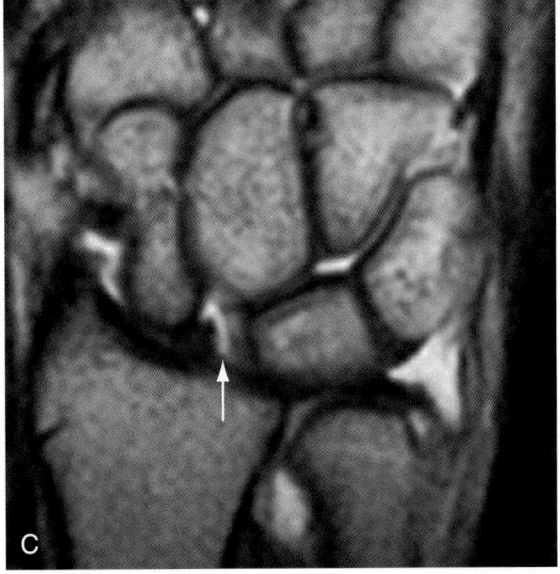

nonspecific finding of ligament tears.[85] In more advanced cases, widening of the scapholunate ligament articulation may be evident, particularly if at least two portions of the ligament are involved. Fluid pooling around a ligament and concomitant bone injury are other clues to injury. Ganglion cysts can also be a secondary finding of ligament derangement.

A partial tear may be diagnosed when there is focal thinning or irregularity and/or fluid signal in a portion of the ligament, more commonly the volar portion (Fig. 101-26) where the weakest ligamentous attachments are.[122] Considerable stretching (elongation) of the scapholunate ligament may also occur prior to or in the absence of a ligament tear,[113] and this may also be observed as an abnormality on MRI examination. Both partial tears and elongated but intact ligaments may be visualized with MRI in the presence of a normal conventional arthrogram (Fig. 101-27).[122] Associated tears of the volar extrinsic radiocarpal ligaments may

also be visualized with MRI (see Fig. 101-26), although less frequently than documented at arthroscopy and surgery.[17,18,53,121] 3D volumetric imaging[16] has been applied with some success in better defining these extrinsic ligament injuries with the aid of obliquely reformatted projections. MR arthrography[3,27,28,111,123,124] may yield an increased sensitivity to scapholunate tears over MRI alone and conventional arthrography, especially in cases of more subtle injuries. This includes partial tears, which may show contrast leak or imbibition into a portion of an injured ligament (Fig. 101-27). MR arthrography may also better outline morphologic alterations or stretching. Instillation of intra-articular contrast may also help outline dysfunctional ligaments that may have healed over with fibrosis and be scarred (Fig. 101-28). This latter process may be evident clinically but difficult to document with conventional MRI. MR arthrography may better outline the surfaces of the ligament, thus improving the detectability of this lesion.

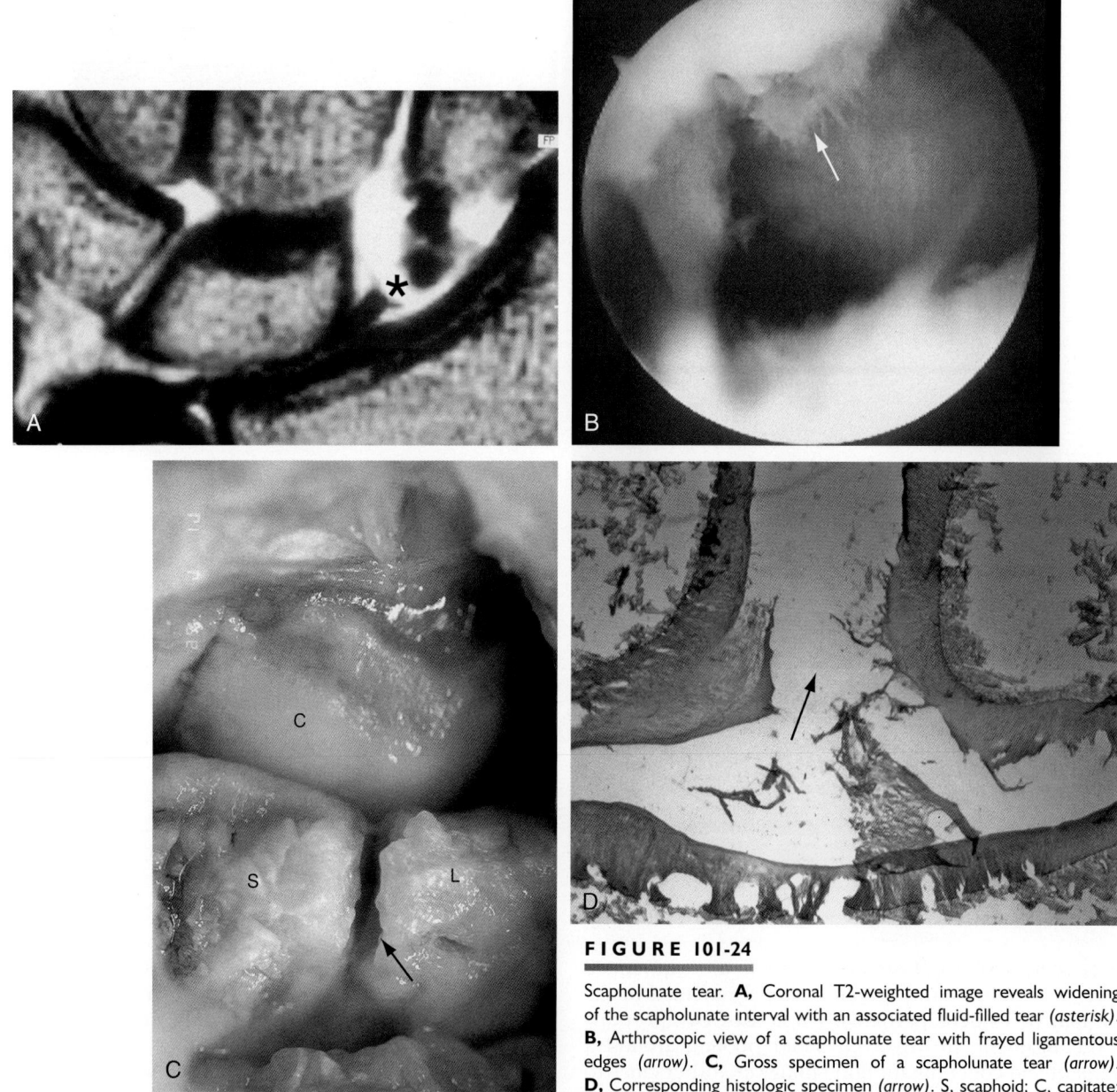

FIGURE 101-24

Scapholunate tear. **A,** Coronal T2-weighted image reveals widening of the scapholunate interval with an associated fluid-filled tear *(asterisk)*. **B,** Arthroscopic view of a scapholunate tear with frayed ligamentous edges *(arrow)*. **C,** Gross specimen of a scapholunate tear *(arrow)*. **D,** Corresponding histologic specimen *(arrow)*. S, scaphoid; C, capitate; L, lunate. *(B and C, Courtesy of EA Ouellette MD, Miami, Fla)*.

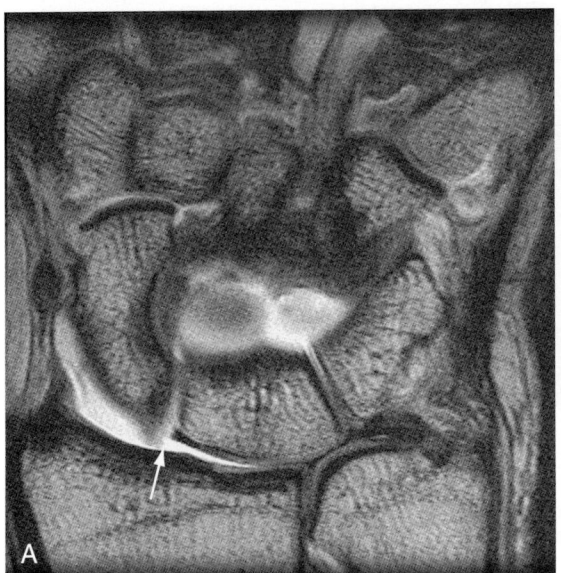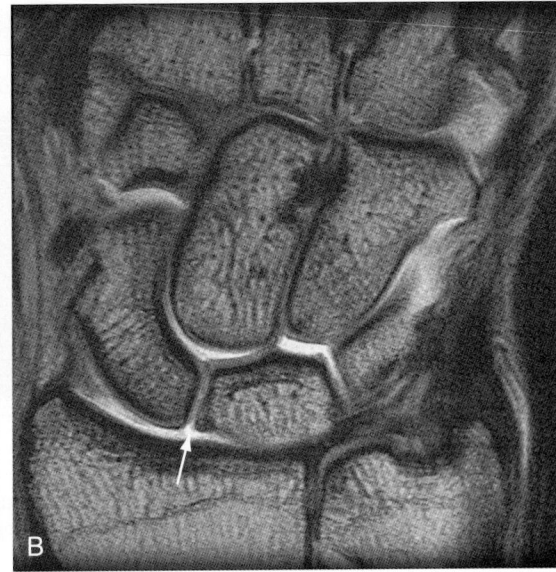

FIGURE 101-25

Scapholunate tear. MR arthrography. Coronal T1-weighted MR arthrograms. Note contrast outlining a tear in the volar (**A**) and mid (**B**) portion of the scapholunate ligament *(arrows)*.

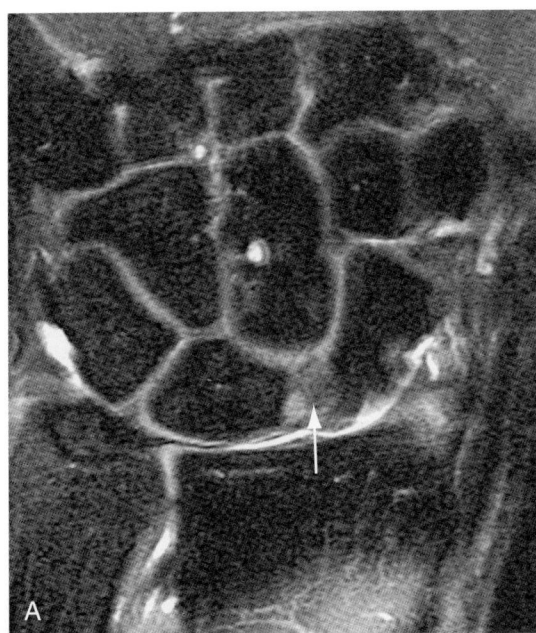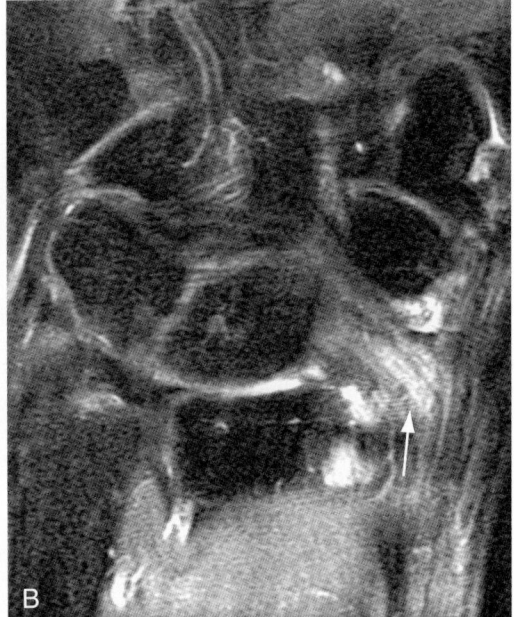

FIGURE 101-26

Scapholunate injury/partial tear. **A,** Coronal T2-weighted FSE image with fat saturation. Note the increased signal and altered morphology of the volar portion of the scapholunate ligament *(arrow)*. **B,** Coronal T2-weighted FSE image with fat saturation. Altered signal and morphology outlines an injury to the volar radiocarpal ligaments *(arrow)*.

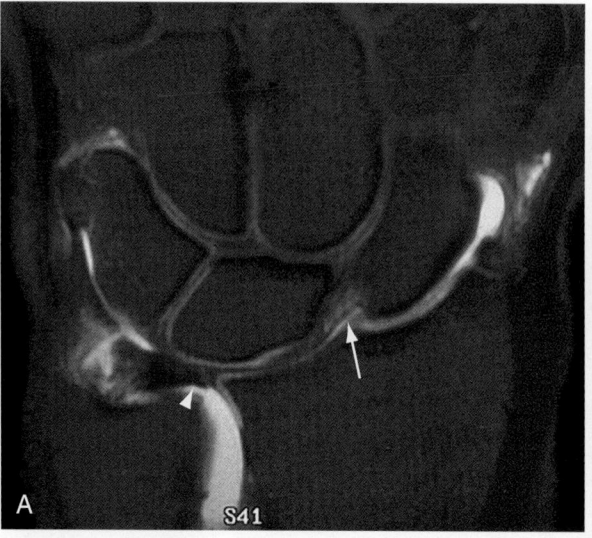
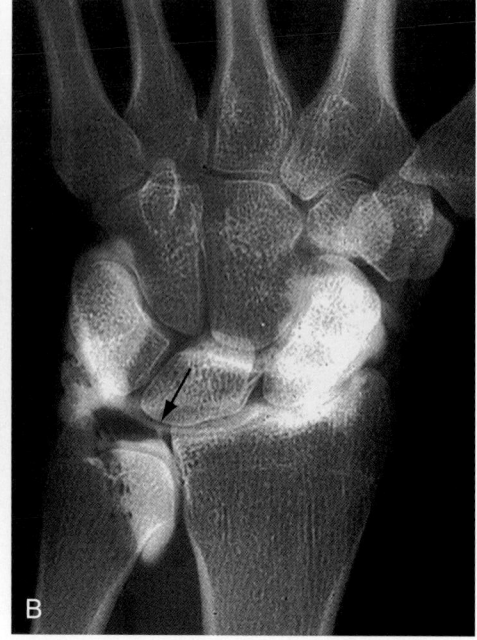

FIGURE 101-27

A, Coronal T1-weighted image after intra-articular contrast injection, with fat saturation. High-signal contrast is imbibed into the scapholunate ligament *(arrow)*. A small defect in the triangular fibrocartilage (TFC) was also noted *(white arrowhead)*. **B,** Radiocarpal wrist arthrogram. The tear in the scapholunate ligament was not identified on the conventional arthrogram in this patient. The TFC tear is seen *(arrow)*.

There is controversy as to which portions of the ligament need to be injured for instability to occur. Mayfield has shown that the volar portion is injured first.[10,112,113] Most authors believe that either the dorsal portion or both the volar and dorsal portions must be injured for instability to occur.[125,126] Complete scapholunate dissociation, seen on plain radiographic examination as a widened scapholunate interval, requires a tear of the radioscaphoid as well as the volar and dorsal portions of the scapholunate ligament. MRI thus has the ability to show scapholunate injuries at an earlier stage than plain radiographs. Additionally, MRI has the ability to diagnose the site and the extent of involvement of these lesions (see Figs. 101-23, 101-24, and 101-25) and thus differentiate those lesions that may involve only the central membranous portion and may be of degenerative origin. These central lesions may be painful, but may not be indicative of instability in the way that involvement of the other portions of the ligament would, particularly the dorsal portion. In this regard MRI is of greater value than conventional arthrography, which cannot make this distinction. MR arthrography may be of significant benefit in establishing the location and extent of such lesions (see Fig. 101-25).[3,4,111,123,127] In addition, 3D volumetric imaging may aid in this diagnosis.[15,21]

Disruption of the scapholunate articulation can be associated with DISI. The scaphoid and lunate are no longer linked, the lunate may collapse in a dorsiflexed posture, and the capitate will migrate proximally into the widened gap now present between the scaphoid and lunate. This is best demonstrated on a midplane sagittal MR image (Fig. 101-29). The radius, lunate, and capitate are no longer co-linear, but are shortened in a Z-like configuration.[39] The scaphoid also rotates volarly. The advantage of MRI over plain radiographs is its tomographic nature: overlap from other carpal bones, as would be present on plain radiographs, is avoided and associated ligament pathology is demonstrated. Measurement of scapholunate angles and capitolunate angles can be performed by evaluating successive sagittal sections. The scapholunate angle will increase to greater than 70° (normal 30 to 60°) and the capitolunate angle will be increased to greater than 30° (normal 0 to

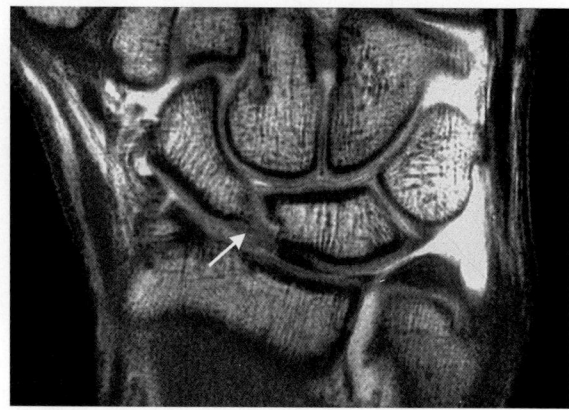

FIGURE 101-28

Scapholunate injury, healed with "scar" formation. Intermediate signal intensity is identified in the volar portion of a thickened scapholunate ligament *(arrow)*. These findings can be likened to those seen in a healed partial anterior cruciate ligament (ACL) tear.

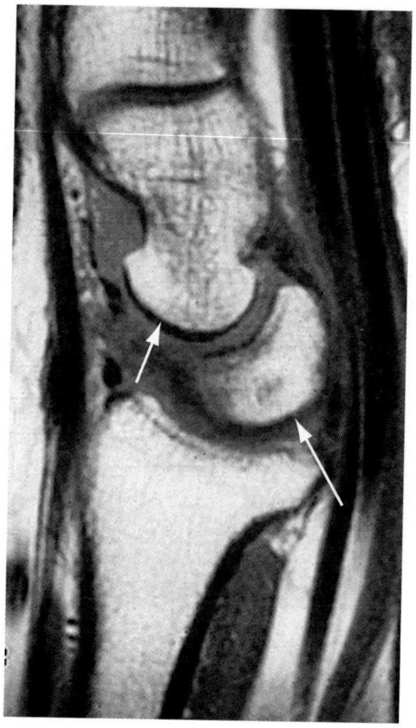

FIGURE 101-29

Dorsal intercalated segmental instability (DISI). Sagittal T1-weighted image shows the dorsal tilt of the lunate (long arrow) and proximal migration of the capitate (short arrow).

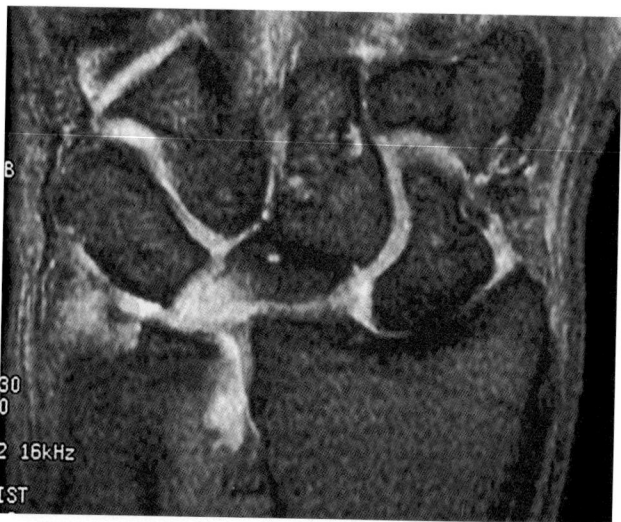

FIGURE 101-30

Scapholunate advance collapse (SLAC): endstage scapholunate instability. The scapholunate ligament is torn and there is widening of the interval. There is advanced radiocarpal arthritis, proximal migration of the capitate, and midcarpal arthritis.

30°).[128,129] It should be noted that the lunate appears more dorsally tilted on MR images than on lateral radiographs, such that a DISI configuration may be simulated.[129] This occurred in subjects with neutrally positioned and ulnarly deviated wrists. Subtle errors in the selection of the imaging plane did not substantially influence measurements. Thus caution must be taken in making this diagnosis based on MR images alone; correlation with plain radiographs and the clinical status of the patient is necessary. Wrist positioning on MRI examination is also critical.

Scapholunate advanced collapse (SLAC) represents the endstage degenerative pattern in scapholunate insufficiency[130-133] (Fig. 101-30). It may also be seen in similar fashion in nonunion of the scaphoid, where it is known as scaphoid nonunion advanced collapse (SNAC).[134]

Lunate-Triquetral Instability

There are different proposed etiologies for lunate-triquetral instability.[135] Disruption of the lunotriquetral ligament may occur in the latter stages of perilunar instability. It may also present as an isolated injury in situations of perilunar instability, where the scapholunate component has healed, leaving only the lunotriquetral tear. Alternatively it may present as a result of loading in maximal extension, radial deviation, and possibly pronation, indicating reverse perilunar insta-

bility. Finally it may occur as part of the ulnocarpal abutment syndrome. Patients with lunate-triquetral instability present with ulnar-sided pain.

The lunotriquetral ligament is smaller than the scapholunate ligament, and tears of this ligament are therefore more difficult to detect,[33,53] but these lesions are less common. The most specific finding for a lunotriquetral tear is discontinuity of the ligament with increased signal intensity on imaging sequences with T2 type contrast (Fig. 101-31). High signal contrast with MR arthrography may also outline a defect in the lunotriquetral ligament (Fig. 101-31). Absence of the ligament is a less useful finding[85] as the lunotriquetral ligament may be less reliably observed on MRI than the scapholunate ligament, although on thin-section 3D volumetric images, this may be a more useful finding owing to the thinner sections that can be obtained.[15,38] Changes in morphology are also less useful than they are in evaluating the scapholunate ligament. Fluid in the midcarpal joint is said to be a sensitive finding for lunotriquetral tears.[85] The volar portion of the ligament attaches to the TFC and may appear discontinuous, representing a diagnostic pitfall to be avoided. Widening of the lunate-triquetral articulation is not usually evident even in advanced cases.[128]

Tears of the lunotriquetral ligament may coexist with static and dynamic patterns of palmar midcarpal instability (VISI; Fig. 101-32). In patients with VISI the lunate is no longer linked to the triquetrum and follows the scaphoid. In this situation the lunate tends to be volar-flexed with the wrist in a neutral position and there is proximal and volar migration of the bones in the distal carpal row. Sagittal MR images show the palmar tilting of the lunate and scaphoid (Fig. 101-32). The scapholunate angle is less than 30° and the capitolunate angle may measure up to 30°.

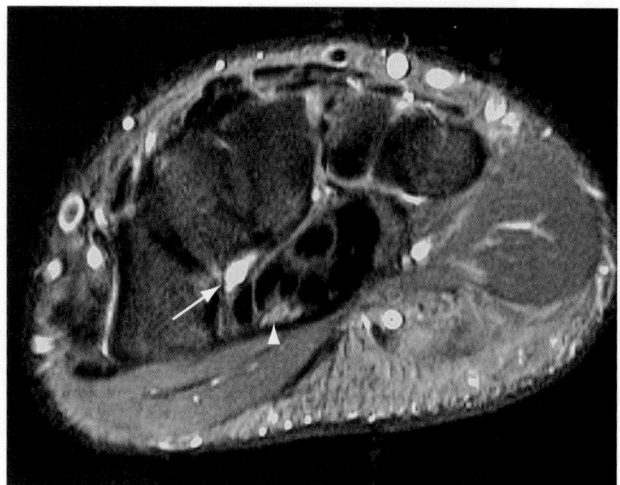

FIGURE 101-33

Axial STIR image. A small ganglion cyst is seen in the posterior aspect of the carpal tunnel (arrow). The median nerve is mildly enlarged and reveals high signal intensity (arrowhead).

MR Imaging

MRI provides good delineation of the structures within the carpal tunnel. Although in the vast majority of patients, CTS is a clinical diagnosis, MRI is a less invasive alternative to electromyographic studies in patients in whom the symptoms and history point to a diagnosis of CTS but in whom objective findings are absent.[151-153,156,157] MRI may also help to determine a specific cause of CTS such as a ganglion (Fig. 101-33) or bony fracture. Finally, MRI has been found useful in the postoperative evaluation of patients with persistent or recurrent symptoms.[157-161]

Four consistent findings of CTS have been found on MR imaging. They include: 1. diffuse swelling of the median nerve; 2. flattening of the median nerve at the level of the hamate; 3. palmar bowing of the flexor retinaculum; and 4. increased signal of the median nerve on long TR/TE images.[157,159] The median nerve may be diffusely enlarged, or segmentally enlarged such as at the level of the pisiform.[162] Mesgarzadeh et al[157,159] established an internal control for each patient. Specifically, pisiform-to-radius and hamate-to-radius "swelling ratios" were determined for normal subjects and for patients with CTS. These were ratios of the cross-sectional area of the median nerve at these levels. In normal subjects, the mean pisiform-to-radius and hamate-to-radius ratios were both 1.1. In patients with CTS the pisiform-to-radius and hamate-to-radius ratios were 2.4:1 and 2.1:1 respectively.[157,159] These workers also established a flattening ratio of the median nerve in carpal tunnel syndrome that was statistically significant only at the level of the hamate, as well as a palmar bowing ratio of the flexor retinaculum at the level of the trapezium and hamate (18% versus 5.8% for normal subjects). Cobb et al[163,164] describe using MRI to establish carpal tunnel contents (CTC) to carpal tunnel volume (CTV) ratios as another objective means of aiding in establishing a diagnosis of CTS. In their more recent study 7 asymptomatic volunteers and 7 patients with symptoms of CTS underwent MRI so that the CTC/CTV ratios could be determined. Standard radiographs were analyzed to identify plain radiographic variables that differed between patients with CTS and control subjects, and no differences were found. On MRI, however, CTC/CTV ratios were noted to be higher for patients with CTS than for matched control subjects.[163]

One early study stated that the most important MRI findings in patients with CTS appeared to be enlargement of the median nerve at the level of the pisiform to a size two to three times that at the level of the distal radius, and increased signal intensity of the edematous median nerve on long TR/TE images (Fig. 101-34).[159] This swelling of the median nerve as it enters the carpal tunnel at the level of the pisiform has been designated a

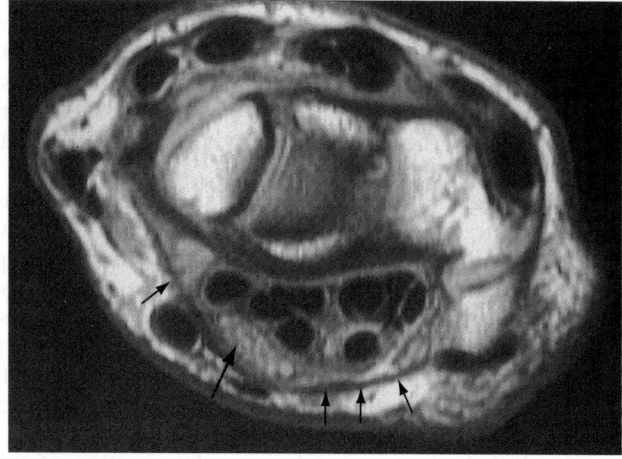

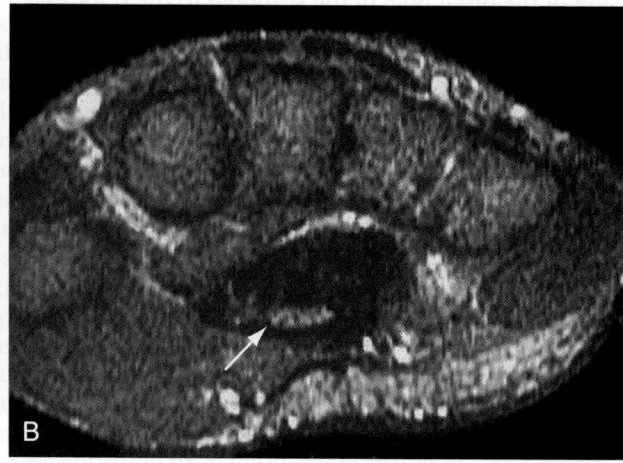

FIGURE 101-34

Carpal tunnel syndrome. **A**, Axial image (TR/TE 2500/25) through the proximal carpal tunnel at the level of the pisiform. The median nerve is markedly enlarged (large arrow). The flexor retinaculum is bowed volarly (small arrows). **B**, Axial image (TR/TE 2500/25). The median nerve is flattened distally and shows increased signal (arrow).

"false neuroma"[146,165] in the surgical literature. In cases of chronic CTS, however, the median nerve may either show no increase in signal or be paradoxically decreased in signal. This may reflect the development of fibrosis of the nerve.[166]

Howe and co-authors[167] have described a method whereby fat and flow suppression combined with T2 weighting provided high-conspicuity images of the median nerve. Standard maximum-intensity projection techniques were then used to produce 3D reconstructions of the nerve (MR neurography). These may prove useful in more direct evaluation of the extent and degree of localized compression of the nerve. Gadolinium enhancement has been studied as a means of establishing an objective diagnosis. Sugimoto et al[168] studied patients with known CTS in flexed, extended, and neutral positions. Two enhancement patterns were noted: marked enhancement attributed to nerve edema, and no enhancement attributed to nerve ischemia.

Thickening or inflammation of the flexor tendon sheaths as the etiologic mechanism of CTS is commonly encountered at surgery[169] and may be documented by MRI[65,157,170-172] but less commonly than would be expected based on what is described in the surgical literature.[169] MRI findings include enlargement of individual tendon sheaths and increased separation between adjacent tendons within the carpal tunnel. Increased signal intensity resulting from fluid in the enlarged tendon sheaths may be seen on images with T2 type contrast (Fig. 101-35). Volar bowing of the flexor retinaculum may be a secondary result of the synovial thickening as well. MRI is most sensitive in detecting thickening of the synovial sheaths when comparison to a contralateral normal wrist can be made,[162] although it may not be necessary to perform this in most cases. Gadolinium enhancement may also be helpful in depict-

ing these findings (Fig. 101-35). When this thickening is the result of certain systemic disorders such as rheumatoid arthritis, gout, or calcium pyrophosphate dihydrate crystal deposition disease (CPPD), the tenosynovitis may appear similar but other bone and joint findings characteristic of these diseases may be evident.[157,170,172] Gout or amyloid can cause regions of persistent low signal intensity within the carpal tunnel on images with T2 type contrast.[70,170]

In spite of the descriptions above of the MRI findings associated with CTS there have been questions regarding their true sensitivity as well as their specificity to CTS. However, one study comparing MRI to intraoperative findings found that MRI correctly diagnosed median nerve compression in 91% of cases.[173] The authors also showed an ability to differentiate between early and advanced CTS by showing differences in the pattern of flattening, swelling, and signal intensity of the median nerve, and showed the effectiveness of MRI in revealing additional lesions such as masses in the carpal tunnel. Other studies have found that many of the aforementioned signs may have limited sensitivity and specificity to CTS. In the study by Radack et al[174] the previously described MRI signs of CTS were said to be insensitive and nonspecific. Exceptions include flexor retinacular bowing, median nerve flattening, and deep palmar bursitis, which had specificities greater than or equal to 94%. In a study by Monagle et al,[175] the only statistically significant difference found between patients with CTS and asymptomatic patients was that the median nerve was 50% larger within and proximal to the carpal tunnel in patients with CTS, and palmar bowing of the flexor retinaculum occurred in patients only at the level of the hamate. Additional study is thus necessary to validate these findings on MRI for their utilization in the routine diagnosis of CTS on MRI.[151-153,176-181]

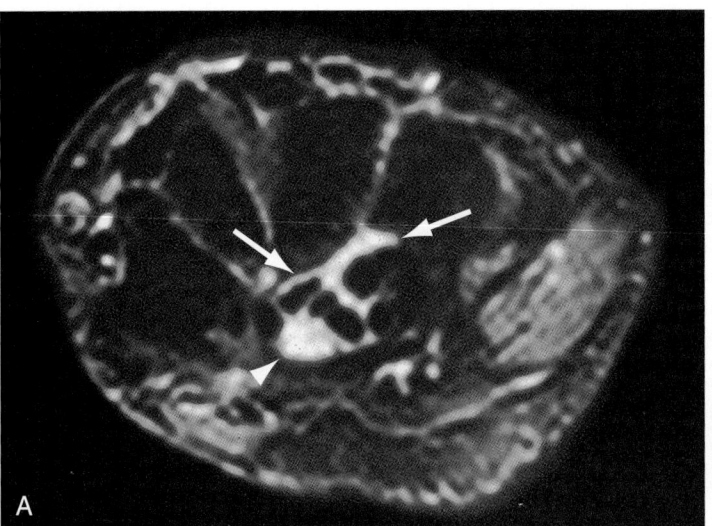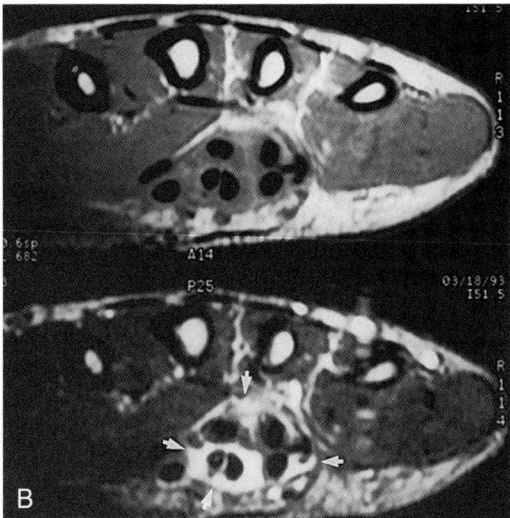

FIGURE 101-35

A, Axial T2 FSE image with fat saturation in the carpal tunnel. There is tissue of increased signal intensity and thickening of the flexor tendon sheaths *(arrows)*. The median nerve is increased in signal intensity *(arrowhead)*. **B,** Axial short TR/TE images before and after gadolinium injection in another patient. High signal intensity reflective of enhancement is seen in the tendon sheaths on the post-contrast images *(arrows)*.

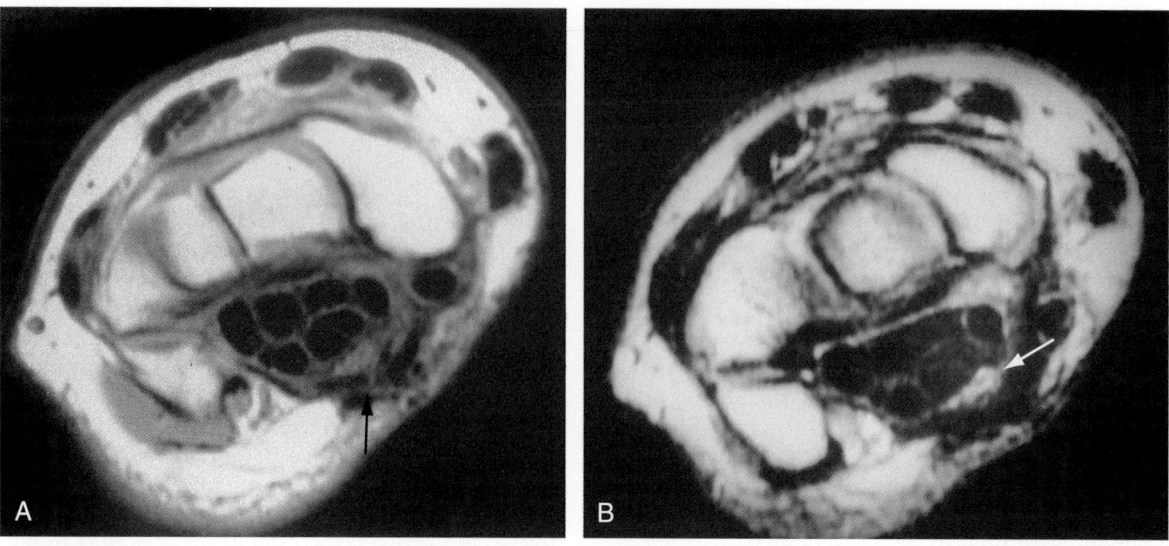

FIGURE 101-36

Postoperative carpal tunnel syndrome. **A,** Axial image (TR/TE 800/20) through the proximal carpal tunnel. The patient remained symptomatic after incision of the flexor retinaculum. The retinaculum retains its integrity likely due to fibrosis *(arrow)*. **B,** Long TR/TE (2500/70) image. Persistent enlargement and increased signal intensity in the median nerve is seen *(arrow)*.

Postoperative Studies

In postoperative patients, the carpal tunnel loses its normal elliptic shape and becomes disorderly. The retinaculum is incised at its ulnar aspect[39] at its insertion into the hamate hook. The flexor tendons appear spread out.[157,160,182-184] The flexor retinaculum is displaced volarly and the carpal tunnel contents may migrate volarly as well. Carpal tunnel release can be performed both surgically and endoscopically. One cause of persistent or recurrent CTS is inadvertent subtotal incision of the flexor retinaculum. This is documented by visualizing a persistently intact retinaculum. Alternatively the retinaculum may have been adequately incised but may remain unchanged due to scar formation (Fig. 101-36). In these cases proximal enlargement and distal flattening of the median nerve may persist. In contrast, persistent increased signal in the median nerve after surgery may not be a useful sign. Nerve signal intensity will only decrease in 33% of cases in spite of symptomatic relief.[184] In other situations flexor tenosynovitis may persist (Fig. 101-37). Fibrous tissue impinging upon and flattening the median nerve, and multiple neuromas in the distribution of the median nerve, are other findings that have been documented by MRI in the symptomatic postoperative patient.[157,159]

Ulnar Tunnel Syndrome

The ulnar nerve may become entrapped at the wrist within Guyon's canal[67,185] due to trauma (including hook of hamate fractures; Fig. 101-38), lipoma,[186] or false aneurysm of the ulnar artery. The ulnar nerve may also be compressed by a mass such as a ganglion cyst.[187,188]

Anatomic variants such as the presence of the abductor digiti minimi coursing within the canal, muscle hypertrophy of the palmaris brevis, and hypertrophy of the flexor retinaculum may also cause entrapment.[66,189] Distal entrapment at the hamate may involve the superficial branch of the ulnar nerve and cause paraesthesias or entrap the deep branch and produce motor deficits. Proximal entrapment at the pisiform causes the whole ulnar nerve to produce both sensory and motor deficits.

Findings similar to those of median nerve entrapment may be expected in patients with ulnar nerve entrapment, including enlargement and/or flattening and increased signal on imaging sequences with T2 contrast.

Injuries of the Scaphoid

Scaphoid Fractures

Scaphoid fractures are the most common carpal fracture, comprising more than 60% of all carpal injuries, and are most common in young adult males. The injury usually occurs from a fall on a dorsiflexed wrist. Fractures of the scaphoid can be seen in three locations: 1. the tuberosity, 2. the waist, and 3. the proximal pole.[190,191] Fractures through the waist are the most common, and make up 70% of scaphoid fractures.

Although most evaluation of acute scaphoid fractures in clinical practice is with plain radiographs, MRI can be helpful in cases of uncertainty due to its depiction of the low-signal-intensity fracture line and its sensitivity to the adjacent marrow edema.[191-196] T1 and STIR imaging may be particularly helpful in such cases (Fig. 101-39). Sagittal images are also helpful in depicting abnormal morphology of the scaphoid such as the humpback

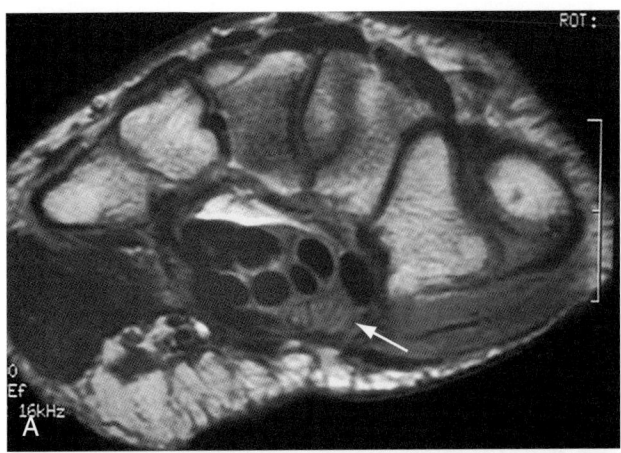

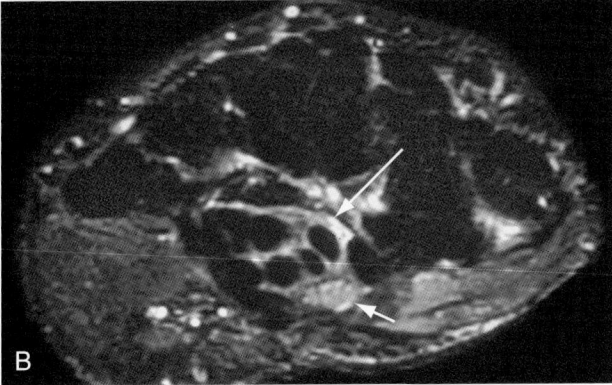

FIGURE 101-37

Postoperative carpal tunnel syndrome. **A,** Axial FSE proton density–weighted image through the proximal carpal tunnel. Note the incision of the flexor retinaculum (white arrow). **B,** Axial FSE T2-weighted image. There is persistent thickening and increased signal of the flexor tendon sheaths (long arrow), reflecting persistent or recurrent tenosynovitis. Persistent enlargement and increased signal intensity of the median nerve is also seen (short arrow).

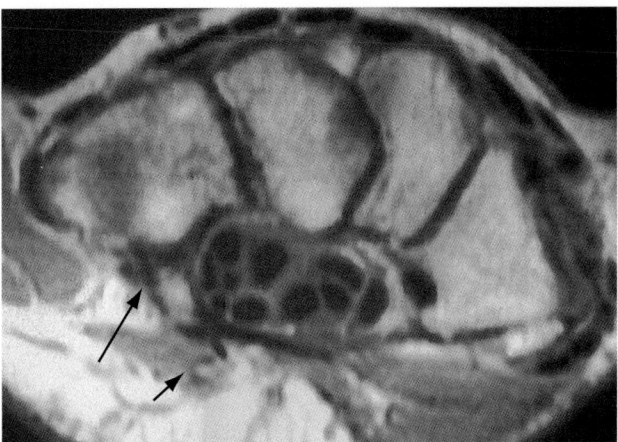

FIGURE 101-38

Axial short TR/TE image. There is a hook of hamate fracture nonunion (long arrow) which is volarly displaced and impinging on the region of the ulnar nerve in Guyon's canal (short arrow).

deformity, which may also be identified in situations of suboptimal healing[197] (Fig. 101-39) in subacute and chronic cases. Foreshortening of the scaphoid in this manner can also lead to a DISI deformity. The presence of an intact cortex is said to imply a chronic fracture. MRI may also be helpful in excluding suspected scaphoid fractures and in depicting other injuries that may mimic them clinically, such as contusions or fractures in other carpal bones, as well as in the distal radius (Fig. 101-40).

Dedicated extremity MRI has been used in this application.[192,198,199] T1-weighted and STIR sequences are most often utilized. In one study of 52 patients using dedicated extremity MRI, occult fractures of the scaphoid were found in 9 patients. All were confirmed on follow-up radiographs.[199] Other occult fractures of the distal radius and other carpal bones were also found (Fig. 101-40). In the study by Brydie and Raby,[192] the incidence of MRI-detected scaphoid and other wrist fractures was determined in a clinical setting in 195 patients with suspected scaphoid injury and negative initial radiographs. The influence on subsequent patient

management was examined. Scans comprising T1 and STIR coronal sequences were performed in a dedicated extremity low-field MRI scanner within 14 days of injury. Occult fractures were present in almost two fifths of patients with suspected scaphoid fracture and normal initial plain films. Half of these were scaphoid fractures. MRI allowed an early definitive diagnosis to be made, and was determined to have changed patient management in over 90% of cases.

Treatment of scaphoid injuries is controversial since most scaphoid fractures are not displaced and will heal with simple immobilization. Despite the success of treatment with conservative management, some authors advocate open reduction and internal fixation in the athletic patient population to expedite recovery and to allow earlier resumption of athletic activity.[191,200]

Complications of Scaphoid Fractures

Avascular Necrosis

The location of the fracture influences the rate of healing and the development of avascular necrosis (AVN) in patients with scaphoid fractures. The scaphoid is second only to the hip in its incidence of post-traumatic AVN.[201-203] The blood supply to the scaphoid is from the radial artery. The major dorsal and volar vessels enter through the distal half of the bone.[204-206] Hence, 30% of fractures through the middle third of the scaphoid, and approximately 100% of fractures through the proximal fifth of the scaphoid, result in AVN of the proximal fragment.[207,208] Plain radiographic criteria of increased density in the proximal pole have been traditionally used for diagnosis of AVN. Plain-film findings lag behind the onset of the disease. Plain-film findings of increased density of the proximal pole may also not be reliable in predicting viability.[209]

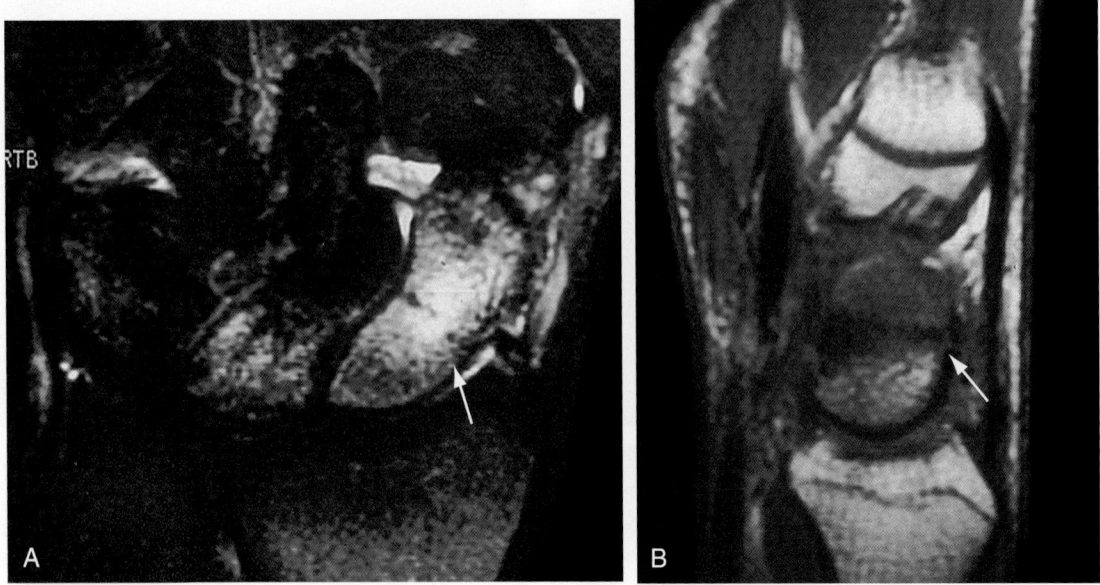

FIGURE 101-39

Scaphoid fracture. **A,** Coronal T2-weighted FSE image with fat saturation. Note the low-signal-intensity fracture line and subjacent marrow edema *(arrow)*. There is edema in the subjacent lunate, reflecting a contusion. **B,** Sagittal short TR/TE image reveals a mild deformity associated with the scaphoid fracture *(arrow)*.

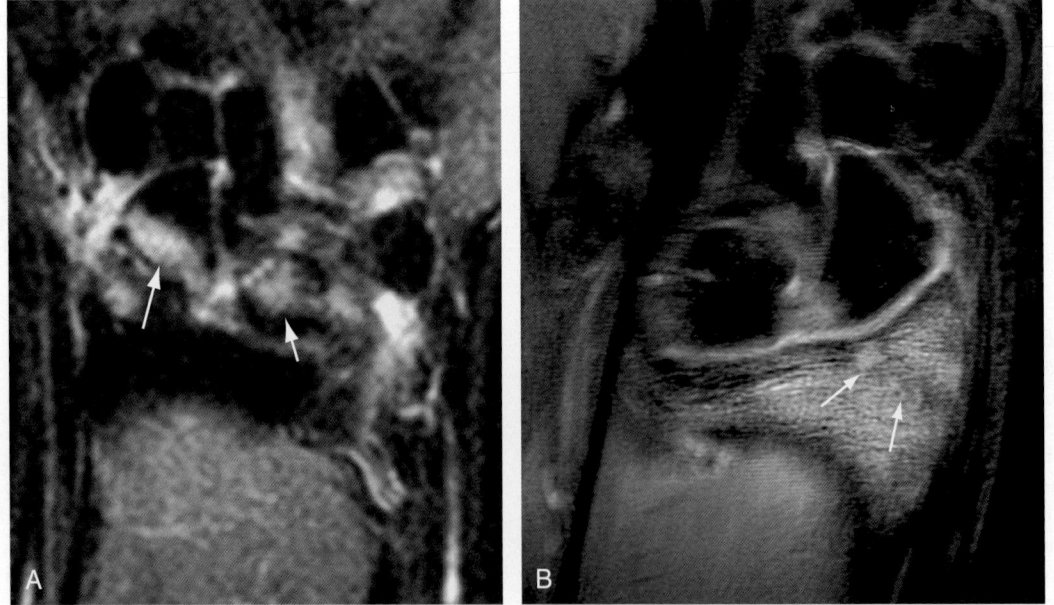

FIGURE 101-40

Scaphoid fracture mimics. **A,** Coronal STIR image, performed on a 0.2 T extremity magnet. Contusions are seen in the scaphoid *(larger arrow)* and lunate *(smaller arrow)*. Fluid is seen in the radiocarpal joint, and there is also edema, reflecting injury to the scapholunate ligament. **B,** Coronal STIR image. A fracture line with subjacent edema identifies an occult, nondisplaced fracture of the radial styloid process *(arrows)*.

Early AVN of the scaphoid has been documented on MRI examination in patients with negative plain radiographs. The results of MRI in assessment of scaphoid AVN have been good.[202,209-213] MR findings in this abnormality include uniform loss of signal intensity within the proximal pole of the scaphoid on T1-weighted images (Figs 101-41 and 101-42)[214] which may be due to fibrosis, sclerosis, or edema. On images with T2 type contrast, a relative increase in signal intensity may be seen. This probably reflects marrow edema and may indicate an earlier stage in the disease process (Fig. 101-42). It may be secondary evidence of viability. Long TR/TE images may also reveal diffuse low signal intensity (Fig. 101-41), which again presumably represents fibrosis and a more chronic phase. Imaging with gadolinium enhancement may help document viability, if enhancement of the proximal pole is present.[211,215-218]

Although almost all cases of AVN of the scaphoid occur after a fracture, occasionally AVN of the scaphoid may occur in the absence of that event and may be secondary to corticosteroids or idiopathic. AVN of the scaphoid in the absence of a fracture is also known as Preiser's disease.[211,219-223] Kalainov et al[220] described two patterns of scaphoid involvement in Preiser's disease. Type 1 cases are characterized by MR signal changes of necrosis and/or ischemia involving the entire scaphoid bone. Patients in this group have a propensity for scaphoid deterioration. Type 2 cases have MR signal changes involving only part of the scaphoid. These patients commonly report a history of wrist trauma, show fewer tendencies toward scaphoid fragmentation, and may have a more favorable clinical outcome.

Scaphoid Nonunion

Another complication of scaphoid fractures is nonunion,[134,197,207,224-227] usually due to delay in diagnosis and inadequate immobilization. The rate of nonunion may be up to 12%. Other causes include rotation or displacement at the fracture site, interposition of soft-tissue in the fracture gap, and a tenuous blood supply. In general, the more proximal the fracture, the longer the rate of healing. This is particularly evident in the proximal one third. Vertical oblique fractures in the middle third may also be at risk. The consequences of nonunion are significant with advanced degenerative arthritis developing in nearly all cases over time (SNAC). The degenerative changes involve the radioscaphoid joint, followed by the scaphocapitate and then the radiolunate joints. Scaphoid nonunion may also result in a DISI deformity.

Radiographic signs of nonunion include bone resorption along the fracture margins within a few weeks, with further resorption producing cyst-like lucencies within 2 to 3 months. Sclerotic edges only appear after several months or years. Nonunion is said to be present when there is no evidence of healing on three progressive sets of radiographs at 1-month intervals. If plain radiographs are insufficient to make a diagnosis then CT may be used. MRI may be useful in the diagnosis of delayed union or nonunion of scaphoid fractures. It is tomographic and images can be obtained in the coronal, sagittal, and axial planes. Oblique coronal images in the plane of the scaphoid also may be useful. The fracture line can be readily identified and the degree of displacement or angulation of fracture fragments determined. In general, CT may be best for detection of fracture healing

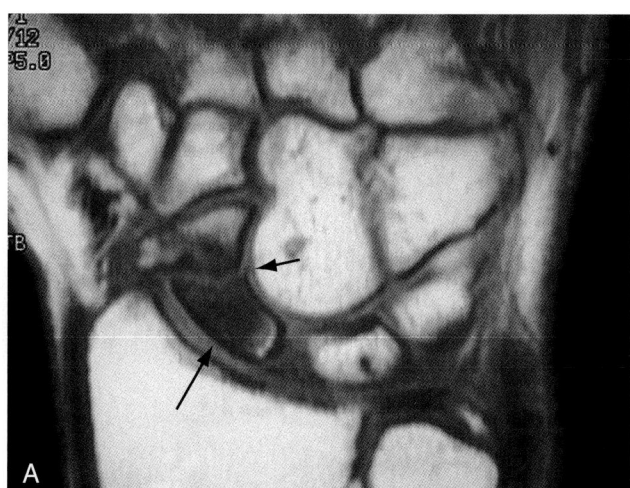 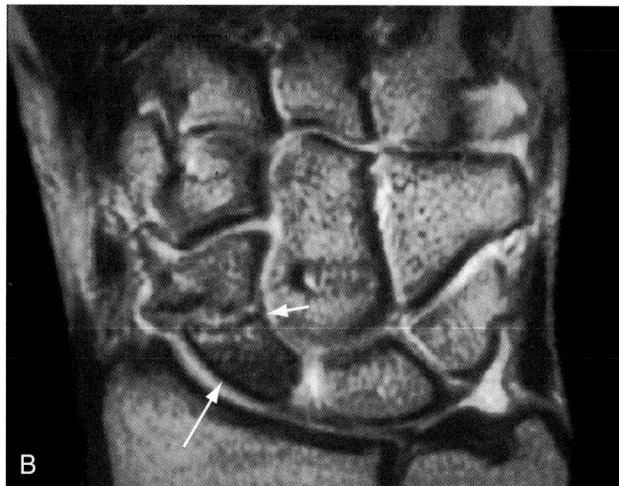

FIGURE 101-41

Avascular necrosis of the scaphoid. **A,** Coronal image (TR/TE 800/20) demonstrates homogeneous low signal intensity in the proximal half of the scaphoid *(long arrow)*, consistent with avascular necrosis, in a patient with a scaphoid waist fracture. The low signal intensity is nonspecific and may be due to fibrosis, sclerosis, or edema. The fracture line is evident *(smaller arrow)*. Low signal intensity in the distal portion of the fracture is likely marrow edema from fracture healing. **B,** Coronal image (TR/TE 2500/70) shows persistent low signal intensity within the proximal portion *(longer arrow)*. This is probably reflective of marrow fibrosis and may indicate a poorer prognosis for fixation and revascularization procedures. High signal intensity is also present along the fracture line *(shorter arrow)*. This may reflect ongoing fracture healing and the lack of a mature fracture union.

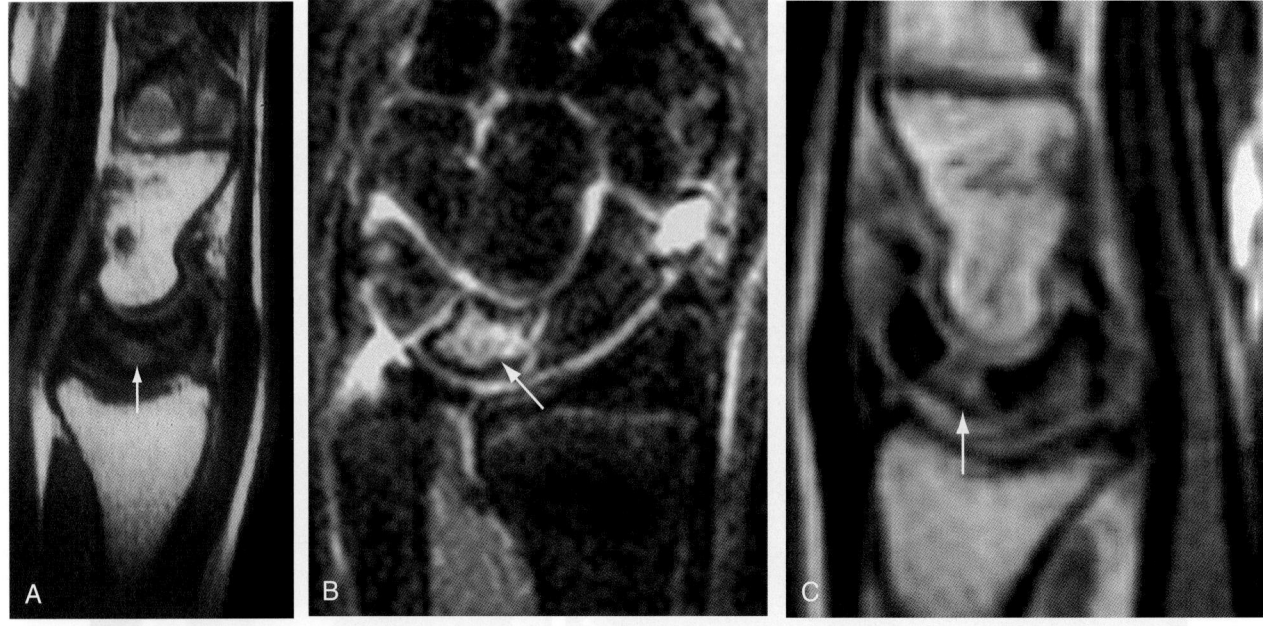

FIGURE 101-45

Avascular necrosis of the lunate (Kienböck's disease). Early stage. **A,** Sagittal short TR/TE image illustrates diffuse low signal intensity in the lunate *(arrow)* without collapse or fragmentation (stage 1). **B,** Coronal STIR image in another patient reveals homogeneous increased signal *(arrow)* in the lunate (stage 1). **C,** Sagittal short TR/TE image. There is diffuse low signal intensity and mild loss of height, reflecting stage 2 disease *(arrow)*.

signal changes are present in approximately half the lunate.[256,260] It should be kept in mind, however, that the extent of involvement can be overestimated since abnormal marrow signal can also be due to reactive granulation tissue and marrow edema. This can be accentuated on fat-saturated T2-weighted images and STIR images.

Although radionuclide studies can be used in the diagnosis of this condition,[261] the better spatial resolution of MR and thus its better depiction of anatomy make it a more useful study. MRI may also evaluate response to treatment in this disease. T2-weighted images may be helpful in determining revascularization. Favorable prognostic signs on T2-weighted MR images for revascularization include a focal area of increased signal intensity within bone that is of diffusely decreased signal intensity, and a return to normal or increased marrow signal on T2-weighted images.[258,262]

Due to its tomographic nature MRI may be able to reveal early lunate collapse, and associated scapholunate dissociation may be visualized[39] (Fig. 101-47). The presence of lunate collapse indicates a transition to stage 3 disease. Scapholunate dissociation differentiates stage 3A from 3B.[202,254,263] Contrast-enhanced MRI may be helpful in the early stages to assess the pattern of vascularity and perfusion.[202,215,257,264]

Capitate Injuries

After the scaphoid and lunate, the capitate is essentially the only other carpal bone with an incidence of AVN.[265,266] Reicher[39] described a case in which MRI showed diffuse low signal throughout the capitate (Fig.

101-48). Capitate fractures, although much less common, are similar to scaphoid fractures as the blood supply of the capitate extends through the waist of the bone, making the proximal pole susceptible to AVN.[204,267] Fractures of the waist and neck are the most common type of capitate fracture (Fig. 101-48). Fractures of the capitate may also be complicated by nonunion.[267,268]

Distal Radius Fractures

MRI may afford better evaluation of the osseous injury accompanying distal radial fractures than conventional radiographs.[269] It adds increased sensitivity to the presence of a fracture and it may detect a fracture when the plain radiographs are negative. Types of fracture include: the Colles fracture with dorsal angulation and displacement, as well as radial shortening; Smith's fracture, which is the reverse of the Colles with palmar angulation; Barton's fracture, which is an intra-articular fracture; and dislocation/subluxation, either volar or dorsal. Melone has also classified distal radius fractures into four types, based on the fracture components.[270]

The best clues to the presence of a fracture are a linear fracture line and associated marrow edema on T2 and STIR images. MRI can better demonstrate extension to the radiocarpal articulation and distal radioulnar joint. It can demonstrate associated occult carpal bone injury. Intra-articular soft-tissue injury accompanies distal radial fractures in almost 50% of cases (Fig. 101-49). In the study by Spence et al,[269] occult carpal bone fractures accompanying fracture of the distal radius were identified in two patients: one of the capitate and the other of the

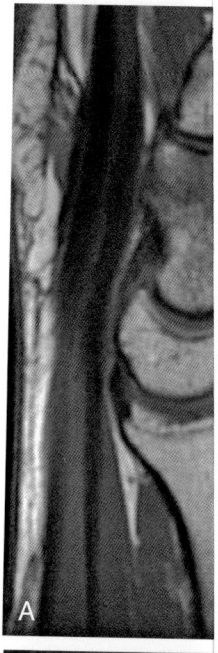

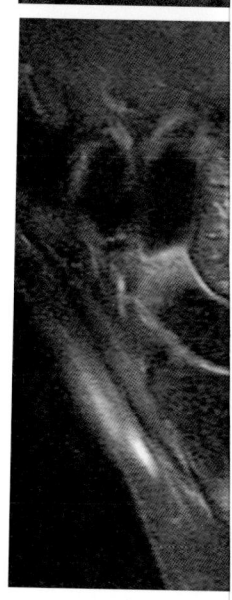

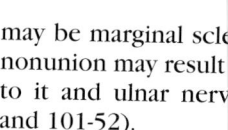

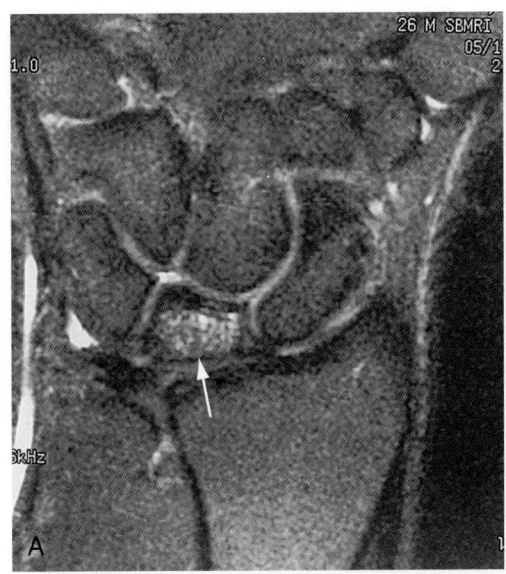

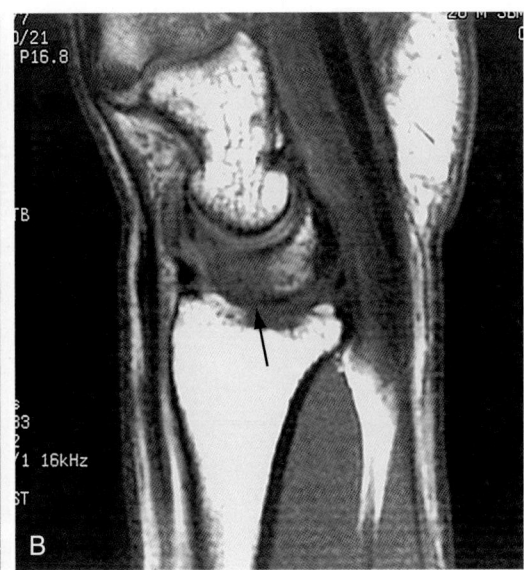

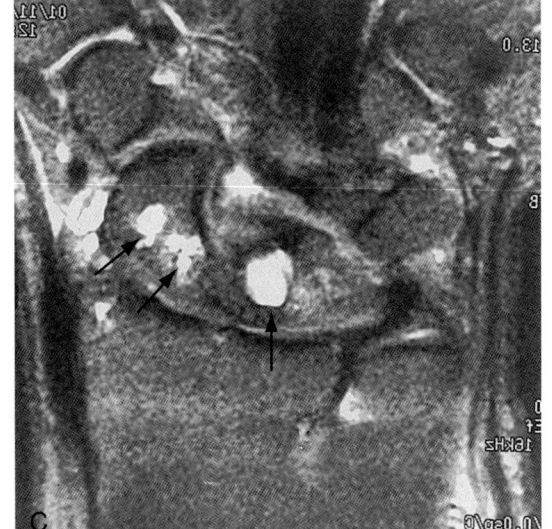

FIGURE 101-46

Kienböck's disease mimics. **A** and **B,** Lunate contusion. Wrist pain developed after injury. **A,** Coronal image (TR/TE 2500/70). High signal in the lunate reflects marrow edema *(arrow)*. **B,** Sagittal image (TR/TE 800/20). Involvement is less than 50% of the lunate on the sagittal view *(arrow)*. This and the clinical history can assist in differentiation from Kienböck's disease, but follow-up is necessary to confirm. **C,** Carpal cysts. Coronal image (TR/TE 2500/70). Cysts are common in the scaphoid and lunate *(arrows)* and may be incidental or post-traumatic or represent intraosseous ganglia.

may be marginal scle
nonunion may result
to it and ulnar nerv
and 101-52).

Wrist Masses

Most (98%) soft-tissu
and approximately 70%
Ganglia are fibrous-w
tain mucinous mate
metaplastic and pro
mately related to join
Ganglia are most free
decade and are equa

second metacarpal base. Ten patients (48%) had associated soft-tissue injury: six patients had scapholunate ligament rupture, two patients had disruption of the TFC, one patient had extensor carpi ulnaris tenosynovitis, and one patient had a tear of a dorsal radiocarpal ligament. Scapholunate ligament disruption commonly accompanies intra-articular fracture through the lunate facet of the distal radius. In this study, although TFC tears were found to be associated with distal radius fractures, fractures of the ulnar styloid were not frequently associated with a tear of the TFCC; however, the study population only included 21 patients.

Die punch fractures of the distal radius[271-273] are intra-articular fractures that occur secondary to lunate impaction, splitting the distal radius into both coronal and sagittal planes. The fracture extends to involve the lunate fossa of the distal radius. MRI is helpful as it can evaluate the extent and nature of the fracture in multiple planes. It can help to assess the degree of diastasis and depression.

Ulnar Styloid Nonunion

Ulnar styloid fractures may occur at the base, mid styloid, or tip of the ulnar styloid process. They may be isolated or occur in relationship to distal radius fractures. Fractures of the base of the ulnar styloid may be related to avulsion of the styloid attachment of the TFC.

Ulnar styloid nonunion is not uncommon following a fracture of this structure,[82] and may occur in 26% of cases. Nonunion of the ulnar styloid process may become symptomatic. The nonunited fragment may act as an irritative loose body or abut the ulnar carpus. A malaligned fibrous nonunion may cause impingement of the extensor carpi ulnaris tendon sheath. Such a nonunion may also be symptomatic because of associated TFCC perforation or be associated with complete rupture of the ulnar attachments of the TFCC and instability of the distal radioulnar joint. Any of these conditions, alone or in combination, may be responsible for painful ulnar styloid nonunion.[82] Type 1 is defined

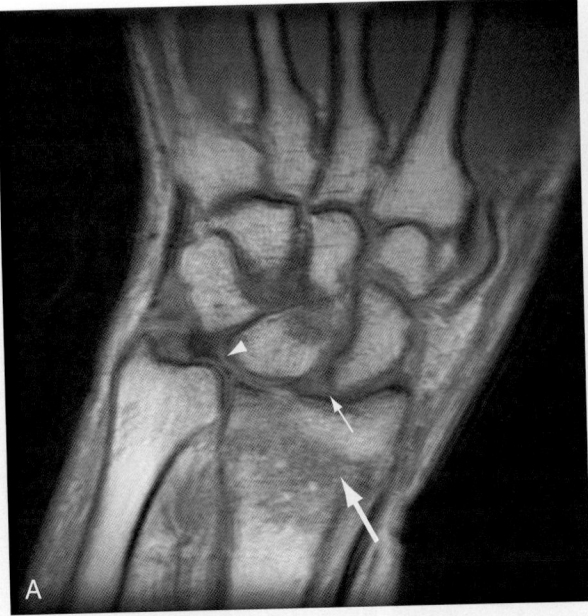
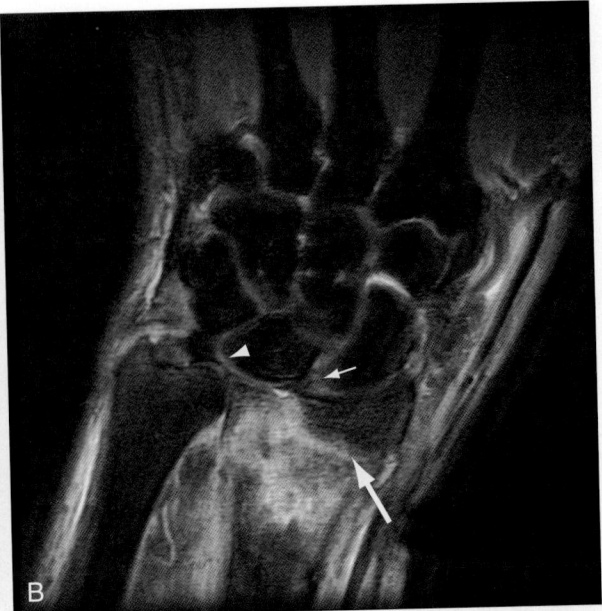

FIGURE 101-49

Coronal T1-weighted (**A**) and fast spin-echo T2-weighted with fat saturation (**B**) images. An occult fracture of the distal radius is identified (*arrow*). Note the scapholunate ligament injury (*smaller arrow*) and small radial tear of the triangular fibrocartilage (*arrowhead*).

FIGUR

Kienböck':
weighted
and fissure
long TR/TI
intensity, c
There is el
of the inter
image in a
deformed.

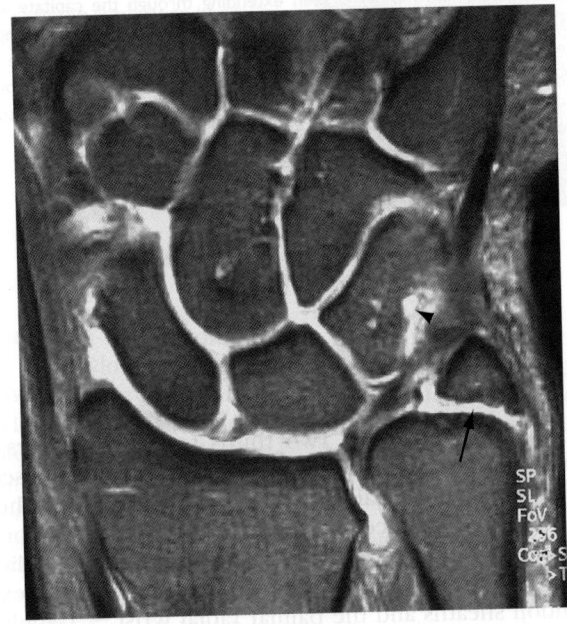

FIGURE 101-50

Ulnar styloid nonunion. MR images reveal nonunion of the ulnar styloid process (*arrow*) associated with ulnar avulsion of the triangular fibrocartilage (TFC) complex (Palmer class IB TFC complex injury). Note the alterations on the inferior margin of the triquetrum (*arrowhead*).

as nonunion ass
joint. It affects
TFC complex re
ments are at the
radioulnar joint
nonunion at the
ciated with dista
the result of avu
TFCC (Palmer cl
patients can visu
its ulnar attachm
fragments, and a:
carpus.[58] Diagnos
the subtypes. If
lacks the norma
derangement of t
nonunion). The u
TFC complex) sl
appropriately fixe
demonstrates the

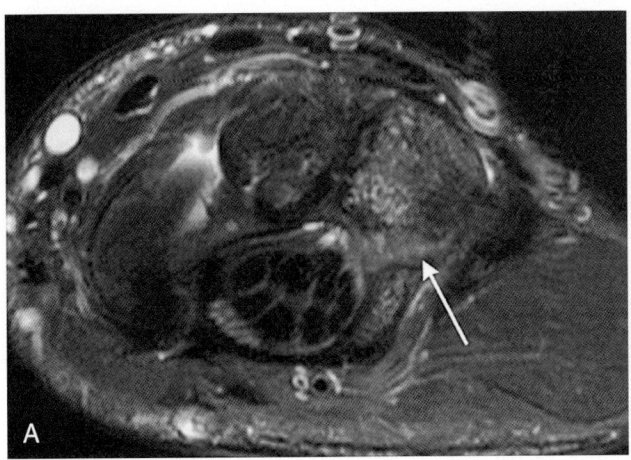

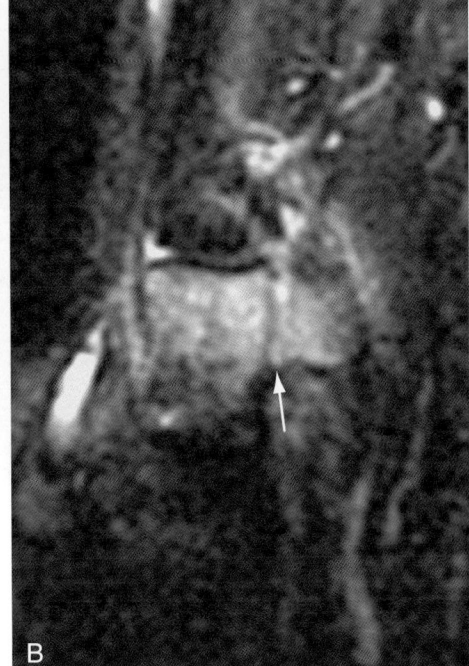

FIGURE 101-51

Hamate fractures. **A,** Axial STIR image. Note the fracture at the base of the hamate hook *(arrow).* **B,** Sagittal STIR images. The hook fracture is manifested by a low-signal-intensity fracture line with subjacent edema *(arrow).*

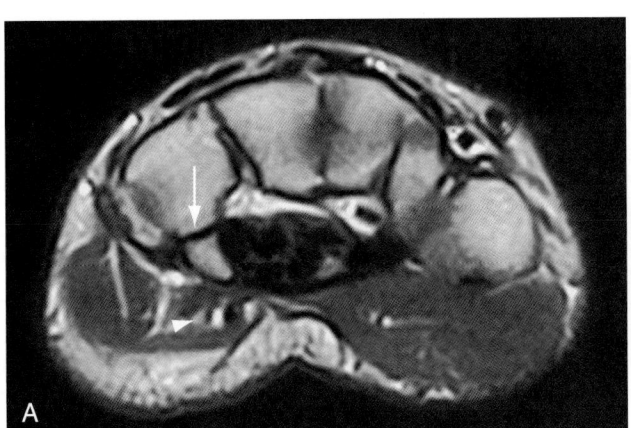

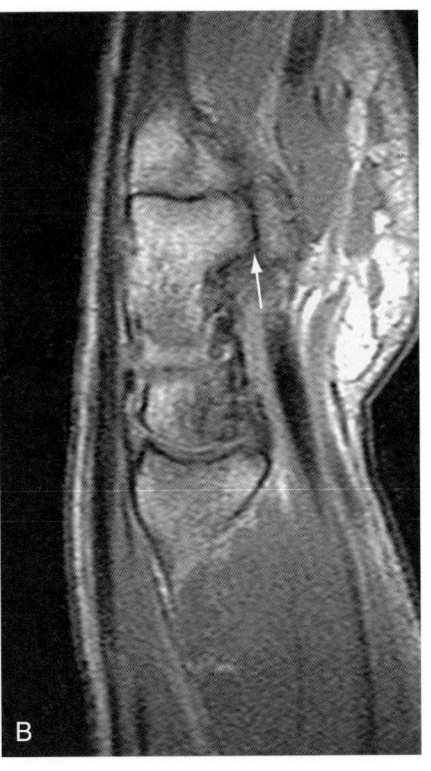

FIGURE 101-52

Hamate hook nonunion. **A,** Axial T1-weighted image. There is marginal sclerosis and absence of edema *(arrow)* reflective of nonunion. Note the close proximity of the ulnar nerve and artery *(arrowhead).* **B,** Sagittal T1-weighted image reveals the presence of the nonunion in a different plane *(arrow).*

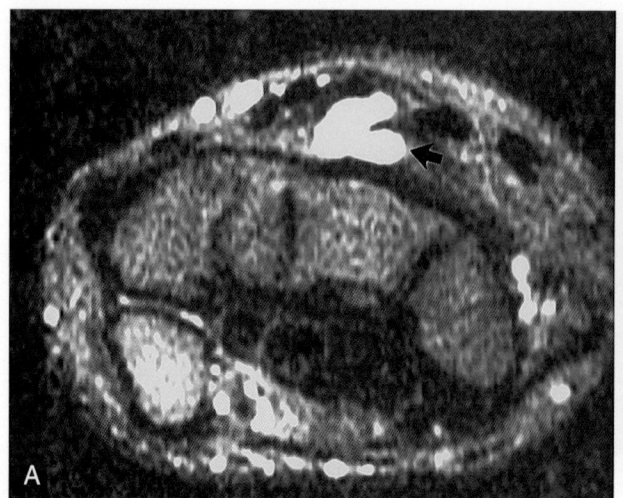

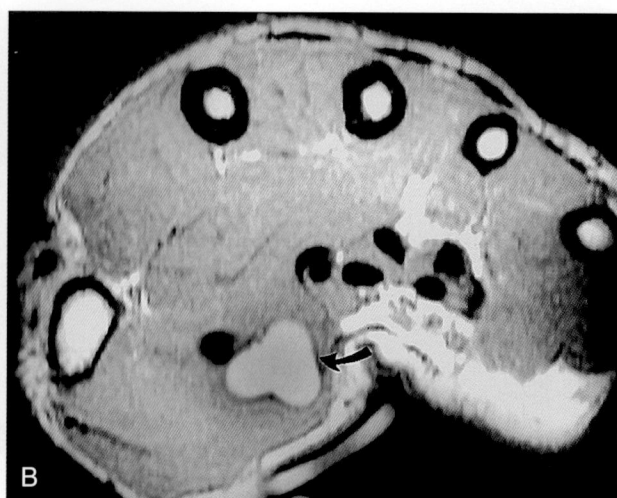

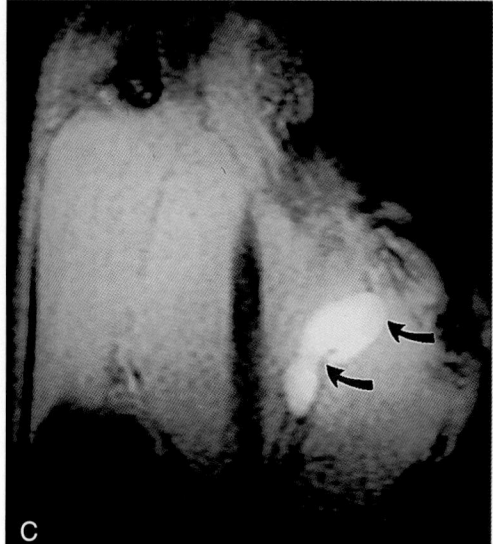

FIGURE 101-53

Wrist masses: ganglion cysts. **A,** Axial image (TR/TE 2500/70) demonstrates a well-circumscribed high-signal-intensity mass in the dorsum of the wrist *(arrow)*, related to the extensor tendons. **B** and **C,** Axial (**B**) and coronal (**C**) images (TR/TE 2500/70). Small ganglion cyst arising from the flexor pollicis longus tendon sheath *(arrows)*. The addition of longitudinal images aids in identifying the lesion neck, which is important in preventing recurrence after surgery.

FIGURE 101-54

Axial long TR/TE fast spin-echo image with fat saturation. A smaller ganglion is seen behind the dorsal scapholunate ligament *(arrowhead)*. Smaller ganglia are more often symptomatic than larger ones.

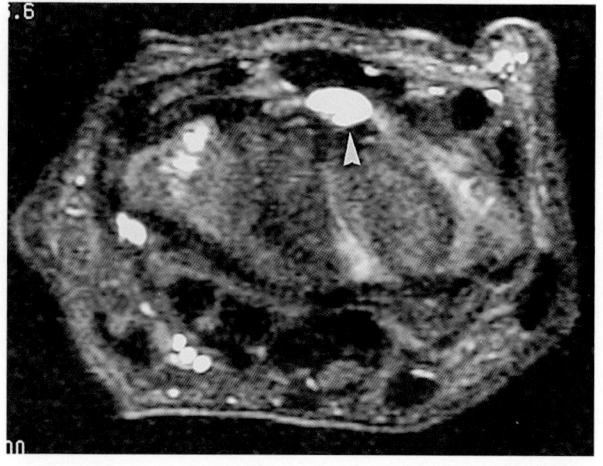

The occult dorsal carpal ganglion is a variant of the dorsal carpal ganglion.[287] It is a small mass that is difficult to palpate. These carpal ganglia have a mean diameter of 4.9 mm and most often originate from the dorsal scapholunate ligament (Fig. 101-54). Although the larger cysts discussed above are usually asymptomatic and present only cosmetic problems, smaller ganglia are more often symptomatic and may be responsible for wrist pain and disability. The pain may be caused by increased ligamentous pressure or by compression of the posterior interosseous nerve.[288] Both MRI and ultrasound have been found effective in detecting these small lesions. Knowledge of their characteristic location helps to differentiate them from fluid in a capsular recess.

Wrist ganglia have been associated, not infrequently, with internal derangements of the wrist (Fig. 101-55). In one study,[289] of the 22 ulnar-sided ganglia, 45% demonstrated associated TFCC tears. Of the 97 radial-sided ganglia, 28% demonstrated ligamentous tears related to the site of the ganglion. The radial-sided tears involved the radial aspect of the TFCC in 12 ganglia; the scapholunate ligament, in isolation, in 8 ganglia; and both the TFCC and the scapholunate ligament in 6 ganglia. Only one of the ganglia demonstrated an associated lunotriquetral ligamentous tear. Surgical findings confirmed the ligamentous tears in 25 patients.

The primary objective of MRI in patients with benign soft-tissue tumors of the wrist is often not to render a definitive diagnosis but to define the anatomic relationship of the mass to the tendons, nerves, and vessels. For example, ganglia which typically have a signal intensity similar to muscle on short TR/TE images and high signal intensity on long TR/TE images and have a tendency to be intimately associated with the tendons (see Fig. 101-53) (especially flexor) and the palmar radial ganglion can circumferentially encompass the radial artery.[283] This information is important to the surgeon preoperatively. The criteria used to distinguish benign from malignant tumors on MRI, particularly margination and homogeneity, are useful rather than specific guidelines.

In general, most soft-tissue masses are nonspecific in nature. In the hand and wrist there is fortunately a preponderance of nonaggressive lesions. In one study[281] these nonaggressive lesions were usually well marginated, did not invade or encase neurovascular or tendinous structures, and had rather uniform signal intensity. There was little or no surrounding tissue reaction. In the hand and wrist fortunately a certain number of these nonaggressive lesions may have a characteristic appearance[280] including ganglion cysts, lipomas (Fig. 101-56), hypertrophic palmaris longus muscle, schwannoma, fibrolipomatous hamartoma of the median nerve, and giant cell tumor of tendon sheath. The fibrolipomatous hamartoma is a rare but distinctive appearing tumor.[154,290-292] It usually presents in childhood or young adulthood as a slowly growing mass on the volar aspect of the hand or wrist. It almost always arises from the median nerve and may give rise to symptoms of pain, paraesthesias, or decreased sensation. In approximately one third of cases it is associated with macrodystrophia lipomatosa of the digits. Pathologically the tumor consists of infiltration of the

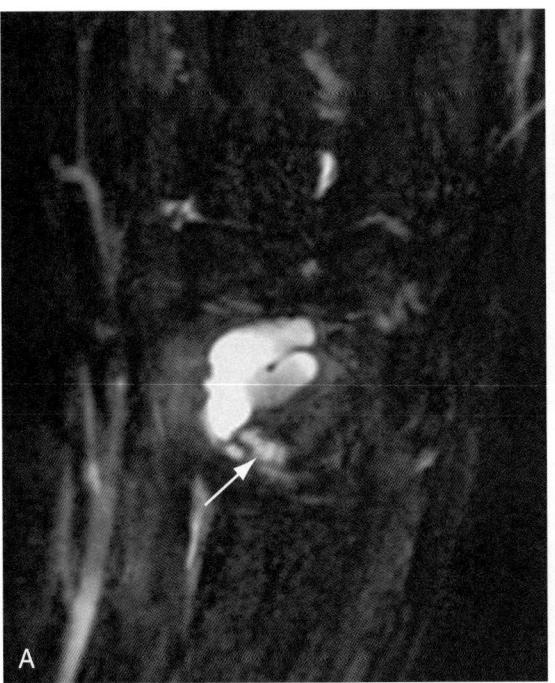
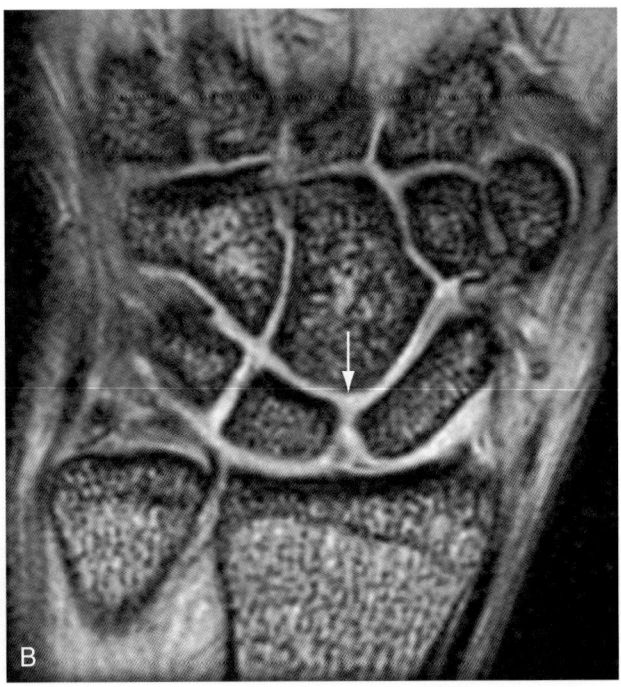

FIGURE 101-55

A, Coronal STIR image. Dorsal ganglion cyst with its neck in the region of the dorsal scapholunate ligament (*arrow*). **B,** Coronal gradient-echo image. Note the accompanying tear in the scapholunate ligament (*arrow*).

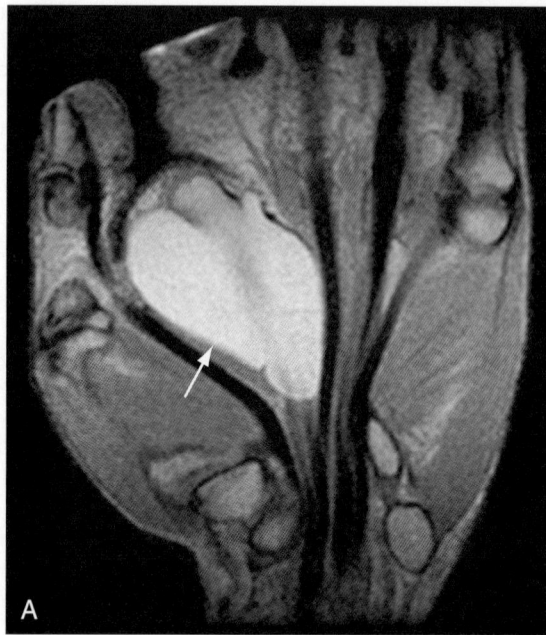

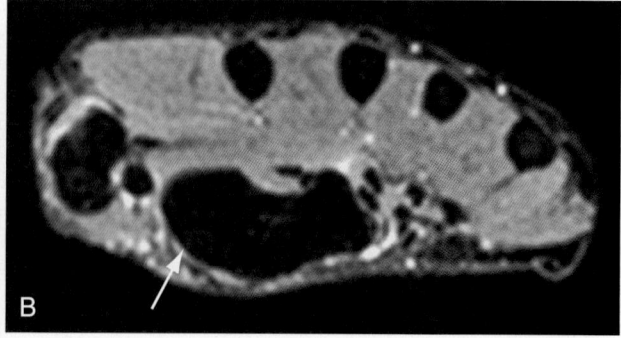

FIGURE 101-56

Lipoma of the hand. **A,** Coronal T1-weighted image. Large lipoma arising in the region of the flexor tendons *(arrow).* **B,** Axial STIR image. Note the homogeneous pattern of fat suppression *(arrow).*

nerve by fibrous and fatty elements, the relative amounts of which may vary. MRI (Fig. 101-57) shows serpiginous or circular low-signal-intensity structures on short and long TR/TE images representing the fibrous component, surrounded by various amounts of fat.

Anomalous muscles may present as pseudo masses on the dorsum or palm of the hand.[66,189,278,293-295] They may cause compression of nerves. In the carpal tunnel in particular, the median nerve may be compressed by an accessory flexor digitorum superficialis or palmaris longus muscle. These anomalous muscles should have a nonaggressive appearance and be isointense to muscle on all pulse sequences.

Pigmented villonodular synovitis may occur in the digits of the hand. When it occurs extra-articularly it may then be known as giant cell tumor of tendon sheath (Fig. 101-58).[277,280,296,297] Histologically it is composed of stromal cells, fibrous tissue giant cells, and hemosiderin. Soft-tissue swelling or a mass with or without erosion of the adjacent bone and without calcification is evident. Typically it has low signal intensity on all pulse sequences. This pattern is not invariable and regions of high signal intensity on T2-weighted spin-echo MR images are encountered,[298] particularly when fat suppression is applied, or with STIR imaging.

Benign vascular lesions are also not uncommon in the hand and wrist.[277,299,300] The most frequent of these is the hemangioma,[39,296] which may have a fairly characteristic appearance on MRI (Fig. 101-59). Hemangiomas may be of low signal intensity on short TR/TE images and of mixed to high signal intensity on long TR/TE sequences. High signal intensity also may be seen on short TR/TE sequences, due to fat or blood. The margins are usually distinct but may be indistinct. The tumors may be inhomogeneous, with a septate appearance due to fibrofatty septa between endothelium-lined vascular channels.

There may be round foci of low signal intensity due to phleboliths, fibrofatty septa, or hyalinized or thrombosed vascular channels. Serpiginous vascular channels of low signal intensity may also be seen.

Malignant bone lesions in the hand and wrist in patients older than 40 years are usually metastases. Primary malignant soft-tissue lesions of the hand and wrist are rare.[277,281] They may have a better prognosis due to early detection, as in this location they are more superficial. The importance of MRI in the preoperative evaluation of patients with known malignant tumors, in addition to ascertaining if there is neurovascular involvement, is to accurately document the proximal and distal margins of the lesion and, if the tumor is of osseous origin, to determine the presence or lack of involvement of the adjacent soft-tissues.

Synovial Processes

MRI is of value in the early detection of bone and cartilage changes in patients with inflammatory arthritis.[301] Erosions are more extensive and numerous on MR images of the hand and wrist than on plain radiographs. In addition a high proportion of rheumatoid arthritis patients develop MRI-visible erosions very early in their disease, when plain radiographs are negative. The most common site for erosions is the capitate. MRI of the dominant wrist may help identify those requiring early aggressive treatment. Erosions appear as low signal intensity on short TR/TE sequences and as high signal intensity on long TR/TE spin-echo and T2* gradient-echo sequences. Articular cartilage irregularities and thinning may be discerned. MRI may also be helpful in the documentation of the severity and magnitude of pannus formation, joint effusions and synovial proliferation, and

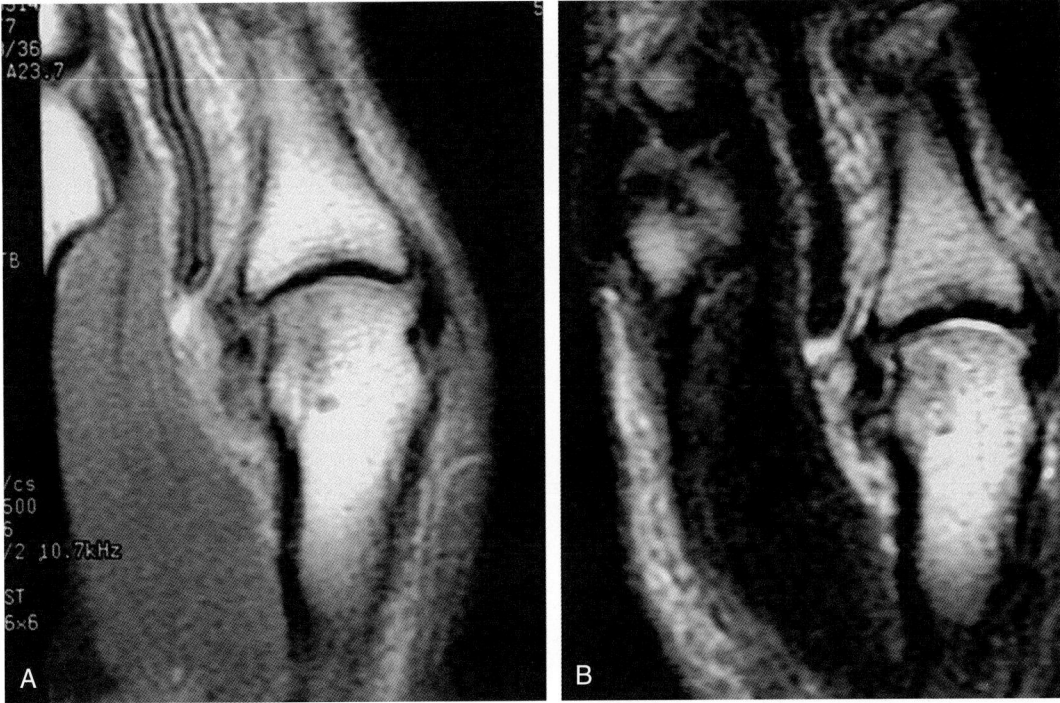

FIGURE 101-64

Gamekeeper's thumb. Coronal proton density–weighted (**A**), and T2-weighted (**B**) images. A nondisplaced tear of the distal ulnar collateral ligament is seen *(long thin arrows)*. The adductor aponeurosis is seen superficial to the ligament *(small thin black arrows)*. Edema reflecting a contusion is present in the adjacent bone *(short black arrows)*.

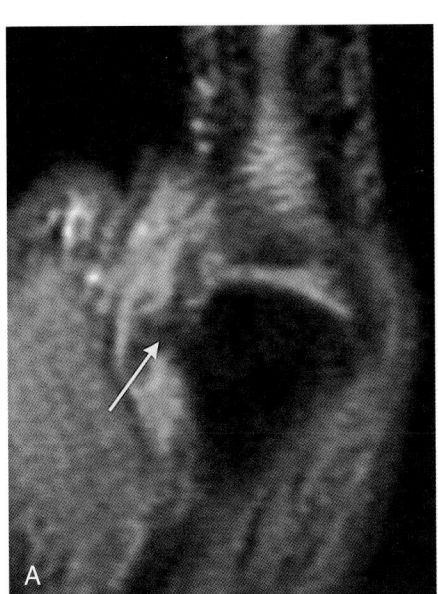
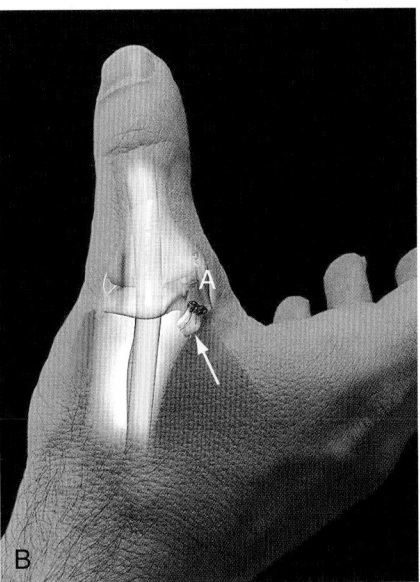

FIGURE 101-65

Gamekeeper's thumb, Stener lesion. **A,** Coronal fat-suppressed T2-weighted image shows a torn, retracted ulnar collateral ligament (UCL) lying superficial to the adductor aponeurosis *(arrow)*. This gives the retracted ligament the appearance of a "yo-yo on a string." **B,** Diagram of a Stener lesion. Note the retracted UCL *(arrow)* outside the aponeurosis (A). (**B,** *Courtesy of Mark Awh MD and Michael Stadnick, Nashville, Tenn).*

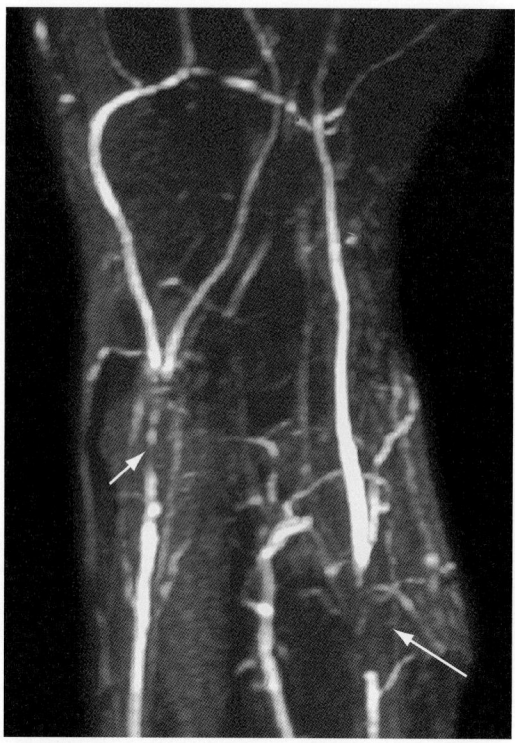

FIGURE 101-66

Hypothenar hammer syndrome. Intravenous MR angiogram in a professional tennis player. Note the occluded ulnar artery *(long arrow)* and narrowed irregular radial artery *(short arrow)*.

REFERENCES

1. Hobby JL, Dixon AK, Bearcroft PW, et al: MR imaging of the wrist: effect on clinical diagnosis and patient care. Radiology 220:589-593, 2001.
2. Morley J, Bidwell J, Bransby-Zachary M: A comparison of the findings of wrist arthroscopy and magnetic resonance imaging in the investigation of wrist pain. J Hand Surg [Br] 26:544-546, 2001.
2a. Weinberg EP, Hollenberg GM, Adams MJ, et al: High-resolution outpatient imaging of the wrist. Semin Musculoskeletal Radiol 5:227-234, 2001.
3. Steinbach LS, Palmer WE, Schweitzer ME: Special focus session. MR arthrography. Radiographics 22:1223-1246, 2002.
4. Beaulieu CF, Ladd AL: MR arthrography of the wrist: scanning-room injection of the radiocarpal joint based on clinical landmarks. Am J Roentgenol 170:606-608, 1998.
5. Bergin D, Schweitzer ME: Indirect magnetic resonance arthrography. Skeletal Radiol 32:551-558, 2003.
6. Schweitzer ME, Natale P, Winalski CS, et al: Indirect wrist MR arthrography: the effects of passive motion versus active exercise. Skeletal Radiol 29:10-14, 2000.
7. Vahlensieck M, Peterfy CG, Wischer T, et al: Indirect MR arthrography: optimization and clinical applications. Radiology 200:249-254, 1996.
8. Weishaupt D, Schweitzer ME, Rawool NM, et al: Indirect MR arthrography of the knee: effects of low-intensity ultrasound on the diffusion rate of intravenously administered Gd-DTPA in healthy volunteers. Invest Radiol 36:493-499, 2001.
9. Haims AH, Schweitzer ME, Morrison WB, et al: Internal derangement of the wrist: indirect MR arthrography versus unenhanced MR imaging. Radiology 227:701-707, 2003.
10. Mayfield JK: Wrist ligamentous anatomy and pathogenesis of carpal instability. Orthop Clin North Am 15:209-216, 1984.
11. Taleisnik J: The ligaments of the wrist. J Hand Surg [Am] 1:110-118, 1976.
12. Berger RA, Linscheid RL, Berquist TH: Magnetic resonance imaging of the anterior radiocarpal ligaments. J Hand Surg [Am] 19:295-303, 1994.
13. Berger RA: The ligaments of the wrist. A current overview of anatomy with considerations of their potential functions. Hand Clin 13:63-82, 1997.
14. Berger RA, Landsmeer JM: The palmar radiocarpal ligaments: a study of adult and fetal human wrist joints. J Hand Surg [Am] 15:847-854, 1990.
15. Smith DK: MR imaging of normal and injured wrist ligaments. Magn Reson Imaging Clin N Am 3:229-248, 1995.
16. Smith DK: Volar carpal ligaments of the wrist: normal appearance on multiplanar reconstructions of three-dimensional Fourier transform MR imaging. Am J Roentgenol 161:353-357, 1993.
17. Adler BD, Logan PM, Janzen DL, et al: Extrinsic radiocarpal ligaments: magnetic resonance imaging of normal wrists and scapholunate dissociation. Can Assoc Radiol J 47:417-422, 1996.
18. Timins ME, Jahnke JP, Krah SF, et al: MR imaging of the major carpal stabilizing ligaments: normal anatomy and clinical examples. Radiographics 15:575-587, 1995.
19. Johnston RB, Seiler JG, Miller EJ, et al: The intrinsic and extrinsic ligaments of the wrist. A correlation of collagen typing and histologic appearance. J Hand Surg [Br] 20:750-754, 1995.
20. Theumann NH, Pfirrmann CW, Antonio GE, et al: Extrinsic carpal ligaments: normal MR arthrographic appearance in cadavers. Radiology 226:171-179, 2003.
21. Totterman SM, Miller R, Wasserman B, et al: Intrinsic and extrinsic carpal ligaments: evaluation by three-dimensional Fourier transform MR imaging. Am J Roentgenol 160:117-123, 1993.
22. Berger RA: The anatomy of the scaphoid. Hand Clin 17:525-532, 2001.
23. Berger RA, Blair WF: The radioscapholunate ligament: a gross and histologic description. Anat Rec 210:393-405, 1984.
24. Berger RA, Kauer JM, Landsmeer JM: Radioscapholunate ligament: a gross anatomic and histologic study of fetal and adult wrists. J Hand Surg [Am] 16:350-355, 1991.
25. Mayfield JK, Johnson RP, Kilcoyne RF: The ligaments of the human wrist and their functional significance. Anat Rec 186:417-428, 1976.
26. Gelberman RH, Cooney WP III, Szabo RM: Carpal instability. Instr Course Lect 50:123-134, 2001.
27. Brown RR, Fliszar E, Cotten A, et al: Extrinsic and intrinsic ligaments of the wrist: normal and pathologic anatomy at MR arthrography with three-compartment enhancement. Radiographics 18:667-674, 1998.
28. Zlatkin MB, Ouellette EA, Needell S: MR and MR arthrography of the intercarpal ligaments of the wrist. Histopathologic correlation. In: Society of Magnetic Resonance Annual Meeting, 1996, New York.
29. Smith DK: Dorsal carpal ligaments of the wrist: normal appearance on multiplanar reconstructions of three-dimensional Fourier transform MR imaging. Am J Roentgenol 161:119-125, 1993.
30. Viegas SF: The dorsal ligaments of the wrist. Hand Clin 17:65-75, vi, 2001.
31. Mizuseki T, Ikuta Y: The dorsal carpal ligaments: their anatomy and function. J Hand Surg [Br] 14:91-98, 1989.
32. DiMarcangelo MT, Smith PA: Use of magnetic resonance imaging to diagnose common wrist disorders. J Am Osteopath Assoc 100:228-231, 2000.
33. Zlatkin MB, Greenan T: Magnetic resonance imaging of the wrist. Magn Reson Q 8:65-96, 1992.
34. Berger RA: The anatomy of the ligaments of the wrist and distal radioulnar joints. Clin Orthop 383:32-40, 2001.
35. Berger RA: The gross and histologic anatomy of the scapholunate interosseous ligament. J Hand Surg [Am] 21:170-178, 1996.
36. Bogumill G: Anatomy of the wrist. In Lichtman DM, Alexander AH (ed): The Wrist and its Disorders, 2nd ed. Philadelphia: WB Saunders, 1997, pp 34-48.
37. Smith DK: Scapholunate interosseous ligament of the wrist: MR appearances in asymptomatic volunteers and arthrographically normal wrists. Radiology 192:217-221, 1994.
38. Smith DK, Snearly WN: Lunotriquetral interosseous ligament of the wrist: MR appearances in asymptomatic volunteers and arthrographically normal wrists. Radiology 191:199-202, 1994.
39. Reicher MA, Kellerhouse LE: MRI of the wrist and hand. New York: Raven Press, 1990.
40. Totterman SM, Miller RJ: Scapholunate ligament: normal MR appearance on three-dimensional gradient-recalled-echo images. Radiology 200:237-241, 1996.
41. Palmer AK, Werner FW: The triangular fibrocartilage complex of the wrist—anatomy and function. J Hand Surg [Am] 6:153-162, 1981.
42. Loftus JB, Palmer AK: Disorders of the distal radioulnar joint and TFCC. An overview. In Lichtman DM, Alexander AH (ed): The Wrist and its Disorders, 2nd ed. Philadelphia: WB Saunders, 1997.
43. Benjamin M, Evans EJ, Pemberton DJ: Histological studies on the triangular fibrocartilage complex of the wrist. J Anat 172:59-67, 1990.
44. Prendergast N, Rauschning W: Normal anatomy of the hand and wrist. Magn Reson Imaging Clin N Am 3:197-212, 1995.
45. Totterman SM, Miller RJ: Triangular fibrocartilage complex: normal appearance on coronal three-dimensional gradient-recalled-echo MR images. Radiology 195:521-527, 1995.
46. Totterman SM, Miller RJ: MR imaging of the triangular fibrocartilage complex. Magn Reson Imaging Clin N Am 3:213-228, 1995.
47. Palmer AK, Werner FW: The triangular fibrocartilage complex of the wrist—anatomy and function. J Hand Surg [Am] 6:153-162, 1981.
48. Palmer AK, Glisson RR, Werner FW: Relationship between ulnar variance and triangular fibrocartilage complex thickness. J Hand Surg [Am] 9:681-682, 1984.
49. De Smet L: Ulnar variance: facts and fiction review article. Acta Orthop Belg 60:1-9, 1994.
50. Bednar MS, Arnoczky SP, Weiland AJ: The microvasculature of the triangular fibrocartilage complex: its clinical significance. J Hand Surg [Am] 16:1101-1105, 1991.

51. Kang HS, Kindynis P, Brahme SK, et al: Triangular fibrocartilage and inter-carpal ligaments of the wrist: MR imaging. Cadaveric study with gross pathologic and histologic correlation. Radiology 181:401-404, 1991.
52. Mikic Z: Age changes in the triangular fibrocartilage of the wrist joint. J Anat 126:367-384, 1978.
53. Zlatkin MB, Chao PC, Osterman AL: Chronic wrist pain: evaluation with high-resolution MR imaging. Radiology 173:723-729, 1989.
54. Totterman SM, Seo GS: MRI findings of scapholunate instabilities in coronal images: a short communication. Semin Musculoskelet Radiol 5:251-256, 2001.
55. af Ekenstam F: Anatomy of the distal radioulnar joint. Clin Orthop 275:14-18, 1992.
56. Drobner WS, Hausman MR: The distal radioulnar joint. Hand Clin 8:631-644, 1992.
57. Chiang CC, Chang MC, Lin CF, et al: Computerized tomography in the diagnosis of subluxation of the distal radioulnar joint. Zhonghua Yi Xue Za Zhi (Taipei) 61:708-715, 1998.
58. Cerezal L, del Pinal F, Abascal F, et al: Imaging findings in ulnar-sided wrist impaction syndromes. Radiographics 22:105-121, 2002.
59. De Smet L: Ulnar variance and its relationship to ligament injuries of the wrist. Acta Orthop Belg 65:416-417, 1999.
60. Escobedo EM, Bergman AG, Hunter JC: MR imaging of ulnar impaction. Skeletal Radiol 24:85-90, 1995.
61. Adolfsson L: Arthroscopic diagnosis of ligament lesions of the wrist. J Hand Surg [Br] 19:505-512, 1994.
62. Friedman SL, Palmer AK: The ulnar impaction syndrome. Hand Clin 7:295-310, 1991.
63. Oneson SR, Scales LM, Timins ME, et al: MR imaging interpretation of the Palmer classification of triangular fibrocartilage complex lesions. Radiographics 16:97-106, 1996.
64. Rotman MB, Donovan JP: Practical anatomy of the carpal tunnel. Hand Clin 18:219-230, 2002.
65. Mesgarzadeh M, Schneck CD, Bonakdarpour A: Carpal tunnel: MR imaging. Part I. Normal anatomy. Radiology 171:743-748, 1989.
66. Zeiss J, Jakab E, Khimji T, et al: The ulnar tunnel at the wrist (Guyon's canal): normal MR anatomy and variants. Am J Roentgenol 158:1081-1085, 1992.
67. Netscher D, Polsen C, Thornby J, et al: Anatomic delineation of the ulnar nerve and ulnar artery in relation to the carpal tunnel by axial magnetic resonance imaging scanning. J Hand Surg [Am] 21:273-276, 1996.
68. Glajchen N, Schweitzer M: MRI features in de Quervain's tenosynovitis of the wrist. Skeletal Radiol 25:63-65, 1996.
69. Tehranzadeh J, Kerr R, Amster J: Magnetic resonance imaging of tendon and ligament abnormalities: Part I. Spine and upper extremities. Skeletal Radiol 21:1-9, 1992.
70. Resnick D: Internal derangement of joints. In Resnick D (ed): Diagnosis of Bone and Joint Disorders, 4th ed. Philadelphia: WB Saunders, 2002, pp 3017-3376.
71. Clavero JA, Golano P, Farinas O, et al: Extensor mechanism of the fingers: MR imaging–anatomic correlation. Radiographics 23:593-611, 2003.
72. Gilula LA, Palmer AK: Is it possible to diagnose a tear at arthrography or MR imaging? Radiology 187:582, 1993.
73. Steinborn M, Schurmann M, Staebler A, et al: MR imaging of ulnocarpal impaction after fracture of the distal radius. Am J Roentgenol 181:195-198, 2003.
74. Tomaino MM: Ulnar impaction syndrome in the ulnar negative and neutral wrist. Diagnosis and pathoanatomy. J Hand Surg [Br] 23:754-757, 1998.
75. Imaeda T, Nakamura R, Shionoya K, et al: Ulnar impaction syndrome: MR imaging findings. Radiology 201:495-500, 1996.
76. Manaster BJ: The clinical efficacy of triple-injection wrist arthrography. Radiology 178:267-270, 1991.
77. Chidgey L: Histologic anatomy of the triangular fibrocartilage. Hand Clin 14:624-627, 1991.
78. Golimbu CN, Firooznia H, Melone CP Jr, et al: Tears of the triangular fibrocartilage of the wrist: MR imaging. Radiology 173:731-733, 1989.
79. Melone CP Jr, Nathan R: Traumatic disruption of the triangular fibrocartilage complex. Pathoanatomy. Clin Orthop 275:65-73, 1992.
80. Millants P, De Smet L, Van Ransbeeck H: Outcome study of arthroscopic suturing of ulnar avulsions of the triangular fibrocartilage complex of the wrist. Chir Main 21:298-300, 2002.
81. Corso SJ, Savoie FH, Geissler WB, et al: Arthroscopic repair of peripheral avulsions of the triangular fibrocartilage complex of the wrist: a multicenter study. Arthroscopy 13:78-84, 1997.
82. Hauck RM, Skahen J III, Palmer AK: Classification and treatment of ulnar styloid nonunion. J Hand Surg [Am] 21:418-422, 1996.
83. Mikic ZD: Treatment of acute injuries of the triangular fibrocartilage complex associated with distal radioulnar joint instability. J Hand Surg [Am] 20:319-323, 1995.
84. Fellinger M, Peicha G, Seibert FJ, et al: Radial avulsion of the triangular fibrocartilage complex in acute wrist trauma: a new technique for arthroscopic repair. Arthroscopy 13:370-374, 1997.
85. Schweitzer ME, Brahme SK, Hodler J, et al: Chronic wrist pain: spin-echo and short tau inversion recovery MR imaging and conventional and MR arthrography. Radiology 182:205-211, 1992.
86. Metz VM, Schratter M, Dock WI, et al: Age-associated changes of the triangular fibrocartilage of the wrist: evaluation of the diagnostic performance of MR imaging. Radiology 184:217-220, 1992.
87. Haims AH, Schweitzer ME, Morrison WB, et al: Limitations of MR imaging in the diagnosis of peripheral tears of the triangular fibrocartilage of the wrist. Am J Roentgenol 178:419-422, 2002.
88. Oneson SR, Timins ME, Scales LM, et al: MR imaging diagnosis of triangular fibrocartilage pathology with arthroscopic correlation. Am J Roentgenol 168:1513-1518, 1997.
89. Topper SM, Wood MB, Ruby LK: Ulnar styloid impaction syndrome. J Hand Surg [Am] 22:699-704, 1997.
90. Potter HG, Asnis-Ernberg L, Weiland AJ, et al: The utility of high-resolution magnetic resonance imaging in the evaluation of the triangular fibrocartilage complex of the wrist. J Bone Joint Surg Am 79:1675-1684, 1997.
91. Johnstone DJ, Thorogood S, Smith WH, et al: A comparison of magnetic resonance imaging and arthroscopy in the investigation of chronic wrist pain. J Hand Surg [Br] 22:714-718, 1997.
92. Herold T, Lenhart M, Held P, et al: [Indirect MR Arthrography of the wrist in the diagnosis of TFCC-Lesions]. Rofo Fortschr Geb Rontgenstr Neuen Bildgeb Verfahr 173:1006-1011, 2001.
93. Osterman AL: Arthroscopic debridement of triangular fibrocartilage complex tears. Arthroscopy 6:120-124, 1990.
94. Baehser-Griffith P, Bednar JM, Osterman AL, et al: Arthroscopic repairs of triangular fibrocartilage complex tears. AORN J 66:101-102, 105-111, quiz 112, 115, 117-108, 1997.
95. Zachee B, De Smet L, Fabry G: Arthroscopic suturing of TFCC lesions. Arthroscopy 9:242-244, 1993.
96. Bednar JM, Osterman AL: The role of arthroscopy in the treatment of traumatic triangular fibrocartilage injuries. Hand Clin 10:605-614, 1994.
97. Minami A, Kato H: Ulnar shortening for triangular fibrocartilage complex tears associated with ulnar positive variance. J Hand Surg [Am] 23:904-908, 1998.
98. Buterbaugh GA, Brown TR, Horn PC: Ulnar-sided wrist pain in athletes. Clin Sports Med 17:567-583, 1998.
99. Theumann NH, Pfirrmann CW, Chung CB, et al: Pisotriquetral joint: assessment with MR imaging and MR arthrography. Radiology 222:763-770, 2002.
100. Thurston AJ, Stanley JK: Hamato-lunate impingement: an uncommon cause of ulnar-sided wrist pain. Arthroscopy 16:540-544, 2000.
101. Nathan R, Schneider LH: Classification of distal radioulnar joint disorders. Hand Clin 7:239-247, 1991.
102. Nicolaidis SC, Hildreth DH, Lichtman DM: Acute injuries of the distal radioulnar joint. Hand Clin 16:449-459, 2000.
103. Mino DE, Palmer AK, Levinsohn EM: The role of radiography and computerized tomography in the diagnosis of subluxation and dislocation of the distal radioulnar joint. J Hand Surg [Am] 8:23-31, 1983.
104. King GJ, McMurtry RY, Rubenstein JD, et al: Computerized tomography of the distal radioulnar joint: correlation with ligamentous pathology in a cadaveric model. J Hand Surg [Am] 11:711-717, 1986.
105. Wechsler RJ, Wehbe MA, Rifkin MD, et al: Computed tomography diagnosis of distal radioulnar subluxation. Skeletal Radiol 16:1-5, 1987.
106. Steinbach LS, Smith DK: MRI of the wrist. Clin Imaging 24:298-322, 2000.
107. Daunt N: Magnetic resonance imaging of the wrist: anatomy and pathology of interosseous ligaments and the triangular fibrocartilage complex. Curr Probl Diagn Radiol 31:158-176, 2002.
108. Manton GL, Schweitzer ME, Weishaupt D, et al: Partial interosseous ligament tears of the wrist: difficulty in utilizing either primary or secondary MRI signs. J Comput Assist Tomogr 25:671-676, 2001.
109. Oneson SR, Scales LM, Erickson SJ, et al: MR imaging of the painful wrist. Radiographics 16:997-1008, 1996.
110. Schadel-Hopfner M, Iwinska-Zelder J, Braus T, et al: MRI versus arthroscopy in the diagnosis of scapholunate ligament injury. J Hand Surg [Br] 26:17-21, 2001.
111. Scheck RJ, Kubitzek C, Hierner R, et al: The scapholunate interosseous ligament in MR arthrography of the wrist: correlation with non-enhanced MRI and wrist arthroscopy. Skeletal Radiol 26:263-271, 1997.
112. Mayfield JK: Mechanism of carpal injuries. Clin Orthop 149:45-54, 1980.
113. Mayfield JK: Patterns of injury to carpal ligaments. A spectrum. Clin Orthop 187:36-42, 1984.
114. Wright TW, Dobyns JH, Linscheid RL, et al: Carpal instability non-dissociative. J Hand Surg [Br] 19:763-773, 1994.
115. Cooney WP, Dobyns JH, Linscheid RL: Arthroscopy of the wrist: anatomy and classification of carpal instability. Arthroscopy 6:133-140, 1990.
116. Cassidy C, Ruby LK: Carpal instability. Instr Course Lect 52:209-220, 2003.
117. Miller RJ: Wrist MRI and carpal instability: what the surgeon needs to know, and the case for dynamic imaging. Semin Musculoskelet Radiol 5:235-240, 2001.
118. Taleisnik J: Classification of carpal instability. Bull Hosp Jt Dis 44:511-531, 1984.
119. Taleisnik J: Current concepts review. Carpal instability. J Bone Joint Surg Am 70:1262-1268, 1988.
120. Farooki S, Seeger LL: Magnetic resonance imaging in the evaluation of ligament injuries. Skeletal Radiol 28:61-74, 1999.
121. Rominger MB, Bernreuter WK, Kenney PJ, et al: MR imaging of anatomy and tears of wrist ligaments. Radiographics 13:1233-1246; discussion 1247-1238, 1993.
122. Schofield BA, Ouellette EA, Zlatkin MB, Murphy B: MRI correlation with scapholunate ligament tears. In: American Academy of Orthopedic Surgeons. Orlando, Fla, 1995.

123. Scheck RJ, Romagnolo A, Hierner R, et al: The carpal ligaments in MR arthrography of the wrist: correlation with standard MRI and wrist arthroscopy. J Magn Reson Imaging 9:468-474, 1999.

124. Zanetti M, Bram J, Hodler J: Triangular fibrocartilage and intercarpal ligaments of the wrist: does MR arthrography improve standard MRI? J Magn Reson Imaging 7:590-594, 1997.

125. Linscheid RL, Dobyns JH, Beabout JW, et al: Traumatic instability of the wrist: diagnosis, classification, and pathomechanics. J Bone Joint Surg Am 84-A:142, 2002.

126. Ruby LK, An KN, Linscheid RL, et al: The effect of scapholunate ligament section on scapholunate motion. J Hand Surg [Am] 12:767-771, 1987.

127. Kovanlikaya I, Camli D, Cakmakci H, et al: Diagnostic value of MR arthrography in detection of intrinsic carpal ligament lesions: use of cine-MR arthrography as a new approach. Eur Radiol 7:1441-1445, 1997.

128. Brody G, Stillee D: The wrist and hand. In Stoller D (ed): Magnetic Resonance Imaging in Orthopedics and Sports Medicine. Philadelphia: JP Lippincott, 1993, pp 683-807.

129. Zanetti M, Hodler J, Gilula LA: Assessment of dorsal or ventral intercalated segmental instability configurations of the wrist: reliability of sagittal MR images. Radiology 206:339-345, 1998.

130. Stabler A, Heuck A, Reiser M: Imaging of the hand: degeneration, impingement and overuse. Eur J Radiol 25:118-128, 1997.

131. Resnick D: SLAC wrist. J Hand Surg [Am] 10:154-155, 1985.

132. Watson HK, Ballet FL: The SLAC wrist: scapholunate advanced collapse pattern of degenerative arthritis. J Hand Surg [Am] 9:358-365, 1984.

133. O'Meeghan CJ, Stuart W, Mamo V, et al: The natural history of an untreated isolated scapholunate interosseus ligament injury. J Hand Surg [Br] 28:307-310, 2003.

134. Osterman AL, Mikulics M: Scaphoid nonunion. Hand Clin 4:437-455, 1988.

135. Weiss LE, Taras JS, Sweet S, et al: Lunotriquetral injuries in the athlete. Hand Clin 16:433-438, 2000.

136. Brown DE, Lichtman DM: Midcarpal instability. Hand Clin 3:135-140, 1987.

137. Lichtman DM, Bruckner JD, Culp RW, et al: Palmar midcarpal instability: results of surgical reconstruction. J Hand Surg [Am] 18:307-315, 1993.

138. Ton ER, Pattynama PM, Bloem JL, et al: Interosseous ligaments: device for applying stress in wrist MR imaging. Radiology 196:863-864, 1995.

139. Osterman AL, Zlatkin MB: Magnetic resonance imaging in patients with chronic wrist pain. In: 45th Annual Meeting of the American Society for Surgery of the Hand, Toronto, Canada, 1990.

140. Walsh JJ, Berger RA, Cooney WP: Current status of scapholunate interosseous ligament injuries. J Am Acad Orthop Surg 10:32-42, 2002.

141. Watson HK, Ryu J, Akelman E: Limited triscaphoid intercarpal arthrodesis for rotatory subluxation of the scaphoid. J Bone Joint Surg Am 68:345-349, 1986.

142. Watson HK, Weinzweig J, Zeppieri J: The natural progression of scaphoid instability. Hand Clin 13:39-49, 1997.

143. Lavernia CJ, Cohen MS, Taleisnik J: Treatment of scapholunate dissociation by ligamentous repair and capsulodesis. J Hand Surg [Am] 17:354-359, 1992.

144. Moskal MJ, Savoie FH III, Field LD: Arthroscopic capsulodesis of the lunotriquetral joint. Clin Sports Med 20:141-153, ix-x, 2001.

145. Viegas SF: Ulnar-sided wrist pain and instability. Instr Course Lect 47:215-218, 1998.

146. Phalen GS: The carpal-tunnel syndrome. Clinical evaluation of 598 hands. Clin Orthop 83:29-40, 1972.

147. Phalen GS: Reflections on 21 years' experience with the carpal-tunnel syndrome. JAMA 212:1365-1367, 1970.

148. Phalen GS: The diagnosis of carpal tunnel syndrome. Cleve Clin Q 35:1-6, 1968.

149. Tanzer RC: The carpal-tunnel syndrome; a clinical and anatomical study. J Bone Joint Surg Am 41-A:626-634, 1959.

150. Skie M, Zeiss J, Ebraheim NA, et al: Carpal tunnel changes and median nerve compression during wrist flexion and extension seen by magnetic resonance imaging. J Hand Surg [Am] 15:934-939, 1990.

151. Fleckenstein JL, Wolfe GI: MRI vs EMG: which has the upper hand in carpal tunnel syndrome? Neurology 58:1583-1584, 2002.

152. Britz GW, Haynor DR, Kuntz C, et al: Carpal tunnel syndrome: correlation of magnetic resonance imaging, clinical, electrodiagnostic, and intraoperative findings. Neurosurgery 37:1097-1103, 1995.

153. Deryani E, Aki S, Muslumanoglu L, et al: MR imaging and electrophysiological evaluation in carpal tunnel syndrome. Yonsei Med J 44:27-32, 2003.

154. Canga A, Abascal F, Cerezal L, et al: Fibrolipomatous hamartoma of the median nerve. Case illustration. J Neurosurg 89:683, 1998.

155. Pierre-Jerome C, Bekkelund SI, Mellgren SI, et al: Quantitative MRI and electrophysiology of preoperative carpal tunnel syndrome in a female population. Ergonomics 40:642-649, 1997.

156. Bak L, Bak S, Gaster P, et al: MR imaging of the wrist in carpal tunnel syndrome. Acta Radiol 38:1050-1052, 1997.

157. Mesgarzadeh M, Triolo J, Schneck CD: Carpal tunnel syndrome. MR imaging diagnosis. Magn Reson Imaging Clin N Am 3:249-264, 1995.

158. Cudlip SA, Howe FA, Clifton A, et al: Magnetic resonance neurography studies of the median nerve before and after carpal tunnel decompression. J Neurosurg 96:1046-1051, 2002.

159. Mesgarzadeh M, Schneck CD, Bonakdarpour A, et al: Carpal tunnel: MR imaging. Part II. Carpal tunnel syndrome. Radiology 171:749-754, 1989.

160. Murphy RX Jr, Chernofsky MA, Osborne MA, et al: Magnetic resonance imaging in the evaluation of persistent carpal tunnel syndrome. J Hand Surg [Am] 18:113-120, 1993.

161. Netscher D, Mosharrafa A, Lee M, et al: Transverse carpal ligament: its effect on flexor tendon excursion, morphologic changes of the carpal canal, and on pinch and grip strengths after open carpal tunnel release. Plast Reconstr Surg 100:636-642, 1997.

162. Middleton WD, Kneeland JB, Kellman GM, et al: MR imaging of the carpal tunnel: normal anatomy and preliminary findings in the carpal tunnel syndrome. Am J Roentgenol 148:307-316, 1987.

163. Cobb TK, Bond JR, Cooney WP, et al: Assessment of the ratio of carpal contents to carpal canal volume in patients with carpal tunnel syndrome: a preliminary report. J Hand Surg [Am] 22:635-639, 1997.

164. Cobb TK, Dalley BK, Posteraro RH, et al: Establishment of carpal contents/canal ratio by means of magnetic resonance imaging. J Hand Surg [Am] 17:843-849, 1992.

165. Phalen GS: The birth of a syndrome, or carpal tunnel revisited. J Hand Surg [Am] 6:109-110, 1981.

166. Kleindienst A, Hamm B, Lanksch WR: Carpal tunnel syndrome: staging of median nerve compression by MR imaging. J Magn Reson Imaging 8:1119-1125, 1998.

167. Howe FA, Saunders DE, Filler AG, et al: Magnetic resonance neurography of the median nerve. Br J Radiol 67:1169-1172, 1994.

168. Sugimoto H, Miyaji N, Ohsawa T: Carpal tunnel syndrome: evaluation of median nerve circulation with dynamic contrast-enhanced MR imaging. Radiology 190:459-466, 1994.

169. Phalen GS: The carpal-tunnel syndrome. Seventeen years' experience in diagnosis and treatment of six hundred and fifty-four hands. J Bone Joint Surg Am 48:211-228, 1966.

170. Gonzalez MH, Cooper ME: Gouty tenosynovitis of the wrist. Am J Orthop 30:562-565, 2001.

171. Ham SJ, Kolkman WF, Heeres J, et al: Changes in the carpal tunnel due to action of the flexor tendons: visualization with magnetic resonance imaging. J Hand Surg [Am] 21:997-1003, 1996.

172. Sueyoshi E, Uetani M, Hayashi K, et al: Tuberculous tenosynovitis of the wrist: MRI findings in three cases. Skeletal Radiol 25:569-572, 1996.

173. Kleindienst A, Hamm B, Hildebrandt G, et al: Diagnosis and staging of carpal tunnel syndrome: comparison of magnetic resonance imaging and intra-operative findings. Acta Neurochir (Wien) 138:228-233, 1996.

174. Radack DM, Schweitzer ME, Taras J: Carpal tunnel syndrome: are the MR findings a result of population selection bias? Am J Roentgenol 169:1649-1653, 1997.

175. Monagle K, Dai G, Chu A, et al: Quantitative MR imaging of carpal tunnel syndrome. Am J Roentgenol 172:1581-1586, 1999.

176. Rosenbaum RB: The role of imaging in the diagnosis of carpal tunnel syndrome. Invest Radiol 28:1059-1062, 1993.

177. Aagaard BD, Maravilla KR, Kliot M: MR neurography. MR imaging of peripheral nerves. Magn Reson Imaging Clin N Am 6:179-194, 1998.

178. Barnes DE: MRI's role uncertain in carpal tunnel syndrome. Diagn Imaging (San Franc) 14:75-77, 1992.

179. Jarvik JG, Yuen E: Diagnosis of carpal tunnel syndrome: electrodiagnostic and magnetic resonance imaging evaluation. Neurosurg Clin N Am 12:241-253, 2001.

180. Pasternack II, Malmivaara A, Tervahartiala P, et al: Magnetic resonance imaging findings in respect to carpal tunnel syndrome. Scand J Work Environ Health 29:189-196, 2003.

181. Seyfert S, Boegner F, Hamm B, et al: The value of magnetic resonance imaging in carpal tunnel syndrome. J Neurol 242:41-46, 1994.

182. Kato T, Kuroshima N, Okutsu I, et al: Effects of endoscopic release of the transverse carpal ligament on carpal canal volume. J Hand Surg [Am] 19:416-419, 1994.

183. Richman JA, Gelberman RH, Rydevik BL, et al: Carpal tunnel syndrome: morphologic changes after release of the transverse carpal ligament. J Hand Surg [Am] 14:852-857, 1989.

184. Ablove RH, Peimer CA, Diao E, et al: Morphologic changes following endoscopic and two-portal subcutaneous carpal tunnel release. J Hand Surg [Am] 19:821-826, 1994.

185. Cobb TK, Carmichael SW, Cooney WP: Guyon's canal revisited: an anatomic study of the carpal ulnar neurovascular space. J Hand Surg [Am] 21:861-869, 1996.

186. Sakai K, Tsutsui T, Aoi M, et al: Ulnar neuropathy caused by a lipoma in Guyon's canal—case report. Neurol Med Chir (Tokyo) 40:335-338, 2000.

187. Shu N, Uchio Y, Ryoke K, et al: Atypical compression of the deep branch of the ulnar nerve in Guyon's canal by a ganglion. Case report. Scand J Plast Reconstr Surg Hand Surg 34:181-183, 2000.

188. Subin GD, Mallon WJ, Urbaniak JR: Diagnosis of ganglion in Guyon's canal by magnetic resonance imaging. J Hand Surg [Am] 14:640-643, 1989.

189. Zeiss J, Jakab E: MR demonstration of an anomalous muscle in a patient with coexistent carpal and ulnar tunnel syndrome. Case report and literature summary. Clin Imaging 19:102-105, 1995.

190. Allan CH, Joshi A, Lichtman DM: Kienbock's disease: diagnosis and treatment. J Am Acad Orthop Surg 9:128-136, 2001.

191. Cooney WP III: Scaphoid fractures: current treatments and techniques. Instr Course Lect 52:197-208, 2003.

192. Brydie A, Raby N: Early MRI in the management of clinical scaphoid fracture. Br J Radiol 76:296-300, 2003.

193. Fowler C, Sullivan B, Williams LA, et al: A comparison of bone scintigraphy and MRI in the early diagnosis of the occult scaphoid waist fracture. Skeletal Radiol 27:683-687, 1998.

194. Gabler C, Kukla C, Breitenseher MJ, et al: Diagnosis of occult scaphoid fractures and other wrist injuries. Are repeated clinical examinations and plain radiographs still state of the art? Langenbecks Arch Surg 386:150-154, 2001.

195. Gaebler C, Kukla C, Breitenseher M, et al: Magnetic resonance imaging of occult scaphoid fractures. J Trauma 41:73-76, 1996.

196. Thorpe AP, Murray AD, Smith FW, et al: Clinically suspected scaphoid fracture: a comparison of magnetic resonance imaging and bone scintigraphy. Br J Radiol 69:109-113, 1996.

197. Topper SM: Magnetic resonance imaging of the humpback scaphoid: the technique and a mathematical performance evaluation. Am J Orthop 28:639-643, 1999.

198. Raby N: Magnetic resonance imaging of suspected scaphoid fractures using a low field dedicated extremity MR system. Clin Radiol 56:316-320, 2001.

199. Bretlau T, Christensen OM, Edstrom P, et al: Diagnosis of scaphoid fracture and dedicated extremity MRI. Acta Orthop Scand 70:504-508, 1999.

200. Muramatsu K, Doi K, Kuwata N, et al: Scaphoid fracture in the young athlete—therapeutic outcome of internal fixation using the Herbert screw. Arch Orthop Trauma Surg 122:510-513, 2002.

201. Mazet R Jr, Hohl M: Conservative treatment of old fractures of the carpal scaphoid. J Trauma 1:115-127, 1961.

202. Schmitt R, Heinze A, Fellner F, et al: Imaging and staging of avascular osteonecroses at the wrist and hand. Eur J Radiol 25:92-103, 1997.

203. Mazet R, Hohl M: Fractures of the carpal navicular. J Bone Joint Surg Am 45:82-111, 1963.

204. Gelberman RH, Gross MS: The vascularity of the wrist. Identification of arterial patterns at risk. Clin Orthop 202:40-49, 1986.

205. Panagis JS, Gelberman RH, Taleisnik J, et al: The arterial anatomy of the human carpus. Part II: The intraosseous vascularity. J Hand Surg [Am] 8:375-382, 1983.

206. Gelberman RH, Menon J: The vascularity of the scaphoid bone. J Hand Surg [Am] 5:508-513, 1980.

207. Cooney WP, Linscheid RL, Dobyns JH: Scaphoid fractures. Problems associated with nonunion and avascular necrosis. Orthop Clin North Am 15:381-391, 1984.

208. Cave E: The carpus with reference to the fractured navicular bone. Arch Surg 40:54-76, 1940.

209. Trumble TE: Avascular necrosis after scaphoid fracture: a correlation of magnetic resonance imaging and histology. J Hand Surg [Am] 15:557-564, 1990.

210. Schimmerl-Metz SM, Metz VM, Totterman SM, et al: Radiologic measurement of the scapholunate joint: implications of biologic variation in scapholunate joint morphology. J Hand Surg [Am] 24:1237-1244, 1999.

211. Golimbu CN, Firooznia H, Rafii M: Avascular necrosis of carpal bones. Magn Reson Imaging Clin N Am 3:281-303, 1995.

212. Cristiani G, Cerofolini E, Squarzina PB, et al: Evaluation of ischaemic necrosis of carpal bones by magnetic resonance imaging. J Hand Surg [Br] 15:249-255, 1990.

213. Reinus WR, Conway WF, Totty WG, et al: Carpal avascular necrosis: MR imaging. Radiology 160:689-693, 1986.

214. Perlik PC, Guilford WB: Magnetic resonance imaging to assess vascularity of scaphoid nonunions. J Hand Surg [Am] 16:479-484, 1991.

215. Dawson JS, Martel AL, Davis TR: Scaphoid blood flow and acute fracture healing. A dynamic MRI study with enhancement with gadolinium. J Bone Joint Surg Br 83:809-814, 2001.

216. Cerezal L, Abascal F, Canga A, et al: Usefulness of gadolinium-enhanced MR imaging in the evaluation of the vascularity of scaphoid nonunions. Am J Roentgenol 174:141-149, 2000.

217. Munk PL, Lee MJ: Gadolinium-enhanced MR imaging of scaphoid nonunions. Am J Roentgenol 175:1184-1185, 2000.

218. Munk PL, Lee MJ, Janzen DL, et al: Gadolinium-enhanced dynamic MRI of the fractured carpal scaphoid: preliminary results. Australas Radiol 42:10-15, 1998.

219. Dreant N, Dautel G: [Development of a arthroscopic severity score for scapholunate instability]. Chir Main 22:90-94, 2003.

220. Kalainov DM, Cohen MS, Hendrix RW, et al: Preiser's disease: identification of two patterns. J Hand Surg [Am] 28:767-778, 2003.

221. Martini G, Valenti R, Giovani S, et al: Idiopathic avascular necrosis of the scaphoid. A case report. Recenti Prog Med 86:238-240, 1995.

222. Dossing K, Boe S: Idiopathic avascular necrosis of the scaphoid. Case report. Scand J Plast Reconstr Surg Hand Surg 28:155-156, 1994.

223. De Smet L, Aerts P, Walraevens M, et al: Avascular necrosis of the carpal scaphoid: Preiser's disease: report of 6 cases and review of the literature. Acta Orthop Belg 59:139-142, 1993.

224. Trumble T, Nyland W: Scaphoid nonunions. Pitfalls and pearls. Hand Clin 17:611-624, 2001.

225. Kulkarni RW, Wollstein R, Tayar R, et al: Patterns of healing of scaphoid fractures. The importance of vascularity. J Bone Joint Surg Br 81:85-90, 1999.

226. Morgan WJ, Breen TF, Coumas JM, et al: Role of magnetic resonance imaging in assessing factors affecting healing in scaphoid nonunions. Clin Orthop 336:240-246, 1997.

227. Peterson DA, Brandser EA, Steyers CM: Imaging scaphoid fractures and nonunions: familiar methods and newer trends. Iowa Orthop J 16:97-103, 1996.

228. Peltier LF: The classic. Concerning traumatic malacia of the lunate and its consequences: degeneration and compression fractures. Privatdozent Dr. Robert Kienbock. Clin Orthop 149:4-8, 1980.

229. Weiss K: Professor Robert Kienbock. Wien Klin Wochenschr 65:883-884, 1953.

230. Yoshida T, Tada K, Yamamoto K, et al: Aged-onset Kienbock's disease. Arch Orthop Trauma Surg 109:241-246, 1990.

231. Almquist EE: Kienbock's disease. Clin Orthop 202:68-78, 1986.

232. Goldfarb CA, Hsu J, Gelberman RH, et al: The Lichtman classification for Kienbock's disease: an assessment of reliability. J Hand Surg [Am] 28:74-80, 2003.

233. Amadio PC, Hanssen AD, Berquist TH: The genesis of Kienbock's disease: evaluation of a case by magnetic resonance imaging. J Hand Surg [Am] 12:1044-1049, 1987.

234. Mjoberg B: Kienbock disease and negative ulnar variance. J Bone Joint Surg Am 82:144, 2000.

235. Chen WS: Kienbock disease and negative ulnar variance. J Bone Joint Surg Am 82:143-144, 2000.

236. Bonzar M, Firrell JC, Hainer M, et al: Kienbock disease and negative ulnar variance. J Bone Joint Surg Am 80:1154-1157, 1998.

237. Szabo RM, Greenspan A: Diagnosis and clinical findings of Kienbock's disease. Hand Clin 9:399-408, 1993.

238. Linscheid RL: Kienbock's disease. Instr Course Lect 41:45-53, 1992.

239. Almquist EE: Kienbock's disease. Hand Clin 3:141-148, 1987.

240. Alexander AH, Lichtman DM: Kienbock's disease. Orthop Clin North Am 17:461-472, 1986.

241. Gelberman RH, Szabo RM: Kienbock's disease. Orthop Clin North Am 15:355-367, 1984.

242. Kuhlmann JN, Kron C, Boabighi A, et al: Vascularised pisiform bone graft. Indications, technique and long-term results. Acta Orthop Belg 69:311-316, 2003.

243. Minami A, Kato H, Suenaga N, et al: Scaphotrapeziotrapezoid fusion: long-term follow-up study. J Orthop Sci 8:319-322, 2003.

244. Leblebicioglu G, Doral MN, Atay AA, et al: Open treatment of stage III Kienbock's disease with lunate revascularization compared with arthroscopic treatment without revascularization. Arthroscopy 19:117-130, 2003.

245. Nagelvoort RW, Kon M, Schuurman AH: Proximal row carpectomy: a worthwhile salvage procedure. Scand J Plast Reconstr Surg Hand Surg 36:289-299, 2002.

246. Takase K, Imakiire A: Lunate excision, capitate osteotomy, and intercarpal arthrodesis for advanced Kienbock disease. Long-term follow-up. J Bone Joint Surg Am 83-A:177-183, 2001.

247. Salmon J, Stanley JK, Trail IA: Kienbock's disease: conservative management versus radial shortening. J Bone Joint Surg Br 82:820-823, 2000.

248. Menth-Chiari WA, Poehling GG, Wiesler ER, et al: Arthroscopic debridement for the treatment of Kienbock's disease. Arthroscopy 15:12-19, 1999.

249. Rhee SK, Kim HM, Bahk WJ, et al: A comparative study of the surgical procedures to treat advanced Kienbock's disease. J Korean Med Sci 11:171-178, 1996.

250. Begley BW, Engber WD: Proximal row carpectomy in advanced Kienbock's disease. J Hand Surg [Am] 19:1016-1018, 1994.

251. Weiss AP, Weiland AJ, Moore JR, et al: Radial shortening for Kienbock disease. J Bone Joint Surg Am 73:384-391, 1991.

252. Sundberg SB, Linscheid RL: Kienbock's disease. Results of treatment with ulnar lengthening. Clin Orthop 187:43-51, 1984.

253. Ingle DJ, Sebes JI, Salazar JE, et al: Early detection of Kienbock's disease with MRI treated by revascularization with a distal radius bone graft. Orthopedics 26:91-93, 2003.

254. Lichtman DM, Degnan GG: Staging and its use in the determination of treatment modalities for Kienbock's disease. Hand Clin 9:409-416, 1993.

255. Hashizume H, Asahara H, Nishida K, et al: Histopathology of Kienbock's disease. Correlation with magnetic resonance and other imaging techniques. J Hand Surg [Br] 21:89-93, 1996.

256. Trumble TE, Irving J: Histologic and magnetic resonance imaging correlations in Kienbock's disease. J Hand Surg [Am] 15:879-884, 1990.

257. Jackson MD, Barry DT, Geiringer SR: Magnetic resonance imaging of avascular necrosis of the lunate. Arch Phys Med Rehabil 71:510-513, 1990.

258. Viegas SF, Amparo E: Magnetic resonance imaging in the assessment of revascularization in Kienbock's disease. A preliminary report. Orthop Rev 18:1285-1288, 1989.

259. Sowa DT, Holder LE, Patt PG, et al: Application of magnetic resonance imaging to ischemic necrosis of the lunate. J Hand Surg [Am] 14:1008-1016, 1989.

260. Desser TS, McCarthy S, Trumble T: Scaphoid fractures and Kienbock's disese of the lunate: MR imaging with histopathologic correlation. Magn Reson Imaging 8:357-361, 1990.

261. Stuckey SL, Kalff V, Hoy G: Bone scan findings in Kienbock's disease. A case report with atypical findings and literature review. Clin Nucl Med 22:481-483, 1997.

262. Imaeda T, Nakamura R, Miura T, et al: Magnetic resonance imaging in Kienbock's disease. J Hand Surg [Br] 17:12-19, 1992.

263. Jafarnia K, Collins ED, Kohl HW III, et al: Reliability of the Lichtman classification of Kienbock's disease. J Hand Surg [Am] 25:529-534, 2000.

264. Tomczak R, Mergo P, Aschoff AJ, et al: MRI follow-up of pisiform bone transposition for treatment of lunatomalacia. Skeletal Radiol 27:26-29, 1998.

265. Arcalis Arce A, Pedemonte Jansana JP, Massons Albareda JM: Idiopathic necrosis of the capitate. Acta Orthop Belg 62:46-48, 1996.

266. Murakami S, Nakajima H: Aseptic necrosis of the capitate bone in two gymnasts. Am J Sports Med 12:170-173, 1984.

267. Yoshihara M, Sakai A, Toba N, et al: Nonunion of the isolated capitate waist fracture. J Orthop Sci 7:578-580, 2002.

268. Mullett H, Shannon F, Syed A, et al: Non-union of the capitate with associated triangular fibrocartilage tear. Arch Orthop Trauma Surg 121:362-363, 2001.

269. Spence LD, Savenor A, Nwachuku I, et al: MRI of fractures of the distal radius: comparison with conventional radiographs. Skeletal Radiol 27:244-249, 1998.

270. Melone CP Jr: Articular fractures of the distal radius. Orthop Clin North Am 15:217-236, 1984.

271. Freeland AE, Geissler WB: The arthroscopic management of intra-articular distal radius fractures. Hand Surg 5:93-102, 2000.

272. Baratz ME, Des Jardins J, Anderson DD, et al: Displaced intra-articular fractures of the distal radius: the effect of fracture displacement on contact stresses in a cadaver model. J Hand Surg [Am] 21:183-188, 1996.

273. Melone CP Jr: Distal radius fractures: patterns of articular fragmentation. Orthop Clin North Am 24:239-253, 1993.

274. Guha AR, Marynissen H: Stress fracture of the hook of the hamate. Br J Sports Med 36:224-225, 2002.

275. Geissler WB: Carpal fractures in athletes. Clin Sports Med 20:167-188, 2001.

276. Rettig ME, Dassa GL, Raskin KB, et al: Wrist fractures in the athlete. Distal radius and carpal fractures. Clin Sports Med 17:469-489, 1998.

277. Capelastegui A, Astigarraga E, Fernandez-Canton G, et al: Masses and pseudomasses of the hand and wrist: MR findings in 134 cases. Skeletal Radiol 28:498-507, 1999.

278. Zeiss J, Guilliam-Haidet L: MR demonstration of anomalous muscles about the volar aspect of the wrist and forearm. Clin Imaging 20:219-221, 1996.

279. Steiner E, Steinbach LS, Schnarkowski P, et al: Ganglia and cysts around joints. Radiol Clin North Am 34:395-425, xi-xii, 1996.

280. Miller TT, Potter HG, McCormack RR Jr: Benign soft tissue masses of the wrist and hand: MRI appearances. Skeletal Radiol 23:327-332, 1994.

281. Binkovitz LA, Berquist TH, McLeod RA: Masses of the hand and wrist: detection and characterization with MR imaging. Am J Roentgenol 154:323-326, 1990.

282. Sanders WE: The occult dorsal carpal ganglion. J Hand Surg [Br] 10:257-260, 1985.

283. Johnson J, Kilgore E, Newmeyer W: Tumorous lesions of the hand. J Hand Surg [Am] 10:284-286, 1985.

284. Nelson CL, Sawmiller S, Phalen GS: Ganglions of the wrist and hand. J Bone Joint Surg Am 54:1459-1464, 1972.

285. Feldman F, Singson RD, Staron RB: Magnetic resonance imaging of para-articular and ectopic ganglia. Skeletal Radiol 18:353-358, 1989.

286. Hollister AM, Sanders RA, McCann S: The use of MRI in the diagnosis of an occult wrist ganglion cyst. Orthop Rev 18:1210-1212, 1989.

287. Cardinal E, Buckwalter KA, Braunstein EM, et al: Occult dorsal carpal ganglion: comparison of US and MR imaging. Radiology 193:259-262, 1994.

288. Gunther SF: Dorsal wrist pain and the occult scapholunate ganglion. J Hand Surg [Am] 10:697-703, 1985.

289. el-Noueam KI, Schweitzer ME, Blasbalg R, et al: Is a subset of wrist ganglia the sequela of internal derangements of the wrist joint? MR imaging findings. Radiology 212:537-540, 1999.

290. Lowenstein J, Chandnani V, Tomaino MM: Fibrolipoma of the median nerve: a case report and review of the literature. Am J Orthop 29:797-798, 2000.

291. Meyer BU, Roricht S, Schmitt R: Bilateral fibrolipomatous hamartoma of the median nerve with macrocheiria and late-onset nerve entrapment syndrome. Muscle Nerve 21:656-658, 1998.

292. Walker CW, Adams BD, Barnes CL, et al: Case report 667. Fibrolipomatous hamartoma of the median nerve. Skeletal Radiol 20:237-239, 1991.

293. Ragoowansi R, Adeniran A, Moss AL: Anomalous muscle of the wrist. Clin Anat 15:363-365, 2002.

294. Pierre-Jerome C, Bekkelund SI, Husby G, et al: MRI of anatomical variants of the wrist in women. Surg Radiol Anat 18:37-41, 1996.

295. Coenen L, Biltjes I: Pseudotumor of the palm due to an anomalous flexor digitorum superficialis muscle belly. J Hand Surg [Am] 16:1046-1051, 1991.

296. Peh WC, Truong NP, Totty WG, et al: Pictorial review: magnetic resonance imaging of benign soft tissue masses of the hand and wrist. Clin Radiol 50:519-525, 1995.

297. Phalen GS, McCormack LJ, Gazale WJ: Giant-cell tumor of tendon sheath (benign synovioma) in the hand. Evaluation of 56 cases. Clin Orthop 15:140-151, 1959.

298. Jelinek JS, Kransdorf MJ, Shmookler BM, et al: Giant cell tumor of the tendon sheath: MR findings in nine cases. Am J Roentgenol 162:919-922, 1994.

299. Parrini M, Bergamaschi R, Azzoni R: Synovial hemangioma. Description of a case. Chir Organi Mov 87:249-253, 2002.

300. Greenspan A, Azouz EM, Matthews J II, et al: Synovial hemangioma: imaging features in eight histologically proven cases, review of the literature, and differential diagnosis. Skeletal Radiol 24:583-590, 1995.

301. Foley-Nolan D, Stack JP, Ryan M, et al: Magnetic resonance imaging in the assessment of rheumatoid arthritis—a comparison with plain film radiographs. Br J Rheumatol 30:101-106, 1991.

302. Stewart NR, McQueen FM, Crabbe JP: Magnetic resonance imaging of the wrist in early rheumatoid arthritis: a pictorial essay. Australas Radiol 45:268-273, 2001.

303. Meske S, Friedburg H, Hennig J, et al: Rheumatoid arthritis lesions of the wrist examined by rapid gradient-echo magnetic resonance imaging. Scand J Rheumatol 19:235-238, 1990.

304. Rubens DJ, Blebea JS, Totterman SM, et al: Rheumatoid arthritis: evaluation of wrist extensor tendons with clinical examination versus MR imaging—a preliminary report. Radiology 187:831-838, 1993.

305. Tan AL, Tanner SF, Conaghan PG, et al: Role of metacarpophalangeal joint anatomic factors in the distribution of synovitis and bone erosion in early rheumatoid arthritis. Arthritis Rheum 48:1214-1222, 2003.

306. Ostendorf B, Peters R, Dann P, et al: Magnetic resonance imaging and miniarthroscopy of metacarpophalangeal joints: sensitive detection of morphologic changes in rheumatoid arthritis. Arthritis Rheum 44:2492-2502, 2001.

307. Savnik A, Malmskov H, Thomsen HS, et al: Magnetic resonance imaging of the wrist and finger joints in patients with inflammatory joint diseases. J Rheumatol 28:2193-2200, 2001.

308. Bonel HM, Schneider P, Seemann MD, et al: MR imaging of the wrist in rheumatoid arthritis using gadobenate dimeglumine. Skeletal Radiol 30:15-24, 2001.

309. Sugimoto H, Takeda A, Hyodoh K: Early-stage rheumatoid arthritis: prospective study of the effectiveness of MR imaging for diagnosis. Radiology 216:569-575, 2000.

310. Klarlund M, Ostergaard M, Lorenzen I: Finger joint synovitis in rheumatoid arthritis: quantitative assessment by magnetic resonance imaging. Rheumatology (Oxford) 38:66-72, 1999.

311. Klarlund M, Ostergaard M, Gideon P, et al: Wrist and finger joint MR imaging in rheumatoid arthritis. Acta Radiol 40:400-409, 1999.

312. Lee J, Lee SK, Suh JS, et al: Magnetic resonance imaging of the wrist in defining remission of rheumatoid arthritis. J Rheumatol 24:1303-1308, 1997.

313. Jevtic V, Watt I, Rozman B, et al: Contrast enhanced Gd-DTPA magnetic resonance imaging in the evaluation of rheumatoid arthritis during a clinical trial with DMARDs. A prospective two-year follow-up study on hand joints in 31 patients. Clin Exp Rheumatol 15:151-156, 1997.

314. Nakahara N, Uetani M, Hayashi K, et al: Gadolinium-enhanced MR imaging of the wrist in rheumatoid arthritis: value of fat suppression pulse sequences. Skeletal Radiol 25:639-647, 1996.

315. Sugimoto H, Takeda A, Masuyama J, et al: Early-stage rheumatoid arthritis: diagnostic accuracy of MR imaging. Radiology 198:185-192, 1996.

316. Gubler FM, Algra PR, Maas M, et al: Gadolinium-DTPA enhanced magnetic resonance imaging of bone cysts in patients with rheumatoid arthritis. Ann Rheum Dis 52:716-719, 1993.

317. Yanagawa A, Takano K, Nishioka K, et al: Clinical staging and gadolinium-DTPA enhanced images of the wrist in rheumatoid arthritis. J Rheumatol 20:781-784, 1993.

318. Rominger MB, Bernreuter WK, Kenney PJ, et al: MR imaging of the hands in early rheumatoid arthritis: preliminary results. Radiographics 13:37-46, 1993.

319. Crues JV SF, Dardashti S, James TW, et al: Identification of wrist and meta-carpophalangeal joint erosions using a portable magnetic resonance imaging system compared to conventional radiographs. J Rheumatol 31:676-685, 2004.

320. Carpintero P, Serrano J, Garcia-Frasquet A: Pigmented villonodular synovitis of the wrist invading bone—a report of 2 cases. Acta Orthop Scand 71:424-426, 2000.

321. Schmitt R, Christopoulos G, Meier R, et al: [Direct MR arthrography of the wrist in comparison with arthroscopy: a prospective study on 125 patients]. Rofo Fortschr Geb Rontgenstr Neuen Bildgeb Verfahr 175:911-919, 2003.

322. Valeri G, Ferrara C, Ercolani P, et al: Tendon involvement in rheumatoid arthritis of the wrist: MRI findings. Skeletal Radiol 30:138-143, 2001.

323. Xarchas KC, Leviet D: Non rheumatoid closed rupture of extensor carpi ulnaris tendon. Report of a case in a professional athlete. Acta Orthop Belg 68:399-402, 2002.

324. Heim D: The skier's thumb. Acta Orthop Belg 65:440-446, 1999.

325. Plancher KD, Ho CP, Cofield SS, et al: Role of MR imaging in the management of "skier's thumb" injuries. Magn Reson Imaging Clin N Am 7:73-84, viii, 1999.

326. Engkvist O, Balkfors B, Lindsjo U: Thumb injuries in downhill skiing. Int J Sports Med 3:50-55, 1982.

327. Kaplan SJ: The Stener lesion revisited: a case report. J Hand Surg [Am] 23:833-836, 1998.

328. Haramati N, Hiller N, Dowdle J, et al: MRI of the Stener lesion. Skeletal Radiol 24:515-518, 1995.

329. Stener B: Skeletal injuries associated with rupture of the ulnar collateral ligament of the metacarpophalangeal joint of the thumb. A clinical and anatomical study. Acta Chir Scand 125:583-586, 1963.

330. Fairhurst M, Hansen L: Treatment of "Gamekeeper's Thumb" by reconstruction of the ulnar collateral ligament. J Hand Surg [Br] 27:542-545, 2002.

331. Melone CP Jr, Beldner S, Basuk RS: Thumb collateral ligament injuries. An anatomic basis for treatment. Hand Clin 16:345-357, 2000.

332. Salvi V: Rupture of the ulnar collateral ligament of the metacarpophalangeal joint of the thumb (Stener's lesion). Panminerva Med 10:159-163, 1968.

333. Kozin SH, Bishop AT: Gamekeeper's thumb. Early diagnosis and treatment. Orthop Rev 23:797-804, 1994.

334. Hintermann B, Holzach PJ, Schutz M, et al: Skier's thumb—the significance of bony injuries. Am J Sports Med 21:800-804, 1993.

335. Vasenius J, Nieminen O, Lohman M: Late reconstruction of the ulnar collateral ligament of the thumb MP joint with free tendon graft—A new technique. J Hand Surg [Am] 28 Suppl 1:44, 2003.

336. Engel J, Ganel A, Ditzian R, et al: Arthrography as a method of diagnosing tear of the ulnar collateral ligament of the metacarpophalangeal joint of the thumb ("gamekeeper's thumb"). J Trauma 19:106-109, 1979.

337. Bowers WH, Hurst LC: Gamekeeper's thumb. Evaluation by arthrography and stress roentgenography. J Bone Joint Surg Am 59:519-524, 1977.

338. Resnick D, Danzig LA: Arthrographic evaluation of injuries of the first metacarpophalangeal joint: gamekeeper's thumb. Am J Roentgenol 126:1046-1052, 1976.

339. Romano WM, Garvin G, Bhayana D, et al: The spectrum of ulnar collateral ligament injuries as viewed on magnetic resonance imaging of the metacarpophalangeal joint of the thumb. Can Assoc Radiol J 54:243-248, 2003.

340. Lohman M, Vasenius J, Kivisaari A, et al: MR imaging in chronic rupture of the ulnar collateral ligament of the thumb. Acta Radiol 42:10-14, 2001.

341. Ahn JM, Sartoris DJ, Kang HS, et al: Gamekeeper thumb: comparison of MR arthrography with conventional arthrography and MR imaging in cadavers. Radiology 206:737-744, 1998.

342. Hinke DH, Erickson SJ, Chamoy L, et al: Ulnar collateral ligament of the thumb: MR findings in cadavers, volunteers, and patients with ligamentous injury (gamekeeper's thumb). Am J Roentgenol 163:1431-1434, 1994.

343. Howse C: Wrist injuries in sport. Sports Med 17:163-175, 1994.

344. Taylor LM Jr: Hypothenar hammer syndrome. J Vasc Surg 37:697, 2003.

345. Lorelli DR, Shepard AD: Hypothenar hammer syndrome: an uncommon and correctable cause of digital ischemia. J Cardiovasc Surg (Torino) 43:83-85, 2002.

346. Noel B, Hayoz D: A tennis player with hand claudication. Vasa 29:151-153, 2000.

347. Liskutin J, Dorffner R, Resinger M, et al: Hypothenar hammer syndrome. Eur Radiol 10:542, 2000.

348. Nakamura T, Kambayashi J, Kawasaki T, et al: Hypothenar hammer syndrome caused by playing tennis. Eur J Vasc Endovasc Surg 11:240-242, 1996.

349. Muller LP, Rudig L, Kreitner KF, et al: Hypothenar hammer syndrome in sports. Knee Surg Sports Traumatol Arthrosc 4:167-170, 1996.

350. Winterer JT, Ghanem N, Roth M, et al: Diagnosis of the hypothenar hammer syndrome by high-resolution contrast-enhanced MR angiography. Eur Radiol 12:2457-2462, 2002.

102

HIP

John D. Reeder

INTRODUCTION

From a clinical perspective, hip pain and functional impairment often represent a diagnostic challenge, as the patient's symptoms may arise from pathology affecting the hip joint, the proximal thigh, the pelvis, the sacrum, or even the lumbar spine through a radicular referral of pain. History and physical examination remain limited in localizing the anatomic origin and in differentiating the osseous, muscular, and synovial components of an injury or an inflammatory process. Determining the site and nature of the abnormality responsible for the patient's symptoms is critical in directing appropriate management and in assessing prognosis for functional recovery. Diagnostic imaging techniques have established an essential role in the evaluation of patients with hip pain.

For the acutely injured patient, conventional radiography maintains relevance in detecting and characterizing fractures and dislocations. However, subcapital femoral neck fractures often remain radiographically occult and nondisplaced fractures of the pelvis can be notoriously subtle. Conventional radiography offers limited information concerning soft-tissue injury. Computed tomographic (CT) studies assist in the detection of cortical disruption and periosteal reaction in cases of osseous neoplasm and infection. CT is also useful in assessing fracture complexity and alignment and in evaluating congenital abnormalities of the hip. Ultrasound has established an important role in detecting congenital hip dislocation but otherwise remains limited in evaluating hip pain in adults. Nuclear medicine, as a physiologic test, offers sensitivity is detecting heightened osseous metabolic activity but remains relatively nonspecific as to the cause and is insensitive to most soft-tissue pathology. MRI provides a uniquely comprehensive assessment of bone and soft-tissue abnormalities in patients with hip pain, identifying the anatomic site and tissue complexity of the pathology. Recognition of abnormal signal intensity patterns involving bone and soft-tissue promotes accurate diagnosis of osteonecrosis, stress injury, acute traumatic injury, neoplasm, and arthropathy.

NORMAL ANATOMY

The hyaline cartilage-covered femoral head and acetabulum form a ball-and-socket joint, reinforced by the fibrocartilaginous acetabular labrum and joint capsule. The iliofemoral, pubofemoral, and ischiofemoral ligaments represent thickened portions of the capsule. The transverse acetabular ligament bridges the acetabular notch and connects the antero- and postero-inferior margins of the fibrocartilaginous acetabular labrum. The labrum deepens the anterior, posterior, and superior aspects of the osseous acetabular fossa. The ligamentum teres, with its associated vasculature, extends across the hip joint to attach to the central fovea of the femoral head. Bursae located adjacent to the hip joint include the trochanteric bursal complex, related to the greater trochanter and the insertions of the gluteus minimus and gluteus medius tendons, the iliopsoas bursa, related to the iliopsoas muscle-tendon complex and communicating with the anterior aspect of the hip joint in approximately 15% of patients, and the obturator externus bursa, related to the obturator externus muscle and communicating with the inferior aspect of the hip joint.

The large muscle groups surrounding the hip joint contribute to its stability. In the athlete, pelvic and proximal femoral sites of musculotendinous attachment are susceptible to stress injury. Therefore, knowledge of the specific origins and insertions of the muscles responsible for hip movement, strength, and stability contributes to the accurate interpretation of MRI studies in the context of sports medicine and athletic injury.

The hip flexors include the iliopsoas, the sartorius, the tensor fascia lata, and the rectus femoris muscles. The iliopsoas, typically the strongest of the flexors, arises from the junction of the iliacus muscle, deep to the iliac bone, and the psoas muscle, which occupies a paraspinal position. The muscle inserts upon the lesser trochanter of the proximal femur. The sartorius arises from the anterior superior iliac spine and inserts with the pes anserine tendon group upon the proximal medial tibia. The tensor fascia lata originates from the anterior lateral aspect of the iliac crest and inserts upon the tubercle of Gerdy at the anterior lateral margin of the lateral tibial plateau. The rectus femoris tendon arises from the anterior inferior iliac spine and, distally, represents the anterior component of the quadriceps tendon.

The hip extensors are primarily comprised of the hamstring muscle group and the gluteus maximus. The hamstrings include the semimembranosus, which arises from the lateral aspect of the ischium, proximal to the ischial tuberosity, and the semitendinosus and biceps femoris will originate from the ischial tuberosity. The semimembranosus inserts upon the posterior medial aspect of the medial tibial plateau and the semitendinosus inserts with the pes anserine group on the proximal medial tibia. The biceps femoris tendon joins the fibular collateral ligament to attach to the fibular head. Although the gluteus maximus is also considered a hip extensor, in comparison to the hamstrings, it contributes considerably less to hip movement. It originates from the posterior ilium and inserts on the iliotibial band.

Abductors of the hip include the gluteus medius and minimus, which originate from the ilium and insert upon the greater trochanter. The gluteal muscles also contribute to external rotation of the hip. Other external rotators include the piriformis, the obturator externus and internus, the superior and inferior gemelli muscles, and the quadratus femoris. The piriformis extends from the sacrum and adjacent sciatic notch to the greater trochanter. The obturator muscles arise from the ischiopubic rami. The obturator externus inserts upon the trochlear fossa of the superior lateral aspect of the femoral neck and the obturator internus inserts on the greater trochanter. The gemelli originate from the ischium and insert on the greater trochanter. The quadratus femoris arises from the ischial tuberosity and inserts upon the quadrate line of the femur. Adductors of

the hip include the adductor magnus, longus, and brevis, the pectineus, and the gracilis. The adductor group arises from the inferior pubic ramus and attaches distally to the linea aspira of the femur. The pectineus originates from the pubis and inserts on the proximal femur. The gracilis arises from the parasymphyseal region and attaches to the medial aspect of the proximal tibia with the other pes anserine tendons.

MRI TECHNIQUE

A typical imaging protocol, applied to the evaluation of hip pathology, includes axial and coronal T1-weighted and fast spin-echo, fat-saturated T2-weighted acquisitions. If field strength limitations preclude spectral fat suppression, short tau inversion recovery (STIR) sequences may be substituted. Either fat-saturated T2-weighted or STIR imaging is critical in detecting the subtle marrow edema associated with acute trauma and stress-related injury, and in identifying intramuscular edema associated with strain or contusion. With coronal imaging, the symphysis pubis and the sacrum should be included within the imaging field of view, as pathology involving these sites may, clinically, present as hip pain. Sagittal T2-weighted imaging is helpful in determining the extent of femoral head pathology and in assessing anterior and posterior acetabular labral integrity. Three-dimensional (3D) gradient-echo acquisitions have also been applied to labral and articular cartilage evaluation. Direct MRI arthrography with T1-weighted fat-saturated images obtained following the intra-articular administration of gadolinium contrast improves sensitivity in identifying acetabular labral tears and chondral defects involving the articular surfaces. Indirect arthrography, using fat-saturated T1-weighted imaging following the intravenous administration of gadolinium contrast, also improves recognition of labral and articular cartilage pathology.

FEMORAL HEAD PATHOLOGY

Osteonecrosis

Impairment of arterial blood flow represents the common pathophysiologic pathway in the development of femoral head osteonecrosis. The arterial vasculature of the femoral head is supplied from medial circumflex branches that enter the proximal femoral neck and traverse the proximal femoral growth plate to the femoral head. Traumatic interruption of arterial supply of the femoral head secondary to fracture has been implicated as a cause of femoral head ischemia. Nontraumatic risk factors are more frequently associated with femoral head osteonecrosis and the etiologic mechanisms are more complex.[1] Diminished blood flow occurs with vasculitis, chronic renal failure, and diabetes. Vascular occlusion is also observed with hemoglobinopathy, particularly sickle cell disease, with fat embolism, and with nitrogen embolism associated with dysbaric states. Diseases that result in increased intramedullary pressure, venous congestion, and secondary arterial compromise are also implicated in the development of femoral head osteonecrosis. Steroid administration, a common antecedent exposure associated with osteonecrosis, increases fat content of the femoral head, resulting in sinusoidal compression, impaired venous drainage, and a back-pressure–related decrease in arterial flow.[2,3] An increase in osteocyte fat may also represent a primary cause of cell death.[4] Steroids also inhibit angiogenesis, a factor that may further impact the development and extent of femoral head osteonecrosis.[5] Other conditions that may result in osteonecrosis through the mechanism of elevated intramedullary pressure include Gaucher disease, Fabry disease, Cushing disease, and marrow proliferative disorders. Arthropathies associated with hip joint effusions may also result in increased intraosseous pressure. Additional risk factors for the development of osteonecrosis include alcoholism, chronic pancreatitis, pregnancy, inflammatory bowel disease, and burns. Approximately 90% of osteonecrosis cases are related to either steroid administration or alcoholism.[1]

Regardless of the specific pathophysiologic mechanism, the common endpoint is subchondral bone death. Hemopoietic cells are most sensitive to ischemia, with cell death occurring within 6 to 12 hours. Osteocytes, osteoclasts, and osteoblasts may survive up to 48 hours. Marrow fat cells are more resistant, succumbing in 2 to 5 days.[6] The reparative phase of osteonecrosis begins at the peripheral margin between normal and abnormal bone with increased blood flow and osseous resorption. Structural weakening may result in microfractures and osseous collapse. Eventually, reactive sclerosis and chronic fibrovascular proliferation develop.[1,7] Initially, articular cartilage integrity is preserved because of its dependence on synovial fluid rather than femoral head vascularity for nutritional support. However, if femoral head collapse occurs, altered joint mechanics can result in articular cartilage fracture and chondromalacia. Approximately 10% of total hip replacements are performed because of osteoarthritis secondary to osteonecrosis of the femoral head.[8]

The Ficat classification system describes four stages of femoral head osteonecrosis, based on the conventional radiographic findings observed in patients with hip pain and biopsy-confirmed osteonecrosis.[9] In stage I disease, the radiographic appearance of the hip is normal. In stage II osteonecrosis, subtle sclerosis, cyst formation, and/or osteopenia become present, indicative of osseous reaction and repair adjacent to the region of bone necrosis. In patients with stage III pathology, findings correspond with subchondral osseous collapse with flattening of the femoral head. The crescent sign, linear subchondral lucency, reflects early subchondral osseous collapse. In stage IV disease, secondary osteoarthritis is evident with periarticular reactive cyst formation and fibrovascular reaction, marginal hypertrophic osteophyte formation, and joint narrowing. Steinberg et al[10] subsequently modified this classification system, describing stage III as subchondral osseous collapse with flattening (crescent sign), stage IV as flattening of the femoral head,

stage V as joint narrowing with or without acetabular involvement, and stage VI as advanced hypertrophic arthopathy and chondromalacia. They also considered the extent of femoral head pathology with mild involvement classified as less than 15% of the articular surface, moderate involvement representing 15% to 30%, and severe involvement indicating greater than 30%.[10] With the advent of MRI, the classification system was further modified to include a stage 0, representing asymptomatic patients with normal radiographs and a positive MRI examination.

MRI findings in femoral head osteonecrosis reflect the cellular and extracellular events which characterize the process of ischemic bone necrosis and secondary osseous reaction. Recognition of the patterns of marrow signal alteration observed in femoral head osteonecrosis permits early and accurate diagnosis and appropriate therapeutic intervention.[11-15] Clinical management options include protected weight bearing, core decompression, and rotational osteotomy. In cases of Ficat stage IV osteonecrosis with advanced osteoarthritis, total hip replacement may be offered. In greater than 50% of cases of femoral head osteonecrosis, the process is bilateral and MRI provides a sensitive means to determine if both femoral heads are involved, even if the process remains clinically occult. Extent of femoral head involvement, as demonstrated on MRI studies, may suggest the relative likelihood of eventual loss of femoral head structural integrity. In one study, a preoperative MRI examination was performed on patients undergoing core decompression for osteonecrosis.[16] The group was evaluated for subsequent femoral head collapse at a mean time interval of 23 months. If the initial MRI study demonstrated 0% to 25% involvement of the weight-bearing surface of the femoral head, no subsequent osseous collapse occurred. In cases with 25% to 50% involvement, collapse was observed in 43%, and in patients with greater than 50% involvement, follow-up revealed osseous collapse in 87%.

The specific MRI signal intensity patterns identified in patients with femoral head osteonecrosis have been grouped into four categories.[17] Most commonly, the necrotic zone remains relatively isointense with normal bone marrow but a well-demarcated rim defines the border between normal and pathologic marrow. This reactive margin represents the "double-line sign," which, on T2-weighted images, exhibits a high signal intensity inner component corresponding with fibrovascular proliferation and granulation tissue and an outer low signal intensity component corresponding histologically with fibrosis and osseous sclerosis (Fig. 102-1).[18,19] In the frequency-encoding plane, chemical shift artifact may exaggerate the two zones. A second pattern reflects the presence of subacute marrow hemorrhage with increased marrow signal intensity identified on both T1-and T2-weighted images. With a third MRI pattern, the necrotic bone appears decreased in signal intensity on T1-weighted images and increased on T2-weighted images, exhibiting features characteristic of fluid or edema (Fig. 102-2). A fourth category corresponds with marrow fibrosis and sclerosis with the necrotic zone demonstrating decreased signal intensity on both T1- and

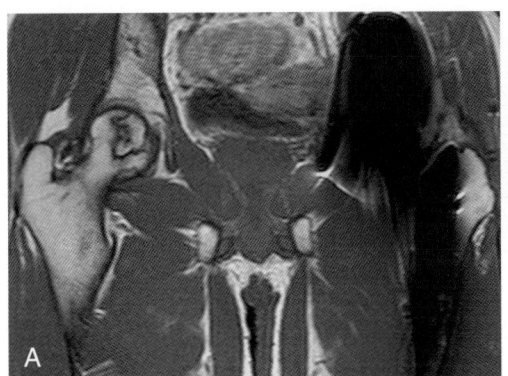

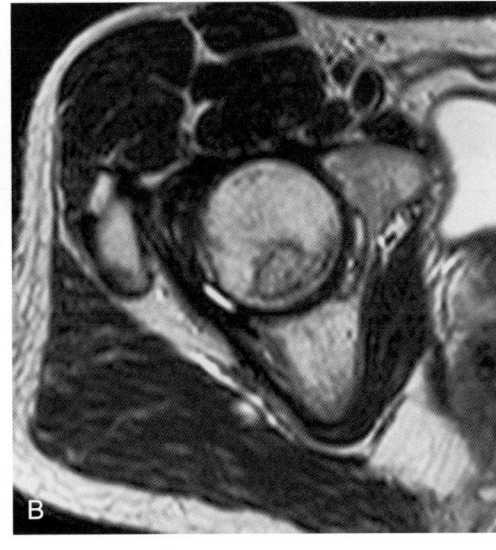

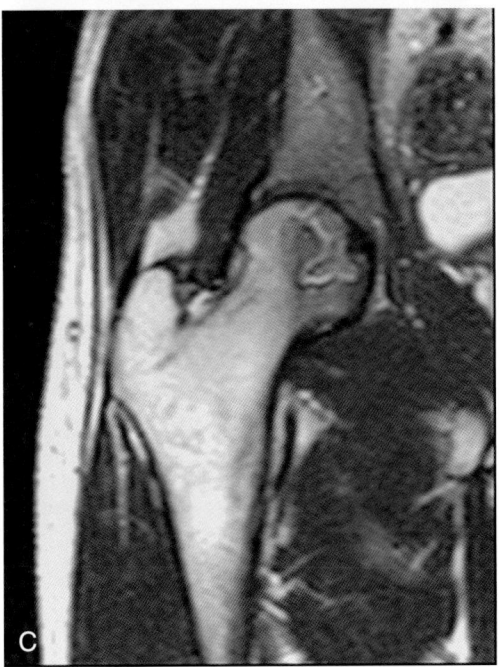

FIGURE 102-1

Osteonecrosis of the right hip in a 35-year-old male. A left hip replacement was performed because of advanced osteonecrosis and secondary osteoarthritis. **A,** Coronal T1-weighted image. A well-defined reactive rim surrounds a zone of osteonecrosis that appears isointense with normal fatty marrow. **B,** Axial T2-weighted image. The region of femoral head osteonecrosis remains relatively isointense with normal marrow. **C,** Coronal fat-saturated T2-weighted image. The double line sign represents an inner hyperintense component, corresponding with hypervascular granulation tissue and fibrovascular proliferation, and an outer, hypointense, fibrotic band.

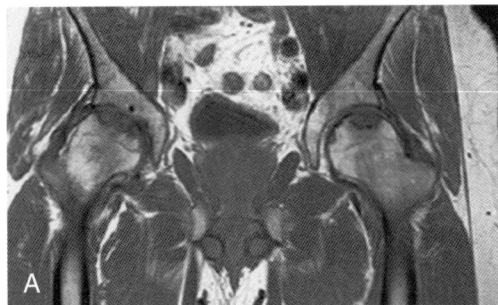

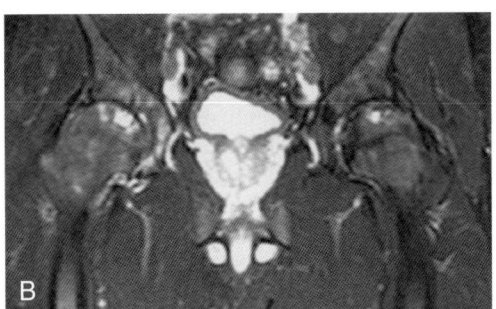

FIGURE 102-2

Bilateral femoral head osteonecrosis, exhibiting a pattern characterized by replacement of subchondral marrow by fluid or cyst formation. **A,** Coronal T1-weighted image. The foci of osteonecrosis are decreased in signal intensity relative to normal marrow. **B,** Coronal, fat-saturated T2-weighted image. The necrotic marrow becomes markedly hyperintense relative to normal marrow, indicative of subchondral fluid accumulation or cyst formation.

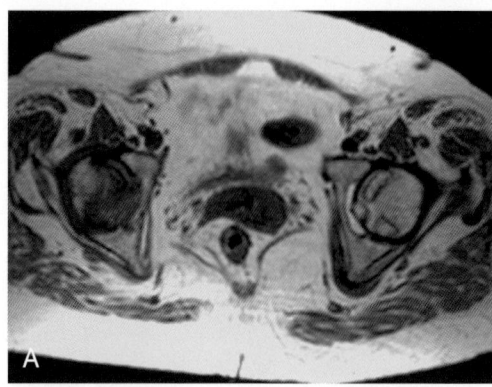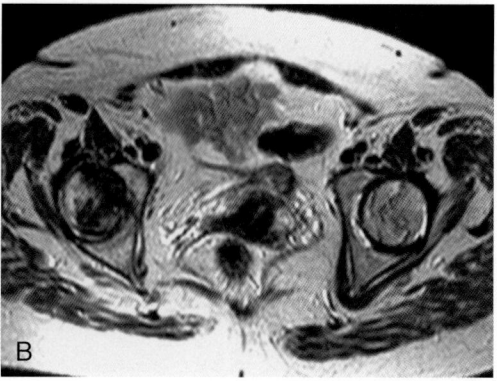

FIGURE 102-3

Osteonecrosis of both hips in a 61-year-old female. **A,** Axial T1-weighted image. On the right, osteonecrosis manifests a hypointense signal pattern, whereas on the left, the regions of osteonecrosis remain isointense with normal marrow. **B,** Axial T2-weighted image. The pattern of osteonecrosis involving the right hip continues to exhibit decreased signal intensity, compatible with marrow sclerosis and fibrosis. On the left, the femoral head osteonecrosis again appears isointense with normal fat, similar to the findings illustrated in Figure 102-1.

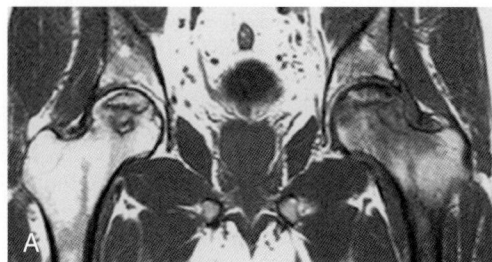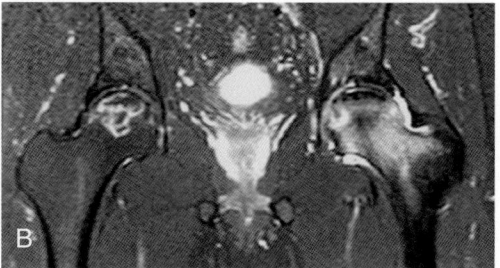

FIGURE 102-4

Bilateral osteonecrosis with unilateral bone marrow edema. **A,** Coronal T1-weighted image. Conspicuous foci of osteonecrosis involve both femoral heads but on the left a diffuse pattern of adjacent decreased marrow signal intensity extends into the femoral neck. **B,** Coronal fat-saturated T2-weighted image. The diffuse signal abnormality involving the left femoral neck becomes markedly hyperintense relative to normal marrow, consistent with reactive marrow edema. The patient was only symptomatic on the left. Identification of marrow edema in association with osteonecrosis often correlates with the presence of hip pain and may portend an increased likelihood of eventual osseous collapse.

T2-weighted imaging (Fig. 102-3). In many instances, a combination of these categories is identified with a necrotic zone exhibiting foci which remain isointense with marrow fat, regions of cyst formation, and hypointense fibrotic components. Additionally, the pattern of osteonecrosis, identified in a specific patient with MRI, may change over time, reflecting the evolving histopathology of osseous ischemia and subsequent reaction and/or relating to marrow changes associated with surgical intervention.

Additional findings identified on MRI in patients with femoral head osteonecrosis include hip joint effusion and the presence of a diffuse bone marrow edema pattern adjacent to the focal subchondral lesion. The identification of marrow edema extending to a variable extent from the femoral head to the intertrochanteric level of the proximal femur often correlates with the severity of the patients symptoms, especially hip pain (Fig. 102-4).[20] In one study, proximal femurs exhibiting the diffuse bone marrow edema pattern in association with focal subchondral necrosis were more likely to experience osseous collapse and progression to an advanced stage of osteonecrosis (Fig. 102-5).[21] The marrow edema pattern probably reflects a multifactorial process involving hyperemia with increased capillary permeability, vascular congestion, inflammatory cellular infiltration, and edema associated with stress-related microfractures related to bone resorption and altered weight-bearing mechanics. In some cases, the marrow edema pattern is considerably more conspicuous than the subchondral necrotic component and the appearance may mimic the pattern of marrow signal alteration observed in patients with transient osteoporosis (Fig. 102-6).

approximate
pain associz
ache, exace
rapid onset.
pain is typi
bearing and

On MRI
edema deve
focal subch
indicative o
from the su
102-8). The
conspicuou
patients wi
marrow ed
femoral he
osteoporos
may develc
mimic the
osteonecro:
patterns ma
osteonecro
head corres
the site, w
increased p
gadolinium
ing femor:
Following
tration, an
images cha
emic react
marrow m;
normal ma

Some a
porosis m
osteonecro
diffuse bc
proximal f
follow-up
healing or
necrosis (F

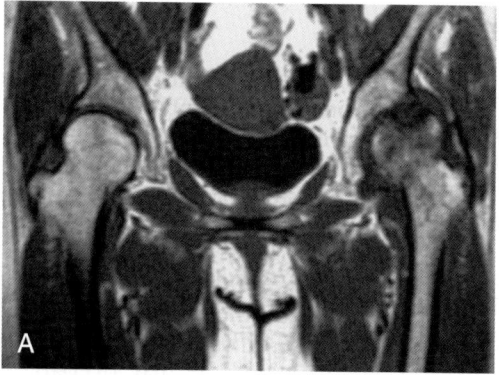
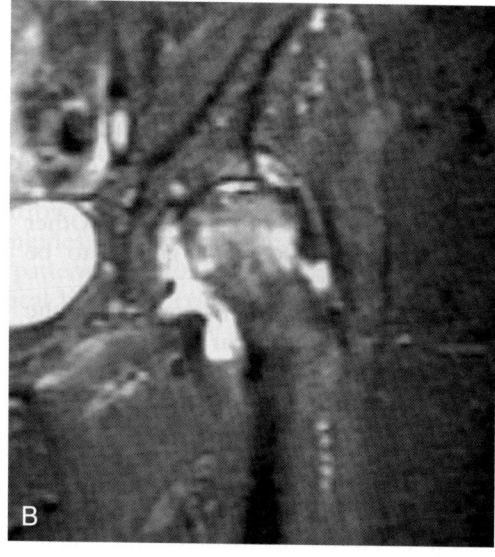

FIGURE 102-5

Osteonecrosis of the left hip with subchondral osseous collapse and osteoarthritis. **A,** Coronal T1-weighted image. Decreased marrow signal intensity is identified within the superior lateral aspect of the left femoral head and the adjacent lateral aspect of the acetabulum. Lateral subluxation of the femoral head is also present. **B,** Coronal fat-saturated T2-weighted image. Flattening of the articular surface of the superior lateral portion of the left femoral head is evident, indicative of subchondral osseous collapse. Increased marrow signal intensity involving the lateral acetabulum and the proximal femur is observed, which is compatible with reactive edema and fibrovascular proliferation. A large left hip joint effusion is also present.

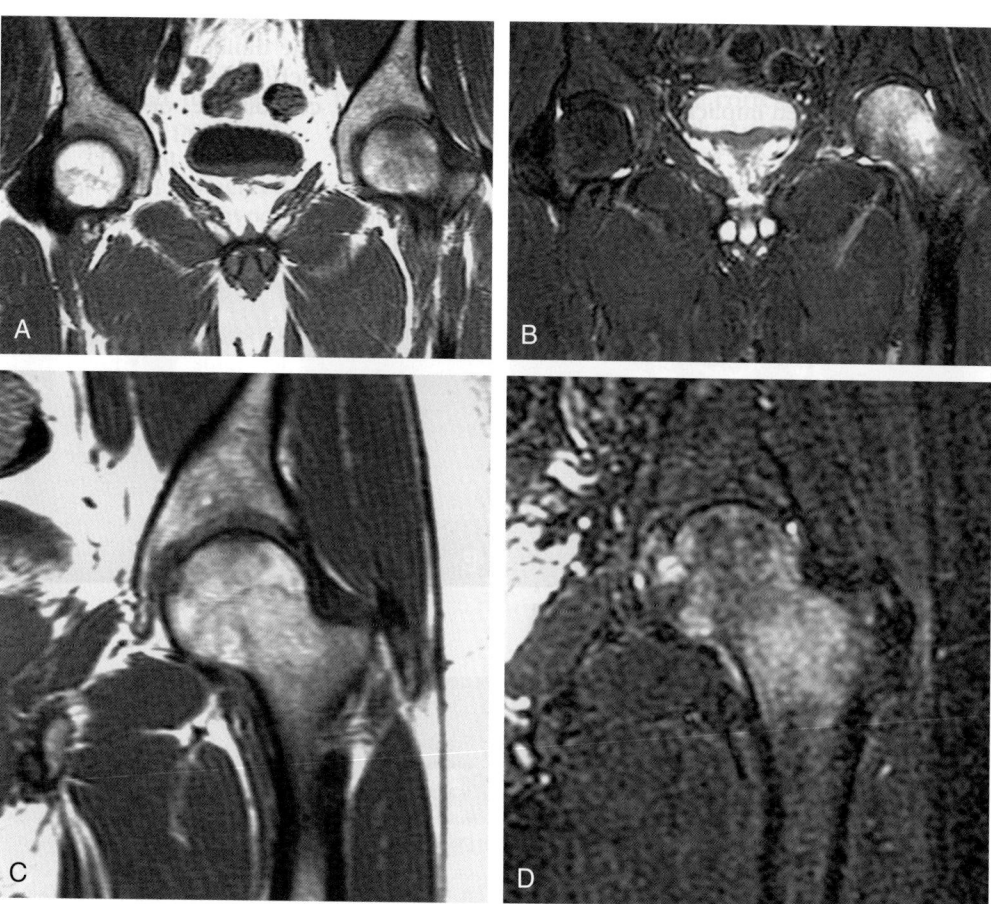

FIGURE 102-6

Osteonecrosis of the left hip with bone marrow edema and follow-up MRI. **A,** Coronal T1-weighted image. A region of decreased subchondral marrow signal intensity involves the anterior aspect of the left femoral head. **B,** Coronal fat-saturated T2-weighted image. The extensive reactive marrow edema pattern involving the left femoral head and neck represents a considerably more conspicuous finding than the focal region of subchondral osteonecrosis. **C,** Coronal T1-weighted image obtained 2 months later. A small but now sharply-marginated zone of subchondral osteonecrosis is identified within the superior segment of the left femoral head. **D,** Coronal fat-saturated T2-weighted follow-up image. The reactive marrow edema has decreased since the initial study.

Trans

Transie
typical
the thi
is invo
than p
associa
Con
affecte
scans,
tified.
extend
ing ma
weight
T2-wei
hip joi
When
but os
radiog
proces
Tra
reflex
With p
the fe
resulti
the pr

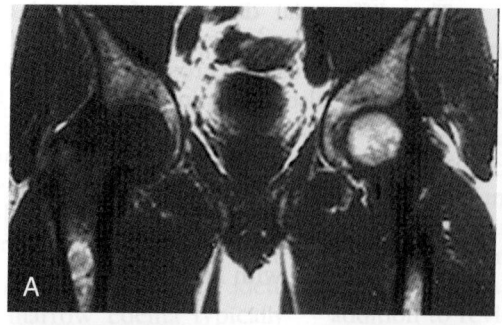

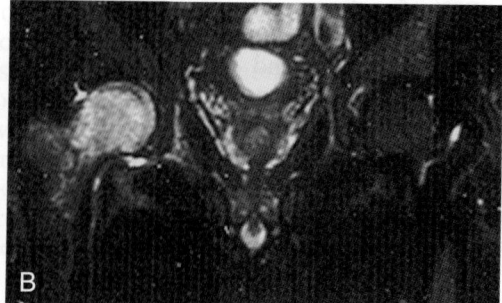

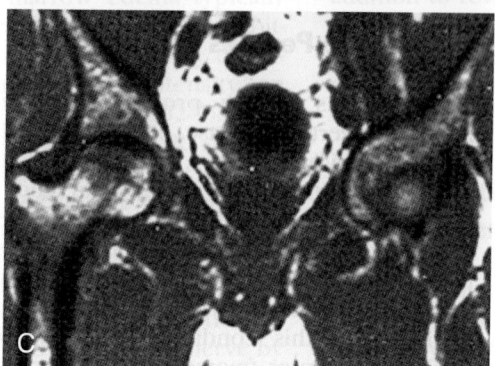

FIGURE 102-9

Osteonecrosis of the right hip with MRI follow-up. **A,** Coronal T1-weighted image. A diffuse decrease in marrow signal intensity involves the right femoral head and neck and differentiation of osteonecrosis and reactive edema is difficult. **B,** Coronal fat-saturated T2-weighted image. In addition to the diffuse hyperintense edema pattern, a linear subchondral hypointense lesion is observed, equivalent to the radiographic crescent sign. **C,** Coronal T1-weighted image obtained 2 months later. The diffusely abnormal signal intensity pattern has decreased, indicative of resolving edema, and a focal subchondral osteonecrotic lesion involving the superior lateral aspect of the femoral head is now more apparent.

only the anterior portion of the epiphysis is involved and no collapse is identified. In group II, partial collapse of the epiphyseal ossification center is identified with formation of a subchondral fissure. Focal metaphyseal reaction is noted. In group III, extensive epiphyseal and diffuse metaphyseal involvement is present. In group IV, the entire epiphysis is abnormal with pronounced collapse and diffuse metaphyseal reaction. In general, the prognosis is better for groups I and II.

Conventional radiographic findings described in the detection and staging of Legg-Calvé-Perthes disease include an asymmetric decrease in size and/or lateral displacement of the affected femoral head ossification center and development of a linear radiolucency involving the epiphyseal ossification indicative of early structural failure and fracture. In older children and in more advanced stages, flattening of the femoral head, widening and shortening of the femoral neck, and lateral subluxation of the femoral head are observed.

With MRI, earlier detection of Legg-Calvé-Perthes disease is possible as internal epiphyseal ossification signal intensity changes precede radiographically-apparent findings. On T1-weighted images, the epiphyseal marrow becomes decreased in signal intensity. The T2-weighted imaging appearance demonstrates more variability but decreased signal intensity is often identified (Fig. 102-11A and B). Whereas the epiphyseal changes are typically more conspicuous on the T1-weighted imaging series, the secondary findings (including hip joint effusion and metaphyseal reaction with cyst formation, marrow edema, and fibrovascular proliferation) are better appreciated on the fat-saturated

T2-weighted or STIR acquisitions. Physeal abnormalities, especially bridging of the growth plate, identified on MRI studies are associated with subsequent growth arrest.[34] In patients with Legg-Calvé-Perthes disease, a phase of transient synovitis may precede the development of recognizable epiphyseal pathology.[35] Therefore, when an isolated hip joint effusion is detected on MRI in a child aged 4 to 9 years with hip pain, performing a follow-up MRI study may be advisable, especially if hip

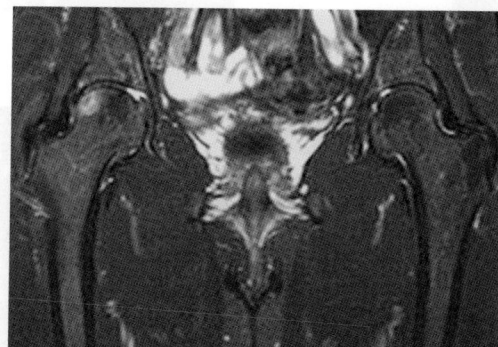

FIGURE 102-10

Femoral head bone bruise. Coronal fat-saturated T2-weighted image. The patient experienced right hip pain after a fall and the MRI study reveals bone marrow edema involving the superior lateral aspect of the right femoral head and the adjacent lateral aspect of the right acetabulum. A subsequent MRI examination revealed partial resolution of the signal abnormality, compatible with a healing bone bruise.

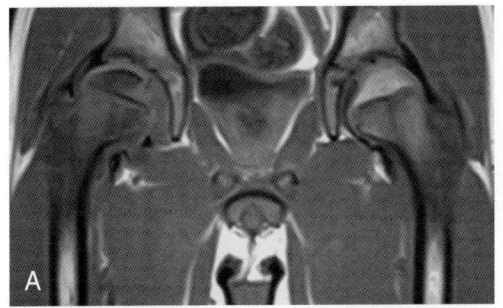
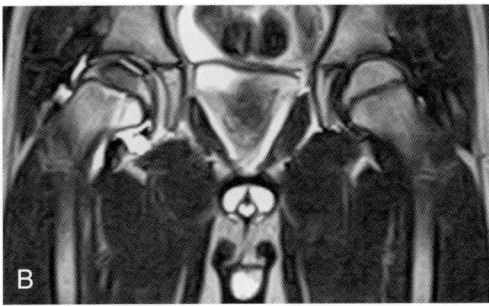
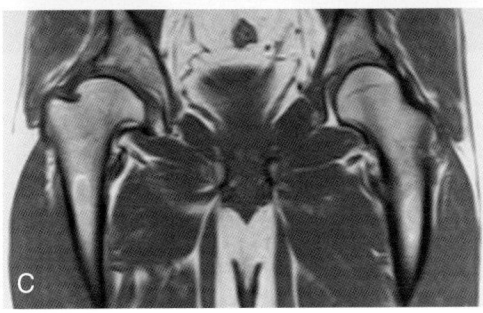

FIGURE 102-11

Legg-Calvé-Perthes disease in a 10-year-old male. **A,** Coronal T1-weighted image. Decreased marrow signal intensity involves the central portion of the right femoral head epiphyseal ossification center and the medial aspect of the proximal right femoral metaphysis. **B,** Coronal T2-weighted image. A central zone of decreased marrow signal intensity is identified within the right femoral head ossification center with evidence of adjacent reactive, hyperintense marrow edema. Reactive marrow changes also involve the medial aspect of the proximal right femoral metaphysis and an effusion is present. **C,** Coronal T1-weighted image in a 48-year-old male with a history of Legg-Calvé-Perthes on the right as a child. Flattening of the femoral head and shortening of the femoral neck are associated with slight lateral subluxation of the femoral head and widening of the acetabulum.

pain persists for 4 to 6 weeks. As with femoral head osteonecrosis in adults, diminished or absent femoral head enhancement following the intravenous administration of gadolinium contrast has been reported in patients with Legg-Calvé-Perthes disease.[36] In later stages of the disease, MRI may reveal compression and fracture of the ossification center, lateral displacement of the ossification center, and metaphyseal reaction. When flattening of the femoral head and shortening of the femoral neck exist, MRI contributes to the assessment of acetabulum-femoral head congruence and containment (Fig. 102-11C).[37] Performing MRI in both neutral position and with hip abduction has been recommended to detect hinge abduction, an abnormal alignment configuration elicited by hip abduction that represents a contraindication to standard treatment approaches.[38]

Treatment of Legg-Calvé-Perthes disease focuses on maintaining hip joint alignment, permitting normal hip movement and structurally-appropriate transmission of loading forces. Application of an external brace or cast and rotational osteotomy represent management approaches to achieve this purpose.

Slipped Capital Femoral Epiphysis

Posteroinferomedial slippage of the femoral head epiphysis occurs in children and adolescents aged 8 to 17 years. Girls are typically affected at a younger age than boys. Boys are slightly more often affected than girls. Approximately 20% to 37% of cases involve both hips.

Patients present with hip or groin pain and limp. Associated risk factors include trauma with Salter I fracture, obesity, and the adolescent growth spurt, particularly when associated with increased physical activity involving repetitive abduction and external rotation of the hip.[39] Premature growth plate fusion and resultant shortening of the femoral neck, femoral head osteonecrosis, and accelerated osteoarthritis represent sequelae of slipped capital femoral epiphysis.[40,41] Treatment options include open reduction and internal fixation and epiphysiodisis with bone graft placement.

MRI findings identified in patients with slipped capital femoral epiphysis include asymmetric widening of the growth plate and reactive marrow edema involving the adjacent epiphyseal and metaphyseal marrow. The physeal widening can be appreciated on T1- and T2-weighted imaging series (Fig. 102-12). Increased marrow signal intensity indicative of edema and fibrovascular proliferation involving the epiphysis and metaphysis is most conspicuous on STIR and fat-saturated T2-weighted images. With multiplanar MRI, the direction and extent of slippage can be accurately characterized and, if present, secondary femoral head osteonecrosis can be detected.

FRACTURES AND STRESS INJURIES

Nondisplaced fractures of the proximal femur are a relatively common traumatic injury in elderly patients experiencing a fall. Radiographic findings are often

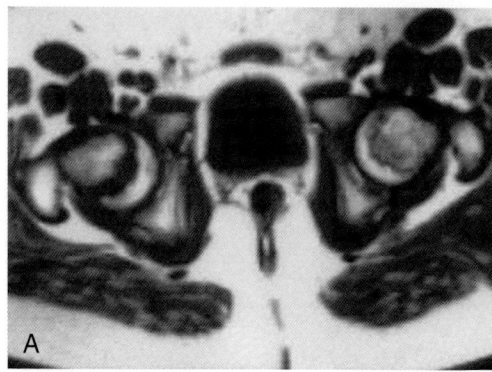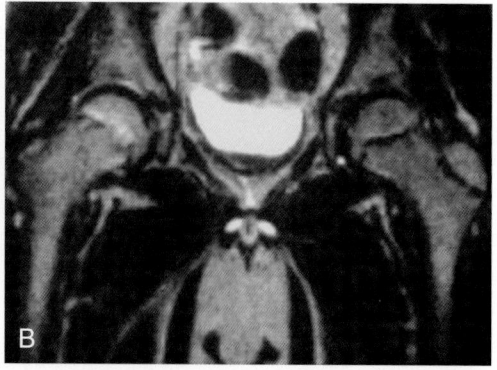

FIGURE 102-12

Slipped capital femoral epiphysis of the right hip in a 10-year-old overweight male. **A,** Axial T1-weighted image. Widening of the right proximal femoral physis is identified and posterior displacement of the right femoral head epiphysis is present. **B,** Coronal T2-weighted image. Minimal medial slippage of the right femoral head epiphysis is noted and a hyperintense reactive zone is observed adjacent to the physis.

subtle and subcapital fractures, in particular, may remain initially undetectable on conventional radiographs (Fig. 102-13). If appropriate clinical management is not instituted, the fracture may displace with weight bearing, complicating subsequent treatment, diminishing the prognosis for a favorable outcome, and increasing the likelihood of sequelae which negatively impact outcome, including osteonecrosis.[42]

MRI facilitates the prompt diagnosis of proximal femoral fractures with the marrow edema which accompanies the fracture appearing conspicuously hyperintense on STIR and fat-saturated T2-weighted imaging series, providing excellent contrast with the suppressed fat of normal marrow. On T1- and T2-weighted images, the fracture exhibits a linear low signal intensity pattern (Fig. 102-14).[43]

Osseous stress injuries develop when the elastic resistance of bone is exceeded by forces of repetitive compression, distraction, and/or rotation.[44] In response to stress, osteoclastic and osteoblastic remodeling of bone occurs. If bone resorption surpasses bone replacement because of excessive physical stress or because of metabolic insufficiency, osseous structural integrity becomes compromised. Microtrabecular fractures and adjacent marrow edema and hemorrhage characterize early stress injury. As the microtrabecular injuries accumulate and coalesce, in the absence of sufficient healing, catastrophic structural failure occurs and a completed stress fracture develops.[44,45]

Stress fractures associated with excessive stress and metabolically normal bone (fatigue fractures) are common injuries in athletes and are usually related to a sudden

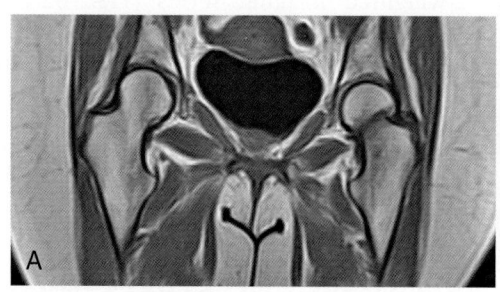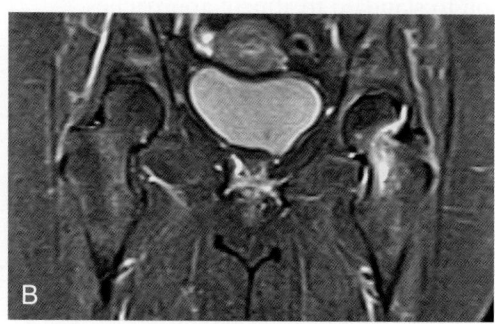

FIGURE 102-13

Subcapital left femoral neck fracture in a 57-year-old female. **A,** Coronal T1-weighted image. Decreased marrow signal intensity corresponds to the fracture and adjacent edema involving the left femoral neck. **B,** Coronal fat-suppressed image. The fracture line and the adjacent marrow edema become hyperintense relative to normal marrow.

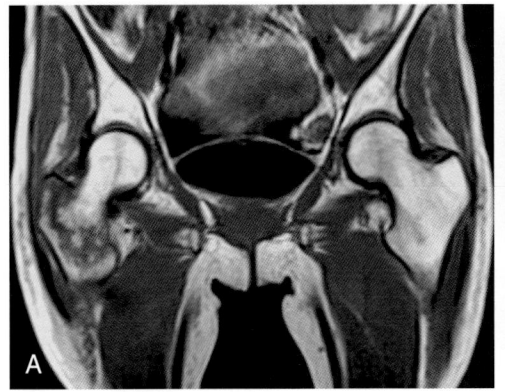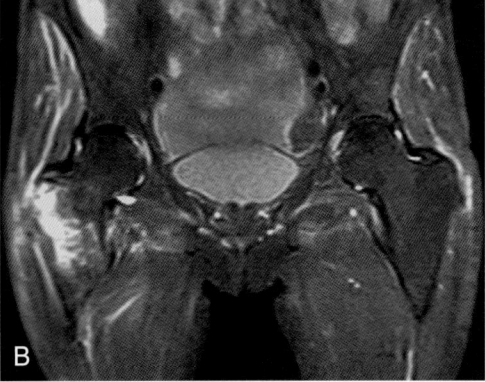

FIGURE 102-14

Nondisplaced intertrochanteric fracture of the right hip in a 79-year-old female. **A,** Coronal T1-weighted image. The oblique fracture line, extending from the right greater trochanter to the lesser trochanter, appears hypointense. The fracture was not detected on conventional radiographs. **B,** Coronal STIR image. Markedly hyperintense marrow edema is observed at the fracture site. Intramuscular edema, compatible with strain, particularly involving the right gluteus medius muscle is also indentified.

increase in training duration or intensity, a change in the shock absorption capacity of running surface or footwear, or the presence of coexistant injuries which alter gait or create a load-bearing imbalance. Insufficiency stress injuries, which occur in patients with impaired osseous metabolism and decreased bone mineralization, are observed in association with osteoporosis, osteomalacia, hyperparathyroidism, osteogenesis imperfecta, multiple myeloma, inflammatory arthritis, and neuromuscular disease.

Early detection of stress injuries is associated with a more rapid recovery. Treatment of low-grade stress reaction involves rest, protected or limited weight bearing, and, in athletes, temporary implementation of an alternative training regimen and a critical examination of training biomechanics. A completed stress fracture often requires immobilization and more prolonged rehabilitation.

With MRI, early or mild stress reaction exhibits a marrow edema pattern, appearing decreased in signal intensity on T1-weighted imaging and hyperintense relative to normal marrow on T2-weighted and STIR imaging.[45,46] Stress injuries can usually be differentiated from bone bruises on the basis of clinical history and anatomic location. Stress injuries typically occur at specific sites of load bearing or at sites of musculotendinous attachment susceptible to traction stress. Completed stress fractures, appreciated best on STIR or fat-saturated T2-weighted imaging series, manifest linear hypointensity, classically oriented perpendicular to the vector of applied stress, surrounded by a zone of marrow edema.[46] Adjacent soft-tissue edema is often present and if the location of the stress injury is periarticular, an effusion may be identified.

The hips and pelvis are particularly vulnerable to stress injuries resulting from either excessive physical stress or metabolic insufficiency. Common locations for stress reaction and fractures include the femoral neck, greater and lesser trochanters, supra-acetabular region, pubic rami, iliac spines, ischial tuberosity, and sacrum.

Femoral Neck

Stress injuries of the femoral neck are categorized as medial compression injuries or lateral distraction injuries. Medial femoral neck stress fractures are more often observed in younger patients and are associated with increased athletic activity (Figs. 102-15 and 102-16).[47,48] They usually respond to conservative treatment without the necessity of surgical intervention. Lateral femoral neck stress fractures develop in older patients and result from tension forces applied to bone which is often metabolically deficient (Fig. 102-17). These fractures often require internal fixation because the distraction rather than impaction mechanics may result in fracture displacement.[42]

The patient usually presents with a history of groin pain. MRI reveals a marrow edema pattern corresponding with the stress reaction and, depending on the severity and/or chronicity of the reaction, a hypointense linear fracture may be evident. The marrow edema which accompanies the medial type of femoral neck injury is usually more conspicuous than the edema associated with the lateral stress injury because the microtrabecular injuries tend to be more extensive with an impaction as opposed to a distraction mechanism of injury. Herniation pits, which frequently develop within the proximal lateral aspect of the femoral neck, should not be mistaken for lateral stress injury. Although adjacent osseous reaction may be identified, a well-defined cystic component is characteristic of a herniation pit (Fig. 102-18). Evaluation of healing of femoral neck stress injuries represents an additional MRI application.[49]

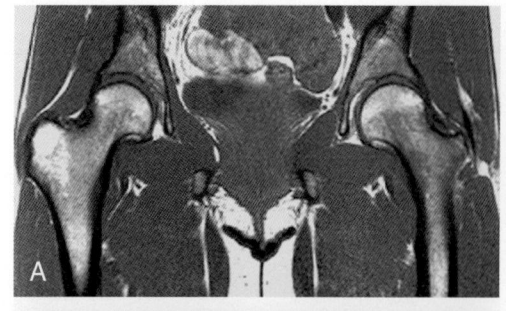
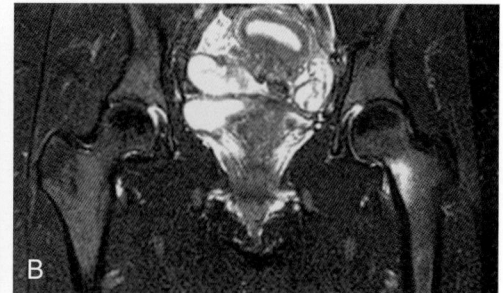
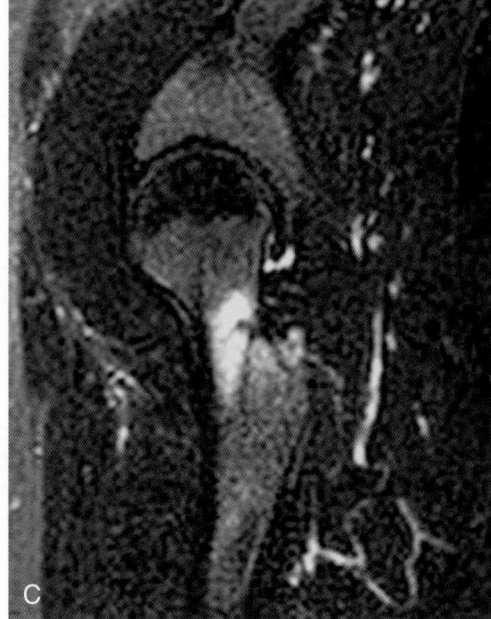

FIGURE 102-15

Medial femoral neck stress injury. **A,** Coronal T1-weighted image. A subtle region of decreased marrow signal intensity involves the medial aspect of the left femoral neck. **B,** Coronal fat-saturated T2-weighted image. Marrow edema, indicative of stress reaction, involves the medial portion of the left femoral neck. **C,** Sagittal fat-saturated T2-weighted image. A hypointense linear stress fracture is surrounded by hyperintense edema.

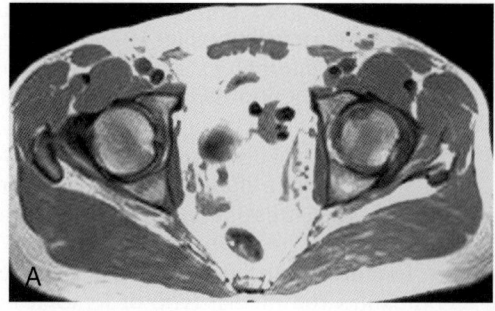
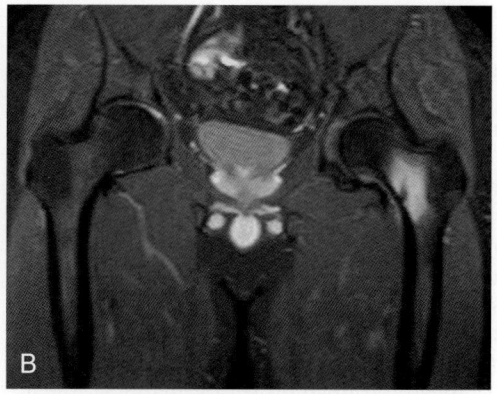

FIGURE 102-16

Medial femoral neck stress injury in a patient with osteonecrosis. **A,** Axial T1-eighted image. A subtle region of subchondral osteonecrosis is identified within the anterior superior aspect of the left femoral head. **B,** Coronal fat-saturated T2-weighted image. A linear hypointense medial femoral neck stress fracture is oriented roughly perpendicular to the vector of applied stress and is surrounded by hyperintense marrow edema, rendered particularly conspicuous by fat signal suppression.

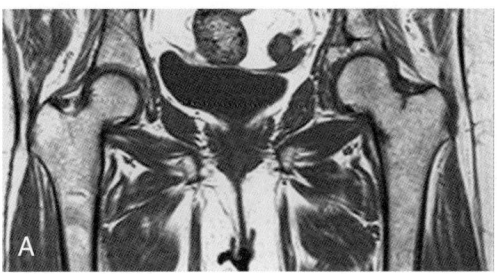

FIGURE 102-17

Lateral left femoral neck stess fracture in an elderly patient. **A,** Coronal T1-weighted image. Decreased linear marrow signal intensity is noted at the proximal lateral margin of the left femoral neck. **B,** Coronal fat-saturated T2-weighted image. The focal marrow signal abnormality becomes hyperintense, indicative of edema associated with stress reaction. The edema related to distraction or tension stress injury is often less extensive and considerably more subtle than the marrow edema which accompanies impaction or compression stress forces.

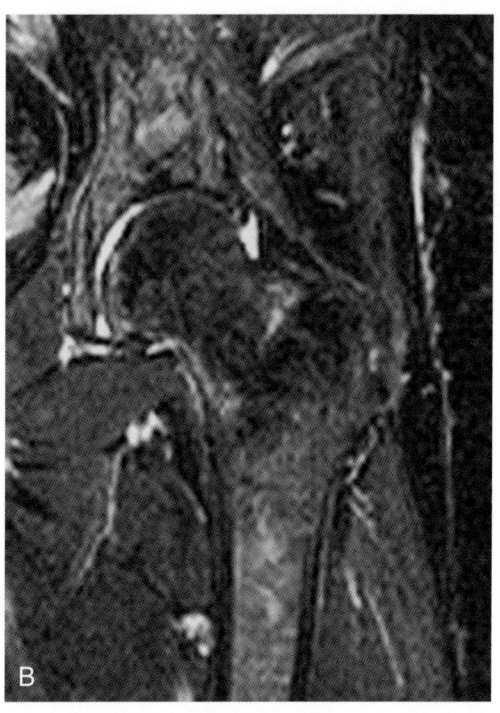

Greater and Lesser Trochanters

The greater trochanter represents the insertion site for the gluteus medius, gluteus minimus, the obturators, and the gemelli muscles responsible for abduction and external rotation of the hip. Stress injuries involving the greater trochanter are particularly observed in athletic activities that require a rapid change in direction when running, such as football and soccer. Patients typically present with pain and tenderness related to the greater

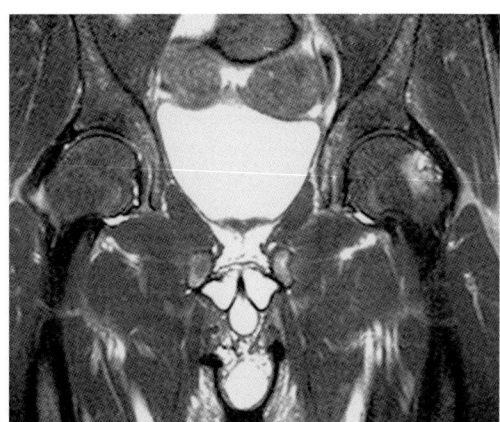

FIGURE 102-18

Herniation pit of the left femoral neck with osseous reaction. Coronal fat-saturated T2-weighted image. Herniation pits typically develop within the proximal lateral aspect of the femoral neck and may be associated with adjacent osseous reaction. The cystic component differentiates it from primary stress injury. Similar findings have been reported in cases of femoroacetabular impingement.

trochanter with painful active abduction and passive adduction.[50] In patients with traction-related osseous stress injury involving the greater trochanter, a marrow edema pattern is identified on MRI (Fig. 102-19).

Lesser trochanteric stress injuries are more common than greater trochanteric injuries and are related to traction stress arising from the insertion of the iliopsoas tendon. Activities that require repetitive hip flexion, such as running, stair climbing, step aerobics, and cheerleading, are often responsible.[50] MRI reveals marrow edema involving the lesser trochanter, often extending into the adjacent medial femoral neck (Figs. 102-20 and 102-21).

Supra-Acetabular Region

Supra-acetabular stress injuries often represent insufficiency fractures in elderly patients but fatigue fractures in athletes and military recruits may also involve this site (Fig. 102-22).[51,52] MRI studies demonstrate the typical marrow edema pattern. In patients with supra-acetebular stress reaction related to metabolic factors such as osteoporosis, additional foci of marrow edema are often identified on MRI, particularly involving the pubic rami and the sacrum.

Parasymphyseal Region and Pubic Rami

Stress injuries adjacent to the symphysis pubis and extending into the superior and inferior pubic rami are commonly related to osseous metabolic insufficiency and associated with stress fractures of the sacrum.[52] As structural failure of the posterior pelvic arch occurs,

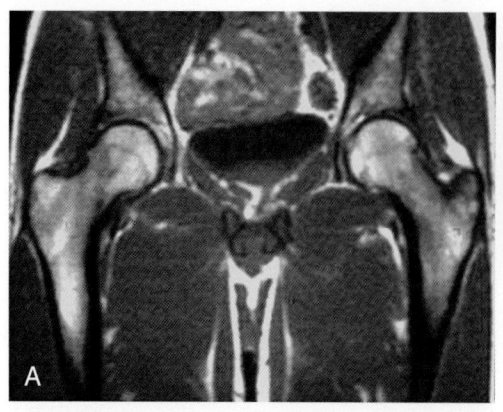
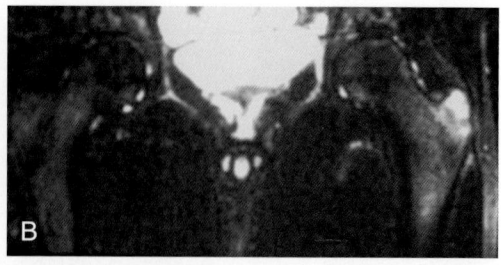

FIGURE 102-19

Greater trochanteric stress injury in a 16-year-old football player. **A,** Coronal T1-weighted image. The left greater trochanter is decreased in signal intensity with a horizontal linear, hypointense fracture. **B,** Coronal fat-saturated T2-weighted image. The marrow edema, associated with abduction and external rotation traction stress on the greater trochanter, appears hyperintense.

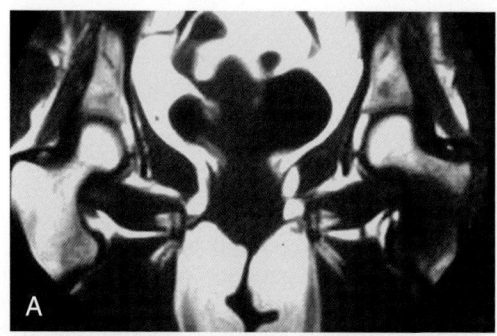
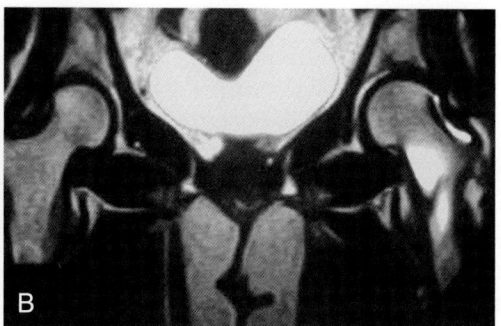
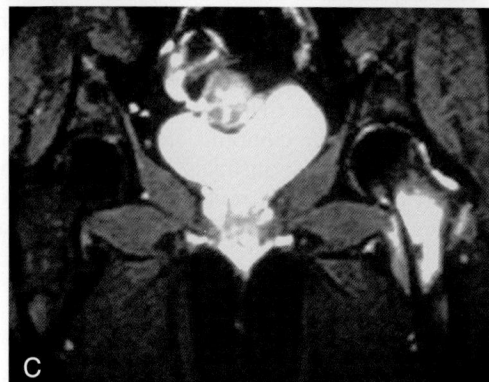

FIGURE 102-20

Lesser trochanteric stress injury in a 45-year-old female. **A,** Coronal T1-weighted image. Markedly decreased marrow signal intensity extends from the lesser trochanter into the intertrochanteric region. **B,** Coronal T2-weighted image. A hypointense stress fracture is identified at the base of the lesser trochanter, surrounded by hyperintense marrow edema. **C,** Coronal STIR image. The marrow edema pattern becomes especially conspicuous with fat-suppressed imaging. Stress injury at the insertion of the iliopsoas muscle is often associated with activity which demands repetitive hip flexion.

FIGURE 102-21

Lesser trochanteric stress injury. Coronal fat-saturated T2-weighted image. Hyperintense marrow edema, indicative of stress injury, extends from the lesser trochanter into the medial intertrochanteric region.

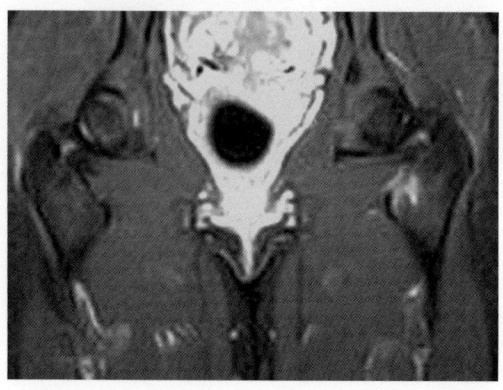

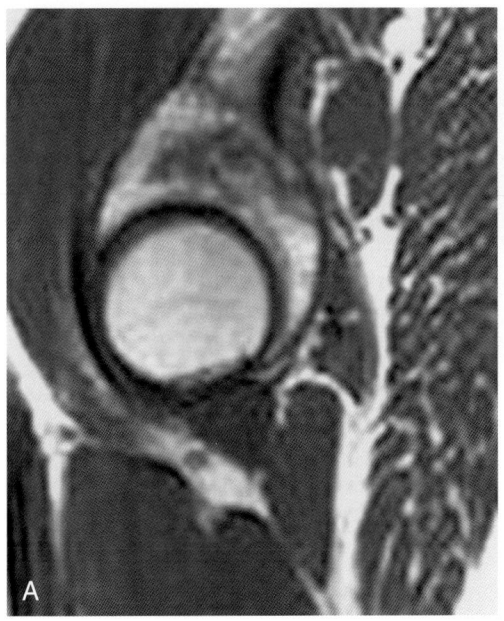

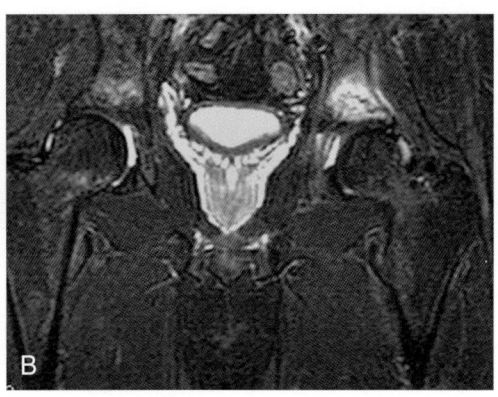

FIGURE 102-22

Supra-acetabular stress injury in a military recruit. **A,** Sagittal T1-weighted image of the left hip. A linear hypointense fracture, predominantly horizontal in orientation, involves the supra-acetabular region of the iliac bone. **B,** Coronal fat-saturated T2-weighted image. The linear fatigue fracture of the left supra-acetabular region is surrounded by hyperintense marrow edema. To a lesser extent, stress injury of the right supra-acetabular marrow and the medial aspect of the right femoral neck is also identified.

increased stress is distributed to the anterior pelvic arch. Acute traumatic injuries of the anterior pelvis are also associated with posterior pelvic injuries. Because the pelvis functions as a ring in terms of force distribution, external forces applied to the pelvis that exceed the capacity of the pelvis to absorb the energy, tend to exhibit fractures that reflect both an entry and an exit site. Inclusion of both the sacrum and the anterior osseous pelvis within the imaging field of view is particularly important on T2-weighted fat-saturated and STIR imaging series to detect the marrow edema pattern which develops in response to stress-related or acute traumatic injury at these sites. Fractures involving the pubic ramus are typically vertical in orientation. Traction stress injury also represents a mechanism of para-symphyseal stress fracture (Fig. 102-23).[53] The adductor

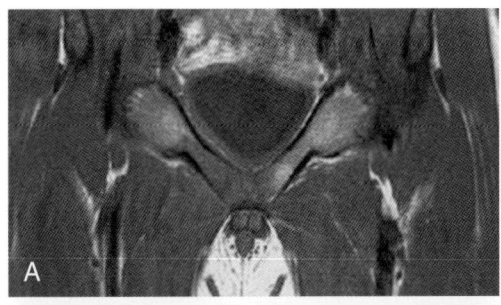

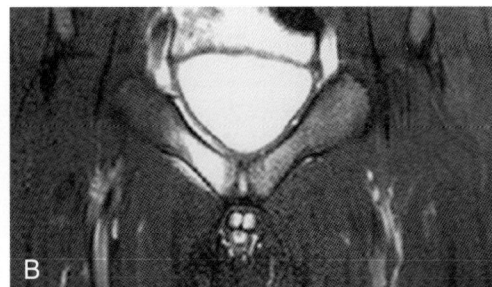

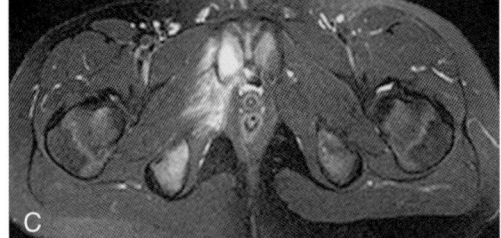

FIGURE 102-23

Parasymphyseal osseous and muscular stress injury in an 11-year-old male. **A,** Coronal T1-weighted image. Decreased marrow signal intensity involving the para-symphyseal portion of the right superior pubic ramus is identified. **B,** Coronal fat-saturated T2-weighted image. The stress-related marrow edema involving the right superior pubic ramus becomes conspicuously hyper-intense. **C,** Axial, fat-saturated T2-weighted image. A marrow edema pattern also involves the parasymphyseal region of the right inferior pubic ramus, with adjacent obturator externus intramuscular edema. Evidence of anterior pelvic muscle injury and additional pelvic foci of osseous stress injury are commonly observed in patients with parasymphyseal stress injury, whether related to metabolic insufficiency or athletic stress.

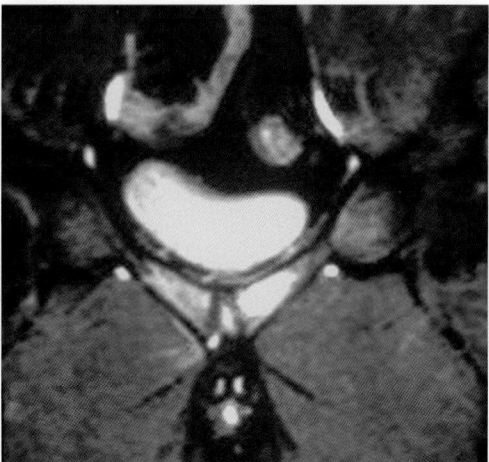

FIGURE 102-24

Parasymphyseal stress injury in a male athlete with groin pain. Coronal STIR image. Marrow edema involves both superior pubic rami, left greater than right.

longus and brevis and the gracilis muscle originate from the parasymphyseal region and may result in stress injury related to athletic activity that requires sprinting, such as soccer, basketball, and track (Fig. 102-24).

Sacrum

The sacrum represents a common site for pelvic stress injury, most frequently encountered in post-menopausal women (Fig. 102-25).[54,55] However, sacral stress fractures are also identified in athletes, particularly long-distance runners (Fig. 102-26).[56] Pain related to the sacral stress injury may be misdiagnosed as radiculopathy associated with lumbar disk disease. MRI provides a means to accurately identify sacral stress injury, determine the

extent and severity of sacral involvement, differentiate osseous stress injury from other causes of sacral pain, such as sacroiliitis, and detect any additional sites of pelvic stress reaction (Fig. 102-27).[52,57]

Anterior Inferior and Anterior Superior Iliac Spines

The anterior inferior iliac spine represents the origin of the rectus femoris muscle and traction injury may develop in association with athletic activities that require repetitive and/or rapid hip flexion, such as sprinting or kicking.[50] Patients present with anterior hip and groin pain and, on physical examination, experience pain with passive extension and active flexion of the hip. MRI reveals focal marrow edema involving the anterior inferior iliac spine and, if a completed fracture is present, the orientation of the hypointense fracture line is typically perpendicular to the axis of the iliac spine (Fig. 102-28).

The anterior superior iliac spine is the origin of the sartorius muscle and traction injuries involving this site are also observed in runners, especially sprinters. Hurdling also results in stretching of the sartorius muscle with the hip in extension and the knee in flexion. Patients present with pain and tenderness to palpation involving the anterior superior iliac spine.[50] MRI reveals a marrow edema pattern involving the osseous origin of the sartorius muscle and, with both anterior superior and anterior inferior iliac spine stress injuries, adjacent muscle edema may be present, indicative of strain or overuse injury (Fig. 102-29).

Traction stress injuries involving the iliac crest may also be identified in athletes. The tensor fascia lata, gluteus medius and maximus, transverse abdominus, internal and external obliques, and latissimus dorsi attach to the iliac crest. Long-distance running is associated with stress reaction involving this site.

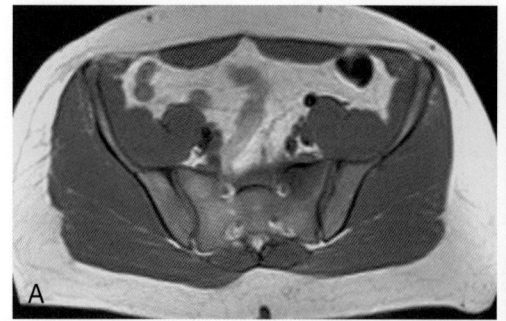

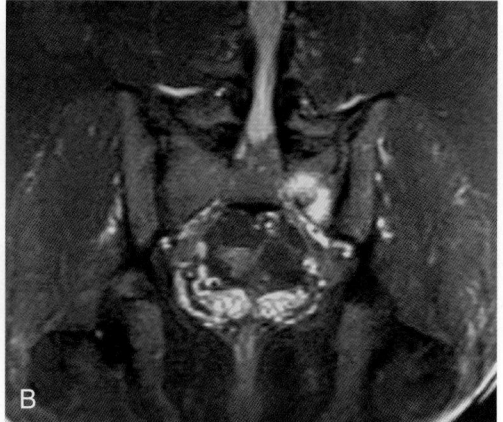

FIGURE 102-25

Sacral stress fracture. **A,** Axial T1-weighted image. Focal, asymmetric decreased marrow signal intensity of the anterior aspect of the left sacral ala is noted. **B,** Coronal T2-weighted image. An obliquely oriented, linear hypointense stress fracture of the left sacral ala is identified with adjacent hyperintense marrow edema. The patient presented with "left hip pain," reinforcing the necessity of including the sacrum as well as the anterior osseous pelvis within the imaging field of view when evaluating patients for hip pathology.

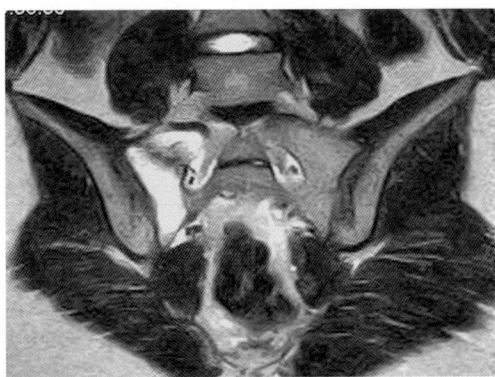

FIGURE 102-26

Sacral stress injury in a 15-year-old female. Coronal T2-weighted image. An obliquely oriented fatigue stress fracture of the right sacral ala is surrounded by an extensive hyperintense marrow edema pattern.

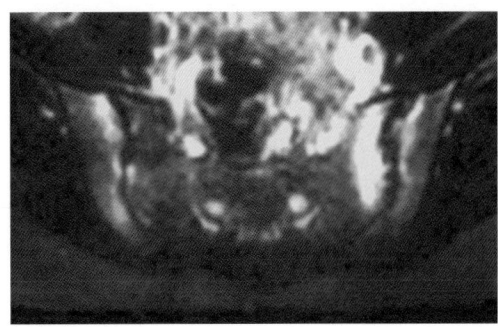

FIGURE 102-27

Sacroiliitis in an 18-year-old female. Axial fat-saturated T2-weighted image. Although this patient was a competitive volleyball player, the periarticular pattern of marrow edema favors inflammatory arthropathy rather than stress injury. Subsequent testing revealed the patient to be HLA B27 positive.

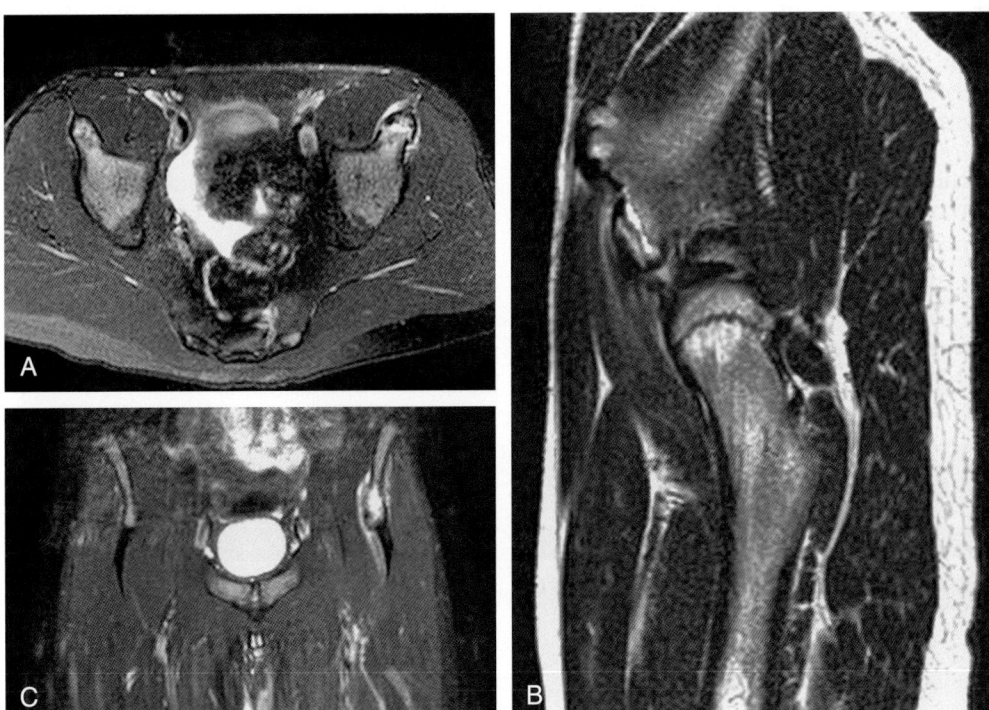

FIGURE 102-28

Anterior inferior iliac spine stress injury in a 15-year-old athlete. **A,** Axial fat-saturated T2-weighted image. Marrow edema and slight avulsion of the left anterior inferior iliac spine have developed secondary to traction stress at the rectus femoris origin. **B,** Sagittal T2-weighted image. Partial avulsion of the anterior inferior iliac spine is noted. **C,** Coronal fat-saturated T2-weighted image. Marrow edema is identified adjacent to the origin of the left rectus femoris tendon.

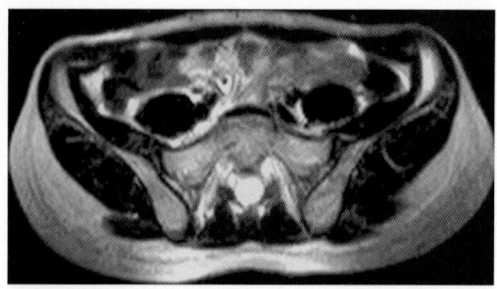

FIGURE 102-29

Anterior superior iliac spine stress injury. Axial T2-weighted image. An asymmetric, hyperintense marrow edema pattern involves the left anterior superior iliac spine, corresponding to the site of the patient's pain and the osseous origin of the sartorius muscle.

Ischial Tuberosity

The hamstring muscle group originates from the ischial tuberosity and traction stress injury involving the ischial tuberosity represents a relatively common occurrence in young athletes involved in sports that require hamstring contraction with the hip in flexion and the knee in extension, such as hurdling and long jumping (Fig. 102-30).[50] Performing the splits in cheerleading and gymnastics also applies repetitive traction stress to the hamstring origin. MRI reveals marrow edema involving the ischial tuberosity and, because the semimembranosus origin involves the lateral aspect of the

ischium proximal to the tuberosity, diffuse edema of the ischium may be encountered and should not be mistaken for infiltrating neoplastic marrow pathology (Fig. 102-31).

BONE MARROW EDEMA ASSOCIATED WITH NEOPLASM

In children and young adults, a marrow edema pattern identified on MRI studies of the hips and pelvis frequently correlates with osseous stress injury related to athletic activity. However, if a history suggestive of excessive stress exposure is not elicited or the process remains refractory to conservative clinical management, other diagnostic possibilities must be considered. In particular, osteoid osteoma and chondroblastoma occur in the same young age group as fatigue stress injuries and are often associated with reactive marrow edema.

Osteoid Osteoma

Osteoid osteomas occur in children and young adults aged 10 to 20 years, and patients often present with a history of nocturnal extremity pain relieved by aspirin and other non-steroidal anti-inflammatory medications.[58]

With most osteoid osteomas, conventional radiographs reveal cortical thickening at the site of the lesion. Nuclear medicine bone scans demonstrate markedly increased radiotracer uptake. On CT examinations, cortical thickening is evident and, frequently, the

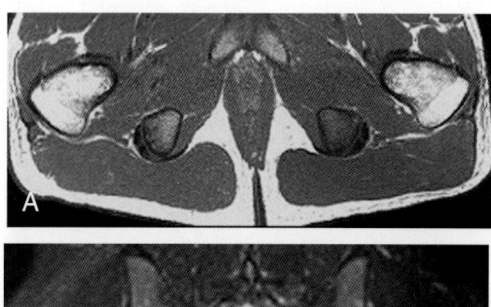

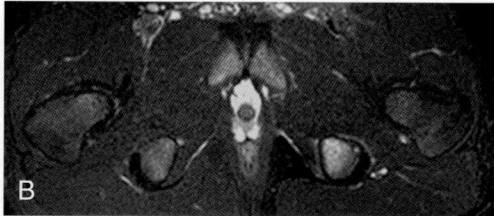

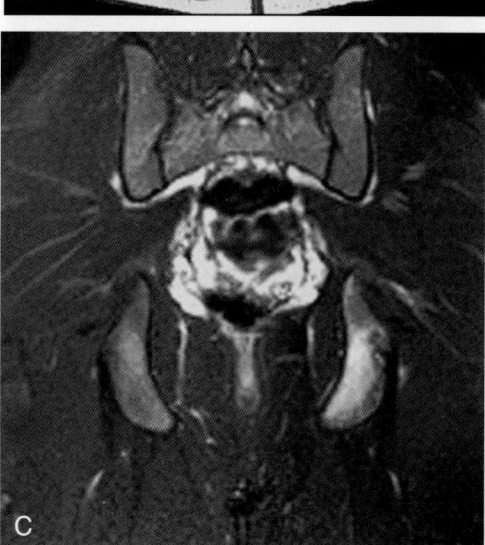

FIGURE 102-30

Ischial tuberosity stress injury in a 14-year-old male athlete with left posterior hip and buttock pain. **A,** Axial T1-weighted image. Asymmetric decreased marrow signal intensity involves the left ischial tuberosity. **B,** Axial fat-saturated T2-weighted image. Marrow edema of the left ischial tuberosity appears hyperintense, with stress injury developing in response to traction at the origin of the hamstring muscle group. **C,** Coronal fat-saturated image. Marrow edema, corresponding to the origin of the hamstring tendon group, involves the left ischium.

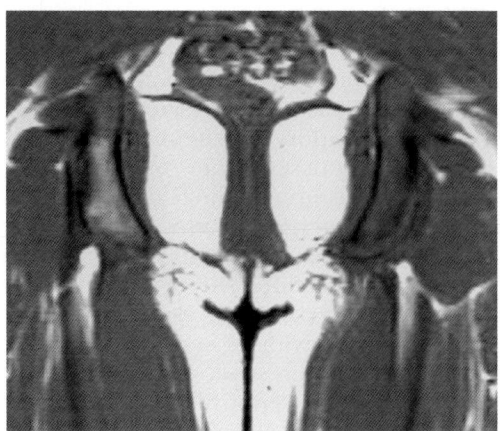

FIGURE 102-31

Ischial stress injury in a 16-year-old female athlete. Coronal T1-weighted image. Asymmetric decreased marrow signal intensity extensively involves the left ischium. Because the semimembranosus component of the hamstring muscle group originates along the lateral margin of the ischium, proximal to the tuberosity, stress injury related to hamstring traction may exhibit a relatively diffuse edema pattern.

nidus can be localized. On MRI studies, marrow edema represents the most conspicuous imaging finding.[59] For this reason, the pattern may be mistaken for stress injury, acute traumatic bone bruise, infection, or malignant neoplasm.[60] If the anatomic location of the lesion is not typical for stress injury and if no history of excessive physical stress is elicited, other diagnostic possibilities,

including osteoid osteoma, should be considered. The nidus can usually be detected with MRI but it may be more conspicuous with CT (Fig. 102-32).[59] Therefore, if the MRI study detects a focal marrow edema pattern without a definite nidus, performing correlative CT may prove helpful in establishing the correct diagnosis. Dynamic gadolinium-enhanced MRI has also been suggested as a means to improve detection of the nidus.[61] Additional findings associated with osteoid osteoma, identified on MRI, include cortical thickening, adjacent soft-tissue edema, and, with intra-articular cases, effusion. An intracapsular osteoid osteoma, involving the hip joint, will not result in cortical thickening. These lesions, however, remain conspicuous on MRI studies because of the extensive marrow edema and reactive synovitis (Fig. 102-33).

Chondroblastoma

Chondroblastomas most frequently occur in patients 10 to 30 years in age and present with focal pain and tenderness to palpation. Again, in this age range stress injuries are common with identical clinical complaints. Chondroblastomas involve epiphyses and apophyses and the apophyseal portion of a long bone represents a common anatomic site for traction stress reaction associated with tendon attachment. The male-to-female ratio for development of a chondroblastoma is 2:1.[62]

Conventional radiographs and CT studies often reveal an expansile lesion. On MRI studies, the focal osseous lesion is evident but it may remain less conspicuous than an adjacent region of marrow edema, which in a patient

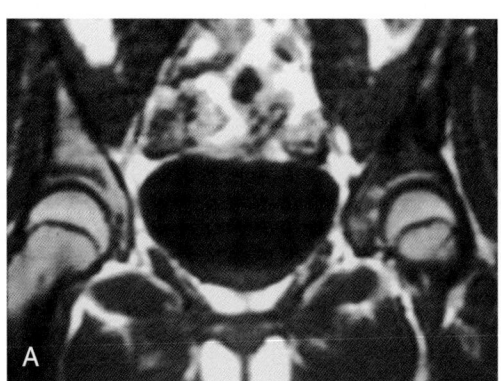

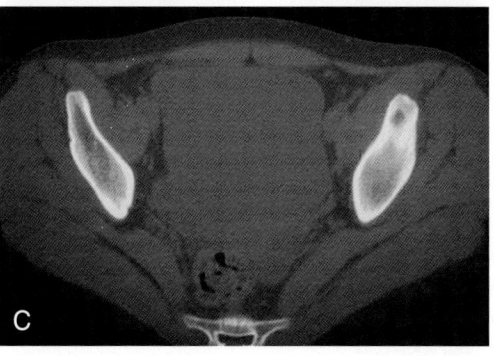

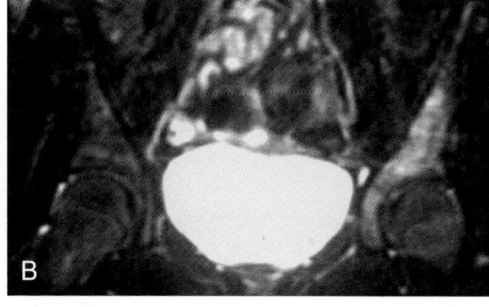

FIGURE 102-32

Osteoid osteoma of the iliac bone in a 13-year-old female. **A,** Coronal T1-weighted image. Decreased marrow signal intensity involves the supra-acetabular portion of the left iliac bone. **B,** Coronal fat-saturated T2-weighted image. The left supra-acetabular region appears markedly increased in signal intensity, compatible with extensive marrow edema. The patient reported no history to suggest excessive athletic stress or metabolic osseous insufficiency. **C,** Axial CT image. The lucent nidus of the osteoid osteoma and adjacent sclerosis involve the left anterior inferior iliac spine. Although the reactive marrow edema associated with an osteoid osteoma is conspicuous on MRI studies, the nidus is often better appreciated with CT.

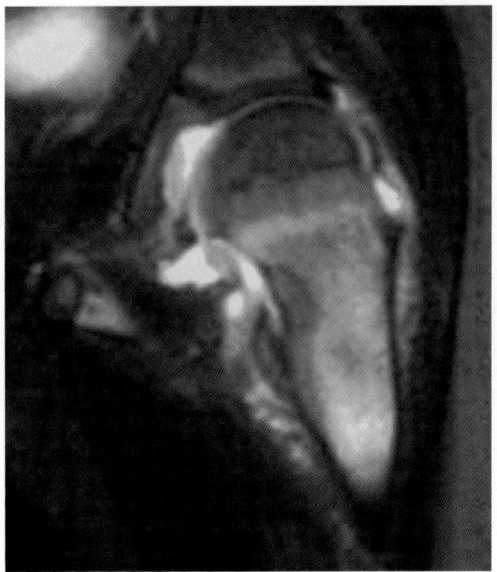

FIGURE 102-33

Osteoid osteoma with synovitis in a 5-year-old patient. Coronal T2-weighted image. The nidus is located within the medial aspect of the left femoral neck. Marked adjacent hyperintense marrow edema is identified and a large reactive hip joint effusion is present.

of this age could be mistaken for osseous stress injury or aggressive osseous malignancy.[60] The marrow edema associated with a chondroblastoma probably arises from the release of enzymes by the tumor which result in hyperemia and adjacent osseous reaction.[63] The diagnosis of chondroblastoma should be suspected on MRI studies whenever a focal apophyseal lesion is accompanied by a marrow edema pattern (Fig. 102-34). Conventional radiographic correlation often provides confirmation of the typical features of this tumor.

MUSCLE INJURIES

Common muscle injuries include acute strain, contusion, and repetitive, overuse injury. Characterizing the extent and anatomic location of the muscle injury and differentiating soft-tissue from osseous injury are critically important in directing appropriate clinical management and determining prognosis for functional recovery. Conventional radiography, CT, and nuclear medicine studies remain relatively insensitive in the evaluation of muscle pathology. Because muscle injury typically is associated with an increase in muscle water content and/or the presence of hemorrhage, MRI represents a uniquely sensitive and specific imaging technique in detecting, localizing, and categorizing muscle injuries.[64]

With acute muscle strain, contusion, delayed-onset muscle soreness, and overuse injury, MRI demonstrates an intramuscular edema pattern characterized by increased signal intensity that is particularly conspicuous on fat-saturated T2-weighted and STIR imaging series.[64,65] In the case of muscle contusion the edema is often more focal and less diffuse than the pattern that accompanies muscle strain. Signal alteration in conjunction with nonhemorrhagic muscle pathology may not be apparent on T1-weighted images but the muscle may appear asymmetrically enlarged because of the interstitial edema. With intramuscular hemorrhage, associated with strain or contusion, T1-weighted imaging series often reveal a focal hyperintense mass, representing the methemaglobin component of a subacute hematoma.[66] On T2-weighted imaging, the hematoma may exhibit a complex signal intensity pattern, with the central portion of the hematoma showing increased signal intensity which is indicative of partial liquifaction (Fig. 102-35). With high-grade muscle tears, muscle discontinuity may be identified on MRI studies and with musculoteninous avulsions the extent of tendon retraction can be accurately measured.

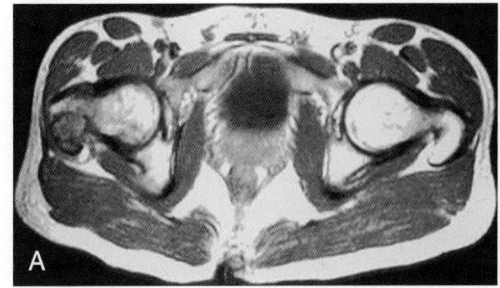
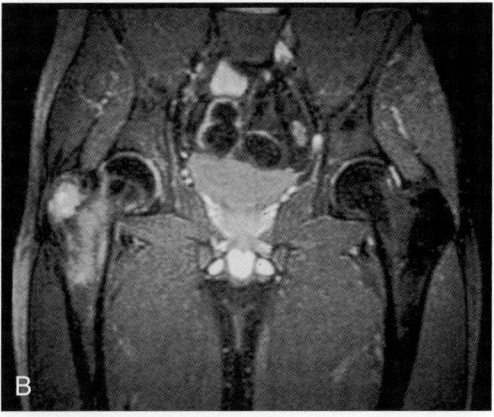

FIGURE 102-34

Chondroblastoma of the right greater trochanter. **A,** Axial T1-weighted image. An expansile lesion of the right greater trochanter is identified. **B,** Coronal fat-saturated T2-weighted image. A hyperintense marrow edema pattern extends medial to the focal chondroblastoma of the greater trochanteric apophysis.

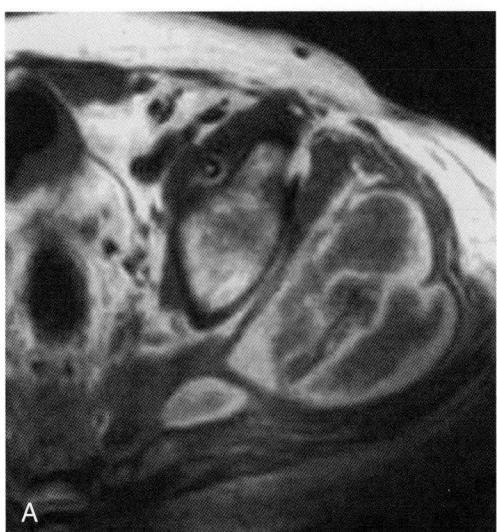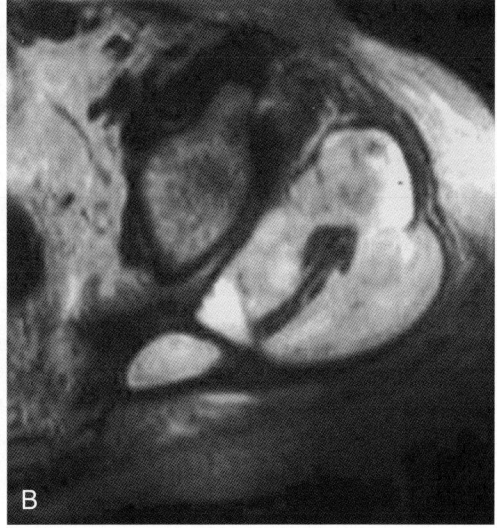

FIGURE 102-35

Gluteal intramuscular hematoma. **A,** Axial T1-weighted image. A subacute left gluteal region hematoma manifests a hyperintense rim, consistent with the presence of methemaglobin. **B,** Axial T2-weighted image. The left gluteal hematoma exhibits a hyperintense signal pattern.

Relatively common sites of muscle injury involving the hips and pelvis include the gluteus maximus, gluteus medius, iliopsoas, adductors and obturator externus, rectus femoris, and hamstring musculotendinous complex. The mechanism for gluteus maximus injuries often involves application of an external force resulting in a contusion rather than a strain related to an intrinsic stretching injury. A fall onto an inelastic surface is a common history in these patients. MRI studies reveal intramuscular edema and/or hemorrhage involving the gluteus maximus muscle (Fig. 102-36). Near-falls result in muscle strains, particularly involving the gluteus medius in elderly patients.[67] Clinically, these injuries may mimic proximal femoral fractures. MRI demonstrates edema, particularly apparent on fat-saturated T2-weighted and STIR acquisitions, involving the gluteus medius muscle-tendon complex near its greater trochanteric insertion (Fig. 102-37). A traction-related bone bruise of the greater trochanter may also be identified on these imaging series

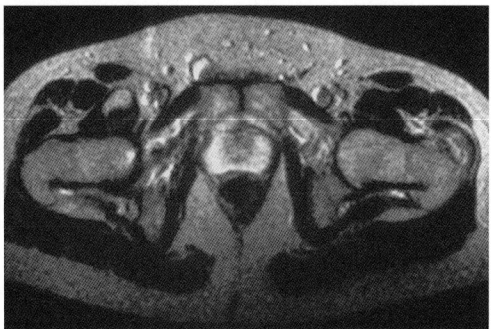

FIGURE 102-37

Gluteus medius strain on the left in a male golfer. Axial T2-weighted image. The distal portion of the left gluteus medius muscle-tendon complex, anterior to its greater trochanteric insertion, appears expanded and increased in signal intensity, consistent with edema associated with strain. The right distal gluteus medius muscle is normal in contour and signal intensity.

FIGURE 102-36

Gluteus maximus contusion. Coronal fat-saturated T2-weighted image. Markedly increased signal intensity involves the left gluteus maximus muscle, indicative of intramuscular edema secondary to contusion experienced in a fall on to the left buttock.

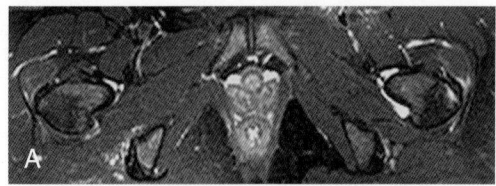
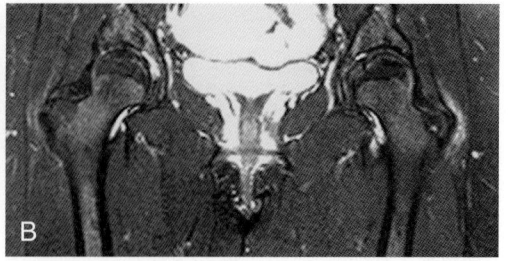

FIGURE 102-38

Gluteus medius strain with bone marrow edema. **A,** Axial fat-saturated T2-weighted image. Increased signal intensity compatible with musculotendinous edema involves the distal left gluteus medius muscle-tendon complex with evidence of hyperintense osseous reaction at the tendon insertion on the greater trochanter. **B,** Coronal fat-saturated T2-weighted image. Left gluteus medius musculotendinous edema is present adjacent to its greater trochanteric insertion, indicative of strain or overuse injury, a pattern that may be observed in patients with greater trochanteric pain syndrome.

(Fig. 102-38). In patients with repetitive overuse injury or greater trochanteric pain syndrome, intramuscular and peritendinous edema involving the gluteus medius insertional complex may also be identified.[68] The appearance of the tendon and mechanism of injury are similar to the pattern observed with overuse tendinosis and peritendinitis affecting the rotator cuff of the shoulder. A near-fall resulting in rapid hip flexion or forcible extension may cause iliopsoas musculoten-dinous strain, with diffuse intramuscular edema evident with MRI (Fig. 102-39). Muscle strain involving the adductors and obturator externus may also be observed in the context of a near-fall in an elderly patient or may be associated with anterior pelvic and parasymphyseal stress injury in both older patients with osseous metabolic insufficiency and in young athletes who make excessive physical demands on the muscles and their osseous origins. Acute muscle strain involving the rectus

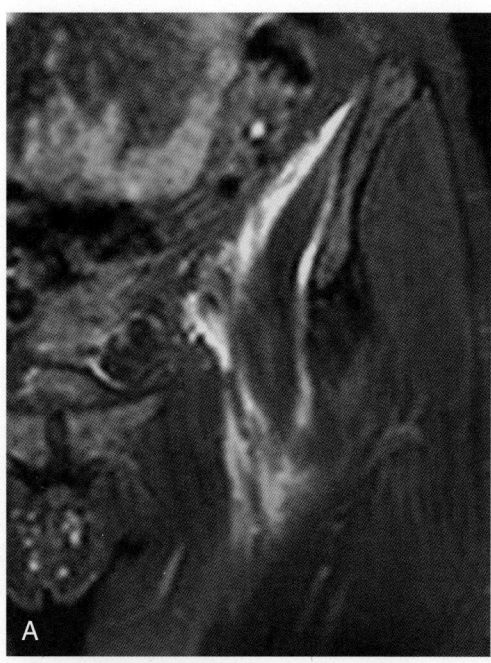
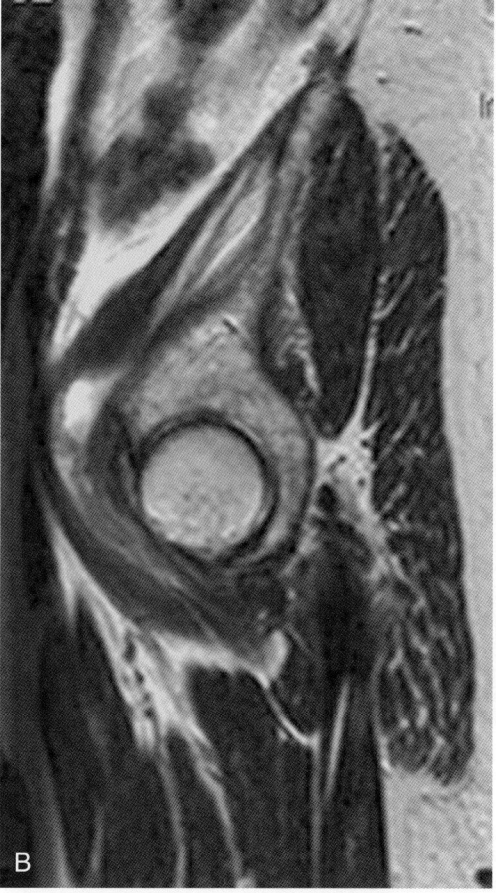

FIGURE 102-39

Iliopsoas strain secondary to a near-fall in an elderly female. **A,** Coronal fat-saturated T2-weighted image. Hyperintense intramuscular edema involves the iliacus muscle and the iliopsoas junction. **B,** Sagittal T2-weighted image. Intramuscular and perimuscular edema associated with acute strain of the iliopsoas muscle complex are identified.

femoris also represents a relatively common athletic injury, particularly found in sprinters and kickers. Hamstring musculotendinous strains represent common athletic injuries, related to running, jumping, and in gymnastics.[69] They usually result from excessive stretching force and tendinous avulsion from the ischium and ischial tuberosity may occur in severe cases. The biceps femoris musculotendinous complex represents the most frequently injured component of the hamstring muscle group.[70] With quadriceps and hamstring injuries, MRI identifies the specific component of muscle group involvement, the extent of intramuscular edema and/or hemorrhage, and, if present, the degree of tendon retraction (Fig. 102-40). Again, particularly in the athlete, this information helps to develop an appropriate treatment and rehabilitation plan, and to determine the prognosis for a successful return to athletic competition.[71]

Piriformis syndrome represents a symptom complex that includes pain and tenderness to palpation involving the region of the sacroiliac joint and sciatic notch, the presence of a palpable mass near the piriformis muscle, and gluteal atrophy.[72] The pain often radiates to the leg and may mimic lumbar radiculopathy. The condition is thought to be post-traumatic in origin, related to gluteal

trauma and the subsequent development of fibrosis between the piriformis muscle and the sciatic nerve.[72,73] The diagnosis is primarily based on history, physical examination, and electromyography results. Because symptoms may mimic radicular pain, performing MRI of the lumbar spine in patients with suspected piriformis syndrome is helpful in detecting or excluding lumbar disk pathology. When CT was performed on a group of patients undergoing evaluation for piriformis syndrome, the size of the piriformis muscle on the affected side was variable.[73] In some patients, it appeared symmetrically normal and in others it was either enlarged or decreased in size. If MRI of the pelvis is performed in the assessment of a patient experiencing symptoms consistent with piriformis syndrome, the piriformis muscle and sciatic notch region should be examined for muscle atrophy or hypertrophy, muscle edema evident on T2-weighted fat-saturated or STIR imaging series, and the presence of a hematoma, seroma, or mass. However, the absence of recognizable pathology involving the piriformis muscle on MRI evaluation does not exclude the clinical diagnosis of piriformis syndrome. Release of the piriformis muscle-tendon complex and sciatic neurolysis have demonstrated success in treating patients with this condition.[73]

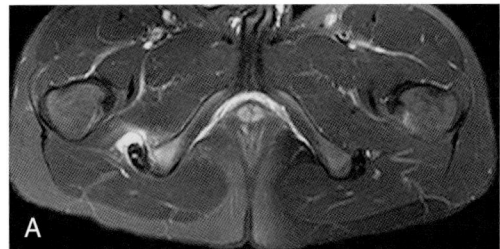
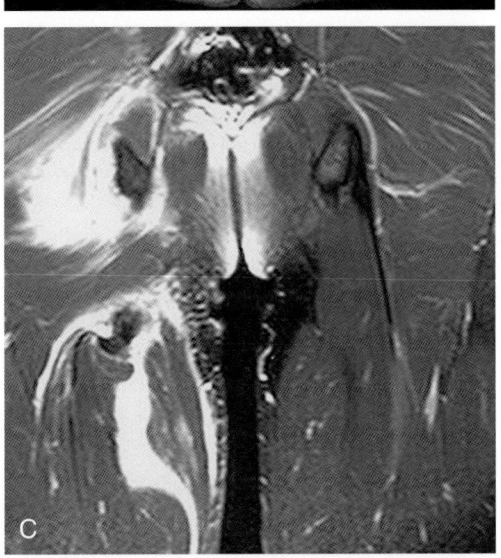
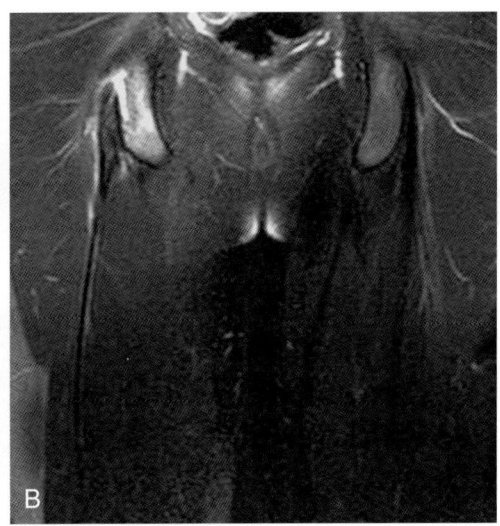

FIGURE 102-40

Hamstring musculotendinous injury. **A,** Axial fat-saturated T2-weighted image in a 14-year-old male with right posterior proximal thigh pain. The biceps femoris and semitendinosus components of the hamstring group on the right remain in continuity with their ischial tuberosity origin. A fluid collection compatible with a seroma is identified immediately anterior to the tendons and a traction-related bone bruise of the ischial tuberosity is present. **B,** Coronal fat-saturated T2 image in the same patient. Partial avulsion of the proximal portion of the semimembranosus tendon at its origin along the lateral aspect of the ischium is observed. The ischial marrow edema is again noted and edema surrounds the proximal muscle-tendon complex. **C,** Coronal, fat-saturated T2-weighted image in a hockey player with a sudden onset of right posterior thigh pain, swelling, and weakness. Hamstring avulsion at the ischial tuberosity on the right is identified, with distal retraction of the muscle-tendon complex.

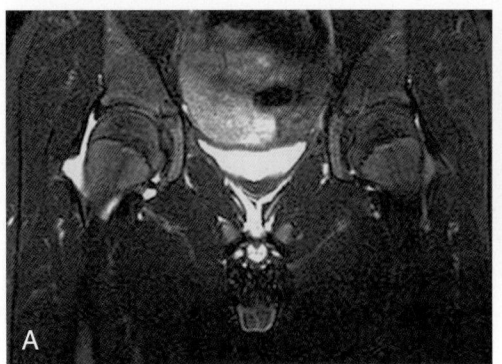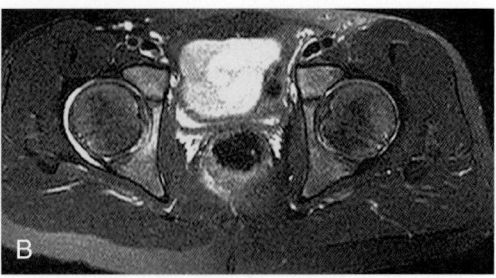

FIGURE 102-41

Synovitis of the right hip in a 12-year-old male. **A,** Coronal fat-saturated T2-weighted image. An effusion of the right hip joint is identified in this patient with an acute onset of hip pain. **B,** Axial fat-saturated T2-weighted image. The right hip joint effusion is again evident and marrow edema involving the central portion of the acetabulum is observed. The patient's family had recently purchased a trampoline and the synovitis and marrow edema probably reflect repetitive impaction and capsular stretching injury.

SYNOVIAL DISORDERS

Transient Synovitis

Transient or toxic synovitis represents a cause of irritable hip syndrome in children. Patients experience an acute onset of hip pain and a decreased range of hip motion, particularly abduction and external rotation. Boys are more frequently affected than girls. Spontaneous resolution of symptoms typically occurs within 48 hours. Etiology is uncertain but may be related to viral infection or trauma.[74,75] Differential diagnostic considerations include synovitis associated with Legg-Calvé-Perthes disease, intra-articular osteoid osteoma, septic arthritis, or juvenile rheumatoid arthritis. MRI studies reveal the presence of a hip joint effusion, most conspicuous on fat-saturated T2-weighted or STIR imaging series (Fig. 102-41). Careful inspection of the size and signal intensity of the femoral head ossification center is necessary to exclude osteonecrosis and, in the absence of demonstrable femoral head pathology on

the initial MRI examination, performing follow-up MRI is recommended, particularly if hip pain persists. The identification of periarticular marrow signal changes suggests the diagnosis of septic arthritis rather than transient synovitis.[76]

Septic Arthritis

In children, septic arthritis, like transient synovitis, presents with hip pain and stiffness. Systemic signs and symptoms, including fever, are often present. *Staphylococcus aureus* or *Haemophilus influenzae* represent bacteriologic organisms commonly responsible for joint infection but septic arthritis may also develop secondary to tuberculosis and other chronic infections. In addition to an effusion, MRI studies may reveal a bone marrow edema pattern involving the acetabulum and femoral head, manifesting decreased signal intensity on T1-weighted imaging and markedly increased signal intensity on fat-saturated T2-weighted or STIR imaging series (Fig. 102-42).[76] Later in the course of

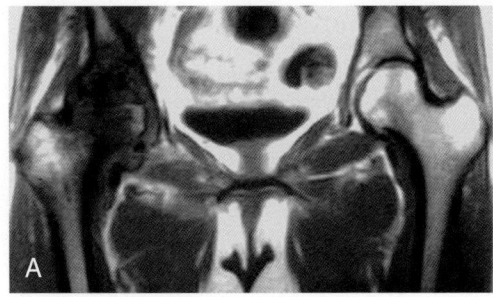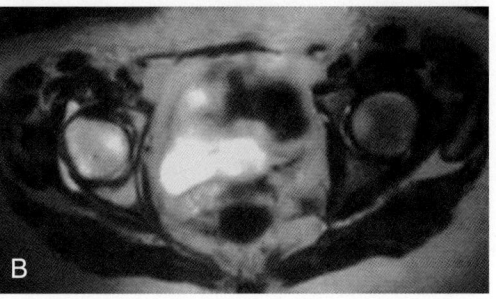

FIGURE 102-42

Septic arthritis. **A,** Coronal T1-weighted image. Both the femoral head and the acetabular components of the right hip joint are markedly decreased in signal intensity. **B,** Axial T2-weighted image. A hyperintense, periarticular marrow edema pattern involves the right hip and an effusion is observed lateral to the right femoral head.

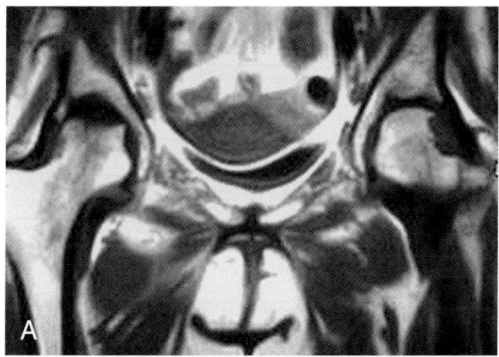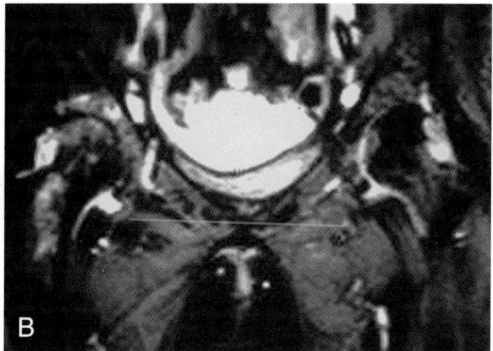

FIGURE 102-43

Rheumatoid arthritis. **A,** Coronal T1-weighted image. Hypointense osseous erosions involve the superior lateral aspects of both femoral head and the left femoral neck. **B,** Coronal STIR image. Bilateral head and neck erosions are present with bilateral effusions. A reactive, periarticular marrow edema pattern is particularly conspicuous on the right.

the disease, joint narrowing and periarticular osseous erosions may be apparent. Osseous erosions also occur in children with juvenile rheumatoid arthritis and in adults with inflammatory arthritis, including rheumatoid arthritis and gout.[77,78]

Rheumatoid Arthritis

When bilateral hip joint effusion and periarticular osseous erosions are identified on MRI, rheumatoid arthritis should be suspected (Fig. 102-43).[78] In addition to an effusion, synovial membrane thickening may be identified, related to villous hypertrophy and pannus formation. The synovial proliferation and hyperemia are particularly pronounced on MRI studies performed following gadolinium contrast administration. T1-weighted fat-saturated images obtained immediately following intravenous injection of gadolinium contrast differentiate inflammatory capsular thickening and pannus from effusion.[79,80]

Pigmented Villonodular Synovitis

Pigmented villonodular synovitis (PVNS) may manifest either as a monoarticular, proliferative synovitis or as a focal, nodular synovial mass. Although osseous erosions are identified in approximately 50% of diffuse synovitis cases, joint narrowing is less common. Histologically, fibroblasts, lipid-laden macrophages, and multinucleated giant cells are present and extensive hemosiderin deposition is identified.[81] These pathologic features account for the characteristic MRI appearance of PVNS. Because of the hemosiderin component, both the diffuse synovial proliferative and the focal nodular forms of PVNS tend to exhibit decreased signal intensity on all standard pulse sequences. On T2*-weighted gradient-echo acquisitions, magnetic susceptibility effects are often identified. Evidence of osseous erosion is also frequently observed.[82,83]

Synovial Osteochondromatosis

Synovial osteochondromatosis manifests as a solitary synovial mass, like nodular PVNS, or as multiple intra-articular loose bodies. These lesions result from synovial metaplasia, forming cartilaginous foci that may calcify or ossify. The nodules may remain attached to the synovial membrane or they may detach and migrate within the joint, contributing to the development of chondral injury and osteoarthritis. On MRI, cartilaginous and calcified nodules exhibit decreased signal intensity on both T1- and T2-weighted imaging, whereas ossified lesions manifest a signal intensity pattern isointense with bone marrow (Fig. 102-44).[84]

Bursitis

The trochanteric bursa is located adjacent to the greater trochanter and covers the lateral aspect of the gluteus medius insertion. The subgluteus medius bursa and subgluteus minimus bursa also contribute to the trochanteric bursal complex.[85] These bursae facilitate the action of the abductors and external rotators of the hip. Trochanteric bursitis may result from acute or repetitive trauma. In the case of acute trauma, bursal fluid accumulation may develop secondary to the application of an external force or contusion (e.g., fall onto the hip) or secondary to internal traction stress associated with an acute gluteus medius strain (Fig. 102-45).[67] Just as subacromial and subdeltoid bursitis may occur in the context of supraspinatus tendinosis and peritendinitis, overuse tendinopathy of the gluteus medius may be associated with fluid accumulation involving the trochanteric bursa. Trochanteric bursitis frequently represents a component of the pathology related to greater trochanteric pain syndrome, a condition with a predilection for middle-aged and elderly women (Fig. 102-46).[68] Patients present with lateral hip pain and tenderness and treatment often involves local injection of steroids. MRI studies reveal distension of the bursal

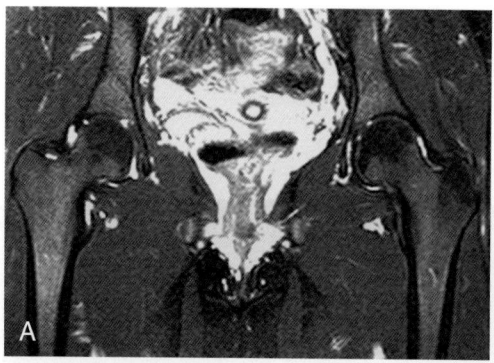

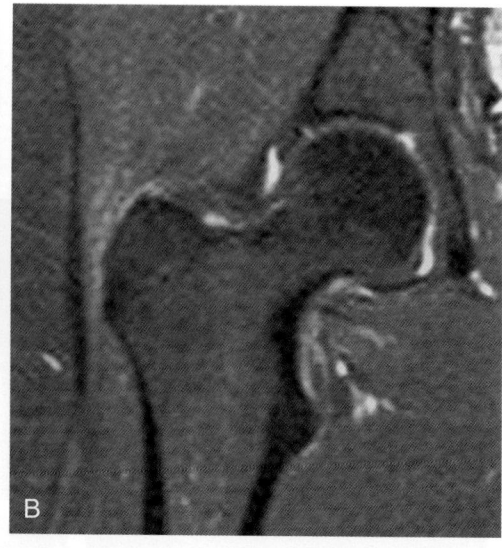

FIGURE 102-54

Acetabular labral tear involving the right hip in a 27-year-old female with groin pain, surgically proven. **A,** Coronal fat-saturated T2-weighted image. Hyperintense synovial fluid penetrates into the undersurface of the right acetabular labrum. A small right hip joint effusion is present. Note the normal left acetabular labrum for comparison. **B,** Coronal fat-saturated T1-weighted image obtained following the intravenous administration of gadolinium contrast material. The tear of the undersurface of the right acetabular labrum is defined by diffusion of gadolinium into the synovial fluid.

REFERENCES

1. Mont MA, Hungerford DS: Non-traumatic avascular necrosis of the femoral head. J Bone Joint Surg Am 77:459-474, 1995.
2. Jaffe WL, Epstein M, Heyman N, et al: The effect of cortisone on femoral and humeral heads in rabbits. An experimental study. Clin Orthop 82:221-228, 1972.
3. Wang GJ, Rawles JG, Hubbard SL, et al: Steroid-induced femoral head pressure changes and their response to lipid-clearing agents. Clin Orthop 174:298-302, 1983.
4. Kawai K, Tamaki A, Hirohata K: Steroid-induced accumulation of lipid in the osteocytes of the rabbit femoral head. A histochemical and electron microscopic study. J Bone Joint Surg Am 67:755-763, 1985.
5. Smith DW: Is avascular necrosis of the femoral head the result of inhibition of angiogenesis? Med Hypotheses 49:497-500, 1997.
6. Vogler III JB, Murphy WA: Bone marrow imaging. Radiology 168:679-693, 1988.
7. Glimcher MJ, Kenzora JE: The biology of osteonecrosis of the human femoral head and its clinical implications. Clin Orthop 138:284-309, 139:283-312, 140:273-312, 1979.
8. Mankin HJ: Nontraumatic necrosis of bone (osteonecrosis). N Engl J Med 326:1473-1479, 1992.
9. Ficat RP: Idiopathic bone necrosis of the femoral head. Early diagnosis and treatment. J Bone Joint Surg Br 67:3-9, 1985.
10. Steinberg ME, Hayken GD, Steinberg DR: A quantitative system for staging avascular necrosis. J Bone Joint Surg Br 77:34-41, 1995.
11. Totty WG, Murphy WA, Ganz WI, et al: Magnetic resonance imaging of the normal and ischemic femoral head. Am J Roentgenol 143:1273-1280, 1984.
12. Robinson HJ, Hartleben PD, Lund G, et al: Evaluation of magnetic resonance imaging in the diagnosis of osteonecrosis of the femoral head. J Bone Joint Surg Am 71:650-663, 1989.
13. Mitchell DG, Kressel HY, Arger PH, et al: Avascular necrosis of the femoral head: morphologic assessment by MR imaging, with CT correlation. Radiology 161:739-742, 1986.
14. Beltran J, Herman LJ, Burk JM, et al: Femoral head avascular necrosis: MR imaging with clinical-pathologic and radionuclide correlation. Radiology 166:215-220, 1988.
15. Hauzeur JP, Pasteels JL, Schoutens A, et al: The diagnostic value of magnetic resonance imaging in non-traumatic osteonecrosis of the femoral head. J Bone Joint Surg Am 71:641-649, 1989.
16. Beltran J, Knight CT, Zuelzer WA, et al: Core decompression for avascular necrosis of the femoral head: correlation between long-term results and preoperative MR staging. Radiology 174:533-536, 1990.
17. Mitchell DG, Rao VM, Kalinka MK, et al: Femoral head avascular necrosis: correlation of MR imaging, radiographic staging, radionuclide imaging, and clinical findings. Radiology 162:709-715, 1987.
18. Mitchell DG, Kressel HY, Rao VM, et al: The unique MRI appearance of the reactive interface in avascular necrosis: the double-line sign. Magn Reson Imaging 5(Suppl 1):41, 1987.
19. Zurlo JV: The double-line sign. Radiology 212:541-542, 1999.
20. Koo K, Ahn I, Kim R, et al: Bone marrow edema and associated pain in early stage osteonecrosis of the femoral head: prospective study with serial MR images, Radiology 213:715-722, 1999.
21. Iida S, Harada Y, Shimizu K, et al: Correlation between bone marrow edema and collapse of the femoral head in steroid-induced osteonecrosis. Am J Roentgenol 174:735-743, 2000.
22. Hayes CW, Conway WF, Daniel WW: MR imaging of bone marrow edema pattern: transient osteoporosis, transient bone marrow edema syndrome, or osteonecrosis, RadioGraphics 13:1001-1011, 1993.
23. Wilson AJ, Murphy WA, Hardy DC, et al: Transient osteoporosis: transient bone marrow edema? Radiology 167:757-760, 1988.
24. Bloem JL: Transient osteoporosis of the hip: MR imaging. Radiology 167:753-755, 1988.
25. Vande Berg BE, Malghem JJ, Labaisse MA, et al: MR imaging of avascular necrosis and transient marrow edema of the femoral head. RadioGraphics 13:501-520, 1993.
26. Guerra JJ, Steinberg ME: Distinguishing transient osteoporosis from avascular necrosis of the hip. J Bone Joint Surg Am 77:616-624, 1995.
27. Vande Berg BC, Malghem JJ, Lecouvet FE, et al: Idiopathic bone marrow edema lesions of the femoral head: predictive value of MR imaging findings. Radiology 212:527-535, 1999.
28. Rafii M, Mitnick H, Klug J, et al: Insufficiency fracture of the femoral head: MR imaging in three patients. Am J Roentgenol 168:159-163, 1997.
29. Lang P, Mauz M, Schörner W, et al: Acute fracture of the femoral neck: assessment of femoral head perfusion with gadopentetate demeglumine-enhanced MR imaging. Am J Roentgenol 160:335-341, 1993.
30. MacDougall L, Conway WF: Controversies in magnetic resonance imaging of the hip. Top Magn Reson Imag 8:44-50, 1996.
31. Nadel SN, Debatin JF, Richardson WJ, et al: Detection of acute avascular necrosis of the femoral head in dogs: dynamic contrast-enhanced MR imaging vs spin-echo and STIR sequences. Am J Roentgenol 159:1255-1261, 1992.
32. Weinstein SL: Legg-Calvé-Perthes syndrome. In Pediatric Orthopedics, vol 2. Lippincott-Raven, Philadelphia, 1996.
33. Catterall A: The natural history of Perthes disease. J Bone Joint Surg Br 53:37-53, 1971.
34. Jaramillo D, Kasser JR, Villegas-Medina OL, et al: Cartilaginous abnormalities and growth disturbances in Legg-Calvé-Perthes disease: evaluation with MR imaging, Radiology 197:767-773, 1995.
35. Rush BH, Bramson RT, Ogden JA: Legg-Calvé-Perthes disease: detection of cartilaginous and synovial change with MR imaging. Radiology 167:473-476, 1988.
36. Ducou le Pointe H, Haddad S, Silberman B, et al: Legg-Calvé-Perthes disease: staging by MRI using gadolinium. Pediatr Radiol 24:88-91, 1994.

37. Egund N, Wingstrand H: Legg-Calvé-Perthes disease: imaging with MR. Radiology 179:89-92, 1991.
38. Jaramillo D, Galen TA, Winalski CS, et al: Legg-Calve-Perthes disease: MR imaging evaluation during manual positioning of the hip—comparison with conventional arthrography. Radiology 212:519-525, 1999.
39. Boles CA, El-Khoury GY: Slipped capital femoral epiphysis. RadioGraphics 17:809-823, 1997.
40. Borsa JJ, Peterson HA, Ehman RL: MR imaging of physeal bars. Radiology 199:683-687, 1996.
41. Jaramillo D, Laor T, Zaleske DJ: Indirect trauma to the growth plate: results of MR imaging after epiphyseal and metaphyseal injury in rabbits. Radiology 187:171-178, 1993.
42. May DA, Purins JL, Smith DK: MR imaging of occult traumatic fractures and muscular injuries of the hip and pelvis in elderly patients. Am J Roentgenol 166:1075-1078, 1996.
43. Deutsch AL, Mink JH, Waxman AD: Occult fractures of the proximal femur: MR imaging. Radiology 170:113-116, 1989.
44. Daffner RH, Pavlov H: Stress fractures: current concepts. Am J Roentgenol 159: 245-252, 1992.
45. Anderson MW, Greenspan A: Stress fractures. Radiology 199:1-12, 1996.
46. Lee JK, Yao L: Stress fractures: MR imaging. Radiology 169:217-220, 1988.
47. Blickenstaff LD, Morris JM: Fatigue fracture of the femoral neck. J Bone Joint Surg Am 48:1031-1047, 1966.
48. Fullerton LR, Snowdy HA: Femoral neck stress fractures. Am J Sports Med 16:365-377, 1988.
49. Slocum KA, Gorman JD, Puckett ML, et al: Resolution of abnormal MR signal intensity in patients with stress fractures of the femoral neck. Am J Roentgenol 168:1295-1299, 1997.
50. Paletta Jr GA, Andrish JT: Injuries about the hip and pelvis in the young athlete. Clin Sports Med 14:591-628, 1995.
51. Cooper KL, Beabout JW, McLeod RA: Supra-acetabular insufficiency fractures. Radiology 157:15-17, 1985.
52. Peh WCG, Pek-Lan K, Yin Y, et al: Imaging of pelvic insufficiency fractures. RadioGraphics 16:335-348, 1996.
53. Gibbon WW, Hession PR: Diseases of the pubis and pubic symphysis: MR imaging appearances. Am J Roentgenol 169:849-853, 1997.
54. Cooper KL, Beabout JW, Swee RG: Insufficiency fractures of the sacrum. Radiology 156:15-20, 1985.
55. Diel J, Ortiz O, Losada RA, et al: The sacrum: pathologic spectrum, multi-modality imaging, and subspecialty approach. RadioGraphics 21:83-104, 2001.
56. Major NM, Helms CA: Sacral fractures in long-distance runners. Am J Roentgenol 174:727-729, 2000.
57. Murphy MD, Wetzel LH, Bramble JM, et al: Sacroiliitis: MR imaging findings. Radiology 180:239-244, 1991.
58. Kransdorf MJ, Stull MA, Gilkey FW, et al: Osteoid osteoma. RadioGraphics 11:671-696, 1991.
59. Assoun J, Richardi G, Railhac JJ, et al: Osteoid osteoma: MR imaging vs CT. Radiology 191:217-223, 1994.
60. Hayes CW, Conway WF, Sundaram M: Misleading aggressive MR imaging appearance of some benign musculoskeletal lesions. RadioGraphics 12:1119-1134, 1992.
61. Liu PT, Chivers FX, Roberts CC, et al: Imaging of osteoid osteoma with dynamic gadolinium-enhanced MR imaging. Radiology 227:691-7000, 2003.
62. Bloem JL, Mulder JD: Chondroblastoma: a clinical and radiological study of 104 cases. Skeletal Radiol 14:1-9, 1985.
63. Weatherall PT, Maale GE, Mendelsohn DB, et al: Chondroblastoma: classic and confusing appearance at MR imaging. Radiology 190:467-474, 1994.
64. Fleckenstein JL, Weatherall PT, Parkey RW, et al: Sports-related muscle injuries: evaluation with MR imaging. Radiology 172:793-798, 1989.
65. Palmer WE, Kuong SJ, Elmadbouh HM: MR imaging of myotendinous strain. Am J Roentgenol 173:703-709, 1999.
66. De Smet AA: Magnetic resonance findings in skeletal muscle tears. Skeletal Radiol 22:479-484, 1993.
67. Chung CB, Robertson JE, Cho GJ, et al: Gluteus medius tendon tears and avulsive injuries in elderly women: imaging findings in six patients. Am J Roentgenol 173:351-353, 1999.
68. Kingzett-Taylor A, Tirman PFJ, Feller J, et al: Tendinosis and tears of gluteus medius and minimus muscles as a cause of hip pain: MR imaging findings. Am J Roentgenol 173:1123-1126, 1999.
69. Brandser EA, El-Khoury GY, Kathol MH, et al: Hamstring injuries: radiographic, conventional tomography, CT, and MR imaging characteristics. Radiology 197:257-262, 1995.
70. De Smet AA, Best TM: MR imaging of the distribution and location of acute hamstring injuries in athletes. Am J Roentgenol 174:393-399, 2000.
71. Pomeranz SJ, Heidt, Jr RS: MR imaging in the prognostication of hamstring injury. Radiology 189:879-900, 1993.
72. Robinson DR: Piriformis syndrome in relation to sciatic pain. Am J Surg 73:355-358, 1947.
73. Benson ER, Schutzer SF: Posttraumatic piriformis syndrome: diagnosis and results of operative treatment. J Bone Joint Surg Am 81:941-949, 1999.
74. Spock A: Transient synovitis of the hip in children. Pediatrics 24:1042-1049, 1959.
75. Adams JA: Transient synovitis of the hip joint in children. J Bone Joint Surg Br 45: 471-476, 1963.
76. Lee SK, Suh KJ, Kim YW, et al: Septic arthritis versus transient synovitis at MR imaging: preliminary assessment with signal intensity alterations in bone marrow. Radiology 211:459-465, 1999.
77. Yulish BS, Liberman JM, Newman AJ, et al: Juvenile rheumatoid arthritis: assessment with MR imaging. Radiology 165:153-157, 1987.
78. Beltran J, Caudill JL, Herman LA: Rheumatoid arthritis: MR imaging manifestations. Radiology 165:153-157, 1987.
79. Adam G, Dammer M, Bohndorf K, et al: Rheumatoid arthritis of the knee: value of gadopentetate dimeglumine-enhanced MR imaging. Am J Roentgenol 56:125-129, 1991.
80. Hervé-Somma CMP, Sebag GH, Prieur AM, et al: Juvenile rheumatoid arthritis of the knee: MR evaluation with Gd-DOTA. Radiology 182:93-98, 1992.
81. Dorwart RH, Genant HK, Johnston WH, et al: Pigmented villonodular synovitis of synovial joints: clinical, pathologic, and radiologic features. Am J Roentgenol 143:877-885, 1984.
82. Bravo SM, Winalski CS, Weissman BN: Pigmented villonocular synovitis. Radiol Clin North Am 34:311-326, 1996.
83. Lin J, Jacobson JA, Jamadar DA, et al: Pigmented villonodular synovitis and related lesions: the spectrum of imaging findings. Am J Roentgenol 172:191-197, 1999.
84. White EM: Magnetic resonance imaging in synovial disorder and arthropathy of the knee. MRI Clin North Am 2:451-461, 1994.
85. Pfirrmann CWA, Chung CB, Theumann NH, et al: Greater trochanter of the hip: attachment of the abductor mechanism and a complex of three bursae—MR imaging and MR bursography in cadavers and MR imaging in asymptomatic volunteers. Radiology 221:469-477, 2001.
86. Robinson P, White LM, Agur A, et al: Obturator externus bursa: anatomic origin and MR imaging features of pathologic involvement. Radiology 228:230-234, 2003.
87. Varma DGK, Richli WR, Charnsangavej C, et al: MR appearance of the distended iliopsoas bursa. Am J Roentgenol 156:1025-1028, 1991.
88. Vaccaro JJP, Sauser DD, Beals RK: Iliopsoas bursa imaging: efficacy in depicting abnormal iliopsoas tendon motion in patients with internal snapping hip syndrome. Radiology 197:853-856, 1995.
89. Hodler J, Yu JS, Goodwin D, et al: MR arthrography of the hip: improved imaging of the acetabular labrum with histologic correlation in cadavers. Am J Roentgenol 165:887-891, 1995.
90. Steinbach LS, Palmer WE, Schweitzer ME: MR arthrography. RadioGraphics 22: 1223-1246, 2002.
91. Czerny C, Hofmann S, Neuhold A, et al: Lesions of the acetabular labrum: accuracy of MR imaging and MR arthrography in detection and staging. Radiology 200:225-230, 1996.
92. Drapé, JL, Thelen P, Gay-Depassier P, et al: Intraarticular diffusion of Gd-DOTA after intravenous injection in the knee: MR imaging evaluation. Radiology 188:227-234, 1993.
93. Winalski CS, Aliabadi P, Wright RJ, et al: Enhancement of joint fluid with intravenously administered gadopentetate dimeglumine: technique, rationale, and implications. Radiology 187:179-185, 1993.
94. Magee T, Hinson G: Association of paralabral cysts with acetabular disorders. Am J Roentgenol 174:1381-1384, 2000.
95. Petersilge CA, Haque MA, Petersilge WJ, et al: Acetabular labral tears: evaluation with MR arthrography. Radiology 200:231-235, 1996.
96. Lage LA, Patel JV, Villar RN: The acetabular labral tear: an arthroscopic classification. Arthroscopy 12:269-272, 1996.
97. Mason JB: Acetabular labral tears in the athlete. Clin Sports Med 20:779-790, 2001.

CHAPTER 103

KNEE

Carolyn M. Sofka ● Hollis G. Potter

TECHNICAL CONSIDERATIONS

Technical specifications for magnetic resonance (MR) imaging of the knee will depend largely on the hardware and software available (high versus low field strength units) as well as clinical familiarity with various pulse sequences. Most clinical MR units are traditional, closed high field strength (1.0-1.5 T) magnets and provide higher signal-to-noise ratios than their lower field strength counterparts. Open, low field strength units, however, are becoming more popular in the outpatient setting, especially with patients who have varying degrees of claustrophobia. Satisfactory diagnostic accuracy can be achieved with these lower field strength units, although the need to increase the number of excitations to produce acceptable diagnostic images can result in longer exam times.[1] A recent study demonstrated 91-93% accuracy for diagnosing medial meniscal tears, 88-90% accuracy for diagnosing lateral meniscal tears and 93-96% accuracy for diagnosing anterior cruciate ligament tears on a 0.2 T MR unit.[2] In another series of 114 patients evaluated with both 1.5 T and 0.5 T, no difference in accuracy, sensitivity or specificity for diagnosing anterior cruciate ligament tears was encountered between different field strengths, although there was a slightly longer imaging time with the 0.5 T unit.[3] The largest pitfall in the use of open constructs for standardized knee evaluation has been the limited ability to detect articular cartilage lesions, particularly if they are partial thickness.[4]

The knee is imaged with the patient supine and knee extended and in slight external rotation. A quadrature or phased array coil is typically recommended to maximize signal to noise. Early studies with a solenoid surface coil led to marked improvement in spatial resolution and diagnostic abilities.[5] The dynamic behavior of the ligamentous stabilizers of the knee can be demonstrated with kinematic MR imaging, although specialized coil designs are required.[6,7]

In general, three planes of imaging (axial, sagittal, and coronal) are obtained. Other tomographic imaging planes, such as the oblique sagittal projection for evaluating the anterior cruciate ligament, can be prescribed as desired.[8] At least one fat suppression sequence should be performed to "rescale" the contrast range and increase conspicuity of soft-tissue edema, fluid collections, and bone marrow edema. In a high field strength system, acceptable fat suppression can be achieved with either frequency-selective fat suppression or short tau inversion recovery (STIR). Sensitivity and specificity for bone marrow contusions utilizing fast spin-echo fat suppression and fast spin-echo STIR have been shown to be equal if not slightly superior to conventional STIR and the long imaging times of conventional STIR sequences limit their practical usefulness in a clinical setting.[9]

Conventional and fast spin-echo imaging may be utilized in clinical MR imaging of the knee (Box 103-1). The longer imaging times for conventional spin-echo sequences, in general, prohibit their utility in a busy clinical practice and this, combined with the superior signal-to-noise ratio achieved with fast spin-echo techniques (due to the stimulated echo contribution), has resulted in the faster techniques serving as the mainstay for most knee protocols. Parameter modifications with fast spin-echo imaging can result in competitive diagnostic image quality compared with conventional spin-echo

Box 103-1	Suggested Protocol for Routine Imaging of the Knee
Coronal fast spin-echo	TR 4000-4500/TE 34 (effective); FOV 11-13 cm; matrix 512 × 256; ETL 8-16; THK 3.0 mm; skip 0 mm; NEX 2; frequency right to left; BW 32 kHz
Sagittal fast spin-echo (fat suppression)	TR 3500-4000/TE 40 (effective); FOV 16 cm; matrix 256 × 224; ETL 8-14; THK 3.5-4 mm; skip 0 mm; NEX 2; frequency anterior to posterior; fat suppression; BW 20.8 kHz
Sagittal fast spin-echo	TR 4000-4500/TE 34-40 (effective); FOV 16 cm; matrix 512 × 288-384; ETL 8-16; THK 3.5 mm; skip 0 mm; NEX 2; frequency anterior to posterior; BW 32 kHz
Axial fast spin-echo	TR 4500/TE 34-40 (effective); FOV 14 cm; matrix 512 × 256-384; ETL 10-12; THK 3.5 mm; skip 0 mm; NEX 2; frequency anterior to posterior; SAT pulse; BW 32 kHz
Sagittal fast spin-echo (for the menisci)	TR 2300/TE 13 (effective); matrix 256 × 224; ETL 4-5; NEX 2; magnification factor 1.5; BW 20.8 kHz

BW, bandwidth (kHz); ETL, echo train length; TR, repetition time (ms); TE, echo time (ms); FOV, field of view (cm); THK, slice thickness (mm); NEX, number of excitations.

images. The faster *k*-space filling of the fast spin-echo techniques, combined with tight interecho spacing, allows for improved spatial resolution and limited blurring within acceptable imaging times. Clinical applications of fast spin-echo imaging of the knee have been demonstrated in the evaluation of a variety of pathologies of internal derangement of the knee, including cruciate ligament tears, meniscal, and cartilage lesions.[10-12]

Several authors have noted improved diagnostic accuracy of internal derangement of the knee with intra-articular injection of gadolinium (MR arthrography). A concentration of 2 mM of gadolinium is suggested for maximum signal intensity.[13,14] A small test injection of non-ionic contrast is suggested to confirm accurate needle placement under fluoroscopy followed by injection of approximately 20-30 mL total fluid in the knee.[14] Post-contrast administration, T1 fat suppression images are acquired, taking advantage of the T1-shortening effects of the gadolinium.

THE POSTOPERATIVE KNEE

Imaging the postoperative patient with indwelling orthopedic hardware can present a challenge. A working knowledge of orthopedic fixation hardware is necessary for appropriate image interpretation, technical parameter modification, and recognition of complications. Appropriate technical parameter modifications can result in diagnostic images in the postoperative setting, even in the presence of bulky metal components such as total knee arthroplasty.[15] The composition and relative ferromagnetism of the hardware have important implications for the ultimate artifact generated. Titanium, for example, results in minimal detectable artifact compared with other metallic substances such as cobalt, chrome or stainless steel.

The biologic behavior of bioabsorbable fixation materials, in addition to metal, results in a variety of MR appearances. A prospective study evaluating bioabsorbable interference screws in the setting of anterior cruciate ligament reconstruction demonstrated a morphologic change in the appearance of the screws and the adjacent bone over time.[16] The bioabsorbable screw was noted to be present in the immediate postoperative time frame (1-3 months) and was no longer visible as a discrete hypointense structure by 6 months. Adjacent bone marrow edema and, in some cases, small fluid collections about the femoral surgical site lasted longer, up to approximately 12 months.[16] A temporal change has also been demonstrated with polydioxanone biodegradable pins, with complete resorption of the pins taking up to 24 months or longer.[17]

The presence of metal yields characteristic artifacts including geometric distortion in the frequency-encoding direction, signal intensity loss due to diffusion and intravoxel dephasing in gradient-echo imaging.[18] Gradient-echo imaging, advocated by some for routine imaging of the menisci and cartilage, is of limited utility in the postoperative setting. The absence of 180° refocusing pulses results in marked signal loss due to diffusion and extensive image distortion. Increased intravoxel dephasing (T2* decay) then results in large areas of signal void.[19]

Additional imaging considerations include the selection of a water-sensitive pulse sequence. Fast inversion recovery is suggested as opposed to frequency-selective fat suppression, as it is less susceptible to regional magnetic field inhomogeneities, such as those encountered in the presence of metal.

Fast spin-echo imaging is favored over conventional spin-echo imaging in the postoperative patient with metal. Decreased interecho spacing allows for less time for spin dephasing and resultant increased signal.[20,21] Longer echo train lengths combined with shorter interecho spacing result in less image distortion in the presence of magnetic field inhomogeneities by decreasing the chance of spins being incorrectly mapped.[22] Conventional spin-echo imaging produces relatively long segments of time between 180° refocusing

Box 103-2	Suggested Protocol for Imaging the Postoperative Knee
Coronal fast spin-echo	TR 4000-5000/TE 34 (effective); ETL 12-18; FOV 16 cm; BW 62 kHz; THK 3 mm; skip 0 mm; matrix 512 × 288; NEX 4-5
Sagittal inversion recovery	TR 4000-5000/TE 17 (effective); inversion time 150 ms; FOV 20-22 cm; BW 32 kHz; THK 4 mm; skip 0 mm; matrix 256 × 224; NEX 2
Sagittal fast spin-echo	TR 4000-5000/TE 34 (effective); ETL 12-18; FOV 18 cm; BW 62 kHz; THK 3.5 mm; skip 0 mm; matrix 512 × 288; NEX 4-5
Axial fast spin-echo	TR 4000-5000/TE 34 (effective); ETL 12-18; FOV 16 cm; BW 62 kHz; THK 3 mm; skip 0 mm; matrix 512 × 288; NEX 4-5

BW, bandwidth (kHz); ETL, echo train length; TR, repetition time (ms); TE, echo time (ms); FOV, field of view (cm); THK, slice thickness (mm); NEX, number of excitations.

pulses, allowing for increased dephasing and increased image distortion.

Increased readout bandwidths (62.5 kHz) are suggested to decrease the degree of linear misregistration artifact. Higher receiver bandwidths (82 kHz) have traditionally been of limited usefulness due to the large fields of view required to maintain acceptable signal to noise; however, new high speed gradients and improved software platforms may make the utility of such higher readout gradient strengths more feasible in a busy clinical practice. A suggested protocol for imaging the postoperative knee is given in Box 103-2.

MAGNETIC RESONANCE ANGIOGRAPHY

Magnetic resonance angiography of the knee in the orthopedic patient is generally performed in the post-traumatic setting, often in the case of reported knee dislocation. In the absence of orthopedic hardware, a general overview of the popliteal artery and proximal trifurcation vessels can be obtained with a noncontrast two-dimensional time-of-flight technique.[23] If more detailed evaluation of the branch vessels, such as the geniculate arteries, is required or if orthopedic hardware is present in the knee, contrast-enhanced technique is necessary.

Contrast-enhanced angiography of the knee has proven to be clinically useful in the setting of acute or subacute knee dislocation.[24] Small intimal flaps in the popliteal artery can be demonstrated at the same time as the diagnostic MR scan is being performed.[24] In the acute or subacute post-traumatic setting, capsular and meniscocapsular hyperemia from the geniculate vessels can be visualized.

Anatomically, the location of the major vessels in the posterior aspect of the knee provides an advantage when performing magnetic resonance angiography of the knee in the patient with orthopedic hardware, as the hardware is not directly adjacent to the neurovascular bundle (Fig. 103-1). Slice and slab thickness should be adjusted to provide maximum resolution, giving thought

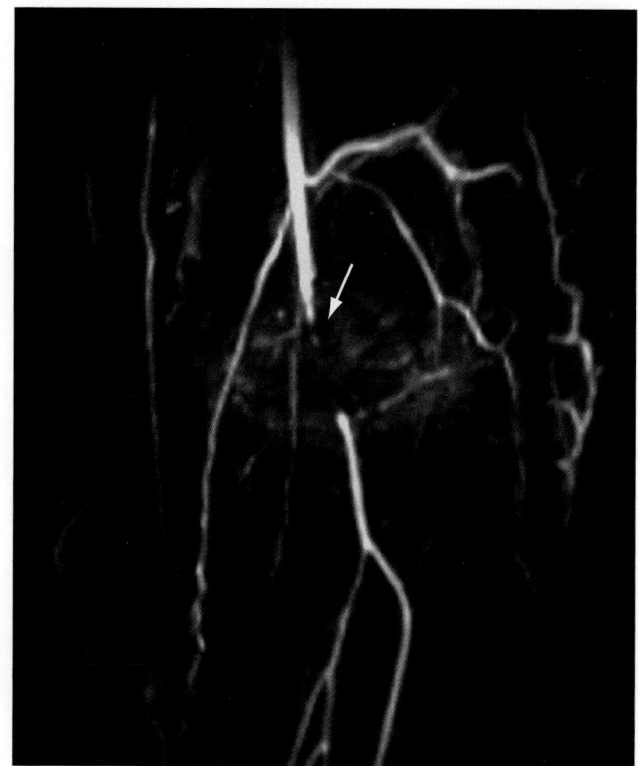

FIGURE 103-1

Three-dimensional contrast-enhanced magnetic resonance angiogram in a patient post primary vascular repair for popliteal artery laceration during total knee arthroplasty placement and subsequent loss of distal pulses. Contrast-enhanced MR angiogram with the prosthetic cement spacer in place demonstrates abrupt tapering of the proximal aspect of the popliteal artery (*arrow*) with a several centimeter segment of absent flow, consistent with thrombosis of the venous patch graft. Note the intact distal run-off vessels.

to the total scan time; each run should be as short as possible (approximately 25-35 seconds), in order to achieve maximum contrast intensity in the arterial system. A suggested protocol for MR angiography of the popliteal fossa is given in Box 103-3.

Box 103-3	Suggested Protocol for MR Angiography of the Popliteal Fossa
Three-dimensional contrast-enhanced fast SPGR	TE min; FOV 22-24 cm; matrix 256 × 128; THK 1.3-2 mm; skip 0 mm; slices per slab 30-36; flip angle 30°; NEX 1-2; BW 31.2 kHz; VBW; NPW; ED 30 cc gadolinium; 10-15 s delay; 3 runs

BW, bandwidth (kHz); TE, echo time; FOV, field of view; THK, slice thickness; NEX, number of excitations; VBW, variable bandwidth; NPW, no phase wrap; ED, extended dynamic range.

LIGAMENTS

In general, a high field strength closed magnet is used to evaluate the knee. Lower field strength open units are, however, increasing in popularity. Equivocal sensitivity, specificity, and accuracy for diagnosing anterior cruciate ligament tears have been demonstrated between 1.5 T and 0.5 T units.[25]

Variations in tomographic multiplanar imaging sequences have been used with varying success in the diagnosis of anterior cruciate ligament (ACL) tears. Oblique sagittal sequences in the plane of the anterior cruciate ligament have been shown to be more reliable in the diagnosis of intact anterior cruciate ligament fibers compared with direct parasagittal images in some centers.[26] Most often, sagittal images are inspected with the most scrutiny to evaluate for ACL tears. As the ACL can be very obliquely oriented and may not be imaged completely in one sagittal plane, utilizing axial and coronal sequences to supplement diagnostic evaluation is suggested.[27] Utilizing sagittal T1 images alone, 94% sensitivity for diagnosing ACL tears was demonstrated in one study, with improved sensitivity of 98% and specificity of 93% utilizing combined multiplanar imaging sequences.[27] Imaging the knee in a mild degree of flexion has also demonstrated improved conspicuity of the anterior cruciate ligament, although specialized coils are needed.[28]

The anterior and posterior cruciate ligaments are the major internal ligamentous stabilizers against anteroposterior translation and rotation of the knee. The anterior cruciate ligament arises at the inner margin of the lateral femoral condyle and courses in a somewhat oblique direction to insert at the anterior margin of the tibia, just medial to the midline. The posterior cruciate ligament arises from the posteromedial margin of the femur and inserts at the posterior margin of the tibia near the midline.

Normally, both the anterior and posterior cruciate ligaments should be hypointense on all MR pulse sequences due to their composition of predominantly type I collagen, which has a highly organized ultrastructure that limits the motion of water dipoles and accentuates dipole interactions, yielding rapid T2 decay (Fig. 103-2).[29] MRI and histologic correlation of the cruciate ligaments, however, have demonstrated that a

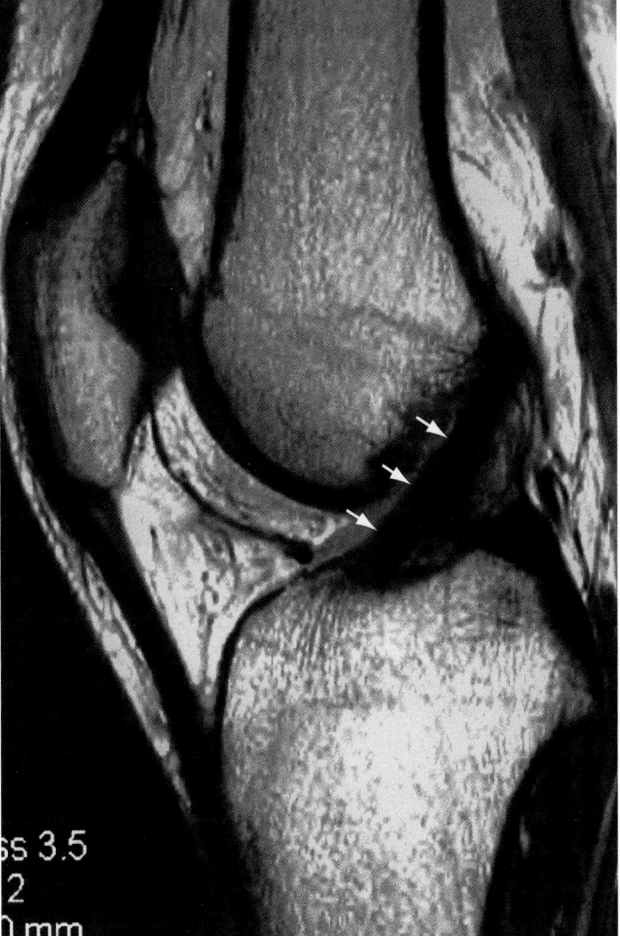

FIGURE 103-2

Sagittal fast spin-echo proton density-weighted image through the midline of the knee demonstrates the normal MR appearance of the anterior cruciate ligament. Note the normal homogeneously hypointense ligament fibers (*arrows*).

normal anterior cruciate ligament occasionally has linear areas of increased signal intensity within the ligament fibers.[30] Histologic examination of cadaver knees has demonstrated a complex intraligamentous architecture of the anterior cruciate ligament with some areas that are thinner than others, likely contributing to the generally observed high linear signal intensity within the anterior cruciate ligament, particularly due to intravoxel signal averaging from the adjacent intercondylar fat.[30] Complex synovial reflections exist around the cruciate ligaments, the integrity of which was of utmost importance in the practice of conventional arthrography. For MR imaging, it has been demonstrated that joint fluid, either native joint fluid or that introduced by MR arthrography, should not enter the deep triangular space between the anterior and posterior cruciate ligaments or either of the ligaments themselves.[31] The presence of fluid within either of these spaces is highly suggestive of injury to the cruciate ligaments.[31]

The most reliable, direct sign of an acute, complete anterior cruciate ligament tear is visualizing a discrete

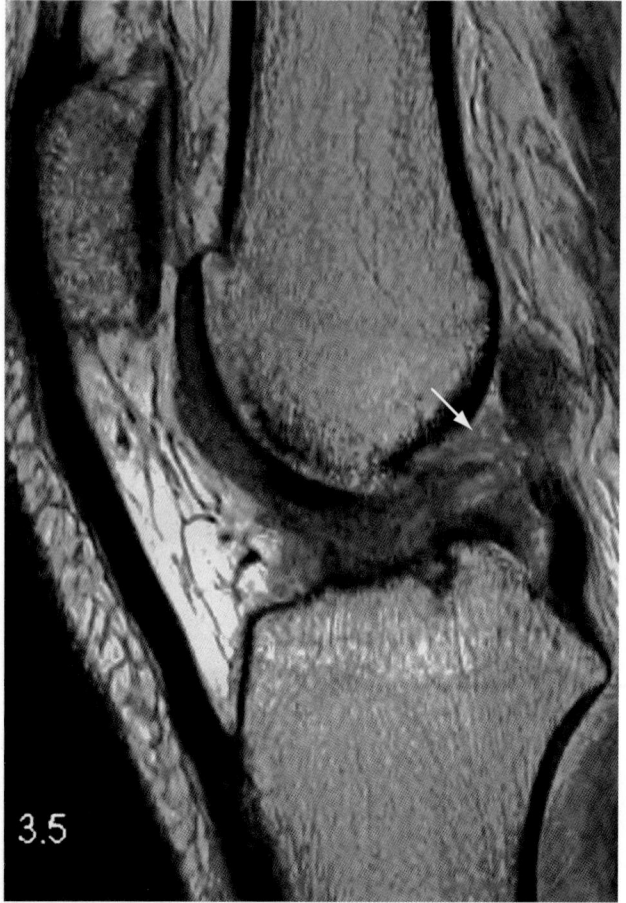

3.5

FIGURE 103-3

Sagittal fast spin-echo proton density-weighted sequence demonstrates complete tear of the junction of the proximal and middle thirds of the anterior cruciate ligament (*arrow*). Note the focal full-thickness ligamentous discontinuity (*arrow*) and the hyperintensity and inhomogeneity of the remaining fibers.

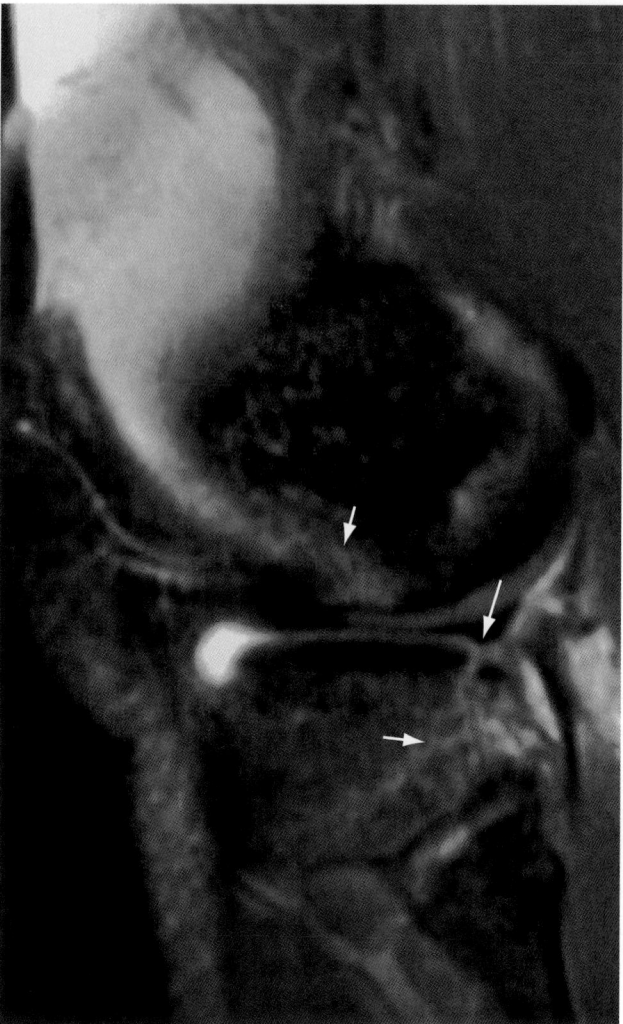

FIGURE 103-4

Sagittal fast spin-echo frequency-selective fat-suppressed image through the lateral femorotibial joint in a patient with a complete anterior cruciate ligament tear. Note the characteristic edema pattern in the anterolateral femoral condyle and the posterolateral tibial plateau (*short arrows*) as well as the frank transchondral fracture line through the posterior lateral tibial plateau (*long arrow*).

area of ligamentous discontinuity, often with a fluid-filled gap, where no hypointense ligament fibers can be traced in continuity (Fig. 103-3). Identifying this focal morphologic abnormality has a sensitivity of 96% and specificity of 94%.[32]

Multiple secondary signs, however, of varying specificities and sensitivities, can also be seen in cases of anterior cruciate ligament injury. These, in general, are a result of the mechanism of injury incurred during the initial insult. One study of 68 patients with anterior cruciate ligament injuries and arthroscopic correlation demonstrated a high specificity between the presence of bone bruising in the posterolateral tibial plateau and posterior displacement of the posterior horn of the lateral meniscus in cases of complete anterior cruciate ligament tears (Fig. 103-4).[33] Similarly, Brandser et al found the characteristic bone marrow contusion pattern in the posterolateral margin of the tibia and lateral femoral condyle to be the most helpful secondary sign of complete anterior cruciate ligament tears.[34] In yet another clinical series, 94% of patients with anterior

cruciate ligament tears had edema in the posterolateral tibial plateau and 91% in the lateral femoral condyle.[35] This characteristic edema pattern in the lateral compartment is caused by anterior subluxation of the tibia with respect to the femur with impaction against the posterolateral margin of the tibia after sufficient force is applied to an extended knee to injure the ACL, creating the pivot shift associated with an ACL disruption. This bone marrow edema pattern is reflective of a transchondral fracture and the presence of these contusions is not without clinical significance. It has been demonstrated that patients can have long-term progressive articular cartilage abnormalities after these injuries.[36] After acute subchondral fractures, osteochondral abnormalities, including cartilage thinning, full-thickness cartilage, and osteochondral defects, have been

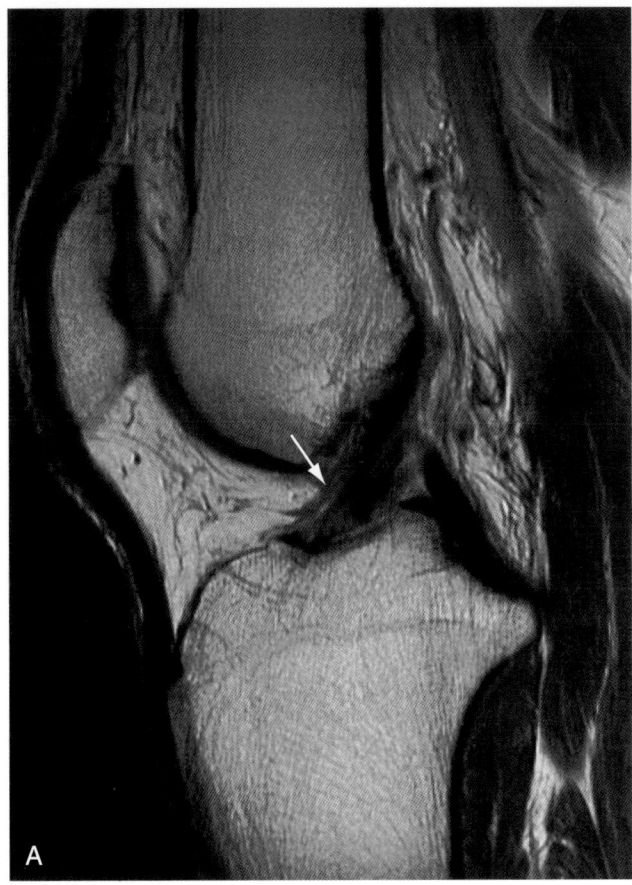

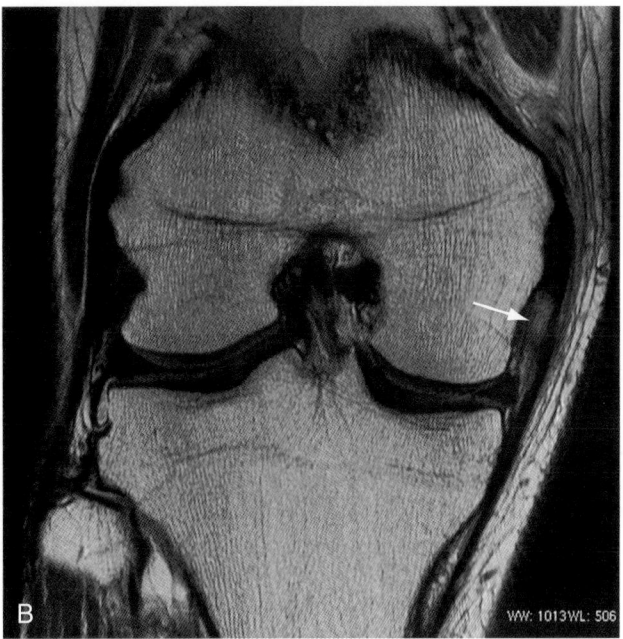

FIGURE 103-5

A, Sagittal fast spin-echo image demonstrates a partial tear of the distal anterior cruciate ligament, confirmed at arthroscopy (*arrow*). **B,** Coronal fast spin-echo image in the same patient demonstrates a partial deep surface tear of the medial collateral ligament (*arrow*).

seen at 6-12 months after injury.[37,38] Johnson et al obtained biopsies of these areas at the time of arthroscopy and noted chondrocyte degeneration, loss of proteoglycan, osteocyte necrosis, and empty lacunae degeneration, indicating that these injuries are not innocuous "bone bruises" but rather transchondral fractures of variable severity.[39] A variety of other secondary signs of anterior cruciate ligament injuries can be identified on MR images, of varying specificities and positive predictive values. Uncovering of the posterior horn of the lateral meniscus and anterior tibial translation, abnormal curvature (buckling) of the posterior cruciate ligament, abnormal posterior cruciate ligament line (drawing a tangent line to the posterior margin of the PCL and evaluating the relationship between it and the posterior cortex of the femur), and a deep lateral femoral notch due to osteochondral impaction have all been described in the setting of anterior cruciate ligament injuries.[34,40-44] Concomitant ligamentous injuries such as medial collateral and posterolateral corner injuries occur quite frequently in the setting of anterior cruciate ligament tears.[45]

The Segond fracture, typically identified on conventional radiographs, is an avulsion fracture of the lateral tibial rim, due to lateral capsular avulsion.[46] Geographic edema at the lateral capsular insertion in the presence of a complete anterior cruciate ligament tear should raise high suspicion for a Segond fracture on MR images, even if a discrete cortical fragment is not seen.[47] Anatomic studies, of note, have demonstrated that slips from the iliotibial band and anterior oblique band, extending from the fibular collateral ligament to the midportion of the lateral tibia, may also be partly responsible for the observed Segond fracture, suggesting the injury may be more complex.[48]

Other sites of bone marrow edema can be seen in the setting of anterior cruciate ligament injuries, likely due to the severe rotational forces encountered, such as posteromedial tibial plateau avulsion fractures at the insertion of the semimembranosus tendon or avulsion of the tibial attachment of the deep medial collateral ligament.[49,50]

In the pediatric patient, evaluation of the status of the physes should be performed as both transphyseal and physeal-sparing anterior cruciate ligament reconstructions can be performed.[51] At our institution, a fast spoiled gradient-echo sequence with fat suppression is typically performed in skeletally immature patients with a history of trauma.

A lower sensitivity (40-75%) and specificity (62-89%) have been reported for the MR diagnosis of partial anterior cruciate ligament tears; however, these results may reflect choice of parameters with relatively low spatial resolution (Fig. 103-5).[52] The presence of concomitant osseous injury in the lateral compartment is highly suggestive of high-grade partial ACL injury and the

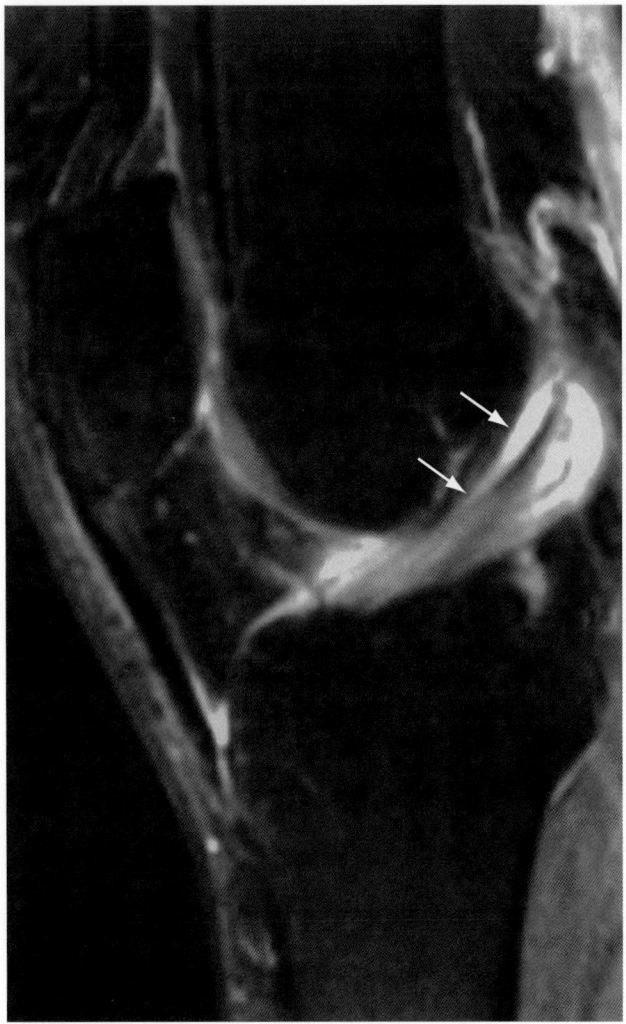

FIGURE 103-6

Sagittal fast spin-echo frequency-selective fat suppression image through the midline of the knee demonstrates ganglion formation of the anterior cruciate ligament (*arrows*). Note the smooth, linear intrasubstance hyperintensity with thickening of the ligament without fiber discontinuity.

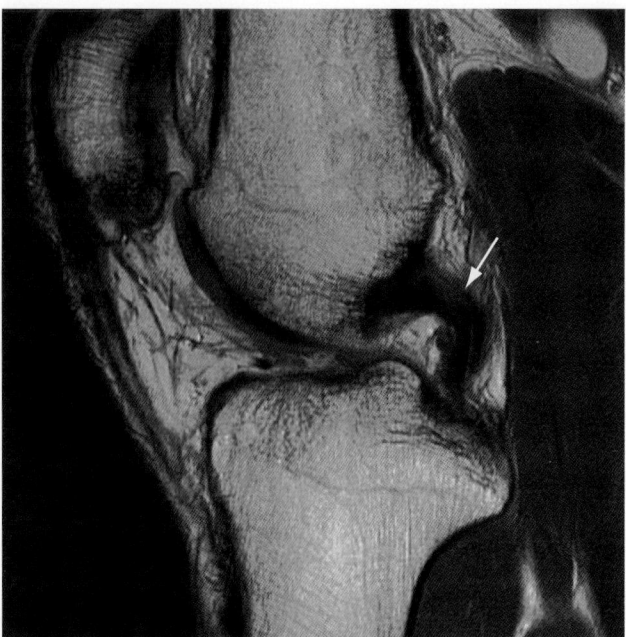

FIGURE 103-7

Sagittal fast spin-echo image in a patient post knee dislocation demonstrates tear of the posterior cruciate ligament from its insertion with retraction, buckling and hyperintensity of the more proximal ligament fibers (*arrow*).

identification of such an edema pattern should indicate that meticulous inspection of the anterior cruciate ligament is needed.[53] The alignment of the anterior cruciate ligament can suggest partial ACL injury, with decreased angle of inclination of the anterior cruciate ligament with respect to the articular surface of the tibial plateau in the setting of ACL injuries.[53]

Chronically torn anterior cruciate ligaments may be more difficult to diagnose. A large joint effusion and characteristic transchondral impaction fractures may not be present. The morphology of the anterior cruciate ligament becomes of utmost importance when diagnosing complete anterior cruciate ligament tears, with horizontal orientation of the distal fibers and fibrous scar formation.[54] Alternatively, the ligament may resorb, leading to excessive fat in the intercondylar notch.

Myxoid or mucoid degeneration of the anterior cruciate ligament can occur, resulting in inhomogeneity,

and hyperintensity of the ligament and should not be confused with a tear (Fig. 103-6).[55,56] In general, secondary signs of anterior cruciate ligament injury are not present and the ligament generally is much thicker than the morphology associated with a tear. Frank ganglion cyst formation within the cruciate ligaments can also occur and occasionally may result in mechanical symptoms requiring arthroscopic debridement.[57,58]

The posterior cruciate ligament is injured much less commonly than the anterior cruciate ligament. Generally, three mechanisms of injury can be implicated in cases of posterior cruciate ligament injury. These include:

1. a direct impaction on the anterior tibia with the knee flexed, forcing the tibia posteriorly
2. a hyperextension force (typically following initial anterior cruciate ligament failure), and
3. severe twisting or rotational forces, injuring the cruciate ligaments after the collateral ligaments have failed (Fig. 103-7).[59]

Associated findings such as cortical avulsion of the medial tibial plateau (medial "Segond" fracture) have been seen with injuries of the posterior cruciate ligament.[60] Abnormal morphology and signal intensity can persist in the injured posterior cruciate ligament both in the native as well as the postoperative state.[61,62] The intensity of the signal abnormality is a reflection of the pulse sequences utilized. Both conservatively treated PCL-injured knees and posterior cruciate ligament graft reconstructions can remain thickened and hyperintense at 1 year, particularly on short TE MR sequences, with the

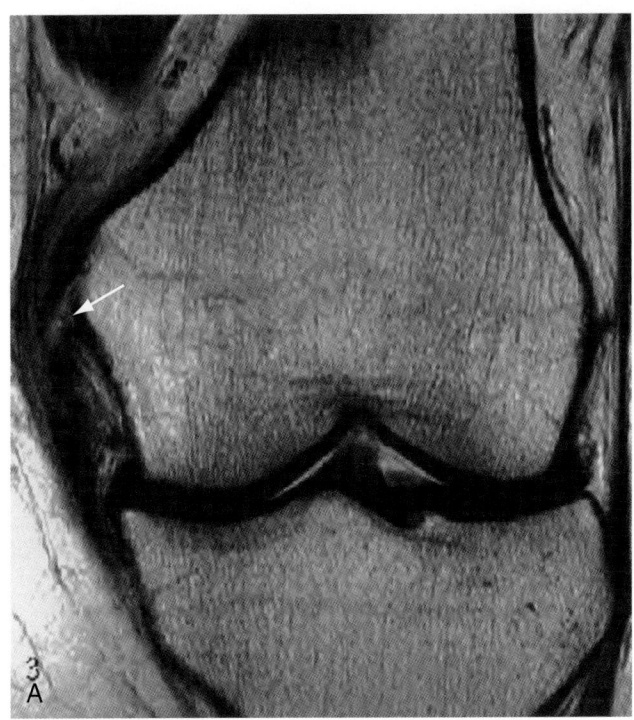
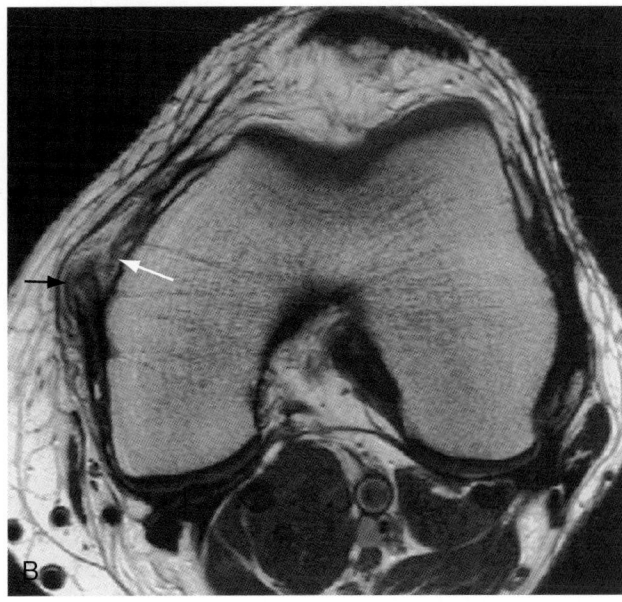

FIGURE 103-8

A, Coronal fast spin-echo MR image demonstrates high-grade proximal medial collateral ligament tear (*arrow*). Note the surrounding infiltration of the periligamentous fat and the thickening and hyperintensity of the ligament fibers. **B,** Axial fast spin-echo image in the same patient demonstrates the tear of the medial collateral ligament from the femur (*black arrow*). Note also the tear of the femoral origin of the medial patellofemoral ligament (*white arrow*). Potential extension of anterior medial collateral ligament tears into the medial patellofemoral ligament and/or retinaculum should be investigated in all cases.

MR imaging findings often lagging behind clinical improvement.[63,64] Following reconstruction, the variable signal intensity changes likely reflect the histologic progression of graft incorporation and are not necessarily indicative of functional failure.

Collateral Ligaments

The medial collateral ligament is composed of both deep and superficial fibers, with the deep portion of the ligament blending with the joint capsule. Three distinct layers of tissue can be identified along the medial joint line including the deep crural fascia, the superficial portion of the medial collateral ligament and the deepest layer, composed of the capsule, the deep portion of the medial collateral ligament, the meniscofemoral and meniscotibial extensions of the deep portion of the MCL and the patellomeniscal ligament.[65,66] The medial collateral ligament resists internal rotation and valgus stress with the knee in extension and anterior displacement of the tibia in cases of complete anterior cruciate ligament insufficiency.[67,68]

For the detection of medial collateral ligamentous injuries, Yao et al found edema in the subcutaneous fat adjacent to the medial collateral ligament, discontinuity or focal non-visualization of the medial collateral ligament, increased signal intensity within or deep to the medial collateral ligament, and longitudinal increased striations within the medial collateral ligament to be the most important morphologic criteria (Fig. 103-8).[69] These authors found that coronal T2-weighted sequences were the most helpful in evaluating medial collateral ligament injuries. Schweitzer et al similarly demonstrated high sensitivity of soft-tissue edema and ill definition of the ligament fibers contrasted with adjacent subcutaneous fat when evaluating for medial collateral ligament pathology.[70] Complete tears of the medial collateral ligament displaced into the medial femorotibial joint compartment can be mistaken for a displaced meniscal tear.[71]

In addition to the collateral ligaments, the multiple periarticular bursae around the knee can be visualized with MR. The semimembranosus-tibial collateral bursa is anatomically located between the semimembranosus tendon and the medial tibia, with the more distal superficial pocket between the semimembranosus tendon and the tibial collateral ligament anterior to the typical location of a popliteal cyst.[72,73] The tibial collateral bursa, located along the medial joint line, is not directly adherent to the medial meniscus but is located slightly more posteriorly.[74,75]

The posterolateral corner is an important yet often overlooked anatomic region about the knee. Generally patients with posterolateral corner injuries have sustained a twisting and/or hyperextension event of the knee and present with clinical symptoms of instability and feeling that the knee is "giving way" even without significant force.[76] While the standing apprehension test has high sensitivity for posterolateral corner injury and instability (typically examined at 30° and 90° with the patient prone and supine), occasionally posterolateral corner injuries can be subtle and unsuspected prior to MR diagnosis.[76] Prompt identification of posterolateral corner injuries is extremely important as optimal surgical repair (rare) or reconstruction (the standard) is done within 3 weeks of injury.[77]

Anatomic and MR imaging correlation has demonstrated in detail the anatomic structures comprising the posterolateral corner, including the medial and lateral limbs of the arcuate ligament, the fabellofibular ligament, popliteofibular ligament, popliteus tendon, fibular collateral ligament, and biceps femoris.[78,79] The popliteus is a thick, fan-shaped muscle that runs in an oblique course along the posterior aspect of the knee. As its course is oblique, that is, posteromedial to anterolateral, it serves as a rotatory stabilizer of the knee. The tendon, curving around the posterolateral margin of the knee, inserts onto the lateral femoral condyle. Injuries to the popliteus in the absence of a high-velocity injury or complete knee dislocation have been reported to most frequently involve the muscle; however, Westrich et al have demonstrated a not infrequent incidence of isolated popliteus tendon avulsions with a significant knee injury.[24,80,81] Proximal popliteus avulsion is typically associated with a bone marrow edema pattern in the central aspect of the femur, posterior to that seen in association with a patella dislocation (adjacent to the trochlea) or an ACL transchondral fracture (above the anterior horn of the lateral meniscus).

Plain film radiographs demonstrating a small avulsion fracture of the fibula can reflect severe soft-tissue damage to the posterolateral corner, including the fibular collateral ligament and biceps femoris, as well as other internal derangement of the knee including collateral ligament and meniscal tears (Fig. 103-9).[82,83]

Injury to the iliotibial band, located at the anterior margin of the lateral aspect of the knee, can result in localized anterolateral knee pain. Iliotibial band friction syndrome, often seen in runners with irritation of the tendon against the anterolateral femur, can be suggested on MR imaging by observing abnormal thickening and hyperintensity of the tendon, occasionally with fluid or debris within a bursa or posterior extension of the joint capsule just deep to the tendon.[84]

The Postoperative Anterior Cruciate Ligament

Knowledge of the surgical technique utilized in the setting of anterior cruciate ligament reconstruction is important when evaluating the postoperative knee. The completely disrupted anterior cruciate ligament may remodel over time, but has little capacity for self-restoration of its innate biomechanical properties. Rarely, a primary surgical repair of the disrupted ligament is performed; in most cases, the ligament is reconstructed

with tendon graft. The most common graft choices are currently central third patellar bone-tendon-bone autograft, hamstring (semitendinosus and gracilis) tendon autograft and, less commonly, quadriceps autograft or tendon allograft (cadaveric tissue). In revision cases, iliotibial band and prosthetic grafts may be encountered, although these have largely been replaced as a primary or revision graft of choice.[85] The technique utilized will depend largely on the surgeon's preference as well as, in the case of revision surgery, the graft source utilized in the index surgery, the bone tunnel size, and the presence of associated ligamentous trauma.[86] While treatment of anterior cruciate ligament injuries with radiofrequency thermal ablation has been reported, with abnormal morphology of the ACL persisting at 1 year, more long-term follow-up studies are necessary to more critically evaluate these techniques.[87]

Central third patellar bone-tendon-bone autograft is usually the most common construct encountered. With this procedure, the central third of the patellar tendon is harvested with bone plugs from the inferior pole of the patella and tibial tubercle and then fixed with interference screws.[85] When patients are imaged after surgery, it should be noted that the patellar tendon might not be completely normal in morphology, even after 1 year.[88] The presence of bone marrow edema usually dissipates by 15 months.[89]

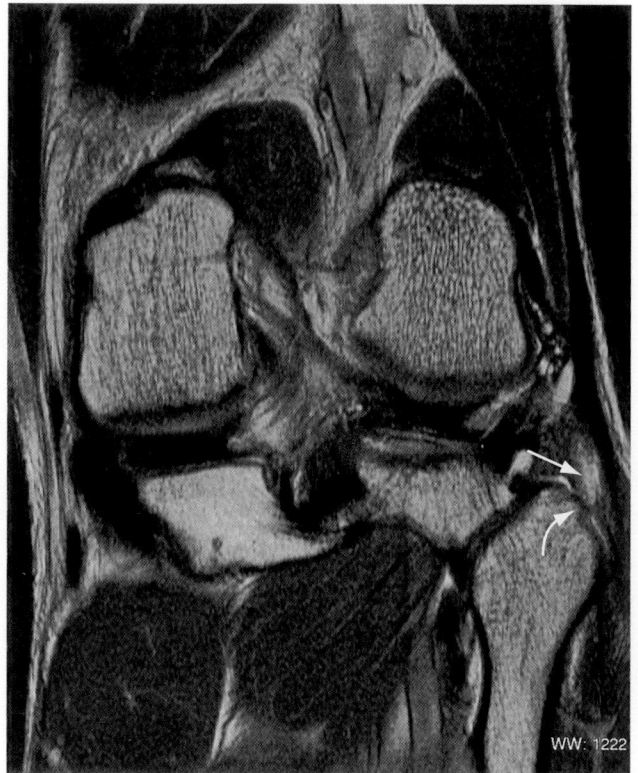

WW: 1222

FIGURE 103-9

Coronal fast spin-echo image demonstrates partial avulsion of the biceps femoris from the fibula (*arrow*) with associated non-displaced cortical avulsion fracture (*curved arrow*).

The femoral tunnel should ideally be placed posterosuperior to the origin of the native ACL origin, at the intersection of Blumensaats's line and the posterior margin of the lateral femoral cortex, and the tibial tunnel is 2-3 mm posterior to the epicenter of the tibial tunnel of the native ACL.[85,90] Evaluation of the morphology and alignment of the anterior cruciate ligament graft is commonly performed with MR imaging.[91] Abnormal signal within the graft may persist for months after surgery as well as thickening of the graft, which likely reflects the histologic continuum of "ligamentization" demonstrated by Jackson et al, including cellular necrosis, repopulation, revascularization, cellular proliferation, and collagen remodeling.[92] A knowledge of this progression is important in the interpretation of the reconstructed ligament for the first year following placement.

The anterior cruciate ligament construct should assume a smooth linear course without focal kinking or angulation (Fig. 103-10). Clinically stable grafts without impingement have been shown to have a steeper angle of obliquity on sagittal MR images compared with normal controls (67° compared with 51°).[93] As with the native anterior cruciate ligament, focal tears of the ACL construct are best diagnosed by observing discrete areas of graft discontinuity, often with characteristic transchondral fractures of the lateral compartment.[94] The secondary signs of ACL tear used in the evaluation of the native ACL (such as anterior tibial translation and uncovering of the posterior horn of the lateral meniscus) are less reliable following reconstruction due to the altered biomechanics of a reconstructed ligament that do not duplicate the optimized condition of an intact, native ligament. The method of fixation will have an impact on the MR appearance of the graft. Some bioabsorbable interference screws have been shown to disappear from magnetic resonance images by 6 months after surgery while other polylactic acid interference screws can persist at 16 and 24 months.[89,95] Bach et al found that interference screws made of polyglycolic acid and trimethylene carbonate had completely resorbed at 1 year with associated remodeling of the tunnels with mild, but stable, enlargement.[96]

Decreased range of motion after ACL reconstruction can be because of ACL tears, impingement or arthrofibrosis. The "Cyclops" lesion has been described, whereby a globular mass-like form of fibrous scar tissue impinges against the anterior cruciate ligament; however, more commonly, a more ill-defined infiltrative fibrotic process is encountered.[85,97,98] The focal deposition of fibrous tissue against the anterior synovial reflection of the ACL often indicates excessive anterior placement of the femoral tunnel, allowing the graft to impinge against the roof of the intercondylar notch. The local deposition of fibrous tissue should be differentiated from a global, cytokine-mediated arthrofibrosis.[99] In the latter setting, fibrosis of all capsular reflections is noted, including contraction of the posterior capsule and scarring of the deep infrapatellar fat pad. Identification of arthrofibrosis is important as it may be a severe impedance to knee function and can be treated surgically with debridement.[100] If untreated, arthrofibrosis can result in increased contact pressures and resultant osteoarthritis.

The Multiple Ligament-Injured Knee

After a complete knee dislocation, multiple ligamentous stabilizers can be damaged (Fig. 103-11). One series of 21 patients demonstrated multiple high grade as well as complete tears of the anterior and posterior cruciate ligaments, the medial collateral ligament, and the posterolateral corner structures.[24] One study of 17 patients with documented complete knee dislocation demonstrated all to have complete tears of the anterior cruciate ligament, while 15 had complete tears of the posterior cruciate ligament, nine had complete tears of the medial collateral ligament, and 12 had tears of the fibular collateral ligament.[101] Six patients had complete tears of the popliteus tendon.[101]

The range of injury to the neurovascular structures ranges from 4.8% in the popliteal artery in low-velocity dislocation to 45% in high-velocity injuries.[102,103] Peroneal nerve injury occurs with an incidence of 25-35%.[104,105] High-resolution magnetic resonance imaging after a knee dislocation can provide detailed

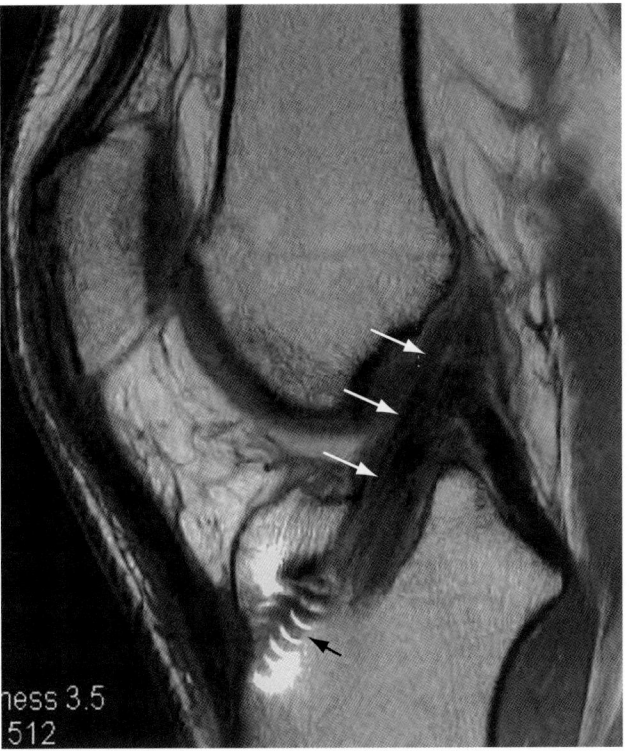

F I G U R E 103-10

Sagittal fast spin-echo image demonstrates a normal postoperative appearance of anterior cruciate ligament reconstruction (*white arrows*). Note the fairly uniformly hypointense fibers of the graft construct with a smooth linear course, without focal angulation or kinking. Note also the interference screw in the proximal tibia, demonstrating minimal susceptibility artifact in the presence of appropriately tailored protocols (*black arrow*).

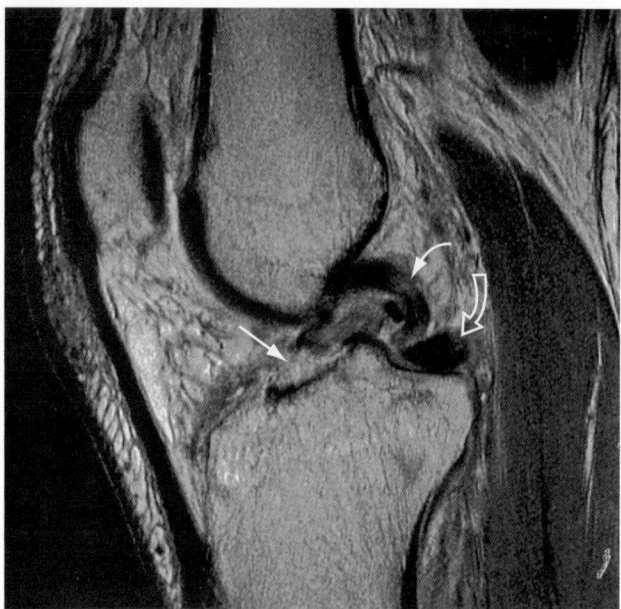

FIGURE 103-11

Sagittal fast spin-echo image in a patient post knee dislocation demonstrates complete avulsion of the anterior cruciate ligament footprint (*straight arrow*) and distal tear with retraction of the posterior cruciate ligament; the more proximal fibers demonstrate abnormal morphology and signal (*curved solid arrow*). Note the displaced fragment of the meniscus (*curved open arrow*) from a large radial split tear.

information as to the status of the regional neurovascular structures, including the peroneal nerve and the popliteal artery. Nerve injuries span from frank distraction of the fascicles, leading to partial disruption, to hematoma encasement and neuroma formation. With appropriate in-plane resolution, the architecture of the nerve is well visualized; the presence of edema in the epineurium and hematoma encasement may reflect a subclinical nerve injury that may not present with clinical evidence of nerve malfunction (Fig. 103-12).[24,106] Contrast-enhanced three-dimensional magnetic resonance angiography can demonstrate small injuries to the popliteal artery, including intimal flaps.[24]

MENISCI

Technical Considerations

One of the most common indications for MR evaluation of the knee is for characterization of meniscal pathology. A variety of pulse sequence parameters have been described in the literature for the evaluation of meniscal pathology with an equally varied combination of sensitivity, specificity, and accuracy.[107-110] Early reports utilizing fast spin-echo imaging yielded disappointing results in the diagnosis of meniscal pathology.[111] Rubin et al evaluated a series of knees utilizing a multiecho fast spin-echo sequence (echo train length 4-6, effective echo

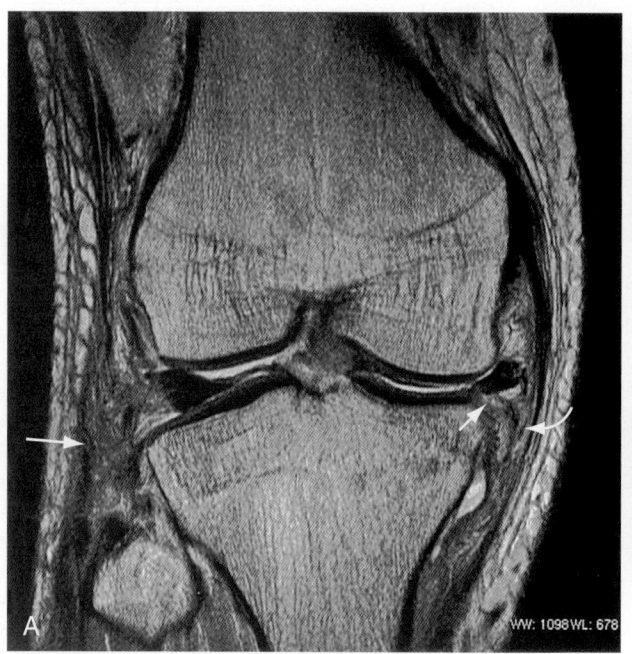

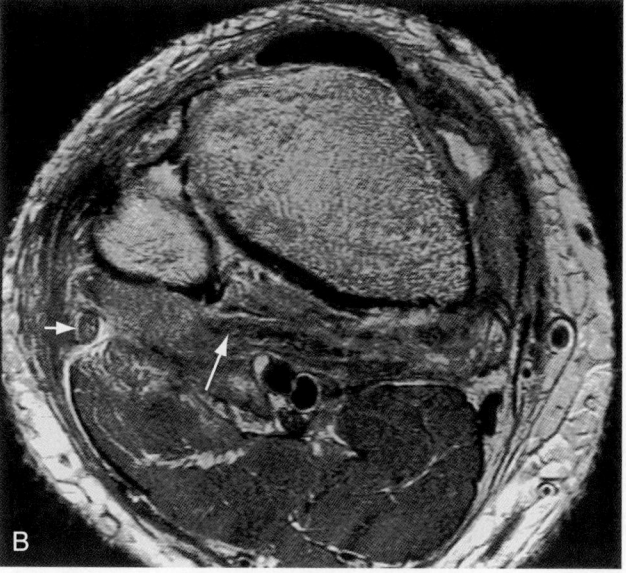

FIGURE 103-12

A, Coronal fast spin-echo image in a patient post subacute knee dislocation. Note the displaced flap tear of the medial meniscus (*short thick arrow*) and high-grade tear of the deep distal fibers of the medial collateral ligament (*curved arrow*). There has been complete disruption of the posterolateral corner structures with avulsion of the biceps femoris (*long arrow*). Radial tear of the medial meniscus is also noted. **B,** Axial fast spin-echo image in the same patient demonstrates marked enlargement and swelling of the peroneal nerve (*short arrow*). Note the high-grade muscle tendon junction injury of the popliteus (*long arrow*).

time 13-16 milliseconds (ms)/64-65ms), correlating with conventional spin-echo imaging as the gold standard, and found the fast spin-echo images only demonstrated 65% of those lesions seen on conventional spin-echo imaging.[111] Interestingly, only seven patients in their series had arthroscopic correlation and of these seven (14 menisci), both the spin-echo and fast spin-echo images were concordant with five positive MR scans and arthroscopically proven tears, and nine normal MR images, only one of which was found to be torn at arthroscopy.[111]

Subsequent evaluations have demonstrated improvements in diagnostic accuracy utilizing fast spin-echo imaging for diagnosing meniscal tears, both in the native as well as the postoperative setting.[112-116] Effective echo times have varied between 16 ms and 34 ms, depending on the desired T2 effect.[113,116] Caution should be exercised, however, in choosing relatively short effective echo times while attempting to maintain high signal to noise. Peh et al have demonstrated in a porcine model that below a threshold TE level of 16 ms, spurious intrameniscal high signal can be seen within histologically normal menisci when imaged on a clinical high field strength (1.5 T) magnet.[117] High performance gradients have resulted in improvements in technical parameter applications in meniscal imaging, in part, by allowing shorter interecho spacing, which helps to reduce blurring.[114] With increasing echo train length, sampling of late low signal intensity echoes occurs, resulting in blurring.[112] Generally speaking, fast spin-echo techniques have replaced spin-echo techniques in meniscal evaluation, provided that interecho spacing is kept to a minimum and the effective echo is maintained around 20 ms.

The acquisition matrix and phase-encoding direction must also be considered when designing appropriate sequences for diagnosing meniscal tears. Truncation artifact is the appearance of thin bands of hyperintensity paralleling the surfaces of the menisci, only a few pixels distance from the overlying articular cartilage, that can be falsely interpreted as a tear. Truncation artifact is due to signal misregistration during the Fourier integral, encountered at high signal interfaces (such as that encountered between the low signal of the fibrocartilaginous menisci and the higher signal of the adjacent hyaline articular cartilage).[118] A larger acquisition matrix can help reduce truncation artifact, but will result in an overall longer scan time.[119] As with any other imaging parameter, the trade-off between total scan time and image quality must be considered. A benefit of fast spin-echo techniques is that they permit the use of a higher resolution matrix that helps to circumvent such artifacts, but yet function within acceptable scan times.

A variety of tomographic modifications have been proposed to increase diagnostic accuracy in diagnosing meniscal tears. Radial MR scanning of the menisci, whereby multiple planes perpendicular to the long axis of the menisci are obtained, has yielded equivocal results in improving diagnostic accuracy.[120] While the sagittal and coronal planes are often of most benefit in diagnosing meniscal pathology, axial images should not be ignored as they can demonstrate vertical (especially radial) tears and displaced meniscal fragments.[121,122] A suggested protocol for imaging the menisci is outlined in Box 103-1.

Post-processing software has allowed for more detailed analysis and depiction of the menisci. The advent of filmless and soft-copy MR reading stations has made window levels on printed images less important; however, when printing hard-copy images, care should be taken to note one's diagnostic accuracy with either conventional soft-tissue or narrow window photography.[123] Other post-processing applications have allowed for accurate volumetric measurements of the meniscal fibrocartilage, potentially useful in evaluating patients following meniscal allograft transplantation.[124]

Anatomic Considerations

The menisci are fibrocartilaginous bands of tissue cushioning approximately 40-70% of the mechanical load across the knee.[125] Normally, the menisci are homogeneously hypointense on all pulse sequences due to their composition largely of type I collagen that allows for the relative restriction of water in its normal state. Both the medial and lateral menisci form a "bowtie" appearance when imaged through their periphery on sagittal images.[126,127] The anterior and posterior horns of the lateral meniscus are generally equal in size, and the posterior horn of the medial meniscus is larger than the anterior horn as visualized in the sagittal projection (Figs. 103-13 and 103-14). The medial meniscus is attached to the medial capsule at its periphery while the lateral meniscus is separated from the posterolateral capsule by the popliteus sleeve. The meniscocapsular attachments (coronary ligaments on the medial side and fascicular attachments on the lateral side) can be seen with high-resolution MR imaging.[128] Some authors have found that evaluating the fascicular attachments on the lateral side with T2-weighted images is most diagnostic, due to fluid contrast from the popliteus sleeve.[129]

The anatomy of the lateral meniscus endows it with more mobility than the medial meniscus, making it potentially less likely to sustain tears. A statistically significant translational movement of the anterior horn of the lateral meniscus has been demonstrated using dynamic magnetic resonance imaging.[130] Such motion may account for the presence of increased signal within the anterior horn of the lateral meniscus. Shankman et al found that the punctate increased signal intensity on MRI within the anterior horn of the lateral meniscus in 22 symptomatic patients did not represent a tear at arthroscopy, and similar intensity was noted in 11 volunteers.[131] These authors proposed that this finding was due to an anatomic variation of the insertion of the anterior horn of the lateral meniscus with fibers of the anterior cruciate ligament. Taken in concert with the dynamic MRI study of Vedi et al, abnormal signal in the anterior horn of the lateral meniscus should be interpreted with caution, particularly if noted as an isolated finding in the knee.

Discoid menisci are enlarged, anatomic variants that usually involve the lateral side. The visibility of

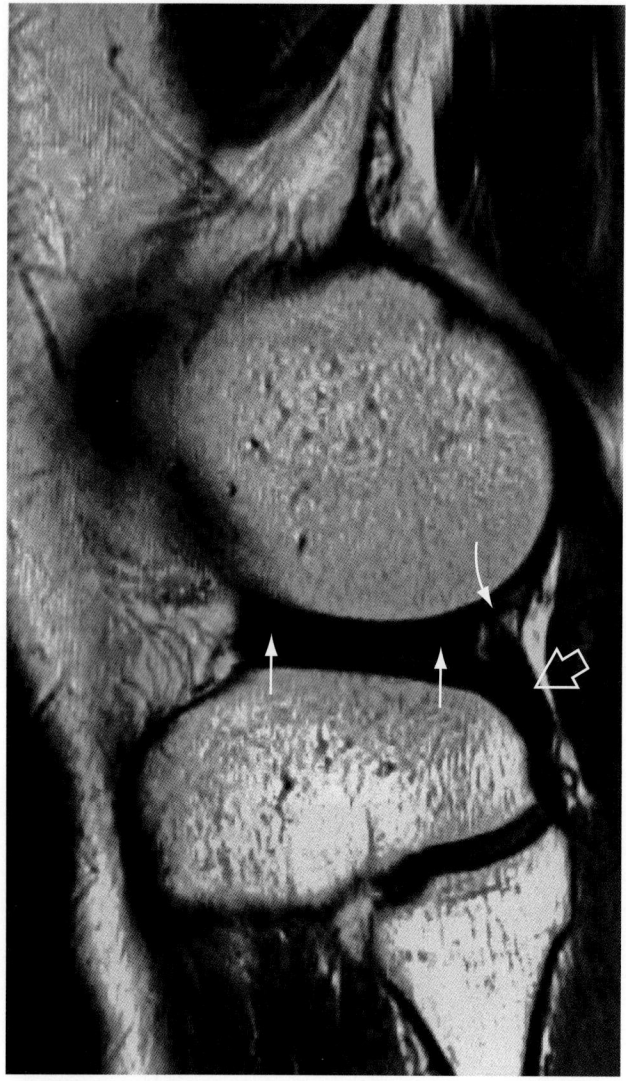

FIGURE 103-13

Sagittal fast spin-echo image demonstrates the normal appearance of the lateral meniscus. The anterior and posterior horns are relatively symmetric in size (*straight arrows*). Observe the normal superior fascicular attachment (*curved arrow*) and the interposition of the popliteus tendon (*open arrow*).

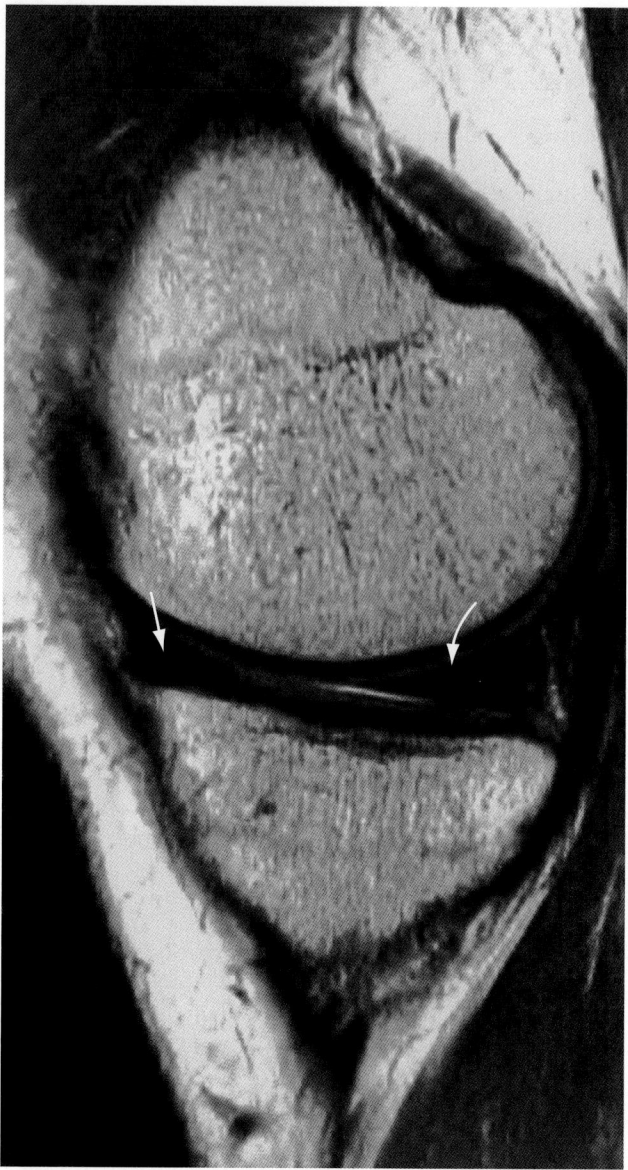

FIGURE 103-14

Sagittal fast spin-echo image demonstrates the normal appearance of the medial meniscus. Note the posterior horn (*curved arrow*) is slightly larger than the anterior horn (*straight arrow*).

hypointense meniscal tissue on multiple images can be suggestive of a discoid meniscus. Silverman et al define the MR imaging criteria of discoid meniscus as meniscal tissue connecting the anterior and posterior horns visualized on three or more 5 mm thick contiguous sagittal images.[132] The incidence of tears in discoid menisci is greater than in normal menisci. One series of 1250 knee MRIs demonstrated an overall incidence of 4.5% of discoid lateral meniscus, with 71% of discoid menisci having one or more tears.[133] Intrasubstance signal not reaching an articular surface can be seen within discoid lateral menisci and the clinical significance of this signal has been debated. Hamada et al found MRI to be more sensitive than arthroscopy in diagnosing tears of discoid menisci by histologic correlation of specimens demonstrating intrameniscal

high signal and slight alteration in morphology correlated with an intrasubstance tear at histologic inspection.[134] These authors propose that identification of Grade 2 signal within discoid menisci holds more clinical significance than in normal menisci.[134]

The meniscofemoral ligaments have been shown to have considerable anatomic variation. Most commonly, the meniscofemoral ligament is seen as a thick, hypointense band of tissue arising from the posterior horn of the lateral meniscus, coursing in an oblique direction and often dividing into two fascicles, one posterior to the posterior cruciate ligament (the ligament of Wrisberg) and another anterior (ligament of Humphrey).[135] The ligament of Wrisberg inserts on the lateral aspect of the medial femoral condyle posterior and inferior to the posterior cruciate ligament insertion while the ligament of Humphrey inserts anterior and inferior to the posterior cruciate ligament and quite often may completely blend with the ligament.[135] The proximal insertion of the meniscofemoral ligament, however, has been shown to range between partially and completely inserting onto the posterior cruciate ligament.[136,137] Variations in anterior ligamentous fixation can also occur, such as the anteromedial meniscofemoral ligament inserting on the posterolateral wall of the femoral intercondylar notch.[138] Intermeniscal supporting ligaments can be encountered as well, such as the oblique meniscomeniscal ligament.[139] Knowledge of these anatomic variations is important so as not to misdiagnose these low signal intensity structures as intra-articular bodies or displaced meniscal fragments, especially on coronal or sagittal images. Confirming the course of the ligaments in the axial projection is useful in confirming the diagnosis of an anatomic variation in meniscal ligamentous fixation.

The blood supply to the meniscus is provided at the periphery ("red zone") by the meniscocapsular plexus supplied by the geniculate arteries.[140] Peripheral tears are more amenable to surgical repair than those in the avascular portion of the meniscus ("white zone"). Evaluation of cadaver specimens with conventional and contrast-enhanced MR imaging demonstrated blood vessels to be only in the outer 10-15% of the meniscal periphery as seen on a sagittal image.[141] This relates to the meniscal classification system described by Cooper et al, with tears in the periphery (0-1 segments) being more amenable to surgical repair than those located more centrally (2-3).[142] Fast spin-echo MR imaging has been shown to have high sensitivity, specificity, and accuracy for predicting repairability of meniscal tears.[115,143]

Meniscal Pathology

The menisci are normally seen in the sagittal projection as well-defined, hypointense triangular bands of tissue. Observation of both abnormal intrameniscal signal as well as altered morphology of the meniscus should indicate the possibility of meniscal pathology (Fig. 103-15).

The most widely utilized grading system, introduced by Crues et al, classified abnormal meniscal signal (not tears) as follows.

Grade 0: normal; homogeneously hypointense
Grade 1: globular increased signal intensity within the substance of the meniscus, not reaching an articular surface
Grade 2: linear high signal intensity within the meniscus, not reaching an articular surface
Grade 3A: increased signal intensity with separation of the meniscal structure
Grade 3B: increased signal intensity extending to at least one articular surface[144]

An advantage of MRI lies in its ability to visualize lesions that do not reach an articular surface and provide insight

into the degree of degeneration of the middle collagenous elements of the fibrocartilage. The above-described so-called Grade 3A signal is thought to be a precursor to a degenerative cleavage tear. Grade 2 signal, however, is not predictive of the future development of a meniscal tear; no progression was noted in a 3-year follow-up study.[145]

Additional subdivisions of Grade 2 intrameniscal signal have been defined. Grade 2A is linear signal not reaching an articular surface, Grade 2B is abnormal signal reaching an articular surface but seen on only one image, and Grade 2C signal is a triangular or wedge-shaped focus of intrameniscal signal that does not extend to the articular surface.[145] McCauley et al retrospectively reviewed 88 patients with Grade 2C signal, seven of whom had subsequent arthroscopic correlation.[146] Half of these patients were found to have tears at arthroscopy and no statistically significant difference in the MR appearance of the signal abnormality was noted, including the extent and volume area of the abnormality.[146]

It is generally accepted that meniscal signal extending to an articular surface is indicative of a tear; however,

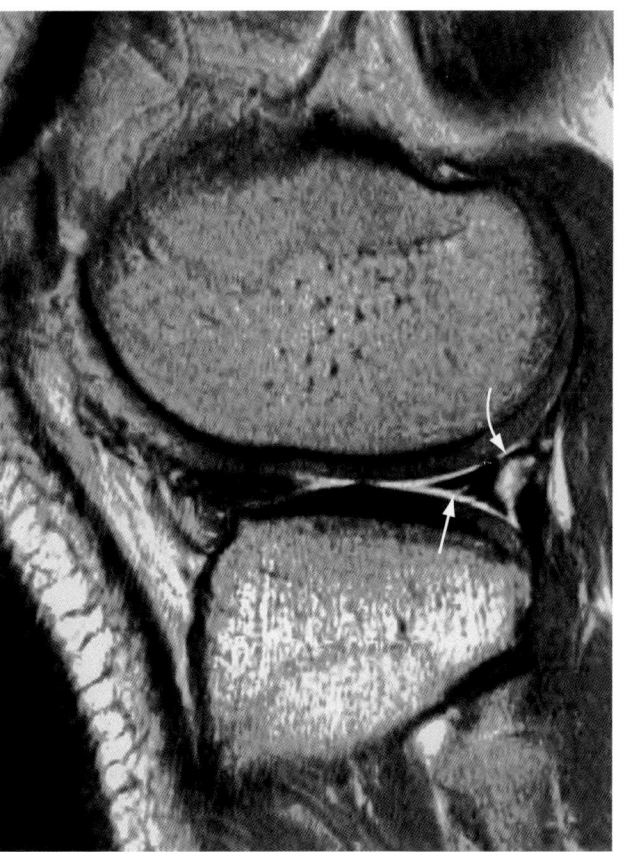

FIGURE 103-15

Sagittal fast spin-echo image demonstrates an undersurface traumatic tear of the posterior horn of the lateral meniscus (*straight arrow*). Note the high signal intensity (fluid signal) abutting the tibial articular surface to define a tear (*straight arrow*). Note the normal appearance of the superior fascicular attachment (*curved arrow*).

care should be taken when interpreting MR images in the absence of clinical symptoms. Intrameniscal signal, even that reaching an articular surface, may arise from mucoid and collagen degeneration and not reflect a traumatic tear. Analysis of both signal and morphology of the menisci is necessary to decrease the number of false-positive MRI interpretations of meniscal tears. De Smet et al evaluated the significance of intrameniscal signal reaching an articular surface with arthroscopy and found that the extent of the area on which the signal abnormality contacted the articular surface was helpful in predicting tears; more than 90% of menisci with signal contacting the articular surface on more than one image were confirmed to be torn at arthroscopic inspection, compared with 30-55% of those with signal reaching the articular surface on only one image.[147]

Degenerative changes of the menisci can result in Grade 1, 2 and 3 signal abnormalities and may not always be associated with a tear (Fig. 103-16). Histologic and MRI correlation of 20 elderly knees demonstrated mucoid and eosinophilic degeneration of the menisci in all grades of MR signal abnormality.[148] The degree of histologic change (mild, moderate, and severe) did not correlate with MRI signal abnormality. Other factors

contributing to MRI signal abnormality in these elderly specimens were fibrosis, chondrocyte proliferation, and dystrophic calcification.[148] The presence of meniscal degeneration, with or without associated tears, should be considered in concert with the patient's clinical symptoms. A high incidence of meniscal tears was found in a large series of 154 patients with osteoarthritis of the knee (Fig. 103-17).[149] Moreover, the degree of arthrosis, determined by Kellgren-Lawrence radiographic grade, correlated with a higher incidence of meniscal tears in the ipsilateral compartment and was not necessarily associated with clinical symptoms (Fig. 103-18).

Meniscal contusions, occurring in the setting of acute trauma, can be seen as areas of high signal intensity reaching an articular surface.[150] These are usually globular, less well defined than a discrete tear and are typically associated with adjacent bone marrow contusions.

Abnormal signal within the menisci can be seen across all groups and in the absence of symptoms. One series of 64 asymptomatic patients demonstrated Grades 1, 2, and 3 signal abnormalities distributed throughout the patient population studied.[151] Zanetti et al found a high percentage of asymptomatic horizontal or oblique meniscal tears in both symptomatic as well as asymptomatic knees; however, radial, vertical or other complex meniscal tears were nearly always associated with clinical symptomatology.[152]

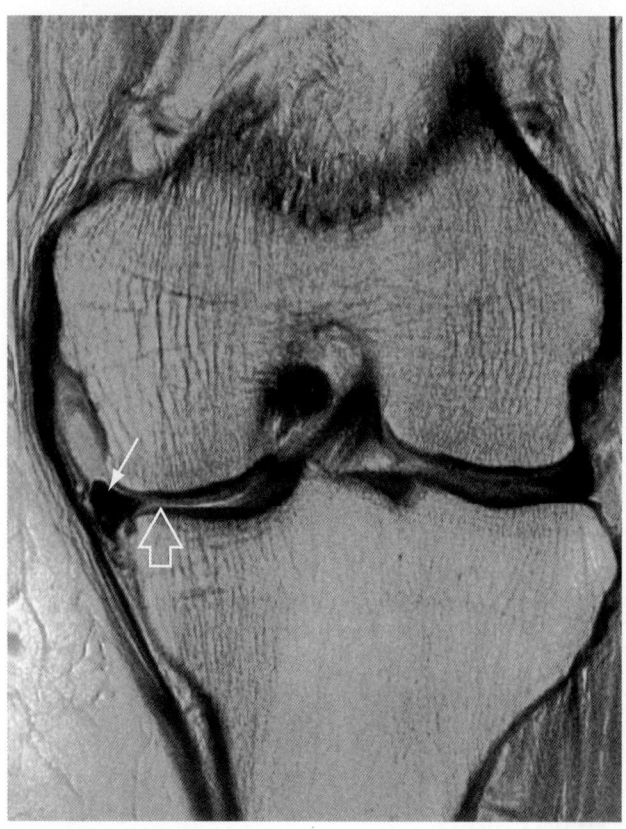

FIGURE 103-16

Coronal fast spin-echo image demonstrates degeneration of the medial meniscus with extrusion of the body segment out of the medial joint line (*straight arrow*). Observe the associated cartilage wear in the medial compartment (*open arrow*). (*Reprinted with permission from reference 29.*)

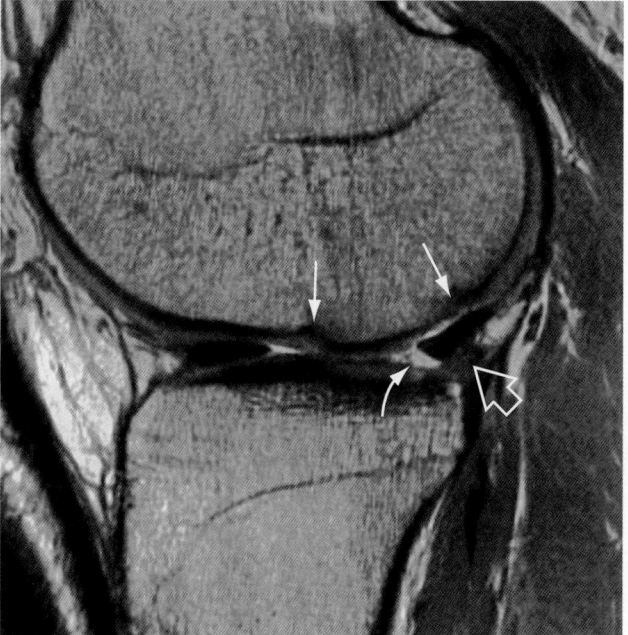

FIGURE 103-17

Sagittal fast spin-echo image demonstrates a degenerative tear of the apex of the posterior horn of the lateral meniscus (*curved arrow*). Note the abnormal morphology with truncation and high signal intensity reaching the tibial articular surface to define a tear. Note the scarring about the inferior fascicular attachment (*open arrow*) and the associated cartilage wear with subchondral osseous changes involving the lateral femoral condyle (*thin white arrows*).

Meniscal tears can be classified in terms of their morphologic appearance and pattern of injury: horizontal, radial, and vertical. A horizontal tear is one that extends parallel to the long axis of the meniscus; degenerative tears are most often horizontal and may be associated with meniscal cyst formation (Fig. 103-19). A radial tear is a specific type of vertical tear that usually occurs at the body/anterior horn interface and is oriented perpendicular to the long axis of the meniscus (Fig. 103-20). Depending on the plane of imaging, the appearance will vary; for example, in the coronal plane, the tear will be oriented in a vertical (superior to inferior) direction. If imaged through the plane of the tear, there will be apparent "absence" of the meniscus.[153] Compared with arthroscopy, prospective sensitivity for diagnosing radial tears of 89% has been reported with the use of fat-saturated proton-density and T2-weighted images.[154]

Meniscal tears can become unstable and displaced, resulting in pain, swelling, and mechanical symptoms. Using arthroscopic findings of a displaced fragment and flap formation as indicative of unstable meniscal lesions, Vande Berg et al found MR to have high specificity in predicting unstable meniscal lesions.[155] Identification of a displaced fragment and a complex meniscal tear had a high positive predictive value for unstable meniscal lesions, as well as a large tear, defined as one spanning

more than three 3 mm thick coronal and two 4 mm thick sagittal images. Flap tears of the menisci, typically involving the undersurface of the menisci, can become displaced and extend into the medial and lateral joint recesses (Fig. 103-21).[156] The preoperative identification of displaced fragments is important, as they might not be readily visualized during routine arthroscopic inspection.

A specific type of displaced meniscal tear is the so-called "bucket-handle" tear which is a vertical tear of the meniscus with a displaced fragment that remains in continuity with the parent meniscus in the periphery (Fig. 103-22). Various sensitivities and specificities for MR diagnosis of bucket-handle tears have been reported.[157,158] The double PCL sign, with two parallel low signal intensity bands in the intercondylar notch on the sagittal and coronal MR images, is highly suggestive of a bucket-handle tear, with a reported specificity of 100% (Fig. 103-23).[158,159] Using a combination of signs, including the double PCL sign, flipped meniscus in the anteroposterior plane and/or a fragment in the intercondylar notch, and areas of increased signal within either meniscus with a displaced fragment on coronal STIR images resulted in an overall sensitivity of 93% compared with arthroscopy.[160] While most bucket-handle tears are on the medial side, lateral meniscal bucket-handle tears are not uncommon and occasionally, bucket-handle tears of both menisci can occur simultaneously.[160,161] Interpretation of the vascular zone of cleavage of the vertical tear, as well as the degree of degeneration of the peripheral remnant, has important implications for predicting the repairability of the tear.

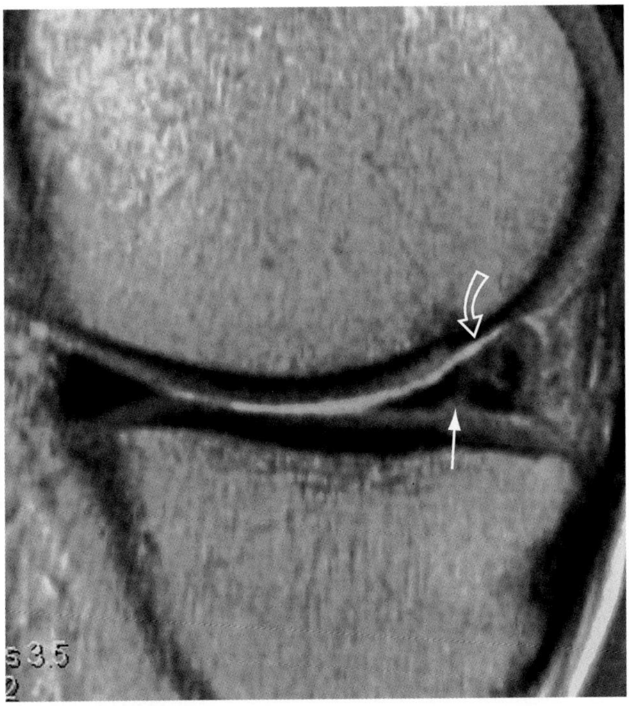

FIGURE 103-18

Sagittal fast spin-echo image demonstrates a degenerative tear of the posterior horn of the medial meniscus. Note the irregular intrasubstance signal in the posterior horn of the medial meniscus reaching the tibial articular surface (*arrow*). Note the full-thickness cartilage abnormality superior to the posterior horn of the medial meniscus with associated subchondral osseous changes (*open arrow*).

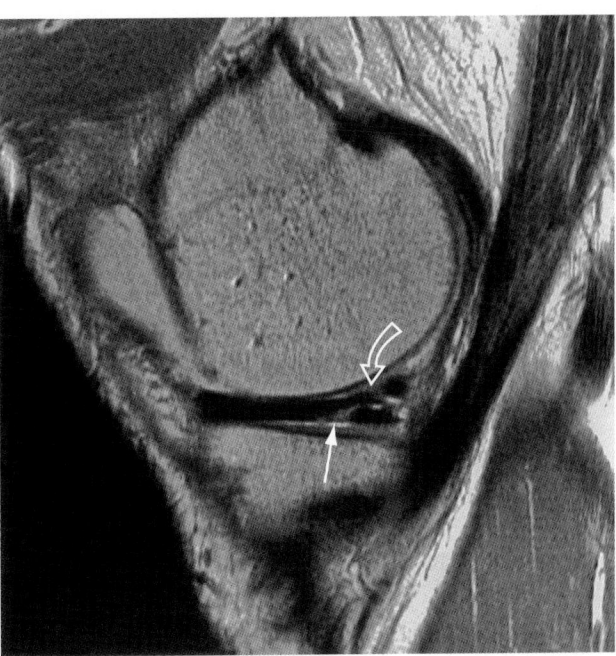

FIGURE 103-19

Sagittal fast spin-echo image through the medial meniscus demonstrates a horizontal tear in the posterior horn reaching both the tibial (*arrow*) as well as the femoral (*open arrow*) articular surfaces.

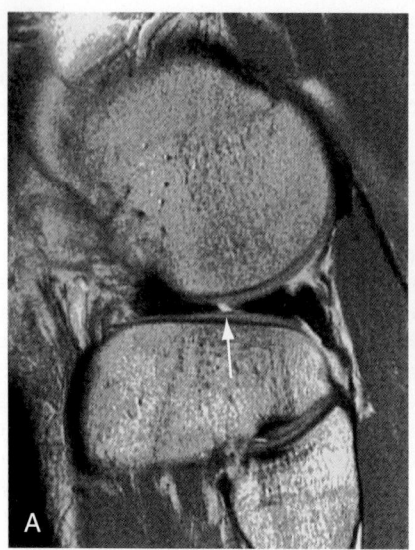
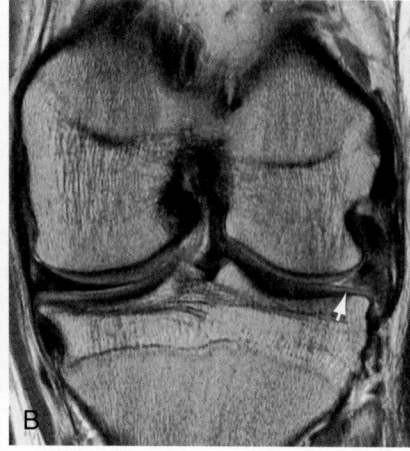
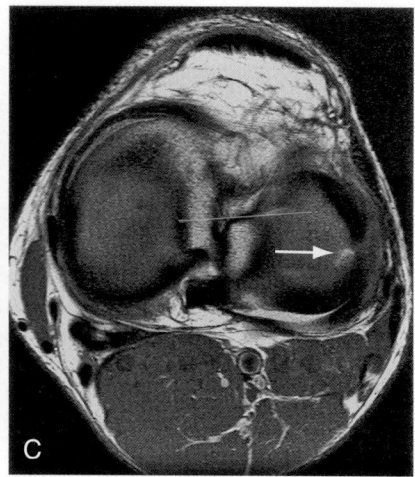

FIGURE 103-20

A, Sagittal fast spin-echo image demonstrates a radial split tear in the body of the lateral meniscus (*arrow*). **B,** Coronal fast spin-echo image in the same patient demonstrates the radial tear (*arrow*). Note the morphology of radial tears as visualized in the coronal plane with subtle truncation and high signal at the inner margin of the body segment of the lateral meniscus. **C,** Axial fast spin-echo image in the same patient demonstrates a radial tear as visualized in the transaxial plane. If the axial images are thin enough and cut through the plane of the menisci, the tear can be visualized as a linear high signal intensity focus through the normally hypointense fibrocartilage of the meniscus (*arrow*). (*Reprinted with permission from reference 29.*)

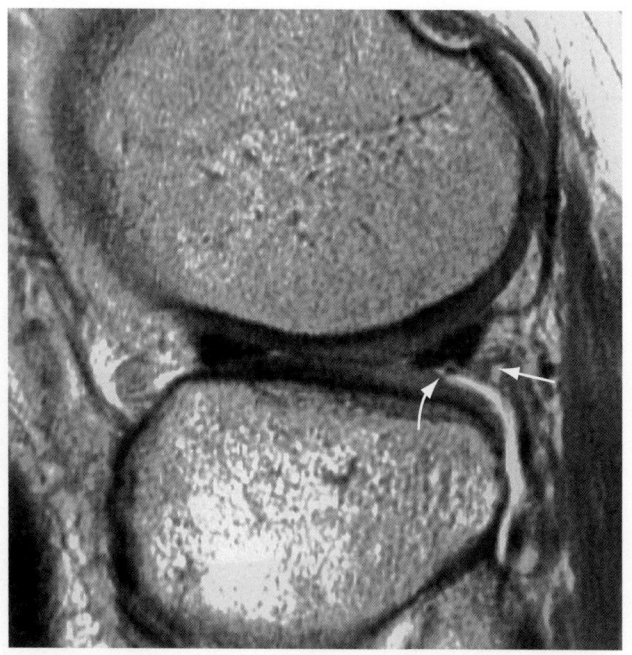

FIGURE 103-21

Sagittal fast spin-echo image in a patient approximately 1 year post anterior cruciate ligament reconstruction with a recent twisting injury. Note the undersurface flap tear of the posterior horn on the lateral meniscus (*curved arrow*) with subacute injury to the inferior fascicular attachment of the posterior horn of the lateral meniscus (*arrow*).

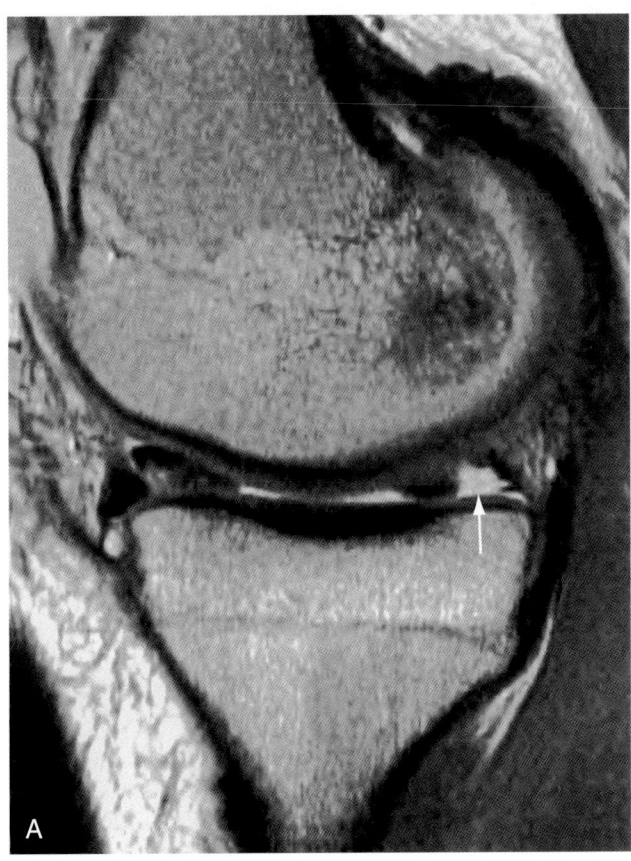

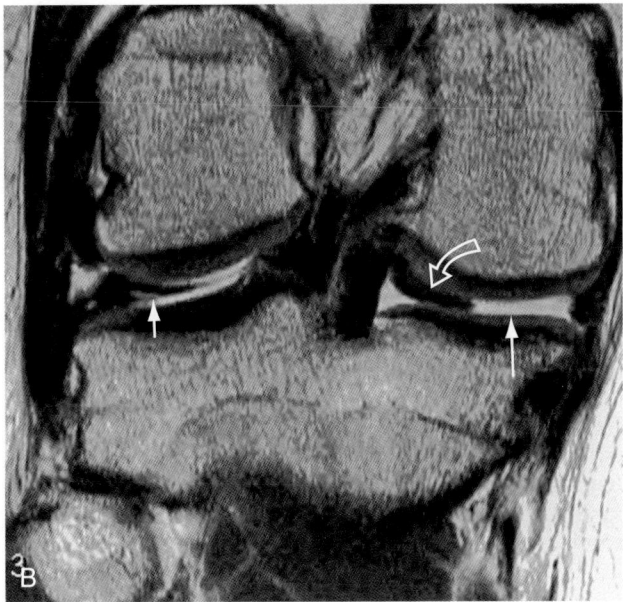

FIGURE 103-22

A, Sagittal fast spin-echo image through the medial femorotibial joint compartment in a patient with a bucket-handle tear of the medial meniscus. In the sagittal plane, a bucket-handle tear is often visualized as a large fluid-filled defect in the substance of the meniscus (*arrow*).

B, Coronal fast spin-echo image in the same patient demonstrates the distracted fragment of fibrocartilage (*open arrow*) into the intercondylar notch. The tear is identified as a large fluid-filled defect (*long arrow*) in the substance of the medial meniscus. Note the tear in the lateral meniscus as well (*short arrow*).

FIGURE 103-23

Sagittal fast spin-echo image through the midline of the knee demonstrates bucket-handle tear of the medial meniscus with a "double posterior cruciate ligament" sign. Note the displaced fragment (*arrow*) of hypointense fibrocartilage into the intercondylar notch, lying just deep to the posterior cruciate ligament. *(Reprinted with permission from reference 29.)*

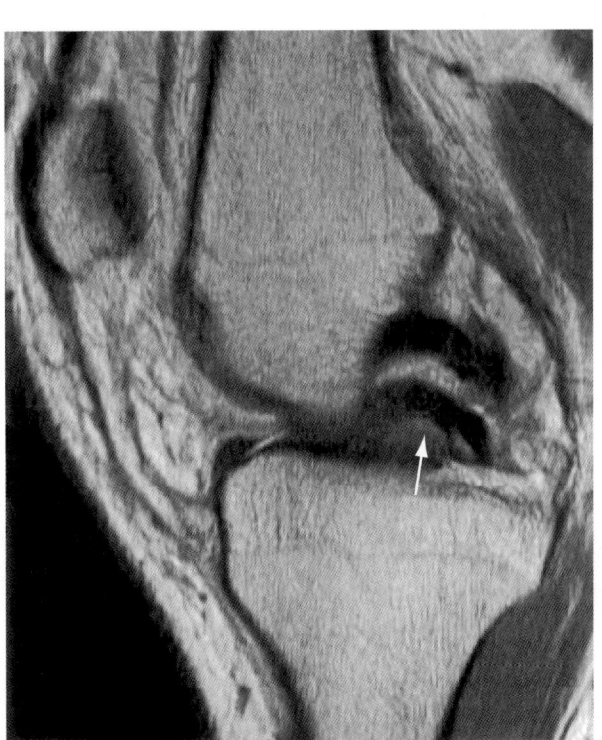

Meniscal cysts, thought to occur from extrusion of synovial fluid through a meniscal tear, are not uncommon lesions (Fig. 103-24).[162] An overall incidence of 4% was found in a series of 2572 knees; 66% of these were associated with abnormalities of the medial meniscus.[162]

Postoperative Meniscal Evaluation

Arthroscopic repair of peripheral meniscal tears is an important alternative to partial meniscectomy, which can lead to degenerative arthrosis of the affected compartment (Fig. 103-25).[163] Tears in the peripheral, vascular zone of the menisci have a strong healing response and are amenable to surgical repair.[164] MR imaging of meniscal repair, however, can be confusing due to persistent signal abnormalities long after the surgery is performed, and often complicated by clinical history of new trauma and clinical concern about re-tear through the repair site or new tear (Fig. 103-26).

Deutsch et al studied 18 menisci with known meniscal tears with serial magnetic resonance imaging.[165] Eleven of the 18 menisci were treated with surgical repair. Persistent Grade 3 signal was noted in 15 menisci (seen on preoperative as well as postoperative MR imaging), as well as in three of four menisci that were confirmed by second-look arthroscopy to have healed at 3-37 months.[165] Farley et al similarly found persistent signal abnormalities in both surgically repaired and conservatively treated menisci that were interpreted as "healed" on conventional arthrography.[166] These authors did suggest, however, that increased signal on T2-weighted images (that approaching joint fluid) was more suggestive of a tear as opposed to routine postoperative change, and this was confirmed on two of the cases that had arthroscopic correlation.[166] Some authors have found that intra-articular administration of gadolinium increases accuracy in diagnosing meniscal tears following surgical intervention.[167,168]

Histologic analysis of healing menisci in dogs harvested at 8, 12, and 26 weeks have demonstrated transformation from highly cellular, fibrovascular scar tissue to fibrocartilage.[169] Correlation of these specimens with MR images obtained on a 4.7 T unit demonstrated persistent high signal intensity in the menisci at 26 weeks, when histologically the injured material was classified as fibrocartilage.[169]

Traditionally, conventional arthrography and, more recently, MR arthrography have been utilized to diagnose meniscal tears in the postoperative patient. Both of these modalities are invasive and the application of an invasive

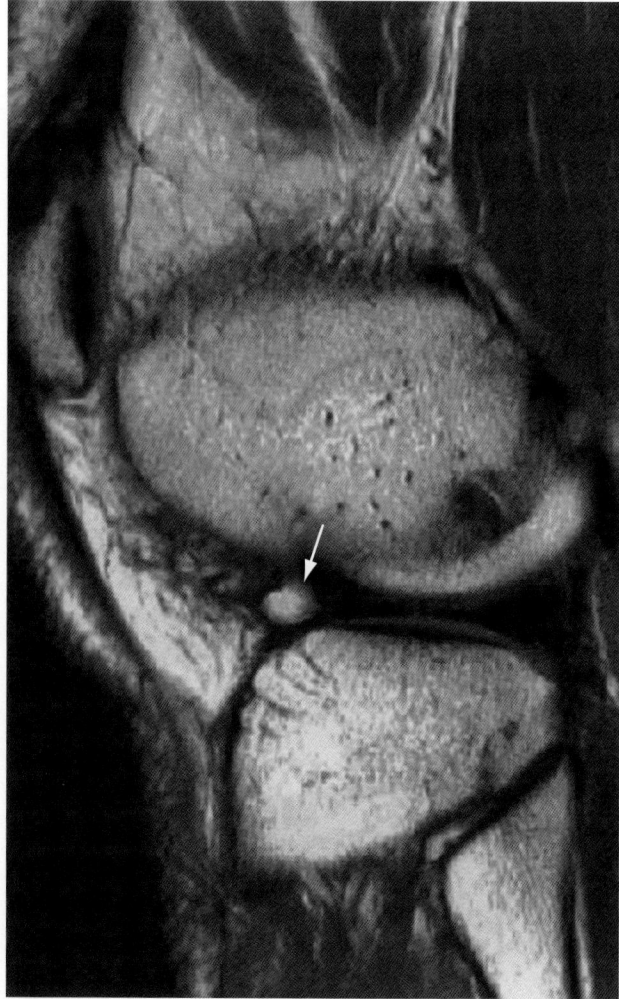

FIGURE 103-24

Sagittal fast spin-echo image through the lateral femorotibial joint compartment demonstrates a meniscal cyst arising from the anterior horn of the lateral meniscus (*arrow*).

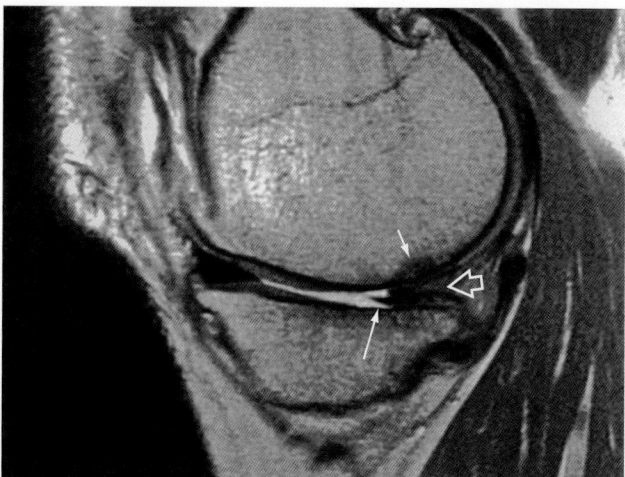

FIGURE 103-25

Sagittal fast spin-echo image demonstrates postoperative changes in the medial meniscus. Note the truncation of the apex of the posterior horn of the medial meniscus with relative equivalent sizes of the anterior and posterior horns, consistent with partial meniscectomy (*long arrow*). Note the associated degenerative signal in the posterior horn remnant (*open arrow*) and degeneration of the articular cartilage over the medial compartment (*short arrow*).

procedure to a potentially time-consuming MR examination detracts from one of the major advantages of MR imaging. One large series of 364 patients who had had meniscal repair surgery were prospectively evaluated with MR arthrography, indirect MR arthrography, and conventional MR imaging.[170] No statistically significant difference between the imaging modalities was noted. These authors evaluated the following morphologic changes in the menisci: intrameniscal signal abnormality reaching an articular surface on T1- and T2-weighted images, morphologic changes in the meniscus, joint effusion, and presence of an obvious meniscal tear. Similar to other authors, White et al found that a linear high signal abnormality approaching fluid signal extending to an articular surface was most sensitive in diagnosing a tear in the postoperative setting.[115,170,171] Noncontrast fast spin-echo imaging has also been validated in diagnosing re-tears in the postoperative patient following primary repair (Fig. 103-27).[115]

More recent advances in meniscal surgery include meniscal transplantation (Fig. 103-28). Arthroscopically transplanted fresh meniscal allografts are performed in certain clinical settings. Candidate selection is of paramount importance for clinical success, as both subjective (clinical) and objective (MRI) failure are associated with high degrees of arthrosis at the time of implantation (Fig. 103-29).[116,163] In addition to the degradation in the articular cartilage, associated condylar remodeling with subchondral flattening and osteophyte formation is associated with poor outcome (Fig. 103-30).[116,172] Noncontrast high-resolution fast spin-echo MR imaging of meniscal allografts has been demonstrated to correlate well with clinical symptoms such as locking, as well as histologic changes of myxomatous degeneration.[116] Some authors have also found MR helpful in estimating meniscal allograft volume in the postoperative period, which can be helpful in assessing the amount of allograft shrinkage.[173]

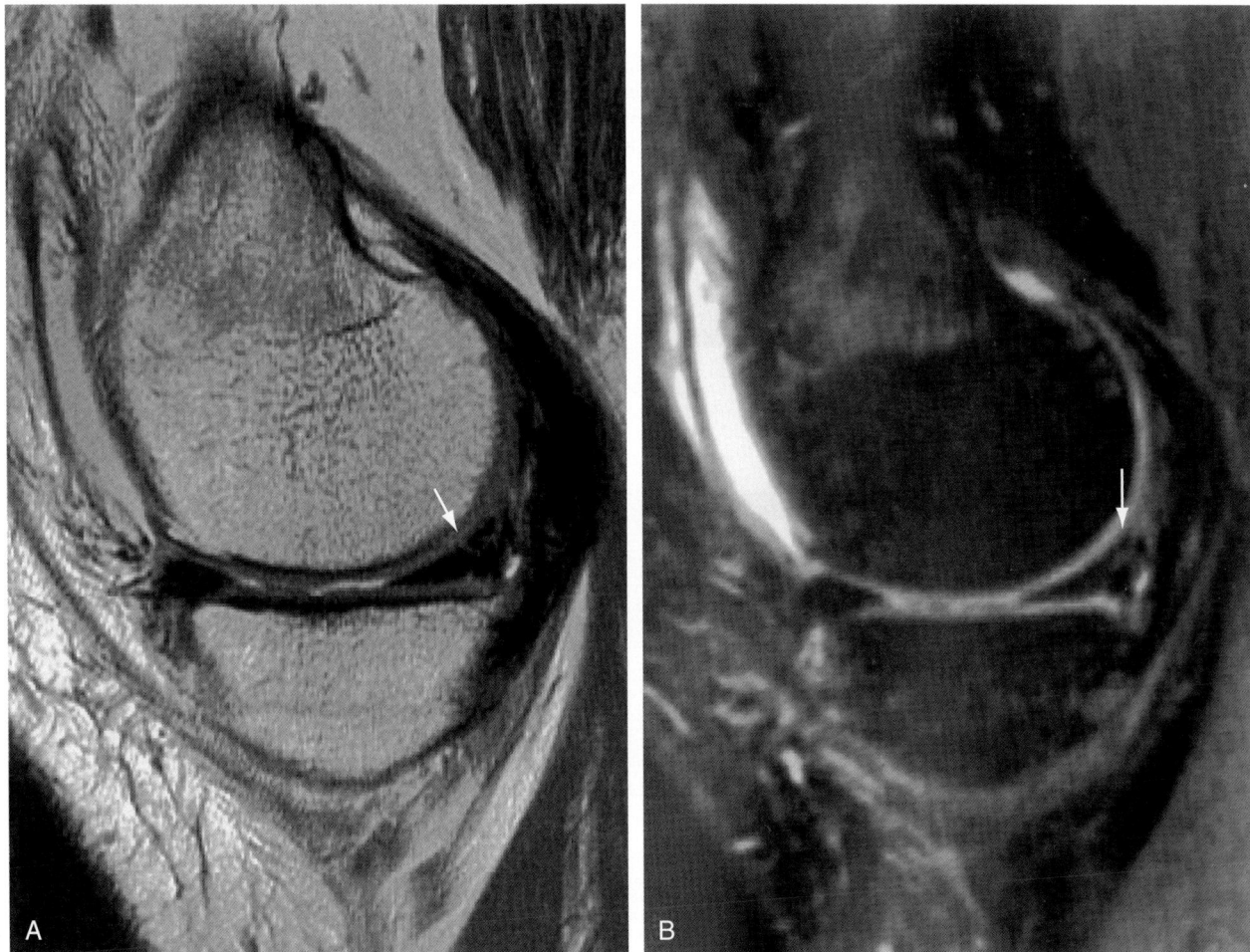

FIGURE 103-26

A, Sagittal fast spin-echo image in a patient post meniscal repair with bioabsorbable tack demonstrates irregular intermediate signal reaching the femoral articular surface (*arrow*). Observe that this is not fluid signal and is therefore consistent with meniscal healing and not a new tear. **B,** Sagittal frequency-selective fat suppression image in the same patient demonstrates minimally high signal in the posterior horn of the medial meniscus, which is not fluid signal to define a tear (*arrow*). (*Reprinted with permission from reference 29.*)

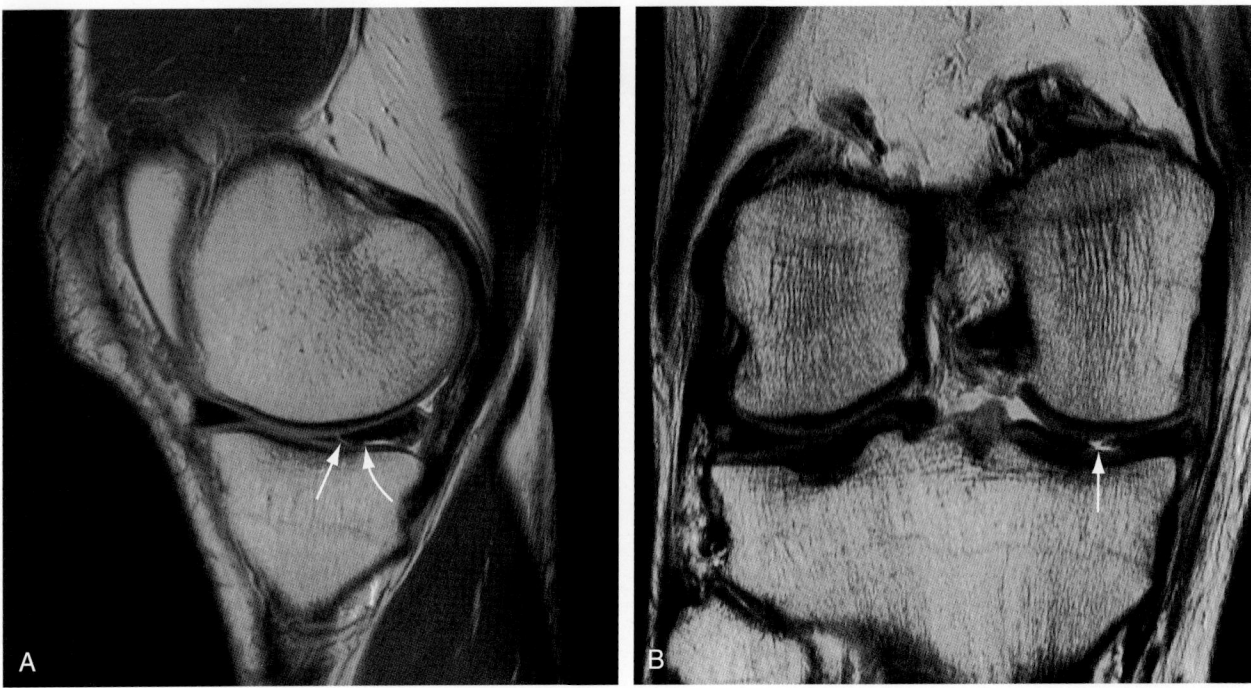

FIGURE 103-27

A, Sagittal fast spin-echo image demonstrates postoperative changes from a primary medial meniscal repair with a superimposed acute tear. Note the sharp, obliquely oriented signal at the medial meniscal apex at the site of primary repair (*arrow*). In addition, there is an acute undersurface flap tear (*curved arrow*) of the posterior horn of the medial meniscus. **B,** Coronal fast spin-echo image in the same patient demonstrates the acute tear as an irregular vertical focus of fluid signal (*arrow*), extending to both the femoral and tibial articular surfaces.

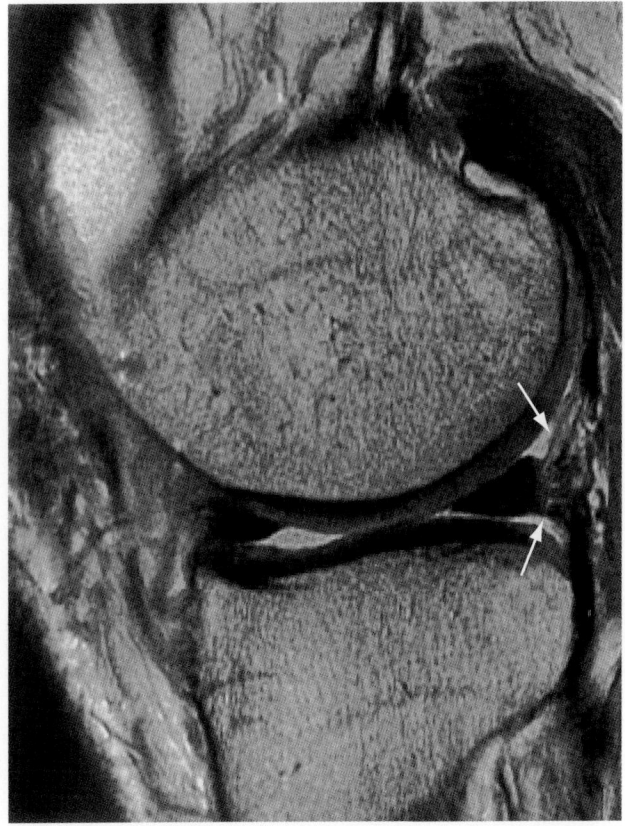

FIGURE 103-28

Sagittal fast spin-echo image of a clinically successful lateral meniscal allograft. Note the normal morphology and signal of the lateral meniscus as well as the integrity of the adjacent articular cartilage. There is only mild scarring of the peripheral capsular attachments (*arrows*). *(Reprinted with permission from reference 29.)*

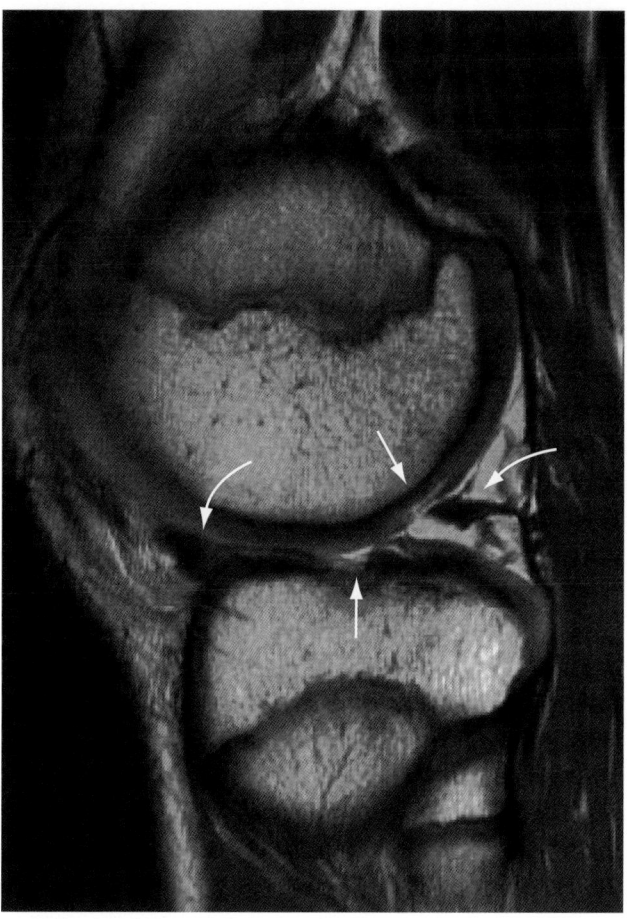

FIGURE 103-29

Sagittal fast spin-echo image in a 15-year-old patient under consideration for meniscal transplant. There are multifocal areas of full-thickness cartilage loss along both sides of the joint (*straight arrows*) as well as abnormal morphology of the lateral meniscus with a small posterior horn remnant (*right curved arrow*) and extrusion of the anterior horn (*left curved arrow*). (*Reprinted with permission from reference 29.*)

OSTEOCHONDRITIS DISSECANS

The term osteochondritis dissecans (OCD) of the knee has, in general, been expanded to encompass an osteochondral injury of varying severity, typically affecting the lateral margin of the medial femoral condyle in young adolescents.[174] The characteristically described lesion can in some cases be visualized on conventional radiographs as a round, well-defined radiolucency, often with an associated lucency or sclerosis undermining the interface between the osteochondral abnormality and the native femoral condyle. The advent of MR imaging has allowed more detailed evaluation of these lesions, including their biologic behavior such as stage of healing and stability.

These lesions can affect articular surfaces other than the medial femoral condyle, including the lateral femoral condyle and the trochlea; the latter location may be best

evaluated using axial images, tangential to the articular surface.[175] Magnetic resonance imaging has been demonstrated to be helpful in preoperative planning as well as a prognostic indicator. A frank transchondral fracture line and incongruity of the articular cartilage surface are generally associated with a poorer prognosis than a smaller, well-defined, stable lesion.[176] Correlation with arthroscopy has suggested that a high signal intensity (fluid) line undermining the osteochondral lesion is an indicator of lesion instability (Fig. 103-31).[177] The overall morphology of the lesion should be evaluated, however, as this finding may in some cases represent a healing response and granulation tissue.[178] O'Connor et al report a higher accuracy rate of grading OCD lesions as stable or unstable if the observed high signal intensity line extends through the subchondral plate and through the articular cartilage (unstable lesion) as opposed to a high signal line isolated to the interface between the OCD lesion and the native femur (healing response).[178] In terms of conservatively treated OCD lesions, a younger patient population generally responds better to conservative treatment than an older age group (Fig. 103-32).[179,180]

CARTILAGE

Conventional radiographs remain the imaging mainstay for assessment of the joint space. As they do not directly depict the articular cartilage, however, they provide an indirect measure of cartilage loss. In addition, assessment of joint space narrowing alone is an inaccurate indication of the structural integrity of articular cartilage.[181] Due to its direct multiplanar capabilities and superior soft-tissue contrast, MR imaging allows for direct visualization of articular cartilage. This permits detection of both traumatic and degenerative chondral lesions, provides a reproducible measurement for cartilage thickness, and assesses for morphologic change in prospective evaluation of cartilage lesions. With appropriate in-plane resolution and tissue contrast, MR imaging will detect focal chondral lesions and subchondral bony abnormalities prior to appearance of abnormalities on plain radiographs.

The signal characteristics of articular cartilage are dependent on the MR pulse sequence utilized, the cellular composition of collagen, proteoglycans and free water, and the orientation of the collagen in different lamina of cartilage.[182]

Multiple options for MR imaging of cartilage are available, including traditional fat-suppressed 3D T1-weighted gradient-echo techniques, fat-suppressed fast spin-echo, high in-plane resolution non-fat suppressed moderate TE fast spin-echo, indirect MR arthrography via the intravenous injection of gadolinium, and direct MR arthrography, using intra-articular gadolinium contrast agents.[183-187] More recently, additional pulse sequences have become available, including 3D steady-state free precession imaging utilizing multipoint fat and water suppression and driven equilibrium Fourier transform (DEFT).[188,189] Each pulse sequence suitable for cartilage

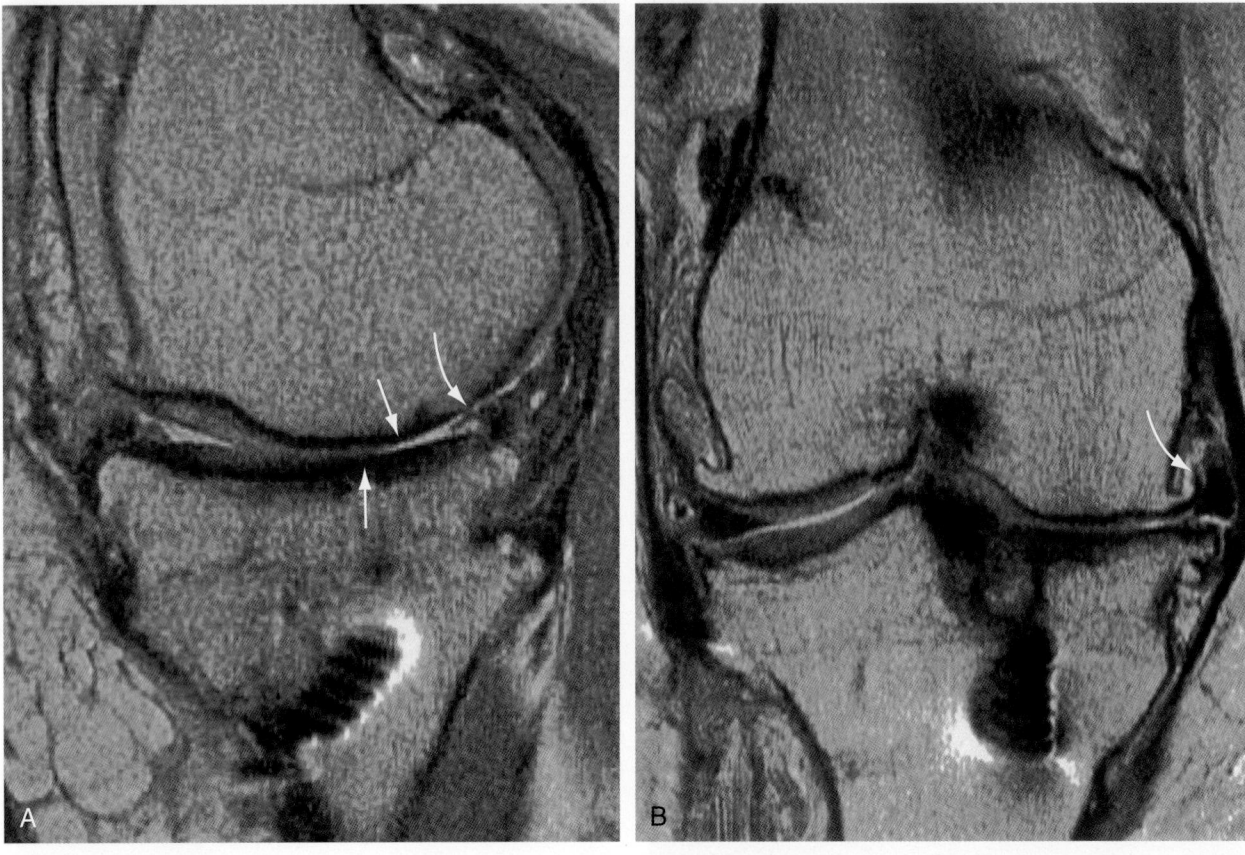

FIGURE 103-30

A, Sagittal fast spin-echo image demonstrates failed medial meniscal allograft in a 39-year-old female. Note the degenerated medial meniscal remnant (*curved arrow*) with full-thickness cartilage loss along both sides of the medial compartment (*straight arrows*). Note also the interference screw in the proximal tibia for prior anterior cruciate ligament reconstruction. **B,** Coronal fast spin-echo image in the same patient demonstrates extrusion of the medial meniscal allograft (*arrow*) out of the medial joint line with degenerative arthrosis in the medial compartment with condylar remodeling and marginal osteophyte formation. *(Reprinted with permission from reference 29.)*

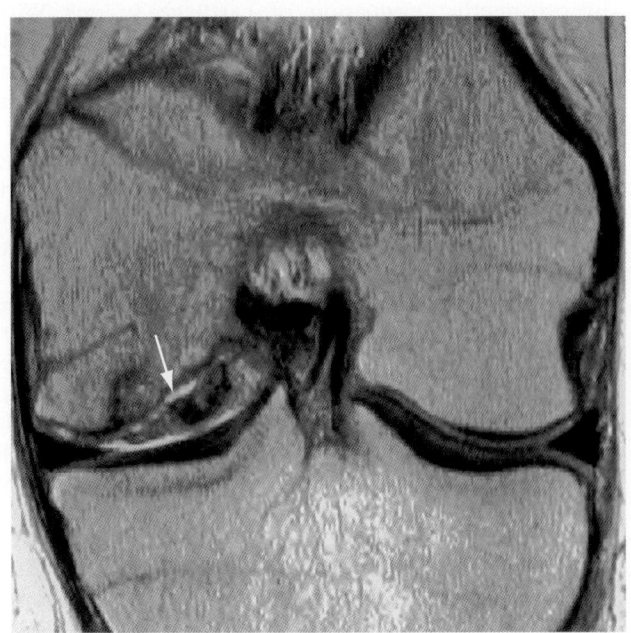

FIGURE 103-31

Coronal fast spin-echo image in a patient with osteochondritis dissecans of the medial femoral condyle (*arrow*) with fluid at the interface between the devitalized subchondral bone and adjacent cartilage. Note the mature bed of donor subchondral bone.

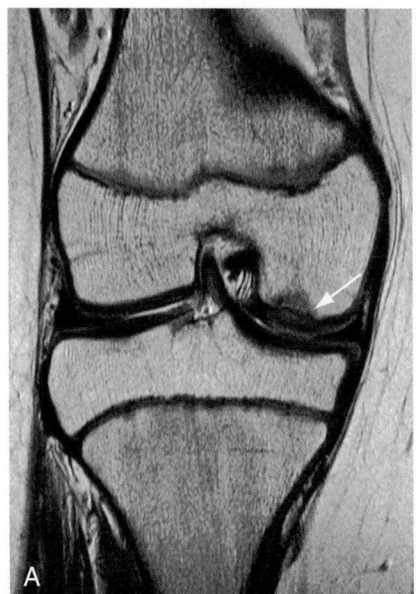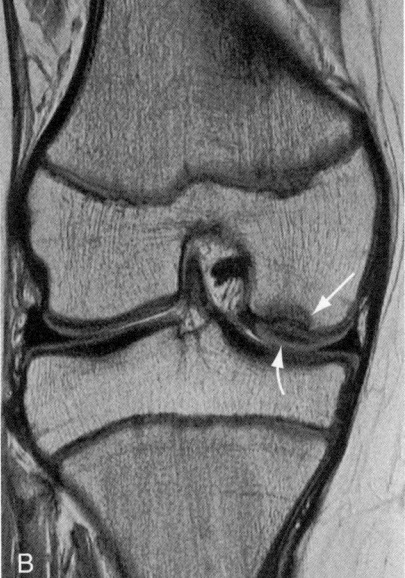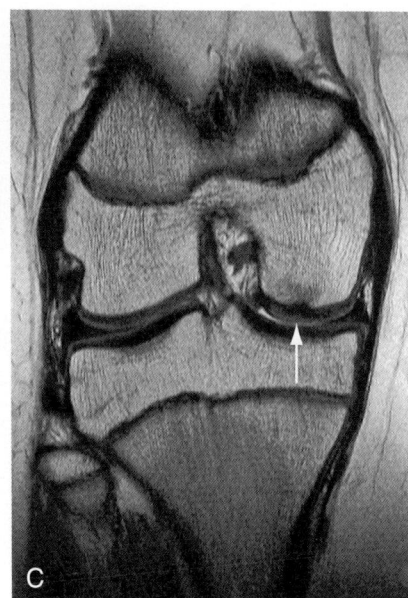

FIGURE 103-32

A, Coronal fast spin-echo image in a 10-year-old girl demonstrating stable osteochondritis dissecans of the medial femoral condyle. Note the minimal inhomogeneity of the overlying articular cartilage with mild irregularity of the subchondral plate and subchondral sclerosis, without any subchondral fluid imbibition to suggest it is unstable (*arrow*). **B,** Coronal fast spin-echo image in the same patient 8 months later demonstrates some interval remodeling of the subchondral bone (*straight arrow*). Note the smooth, homogeneous overlying articular cartilage (*curved arrow*). **C,** Coronal fast spin-echo image in the same patient 11 months later (19 months after initial presentation) demonstrates minimal subchondral changes with normal-appearing overlying articular cartilage (*arrow*).

carries its own advantages and disadvantages, but some validated standardized form of cartilage imaging is necessary on all standard MR imaging of the knee. Field strength is an additional issue in the ability to detect chondral lesions. Higher field strength (1.0-1.5 T) units have been shown to be superior in detecting partial-thickness articular cartilage lesions compared with a low field strength 0.18 T unit, likely due to the lower signal to noise and spatial resolution capabilities of the lower field strength magnet (Fig. 103-33).[4]

In order to obtain acceptance amongst clinicians, validation of cartilage pulse sequence against the surgical standard is necessary and has been performed on both the standard gradient-echo and fast spin-echo techniques.[184,186] There is a correlation between findings noted at MR examination and those found at arthroscopy and indeed, on histologic evaluation. A modified Outerbridge classification may be used to detect the degree of cartilage loss:

● Grade I, which is deemed at arthroscopy to be "soft cartilage", is manifest as increased signal intensity on MRI
● Grade II reflects fissures or fibrillation involving <50% of the thickness
● Grade III, with >50% cartilage thickness loss, is manifest as variable foci of partial-thickness cartilage loss with irregular surface change

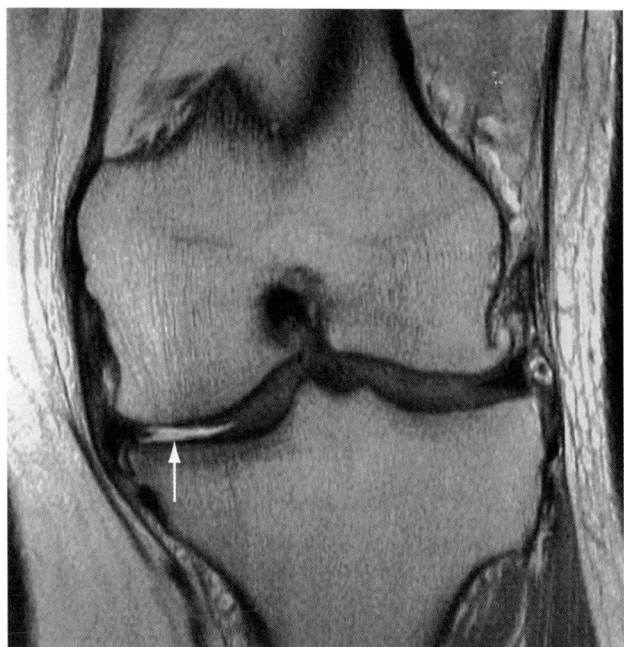

FIGURE 103-33

Coronal fast spin-echo image on a high field strength (0.7 T) open MR system demonstrates focally severe cartilage wear in the medial femorotibial joint compartment with full-thickness cartilage loss along both sides of the joint (*arrow*).

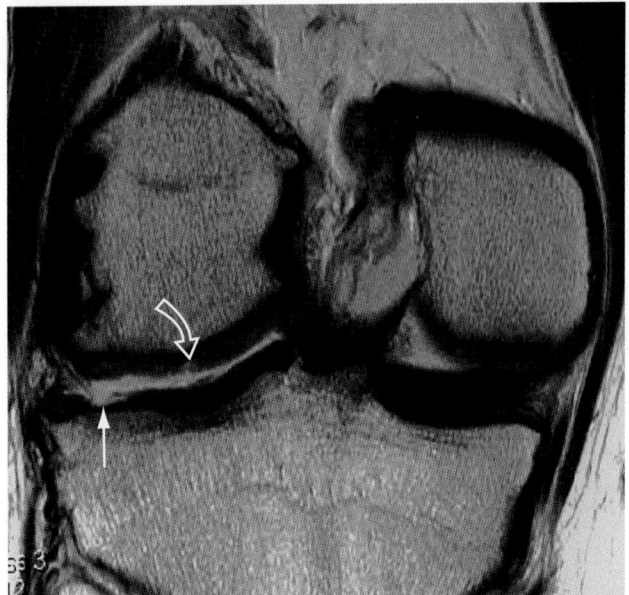

FIGURE 103-34

Coronal fast spin-echo image demonstrates a focal area of full-thickness cartilage loss in the lateral tibial plateau (*white arrow*) as well as a full-thickness fissure in the mirroring surface of the lateral femoral condyle (*curved open arrow*) in this patient with mild to moderate degenerative arthrosis in the lateral compartment.

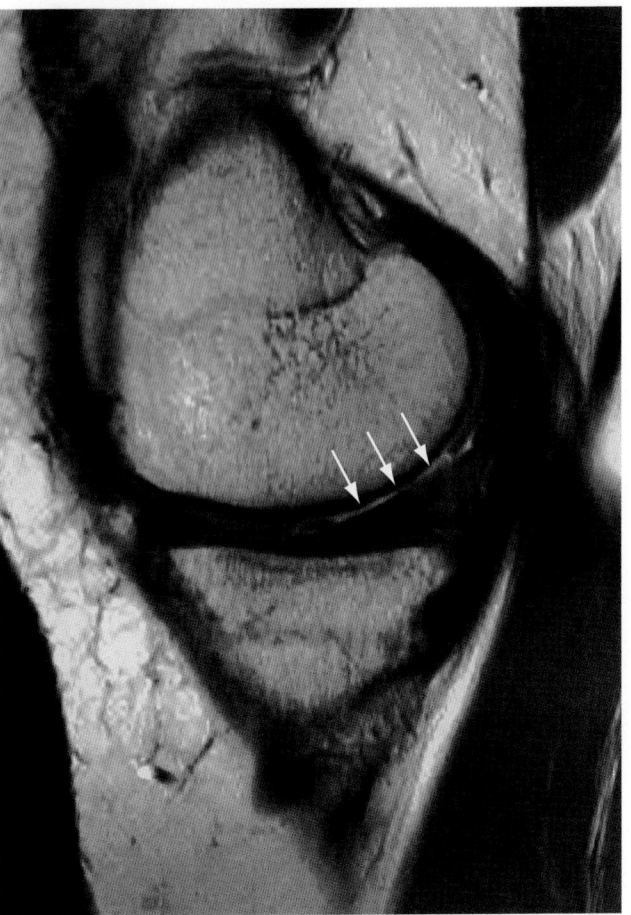

FIGURE 103-35

Sagittal fast spin-echo image through the medial femorotibial joint compartment demonstrates traumatic delamination of cartilage of the medial femoral condyle (*arrows*).

● Grade IV reflects exposed subchondral bone and is noted on MRI evaluation to reflect a surface flap extending down to subchondral bone or focal complete loss of the articular cartilage signal (Figs.103-34 and 103-35).[186,190]

In degenerative osteoarthrosis, MR imaging can be efficacious in detecting the degree of articular cartilage loss as well as the reaction of the subchondral bone (Fig. 103-36). The presence of bone marrow edema pattern in load-bearing joints with concomitant osteoarthritis is not an uncommon finding. Surprisingly, a histologic study of explants obtained from patients referred for total knee arthroplasty and who demonstrated a bone marrow edema pattern on preoperative MRI disclosed that bone marrow edema was not a major contributor to the signal abnormality. Rather, marrow necrosis, remodeled trabeculae, and bone marrow fibrosis were additionally demonstrated with greater proportions (Fig. 103-37).[191] The bone marrow edema pattern is thus more likely a reflection of the continuous subchondral remodeling that occurs in the presence of osteoarthrosis.

While standardized validated MR pulse sequences suitable for cartilage can detect moderate degrees of cartilage loss, they are relatively insensitive in detecting early structural alterations in the extracellular matrix that proceed morphologic loss of cartilage thickness.[192] Recent techniques utilized in an attempt to visualize matrix alterations studied two distinct pools of protons within the matrix: specifically, those hydrostatically bound to proteoglycan and those structurally bound to collagen. Osteoarthrosis is associated with negatively charged glycosaminoglycans in the proteoglycan component. This process may be tracked on MRI using high field strength (4 T) systems to detect the depletion of the fixed negative charge of proteoglycans, as they attract to the positively charged sodium MR species.[193] These studies, however, are limited by long scan times and special coil requirements. Additional investigators have utilized negatively charged gadolinium compounds to detect areas of proteoglycan depletion in cartilage by performing quantitative T1 mapping. These techniques use T1 relaxation maps to monitor the diffusion of gadolinium contrast, which is tagged to the negatively charged salt, in the synovial fluid and through the subchondral bone to the cartilage as a function of fixed charged density. This allows for the qualitative assessment of the relative distribution of negatively charged glycosaminoglycan as it reflects changes in the proteoglycan of the cartilage matrix.[194]

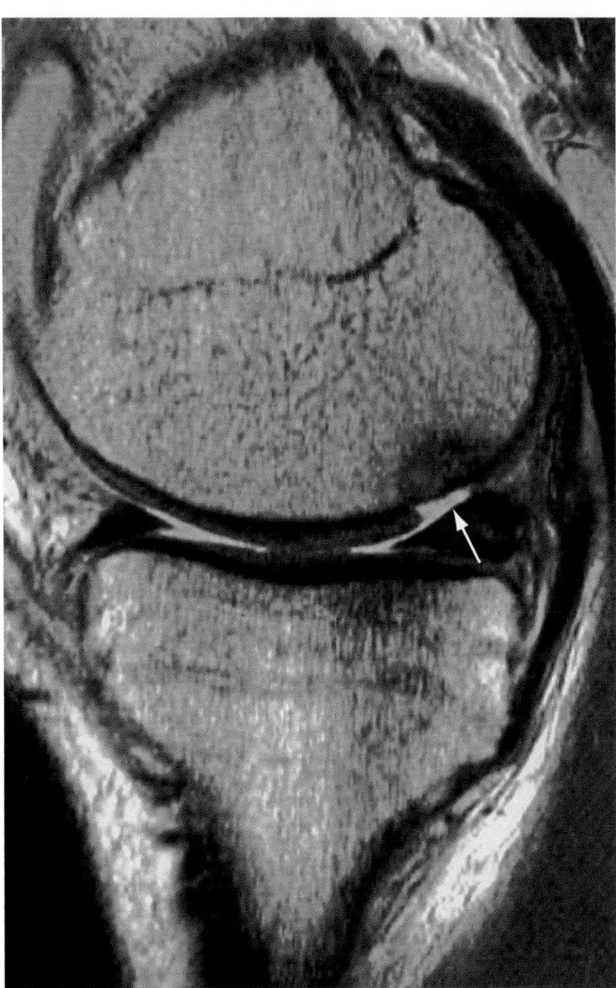

FIGURE 103-36

Sagittal fast spin-echo image through the medial joint line demonstrates focal full-thickness chondral injury with associated subchondral osseous changes (*arrow*).

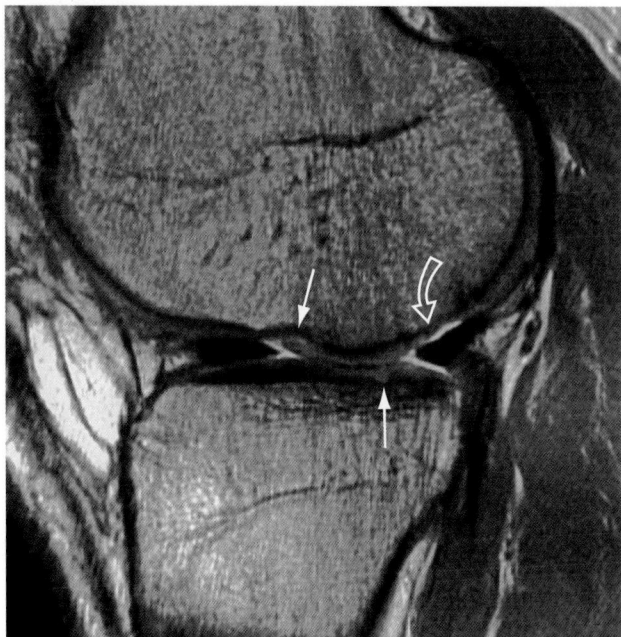

FIGURE 103-37

Sagittal fast spin-echo image in a 38-year-old patient demonstrating moderate cartilage loss with chronic anterior cruciate ligament insufficiency. Note the subacute characteristic transchondral fractures (*long arrows*) and additional non-acute chondral injury (*open arrow*).

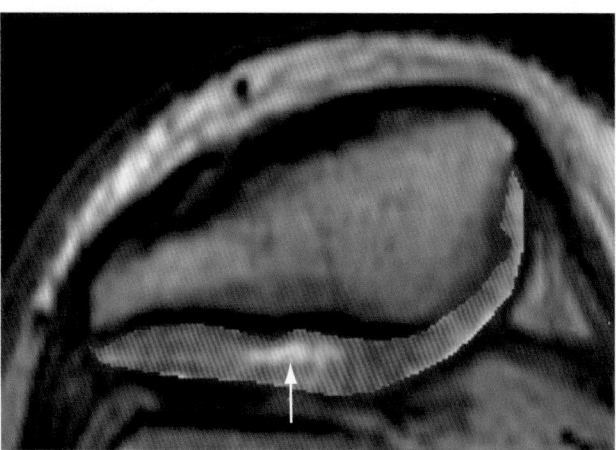

FIGURE 103-38

Axial quantitative T2 relaxation color map in an asymptomatic 31-year-old female demonstrates focal T2 prolongation in the radial zone of the dominant lateral facet (*arrow*), suggesting disorganization of the collagen in the radial zone.

Assessment of collagen is largely based on T2 mapping, which takes advantage of the expected stratification of T2 relaxation time as a function of the collagen orientation (Fig. 103-38).[195] Within the basilar components, where the collagen is highly ordered and perpendicular to the subchondral plate, there is relative restriction of water, accounting for the shorter T2 relaxation times encountered, as opposed to that in the transitional zone where the collagen is more randomly oriented and the T2 relaxation time is prolonged. A laminar appearance of articular cartilage has been noted on MRI in bovine explants at 1.5 T and these laminae reflect the preferential alignment of water associated with the orientation of collagen component of the matrix, relative to the long axis of the external field (B_0).[196] Using both MRI at 7 T and polarized light microscopy, Xia et al provided quantitative correlation between T2 profiles and histologic zones based on collagen fiber orientation.[197] Care must be taken when transporting these techniques to clinical field strengths, as errors may be introduced by the use of standard multiecho, multislice pulse sequences.[198] The ability to detect early alterations in the structure of collagen is intriguing as it would provide a noninvasive means of assessing early changes in the matrix that precede morphologic degradation and degenerative joint disease.

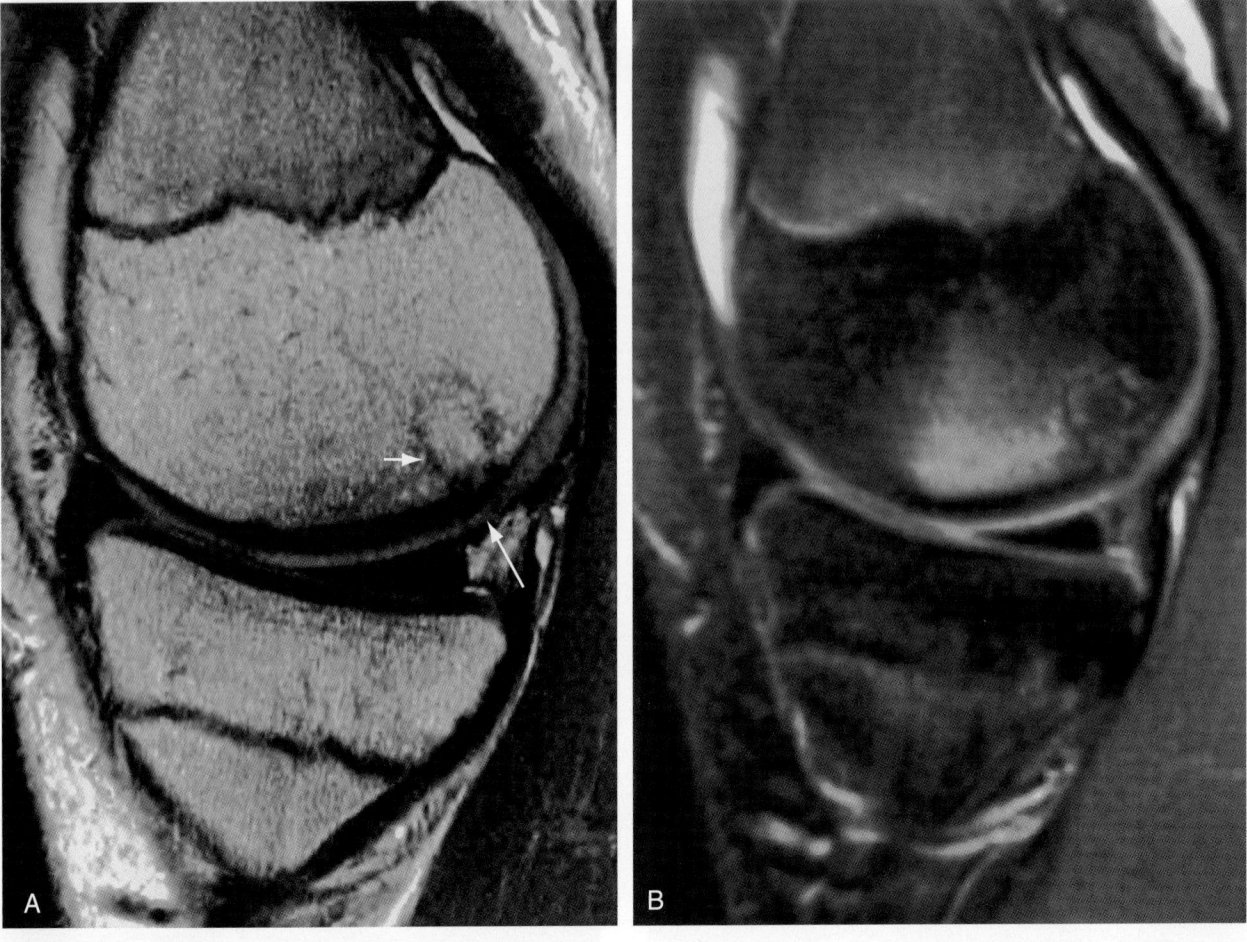

FIGURE 103-39

A, Sagittal fast spin-echo image in a patient 7 months post mosaicplasty. Note the partial incorporation of the plug (*short arrow*) with congruity and healing of the articular cartilage (*long arrow*). **B,** Sagittal fast spin-echo image in the same patient demonstrates persistent subchondral edema.

Assessment of Repair Cartilage

Both morphologic MRI assessment and the above matrix assessment techniques will be necessary to provide a comprehensive, objective assessment of cartilage repair techniques. Hyaline cartilage has little ability to undergo self-repair following traumatic and degenerative degradation. Many techniques have been suggested to resurface the degenerative joint, including microfracture, autologous cartilage implantation, fresh osteochondral allografts, and autologous osteochondral grafting.[199-203] Many components of the repair cartilage morphology may be measured, including signal characteristics relative to hyaline cartilage, morphology of the repair, interface with the native cartilage, as well as the integrity of the periosteal flap in the setting of those techniques using periosteum to stabilize the repair matrix.[204] In an observational study of 180 MR examinations obtained in 112 patients who had a variety of cartilage resurfacing techniques, autologous cartilage implantation (ACI) consistently demonstrated better fill of the defects at all times compared to microfracture.[204] The periosteal graft

of ACI, however, was hypertrophied in 63% of surgeries. Propensity for bony overgrowth was most marked in the microfracture group, with loss of adjacent cartilage evident in progressive follow-up MR examination.[204]

Early reports of the MR imaging findings following mosaicplasty have demonstrated healing of the osteochondral plugs with visualization of an intact layer of cartilage at the interface between the plug and the articular surface interface (Fig. 103-39).[205] The presence of fluid about the plugs suggested non-incorporation as well as frank necrosis of the plugs.[205] Surgical restoration of the articular surface is paramount to healing of the graft. Jakob et al note that if the plug is placed too high, it will bear a large proportion of the mechanical load, leading to abrasion of the surface as well as damage to the opposite articular surface; conversely, if the plug is placed too low, the surface may be predisposed to degradation.[206]

Standardized validated cartilage sequences are now available for all joints and the sequences ideally should not be limited in the postoperative setting or in the presence of orthopedic instrumentation. Such techniques

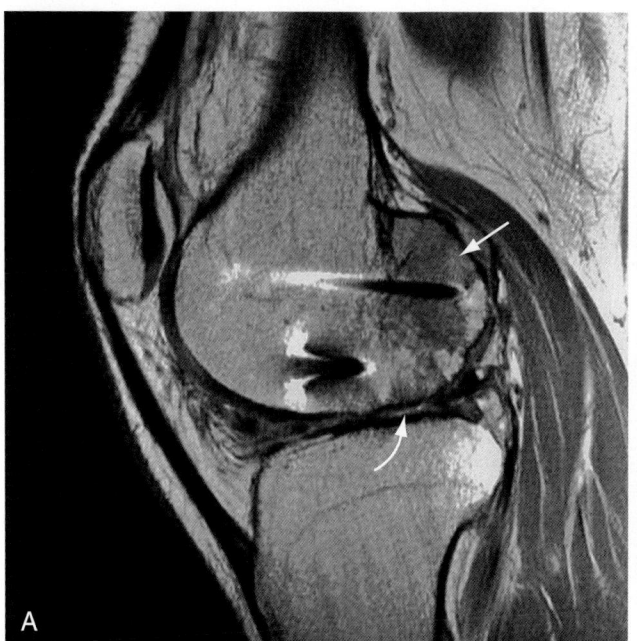 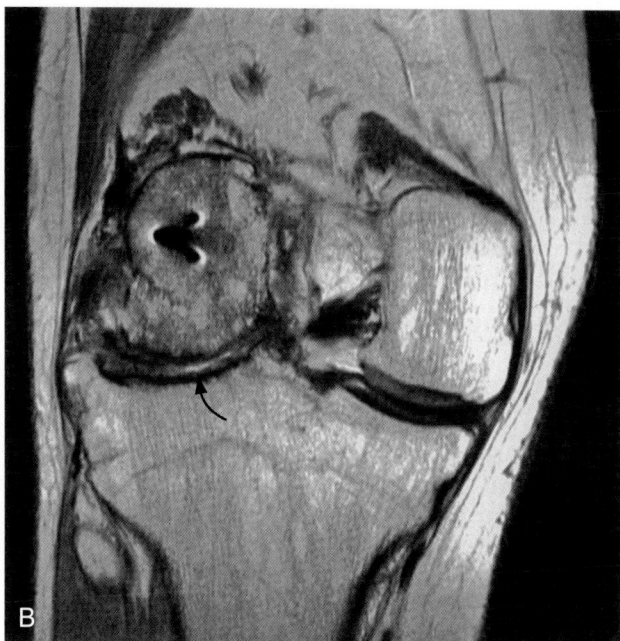

FIGURE 103-40

A, Sagittal fast spin-echo image in a 28-year-old male 9 years post hemicondylar fresh frozen allograft (*straight arrow*) for avascular necrosis. Note the loss of cartilage over the plateau (*curved arrow*), typical of frozen allograft tissue. **B,** Coronal fast spin-echo image in the same patient demonstrates cartilage loss over the tibial plateau (*curved arrow*).

provide noninvasive detection of traumatic injury as well as the ability to monitor progression of cartilage degeneration, and osteoarthrosis and disease status in the inflammatory arthritides. Lastly, they provide objective outcome assessment of cartilage repair techniques (Fig. 103-40). Future development will allow for detection of early changes in the extracellular matrix prior to morphologic alteration.

A more comprehensive discussion of cartilage is provided in Chapter 109.

PATELLOFEMORAL JOINT

Magnetic resonance imaging of the patellofemoral joint is often used to evaluate patellar tracking and sequela of patellar dislocation. In the setting of acute/subacute patellar dislocation, MR imaging is often requested to evaluate the extent of soft-tissue injury as well as possible cartilaginous or osteochondral injuries and intra-articular bodies. A characteristic osseous edema pattern in the setting of patellar dislocation and subsequent relocation is found in the anterolateral femoral condyle and inferomedial patella.[207,208] In a series of patellar dislocations reported by Elias et al, 15% of cases had intra-articular bodies.[207]

MRI has been shown to demonstrate various soft-tissue injuries in the setting of lateral patellar dislocation, including medial patellofemoral ligament injuries and edema in the inferior margin of the vastus medialis obliquus.[207] Injury to the medial patellofemoral ligament

was identified in 49% of cases of lateral patellar dislocation in one series; of these, complete tears were present in 40%. The medial patellofemoral ligament and the superficial medial collateral ligament have been demonstrated in cadaver studies to be extracapsular structures.[209] The medial patellofemoral ligament attaches at the superomedial aspect of the patella and attaches to the femur just anterior to the medial epicondyle and is contiguous with the deep retinacular layer of the vastus medialis obliquus.[210] Cadaver studies have demonstrated that the medial patellofemoral ligament contributes to 60% of the total force restraining lateral patellar subluxation.[211] The medial patellofemoral ligament usually tears from the femur; one series of acute patellar dislocation with arthroscopic correlation demonstrated avulsion of the medial patellofemoral ligament from the femur in 94% of cases.[212] The presence of medial collateral ligament injury affecting the anterior margin at the femur should prompt a more thorough evaluation of the medial patellofemoral ligament, as 89% of medial collateral ligament injuries were associated with injuries to the medial patellofemoral ligament.[207]

Some authors have studied the lateral trochlear inclination on axial magnetic resonance images to evaluate for trochlear dysplasia in cases of patellar instability.[213] The lateral trochlear index has been defined on axial fat-suppressed T2-weighted images by a line tangential to the subchondral plate of the posterior margin of the femoral condyles, crossed with a line drawn tangential to the subchondral plate of the lateral trochlear facet.[213] The mean lateral trochlear index was 6.17° in symptomatic patients and 16.93° in asymptomatic controls; patients with patellar instability were found to have a more horizontally oriented lateral trochlear facet compared with controls with an average lateral trochlear index of less than 11°.[213] Dynamic magnetic resonance imaging may also be used to evaluate patellar tracking with specialized coil designs.[214]

Synovial Disorders

Magnetic resonance imaging provides excellent anatomic depiction of the various synovial reflections of the knee. Even the presence of a small joint effusion can be clearly delineated with the use of fast inversion recovery or fat-suppressed T2-weighted images.

One of the most common synovial disorders diagnosed with magnetic resonance imaging is pigmented villonodular synovitis (PVNS). One of the advantages of magnetic resonance imaging is its ability to demonstrate the entire regional involvement of PVNS, with both intra- as well as extra-articular spread. PVNS can occur in diffuse or nodular form, the latter most commonly occurring in the deep infrapatellar fat pad and the suprapatellar pouch. PVNS is heterogeneously intermediate signal intensity or heterogeneously low signal intensity on proton-density or T1-wighted sequences, respectively. The addition of a gradient recalled echo sequence can help increase the conspicuity of small nodular foci of PVNS, taking advantage of the hemosiderin effect and resultant dephasing caused by such lesions (Fig. 103-41). These sequences, however, are of limited use in the postoperative setting and meticulous inspection of the various synovial reflections for small nodular foci of recurrence on routine sequences is necessary.

A high recurrence rate of PVNS foci has been demonstrated with incomplete excision of the primary lesions, which underscores the importance of preoperative evaluation with magnetic resonance imaging to visualize both intra- as well as extracapsular foci of disease.[215] Preoperative localization of tumor bulk with MR imaging is important as well, as patients' clinical presentation may not always correlate with the extent of disease.[216]

Extensor Mechanism

Anterior knee pain is a not uncommon complaint in athletes, particularly in those sports that involve jumping, such as basketball. Patients with anterior knee pain may develop pathology of the quadriceps tendon, patellar tendon or the patella itself or sustain cartilage damage in the patellofemoral joint. MR imaging can aid in establishing the correct diagnosis and direct treatment to the appropriate area.[217] MR imaging is often needed to diagnose injuries to the extensor mechanism as, in the acute stage, regional soft-tissue hematoma and swelling may preclude detailed clinical examination.[218]

The quadriceps mechanism is composed of the conjoined tendons of the rectus femoris and the three vasti: the vastus medialis, the vastus intermedius, and the vastus lateralis. The normal quadriceps tendon appears as a low signal intensity structure, often with an internal mildly hyperintense laminated appearance.[218] Complete tears of the quadriceps mechanism are seen as focal, complete areas of full-thickness tendinous discontinuity, often with caudal retraction of the patella, due to unopposed pull of the patellar tendon. Partial tears of the quadriceps, however, are not uncommon and these lesions should be graded by the degree of cross-sectional area of involvement of the tear. The degree of pre-existing tendinosis should also be assessed, as this has implications for primary repair capacity versus tissue augmentation techniques.

The patellar tendon is a thick, homogeneously low signal intensity band connecting the distal two-thirds of the patella to the anterior margin of the tibial tubercle.[219] The patellar tendon fibers are not uniformly oriented as the internal fibers are somewhat more obliquely oriented near the tibial attachment, similar to the supraspinatus tendon in the shoulder, resulting in a moderately anisotropic tissue, exhibiting the magic angle phenomenon.[219,220] Karantanas et al found spurious high signal intensity within clinically normal patellar tendons on three-dimensional T1-weighted pulse sequences with fat suppression, which were normal on routine T2 turbo spin-echo images.[220] Normal patellar tendons on gradient-echo sequences have also demonstrated mild foci of increased signal intensity at both the proximal and distal ends.[221] Schweitzer et al have also found that 74% of clinically asymptomatic patients in one series had areas of abnormal signal within the patellar tendon, possibly reflecting early subclinical degeneration.[222]

Not truly an inflammatory state, patellar "tendinitis" or tendinosis has been shown histologically to reflect angiofibroblastic tissue[223] (Fig. 103-42). This is consistent with contrast-enhanced MR imaging studies demonstrating areas of variable enhancement correlating with degrees of fibrovascular repair.[224] MR findings of patellar tendinosis include thickening of the tendon as well as abnormal intrasubstance signal abnormality.[225]

The relationship between patellar tendon abnormalities and Osgood-Schlatter disease has been debated. Rosenberg et al reviewed the clinical, MR, CT, and scintigraphic data of 20 patients and concluded that Osgood-Schlatter disease results from trauma to the patellar tendon and adjacent soft-tissues, as opposed to a primary apophyseal fracture of the tibial tubercle.[226] The stages of Osgood-Schlatter disease can be followed with MR imaging, with regional soft-tissue edema around the tibial tuberosity present in the earliest stage, followed by partial avulsion of the ossification center, and finally by complete avulsion of the tibial tubercle apophysis, often with retraction.[227]

Plicae

Synovial plicae are remnants of partitions that exist in the fetal knee. Rarely these synovial folds may become thickened and symptomatic. "Plicae syndrome" is usually a diagnosis of exclusion, in which the only MR finding

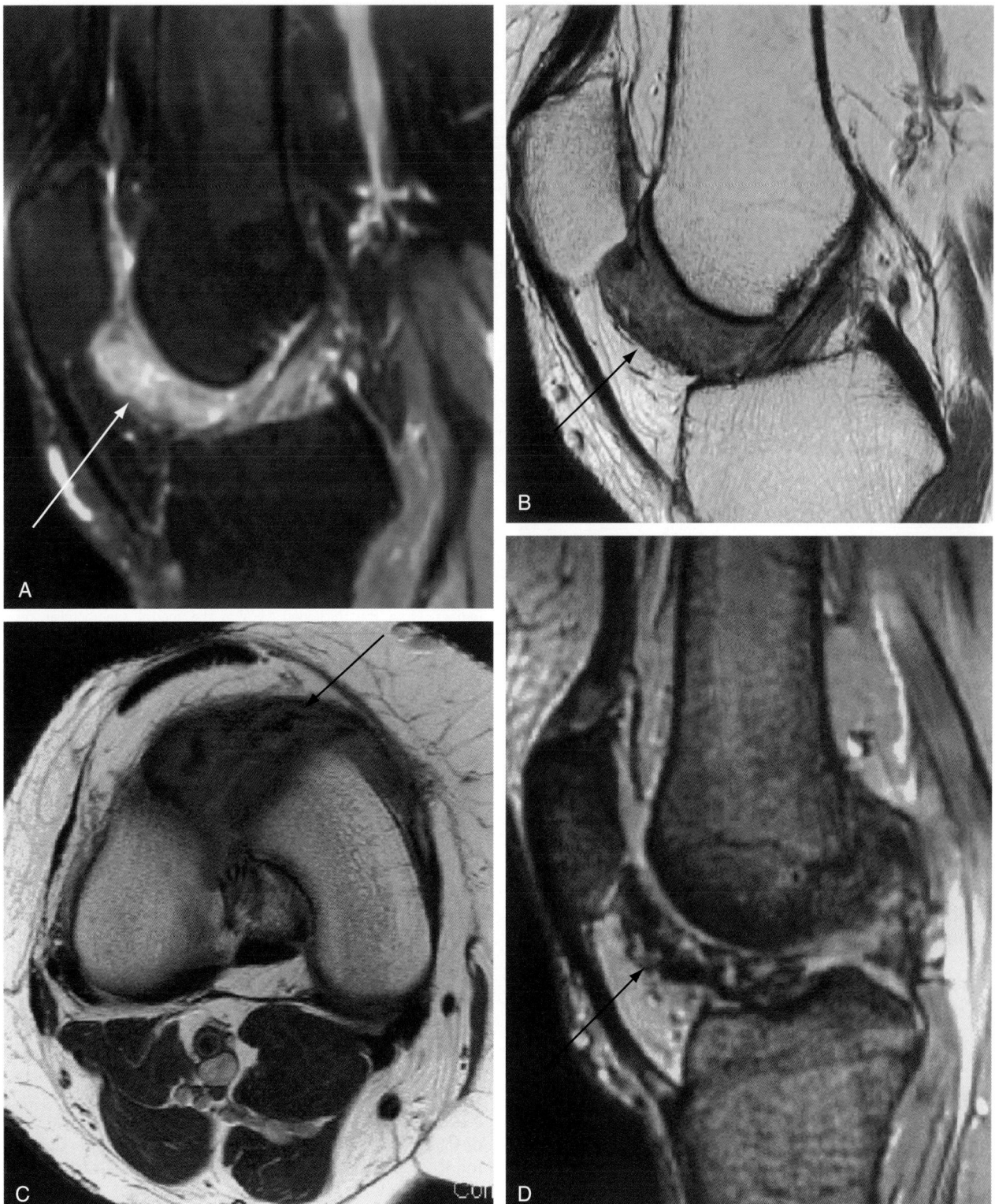

FIGURE 103-41

A, Sagittal frequency-selective fat-suppressed image demonstrating a heterogeneous hyperintense nodular mass in the infrapatellar fat (*arrow*). **B,** Sagittal fast spin-echo proton density-weighted image in the same patient demonstrating a heterogeneously intermediate signal intensity to low signal intensity mass (*arrow*). **C,** Axial fast spin-echo image in the same patient demonstrating the heterogeneous intermediate to low signal intensity mass (*arrow*). **D,** Sagittal gradient-echo image demonstrating focal field dephasing created by the paramagnetic effect of the hemosiderin blood products (*arrow*). Note the erosion of the lateral femoral condyle.

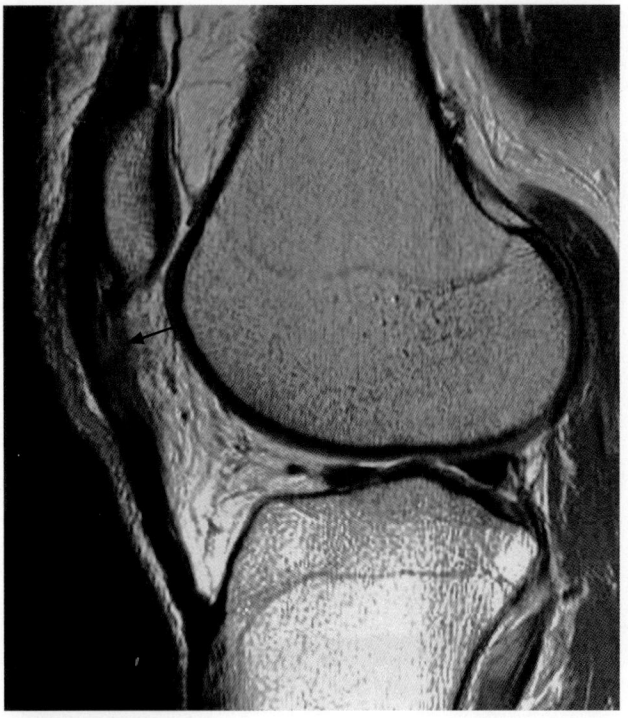

FIGURE 103-42

Sagittal fast spin-echo proton density-weighted image demonstrating moderate proximal patellar tendinosis (*arrow*). Note the abnormal signal intensity, inhomogeneity and fraying of the proximal, deep fibers of the normally hypointense patellar tendon.

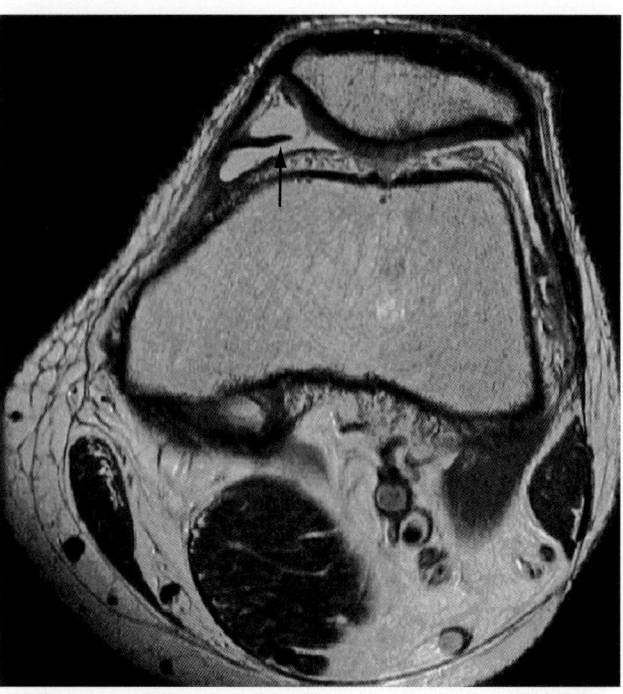

FIGURE 103-43

Axial fast spin-echo image demonstrating a medial parapatellar plica (*arrow*). Note the thickened plica in the medial suprapatellar recess surrounded by fluid. Medial parapatellar plicae are best visualized using axial images.

that can possibly explain the patient's pain is the presence of an enlarged thickened synovial plica surrounded by fluid and typically located in the medial gutter, known as the medial parapatellar plica.[228] Suprapatellar and deep infrapatellar plicae are typically not of clinical significance. Axial images are most helpful in diagnosing the presence of a medial parapatellar plica, while the sagittal sequence will show a supra- or infrapatellar plicae to best advantage[229,230] (Figs. 103-43 and 103-44).

Intra-articular Bodies

The presence of intra-articular fragments, whether they are osseous or cartilaginous, can cause considerable patient symptomatology, with pain, locking, and clicking. These fragments must be meticulously screened for, especially in a severely arthritic knee or one with a complex meniscal tear, in which a small fragment of fibrocartilage may be displaced. Unless high signal intensity fluid surrounds such fragments, they should not be described as "loose" as they may be attached to the capsule and less amenable to prompt arthroscopic removal. The bodies may not always be near their donor site and often migrate. Common locations for these intra-articular bodies include the intercondylar notch, the far

posterosuperior joint recess, behind the distal femoral metaphysis, in the popliteus hiatus or bursa, the meniscosynovial recesses and in the medial or lateral suprapatellar bursae. It should be noted that these bodies may be nourished by the synovial tissue and may grow over time, resulting in hypertrophy and occasionally ossification.[231]

Osteonecrosis

Osteonecrosis usually occurs as a result of a systemic process such as steroid use, alcohol abuse, collagen vascular disorders, human immunodeficiency virus (HIV) infection, renal transplantation, and sickle cell disease.[232-236] There have been reports of the development of osteonecrosis after arthroscopic intervention, usually in older patients with chondral or meniscal lesions.[237-241] This has been proposed to be a result of altered mechanical forces in cases of meniscal pathology.[238] The true incidence of postarthroscopy avascular necrosis (AVN) is unknown, as the temporal relationship between clinical symptoms, preoperative and postoperative MR examinations in the large majority of these studies is quite variable. Johnson et al attempted to standardize the duration of clinical symptoms, preoperative and postoperative MR examinations and

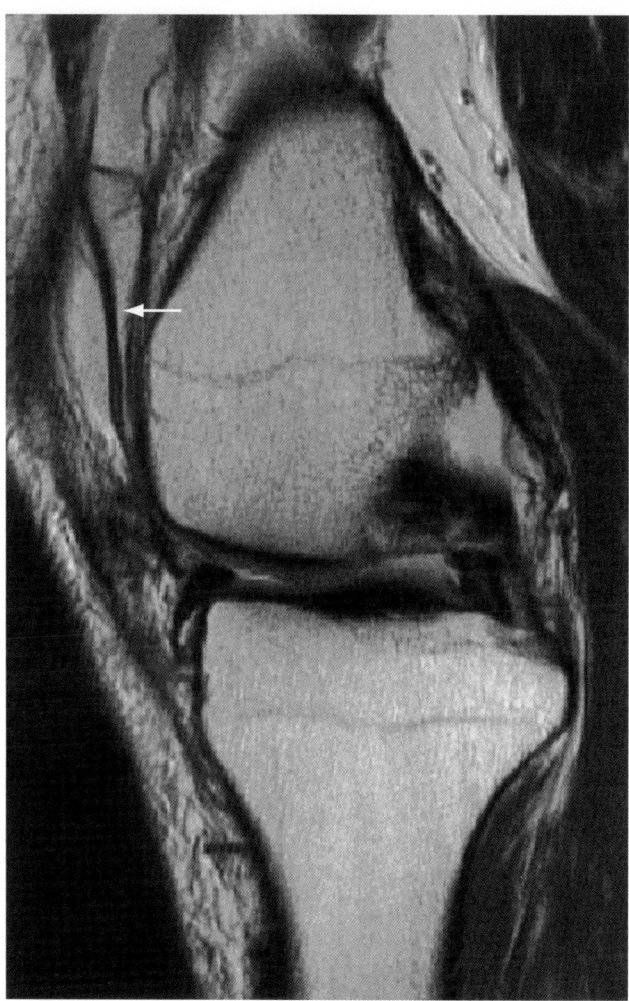

FIGURE 103-44

Sagittal fast spin-echo proton density-weighted image demonstrating a prominent suprapatellar plica (*arrow*) surrounded by fluid. Infrapatellar and suprapatellar plicae are seen to best advantage on sagittal images.

found seven patients with postarthroscopy AVN.[238] All seven patients had pre-existing pathology in the ipsilateral compartment (meniscal tears, chondral lesions); however, only one case had pathologically proven necrosis. It is possible that some of these suspected cases of postarthroscopy AVN actually have reflected subchondral insufficiency fractures, as the early MR appearances of both can be similar.

Distinguishing spontaneous osteonecrosis from subchondral insufficiency fracture may be difficult and, in fact, histologically, the two have been shown to be related.[242,243] Yamamoto and Bullough have proposed that in some cases, a subchondral insufficiency fracture is the inciting event in the development of osteonecrosis.[243] Other authors similarly have suggested a traumatic etiology for "spontaneous" osteonecrosis on the knee.[242]

MR imaging can diagnose clinically unsuspected cases of osteonecrosis and thus can direct appropriate intervention, depending on the degree of areas of involvement. The relationship of the necrotic bone to the articular surface is an important prognostic indicator, often indicating the knee for aggressive surgical intervention such as core decompression, high tibial osteotomy or total knee arthroplasty.[234,244] Fibrotic, non-viable bone is low signal intensity on all pulse sequences. In general, osteonecrosis is seen as a focal area of signal abnormality, involving either the subchondral surface or intramedullary cavity, often having a peripheral "serpiginous" high signal intensity rim around a low signal intensity core. The degree of involvement should be reported and if the lesion involves an articular surface, the amount of involvement or cross-sectional area of the necrotic fragment should be noted. The appearance of the adjacent articular cartilage, in cases of subchondral lesions, and the presence, if any, of subchondral collapse should be noted.

CONCLUSION

Magnetic resonance imaging is an indispensable imaging method for diagnosing various causes of internal derangement in the knee. Its importance as a clinical diagnostic imaging tool lies in its ability to identify and characterize possible causes of internal derangement as well as to identify the extent of disease, often clinically unsuspected by the referring orthopedic surgeon or rheumatologist. The ability to "look into" the knee noninvasively prior to arthroscopic inspection can direct the orthopedic surgeon to the location of meniscal fragments, cartilage defects, and ligament tears. In addition, appropriate modification of pulse sequence parameters allows an accurate, reliable method of diagnosing possible internal derangement in the postoperative setting, with or without orthopedic hardware in place, including bulky metallic hardware such as total knee arthroplasty. Meticulous attention to pulse sequence parameters also allows a noninvasive method of monitoring both hyaline and fibrocartilage repair procedures, sometimes obviating the need for second-look arthroscopy.

REFERENCES

1. Langer JE, Meyer SJF, Dalinka MK: Imaging of the knee. Radiol Clin North Am 28:975-990, 1990.
2. Cotton A. Delfaut E, Demondion X, et al: MR imaging of the knee at 0.2 and 1.5T: correlation with surgery. Am J Roentgenol 174:1093-109, 2000.
3. Vellet AD, Lee DH, Munk PL, et al: Anterior cruciate ligament tear: prospective evaluation of diagnostic accuracy of middle and high-field strength MR imaging at 1.5 and 0.5T. Radiology 197:826-830, 1995.
4. Woertler K, Strothmann M, Tombach B, et al: Detection of articular cartilage lesions: experimental evaluation of low and high field strength MR imaging at 0.18 and 1.0 T. J Magn Reson Imaging 11:678-685, 2000.
5. Reicher MA, Bassett LW, Gold RH: High-resolution magnetic resonance imaging of the knee joint: pathologic correlations. Am J Roentgenol 145:903-909, 1985.
6. Niitsu M, Akisada M, Anno I, et al: Moving knee joint: technique for kinematic MR imaging. Radiology 174:569-570, 1990.
7. Niitsu M, Anno I, Fukubayashi T, et al: Tears of cruciate ligaments and menisci: evaluation with cine MR imaging. Radiology 178:859-864, 1991.
8. Buckwalter KA, Pennes DR: Anterior cruciate ligament: oblique sagittal MR imaging. Radiology 175:276-277, 1990.

9. Arndt WF, Truax AL, Barnett FM, et al: MR diagnosis of bone contusions of the knee: comparison of coronal T2-weighted fast spin-echo with fat saturation and fast spin-echo STIR images with conventional STIR images. Am J Roentgenol 166:119-124, 1996.

10. Eustace S, Hentzen P, Adams J, et al: Comparison of conventional and turbo spin-echo T1-weighted MR imaging in acute knee trauma. Am J Roentgenol 172:1393-1395, 1999.

11. Ha TPT, Li KCP, Beaulieu CF, et al: Anterior cruciate ligament injury: fast spin-echo MR imaging with arthroscopic correlation in 217 examinations. Am J Roentgenol 170:1215-1219, 1998.

12. Sonin AH, Pensy RA, Mulligan ME, et al: Grading articular cartilage of the knee using fast spin-echo proton density-weighted MR imaging without fat suppression. Am J Roentgenol 179:1159-1166, 2002.

13. Hajek PC, Sartorius DJ, Neumann CH, et al: Potential contrast agents for MR arthrography: in vitro evaluation and practical observations. Am J Roentgenol 149:97, 1987.

14. Coumans JM, Palmer WE: Knee arthrography: evolution and current status. Radiol Clin North Am 36:703-728, 1998.

15. Sofka CM, Potter HG, Figgie M, et al: Magnetic resonance imaging of total knee arthroplasty. Clin Orthop 406:129-135, 2003.

16. Lajtai G, Humer K, Aitzetmuller G, et al: Serial magnetic resonance imaging evaluation of a bioabsorbable interference screw and the adjacent bone. Arthroscopy 15:481-488, 1999.

17. Sirlin CB, Boutin RD, Brossmann J, et al: Polydioxanone biodegradable pins in the knee; MR imaging. Am J Roentgenol 176:83-90, 2001.

18. White LM, Kim JK, Mehta M, et al: Complications of total hip arthroplasty: MR imaging—initial experience. Radiology 215:254-262, 2000.

19. Sofka CM, Potter HG: MR imaging of joint arthroplasty. Semin Musculoskeletal Radiol 6:79-85, 2002.

20. Eustace S, Jara H, Goldberg R, et al: A comparison of conventional spin-echo and turbo spin-echo imaging of soft tissues adjacent to orthopedic hardware. Am J Roentgenol 170:455-458, 1998.

21. Tartaglino LM, Flanders AE, Vinitski S, et al: Metallic artifacts on MR images of the postoperative spine: reduction with fast spin-echo techniques. Radiology 190:565-569, 1994.

22. Henck CB, Brodner W, Grampp S, et al: The postoperative spine. Top Magn Reson Imaging 10:247-29, 1999.

23. Cortell ED, Kaufman JA, Geller SC, et al: MR angiography of tibial runoff vessels: imaging with the head coil compared with conventional arteriography. Am J Roentgenol 167:147-151, 1996.

24. Potter HG, Weinstein M, Allen AA, et al: Magnetic resonance imaging of the multiple-ligament injured knee. J Orthop Trauma 16:330-339, 2002.

25. Barnett MJ: MR diagnosis of internal derangements of the knee: effect of field strength on efficacy. Am J Roentgenol 161:115-118, 1993.

26. Smith DK, May DA, Phillips P: MR imaging of the anterior cruciate ligament: frequency of discordant findings on sagittal-oblique images and correlation with arthroscopic correlation. Am J Roentgenol 166:411-413, 1996.

27. Fitzgerald SW, Remer EM, Friedman H, et al: MR evaluation of the anterior cruciate ligament: value of supplementing sagittal images with coronal and axial images. Am J Roentgenol 160:1233-1237, 1993.

28. Niitsu M, Ikeda K, Itai Y: Slightly flexed knee position within a standard knee coil: MR delineation of the anterior cruciate ligament. Eur Radiol 8:113-115, 1998.

29. Potter HG, Sofka CM, Hooper T: Imaging the knee. In: Callaghan J, Rosenberg A, Rubash H, et al (eds) The Adult Knee. New York: Lippincott, Williams and Wilkins, 2003.

30. Hodler J, Haghighi P, Trudell D, et al: The cruciate ligaments of the knee: correlation between MR appearance and gross and histologic findings in cadaveric specimens. Am J Roentgenol 159:357-360, 1992.

31. Lee SH, Peterslige CA, Trudell DJ, et al: Extrasynovial spaces of the cruciate ligaments: anatomy, MR imaging, and diagnostic implications. Am J Roentgenol 166:1433-1437, 1996.

32. Tung GA, Davis LM, Wiggins ME, et al: Tears of the anterior cruciate ligament: primary and secondary signs at MR imaging. Radiology 188:661-667, 1993.

33. McCauley TR, Moses M, Kier R, et al: MR diagnosis of tears of anterior cruciate ligament of the knee: importance of ancillary findings. Am J Roentgenol 162:115-119, 1994.

34. Brandser EA, Riley MA, Berbaum KS, et al: MR imaging of anterior cruciate ligament injury: independent value of primary and secondary signs. Am J Roentgenol 167:121-126, 1996.

35. Murphy BJ, Smith RL, Uribe JW, et al: Bone signal abnormalities in the posterolateral tibia and lateral femoral condyle in complete tears of the anterior cruciate ligament: a specific sign? Radiology 182:221-224, 1992.

36. Stein LN, Fischer DA, Fritts HM, et al: Occult osseous lesions associated with anterior cruciate ligament tears. Clin Orthop 313:187-193, 1995.

37. Vellet AD, Marks PH, Fowler PJ, et al: Occult posttraumatic osteochondral lesions of the knee: prevalence, classification, and short-term sequelae evaluated with MR imaging. Radiology 178:271-276, 1991.

38. Lahm A, Erggelet C, Steinwachs M, et al: Articular and osseous lesions in recent ligament tears: arthroscopic changes compared with magnetic resonance imaging findings. Arthroscopy 14:597-604, 1998.

39. Johnson DL, Urban Jr WP, Caborn DNM, et al: Articular cartilage changes seen with magnetic resonance imaging-detected bone bruises associated with acute anterior cruciate ligament rupture. Am J Sports Med 26:409-414, 1998.

40. Vahey TN, Hunt JE, Shelbourne KD: Anterior translocation of the tibia at MR imaging: a secondary sign of anterior cruciate ligament tear. Radiology 187:817-81, 1993.

41. Remer EM, Fitzgerald SW, Friedman H, et al: Anterior cruciate ligament injury: MR imaging diagnosis and pattens of injury. Radiographics 12:901-915, 1992.

42. Robertson PL, Schweitzer ME, Bartolozzi AR, et al: Anterior cruciate ligament tears: evaluation of multiple signs with MR imaging. Radiology 193:829-834, 1994.

43. Gentilli A, Seeger LL, Yao L, et al: Anterior cruciate ligament tear: indirect signs at MR imaging. Radiology 193:835-840, 1994.

44. Moore SL: Imaging the anterior cruciate ligament. Orthop Clin North Am 33:663-674, 2002.

45. Staron RB, Haramati N, Feldman F, et al: O'Donoghue's triad: magnetic resonance imaging evaluation. Skeletal Radiol 23:633-636, 1994.

46. Goldman AB, Pavlov H, Rubenstein D. The Segond fracture of the proximal tibia: a small avulsion that reflects major ligamentous damage. Am J Roentgenol 151:1163-1167, 1988.

47. Weber WN, Neumann CH, Barakos JA, et al: Lateral tibial rim (Segond) fractures: MR imaging characteristics. Radiology 180:731-734, 1991.

48. Campos JC, Chung CB, Lektrakul N, et al: Pathogenesis of the Segond fracture: anatomic and MR imaging evidence of an iliotibial tract or anterior oblique band avulsion. Radiology 219:381-386, 2001.

49. Escobedo EM, Mills WJ, Hunter JC: The "reverse Segond" fracture: association with a tear of the posterior cruciate ligament and medial meniscus. Am J Roentgenol 178:979-983, 2002.

50. Chan KK, Resnick D, Goodwin D, et al: Posteromedial tibial plateau injury including avulsion fracture of the semimembranosus tendon insertion site: ancillary sign of anterior cruciate ligament tear at MR imaging. Radiology 211:754-758, 1999.

51. Paletta G: Special considerations: anterior cruciate ligament reconstruction in the skeletally immature. Orthop Clin North Am 34:65-77, 2003.

52. Umans H, Wimpfheimer O, Haramati N, et al: Diagnosis of partial tears of the anterior cruciate ligament of the knee: value of MR imaging. Am J Roentgenol 165:893-897, 1995.

53. Yao L, Gentilli A, Petrus L, et al: Partial ACL rupture: an MR diagnosis? Skeletal Radiol 24:247-251, 1995.

54. Vahey TN, Broome DR, Kayes KJ, et al: Acute and chronic tears of the anterior cruciate ligament: differential features at MR imaging. Radiology 181:251-253, 1991.

55. Kumar A, Bickerstaff DR, Grimwood JS, et al: Mucoid cystic degeneration of the cruciate ligament. J Bone Joint Surg 81-B:304-305, 1999.

56. McIntyre J, Moelleken S, Tirman P: Mucoid degeneration of the anterior cruciate ligament mistaken for ligamentous tears. Skeletal Radiol 30:312-315, 2001.

57. Zantop T, Rusch A, Hassenpfug J, et al: Intra-articular ganglion cysts of the cruciate ligaments: case report and review of the literature. Arch Orthop Trauma Surg 123:195-198, 2003.

58. Deutsch A, Veltri DM, Altchek DW, et al: Symptomatic intraarticular ganglia of the cruciate ligaments of the knee. Arthroscopy 10(2):219-22, 1994.

59. Sonin AH, Fitzgerald SW, Friedman H, et al: Posterior cruciate ligament injury: MR imaging diagnosis and patterns of injury. Radiology 190:455-458, 1994.

60. Hall FM, Hochman MG: Medial Segond-type fracture: cortical avulsion off the medial tibial plateau associated with tears of the posterior cruciate ligament and medial meniscus. Skeletal Radiol 26:553-555, 1997.

61. Grover JS, Bassett LW, Gross ML, et al: Posterior cruciate ligament: MR imaging. Radiology 174:527-530, 1990.

62. Mariani PP, Adriani E, Bellelli A, et al: Magnetic resonance imaging of tunnel placement in posterior cruciate ligament reconstruction. Arthroscopy 15:733-740, 1999.

63. Tewes D, Fritts H, Fields R, et al: Chronically injured posterior cruciate ligament: magnetic resonance imaging. Clin Orthop 335:224-232, 1997.

64. Sherman PM, Sanders TG, Morrison WB, et al: MR imaging of the posterior cruciate ligament graft: initial experience in 15 patients with clinical correlation. Radiology 221:191-198, 2001.

65. de Maeseneer M, van Roy F, Lenchik L, et al: Three layers of the medial capsular and supporting structures of the knee: MR imaging—anatomic correlation. Radiographics 20:S83-S89, 2000.

66. Loredo R, Hodler J, Pedowitz R, et al: Posteromedial corner of the knee: MR imaging with gross anatomic correlation. Skeletal Radiol 28:305-311, 1999.

67. Inoue MI, McGurk-Burleson E, Hollis JM, et al: Treatment of the medial collateral ligament injury. I: The importance of anterior cruciate ligament on the varus-valgus knee laxity. Am J Sports Med 15:15-21, 1987.

68. Shoemaker SC, Markolf KL: Effects of joint load on the stiffness and laxity of ligament-deficient knees: an in vivo study of the anterior cruciate and medial collateral ligaments. J Bone Joint Surg 67-A:136-146, 1985.

69. Yao L, Dungan D, Seeger LL: MR imaging of tibial collateral ligament injury: comparison with clinical examination. Skeletal Radiol 23:521-524, 1994.

70. Schweitzer ME, Tran D, Deely DM, et al: Medial collateral ligament injuries: evaluation of multiple signs, prevalence, and location of associated bone bruises and assessment with MR imaging. Radiology 194:825-829, 1995.

71. Patel JJ: Intra-articular entrapment of the medial collateral ligament: radiographic and MRI findings. Skeletal Radiol 28:658-660, 1999.

72. Hennigan SP, Schneck CD, Mesgarzadeh M, et al: The semimembranosus-tibial collateral bursa: anatomical study and magnetic resonance imaging. J Bone Joint Surg 76-A:1322-1327, 1994.

73. Rothstein CP, Laorr A, Helms CA, et al: Semimembranosus-tibial collateral ligament bursitis: MR imaging findings. Am J Roentgenol 166:875-87, 1996.

74. de Maeseneer M, Shahabpour M, van Roy F, et al: MR imaging of the medial collateral ligament bursa: findings in patients and anatomic data derived from cadavers. Am J Roentgenol 177:911-917, 2001.

75. Lee JK, Yao L: Tibial collateral ligament bursa: MR imaging. Radiology 178:855-857, 1991.

76. Ferrari DA, Ferrari JD, Coumans J: Posterolateral instability of the knee. J Bone Joint Surg 76-B:187-192, 1994.

77. Covey DC. Injuries of the posterolateral corner of the knee. J Bone Joint Surg 83-A:106-118, 2001.

78. Munshi M, Pretterklieber ML, Kwak S, et al: MR imaging, MR arthrography, and specimen correlation of the posterolateral corner of the knee: an anatomic study. Am J Roentgenol 180:1095-1101, 2003.

79. Recondo JA, Salvador E, Villanua JA, et al: Lateral stabilizing structures of the knee: functional anatomy and injuries assessed with MR imaging. Radiographics 20:S91-S102, 2000.

80. Brown TR, Quinn SF, Wensel JP, et al: Diagnosis of popliteus injuries with MR imaging. Skeletal Radiol 24:511-514, 1995.

81. Westrich GH, Hannafin JA, Potter HG: Isolated rupture and repair of the popliteus tendon. Arthroscopy 11(5):628-632, 1995.

82. Huang GS, Yu JS, Munshi M, et al: Avulsion fracture of the head of the fibula (the "arcuate" sign): MR imaging findings predictive of injuries to the posterolateral ligaments and posterior cruciate ligament. Am J Roentgenol 180:381-387, 2003.

83. Juhng SK, Lee JK, Choi SS, et al: MR evaluation of the "arcuate" sign of posterolateral knee instability. Am J Roentgenol 178:583-588, 2002.

84. Muhle C, Ahn JM, Yeh L, et al: Iliotibial band friction syndrome: MR imaging findings in 16 patients and MR arthrographic study of six cadaver knees. Radiology 212:103-110, 1999.

85. Schatz J, Potter HG, Rodeo SA, et al: MR imaging of anterior cruciate ligament reconstruction. Am J Roentgenol 169:223-228, 1997.

86. Harner CD, Giffin JR, Dunteman RC, et al: Evaluation and treatment of recurrent instability after anterior cruciate ligament reconstruction. J Bone Joint Surg 82-A:1652-1664, 2000.

87. Khan AS, Sherman OH, DeLay B: Thermal treatment of anterior cruciate ligament injury and laxity with its imaging characteristics. Clin Sports Med 21:701-711, 2002.

88. Bernicker JP, Haddad JL, Lintner DM, et al: Patellar tendon defect during the first year after anterior cruciate ligament reconstruction: appearance on serial magnetic resonance imaging. Arthroscopy 14:804-809, 1998.

89. Lajtai G, Noszian I, Humer K, et al: Serial magnetic resonance imaging evaluation of operative site after fixation of patellar tendon graft with bio-absorbable interference screws in anterior cruciate ligament reconstruction. Arthroscopy 15:709-718, 1999.

90. Tomczak RJ, Hehl G, Mergo PJ, et al: Tunnel placement in anterior cruciate ligament reconstruction: MRI analysis as an important factor in the radiological report. Skeletal Radiol 26:409-413, 1997.

91. Rak KM, Gillogly SD, Schaefer RA, et al: Anterior cruciate ligament reconstruction: evaluation with MR imaging. Radiology 178:553-556, 1991.

92. Jackson DW, Grood ES, Goldstein JD, et al: A comparison of patellar tendon autograft and allograft used for anterior cruciate ligament reconstruction in the goat model. Am J Sports Med 21:176-185, 1993.

93. Ayerza MA, Muscolo DL, Costa-Paz M, et al: Comparison of sagittal obliquity of the reconstructed anterior cruciate ligament with native anterior cruciate ligament using magnetic resonance imaging. Arthroscopy 19:257-261, 2003.

94. Horton LK, Jacobson JA, Lin J, et al: MR imaging of anterior cruciate ligament reconstruction graft. Am J Roentgenol 175:1091-1097, 2000.

95. Warden WH, Friedman R, Teresi LM, et al: Magnetic resonance imaging of bioabsorbable polylactic acid interference screws during the first 2 years after anterior cruciate ligament reconstruction. Arthroscopy 15:474-480, 1999.

96. Bach FD, Carlier RY, Elis JB, et al: Anterior cruciate ligament reconstruction with bioabsorbable polyglycolic acid interference screws: MR imaging follow-up. Radiology 225:541-550, 2002.

97. Bradley DM, Bergman AG, Dillingham MF: MR imaging of Cyclops lesions. Am J Roentgenol 174:719-726, 2000.

98. Recht MP, Piraino DW, Cohen MAH, et al: Localized anterior arthrofibrosis (Cyclops lesion) after reconstruction of the anterior cruciate ligament: MR imaging findings. Am J Roentgenol 165:383-385, 1995.

99. Rodeo SA, Hannafin JA, Tom J, et al: Immunolocalization of cytokines and their receptors in adhesive capsulitis of the shoulder. J Orthop Res 15:427-436.

100. Lindenfeld TN, Wojtys EM, Husain A: Operative treatment of arthrofibrosis of the knee. J Bone Joint Surg 81-A:1772-1784, 1999.

101. Yu JS, Goodwin D, Salonen D, et al: Complete dislocation of the knee: spectrum of associated soft-tissue injuries depicted by MR imaging. Am J Roentgenol 164:135-139, 1995.

102. Green NE, Allen BL. Vascular injuries associated with dislocation of the knee. J Bone Joint Surg Am 59:236-23, 1997.

103. McCoy GF, Hannon DG, Barr RJ, et al: Vascular injury associated with low velocity dislocations of the knee. J Bone Joint Surg Br 69:285-287, 1987.

104. Hill JA, Rana NA: Complications of posterolateral dislocation of the knee. Clin Orthop 154:212-215, 1981.

105. Shields L, Mital M, Cave EF: Complete dislocation of the knee: experience at the Massachusetts General Hospital. J Trauma 9:192-212, 1969.

106. Potter HG, Montgomery KD, Heise CW, et al: MR imaging of acetabular fractures: value in detecting femoral head injury, intraarticular fragments and sciatic nerve injury. Am J Roentgenol 163(4):881-88, 1994.

107. Cheung LP, Li KC, Hollett MD, et al: Meniscal tears of the knee: accuracy of detection with fast spin echo MR imaging and arthroscopic correlation in 293 patients. Radiology 203(2):508-512, 1997.

108. Kirkley S: A comparison of accuracy between clinical examination and magnetic resonance imaging in the diagnosis of meniscal and anterior cruciate ligament tears. Arthroscopy 13(2):279-280, 1997.

109. Rose NE, Gold SM: A comparison of accuracy between clinical examination and magnetic resonance imaging in the diagnosis of meniscal and anterior cruciate ligament tears. Arthroscopy 12(4):398-405, 1996.

110. De Smet AA, Norris MA, Yandrow DR, et al: Diagnosis of meniscal tears of the knee with MR imaging: effect of observer variation and sample size on sensitivity and specificity. Am J Roentgenol 160(3):555-559, 1993.

111. Rubin DA, Kneeland JB, Listerud J, et al: MR diagnosis of meniscal tears of the knee: value of fast spin-echo vs conventional spin-echo pulse sequences. Am J Roentgenol 162:1131-1135, 1994.

112. Escobedo EM, Hunter JC, Zink-Broday GC, et al: Usefulness of turbo spin-echo MR imaging in the evaluation of meniscal tears: comparison with a conventional spin-echo sequence. Am J Roentgenol 167:1223-1227, 1996.

113. Cheung LP, Li KCP, Hollett MD, et al: Meniscal tears of the knee: accuracy of detection with fast spin-echo MR imaging and arthroscopic correlation in 293 patients. Radiology 203:508-512, 1997.

114. Kowalchuk RM, Kneeland JB, Dalinka MK, et al: MRI of the knee: value of short echo time fast spin-echo using high performance gradients versus conventional spin-echo imaging for the detection of meniscal tears. Skeletal Radiol 29:520-524, 2000.

115. van Trommel MF, Potter HG, Ernberg LA, et al: The use of noncontrast magnetic resonance imaging in evaluating meniscal repair: comparison with conventional arthrography. Arthroscopy 14:2-8, 1998.

116. Potter HG, Rodeo SA, Wickiewicz TL, et al: MR imaging of meniscal allografts: correlation with clinical and arthroscopic outcomes. Radiology 198:509-514, 1996.

117. Peh WCG, Chan JHM, Shek TWH, et al: The effect of using shorter echo times in MR imaging of knee menisci: a study using a porcine model. Am J Roentgenol 172:485-488, 1999.

118. Wood ML, Henkelman RM: Truncation artifacts in magnetic resonance imaging. Magn Reson Med 2(6):517-526, 1985.

119. Turner DA, Rapoport MI, Erwin WD, et al: Truncation artifact: a potential pitfall in MR imaging of the menisci of the knee. Radiology 179:629-633, 1991.

120. Quinn SF. Brown TR, Szumowski J: Menisci of the knee: radial MR imaging correlated with arthroscopy in 259 patients. Radiology 185:577-580, 1992.

121. Lee JHE, Singh TT, Bolton G: Axial fat-saturated FSE imaging of knee: appearance of meniscal tears. Skeletal Radiol 31:384-395, 2002.

122. Araki Y, Ootani F, Tsukaguchi I, et al: MR diagnosis of meniscal tears of the knee: value of axial three-dimensional Fourier transformation GRASS images. Am J Roentgenol 158:587-590, 1992.

123. Buckwalter KA, Braunstein EM, Janizek DB, et al: MR imaging of meniscal tears: narrow versus conventional window width photography. Radiology 187:827-830, 1993.

124. Stone KR, Stoller DW, Irving SG, et al: 3D MRI volume sizing of knee meniscus cartilage. Arthroscopy 10:641-644, 1994.

125. Walker PS, Erkman MJ: The role of the menisci in force transmission across the knee. Clin Orthop 109:184-192, 1975.

126. Beltran J, Noto AM, Mosure JC, et al: The knee: surface-coil imaging at 1.5T. Radiology 159:747-751, 1986.

127. Deutsch AL, Mink JH: Articular disorders of the knee. Top Magn Reson Imaging 1:43-56, 1989.

128. Simonian PT, Sussman PS, van Trommel M, et al: Popliteomeniscal fasciculi and lateral meniscal stability. Am J Sports Med 25(6):849-853, 1997.

129. Crues JV, Ryu R, Morgan FW: Meniscal pathology: the expanding role of magnetic resonance imaging. Clin Orthop 252:80-8, 1990.

130. Vedi V, Williams A, Tennant SJ, et al: Meniscal movement: an in vivo study using dynamic MRI. J Bone Joint Surg Br 81-B:37-41, 1999.

131. Shankman S, Beltran J, Melamed E, et al: Anterior horn of the lateral meniscus: another potential pitfall in MR imaging of the knee. Radiology 204:181-184, 1997.

132. Silverman JM, Mink JH, Deutsch AL: Discoid menisci of the knee: MR imaging appearance. Radiology 173:351-354, 1989.

133. Rohren EM, Kosarek FJ, Helms CA: Discoid lateral meniscus and the frequency of meniscal tears. Skeletal Radiol 30:316-320, 2001.

134. Hamada M, Shino K, Kawano K, et al: Usefulness of magnetic resonance imaging for detecting intrasubstance tear and/or degeneration of lateral discoid meniscus. Arthroscopy 10:645-65, 1994.

135. Poynton AR. Javadpour SM, Finegan PJ, et al: The meniscofemoral ligaments of the knee. J Bone Joint Surg Br 79-B:327-330, 1997.

136. Cho JM, Suh JS, Na JB, et al: Variations in meniscofemoral ligaments at anatomical study and MR imaging. Skeletal Radiol 28:189-195, 1999.

137. Gupte CM, Smith A, McDermott ID, et al: Meniscofemoral ligaments revisited: anatomical study, age correlation and clinical implications. J Bone Joint Surg Br 84-B:846-851, 2002.

138. Soejima T, Murakami H, Tanaka N, et al: Anteromedial meniscofemoral ligament. Arthroscopy 19:90-95, 2003.
139. Sanders TG, Linares RC, Lawhorn KW, et al: Oblique meniscomeniscal ligament: another potential pitfall for a meniscal tear; anatomic description and appearance at MR imaging in three cases. Radiology 213:213-216, 1999.
140. Arnoczky SP, Warren RF: The microvasculature of the meniscus and its response to injury: an experimental study in the dog. Am J Sports Med 11(3):131-141, 1983.
141. Hauger O, Frank LR, Boutin RD, et al: Characterization of the "red zone" of knee meniscus: MR imaging and histologic correlation. Radiology 217:193-200, 2000.
142. Cooper DE, Arnoczky SP, Warren RF: Arthroscopic meniscal repair. Clin Sports Med 9:589-607, 1990.
143. Jee WH, McCauley TR, Kim JM, et al: Meniscal tear configurations: categorization with MR imaging. Am J Roentgenol 180:93-97, 2003.
144. Crues JV, Mink J, Levy TL, et al: Meniscal tears of the knee: accuracy of magnetic resonance imaging. Radiology 164:445-448, 1987.
145. Dillon EH, Pope CF, Jokl P, et al: The clinical significance of stage 2 meniscal abnormalities on magnetic resonance knee images. Magn Reson Imaging 8:411-415, 1990.
146. McCauley TR, Jee WH, Galloway MT, et al: Grade 2C signal in the meniscus on MR imaging of the knee. Am J Roentgenol 179:645-648, 2002.
147. DeSmet AA, Norris MA, Yandow DR, et al: MR diagnosis of meniscal tears of the knee: importance of high signal in the meniscus that extends to the surface. Am J Roentgenol 161:101-107, 1993.
148. Hodler J, Haghighi P, Pathria MN, et al: Meniscal changes in the elderly: correlation of MR imaging and histologic findings. Radiology 184:221-225, 1992.
149. Bhattacharyya T, Gale D, Dewire P, et al: The clinical importance of meniscal tears demonstrated by magnetic resonance imaging in osteoarthritis of the knee. J Bone Joint Surg 85-A:4-9, 2003.
150. Cothran Jr RL, Major NM, Helms CA, et al: MR imaging of meniscal contusion in the knee. Am J Roentgenol 177:1189-1192, 2001.
151. Kornick J, Trefekner E, McCarthy S, et al: Meniscal abnormalities in the asymptomatic population at MR imaging. Radiology 177:463-465, 1990.
152. Zanetti M, Pfirrmann CWA, Schmid MR, et al: Patients with suspected meniscal tears: prevalence of abnormalities seen on MRI of 100 symptomatic and 100 contralateral asymptomatic knees. Am J Roentgenol 181:635-641, 2003.
153. Tuckman GA, Miller WJ, Remo JW, et al: Radial tears of the menisci: MR findings. Am J Roentgenol 163:395-400, 1994.
154. Magee T, Shapiro M, Williams D: MR accuracy and arthroscopic incidence of meniscal radial tears. Skeletal Radiol 31:686-689, 2002.
155. Vande Berg BC, Poilvache P, Duchateau F, et al: Lesions of the menisci of the knee: value of MR imaging criteria for recognition of unstable lesions. Am J Roentgenol 176:771-776, 2001.
156. Lecas LK, Helms CA, Kosarek FJ, et al: Inferiorly displaced flap tears of the medial meniscus: MR appearance and clinical significance. Am J Roentgenol 174:161-164, 2000.
157. Wright DH, DeSmet AA, Norris M: Bucket-handle tears of the medial and lateral menisci of the knee: value of MR imaging in detecting displaced fragments. Am J Roentgenol 165:621-625, 1995.
158. Dorsay TA, Helms CA: Bucket-handle meniscal tears of the knee: sensitivity and specificity of MRI signs. Skeletal Radiol 32:266-272, 2003.
159. Singson RD, Feldman F, Staron R, et al: MR imaging of displaced bucket-handle tear of the medial meniscus. Am J Roentgenol 156:121-124, 1991.
160. Magee TH, Hinson GW: MRI of meniscal bucket-handle tears. Skeletal Radiol 27:495-499, 1998.
161. Brammer H, Sover E, Erickson S, et al: Simultaneous identification of medial and lateral bucket-handle tears: the Jack and Jill lesion. Am J Roentgenol 173:860-861, 1999.
162. Campbell SE, Sanders TG, Morrison WB: MR imaging of meniscal cysts: incidence, location and clinical significance. Am J Roentgenol 177:409-413, 2001.
163. Veltri DM, Warren RF, Wickiewicz TL, et al: Current status of allograft meniscal transplantation. Clin Orthop 303:44-55, 1994.
164. Rodeo SA: Arthroscopic meniscal repair with use of the outside-in technique. J Bone Joint Surg 82-A:127-141, 2000.
165. Deutsch AL, Mink JH, Fox JM, et al: Peripheral meniscal tears: MR findings after conservative treatment or arthroscopic repair. Radiology 176:485-488, 1990.
166. Farley TE. Howell SM, Love KF, et al: Meniscal tears: MR and arthrographic findings after arthroscopic repair. Radiology 180:517-522, 1991.
167. Applegate GR, Flannigan BD, Tolin BS, et al: MR diagnosis of recurrent tears in the knee: value of intraarticular contrast material. Am J Roentgenol 161:821-825, 1993.
168. Sciulli RL, Boutin RD, Brown RR, et al: Evaluation of the postoperative meniscus of the knee: a study comparing conventional arthrography, conventional MR imaging, MR arthrography with iodinated contrast material and MR arthrography with gadolinium-based contrast material. Skeletal Radiol 28:508-514, 1999.
169. Arnoczky SP, Cooper TG, Stadelmaier DM, et al: Magnetic resonance signals in healing menisci: an experimental study in dogs. Arthroscopy 10:552-557, 1994.
170. White LM, Schweitzer ME, Weishaupt D, et al: Diagnosis of recurrent meniscal tears: prospective evaluation of conventional MR imaging, indirect MR arthrography, and direct MR arthrography. Radiology 222:421-429, 2002.
171. Lim PS, Schweitzer ME, Bhatia M, et al: Repeat tear of postoperative meniscus: potential MR imaging signs. Radiology 210:183-188, 1999.
172. Rodeo SA: Meniscal allografts – where do we stand? Am J Sports Med 29(2):246-261, 2001.
173. Stollsteimer GT, Shelton WR, Dukes A, et al: Meniscal allograft transplantation: a 1 to 5 year follow up of 22 patients. Arthroscopy 16:343-347, 2000.
174. Hefti F, Beguiristain J, Krause R, et al: Osteochondritis dissecans: a multicenter study of the European Pediatric Orthopedic Society. J Pediatr Orthop B 8(4):231-245, 1999.
175. Boutin RD, Januario JA, Newberg AH, et al: MR imaging features of osteochondritis dissecans of the femoral sulcus. Am J Roentgenol 180(3):641-645, 2003.
176. De Smet AA, Ilahi OA, Graf BK: Untreated osteochondritis dissecans of the femoral condyles: prediction of patient outcome using radiographic and MR findings. Skeletal Radiol 26(8):463-467, 1997.
177. De Smet AA, Fisher DR, Graf BK, et al: Osteochondritis dissecans of the knee: value of MR imaging in determining lesion stability and the presence of articular cartilage defects. Am J Roentgenol 155(3):549-553, 1990.
178. O'Connor MA, Palaniappan M, Khan N, et al: Osteochondritis dissecans of the knee in children: a comparison of MRI and arthroscopic findings. J Bone Joint Surg 84(2):258-262, 2002.
179. Jurgensen I, Bachmann G, Schleicher I, et al: Arthroscopic versus conservative treatment of osteochondritis dissecans of the knee: value of magnetic resonance imaging in therapy planning and follow-up. Arthroscopy 18(4):378-386, 2002.
180. Sales de Gauzy J, Mansat C, Darodes PH, et al: Natural course of osteochondritis dissecans in children. J Pediatr Orthop B 8(1):26-28, 1999.
181. Fife RS, Brandt KD, Braunstein EM, et al: Relationship between arthroscopic evidence of cartilage damage and radiographic evidence of joint space narrowing in early osteoarthritis of the knee. Arthritis Rheum 34:377-382, 1991.
182. Xia Y: Heterogeneity of cartilage laminae in MR imaging. J Magn Reson Imaging 11:686-693, 2000.
183. Recht MP, Piraino DW, Paletta GA, et al: Accuracy of fat suppressed three dimensional spoiled gradient echo FLASH MR imaging in the detection of patellofemoral articular cartilage abnormalities. Radiology 198:209-212, 1996.
184. Disler DG, Mc Cauley TR, Wirth CR, et al: Detection of knee hyaline cartilage defects using fat-suppressed three-dimensional spoiled gradient-echo MR imaging: comparison with standard MR imaging and correlation with arthroscopy. Am J Roentgenol 165:377-382, 1995.
185. Bredella MA, Tirman PFJ, Peterfy CG, et al: Accuracy of T2-weighted fast spin echo MR imaging with fat saturation in detecting cartilage defects in the knee: comparison with arthroscopy in 130 patients. Am J Roentgenol 172:1073-1080, 1999.
186. Potter HG, Linklater JM, Allen AA, et al: Magnetic resonance imaging of articular cartilage in the knee: an evaluation with the use of fast spin-echo imaging. J Bone Joint Surg 80-A(9):1276-1284, 1998.
187. Vahlensieck M, Peterfy CG, Wischer T, et al: Indirect MR arthrography: optimization and clinical applications. Radiology 200:249-254, 1996.
188. Reader SB, Pelc NJ, Alley MT, et al: Rapid imaging of articular cartilage with steady state free precession and multipoint fat-water suppression. Am J Roentgeol 180:357-362, 2003.
189. Hargreaves BA, Gold GE, Lang PK, et al: MR imaging of articular cartilage using driven equilibrium. Magn Reson Med 42(4):695-703, 1999.
190. Outerbridge RE: The etiology of chondromalacia patellae. J Bone Joint Surg 43-B:752-757, 1961.
191. Zanetti M, Bruder E, Romero J, et al: Bone marrow edema pattern in osteoarthritic knees: correlation between MR imaging and histologic findings. Radiology 215:835-840, 2000.
192. Rubinstein JD, Li JG, Majumdar S, et al: Image resolution and signal-to-noise ratio requirements for MR imaging of degenerative cartilage. Am J Roentgenol 169:1089-1096, 1997.
193. Reddy R, Insko EK, Noyszewski EA, et al: Sodium MRI of human articular cartilage in vivo. Magn Reson Med 39:697-701, 1998.
194. Bashir A, Gray ML, Hartke J, Burstein D: Nondestructive imaging of human cartilage glycosaminoglycan concentration by MRI. Magn Reson Med 41(5):857-865, 1999.
195. Xia Y, Moody JB, Alhadlaq H: Orientational dependence of T2 relaxation in articular cartilage: a microscopic MRI (MRI) study. Magn Reson Med 48:460-469, 2002.
196. Rubinstein JD, Kim JK, Morava-Protzner I, et al: Effects of collagen orientation on MR imaging characteristics on bovine articular cartilage. Radiology 188:219-226, 1993.
197. Xia Y, Moody JB, Burton-Wurster N, et al: Quantitative in situ correlation between microscopic MRI and polarized light microscopy studies of articular cartilage. Osteoarthritis and Cartilage 9:393-406, 2001.
198. Maier CF, Tan SG, Hariharan H, et al: T2 quantitation of articular cartilage at 1.5T. J Magn Reson Imaging 17:358-364, 2003.
199. Steadman JR, Rodkey WG, Rodrigo JJ: Microfracture: surgical technique and rehabilitation to treat chondral defects. Clin Orthop 391 Suppl:S362-36, 2001.

200. Peterson L, Minas T, Brittberg M, et al: Treatment of osteochondritis dissecans of the knee with autologous chondrocyte transplantation: results at two to ten years. J Bone Joint Surg Am 85-A Suppl 2:17-24, 2003.

201. Brittberg M, Lindahl A, Nilsson A, et al: Treatment of deep cartilage defects in the knee with autologous chondrocyte transplantation. N Engl J Med 331:889-895, 1994.

202. Gross AE, Aubin P, Cheah HK, et al: A fresh osteochondral allograft alternative. J Arthroplasty 17:50-53, 2002.

203. Hangody L, Kish G, Karpati Z, et al: Mosaicplasty for the treatment of articular cartilage defects: application in clinical practice. Orthopedics 21:751-756, 1998.

204. Brown WE, Potter HG, Marx RG, et al: Magnetic resonance imaging appearance of cartilage repair in the knee. Clin Orthop 422:214-223, 2004.

205. Berlet GC, Mascia A, Miniaci A: Treatment of unstable osteochondritis dissecans lesions of the knee using autogenous osteochondral grafts (mosaicplasty). Arthroscopy 15(3):312-316, 1999.

206. Jakob RP, Franz T, Gautier E, et al: Autologous osteochondral grafting in the knee: indication, results and reflections. Clin Orthop Rel Res 401:170-184, 2002.

207. Elias DA, White LM, Fithian DC: Acute lateral patellar dislocation at MR imaging: injury patterns of medial patellar soft-tissue restraints and osteochondral injuries of the inferomedial patella. Radiology 225:736-743, 2002.

208. Kirsch MD, Fitzgerald SW, Friedman H, et al: Transient lateral patellar dislocation: diagnosis with MR imaging. Am J Roentgenol 161:109-113, 1993.

209. Warren RF, Marshall JL: The supporting structures and layers on the medial side of the knee. J Bone Joint Surg 61-A:56-62, 1979.

210. Warren LF, Marshall JL, Girgis F: The prime static stabilizer of the medial side of the knee. J Bone Joint Surg 56-A:665-674, 1974.

211. Desio SM, Burks RT, Buchus KN: Soft tissue restraints to lateral patellar translation in the human knee. Am J Sports Med 26:59-65, 1998.

212. Sallay PI: Acute dislocation of the patella: a correlative pathoanatomic study. Am J Sports Med 24:52-60, 1996.

213. Carillon Y, Abidi H, Dejour D, et al: Patellar instability: assessment on MR images by measuring the lateral trochlear inclination: initial experience. Radiology 216:582-585, 2000.

214. Ward SR, Shellock FG, Terk MR, et al: Assessment of patellofemoral relationships using kinematic MRI: comparison between qualitative and quantitative methods. J Magn Reson Imaging 16:69-74, 2002.

215. Ohnuma M, Sugita T, Kawamata T, et al: Pigmented villonodular synovitis of the knee with lesions of the bursae. Clin Orthop 414:212-218, 2003.

216. Chin KR, Barr SJ, Winalski C, et al: Treatment of advanced primary and recurrent diffuse pigmented villonodular synovitis of the knee. J Bone Joint Surg Am 84-A (12):2192-2202, 2002.

217. Sonin AH: Magnetic resonance imaging of the extensor mechanism. Magn Reson Imaging Clin North Am 2(3):401-411, 1994.

218. Yu JS, Petersilge C, Sartoris DJ, et al: MR imaging of injuries of the extensor mechanism of the knee. Radiographics 14(3):541-551, 1994.

219. Basso O, Johnson DP, Amis AA: The anatomy of the patellar tendon. Knee Surg Sports Traumatol Arthrosc 9(1):2-5, 2001.

220. Karantanas AH, Zibis AH, Papanikolaou N: Increased signal intensity on fat-suppressed three-dimensional T1-weighted pulse sequences in patellar tendon: magic angle effect? Skeletal Radiol 30(2):67-71, 2001.

221. Reiff DB, Heenan SD, Heron CW: MRI appearances of the asymptomatic patellar tendon on gradient echo imaging. Skeletal Radiol 24(2):123-126, 1995.

222. Schweitzer ME, Mitchell DG, Ehrlich SM: The patellar tendon: thickening, internal signal buckling, and other MR variants. Skeletal Radiol 22(6):411-416, 1993.

223. Popp JE, Yu JS, Kaeding CC: Recalcitrant patellar tendinitis: magnetic resonance imaging, histologic evaluation, and surgical treatment. Am J Sports Med 25(2):218-222, 1997.

224. McLoughlin RF, Raber EL, Vellet AD, et al: Patellar tendinitis: MR imaging features, with suggested pathogenesis and proposed classification. Radiology 197(3):843-848, 1995.

225. Johnson DP, Wakeley CJ, Watt I: Magnetic resonance imaging of patellar tendonitis. J Bone Joint Surg Br 78(3):452-257, 1996.

226. Rosenberg ZS, Kawelblum M, Cheung YY, et al: Osgood-Schlatter lesion: fracture or tendinitis? Scintigraphic, CT, and MR imaging features. Radiology 185(3):853-858, 1992.

227. Hirano A, Fukubayashi T, Ishii T, Ochiai N: Magnetic resonance imaging of Osgood-Schlatter disease: the course of the disease. Skeletal Radiol 31(6):334-342, 2002.

228. Garcia-Valtuille R, Abascal F, Cerezal L, et al: Anatomy and MR imaging appearances of synovial plicae of the knee. Radiographics 22(4):775-784, 2002.

229. Jee WH, Choe BY, Kim JM, et al: The plica syndrome: diagnostic value of MRI with arthroscopic correlation. J Comput Assist Tomogr 22(5):814-81, 1998.

230. Kosarek FJ, Helms CA: The MR appearance of the infrapatellar plica. Am J Roentgenol 172(2): 481-484, 1999.

231. Attarian DE, Guilak F: Observations on the growth of loose bodies in joints. Arthroscopy 18(8):930-934, 2002.

232. Low K, Mont MA, Hungerford DS: Instructional Course Lecture. American Academy of Orthopedic Surgeons, 2001:489-493.

233. Baumgarten KM, Mont MA, Rifai A, Hungerford DS: Atraumatic osteonecrosis of the patella. Clin Orthop 383:191-196, 2001.

234. Mont MA, Baumgarten KM, Rifai A, et al: Atraumatic osteonecrosis of the knee. J Bone Joint Surg 82-A(9):1279-1290, 2000.

235. Llauger J, Palmer J, Roson N, et al: Osteonecrosis of the knee in an HIV-infected patient. Am J Roentgenol 171(4):987-988, 1998.

236. Pollack MS, Dalinka MK, Kressel HY, et al: Magnetic resonance imaging in evaluation of suspected osteonecrosis of the knee. Skeletal Radiol 16(2):121-12, 1987.

237. Athanasian EA, Wickiewicz TL, Warren RF: Osteonecrosis of the femoral condyle after arthroscopic reconstruction of a cruciate ligament: report of two cases. J Bone Joint Surg 77-A:1418-1422, 1995.

238. Johnson TC, Evans JA, Gilley JA, DeLee JC: Osteonecrosis of the knee after arthroscopic surgery for meniscal tears and chondral lesions. Arthroscopy 16(3):254-261, 2000.

239. Muscolo DL, Costa-Paz M, Makino A, Ayerza MA: Osteonecrosis of the knee following arthroscopic meniscectomy in patients over 50-years old. Arthroscopy 12(3):273-279, 1996.

240. Brahme SK, Fox JM, Ferkel RD, et al: Osteonecrosis of the knee after arthroscopic surgery: diagnosis with MR imaging. Radiology 178(3):851-853, 1991.

241. Rozbruch SR, Wickiewicz TL, DiCarlo EF, Potter HG: Osteonecrosis of the knee following arthroscopic laser meniscectomy. Arthroscopy 12:245-250, 1996.

242. Narvaez JA, Narvaez J, DeLama E, Sanchez A: Spontaneous osteonecrosis of the knee associated with tibial plateau and femoral condyle insufficiency stress fractures. Eur Radiol 13(8):1843-1848, 2003.

243. Yamamoto T, Bullough PG: Spontaneous osteonecrosis of the knee: the result of subchondral insufficiency fracture. J Bone Joint Surg 82-A(6):858-866, 2000.

244. Marti CB, Rodriguez M, Zanetti M, Romero J: Spontaneous osteonecrosis of the medial compartment of the knee: a MRI follow-up after conservative and operative treatment, preliminary results. Knee Surg Sports Traumatol Arthrosc 8(2):83-88, 2000.

ANKLE AND FOOT

Javier Beltran

IMAGING TECHNIQUES

High-quality magnetic resonance imaging (MRI) of the ankle and foot can be performed using intermediate- or high-field-strength magnets (0.5 to 1.5 T). In general, high-field-strength magnets are preferred because of their higher signal-to-noise ratio (SNR) compared with those of intermediate field strength.[1] Surface coils are essential for imaging of the ankle and foot. Most manufacturers provide transmit-receive extremity coils, which are adequate for ankle and hindfoot imaging (Fig. 104-1). With the patient in a comfortable supine position, the ankle to be examined is placed within the extremity coil in neutral position and taped to prevent involuntary motion. Some investigators have proposed the use of a head coil and imaging of both ankles simultaneously with the patient in the prone position and feet plantar flexed.[2] The advantages of this technique are that it allows comparison of the anatomy of both ankles and helps to prevent the patient's motion. The main disadvantage is that it significantly decreases image resolution. For imaging of the forefoot, smaller, circular receive-only coils (3 to 5 inches [approx. 7 to 12 cm] in diameter) or small flexible phase array coils can be used. However, in most circumstances the extremity coil is sufficient for adequate imaging of the forefoot. For suspected Achilles tendon ruptures, sagittal images obtained with the foot in plantar flexion can provide information regarding approximation of the tendon ends when conservative treatment is contemplated.

As in most joints, imaging in three orthogonal planes is mandatory. The coronal plane is oriented parallel to the bimalleolar line as prescribed in the axial localizer. The sagittal plane is oriented perpendicular to the bimalleolar line. When the foot is imaged, it should be noted that coronal plane refers to the short axis of the foot, perpendicular to the metatarsal, and the axial plane refers to the long axis of the foot, parallel to the

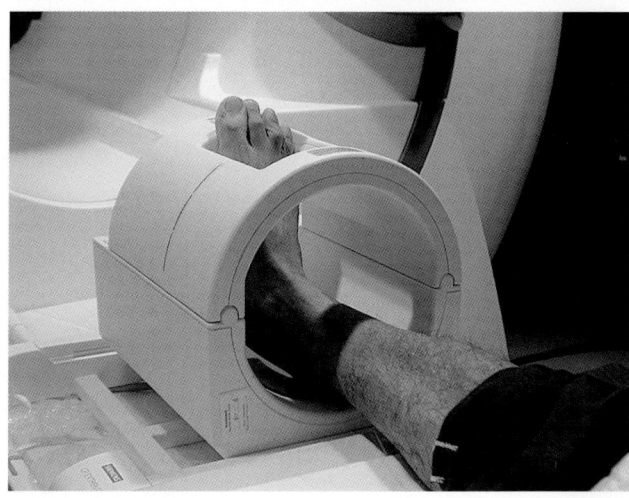

FIGURE 104-1

Ankle imaging using a phase array extremity coil. Note the neutral position of the foot.

metatarsals. In some instances, an oblique axial plane may be useful to study the integrity of the tendons as they turn around the malleoli.[3] Some authors recommend placement of the foot in plantar flexion for the axial images. This position allows improved visualization of the tendons in cross section as well as the calcaneofibular ligament.[4] A small field of view, in the range of 12 to 16 cm, and thin (3 to 4 mm) sections, with one or two excitations, provide excellent image quality of the ankle and hindfoot. Smaller fields of view may be necessary for imaging the forefoot.

Selection of specific pulse sequences for imaging the ankle and foot depends on the suspected pathologic process, user preference, and experience. Using a limited number of pulse sequences, such as T1- and T2-weighted two-dimensional multisection spin-echo techniques and short tau inversion recovery (STIR) sequences, most ankle and foot MRI studies can be performed. The short repetition time (TR) and echo time (TE) technique provides excellent depiction of the normal and abnormal anatomy of the tendons, ligaments, cortical bone, and bone. STIR sequences are very useful for detecting pathology in the bone marrow and soft-tissues. Long TR/TE spin-echo pulse sequences provide detection of pathologic processes such as ligamentous injuries, soft-tissue tumors, edema, and bone marrow abnormalities. The use of a low-bandwidth option available in some scanners provides improved SNR, but it creates prominent chemical-shift artifact. The main inconvenience of conventional spin-echo techniques is the prolonged acquisition time.

Fast spin-echo pulse sequences allow generation of images with contrast characteristics similar to those of conventional spin-echo imaging with reduced imaging time. One of the disadvantages of fast spin-echo imaging is that the signal intensity of fat remains high on long TR/TE techniques and, theoretically, hyperintense bone marrow lesions could be missed. This can be solved by using an effective TE of 120 ms or greater,[5] or by combining fast spin-echo sequences with fat-saturation techniques. A second disadvantage of fast spin-echo imaging is the loss of resolution, especially when using a long echo-train length, longer interecho spacing, and a small acquisition matrix.[1] High contrast between normal bone marrow and bone marrow lesions such as tumors and osteomyelitis can also be achieved by using other strategies such as short-tau inversion recovery (STIR or fast STIR) or fat saturation with short TR/TE spin-echo imaging after intravenous injection of gadolinium. Disadvantages of these techniques include decreased SNR, dependence on uniformity of the radiofrequency pulses when using STIR, and the relative invasiveness and increased expense when using intravenous gadolinium.

Gradient-echo pulse sequences with two- or three-dimensional acquisitions can be used to obtain images with T2* contrast in a relatively short acquisition time. My colleagues and I have found these techniques most useful in the ankle for the evaluation of articular cartilage and ligaments.[6] True contiguous sections of less than 3 mm with a high SNR can be obtained with three-dimensional acquisition. The major disadvantage of gradient-echo techniques is the loss of signal within the

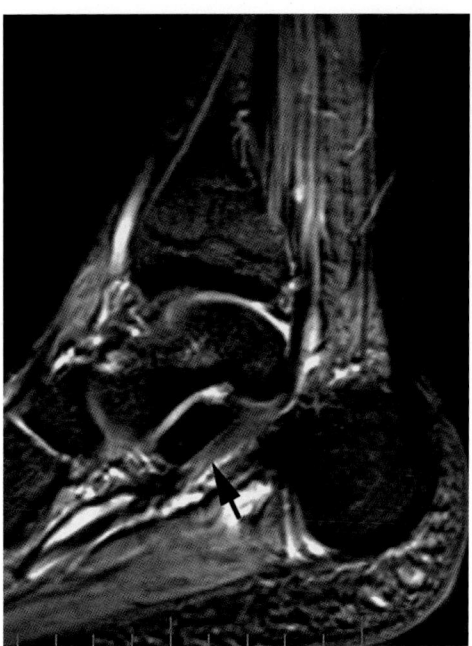

FIGURE 104-2

Magic angle artifact. Sagittal gradient-echo image (GRE 400/20, 15° flip angle) through the flexor hallucis longus tendon (arrow). Note the hyperintensity of the tendon as it takes a 55° turn in relationship with the main magnetic field.

bone marrow due to susceptibility artifacts. Another problem with gradient-echo sequences is the so-called magic angle artifact. Ligaments and tendons oriented about 55-degrees with the main magnetic field demonstrate signal intensity when using a TE of less than 20 ms[7,8] (Fig. 104-2).

NORMAL ANATOMY

Knowledge of the normal anatomy of the ankle and foot and its MRI representation is essential for accurate interpretation. In this chapter, the normal anatomy is discussed following a regional approach rather than using the more traditional method of discussion of the anatomy as it is represented in different orthogonal planes.

The normal signal intensity of the different tissues of the ankle and foot depends on the pulse sequence. Tendons, ligaments, and cortical bone are hypointense in practically any pulse sequence.[8] However, when using short-TE techniques, focal hyperintensity of ligaments and tendons can be seen, depending on their orientation (magic angle artifact).[9] Muscles and nerves are seen as intermediate signal intensity structures on all pulse sequences. On spin-echo images, arteries demonstrate hypointensity due to flow void and veins show hyperintensity due to slow flow. On gradient-echo images, both arteries and veins are hyperintense. Depending on the percentage of fat, hematopoietic marrow, and trabecular bone, the bone marrow has signal intensity similar to that of the subcutaneous fat. In young individuals, islands of hematopoietic marrow can be present in the distal tibia. Hematopoietic red marrow is relatively hypointense on T1- and T2-weighted spin-echo pulse sequences and is hyperintense on STIR images and T2 fat-saturated sequences.

In the pediatric population, hematopoietic marrow is more prevalent in the metatarsals and hindfoot. At the junction between bone and cartilage, at the periphery of the ossification centers, there is also increased red marrow, which provides high signal intensity on the T2 fat-saturated and STIR images. Additionally, increased vascularization of these areas, also known as the "metaphyseal-equivalent zone," produce enhancement after administration of gadolinium.[10] Heterogeneous hyperintense foci on T2 fat-saturated and STIR sequences in the bone marrow of the tarsal and metatarsal bones are often seen in the normal pediatric population, representing a normal variant.[11]

Ligaments

The ligaments of the tibiofibular syndesmosis include the anterior inferior tibiofibular ligament, the posterior inferior tibiofibular ligament, and the interosseous tibiofibular ligament or posterior intermalleolar ligament.

The anterior inferior tibiofibular ligament may have a separate distal fascicle that has been implicated in talar impingement syndrome.[10] This normal variant is also known as the ligament of Basset or the ligament of Duke.[12] The posterior inferior tibiofibular ligament contains a deep and more inferior fascicle called the transverse inferior tibiofibular ligament or deep inferior posterior tibiofibular ligament. It has been postulated that the transverse inferior tibiofibular ligament provides increased depth to the tibial plafond posteriorly, in a way similar to the glenoid labrum. These ligaments may have striated appearance when imaged in their longitudinal axis. Use of axial and coronal planes is the best for their evaluation (Figs. 104-3 and 104-4).

The lateral collateral ligaments of the ankle include the anterior talofibular, posterior talofibular, and calcaneofibular ligaments. The anterior talofibular ligament is better seen in the axial plane, extending from the anterior aspect of the lateral malleolus to the talar neck (Fig. 104-5). The posterior talofibular ligament is well identified in the axial or coronal planes. It extends from the malleolar fossa of the distal fibula to the posterior talar tubercle (Fig. 104-6). The calcaneofibular ligament is better seen in the oblique coronal plane or axial plane with the foot in plantar flexion.[4,13,14]

Four superficial and two deep ligaments form the medial collateral ligament or deltoid ligament. The superficial ligaments originate from the tip of the medial

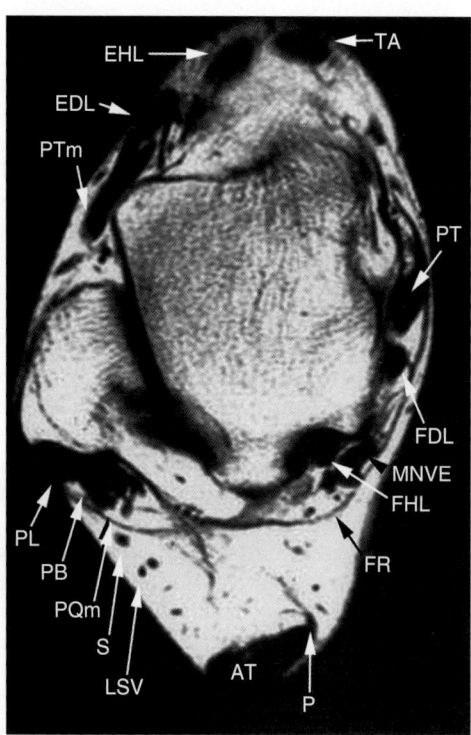

FIGURE 104-3

Normal anatomy. Axial T1-weighted image through the distal tibiofibular syndesmosis. AT, Achilles tendon; EHL, Extensor hallucis longus tendon; EDL, Extensor digitorum longus tendon; FDL, Flexor digitorum longus tendon; FHL, Flexor hallucis longus tendon; FR, Flexor retinaculum; LSV, Lesser saphenous vein; MNVB, Medial neurovascular bundle; P, Plantaris tendon; PB, Peroneus brevis tendon; PL, Peroneus longus tendon; PQm, Peroneus quartus muscle; PT, Posterior tibialis tendon; PTm, Peroneus tertius muscle; S, Sural nerve; TA, Tibialis anterior tendon.

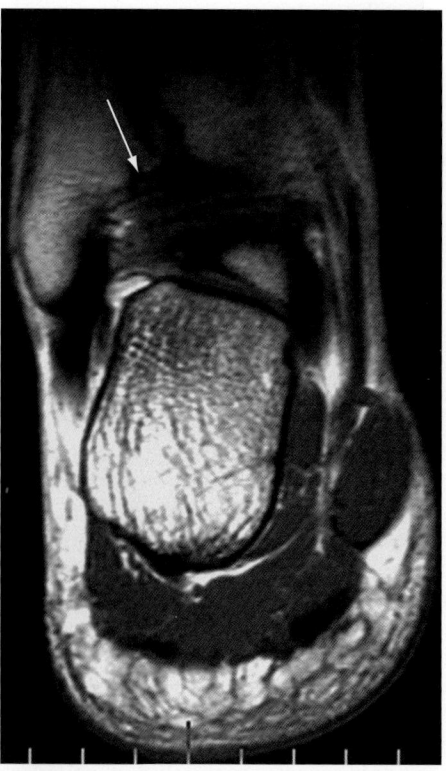

FIGURE 104-4

Normal anatomy. Coronal T1-weighted image through the posterior aspect of the distal tibiofibular joint. Note the posterior tibiofibular ligament (arrow).

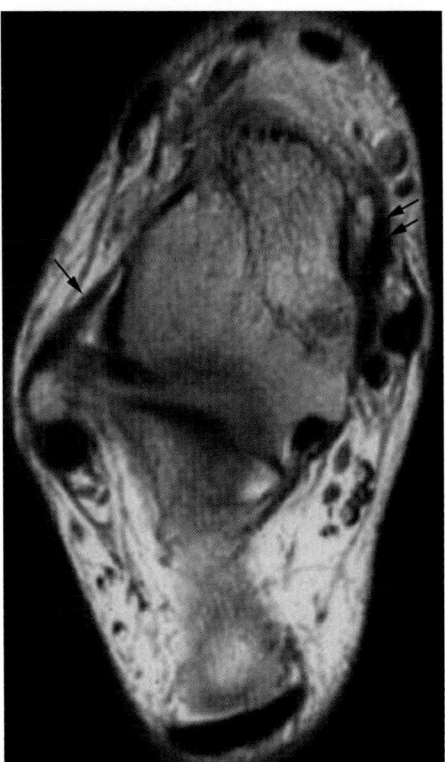

FIGURE 104-5

Normal anatomy. Axial T1-weighted image through the talus. Note the anterior talofibular ligament (arrow) and the deltoid ligament (double arrow).

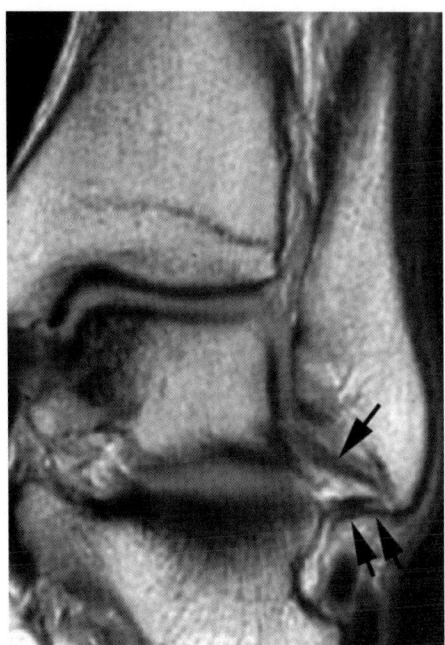

FIGURE 104-6

Normal anatomy. Coronal T1-weighted image. Note the posterior talofibular ligament (arrow) and the calcaneofibular ligament (double arrow).

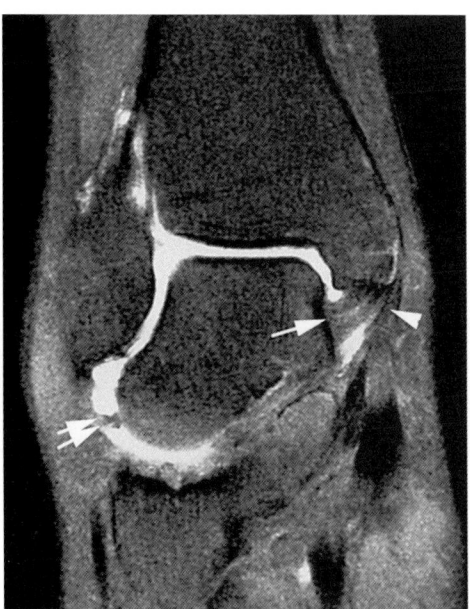

FIGURE 104-7

Normal anatomy. Coronal T1-weighted image with fat suppression, following intra-articular injection of contrast material. Note the superficial (arrowhead) and deep fibers (arrow) of the deltoid ligament (double arrow, anterior talofibular ligament).

malleolus (anterior colliculus) and extend distally to insert into the navicular (tibionavicular ligament), into the spring ligament (tibiospring ligament), into the sustentaculum tali of the calcaneus (tibiocalcaneal ligament), and into the medial tubercle of the talus (superficial tibiotalar ligament). The deep ligaments originate from the posterior colliculus of the tibial malleolus and insert into the anterior and posterior aspects of the talus (anterior and posterior deep tibiotalar ligaments). Axial and coronal images demonstrate these ligaments adequately (Fig. 104-7; see Fig. 104-5).

The spring ligament or plantar calcaneonavicular ligament contributes to the stability of the longitudinal arch of the foot. It originates in the undersurface of the sustentaculum tali and inserts into the medial inferior portion of the navicular bone. Medially, its fibers merge with the deltoid ligament (the tibiospring ligament) and laterally with the bifurcate ligament or ligament of Chopart. The bifurcate ligament is a Y-shaped ligament extending from the anterior process of the calcaneus to the navicular and cuboid bones.

The long plantar ligament also contributes to the stability of the plantar arch. It originates in the plantar surface of the calcaneus and cuboid bones and inserts into the second through the fifth metatarsals. The short plantar ligament or plantar calcaneocuboid ligament is a striated ligament extending from the anterior inferior aspect of the calcaneus to the inferior aspect of the cuboid.

Another important ligament is the Lisfranc ligament, which extends from the medial cuneiform to the base of the second metatarsal and is made of a dorsal and a plantar band. The dorsal band is weaker and is the first to become inured.

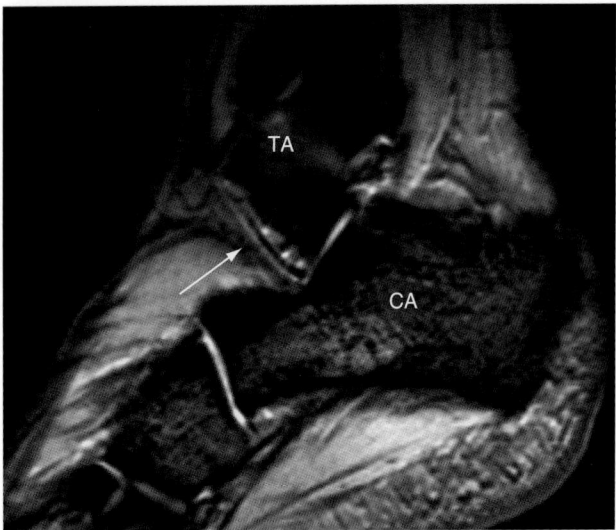

FIGURE 104-8

Normal anatomy. Sagittal gradient-echo image through the peripheral region of the sinus tarsi, demonstrating the inferior extensor retinaculum (*arrow*). (CA, calcaneus; TA, talus.)

The sinus tarsi is an anatomic space located between the talus and calcaneus, and it contains fat, neurovascular structures, and two ligaments, the talocalcaneal or interosseous ligament and the cervical ligament. The talocalcaneal ligament is broad and strong, contributing significantly to the stability of the subtalar joints. The cervical ligament is located more anteriorly and is sometimes considered as an anterior extension of the talocalcaneal ligament.[3,6,15]

Another structure identified in the more superficial region of the sinus tarsi is the inferior extensor retinaculum. This structure turns downward in the lateral aspect in the neck of the talus and enters the sinus tarsi, where it divides into three roots: the lateral, intermediate, and medial fibers. The lateral root becomes incorporated with the deep fascia of the lateral aspect of the foot, and the intermediate root inserts in the calcaneus. The medial root enters the sinus tarsi and inserts into the superior surface of the calcaneus.

Normal MRI anatomy of the sinus tarsi and tarsal canal is well displayed on coronal and sagittal images. The most superficial fibers of the inferior extensor retinaculum are better seen on peripheral sagittal MR images as low-signal-intensity lines crossing over the region of the sinus tarsi and talar neck and inserting into the superior aspect of the calcaneus (Fig. 104-8). Sagittal images obtained more medially demonstrate the cervical ligament as a low–signal-intensity band extending from the inferior aspect of the talus to the superior aspect of the calcaneus anteriorly (Fig. 104-9). Deeper sagittal images within the tarsal canal show the interosseous ligament as a fanlike structure sometimes seen as individual fibers separated by high–signal-intensity bands.

Coronal MRI, obtained through the anterior portion of the sinus tarsi, demonstrates the cervical ligament extending in a vertical course from the talus to the

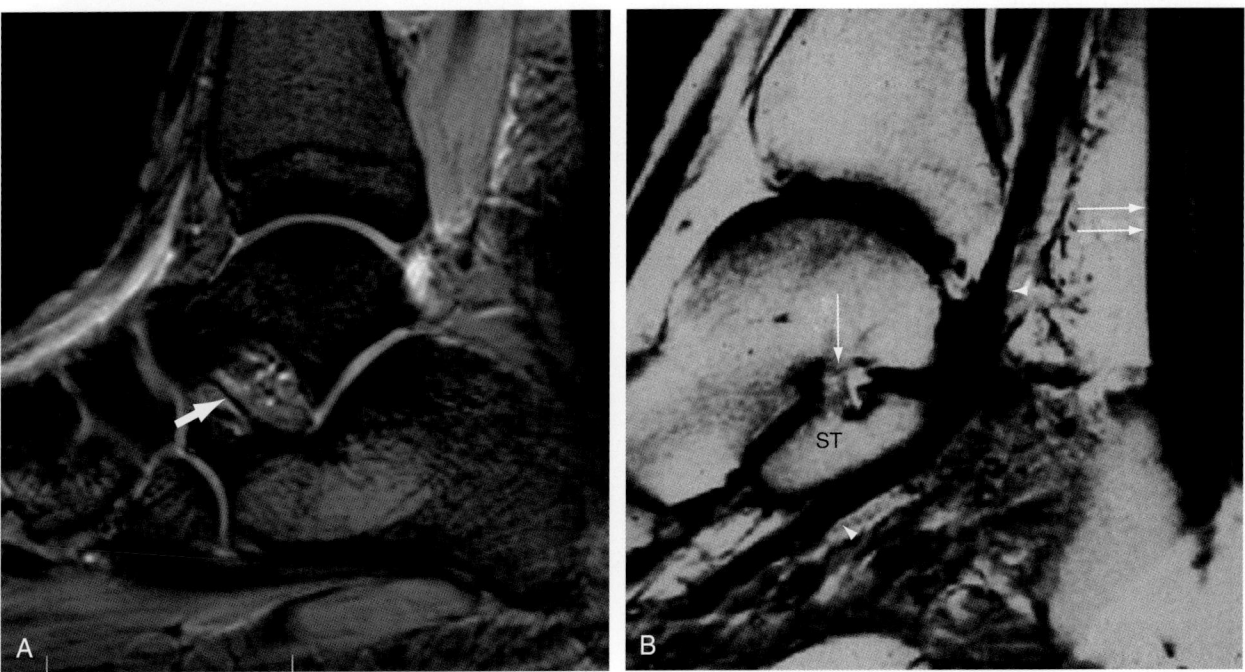

FIGURE 104-9

Normal anatomy. Sagittal gradient-echo image through the sinus tarsi (**A**), demonstrating the cervical ligament (*arrow*). A more medial T1 weighted image (**B**) through the sustentaculum tali (ST), shows the deepest fibers of the tarsal canal (*arrow*). Note the flexor hallucis longus tendon (*arrowheads*) and the distal Achilles tendon (*double arrow*).

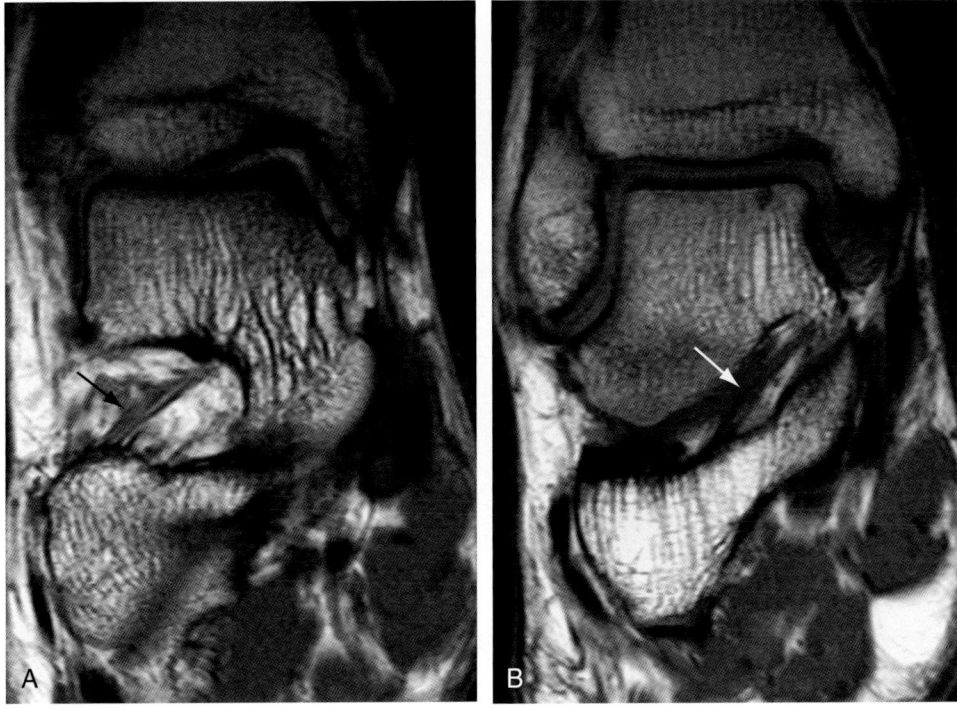

FIGURE 104-10

Normal anatomy. Coronal T1-weighted images through anterior (**A**) and posterior (**B**) aspect of the sinus tarsi and tarsal canal, demonstrating the cervical ligament (*arrow* in **A**) and the interosseous ligament (*arrow* in **B**).

calcaneus. Coronal images obtained through the middle portion of the sinus tarsi demonstrate the interosseous ligament extending obliquely from the inferior surface of the talus to the superior surface of the calcaneus (Fig. 104-10).

Muscles and Tendons

Tendons of the ankle can be divided into lateral tendons (peroneus longus and peroneus brevis), medial tendons (tibialis posterior, flexor digitorum longus, and flexor hallucis longus), posterior tendons (Achilles and plantaris), and anterior tendons (tibialis anterior, extensor hallucis longus, extensor digitorum longus, and peroneus tertius).

Lateral Tendons

The peroneus longus muscle belly is attached to the head and proximal fibula and lateral tibial condyle. Its tendon descends behind the lateral malleolus in a groove shared with the tendon of the peroneus brevis muscle. Both tendons are covered by the superior peroneal retinaculum and share a common synovial sheath proximally. Distal to the peroneal retinaculum, the peroneus longus tendon is covered by its own tendon sheath for a short segment. It then curves at the level of the cuboid bone and crosses the plantar aspect of the foot, obliquely

inserting at the base of the first metatarsal and adjacent medial cuneiform. Occasionally, a third attachment can be found in the base of the second metatarsal. A second synovial sheath covers the tendon where it crosses the sole of the foot.

The peroneus brevis muscle is attached to the distal two thirds of the lateral aspect of the fibular surface, anterior to the peroneus longus. It also descends vertically, behind the lateral malleolus, and anterior to the peroneus longus tendon. Below the lateral malleolus, it turns anteriorly and its own synovial sheath covers it. It passes lateral to the calcaneus above the peroneal trochlea and inserts onto the base of the fifth metatarsal.

The function of the peroneus longus is to evert and plantar flex the foot. The peroneus brevis action is to limit inversion and also aid in eversion.

At axial MRI performed proximal to the lateral malleolus, both peroneal tendons are shown in close apposition, and it is sometimes difficult to separate them (see Fig. 104-3). Just below the lateral malleolus, they can be seen as two separate black structures covered by the peroneal retinaculum and superficial to the calcaneofibular ligament. On sagittal images, the peroneus brevis is seen anterior to the peroneus longus, extending distally to reach the base of the fifth metatarsal (Fig. 104-11). The peroneus longus is located medially and posteriorly to the peroneus brevis, and it thickens when it turns medially at the level of the cuboid. MRI does not demonstrate the tendon sheaths unless they are distended by fluid.[16-20]

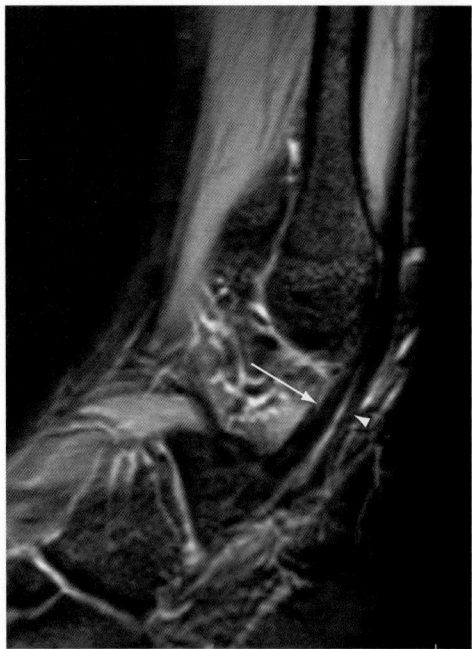

FIGURE 104-11

Normal anatomy. Sagittal gradient-echo image through the lateral malleolus demonstrating the peroneus brevis *(arrow)* and longus *(arrowhead)* tendons. The distal portion of the peroneus longus is not seen in this image.

Medial Tendons

The tibialis posterior muscle is attached between the flexor hallucis longus and flexor digitorum longus in the proximal tibia and fibula. Its tendon extends distally, just posterior to the medial malleolus. At this level its own synovial sheath covers it. It turns anteriorly below the medial malleolus and is located superficial to the deltoid ligament. Distally, the tibialis posterior tendon is attached to the navicular tuberosity. A second group of fibers extends to the anterior surface of the medial cuneiform and base of the first metatarsal. Tendon slips also extend to the middle and lateral cuneiform. The tibialis posterior muscle provides inversion of the foot and assists in plantar flexion. It also contributes to elevation of the longitudinal arch through its attachments in the cuneiform bones and metatarsal base. The tibialis posterior tendon is seen at axial MRI, just anterior to the flexor digitorum longus, behind the medial malleolus (see Fig. 104-3). It is the thickest of the three medial tendons, and it is located in a superficial position. Occasionally, a sesamoid bone, the os tibialis externus, is seen in its more distal area, just proximal to its insertion. Slight increase in signal intensity of the substance of the tendon is noted just proximal to its insertion. This is better seen on axial views and should not be interpreted as a lesion.[19]

The flexor digitorum longus muscle is attached to the posterior surface of the tibia, medial to the tibialis posterior. Its tendon passes behind the medial malleolus, posterior to the tibialis posterior tendon, with its own synovial sheath. The flexor digitorum longus tendon

curves anteriorly and comes in contact with the medial aspect of the sustentaculum tali and is superficial to the flexor hallucis longus tendon. More distally, it crosses the sole of the foot, dividing into four tendon slips, which insert into the base of the distal phalanx of the second, third, fourth, and fifth toes. At axial MRI, the tendon is located deeper and posterior to the tibialis posterior tendon (see Fig. 104-3). Its distal extensions can be followed with transverse imaging through the midfoot and forefoot.

The flexor hallucis longus muscle is attached to the distal two thirds of the posterior fibular surface, interosseous membrane, and intermuscular septum. Its tendon descends in the posterior aspect of the tibia through a groove and then crosses the posterior aspect of the talus and inferior surface of the sustentaculum tali. Fibrous bands cover the grooves of the talus and calcaneus. A synovial sheath lines the tendon. In the distal portion, it crosses the flexor digitorum longus obliquely, from the lateral to the medial side. At the crossing point, the long digital flexor receives a fiber slip from the flexor hallucis longus tendon, and the latter then extends distally between the sesamoid bones of the hallux to insert into the base of the distal phalanx of the great toe. Axial and sagittal images can demonstrate the entire extent of the tendon (see Figs. 104-3 and 104-9B). As in other tendons, the synovial sheath is not identified unless it is distended by fluid. This is a frequent occurrence in the flexor hallucis longus because it communicates directly with the ankle joint.[20,21]

Posterior Tendons

The Achilles tendon is formed by the junction of the gastrocnemius and soleus tendons and is the largest and strongest human tendon. It measures about 15 cm in length. Proximally it is oval, and more distally it is flattened. It flares off at the level of its insertion in the dorsal aspect of the calcaneus. Axial and sagittal MR images demonstrate the tendon in its entirety (see Figs. 104-3 and 104-9B). The soleus and gastrocnemius muscles are the major plantar flexors.

The plantaris muscle is attached in the lateral supracondylar area of the distal femur. Its belly is fusiform and small (7 to 10 cm long), and it ends in a long slender tendon crossing obliquely between the gastrocnemius and soleus. It descends along the medial border of the Achilles tendon, gradually fusing with it. It is absent in about 10% of the population. At MRI, it is identified only on axial images as a small black dot medial and anterior to the Achilles tendon (see Fig. 104-3). The plantaris is a rudimentary muscle, and it probably acts with the gastrocnemius muscles.[21]

Anterior Tendons

The tibialis anterior muscle arises from the lateral tibial condyle, and its tendon descends vertically in the anterior surface of the tibia, runs through the medial compartment of the superior and inferior extensor retinaculum, and attaches distally to the medial and inferior surfaces of the medial cuneiform and the base of the first metatarsal. The tibialis anterior muscle is a dorsiflexor. Sagittal and axial MR images can demonstrate the normal anatomy and pathology of the tibialis anterior tendon (see Fig. 104-3).

The extensor digitorum longus muscle attaches to the lateral tibial condyle, proximal fibula, interosseous membrane, and intermuscular septum. The tendon passes behind the superior extensor retinaculum and within a loop of the inferior retinaculum, where it divides into four slips extending distally to the bases of the distal phalanges of the second, third, fourth, and fifth toes. Its integrity is better assessed with axial MRI (see Fig. 104-3). The distal extensions can be evaluated by means of transverse imaging through the midfoot and forefoot.

The peroneus tertius tendon is attached to the distal third of the medial fibular surface. The tendon passes behind the superior and inferior extensor retinaculum with the extensor digitorum longus tendons, and it inserts distally in the proximal fifth metatarsal. It is absent in about 5% of the population. Its action is to dorsiflex the foot. When present, it can be identified on transverse MR images through the midfoot area in the dorsomedial aspect of the fifth metatarsal.

Intrinsic Muscles and Tendons of the Foot

Intrinsic muscles and tendons of the plantar aspect of the foot can be divided into four layers. The first and most superficial layer contains the adductor hallucis muscle, the flexor digitorum brevis muscle, and the abductor digiti minimi. All three muscles originate in the inferior surface of the calcaneus. The abductor hallucis tendon inserts in the base of the proximal phalanx of the great toe medially. The flexor digitorum brevis tendon inserts into the inferior proximal aspect of the middle phalanges of the second, third, fourth, and fifth toes. The tendons of the abductor digiti minimi insert in the lateral aspect of the base of the proximal phalanx of the fifth toe. The second layer is composed of the tendons of the flexor digitorum longus, the flexor hallucis longus, the quadratus plantae muscle, and lumbricalis muscles and tendons. The third layer is composed of 1. the flexor hallucis brevis, which extends from the inferior aspect of the cuboid to the medial sesamoid bone; 2. the abductor hallucis muscle, which originates from the base of the cuboid, base of the third and fourth metatarsal, and distal ends of the second through fourth metatarsal extending medially to insert in the lateral sesamoid; and finally 3. the flexor digiti minimi brevis extending from the base of the fifth metatarsal to the base of the proximal phalanx of the fifth toe. The fourth layer is the deepest, and it is composed, from posterior to anterior, by the insertion of the tibialis posterior tendon, tibialis anterior tendon, and peroneus longus tendon, all of them inserting into the base of the fifth metatarsal, and the interosseous muscles and tendons extending from the metatarsal to the base of the proximal phalanges of the second, third, fourth, and fifth toes.

The anatomy of the plantar aspect of the foot can also be divided into four compartments (medial, lateral, central, and interosseous), separated by interosseous fascia, and the medial and lateral intermuscular septa. Coronal imaging through the midfoot and forefoot demonstrates the detailed anatomy of this arrangement[12,21,22] (Fig. 104-12). The medial compartment is occupied by the following structures: abductor hallucis muscle, flexor hallucis brevis muscle, flexor hallucis longus tendon, medial plantar neurovascular bundle, peroneus longus tendon, and tibialis posterior tendon. The central compartment contains the flexor digitorum

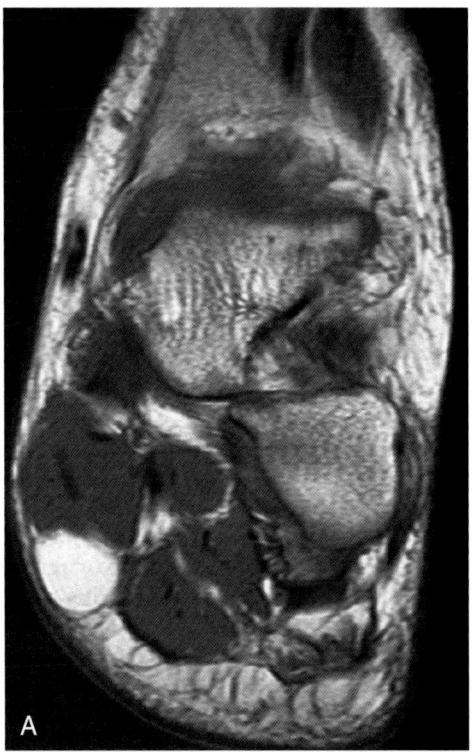

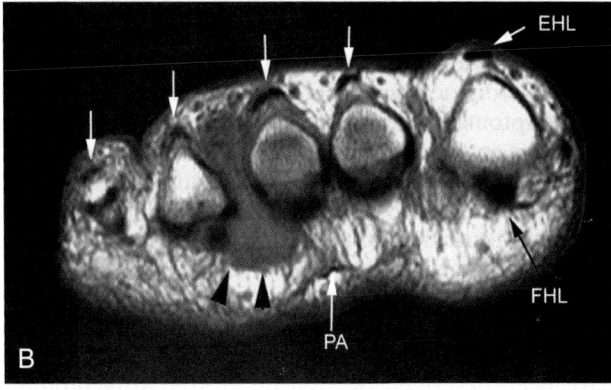

FIGURE 104-12

Normal anatomy. Coronal T1-weighted images through the midfoot (**A**) and forefoot (**B**), demonstrating the normal distribution of muscles and tendons. Note the presence of a Morton's neuroma (*arrowheads* in **B**) (see also Fig. 104-33). Extensor digitorum tendons are shown by arrows. EHL, Extensor hallucis longus tendon; FHL, Flexor hallucis longus tendon; PA, Plantar aponeurosis.

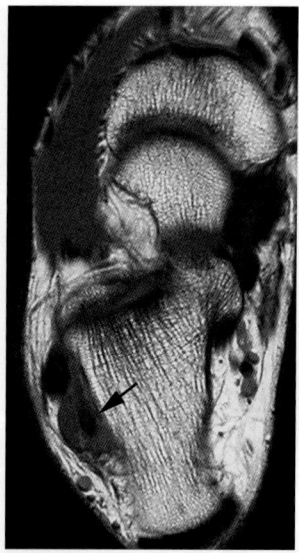

FIGURE 104-15

Calcaneofibular ligament tear. Axial T1-weighted image showing a calcaneofibular ligament *(arrow)*, with surrounding edema.

Chandnani and associates[34] indicated that MR arthrography is superior to plain MRI for the assessment of lateral collateral ligament injuries.

Spring Ligament Injuries

Acute injuries to the calcaneonavicular ligament or spring ligament are unusual. Chronic attrition is associated with posterior tibial tendon degeneration and failure. When the posterior tibial tendon ruptures, the spring ligament becomes the only support to the head of the talus, and eventually chronic loading leads to its degeneration and tear.[13] MRI shows irregular thickening and heterogeneous signal intensity.

Sinus Tarsi Syndrome

Sinus tarsi syndrome is a condition presenting clinically with pain in the lateral aspect of the foot, over the sinus tarsi region, and a sensation of hindfoot instability. Symptoms are often relieved by injection of local anesthetics. The most frequent cause of sinus tarsi syndrome is trauma (70%). Inflammatory conditions, such as rheumatoid arthritis and ankylosing spondylitis, and foot deformities (pes cavus, pes planus) can also produce the syndrome.

Inversion injuries to the ankle induce tears of the lateral collateral ligament, beginning with the anterior talofibular ligament and followed by the calcaneofibular ligament. With increasing inversion, the interosseous ligament of the sinus tarsi can be torn. This leads to instability of the subtalar joint and subsequently to a chronic inflammatory synovial reaction.

The MRI manifestations of sinus tarsi syndrome include loss of the signal intensity of fat within the sinus tarsi and tarsal canal, with hypointensity on T1-weighted images and hyperintensity on T2-weighted images, associated with lack of visualization of the ligaments.[6,15] Other ligamentous and tendon lesions can be seen in association with sinus tarsi syndrome. Lateral collateral ligament tears have been found in about 79% of cases of sinus tarsi syndrome, and 39% of patients with lateral collateral ligament injuries had an abnormal signal intensity pattern within the region of the sinus tarsi.[15] Tibialis posterior tendon tears can also be seen in association with sinus tarsi syndrome[15] (Fig. 104-16). Osteoarthritis of the subtalar joint and subchondral cysts may be present in advanced cases.

Lisfranc Ligament Injuries

The Lisfranc ligament is one of the structures contributing to the stability of the tarsometatarsal joint, along with the intertarsal ligaments, the tarsometatarsal ligaments, and the normal proximal recession of the second metatarsal. This ligament may be injured in high-energy trauma or axial loading with the foot in plantar flexion. Most commonly lesions occur at the insertion of the ligament in the base of the second metatarsal, producing an avulsion fracture and malalignment, better seen on CT. MRI may demonstrate focal areas of edema, ligament disruption and bone marrow bruise.

Soft-Tissue Impingement Syndromes

Altered joint biomechanics often secondary to ligamentous injuries may produce chronic painful conditions around the ankle, known as ankle impingement syndromes. Five syndromes have been described, depending on their location and clinical manifestations: anterolateral, anterior, anteromedial, posteromedial, and posterior.

Anterolateral Impingement Syndrome

Also known as anterolateral gutter syndrome or Wolin syndrome,[35,36] the anterolateral impingement syndrome is defined clinically as chronic ankle pain produced by entrapment of hypertrophied synovial tissue and fibrosis as a result of an acute anterolateral capsuloligamentous lesion or repetitive microtrauma. The hypertrophied soft-tissues may mold to a hyalinized meniscoid lesion as described by Wolin.[36] Hypertrophy of the accessory fascicle of the anterior tibiofibular ligament and osteophyte formation may also be contributing factors. The MRI findings of anterolateral impingement syndrome include a hypointense mass in the anterolateral ankle gutter, hypertrophy of the accessory fascicle of the anterior inferior tibiofibular ligament and a joint effusion.[35,37] Lack of distension of the anterolateral recess of the joint due to scarring can be seen in the presence of an effusion or during MR arthrography.[35,38]

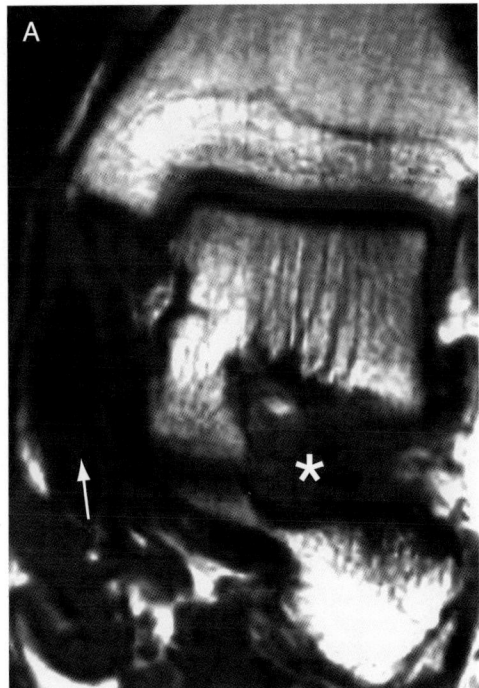

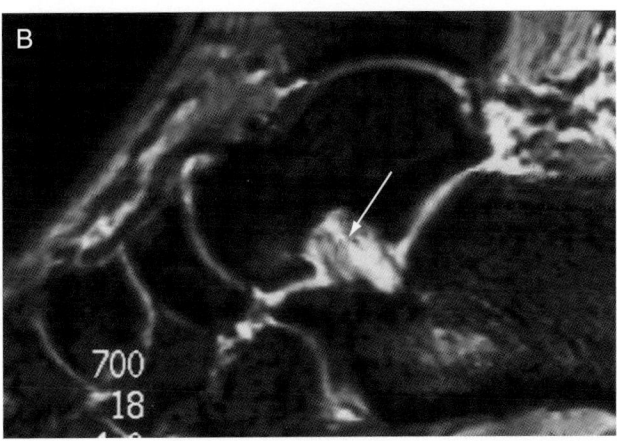

FIGURE 104-16

Sinus tarsi syndrome. Coronal T1-weighted (**A**) and sagittal gradient-echo (**B**) images demonstrating loss of the normal signal intensity of the fat in the subtalar area (*asterisk* in **A**). The cervical ligament is seen in the sagittal image (*arrow*). Note also severe tendinosis of the posterior tibialis tendon (*arrow* in **A**).

Anterior Impingement Syndrome

Repeated stress in ankle dorsiflexion may produce osteophyte formation in the anterior rim of the tibial plafond and the dorsal aspect of the talar neck, within the joint capsule, resulting in soft-tissue impingement, pain and limited motion.[35,39,40] Anterior impingement syndrome is frequently seen in athletes such as soccer players. MRI may demonstrate cartilage damage, bone marrow edema, and synovitis in the anterior capsule, in addition to the anterior osteophytes.

Anteromedial Impingement Syndrome

Anteromedial impingement syndrome also may result in the formation of a meniscoid lesion in the anteromedial aspect of the ankle, anterior to the deltoid ligament. A tear of the deep fibers of the deltoid ligament may or may not be associated with this syndrome.[41] Thickening of the anterior tibiotalar ligament, osteophyte formation, and a chondral lesion of the anterior medial talar dome may be present. This syndrome is most frequently associated with inversion and medial ligamentous injuries. MR arthrography may demonstrate the meniscoid lesion, thickening of the anterior tibiotalar ligament, and the chondral lesions.[41]

Posteromedial Impingement Syndrome

Posteromedial ankle pain after severe ankle inversion may be due to injury of the deep posterior fibers of the deltoid ligament, crushed between the medial talus and the medial malleolus.[42] This injury may lead to chronic hypertrophy and scar formation, shown on MRI with associated bone marrow edema of the medial talus and medial malleolus.[42]

Posterior Impingement Syndrome

Also known as the *os trigonum* syndrome, talar compression syndrome, and posterior block of the ankle, posterior impingement syndrome is produced by forced plantar flexion with resulting injury to the soft-tissues and the posterior talus located between the distal tibia and calcaneus.[43] This syndrome is frequent in ballet dancers and also in other sportspeople. Contributing factors to the syndrome are variations of the normal osseous anatomy including the presence of an os trigonum, an elongated lateral tubercle of the talus (the Stieda process), a downwards sloping of the posterior lip of the tibia, a prominent posterior process of the calcaneus, and the presence of loose bodies. Osseous and soft-tissue injury may result, including fracture, fragmentation, and pseudoarthrosis of the os trigonum or lateral tubercle of the talus, posterior ankle and subtalar joint synovitis, hypertrophy of the intermalleolar ligament, and flexor hallucis longus tenosynovitis.[40,43] MRI may demonstrate signal changes in the corresponding bony structures, with or without fractures and inflammatory changes of the tibiotalar joint, posterior subtalar joint, and flexor hallucis longus tendon sheath.

TENDON LESIONS

Tendon lesions can be classified as tenosynovitis, rupture, entrapment, and dislocation.[3,8,17-22,44] In tenosynovitis, MRI can demonstrate distention of the tendon sheath with or without thickening of the tendon. Focal hyperintense areas within the tendon can also be seen. Tendon ruptures can be complete or partial. In complete ruptures, MRI shows interruption of the tendon fibers with irregularity of the ends of the ruptured tendon,

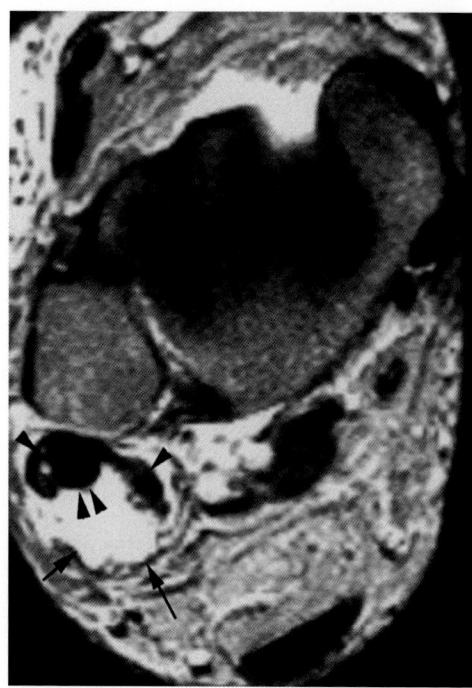

FIGURE 104-17

Peroneal tenosynovitis and chronic tear of the peroneus brevis tendon. Axial T2-weighted image showing distension of the tendon sheaths of the peroneal and extensor digitorum tendons *(arrows)*, with extensive flattening and chronic tearing of the peroneus brevis tendon *(single arrowhead)*. Note the peroneus longus tendon located posterior to the presoneus brevis tendon *(double arrowhead)*.

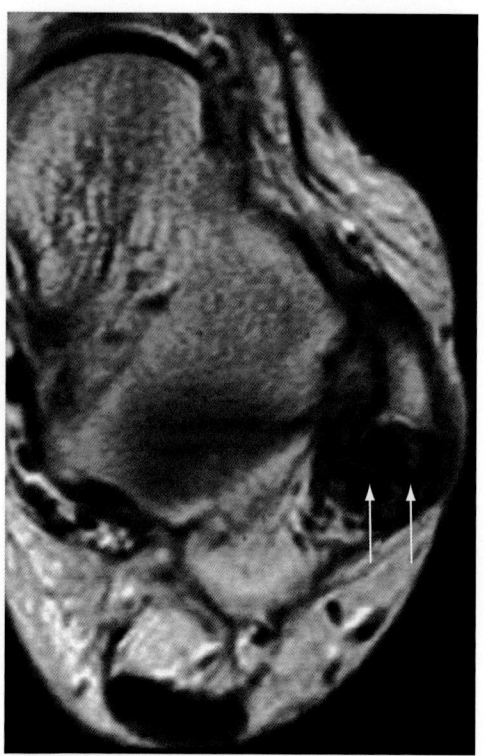

FIGURE 104-18

Peroneal tendon rupture. Axial T1-weighted image demonstrating complete tears of both peroneal tendons *(arrows)*, with discontinuity of the tendon fibers.

associated with abnormal signal intensity in the surrounding tissues and within the gap created by the rupture, reflecting edema or hematoma. Incomplete tendon ruptures, such as longitudinal tears, are seen on MR images as focal tendon thickening or attenuation and as focal or longitudinal hyperintense areas corresponding to the actual tears. Tendon entrapment occurs as a consequence of callus formation and fibrous tissue forming after a fracture and involving the adjacent tendons. Tenosynovitis and partial or complete tears are often associated with entrapment. MRI shows the callus and surrounding hypointense scar tissue in the expected location of the tendon. Dislocation of a tendon can be diagnosed with MRI when the tendon is not found in its exact anatomic location. Subluxations occur more often than dislocations. Tenosynovitis may also accompany tendon dislocation.

Peroneal Tendons

Peroneal tenosynovitis can occur as a result of entrapment after calcaneal fracture, inflammatory or infectious arthritis (Fig. 104-17), hypertrophy of the peroneal tubercle, or abnormal foot mechanics (pes planus, tarsal coalition); or it can be idiopathic. In mild cases, the tendons may have normal appearance at MRI and only synovitis with tendon sheath distention may be seen. In

advanced cases, MRI may also demonstrate tendon signal abnormalities and changes in contour.

Mechanical stress can lead to peroneal tendon tears. Lack of visualization of the ruptured peroneal tendon with surrounding inflammatory changes is well demonstrated on axial MR images (Fig. 104-18). Partial longitudinal tears (splits) occur more often than complete peroneal tendon tears, and the peroneus brevis tendon is frequently involved (Fig. 104-19).

Peroneal tendon dislocation occurs as a result of a violent contraction of the peroneal muscles during sports activities, with disruption of the retinaculum and lateral subluxation or dislocation of the tendons (Fig. 104-20). Congenital laxity of the peroneal retinaculum can predispose to recurrent dislocations and even longitudinal tears.[3]

Posterior Tibial Tendon Lesions

Partial or complete rupture of the posterior tibial tendon is a relatively frequent syndrome in women in their fifth or sixth decade. It has also been described in young athletes playing soccer, tennis, or ice hockey and in young girls involved in gymnastic activities requiring excessive pointing of their toes. A painful mass in the medial aspect of the foot, associated with progressive flat-foot deformity, may be the presenting clinical feature.

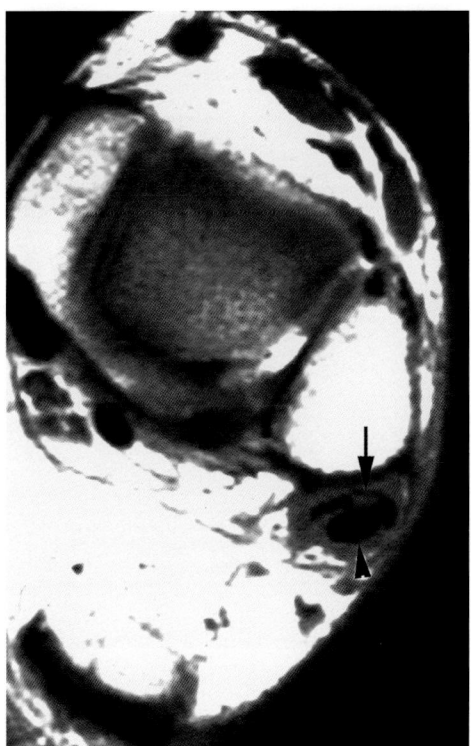

FIGURE 104-19

Longitudinal tear of the peroneus brevis tendon. Axial T1-weighted image showing splitting of the peroneus brevis tendon *(arrow)*, with an intact peroneus longus tendon *(arrowhead)*.

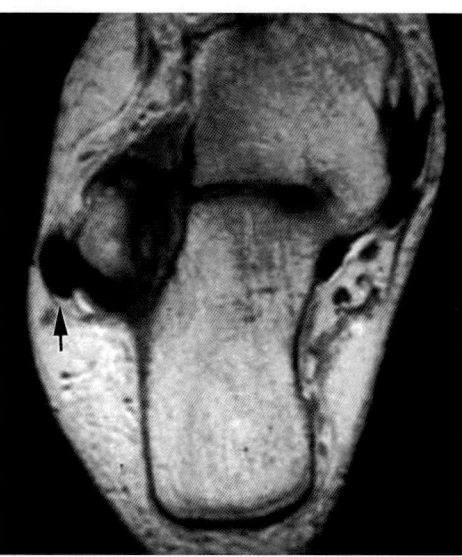

FIGURE 104-20

Dislocation of the peroneal tendons. Axial T1-weighted image demonstrating anterior dislocation of both peroneal tendons *(arrow)*, without associated tear. Note the presence of tarsal coalition. *(Reprinted from The Ankle and foot. MRI Clinics of North America. Beltran J. Guest ed. WB Saunders Co. Philadelphia, 1994.)*

Inflammatory arthritis, such as rheumatoid arthritis, and seronegative spondyloarthropathies can also cause posterior tibial tendon rupture.

Three types of posterior tibial tendon rupture have been described.[17,45,46] In type I lesions, the tendon is thickened, with longitudinal tears producing a striated appearance on sagittal MR images and splits shown in axial images (Fig. 104-21). In type II lesions, the tendon is markedly attenuated, and in type III lesions a complete tear with discontinuity of the tendon is seen on MR images (Fig. 104-22). Associated peritendinous inflammatory changes can be present in all three types.

Flexor Hallucis Longus Lesions

Tenosynovitis of the flexor hallucis longus occurs in athletes and dancers performing repeated plantar flexion of their forefoot in weight-bearing exercise. Compression of the tendon in forced plantar flexion in patients with a prominent os trigonum has been termed *os trigonum syndrome*, described earlier in the chapter. Inflammatory arthritis may also produce tenosynovitis of this tendon. MRI demonstrates fluid distending the synovial sheath, more often in the posterior aspect of the ankle where the tendon passes through a fibro-osseous tunnel created between the medial and lateral tubercles

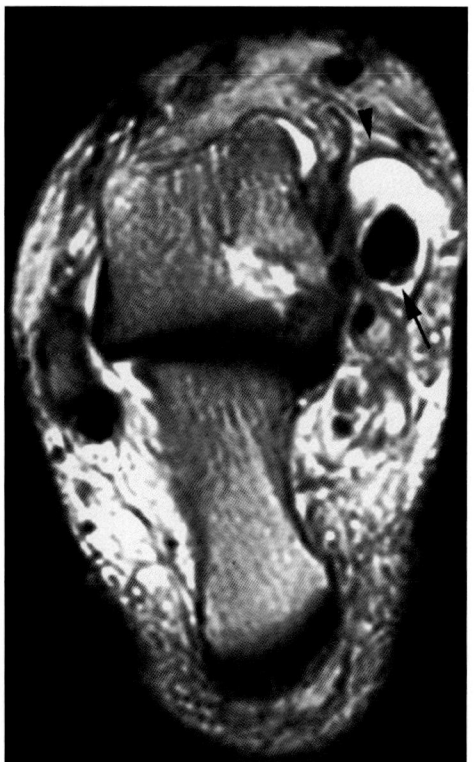

FIGURE 104-21

Type I posterior tibialis tendon tear. Axial T2-weighted image showing increased thickness and inhomogeneous signal of the posterior tibialis tendon *(arrow)*, with fluid distending the synovial sheath *(arrowhead)*.

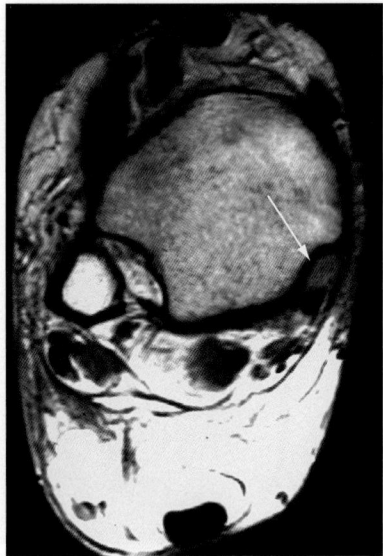

FIGURE 104-22

Type III posterior tibialis tendon tear. Axial T1-weighted image demonstrating complete absence of the fibers of the posterior tibialis tendon (*arrow*) in the retromalleolar area.

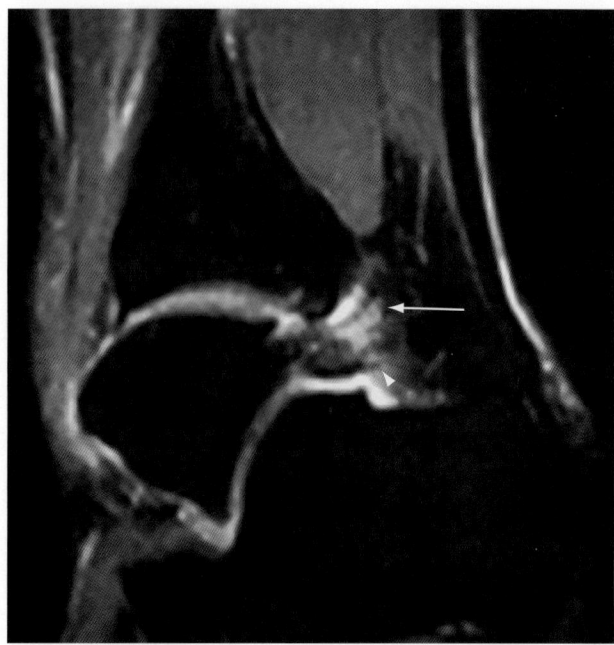

FIGURE 104-23

Os trigonum syndrome. Sagittal STIR image demonstrates an os trigonum (*arrowhead*) with bone marrow edema and surrounding inflammatory changes (*arrow*).

of the talus (Fig. 104-23). One can expect to see small amounts of fluid in this region in asymptomatic cases,[20] and also in patients with effusion of the ankle joint due to the normal communication between this joint and the synovial sheath of the flexor hallucis longus tendon, which is present in about 20% of the population. A large amount of fluid distending the tendon sheath is abnormal. Continued stress of the tendon can lead to longitudinal tendon tears (Fig. 104-24). Complete tears of the flexor hallucis longus tendon are rare.

A second site of injury with tenosynovitis or tears of the flexor hallucis longus may occur with repetitive trauma at the level of the head of the first metatarsal ("turf toe").

Achilles Tendon Lesions

Acute tendinitis and peritendinitis of the Achilles tendon develop as a result of athletic overuse. It has been suggested that ischemia might play a significant role in the production of inflammatory changes in the tendon. On MR images, linear or irregular areas of abnormal signal intensity in the pre-Achilles fat pad may be seen in peritendinitis. In tendinitis, MRI can demonstrate focal or diffuse swelling of tendon, with linear or irregular areas of increased signal intensity within the tendon substance. This is more frequently seen in chronic tendinitis. With more continued inflammatory changes, focal areas of mucoid degeneration develop, eventually leading to tendon tears (Fig. 104-25). Focal swelling of the Achilles tendon at its calcaneal insertion has been termed *insertional tendinitis,* a condition associated

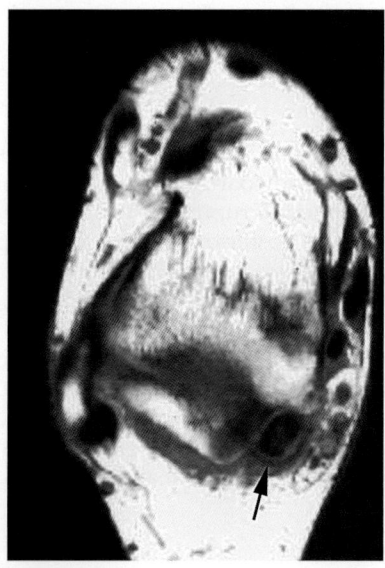

FIGURE 104-24

Partial tear of the flexor hallucis tendon. Axial T1-weighted image demonstrating thickening and partial tear of the flexor hallucis longus tendon (*arrow*), with synovitis and thickening of the synovial sheath.

with Haglund's syndrome (Fig. 104-26). In Achilles tendon ruptures, MRI demonstrates partial or complete disruption of the tendon either at the musculotendinous interface or more distally (Fig. 104-27), or at its insertion into the posterior aspect of the calcaneus.[3,16] Achilles tendon rupture typically occurs in unconditioned

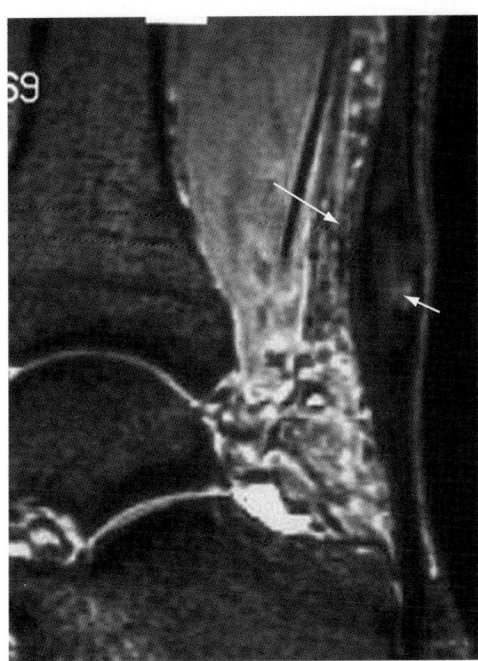

FIGURE 104-25

Chronic Achilles tendinosis. Sagittal STIR image sowing fusiform thickening of the Achilles tendon *(long arrow)*, with a focal area of increased signal intensity *(short arrow)*. Note diffuse peritendinitis of the Kager's fat triangle.

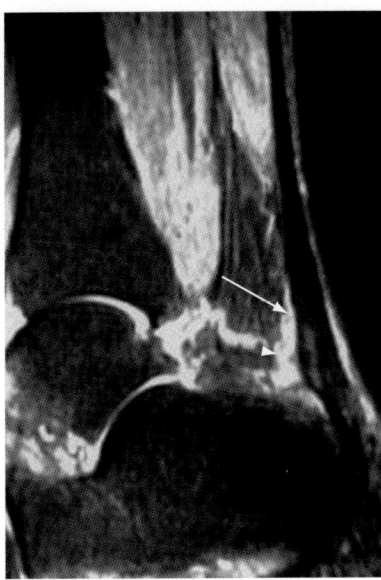

FIGURE 104-26

Insertional Achilles tendinosis. Sagittal STIR image showing focal thickening of the Achilles tendon at its insertion *(arrow)*, associated with peritendinitis *(arrowhead)*. Note also reactive edema of the calcaneus at the tendon attachment.

individuals, but it is also found in professional athletes. It is more frequent in men than in women, and occasionally it can be bilateral. Systemic disorders (rheumatoid arthritis, gout, hyperthyroidism, chronic renal failure, diabetes), and corticosteroid injection may predispose to tendon ruptures. Clinical history and physical examination are characteristic for Achilles tendon rupture, but occasionally the distinction between complete and incomplete tears may be difficult, and MRI can provide further assessment.

Internal degeneration of the Achilles tendon can occasionally be seen in patients with renal failure. This is demonstrated on MR images as large areas of high signal intensity on proton density- and T2-weighted images, presumably representing focal regions of degeneration and fluid accumulation.

Tendinous xanthomas occur in patients with hyperlipoproteinemia. MRI demonstrates massive thickening of the Achilles tendon with irregular signal intensity[44] (Fig. 104-28).

Anterior Tibial Tendon Lesions

Anterior tibial tendon tears are relatively rare and occur more frequently in elderly patients or in athletes with forced plantar flexion of the foot. Tenosynovitis may occur associated with inflammatory conditions such as rheumatoid arthritis or even infectious conditions (diabetic foot). Distention of the synovial sheath is easily demonstrated with MRI.

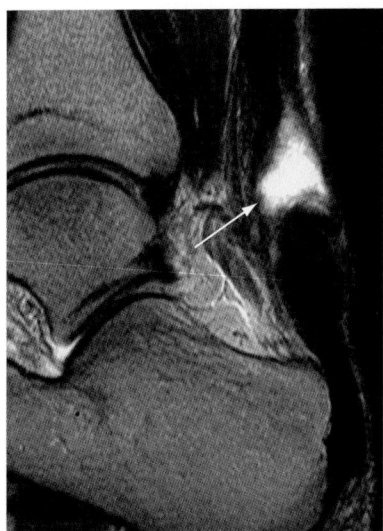

FIGURE 104-27

Complete Achilles tendon tear. Sagittal T2-weighted image demonstrating discontinuity of the fibers *(arrow)*, and hematoma/edema at the rupture site.

BONE LESIONS

Bone contusions or "bruises" are manifested on MR images as reticular and ill-defined areas of decreased signal intensity on T1-weighted images, with increased signal intensity on T2-weighted and fat-suppressed images (STIR, fat saturation). They are apparently related to microfractures of the trabecular bone and to edema or

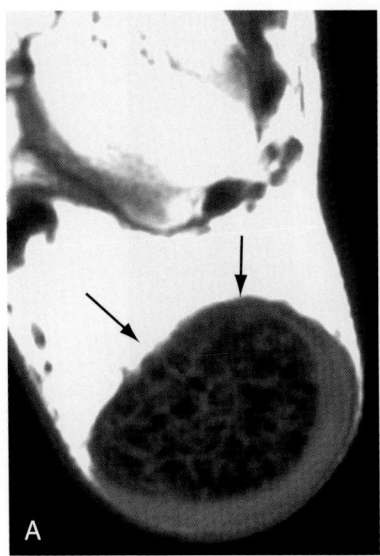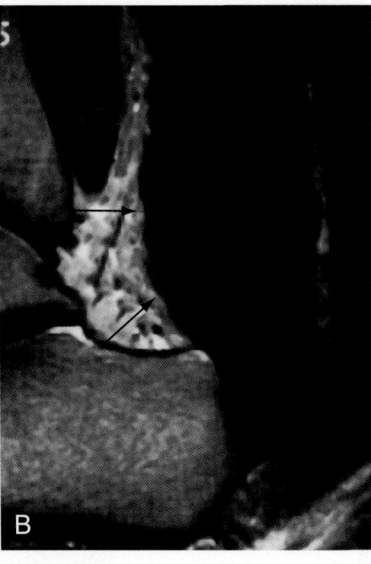

FIGURE 104-28

Achilles tendon xanthoma. Axial T1-weighted image (**A**) and sagittal T2-weighted image (**B**), showing massive tendon thickening with markedly heterogeneous signal (*arrows*).

hemorrhage within the bone marrow. Normally, they resolve within 4 to 6 weeks (Fig. 104-29).

Stress fractures and insufficiency fractures are frequent occurrences in the ankle and foot, involving predominantly the second metatarsal, the calcaneus, and, less frequently, the navicular bone. Before a stress fracture takes place, a condition termed *stress response* occurs.[3] During this period, edema, hyperemia, and osteoclastic activity develop within the stressed area of the bone, shown on MR images as poorly defined abnormal signal intensity of the bone marrow, similar to a bone contusion. As the stress persists and a fracture develops, MRI then shows a hypointense irregular line within the area of edema and hyperemia. Acute post-traumatic fractures have similar MRI manifestations. Although plain-film radiography often provides most of the necessary information for the diagnosis of fractures, MRI has been found more sensitive than conventional radiography and more specific than bone scintigraphy for this diagnosis.[3]

Osteochondritis dissecans or osteochondral fractures of the ankle occur primarily in the talar dome, most frequently in the middle third of the lateral border and in the posterior third of the medial border.[3] Treatment is aimed at revascularization, healing, and prevention of detachment of the osteochondral fragment. The size, signal intensity, and alignment of the osteochondral fragment are important MRI data for management of these lesions. Based on cadaveric studies,[47] four stages of osteochondritis dissecans of the talar dome have been proposed. In stage I, the injury is confined to the subchondral bone, with preservation of the articular surface. In stage II, the articular cartilage is involved by the fracture, but the articular surface is still smooth and congruent. In stage III, the osteochondral fragment is partially displaced, and, in stage IV, the fragment has become an intra-articular loose body. Details of the condition and alignment of the articular cartilage can be gained with the use of MRI, allowing accurate classi-fication of the type of injury for treatment planning

(Fig. 104-30). The signal intensity of the interface between the normal bone and the osteochondral fragment has received attention in the MRI literature. Hypointensity of the interface on T2-weighted pulse sequences would indicate healing and stability, whereas hyperintensity could indicate fluid interposed between the fragment and the donor site, and therefore insta-bility.[3,48,49] A potential pitfall is a hyperintense signal pat-tern at the interface related to healing granulation tissue.[3]

Osteonecrosis of the ankle and foot occurs more often in the talus, as a consequence of talar neck fractures.

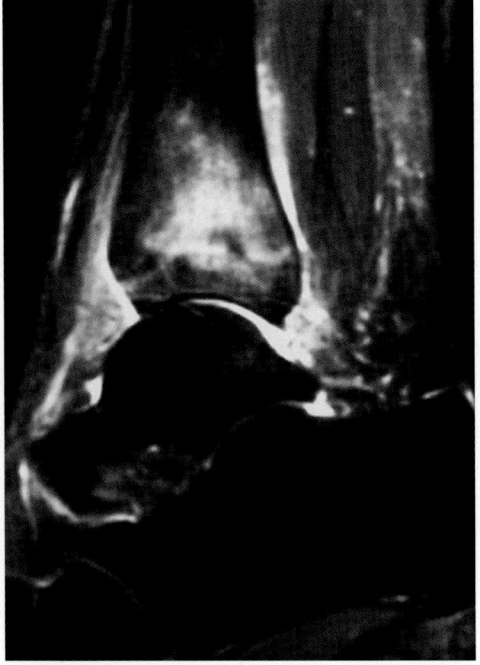

FIGURE 104-29

Bone contusion. Sagittal STIR image demonstrating an irregular area of increased signal intensity in the distal tibia, without associated fracture.

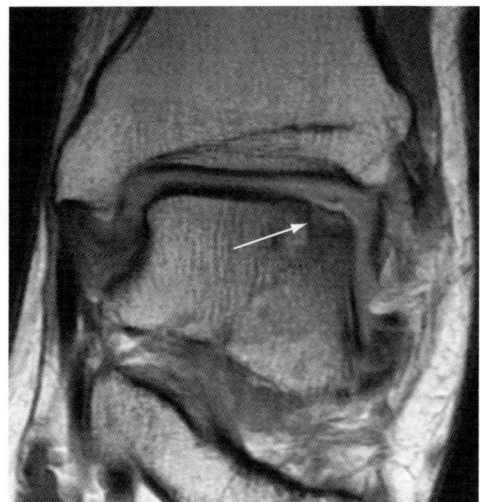

FIGURE 104-30

Osteochondritis dissecans, type II. Coronal T1-weighted image demonstrates a small osteochondral fracture in the lateral aspect of the talar dome *(arrow)*. The fragment is slightly depressed and there is an area of decreased signal intensity at the base of the fragment, probably indicating reactive sclerosis. There is some signal within the fragment itself, probably indicating viable bone.

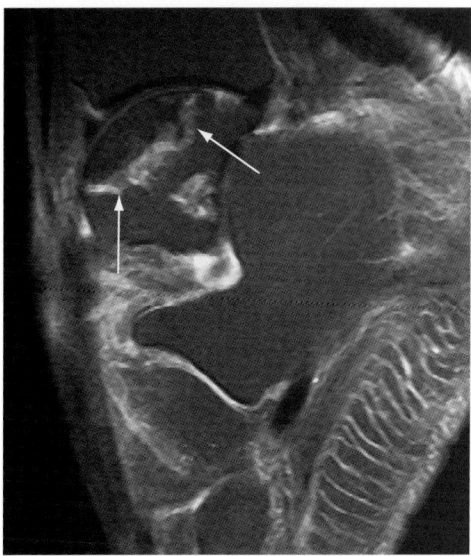

FIGURE 104-31

Osteonecrosis of the talus. Sagittal T1-weighted image with fat saturation following intravenous injection of contrast material showing an enhancing serpiginous band *(arrows)*, representing the reactive interface. Note the non-enhancing low signal intensity of the talar dome, indicating non-viable bone.

MRI is valuable for assessment of the presence, size, and fragment viability of post-traumatic osteonecrosis (Fig. 104-31). Osteonecrosis of the tarsal navicular can occur in children (Kohler's disease) or in adults, more frequently in females, with deformity and collapse of the bone. MRI can be valuable in showing the morphologic and signal intensity changes of the necrotic bone.

Osteonecrosis of the second metatarsal head (Freiberg's disease) can be diagnosed with MRI when questionable flattening of the metatarsal head is seen on plain radiographs.

Transient bone marrow edema is an entity seen more often in the femoral head and neck (transient osteoporosis of the hip), but it can appear also in the tarsal bones as a part of the syndrome of transient migratory osteoporosis.[50,51] Only anecdotal cases of this entity involving the tarsal bones have been described using MRI, which shows changes compatible with bone marrow edema.[3]

COMPRESSIVE NEUROPATHIES

The most frequent compressive neuropathies of the ankle and foot are tarsal tunnel syndrome and Morton's neuroma. Less frequent compressive neuropathies include deep peroneal nerve entrapment and sural nerve entrapment.[52]

Tarsal Tunnel Syndrome

Tarsal tunnel syndrome is the most common compressive neuropathy involving the foot and is charac-

terized by pain and paresthesia in the plantar aspect of the foot and toes. Nerve entrapment or compression can occur at the level of the posterior tibial nerve or its branches (medial calcaneal nerve, lateral plantar nerve, and medial plantar nerve), producing different symptoms depending on the site of compression[32] (see Fig. 104-3). Ganglion cysts, nerve origin tumors, varicosities, lipomas, synovial hypertrophy, and scar tissue are some of the frequent intrinsic lesions producing tarsal tunnel syndrome. Foot deformities, hypertrophied and accessory muscles (Fig. 104-32), and excessive pronation during the practice of some sports are just a few of the extrinsic causes of this syndrome.

Only a few cases of tarsal tunnel syndrome evaluated with MRI have been published in the literature.[53-55] These reports emphasize the use of MRI to determine the presence of a tarsal tunnel lesion preoperatively.

Morton's Neuroma

Morton's neuroma is actually a fibrosing and degenerative process produced by compression of the plantar digital nerve, more frequently between the heads of the third and fourth metatarsal. The nerve becomes thickened, and an associated bursitis is often present.[56] Exquisite tenderness is elicited on lateral compression of the metatarsal. MRI can demonstrate the "neuroma" as a dumbbell-shaped mass located between the metatarsal heads, with intermediate-to-low signal intensity on T1- and T2-weighted images (Fig. 104-33). Enhancement after intravenous injection of gadolinium has been described in some cases. Morton's neuroma is an entity different from true plantar neuromas. Plantar neuromas

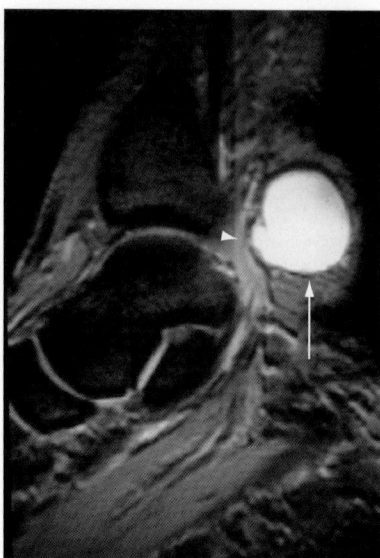

FIGURE 104-32

Tarsal tunnel syndrome. Sagittal STIR image showing a ganglion cyst *(arrow)*, producing compression of the neurovascular bundle in the tarsal tunnel *(arrowhead)*.

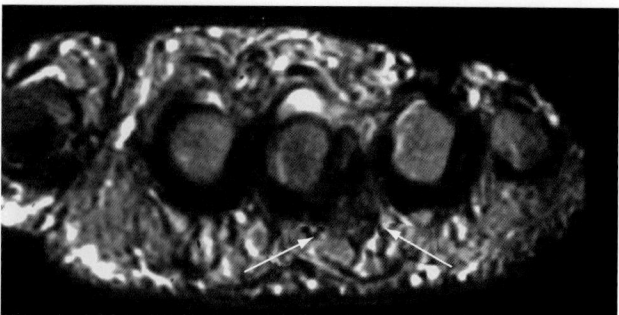

FIGURE 104-33

Morton's neuroma. Coronal (short axis) T2-weighted image through the forefoot demonstrating a hypointense lesion located between the third and fourth metatarsal heads *(arrows)*.

are hyperintense on T2-weighted pulse sequences and, unlike Morton's neuroma, they are found more often in the plantar aspect of the foot.

SYNOVIAL DISORDERS

Pigmented Villonodular Synovitis

Pigmented villonodular synovitis is a condition characterized by inflammatory proliferation of the synovium associated with deposits of hemosiderin. It can be present in any joint, tendon sheath, or bursa but is seen more frequently in the knee, hip, ankle, and elbow. It can present as a focal lesion, or it may involve the joint diffusely. Pressure erosions may be present in the diffuse form. The MRI manifestations of pigmented villonodular synovitis are characteristic owing to the paramagnetic effect of hemosiderin. Focal areas of decreased signal intensity are produced on practically any pulse sequence, mixed with other areas of decreased signal intensity on T1-weighted images and increased signal intensity on T2-weighted images (Fig. 104-34).

Inflammatory Arthritis

The characteristic radiographic manifestations of seropositive and seronegative inflammatory arthritis involving the ankle and foot include articular erosions, bony erosions, retrocalcaneal bursitis, tendon ruptures, and, in the late stages, bony ankylosis. MRI can be used to better depict the soft-tissue lesions such as ligamentous and tendon ruptures, bursitis, and synovial proliferation

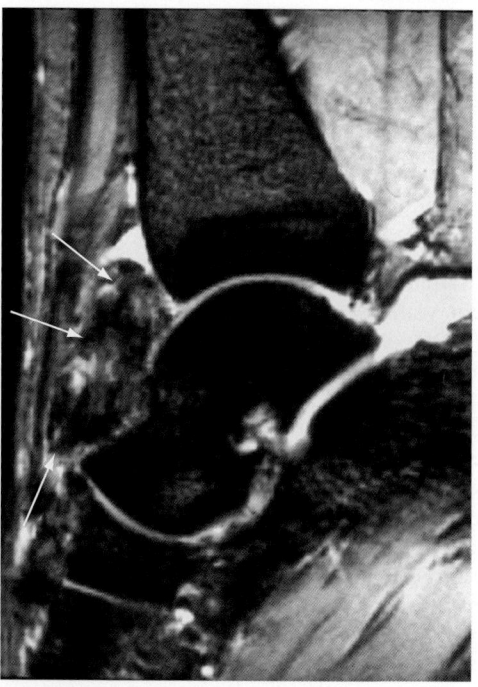

FIGURE 104-34

Pigmented villonodular synovitis. Sagittal gradient-echo image showing a nodular area of decreased signal intensity *(arrows)* in the anterior aspect of the ankle joint representing a nodular form of pigmented villonodular synovitis.

(Fig. 104-35). Intravenous injection of gadolinium has been used to define the size of proliferative pannus in patients with rheumatoid arthritis.[57,58]

Hemophilic Arthropathy

Hypertrophy and inflammation develop in the synovium in patients with hemophilia suffering repeated episodes of hemarthrosis and lead to a severe, disabling arthropathy. The elbow, knee, and ankle are the most

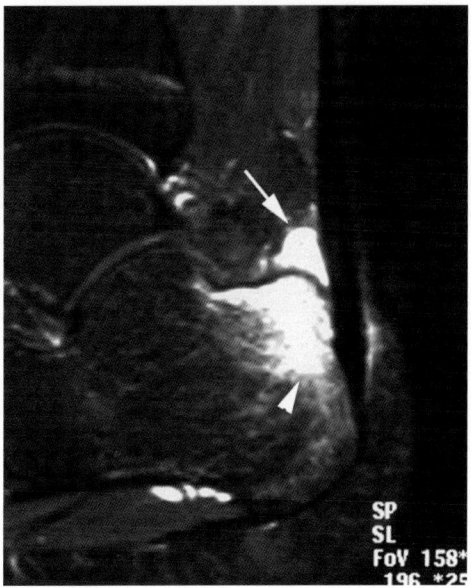

FIGURE 104-35

Juvenile rheumatoid arthritis. Sagittal STIR image showing retrocalcaneal bursitis *(arrow)* and bone marrow edema of the calcaneus *(arrowhead)*.

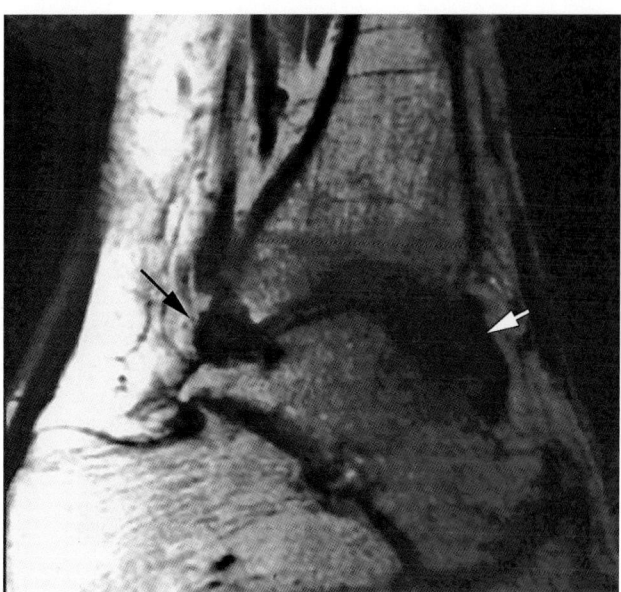

FIGURE 104-36

Hemophilic arthropathy. Sagittal T1-weighted image demonstrating low signal intensity material *(arrows)* in the tibiotalar joint, representing hemosiderin deposition within hypertrophied synovium.

commonly affected joints. Because of the hemosiderin deposition in the hypertrophied synovium, MRI demonstrates areas of signal intensity loss, associated with other signs of arthritis, such as joint space narrowing, cysts, erosions, and sclerosis (Fig. 104-36). These findings are not specific and can also be seen in pigmented villonodular synovitis, but in the proper clinical setting they suggest hemophilic arthropathy. Other joint conditions that can be associated with hypointensity on T1- and T2-weighted sequences include gout and amyloid arthropathy. In severe cases, the MRI assessment of the degree of synovial hypertrophy can be used to plan synovectomy.

MISCELLANEOUS CONDITIONS

Diabetic Foot

The combination of vasculitis, infection, and neuroarthropathy in the feet of diabetic patients leads to an entity termed *diabetic foot,* characterized clinically by ulcerations, tissue necrosis, draining sinuses, and cellulitis. In many patients, amputation is required to control the process. The radiographic manifestations include atrophic or hypertrophic neuroarthropathy, bone destruction secondary to osteomyelitis, soft-tissue swelling, and skin ulcerations. Combinations of scintigraphic techniques including those using technetium, indium, and gallium detect the presence of infection.[59-61] MRI is helpful in assessing the extent of the infection in the bone, joints, tendons, and surrounding soft-tissues, thus allowing accurate surgical planning [62-64] (Fig. 104-37).

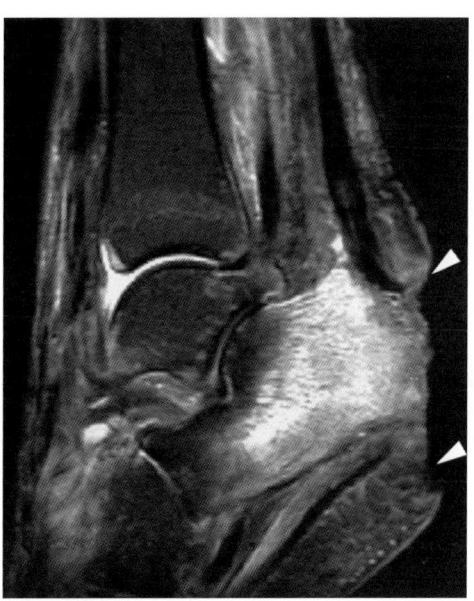

FIGURE 104-37

Diabetic foot. Sagittal STIR image demonstrating a large heel ulcer *(arrowheads)* with destruction of the cortex of the posterior process of the calcaneus and extensive osteomyelitis. Note the associated inflammatory changes in the distal Achilles tendon and a torn plantar fascia.

Distinction between neuroarthropathy and infection may be difficult with any imaging technique. With MRI, neuroarthropathy exhibits the characteristic findings of bone fragmentation, dislocations, cortical and periosteal thickening, joint effusion, and soft-tissue swelling.

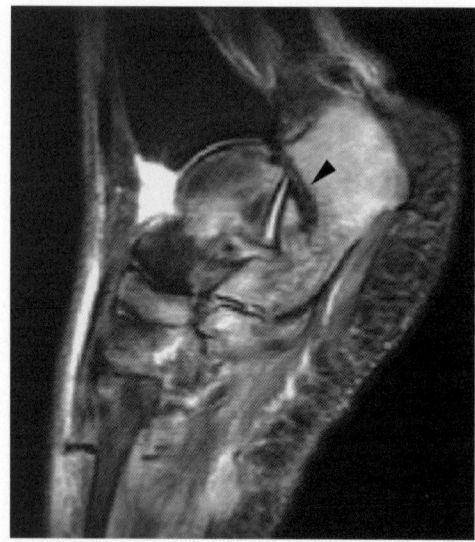

FIGURE 104-38

Neuroarthropathy in a diabetic patient. Sagittal STIR image demonstrating extensive bone edema of the tarsal bones with a fracture of the sustentaculum tali, with central depression (arrowhead). A joint effusion and soft-tissue edema is also present.

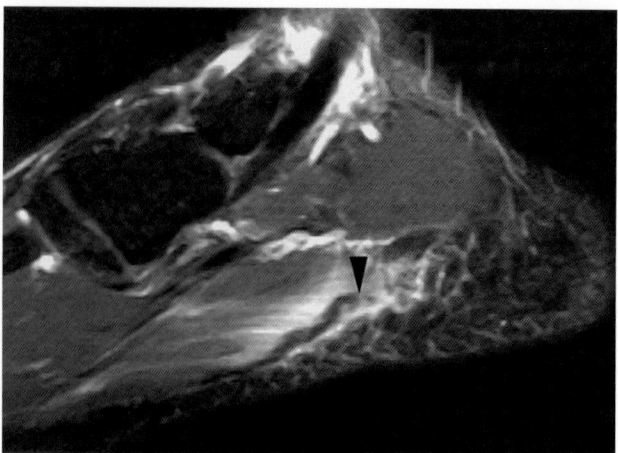

FIGURE 104-39

Rupture of the central cord of the plantar fascia. Sagittal STIR image demonstrating discontinuity of the plantar fascia, with extensive edema of the flexor digitorum brevis muscle (arrowhead).

Despite all the bone and articular changes, in most cases the bone marrow displays hypointensity on T1- and T2-weighted pulse sequences (Fig. 104-38), in contrast to osteomyelitis, which shows hypointensity of the bone marrow on T1-weighted images and hyperintensity on T2-weighted images. In some circumstances, however, the bone marrow signal intensity changes with neuroarthropathy and osteomyelitis are similar, making distinction between the two entities difficult.[62,65]

Plantar Fasciitis

The plantar fascia is a fibrous aponeurosis that extends from the posteromedial calcaneal tuberosity to the proximal phalanx and into the skin centrally. Laterally it covers the abductor digiti quinti muscle, and medially it covers the abductor hallucis muscle.[66] Patients with plantar fasciitis present with pain in the anteromedial aspect of the calcaneus. This entity can be related to repetitive trauma or inflammatory conditions. On sagittal and coronal MR images, the normal plantar fascia can be identified as a thin hypointense structure extending anteriorly from the calcaneal tuberosity. When inflammatory changes take place, the plantar fascia becomes thickened and hyperintense on proton density-weighted and T2-weighted images.[66] Occasionally, rupture of the plantar fascia can be seen (Fig. 104-39).

BONE AND SOFT-TISSUE TUMORS

Simple bone cyst, aneurysmal bone cyst, intraosseous lipoma, giant cell tumor, enchondroma, and osteoid osteoma are among the relatively frequent benign bone tumors involving the ankle and foot.[67] Malignant bone tumors of the foot and ankle are rare, but metastasis, Ewing's sarcoma, chondrosarcoma, and osteosarcoma are occasionally seen in this region. The diagnostic approach to benign and malignant bone tumors is made radiographically, and MRI or CT is used to determine the extension of the tumor before surgery.

The detection of soft-tissue tumors is elusive with routine radiographic techniques, and MRI is used to ascertain their presence and determine their extent. In most cases, signal intensity characteristics are not specific for any type of tumor or even for discrimination between malignant or benign lesions. However, a few morphologic and signal intensity characteristics occasionally allow a more specific diagnosis in a few soft-tissue neoplasms, such as the striated pattern of hemangiomas, the hypointensity on T1- and T2-weighted pulse sequences seen in some cases of fibromatosis, or the fatty characteristics of lipoma. Relatively common soft-tissue tumors of the ankle and foot include synovial sarcoma, fibromatosis, nerve origin tumors, and lipomas (Fig. 104-40).

CONCLUSION

MRI is a powerful technique for evaluation of the normal anatomy and pathology of the ankle and foot, and clinicians involved in the treatment of patients with ankle and foot conditions are increasingly depending on this modality. The most frequent indications of MRI in this area include suspected tendon lesions, palpable masses, chronic post-traumatic ankle instability, and ankle or foot pain of unknown etiology. MRI is also gaining rapid acceptance as the modality of choice to estimate the extent of infection in patients with diabetic foot. In tendon lesions, MRI is valuable in discriminating between partial and complete tears and in assessing the

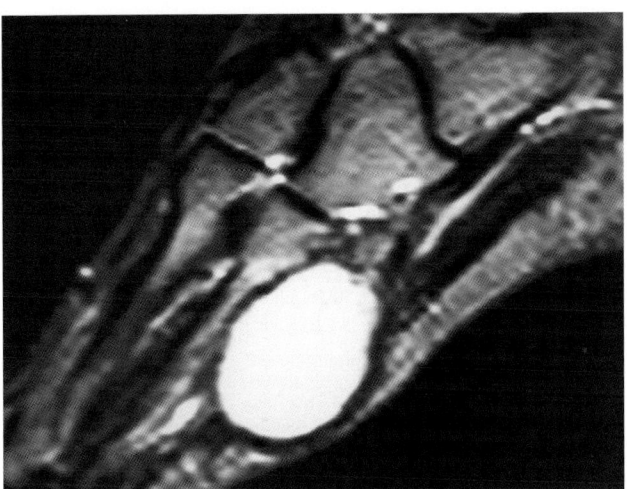

FIGURE 104-40

Synovial sarcoma. Sagittal T2-weighted image demonstrating a large soft-tissue mass in the plantar aspect of the foot. The mass is very homogeneous and exhibits a thick capsule, simulating a fluid collection.

size and location of a complete tendon rupture. In palpable masses, MRI can accurately demonstrate the size and location of the tumor and its relationship with neurovascular bundles, but only in a few circumstances can it provide sufficient data to make a tissue-specific diagnosis. In chronic ankle instability, MRI can depict ligamentous lesions, but its sensitivity and specificity have yet to be determined. Reports indicate that MR arthrography may be needed to establish the presence of a ligamentous tear. Finally, although MRI is highly sensitive, its specificity is relatively low when assessing bone and soft-tissue tumors, infection, and inflammatory joint disorders.

REFERENCES

1. Kneeland JB: Technical considerations for magnetic resonance imaging of the ankle and foot. MRI Clin North Am 2:23-28, 1994.
2. Sartoris DJ, Mitchell MJ, Resnick D: MR imaging of the ankle and foot. In Edelman RR, Hesselink JR (eds): Clinical Magnetic Resonance Imaging. Philadelphia: WB Saunders, 1990, pp1076-1096.
3. Mink JH: Tendons. In Deutch AL, Mink JH, Kerr R (eds): MRI of the Foot and Ankle. New York: Raven Press, 1993, pp135-172.
4. Mesgarzadeh M, Schneck CD, Tehranzadeh J, et al: Magnetic resonance imaging of ankle ligaments. Emphasis on anatomy and injuries to lateral collateral ligaments. MRI Clin North Am 2:39-58, 1994.
5. Listerud J, Einstein S, Outwater E, et al: First principles of fast spin echo. Magn Reson Q 2:199-224, 1992.
6. Beltran J, Munchow AM, Khabiri Hoonan K, et al: Ligaments of the lateral aspect of the ankle and sinus tarsi: an MR imaging study. Radiology 177:455-458, 1990.
7. Fullerton GD, Cameron IL, Ord VA: Orientation of tendons in the magnetic field and its effects on T2 relaxation times. Radiology 155:433-435, 1985.
8. Beltran J: The ankle and foot. In Beltran J (ed): MRI: Musculoskeletal System. Philadelphia: JB Lippincott, 1990, pp8.2-8.30.
9. Erickson SJ, Cox IH, Hyde JS, et al: Effect of tendon orientation on MR imaging SI: a manifestation of the "magic angle" phenomenon. Radiology 181:389-392, 1991.
10. Vallejo JM, Jaramillo D: Normal MR Imaging anatomy of the ankle and foot in the pediatric population. MRI Clin North Am 9:435-446, 2001.
11. Harty MP, Hubbard AM: MR Imaging of pediatric abnormalities in the ankle and foot. MRI Clin North Am 9:579-602, 2001.
12. Kirch MD, Erickson SJ: Normal magnetic resonance imaging of the ankle and foot. MRI Clin North Am 2:1-22, 1994.
13. Cheung I, Rosenberg ZS: MR Imaging of ligamentous abnormalities of the ankle and foot. MRI Clin North Am 9:507-532, 2001.
14. Schneck CD, Mesgarzadeh M, Bonakdarpour A: MR imaging of the most commonly injured ankle ligaments. Part 2. Ligament injuries. Radiology 184:507-512, 1992.
15. Klein MA, Spreitzer AM: MR imaging of the tarsal sinus and canal: normal anatomy, pathologic findings and features of the sinus tarsi syndrome. Radiology 226:169-173, 1993.
16. Beltran J, Noto AM, Mosure JC, et al: Ankle: surface coil MR imaging at 1.5 T. Radiology 161:203-209, 1986.
17. Rosenberg ZS, Cheung Y, Jahss M: Computed tomography and magnetic resonance imaging of ankle tendons: an overview. Foot Ankle 8:297-307, 1988.
18. Kneeland JB, Macrander S, Middleton WD, et al: MR imaging of the normal ankle: correlation with anatomic sections. Am J Roentgenol 151:117-123, 1988.
19. Noto AM, Cheung Y, Rosenberg ZS, et al: MR imaging of the ankle: normal variants. Radiology 170:121-124, 1989.
20. Schweitzer ME, van Leersum M, Ehrlich SS, Wapner K: Fluid in normal and abnormal ankle joints: amount and distribution as seen on MR images. Am J Roentgenol 162:111-114, 1994.
21. Williams PL, Warwick R, Dyson M, Bannister LH: Arthrology. In Williams PL, Warwick R, Dyson M, Bannister LH (eds): Gray's Anatomy of the Human Body, 37th ed. New York: Churchill Livingstone, 1989, pp485-489.
22. Erickson SJ, Rosengarten JL: MR imaging of the forefoot. Normal anatomic findings. Am J Roentgenol 169:567-571, 1993.
23. Cheung I, Rosenberg ZS: MR Imaging of the accessory muscles around the ankle. MRI Clin North Am 9:465-474, 2001.
24. Peterson DA, Stinson W, Carter J: Bilateral accessory soleus: A report of four patients with partial fasciectomy. Foot Ankle 14:284-288, 1993.
25. Wu KK: Accessory soleus muscle simulating a soft tissue tumor of the posteromedial ankle region. J Foot Surg 30:470-472, 1991.
26. Lewis O: The comparative morphology of m. flexor accessorius and the associated long flexor tendons. J Anat 96:321, 1962.
27. Nathan H, Gloobe H, Yosipovitch Z: Flexor digitorum accessorius longus. Clin Orthop 113:158-161, 1975.
28. VanCourt RB, Siessel KJ: Flexor digitorum accessorius longus muscle. J Am Podiatr Med Assoc 86:559, 1996.
29. Cheung I, Rosenberg ZS, Ramsingani R, et al: Peroneus quartus muscle: MR imaging features. Radiology 202:745, 1997.
30. Mellado JM, Rosenberg ZS, Beltran J, et al: The peroneocalcaneus internus muscle: MR imaging features. Am J Roentgenol 169:585, 1997.
31. Sarrafian S: Mycology: Anatomy of the foot and ankle, Vol 2. Philadelphia, JB Lippincott, 1993, pp218-226.
32. Finkel JE: Tarsal tunnel syndrome. MRI Clin North Am 2:67-78, 1994.
33. Kerr R, Frey C: MR imaging in tarsal tunnel syndrome. J Comput Assist Tomogr 15:280-286, 1991.
34. Chandnani VP, Harper MT, Ficke JR, et al: Chronic ankle instability: evaluation with MR arthrography. Radiology 192:189-194, 1994.
35. Cerezal L, Abascal F, Canga A, et al: MR Imaging of ankle impingement syndromes. Am J Roentgenol 181:551-559, 2003.
36. Wolin I, Glassman F, Sideman S, et al: Internal derangement of the talofibular component of the ankle. Surg Gynocol Obstet 91: 193-200, 1950.
37. Rubin DA, Tishkoff NW, Britton CA, et al: Anterolateral soft-tissue impingement in the ankle: Diagnosis using MR imaging. Am J Roentgenol 169:829-835, 1997.
38. Robinson P, White LM, Salonen DC, et al: Anterolateral ankle impingement: MR arthrographic assessment of the anterolateral recess. Radiology 221:186-190, 2001.
39. Umans H: Ankle impingement syndromes. Semin Musculoskelet Radiol 6:133-139, 2002.
40. Robinson P, White LM: Soft-tissue and osseous impingement syndromes of the ankle: role of imaging in diagnosis and management. RadioGraphics 22:1457-1469, 2002.
41. Robinson P, White LM, Salonen DC, et al: Anteromedial impingement of the ankle: using MR arthrography to assess the anteromedial recess. Am J Roentgenol 178:601-604, 2002.
42. Paterson RS, Brown JN: the posteromedial impingement lesion of the ankle: a series of six cases. Am J Sports Med 29:550-557, 2001.
43. Bureau NJ, Cardwinal E, Hobden R, et al: Posterior ankle impingement syndrome: MR imaging findings in seven patients. Radiology 215:497-503, 2000.
44. Liem MSL, Gevers Leuven JA, Bloem JL, Schipper J: Magnetic resonance imaging of Achilles tendon xanthomas in familial hypercholesterolemia. Skeletal Radiol 21:453-457, 1992.
45. Rosenberg ZS: Chronic rupture of the posterior tibial tendon. MRI Clin North Am 2:79-87, 1994.
46. Rosenberg ZS, Cheung Y, Jahss MH, et al: Rupture of posterior tibial tendon: CT and MR imaging with surgical correlation. Radiology 169:229-236, 1988.
47. Berndt AL, Harty M: Transchondral fractures (osteochondritis dissecans) of the talus. J Bone Joint Surg Am 41:988-1020, 1959.
48. De Smet AA, Fisher DR, Bernstein MI, et al: Value of MR imaging in staging osteochondral lesions of the talus (osteochondritis dissecans): results in 14 patients. Am J Roentgenol 154:555-558, 1990.

49. Mesgarzadeh M, Sapega AA, Bonakdarpour A, et al: Osteochondritis dissecans: analysis of mechanical stability with radiography, scintigraphy and MR imaging. Radiology 165:775-780, 1987.

50. Bloem JL: Transient osteoporosis of the hip: MR imaging. Radiology 167:753-757, 1988.

51. Wilson AJ, Murphy WA, Hardy DC, Totty WG: Transient osteoporosis: transient bone marrow edema? Radiology 167:757-760, 1988.

52. Delfaut E, Demondion X, Bieganski A, et al: Imaging of foot and ankle nerve entrapment syndromes: from well-demonstrated to unfamiliar sites. RadioGraphics 23:613-623, 2003.

53. Erickson SJ, Quinn SF, Kneeland JB, et al: MR imaging of the tarsal tunnel and related spaces: normal and abnormal findings with anatomic correlation. Am J Roentgenol 155:323-328, 1990.

54. Myerson M, Soffer S: Lipoma as an etiology of the tarsal tunnel syndrome: a report of two cases. Foot Ankle 10:176-179, 1990.

55. Zeiss J, Ebraheim N, Rusin J: Magnetic resonance imaging in the diagnosis of tarsal tunnel syndrome: case report. Clin Imaging 14:123-126, 1990.

56. Erickson SJ, Canale PB, Carrera GF, et al: Interdigital (Morton) neuroma: high-resolution MR imaging with a solenoid coil. Radiology 181:833-836, 1991.

57. Kursunoglu-Brahme S, Riccio T, Weisman MH, et al: Rheumatoid knee: role of gadopentetate-enhanced MR imaging. Radiology 176:831-835, 1990.

58. Bergman AG: Magnetic resonance imaging manifestations of synovial lesions of the ankle and foot. MRI Clin North Am 2:131-138, 1994.

59. Wheat J: Diagnostic strategies in osteomyelitis. Am J Med 78:218-223, 1985.

60. Seabold JE, Flickinger FW, Kao SCS, et al: Indium-111-leukocyte/technetium-99m-MDP bone and magnetic resonance imaging: difficulty of diagnosing osteomyelitis in patients with neuropathic osteoarthropathy. J Nucl Med 31:549-556, 1990.

61. Yuh WTC, Corson JD, Baraniewski HM, et al: Osteomyelitis of the foot in diabetic patients: evaluation with plain film, ^{99m}Tc-MDP bone scintigraphy, and MR imaging. Am J Roentgenol 152:759-782, 1989.

62. Beltran J, Campanini DS, Knight C, et al: The diabetic foot: magnetic resonance imaging evaluation. Skeletal Radiol 19:37-40, 1990.

63. Beltran J, McGhee RB, Schaffer PB, et al: Experimental infections of the musculoskeletal system: evaluation with MR imaging, Tc-99m MDP, and Ga-67 scintigraphy. Radiology 167:167-172, 1988.

64. Beltran J, Noto AM, McGhee RB, et al: Infections of the musculoskeletal system: high-field-strength MR imaging. Radiology 164:449-454, 1987.

65. Erdman WA, Tamburro F, Jayson HT, et al: Osteomyelitis: characteristics and pitfalls of diagnosis with MR imaging. Radiology 180:533-539, 1991.

66. Kier R: Magnetic resonance imaging of plantar fasciitis and other causes of heel pain. MRI Clin North Am 2:97-108, 1994.

67. Shankman S, Cisa J, Present D: Tumors of the ankle and foot. MRI Clin North Am 2:139-154, 1994.

105

TEMPOROMANDIBULAR JOINT

Steven M. Cohen ● Gregory Eckel

ANATOMY

The temporomandibular joint (TMJ) is a synovial, diarthroidal joint formed by the articulation of the mandibular condyle and the articular fossa of the temporal bone (Fig. 105-1). Although generally thought of as a "hinge" joint, the loose fibrous capsule of the TMJ allows for lateral movement, mandibular protrusion, and rotation. These are essential movements for mastication, as well as simple opening and closing of the mouth.

The TMJ, unlike most other joints, is lined by fibrocartilidge, rather than hyaline cartilage.[1] The articular disc (meniscus) divides it into superior and inferior compartments, which do not communicate. The inferior compartment is further subdivided into an anterior and a posterior recess by the mandibular condyle. The meniscus is a fibrocartilage bow-tie–shaped structure. The thick posterior portion is called the posterior band and is separated by a thin intermediate zone from the anterior band. The meniscus is anchored posteriorly by the bilaminar zone. Consisting of collagen, elastin, and fat, the bilaminar zone is composed of two segments: a posterior superior ligament attaching to the temporal bone just above the glenoid fossa; and a posterior inferior ligament, which attaches to the posterior subcondylar area. Tearing of the former structure facilitates meniscal displacement.[2] Anteriorly, the meniscus attaches to the inferior head of the lateral pterygoid muscle, one of the four muscles of mastication. The other three muscles of mastication, the medial pterygoid, masseter, and temporalis muscles, do not directly attach to the TMJ. The lateral pterygoid muscle is responsible for opening of the mouth. It consists of a superior and an inferior head. The superior head attaches separately from the meniscus with fibers blending into the anterior TMJ capsule. The inferior head, which attaches directly to the meniscus, is responsible for

anterior translation of both the mandibular condyle and the meniscus during opening of the mouth.

When the mouth is closed, the meniscus is located in the anterior aspect of the articular fossa (Fig. 105-2), with the posterior band near the apex and the intermediate zone and anterior band resting along the anterior margin of the fossa. The mandibular condyle rests directly below the posterior zone at the 12 o'clock position.[3] On opening the mouth, there is progressive anterior translation of the meniscus and condyle, controlled by the lateral pterygoid muscle. When the mouth is fully open, the mandibular condyle comes to rest beneath the intermediate zone of the meniscus, which, in turn, is at a relative 12 o'clock position to the articular eminence.

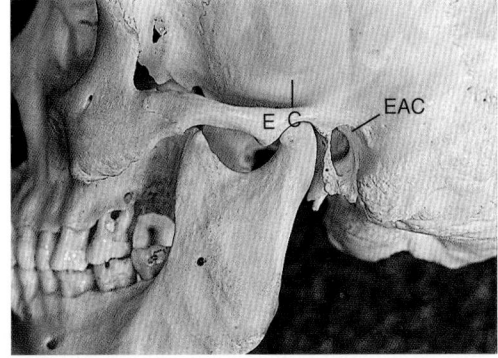

FIGURE 105-1

Bony landmarks of the temporomandibular joint. The condyle (C) rests on the condylar fossa (F). The fossa is bounded anteriorly by the temporal eminence (E) and posteriorly by the external auditory canal (EAC). *(Reproduced with permission from Harms SE: The temporomandibular joint. In Stark DD, Bradley WG JR (eds): Magnetic Resonance Imaging, 3rd ed. St Louis, Mosby, 1999, pp 673-690.)*

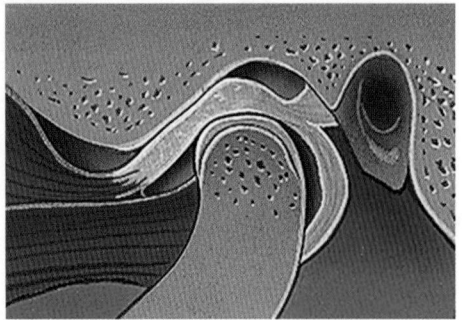

FIGURE 105-2

Normal temporomandibular motion. The posterior band of the disk is seen to move toward the apex of the condyle (12 o'clock) in the resting position. With mouth opening, the disk and condyle translate anteriorly. The intermediate zone is the weight-bearing portion of the disk for most of the normal functional cycle. *(Reproduced with permission from Harms SE: The temporomandibular joint. In Stark DD, Bradley WG JR (eds): Magnetic Resonance Imaging, 3rd ed. St Louis, Mosby, 1999, pp 673-690.)*

IMAGING METHODS

Plain Radiographs

Plain radiographs are of limited value in evaluating TMJ pathology, primarily due to overlying bone obscuring visualization of the joint. On proper patient positioning however, the joints can be visualized and gross displacements and fractures demonstrated. Most radiographic examinations of the TMJ include anteroposterior, lateral, oblique, open mouth, oblique closed-mouth, and Towne views.

Tomography

Plain tomography has an advantage over plain radiographic examination as it blurs overlying structures, allowing for better visualization of the joint. Soft-tissues, however, are not visualized, limiting the role of this method in evaluating TMJ disorders.

Arthrography

Formerly a widely used procedure, this method of TMJ assessment is seldom performed today as MRI is superior to arthrography for most TMJ pathology, with the exception of joint capsule adhesions and small perforations of the meniscus.[4] Arthrography is performed using a 27-gauge needle to inject iodinated contrast into the joint space, the lower joint compartment being opacified first under fluoroscopy to identify meniscal perforations. There is normally no communication between the superior and inferior compartments of the joint. Demonstration of contrast material in the superior compartment after inferior compartment injection is indicative of meniscal perforation. False-positive results are possible if the initial injection inadvertently punctures the lateral recess of the superior compartment, creating an iatrogenic communication.[4] After evaluating for perforations, the superior compartment is opacified to identify the meniscal surfaces and to evaluate for loose bodies and adhesions. Capsular adhesions appear as small filling defects within the opacified joint space. Other factors discouraging the use of arthrography of the TMJ are its invasiveness, morbidity related to contrast injection, and level of expertise required for proper TMJ injection.

Computed Tomography

CT has a very limited role in the evaluation of TMJ pathology. It is excellent for demonstrating bone detail and may be useful for evaluating trauma and arthritis. However, lack of soft-tissue detail makes CT of little value as a diagnostic procedure for most TMJ disorders. In addition, joint motion is difficult to evaluate by CT.[5]

Magnetic Resonance Imaging

MRI has replaced arthrography and tomography as the imaging modality of choice in the evaluation of TMJ pathology. MRI, with its superior soft-tissue contrast resolution, provides excellent detail of the components of the TMJ, including detailed anatomy and position of the meniscus, the marrow of surrounding osseous structures, the articular cartilage, and the musculature. Joint motion can be assessed using fast scanning techniques. Satisfactory MRI images of the TMJ can be obtained in most patients, except in the presence of nonremovable metallic dental work and severe claustrophobia.

MRI IMAGING PROTOCOL

Imaging of the TMJ is best performed using a high field strength MRI scanner, generally 1.5 T, and a small surface coil placed over the area of interest should be used to maximize the signal-to-noise ratio (SNR). Dedicated TMJ coils cover both joints, allowing bilateral imaging.[6] Using a 12 cm field of view and 256×256 matrix, and one or two excitations (NEX), 3 mm images are generally obtained. Thinner images can be obtained but then decreased SNR degrades image quality. Axial localizer images using fast scanning technique (gradient-echo imaging) allow accurate localization of subsequent diagnostic images. Sagittal oblique images with the mouth closed are obtained parallel to the axis of the TMJ using T1 weighting with a repetition time (TR) of 600 ms and a time to echo (TE) of 20 ms. T2-weighted images are then obtained using a fast spin-echo technique to help identify joint effusions (Fig. 105-3). Closed-mouth T1-weighted coronal oblique images are obtained to evaluate medial or lateral meniscal displacement, which is not well seen in the sagittal plane.[7] Open-mouth sagittal oblique images are then obtained to assess the extent of meniscal and condylar anterior translation.

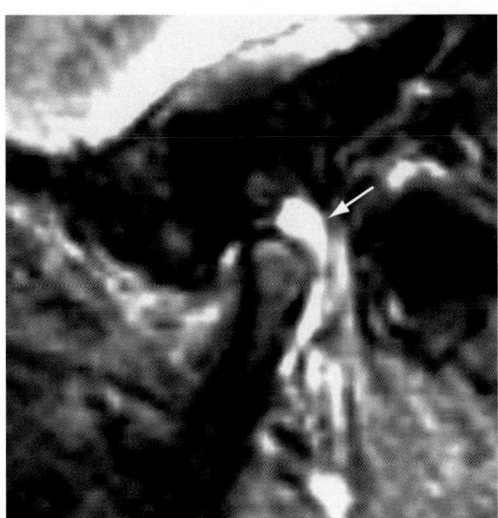

FIGURE 105-3

T2-weighted sagittal oblique closed-mouth image shows high signal intensity distending the joint capsule, consistent with a temporomandibular effusion (*arrow*).

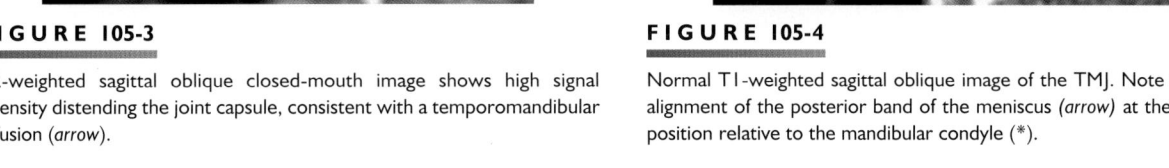

FIGURE 105-4

Normal T1-weighted sagittal oblique image of the TMJ. Note the normal alignment of the posterior band of the meniscus (*arrow*) at the 12 o'clock position relative to the mandibular condyle (*).

An aid such as a Burnett mouth-positioning device should be used to help prevent patient movement during the open-mouth portion of the examination.

Kinematic imaging of the TMJ can also be performed. Gradient-echo three-dimensional (3D) Fourier transformation imaging is used. A series of sagittal oblique images are obtained during progressive points of opening of the mouth. A Burnett device is used to assist in maintaining the mouth position for each acquisition. The images obtained can be viewed as a series demonstrating the anterior translation of the meniscus and the condyle, as well as "recapture" of the meniscus.[7]

NORMAL ANATOMY ON MRI

Using MRI, the TMJ is evaluated in the sagittal plane in both the open- and closed-mouth position, as well as coronal images (Fig. 105-4). The bony components of the TMJ include the condyle of the mandible, articular fossa, and articular eminence. The bone marrow of these structures is predominantly fatty, resulting in high signal intensity on T1- and T2-weighted images. The surrounding cortical bone demonstrates low signal on all sequences. The synovium of the joint is intermediate in signal on both T1- and T2-weighted images and is 1 to 2 mm in thickness.

The bow-tie–shaped meniscus is best evaluated on sagittal images. It is composed of collagen, elastin, and glycosaminoglycans.[1] As a result, the normal meniscus demonstrates low signal intensity on both T1- and T2-weighted images. Normally, in the closed-mouth position, the meniscus should be positioned slightly anterior within the articular fossa, with the thick, posterior band located approximately at the 12 o'clock

position in relation to the mandibular condyle. When making this determination, it is important to identify the junction of the posterior band of the meniscus and the bilaminar zone, which anchors the meniscus to the temporal bone. The junction is seen as a vertically oriented band of intermediate signal intensity. If this point is within 10 degrees of vertical, the meniscal position is considered normal in the sagittal plane (Fig. 105-4).[8] Identification of the transition point helps avoid the pitfall of confusing the low-signal bilaminar zone with the posterior band. This type of error could result in a false-negative interpretation in patients with mild anterior displacement of the meniscus.[8] In the open-mouth position, there is anterior translation of the mandibular condyle and the meniscus. The articular eminence, thin intermediate zone of the meniscus, and mandibular condyle should be in vertical alignment with the mouth fully opened.

Coronal images are useful to confirm the normal medial and lateral margins of the meniscus. The central axis of the meniscus should be in vertical alignment with the medial and lateral margins of the condyle. Extension of the margin of the meniscus beyond the medial or lateral margins is consistent with meniscal displacement.[7]

INTERNAL DERANGEMENTS

Clinically, internal derangement of the TMJ is associated with focal pain, a limited range of motion of the TMJ, and a "click" during opening and/or closing of the mouth. The most common form of internal derangement of the TMJ is displacement of the meniscus. Meniscal displacement is often the result of laxity of the supporting

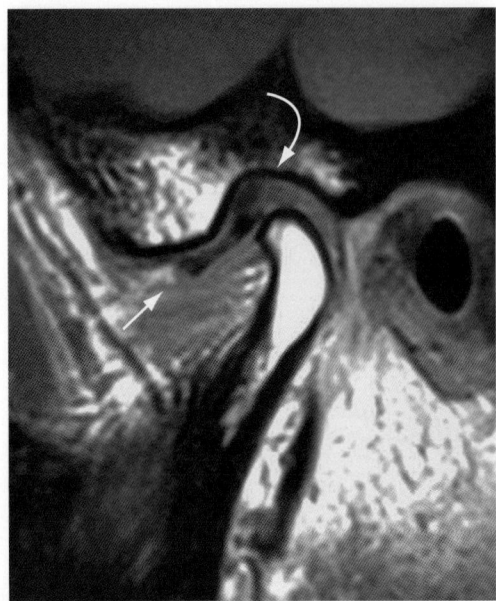

FIGURE 105-5

T1-weighted, sagittal oblique closed-mouth image shows anterior displacement of the TMJ meniscus (*arrow*). Note the slight anterior position of the bilaminar zone (*curved arrow*) relative to the 12 o'clock position.

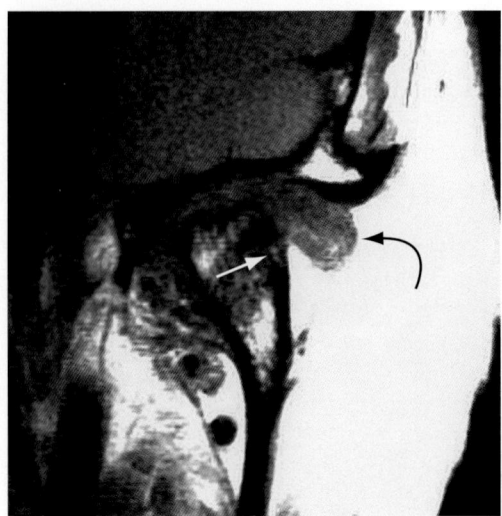

FIGURE 105-6

T1-weighted coronal image demonstrates lateral meniscal displacement. The lateral edge of the meniscus (*arrow*) protrudes far beyond the lateral cortical margin of the mandibular condyle (*curved arrow*).

attachments from degeneration or trauma. The position of the posterior band is used to define the location and degree of disk displacement (Fig. 105-5). Meniscal displacement is most common in the anteromedial direction[9]; however, displacements can be partial or complete and may be lateral (Fig. 105-6) or posterior (rarely), as well as anteromedial. The meniscus may retain its normal configuration or become deformed due to repetitive microtrauma during opening and closing of the mouth (Fig. 105-7). Abnormal meniscal displacement increases loading, which can result in complete disruption of the posterior attachments, leading to worsening meniscal degeneration, increased signal abnormalities, and deformity. Helms et al[10] proposed a grading system for characterizing meniscal displacements by morphology. Normal morphology and position of the meniscus is defined as grade 0. In a grade 1 meniscal displacement, the meniscus is no longer located in its normal position, as defined by the position of the posterior band relative to the articular fossa of the TMJ but the morphology of the disc remains normal. A grade 2 displacement shows as abnormal disc position and morphology, commonly associated with degenerative change of the entire TMJ (Fig. 105-8).

Other types of internal derangements of the TMJ include "stuck" or adherent disc, meniscal perforation, and degenerative disease. A stuck disc is fixed in its position relative to the articular eminence and the articular fossa, and does not demonstrate normal anterior translation with opening of the mouth.[11] Stuck discs result from intra-articular adhesions and manifest as clinical TMJ dysfunction with limitation of the range of motion of the TMJ and limited anterior translation of the mandibular condyle. According to Rao et al[11] the meniscus may be fixed in a normal or displaced position.

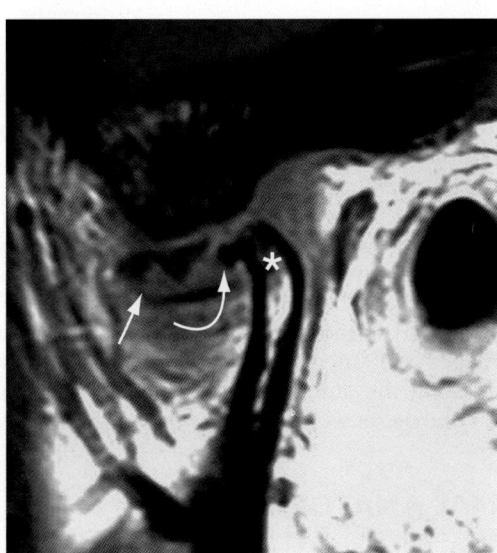

FIGURE 105-7

Severe anterior displacement of the temporomandibular meniscus. T1-weighted sagittal oblique open-mouth image demonstrates severe displacement of the meniscus (*arrow*), which contains slightly increased signal intensity and deformity. Additionally, there is restricted anterior translation of the mandibular condyle (*) by the displaced disc, giving the patient a sensation of "locking" of the joint. The degree of displacement and the morphologic changes of the meniscus is consistent with grade 2 displacement. Also note the flattening of the condyle and the small anterior osteophyte (*curved arrow*), consistent with osteoarthritis.

Disc perforations are difficult to identify on MRI images and are more easily seen by arthrography as communication of the superior and inferior compartments of the TMJ during arthrographic injection. However, false-positive rates of up to 20% have been reported. False positives result from inadvertent

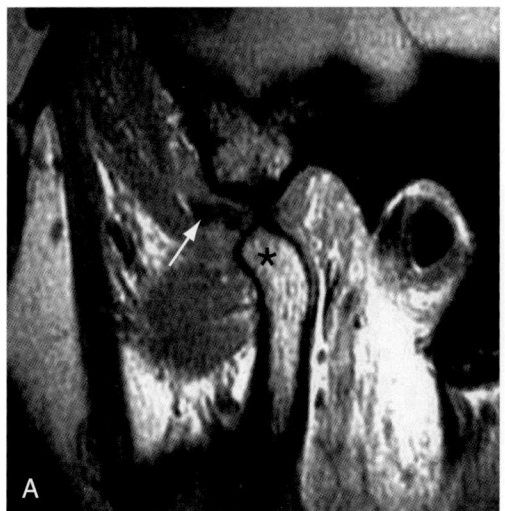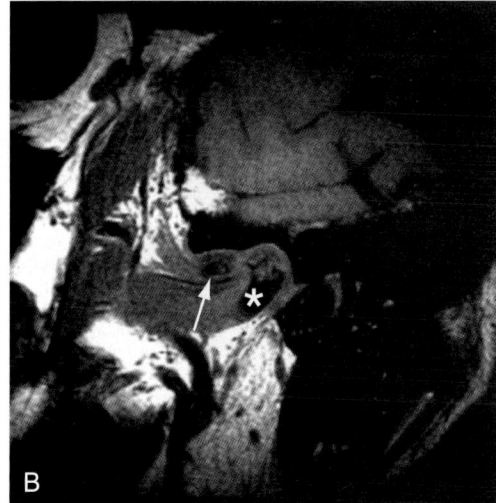

FIGURE 105-8

Anterior displacement of the temporomandibular (TMJ) meniscus. **A,** T1-weighted open-mouth image demonstrates grade 2 displacement of the TMJ meniscus (*arrow*). Note the position of the meniscus, as well as the loss of the normal bow-tie configuration. Anterior translation of the condyle (*) is normal. **B,** T1-weighted closed-mouth image of a different patient shows more severe, chronic, grade 2 anterior meniscal displacement. The position of the meniscus (*arrow*) is abnormal and it is severely deformed, with markedly increased internal signal intensity. Deformity of the condyle (*) is noted as well, consistent with degenerative osteoarthritis.

puncture of both joint compartments during the procedure, creating an iatrogenic, temporary communication.[4] Although perforations are often not seen on MRI, they are usually associated with abnormal disc motion or displacement, which is well demonstrated.

Degenerative changes of the TMJ manifest similar to changes related to osteoarthritis in other joints (Fig. 105-9). Flattening and deformity of the mandibular condyle may occur, as well as deformity of the articular fossa. Normal fatty marrow signal may be replaced by decreased signal on T1- and T2-weighted images, indicating subchondral sclerosis. Increased subchondral signal may be seen on STIR and fat-saturated T2-weighted images, indicating edema or inflammation of the affected joint. In advanced cases, ankylosis of the joint, or subluxation with pseudarthrosis can occur.

TRAUMA

Trauma to the mandible may result in intra- or extracapsular fracture. Intracapsular fractures are far more likely to affect the TMJ, though extracapsular fractures may also result in internal derangement of the TMJ via transmitted forces to the joint. Intracapsular fractures are more likely to result in long-term osteoarthritis or avascular necrosis of the condyle, causing TMJ dysfunction. Extracapsular fractures may lead to meniscal displacement, though this can occur in direct trauma to the mandible without fracture. Whiplash-type injuries may also be associated with an increased risk of disc displacement, though this point is controversial.[2,12]

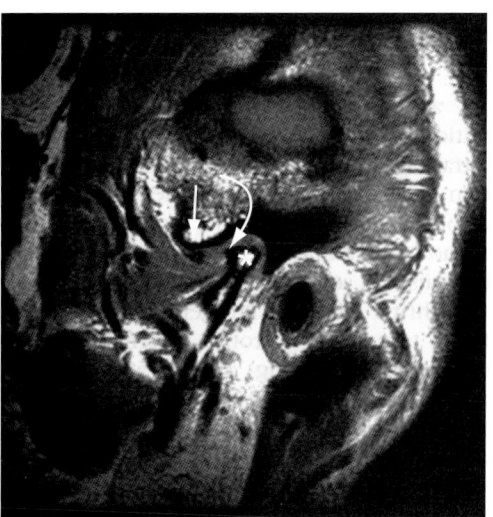

FIGURE 105-9

Secondary osteoarthritis of the temporomandibular joint (TMJ). The TMJ meniscus (*arrow*) is anteriorly displaced. The mandibular condyle (*) is flattened superiorly, with subchondral marrow signal loss, consistent with sclerosis, and anterior osteophyte formation (*curved arrow*).

ARTHRITIS

Patients with rheumatoid arthritis may have TMJ involvement (Fig. 105-10). Rheumatoid arthritis of the TMJ is similar to its involvement in other joints, including synovial proliferation, cortical osseous erosions, joint

106

Muscle

Robert D. Boutin ● Mini N. Pathria

Muscular activity is the visible manifestation of being alive. Indeed, life's essential activities are expressed through muscular activity, including respiration, speech, eating, digestion, and, of course, mobility.[1] This chapter focuses on striated muscle that is specialized for repeated contraction under voluntary control: skeletal muscle.

Although skeletal muscle was once a subject for anatomists only, MRI has become the most sophisticated tool for the noninvasive study of anatomy and pathology. After reviewing imaging techniques and fundamental anatomic considerations, this chapter focuses on the most important abnormalities evaluated by MRI, including neuromuscular diseases; metabolic myopathies; infectious, inflammatory, and idiopathic acquired myopathies; muscle ischemia and necrosis; traumatic muscle injuries; and muscle denervation.

OVERVIEW OF TECHNIQUES FOR IMAGING MUSCLE

MRI facilitates the diagnostic process by detecting alterations in muscle size, shape, or signal intensity. Commonly accepted advantages of MRI include excellent soft-tissue contrast resolution, multiplanar tomographic image display, and the lack of ionizing radiation. In some cases other imaging techniques (particularly radiography, CT, sonography, and scintigraphy) may play complementary roles in achieving the correct diagnosis.

Radiography is a relatively inexpensive means of screening patients for abnormal radiodensity in muscle (e.g., a phlebolith, heterotopic ossification). CT provides for cross-sectional assessment of abnormalities like those detected by radiography (e.g., characterization of mineralized matrix). Potential disadvantages of CT include radiation exposure and limited contrast resolution for examining muscle (which may result in a need for intravenous iodinated contrast material).

Sonography allows dynamic examination of musculotendinous structures, differentiation between cystic and solid lesions, and interrogation of soft-tissue vascularity.[2] However, sonography is regarded as an operator-dependent technique that commonly has substantial limitations in field of view, contrast resolution, and soft-tissue penetration.

Scintigraphy has been used in an effort to diagnose various muscle derangements. However, soft-tissue uptake of a radiopharmaceutical such as technetium-99m methylene diphosphonate is nonspecific, and may be seen with neoplastic, inflammatory, ischemic, traumatic (e.g., heterotopic ossification), or metabolic (e.g., hyperparathyroidism) abnormalities.[3]

TECHNICAL CONSIDERATIONS FOR MRI

Routine Clinical "Screening" MRI Protocol

MRI protocols used to assess muscle disorders vary considerably, depending on factors such as the available MR equipment, clinical context, and goal of the examination. Routine clinical assessment of muscle disorders commonly utilizes a combination of pulse sequences in both long- (sagittal or coronal) and short-axis (axial) planes. For example, a routine "screening" clinical examination might include five pulse sequences: long-axis T1-weighted and fast spin-echo (FSE) short-tau inversion recovery (STIR) images, as well as axial T1-weighted, FSE T2-weighted, and FSE fat-suppressed T2-weighted images.

Long-axis images (parallel to long bones) are prescribed with a field of view sufficient to display the proximal-to-distal extent of a muscle disorder. Sagittal images are particularly advantageous for showing anterior and posterior muscle abnormalities, while simultaneously showing the adjacent bone for anatomic reference. Similarly, coronal images are especially helpful for evaluating abnormalities at the medial and lateral derangements. Axial images enable cross-sectional evaluation of individual muscles, compartments, and neurovascular structures.

T1-weighted images tend to have a favorable acquisition time and signal-to-noise ratio, while aiding in specific characterization of certain abnormalities. Muscle derangements associated with high T1 signal intensity commonly contain methemoglobin (e.g., hematoma, hemorrhagic neoplasm), abnormal accumulations of fat (e.g., lipomatous tumor, muscle atrophy, mature heterotopic ossification), proteinaceous material (e.g., proteinaceous debris in a necrotic neoplasm),[4] or certain paramagnetic materials (e.g., melanin in a metastatic melanoma,[5,6] enhancement with gadolinium-based contrast material).

T2-weighted images are considered "fluid sensitive." The differential diagnosis for high T2 signal intensity in muscle includes: muscular exertion; direct or indirect trauma; inflammation; infection; subacute denervation; infiltrative neoplasm; ischemia; and myonecrosis. The differential diagnosis for low T2 signal intensity in muscle includes calcification, foreign bodies, gas, and hemosiderin. Compared to conventional spin-echo techniques, it is commonly recognized that images acquired with a FSE technique tend to result in shortened image acquisition time, decreased motion artifact, diminished metallic susceptibility artifact at postoperative sites, and increased patient throughput.

Fat-suppressed T2-weighted and *IR-FSE* images are exquisitely sensitive to the presence of fluid, edema, the most common stages of hemorrhage, and most neoplasms (Fig. 106-1). However, compared to T2-weighted images, the altered dynamic range on fat-suppressed T2 and IR-FSE images may make specific diagnosis of soft-tissue masses more difficult.[7] Potential disadvantages of the frequency-selective fat-suppression method can include sensitivity to magnetic field nonuniformity,[8] unreliability of low-field scanners,[8] misregistration artifacts,[8] and a relatively low signal-to-noise ratio.[9] The IR-FSE technique allows for relatively reliable and uniform fat suppression. However, the suppression of signal is not entirely specific with an IR-FSE technique (e.g., may be seen in some subacute hematomas).[8]

Supplemental Clinical Pulse Sequences

In addition to the routine "screening" pulse sequences, supplemental or "trouble shooting" scanning techniques may prove helpful, including gradient-echo imaging and gadolinium enhancement. For example, T2*-weighted gradient-echo sequences can be used to intentionally accentuate certain paramagnetic effects. This "blooming" effect may call attention to the presence of hemosiderin,

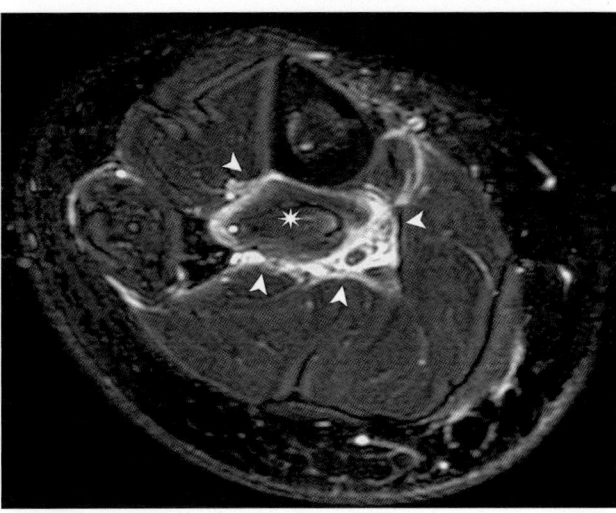

FIGURE 106-1

Axial T2-weighted fat-suppressed fast spin-echo MR image through the calf shows increased signal intensity within the tibialis posterior muscle (*) consistent with a muscle strain. High signal intensity fluid is seen along the fascial planes surrounding the muscle (*arrowheads*).

gas, metallic foreign bodies, or prior surgery, and thus help in honing a differential diagnosis. Alternatively, fast gradient-echo images can be used to provide high temporal resolution for assessing anatomic and pathologic changes in muscle (Fig. 106-2). For example, muscle contraction during the MR examination may demonstrate retraction of a torn muscle, herniation of a muscle through a fascial defect, or nerve entrapment that may occur dynamically during muscle activation (e.g., tarsal tunnel syndrome caused by a hypertrophied accessory soleus muscle).[10]

Gadolinium-based contrast material does not add substantial diagnostic information in the detection of most muscle disorders, but may prove helpful under several circumstances. Major indications for gadolinium-based contrast material include:

1. Characterization of certain mass lesions (e.g., differentiation of solid lesions versus lesions that are cystic or necrotic);
2. Assessment of soft-tissue for areas of necrosis (e.g., gangrene, diabetic myonecrosis);
3. Identifying optimal biopsy sites (e.g., active areas of inflammation, non-necrotic areas of tumor);
4. Evaluating the operative bed for recurrence after sarcoma resection (Fig. 106-3).

Experimental Techniques

Dynamic and functional MR techniques are promising additions to the usual static MR examination of muscle.[11] Dynamic techniques now allow realtime imaging at several frames per second and may prove useful in both biomechanical and clinical analysis of muscle contraction in vivo.[12] Combination of realtime techniques

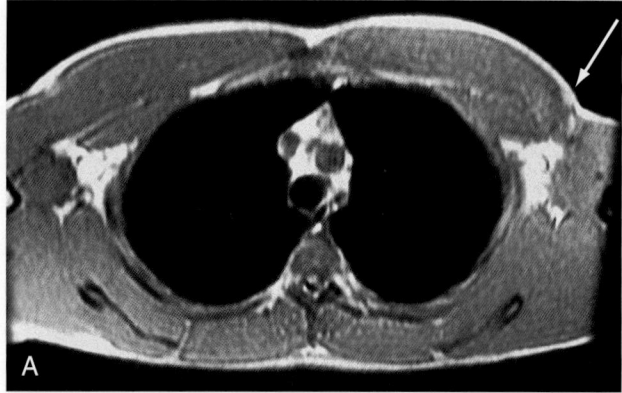

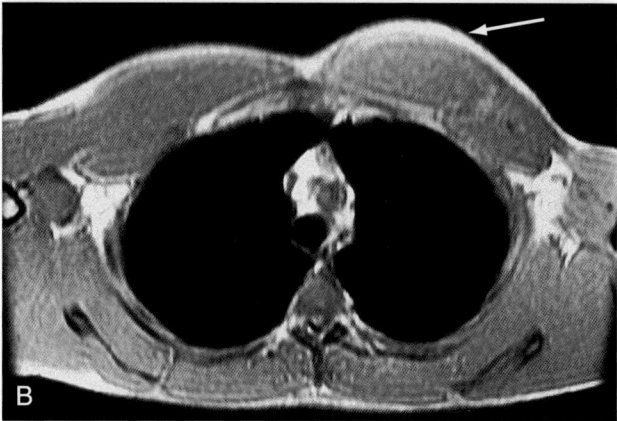

FIGURE 106-2

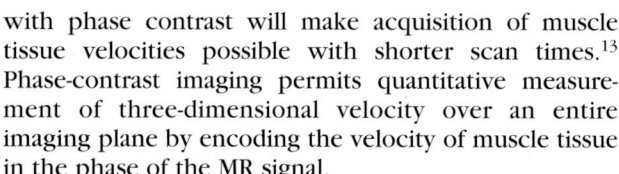

A, Resting axial gradient-recalled echo (GRE) MR image obtained in a patient with a known pectoralis tendon tear adjacent to the left humerus at rest shows mild asymmetry of the pectoralis major muscles, with apparent discontinuity of the left pectoralis major muscle at the axillary line (*arrow*). **B,** Axial GRE MR image obtained in the same patient with sustained maximal contraction of the injured muscle shows a prominent bulge in the medial aspect of the left pectoralis major muscle (*arrow*).

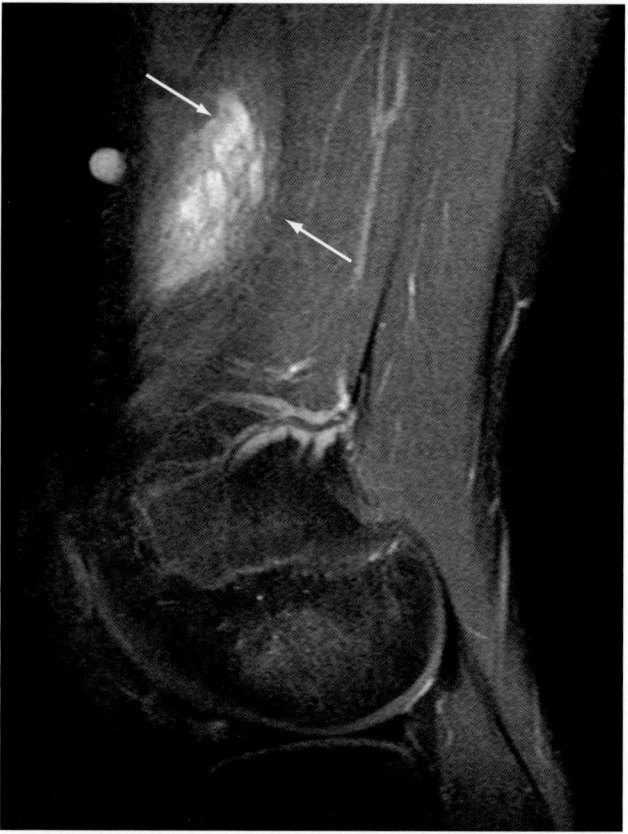

FIGURE 106-3

Sagittal T1-weighted fat-suppressed image of the knee acquired after intravenous administration of a gadolinium-based contrast material shows a high signal intensity skin surface marker indicating the location of a palpable mass. The use of contrast helps to characterize the enhancing, tubular nature (*arrows*) of this soft-tissue hemangioma.

with phase contrast will make acquisition of muscle tissue velocities possible with shorter scan times.[13] Phase-contrast imaging permits quantitative measurement of three-dimensional velocity over an entire imaging plane by encoding the velocity of muscle tissue in the phase of the MR signal.

Functional information on muscle can be provided with techniques such as blood-oxygenation-level-dependent (BOLD) imaging and T2 mapping. BOLD imaging produces MRI contrast from changes in the microvascular ratio of oxyhemoglobin (a diamagnetic substance) to deoxyhemoglobin (a paramagnetic substance). BOLD contrast results from focal increase in oxygenated blood from maneuvers such as exercise, oxygen administration, or certain medications (e.g., vasodilators) that are visible with T2*-weighted functional scans.[14] Evaluation of the microcirculation of normal and diseased skeletal muscle may provide insights into such diverse topics as muscle fiber composition in athletes, vascular insufficiency, tumor oxygenation, and even oxygen-limited thermal tolerance in Antarctic fish.[15]

T2 mapping refers to the transient activity-induced increase in T2 signal intensity that occurs after as few as two contractions and normally resolves within 30 minutes.[16] This technique literally "maps" the spatial patterns of muscle recruitment and the intensity of muscle activation immediately after exercise. The signal intensity changes are most strongly related to exercise intensity when intensity is quantified as peak force, power (force × rate), or rate of energy use. Increased T2 signal is thought to result from osmotically driven shifts of muscle water that increase the volume of the intracellular space and from metabolic endproducts that cause postexercise intracellular acidosis.[16] This MRI technique is considered complementary to electromyography (EMG). Surface EMG detects electrical activity (rather than metabolic activity) in muscle and is biased by activity in muscles located superficially.[17]

T2 mapping techniques can be used experimentally to study in vivo the muscle activation patterns associated with optimal sports performance, overuse injuries, metabolic myopathies (e.g., McArdle's disease), and various treatment interventions (e.g., physical therapy programs).[18,19] For example, after completion of a training program, MRI demonstrates that individuals performing a given exercise use less muscle volume,[20] and that the exercise-induced T2 hyperintensity in muscle is reduced.[21] In patients with peripheral vascular disease, alterations in T2 relaxation time in muscle correlate well with clinical findings of intermittent claudication and with successful treatment using bypass surgery or percutaneous angioplasty.[22]

NORMAL ANATOMY

Microscopic Anatomy

The basic structural element of skeletal muscle is the muscle fiber. A single pixel on a standard MR image includes approximately 100 muscle fibers.[16] The architecture of the fibers in any particular muscle is directly related to the muscle's function. For example, the maximal force that can be produced by a muscle is proportional to the physiologic cross-sectional area of that muscle. On the other hand, the speed and amount of shortening in any given muscle is proportional to the length of its fibers. When studying skeletal muscle biomechanics with ciné phase-contrast MRI, it is generally assumed that the maximum velocity of muscle tissue is at the myotendinous junction closest to the joint that is moving, whereas the tendon is relatively inextensible.[13]

Muscle contraction is explained by the "sliding filament model," which describes the interactions between the thin filaments of the protein actin and the thick filaments of the protein myosin. Mechanical force is generated when the energy source adenosine triphosphate (ATP) fuels movement of the myosin relative to actin.

Muscle fibers in a single motor unit have the same contractile and metabolic properties. Two general types of motor units are recognized. Type I (slow twitch) fibers are relatively slow to contract and relax, but are relatively fatigue resistant. Type II (fast twitch) fibers have the fastest contraction time, but are the least resistant to fatigue. Motor unit loss is considered the hallmark of aging and several neuromuscular disorders (e.g., post-polio syndrome).[16]

A typical motor neuron in the lower extremity innervates approximately 400 muscle fibers which are heterogeneously distributed in a muscle. Thus, with routine clinical MRI, the single motor unit territory is spread over several dozen pixels and cannot be adequately resolved in isolation. However, advances in MRI spatial and contrast resolution may improve the ability to resolve motor unit activation patterns in normal and pathologic states.[16]

Compartmental Anatomy

Compartments are distinct domains bordered by tissues (e.g., fascia, cortical bone) that act to constrain the spread of pathologic processes (e.g., infection, neoplasm). Given that there are hundreds of muscles in the body, the easiest way to conceptualize the location and function of muscles is to become familiar with compartmental anatomy. For example, in the mid thigh, three compartments are present: anterior (quadriceps and sartorius); posterior (hamstrings); and medial (adductors and gracilis). Four compartments are present in the leg: anterior; lateral; superficial posterior; and deep posterior. Knowledge of such compartmental anatomy is of particular importance in the proper staging, biopsy, and treatment of musculoskeletal neoplasms.

NORMAL VARIATIONS IN MUSCLES

Normal anatomic variations in muscle are commonplace.[1] For example, in one study examining the volar aspect of 42 normal wrists,[23] MRI demonstrated a total of 23 muscle variations. The multitudinous anomalies in muscle may be divided conceptually into seven fundamental types.[24] A muscle may be:

1. Absent;
2. Doubled;
3. Divided into two or more parts;
4. Deviant in its course;
5. Joined to a neighboring muscle;
6. Altered in size or shape (e.g., the distribution of the fleshy and tendinous portions); or
7. A completely new, "extra" muscle.

Muscle variations usually are of no clinical significance *per se,* but can become clinically important.[25] Just as with other muscles, anomalous muscles may be affected by various derangements (e.g., strain injury) and their particular anatomy may have surgical implications. Furthermore, anomalous muscles can be mistaken for neoplasms or torn, retracted muscles. Finally, anomalous muscles may result in neurovascular entrapment, particularly when such a muscle is hypertrophied.[1,26]

Anomalous muscles and consequent compressive neuropathy are particularly common about the wrist and ankle regions, and may be underdiagnosed with MRI in daily practice (Fig. 106-4). For example, in a report of four patients with an anomalous palmaris longus muscle causing effort-related median nerve compression,[27] the diagnosis was missed during initial interpretation of each MRI examination.

MRI facilitates the diagnosis of an anomalous muscle by demonstrating its characteristic morphology, origin, insertion, and course relative to adjacent anatomic structures. When undisturbed by trauma or other insults, an anomalous muscle has the same signal intensity as neighboring skeletal muscles. Two of the most studied muscle variations seen on MRI are found in the popliteal fossa and the pre-Achilles fat pad regions.

Popliteal Artery Entrapment

In the popliteal fossa, compression of the popliteal artery can result from an anomalous anatomic relationship between the popliteal artery and its neighboring muscles. Popliteal artery entrapment typically presents as progressive intermittent leg claudication in active

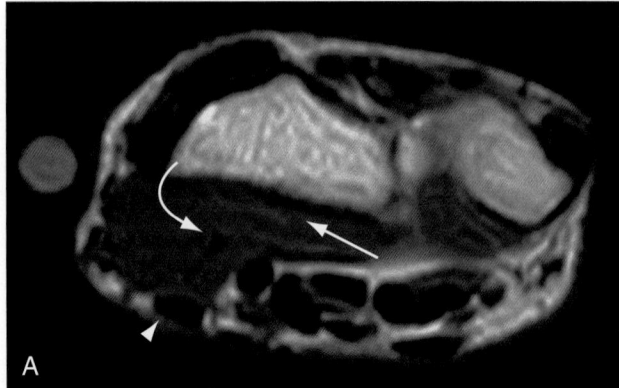

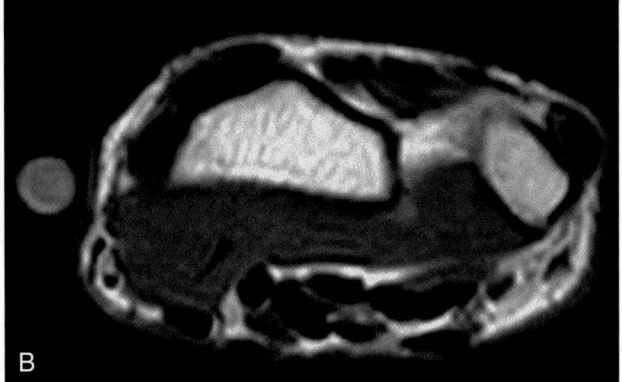

FIGURE 106-4

Sequential **A,** distal and **B,** proximal axial T1-weighted MR images through the wrist show a skin marker indicating the region of a palpable mass on physical examination. The MR images reveal that the mass is located between the pronator quadratus (*arrow*) and the flexor carpi radialis tendon (*arrowhead*) and shows both signal intensity and architecture consistent with muscle. The presence of a centrally located tendon (*curved arrow*) further supports the diagnosis of anomalous musculature about the wrist.

young adults with anomalous, hypertrophied popliteal musculature. The pathogenesis of this condition is thought to relate to repeated arterial microtrauma caused by muscle compression during exercise that eventually may result in stenosis, post-stenotic aneurysm, and thrombosis.

Several different muscle variations can cause neurovascular entrapment in the popliteal fossa. For example, in one series of 31 cases,[28] 10 different anatomic variants were observed in the popliteal fossa. Most commonly, a third head of the gastrocnemius is cited as the cause of neurovascular entrapment. (A third head of the gastrocnemius arises from the popliteal surface of the femur in approximately 3% to 5% of individuals.[1]) Variations in the popliteus and plantaris muscles also may cause popliteal artery compression.[29-32]

MRI can be used to diagnose the presence of arterial stenosis and to identify the anatomic structure compressing the popliteal artery (Fig. 106-5). MR arteriography allows direct visualization of the popliteal artery (e.g., for thrombus and post-stenotic aneurysm). Treatment may include thromboendarterectomy, operative

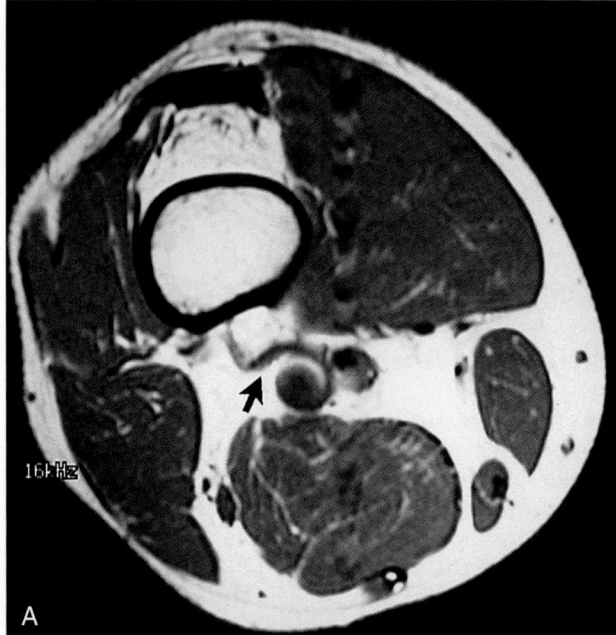

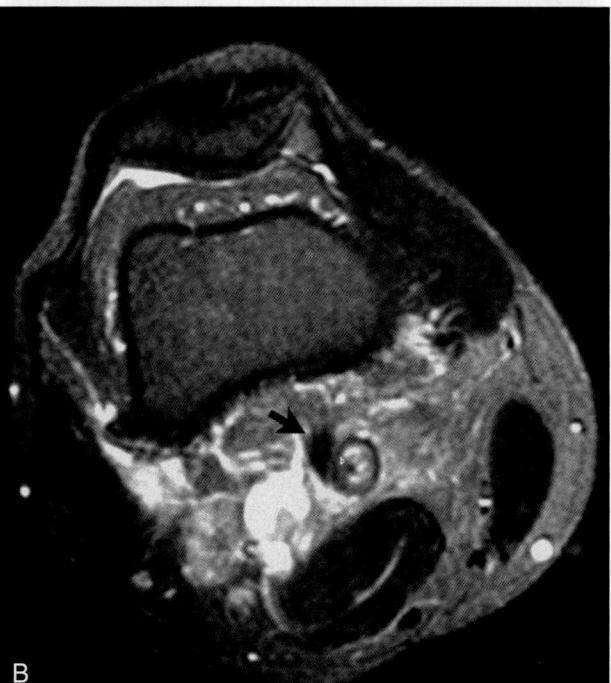

FIGURE 106-5

A, Axial T1-weighted MR image at the level of the distal femur shows a curvilinear low signal intensity structure (*arrow*) emanating from the posterior aspect of the femur, extending between the popliteal artery and vein. Note the presence of pulsation artifact within the artery. **B,** Axial T2-weighted fat-suppressed fast spin-echo MR image through the superior aspect of the knee shows a low signal intensity structure (*arrow*) interposed between the artery and vein. The structure ultimately extends to the gastrocnemius muscle and represents an anomalous tendon slip attachment with entrapment of the popliteal artery at the level of the knee. At this level, no pulsation artifact is present, suggesting compromised vascular flow.

decompression of the popliteal artery (by releasing or resecting the aberrant muscle that may be present),[32] or bypass grafting.[33]

Accessory Soleus

The soleus muscle originates primarily from the upper third of the tibial and fibular shafts, and inserts into the Achilles tendon. The accessory soleus muscle originates proximally from the adjacent tibia, fibula, or anterior portion of the soleus; it inserts distally into the Achilles tendon, the superior surface of the calcaneus, or the medial surface of the calcaneus.[34-37] MRI may be used to document the variable distal insertion site, which may impact surgical planning.[38]

The accessory soleus muscle may come to clinical attention when it is strained,[39] causes an entrapment neuropathy,[40] or presents as a mass lesion.[41,42] Furthermore, this muscle can become painful with exercise,[37,43] which may be due to closed-compartment ischemia.[41,44] MRI is considered the preferred diagnostic technique, usually providing an explanation for symptoms caused by an accessory soleus muscle, based on its characteristic location, morphology, and signal intensity (Fig. 106-6). The accessory soleus is most easily identified as it courses anterior to the Achilles tendon and superficial to the flexor retinaculum (outside of the tarsal tunnel).

PATHOLOGIC CONDITIONS

Neuromuscular Diseases

Neuromuscular diseases may be defined as disorders that primarily involve the cranial nerves (motor nuclei) and spinal cord (anterior horn cells), the peripheral nerves, the neuromuscular junction, and/or the muscle itself.[45,46] The daunting array of neuromuscular diseases may be classified according to numerous features, including the mode of acquisition (e.g., hereditary versus acquired); the time of onset (e.g., congenital, childhood, adulthood); duration (e.g., acute versus chronic); molecular genetics (e.g., ion channel dysfunction in the muscle cell membrane);[47] and the site of primary disorder (e.g., neuropathies versus myopathies). After a general overview of neuromuscular disease, this section focuses on inherited and acquired *myopathies* (primary disorders of muscle), including muscular dystrophies, metabolic myopathies, and various infectious and inflammatory myopathies. [A detailed discussion of *neuropathies* (primary disorders of the nervous system) is beyond the scope of this chapter.]

Clinical Presentation

Patients with neuromuscular diseases commonly present with the nonspecific complaints of muscle pain and abnormal fatigability.[46] Findings on physical examination may include other important but nonspecific findings: abnormal muscle tone, fasciculation, spasm, weakness,

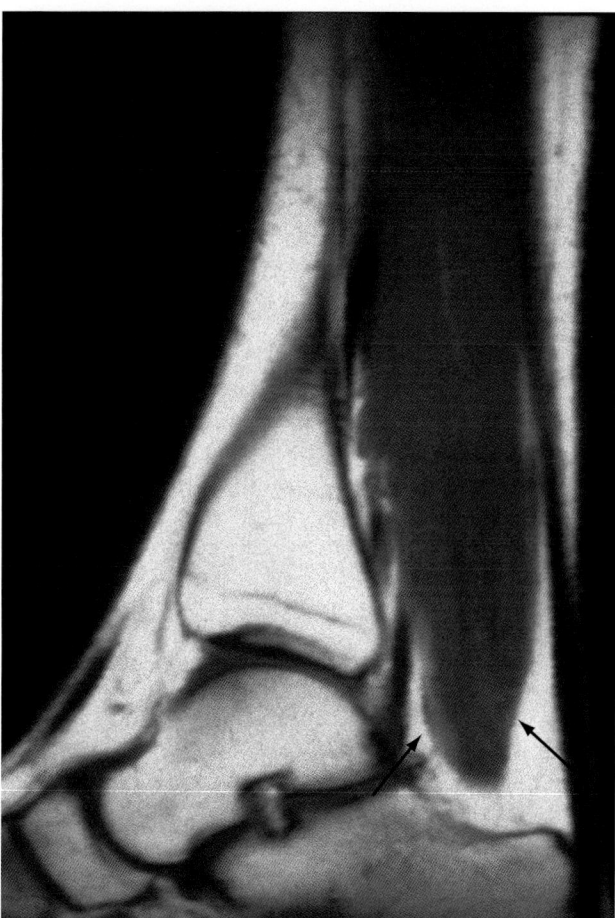

FIGURE 106-6

Sagittal T1-weighted MR image through the ankle shows the classic location of the accessory soleus muscle (*arrows*) anterior to the Achilles tendon at the level of the tibiotalar joint.

and abnormal tendon reflexes. Neuromuscular diseases tend to have a chronic course, and may progress at highly variable rates.

Ancillary testing commonly focuses on laboratory evaluation for elevated levels of serum muscle enzymes (e.g., creatine kinase) and myoglobinuria. Highly elevated enzyme levels (i.e., >10 times normal) are indicative of primary myopathic disease.[48] However, muscle enzymes are of limited diagnostic utility. Normal muscle enzyme levels do not exclude muscle disease, and moderate enzyme elevations may be due to primary myopathies or neuropathies.

Electrodiagnostic testing facilitates differentiation between primary myopathic versus primary neuropathic disorders. Limitations of EMG include that it is subjective, subject to sampling error, mildly invasive, and rarely generates a specific diagnosis.

Biopsy allows for detailed structural and biochemical histopathologic examination. Since the location and extent of neuromuscular disorders may be difficult to predict clinically, limitations of biopsy include its small sample size and the potential for sampling error. In addition, advanced muscle derangements (e.g., chronic fibrosis, fatty replacement) may result in a nondiagnostic sample. Muscle biopsy may not be appropriate for certain patients, such as those with heritable motor and sensory neuropathies who tend to have nonspecific histologic muscle biopsy findings. Finally, because of its invasive nature and cost, biopsy is impractical for frequent serial evaluations.

Imaging

MRI is considered the preeminent imaging technique for evaluating patients with suspected neuromuscular diseases. MRI can contribute to the diagnostic work-up in numerous ways, including rapidly defining the presence, distribution, severity, and chronicity of muscle disease. In so doing, MRI can help limit the differential diagnosis, provide prognostic information, direct subsequent invasive procedures (e.g., biopsy, if indicated), and establish an objective baseline for subsequent comparison.[46]

Neuropathic conditions are generally highly asymmetric, whereas primary myopathies tend to be highly symmetrical in any given patient.[46] Neuropathies may be demonstrated as patchy or particular distributions of muscle volume loss. In contrast, noninflammatory myopathies tend to progress more slowly, with prominent fat deposition that may preserve the net volume of a muscle. However, MRI does not usually allow for a specific diagnosis. Indeed, many different neuromuscular diseases may share the same distribution and signal intensity characteristics. Furthermore, a single type of neuromuscular disease may have a variable distribution in different patients.

Muscular Dystrophies

The muscular dystrophies are the largest and most common group of hereditary neuromuscular diseases. *Muscular dystrophy* refers to a heterogeneous group of heritable muscle disorders characterized by progressive muscle wasting and weakness (without spinal cord or peripheral nervous system involvement). Traditionally, the numerous forms of muscular dystrophy have been classified empirically on the basis of several clinical factors, including the age when symptoms appear; the types of symptoms that develop; the muscles that are affected; the expected prognosis; and the type of inheritance (e.g., via autosomal-dominant genes).

Advances in genetics are expected to result in modifications to the traditional clinical classification of the muscular dystrophies.[49-53] More than 30 different forms of muscular dystrophy now can be diagnosed and molecularly characterized.[54] For example, the gene encoding the muscle membrane protein *dystrophin* is the fundamental defect in patients with both Duchenne and Becker muscular dystrophy, leading to the term to describe both diseases: *dystrophinopathies*.

Duchenne Muscular Dystrophy

Duchenne muscular dystrophy, the most common type of muscular dystrophy, is an X-linked recessive disorder with a worldwide prevalence of 1 in 3500 live male births.[55] Females may carry the gene for this disorder, but rarely develop substantial symptoms. Symptoms of Duchenne muscular dystrophy generally arise in children before the age of 6 years. Muscle weakness, wasting, and contractures preferentially tend to affect muscles in the pelvis and lower extremities, especially the hip and knee extensors. In the calf muscles, characteristic replacement of muscle tissue by fat and connective tissue results in "pseudohypertrophy." By the age of 12 years, most patients with Duchenne muscular dystrophy are confined to a wheelchair. Skeletal muscle weakness is frequently accompanied by smooth muscle and myocardial dysfunction (e.g., cardiomyopathy), as well as cognitive deficits.[55] This rapidly progressive form of muscular dystrophy usually results in death from cardiac or respiratory complications by the age of about 20 years.

Becker Muscular Dystrophy

Becker muscular dystrophy is a less common and less severe dystrophinopathy than Duchenne muscular dystrophy. Although the symptoms and signs of Becker muscular dystrophy are similar to those of Duchenne, they begin later (average age, 11 years) and progress more slowly. Death due to cardiopulmonary complications typically occurs in the fourth decade.

Imaging

MRI may be helpful to monitor the presence, location, extent, and progression of muscular dystrophy. These features can be helpful for several reasons. For example, muscle atrophy may be underestimated on clinical inspection because of the accumulation of fat and connective tissue, while MRI can show this progressive muscle deterioration which is subclinical in one half of patients.[56] In addition, the degree of fatty infiltration shown by MRI has a statistically significant correlation with clinical function and disease duration.[57] Finally, MRI also may prove helpful in assessing new therapeutic regimens as they become available.[58,59]

MRI characteristically shows fatty infiltration of muscle on T1-weighted images, especially in proximal muscles. Fatty replacement of muscle may be symmetric or asymmetric, and parallels declination in muscle strength.[57,60] With Duchenne muscular dystrophy, early involvement tends to target the gastrocnemius, quadriceps, biceps femoris, and gluteus maximus and medius muscles (Fig. 106-7). Thigh muscles that tend to be spared are the gracilis, followed by the sartorius, semitendinosus, and semimembranosus muscles,[57,60] and in Becker muscular dystrophy, as well as these muscles, the rectus femoris and adductor longus are also reportedly resistant to fatty infiltration. MRI of the spine may show atrophy in the paraspinal muscles in many types of muscular dystrophy.[46]

MRI is considered the premier method for determining the volume and location of muscle and fat in patients with muscular dystrophy.[58,59] MRI, however, is not considered highly sensitive or specific for the

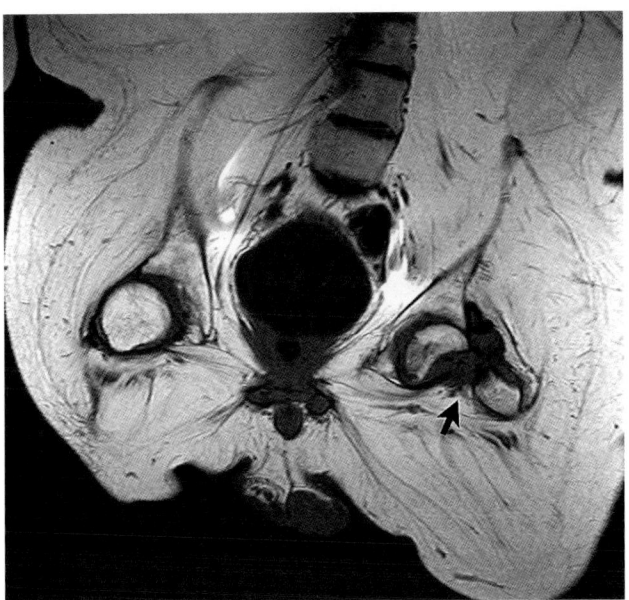

FIGURE 106-7

Coronal T1-weighted MR image through the pelvis in a patient with Duchenne muscular dystrophy shows diffuse atrophy of every muscle group about the pelvic girdle. Note the intermediate signal intensity material in the area of the left femoral neck (*arrow*), which is related to a chronic nonunited femoral neck fracture.

diagnosis of muscular dystrophy. In the first few years of the disease, MRI findings may be normal until fatty deterioration becomes apparent.[46] This feature is unlike idiopathic inflammatory myopathies and most neuromuscular disorders, in which conspicuous edema-like signal is observed on IR-FSE images before fatty infiltration is displayed on T1-weighted images.

Experimental MR techniques have been applied to the study of muscular dystrophies, including: T1-weighted MRI with magnetization transfer (to gain a quantitative measure of disease extent, progression, and therapeutic response);[61] spin-lock MRI (to quantify microstructural changes of muscle);[62] and ^{23}Na-MRI (to facilitate understanding of the role of the Na^+/K^+ pump and perfusion in normal and diseased muscle).[63,64]

Treatment

Despite this enormous progress in our understanding of muscular dystrophy, there is still no cure.[65] Treatment with gentamicin,[66] gene therapy,[54] and stem cells[65] are all active areas of research.

Metabolic Myopathies

The metabolic myopathies (MMs) are a heterogeneous group of diseases characterized by the inability of skeletal muscle to produce adequate levels of energy (ATP).[67] Defects in almost every step of carbohydrate and lipid metabolism leading to energy production have been identified and are known to cause myopathy. MMs are classified generally as glycogen storage diseases (glycogenoses), lipid metabolism disorders, and mitochondrial myopathies. Most MMs are inherited, though some are acquired.

Clinical Presentation

The clinical presentation of MMs varies widely, but often is initially indistinguishable from polymyositis. Symptoms commonly include progressive muscle weakness, premature fatigue, and myalgias. Most MMs present in childhood or the teenage years, but symptoms may begin at any age. MMs are generally different from idiopathic inflammatory myopathies (IIMs) in several important ways:[67]

● Most MMs are inherited and therefore the family history may be positive for symptoms of MM (such as muscles weakness)
● Systemic manifestations in organ systems other than muscle differ between MMs and IIMs
● Severe rhabdomyolysis, though uncommon, is much more likely to portend a MM than an IIM
● Patients with MM are refractory to immunosuppressive therapy.

Imaging

MRI can play an important role in suggesting the diagnosis of MM. In contrast to active IIM, inflammation usually is not detected in the muscles of patients with MM. Rather, established MM commonly causes muscle atrophy and fatty infiltration, without associated edema-like signal.[48,67] MRI of patients with MM demonstrates that fatty replacement in lower extremity muscles often correlates well with patient age,[68] and may be absent in young infants.[60] ^{31}P-MR spectroscopy with exercise reportedly performs well in detecting muscle glycogenoses.[69]

Infectious, Inflammatory, and Idiopathic Acquired Myopathies

Myositis is defined as inflammation of muscle. Muscle inflammation, of course, may be caused by infectious or noninfectious etiologies. Infectious causes of myositis include a wide variety of bacterial, viral, parasitic, and fungal pathogens. Specific infectious entities affecting muscle include pyomyositis, necrotizing fasciitis, and various HIV-related infections. Noninfectious inflammation of muscle may be caused by autoimmune or idiopathic mechanisms, including sarcoid myopathy, polymyositis, dermatomyositis, and inclusion body myositis.

Pyomyositis

Primary pyomyositis is an acute or subacute bacterial infection of skeletal muscle that usually results after an episode of transient bacteremia.[70-80] Bacteremia in the absence of certain risk factors usually is not sufficient to cause pyomyositis. Common risk factors for pyomyositis include immunosuppression (e.g., HIV infection), malnutrition, diabetes, malignancy, intravenous drug use, and trauma (e.g., muscle contusion). Muscle contusion may be a risk factor because muscle damage, hematoma formation, and hyperemia may create a fertile ground for infection. Pyomyositis may affect individuals in both tropical (more common) and temperate (less common) climates.

CLINICAL PRESENTATION. As observed in a recent review of 676 patients,[78] primary pyomyositis is most common in children and young adults (mean age, 28 years). A single site usually is affected (83% of cases). Primary pyomyositis is most common in the largest muscle groups in the pelvis and lower extremities, including the quadriceps (26%), iliopsoas (14%), gluteal (11%), and calf (7%) musculature.

The most commonly reported symptoms and signs of primary pyomyositis are progressive myalgia, pain, swelling, erythema, tenderness, and fever. Pyomyositis may evolve over time through three general stages: 1. insidious onset of poorly localized diffuse inflammation, often over a 1 to 2 week period; 2. focal muscle abscess formation; and (if untreated) 3. extension of infection and systemic sepsis.

The clinical differential diagnosis may include entities such as cellulitis, septic arthritis, osteomyelitis, thrombophlebitis, contusion, muscle strain, compartment syndrome, neoplasm, and diabetic muscle infarction.

Laboratory analysis reveals leukocytosis in approximately 75% of patients. The most commonly identified bacterium is *Staphylococcus aureus* (77%).[78] Less commonly, other species are found, including streptococci, Gram-negative microorganisms (e.g., *Escherichia coli*), and *Mycobacterium tuberculosis*. Cultures of blood and purulent material are positive in only approximately one third of cases. Consequently, the diagnosis of pyomyositis is based commonly on clinical and imaging findings.

IMAGING. Diagnostic imaging helps in delineating the location(s) and extent of pyomyositis.[70,73,76,81,82] Imaging findings commonly include muscle edema, muscle enlargement, effacement of intra- and inter-muscular fat, enhancement in the inflamed region after contrast administration, and focal collection of fluid that may contain septations. A purulent fluid collection usually is detected, but this is not invariably the case.

MR images of areas affected by pyomyositis demonstrate hyperintense signal on fluid-sensitive pulse sequences.[80] Post-gadolinium images show enhancement in affected muscles, including around any abscess that may be present (Fig. 106-8). MR images also may show abnormal signal in the adjacent bone marrow, either owing to the presence of reactive inflammatory changes or the presence of coexisting osteomyelitis. Uncommon imaging findings are soft-tissue gas and lymph node enlargement.

MRI is regarded as the preferred imaging modality[78] to demonstrate muscle inflammation that may be accompanied by abscess formation or complications of pyomyositis (e.g., osteomyelitis). CT may show asymmetric muscle enlargement, gas formation, or contrast enhancement at the periphery of an abscess. However, early muscle inflammation may be difficult to diagnose

by CT, particularly in children with a paucity of adipose tissue. Sonography typically reveals abnormal echotexture in affected musculature, as well as focal hypoechogenicity from abscess formation.[79] However, sonography may have difficulty demonstrating involvement in the pelvis and does not reliably allow for the diagnosis of osteomyelitis.[78,79]

The imaging differential diagnosis (depending on the clinical context) may include other types of infectious or noninfectious inflammation (e.g., necrotizing fasciitis), muscle ischemia or necrosis (e.g., compartment syndrome, diabetic muscle infarction), venous insufficiency, soft-tissue neoplasm, and muscle trauma (e.g., contusion).

TREATMENT. Treatment of pyomyositis consists of antibiotics and, if an abscess has formed, abscess drainage.[78] Most patients respond well to this treatment and have no long-term sequelae. However, delay in diagnosis may be accompanied by pyomyositis complications, including compartment syndrome, extensive muscle necrosis, septic arthritis, osteomyelitis, and occasionally death.

Human Immunodeficiency Virus Infection

HIV has infected 40 million people globally.[83] Acutely after infection with HIV, most patients (50-75%) experience a mononucleosis-like illness, with symptoms that may include myalgias, arthralgias, and paresthesias.[84]

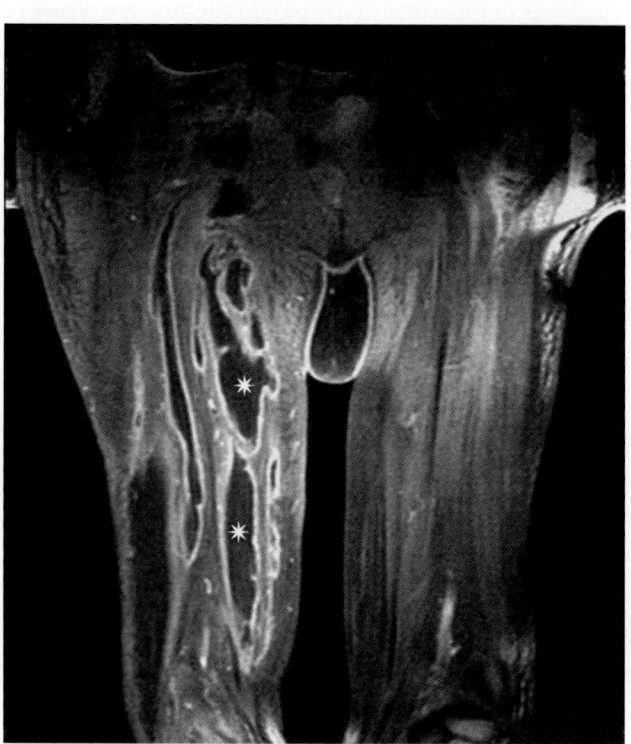

FIGURE 106-8

Coronal T1-weighted fat-suppressed MR image of the thigh acquired after administration of a gadolinium-based contrast material shows multiple abscesses in the quadriceps muscle of this diabetic patient, establishing the diagnosis of pyomyositis. The collections demonstrate central low signal intensity (*), with a thick surrounding rim of enhancement.

TABLE 106-1 HIV-Associated Muscle Derangements and Various Treatments

HIV-associated muscle derangement	Treatment
Infectious myositis	
Pyomyositis[84]	Antibiotics
Toxoplasmic myositis[86]	Antiprotozoal therapy
Direct HIV infection[382]	Antiretroviral therapy
Noninfectious myositis	
HIV-associated polymyositis[87]	Corticosteroids
	Immunosuppressive therapy (e.g., methotrexate, intravenous immunoglobulin)
Proliferative myositis[383]	None (heals spontaneously)
Neoplastic	
HIV-associated malignancies[384]	Oncologic therapy
Drug-associated myopathy	
AZT-associated myopathy[385]	AZT discontinuation
	L-carnitine
Miscellaneous	
HIV-associated rhabdomyolysis[98]	Supportive care
	Discontinue any offending drug
HIV-wasting syndrome[386]	Anabolic steroids, exercise
	Recombinant human growth hormone

Years later, more serious complications of HIV infection commonly develop in skeletal muscle. These conditions ultimately may need to be differentiated definitively by biopsy, because treatments and outcomes vary substantially (Table 106-1). HIV-associated muscle derangements include: infectious myositis [e.g., pyomyositis[85] (see earlier discussion), toxoplasmosis[86]]; noninfectious myositis (e.g., HIV-associated polymyositis, proliferative myositis); HIV-associated malignancies (e.g., lymphoma, Kaposi sarcoma); drug-associated myopathies [e.g., zidovudine (AZT)-associated myopathy]; and miscellaneous other myopathies (e.g., HIV-associated rhabdomyolysis, HIV-wasting syndrome).

NONINFECTIOUS MYOSITIS. HIV-associated polymyositis is characterized by symptoms similar to those of polymyositis (idiopathic inflammatory myositis) seen in HIV-negative patients.[87] Patients typically present with bilateral, symmetric, proximal muscle weakness and elevated serum creatine kinase levels.[73] As with other types of active myositis, MRI demonstrates high signal intensity on fat-suppressed T2-weighted and IR-FSE images, particularly in the hip and shoulder girdle regions (Fig. 106-9). Differentiating this type of inflammatory myopathy from certain other myopathies allows appropriate treatment with corticosteroids.[88]

NEOPLASMS. HIV-associated malignancies that may infiltrate muscle are well displayed with MRI, including non-Hodgkin lymphoma and Kaposi sarcoma.[73,89,90,91]

DRUG-ASSOCIATED MYOPATHY. Zidovudine (also referred to as azidodideoxythymidine or AZT) may be associated with myopathy.[92] AZT-associated myopathy is a progressive, usually painful condition causing pronounced muscle wasting, especially in the proximal appendicular skeleton. Patients may have normal-to-moderately elevated creatine kinase levels, and a myopathic pattern on EMG.[93] MRI may show nonspecific, abnormally increased T2 signal intensity in affected muscle. Symptoms typically resolve within 6 weeks of discontinuing AZT.

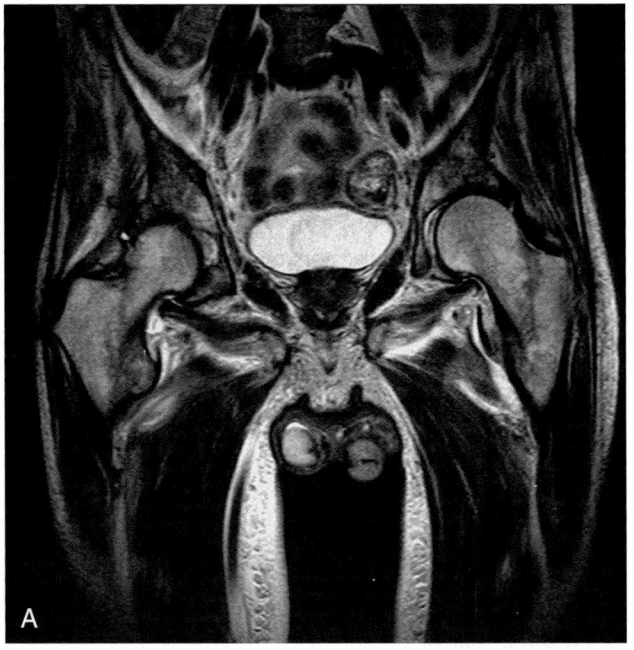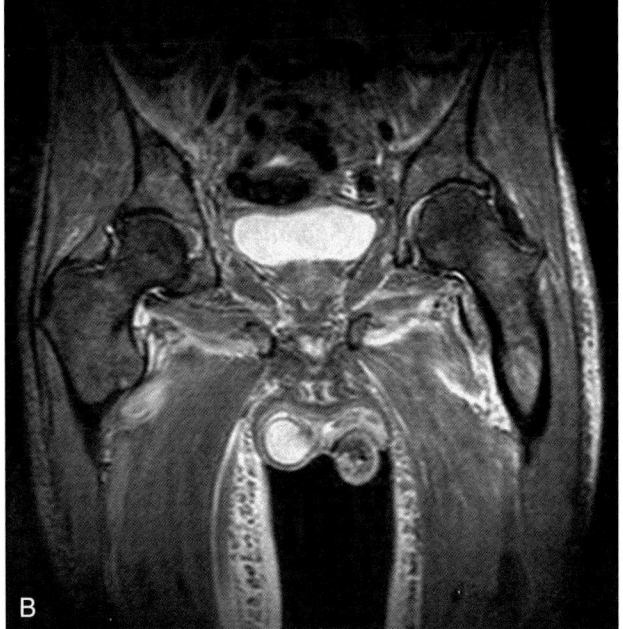

FIGURE 106-9

A, Coronal T2-weighted fast spin-echo and **B,** T2-weighted fat-suppressed fast spin-echo MR images through the pelvis and proximal thighs in an HIV-positive patient shows abnormal high signal intensity in and about the fascial planes of the obturator externus and adductor brevis muscles.

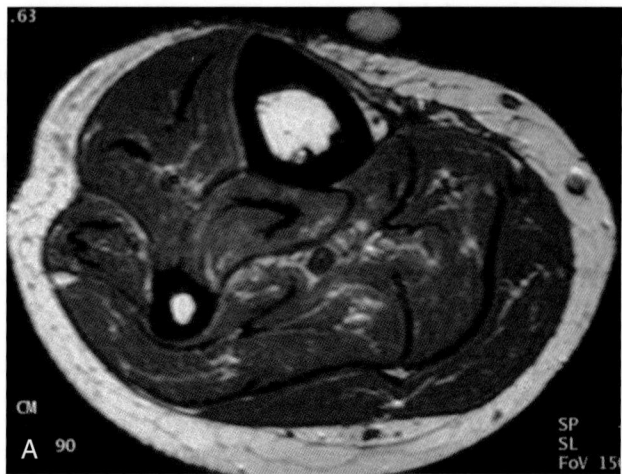

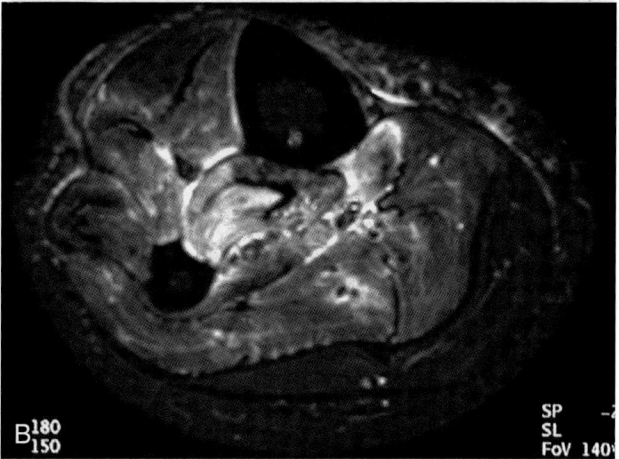

FIGURE 106-11

A, Axial T1-weighted MR image through the calf shows mild fatty infiltration in the anterior, posterior, and lateral compartments of the calf, sparing only the gastrocnemius muscles. **B,** Corresponding axial inversion recovery MR image shows diffuse high signal intensity throughout the muscles of the calf in the same muscular distribution. This T2 hyperintensity or muscle edema indicates active polymyositis.

edema-like signal and the least atrophy.[127] These areas usually have active disease and the best diagnostic yield on histopathologic examination. When MRI is not used, blind biopsy is associated with false-negative results in 10% to 15% of cases because of the patchy nature of the inflammatory infiltrate.[126]

Biopsy may be performed with incisional or percutaneous biopsy techniques. Some experts strongly prefer an open biopsy to a needle biopsy of muscle, because it allows for a larger sample.[118] Other investigators maintain that percutaneous needle biopsy of muscle is a safe, convenient, and relatively inexpensive method of muscle biopsy, with a good diagnostic yield for the confirmation of IIM.[149]

TREATMENT. Treatment of IIMs generally begins with corticosteroids. Before the availability of corticosteroids, mortality from DM and PM was up to 50%.[116] Now, 5- and 10-year survival rates are 95% and 84%, respectively.[150] Although most patients respond at least partially to cor-

ticosteroids, second-line agents may become necessary when progressive disease is observed clinically and displayed objectively (e.g., persistent hyperintense signal on IR-FSE images).[116] Second-line agents include methotrexate, cyclosporine, intravenous immune globulin, and antitumor necrosis factor agents. ^{31}P-MR spectroscopy has been used to evaluate noninvasively the beneficial effects of prednisone and immunosuppression therapy in elevating low levels of magnesium in the muscles of patients with IIM.[151]

Childhood Idiopathic Inflammatory Myopathies

IIM in children has both similarities and differences compared to IIM in adults.[152] The vast majority of children with IIM have juvenile dermatomyositis (JDM). Like its adult counterpart, JDM is characterized by perivascular inflammation causing capillary destruction in muscle and skin. This uncommon disease is diagnosed in two to three children per million population annually.

CLINICAL PRESENTATION. The hallmark of JDM is its characteristic cutaneous presentation (e.g., heliotrope rash, Gottron sign). Other organ systems can be affected, including the gastrointestinal tract and lungs. Common features at the time of diagnosis in 79 children were: skin rash (100%), proximal muscle weakness (100%), muscle pain (73%), fever (65%), dysphagia (44%), arthritis (35%), and calcinosis (23%).[153]

IMAGING. Radiography and CT may show scattered or diffuse calcifications, particularly around the thighs and knees bilaterally.[154] JDM is complicated eventually by the development of calcinosis in 30% to 70% of all patients.[152,155-157] *Calcinosis* refers to calcium-laden fluid collections in the subcutaneous and intermuscular tissues. Gadolinium-enhanced images facilitate differentiation of these fluid collections (which have negligible peripheral enhancement) from abscesses (which often display more avid peripheral enhancement) in these children who are often on corticosteroids.[60,158,159]

MRI is regarded as helpful for assessing disease activity and guiding the treatment of JDM. Hyperintense signal indicative of edema is seen in the fascia, subcutaneous tissues, and skin in up to 85% of JDM patients at baseline evaluation on IR-FSE images of the thighs and buttocks.[160] T2 relaxation times correlate with disease activity (including muscle function) and can be used as a quantitative measure of muscle inflammation.[161] Prompt diagnosis and treatment may help prevent the formation of fistulas and contractures.[162] In addition to these signs of acute inflammation, sequelae of chronic disease are well displayed, including muscular atrophy, fibrotic tissue, and lipodystrophy (slow, progressive, symmetrical loss of subcutaneous soft-tissue).[152,163]

TREATMENT. Treatment of JDM begins with corticosteroids, though second-line agents like methotrexate are used increasingly.[152,156,164] Prior to the use of corticosteroids, patient outcome was guarded (approximately one third of patients died of JDM, one third developed severe physical limitations, and only one third recovered completely[152]). Since that time, functional outcomes have improved substantially, and the mortality of JDM has decreased to approximately 10%.

Muscle Ischemia and Necrosis

Compartment Syndrome

Compartment syndrome is defined as elevated pressure in a relatively noncompliant anatomic space that causes ischemia, pain, and potentially neuromuscular injury.[165-168] Potential complications of compartment syndrome include myonecrosis, rhabdomyolysis, renal failure, and even death.[168-170]

When elevated intracompartmental pressure exceeds the intravascular pressure of thin-walled small vessels in muscle, these vessels may collapse, thereby decreasing the arteriovenous pressure gradient, impeding blood flow,[171] and potentially resulting in tissue ischemia. Risk factors for compartment syndrome include a history of trauma, external compression, loss of compartment elasticity (e.g., fibrotic, constricted fascia), systemic hypotension, and increased intracompartmental volume (e.g., hemorrhage in patients with bleeding disorders or taking anticoagulant medications, muscle hypertrophy in athletes).[172-174] Compartment syndrome is classified generally as acute or chronic.

Acute Compartment Syndrome

Acute compartment syndrome occurs most commonly in association with fractures, particularly of the tibia. The second most common cause is soft-tissue injury (e.g., severe contusion, crush injury) without fracture.[174] Compartments commonly affected by this syndrome are in the forearm (volar compartment) and leg (anterior and deep posterior compartments), though compartment syndrome may affect virtually any noncompliant anatomic compartment.

Chronic Compartment Syndrome

Chronic compartment syndrome results most commonly from exertional causes (e.g., exercise, occupational overuse); "nonexertional" causes (e.g., mass lesion, infection) are considered uncommon. Chronic compartment syndrome occurs secondary to exertion because chronic muscle activity causes muscle hypertrophy and transiently can swell muscle fibers up to 20 times their resting size, thus causing increased pressure in noncompliant compartments.[167,175] The most frequent sites of chronic compartment syndrome in athletes are the leg, thigh, and forearm.[176]

Clinical Presentation

The typical chief complaint is pain that worsens with palpation and passive stretching of the affected muscles. With acute compartment syndrome, the most important early symptom is pain out of proportion to that expected for the given injury.[177] With chronic exertional compartment syndrome, aching or cramping pain typically begins during or immediately after exercise, and tends to resolve at rest after a variable period. With both acute and chronic compartment syndrome, deficits in nerve function and arterial pulses are considered late findings.[167,168,178]

Diagnostic tests used to evaluate for compartment syndrome include percutaneous measurements of compartment pressure,[179] near-infrared spectroscopy measurements of oxygen saturation,[180-183] and MRI.

Direct pressure measurement with various types of percutaneous catheters is considered the gold standard for the diagnosis of compartment syndrome. Normally, compartment pressures measure approximately less than 15 mmHg at rest, increase with exercise, and return to less than 20 to 25 mmHg within 5 minutes after exercise.[167,176,184,185] Limitations of percutaneous pressure measurements include inconsistent use of the equipment, improper catheter insertion into an unintended compartment, and inadvertent damage to neurovascular structures.[167,186,187] Despite these limitations, the emergent diagnosis of acute compartment syndrome is made routinely using percutaneous pressure measurements, without MRI.

Imaging

MRI can be used to clarify the location and extent of ischemic damage to muscle.[188-191] Particularly in the nonemergent setting, potential indications for MRI include the diagnostic assessment of atypical cases (e.g., uncommon location or cause for compartment syndrome, borderline pressure measurements), guidance for percutaneous catheter placement, and evaluation for an underlying lesion (e.g., hematoma, neoplasm) that may contribute to compartment hypertension and need to be addressed at surgery.

ACUTE COMPARTMENT SYNDROME. With acute compartment syndrome, diffuse edema-like signal and mildly increased muscle girth are common, occasionally with foci of hemorrhage[192,193] (Fig. 106-12). With impending compartment syndrome, gadolinium-enhanced T1-weighted images typically show avid contrast enhancement in the affected muscles.[191]

CHRONIC COMPARTMENT SYNDROME. With chronic exertional compartment syndrome, diffuse edema-like signal and mildly increased muscle girth are common after exercise. The change in T2 signal intensity between pre- and post-exercise images is significantly greater in compartments with postexercise hypertension.[194,195] MRI findings of chronic exertional compartment syndrome may be accompanied by bone stress injury and traction periostitis,[196] as well as occasionally muscle herniation.

After an episode of compartment syndrome, hyperintense signal on T2-weighted images tends to resolve in parallel with the clinical course. After successful surgery, signal intensity derangements in muscle may normalize within 4 months.[197] However, even after resolution of acute symptoms, sequelae of muscle injury may persist,[198] including findings of muscle volume loss, fatty infiltration, fibrosis, and/or dystrophic calcification.

The imaging differential diagnosis (depending on the clinical context) may include other causes of painful,

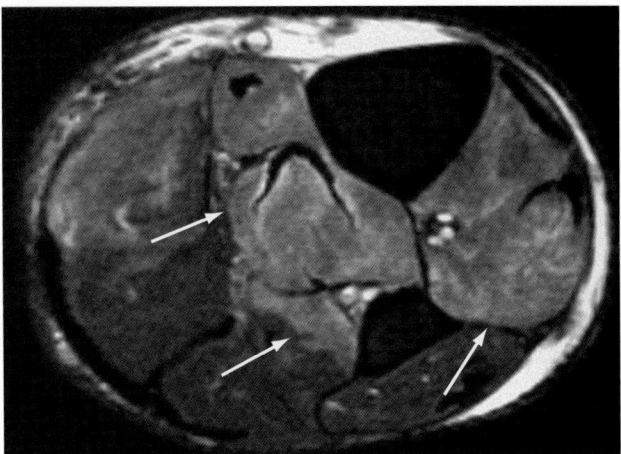

FIGURE 106-12

Axial T1-weighted fat-suppressed MR image acquired after the administration of a gadolinium-based contrast material in a patient after total knee replacement shows abnormal enhancement (*arrows*) in the anterior and posterior compartments of the calf. In the areas of abnormal enhancement, there is loss of normal muscle architecture and a subtle increase in muscle girth consistent with muscle swelling and the imaging diagnosis of compartment syndrome.

swollen extremities, including muscle contusion, myositis, deep venous thrombosis, and delayed-onset muscle soreness. Although MRI can be helpful in the evaluation of compartment syndrome, imaging findings by themselves generally are not specific.

Experimentally, diffusion-weighted echo-planar MRI can depict alterations in the circulating blood volume in muscle induced by exercise and changes in compartment pressure.[199] ^{31}P-MR spectroscopy may permit assessment of the pressure threshold for metabolic deterioration of skeletal muscle after an ischemic insult and subsequent healing after fasciotomy.[189]

Treatment

ACUTE COMPARTMENT SYNDROME. For acute compartment syndrome, surgical decompression has been recommended when compartment pressures rise to 30 to 80 mmHg[200-203] or to within 20 to 30 mmHg of the diastolic pressure.[168,204] Findings favoring surgical decompression include increasing compartment pressures over time, paresthesia, and paresis. When fasciotomy is performed within 12 hours after the onset of acute compartment syndrome, two thirds of all extremities will have normal function.[205] Contrarily, fasciotomy more than 12 hours after acute onset of compartment syndrome results in normal limb function in only 8% of cases. Prompt fasciotomy also is strongly associated with successful defense against malpractice claims involving compartment syndrome.[206]

CHRONIC COMPARTMENT SYNDROME. Initial treatment of chronic exertional compartment syndrome is generally nonoperative. Conservative treatment commonly fails if the precipitating activity is not discon-

tinued. If symptoms persist for longer than 6 months despite conservative therapy, fasciotomy generally is recommended.

Calcific Myonecrosis

Calcific myonecrosis refers to dystrophic calcification and necrosis in skeletal muscle that occurs as an uncommon late sequela of trauma and ischemic injury (compartment syndrome).[207-216] It is postulated that unrecognized, untreated compartment syndrome results in muscle necrosis that may be associated ultimately with pathologic findings of fibrosis, hematoma, liquefaction, and calcification. This entity may be in the continuum of pathologic processes that includes post-traumatic cystic change in soft-tissue, chronic expanding hematoma,[217-219] and calcific myonecrosis.

Clinical Presentation

Patients present decades after trauma, typically with pain, nerve palsy, and/or a soft-tissue mass in the leg. The time interval between the traumatic event and the diagnosis of calcific myonecrosis averages 36 years (range 10-64 years), with an average patient age at diagnosis of 54 years (range 34-80 years).[215]

Imaging

Radiography and CT show a soft-tissue mass with dystrophic calcifications that characteristically are plaquelike and oriented longitudinally in the affected compartment (Fig. 106-13). MRI demonstrates a fusiform mass of heterogeneous signal intensity, most commonly in the anterior compartment of the leg. Other imaging features may include heterogeneous signal intensity, cystic-appearing contents, eccentric erosion of bone, and peripheral enhancement. The imaging differential diagnosis generally includes soft-tissue sarcoma and chronic infection.

Treatment

The optimal treatment regimen is debated, but may include aggressive debridement of necrotic tissue. Potential treatment complications include chronic sinus tract formation and secondary infection.

Rhabdomyolysis

Rhabdomyolysis refers to the breakdown of skeletal muscle and leakage of muscle contents into the circulation.[220-222] This process releases myoglobin and other metabolites from damaged muscle that potentially can result in acute renal failure (in 15-30% of patients), electrolyte imbalance with cardiac arrest, and disseminated intravascular coagulation.[223-225] The insults causing rhabdomyolysis are numerous, including compartment syndrome, ischemia, trauma (e.g., crush, electrical, and

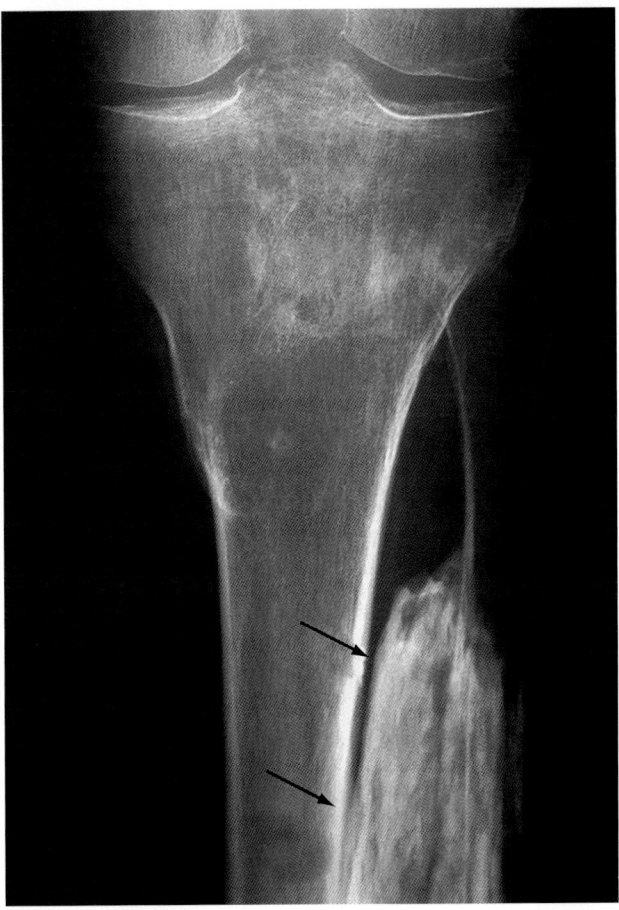

FIGURE 106-13

Frontal radiograph of the proximal tibia demonstrates a sheetlike region of calcification (*arrows*) in the distribution of the peroneal musculature, oriented along the longitudinal axis of the lateral compartment of the calf consistent with calcific myonecrosis and previous compartment syndrome. Note the deformity of the proximal tibia from a healed fracture.

thermal injury), excessive muscle activity, drugs (e.g., statin medications), toxins, myositis, and genetic metabolic derangements.

Clinical Presentation

The diagnosis of rhabdomyolysis can be defined clinically as muscle pain or weakness associated with myoglobinuria and creatine kinase levels higher than 10 times the upper limit of normal.[226] The classic, complete triad of muscle pain, weakness, and dark brown urine is not observed in the majority of patients (particularly early in the disease course, when patients may complain only of nonspecific muscle weakness or myalgia).[227]

Imaging

MRI is considered the most sensitive imaging test to evaluate patients with rhabdomyolysis. In a prospective study of 15 patients with acute rhabdomyolysis,[228] abnormal muscles were demonstrated by sonography in

42% of patients, by CT in 62% of patients, and by MRI in 100% of patients. Consequently, MRI has been used to document the location and extent of muscle involvement in patients with rhabdomyolysis.[229]

The principal MRI finding of rhabdomyolysis is edema-like signal diffusely in the involved muscle. This nonspecific finding is thought to reflect the presence of increased water content and increased mobility of water molecules. The severity of the signal alterations correlates with the severity of the injury. In milder cases, repeat MR examinations show that the edema-like signal resolves in parallel with the clinical course. This reversibility suggests that the high intensity areas do not reflect permanent myopathic changes, but probably represent transient edema in the acute phase of rhabdomyolysis.[230]

Treatment

Rhabdomyolysis is treated with immediate intravenous volume replacement. This commonly is followed by mannitol-induced diuresis and alkalinization of the patient's urine[225] and, in some advanced cases, hemodialysis.[231]

Diabetic Muscle Infarction

Skeletal muscle has a relatively rich vascular supply and a relatively low metabolic demand when at rest. Consequently, skeletal muscle infarction is generally uncommon. However, in patients with diabetes, diseased vascular endothelium and relative hypercoagulability may result in thrombosis of small and medium-sized arterioles.[232-234] Most patients with diabetic muscle infarction have known microvascular complications of poorly controlled or longstanding diabetes (e.g., neuropathy, retinopathy, or nephropathy) (94%).[235] Type I diabetes is a more common risk factor than type II diabetes.[236]

Clinical Presentation

Patients are typically adults of middle age (mean age, 42 years; range, 19-81 years).[235] They commonly present with abrupt onset of muscle pain that occurs at rest and is exacerbated by movement.[237,238] The affected area usually is enlarged and exquisitely tender, sometimes with a palpable mass (44%).[235] Diabetic muscle infarction commonly involves multiple muscles and may be bilateral (approximately 40%).[237] The most commonly affected muscles are in the thigh (>80% of patients) and calf (approximately 15% of patients) (Fig. 106-14).[235,237] Laboratory evaluations generally are not helpful in establishing the diagnosis of diabetic muscle infarction.[235,238,239]

Imaging

MRI generally is the imaging test of choice for evaluating patients with suspected diabetic muscle infarction.[236,237] Findings on fluid-sensitive images include diffuse edema-like signal in the subcutaneous and intermuscular

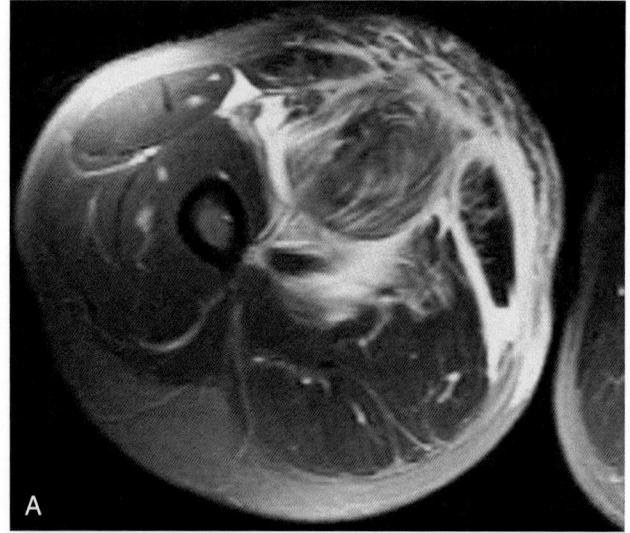

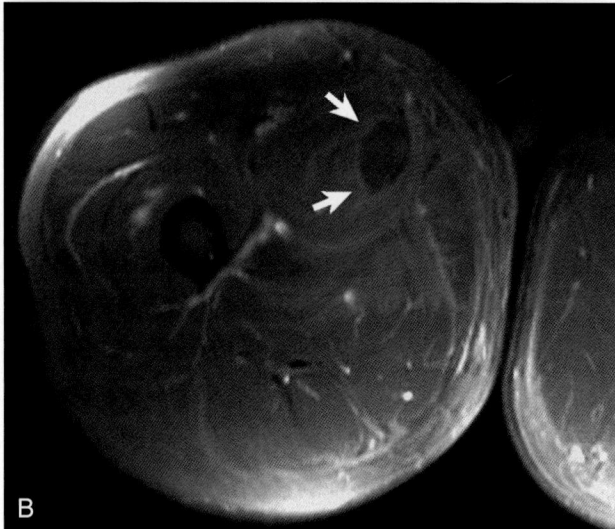

FIGURE 106-14

A, Axial T2-weighted MR image through the proximal thigh in a diabetic patient shows areas of heterogeneous high signal intensity in the distribution of the sartoris, adductor longus, adductor brevis, and gracilis muscles, as well as diffuse high signal intensity between the fascial planes of these muscles. **B,** Corresponding axial T1-weighted fat-suppressed MR image acquired after the administration of a gadolinium-based contrast material shows mild enhancement in the muscles of the proximal thigh with focal areas of nonenhancement most notable in the adductor longus and brevis (*arrows*), establishing the presence of diabetic muscle infarcts.

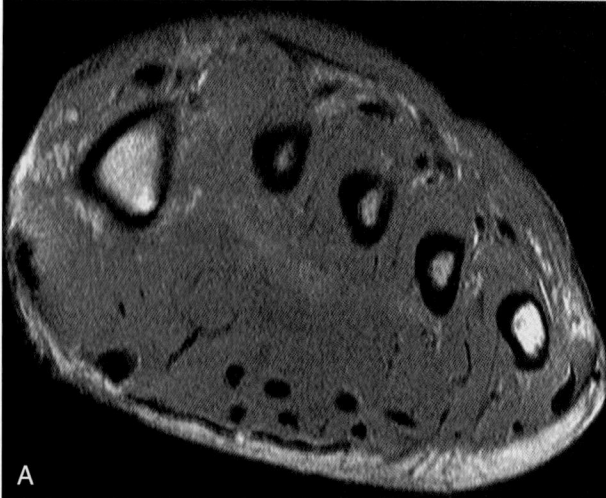

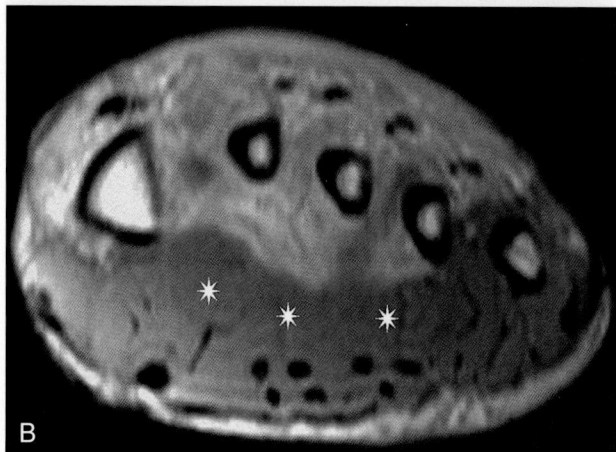

FIGURE 106-15

A, Coronal T1-weighted MR image through the forefoot in a diabetic patient with gangrene shows very subtle differential signal intensity dividing the visualized musculature of the foot into plantar and dorsal halves, the plantar side with slightly lower signal intensity than the dorsal side. **B,** Corresponding coronal T1-weighted MR image acquired after the administration of a gadolinium-based contrast material accentuates the differential signal intensity in the muscles of the forefoot. The lack of enhancement in the plantar-sided muscles (*) establishes a lack of blood supply, supporting the clinical diagnosis of dry gangrene.

soft-tissues, subfascial fluid, and swelling in the side of the affected muscles. After the administration of gadolinium contrast material, enhancement may be seen due to cell membrane breakdown. This pattern of contrast enhancement can be diffuse, often with focal areas of nonenhancement (corresponding to macroscopic areas of muscle infarction) (Fig. 106-15).[235] Although these findings are not entirely specific, MRI is considered essentially 100% sensitive.[235,240,241]

The imaging differential diagnosis (depending on the clinical context) may include entities such as trauma, pyomyositis, noninfectious forms of myositis, and neoplasm.[70,237] Clinical history is often helpful, particularly considering the wide array of muscle abnormalities causing edema-like signal in muscle. In patients with characteristic clinical and imaging manifestations, expectant management can be pursued and percutaneous core needle biopsy may be obviated.[235-237,240,242]

Treatment

Treatment for uncomplicated diabetic muscle infarction typically includes rest, analgesics, and sometimes anticoagulation.[236,243,244] Symptoms routinely resolve over a period of 2 weeks to 2 months, though recurrent episodes of infarction reportedly occur in up to approximately 50% of patients.[235,236,238,244,245]

Traumatic Derangements of Muscle

Traumatic insults to muscle may occur by a variety of mechanisms and have a variety of manifestations. Categories of traumatic insults include biomechanical overload during muscle contraction (e.g., strain, delayed-onset muscle soreness), penetrating trauma (e.g., laceration), muscle herniation, blunt trauma (e.g., contusion), hemorrhage, and heterotopic ossification. MRI impacts the care of patients by providing meaningful information regarding the location, extent, severity, and acuity of muscular disorders.

Muscle Strain

Clinical Presentation

Strain injuries commonly occur when a powerful muscle contraction is combined simultaneously with forced lengthening of the myotendinous unit. Muscle fatigue may play an important role in the pathogenesis of some strain injuries.[246] Strains often are located in muscles undergoing eccentric contraction, that cross two joints, or have a high proportion of fast twitch fibers. The most commonly strained muscles in the extremities include the hamstrings, hip adductors, rectus femoris, and gastrocnemius.[247-249] Trunk muscles associated with the spine[250] and abdominal wall[251] also may be strained.

Within any given muscle, strain injuries are centered most commonly at the intramuscular myotendinous junction in young adults.[252,253] For example, in one study of 179 acute athletic hamstring injuries, only 21 occurred at the proximal tendon (five partial tears and 16 avulsions) and only four occurred at the distal tendon attachment (all avulsions).[254]

Muscle strains may be graded along a spectrum of injury, from mild (first-degree, microscopic injury) to moderate (second-degree, macroscopic partial tear) to severe (third-degree, complete tear). Low-grade injuries are more common than severe injuries. For example, in a study of 431 professional football players,[255] 324 (75%) injuries were first-degree strains. Second- or third-degree injuries were observed in 107 players (25%), with 58 players (13%) sustaining severe injuries with a discrete, palpable defect in the muscle. In another study of 65 patients with strain injuries in the calf,[256] 51 partial and 14 complete tears were diagnosed.

Imaging

Mild strains are characterized by microscopic injury to the muscle or tendon (<5% fiber disruption). No significant loss in strength or range of motion is observed clinically. In the acute setting, strain injuries result in edema and hemorrhage at the myotendinous junction that creates high signal intensity on fluid-sensitive images. This edema and hemorrhage may be seen focally or diffusely in muscle, and reflects the severity of the injury. Edema-like signal characteristically tracks along muscle fascicles creating a feathery margin (Fig. 106-16). With mild (first-degree) strains, no muscle fiber discontinuity or laxity is seen.

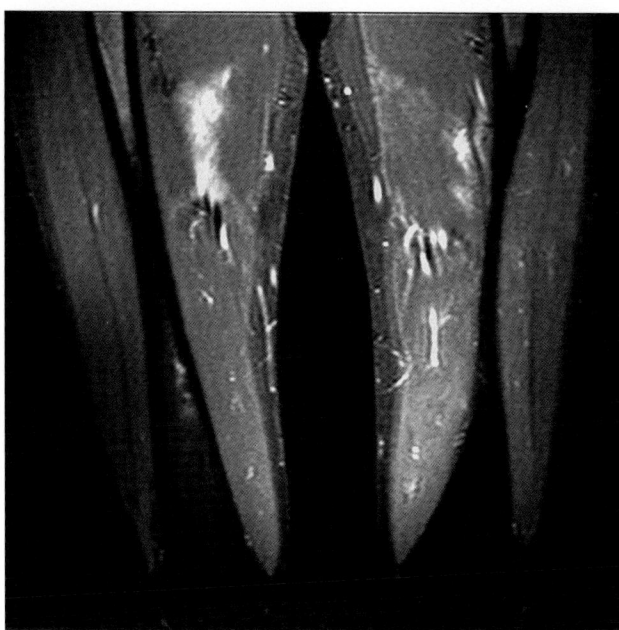

FIGURE 106-16

Coronal T2-weighted MR image through the proximal thighs shows feathery, abnormal high signal intensity along the bilateral fascicles of the adductor longus muscles consistent with mild muscle strain. No muscle fiber discontinuity can be identified.

With moderate (second-degree) strains, some muscle fibers are torn, but there is continuity of some fibers near the site of injury. The presence of a hematoma at the myotendinous junction is regarded as essentially pathognomic of a second-degree strain injury.[257,258] In addition, a rim of hyperintense perifascial fluid may track around a muscle belly or group of muscles. Perifascial edema or blood is common, occurring in up to 87% of athletes with acute partial tears.[252]

With a complete tear, MRI displays discontinuity of all fibers at the level of injury, with or without retraction of the torn fibers (Fig. 106-17). With even mild retraction, fibers adjacent to the tear may appear lax or bunched. Focal collection of fluid or hematoma typically is identified in the gap created by the acute tear.

In the chronic setting, hemosiderin and fibrosis commonly cause low signal intensity on T2-weighted images. Diminished caliber of the myotendinous unit at the site of injury also may be observed if healing has been incomplete.

Prognosis

Rehabilitation time may be predicted by the volume[259] or longitudinal length[260] of the hamstring injury shown by MRI. Furthermore, an abnormal scan at 6 weeks after injury may predict an increased risk of reinjury.[260] Convalescence periods reportedly vary from less than 1 week to more than 1 year.[246,254] Recurrent injuries are relatively common, occurring in one quarter of athletes.[261] Even minor hamstring injuries may double the risk of a more severe injury within 2 months.[262]

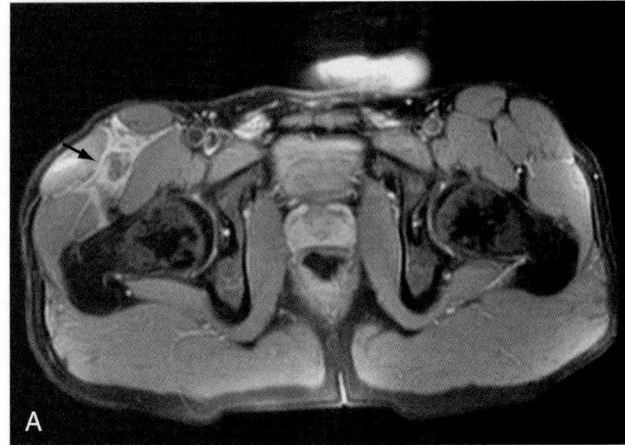

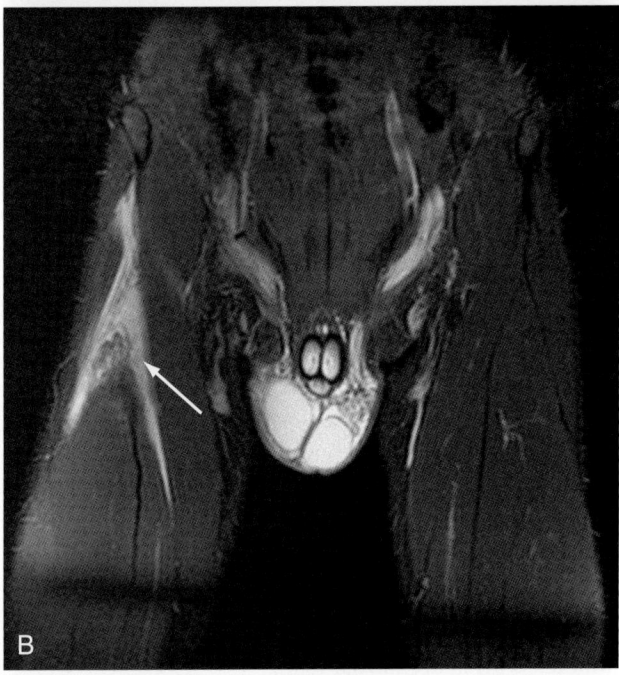

FIGURE 106-17

A, Axial proton-density–weighted fat-suppressed MR image through the hips shows abnormal high signal intensity within the substance of the rectus femoris muscle (*arrow*) consistent with muscle tear. High signal intensity is also present within the fascial planes surrounding the muscle. **B,** Corresponding coronal T2-weighted fat-suppressed MR image verifies the presence of discontinuous and retracted muscle fibers of the rectus femoris (*arrow*). High signal intensity fluid fills the gap between the retracted musculotendinous junction and its site of attachment on the ilium.

Treatment

Treatment varies with the severity of the strain and the patient's lifestyle. Management may include activity modification, physical therapy, ice, massage, therapeutic ultrasound, electrical stimulation, nonsteroidal anti-inflammatory medications, and intramuscular injection of corticosteroid with lidocaine.[263-265] Controversial or experimental treatments include hyperbaric oxygen and use of growth factors (e.g., insulin-like growth factor).[266,267] Surgery occasionally may be indicated for

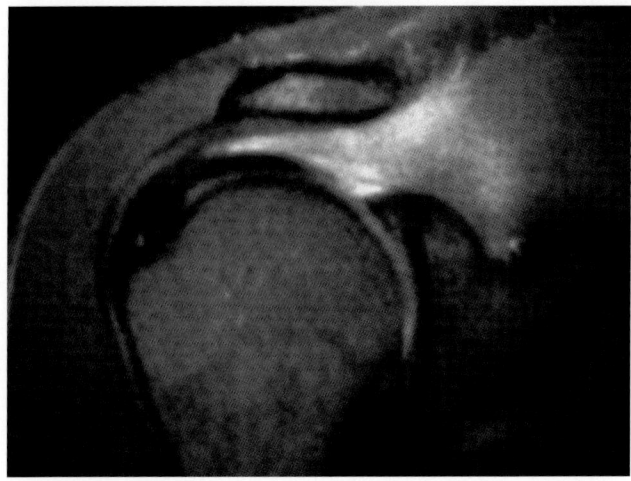

FIGURE 106-18

Coronal proton-density–weighted fat-suppressed MR image through the shoulder of a competitive weightlifter complaining of muscle soreness after prolonged training shows diffuse high signal intensity throughout the visualized supraspinatus muscle. The lack of a history of a recent acute injury, coupled with the nonspecific MR imaging finding of muscle edema, are consistent with delayed-onset muscle soreness.

loss of function after a complete rupture or avulsion in the acute setting, or for persistent pain and functional limitations that may be due to scarring and adhesions in the chronic setting.[268-270]

Delayed-Onset Muscle Soreness

Clinical Presentation

Delayed-onset muscle soreness (DOMS) refers to the pain and soreness in muscles that follows unaccustomed exertion.[271] Unlike strain injuries, patients with DOMS do not recall any one particular moment of trauma or experience an acute onset of pain. Rather, soreness typically begins the day after exertion and then subsides within 1 week. Activities requiring eccentric muscle contractions are common culprits, such as downhill hiking or certain types of manual labor. Muscle affected by DOMS shows good correlation between the ultra-structural remodeling seen on electron microscopy[272] (e.g., loss of regular orientation of the Z bands in muscle) and the signal intensity increases seen on fluid-sensitive MR images.[273]

Imaging

MRI displays high T2 signal intensity indicative of interstitial edema, and is reported to have an MR appearance similar to a first-degree strain (Fig. 106-18). Clinical history can allow for easy differentiation between these two entities in most instances. However, since abnormal signal intensity caused by DOMS may remain for up to 80 days,[274] the history of a provocative event may not be forthcoming in all cases.

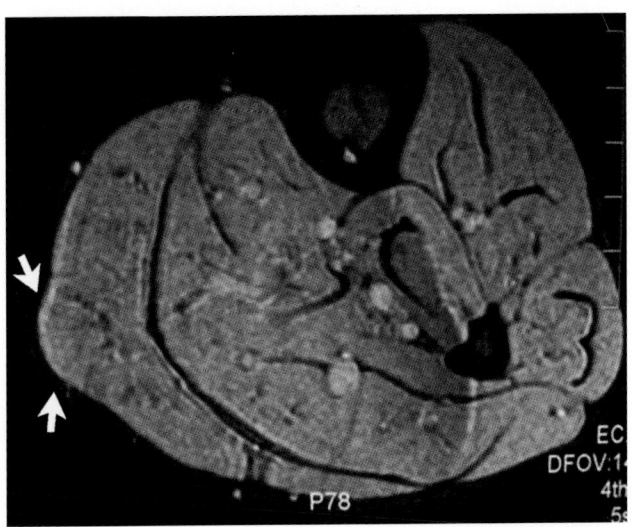

FIGURE 106-19

Axial gradient-recalled echo MR image through the calf acquired during active contraction of the muscles reveals a subtle contour change (*arrows*) along the medial border of the gastrocnemius muscle that resolved in the resting state. On physical examination, there is a palpable mass in this region during active muscle contraction consistent with muscle herniation.

Muscle Laceration

Lacerations are produced by a penetrating injury, such as a knife. MRI demonstrates the acute laceration as a sharply marginated zone of fiber discontinuity with associated T2 hyperintensity caused by hemorrhage and edema. In the chronic setting, volume loss in the muscle may be seen. Fibrotic tissue in the affected muscle is displayed as low T2 signal intensity and any deposition of fat associated with atrophy is manifested as high T1 signal intensity. Interestingly, scar tissue has been found to be mechanically stronger than adjacent atrophic muscle.[275]

Treatment of acutely lacerated muscle by suturing reportedly results in improved functional healing compared to immobilization.[276] Novel, experimental treatments show promise in enhancing muscle recovery,[277] including growth factors (e.g., basic fibroblast growth factor)[276] and the antifibrosis agent decorin,[278] and stem cells[279] show substantial promise.

Muscle Herniation

Clinical Presentation

Muscle herniation refers to protrusion of muscle tissue through a focal fascial defect.[280] These fascial defects occur due to increased intracompartmental pressure (e.g., due to muscle hypertrophy associated with chronic exertional compartment syndrome) or due to traumatic disruption of the fascial sheath.

Although virtually any muscle can be affected, muscle hernias most commonly occur in the middle-to-lower portions of the leg, and involve the tibialis anterior muscle.[281] Herniations of muscle are seen typically as a small, superficial, soft-tissue bulge that becomes more prominent and firm with muscle contraction. Most muscle herniations are asymptomatic, but they can cause substantial pain, cramping, and tenderness.[282,283] Muscle herniations may enlarge over time,[283] become incarcerated,[284] and rarely impinge upon an adjacent nerve.[285]

Imaging

MRI can display herniation of muscle (that typically appears normal in signal intensity) through discontinuous overlying fascia, thus allowing differentiation from a soft-tissue neoplasm (Fig. 106-19).[280,286,287] The outward bulging of muscle is often subtle, and may be elicited dynamically with muscle contraction during MRI or sonography.[282,288]

Treatment

Conservative management is usually adequate, but treatment options reportedly include local injection of botulinum toxin,[283] fasciotomy,[289,290] and fascial repair.[281,291]

Muscle Contusion

Clinical Presentation

Contusion of muscle is produced by direct, blunt trauma. The consequent hemorrhage and edema result in varying degrees of pain, swelling, ecchymosis, hematoma formation, and (in some cases) heterotopic ossification.[292]

Imaging

Fluid-sensitive images demonstrate hyperintense signal that may have a diffuse or geographic appearance, often with feathery margins. Unlike a muscle tear, no gross discontinuity or laxity in muscle fibers is observed. The muscle volume typically appears increased. Although contusion injuries usually appear larger in size than strain injuries, the recovery time for contusions tends to be significantly shorter than for strain injuries (mean time, 19 ± 9 days versus 26 ± 22 days).[293]

Hemorrhage and Hematoma

Clinical Presentation

Hemorrhage may occur interstitially in a nonfocal fashion within the substance of muscle (yielding edema-like signal in the acute setting) or may accumulate focally in the form of a hematoma. Bleeding in the extremities occurs in association with a wide variety of disorders, including trauma, anticoagulation (e.g., heparin), bleeding diathesis (e.g., hemophilia), and focal vascular disorders (e.g., vascular malformation). Hemorrhage into muscle may result in pain,[294] anemia,[295,296] a soft-tissue mass,[296] or a compressive neuropathy.[294,297] For example, a hematoma in the iliacus muscle may cause a femoral nerve neuropathy with associated quadriceps muscle fasciculations[298] or paralysis.[299]

Imaging

The pathophysiology and MR appearances of brain hemorrhage are detailed in Chapter 45. Just as in the brain, sequential formation of specific iron compounds influences the MR appearance of a hematoma in the various stages: oxyhemoglobin, deoxyhemoglobin, intracellular methemoglobin, extracellular methemoglobin, and hemosiderin.[300-302] In addition to the state of hemoglobin breakdown products, other variables potentially influencing the appearance of hemorrhage in the extremities include differences in MR technique (e.g., field strength, echo time) and variables in the hematoma itself (e.g., clot retraction, location, and size of hematoma).

The normal erythrocyte contains hemoglobin that binds oxygen (oxyhemoglobin) and releases oxygen (deoxyhemoglobin). Although active ("hyperacute") hemorrhage in muscle rarely is observed,[300] it is characterized by the presence of oxyhemoglobin, which is diamagnetic (not paramagnetic), and therefore does not produce any substantial T1 or T2 shortening. The "acute" hematoma forms rapidly as oxyhemoglobin is converted to (intracellular) deoxyhemoglobin in the relatively hypoxic environment of a hematoma.[300] Deoxyhemoglobin can cause hypointensity in the center of acute hematomas on T2-weighted images, but does not substantially influence T1 signal intensity.[301]

The "early subacute" hematoma forms as deoxyhemoglobin is oxidized to intracellular methemoglobin. (This oxidation occurs because the metabolic pathways that require oxygen in erythrocytes grind to a halt.) Paramagnetic properties of methemoglobin cause hyperintense signal on T1-weighted images. This T1 hyperintensity often is recognized first at the periphery of a subacute hematoma, producing a "concentric ring" sign (Fig. 106-20).[300,303] T2 shortening caused by intracellular methemoglobin tends to appear similar to that observed with intracellular deoxyhemoglobin. The "late subacute" hematoma forms with the passage of time as lysis of erythrocytes containing methemoglobin occurs. This extracellular methemoglobin remains hyperintense on T1-weighted images, while becoming heterogeneous and often predominantly hyperintense on T2-weighted images.

Finally, the "chronic" hematoma forms as macrophages produce the last iron-containing product of hemoglobin degradation, hemosiderin.[300] Both hemosiderin and the fibrous tissue may contribute to very low signal intensity that may be most conspicuous at the margin of chronic hematomas on T1- and T2-weighted spin-echo images (Fig. 106-21). Hemosiderin characteristically is associated with susceptibility ("blooming") artifact on gradient-echo images.

Intramuscular hematomas often resorb substantially over a period of 6 to 8 weeks,[304] but they may linger for many months.[305] Most of the intramuscular hematomas that have been evaluated with MRI between 2 days[306] and 5 months[307] after injury display characteristics of methemoglobin, with increased signal intensity on both T1- and T2-weighted images.[308] Serous-appearing fluid from a hematoma occasionally may persist to form an

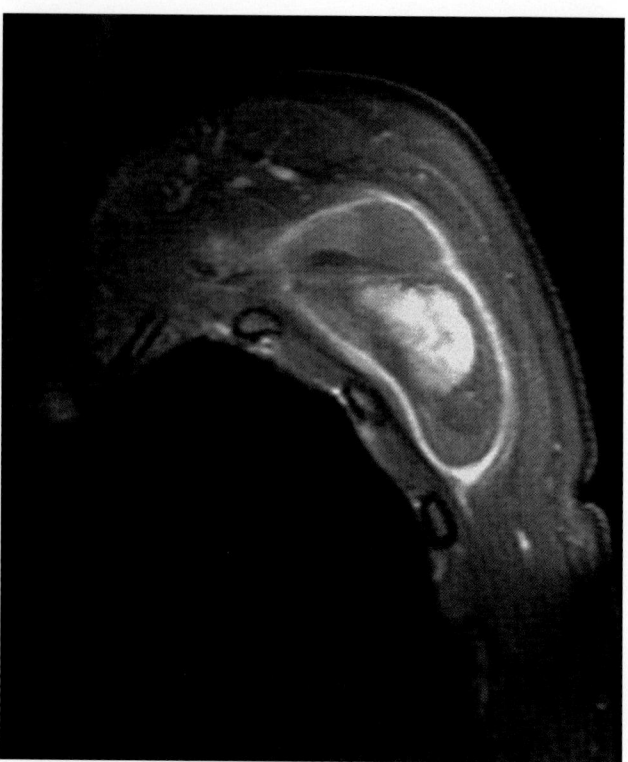

FIGURE 106-20

Sagittal fat-suppressed T1-weighted image of the right chest wall with a history of trauma 3 months earlier demonstrates a heterogenous mass in the posterosuperior soft-tissues superficial to the ribs. Note the high signal rim and the high signal material within the lesion, consistent with methemoglobin.

intramuscular pseudocyst.[309] Pseudotumors after a muscle strain are centered characteristically at the myotendinous junction and composed histologically of blood products, fibrosis, muscle fiber degeneration, and chronic inflammatory cells.[310-313] These pseudotumors are most commonly reported in the rectus femoris, but may be observed at other sites.

Differential Diagnosis

The clinical and imaging differential diagnosis of a benign hematoma sometimes includes a hemorrhagic neoplasm. When the lesion in question shows no contrast enhancement, this generally aids in excluding a neoplasm. Like neoplasms, however, post-traumatic hematomas may show variable contrast enhancement. Therefore, follow-up clinical and MRI evaluation may be indicated when the diagnosis of a probably benign hematoma is in doubt.

Heterotopic Ossification

Heterotopic ossification may be defined as the formation of non-neoplastic bonelike tissue in the soft-tissues. A common location for heterotopic ossification is muscle, and here it is referred to frequently as *myositis ossificans* (even though this is not a primary inflammatory process[314]).

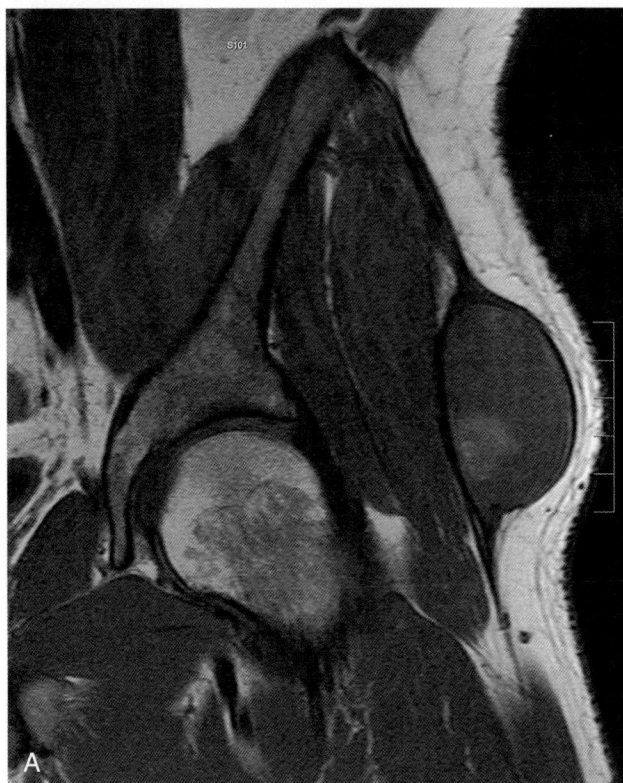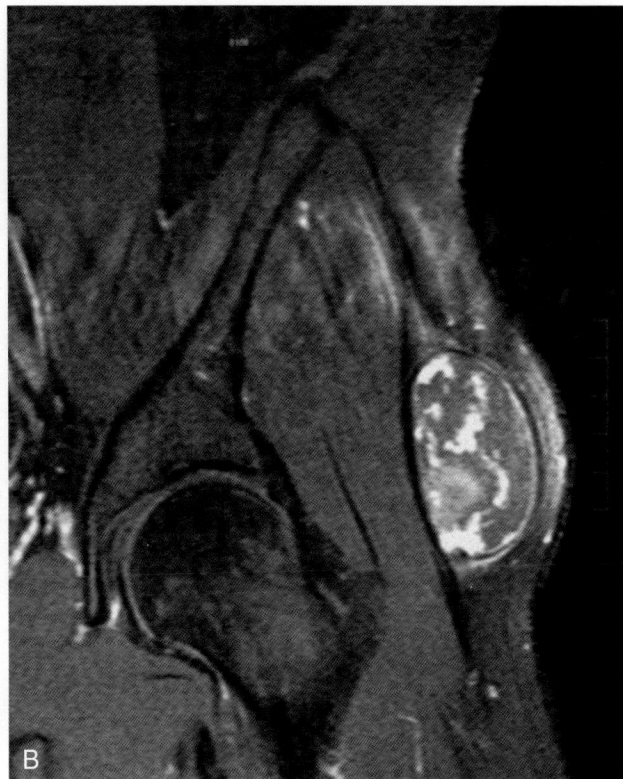

FIGURE 106-21

A, Coronal T1-weighted MR image through the left hip in a patient with prior trauma shows a heterogenous well circumscribed, intermediate signal intensity oval mass superficial to the gluteus medius muscle with a low signal intensity rim. Note the hazy high signal material in the inferior aspect of the lesion, consistent with methemoglobin within a subacute or chronic hematoma. The low intensity rim is indicative of hemosiderin lining a chronic hematoma. **B,** Corresponding coronal T2-weighted MR image demonstrates heterogeneous signal intensity within the mass consistent with blood products in varying stages of organization. The low signal intensity margin on both the T1- and T2-weighted images supports a more chronic stage within the spectrum of hematoma formation.

Heterotopic ossification is acquired most commonly in patients with certain predisposing factors (found in 37-75% of patients[315-318]), including: trauma (e.g., contusion,[319] surgery,[320-322] burns[323]); neurologic insults (e.g., spinal cord injury,[324] traumatic brain injury,[325] stroke[326]); and conditions associated with a propensity for bone formation (e.g., diffuse idiopathic skeletal hyperostosis, ankylosing spondylitis[327]). Rarely, heterotopic ossification occurs in a heritable form, such as fibrodysplasia ossificans progressiva or progressive osseous heteroplasia.[328]

Heterotopic ossification classically may evolve through three histologic, clinical, and radiologic phases: 1. an acute or pseudoinflammatory phase; 2. a subacute or pseudotumoral phase; and 3. a mature, self-limited phase.[329] Although the pathogenesis is not entirely understood, it is hypothesized that certain insults to soft-tissue may trigger an early inflammatory cell reaction,[330] as well as mesenchymal cell metaplasia that results in highly cellular areas of pleomorphic fibroblasts and osteoblasts. Osteoblasts then deposit osteoid in a centripetal fashion. With time, this gives rise to the recognizable zonal architecture that approximates native bone: a mature shell of compact bone peripherally surrounding cancellous bone centrally.

Clinical Presentation

The most common symptoms and signs are pain, tenderness, swelling, and a palpable mass.[331-334] Substantial functional limitations develop in up to 10% of patients.[335] For example, heterotopic ossification may result in nerve impingement, including on the ulnar,[336,337] median,[337] radial,[338] and sciatic nerves.[339] Heterotopic ossification typically targets the large muscles in the hip, thigh, upper arm, and elbow regions.[340-341]

Imaging

In the acute and subacute stages of heterotopic ossification, imaging examinations have a notoriously nonspecific appearance, and therefore serial examinations may be indicated. During the first week, imaging examinations commonly show only vague swelling. Within approximately 2 to 6 weeks after the onset of symptoms, radiography and CT demonstrate foci of nonspecific mineralization.[314,342] Both CT and MRI typically show an ill-defined mass that may be confused with a soft-tissue sarcoma (e.g., osteosarcoma[343]) or infection (e.g., abscess[344]) (Fig. 106-22). Although adjacent osseous destruction is absent, periostitis may be present.

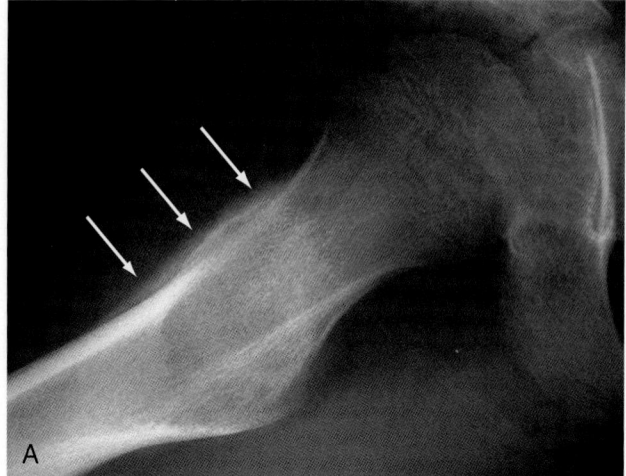

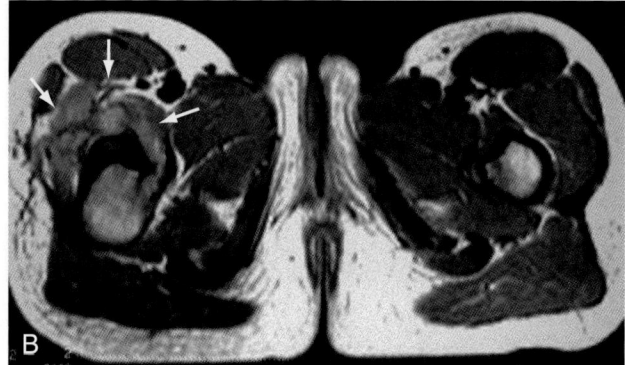
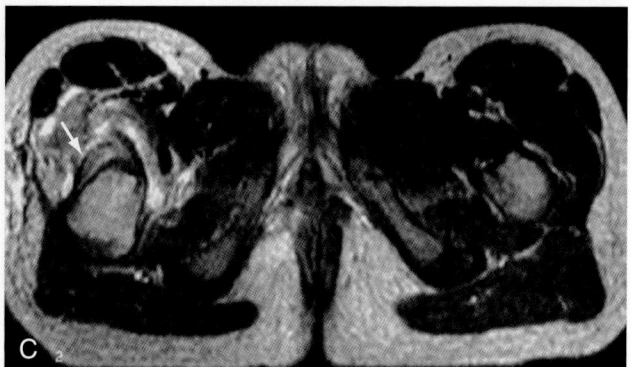

FIGURE 106-22

A, Frog-leg lateral view of the femur of a skeletally immature patient shows subtle increased density (*arrows*) emanating from the anterior femoral shaft, inferior to the anterior facet of the greater trochanter. Corresponding **B,** T1-weighted and **C,** T2-weighted axial MR images through the hips show a soft-tissue mass encircling the anterior half of the femur (*arrows*) in the distribution of the iliopsoas and vastus lateralis muscles. There is intermediate signal on T1-weighted, and heterogeneous signal intensity on T2-weighted images. There is thickening of the anterior cortical margin of the femur (*arrows*) consistent with a periosteal reaction. A recent history of trauma and the absence of adjacent osseous destruction helped establish the diagnosis of myositis ossificans.

Given that this early, immature mineralization is not diagnostic, short-term follow-up radiography or CT (repeated at an interval of 3-4 weeks) is commonly used to confirm suspected heterotopic ossification. By 1 to 2 months after the onset of symptoms, CT typically shows a peripheral rind of mineralization. The diagnostic specificity of CT is higher than MRI (because mineralization is not demonstrated as reliably by MRI), though MRI is the most sensitive technique for identifying small, early lesions.[345]

With MRI, prior to lesion maturity, most heterotopic ossification is displayed as nonspecific intermediate T1 signal intensity and hyperintense T2 signal intensity.[333,344] In the adjacent muscle and bone marrow,[332] nonspecific areas of high T2 signal intensity and contrast enhancement also may be observed. Intralesional fluid-fluid levels may be present in some cases, a nonspecific feature that also may be seen with certain soft-tissue neoplasms (e.g., synovial sarcomas).[334,346] Gadolinium contrast material does not tend to aid in achieving a specific diagnosis. Immature heterotopic ossification may show enhancement centrally or peripherally, while mature lesions show such variable enhancement in 20% of cases.[344] With mature heterotopic ossification, T2 hyperintensity is uncommon and approximately 85% of sites have signal intensity that is equivalent to fat and cortical bone.[344] For detecting areas of soft-tissue

mineralization, gradient-echo pulse sequences can be more sensitive than spin-echo pulse sequences.

In the mature form, the imaging findings that allow confident differentiation of heterotopic ossification from neoplasm include that the well-defined ossific mass is more mature peripherally than centrally, is not associated with underlying bone destruction, and does not grow over time. Heterotopic ossification matures over a period that is usually reported as 6 months to 1.5 years,[347-350] but ranges widely from 3.5 months to longer than 5 years.[344] Resorption of the osseous mass may occur in some patients over a period of 1 year to longer than 5 years.[342,344,351]

Treatment

In high-risk patients, strategies for prevention of heterotopic ossification may include nonsteroidal anti-inflammatory agents (e.g., indomethacin, celecoxib),[352] biphosphonates (e.g., alendronate),[353] and low-dose irradiation therapy.[354] Surgical excision occasionally may be indicated for heterotopic ossification that causes unremitting pain, restricted range of motion, or nerve entrapment.[323,332,355,356] Although much has been written regarding the use of bone scintigraphy to determine lesion maturity preoperatively, this test does not influence operative treatment for many surgeons at present.[323,325]

Muscle Denervation

Clinical Presentation

Denervation of muscle can be associated with pain, weakness, and disability. Muscle denervation may be caused by various insults to nerves, including: entrapment (e.g., by a mass or anomalous muscle); trauma (e.g., mechanical stretch); inflammation (e.g., autoimmune); infection; vascular compromise; and idiopathic causes.[357-359] EMG is used most commonly to evaluate for denervation, but some regard it as painful, operator dependent, and potentially limited in its assessment of small areas of deep muscle.[360]

Imaging

MRI is used increasingly as an adjunct to diagnose the presence of muscle denervation, as well as its cause and location in many cases.[361-366] For example, in a study of 90 patients with clinical evidence of peripheral nerve injury or radiculopathy,[362] the sensitivity and specificity of IR-FSE MRI relative to EMG were 84% and 100%, respectively. In another study prospectively evaluating 40 consecutive patients with foot drop,[367] MRI and EMG were in agreement in 37 (92%) of the patients. In three patients, MRI demonstrated more widespread involvement than EMG, and there were no false-negative MRI results.

The signal intensity and morphology of muscle undergo well-described changes with subacute and chronic denervation.[359-361,368-372] After a nerve insult, changes generally are seen in muscle using MRI within 2 to 3 weeks (though changes have been reported as early as 1 day in animals). In particular, these "subacute" changes in muscle are displayed as high signal intensity on fluid-sensitive images and normal signal intensity on T1-weighted images (Fig. 106-23). T2 hyperintensity in muscle reportedly occurs because of an increase in the extracellular fluid volume or capillary enlargement.[360,370,371]

Although hyperintense T2 signal in muscle is not a specific finding in itself, a specific diagnosis is suggested in the appropriate clinical setting by involvement of a specific nerve territory and substantially hyperintense T2 signal in a peripheral nerve.[361,373] (Normally, peripheral nerves are similar in signal intensity to the normal muscle on T2-weighted images and only mildly hyperintense to normal muscle on fat-suppressed T2-weighted or IR-FSE MR images.[361,373]) In addition, unlike a muscle strain injury, the hyperintense T2 signal in denervated muscles is not associated with perifascial edema.

With chronic denervation, diminished bulk and fatty infiltration occur in muscle. These atrophic changes are best displayed on T1-weighted MR images (Fig. 106-24). The atrophic changes from denervation are not specific, and may be seen with conditions as diverse as motor neuron diseases (e.g., poliomyelitis[374]) and demyelination (e.g., hereditary motor and sensory neuropathies[375]).

The signal intensity changes of subacute muscle denervation can increase until at least 2 months (in an animal model[360,370]) and are reversible. After reinnervation occurs, T2 hyperintensity peaks approximately 2 to 3 weeks later and normalizes by 6 to 10 weeks.[360-371] Profound atrophic changes seen after chronic denervation may be irreversible.[376]

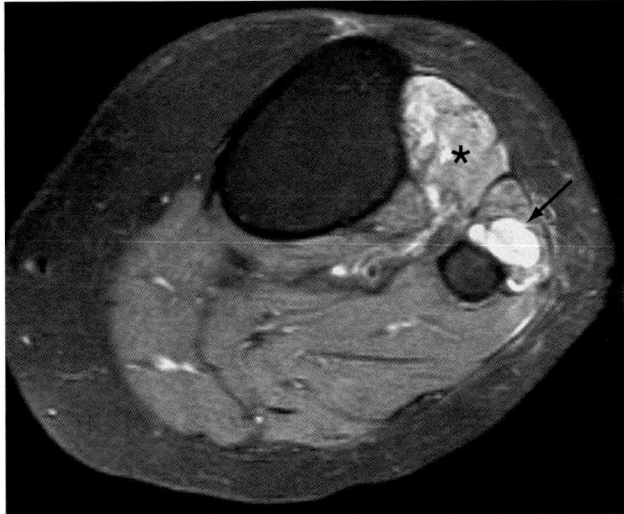

FIGURE 106-23

Axial proton-density–weighted fat-suppressed MR image through the calf shows a well-defined polylobulated fluid collection (arrow) anterior to the proximal fibula, with high signal intensity in the distribution of the tibialis anterior, extensor digitorum longus and peroneus longus muscles (*). This constellation of findings suggests subacute denervation-type injury of the muscle due to a mass effect on the nerve from the ganglion.

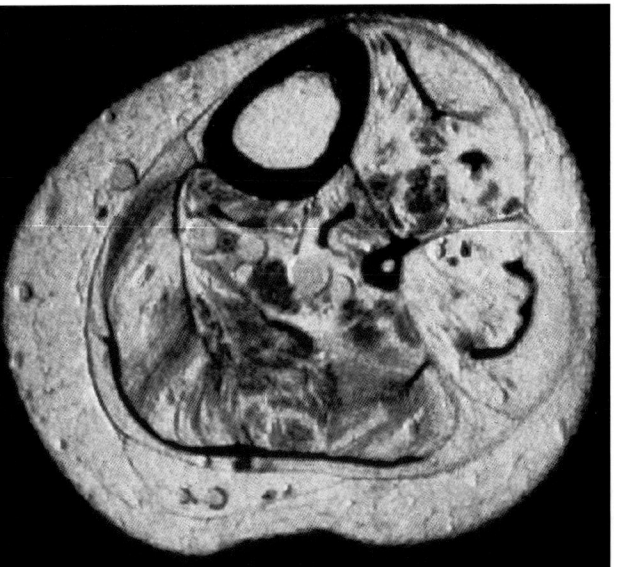

FIGURE 106-24

Axial T1-weighted MR image through the calf of a patient with Charcot-Marie-Tooth disease demonstrates the nonspecific findings of diffuse muscle atrophy, with loss of muscle bulk and fatty infiltration.

Chronic denervation results most commonly in muscle atrophy, but pseudohypertrophy and true hypertrophy may occur in the affected extremity.[377-381] Both pseudohypertrophy and true hypertrophy may result in a palpable soft-tissue mass that serves as an indication for MRI. *Pseudohypertrophy* may occur in denervated muscle when accumulation of fat and connective tissue causes paradoxical muscle enlargement and hyperintense T1 signal intensity due to adipose tissue. *True hypertrophy* may occur in synergistic muscles adjacent to the area of denervation; hypertrophied muscle is isointense with normal muscle.

DIFFERENTIAL DIAGNOSIS

MRI facilitates the diagnostic process primarily by detecting alterations in muscle morphology or signal intensity. Although these alterations may be diagnostic in the appropriate clinical setting, a wide array of focal and systemic pathologic conditions affecting muscle may have a similar appearance. Indeed, skeletal muscle may be afflicted by a spectacular array of primary and systemic disorders. This myriad of insults, however, commonly results in a limited number of biologic responses in muscle. In other words, similar gross pathologic features may be caused by many different disorders. Given that the potential causes for abnormal signal intensity in muscle are diverse, the MRI differential diagnosis may be simplified by recognizing one of three basic patterns on MR images.[357]

The "muscle edema pattern" may be seen with recent trauma (e.g., strain injury), as well as with subacute denervation, infectious or autoimmune myositis, rhabdomyolysis, vascular insult (e.g., diabetic muscle infarction, deep venous thrombosis), or recent iatrogenic insults (e.g., surgery, radiation therapy).

The "fatty infiltration pattern" may be observed in the chronic setting after a high-grade myotendinous injury, as well as with other insults causing chronic muscle disuse or chronic denervation.

The "mass lesion pattern" can be seen with traumatic injuries (e.g., myositis ossificans), as well as with neoplasm, infection (e.g., pyomyositis, parasitic infection), and muscular sarcoidosis.

CONCLUSION

Knowledge of anatomy and the capabilities of various radiologic techniques serves as a prerequisite for interpreting pathologic changes seen on imaging examinations. Muscle disorders have a wide variety of causes, treatments, and prognoses. Given that the cause and severity of musculoskeletal disorders may be difficult to determine clinically, MRI commonly aids in identifying the location, severity, and extent of the pain generator. In so doing, MRI is increasingly playing a key role in influencing treatment, predicting prognosis, guiding invasive procedures, assessing therapeutic response, and monitoring for potential treatment complications.

REFERENCES

1. Bergman RA, Afifi AK, Miyauchi R: Illustrated Encyclopedia of Human Anatomic Variation. Iowa City, IA, Virtual Hospital, University of Iowa, Revised June 2002. Available at http://www.vh.org/Providers/Textbooks/AnatomicVariants/AnatomyHP.html/
2. Newman JS, Adler RS, Rubin JM: Power Doppler sonography: use in measuring alterations in muscle blood volume after exercise. Am J Roentgenol 168:1525-1530, 1997.
3. Love C, Din AS, Tomas MB, et al: Radionuclide bone imaging: an illustrative review. Radiographics 23:341-358, 2003.
4. White LM, Schweitzer ME: MR imaging of musculoskeletal tumors. In Maier CF (ed): Introduction to Orthopedic MR Imaging: A Practical Guide to Orthopedic MRI. Milwaukee, WI, GE Medical Systems, 2000.
5. Yoshioka H, Itai Y, Niitsu M, et al: Intramuscular metastasis from malignant melanoma: MR findings. Skeletal Radiol 28:714-716, 1999.
6. Isiklar I, Leeds NE, Fuller GN, et al: Intracranial metastatic melanoma: correlation between MR imaging characteristics and melanin content. Am J Roentgenol 165:1503-1512, 1995.
7. Hwangbo S: Can we determine T2 signal of musculoskeletal tumorous conditions on fat-suppressed fast spin-echo MR imaging [abstract]? Am J Roentgenol 178(Suppl):68, 2002.
8. Delfaut EM, Beltran J, Johnson G, et al: Fat suppression in MR imaging: techniques and pitfalls. Radiographics 19:373-382, 1999.
9. Rubin DA, Kneeland JB: MR imaging of the musculoskeletal system: technical considerations for enhancing image quality and diagnostic yield. Am J Roentgenol 163:1155-1163, 1994.
10. Pla ME, Dillingham TR, Spellman NT, et al: Painful legs and moving toes associate with tarsal tunnel syndrome and accessory soleus muscle. Mov Disord 11:82-86, 1996.
11. Gold GE: Dynamic and functional imaging of the musculoskeletal system. Semin Musculoskelet Radiol 7:245-248, 2003.
12. Quick HH, Ladd ME, Hoevel M, et al: Real-time MRI of joint movement with true FISP. J Magn Reson Imaging 15:710-715, 2002.
13. Asakawa DS, Pappas GP, Blemker SS, et al: Cine phase-contrast magnetic resonance imaging as a tool for quantification of skeletal muscle motion. Semin Musculoskelet Radiol 7:287-295, 2003.
14. Noseworthy MD, Bulte DP, Alfonsi J: BOLD magnetic resonance imaging of skeletal muscle. Semin Musculoskelet Radiol 7:307-315, 2003.
15. Mark FC, Bock C, Portner HO: Oxygen-limited thermal tolerance in Antarctic fish investigated by MRI and ^{31}P-MRS. Am J Physiol Regul Integr Comp Physiol 283:R1254-R1262, 2002.
16. Patten C, Meyer RA, Fleckenstein JL: T2 mapping of muscle. Semin Musculoskelet Radiol 7:297-305, 2003.
17. Price TB, Kamen G, Damon BM, et al: Comparison of MRI with EMG to study muscle activity associated with dynamic plantar flexion. Magn Reson Imaging 21:853-861, 2003.
18. Warfield SK, Mulkern RV, Winalski CS, et al: An image processing strategy for the quantification and visualization of exercise-induced muscle MRI signal enhancement. J Magn Reson Imaging 11:525-531, 2000.
19. Yanagisawa O, Niitsu M, Yoshioka H, et al: MRI determination of muscle recruitment variations in dynamic ankle plantar flexion exercise. Am J Phys Med Rehabil 82:760-765, 2003.
20. Ploutz LL, Tesch PA, Biro RL, et al: Effect of resistance training on muscle use during exercise. J Appl Physiol 76:1675-1681, 1994.
21. Conley MS, Stone MH, Nimmons M, et al: Resistance training and human cervical muscle recruitment plasticity. J Appl Physiol 83:2105-2111, 1997.
22. Yoshioka H, Anno I, Kuramoto K, et al: Acute effects of exercise on muscle MRI in peripheral arterial occlusive disease. Magn Reson Imaging 13:651-659, 1995.
23. Zeiss J, Guilliam-Haidet L: MR demonstration of anomalous muscles about the volar aspect of the wrist and forearm. Clin Imaging 20:219-221, 1996.
24. Kopsch F: Rauber's Lehrbuch der Anatomie des Menschen. Leipzig, Germany, Thieme, 1908.
25. Boutin RD: Anatomy and MR imaging of sports-related muscle injuries. In RSNA Categorical Course in Diagnostic Radiology: Musculoskeletal Imaging—Exploring New Limits. Oak Brook, IL, Radiological Society of North America, 2003, pp 25-35.
26. Zeiss J, Jakab E: MR demonstration of an anomalous muscle in a patient with coexistent carpal and ulnar tunnel syndrome. Case report and literature summary. Clin Imaging 19:102-105, 1995.
27. Schuurman AH, van Gils AP: Reversed palmaris longus muscle on MRI: report of four cases. Eur Radiol 10:1242-1244, 2000.
28. di Marzo L, Cavallaro A, Sciacca V, et al: Surgical treatment of popliteal artery entrapment syndrome: a ten-year experience. Eur J Vasc Surg 5:59-64, 1991.
29. Atilla S, Akpek ET, Yucel C, et al: MR imaging and MR angiography in popliteal artery entrapment syndrome. Eur Radiol 8:1025-1029, 1998.
30. Takase K, Imakita S, Kuribayashi S, et al: Popliteal artery entrapment syndrome: aberrant origin of gastrocnemius muscle shown by 3D CT. J Comput Assist Tomogr 21:523-528, 1997.
31. Goebel N, Brunner U, Schneider E: CT demonstration of an entrapment syndrome of the popliteal artery. Digitale Bilddiagn 6:28-30, 1986.
32. Radonic V, Koplic S, Giunio L, et al: Popliteal artery entrapment syndrome: diagnosis and management, with report of three cases. Tex Heart Inst J 27:3-13, 2000.

33. Elias DA, White LM, Rubenstein JD, et al: Clinical evaluation and MR imaging features of popliteal artery entrapment and cystic adventitial disease. Am J Roentgenol 180:627-632, 2003.
34. Grasso A, Dini P, Allegra M: An accessory musculus soleus (symptomatic and asymptomatic). The CT findings. Radiol Med (Torino) 84:22-25, 1992.
35. Buschmann WR, Cheung Y, Jahss MH: Magnetic resonance imaging of anomalous leg muscles: accessory soleus, peroneus quartus and the flexor digitorum longus accessories. Foot Ankle 12:109-116, 1991.
36. Lorentzon R, Wirell S: Anatomic variations of the accessory soleus muscle. Acta Radiol 28:627-629, 1987.
37. Romanus B, Lindahl S, Stener B: Accessory soleus muscle. A clinical and radiographic presentation of eleven cases. J Bone Joint Surg Am 68:731-734, 1986.
38. Hallock GG, Lutz DA, Osborne MA: Nonoperative estimation of the soleus musculotendinous junction using magnetic resonance imaging. Plast Reconstr Surg 100:896-899, 1997.
39. Featherstone T: MRI diagnosis of accessory soleus muscle strain. Br J Sports Med 29:277-278, 1995.
40. DosRemedios ET, Jolly GP: The accessory soleus and recurrent tarsal tunnel syndrome: case report of a new surgical approach. J Foot Ankle Surg 39:194-197, 2000.
41. Yu JS, Resnick D: MR imaging of the accessory soleus muscle appearance in six patients and a review of the literature. Skeletal Radiol 23:525-528, 1994.
42. Ekstrom JE, Shuman WP, Mack LA: MR imaging of accessory soleus muscle. J Comput Assist Tomogr 14:239-242, 1990.
43. Travis MT, Pitcher JD: Accessory soleus presenting as a posterior ankle mass: a case report and literature review. Foot Ankle Int 16:651-654, 1995.
44. Gordon SL, Matheson DW: The accessory soleus. Clin Orthop 97:129-132, 1973.
45. Reimers CD, Fischer P, Pongratz DE: Histopathological basis of muscle imaging. In Fleckenstein JL, Crues JV, Reimers CD (eds): Muscle Imaging in Health and Disease. New York, Springer, 1996.
46. Fleckenstein JL: MRI of neuromuscular disease: the basics. Semin Musculoskelet Radiol 4:393-419, 2000.
47. Davies NP, Hanna MG: The skeletal muscle channelopathies: distinct entities and overlapping syndromes. Curr Opin Neurol 16:559-568, 2003.
48. Reimers CD: Imaging in myology: a neurologist's perspective. Semin Musculoskelet Radiol 4:367-373, 2000.
49. Kissel JT, Mendell JR: Muscular dystrophy: historical overview and classification in the genetic era. Semin Neurol 19:5-7, 1999.
50. Toniolo D, Minetti C: Muscular dystrophies: alterations in a limited number of cellular pathways? Curr Opin Genet Dev 9:275-282, 1999.
51. Bushby KM: The limb-girdle muscular dystrophies—multiple genes, multiple mechanisms. Hum Mol Genet 8:1875-1882, 1999.
52. Brown RH Jr: Dystrophin-associated proteins and the muscular dystrophies. Annu Rev Med 48:457-466, 1997.
53. Fadic R, Waclawik AJ, Lewandoski PJ, et al: Muscle pathology and clinical features of the sarcolemmopathies. Pediatr Neurol 16:79-82, 1997.
54. Engvall E, Wewer UM: The new frontier in muscular dystrophy research: booster genes. FASEB J 17:1579-1584, 2003.
55. Wagner KR: Genetic diseases of muscle. Neurol Clin 20:645-678, 2002.
56. DeVisser M, Schalke BCG, Reimers CD: Muscular dystrophies. In Fleckenstein JL, Crues JV, Reimers CD (eds): Muscle Imaging in Health and Disease. New York, Springer, 1996, pp 219-236.
57. Liu GC, Jong YJ, Chiang CH, et al: Duchenne muscular dystrophy: MR grading system with functional correlation. Radiology 186:475-480, 1993.
58. Gong QY, Phoenix J, Kemp GJ, et al: Estimation of body composition in muscular dystrophy by MRI and stereology. J Magn Reson Imaging 12:467-475, 2000.
59. Leroy-Willig A, Willig TN, Henry-Feugeas MC, et al: Body composition determined with MR in patients with Duchenne muscular dystrophy, spinal muscular atrophy, and normal subjects. Magn Reson Imaging 15:737-744, 1997.
60. Chan WP, Liu GC: MR imaging of primary skeletal muscle diseases in children. Am J Roentgenol 179:989-997, 2002.
61. McDaniel JD, Ulmer JL, Prost RW: Magnetization transfer imaging of skeletal muscle in autosomal recessive limb girdle muscular dystrophy. J Comput Assist Tomogr 23:609-614, 1999.
62. Franczak MB, Ulmer JL, Jaradeh S, et al: Spin-lock magnetic resonance imaging of muscle in patients with autosomal recessive limb girdle muscular dystrophy. J Neuroimaging 10:73-77, 2000.
63. Constantinides CD, Gillen JS, Boada FE, et al: Human skeletal muscle: sodium MR imaging and quantification—potential applications in exercise and disease. Radiology 216:559-568, 2000.
64. Kushnir T, Knubovets T, Itzchak Y, et al: In vivo 23Na NMR studies of myotonic dystrophy. Magn Reson Med 37:192-196, 1997.
65. Sohn RL, Gussoni E: Stem cell therapy for muscular dystrophy. Expert Opin Biol Ther 4:1-9, 2004.
66. Politano L, Nigro G, Nigro V, et al: Gentamicin administration in Duchenne patients with premature stop codon. Preliminary results. Acta Myol 22:15-21, 2003.
67. Wortmann RL, DiMauro S: Differentiating idiopathic inflammatory myopathies from metabolic myopathies. Rheum Dis Clin North Am 28:759-778, 2002.
68. De Kerviler E, Leroy-Willig A, Duboc D, et al: MR quantification of muscle fatty replacement in McArdle's disease. Magn Reson Imaging 14:1137-1141, 1996.
69. Laforet P, Wary C, Duteil S, et al: Exploration of exercise intolerance by 31P NMR spectroscopy of calf muscles coupled with MRI and ergometry. Rev Neurol (Paris) 159:56-67, 2003.
70. Gordon BA, Martinez S, Collins AJ: Pyomyositis: characteristics at CT and MR imaging. Radiology 197:279-286, 1995.
71. Hall RL, Callaghan JJ, Moloney E, et al: Pyomyositis in a temperate climate. Presentation, diagnosis, and treatment. J Bone Joint Surg Am 72:1240-1244, 1990.
72. Chiedozi LC: Pyomyositis. Review of 205 cases in 112 patients. Am J Surg 137:255-259, 1979.
73. Steinbach LS, Tehranzadeh J, Fleckenstein JL, et al: Human immuno-deficiency virus infection: musculoskeletal manifestations. Radiology 186:833-838, 1993.
74. Martinez-de Jesus FR, Mendiola-Segura I: Clinical stage, age and treatment in tropical pyomyositis: a retrospective study including forty cases. Arch Med Res 27:165-170, 1996.
75. Patel SR, Olenginski TP, Perruquet JL, et al: Pyomyositis: clinical features and predisposing conditions. J Rheumatol 24:1734-1738, 1997.
76. Spiegel DA, Meyer JS, Dormans JP, et al: Pyomyositis in children and adolescents: report of 12 cases and review of the literature. J Pediatr Orthop 19:143-150, 1999.
77. Ameh EA: Pyomyositis in children: analysis of 31 cases. Ann Trop Paediatr 19:263-265, 1999.
78. Bickels J, Ben-Sira L, Kessler A, et al: Primary pyomyositis. J Bone Joint Surg Am 84-A:2277-2286, 2002.
79. Trusen A, Beissert M, Schultz G, et al: Ultrasound and MRI features of pyomyositis in children. Eur Radiol 13:1050-1055, 2003.
80. Hernandez RJ, Strouse PJ, Craig CL, et al: Focal pyomyositis of the perisciatic muscles in children. Am J Roentgenol 179:1267-1271, 2002.
81. Wilson DJ: Soft tissue and joint infection. Eur Radiol 14:E64-E71, 2004.
82. Tsirantonaki M, Michael P, Koufos C: Pyomyositis. Clin Rheumatol 17:333-334, 1998.
83. UNAIDS: Epidemiological software and tools. Available at http://www.unaids.org/en/resources/epidemiology.
84. Biviji AA, Paiement GD, Steinbach LS: Musculoskeletal manifestations of human immunodeficiency virus infection. J Am Acad Orthop Surg 10:312-320, 2002.
85. Tehranzadeh J, Ter-Oganesyan RR, Steinbach LS: Musculoskeletal disorders associated with HIV infection and AIDS. Part I: infectious musculoskeletal conditions. Skeletal Radiol 33:249-259, 2004.
86. Plonquet A, Bassez G, Authier FJ, et al: Toxoplasmic myositis as a presenting manifestation of idiopathic CD4 lymphocytopenia. Muscle Nerve 27:761-765, 2003.
87. Johnson RW, Williams FM, Kazi S, et al: Human immunodeficiency virus-associated polymyositis: a longitudinal study of outcome. Arthritis Rheum 49:172-178, 2003.
88. Masanes F, Pedrol E, Grau JM, et al: Symptomatic myopathies in HIV-1 infected patients untreated with antiretroviral agents—a clinico-pathological study of 30 consecutive patients. Clin Neuropathol 15:221-225, 1996.
89. Fleckenstein JL, Burns DK, Murphy FK, et al: Differential diagnosis of bacterial myositis in AIDS: evaluation with MR imaging. Radiology 179:653-658, 1991.
90. Beggs I: Primary muscle lymphoma. Clin Radiol 52:203-212, 1997.
91. Chevalier X, Amoura Z, Viard JP, et al: Skeletal muscle lymphoma in patients with the acquired immunodeficiency syndrome: a diagnostic challenge. Arthritis Rheum 36:426-427, 1993.
92. Lewis W, Gonzalez B, Chomyn A, et al: Zidovudine induces molecular, bio-chemical, and ultrastructural changes in rat skeletal muscle mitochondria. J Clin Invest 89:1354-1360, 1992.
93. Mhiri C, Baudrimont M, Bonne G, et al: Zidovudine myopathy: a distinctive disorder associated with mitochondrial dysfunction. Ann Neurol 29:606-614, 1991.
94. Peraldi MN, Maslo C, Akposso K, et al: Acute renal failure in the course of HIV infection: a single-institution retrospective study of ninety-two patients and sixty renal biopsies. Nephrol Dial Transplant 14:1578-1585, 1999.
95. Eustace S, McEnif N, Rastegar J, et al: Acute HIV polymyositis with complicating myoglobinuric renal failure: CT appearance. J Comput Assist Tomogr 19:321-323, 1995.
96. Joshi MK, Liu HH: Acute rhabdomyolysis and renal failure in HIV-infected patients: risk factors, presentation, and pathophysiology. AIDS Patient Care STDS 14:541-548, 2000.
97. McDonagh CA, Holman RP: Primary human immunodeficiency virus type 1 infection in a patient with acute rhabdomyolysis. South Med J 96: 1027-1030, 2003.
98. Mah Ming JB, Gill MJ: Drug-induced rhabdomyolysis after concomitant use of clarithromycin, atorvastatin, and lopinavir/ritonavir in a patient with HIV. AIDS Patient Care STDS 17:207-210, 2003.
99. Mendila M, Walter GF, Stoll M, et al: Rhabdomyolysis in antiretroviral therapy with Lamivudin. Dtsch Med Wochenschr 122:1003-1006, 1997.
100. Kotler DP: Body composition studies in HIV-infected individuals. Ann N Y Acad Sci 904:546-552, 2000.

101. Engelson ES, Kotler DP, Tan Y, et al: Fat distribution in HIV-infected patients reporting truncal enlargement quantified by whole-body magnetic resonance imaging. Am J Clin Nutr 69:1162-1169, 1999.

102. Zinna EM, Yarasheski KE: Exercise treatment to counteract protein wasting of chronic diseases. Curr Opin Clin Nutr Metab Care 6:87-93, 2003.

103. Barnard J, Newman LS: Sarcoidosis: immunology, rheumatic involvement, and therapeutics. Curr Opin Rheumatol 13:84-91, 2001.

104. Otake S, Ishigaki T: Muscular sarcoidosis. Semin Musculoskelet Radiol 5:167-170, 2001.

105. Baydur A, Pandya K, Sharma OP, et al: Control of ventilation, respiratory muscle strength, and granulomatous involvement of skeletal muscle in patients with sarcoidosis. Chest 103:396-402, 1993.

106. Otake S: Sarcoidosis involving skeletal muscle: imaging findings and relative value of imaging procedures. Am J Roentgenol 162:369-375, 1994.

107. Yamamoto T, Nagira K, Akisue T, et al: Aspiration biopsy of nodular sarcoidosis of the muscle. Diagn Cytopathol 26:109-112, 2002.

108. Andonopoulos AP, Papadimitriou C, Melachrinou M, et al: Asymptomatic gastrocnemius muscle biopsy: an extremely sensitive and specific test in the pathologic confirmation of sarcoidosis presenting with hilar adenopathy. Clin Exp Rheumatol 19:569-572, 2001.

109. Moore SL, Teirstein AE: Musculoskeletal sarcoidosis: spectrum of appearances at MR imaging. Radiographics 23:1389-1399, 2003.

110. Sohn HS, Kim EN, Park JM, et al: Muscular sarcoidosis: Ga-67 scintigraphy and magnetic resonance imaging. Clin Nucl Med 26:29-32, 2001.

111. Senju R, Sakito O, Fukushima K, et al: MRI findings of muscular sarcoidosis. Rinsho Hoshasen 35:703-708, 1990.

112. Oddis CV: Idiopathic inflammatory myopathies. In Wortmann RL (ed): Diseases of Skeletal Muscle. Philadelphia, Lippincott Williams & Wilkins, 2000.

113. Messner RP: Pathogenesis of idiopathic inflammatory myopathies. In Wortmann RL, (ed): Diseases of Skeletal Muscle. Philadelphia, Lippincott Williams & Wilkins, 2000.

114. Yazici Y, Kagen LJ: Clinical presentation of the idiopathic inflammatory myopathies, Rheum Dis Clin North Am 28:823-832, 2002.

115. Mastaglia FL, Phillips BA: Idiopathic inflammatory myopathies: epidemiology, classification, and diagnostic criteria. Rheum Dis Clin North Am 28:723-741, 2002.

116. Oddis CV: Idiopathic inflammatory myopathy: management and prognosis. Rheum Dis Clin North Am 28: 979-1001, 2002.

117. Reed AM, Ytterberg SR: Genetic and environmental risk factors for idiopathic inflammatory myopathies. Rheum Dis Clin North Am 28:891-916, 2002.

118. Dalakas MC: Muscle biopsy findings in inflammatory myopathies. Rheum Dis Clin North Am 28:779-798, 2002.

119. Akira M, Hara H, Sakatani M: Interstitial lung disease in association with polymyositis-dermatomyositis: long-term follow-up CT evaluation in seven patients. Radiology 210:333-338, 1999.

120. Maugars YM, Berthelot JM, Abbas AA, et al: Long-term prognosis of 69 patients with dermatomyositis or polymyositis. Clin Exp Rheumatol 14:263-274, 1996.

121. Dourmishev LA: Dermatomyositis associated with malignancy. 12 case reports. Adv Exp Med Biol 455:193-199, 1999.

122. Maoz CR, Langevitz P, Livneh A, et al: High incidence of malignancies in patients with dermatomyositis and polymyositis: an 11-year analysis. Semin Arthritis Rheum 27:319-324, 1998.

123. Sigurgeirsson B, Lindelof B, Edhag O, et al: Risk of cancer in patients with dermatomyositis or polymyositis. A population-based study. N Engl J Med 326:363-367, 1992.

124. Buchbinder R, Forbes A, Hall S, et al: Incidence of malignant disease in biopsy-proven inflammatory myopathy. A population-based cohort study. Ann Intern Med 134:1087-1095, 2001.

125. Buchbinder R, Hill CL: Malignancy in patients with inflammatory myopathy. Curr Rheumatol Rep 4:415-426, 2002.

126. Bohan A, Peter JB: Polymyositis and dermatomyositis. N Engl J Med 292:344-407, 1975.

127. Schweitzer ME, Fort J: Cost-effectiveness of MR imaging in evaluating polymyositis. Am J Roentgenol 165:1469-1471, 1995.

128. Hausmanowa-Petrusewicz I, Kowalska-Oledzka E, Miller FW, et al: Clinical, serologic, and immunogenetic features in Polish patients with idiopathic inflammatory myopathies. Arthritis Rheum 40:1257-1266, 1997.

129. de Rooij DJ, Van de Putte LB, Habets WJ, et al: Marker antibodies in scleroderma and polymyositis: clinical associations. Clin Rheumatol 8:231-237, 1989.

130. Garcia J: MRI in inflammatory myopathies. Skeletal Radiol 29:425-438, 2000.

131. Targoff IN: Laboratory testing in the diagnosis and management of idiopathic inflammatory myopathies. Rheum Dis Clin North Am 28:859-890, 2002.

132. Adams EM, Chow CK, Premkumar A, et al: The idiopathic inflammatory myopathies: spectrum of MR imaging findings. Radiographics 15:563-574, 1995.

133. Lacomis D: Electrodiagnostic approach to the patient with suspected myopathy. Neurol Clin 20:587-603, 2002.

134. Dion E, Cherin P, Payan C, et al: Magnetic resonance imaging criteria for distinguishing between inclusion body myositis and polymyositis. J Rheumatol 29:1897-1906, 2002.

135. Sekul EA, Chow C, Dalakas MC: Magnetic resonance imaging of the forearm as a diagnostic aid in patients with sporadic inclusion body myositis. Neurology 48:863-866, 1997.

136. Lam WW, Chan H, Chan YL, et al: MR imaging in amyopathic dermatomyositis. Acta Radiol 40:69-72, 1999.

137. Park JH, Olsen NJ, King L Jr, et al: Use of magnetic resonance imaging and P-31 magnetic resonance spectroscopy to detect and quantify muscle dysfunction in the amyopathic and myopathic variants of dermatomyositis. Arthritis Rheum 38:68-77, 1995.

138. Reimers CD, Schedel H, Fleckenstein JL, et al: Magnetic resonance imaging of skeletal muscles in idiopathic inflammatory myopathies of adults. J Neurol 241:306-314, 1994.

139. Hernandez RJ, Keim DR, Chenevert TL, et al: Fat-suppressed MR imaging of myositis. Radiology 182:217-219, 1992.

140. Chung YL, Smith EC, Williams SC, et al: In vivo proton magnetic resonance spectroscopy in polymyositis and dermatomyositis: a preliminary study. Eur J Med Res 2:483-487, 1997.

141. Schedel H, Reimers CD, Vogl T, et al: Muscle edema in MR imaging of neuromuscular diseases. Acta Radiol 36:228-232, 1995.

142. Hargaden G, O'Connell M, Kavanagh E, et al: Current concepts in whole-body imaging using turbo short tau inversion recovery MR imaging. Am J Roentgenol 180:247-252, 2003.

143. O'Connell MJ, Powell T, Brennan D, et al: Whole-body MR imaging in the diagnosis of polymyositis. Am J Roentgenol 179:967-971, 2002.

144. Bartlett ML, Ginn L, Beitz L, et al: Quantitative assessment of myositis in thigh muscles using magnetic resonance imaging. Magn Reson Imaging 17:183-191, 1999.

145. Yao L, Dalakas M, Gahl W, et al: MRI assessment of myopathy: an illustration of analysis driven protocol design. Paper presented at the Radiological Society of North America Annual Meeting, 2003, Chicago.

146. Park JH, Kari S, King LE Jr, et al: Analysis of ^{31}P MR spectroscopy data using artificial neural networks for longitudinal evaluation of muscle diseases: dermatomyositis. NMR Biomed 11:245-256, 1998.

147. Park JH, Olsen NJ: Utility of magnetic resonance imaging in the evaluation of patients with inflammatory myopathies. Curr Rheumatol Rep 3:334-345, 2001.

148. Beese MS, Winkler G, Nicolas V, et al: The diagnosis of inflammatory muscular and vascular diseases using MRT with STIR sequences. Rofo Fortschr Geb Rontgenstr Neuen Bildgeb Verfahr 158:542-549, 1993.

149. Campellone JV, Lacomis D, Giuliani MJ, et al: Percutaneous needle muscle biopsy in the evaluation of patients with suspected inflammatory myopathy. Arthritis Rheum 40:1886-1891, 1997.

150. Sultan SM, Ioannou Y, Moss K, et al: Outcome in patients with idiopathic inflammatory myositis: morbidity and mortality. Rheumatology (Oxford) 41:22-26, 2002.

151. Niermann KJ, Olsen NJ, Park JH: Magnesium abnormalities of skeletal muscle in dermatomyositis and juvenile dermatomyositis. Arthritis Rheum 46:475-488, 2002.

152. Ramanan AV, Feldman BM: Clinical features and outcomes of juvenile dermatomyositis and other childhood onset myositis syndromes. Rheum Dis Clin North Am 28:833-857, 2002.

153. Pachman LM, Hayford JR, Chung A, et al: Juvenile dermatomyositis at diagnosis: clinical characteristics of 79 children. J Rheumatol 25:1198-1204, 1998.

154. Bahner D, Meller J, Stiefel M, et al: Juvenile dermatomyositis—acute recidivism or sepsis? Nervenarzt 70:547-551, 1999.

155. Callen JP: Dermatomyositis. Lancet 355:53-57, 2000.

156. Huber AM, Lang B, LeBlanc CM, et al: Medium- and long-term functional outcomes in a multicenter cohort of children with juvenile dermatomyositis. Arthritis Rheum 43:541-549, 2000.

157. Tabarki B, Ponsot G, Prieur AM, et al: Childhood dermatomyositis: clinical course of 36 patients treated with low doses of corticosteroids. Eur J Paediatr Neurol 2:205-211, 1998.

158. Samson C, Soulen RL, Gursel E: Milk of calcium fluid collections in juvenile dermatomyositis: MR characteristics. Pediatr Radiol 30:28-29, 2000.

159. Hesla RB, Karlson LK, McCauley RG: Milk of calcium fluid collection in dermatomyositis: ultrasound findings. Pediatr Radiol 20:344-346, 1990.

160. Kimball AB, Summers RM, Turner M, et al: Magnetic resonance imaging detection of occult skin and subcutaneous abnormalities in juvenile dermatomyositis. Implications for diagnosis and therapy. Arthritis Rheum 43:1866-1873, 2000.

161. Maillard SM, Jones R, Owens C, et al: Quantitative assessment of MRI T2 relaxation time of thigh muscles in juvenile dermatomyositis. Rheumatology (Oxford) 43:603-608, 2004.

162. Fishel B, Diamant S, Papo I, et al: CT assessment of calcinosis in a patient with dermatomyositis. Clin Rheumatol 5:242-244, 1986.

163. Hilario MO, Yamashita H, Lutti D, et al: Juvenile idiopathic inflammatory myopathies: the value of magnetic resonance imaging in the detection of muscle involvement. Sao Paulo Med J 118:35-40, 2000.

164. Al-Mayouf S, Al-Mazyed A, Bahabri S: Efficacy of early treatment of severe juvenile dermatomyositis with intravenous methylprednisolone and methotrexate. Clin Rheumatol 19:138-141, 2000.

165. Mubarak SJ, Hargens AR, Owen CA, et al: The wick catheter technique for measurement of intramuscular pressure. A new research and clinical tool. J Bone Joint Surg Am 58:1016-1020, 1976.

166. Jobe MT: Compartment syndromes and Volkmann contracture. In Canale ST (ed): Campbell's Operative Orthopaedics. St Louis, Mosby, 1998.

167. Fraipont MJ, Adamson GJ: Chronic exertional compartment syndrome. J Am Acad Orthop Surg 11:268-276, 2003.

168. Elliott KG, Johnstone AJ: Diagnosing acute compartment syndrome. J Bone Joint Surg Br 85:625-632, 2003.

169. Kuklo TR, Tis JE, Moores LK, et al: Fatal rhabdomyolysis with bilateral gluteal, thigh, and leg compartment syndrome after the Army Physical Fitness Test. A case report. Am J Sports Med 28:112-116, 2000.

170. Finkelstein JA, Hunter GA, Hu RW: Lower limb compartment syndrome: course after delayed fasciotomy. J Trauma 40:342-344, 1996.

171. Eaton RG, Green WT: Epimysiotomy and fasciotomy in the treatment of Volkmann's ischemic contracture. Orthop Clin North Am 3:175-186, 1972.

172. Botte MJ, Keenan MA, Gelberman RH: Volkmann's ischemic contracture of the upper extremity. Hand Clin 14:483-497, 1998.

173. Schwartz JT Jr, Brumback RJ, Lakatos R, et al: Acute compartment syndrome of the thigh. A spectrum of injury. J Bone Joint Surg Am 71:392-400, 1989.

174. McQueen MM, Gaston P, Court-Brown CM: Acute compartment syndrome. Who is at risk? J Bone Joint Surg Br 82:200-203, 2000.

175. Fronek J, Mubarak SJ, Hargens AR, et al: Management of chronic exertional anterior compartment syndrome of the lower extremity. Clin Orthop 220:217-227, 1987.

176. Hutchinson MR, Ireland ML: Common compartment syndromes in athletes. Treatment and rehabilitation. Sports Med 17:200-208, 1994.

177. Willis RB, Rorabeck CH: Treatment of compartment syndrome in children. Orthop Clin North Am 21:401-412, 1990.

178. Turnipseed WD, Hurschler C, Vanderby R Jr: The effects of elevated compartment pressure on tibial arteriovenous flow and relationship of mechanical and biochemical characteristics of fascia to genesis of chronic anterior compartment syndrome. J Vasc Surg 21:810-816, 1995.

179. Willy C, Gerngross H, Sterk J: Measurement of intracompartmental pressure with use of a new electronic transducer-tipped catheter system. J Bone Joint Surg Am 81:158-168, 1999.

180. Giannotti G, Cohn SM, Brown M, et al: Utility of near-infrared spectroscopy in the diagnosis of lower extremity compartment syndrome. J Trauma 48:396-399, 2000.

181. Mohler LR, Styf JR, Pedowitz RA, et al: Intramuscular deoxygenation during exercise in patients who have chronic anterior compartment syndrome of the leg. J Bone Joint Surg Am 79:844-849, 1997.

182. Breit GA, Gross JH, Watenpaugh DE, et al: Near-infrared spectroscopy for monitoring of tissue oxygenation of exercising skeletal muscle in a chronic compartment syndrome model. J Bone Joint Surg Am 79:838-843, 1997.

183. van den Brand JG, Verleisdonk EJ, van der Werken C: Near infrared spectroscopy in the diagnosis of chronic exertional compartment syndrome. Am J Sports Med 32:452-456, 2004.

184. Nkele C, Aindow J, Grant L: Study of pressure of the normal anterior tibial compartment in different age groups using the slit-catheter method. J Bone Joint Surg Am 70:98-101, 1988.

185. Pedowitz RA, Hargens AR, Mubarak SJ, et al: Modified criteria for the objective diagnosis of chronic compartment syndrome of the leg. Am J Sports Med 18:35-40, 1990.

186. McCarthy DM, Sotereanos DG, Towers JD, et al: A cadaveric and radiologic assessment of catheter placement for the measurement of forearm compartment pressures. Clin Orthop 312:266-270, 1995.

187. Dominic WJ, Field TO Jr, Hansbrough JF: Comparison of wick and fibreoptic catheters in measurement of interstitial pressures in burned extremities. Burns Incl Therm Inj 14:125-129, 1988.

188. Sievers KW, Hogerle S, Olivier LC, et al: Magnetic resonance tomography evaluation of the lower limb after compartment syndrome. Unfallchirurgie 21:64-69, 1995.

189. Wilke N, Landsleitner B: Monitoring of an acute compartment syndrome of unusual etiology using MRI (magnetic resonance tomography) and MRS. Handchir Mikrochir Plast Chir 22:255-260, 1990.

190. Kumar PR, Jenkins JP, Hodgson SP: Bilateral chronic exertional compartment syndrome of the dorsal part of the forearm: the role of magnetic resonance imaging in diagnosis: a case report. J Bone Joint Surg Am 85-A:1557-1559, 2003.

191. Rominger MB, Lukosch CJ, Bachmann GF: MR imaging of compartment syndrome of the lower leg: a case control study. Eur Radiol 14:1432-1439, 2004.

192. Orava S, Rantanen J, Kujala UM: Fasciotomy of the posterior femoral muscle compartment in athletes. Int J Sports Med 19:71-75, 1998.

193. Geske B, Jerosch J, Reifenrath M: Compartment syndrome after impact trauma from a car bumper. Dtsch Med Wochenschr 116:375-378, 1991.

194. Eskelin MK, Lotjonen JM, Mantysaari MJ: Chronic exertional compartment syndrome: MR imaging at 0.1 T compared with tissue pressure measurement. Radiology 206:333-337, 1998.

195. Ryan M, Eustace S, Brennan D: Pre and post exercise fast spin-echo inversion recovery imaging in the diagnosis of compartment syndrome. Paper presented at the Radiologic Society of North America Annual Meeting, 2003, Chicago.

196. Kiuru MJ, Mantysaari MJ, Pihlajamaki HK, et al: Evaluation of stress-related anterior lower leg pain with magnetic resonance imaging and intracompartmental pressure measurement. Mil Med 168:48-52, 2003.

197. Leppilahti J, Tervonen O, Herva R, et al: Acute bilateral exercise-induced medial compartment syndrome of the thigh. Correlation of repeated MRI with clinicopathological findings. Int J Sports Med 23:610-5, 2002.

198. Amendola A, Rorabeck CH, Vellett D, et al: The use of magnetic resonance imaging in exertional compartment syndromes. Am J Sports Med 18:29-34, 1990.

199. Yao L, Sinha U: Imaging the microcirculatory proton fraction of muscle with diffusion-weighted echo-planar imaging. Acad Radiol 7:27-32, 2000.

200. Myerson MS: Management of compartment syndromes of the foot. Clin Orthop 271:239-248, 1991.

201. Swain R, Ross D: Lower extremity compartment syndrome. When to suspect acute or chronic pressure buildup. Postgrad Med 105:159-168, 1999.

202. Engelund D, Kjersgaard AG: Acute compartment syndrome. Ugeskr Laeger 153:1110-1113, 1991.

203. Schmit-Neuerburg KP: Diagnosis and differential diagnosis of the compartment syndrome. Langenbecks Arch Chir 358:221-226, 1982.

204. Whitesides TE, Heckman MM: Acute compartment syndrome: update on diagnosis and treatment. J Am Acad Orthop Surg 4:209-218, 1996.

205. Sheridan GW, Matsen FA 3rd: Fasciotomy in the treatment of the acute compartment syndrome. J Bone Joint Surg Am 58:112-115, 1976.

206. Bhattacharyya T, Vrahas MS: The medical-legal aspects of compartment syndrome. J Bone Joint Surg Am 86-A:864-868, 2004.

207. Renwick SE, Naraghi FF, Worrell RV, et al: Cystic degeneration and calcification of muscle: late sequelae of compartment syndrome. J Orthop Trauma 8:440-444, 1994.

208. Tuncay IC, Demirors H, Isiklar ZU, et al: Calcific myonecrosis. Int Orthop 23:68-70, 1999.

209. Janzen DL, Connell DG, Vaisler BJ: Calcific myonecrosis of the calf manifesting as an enlarging soft-tissue mass: imaging features. Am J Roentgenol 160:1072-1074, 1993.

210. Ryu KN, Bae DK, Park YK, et al: Calcific tenosynovitis associated with calcific myonecrosis of the leg: imaging features. Skeletal Radiol 25:273-275, 1996.

211. Zohman GL, Pierce J, Chapman MW, et al: Calcific myonecrosis mimicking an invasive soft-tissue neoplasm. A case report and review of the literature. J Bone Joint Surg Am 80:1193-1197, 1998.

212. Mirra JM: Calcific myonecrosis. Clin Orthop 327:308-310, 1996.

213. Snyder BJ, Oliva A, Buncke HJ: Calcific myonecrosis following compartment syndrome: report of two cases, review of the literature, and recommendations for treatment. J Trauma 39:792-795, 1995.

214. O'Keefe RJ, O'Connell JX, Temple HT, et al: Calcific myonecrosis. A late sequela to compartment syndrome of the leg. Clin Orthop 318:205-213, 1995.

215. Holobinko JN, Damron TA, Scerpella PR, et al: Calcific myonecrosis: keys to early recognition. Skeletal Radiol 32:35-40, 2003.

216. Larson RC, Sierra RJ, Sundaram M, et al: Calcific myonecrosis: a unique presentation in the upper extremity. Skeletal Radiol 33:306-309, 2004.

217. Aoki T, Nakata H, Watanabe H, et al: The radiological findings in chronic expanding hematoma. Skeletal Radiol 28:396-401, 1999.

218. Mentzel T, Goodlad JR, Smith MA, et al: Ancient hematoma: A unifying concept for a post-traumatic lesion mimicking an aggressive soft tissue neoplasm. Mod Pathol 10:334-340, 1997.

219. Reid JD, Kommareddi S, Lankerani A, et al: Chronic expanding hematomas. A clinicopathologic entity. JAMA 244:2441-2442, 1980.

220. Sauret JM, Marinides G, Wang GK: Rhabdomyolysis. Am Fam Physician 65:907-912, 2002.

221. Warren JD, Blumbergs PC, Thompson PD: Rhabdomyolysis: a review. Muscle Nerve 25:332-347, 2002.

222. Coco TJ, Klasner AE: Drug-induced rhabdomyolysis. Curr Opin Pediatr 16:206-210, 2004.

223. Visweswaran P, Guntupalli J: Rhabdomyolysis. Crit Care Clin 15:415-428, 1999.

224. Guglielminotti J, Guidet B: Acute renal failure in rhabdomyolysis. Minerva Anestesiol 65:250-255, 1999.

225. Abassi ZA, Hoffman A, Better OS: Acute renal failure complicating muscle crush injury. Semin Nephrol 18:558-565, 1998.

226. Gotto AM Jr: Risks and benefits of continued aggressive statin therapy. Clin Cardiol 26: III3-12, 2003.

227. Moghtader J, Brady WJ Jr, Bonadio W: Exertional rhabdomyolysis in an adolescent athlete. Pediatr Emerg Care 13:382-385, 1997.

228. Lamminen AE, Hekali PE, Tiula E, et al: Acute rhabdomyolysis: evaluation with magnetic resonance imaging compared with computed tomography and ultrasonography. Br J Radiol 62:326-330, 1989.

229. Goubier JN, Hoffman OS, Oberlin C: Exertion induced rhabdomyolysis of the long head of the triceps. Br J Sports Med 36:150-151, 2002.

230. Shintani S, Shiigai T: Repeat MRI in acute rhabdomyolysis: correlation with clinicopathological findings. J Comput Assist Tomogr 17:786-791, 1993.

231. Szumilak D, Sulowicz W, Walatek B: Rhabdomyolysis: clinical features, causes, complications and treatment. Przegl Lek 55:274-279, 1998.

232. Angervall L, Stener B: Tumoriform focal muscle degeneration in two diabetic patients. Diabetologia 1:39-42, 1965.

233. Rocca PV, Alloway JA, Hashel DJ: Diabetic muscle infarction. Semin Arthritis Rheum 22:280-287, 1993.

234. Bjornskov EK, Carry MR, Katz FH, et al: Diabetic muscle infarction: a new perspective on pathogenesis and management. Neuromuscul Disord 5:39-45, 1995.

235. Grigoriadis E, Fam AG, Starok M, et al: Skeletal muscle infarction in diabetes mellitus. J Rheumatol 27:1063-1068, 2000.
236. Trujillo-Santos AJ: Diabetic muscle infarction: an underdiagnosed complication of long-standing diabetes. Diabetes Care 26:211-215, 2003.
237. Jelinek JS, Murphey MD, Aboulafia AJ, et al: Muscle infarction in patients with diabetes mellitus: MR imaging findings. Radiology 211:241-247, 1999.
238. Delaney-Sathy LO, Fessell DP, Jacobson JA, et al: Sonography of diabetic muscle infarction with MR imaging, CT, and pathologic correlation. Am J Roentgenol 174:165-169, 2000.
239. Willenberg HS, Wiefels K, Driesch E, et al: Diabetic muscle infarct. Dtsch Med Wochenschr 125:114-118, 2000.
240. Chason DP, Fleckenstein JL, Burns DK, et al: Diabetic muscle infarction: radiologic evaluation. Skeletal Radiol 25:127-132, 1996.
241. Lafforgue P, Janand-Delenne B, Lassman-Vague V, et al: Painful swelling of the thigh in a diabetic patient: diabetic muscle infarction. Diabetes Metab 25:255-260, 1999.
242. Khoury NJ, El-Khoury GY, Kathol MH: MRI diagnosis of diabetic muscle infarction: report of two cases. Skeletal Radiol 26:122-127, 1997.
243. Aboulafia AJ, Monson DK, Kennon RE: Clinical and radiological aspects of idiopathic diabetic muscle infarction. Rational approach to diagnosis and treatment. J Bone Joint Surg Br 81:323-326, 1999.
244. Madhan KK, Symmans P, Te Strake L, et al: Diabetic muscle infarction in patients on dialysis. Am J Kidney Dis 35:1212-1216, 2000.
245. Umpierrez GE, Stiles RG, Kleinbart J, et al: Diabetic muscle infarction. Am J Med 101:245-250, 1996.
246. Verrall GM, Slavotinek JP, Barnes PG, et al: Diagnostic and prognostic value of clinical findings in 83 athletes with posterior thigh injury: comparison of clinical findings with magnetic resonance imaging documentation of hamstring muscle strain. Am J Sports Med 31:969-973, 2003.
247. Cross TM, Gibbs N, Houang MT, et al: Acute quadriceps muscle strains: magnetic resonance imaging features and prognosis. Am J Sports Med 32:710-719, 2004.
248. Holmich P, Uhrskou P, Ulnits L, et al: Effectiveness of active physical training as treatment for long-standing adductor-related groin pain in athletes: randomised trial. Lancet 353:439-453, 1999.
249. Tuite DJ, Finegan PJ, Saliaris AP, et al: Anatomy of the proximal musculotendinous junction of the adductor longus muscle. Knee Surg Sports Traumatol Arthrosc 6:134-137, 1998.
250. Bono CM: Low-back pain in athletes. J Bone Joint Surg Am 86-A:382-396, 2004.
251. Connell DA, Jhamb A, James T: Side strain: a tear of internal oblique musculature. Am J Roentgenol 181:1511-1517, 2003.
252. De Smet AA, Best TM: MR imaging of the distribution and location of acute hamstring injuries in athletes. Am J Roentgenol 174:393-399, 2000.
253. Weishaupt D, Schweitzer ME, Morrison WB: Injuries to the distal gastrocnemius muscle: MR findings. J Comput Assist Tomogr 25:677-682, 2001.
254. Koulouris G, Connell D: Evaluation of the hamstring muscle complex following acute injury. Skeletal Radiol 32:582-589, 2003.
255. Levine WN, Bergfeld JA, Tessendorf W, et al: Intramuscular corticosteroid injection for hamstring injuries. A 13-year experience in the National Football League. Am J Sports Med 28:297-300, 2000.
256. Bianchi S, Martinoli C, Abdelwahab IF, et al: Sonographic evaluation of tears of the gastrocnemius medial head ("tennis leg"). J Ultrasound Med 17:157-162, 1998.
257. Palmer WE, Kuong SJ, Elmadbouh HM: MR imaging of myotendinous strain. Am J Roentgenol 173:703-709, 1999.
258. Palmer WE: Myotendinous unit: MR imaging diagnosis and pitfalls. In RSNA Categorical Course in Diagnostic Radiology: Musculoskeletal Imaging—Exploring New Limits. Oak Brook, IL, Radiological Society of North America, 2003, pp 25-35.
259. Slavotinek JP, Verrall GM, Fon GT: Hamstring injury in athletes: using MR imaging measurements to compare extent of muscle injury with amount of time lost from competition. Am J Roentgenol 179:1621-1628, 2002.
260. Connell DA, Burke F, Malara F, et al: Comparison of ultrasound and MR imaging in the assessment of acute and healing hamstring injuries. Paper presented at the Society of Skeletal Radiology Annual Meeting, 2003.
261. Heiser TM, Weber J, Sullivan G, et al: Prophylaxis and management of hamstring muscle injuries in intercollegiate football players. Am J Sports Med 12:368-370, 1984.
262. Ekstrand J, Gillquist J: Soccer injuries and their mechanisms: a prospective study. Med Sci Sports Exerc 15:267-270, 1983.
263. Sherry MA, Best TM: A comparison of 2 rehabilitation programs in the treatment of acute hamstring strains. J Orthop Sports Phys Ther 34:116-125, 2004.
264. Beaulieu CF: Sports injury and intervention. In RSNA Categorical Course in Diagnostic Radiology: Musculoskeletal Imaging—Exploring New Limits. Oak Brook, IL, Radiological Society of North America, 2003, pp 37-43.
265. Prisk V, Huard J: Muscle injuries and repair: the role of prostaglandins and inflammation. Histol Histopathol 18:1243-1256, 2003.
266. Walter GA, Cahill KS, Huard J, et al: Noninvasive monitoring of stem cell transfer for muscle disorders. Magn Reson Med 51:273-277, 2004.
267. Huard J, Li Y, Fu FH: Muscle injuries and repair: current trends in research. J Bone Joint Surg Am 84-A:822-832, 2002.
268. Kujala UM, Orava S, Jarvinen M: Hamstring injuries: current trends in treatment and prevention. Sports Med 23:397-404, 1997.
269. Sallay PI, Friedman RL, Coogan PG, et al: Hamstring muscle injuries among water skiers: functional outcome and prevention. Am J Sports Med 24:130-136, 1996.
270. Blasier RB, Morawa LG: Complete rupture of the hamstring origin from a water skiing injury. Am J Sports Med 18:435-437, 1990.
271. Lieber RL, Friden J: Morphologic and mechanical basis of delayed-onset muscle soreness. J Am Acad Orthop Surg 10:67-73, 2002.
272. Yu JG, Carlsson L, Thornell LE: Evidence for myofibril remodeling as opposed to myofibril damage in human muscles with DOMS: an ultrastructural and immunoelectron microscopic study. Histochem Cell Biol 121:219-227, 2004.
273. Nurenberg P, Giddings CJ, Stray-Gundersen J, et al: MR imaging-guided muscle biopsy for correlation of increased signal intensity with ultrastructural change and delayed-onset muscle soreness after exercise. Radiology 184:865-869, 1992.
274. Shellock FG, Fukunaga T, Mink JH, et al: Exertional muscle injury: evaluation of concentric versus eccentric actions with serial MR imaging. Radiology 179:659-664, 1991.
275. Kaariainen M, Kaariainen J, Jarvinen TL, et al: Correlation between biomechanical and structural changes during the regeneration of skeletal muscle after laceration injury. J Orthop Res 16:197-206, 1998.
276. Menetrey J, Kasemkijwattana C, Fu FH, et al: Suturing versus immobilization of a muscle laceration. A morphological and functional study in a mouse model. Am J Sports Med 27:222-229, 1999.
277. Chan YS, Li Y, Foster W, et al: Antifibrotic effects of suramin in injured skeletal muscle after laceration. J Appl Physiol 95:771-780, 2003.
278. Fukushima K, Badlani N, Usas A, et al: The use of an antifibrosis agent to improve muscle recovery after laceration. Am J Sports Med 29:394-402, 2001.
279. Li Y, Huard J: Differentiation of muscle-derived cells into myofibroblasts in injured skeletal muscle. Am J Pathol 161:895-907, 2002.
280. Mellado JM, Perez del Palomar L: Muscle hernias of the lower leg: MRI findings. Skeletal Radiol 28:465-469, 1999.
281. Siliprandi L, Martini G, Chiarelli A, et al: Surgical repair of an anterior tibialis muscle hernia with Mersilene mesh. Plast Reconstr Surg 91:154-157, 1993.
282. Bianchi S, Abdelwahab IF, Mazzola CG, et al: Sonographic examination of muscle herniation. J Ultrasound Med 14:357-360, 1995.
283. Burg D, Schnyder H, Buchmann R, et al: Effective treatment of a large muscle hernia by local botulinum toxin administration. Handchir Mikrochir Plast Chir 31:75-78, 1999.
284. Simon HE, Sacchet HA: Muscle hernias of the leg. Review of literature and report of twelve cases. Am J Surg 67:87-89, 1945.
285. Alhadeff J, Lee CK: Gastrocnemius muscle herniation at the knee causing peroneal nerve compression resembling sciatica. Spine 20:612-614, 1995.
286. Braunstein JT, Crues JV, 3rd: Magnetic resonance imaging of hereditary hernias of the peroneus longus muscle. Skeletal Radiol 24:601-604, 1995.
287. Zeiss J, Ebraheim NA, Woldenberg LS: Magnetic resonance imaging in the diagnosis of anterior tibialis muscle herniation. Clin Orthop 244:249-253, 1989.
288. Beggs I: Sonography of muscle hernias. Am J Roentgenol 180:395-399, 2003.
289. Berglund HT, Stocks GW: Muscle hernia in a recreational athlete. Orthop Rev 22:1246-1248, 1993.
290. Miniaci A, Rorabeck CH: Tibialis anterior muscle hernia: a rationale for treatment. Can J Surg 30:79-80, 1987.
291. Marques A, Brenda E, Amarante MT: Bilateral multiple muscle hernias of the leg repaired with Marlex mesh. Br J Plast Surg 47:444-446, 1994.
292. Beiner JM, Jokl P: Muscle contusion injuries: current treatment options. J Am Acad Orthop Surg 9:227-237, 2001.
293. Thorsson O, Lilja B, Nilsson P, et al: Immediate external compression in the management of an acute muscle injury. Scand J Med Sci Sports 7:182-190, 1997.
294. Holscher RS, Leyten FS, Oudenhoven LF, et al: Percutaneous decompression of an iliopsoas hematoma. Abdom Imaging 22:114-116, 1997.
295. Berna JD, Zuazu I, Madrigal M, et al: Conservative treatment of large rectus sheath hematoma in patients undergoing anticoagulant therapy. Abdom Imaging 25:230-234, 2000.
296. Moreno Gallego A, Aguayo JL, Flores B, et al: Ultrasonography and computed tomography reduce unnecessary surgery in abdominal rectus sheath haematoma. Br J Surg 84:1295-1297, 1997.
297. Giuliani G, Poppi M, Acciarri N, et al: CT scan and surgical treatment of traumatic iliacus hematoma with femoral neuropathy: case report. J Trauma 30:229-231, 1990.
298. Seijo-Martinez M, Castro del Rio M, Fontoira E, et al: Acute femoral neuropathy secondary to an iliacus muscle hematoma. J Neurol Sci 209:119-122, 2003.
299. Tamai K, Kuramochi T, Sakai H, et al: Complete paralysis of the quadriceps muscle caused by traumatic iliacus hematoma: a case report. J Orthop Sci 7:713-716, 2002.
300. Bush CH: The magnetic resonance imaging of musculoskeletal hemorrhage. Skeletal Radiol 29:1-9, 2000.
301. Rubin JI, Gomori JM, Grossman RI, et al: High-field MR imaging of extracranial hematomas. Am J Roentgenol 148:813-817, 1987.

302. Cohen MD, McGuire W, Cory DA, et al: Society for Pediatric Radiology John Caffey Award. MR appearance of blood and blood products: an in vitro study. Am J Roentgenol 146:1293-1297, 1986.
303. Hahn PF, Saini S, Stark DD, et al: Intraabdominal hematoma: the concentric-ring sign in MR imaging. Am J Roentgenol 148:115-119, 1987.
304. El-Khoury GY, Brandser EA, Kathol MH, et al: Imaging of muscle injuries. Skeletal Radiol 25:3-11, 1996.
305. Saotome K, Koguchi Y, Tamai K, et al: Enlarging intramuscular hematoma and fibrinolytic parameters. J Orthop Sci 8:132-136, 2003.
306. Dooms GC, Fisher MR, Hricak H, et al: MR imaging of intramuscular hemorrhage. J Comput Assist Tomogr 9:908-913, 1985.
307. De Smet AA, Fisher DR, Heiner JP, et al: Magnetic resonance imaging of muscle tears. Skeletal Radiol 19:283-286, 1990.
308. De Smet AA: Magnetic resonance findings in skeletal muscle tears. Skeletal Radiol 22:479-484, 1993.
309. Hasselman CT, Best TM, Hughes C, 4th, et al: An explanation for various rectus femoris strain injuries using previously undescribed muscle architecture. Am J Sports Med 23:493-499, 1995.
310. Varela JR, Rodriguez E, Soler R, et al: Complete rupture of the distal semimembranosus tendon with secondary hamstring muscles atrophy: MR findings in two cases. Skeletal Radiol 29:362-364, 2000.
311. Temple HT, Kuklo TR, Sweet DE, et al: Rectus femoris muscle tear appearing as a pseudotumor. Am J Sports Med 26:544-548, 1998.
312. Hughes C 4th, Hasselman CT, Best TM, et al: Incomplete, intrasubstance strain injuries of the rectus femoris muscle. Am J Sports Med 23:500-506, 1995.
313. Rubin SJ, Feldman F, Staron RB, et al: Magnetic resonance imaging of muscle injury. Clin Imaging 19:263-269, 1995.
314. Ackerman LV: Extra-osseous localized non-neoplastic bone and cartilage formation (so-called myositis ossificans). Clinical and pathological confusion with malignant neoplasms. J Bone Joint Surg 40-A:279-298, 1958.
315. Schutte HE, van der Heul RO: Reactive mesenchymal proliferation. J Belg Radiol 75:297-302, 1992.
316. Nuovo MA, Norman A, Chumas J, et al: Myositis ossificans with atypical clinical, radiographic, or pathologic findings: a review of 23 cases. Skeletal Radiol 21:87-101, 1992.
317. Kjaersgaard-Andersen P, Sletgard J, Gjerloff C, et al: Heterotopic bone formation after noncemented total hip arthroplasty. Location of ectopic bone and the influence of postoperative antiinflammatory treatment. Clin Orthop 252:156-162, 1990.
318. Paterson DC: Myositis ossificans circumscripta. Report of four cases without history of injury. J Bone Joint Surg Br 52:296-301, 1970.
319. Beiner JM, Jokl P: Muscle contusion injury and myositis ossificans traumatica. Clin Orthop 403(Suppl):S110-119, 2002.
320. Byrd JW, Jones KS: Prospective analysis of hip arthroscopy with 2-year follow-up. Arthroscopy 16:578-587, 2000.
321. Neal B, Gray H, MacMahon S, et al: Incidence of heterotopic bone formation after major hip surgery. Austral NZ J Surg 72:808-821, 2002.
322. Neal B: Effects of heterotopic bone formation on outcome after hip arthroplasty. Austral NZ J Surg 73:422-426, 2003.
323. Gaur A, Sinclair M, Caruso E, et al: Heterotopic ossification around the elbow following burns in children: results after excision. J Bone Joint Surg Am 85-A:1538-1543, 2003.
324. van Kuijk AA, Geurts AC, van Kuppevelt HJ: Neurogenic heterotopic ossification in spinal cord injury. Spinal Cord 40:313-326, 2002.
325. Melamed E, Robinson D, Halperin N, et al: Brain injury-related heterotopic bone formation: treatment strategy and results. Am J Phys Med Rehab 81:670-674, 2002.
326. DiCaprio MR, Huo MH, Zatorski LE, et al: Incidence of heterotopic ossification following total hip arthroplasty in patients with prior stroke. Orthopedics 27:41-43, 2004.
327. Iorio R, Healy WL: Heterotopic ossification after hip and knee arthroplasty: risk factors, prevention, and treatment. J Am Acad Orthop Surg 10:409-416, 2002.
328. Kaplan FS, Glaser DL, Hebela N, et al: Heterotopic ossification. J Am Acad Orthop Surg 12:116-125, 2004.
329. Bouchardy L, Garcia J: Magnetic resonance imaging in the diagnosis of myositis ossificans circumscripta. J Radiol 75:101-110, 1994.
330. Aro HT, Viljanto J, Aho HJ, et al: Macrophages in trauma-induced myositis ossificans. APMIS 99:482-486, 1991.
331. Gindele A, Schwamborn D, Tsironis K, et al: Myositis ossificans traumatica in young children: report of three cases and review of the literature. Pediatr Radiol 30:451-459, 2000.
332. Hanquinet S, Ngo L, Anooshiravani M, et al: Magnetic resonance imaging helps in the early diagnosis of myositis ossificans in children. Pediatr Surg Int 15:287-289, 1999.
333. Shirkhoda A, Armin AR, Bis KG, et al: MR imaging of myositis ossificans: variable patterns at different stages. J Magn Reson Imaging 5:287-292, 1995.
334. Kransdorf MJ, Meis JM, Jelinek JS: Myositis ossificans: MR appearance with radiologic-pathologic correlation. Am J Roentgenol 157:1243-1248, 1991.
335. Subbarao JV, Garrison SJ: Heterotopic ossification: diagnosis and management, current concepts and controversies. J Spinal Cord Med 22:273-283, 1999.
336. Djurickovic S, Meek RN, Snelling CF, et al: Range of motion and complications after postburn heterotopic bone excision about the elbow. J Trauma 41:825-830, 1996.
337. Munin MC, Balu G, Sotereanos DG: Elbow complications after organ transplantation. Case reports. Am J Phys Med Rehabil 74:67-72, 1995.
338. Fitzsimmons AS, O'Dell MW, Guiffra LJ, et al: Radial nerve injury associated with traumatic myositis ossificans in a brain injured patient. Arch Phys Med Rehabil 74:770-773, 1993.
339. Jones BV, Ward MW: Myositis ossificans in the biceps femoris muscles causing sciatic nerve palsy. A case report. J Bone Joint Surg Br 62-B:506-507, 1980.
340. Garland DE: Clinical observations on fractures and heterotopic ossification in the spinal cord and traumatic brain injured populations. Clin Orthop 233:86-101, 1988.
341. Kransdorf MJ, Murphy MD: Extraskeletal osseous and cartilaginous tumors. In Kransdorf MJ, Murphy MD (eds): Imaging of Soft Tissue Tumors. Philadelphia, WB Saunders, 1997.
342. Renault E, Favier T, Laumonier F: Non-traumatic myositis ossificans circumscripta. Arch Pediatr 2:150-155, 1995.
343. Okada K, Ito H, Miyakoshi N, et al: A low-grade extraskeletal osteosarcoma. Skeletal Radiol 32:165-169, 2003.
344. Ledermann HP, Schweitzer ME, Morrison WB: Pelvic heterotopic ossification: MR imaging characteristics. Radiology 222:189-195, 2002.
345. Parikh J, Hyare H, Saifuddin A: A review of the imaging features of post traumatic myositis ossificans using a multimodality approach with a particular emphasis on MRI. Paper presented at the Radiological Society of North America Annual Meeting, 2003, Chicago.
346. Tsai JC, Dalinka MK, Fallon MD, et al: Fluid-fluid level: a nonspecific finding in tumors of bone and soft tissue. Radiology 175:779-782, 1990.
347. Kluger G, Kochs A, Holthausen H: Heterotopic ossification in childhood and adolescence. J Child Neurol 15:406-413, 2000.
348. Lewallen DG: Heterotopic ossification following total hip arthroplasty. Instr Course Lect 44:287-292, 1995.
349. Tibone J, Sakimura I, Nickel VL, et al: Heterotopic ossification around the hip in spinal cord-injured patients. A long-term follow-up study. J Bone Joint Surg Am 60:769-775, 1978.
350. Shehab D, Elgazzar AH, Collier BD: Heterotopic ossification. J Nucl Med 43:346-353, 2002.
351. Coblentz CL, Cockshott WP, Martin RF: Resolution of myositis ossificans in a hemophiliac. J Can Assoc Radiol 36:161-162, 1985.
352. Romano CL, Duci D, Romano D, et al: Celecoxib versus indomethacin in the prevention of heterotopic ossification after total hip arthroplasty. J Arthroplasty 19:14-18, 2004.
353. Ben Hamida KS, Hajri R, Kedadi H, et al: Myositis ossificans circumscripta of the knee improved by alendronate. Joint Bone Spine 71:144-146, 2004.
354. Padgett DE, Holley KG, Cummings M, et al: The efficacy of 500 CentiGray radiation in the prevention of heterotopic ossification after total hip arthroplasty: a prospective, randomized, pilot study. J Arthroplasty 18:677-686, 2003.
355. Merchan EC, Sanchez-Herrera S, Valdazo DA, et al: Circumscribed myositis ossificans. Report of nine cases without history of injury. Acta Orthop Belg 59:273-277, 1993.
356. Ogilvie-Harris DJ, Fornasier VL: Pseudomalignant myositis ossificans: heterotopic new-bone formation without a history of trauma. J Bone Joint Surg Am 62:1274-1283, 1980.
357. May DA, Disler DG, Jones EA, et al: Abnormal signal intensity in skeletal muscle at MR imaging: patterns, pearls, and pitfalls. Radiographics 20(Suppl):S295-315, 2000.
358. Haig AJ, Weiner JB, Tew J, et al: The relation among spinal geometry on MRI, paraspinal electromyographic abnormalities, and age in persons referred for electrodiagnostic testing of low back symptoms. Spine 27:1918-1925, 2002.
359. Elsayes K, Khosla A, Mukundan G, et al: Value of MR imaging for muscle denervation syndromes of the shoulder girdle. Paper presented at the Radiologic Society of North America Annual Meeting, 2003, Chicago.
360. Kikuchi Y, Nakamura T, Takayama S, et al: MR imaging in the diagnosis of denervated and reinnervated skeletal muscles: experimental study in rats. Radiology 229:861-867, 2003.
361. Fritz RC, Boutin RD: Magnetic resonance imaging of the peripheral nervous system. Phys Med Rehabil Clin N Am 12:399-432, 2001.
362. McDonald CM, Carter GT, Fritz RC, et al: Magnetic resonance imaging of denervated muscle: comparison to electromyography. Muscle Nerve 23:1431-1434, 2000.
363. Bredella MA, Tirman PF, Fritz RC, et al: Denervation syndromes of the shoulder girdle: MR imaging with electrophysiologic correlation. Skeletal Radiol 28:567-572, 1999.
364. Grainger AJ, Campbell RS, Stothard J: Anterior interosseous nerve syndrome: appearance at MR imaging in three cases. Radiology 208:381-384, 1998.
365. Carter GT, Fritz RC: Electromyographic and lower extremity short time to inversion recovery magnetic resonance imaging findings in lumbar radiculopathy. Muscle Nerve 20:1191-1193, 1997.
366. Spinner RJ, Lins RE, Collins AJ, et al: Posterior interosseous nerve compression due to an enlarged bicipital bursa confirmed by MRI. J Hand Surg (Br) 18:753-756, 1993.
367. Bendszus M, Wessig C, Reiners K, et al: MR imaging in the differential diagnosis of neurogenic foot drop. Am J Neuroradiol 24:1283-1289, 2003.

368. Fleckenstein JL, Watumull D, Conner KE, et al: Denervated human skeletal muscle: MR imaging evaluation. Radiology 187:213-218, 1993.

369. Polak JF, Jolesz FA, Adams DF: Magnetic resonance imaging of skeletal muscle. Prolongation of T1 and T2 subsequent to denervation. Invest Radiol 23:365-369, 1988.

370. Bendszus M, Koltzenburg M, Wessig C, et al: Sequential MR imaging of denervated muscle: experimental study. Am J Neuroradiol 23:1427-1431, 2002.

371. Wessig C, Koltzenburg M, Reiners K, et al: Muscle magnetic resonance imaging of denervation and reinnervation: correlation with electrophysiology and histology. Exp Neurol 185:254-261, 2004.

372. Cudlip SA, Howe FA, Griffiths JR, et al: Magnetic resonance neurography of peripheral nerve following experimental crush injury, and correlation with functional deficit. J Neurosurg 96:755-759, 2002.

373. Aagaard BD, Maravilla KR, Kliot M: MR neurography. MR imaging of peripheral nerves. Magn Reson Imaging Clin N Am 6:179-194, 1998.

374. Tollback A, Soderlund V, Jakobsson F, et al: Magnetic resonance imaging of lower extremity muscles and isokinetic strength in foot dorsiflexors in patients with prior polio. Scand J Rehabil Med 28:115-123, 1996.

375. Schalke BCG, Hofmann E, Reiners K, et al: Neuropathies and motor neuron diseases. In Fleckenstein JL, Crues III JV, Reimers CD (eds): Muscle Imaging in Health and Disease. New York, Springer, 1999.

376. Steinbach LS, Fleckenstein JL, Mink JH: MR imaging of muscle injuries. Semin Musculoskelet Radiol 1:127-141, 1997.

377. De Beuckeleer L, Vanhoenacker F, De Schepper A, Jr, et al: Hypertrophy and pseudohypertrophy of the lower leg following chronic radiculopathy and neuropathy: imaging findings in two patients. Skeletal Radiol 28:229-232, 1999.

378. Petersilge CA, Pathria MN, Gentili A, et al: Denervation hypertrophy of muscle: MR features. J Comput Assist Tomogr 19:596-600, 1995.

379. Drozdowski W, Dzieciol J: Neurogenic muscle hypertrophy in radiculopathy. Acta Neurol Scand 89:464-468, 1994.

380. de Visser M, Verbeeten B Jr, Lyppens KC: Pseudohypertrophy of the calf following S1 radiculopathy. Neuroradiology 28:279-280, 1986.

381. Ilaslan H, Wenger DE, Shives TC, et al: Unilateral hypertrophy of tensor fascia lata: a soft tissue tumor simulator. Skeletal Radiol 32:628-632, 2003.

382. Sheikh RA, Yasmeen S, Munn R, et al: AIDS-related myopathy. Med Electron Microsc 32:79-86, 1999.

383. Wlachovska B, Abraham B, Deux JF, et al: Proliferative myositis in a patient with AIDS. Skeletal Radiol 33:237-240, 2004.

384. Berretta M, Cinelli R, Martellotta F, et al: Therapeutic approaches to AIDS-related malignancies. Oncogene 22:6646-6659, 2003.

385. Cupler EJ, Danon MJ, Jay C, et al: Early features of zidovudine-associated myopathy: histopathological findings and clinical correlations. Acta Neuropathol (Berl) 90:1-6, 1995.

386. Hengge UR, Stocks K, Wiehler H, et al: Double-blind, randomized, placebo-controlled phase III trial of oxymetholone for the treatment of HIV wasting. AIDS 17:699-710, 2003.

BONE AND SOFT-TISSUE TUMORS

Paul D. Clifford ● H. Thomas Temple

INTRODUCTION

There has been considerable progress in the surgical management, adjuvant therapy and prognosis of patients with musculoskeletal tumors over the past two decades. From 70% to 85% of all primary malignant musculoskeletal tumors are treated by limb salvage procedures.[1] Magnetic resonance imaging has become an important tool in the evaluation of musculoskeletal masses. Direct multiplanar acquisition, the absence of ionizing radiation and superior soft-tissue contrast resolution have championed use of MR in the detection, staging and posttherapeutic follow-up of musculoskeletal neoplasms.[2-7]

Bone and soft-tissue sarcomas are tumors of mesenchymal origin. Sarcomas account for less than 1% of all malignancies and yet they and their more common benign counterparts present significant diagnostic problems for the orthopedic surgeon, the radiologist, and the pathologist. The incidence of soft-tissue sarcomas in the United States is 2.4/100,000 people while the incidence of primary bone tumors is 0.8/100,000 people.[8] In 2003, an estimated 8300 new soft-tissue sarcomas and 2400 new bone sarcomas will be diagnosed in the United States.[9] Benign soft-tissue masses are 50 to 60 times more common than primary malignant tumors while primary osseous benign tumors and osseous metastases are over 100 times more common than primary osseous malignancies.

Distant metastases to soft-tissue are rarely reported and the prevalence of metastatic disease to soft-tissues is unknown. Most published articles are case reports or small reviews of the subject. Metastatic disease to skeletal muscle has been reported to be three times more common than metastases to subcutaneous tissues[10] (Fig. 107-1). Sudo et al[11] reported their 15 year experience at one institution during which time 147 soft-tissue sarcomas and only four soft-tissue skeletal muscle carcinomatous metastases were encountered, a 37 : 1

ratio of soft-tissue sarcomas to skeletal muscle metastasis from carcinoma. Glockner et al[12] retrospectively evaluated 1421 patients who presented with a solitary soft-tissue mass. Only 25 of these lesions (1.8%) were metastases from a known primary malignancy. The incidence was even lower (0.8%) for soft-tissue metastases whose identification antedated the discovery of the primary malignancy. Autopsy studies have reported soft-tissue metastases in 0.8% to 17% of patients dying of metastatic disease.[10] The autopsy series reporting an incidence of 17% including patients with leukemia and

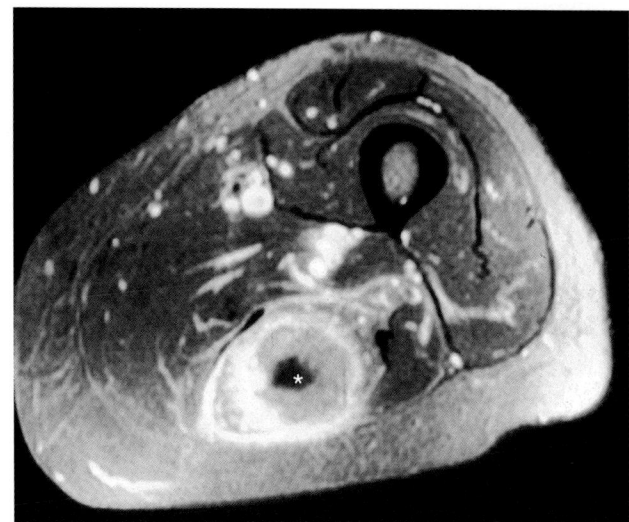

FIGURE 107-1

Skeletal muscle metastasis. Axial fat saturation post-contrast T1-weighted image shows enhancing metastatic soft-tissue mass with associated edema and nonenhancing central necrotic center (*asterisk*) within muscle in this patient with renal adenocarcinoma.

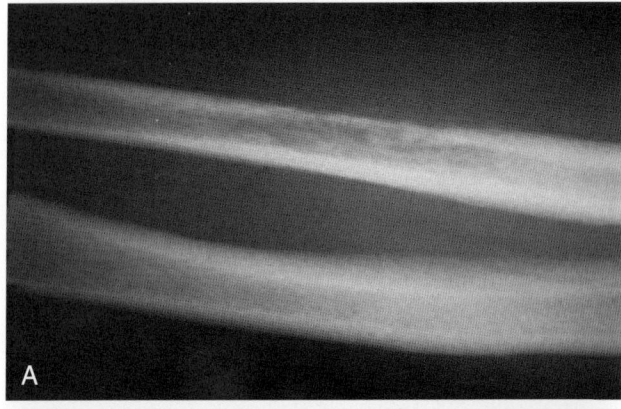

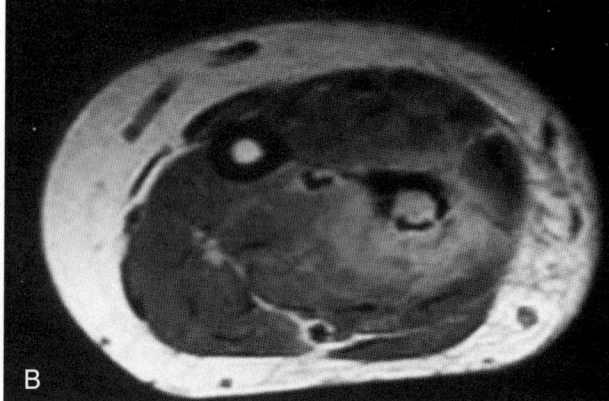

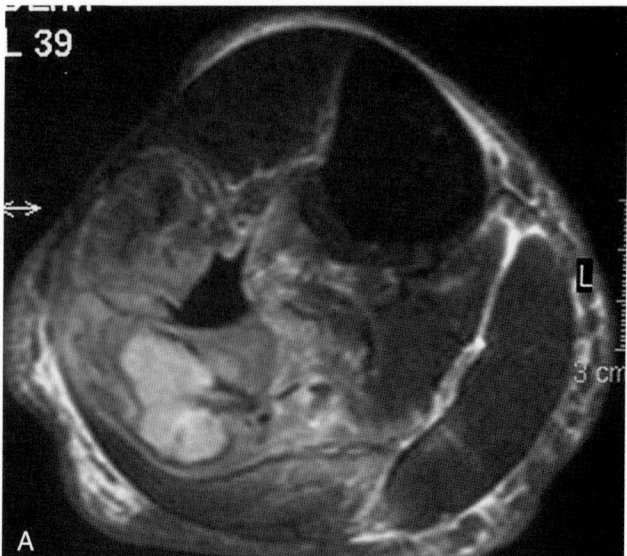

FIGURE 107-2

A 46-year-old woman with pain and swelling in her right dominant forearm. **A,** There is a lesion in the ulnar diaphysis having a permeative pattern and cortical erosion *(arrow)*. **B,** Proton density axial MR shows marrow replacement, cortical destruction, and circumferential soft-tissue mass. This patient had acute streptococcal osteomyelitis.

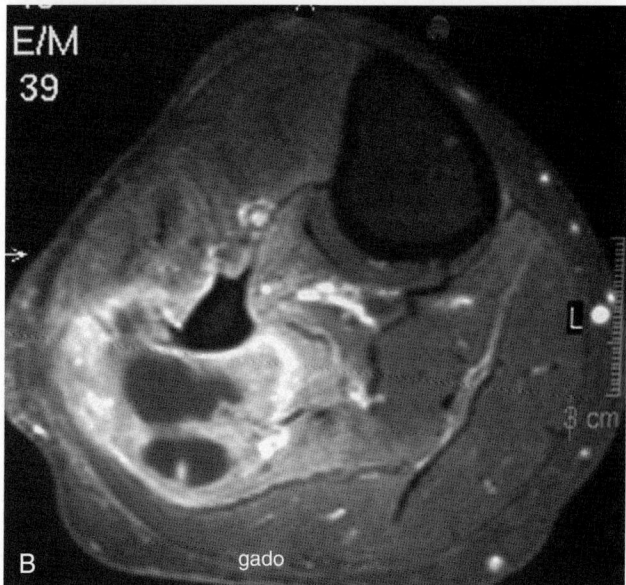

FIGURE 107-3

Patient presents with edema and soft-tissue mass. **A,** Axial T2 fat saturation image shows a heterogeneous high signal intensity mass in the postero-lateral calf with prominent edema in adjacent musculature, intermuscular spaces, and subcutaneous tissues. **B,** Post-contrast fat-saturation T1-weighted image shows prominent peripheral enhancement and a central non-enhancing region in this patient with soft-tissue abscess.

lymphoma, which may have skewed the data as skeletal muscle involvement in patients with leukemia and lymphoma has been reported in up to 52% of patients at autopsy.[13] The number of soft-tissue metastases reported are surprisingly low given the prevalence of carcinomas and the fact that skeletal muscle accounts for at least 50% of body mass. The most common sites of origin of tumors metastatic to soft-tissues are lung followed by kidney, colon, unknown primary carcinoma, and soft-tissue sarcoma.[14] The most common site of soft-tissue metastasis is the thigh followed by the psoas, gluteal area, lumbar and paraspinal muscles, and the leg/calf.[14] Skeletal muscle injury may alter muscle physiology and result in susceptibility to the development of metastatic disease.[15]

APPROACH TO MR IMAGING OF MUSCULOSKELETAL MASSES

An accurate history must first be obtained. Patients may present with pain, mass, or both. The patient may be asymptomatic with the lesion detected on a diagnostic study conducted for other indications. Bone tumors

frequently cause pain whereas soft-tissue masses are frequently painless. Pain is common however with neurogenic tumors or those soft-tissue tumors that impinge upon neural structures or erode bone. In the evaluation of bone and soft-tissue tumors, infection and inflammatory conditions should also be considered in the differential (Fig. 107-2). For this reason, every tumor should be cultured and every infection should undergo biopsy (Fig. 107-3).

Pertinent surgical, medical and family history should be evaluated. Family history is only occasionally helpful

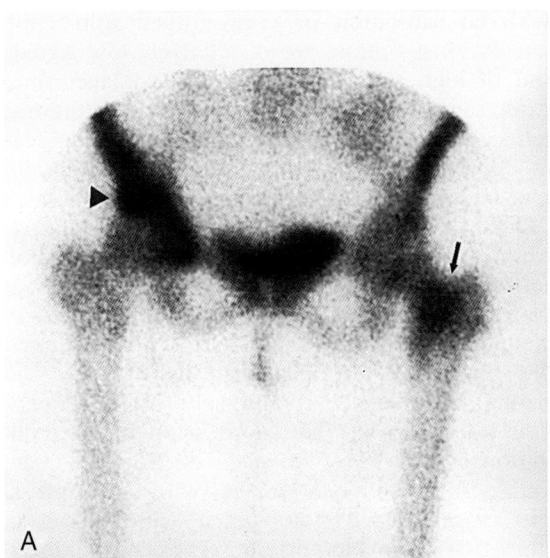

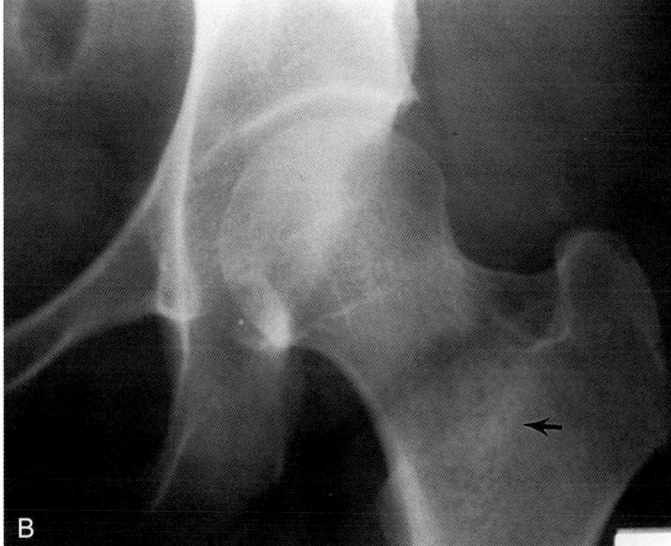

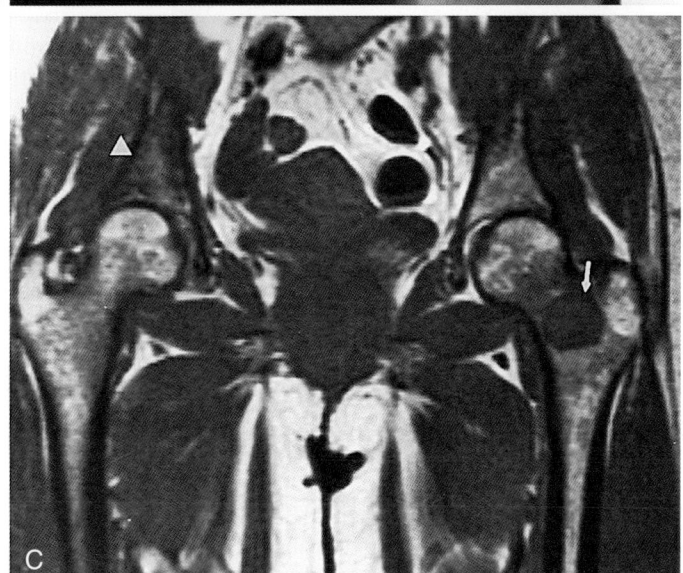

FIGURE 107-4

A 34-year-old woman presented with known breast cancer and left hip pain. **A,** Anterior pelvic view from a radionuclide bone scan reveals increased uptake in the left intertrochanteric region *(arrow)* and right acetabulum *(arrowhead)*. The study was otherwise normal, and the pattern was interpreted as atypical for metastatic disease because the abnormality was confined solely to the hips. **B,** Radiograph of the left femoral neck shows questionable medullary sclerosis in the intertrochanteric region *(arrow)*. Films of the right acetabulum (not shown) were normal. **C,** Coronal T1-weighted (600/20) image clearly shows a focal medullary mass *(arrow)* in the left intertrochanteric region and diffuse marrow replacement in the right acetabulum *(arrowhead)*. The appearance is highly suggestive of metastatic disease, which was confirmed by follow-up imaging.

but is important in diseases such as neurofibromatosis, multiple hereditary exoxtosis, and Gardner's syndrome. A history of trauma or blood dyscrasia or the use of anticoagulants may result in a hematoma mimicking a mass or hemorrhage into a pre-existent mass. Inquiry should be made regarding antecedent trauma or a history of benign or malignant tumor. The presence of multiple bone or soft-tissue lesions narrows the differential considerations (Fig. 107-4).

Plain films are the primary imaging modality in the diagnosis of bone tumors and they are absolutely essential in the complete evaluation of bone lesions. Radiographs are also useful in the initial evaluation and diagnosis of soft-tissue masses and should routinely be obtained (Fig. 107-5). Regions of mineralization evident on radiographs may easily be overlooked when the MR is viewed in isolation. The presence of osteoid deposition or certain characteristic mineralization such as

phleboliths or typical patterns of cartilage mineralization (rings and arcs, stippled calcifications, and flocculation) will limit the differential diagnosis (Fig. 107-6). Previous MR studies, bone scans, CT scans, or other pertinent examinations should be acquired. A close and on-going consultation between the radiologist and the treating surgeon does much to insure an appropriate MR study, diagnostic biopsy, adequate post-therapeutic surveillance, and optimum clinical outcome.

ROUTINE MR MASS PROTOCOL

A baseline MRI study should be obtained prior to biopsy. A skin marker should be placed over a palpable or suspected mass. For follow-up studies, the site of prior surgery should be similarly indicated. Commonly used skin markers include vitamin E capsules; oil-filled vials or

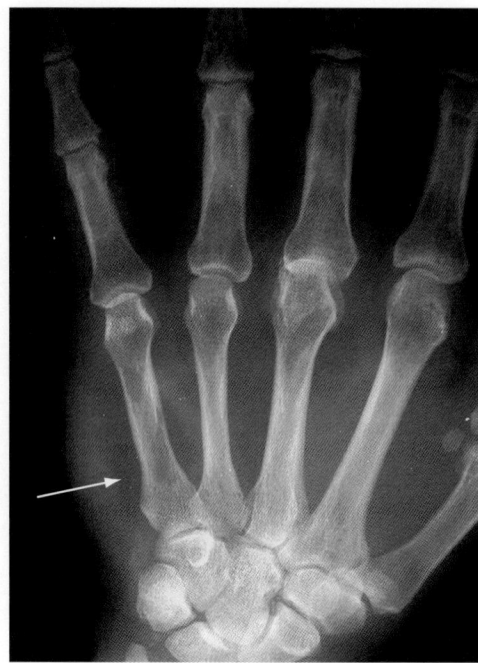

FIGURE 107-5

Low attenuation (arrow) consistent with fat seen over the fifth metacarpal suggests the diagnosis of a lipomatous soft-tissue mass, in this case a benign lipoma.

syringes containing a dilute gadolinium solution. For smaller masses or very superficial lesions where a large marker might distort the mass, a small dab of petroleum jelly placed on the skin will suffice.

Careful attention to proper MR technique is required to adequately evaluate musculoskeletal neoplasms. Initial imaging should include a large field of view T1 sequence utilizing the body coil, visualizing the involved extremity from the joint above to the joint below the lesion in order to evaluate tumor extent and "skip lesions." Skip lesions or skip metastases are intracompartmental metastases occasionally seen in sarcomas where a secondary lesion, the skip lesion, is separated from the primary tumor by normal bone or soft-tissue[16] (Fig. 107-7). A matching large field of view short tau inversion recovery (STIR) sequence may be of aid particularly in the detection of soft-tissue skip lesions. If a mass is anterior or posterior in location, large field of view sagittal sequences are performed. If a mass is primarily medial or lateral in location, we prefer coronal images.

Ideally, a surface coil should then be placed over the mass and the lesion should be imaged in at least two orthogonal planes. The surface coil and the field of view should be large enough to include the entire mass and the normal adjacent tissues. The smallest surface coil adequate to cover the area is preferred in order to optimize signal to noise and spatial resolution. The region to be examined should be placed as close to the isocenter of the magnet as possible. Axial T1- and T2-weighted or STIR sequences should be performed in all cases. Axial T2-weighted sequences may be either fast spin-echo

T2 with fat saturation or conventional spin-echo T2 sequences. Most tumors are of relatively low signal on T1 and of high signal intensity on T2 images due to increased tumor water content. Because most tumors are of high signal intensity on T2 images, there is decreased lesion conspicuity when fast spin-echo T2 sequences without fat saturation are utilized due to the persistent high signal of regional fat in both soft-tissues and bone marrow.[17,18] Fat saturation technique requires a homogeneous field and saturation is optimum at the isocenter. Failure of an attempted fat saturation T2 sequence or marked field heterogeneity may lead to poor delineation of the mass and spurious regions of high signal simulating pathology. Fast spin-echo STIR sequences provide homogeneous fat suppression and excellent lesion conspicuity.[19] Fast spin-echo STIR images may be preferable to fast spin-echo images with fat suppression due to better image homogeneity and lesion conspicuity.[20] STIR signal-to-noise however lags behind that of fast spin-echo and conventional spin-echo imaging and the sequences are somewhat susceptible to motion artifact.[21] The intense high signal on STIR images within tissues of high fluid content may obscure subtle variations in internal signal that could be of aid in tissue characterization.[7] Advocates of conventional spin-echo T2 or dual-echo sequences argue that the sequence is the most reproducible, the most often referenced sequence in tumor imaging, and the standard by which all other sequences must be judged.[7,8] Conventional T2 sequences are time consuming however, and patient motion during the long acquisition may require the sequence to be repeated.

Orthogonal views (either coronal or sagittal) with the patient in the surface coil are desirable. We prefer sagittal orientation if the mass is anterior or posterior and coronal orientation if the mass is medial or lateral. Oblique views may occasionally be helpful to define a mass relative to normal adjacent structures such as the neurovascular bundle. Due to magnetic susceptibility effects, gradient-echo sequences are sensitive to and may be utilized for the detection of calcification, gas, metal, and hemosiderin. Flow-sensitive sequences delineate the patency of vascular structures. Fat saturation T1 sequences may confirm a lipomatous lesion or hemorrhage.

Use of MR Contrast

The pharmacokinetic behavior of gadolinium is similar to that of traditional iodinated contrast utilized in CT, angiographic and other radiographic studies. Following injection, gadolinium is rapidly distributed in the vascular system and eventually excreted via the kidneys. Gadolinium uptake causes a reduction of the T1 relaxation time of the target tissue and relative high signal intensity on postcontrast T1-weighted images. On non-fat-saturated T1 post-gadolinium sequences, it is possible for the enhancing tumor to be obscured by high signal intensity of subcutaneous fat or bone marrow.[22] For this reason, many radiologists use fat saturation on postcontrast T1 sequences. If postcontrast fat saturation

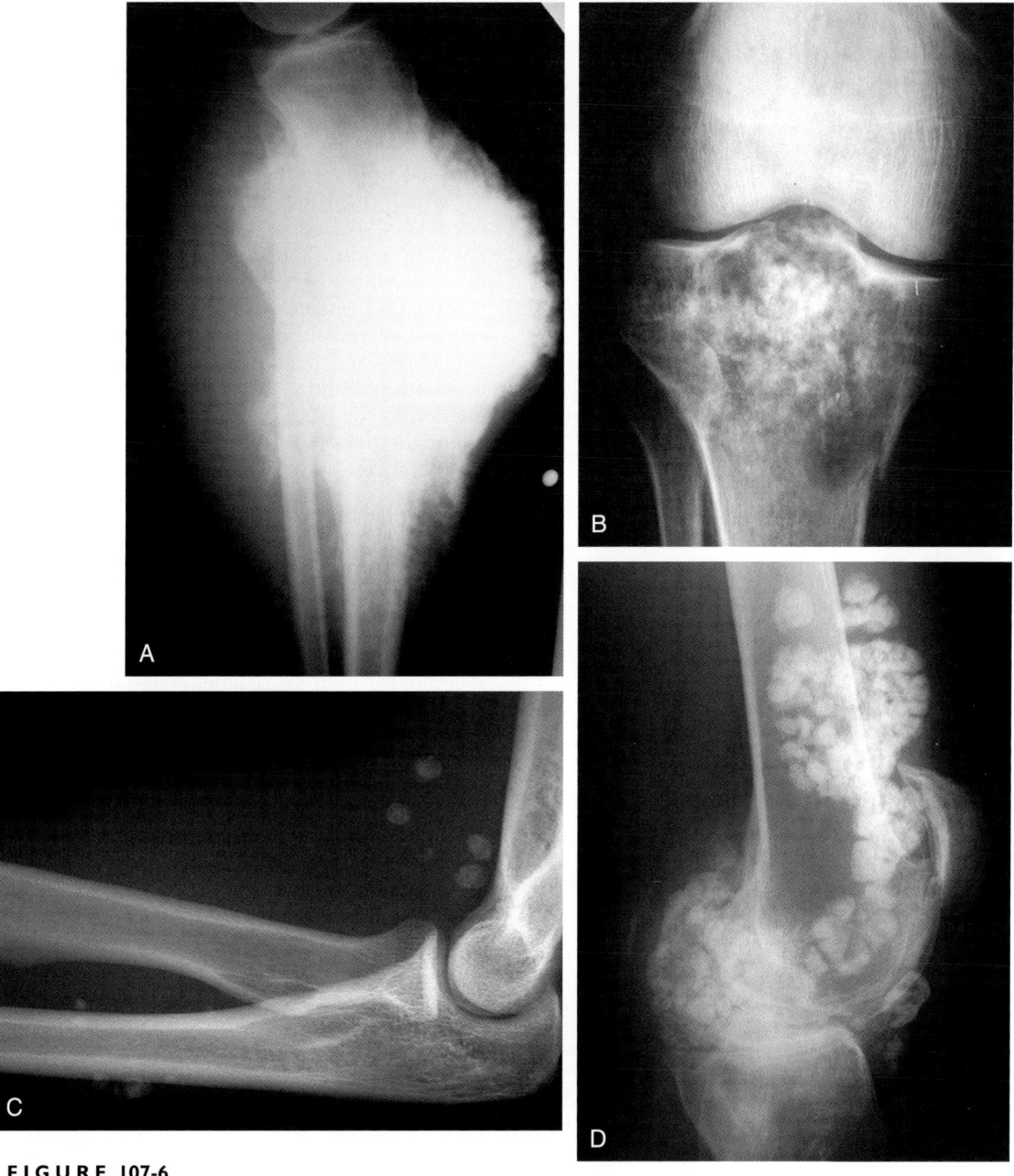

FIGURE 107-6

The value of the radiograph in the MR evaluation of musculoskeletal masses. **A,** Osteosarcoma with dense osteoid. **B,** Chondrosarcoma with characteristic mineralization and pathologic fracture. **C,** Phleboliths within soft-tissues about the elbow consistent with hemangioma. **D,** Multiple mineralized bodies within the knee in a patient with synovial osteochondromatosis.

T1 sequences are to be utilized, the injection should be preceded by a fat saturation T1 sequence to avoid interpretive errors due to a rescaling effect.[23] With this effect, a region of subtle increased signal intensity on routine T1-weighted images will appear markedly increased in signal intensity on fat saturation T1-weighted images. If not preceded by a fat saturation noncontrast sequence, the resultant fat saturation postcontrast images may be erroneously interpreted as showing tumor enhancement.[23]

MR contrast is not routinely required in the evaluation of bone or soft-tissue masses[23] and the use of gadolinium remains controversial. May et al, in a study of 242 patients with musculoskeletal masses, found that gadolinium did not contribute to the differential diagnosis or patient management in 89% of cases.[24] The use of gadolinium entails additional cost, a substantially prolonged examination time and an increased risk, albeit small, of significant and potentially life threatening contrast-induced reaction.[25-27] Gadolinium is clearly useful in

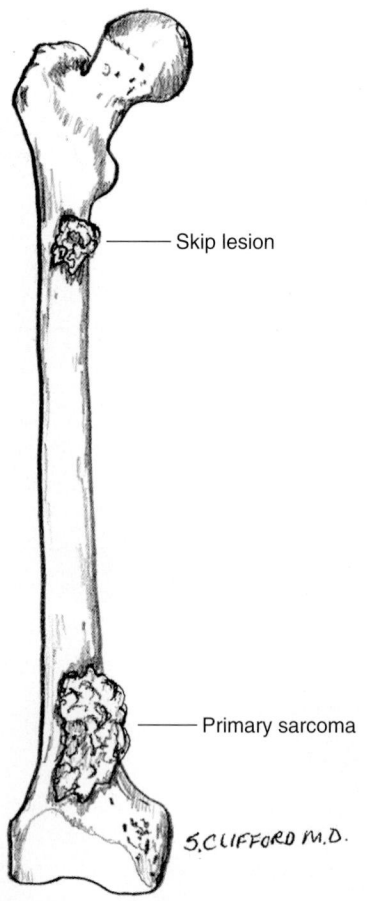

FIGURE 107-7

Sarcoma metastasis within the compartment of tumor origin is known as a skip lesion. The skip lesion here is separated from the primary sarcoma in the distal femur by normal tissue. Limb-sparing procedures performed without evaluation of the entire involved compartment may result in tumor recurrence due to the presence of undetected skip lesions.

differentiating solid from cystic or necrotic lesions. Some solid masses, particularly neural tumors and synovial sarcomas, may appear "cystic" on nonenhanced scans[23] (Fig. 107-8). Some lesions such as intramuscular myxomas,[28,29] myxoid liposarcoma, and hyaline cartilage lesions[19] may show minimal enhancement. Gadolinium is of aid in determining appropriate sites for biopsy in a partially necrotic or cystic mass.[30] Gadolinium has been used to assess chemotherapy-induced necrosis. Dynamic contrast-enhanced MR provides a more accurate assessment of remaining viable tumor[30-33] than static postcontrast images. Gadolinium is valuable in postsurgical surveillance to differentiate postoperative fluid collections and post-therapeutic changes from residual or recurrent tumor.[6,24,34] Contrast is helpful in distinguishing hematoma from tumor with secondary hemorrhage, although it should be kept in mind that fibrovascular proliferation in organized hematomas may also enhance.[19,24,35]

DIFFUSION-WEIGHTED IMAGING

Diffusion-weighted imaging (DWI) is an MR technique that measures intravoxel incoherent motion (IVIM) wherein the contrast of a generated image is based upon the random microscopic motion of water molecules. The freedom of water molecules to move about is decreased for a molecule within an intact cell. Cell membrane disruption allows these water molecules greater freedom to move larger distances. The greater the ability a molecule of water has to move about freely (the higher the diffusion), the more prominent the signal loss on the diffusion-weighted image. The more contained or restricted a molecule of water is (the lower the diffusion), the higher the resultant signal on the diffusion-weighted image on DWI.

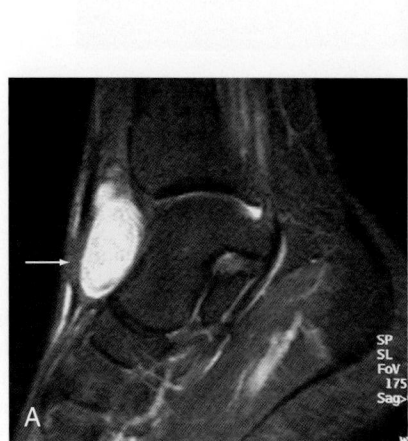
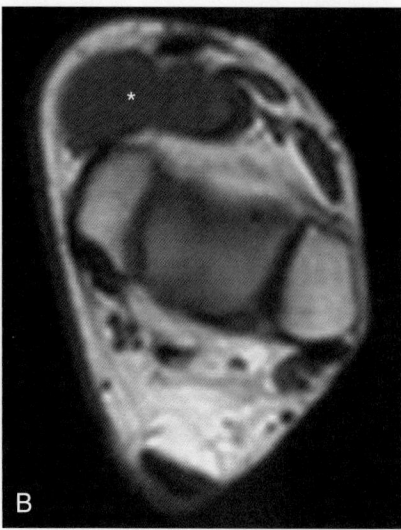
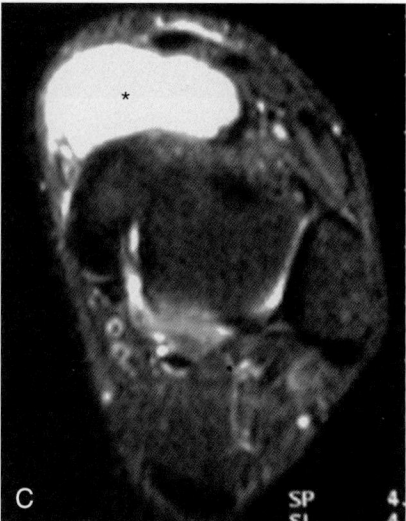

FIGURE 107-8

Solid mass simulating a cystic lesion. **A,** Sagittal STIR shows a nearly homogeneous high signal intensity well-circumscribed mass *(arrow)* in a 29-year-old female complaining of a mass on the dorsum of her foot. **B,** T1-weighted image shows a homogeneous well-defined mass isointense to muscle *(asterisk)*. **C,** Axial STIR shows a "cystic" appearing mass *(asterisk)*. Contrast study or ultrasound was not carried out. The clinician was unsuccessful in the attempted aspiration of the suspected ganglion cyst. Biopsy revealed a synovial sarcoma.

Conventional contrast-enhanced MR images underestimate tumor necrosis in part because the contrast molecules may diffuse into interstitial spaces and into necrotic tissues over time.[36] Properly performed dynamic gadolinium technique is more accurate in differentiating viable tumor from necrosis. DWI allows discrimination between viable tumor and necrotic tissue.[37-39] The random motion of water molecules is greater in areas of necrotic tumor due to disrupted cell membranes compared to viable intact tumor cells. Necrotic tumor tissue is distinguished from viable tumor tissue by the higher diffusion of water within the necrotic regions. Necrotic regions are seen as areas of relative decreased signal on DWI, exhibiting a significantly stronger signal loss than viable tumor. DWI may therefore have a role in monitoring tumor necrosis following treatment.[36]

Routine MR imaging may fail to adequately distinguish post-therapeutic change from tumor recurrence, as all of these processes tend to be of high signal intensity on T2-weighted images. DWI appears to have a role in differentiating postsurgical and postradiation changes from tumor.[36-38] Post-therapeutic changes such as hygromas and muscle edema have a significantly higher diffusion than viable recurrent tumor.[38]

Recent studies indicate that DWI may help in differentiating benign from malignant lesions.[40-42] Spuentrup et al[41] found that diffusion signal characteristics allowed differentiation between edema seen in benign vertebral compression fractures and tumor infiltration with or without fracture. Chan et al[43] reviewed 49 acute benign and malignant vertebral fractures and found (with the exception of two sclerotic metastases) that all benign fractured vertebrae were hypointense and that all malignant lesions were hyperintense with respect to normal marrow on DWI. The apparent diffusion coefficient (ADC) was useful in distinguishing benign from malignant lesions but there was overlap of ADC values between malignancy and tuberculous spondylitis. Zhou et al[44] found quantitative ADC measures provided valuable information in differentiating benign from malignant vertebral fractures.

BONE TUMORS

The differential diagnosis of a primary bone lesion is principally based on plain film analysis. Conventional radiographs are essential for diagnosis and assessment of tumor aggressiveness. These studies should be reviewed in the context of tumor margins, matrix patterns, and periosteal reactions. Bone tumors tend to occur at predictable ages and in common locations, and thus knowledge of the patient's age and the location of the lesion are critical in the differential diagnosis. Many benign lesions have characteristic features on radiographs and require no further imaging or follow-up. Biopsies of these lesions are unnecessary and are sometimes a source of confusion. These "no touch lesions" include fibroxanthoma, periosteal desmoid, intraosseous ganglion, and bone infarct. MRI may play a complimentary role in diagnosis but the modality is of greatest use in evaluating the full anatomic extent of a mass and its relationship to normal surrounding structures. MR image guided percutaneous biopsy of primary bone tumors has proven efficient and safe.[45-47] MRI also plays a role in the post-therapeutic and post-surgical evaluation of bone tumors. The MR characteristics of most bone tumors are nonspecific[48] and there is little correlation between MR appearance and histologic diagnosis of bone tumors.[49] In spite of this, there are some MR features discussed below that are helpful in diagnosing certain tumors and tumor-like conditions of bone.

Bone Tumor Characterization

Hemangioma, intraosseous lipoma, bone infarct, and Paget's disease are bone lesions that frequently exhibit high signal intensity on T1-weighted images. Hemangiomas are benign bone lesions composed of a collection of abnormal and normal vessels with interposed fat. The overgrowth of adipose frequently associated with hemangiomas may be a response to marrow atrophy.[50] It is this interspersed fat that is of high signal intensity seen on T1-weighted images.[51] Hemangiomas are usually solitary and are most common in the spine followed by the skull where they are usually seen in the frontal and parietal bones. Hemangiomas of short and long tubular bones are uncommon.[52] Hemangiomas of the spine usually involve the vertebral body but may affect the posterior elements.[53] Hemangiomas are found in 10% to 11% of spines[50-54] examined at autopsy and are most frequent in the thoracic region.[52] The vertebral lesions are usually asymptomatic but less than 1% may become symptomatic with spinal cord encroachment or compression fracture.[54] Typically hemangiomas are high to intermediate signal intensity on T1- and high signal intensity on T2-weighted image.[55] A coarse low signal trabecular pattern that may be seen on MRI corresponds to the corduroy or honeycomb pattern seen radiographically. Regions of fat are seen as areas of high signal intensity on T1 sequences with vascular channels and edema accounting for high signal intensity on T2-weighted images.[50,51,55]

Lipomas account for less than 0.1% of all intraosseous tumors.[56] Common sites include the intertrochanteric region of the proximal femur followed by the calcaneus, ilium, and proximal tibia.[57] MRI shows varying degrees of high signal fat similar to subcutaneous fat on T1 and T2 sequences.[56,58] The MR appearance of an intraosseous lipoma may vary, depending upon the degree of saponification and subsequent mineralization (Fig. 107-9). A stage 1 intraosseous lipoma is a pure fatty lesion with a fine peripheral rim of reactive bone sclerosis. A similar lesion with central low signal calcification due to fat necrosis is seen in stage 2. Further involution and necrosis (stage 3) shows variable internal signal and calcification often with a thin periphery of preserved fat surrounded by marked reactive bone sclerosis.[56,57]

A mature infarct contains internal fat seen as high signal intensity on T1-weighted sequences. The "double line sign" characterizes the classic infarct.[59] This double

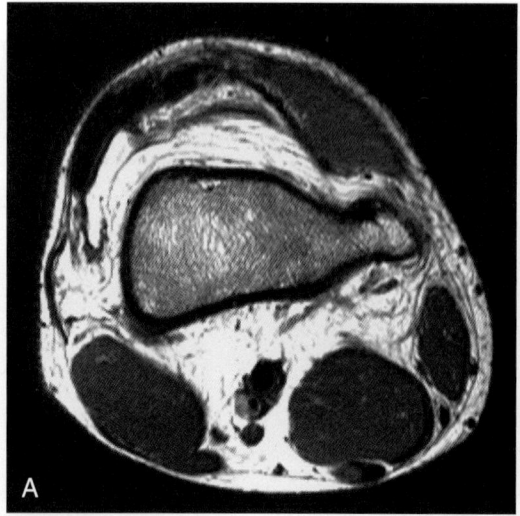

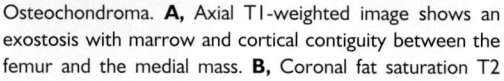

FIGURE 107-11

Osteochondroma. **A,** Axial T1-weighted image shows an exostosis with marrow and cortical contiguity between the femur and the medial mass. **B,** Coronal fat saturation T2 image shows the osteochondroma with a thin cartilage cap (*arrowheads*) and an adjacent fluid collection, the exostosis bursata (*arrow*).

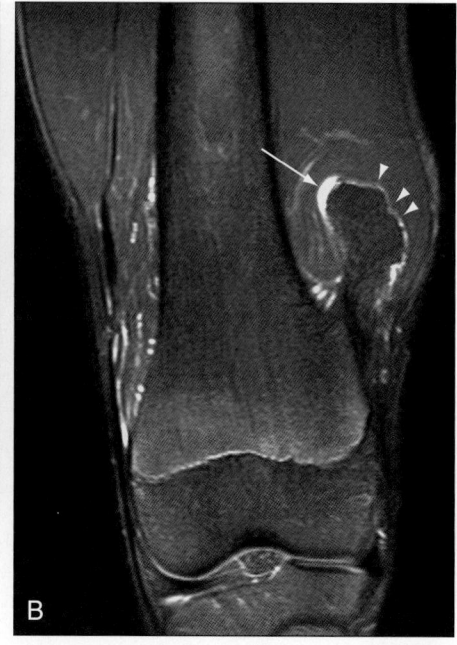

cited as suspicious for malignancy. In a recent review from the Armed Forces Institute of Pathology (AFIP) archives, Murphey et al[72] made a strong case for suspected malignant transformation in lesions with a cartilage cap thickness of greater than 1.5 cm in a skeletally mature individual. Complications of osteochondromas include growth disturbance, cosmetic deformities, fracture, bursitis, tendinosis, osteonecrosis of the cartilage cap, and encroachment on adjacent bones, soft-tissues, neural and vascular structures.

Enchondromas are the second most common chondroid tumor accounting for 12% to 14% of benign bone neoplasms and 3% to 10% of all osseous neoplasms.[77] Enchondromas are usually solitary and arise from cartilaginous rests originating from the growth plate. They are most common in the hands, accounting for 40% to 65% of all solitary enchondromas.[70] Enchondromas have a characteristic MR appearance of low signal intensity on T1, very high signal intensity hyaline cartilage on T2, a lobulated contour and internal low signal septae best appreciated on T2 sequences.[78] A mineralized matrix may be seen as focal areas of low signal on all sequences. Focal islands of normal yellow bone marrow may be interspersed between lobules of chondroid tissue.[70,79,80] Peripheral and septal tumor enhancement is noted with gadolinium administration[70,80,81] (Fig. 107-12). Enchondromatosis or multiple enchondromas occur in multiple syndromes,[55] including Ollier's disease, Mafucci's syndrome and metachondromatosis. Ollier's disease consists of enchondromas exclusively or predominantly on one side of the body.[70] Mafucci's syndrome consists of enchondromas with associated soft-tissue hemangiomas, less often lymphangiomas. Metachondromatosis, an autosomal dominant

disease, is the only hereditary condition of the three and is characterized by multiple enchondromas and osteochondromas. The exostoses are small and, unlike conventional osteochondromas, point toward the joint and may decrease in size or completely resolve over time.[77,82]

Distinction between enchondroma and low-grade chondrosarcoma is difficult and a common dilemma confronting radiologists.[79,83] Enchondromas are common in the hands and feet, involving the metacapals, metatarsals, and phalanges. Sarcomatous transformation of an enchondroma is rare in the hands and the feet and is more commonly seen in the long tubular bones of the appendicular skeleton.[70,80] Chondrosarcomas of the axial skeleton (spine and pelvis) are common while enchondromas are rare in these locations.[80] The diagnostic quandary of enchondroma versus low-grade chondrosarcoma therefore centers on the appendicular skeleton proximal to the metacarpals and metatarsals.

Murphey et al found that clinical and radiographic features can distinguish enchondroma from low-grade chondrosarcoma in 90% of lesions in the appendicular skeleton excluding the hands and feet.[80] The study found statistically significant features suggesting chondrosarcoma to include the presence of pain and deep endosteal scalloping of greater than two-thirds of the cortical thickness. Cortical breakthrough or destruction, soft-tissue mass, epiphyseal location (enchondromas are uncommonly epiphyseal), and lesion size greater than 5-6 cm also favor malignancy. Pathologic fracture, cortical thickening, periosteal reaction, and scintigraphic activity within the lesion exceeding the anterior iliac crest all favor the diagnosis of chondrosarcoma.[80] Abnormal marrow signal around an intramedullary chondroid tumor on STIR sequences suggests chondrosarcoma.[78]

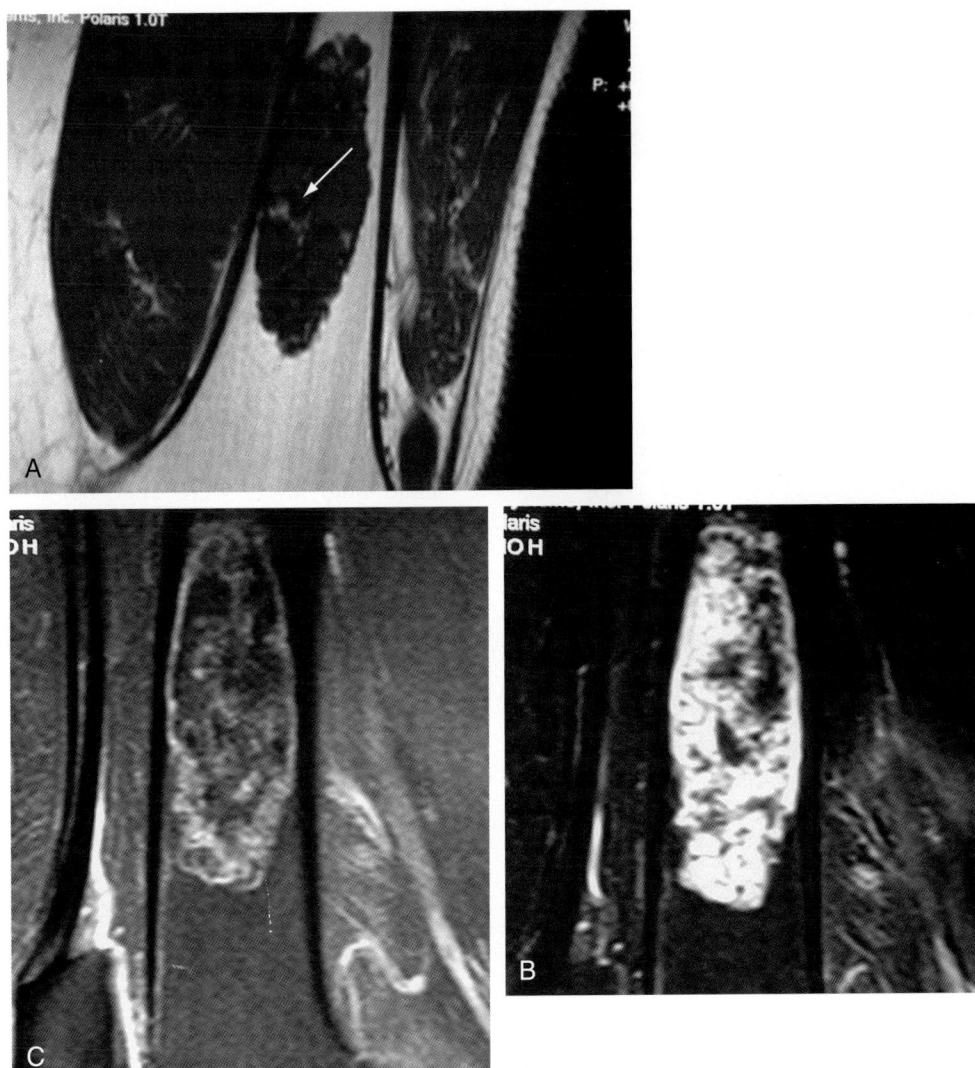

FIGURE 107-12

Enchondroma. **A,** Coronal T1 image of distal femur shows a well-defined lobulated intermediate signal intensity mass with areas of high signal intensity area representing interspersed fat *(arrow)*. **B,** Sagittal STIR shows lobulated high signal chondroid and low signal mineralization and suppressed fat. There is no surrounding marrow edema. **C,** Sagittal post-contrast T1 with evident peripheral and septal enhancement.

Certain bone tumors or tumor-like conditions with internal calcification, osteoid formation, or significant sclerosis may exhibit low signal intensity on T2-weighted sequences. Enostoses or bone islands are hamartomas consisting of cortical bone within cancellous bone exhibiting low signal intensity on all MR sequences.[84] Multiple bone islands may be seen in a periarticular distribution in patients with osteopoikilosis or in the same distribution with slight elongation of the individual lesions with osteopathia striata (Voorhoeve's disease).[85] Melorheostosis is a rare sclerosing dysplasia of bone with cortical hyperostosis, described as having a characteristic radiographic appearance reminiscent of "flowing candle wax." These lesions are of low signal intensity on all imaging sequences[86,87] (Fig. 107-13). Contiguous or adjacent mineralized or nonmineralized soft-tissue masses may be present.[87]

Osteosarcoma is the second most common primary malignancy of bone following multiple myeloma and is characterized by the formation of bone or osteoid by malignant cells. Osteosarcomas are microscopically heterogeneous and have variable clinical and radiographic features. Osteosarcomas may be characterized by the predominant constituent matrix, histologic grade, location within bone (surface vs. intramedullary), distribution (focal vs. multifocal), and by whether the lesion is primary or secondary to malignant transformation.[85] Osteosarcomas and chondroid tumors may exhibit regions of internal low signal intensity on all MR sequences corresponding to areas of mineralization (Fig. 107-14).

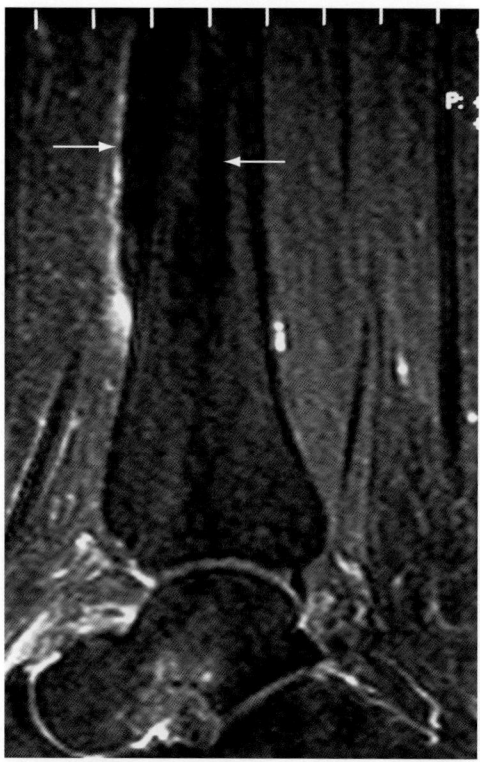

FIGURE 107-13

Melorheostosis. Sagittal STIR image shows low signal cortical hyperostosis (*arrows*) at the anterior tibia. Encroachment on the marrow space may be present resulting from endosteal involvement.

Fibrous lesions have variable signal characteristics but may exhibit low to intermediate signal on long TR images. Fibrous dysplasia, initially described as being of low signal intensity on all sequences, is usually low signal intensity on T1 and of variable signal on T2 sequences[88] and therefore nonspecific in MR appearance. In patients with cystic fibrous dysplasia, signal characteristics are consistent with fluid.[89] Fibroxanthomas usually exhibit a pathognomonic plain film appearance. On MRI these lesions tend to be septated and have low signal on T1 and T2 sequences in approximately 80% of cases[88,90,91] (Fig. 107-15). The signal intensity is related to the amount of fibrous tissue, hemosiderin, hemorrhage, collagen, foamy histiocytes, and bone trabeculae present.[90] Desmoplastic fibroma is a very rare locally aggressive lesion accounting for up to 0.3% of all benign bone tumors.[88,92] The lesion is histologically identical to the desmoid tumor of soft-tissues.[93,94] Desmoplastic fibroma is most common in the second and third decades with a mean age of 21 years.[88,94] Desmoplastic fibroma most commonly involves the mandible (22%) and femur (15%), followed by the pelvic bones, radius, and tibia (13%, 12%, and 9%, respectively).[93] The MR signal is often in whole or in part low on T1 and T2.[88] The presence of low signal intensity areas on T2 is attributed to regions of increased collagen content, while more

cellular areas are responsible for regions of increased signal[93] (Fig. 107-16).

Primary lymphoma of bone accounts for approximately 5% of primary bone tumors and has a variable MR appearance. Most primary bone lymphomas are isointense to hypointense to muscle on T1 sequences with T2 signal being hypointense, isointense, or hyperintense to fat.[95,96] Primary lymphoma of bone may be suspected in patients over 30 years of age when MRI shows extensive marrow involvement with significant extraosseous soft-tissue mass and minimal or no cortical destruction.[97] These tumors spread through the penetrating vascular channels into adjacent soft-tissues with cortical bone being left largely intact.[96] This appearance has been reported with other round cell tumors such as Ewing's sarcoma.

Fluid–fluid levels were once believed to be highly suggestive of an aneurysmal bone cyst[98] (Fig. 107-17). Aneurysmal bone cysts arise in benign antecedent lesions in 29% to 35% of cases.[99] Although most common in aneurysmal bone cysts, fluid–fluid levels have now been noted in multiple bone lesions including giant cell tumor, chondroblastoma, telangiectatic osteosarcoma (Fig. 107-18), fibrous dysplasia, conventional osteosarcoma, malignant fibrous histiocytoma, simple bone cysts with superimposed hemorrhage, osteomyelitis/abscess, necrotic tumors, synovial sarcoma, osteoblastoma, hemophillic pseudotumors, bone metastases, or hemorrhage into a pre-existing lesion.[49,100-103]

SOFT-TISSUE TUMORS

Magnetic resonance imaging has become the primary diagnostic imaging tool in the evaluation of soft-tissue masses.[104] MRI can confirm the presence of a mass, define its anatomic extent and, in some cases, provide a specific diagnosis. MRI aids in the selection of an appropriate site for successful biopsy of soft-tissue lesions. MR image-guided biopsies of soft-tissue lesions have met with some success.[105] MRI also plays a central role in assessing the post-therapeutic response to chemotherapy and local tumor surveillance. A study by the Radiology Diagnostic Oncology Group evaluated patients from four institutions with both primary osseous and soft-tissue tumors and found CT and MRI equally accurate in the local staging of malignant bone and soft-tissue tumors at the anatomic sites studied.[106] Despite this report, most radiologists and orthopedic surgeons believe that MRI is the study of choice for the evaluation of soft-tissue masses.[7] The excellent soft-tissue contrast resolution, direct multiplanar acquisition, and the possibility of tissue characterization through the evaluation of signal characteristics have made MRI the preferred means of staging and evaluation of tumor extent.

Similar to osseous tumors, the radiographic evaluation of a suspected soft-tissue mass should begin with orthogonal radiographs. Radiographs may show phleboliths associated with hemangiomas, stippled or arc-and-ring

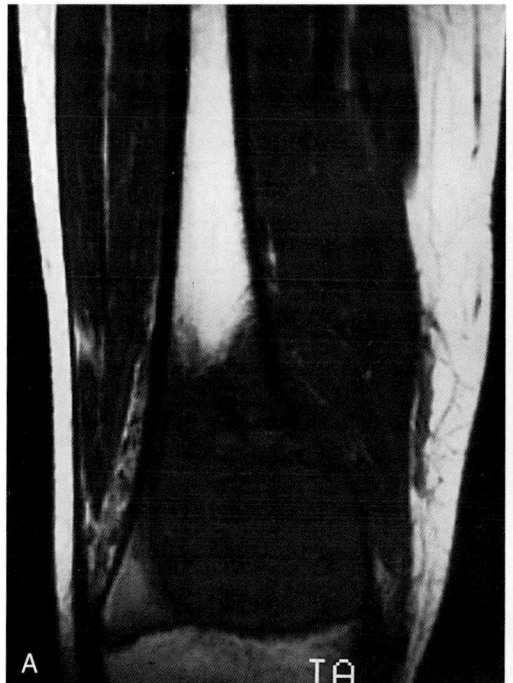

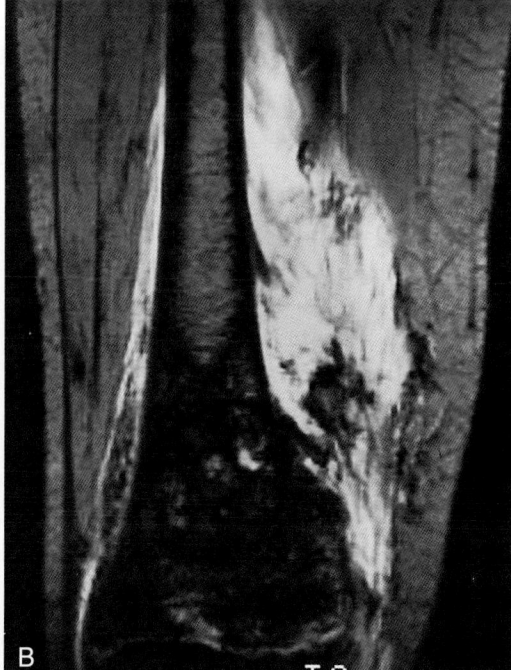

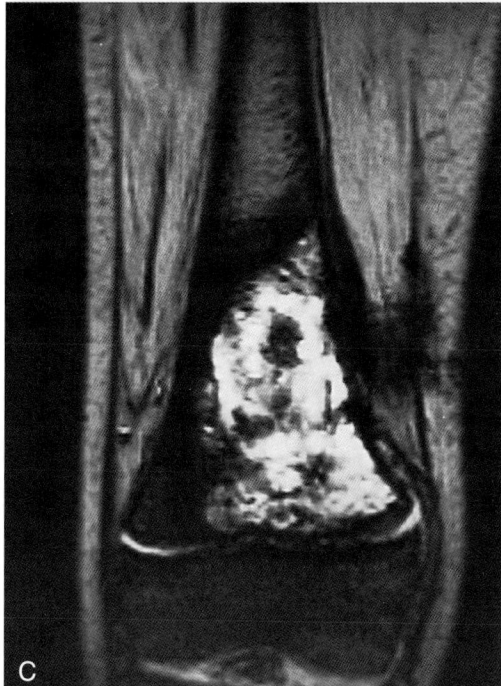

FIGURE 107-14

An 11-year-old girl presented with an osteogenic sarcoma of the distal femur. Coronal T1-weighted (600/20) (**A**) and T2*-weighted gradient-echo (363/30/20°) (**B**) images reveal an aggressive lesion in the distal femoral metaphysis with cortical breakthrough and a large soft-tissue mass. The intramedullary portion is dark on the T2*-weighted image due to ossification. **C,** Coronal T2*-weighted gradient-echo (370/30/20°) image obtained after a 2-month cycle of chemotherapy and irradiation. The soft-tissue component of the tumor and adjacent edema have resolved, but the intramedullary tumor is unchanged in size. The medullary tumor has become more heterogeneous and brighter in signal intensity. This nonspecific change could reflect necrosis, hemorrhage, granulation tissue, or viable tumor. No residual viable tumor was present histologically when the tumor was resected.

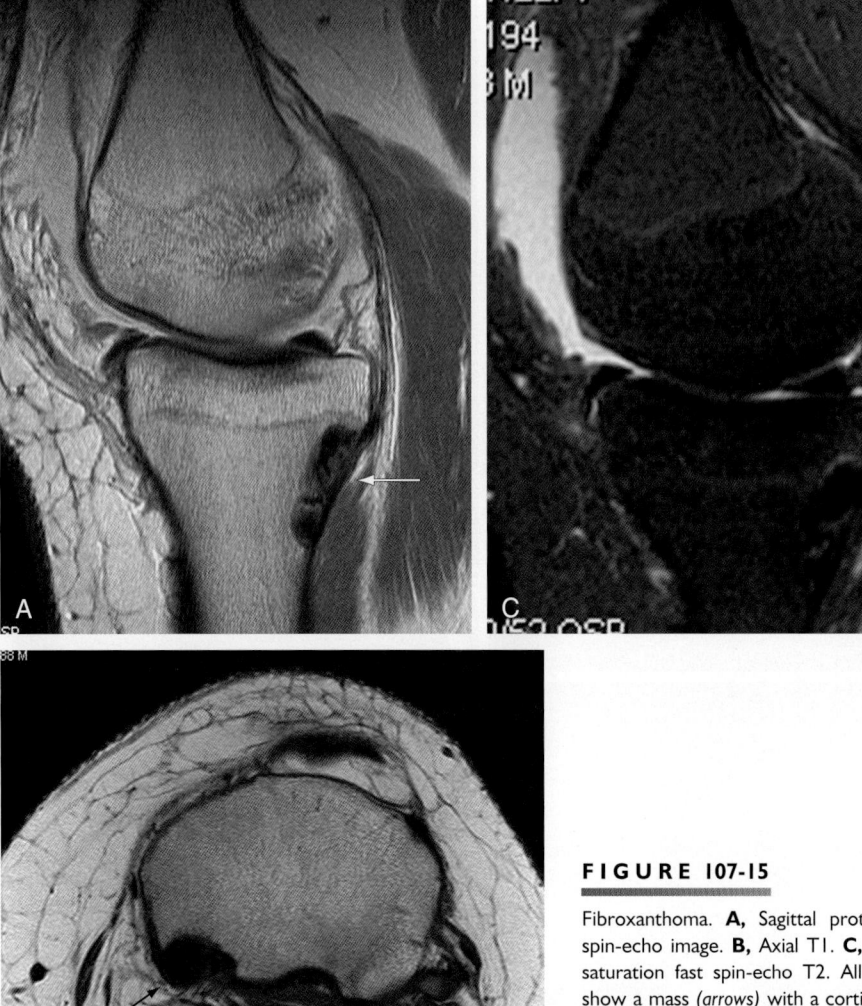

FIGURE 107-15

Fibroxanthoma. **A,** Sagittal proton density spin-echo image. **B,** Axial T1. **C,** Sagittal fat saturation fast spin-echo T2. All sequences show a mass (*arrows*) with a cortical location and a prominent low signal component.

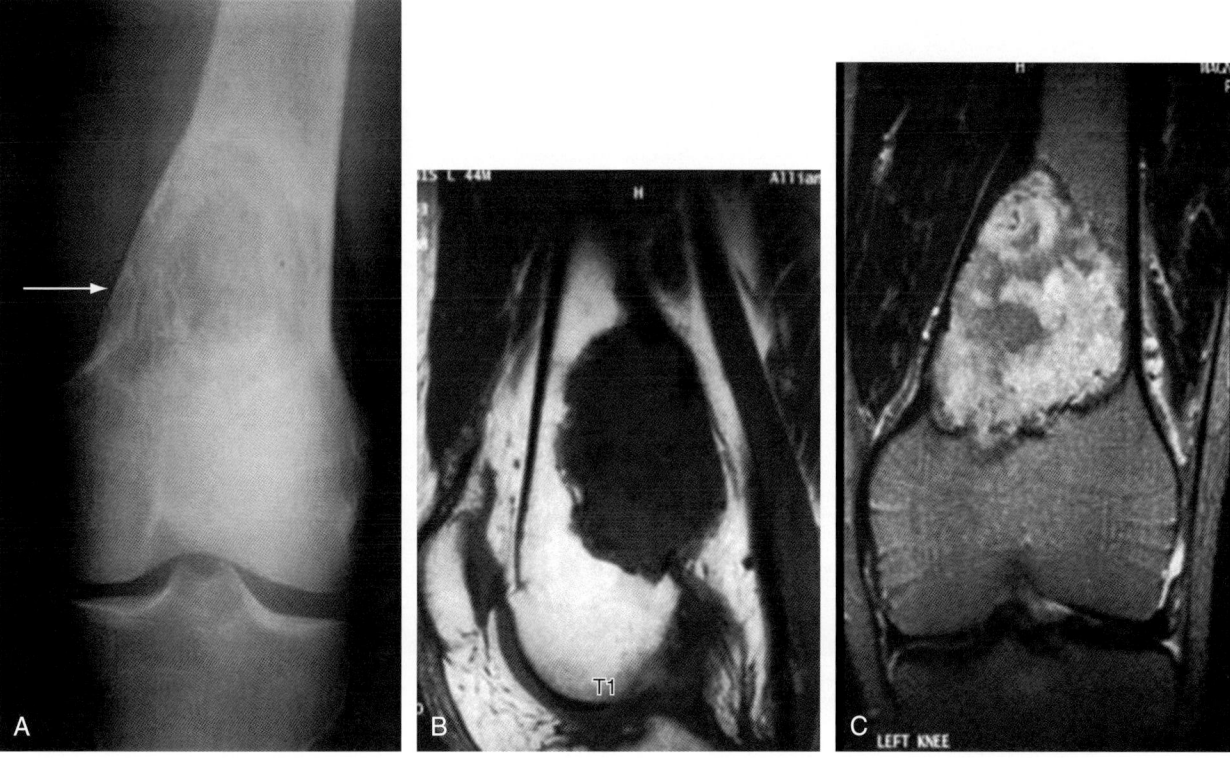

FIGURE 107-16

Desmoplastic fibroma of bone. **A,** Radiograph of this rare tumor shows a lytic, geographic lesion with (*arrow*) somewhat sclerotic borders and no mineralized matrix. **B,** T1 sagittal image shows a mildly heterogeneous lesion, primarily intermediate in signal intensity. **C,** The tumor is heterogeneous on the T2 coronal image with moderate high signal intensity and prominent areas of decreased signal intensity reflecting cellular and collagen content respectively.

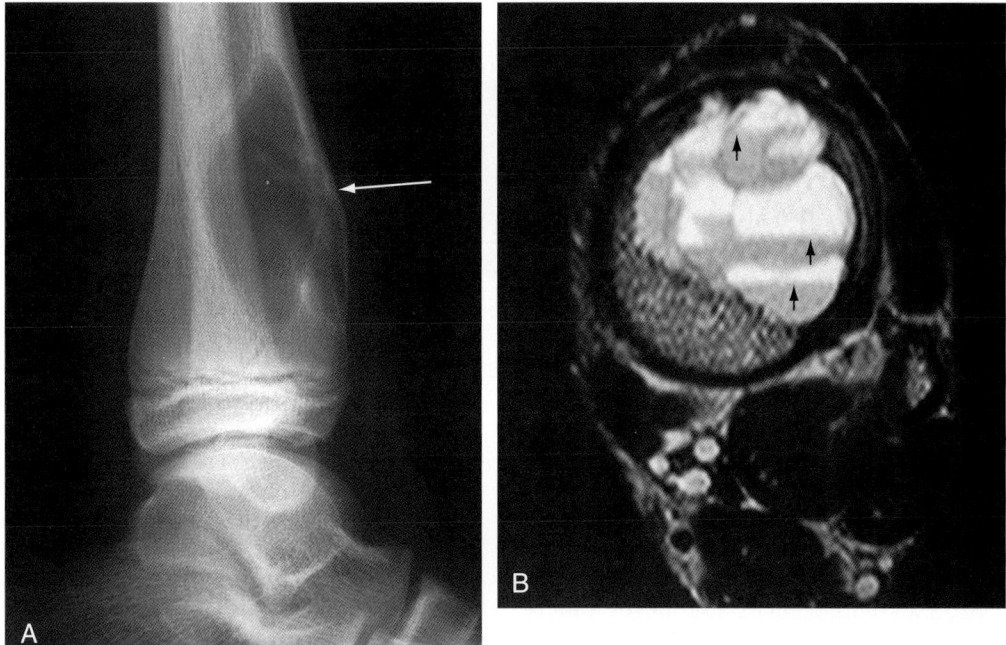

FIGURE 107-17

Aneurysmal bone cyst with fluid–fluid levels. **A,** An eccentrically placed expansile, lytic geographic lesion with somewhat sclerotic margins (*arrow*) is noted in the distal tibia of this 12-year-old patient. **B,** Axial fast spin-echo T2-weighted image of the distal tibial lesion with multiple fluid–fluid levels (*arrows*).

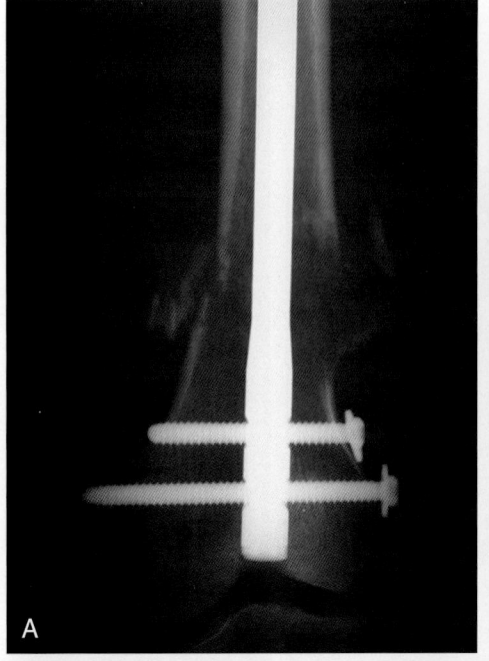

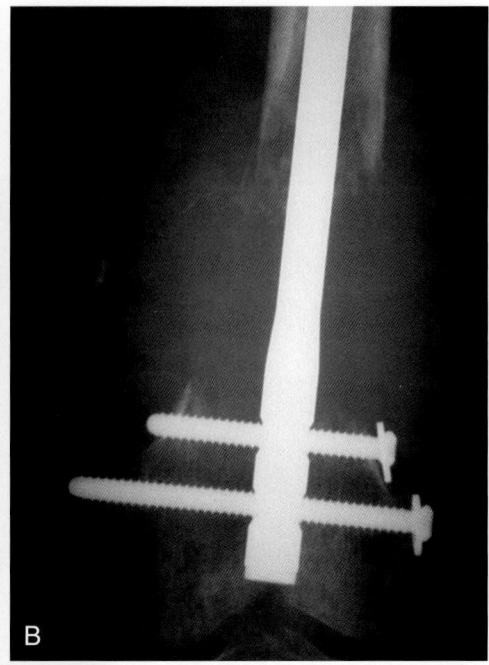

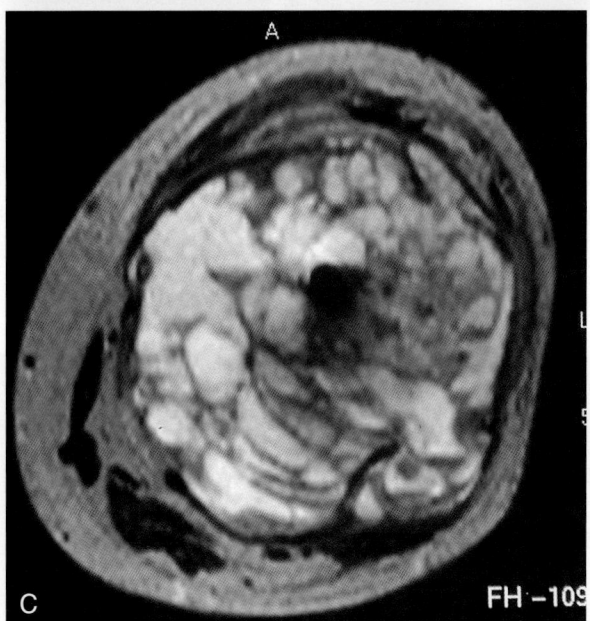

FIGURE 107-18

A 48-year-old female referred from a community medical center with a distal femur fracture treated with intramedullary (IM) rod fixation. **A,** Radiograph taken soon after fixation. Note fracture, IM rod, and underlying permeative pattern in the femur. **B,** Radiograph taken nearly 2 months later showing increased bone destruction. **C,** Axial T2-weighted image exhibits multiple fluid–fluid levels. The patient was imaged with the IM rod in place with little metal artifact due to optimization of fast spin-echo techniques and the avoidance of fat saturation in this patient with telangiectatic osteosarcoma.

chondroid calcifications, osteoid matrix, myositis ossificans, fat elements, or mineralization associated with synovial sarcoma, tumoral calcinosis, gout, or synovial osteochondromatosis. Periosteal reaction, bone remodeling and secondary osseous invasion may also be detected on radiographs.

While MRI plays a complimentary role in the differential diagnosis and evaluation of primary bone lesions, it is the preferred modality for the imaging diagnosis of soft-tissue masses. Under ideal circumstances, however, MRI is able to provide a correct diagnosis of a soft-tissue neoplasm in one quarter to one third of cases.[7,107] Despite this limitation, a significant number of soft-tissue

tumors or tumor-like masses may be diagnosed or strongly suspected on the basis of MR signal characteristics. When a specific diagnosis of a soft-tissue tumor cannot be made on the basis of MR alone, evaluation of the lesion in light of the history, clinical findings, tumor prevalence by age, and anatomic site helps to narrow differential considerations. For those soft-tissue masses with normal radiographs and nonspecific MR signal characteristics, a reasonable differential can be constructed by referring to Tables 107-1 and 107-2. These tables are based on 39,179 benign and malignant soft-tissue lesions collected over a 10-year period by the Armed Forces Institute of Pathology (AFIP).[108,109]

Text continues on page 3519

TABLE 107-1A Distribution of Common Benign Soft-Tissue Tumors by Anatomic Location and Age

Age (yrs)	Hand and wrist	No. (%)	Upper extremity	No. (%)	Axilla and shoulder	No. (%)	Foot and ankle	No. (%)	Lower extremity	No. (%)
0–5	Fibromatosis[a]	21 (22)	Fibrous histiocytoma	6 (6)	Myofibromatosis	6 (8)	Infantile digital fibromatosis	7 (9)	Lipoblastoma	13 (7)
	Hemangioma	15 (15)	Fibrous hamartoma of infancy	15 (16)	Fibrous hamartoma of infancy	23 (29)	Granuloma annulare	23 (30)	Granuloma annulare	42 (23)
	Granuloma annulare	14 (14)	Granuloma annulare	15 (16)	Hemangioma	12 (15)	Fibromatosis	19 (25)	Hemangioma	26 (14)
	Infantile digital fibromatosis	8 (8)	Hemangioma	14 (15)	Lipoblastoma	11 (14)	Hemangioma	8 (11)	Myofibromatosis	16 (9)
	Aponeurotic fibroma	7 (7)	Fibromatosis	13 (14)	Fibrous histiocytoma	7 (9)	Lipoblastoma	6 (8)	Fibrous histiocytoma	15 (8)
	Fibrous histiocytoma	5 (5)	Juvenile xanthogranuloma	6 (6)	Lymphangioma	5 (6)	Lipoma	4 (5)	Lymphangioma	10 (6)
	Nodular fasciitis	5 (5)	Myofibromatosis	6 (6)	Nodular fasciitis	4 (5)	Neurofibroma	3 (4)	Juvenile xanthogranuloma	10 (6)
	Other	22 (23)	Other	19 (20)	Other	12 (15)	Other	6 (8)	Other	48 (27)
6–15	Fibrous histiocytoma	32 (14)	Fibrous histiocytoma	41 (23)	Fibrous histiocytoma	25 (34)	Fibromatosis	37 (23)	Hemangioma	47 (22)
	Hemangioma	31 (13)	Nodular fasciitis	39 (21)	Nodular faciitis	18 (25)	Granuloma annulare	21 (13)	Fibrous histiocytoma	34 (16)
	Aponeurotic fibroma	25 (11)	Hemangioma	24 (13)	Hemangioma	7 (10)	Hemangioma	21 (13)	Nodular fasciitis	22 (10)
	Fibroma of tendon sheath	22 (9)	Granuloma annulare	12 (7)	Granular cell tumor	4 (5)	Fibrous histiocytoma	14 (9)	Granuloma annulare	20 (9)
	GCTTS[b]	17 (7)	Fibromatosis	12 (7)	Neurofibroma	3 (4)	GCTTS	13 (8)	Fibromatosis	15 (7)
	Fibromatosis	14 (6)	Neurofibroma	7 (4)	Lymphangioma	2 (3)	Chondroma	11 (7)	Lipoma	13 (6)
	Neurothekeoma	9 (4)	Lipoma	6 (3)	Myofibromatosis	2 (3)	Lipoma	9 (6)	Neurofibroma	8 (4)
	Other	85 (36)	Other	41 (23)	Other	12 (16)	Other	35 (22)	Other	57 (26)
16–25	GCTTS	84 (20)	Nodular fasciitis	130 (35)	Fibrous histiocytoma	62 (36)	Fibromatosis	46 (22)	Fibrous histiocytoma	118 (24)
	Fibrous histiocytoma	57 (14)	Fibrous histiocytoma	87 (23)	Nodular fasciitis	35 (20)	GCTTS	29 (14)	Nodular fasciitis	61 (13)
	Hemangioma	40 (10)	Hemangioma	36 (10)	Fibromatosis	16 (9)	Granuloma annulare	25 (12)	Hemangioma	55 (11)
	Fibroma of tendon sheath	40 (10)	Neurofibroma	24 (6)	Lipoma	14 (8)	Fibrous histiocytoma	24 (12)	Neurofibroma	48 (10)
	Nodular fasciitis	26 (6)	Granuloma annulare	20 (5)	Neurofibroma	12 (7)	Hemangioma	13 (6)	Fibromatosis	38 (8)
	Granuloma annulare	21 (5)	Granular cell tumor	17 (5)	Hemangioma	4 (2)	PVNS[c]	12 (6)	Lipoma	22 (5)
	Ganglion	20 (5)	Schwannoma	11 (3)	Schwannoma	4 (2)	Neurofibroma	11 (5)	Schwannoma	20 (4)
	Other	132 (31)	Other	51 (14)	Other	25 (15)	Other	45 (22)	Other	122 (25)

Note: No. (%) indicates the number of specified lesions in the indicated location for the given age group (percentage of all malignant tumors in this location and for this age group). For example, 5 (45) indicates that there are five fibrosarcomas in the hand and wrist of patients 0–5 years old, and this represented 45% of all malignant tumors in this location and age group.

[a] 21 (22) indicates there were 21 cases of fibromatosis in the hand and wrist of patients 0–5 years old and this represented 22% of all benign tumors in this location and age group.

[b] Giant cell tumor of tendon sheath.

[c] Pigmented villonodular synovitis.

From Kransdorf MJ, et al: Benign soft-tissue tumors in a large referral population: distribution of specific diagnoses by age, sex, and location. Am J Roentgenol 164:395–402, 1995. Reprinted with permission from the American Journal of Roentgenology.

Continued

TABLE 107-1A Distribution of Common Benign Soft-Tissue Tumors by Anatomic Location and Age—cont'd

Age (yrs)	Hand and wrist	No. (%)	Upper extremity	No. (%)	Axilla and shoulder	No. (%)	Foot and ankle	No. (%)	Lower extremity	No. (%)
26–45	Fibrous histiocytoma	167 (18)	Nodular fasciitis	309 (38)	Lipoma	105 (28)	Fibromatosis	99 (21)	Fibrous histiocytoma	245 (25)
	GCTTS	148 (16)	Fibrous histiocytoma	145 (18)	Fibrous histiocytoma	92 (24)	Fibrous histiocytoma	74 (16)	Nodular fasciitis	229 (23)
	Fibroma of tendon sheath	106 (11)	Angiolipoma	48 (6)	Nodular fasciitis	55 (14)	GCTTS	41 (9)	Lipoma	101 (10)
	Hemangioma	86 (10)	Hemangioma	43 (5)	Fibromatosis	29 (8)	Hemangioma	36 (8)	Neurofibroma	71 (7)
	Nodular fasciitis	79 (8)	Schwannoma	43 (5)	Hemangioma	17 (4)	Schwannoma	30 (6)	Schwannoma	59 (6)
	Fibromatosis	46 (5)	Neurofibroma	37 (5)	Neurofibroma	13 (3)	Neurofibroma	24 (5)	Myxoma	53 (5)
	Chondroma	42 (4)	Lipoma	32 (4)	Schwannoma	12 (3)	Chondroma	23 (5)	Hemangioma	52 (5)
	Other	269 (29)	Other	153 (19)	Other	57 (15)	Other	135 (29)	Other	185 (19)
46–65	GCTTS	143 (23)	Nodular fasciitis	86 (20)	Lipoma	189 (58)	Fibromatosis	83 (25)	Lipoma	157 (23)
	Fibrous histiocytoma	63 (10)	Lipoma	80 (19)	Fibrous histiocytoma	28 (9)	Fibrous histiocytoma	43 (13)	Myxoma	109 (16)
	Hemangioma	61 (10)	Fibrous histiocytoma	44 (10)	Myxoma	16 (5)	Lipoma	35 (11)	Fibrous histiocytoma	93 (14)
	Lipoma	59 (9)	Schwannoma	30 (7)	Fibromatosis	14 (4)	Schwannoma	25 (8)	Nodular fasciitis	40 (6)
	Chondroma	52 (8)	Neurofibroma	24 (6)	Nodular fasciitis	13 (4)	GCTTS	21 (6)	Schwannoma	39 (6)
	Fibromatosis	43 (7)	Myxoma	24 (6)	Schwannoma	12 (4)	Chondroma	21 (6)	Neurofibroma	31 (5)
	Fibroma of tendon sheath	37 (6)	Hemangioma	19 (4)	Granular cell tumor	12 (4)	Hemangioma	16 (5)	Proliferative fasciitis	28 (4)
	Other	172 (27)	Other	125 (29)	Other	44 (13)	Other	89 (27)	Other	186 (27)
66 and over	GCTTS	51 (21)	Lipoma	39 (22)	Lipoma	83 (58)	Fibromatosis	16 (14)	Lipoma	68 (26)
	Hemangioma	24 (10)	Myxoma	19 (11)	Myxoma	14 (10)	Schwannoma	15 (13)	Myxoma	44 (17)
	Schwannoma	24 (10)	Nodular fasciitis	18 (10)	Schwannoma	6 (4)	Fibrous histiocytoma	13 (11)	Fibrous histiocytoma	33 (13)
	Chondroma	24 (10)	Schwannoma	17 (9)	Fibromatosis	5 (3)	Chondroma	11 (9)	Schwannoma	31 (12)
	Neurofibroma	21 (9)	Glomus tumor	12 (7)	Fibrous histiocytoma	5 (3)	Lipoma	10 (8)	Hemangiopericytoma	10 (4)
	Fibromatosis	14 (6)	Neurofibroma	10 (6)	Proliferative fasciitis	5 (3)	Granuloma annulare	8 (7)	Neurofibroma	9 (4)
	Lipoma	13 (5)	Angiolipoma	10 (6)	Hemangioma	4 (3)	GCTTS	6 (5)	Hemangioma	8 (3)
	Other	71 (29)	Other	55 (31)	Other	22 (15)	Other	39 (33)	Other	56 (22)

Note: No. (%) indicates the number of specified lesions in the indicated location for the given age group (percentage of all malignant tumors in this location and for this age group). For example, 5 (45) indicates that there are five fibrosarcomas in the hand and wrist of patients 0–5 years old, and this represented 45% of all malignant tumors in this location and age group.

From Kransdorf MJ, et al: Benign soft-tissue tumors in a large referral population: distribution of specific diagnoses by age, sex, and location. Am J Roentgenol 164:395–402, 1995. Reprinted with permission from the American Journal of Roentgenology.

TABLE 107-1B Distribution of Common Benign Soft-Tissue Tumors by Anatomic Location and Age

Age (yrs)	Hip, groin, and buttocks	No. (%)	Head and neck	No. (%)	Trunk	No. (%)	Retroperitoneum	No. (%)
0–5	Fibrous hamartoma of infancy	14 (20)	Nodular fasciitis	47 (20)	Hemangioma	36 (18)	Lipoblastoma	7 (37)
	Lipoblastoma	14 (20)	Hemangioma	43 (18)	Juvenile xanthogranuloma	24 (12)	Lymphangioma	5 (26)
	Myofibromatosis	8 (11)	Myofibromatosis	27 (11)	Myofibromatosis	24 (12)	Hemangioma	4 (21)
	Lymphangioma	7 (10)	Fibromatosis	30 (13)	Nodular fasciitis	17 (8)	Ganglioneuroma	2 (11)
	Fibrous histiocytoma	5 (7)	Granuloma annulare	14 (6)	Lipoblastoma	17 (8)	Fibrous hamartoma of infancy	1 (5)
	Nodular fasciitis	4 (6)	Fibrous histiocytoma	13 (5)	Fibromatosis	23 (11)		
	Fibromatosis	4 (6)	Lipoblastoma	11 (5)	Fibrous hamartoma of infancy	15 (7)		
	Other	14 (20)	Other	52 (22)	other	55 (27)		
6–15	Nodular fasciitis	15 (27)	Nodular fasciitis	75 (33)	Nodular fasciitis	54 (28)	Lymphangioma	7 (37)
	Fibroma	7 (13)	Fibrous histiocytoma	34 (15)	Fibrous histiocytoma	43 (22)	Ganglioneuroma	4 (21)
	Fibrous histiocytoma	6 (11)	Neurofibroma	23 (10)	Hemangioma	25 (13)	Schwannoma	2 (11)
	Fibromatosis	6 (11)	Hemangioma	21 (9)	Lipoma	9 (5)	Fibromatosis	2 (11)
	Lipoma	5 (9)	Myofibromatosis	14 (6)	Neurofibroma	7 (4)	Paraganglioma	1 (5)
	Lipoblastoma	3 (5)	Fibromatosis	15 (7)	Fibromatosis	8 (4)	Hemangioma	1 (5)
	Neurofibroma	3 (5)	Lipoma	6 (3)	Granular cell tumor	6 (3)	Inflammatory pseudotumor	1 (5)
	Other	10 (18)	Other	40 (18)	Other	43 (22)	Other	1 (5)
16–25	Neurofibroma	20 (16)	Nodular fasciitis	61 (21)	Nodular fasciitis	112 (24)	Fibromatosis	14 (20)
	Fibromatosis	18 (15)	Hemangioma	48 (17)	Fibromatosis	72 (16)	Schwannoma	10 (14)
	Fibrous histiocytoma	18 (15)	Fibrous histiocytoma	45 (16)	Fibrous histiocytoma	71 (15)	Neurofibroma	9 (13)
	Nodular fasciitis	12 (10)	Neurofibroma	37 (13)	Hemangioma	52 (11)	Hemangiopericytoma	8 (11)
	Hemangioma	9 (7)	Schwannoma	19 (7)	Neurofibroma	38 (8)	lymphangioma	8 (11)
	Lipoma	8 (7)	Fibromatosis	11 (4)	Lipoma	21 (5)	Ganglioneuroma	6 (8)
	Hemangiopericytoma	8 (7)	Lipoma	10 (4)	Schwannoma	17 (4)	Hemangioma	4 (6)
	Other	29 (24)	Other	56 (20)	Other	79 (17)	Other	12 (17)

Note: No. (%) indicates the number of specified lesions in the indicated location for the given age group (percentage of all malignant tumors in this location and for this age group). For example, 5 (45) indicates that there are five fibrosarcomas in the hand and wrist of patients 0–5 years old, and this represented 45% of all malignant tumors in this location and age group.

From Kransdorf MJ, et al: Benign soft-tissue tumors in a large referral population: distribution of specific diagnoses by age, sex, and location. Am J Roentgenol 164:395–402, 1995. Reprinted with permission from the American Journal of Roentgenology.

Continued

TABLE 107-1B Distribution of Common Benign Soft-Tissue Tumors by Anatomic Location and Age—cont'd

Age (yrs)	Hip, groin, and buttocks	No. (%)	Head and neck	No. (%)	Trunk	No. (%)	Retroperitoneum	No. (%)
26–45	Lipoma	57 (17)	Lipoma	168 (29)	Lipoma	178 (19)	Schwannoma	38 (23)
	Neurofibroma	38 (12)	Nodular fasciitis	145 (19)	Nodular fasciitis	150 (16)	Fibromatosis	30 (18)
	Fibrous histiocytoma	37 (11)	Fibrous histiocytoma	137 (18)	Fibromatosis	148 (16)	Hemangiopericytoma	25 (15)
	Fibromatosis	36 (11)	Hemangioma	97 (13)	Fibrous histiocytoma	98 (10)	Neurofibroma	13 (8)
	Nodular fasciitis	31 (9)	Neurofibroma	57 (8)	Hemangioma	78 (8)	Angiomyolipoma	10 (6)
	Hemangiopericytoma	24 (7)	Hemangiopericytoma	37 (5)	Neurofibroma	65 (7)	Hemangioma	9 (5)
	Myxoma	22 (7)	Schwannoma	27 (4)	Schwannoma	51 (5)	Sclerosing retroperitonitis	7 (4)
	Other	83 (25)	Other	91 (12)	Other	180 (19)	Other	34 (20)
46–65	Lipoma	76 (35)	Lipoma	306 (46)	Lipoma	290 (44)	Schwannoma	33 (19)
	Myxoma	36 (17)	Nodular fasciitis	66 (10)	Fibromatosis	63 (9)	Fibromatosis	25 (14)
	Fibrous hystiocytoma	17 (8)	Hemangioma	55 (8)	Nodular fasciitis	44 (7)	Sclerosing retroperitonitis	25 (14)
	Schwannoma	17 (8)	Fibrous histiocytoma	42 (6)	Hemangioma	31 (5)	Hemangiopericytoma	21 (12)
	Nodular fasciitis	11 (5)	Neurofibroma	30 (4)	Fibrous histiocytoma	29 (4)	Angiomyolipoma	12 (7)
	Hemangiopericytoma	11 (5)	Schwannoma	25 (4)	Neurofibroma	28 (4)	Lipoma	10 (6)
	Hemangioma	9 (4)	Myxoma	23 (3)	Schwannoma	28 (4)	Paraganglioma	9 (5)
	Other	40 (18)	Other	120 (18)	Other	151 (23)	Other	40 (23)
66 and over	Lipoma	22 (21)	Lipoma	158 (50)	Lipoma	124 (42)	Schwannoma	19 (26)
	Myxoma	16 (15)	Hemangioma	22 (7)	Fibromatosis	26 (9)	Hemangiopericytoma	14 (19)
	Neurofibroma	13 (12)	Schwannoma	18 (6)	Neurofibroma	20 (7)	Lipoma	6 (8)
	Schwannoma	10 (9)	Fibrous histiocytoma	17 (5)	Schwannoma	18 (6)	Mesothelioma	6 (8)
	Hemangiopericytoma	10 (9)	Neurofibroma	16 (5)	Elastofibroma	17 (6)	Sclerosing retroperitonitis	5 (7)
	Hemangioma	8 (8)	Nodular fasciitis	13 (4)	Myxoma	16 (5)	Fibromatosis	4 (6)
	Nodular fasciitis	4 (4)	Myxoma	12 (4)	Hemangioma	14 (5)	Paraganglioma	4 (6)
	Other	23 (22)	Other	58 (18)	Other	61 (21)	Other	14 (19)

Note: No. (%) indicates the number of specified lesions in the indicated location for the given age group (percentage of all malignant tumors in this location and for this age group). For example, 5 (45) indicates that there are five fibrosarcomas in the hand and wrist of patients 0–5 years old, and this represented 45% of all malignant tumors in this location and age group.

From Kransdorf MJ, et al: Benign soft-tissue tumors in a large referral population: distribution of specific diagnoses by age, sex, and location. Am J Roentgenol 164:395-402, 1995. Reprinted with permission from the American Journal of Roentgenology.

TABLE 107-2A Distribution of Common Malignant Soft-Tissue Tumors by Anatomic Location and Age

Age (yrs)	Hand and wrist	No. (%)	Upper extremity	No. (%)	Axilla and shoulder	No. (%)	Foot and ankle	No. (%)	Lower extremity	No. (%)
0–5	Fibrosarcoma	5 (45)	Fibrosarcoma	9 (29)	Fibrosarcoma	9 (56)	Fibrosarcoma	5 (45)	Fibrosarcoma	24 (45)
	Angiosarcoma	1 (9)	Rhabdomyosarcoma	7 (23)	Rhabdomyosarcoma	4 (25)	DFSP	2 (18)	Rhabdomyosarcoma	8 (15)
	Epithelioid sarcoma	1 (9)	Angiomatoid MFH	3 (10)	Angiomatoid MFH	1 (6)	Malignant schwannoma	2 (18)	Giant-cell fibroblastoma	5 (9)
	DFSP	1 (9)	Malignant schwannoma	2 (6)	Chondrosarcoma	1 (6)	Rhabdomyosarcoma	2 (18)	Malignant schwannoma	5 (9)
	Malignant schwannoma	1 (9)	MFH	2 (6)	Malignant schwannoma	1 (6)			DFSP	3 (6)
	Other	2 (18)	Other	8 (26)					Other	8 (15)
6–15	Epithelioid sarcoma	9 (21)	Angiomatoid MFH	30 (33)	Angiomatoid MFH	8 (21)	Synovial sarcoma	11 (21)	Synovial sarcoma	28 (22)
	Angiomatoid MFH	7 (16)	Synovial sarcoma	14 (15)	MFH	5 (13)	DFSP	9 (17)	Angiomatoid MFH	22 (17)
	Synovial sarcoma	5 (12)	Fibrosarcoma	8 (9)	Ewing's sarcoma	4 (10)	Rhabdomyosarcoma	5 (9)	MFH	13 (10)
	MFH	4 (9)	Malignant schwannoma	7 (8)	Malignant schwannoma	4 (10)	Angiosarcoma	4 (8)	Liposarcoma	11 (9)
	Angiosarcoma	3 (7)	MFH	7 (8)	Rhabdomyosarcoma	4 (10)	Clear-cell sarcoma	4 (8)	Malignant schwannoma	9 (7)
	Other	15 (35)	Other	26 (28)	Other	14 (36)	Other	20 (38)	Other	45 (35)
16–25	Epithelioid sarcoma	25 (29)	Synovial sarcoma	32 (23)	Synovial sarcoma	13 (18)	Synovial sarcoma	27 (30)	Synovial sarcoma	76 (22)
	MFH	11 (13)	MFH	19 (14)	DFSP	12 (16)	Clear-cell sarcoma	10 (11)	Liposarcoma	45 (13)
	DFSP	7 (8)	Malignant schwannoma	16 (12)	Malignant schwannoma	11 (15)	Fibrosarcoma	7 (8)	Malignant schwannoma	44 (13)
	Synovial sarcoma	7 (8)	Fibrosarcoma	12 (9)	Fibrosarcoma	8 (11)	DFSP	7 (8)	MFH	36 (11)
	Rhabdomyosarcoma	7 (8)	Angiomatoid MFH	10 (7)	MFH	8 (11)	MFH	6 (7)	Fibrosarcoma	24 (7)
	Other	29 (34)	Other	49 (36)	Other	22 (30)	Other	33 (37)	Other	113 (33)
26–45	MFH	26 (18)	MFH	65 (28)	DFSP	55 (33)	Synovial sarcoma	50 (26)	Liposarcoma	196 (28)
	Epithelioid sarcoma	24 (16)	Malignant schwannoma	29 (12)	MFH	30 (18)	Clear-cell sarcoma	25 (13)	MFH	151 (21)
	Synovial sarcoma	21 (14)	Fibrosarcoma	25 (11)	Liposarcoma	22 (13)	MFH	22 (13)	Synovial sarcoma	78 (11)
	Fibrosarcoma	17 (12)	Synovial sarcoma	23 (10)	Malignant schwannoma	21 (12)	Hemangioendothelioma	14 (7)	Malignant schwannoma	70 (10)
	Clear-cell sarcoma	9 (6)	Liposarcoma	20 (8)	Fibrosarcoma	10 (6)	DFSP	13 (7)	Fibrosarcoma	47 (7)
	Other	49 (34)	Other	74 (31)	Other	31 (18)	Other	62 (33)	Other	166 (23)
46–65	MFH	16 (19)	MFH	133 (46)	MFH	66 (35)	MFH	39 (25)	MFH	399 (43)
	Synovial sarcoma	12 (14)	Liposarcoma	34 (12)	Liposarcoma	39 (21)	Synovial sarcoma	27 (17)	Liposarcoma	232 (25)
	Fibrosarcoma	8 (10)	Leiomyosarcoma	22 (8)	DFSP	22 (12)	Leiomyosarcoma	19 (12)	Leiomyosarcoma	63 (7)
	Epithelioid sarcoma	7 (8)	Fibrosarcoma	18 (6)	Malignant schwannoma	20 (11)	Kaposi's sarcoma	14 (9)	Synovial sarcoma	40 (4)
	Liposarcoma	7 (8)	Malignant schwannoma	17 (6)	Leiomyosarcoma	14 (7)	Liposarcoma	9 (6)	Malignant schwannoma	38 (4)
	Other	34 (40)	Other	68 (23)	Other	15 (14)	Other	47 (30)	Other	148 (16)
66 and over	MFH	28 (35)	MFH	183 (60)	MFH	67 (50)	Kaposi's sarcoma	49 (37)	MFH	455 (55)
	Leiomyosarcoma	10 (13)	Liposarcoma	25 (8)	Liposarcoma	30 (23)	MFH	25 (19)	Liposarcoma	178 (22)
	Synovial sarcoma	6 (8)	Leiomyosarcoma	23 (8)	Malignant schwannoma	12 (9)	Leiomyosarcoma	20 (15)	Leiomyosarcoma	86 (10)
	Kaposi's sarcoma	5 (6)	Malignant schwannoma	20 (7)	DFSP	6 (5)	Fibrosarcoma	9 (7)	Fibrosarcoma	22 (3)
	Fibrosarcoma	5 (6)	Kaposi's sarcoma	10 (3)	Fibrosarcoma	4 (3)	Chondrosarcoma	6 (4)	Chondrosarcoma	16 (2)
	Other	25 (32)	Other	43 (14)	Other	14 (11)	Other	25 (17)	Other	69 (8)

Note: No. (%) indicates the number of specified lesions in the indicated location for the given age group (percentage of all malignant tumors in this location and for this age group). For example, 5 (45) indicates that there are five fibrosarcomas in the hand and wrist of patients 0–5 years old, and this represented 45% of all malignant tumors in this location and age group.

DFSP = dermatofibrosarcoma protuberans, MFH = malignant fibrous histiocytoma.

From Kransdorf MJ, et al: Benign soft-tissue tumors in a large referral population: distribution of specific diagnoses by age, sex, and location. Am J Roentgenol 164:129-134, 1995. Reprinted with permission from the American Journal of Roentgenology.

TABLE 107-2B Distribution of Common Malignant Soft-Tissue Tumors by Anatomic Location and Age

Age (yrs)	Hip, groin, and buttocks	No. (%)	Head and neck	No. (%)	Trunk	No. (%)	Retroperitoneum	No. (%)
0–5	Fibrosarcoma	7 (32)	Fibrosarcoma	22 (37)	Fibrosarcoma	13 (26)	Fibrosarcoma	4 (20)
	Giant-cell fibroblastoma	3 (14)	Rhabdomyosarcoma	20 (33)	Giant-cell fibroblastoma	8 (16)	Neuroblastoma	4 (20)
	Rhabdomyosarcoma	3 (14)	Hemangiopericytoma	3 (5)	Rhabdomyosarcoma	8 (16)	Rhabdomyosarcoma	4 (20)
	DFSP	2 (9)	DFSP	2 (3)	Angiomatoid MFH	6 (12)	Ganglioneuroblastoma	3 (15)
	MFH	2 (9)	Malignant schwannoma	2 (3)	DFSP	4 (8)	Leiomyosarcoma	2 (10)
	Other	5 (23)	Other	11 (18)	Other	11 (22)	Other	3 (15)
6–15	Angiomatoid MFH	8 (21)	Rhabdomyosarcoma	17 (26)	Angiomatoid MFH	14 (15)	Rhabdomyosarcoma	9 (31)
	Synovial sarcoma	7 (19)	Fibrosarcoma	13 (20)	Fibrosarcoma	13 (14)	Malignant schwannoma	5 (17)
	Rhabdomyosarcoma	6 (16)	Synovial sarcoma	7 (11)	Ewing's sarcoma	12 (13)	Neuroblastoma	4 (14)
	MFH	4 (11)	Malignant schwannoma	6 (9)	DFSP	12 (13)	Fibrosarcoma	2 (7)
	Epithelioid sarcoma	2 (5)	MFH	6 (9)	Malignant schwannoma	9 (10)	MFH	2 (7)
	Other	11 (29)	Other	16 (25)	Other	31 (34)	Other	7 (24)
16–25	Synovial sarcoma	15 (18)	MFH	17 (19)	DFSP	37 (23)	Malignant schwannoma	9 (20)
	Malignant schwannoma	13 (16)	DFSP	14 (16)	MFH	21 (13)	Ewing's sarcoma	8 (18)
	Liposarcoma	8 (10)	Malignant schwannoma	8 (9)	Malignant schwannoma	19 (12)	Leiomyosarcoma	6 (14)
	DFSP	6 (7)	Synovial sarcoma	8 (9)	Fibrosarcoma	15 (9)	Ganglioneuroblastoma	4 (9)
	MFH	6 (7)	Rhabdomyosarcoma	8 (9)	Synovial sarcoma	13 (8)	Neuroblastoma	4 (9)
	Other	35 (42)	Other	34 (38)	Other	56 (35)	Other	13 (30)
26–45	Liposarcoma	45 (18)	DFSP	59 (30)	DFSP	129 (30)	Leiomyosarcoma	57 (32)
	DFSP	42 (17)	Malignant schwannoma	27 (14)	MFH	77 (18)	Liposarcoma	52 (29)
	MFH	38 (16)	Liposarcoma	18 (9)	Malignant schwannoma	45 (10)	MFH	22 (12)
	Leiomyosarcoma	26 (11)	MFH	15 (8)	Liposarcoma	41 (9)	Malignant schwannoma	11 (6)
	Malignant schwannoma	15 (6)	Fibrosarcoma	14 (7)	Fibrosarcoma	36 (8)	Fibrosarcoma	7 (4)
	Other	78 (32)	Other	61 (31)	Other	105 (24)	Other	30 (17)
46–65	Liposarcoma	67 (24)	MFH	54 (28)	MFH	131 (31)	Liposarcoma	170 (33)
	MFH	66 (23)	DFSP	28 (15)	Liposarcoma	80 (19)	Leiomyosarcoma	154 (30)
	Leiomyosarcoma	40 (14)	Malignant schwannoma	23 (12)	DFSP	60 (14)	MFH	111 (22)
	DFSP	20 (7)	Liposarcoma	22 (12)	Malignant schwannoma	35 (8)	Malignant schwannoma	23 (5)
	Fibrosarcoma	16 (6)	Angiosarcoma	16 (8)	Leiomyosarcoma	27 (6)	Malignant mesenchymoma	10 (2)
	Other	74 (26)	Other	47 (25)	Other	89 (21)	Other	43 (8)
66 and over	MFH	111 (46)	MFH	82 (34)	MFH	137 (44)	Liposarcoma	164 (39)
	Liposarcoma	49 (20)	Atypical fibroxanthoma	41 (17)	Liposarcoma	56 (18)	Leiomyosarcoma	118 (28)
	Leiomyosarcoma	24 (10)	Angiosarcoma	27 (11)	Leiomyosarcoma	23 (7)	MFH	99 (24)
	Angiosarcoma	11 (5)	Liposarcoma	20 (8)	Malignant schwannoma	20 (6)	Malignant schwannoma	13 (3)
	Malignant schwannoma	11 (5)	Malignant schwannoma	16 (7)	DFSP	17 (5)	Fibrosarcoma	8 (2)
	Other	37 (15)	Other	54 (23)	Other	58 (19)	Other	14 (3)

Note: No. (%) indicates the number of specified lesions in the indicated location for the given age group (percentage of all malignant tumors in this location and for this age group). For example, 5 (45) indicates that there are five fibrosarcomas in the hand and wrist of patients 0–5 years old, and this represented 45% of all malignant tumors in this location and age group.

DFSP = dermatofibrosarcoma protuberans, MFH = malignant fibrous histiocytoma.

From Kransdorf MJ, et al: Benign soft-tissue tumors in a large referral population: distribution of specific diagnoses by age, sex, and location. Am J Roentgenol 164:129-134, 1995. Reprinted with permission from the American Journal of Roentgenology.

Attempts have been made to develop criteria to differentiate benign from malignant soft-tissue lesions utilizing MR signal characteristics and tumor morphology. In general, the larger the mass, the greater is the possibility of malignancy. Only 5% of benign soft-tissue tumors are more than 5 cm in size.[7] Most malignant tumors are deep, being located below the fascia, while only 1% of all benign soft-tissue tumors are similarly located.[7] Most benign soft-tissue lesions have uniform high signal intensity on T1 and T2 sequences.[110] The soft-tissue masses that are small with homogeneous T2 signal intensity, a delayed enhancement pattern and no neurovascular or osseous involvement tend to be benign, whereas ill-defined, heterogeneous, rapidly enhancing lesions with neurovascular encasement or osseous invasion tend to be malignant.[111] De Schepper et al[112] retrospectively studied 141 soft-tissue tumors (84 benign, 57 malignant) and evaluated a wide variety of MRI features. Univariate and multivariate analysis of 10 imaging parameters was carried out to determine the utility of these parameters in predicting malignancy in soft-tissue masses. The highest sensitivities for malignancy included high signal intensity on T2-weighted sequences (100%), mean diameter greater than 33 mm (90%), and heterogeneous signal on T1 (88%). The highest specificity in favor of malignancy was obtained for necrosis (98%), bone or neurovascular involvement or metastases (94%), and mean lesion diameter of greater than 66 mm (87%). The overlap between benign and malignant tumors is greater however, and MRI cannot consistently and reliably distinguish benign from malignant processes.[7]

Most soft-tissue tumors and tumor-like masses exhibit prolonged T1 and T2 relaxation times appearing of relative low signal intensity on T1 and high signal intensity on T2 sequences.[113] The appearance of some soft-tissue tumors may allow a specific diagnosis to be suspected by MRI alone. These imaging characteristics are discussed below.

Tumor Characterization

Soft-tissue Lesions of High Signal Intensity on T1-weighted Sequences

Certain soft-tissue tumors and tumor-like conditions exhibit high signal intensity on T1-weighted sequences. Lesions that may be of high signal intensity on T1 sequences include hemangioma/vascular malformations, hematoma, melanoma, elastofibroma, and lipomatous lesions such as lipoma, liposarcoma, and fibrolipoma.[7,101,104,114-117]

Lipomas exhibit high signal intensity on T1-weighted sequences and are the most common soft-tissue tumor.[118] A lipoma is a benign lesion composed of mature adipose tissue. Lipomas are unusual in the first two decades of life and most commonly are diagnosed between the ages of 40 to 60 years.[118] Approximately 5-8% of patients with lipomas have multiple lesions. The signal intensity of a benign lipoma parallels that of subcutaneous fat on all sequences and exhibits no discernable enhancement with gadolinium administration.[119] Lipomas may be surrounded by a thin fibrous capsule or may blend imperceptibly with surrounding subcutaneous fat. Heterotopic lipomas may occur which are intimately associated with tissues other than fat, and these lesions include angiomyolipoma, lipoma of tendon sheath, lipoma arborescens, neural fibrolipoma (fibrolipomatous hamartoma), periosteal liposarcoma, lumbosacral lipoma as well as intermuscular and intramuscular lipomas.[119]

Intermuscular and intramuscular lipomas are fairly common and are of concern to clinicians given their large size, deep location, and infiltrating nature.[118] Intramuscular lipomas are far more common than lipomas isolated to the areas between musculature (intermuscular lipomas)[118,119] (Fig. 107-19). Lipoma arborescens is composed of hypertrophic synovial villae filled with fat resulting in a characteristic villiform or frond-like appearance of signal intensity consistent with its fatty nature on all imaging sequences.[119,120] This lesion is most common in the knee and is usually visualized in the suprapatellar region[118-120] (Fig. 107-20). Lipoma arborescens has also been described in other areas including the bursae, hip, shoulder, elbow, hand, and ankle.[120] It occurs most often in the elderly and is associated with recurrent joint effusions, degenerative arthritis, meniscal tears, and prior trauma.[120] Synovial lipomas are rare, discrete synovial-based masses occurring less commonly than lipoma arborescens.[119,121] Neural fibrolipoma is a tumor-like infiltration of nerves by lipomatous tissue that typically is usually seen before the age of 30 with most lesions presenting at birth or in infancy.[118] There is a striking predominance in the upper extremity (78-98%) and a predilection for the median nerve (up to 85% of cases in one series).[122] Most patients present with a soft-tissue swelling or mass, with or without associated pain or neurologic symptoms. In 27% to 67% of cases, neural fibrolipoma is associated with macrodactyly (macrodactyly lipomatosa).[122]

Hibernoma is a rare benign tumor of brown fat that most commonly occurs in the periscapular or interscapular area, neck, and axilla.[118,123] Although this tumor exhibits increased signal on T1-weighted sequences, the signal intensity is usually slightly less than that of subcutaneous fat.[123] T2 images commonly exhibit heterogeneous high signal intensity and postcontrast studies may show marked enhancement raising concern for liposarcoma.[123]

Lipoblastoma is a childhood tumor (90% seen under the age of 3 years), which on MRI exhibits predominantly fatty components with associated nonlipomatous elements.[116] There is a 3 : 1 male predominance.[124] The natural history of the lesion is that of progression to a mature lipoma.[119,125] The MR appearance is nonspecific and may be indistinguishable from liposarcoma, the latter an especially rare tumor in children.[119]

Liposarcomas may exhibit discernable high signal fat on T1 sequences or fat may be completely undetected at MRI in high-grade or pleomorphic sarcomas. Liposarcoma, the second most common adult soft-tissue sarcoma after malignant fibrous histiocytoma, accounts for 9.8% to 18% of all malignant soft-tissue tumors.[113,118]

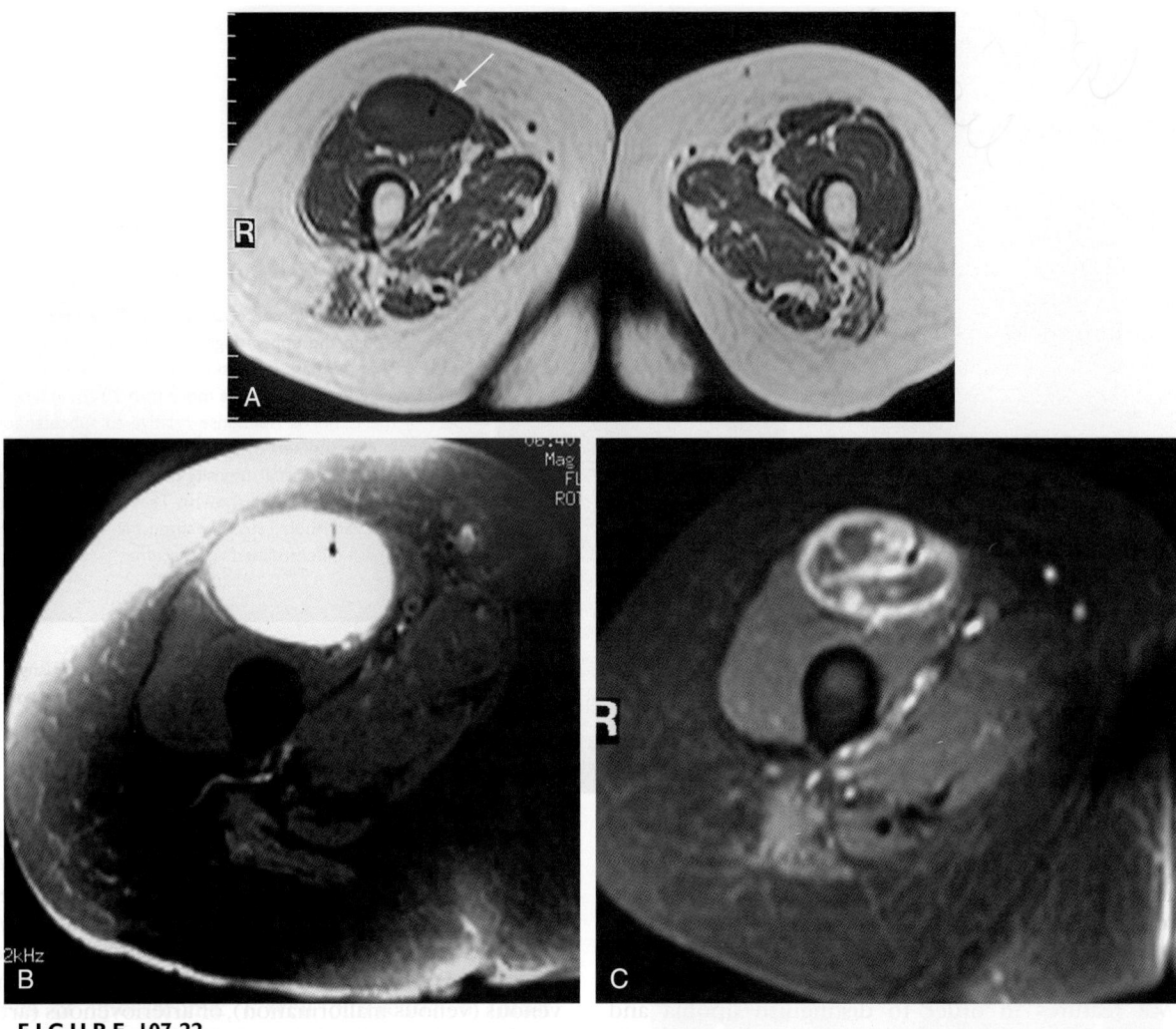

FIGURE 107-22

Myxoid liposarcoma. **A,** Axial T1 shows a hypointense lesion within the rectus femoris muscle of the right thigh *(arrow).* **B,** Axial fat saturation T$_2$ shows the lesion as a high signal "cystic" appearing lesion. Note the lack of uniform fat saturation on this image. **C,** Post-contrast T1 shows heterogeneous enhancement, not compatible with a simple cyst.

gadolinium injection. Fluid–fluid levels may be noted.[49] High flow lesions (arteriovenous malformations) show prominent serpentine vessels, increased flow signal voids, as well as prominent feeding and draining vessels.[132,133]

Hematomas may present as mass-like lesions with high signal intensity on T1 sequences. The MR appearance of extracranial hematomas is variable and dependent upon age-related changes.[135,136] Hyperacute bleeds (1–24 hours) appear fluid-like being hypointense to isointense on T1 and hyperintense on T2. Acute hematomas (1–7 days) are hypointense to isointense on T1 and hypointense on T2 due to the paramagnetic effect of intracellular deoxyhemoglobin. Subacute hemorrhage (1 week to 3 months) shows high signal on T1 due to methemoglobin. T2 during this phase is initially hypointense (due to intracellular methemoglobin) and later, after red cell lysis, hyperintense (due to extracellular methemoglobin). High signal intensity first develops at the periphery of the bleed (Fig. 107-24). Chronic

hematomas exhibit high signal intensity on all spin-echo sequences but eventually develop a peripheral rim of low signal due to fibrosis and the paramagnetic effect of hemosiderin-ladened macrophages. Eventually, over time, the entire collection becomes either "cystic" in nature with a low signal intensity rim or diffusely low signal on all imaging sequences.[132,135,136] Soft-tissue sarcomas may show hemorrhagic components (Fig. 107-25) occasionally forming large hematomas with the blood masking the underlying sarcoma. A clinical history remarkable for the absence of significant trauma or bleeding dyscrasia in such cases should raise the index of suspicion for underlying tumor. Follow-up studies may be required. Focal gadolinium enhancement may detect an underlying neoplasm.[137]

Elastofibroma is a benign fibroelastic pseudotumor located in a characteristic position between the inferior scapular tip and the chest wall in 99% of reported cases.[138] Most elastofibromas are subclinical and bilateral

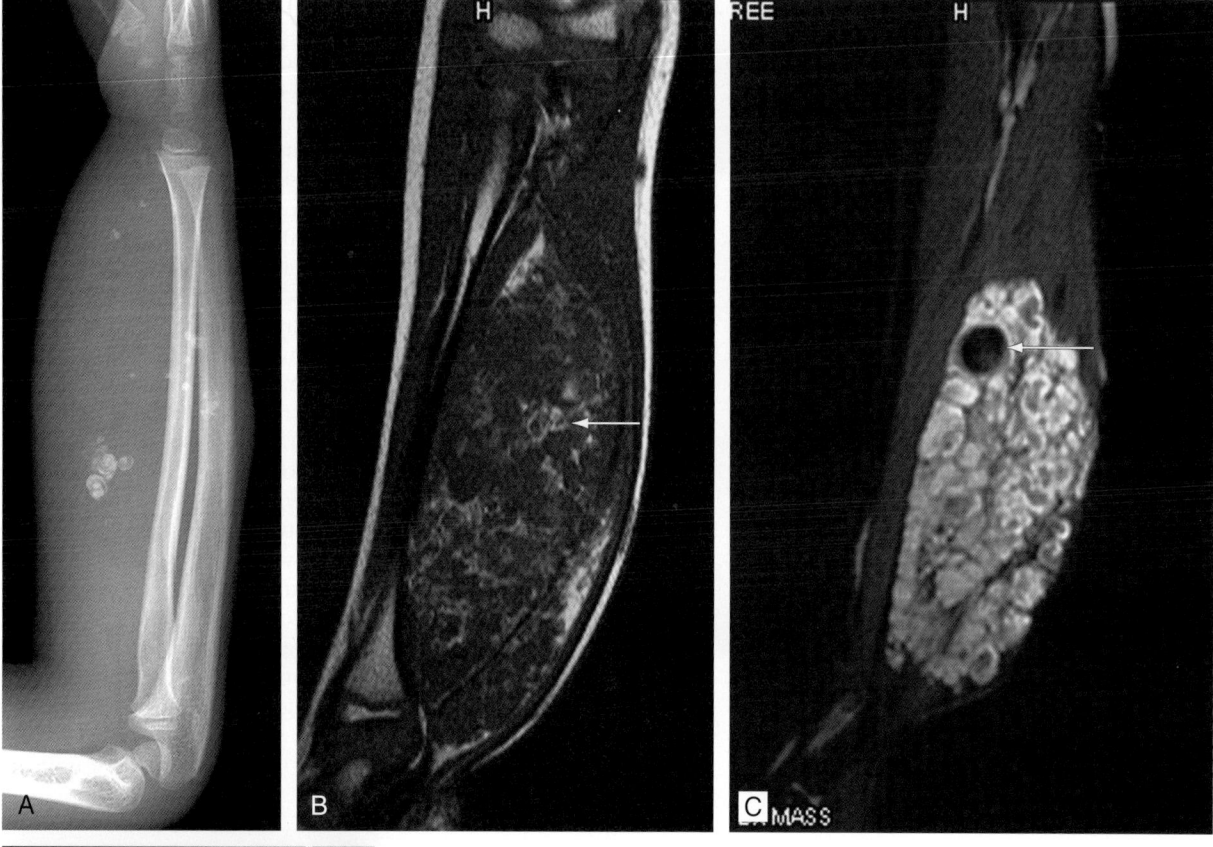

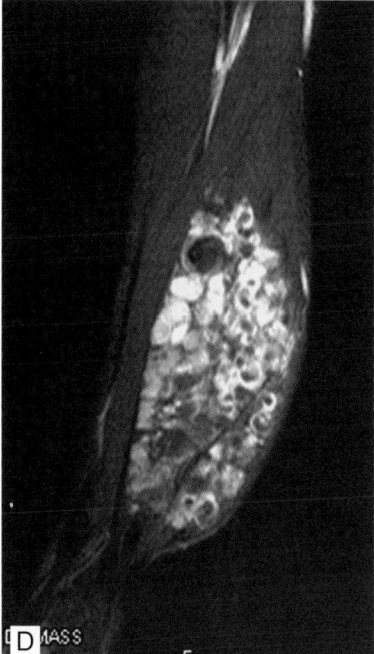

FIGURE 107-23

Hemangioma. **A,** Lateral forearm radiograph shows a volar soft-tissue mass containing phleboliths and scattered area of low attenuation consistent with fat. **B,** Coronal T1-weighted image shows the large mass of a signal intensity approximating muscle with prominent areas of interspersed high signal fat *(arrow)*. Phleboliths are difficult to appreciate on this sequence. **C,** Coronal STIR shows high signal vascular channels, suppressed interstitial fat, and focal low signal phleboliths *(arrow)*. **D,** T1 fat saturation + post contrast image shows marked enhancement of vascular channels.

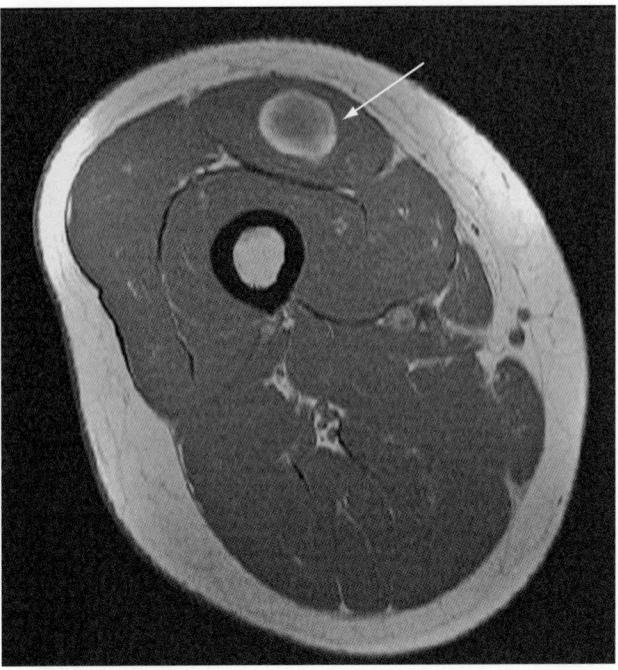

FIGURE 107-24

Subacute hematoma within the rectus femoris muscle. A T1 high signal intensity first develops at the periphery of the bleed *(arrow)*.

lesions are seen in up to 66%.[138,139] MRI reveals a lenticular unencapsulated soft-tissue mass with skeletal muscle signal intensity interspersed with strands of fat, the latter of which are of high signal intensity on T1-weighted images.[138]

Melanoma frequently but not always has high signal intensity on T1-weighted images and may exhibit low signal intensity on T2 sequences.[112,114,140] It is thought that the paramagnetic effects of stable free radicals within melanin pigment leads to shortening of both T1 and T2 relaxation times yielding high signal intensity on T1 and low signal intensity on T2 sequences,[141] although other theories have been proposed.[142]

Several other less commonly encountered tumors may also exhibit short T1 relaxation. Clear cell sarcoma (malignant melanoma of soft parts) is a rare, slow growing malignant tumor showing melanotic differentiation.[143] The lesion may be variable in MR appearance but up to 52% of patients have increased signal intensity relative to muscle on T1-weighted sequences.[144] Clear cell sarcoma presents as an enlarging deep-seated mass arising adjacent to tendons and aponeurotic structures and predominately affects young to middle-aged adults.[143,144] It is most common in the foot and ankle followed by the knee, thigh, and hand.[143] Alveolar soft part sarcoma, another rare soft-tissue sarcoma, is seen in the lower extremities and buttock region in adults and in

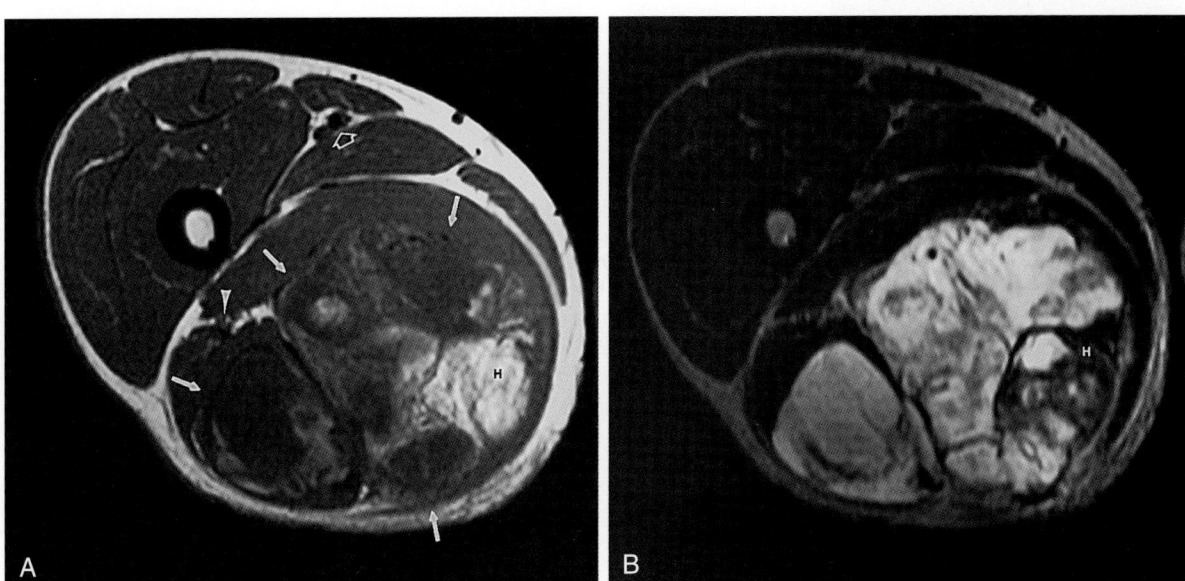

FIGURE 107-25

Malignant fibrous histiocytoma of the thigh in a 45-year-old man. **A,** Axial T1-weighted image reveals a heterogeneous mass *(solid arrows)* in the posteromedial thigh. The mass is of mixed low and high signal intensity. The sciatic nerve *(arrowhead)* and femoral neurovascular bundle *(open arrow)* are spared. **B,** Axial T2-weighted image clearly demonstrates the intramuscular extent of the mass (adductor magnus, semimembranosus, semitendinosus), which was successfully resected after a course of radiation therapy. Viable portions of the tumor appear dark on the T1-weighted image and bright on the T2-weighted image. Area of corresponding high T1-weighted signal intensity and low T2-weighted signal intensity represents hemorrhagic necrosis (H). The heterogeneous signal intensity, necrosis, and ill-defined margination are typical of a malignant sarcoma.

the head and neck region in infants and children.[145] Alveolar soft part sarcoma is a highly vascular tumor that at MRI exhibits characteristic central and marginal vascular flow voids as well as high signal intensity on T1 and T2 sequences.[146] Melanotic schwannomas, most commonly seen in the paravertebral or central nervous system, have high signal intensity on T1.[144]

Lesions of Low Signal Intensity on T2-weighted Sequences

Several tumors and tumor-like conditions may have low signal intensity on T2-weighted images. Lesions exhibiting low signal intensity on T2-weighted sequences include pigmented villonodular synovitis, giant cell tumor of the tendon sheath, fibromatosis, scar tissue, Morton's neuroma, hematoma, amyloid, gout, melanoma, and heavily mineralized masses. High flow arteriovenous malformations will have low signal intensity vessels secondary to flow void on conventional spin-echo images.

Pigmented villonodular synovitis (PVNS) is a benign inflammatory process of unknown origin involving the synovial lining of a joint, bursa, or tendon sheath. Focal and diffuse forms exist.[147,148] The focal form known as giant cell tumor of the tendon sheath most commonly involves the hand (67%) and less commonly the foot.[149] Giant cell tumor of the tendon sheath is the second most common mass of the hand behind ganglion cyst.[150] The diffuse form of PVNS is almost always monoarticular and has a predilection for large joints with 80% of cases involving the knee followed in frequency by the hip, ankle, shoulder, and elbow.[151] Patients typically present in their third or fourth decades and there is a female predominance. Bone erosions are seen in 50% of cases with joint involvement and osseous erosions are more common in joints having tight capsules such as the hip.[113] The MR appearance of PVNS is often characteristic, with lesions being isointense to hypointense relative to skeletal muscle on T1 and T2 sequences (Fig. 107-26). The T2 shortening is secondary to hemosiderin deposition in the lesion and the effect is more pronounced on a high field system. Focal areas of high signal intensity may be seen secondary to lipid-laden macrophages (foam cells). Gradient-echo sequences readily detect the presence of hemosiderin. Recurrence rates following surgery are as high as 50%.[113] The differential diagnosis of synovial-based lesions hypointense on T2 sequences includes PVNS, giant cell tumor of the tendon sheath, synovial chondromatosis, hemophiliac arthropathy, amyloid, longstanding rheumatoid arthritis, gout, and siderotic synovitis.[152]

The fibromatoses are a group of soft-tissue lesions characterized by proliferation of fibroblasts in an abundant collagen matrix.[138] The fibromatoses are prone to recurrence after surgery and may be divided into superficial and deep categories based upon anatomic location.[153] The superficial fibromatoses tend to be small and slow growing and include palmar fibromatosis (Dupytren's disease) and plantar fibromatosis (Ledderhose

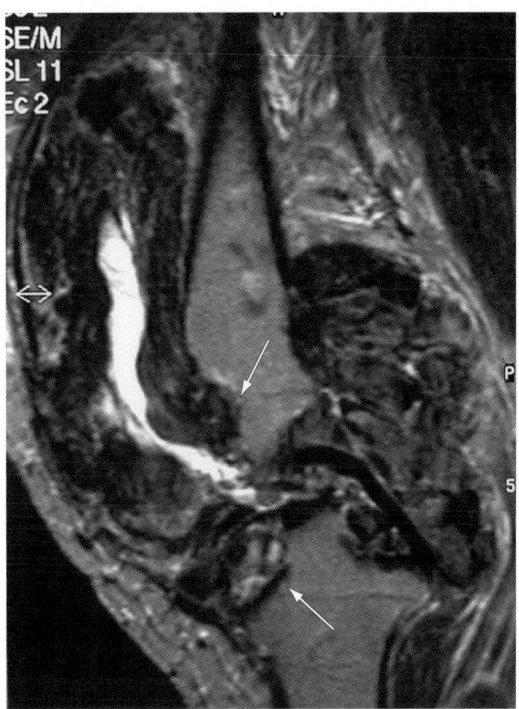

FIGURE 107-26

Pigmented villonodular synovitis (PVNS) of the knee. Sagittal spin-echo T2 image shows thick primarily low signal intensity material diffusely throughout the synovial surfaces of the knee. Note the associated bone erosions at both tibial and femoral components (arrows).

disease) as well as penile fibromatosis (Peyronie's disease) and knuckle pads. The deep fibromatoses or desmoid tumors are larger and more rapid growing. Desmoid tumors include extra-abdominal, abdominal, and intra-abdominal fibromatoses.[153] Robbin et al in a review of musculoskeletal fibromatoses included fibrous lesions of infancy and childhood such as juvenile aponeurotic fibroma and infantile digital fibroma in the superficial group and infantile myofibromatosis, fibromatosis colli, and aggressive infantile fibromatosis in the deep group.[154] Characteristic MR findings include low to intermediate signal intensity on T1 and T2 sequences (Fig. 107-27). The characteristic low signal intensity changes are noted in fibromatoses with abundant collagen, whereas lesions with less collagen and more cellularity show nonspecific high signal intensity on T2 sequences.[154] Intense scar tissue may also present as a low signal intensity mass on T2 sequences due to high collagen content. Fibromatosis typically enhances heterogeneously with gadolinium administration, whereas mass-like low signal intensity scar tissue tends not to enhance.

Morton's neuroma is a non-neoplastic lesion that arises from perineural fibrosis of the plantar digital nerve. This lesion is deep to the plantar transverse metatarsal ligament at the level of the metatarsal heads. Morton's neuroma is more common in women (80%)

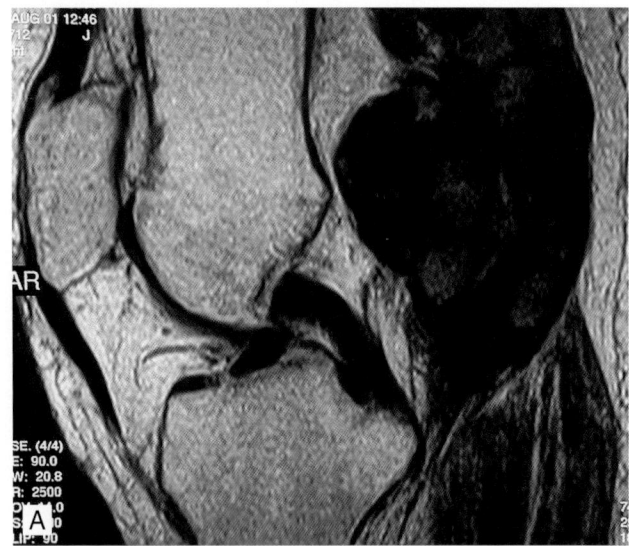
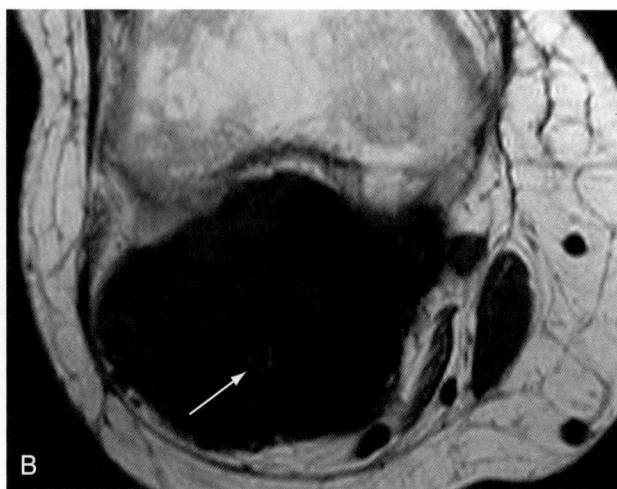

FIGURE 107-27

Desmoid tumor. **A,** Sagittal T2 shows a large posterior mass with dominant low signal intensity. **B,** The mass is isointense to hypointense and surrounding the neurovascular bundle posterior to the knee on the T1 image *(arrow)*.

and occurs most commonly between the third and fourth metatarsals followed by the second intermetatarsal space.[148] Patients often present with numbness, a burning sensation, and shooting pain in the affected digits. Morton's neuroma is of intermediate to low signal intensity on T1 and T2 sequences[155,156] and enhances following contrast administration[157] (Fig. 107-28). Clinical examination involves manually compressing the forefoot in the transverse plane and simultaneously palpating the affected intermetatarsal space between the fingers of the other hand. A positive test (known as Mulder's sign) results in a painful and palpable click that reproduces the patient's symptoms. The characteristic location, signal intensities, and clinical presentation generally make the MR diagnosis straightforward.

Amyloid is a protein that is deposited in an extracellular location within bone and soft-tissues either primarily (primary amyloidosis) or secondary to other diseases (secondary amyloidosis). Secondary amyloidosis is most commonly associated with chronic renal failure since the responsible protein (beta$_2$-microglobulin) is not filtered by standard dialysis membranes, accumulates in the blood and ultimately is deposited within tissues.[158,159] Secondary amyloidosis may also be seen in multiple myeloma and in chronic inflammatory or infectious disease states. Shoulder, hip, wrist, knee, and spine are typical sites of involvement.[159] Shoulder pain and carpel tunnel syndrome are the most common musculoskeletal manifestations. Soft-tissue deposits show heterogeneously low to intermediate signal intensity on T1 and T2 sequences,[152,160] while associated bone lesions may be more variable in appearance.[159] Synovial and peritendinous involvement are typical features of amyloid deposition in joints.[152,159] Low signal synovial involvement may occur with PVNS or

hemosiderin deposition but polyarticular involvement and the conspicuous absence of a paramagnetic effect on gradient-echo sequences help to establish the diagnosis of amyloidosis.[152]

Gout, a disease of calcium urate deposition in bone or in soft-tissues, may manifest as a soft-tissue mass. The MR appearance of tophaceous gout is variable. Most gouty tophi are isointense relative to muscle on T1-weighted images. T2-weighted images usually show low to intermediate heterogeneous signal intensity, although lesions with high signal intensity have been reported.[160,161] The variation in T2 signal characteristics is related to calcium

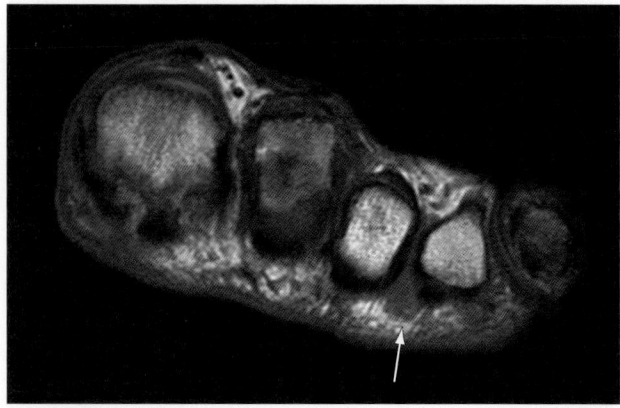

FIGURE 107-28

There is a convex border and soft-tissue prominence at the plantar aspect of the third metatarsal interspace *(arrow)* between the third and fourth metatarsal heads consistent with a Morton's neuroma.

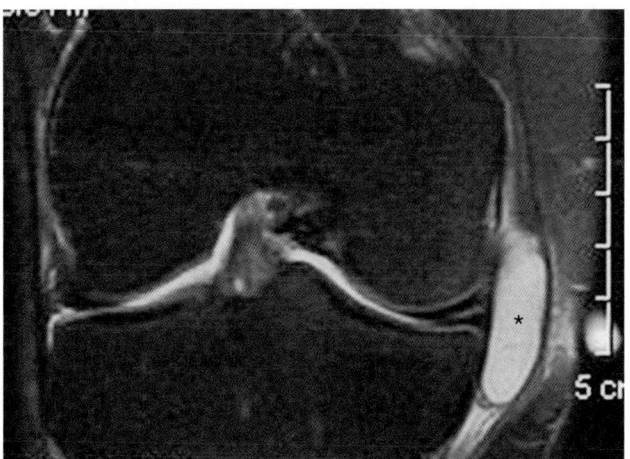

FIGURE 107-29

Para-meniscal meniscal cyst. Coronal fat saturation T2 image of a palpable medial knee mass *(asterisk)* marked with a skin marker. Horizontal posterior horn and body medial meniscal tear was seen with an associated cystic mass intercalating between layers one and two of the three layers of the medial collateral ligament. See also Figure 107-31 below.

concentration within the lesion. Gout should be suspected when a mass shows intermediate signal intensity on T1 and low to intermediate signal on T2 sequences, particularly if adjacent bone erosions are noted or other joints are involved.[161]

"Cystic" Appearing Lesions

Certain soft-tissue masses or mass-like lesions exhibit low signal intensity on T1- and high signal intensity on T2-weighted images MR images, resembling a fluid-filled structure or cyst. Lesions appearing "cyst-like" on MR include synovial/ganglion cysts, paralabral and para-meniscal cysts (Fig. 107-29), bursae, myxomas, myxoid malignancies (Fig. 107-30), synovial sarcoma (Fig. 107-31), nerve sheath tumors, and seromas. Cystic lesions may be differentiated from cystic-appearing tumors utilizing gadolinium-enhanced sequences or ultrasound.

Ganglion cysts are benign masses of uncertain etiology, possibly related to trauma, repetitive stress, myxomatous degeneration, or synovial herniation. Ganglion cysts contain fluid that is more viscous than joint fluid and they are surrounded by fibrous tissue compared to synovial cysts, which have a synovial lining.[162] Although most ganglia are either periarticular or peritendinous in location, they may also be intra-articular,[163] intraosseous[164] or, rarely, intratendinous.[165] Nerve sheath ganglion or intraneural ganglion cyst has been reported most frequently involving the nerves about the knee[122] (Fig. 107-32). Intraneural ganglia may be associated with nerve palsy or other neurologic symptoms related to nerve compression.[166] Seventy percent of all ganglia are located around the wrist. Ganglion cysts demonstrate low signal intensity on T1 and high signal intensity on T2 sequences. Thin internal septae are common. There is no internal enhancement on postcontrast images although the thin wall and septae

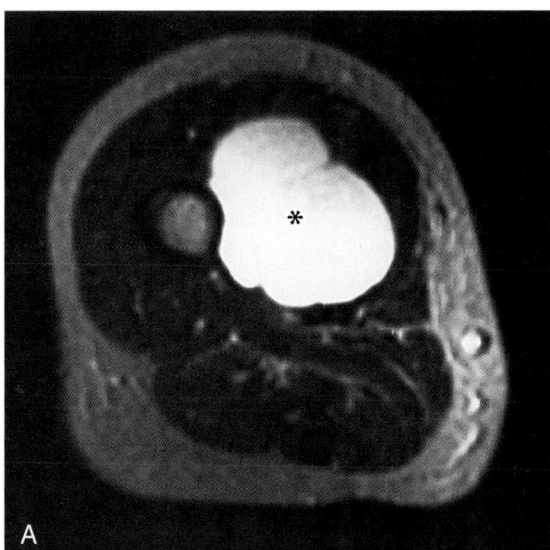
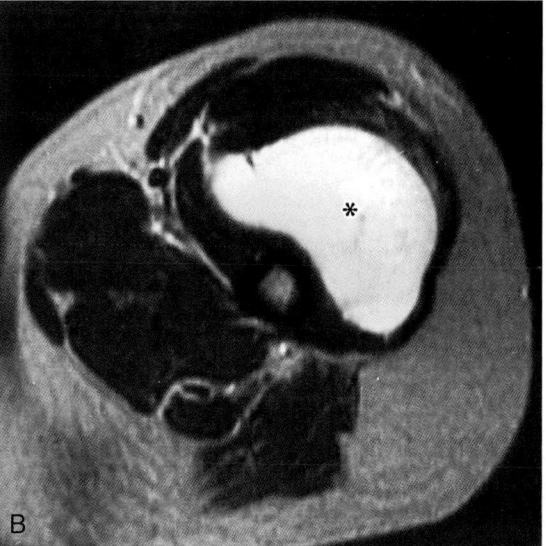

FIGURE 107-30

Myxoid tumors in two different middle-aged women who presented with mass lesions in the thigh. **A,** Axial T2-weighted (2200/80) image demonstrates a well-circumscribed, homogeneously bright mass *(asterisk)* within the vastus intermedius muscle. The pathologic diagnosis was benign myxoma of skeletal muscle. **B,** Axial T2-weighted (2000/80) image shows a well-circumscribed high signal intensity mass *(asterisk)* indistinguishable from that in **A**. The pathologic diagnosis was myxoid liposarcoma. Tumors with a myxoid matrix typically demonstrate homogeneously high signal intensity and may appear "cystic" despite their solid nature. *(From Moulton JS, Braley SE: MRI of soft-tissue tumors. Contemp Diagn Radiol 7[12]:1-6, 1994.)*

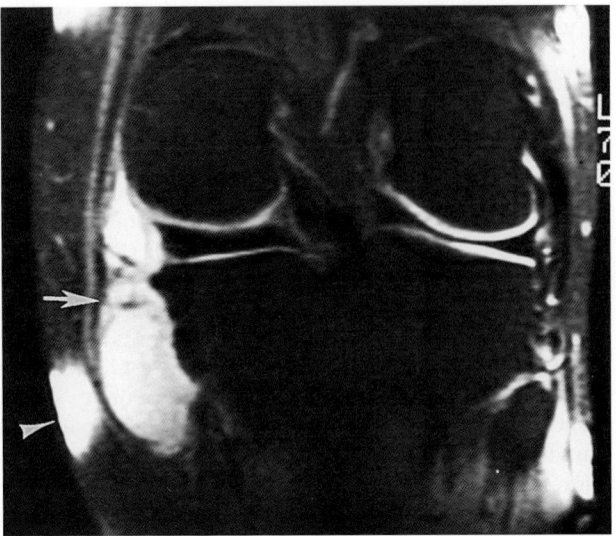

FIGURE 107-31

A 25-year-old man presented with a painful mass along the medial aspect of the knee. Coronal fat-suppressed spin-echo (1500/20) image reveals a lobulated mass *(arrow)* along the medial joint line, deep to the pes anserine tendons. The mass is of markedly high signal intensity, suggesting fluid, with several low signal intensity septa. No meniscal abnormality is seen to suggest a meniscal cyst. The more peripheral high signal intensity *(arrowhead)* represents a coil artifact. The mass was removed because of the patient's symptoms and proved to be a synovial sarcoma. *(Courtesy of Stan Weiss, MD, University of Rochester, Rochester, NY.)*

may enhance (Fig. 107-33). Bursae may clinically present as masses but their characteristic location and cyst-like character on MRI are sufficiently diagnostic.

Mxyomas are benign soft-tissue tumors thought to arise from fibroblasts that produce excess amounts of mucopolysaccharide. The lesions are usually intramuscular (82%), are most common in the thigh (51%), and appear to be "cystic" on noncontrast CT and MR images[167] (Fig. 107-34). MR contrast enhancement can be diffuse and heterogeneous.[11] An intramuscular mass of water signal intensity showing a perilesional fat rind often with increased signal in adjacent muscle on T2-weighted sequences is strongly suggestive of an intramuscular myxoma.[28] The small amount of adjacent fat seen in 71% of myxomas is due to atrophy of adjacent muscle.[167] The latter two findings help to differentiate benign myxoma from other more aggressive myxoid soft-tissue tumors such as myxoid liposarcoma. Sarcomas, particularly those with myxoid elements such as myxoid liposarcoma, myxoid malignant fibrous histiocytoma, and myxoid chondrosarcoma, may have signal characteristics resembling myxoma. The combination of myxomas and fibrous dysplasia is known as Mazabraud's syndrome.[168]

According to the Armed Forces Institute of Pathology, synovial sarcoma is the fourth most common soft-tissue sarcoma following malignant fibrous histiocytoma, liposarcoma, and rhabdomyosarcoma.[169] Synovial sarcoma accounts for 5.6% to 10% of all soft-tissue sarcomas and

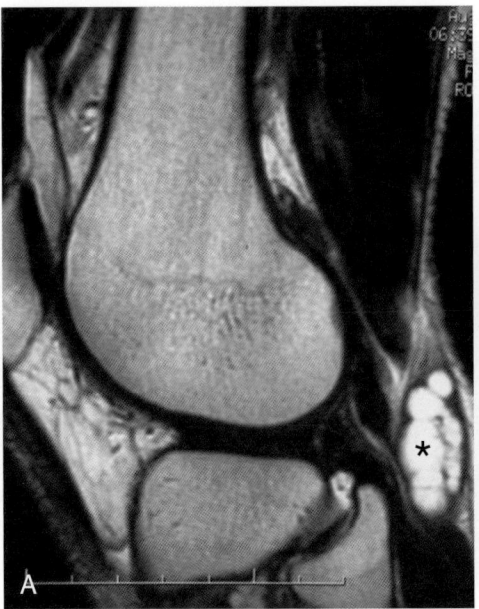
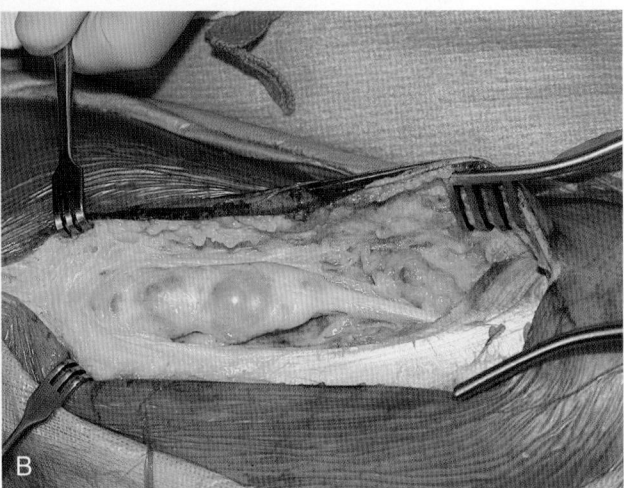

FIGURE 107-32

Intraneural ganglion. **A,** Sagittal T2 shows a lobulated fluid signal intensity mass *(asterisk)* along the course of the peroneal nerve.
B, Intraoperative photograph shows a lobulated mass intimate with the peroneal nerve.

the tumor is most common in individuals 15 to 40 years of age. Approximately 84% of synovial sarcomas are found in patients between 10 and 50 years.[169] Synovial sarcoma is the second most common sarcoma in pediatric patients behind rhabdomyosarcoma.[170] Eighty to ninety five percent of synovial sarcomas occur in the extremities with up to 70% being found in the lower extremity.[169] Synovial sarcoma is the most common sarcoma of the foot. Synovial sarcoma usually occurs near joints, bursae, and tendon sheaths, and less than 10% of the tumors are intra-articular.[171] Up to one third demonstrate radiographically detectable mineralization that is often peripheral.[172] Synovial sarcomas generally have a nonspecific MR appearance being isointense to muscle on T1 and of heterogeneous high signal on T2 sequences. Signal consistent with hemorrhage is present in 44%, fluid–fluid levels in 18%, and cortical erosion or medullary invasion is seen in 21% of patients.[171] Smaller lesions, usually less than 5 cm, can have well-circumscribed margins and a homogeneous appearance resembling a cyst. This "nonaggressive" appearance may lead to inappropriate surgical intervention.[173] Gadolinium administration or ultrasound may be helpful in differentiating a solid from a cystic mass in these cases. Thirty-five percent of synovial sarcomas in one series exhibited "triple signal intensity" with signal that was hyperintense, isointense and hypointense to fat on T2-weighted sequences.[171]

Peripheral nerve sheath tumors may appear "cystic" on MRI in some cases due to their often well-defined margins and high signal intensity on T2 sequences. T1-weighted sequences usually have an intermediate to slightly increased signal intensity relative to muscle. Benign peripheral nerve sheath tumors are divided into two groups: schwannomas (neurilemomas or neurinomas) and neurofibromas. Schwannomas account for less than 5% of all soft-tissue tumors, are usually solitary, and measure less than 5 cm in size.[109] They are most common between the ages of 20 and 50 years and are slightly less common than neurofibromas.[109] Multiple schwannomas may be seen in neurofibromatosis type 2 (NF2). In one study, 90% of schwannomas were sporadic, 3% occurred in patients with NF2, 2% with schwannomatosis without NF2, and 5% in association with multiple meningiomas with or without NF2.[174] Schwannomas rarely occur with NF1. Neurofibromas constitute more than 5% of soft-tissue neoplasms and are most common in young adults between 20 and 30 years.[172] Neurofibromas are of three types: localized, diffuse, and plexiform. Diffuse and plexiform neurofibromas are closely association with neurofibromatosis type 1 (NF1). Ninety percent of neurofibromas are the localized variety and most of these are solitary and not associated with NF1.[113]

Morphologically the MR appearance of benign nerve sheath tumors is fairly typical. These tumors have a

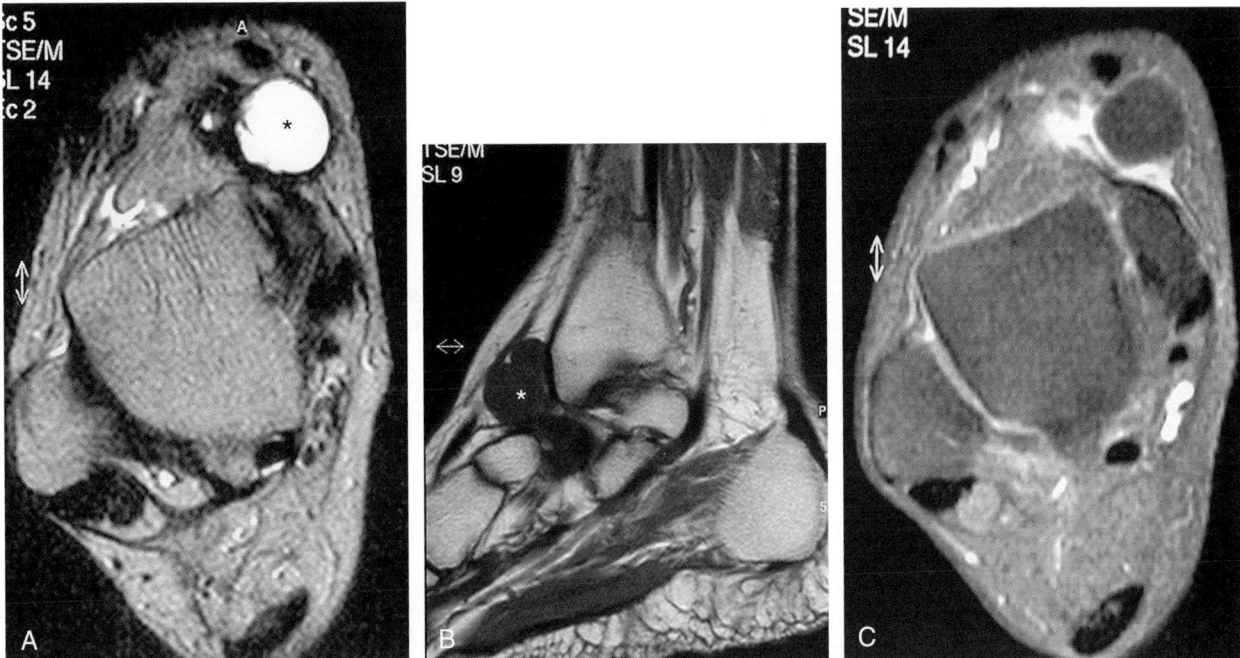

FIGURE 107-33

Ganglion cyst. Axial T2 (**A**) and sagittal T1 (**B**) show a fluid signal intensity mass anterior to the tibiotalar joint (*asterisk*). **C,** Post-contrast fat saturation T1 shows no enhancement of the mass.

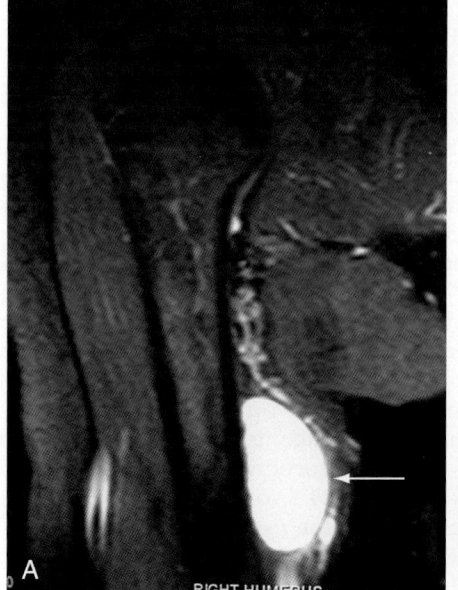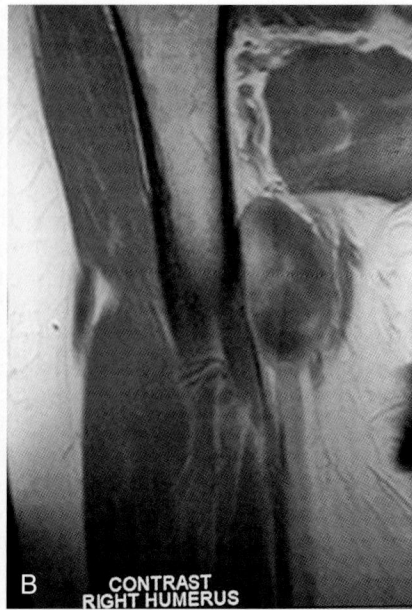

FIGURE 107-34

Myxoma. **A,** Coronal fat saturation T2 show a cystic-appearing mass within soft-tissues medial to the proximal humerus *(arrow).* **B,** Post-contrast T1 show heterogeneous enhancement. **C,** Gross cut specimen.

fusiform shape oriented along the long axis of a nerve with the nerve itself often visualized entering and leaving the mass.[172] Although schwannomas and neurofibromas have overlapping imaging features, schwannomas are eccentric to the involved nerve and neurofibromas tend to obliterate the nerve. At surgery, a schwannoma can be separated from the nerve while neurofibromas are intertwined with the nerve and require nerve sacrifice upon excision. Many nerve sheath tumors exhibit a peripheral rim of fat, the so-called "split-fat" sign. The " split-fat" sign is seen when a tumor arises from a large peripheral nerve and splits the adjacent normal perineural fat; the fat remaining as a high signal intensity rim arrayed about the growing lesion is best seen on T1-weighted sequences.[122] A malignant peripheral nerve sheath tumor (MPNST) frequently lacks the split-fat sign due to its more infiltrative growth. Paraspinal peripheral nerve sheath tumors often have a dumbbell shape and may enlarge the adjacent neural foramen. The "fascicular" sign may be seen in tumors imaged in cross section to the nerve appearing as ring-like areas within the tumor reflecting the fascicular nature of the associated nerve fibers.[122] The " target sign" consists of a hyperintense rim with central decreased signal intensity on T2-weighted images. The hyperintense rim is due to myxomatous elements and the central low signal secondary to fibrous and collagenous tissue[113] (Fig. 107-35). The target sign is more commonly observed in patients with neurofibromas than schwannomas and is uncommonly associated with malignant peripheral nerve sheath tumors. Thus the presence or absence of a target sign on T2-weighted MR images is helpful in differentiating benign from malignant peripheral nerve sheath tumors.[175]

Malignant peripheral nerve sheath tumors typically occur in patients from ages 20 to 50 and account for 5% to 10% of all soft-tissue sarcomas.[122] MPNST is associated with NF1 in 25% to 70% of cases.[122] Three to five percent of individuals with NF1 develop PMNSTs.[169] Therapeutic or occupational irradiation accounts for 10% to 20% of

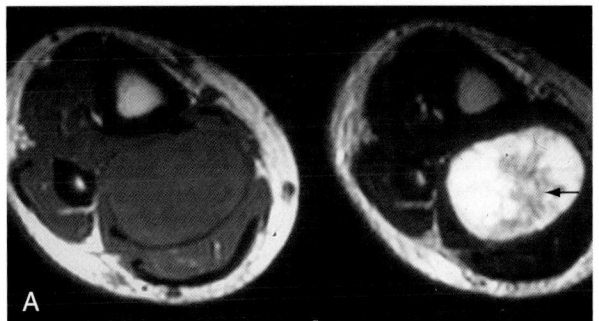

FIGURE 107-35

Neurilemoma posterior tibial nerve. **A,** T1 (*left)* and T2 *(right)*. T1 image shows mildly heterogeneous mass along the course of the posterior tibial nerve. Axial T2 show a high signal mass with a central area of low internal signal *(arrow)*, the "Target Sign." **B,** Sagittal post-contrast T1 shows the mass to heterogeneously enhance. The nerve is seen entering the mass above, the "string sign" *(arrow)*. The mass is seen to cleave the surrounding fat, the " split-fat sign" *(arrowheads)*. **C,** Intraoperative photograph of the posterior calf shows the fusiform mass. Blue tags note the cephalad and caudad tibial nerve. **D,** The gross specimen shows the benign tumor has been separated from the nerve. The nerve was preserved.

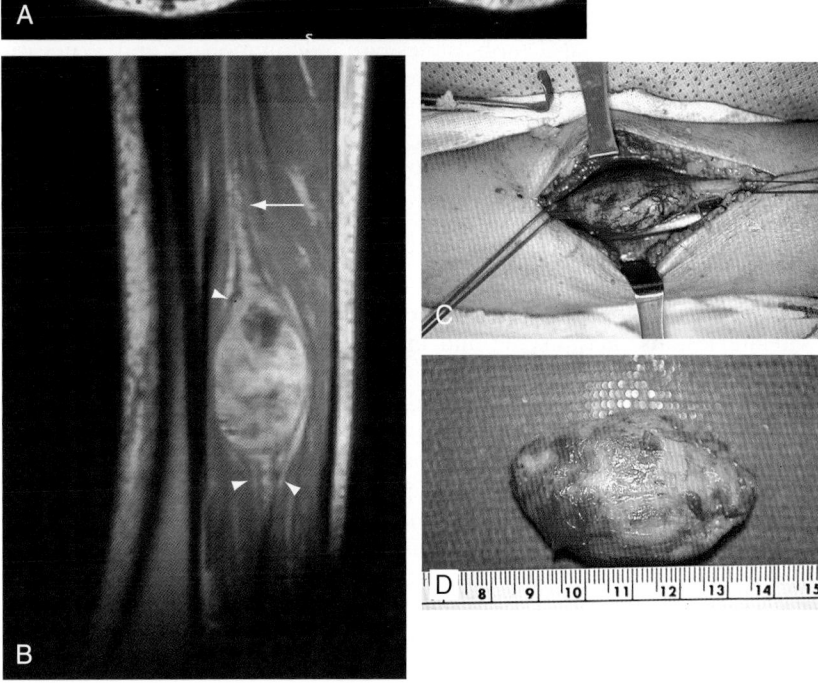

MPNSTs.[169] Differentiating benign from malignant nerve sheath tumors on MRI examination is difficult but features more commonly associated with malignancy are size greater than 5 cm, rapid growth, prominent enhancement, infiltrative margins, and marked heterogeneity with necrosis. Sudden enlargement of a preexisting neurofibroma should raise suspicion for malignant transformation.

TUMOR STAGING

Bone and soft-tissue sarcomas are uncommon and often unsuspected. For these reasons, they are often missed on physical examination resulting in delays in diagnosis and, sometimes, inappropriate treatment. Sarcoma staging is the process of identifying the local anatomic extent and distant spread of tumor. The process involves a thorough history and physical examination, directed radiographic imaging, and biopsy. Biopsy is complicated in about 20% of cases and should be performed only by experienced personnel in a center with a multidisciplinary team that is familiar with sarcoma treatment.

Osseous and soft-tissue sarcomas have a common mesenchymal origin and their behavior varies from that of carcinomas that are of epithelial lineage. Sarcomas grow centripetally along the path of least resistance. Sarcomas tend to respect anatomic borders and usually are confined to a single compartment or muscle group. Certain tissues act as natural relative barriers to sarcoma spread including synovium, articular cartilage, major fascial planes, sites of tendinous insertion or origin as well as cortical bone and periosteum.[176] These barriers separate tissues into anatomic compartments and a tumor arising and confined to one of these compartments is considered intracompartmental. Tumor spread to adjacent compartments or contamination of other compartments either by invasion or pathologic fracture or by an improperly performed biopsy is considered extracompartmental. An extracompartmental tumor requires a more extensive excision compared to a tumor confined to a single compartment. Certain anatomic areas are not confined by distinct anatomic boundaries such as the head and neck, supraclavicular fossa, axilla, antebrachial fossa, wrist and the dorsum of the hand. Extracompartmental sites in the lower extremity include the inguinal region, popliteal fascia, ankle, and dorsum of the foot. There are distinct compartments in the palmar aspect of the hand and plantar aspect of the foot but due to the complex anatomy and compactness of the structures, compartmental resection is difficult to achieve. Understanding compartmental anatomy is crucial for proper staging and biopsy of tumors. Sarcomas spread to distant sites almost exclusively through the hematologic system, with tumors of the extremities metastasizing to lung and tumors of the abdomen and pelvis metastasizing to liver and lung. Metastases to regional lymph nodes are uncommon occurring in 5.9% of soft-tissue sarcomas[177] and under 10% of osteosarcomas at autopsy.[181] Certain tumors such as epitheloid sarcoma, rhabdomyosarcoma, and clear cell sarcoma have a higher incidence of lymph node metastases.[178-180]

Sarcomas are surrounded by a reactive zone or "pseudocapsule" consisting of fibrovascular reactive tissue and compressed normal tissue. Microscopic finger-like tumor extensions or foci of tumor cells referred to as "satellite lesions" may invade and extend beyond this pseudocapsule. High-grade sarcomas generally have a less well defined pseudocapsule and tumor may occasionally spread more readily within the compartment and sometimes into adjacent compartments. Noncontiguous spread of tumor within a compartment is known as a "skip lesion." Rarely, a skip lesion may occur across an adjacent joint when the primary tumor is in a subarticular site (a transarticular skip metastasis).[183] Limb sparing procedures performed distal to a skip metastasis may account for the local recurrence of a tumor despite "adequate" surgical margins. Skip lesions are reported to occur in 1% to 25% of high-grade intramedullary osteosarcomas but the true prevalence is probably at the lower end of the spectrum.[179,184] Five-year survival for patients with skip metastases approximates that of patients with distal metastases. It is imperative that the radiologist includes the entire compartment of tumor origin on at least one sequence to exclude skip lesions.

Basic types of surgical excisions include intralesional, marginal, wide and radical. *Intralesional or intracapsular excisions* are performed within the tumor. The likelihood of recurrence with an intracapsular procedure is 100%. *Marginal excisions* are resections performed through the reactive zone or pseudocapsule surrounding the tumor. Excisional biopsies are marginal excisions. Local recurrence for marginal excision alone is 60% sp 80%. *Wide excisions* are resections done through normal tissue, the specimen being composed of the tumor, the pseudocapsule, and a rim of normal tissue resected en-bloc. *Radical excisions* are en-bloc resections of the entire compartment of tumor origin.

MR is an important imaging modality utilized in the staging of osseous and soft-tissue sarcomas. Radiologists must insure that adequate technique is utilized in evaluating masses. The tumor should be measured in three dimensions. Tumor signal, necrosis, enhancement pattern, and characteristic tumor morphology should be assessed. The location and extent of the lesion should be precisely described with reference to the compartment or compartments involved. Intercompartmental spread should be noted as indicated by tumor involement of adjacent compartments and abnormalities in underlying bone, soft-tissues, or adjacent joints. Intracompartmental metastases or skip lesions should be excluded by a large field of view sequence imaging the entire involved compartment. Lymphadenopathy should be noted and the relationship between the mass and regional neurovascular structures must be defined. Bloem et al[182] found that MRI had a sensitivity of 100%, a specificity of 98%, an accuracy of 98%, a positive predictive value of 91%, and a negative predictive value of 100% in assessing neurovascular involvement.

Staging not only defines the type and anatomic extent of a tumor but it also helps to guide treatment and predict survival. There is no universally accepted staging system for bone and soft-tissue sarcomas, however there are a number of classification schemes that stratify patients into groups based on prognostic factors such as tumor size, grade, depth, and distant spread. The Enneking classification[185] adopted by the Musculoskeletal Tumor Society is a surgical classification utilized for both soft-tissue and bone sarcoma that is based on tumor grade, location (either intra- or extracompartmental) and the presence or absence of metastases (Table 107-3). The TNM classification adopted by the American Joint Committee on Cancer relies on tumor size, grade (low, intermediate, and high), the presence or absence of distant metastases, and the presence or absence of nodal disease.[186] Almost uniformly, grade and size are important factors in predicting survival in patients with soft-tissue sarcomas, with large high-grade tumors presenting the greatest risk for metastases.[187-189] Spiral computed tomography (CT) is the study of choice to evaluate the lungs for potential metastases, the most common site of distant spread. CT of the chest should be done in all patients with known or suspected sarcoma. Bone scintigraphy is most useful in detecting distant disease and can be helpful in assessing response to systemic treatment. Whole body STIR examination at the time of the initial MR study may also detect distant metastases.[190]

Positron-emission tomography (PET) is a rapidly developing imaging technique that provides unique information regarding the metabolism of musculoskeletal lesions through the use of positron-emitting radionuclides. The most commonly used radionuclide for PET imaging, ^{18}F-labeled 2-deoxy-2-fluoro-D-glucose (FDG), is proving of utility in the staging of musculoskeletal tumors. FDG is transported into metabolically active tissues as a glucose analog. After initial phosphorylation into FDG-6-phosphate, a poor substrate for

TABLE 107-3 Sarcoma Staging (Enneking)

Stage	Histologic grade	Compartment	Metastatic
IA	Low	Within	No
IB	Low	Outside	No
IIA	High	Within	No
IIB	High	Outside	No
III	Any	Any	Yes

further glucose metabolism, the compound becomes trapped and subsequently accumulates within the tissue. Uptake of glucose and therefore FDG-6-phosphate accumulation as measured by standard uptake value (SUV) increases in cells with higher metabolic rates. Generally, high-grade sarcomas and aggressive benign lesions tend to have higher SUVs than other benign lesions.[191] While FDG PET is highly sensitive, FDG may accumulate in aggressive benign and inflammatory lesions.[192] There is considerable overlap of SUV values between benign and malignant osseous and soft-tissue processes. FDG PET appears to be insufficient as a screening tool in the differentiation of benign and malignant musculoskeletal lesions.[193] PET has been found useful in the grading of musculoskeletal tumors and as a predictor of survival and disease progression.[194-197] MR and FDG PET have the potential to evaluate the entire body for primary malignancy and metastatic disease in a single study with a sensitivity for detecting bone metastases superior to that of skeletal scintigraphy.[198,199]

Staging of Osseous Tumors

The diagnosis of bone tumors is principally made on radiographs. Patients with osseous sarcomas require a careful history and physical examination, appropriate imaging studies, and formal staging for suspicious masses. The diagnosis is made, the tumor staged and optimum results obtained by utilizing the combined expertise of an experienced musculoskeletal radiologist, pathologist and orthopedic oncologist. Consideration

should be given to referral to centers dedicated and experienced in the medical and surgical management of sarcomas.

Certain bone tumors tend to occur in certain age groups. For example, osteosarcoma is the most common bone tumor of adolescents while malignant fibrous histiocytoma of bone has a peak incidence in individuals over the age of 50.[200] Certain bone tumors have a characteristic location within bone. For example, osteosarcomas arise near the growth plate in the metaphysis (Fig. 107-36) and Ewing's sarcoma typically presents in the metadiaphysis and diaphysis of long bones. Pain is the usual presenting symptom, unlike soft-tissue sarcomas where masses may become quite large before becoming painful.[201] Pathologic fractures are not unusual. Ten percent of osteosarcoma patients have a pathologic fracture at some point during the disease.[202] The presence of a pathologic fracture may influence surgery, impact on local disease control, and possibly affect survival.

The prognosis for osteosarcoma patients with skip lesions, regional lymph node metastases, and distant metastases is uniformly poor.[16] The entire compartment of tumor origin must be imaged from the joint above to the joint below the tumor. If the tumor is subarticular, images should also be obtained across the joint. Large field of view coronal or sagittal T1- and fat saturation T2-weighted or STIR sequences are best suited for this purpose.[203] Several studies have compared sequence accuracy in determining intraosseous tumor extent compared with pathologic specimens.[204-206] Generally T1-weighted images are superior in the evaluation of intramedullary tumor extent. Onikul et al[205] suggested

FIGURE 107-36

A 16-year-old boy presented with an osteosarcoma of the distal tibia. **A,** Anteroposterior radiograph reveals a destructive, expansile lesion of the distal tibial metaphysis with abundant ossification within the tumor matrix. **B,** Sagittal T1-weighted (600/20) image nicely demonstrates the intramedullary extent of the tumor, with sparing of the epiphysis (asterisk). The ossification, visible as foci of low signal intensity, is not as well seen as on the radiograph. In this case, the plain radiograph is adequate for diagnostic purposes. MRI provides a detailed analysis of the local anatomic extent of the mass, which in this case does not exceed that suggested by the radiograph. (**B** from Caron KH, Bisset GS III: Magnetic resonance imaging of pediatric atraumatic musculoskeletal lesions. Top Magn Reson Imaging 3:43-60, 1990.)

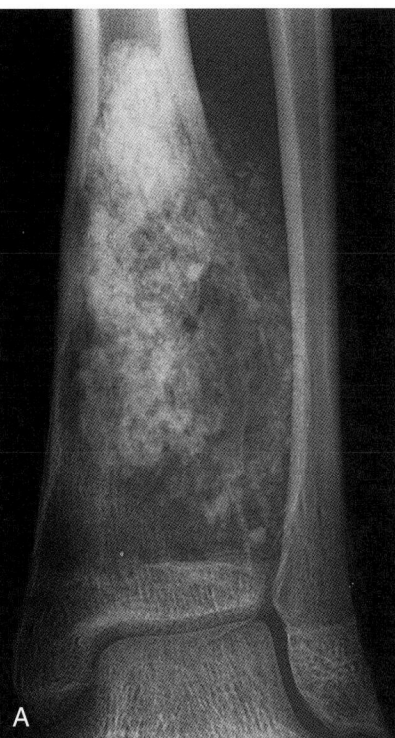
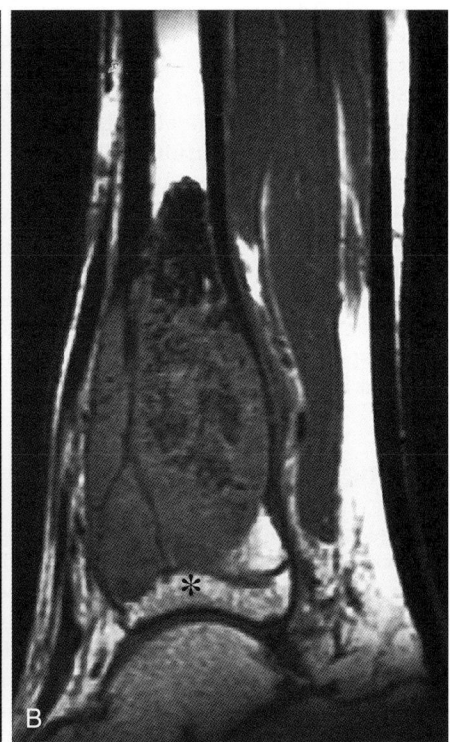

that STIR sequences lead to overestimation of intra-osseous tumor extent in 73% of cases due to STIR sensitivity to marrow edema. In patients undergoing limb-sparing procedures, intramedullary extent determines the appropriate site of bone resection.

The presence or absence of epiphyseal involvement in skeletally immature individuals dictates whether or not joint-sparing surgery can be performed, permitting continued growth of the limb. The epiphyseal plate is not a barrier to tumor extension as was previously surmised (Fig. 107-37). Pathologic studies note physeal and epiphyseal involvement in 75% to 88% of cases of metaphyseal-based osteosarcoma.[207,208] Hoffer et al[206] found T1-weighted images more specific and STIR images more sensitive for detecting epiphyseal involvement, although overall accuracy of the sequences was equivalent. Panuel et al[204] found T1-weighted images alone to be sufficient to evaluate epiphyseal disease.

Extramedullary tumor extension determines the feasibility and type of limb-sparing procedure to be performed.[207] Thinning, absence or focal attenuation of the normal sharply defined low signal of the bone cortex indicates cortical expansion, destruction, or erosion. Periosteal reaction may be detected as cortical thickening or as a low signal intensity line oblique or parallel to the adjacent bone. CT and radiographs are more sensitive than MRI in the evaluation of periosteal reaction. Extramedullary extension and involvement of adjacent muscle and soft compartments are best evaluated with MRI. The relationship of extraosseous extension of a tumor mass relative to neurovascular structures is an important element of appropriate surgical planning. Encasement of the neurovascular bundle is a relative contraindication to limb salvage surgery. Pathologic fractures contaminate adjacent compartments, or if intra-articular, contaminate the associated joint. Criteria for joint involvement are not well established. In a review of 46 osteosarcoma patients, Schima et al[209] utilized disruption of the joint capsule, destruction of articular cortical bone and cartilage, and involvement of the cruciate ligaments as criteria for joint invasion. Often the focus of intra-articular disease will be surrounded and sequestered by abundant synovium making intra-articular resection possible. Utilizing these parameters for joint involvement, sensitivity for joint involvement was 100% (all 10 patients with joint extension were correctly identified). However, there were 11 false positives for joint involvement (specificity, 69%) resulting in unnecessary extra-articular resection or amputation.

Staging of Soft-tissue Tumors

Soft-tissue sarcomas are a diverse group of neoplasms that vary clinically, radiographically, and pathologically. Many patients with soft-tissue sarcomas undergo inappropriate biopsy and inadequate resection prior to referral.[210,211] Because of poorly placed biopsy sites and ill-advised incisions, contamination of normal adjacent tissues may compromise limb salvage and even threaten survival.[212]

Soft-tissue sarcomas occur in a wide age range of individuals, with males affected slightly more than females.[213] Patients usually present between the third and eighth decades and the incidence of sarcoma increases with increasing age. Like bone tumors, tumors of soft-tissue tend to occur in predictable age ranges. Rhabdomyosarcoma occurs in the first two decades of life while synovial sarcomas occur most commonly in the third to fifth decades of life. Malignant fibrous histiocytoma, the most common soft-tissue sarcoma, occurs in the fifth to seventh decades and beyond. Patients with soft-tissue sarcomas usually present with a painless growing mass. A past medical history of malignancy, trauma, radiation or chronic infection is important to note. Soft-tissue sarcomas are not uncommon in patients surviving retinoblastoma[214] as well as patients with neurofibromatosis.[215-217] Patients infrequently present with radiating pain exacerbated by certain positions or activities, findings suggestive of either central or peripheral neural impingement. Vascular claudication or insufficiency is rare, even in patients with neglected tumors that completely encase major vessels. Venous and lymphatic obstruction however may result in swelling of the distal limb. Metastatic or disseminated disease is present in a small number of individuals at initial presentation[218,219] and may manifest as weight loss, anorexia, a nonproductive cough, and skeletal pain in individuals with osseous metastases.

Malignant tumors in general grow more rapidly than benign lesions. Occasionally lipomas, traumatized benign tumors with secondary hemorrhage, and pseudotumors can grow quite rapidly raising the suspicion of malignancy. Conversely, some sarcomas such as synovial sarcoma can grow insidiously over many months and even years.[220] Although certain soft-tissue sarcomas have a predilection for certain locations, this feature is not as predictable as with bone tumors. Epithelioid sarcoma, for example, is common in the hand and upper extremity while synovial sarcoma is the most common deep-seated malignancy of the foot.[220] Pleomorphic rhabdomyosarcomas are more frequent in the thigh and neurogenic tumors arise around nerves.

On physical examination, it is important to assess and record tumor size and depth, as both observations are important prognostic variables for survival. Overlying skin changes can be seen in patients with vascular tumors or in patients with neglected fungating tumors. Dermatofibrosarcoma protruberans is a superficial dermal-based lesion that frequently ulcerates the skin. Skin pigmentation or café-au-lait spots can be seen in patients with neurofibromatosis. If the tumor involves overlying dermis, wide margins of skin must be excised with the mass that would require flap and or split thickness skin graft reconstruction for wound closure. Occasionally, lesions arising within or around nerves will cause dysesthesias when percussing the area on physical examination. Neurologic deficits are uncommon in patients with appendicular tumors but are frequently seen in patients with pelvic sarcomas. Palpation and auscultation can elicit a thrill or bruit respectively in patients with highly vascular tumors, which should evoke caution in performing a biopsy.

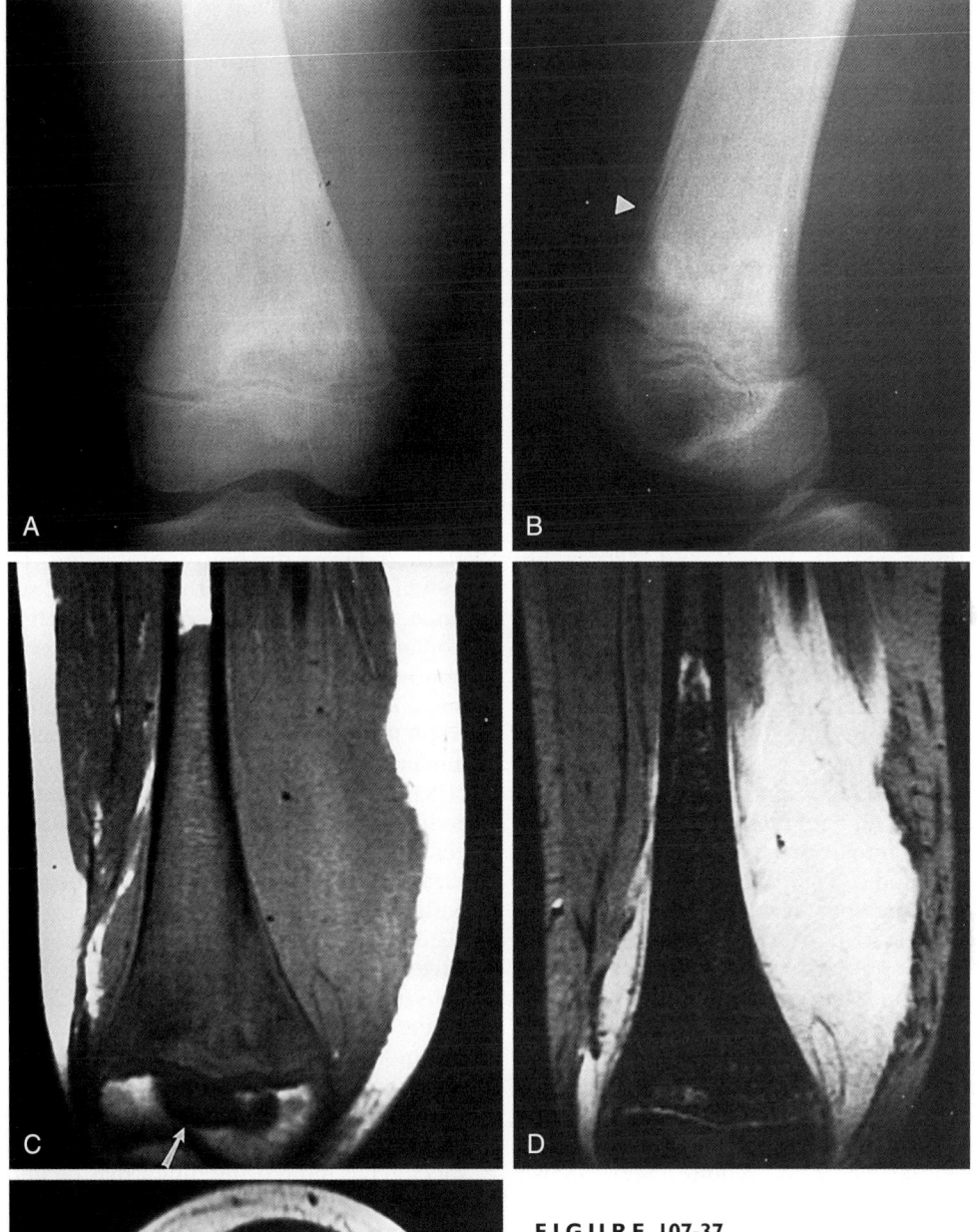

FIGURE 107-37

A 10-year-old boy presented with primary lymphoma of bone. **A,** Anteroposterior radiograph of the distal femur shows diffuse medullary sclerosis within the metaphysis. **B,** Lateral radiograph shows subtle permeative destruction of the anterior cortex *(arrowhead),* suggesting an aggressive lesion. **C,** Coronal T1-weighted (600/20) image better demonstrates the full intramedullary extent of the tumor. Note the epiphyseal invasion *(arrow)* not detectable on plain radiographs. **D,** T2*-weighted gradient-echo (370/30/20°) image better delineates the soft-tissue extent of the tumor. The intramedullary portion of the tumor is dark due to calcification (magnetic susceptibility effect) and is poorly demarcated from adjacent marrow. **E,** Axial T2-weighted (1800/80) spin-echo image demonstrates the extensive multicompartmental soft-tissue mass with neurovascular encasement *(arrowhead).* (**C** from Moore SG, Bisset GS III, Siegel MJ, Donaldson JS: Pediatric musculoskeletal MR imaging. Radiology 179:345-360, 1991.)

Palpation of regional lymph nodes is necessary since a small number of patients with soft-tissue sarcomas will have lymph node metastasis at the time of presentation.[221] Certain tumors including rhabdomyosarcoma, synovial sarcoma, clear cell sarcoma, mesenchymal chondrosarcoma, angiosarcoma and epithelioid sarcoma have a higher rate of lymphatic spread, prompting some investigators to routinely sample lymph nodes at the time of resection.[222] If nodal disease is clinically suspected, imaging of the area in anticipation of nodal sampling is important, although the absence of radiographic findings does not mitigate against nodal disease. In general, nodal sampling for most soft-tissue sarcomas is not recommended since nodal spread of disease is relatively uncommon at presentation.[221]

From a surgical perspective, MRI is critical in assessing the exact location of the tumor. Generally T2 or STIR sequences are best to evaluate soft-tissue extent of a tumor while T1 sequences are best to evaluate intraosseous tumor extent. Vessels and nerves are uninvolved by tumor when a clear plane of muscle or fat is interposed between tumor and neurovascular structures. Often, when tumor effaces or displaces the neurovascular bundle, a subtle fat plain can still be appreciated between the tumor and nerve or vessel. A tumor is said to abut the nerve or vessel when this intervening soft-tissue plane is obliterated. Finally, a tumor may clearly infiltrate or encase the neurovascular bundle. Although this finding does not entirely exclude limb salvage, a more complicated resection coupled with vascular reconstruction is required to achieve tumor-free margins and viable functional results.

Joint involvement is rare and many tumors that appear to extend into the joint are often actually covered by a synovial reflection. This is an important observation because when tumor is covered by synovium, the joint can be preserved without compromising tumor-free margins. An exception to this is the tumor that arises in the popliteal fossa that is closely adherent to or frankly involving bone and capsule. These tumors may extend along the cruciate ligaments and require extra-articular resection to achieve tumor-free margins as the cruciates invest into bone above and below. The observation of tumor within a joint is very important since joint resections and reconstructions are more difficult to perform, have much higher rates of complications, and functionally are less satisfactory than joint preservation. Primary intra-articular sarcomas are rare but have been reported to occur in 5% of patients with synovial sarcomas.[223] Malignant transformation of synovial chondromatosis to chondrosarcoma is rarer still but should be considered when articular bone destruction is detected on radiographs along with associated intramedullary invasion on MRI.[224]

BIOPSY

The staging process culminates with the biopsy for diagnosis. The radiologist's role in managing sarcomas extends beyond diagnostic imaging and involves image-directed needle biopsy. Because percutaneous needle biopsies are common in diagnosing potential sarcomas, practical knowledge of compartments and limb-salvage principals is critical to avoid inappropriate placement of the needle. There is the risk of seeding of malignant cells along the needle track and the track therefore is usually resected at the time of definitive surgery.[225,226] Thus, the biopsy in effect determines surgical options. An ill-advised biopsy approach may have devastating consequences and may necessitate a more radical resection or even an unnecessary amputation.[212] The radiologist must work in concert with the operative surgeon to determine the appropriate biopsy approach. The radiologist must work with the pathologist to ensure that sufficient tissue for diagnosis is obtained so that misdiagnoses and delays in treatment are avoided.

Disease-free margins are more difficult to achieve when tumors occur outside of or involve more than one compartment. Sarcomas, unlike carcinomas, are highly implantable, therefore only one compartment should be violated during the biopsy procedure. The biopsy track should also be in line with the planned surgical resection since it needs to be resected with the specimen. Contamination of more than one compartment by a poorly placed biopsy track or a hematoma will require more extensive surgery and larger radiation fields and result in an increased risk of local disease recurrence and impaired or diminished function.

Sarcomas appear to be radiographically heterogeneous because of intervening trauma and hemorrhage, central tumor necrosis, fibrosis and the presence of variable histologic cell types and degrees of cellularity within a given tumor. For example, liposarcomas are histomorphologically diverse and a single tumor may have areas that contain cytologically well-differentiated liposarcoma, other areas that are clearly myxoid, and others still that have focal areas of round cell or pleomorphic cell types. Unlike carcinomas that are commonly homogeneous, mesenchymal tumors have regional morphologic variation and multiple samples are required to establish a diagnosis.[227] If the biopsy specimen is limited, the tumor may be underestimated or overestimated with regard to grade and, hence, metastatic potential. Treatment options vary according to grade and tumor extent and errors in biopsy will result in inappropriate management of these patients. FDG PET may be of aid in directing the biopsy to the region of the highest grade abnormality.[228] Special studies such as cytogenetic tests, flow cytometry, and immunohistochemistry are often required for particular tumors. Some of these tests require special processing to preserve constituent proteins, RNA, and DNA. These issues should be decided prior to biopsy and adequate tissue obtained to satisfy situational requirements.

The decision to perform an open biopsy or needle biopsy depends on the institutional experience with sarcoma management and the relative expertise of the musculoskeletal radiologist and pathologist. The advantage of open biopsy is that, in general, adequate tissue is obtained for most diagnostic procedures. An experienced pathologist can usually make a diagnosis on frozen section and a decision to proceed to wide local resection can be undertaken, thus avoiding a second operation. The disadvantages are that sometimes the frozen section is not diagnostic but instead reveals only that sufficient and potentially diagnostic tissue was obtained that requires further processing and special staining for definitive diagnosis. Since the open biopsy is done in an operating room, the cost is significantly higher than needle biopsy alone. In addition, the risk of infection and hematoma is increased with consequent greater potential contamination of adjacent tissues.[229]

Needle biopsy is a relatively inexpensive procedure with a low risk of hemorrhage and infection.[229] The diagnostic accuracy of fine needle aspiration ranges between 64% and 96%.[230,231] The fundamental problem with fine needle biopsy and even core needle biopsy is one's confidence in the accuracy of diagnostic interpretation given the small amount of available tissue. There are a number of studies that highlight the diagnostic challenge of differentiating benign from malignant soft-tissue tumors with a small needle specimen with interobserver variability ranging from 16% to 39%.[232-236]

The hazards of biopsy in patients with musculoskeletal tumors are well known and described in two identical studies conducted 14 years apart.[203,237] In the latest report, the rate of error in diagnosis was 17.8% and the overall outcome was altered in 16.6% of patients with soft-tissue tumors.[203] Unnecessary amputation was performed in 3% of patients as a result of a poorly done biopsy. The biopsy-related problems were greater in community hospitals than referral hospitals (by a factor of two to twelve times!). Sadly, the incidence of biopsy-related problems remained essentially unchanged in the 1996 study despite admonitions and recommendations made in light of the original 1982 study.[203] Thus, the authors concluded, biopsy should be done by the surgeon or by the radiologist in careful consultation with the surgeon who will perform the definitive procedure in an institution familiar with the diagnosis and care of patients with bone and soft-tissue sarcomas.

FOLLOW-UP

MR imaging is used to evaluate the tumor after preoperative chemotherapy, radiation therapy, or both (Fig. 107-38). Restaging with MRI is needed after the

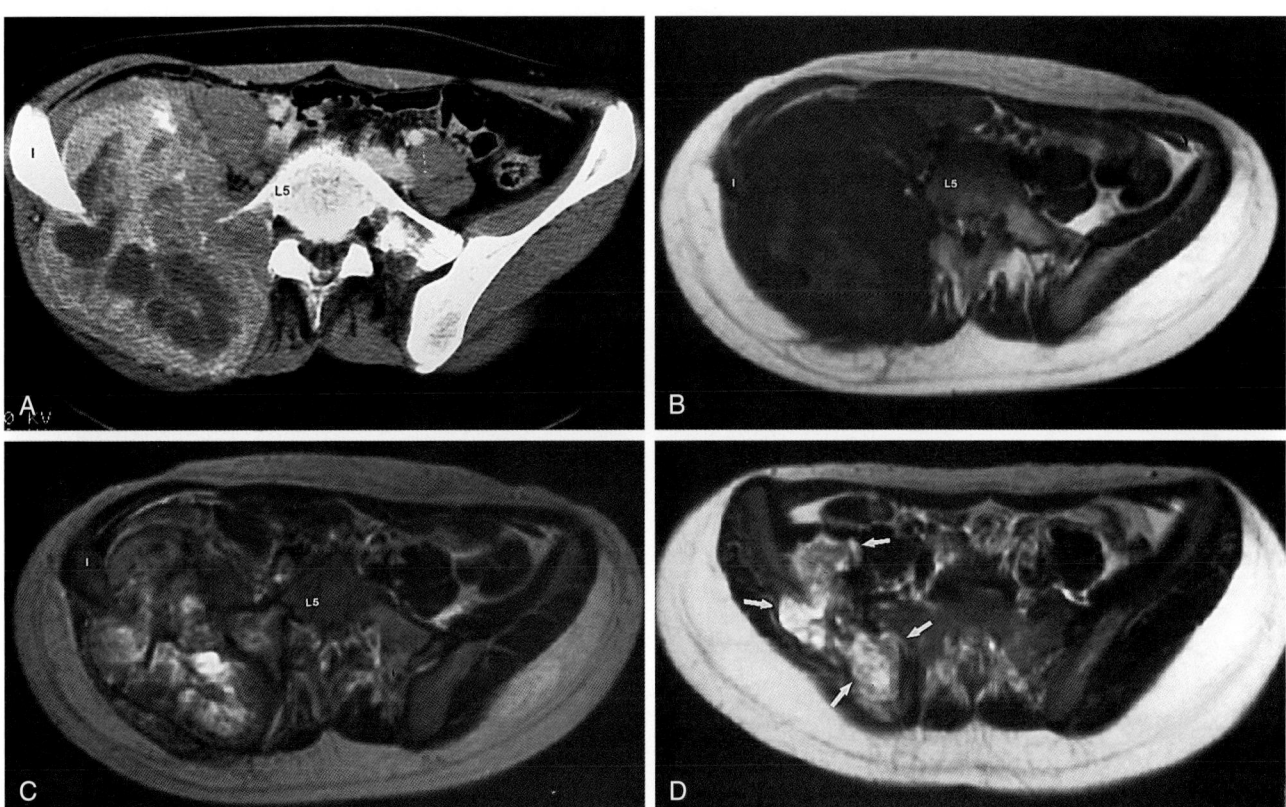

FIGURE 107-38

A 13-year-old girl presented with Ewing's sarcoma of the ilium. **A,** Axial contrast-enhanced CT scan shows a large soft-tissue mass replacing the right iliac crest (I) and invading the L5 vertebral body (L5). Axial T1-weighted (600/12) (**B**) and corresponding T2-weighted (2700/119) (**C**) fast spin-echo images demonstrate the full extent of the tumor but offer no additional information compared with the CT scan. **D,** Axial T2-weighted (2700/85) fast spin-echo image after 6 months of chemotherapy. There has been near-complete resolution of the soft-tissue component of the tumor, with persistence of a smaller, lobulated high signal intensity mass (arrows). The marked decrease in tumor volume suggests a favorable response. The increase in signal intensity of the intramedullary component is nonspecific. No viable tumor was detected histologically after hemipelvectomy. (*A to D courtesy of George S. Bisset, III, MD, Children's Hospital Medical Center, Cincinnati, OH.*)

preoperative therapy to determine tumor response to preoperative treatment (Fig. 107-39). The definition of a good pathologic response is variable, ranging from 60% to 95% necrosis.

Postoperative imaging is difficult because of distorted anatomy and postoperative tissue changes after resection. The use of rotational and or free flaps for soft-tissue coverage can be confused with recurrent tumor. Metallic implants and metal clips along vessels distort MR images. The use of allografts fixed with plates or metal implants in patients requiring bone resection and skeletal reconstruction cause such distortion that the use of routine MR mass protocol sequences for local recurrence are of limited value. MR techniques may be modified to allow acceptable imaging in the face of substantial indwelling hardware. Fast spin-echo imaging with frequency encoding parallel to the long axis of the

hardware, increased receiver bandwidth, increased matrix, and short interecho spacing should be utilized.[238] Gradient-echo imaging, conventional spin-echo sequences, and fat saturation should be avoided.

Tumor recurrence should be suspected with a focal mass or nodule where low to intermediate signal intensity on T1- and high signal intensity on T2-weighted sequences is detected (Fig. 107-40). Recurrent tumor generally exhibits enhancement and associated mass and mass effect. High signal intensity on T2-weighted images without focal mass usually indicates post-therapeutic or postsurgical change. Vanel et al found T2-weighted images were the most useful to evaluate for possible recurrence and that the absence of T2-weighted high signal intensity excluded tumor in 99% of their cases.[239] On T2-weighted images, virtually all areas of low signal intensity do not require biopsy. Exceptions include

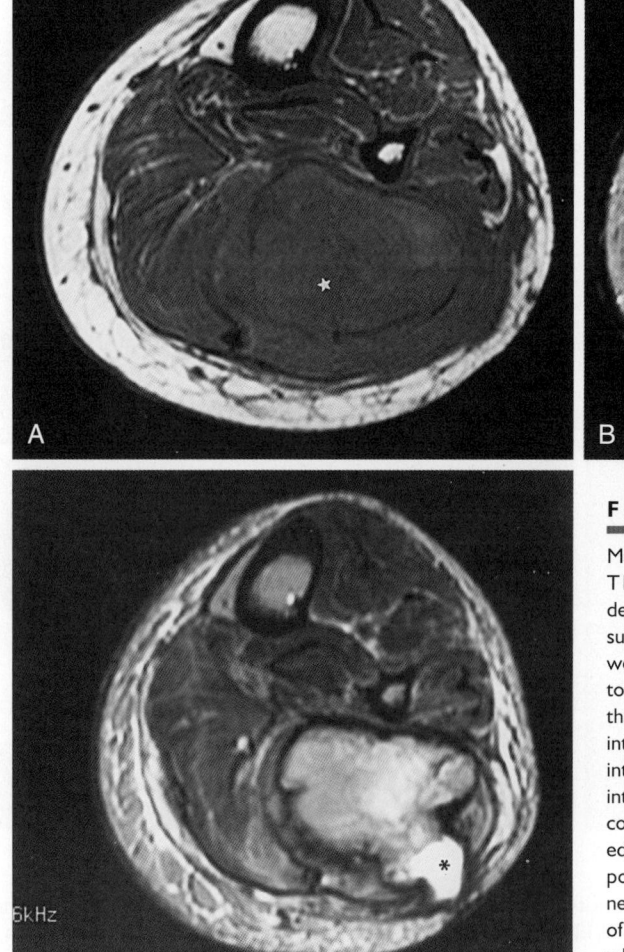

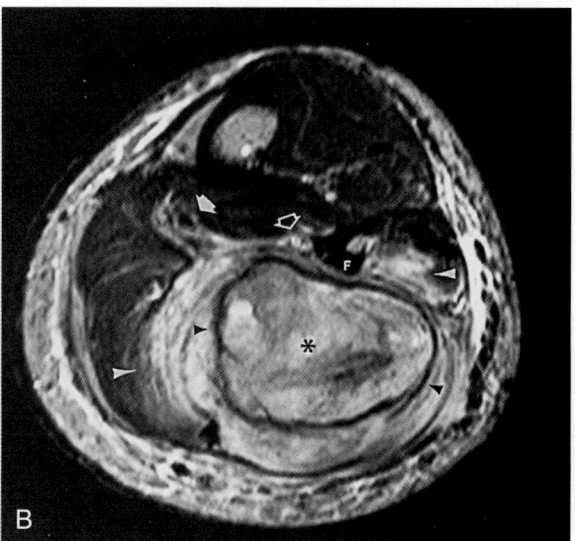

FIGURE 107-39

Malignant fibrous histiocytoma in a 58-year-old woman. **A,** Axial T1-weighted (617/20) image through the middle calf shows an ill-defined mass *(star)* of predominantly low signal intensity, with subtle peripheral regions of brighter signal intensity. **B,** Axial T2-weighted (2000/80) image shows the bulk of the tumor *(asterisk)* to be of heterogeneous high signal intensity. Portions of the mass that were bright on the T1-weighted image are dark, indicative of intratumor hemorrhage. The tumor is surrounded by a low signal intensity pseudocapsule *(black arrowheads)*. There is high signal intensity infiltrating the adjacent posterior and lateral muscle compartments *(white arrowheads)*. This predominantly represents edema but must be considered contaminated with tumor. The posterior tibial *(solid arrow)* and peroneal *(open arrow)* neurovascular bundles are engulfed. There is artifactual thinning of the lateral fibular (F) cortex caused by a chemical-shift artifact, which is less prominent on the T1-weighted image (the fibula was uninvolved at surgery). **C,** Axial T2-weighted (2200/80) image after incisional biopsy and 3 months of chemotherapy and irradiation. There is a superficial postbiopsy fluid collection *(asterisk)*. The edema in the muscles surrounding the tumor largely resolved, and the posterior tibial neurovascular bundle is no longer engulfed, indicating more favorable anatomy for resection.

hypocellular lesions such as fibromatosis and densely mineralized lesions such as osteosarcoma. Knowledge of the preoperative tumor signal characteristics and analysis of recent plain films should be of aid in avoiding these pitfalls.[240] Areas of high signal intensity on T2-weighted sequences without associated mass do not require biopsy. A focal high signal intensity mass on T2-weighted images raises the suspicion of recurrent tumor, however, seroma, hematoma, necrosis, abscess, postradiation changes including radiation-induced pseudomass, surgical hemostatic packing material, or inflammatory changes must also be considered. Gadolinium administration may be of aid in the differential diagnosis (Fig. 107-41). Dynamic gadolinium perfusion imaging shows early enhancement of tumor and delayed enhancement of post-treatment changes.[30] Diffusion imaging may help distinguish between postsurgical/post-therapeutic change and recurrent or residual viable tumor.[37] Biopsy is generally necessary in a region of focal mass-like high signal on T2 sequences that enhance on T1 postcontrast sequences.

FDG PET seems to be a promising tool to evaluate tumor response to chemotherapy.[241] PET allows for detection of metabolic change (in the form of decreased FDG uptake) that may occur within a lesion even prior to visible morphologic change in the mass. CT and MRI excel at defining tumor morphology but in the patient who is status postsurgery, radiation, or chemotherapy, altered tissue planes, inflammation, edema, fibrosis, and scar limit these modalities. These post-therapeutic changes may mimic residual or recurrent tumor on follow-up MR or CT examination. FDG PET is a useful adjunct to MRI in distinguishing viable tumor from postsurgical and post-therapeutic changes in patients with musculoskeletal sarcomas.[242,243]

Radiation causes changes in bone and soft-tissues. Scarring is difficult to separate or distinguish from local recurrence but radiation changes generally have less mass effect than recurrence. Soft-tissue signal intensity in the radiation field seen as high signal intensity on long TR sequences increases over time, peaking at about 6 months for neutron-treated patients and at about 12 to 18 months for photon-treated patients.[244] Postradiation edema resolves in half of the photon-treated patients within 2 to 3 years and in less than 20% of neutron-treated patients by 3 to 4 years post-treatment.[244] Postradiation enhancement may persist in inflammatory masses for longer than 5 years.[245] Radiation osteonecrosis is also a significant problem in patients treated with over 65 Gy and large fields. These patients develop stress fractures and reparative changes in bone that may be confused with secondary sarcoma. Pathologic fractures are very difficult to manage because of the impaired reparative capabilities of radiated bone and extensive soft-tissue fibrosis. Clinical history and serial radiographic follow-up is critical in these patients.

Finally, postoperative imaging is useful to evaluate potential secondary sarcomas that infrequently occur in patients receiving radiation. To qualify as a secondary or radiation-induced sarcoma, a latent period between the administration of radiation and the presence of a secondary sarcoma must be established ranging between

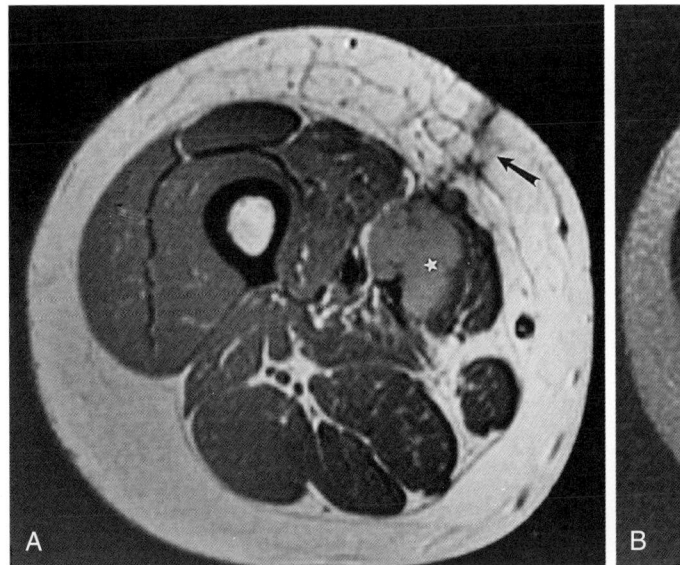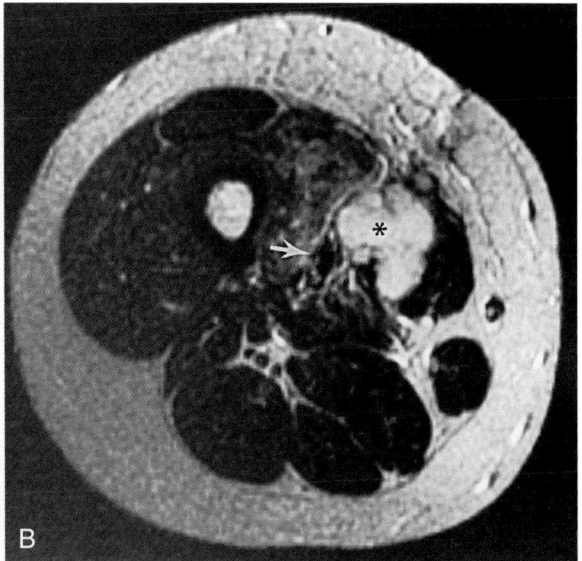

FIGURE 107-40

A 24-year-old woman presented with recurrent pain 6 months after resection of a hemangiopericytoma from the thigh. **A,** Axial proton density-weighted (1800/20) image demonstrates the surgical scar *(arrow)* and a mass *(star)* of homogeneous intermediate signal intensity in the resection bed. **B,** Axial T2-weighted (1800/80) image shows the mass *(asterisk)* to be of fairly homogeneous high signal intensity, clearly separable from the adjacent muscles and abutting the femoral neurovascular bundle *(arrow)*. Recurrent hemangiopericytoma was confirmed at subsequent surgery.

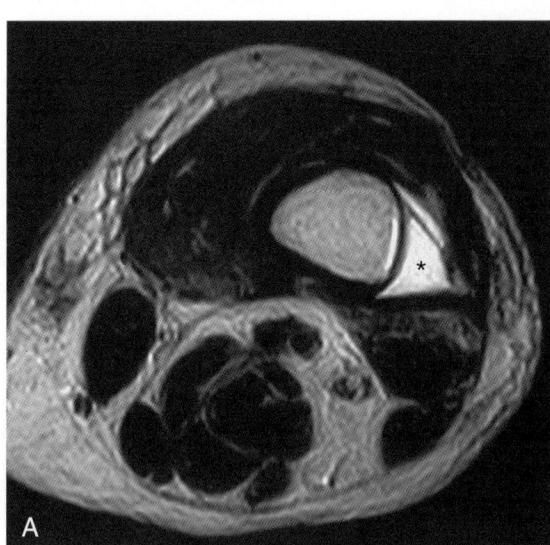
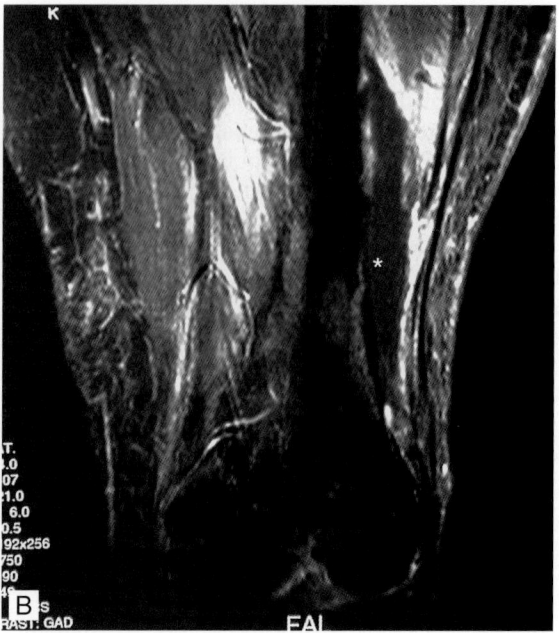

FIGURE 107-41

Postoperative seroma. **A,** Axial T2 shows high signal intensity *(asterisk)* adjacent to the femur in this patient status post sarcoma resection. **B,** Post-contrast fat saturation T1 coronal shows failure of the mass to enhance *(asterisk),* consistent with postoperative seroma. Enhancement adjacent to the seroma is consistent with postoperative and post-therapeutic change.

2 years and 5 years or more. The lesion should occur within the radiated field and must be histologically distinct from the primary tumor.

SUMMARY

MRI has become an important tool in the evaluation of osseous and soft-tissue masses. High contrast resolution, direct multiplanar acquisition, and the capability of tissue characterization through the evaluation of signal characteristics have made MRI the most accurate means of staging and evaluating tumor extent. Plain radiographs remain the primary tool for the diagnosis of bone tumors. MRI is the primary imaging tool for the detection and diagnosis of soft-tissue tumors. Still, MRI is able to determine the histologic diagnosis in only one quarter to one third of cases by evaluation of MR signal characteristics alone. MRI plays its greatest role in the anatomic staging, postchemotherapeutic and postsurgical follow-up of musculoskeletal tumors.

REFERENCES

1. Veth R, Van Hoesel R, Pruszczynski MJ, et al: Limb salvage in musculoskeletal oncology. Lancet Oncology 4:343-50, 2003.
2. Zimmer WD, Berquist TH, McLeodra, et al: Bone tumors: magnetic resonance imaging versus computed tomography. Radiology 155:709-718, 1985.
3. Demas BE, Heelan RT, Lane J, et al: Soft-tissue sarcoma of the extremeties: comparison of MR and CT in determining the extent of disease. Am J Roentgenol 150:615-620, 1988.
4. Moulton JS, Blebea JS, Dunco DM, et al: MR imaging of soft-tissue masses: diagnostic efficiency and value of distinguishing between benign and malignant lesions. Am J Roentgenol 164:1191-1199, 1995.
5. O'Flanagan SJ, Stack JP, McGee HM, et al: Imaging of intramedullary tumour spread in osteosarcoma: a comparison of techniques. J Bone Joint Surg Br 73:998-1001, 1991.
6. Panicek DM, Schwartz LH: MR imaging after surgery for musculoskeletal neoplasm. Semin Musculoskeletal Radiol 6:57-66, 2002.
7. Kransdorf MJ, Murphy MD: Radiologic evaluation of soft-tissue masses: a current perspective. Am J Roentgenol 175:575-87, 2000.
8. United States Cancer Statistics: Incidence. A joint publication of the Centers for Disease Control and the National Cancer Institute in collaboration with the North American Association of Central Cancer Registries, 1999.
9. American Cancer Society Estimate, 2003. Cancer facts and figures 2003, Atlanta.
10. Damron TA, Heiner J: Orthopedic management of metastatic disease: management of metastatic disease to soft tissues. Orthop Clin North Am 31:661-73, 2000.
11. Sudo A, Ogihara Y, Shiokawa Y, et al: Intramuscular metastases of carcinoma. Clin Orthop 296:213-217, 1993.
12. Glockner J, White LM, Sundaram M, et al: Unsuspected metastases presenting as solitary soft-tissue lesions: a fourteen year review. Skeletal Radiol 29:270-274, 2000.
13. Acinas-Garcia O, Fernandez FA, Stane EG, et al: Metastasis of malignant neoplasms to skeletal muscle. Rev Exp Oncol 31:57-67, 1984.
14. Damron TA, Heiner J: Distant soft-tissue metastases: a series of 30 new patients and 91 cases from the literature. Ann Surg Oncol 7:526-534, 2000.
15. Magee T, Rosenthal H: Skeletal muscle metastases at sites of documented trauma. Am J Roentgenol 178:985-988, 2002.
16. Wuisman P, Enneking WF: Prognosis for patients who have osteosarcoma with skip metastases. J Bone Joint Surg 72:60-68, 1990.
17. Mirowitz SA: Fast scanning and fat-suppression MR imaging of musculoskeletal disorders. Am J Roentgenology 161:1147-1157, 1993.
18. Pui MH, Chang SK: Comparison of inversion recovery fast spin-echo (FSE) with T2-weighted fat-saturation FSE and T1-weighted MR imaging in bone marrow lesion detection. Skeletal Radiol 25:149-152, 1996.
19. Dwyer AJ, Frank JA, Sank VJ, et al: Short-Ti inversion-recovery pulse sequence: analysis and initial experience in cancer staging. Radiology 168:827-36, 1988.
20. Hilfiker P, Zanetti M, Debatin F, et al: Fast spin-echo inversion-recovery imaging versus fast T2-weighted spin-echo imaging in bone marrow abnormalities. Invest Radiol 30:110-14, 1995.

21. Rubin DA, Kneeland JB: MR imaging of the musculoskeletal system: technical considerations for enhancing image quality and diagnostic yield. Am J Roentgenol 163:1155-63, 1994.

22. Seeger LL, Widoff BE, Bassett LW, et al: Preoperative evaluation of osteosarcoma: value of gadolinium demeglumine enhanced MR imaging. Am J Roentgenol 157:347-351, 1991.

23. Helms CA: The use of fat suppression in gadolinium-enhanced MR imaging of the musculoskeletal system: a potential source of error. Am J Roentgenol 173:234-236, 1999.

24. May DA, Good RB, Smith DK, et al: MR imaging of musculoskeletal tumors and tumor mimickers with intravenous gadolinium: experience with 242 patients. Skeletal Radiol 26:2-15, 1997.

25. Jordon RM, Mintz RD: Fatal reaction to gadopentetate dimeglumine. Am J Roentgenol 164:743-4, 1995.

26. Unal O, Arslan H: Cardiac arrest caused by IV gadopentetate dimeglumine. Am J Roentgenol 172:1141, 1999.

27. Shellock FG, Hahn HP, Mink JH, et al: Adverse reaction to intravenous gadoteridol. Radiology 189:151-152, 1993.

28. Bancroft LW, Kransdorf MJ, Menke DM, et al: Intramuscular myxoma: characteristic MR imaging features. Am J Roentgenol 178:1255-1259, May 2002.

29. Murphey MD, McRae GA, Fanburg-Smith RC, et al: Imaging of soft-tissue myxoma with emphasis on CT and MR and comparison of radiology and pathologic findings. Radiology 225:215-24, 2002.

30. Shapeero LG, Vanel D, Verstraete KL, et al: Dynamic contrast enhanced MR imaging for soft-tissue sarcomas. Semin Musculoskelet Radiol 3:101-114, 1999.

31. Van Rijswijk CS, Geirnaerdt MJ, Hogendoorn PC, et al: Dynamic contrast-enhanced MR imaging in monitoring response to isolated limb perfusion in high-grade soft-tissue sarcoma: initial results. Eur Radiol 13:1849-58, 2003.

32. Vanderwoude HT, Bloem JL, Verstraete KL, et al: Osteosarcoma and Ewing's sarcoma after neoadjuvant chemotherapy: value of dynamic MR imaging in detecting viable tumor before surgery. Am J Roentgenol 16:593-8, 1995.

33. Shapeero LA, Vanel D, Verstraete KL, et al: Fast magnetic resonance imaging with contrast for soft-tissue sarcoma viability. Clin Orthop 397:212-27, 2002.

34. Poon-chue A, Menedez L, Gerstner MM, et al: MR evaluation of post-operative sarcomas in extremity soft-tissue sarcomas. Skeletal Radiol 28:279-282, 1999.

35. Sundaram M: The use of gadolinium in the MR imaging of bone tumor. Semin Ultrasound CT MR 18:307-11, 1997.

36. Lang PJ, Bradley MM, Fitzsimmons JR, et al: Osteogenic sarcoma: noninvasive in vivo assessment of tumor necrosis with diffusion-weighted MR imaging. Radiology 206:227-235, 1998.

37. Baur A, Reiser MF: Diffusion-weighted imaging of the musculoskeletal system in humans. Skeletal Radiol 29:555-562, 2000.

38. Baur A, Huber A, Arbogast S, et al: Diffusion-weighted imaging of tumor recurrences and post therapeutical soft-tissue changes in humans. Eur Radiol 11:828-833, 2001.

39. Karczmar GS, River JN, Goldman Z, et al: Magnetic resonance imaging of rodent tumors using radiofrequency gradient echoes. Magn Reson Med 12:881-891, 1994.

40. Van Rijswijk CSP, Kunz P, Hogendoom PCW: Diffusion-weighted MRI in the characterization of soft-tissue tumors. Journal of Magn Reson Imaging 15:305-307, 2002.

41. Spuentrup E, Buecker A, Adam G, et al: MR imaging for differentiation of benign fracture edema and tumor infiltration of the vertebral body. Am J Roentgenol 176:351-358, 2001.

42. Baur A, Stabler A, Bruning R, et al: Diffusion-weighted MR imaging of bone marrow: differentiation of benign versus pathologic compression fractures. Radiology 207:349-356, 1998.

43. Chan JH, Peh WC, Tsui EY, et al: Acute vertebral body compression fractures: discrimination between benign and malignant causes using apparent diffusion coefficients. Br J Radiol 75:207-214, 2002.

44. Zhou XJ, Leeds NE, McKinnon GC, et al: Characterization of benign and metastatic vertebral compression fractures with quantitative diffusion MR imaging. Am J Neuroradiol 23:165-170, 2002.

45. Jelinek JS, Murphy MD, Welker JA, et al: Diagnosis of primary bone tumors with image-guided percutaneous biopsy: experience in 110 tumors. Radiology 223:731-7, 2002.

46. Blanco Sequeiros R, Klemula R, Ojala R, et al: MRI-guided trephine biopsy and fine-needle aspiration in the diagnosis of bone lesions in low field (0.23 T) MRI system using optical instrument tracking. Eur Radiol 12:830-835, 2002.

47. Parkkola RK, Mattila KT, Heikkila JT, et al: Dynamic contrast-enhanced MR imaging and MR-guided bone biopsy on a 0.23 T open image. Skeletal Radiol 30:620-4, 2001.

48. Dalinka MK, Zlatkin MB, Chao P, et al: The use of magnetic resonance imaging in the evaluation of bone and soft-tissue tumors. Radiol Clin North Am 28:461-470, 1990.

49. Tsai JC, Dalinka MK, Fallon MD, et al: Fluid-fluid level: a non-specific finding in tumor of bone and soft tissue. Radiology 175:779-782, 1990.

50. Choi JT, Murphy MD: Angiomatous skeletal lesions. Semin Musculoskelet Radiol 491:103-112, 2000.

51. Ross JS, Masaryk TJ, Modic MT, et al: Vertebral hemangiomas: MR imaging. Radiology 165:165-169, 1987.

52. Resnick D: Bone and Joint Imaging, 2nd ed. Philadelphia: WB Saunders, 1039, 1996.

53. Greenspan A, Remagen W: Differential Diagnosis of Tumors and Tumor-like Lesions of Bone and Joint, Philadelphia: Lippincott-Raven, 1998, p 290.

54. Doppman JL, Oldfield KH, Heiss JD: Symptomatic vertebral hemangiomas: treatment by means of direct intralesional injection of ethanol. Radiology 214:341-48, 2000.

55. Baudrez V, Grant C, Vandeberg BC: Benign vertebral hemangioma: MR-histological correlation. Skeletal Radiol 30:442-446, 2001.

56. Propeck T, Bullard MA, Lin J, et al: Radiologic-pathologic correlation of intraosseous lipomas. Am J Roentgenol 175:673-8, 2000.

57. Milgram JW: Intraosseous lipomas: radiologic and pathologic manifestations. Radiology 167:155-160, 1988.

58. Blacksin MF, Encle N, Benevenia J: Magnetic resonance imaging of intraosseous lipomas: a radiologic-pathologic correlation. Skeletal Radiol 24:37-41, 1995.

59. Zurlo JV: The double line sign. Radiology 212:541-542, 1999.

60. Glickstein MF, Burk DL, Schiebler ML, et al: Avascular necrosis versus other diseases of the hip: sensitivity of MR imaging. Radiology 169:213-215, 1988.

61. Abelwahab IF, Klein MJ, Hermann G, et al: Angiosarcoma associated with bone infarcts. Skeletal Radiol 27:546-551, 1998.

62. Vandeburg BC, Malghem J, Lecouvet FE, et al: Magnetic resonance appearance of uncomplicated Paget's disease. Semin Musculoskelet Radiol 5:69-77, 2001.

63. Whitehouse RW: Paget's disease of bone. Semin Musculoskelet Radiol 6:313-322, 2002.

64. Boutin RD, Spitz DJ, Newman JS: Complications in Paget disease at MR imaging. Radiology 209:641-651, 1998.

65. Dorfman HD, Czerniak B: Bone Tumors. St Louis, MO: Mosby, 1997, p 1206.

66. Resnick D: Bone and Joint Imaging, 2nd ed. Philadelphia: WB Saunders, 1996, p 531.

67. Brandolini F, Bacchini P, Moscato M, et al: Chondrosarcoma as a complication factor in Paget's disease of bone. Skeletal Radiol 26:497-500, 1997.

68. Robbins MR, Murphy MD: Benign chondroid neoplasms of bone. Semin Musculoskelet Radiol 4:45-58, 2000.

69. Cohen EK, Kressel HY, Frank TS, et al: Hyaline cartilage origin bone and soft-tissue neoplasms: MR appearance and histologic correlation. Radiology 167:477-481, 1988.

70. Flemming DJ, Murphy MD: Enchondroma and chondrosarcoma. Semin Musculoskelet Radiol 4:59-71, 2000.

71. Mehta M, White LM, Knapp T, et al: MR imaging of symptomatic osteochondromas with pathologic correlation. Skeletal Radiol 27:427-433, 1988.

72. Murphy MD, Choi JF, Kransdorf MJ, et al: Imaging of osteochondroma: variants and complication with radiologic-pathologic correlation. Radiographics 20:1407-37, 2000.

73. Woertler K, Lindner N, Gosheger G, et al: Osteochondroma: MR imaging of tumor-related complications. Eur Radiol 10:832-840, 2000.

74. Vanel D, Picci P, DePaolis M, et al: Osteosarcoma arising in an exostosis: CT and MR imaging. Am J Roentgenol 176:259-260, 2001.

75. Giudici MA, Moser RP, Krandorf MJ: Cartilaginous tumors. Radiol Clin North Am 31:237-259, 1993.

76. Greenspan A, Remagen W: Differential Diagnosis of Tumors and Tumor-like Lesions of Bones and Joints. Philadelphia: Lippincott-Raven, 1998.

77. Resnick D: Bone and Joint imaging, 2nd ed. Philadelphia: WB Saunders, 1996, p 1145.

78. Janzen L, Logan PM, O'Connell JX, et al: Intramedullary chondroid tumors of bone: correlation of abnormal peritumoral marrow and soft-tissue MRI signal with tumor type. Skeletal Radiol 26:100-106, 1997.

79. Brien EW, Mirra JM, Kerr R: Benign and malignant cartilage tumors of bone and joint: their anatomical theoretical basis with emphasis on radiology, pathology and clinical biology. I. The intramedullary cartilage tumors. Skeletal Radiol 26:325-353, 1997.

80. Murphy MD, Flemming DJ, Boyea SR, et al: Enchondroma versus chondrosarcoma in the appendicular skeleton: differentiating features. Radiographics 8:1213-1237.

81. Akoi J, Sone S, Fujioka F, et al: MR enchondroma and chondrosarcoma. RINS and ARCS of GD-DTPA enhancement. J Comput Assist Tomography 15:1011-1015, 1991.

82. Chew FS, Maldjian C: Enchondroma and enchondromatosis. Available at http://www.emedicine.com, May 14, 2002.

83. Wang XL, De Beuckeleer LH, De Schepper AMA, et al: Low grade chondrosarcoma vs. enchondroma: challenges in diagnosis and management. Eur Radiol 11:1054-1057, 2001.

84. Greenspan A: Bone island (enostosis):current concept—a review. Skeletal Radiol 24:111-115, 1995.

85. White LM, Kandel R: Osteoid-producing tumors of bone. Semin Musculoskelet Radiol 4:25-43, 2000.

86. Osgood GM, Lee FY, Parisien MV, et al: Magnetic resonance imaging depiction of tight iliotibial bone in melorheostosis associated with severe external rotation deformity, limb shortening and patellar dislocation in planning surgical correction. Skeletal Radiol 31:49-52, 2002.

87. Judkiewicz AM, Murphey MD, Resnik CS, et al: Advanced imaging of melorheostosis with emphasis on MRI. Skeletal Radiol 30:447-553, 2001.

88. Smith SE, Kransdorf MJ: Primary musculoskeletal tumors of fibrous origin. Semin Musculoskelet Radiol 4:113-125, 2000.

89. Okada K, Yoshida S, Okane K, et al: Cystic fibrous dysplasia mimicking giant cell tumor: MRI appearance. Skeletal Radiol 29:45-4, 2000.

90. Jee WH, Choe BY, Krang HS, et al: Nonossifying fibroma: characteristics at MR imaging with pathologic correlation. Radiology 209:197-202, 1998.

91. Kransdorf MJ, Utz JA, Gilkey FW, et al: MR appearance of fibroxanthoma. J Comput Assist Tomogr 12:612-615, 1998.

92. Taconis WK, Schütte HE, van der Heul RO. Desmoplastic fibroma of bone: a report of 18 cases. Skeletal Radiol 23:283-288, 1994.

93. Vanhoenacker FM, Hauben FC, De Beuckeleer LH, et al: Desmoplastic fibroma of bone: MRI features. Skeletal Radiol 29:171-175, 2000.

94. Dorfman HD, Czerniak B: Bone Tumors. St Louis, MO: Mosby, 1998, pp 514-529.

95. White LM, Schweitzer ME, Khalili K, et al: MR imaging of primary lymphoma of bone. Variability of T2-weighted signal intensity. Am J Roentgenol 170:1243-1247, 1998.

96. Mulligan ME: Myeloma and lymphoma. Semin Musculoskelet Radiol 4:127-135, 2000.

97. Häussler MD, Feustermacher MJ, Johnston DA, et al: MRI of primary lymphoma of bone. Cortical disorder as a criterion for differential diagnosis. J Magn Reson Imaging 9:93-100, 1999.

98. Munk PL, Helms CA, Holt RG: MR imaging of aneurysmal bone cysts. Am J Roentgenol 153:99-101, 1989.

99. Kransdorf MJ, Sweet DR: Aneurysmal bone cyst: concept, controversy, clinical presentation, and imaging. Am J Roentgenol 164:573-580, 1995.

100. Kale HA, Rathod KR, Prasad ST, et al: Mandibular haemophilic pseudotumor containing a fluid–fluid level. Br J Radiol 74:186-188, 2001.

101. Berger FH, Verstraete KL, Gooding CA, et al: MR imaging of musculoskeletal neoplasm. MRI Clin North Am 8:929-51, 2000.

102. Chan KK, Pathria M: The LWW MRI teaching file series: MRI of the musculoskeletal system, 2nd ed. Philadelphia: Lippincott/Williams and Wilkins, 2001, p 189.

103. Vilanova JC, Dolz JL, Maestrodeleon JL, et al: MR imaging of a malignant schwannoma and an osteoblastoma with fluid–fluid levels. Report of two new cases. Eur Radiol 8:1359-1362, 1998.

104. De Schepper AM, De Beuckeleer L, Vandevenne J, et al: Magnetic resonance imaging of soft-tissue tumors. Eur Radiol 10:213-222, 2000.

105. Koenig CW, Duda SH, Truebenbach J, et al: MR-guided biopsy of musculoskeletal lesions in a low-field system. J Magn Res Imaging 13:761-8, 2001.

106. Panicek DM, Garsonis C, Rosenthal DI, et al: CT and MR imaging in the local staging of primary malignant musculoskeletal neoplasms: Report of the Radiology Diagnostic Oncology Group. Radiology 202:237-246, 1997.

107. Kransdorf MJ, Murphey MD: Imaging of Soft Tissue Tumors. Philadelphia: WB Saunders, 1997, p 37.

108. Kransdorf MJ: Malignant soft-tissue tumors in a large referral population: Distribution of diagnosis by age, sex and location. Am J Roentgenol 164:129-134, 1995.

109. Kransdorf MJ: Benign soft-tissue tumors in a large referral population: distribution of specific diagnosis by age, sex and location. Am J Roentgenol 164:395-402, 1995.

110. Petasnick DM, Turner DA, Charles JR, et al: Comparison of MR imaging with CT. Radiology 160:125-133, 1986.

111. Berquist TH, Ehman RL, King BE, et al: Value of MR imaging in differentiating benign from malignant soft-tissue masses: study of 95 lesions. Am J Roentgenol 155:1251-1255, 1990.

112. De Schepper AM, Ramon FA, Degryse HR: Statistical analysis of MRI parameters predicting malignancy in 141 soft-tissue masses. Rofo Fortschr Geb Neuen Bildgeb Verfahr. 156:587-591, 1992.

113. Bancroft LW, Peterson JJ, Kransdorf MJ, et al: Soft-tissue tumors of the lower extremities. Radiol Clin North Am 40:991-1011, 2002.

114. Yoshioka H, Itai Y, Niitsu M, et al: Intramuscular metastasis from malignant melanoma: MR findings. Skeletal Radiol 28:714-716, 1999.

115. Yoshioka H, Kamada R, Kandatsu S, et al: MR of mucosal malignant melanoma of the head and neck. J Comput Assist Tomogr 22:492-497, 1998.

116. Peterson JJ, Kransdorf MJ, Bancroft LW, et al: Malignant fatty tumors. Classification, clinical course, imaging appearance and treatment. Skeletal Radiol 32:493-503, 2003.

117. De Maeseneer M, Jaovisidha S, Lenchik L, et al: Fibrolipomatous hamaroma: MR imaging findings. Skeletal Radiol 26:155-160, 1997.

118. Weiss SW, Goldblum JR: Enzinger and Weiss's Soft Tissue Tumors, 4th ed. St Louis, MO: Mosby, 2001, pp 571-693.

119. Kransdorf MJ, Murphy MD: Imaging of Soft Tissue Tumors. Philadelphia: WB Saunders, 1997.

120. Vilanova JC, Barcelo J, Villalon M, et al: MR imaging of lipoma arborescens and the associated lesions. Skeletal Radiol 32:504-9, 2003.

121. Marui T, Yamamoto T, Kimura T: A true intra-articular lipoma of the knee in a girl. Arthroscopy 18:E24, 2002.

122. Murphy MD, Smith WS, Smith SE, et al: Imaging of musculoskeletal neurogenic tumors: radiologic–pathologic correlation. Radiographics 19:1253-1280, 1999.

123. Anderson SE, Schwab C, Stauffer E, et al: Hibernoma: imaging characteristics of a rare benign soft-tissue tumor. Skeletal Radiol 3:590-595, 2001.

124. Castellote A, Vazquez E, Vera J, et al: Cervicothoracic lesions in infants and children. Radiographics 19:583-600, 1999.

125. O'Donnell KA, Caty MG, Allen JE, et al: Lipoblastoma: better termed infantile lipoma? Pediatr Surg Int 16:458-461, 2000.

126. Evans HL, Soule EH, Winkelmann RK: Atypical lipoma, atypical intramuscular lipoma and well differentiated liposarcoma: a reappraisal of 30 cases formerly classified as well-differentiated liposarcoma. Cancer 43:574-584, 1979.

127. Ohguri T, Aoki A, Hisaoka M, et al: Differential diagnosis of benign peripheral lipoma from well-differentiated liposarcoma on MR imaging: is comparison of margins and internal characteristic useful? Am J Roentgenol 180: 2003.

128. Nascimento AG: Dedifferentiated liposarcoma. Semin Diagn Pathol 18:263-6, 2001.

129. Kransdorf MJ, Bancroft LW, Peterson JJ: Imaging of fatty tumors: distinction of lipoma and well-differentiated liposarcoma. Radiology 224:99-104, 2002.

130. Galant J, Martí-Bonmatí L, Sáez F, et al: The value of fat suppressed T2 or STIR sequences in distinguishing lipoma from well-differentiated liposarcoma. Eur Radiol 13:337-343, 2003.

131. Weiss SW, Guldblum JR: Enzinger and Weiss's Soft Tissue Tumors, 4th ed. Philadelphia: Mosby, 2001, pp 837-887.

132. Siegel M: Magnetic resonance imaging of musculoskeletal soft-tissue masses. Radiol Clin North Am 4:701-720, 2001.

133. Rak KM, Yakes WF, Ray RL, et al: MR imaging of symptomatic peripheral vascular malformations. Am J Roentgenol 159:107-112, 1992.

134. Murphey MD, Fairburn KJ, Parman LM, et al: Musculoskeletal angiomatous lesions: radiologic–pathologic correlation. Radiographs 15:893-917, 1995.

135. Rubin JI, Gomori JM, Grosman RI, et al: High-field MR imaging of extra-cranial hematomas. Am J Roentgenol 148:813-817, 1987.

136. Bush CH: The magnetic resonance imaging of musculoskeletal hemorrhage. Skeletal Radiol 29:1-9, 2000.

137. Imaizumi S, Morita T, Ogose A, et al: Soft-tissue sarcoma mimicking chronic hematoma: value of magnetic resonance imaging in differential diagnosis. J Orthop Sci 7:33-37, 2002.

138. Kransdorf MJ, Murphey MD: Imaging of Soft Tissue Tumors. Philadelphia: WB Saunders, pp 148-186, 1997.

139. Kudo S: Elastofibroma dorsi: CT and MR imaging findings. Semin Musculoskelet Radiol 5:103-105, 2001.

140. Escott EJ: A variety of appearances of malignant melanoma in the head: a review. Radiographics 21:625-39, 2001.

141. Ho LWC, Wong KP, Chan JHM, et al: MR appearance of metastatic melanotic melanoma of the breast. Clin Radiol 55:572-573, 2000.

142. Enochs WS, Petherick P, Bogdanwa A, et al: Paramagnetic metal scavenging by melanin: MR imaging. Radiology 204:417-423, 1997.

143. Isada J, Kuroda M, Saitoh M, et al: MR finding of clear cell sarcoma. Two case reports. J Clin Imaging 27:229-232, 2003.

144. De Beuckeleer LH, De Schepper AM, Vandevenne JE, et al: MR imaging of clear cell sarcoma (malignant melanoma of the soft parts): a multicenter correlative MRI–pathology study of 21 cases and literature review. Skeletal Radiol 29:187-193, 2000.

145. Weiss S, Goldblum JR: Enzinger and Weiss's Soft Tissue Tumors, 4th ed. St Louis, MO: Mosby, 2001, pp 1509-1521.

146. Iwamoto Y, Morimoto N, Chuman H, et al: The role of MR imaging in the diagnosis of alveolar soft part sarcoma: a report of 10 cases. Skeletal Radiol 24:267-270, 1995.

147. Monu JV, Elvey S: Pigmented villonodular synovitis. www.emedicine.com/radio/topic553.htm www.emedicine.com April 2002.

148. Gentili A, Sorenson S, Masih S: MR imaging of soft-tissue masses of the foot. Semin Musculoskelet Radiol 6:141-152, 2002.

149. Peh WCG, Wons Y, Shek TWH, et al: Giant cell tumor of the tendon sheath of the hand: a pictoral essay. Australas Radiol 45:274-280, 2001.

150. Karasick D, Karasick S: Giant cell tumor of tendon sheath: spectrum of radiologic findings. Skeletal Radiol 21:219-224, 1992.

151. Hughes TH, Sartoris DJ, Schweiteer ME, et al: Pigmental villonodular synovitis: MRI characteristics. Skeletal Radiol 24:7-12, 1995.

152. Narvaez JA, Narvaez J, Ortega R, et al: Hypointense synovial lesions on T2-weighted images: differential diagnosis with pathologic correlation. Am J Roentgenol 181:761-769, 2003.

153. Weiss SW, Goldblum JR: Enzinger and Weiss's Soft Tissue Tumors, 4th ed. St Louis, MO: Mosby, 1997, pp 309-346.

154. Robbin MR, Murphy MD, Temple HT, et al: Imaging of musculoskeletal fibromatosis. Radiographics 21:585-600, 2001.

155. Bencardino J, Rosenberg ZS, Beltran J, et al: Morton's neuroma: is it always symptomatic? Am J Roentgenol 175:649-653, 2000.

156. Zanetti M, Ledermann T, Zollinger H, et al: Efficiency of MR imaging in patients suspected of having Morton's neuroma. Am J Roentgenol 168:529-532, 1997.

157. Terk MR, Kwong PN, Suthar M, et al: Morton neuroma: evaluation with MR imaging performed with contrast enhancement and fat suppression. Radiology 189:239-241, 1993.

158. Ross LV, Ros GJ, Mesgarzadeh M, et al: Hemodialysis-related amyloidomas of bone. Radiology 178:263-265, 1991.

159. Slovotinek JP, Coates TH, McDonald SP, et al: Shoulder appearances at MR imaging in long-term dialysis recipients. Radiology 217:539-543, 2000.

160. Llauger J, Palmer J, Rosón N, et al: Nonseptic monoarthritis: imaging feature with clinical and histopathologic correlation. Radiographics 20:S263-278, 2000.
161. Yu TS, Chung C, Recht M, et al: MR imaging of tophaceous gout. Am J Roentgenol 168:523-527, 1997.
162. Resnick D, Kang HS: Internal derangement of joints. Philadelphia: WB Saunders, 1997, pp 451-453.
163. Kim MG, Kim BH, Choi J, et al: Intra-articular ganglion cysts of the knee: clinical and MR imaging features. Eur Radiol 11:834-840, 2001.
164. Pablos JM, Valdes JC, Gavilan F: Bilateral lunate intraosseous ganglia. Skeletal Radiol 27:708-10, 1998.
165. Costa CR, Morrison WB, Carrino JA, et al: MRI of an intratendinous ganglion cyst of the peroneus brevis tendon. Am J Roentgenol 181:890-891, 2003.
166. Yamazaki H, Saitch S, Seki H, et al: Peroneal nerve palsy caused by intraneural ganglion. Skeletal Radiol 28:52-56, 1999.
167. Murphy MD, McRae GA, Fanburg-Smith JC, et al: Imaging of soft-tissue myxoma with emphasis on CT and MR and comparison of radiologic and pathologic findings. Radiology 225:215-224, 2002.
168. Iwasko N, Steinbach LS, Disler D, et al: Imaging findings in Mazabraud's syndrome: seven new cases. Skeletal Radiol 31:81-87, 2002.
169. Weiss S, Goldblum JR: Enzinger and Weiss's Soft Tissue Tumors, 4th ed. 2001, pp 1483-1571.
170. McCarvilla MB, Spunt SL, Skapek SX, et al: Synovial sarcoma in pediatric patients. Am J Roentgenol 179:791-801, 2002.
171. Jones B, Sundaran M, Kransdorf M: Synovial sarcoma: MR imaging findings in 34 patients. Am J Roentgenol 161:827-30, 1993.
172. Kransdorf MJ, Murphey MD: Imaging of soft-tissue tumors. Philadelphia: WB Saunders, 1997, pp 235-274.
173. Blacksin MF, Siegel JR, Benevenia J, et al: Synovial sarcoma: frequency of nonaggressive MR characteristics. J Comput Assist Tomogr 21:785-789, 1997.
174. Antinheimo J, Sankila R, Carpen O, et al: Population based analysis of sporadic and type 2 neurofibromatosis-associated meningiomas and schwannomas. Neurology 54:71, 2000.
175. Bhargava R, Parhan DM, Lasater OE, et al: MR imaging differentiation of benign and malignant peripheral nerve sheath tumors: use of the target sign. Pediatr Radiol 27:124-129, 1997.
176. Anderson MW, Temple HT, Dussault RG, et al: Compartmental anatomy: relevance to staging and biopsy of musculoskeletal tumors. Am J Roentgenol 173:1663-1671, 1999.
177. Mazeron JJ, Suit HD: Lymph nodes as site of metastases from sarcomas of soft tissue. Cancer 60:1800-1808, 1987.
178. Malawer M, Sugarbaker P: Musculoskeletal Cancer Surgery: Treatment of Sarcomas and Allied Diseases. Boston: Kluwer Academic, 2001.
179. Caceres E, Zaharia M, Calderon R: Incidence of regional lymph node metastases in operable osteogenic sarcoma. Semin Surg Oncol 6:231-233, 1990.
180. Weiss SW, Goldblum JR: Enzinger and Weiss's Soft Tissue Tumors, 4th ed. St Louis, MO: Mosby, 2001, p 26.
181. Jeffrey GM, Price CH, Sissons HA: Metastatic patterns of osteosarcoma. Br J Cancer 32:87-107, 1975.
182. Bloem JL, Taminiau AH, Eulderink F, et al: Radiologic staging of primary bone sarcoma: MR imaging, scintigraphy, angiography, and CT correlated with pathologic examination. Radiology 169:805-810, 1988.
183. Enneking WF, Kagan A: The implications of "skip" metastases in osteosarcoma. Clin Orthop 111:33-41, 1975.
184. Murphey MD, Robbin MR, McRae GA, et al: The many faces of osteosarcoma. Radiographics 17:1205-1231, 1997.
185. Enneking WF, Spanier SS, Goodman MA: A system for the surgical staging of musculoskeletal sarcoma. Clin Orthop 153:106-120, 1980.
186. Manual for Staging of Cancer. Chicago: American Joint Committee for Cancer Staging and End-Result Reporting, 1978.
187. Coindre JM, Terrier O, Bui NB, et al: Prognostic factors in adult patients with locally controlled soft-tissue sarcoma. A study of 546 patients from the French Federation of Cancer Centers Sarcoma Group. J Clin Oncol 14:869-877, 1996.
188. Pisters PW, Leung DH, Woodruff J, et al: Analysis of prognostic factors in 1041 patients with localized soft-tissue sarcoma of the extremities. J Clin Oncol 14:1679-1689, 1996.
189. Nakanishi H, Tomita Y, Ohsawa M, et al: Tumor size as a prognostic indicator of histologic grade of soft-tissue sarcoma. J Surg Oncol 65:183-187, 1997.
190. Walker RE, Eustace SJ: Whole-body magnetic resonance imaging: techniques, clinical indications, and future applications. Semin Musculoskelet Radiol 5:5-20, 2001.
191. Feldman F, van Heertum R. Manos C: ^{18}FDG PET scanning of benign and malignant musculoskeletal lesions. Skeletal Radiol 32:201-208, 2003.
192. Akoi J, Watanabe H, Shinozaki J, et al: FDG PET of primary benign and malignant tumors: standardized uptake values in 52 lesion. Radiology 219:774-777, 2001.
193. Akoi J, Watanabe H, Shinozaki T, et al: FDG PET for preoperative differential diagnosis between benign and malignant soft-tissue masses. Skeletal Radiol 32:133-138, 2003.
194. Adler LP, Blair HF, Makley JT, et al: Noninvasive grading of musculoskeletal tumors using PET. J Nucl Med 32:1508-12, 1991.
195. Eary JF, O'Sullivan F, Powitan Y, et al: Sarcoma FDG uptake measured by PET and patient outcome: a retrospective analysis. Eur J Nucl Med 29:1149-1154, 2002.
196. Ioannidis JP, Lau J: ^{18}F-FDG PET for the diagnosis and grading of soft-tissue sarcoma: a meta-analysis. J Nucl Med 44:717-724, 2003.
197. Brenner W, Conrad EU, Eary JF: FDG PET imaging for grading and prediction of outcome in chondrosarcoma patients. Eur J Nucl Med Mol Imaging 31:189-95, 2004.
198. Galdrup-Link HE, Franzius C, Link TM, et al: Whole-body MR imaging for detection of bone metastases in children and young adults: comparison with skeletal scintigraphy and FDG PET. Am J Roentgenol 177:229-236, 2001.
199. Martin WH, Delbeke D, Patton JA, et al: Detection of malignancies with SPECT versus PET, with 2-[fluorine-18]fluro-2-deoxy-D-glucose. Radiology 198:225-231, 1996.
200. Dorfman HD, Czerniak B: Bone Tumors. St Louis, MO: Mosby, 1998, pp 20-21.
201. Temple HT, Bashore CJ: Staging of bone neoplasms: an orthopedic oncologist's perspective. Semin Musculoskelet Radiol 1:17-23, 2000.
202. Scully SP, Temple HT, O'Keefe RJ, et al: The surgical treatment of patients with osteosarcoma who sustain a pathologic fracture. Clin Orthop 324:227-232, 1996.
203. Mirowitz SA, Apicella P, Reinus WR, et al: MR imaging of bone marrow lesions: relative conspicuousness on T1-weighted, fat-suppressed T2-weighted and STIR sequences. Am J Roentgenol 162:215-221, 1994.
204. Panuel M, Gentet JC, Scheiner C: Physeal and epiphyseal extent of primary malignant bone tumors in childhood. Correlation of preoperative MRI and the pathologic specimen. Pediatr Radiol 23:421-4, 1993.
205. Onikul E, Fletcher BD, Parham DM: Accuracy of MR imaging for estimating intraosseous extent of osteosarcoma. Am J Roentgenol 167:1211-15, 1996.
206. Hoffer FA, Kinanovou AY, Reddick WIE: Accuracy of MR for detecting epiphyseal extension of osteosarcoma. Pediatr Radiol 30(5):289-298, May 2000.
207. Saifuddin A: The accuracy of imaging in the local staging of appendicular osteosarcoma. Skeletal Radiol 31:191-201, 2002.
208. Jesus-Garcia R, Scixas MT, Costa SR: Epiphyseal plate involvement in osteosarcoma. Clin Orthop 373:32-38, 2000.
209. Schima W, Amann G, Stiglbauer R: Preoperative staging of osteosarcoma: efficiency of MR imaging in detecting joint involvements. Am J Roentgenol 163:1171-5, 1994.
210. Noria S, Davis A, Kandel R, et al: Residual disease following unplanned excision of a soft-tissue sarcoma of an extremity. J Bone Joint Surg 78A: 650-655, 1996.
211. Guiliano AE, Eilber FR: The rational for planned reoperation after unplanned total excision of soft-tissue sarcomas. J Clin Oncol 3:1344-1348, 1985.
212. Mankin, HJ, Mankin CJ, Simon MA: The hazards of biopsy revisited. J Bone Joint Surg 78A: 656-663, 1996.
213. Parker SL, Tong T, Bolden S, Wingo PA: Cancer statistics 1997. CA Cancer J Clin 46:9-10, 1997.
214. Mall AC, Imhof SM, Bouter LM, Tan KE: Secondary primary tumors in patients with retinoblastoma. A review of the literature. Ophthalmic Genetics 18:27-34, 1997.
215. Hope DG, Mulville JJ: Malignancy in neurofibromatosis. Adv Neurol 29:33-56, 1981.
216. Knight WA III, Murphy WK, Gottleib JA: Neurofibromatosis associated with malignant neurofibromas. Arch Dermatol 107:747-750, 1973.
217. D'Agostino AN, Soule EH, Miller RH: Sarcomas of the peripheral nerves and somatic soft tissues associated with multiple neurofibromatosis (von Recklinghausen's disease). Cancer 16:1015-1027, 1963.
218. Cantin J, McNeer GP, Chu FC, Booher RJ: The problem of local recurrence after treatment of soft-tissue sarcoma. Ann Surg 205:340-348, 1968.
219. Potter DA, Glenn J, Kinsella T, et al: Patterns of recurrence in patients with high-grade soft-tissue sarcomas. J Clin Oncol 3:353-66, 1985.
220. Scully SP, Temple HT, Harrelson JM: Synovial sarcoma of the foot and ankle. The American Orthopaedic Foot and Ankle Society Meeting, Boston, MA, July 24, 1998.
221. Weingrad DN, Rosenberg SA: Early lymphatic spread of osteogenic and soft-tissue sarcomas. Surgery 84 :231-40, 1978.
222. Steinberg BD, Gelberman RH, Mankin HJ, Rosenberg AE: Epithelioid sarcoma in the upper extremity. J Bone Joint Surg 74:28-35, 1992.
223. Enzinger, FM, Weiss: Synovial Sarcoma in Soft Tissue Tumors, 2nd ed. St Louis, MO: Mosby-Yearbook, 1988, p 661.
224. Anract P, Katabi M, Forest M, et al: Synovial chondromatosis and chondrosarcoma. A study of the relationship between these two diseases. Rev Chir Orthop Repartrice Appar Moteur 82:216-224, 1996.
225. Heare TC, Enneking WH, Heare MM: Staging techniques and biopsy of bone tumors. Orthop Clin North Am 20:273-285, 1989.
226. Olsen PN, Everson LI, Griffiths HJ: Staging of musculoskeletal tumors. Radiol Clin North Am 32:151-162, 1994.

water, with fat predominating in both red and yellow marrow.[1-4] The mobile proton densities of fat and water are similar. Because of this, proton density itself does not make a significant contribution to contrast resolution between red and yellow marrow. Thus, chemical shift affects T1 and T2 relaxation times, while selected pulse sequences offer the required contrast resolution to differentiate normal hematopoietic from fatty and abnormal marrow.[5-8]

MR may be utilized to image a particular site for focal bone marrow pathology or may image the marrow more diffusely. In the latter instance, screening with MR would include the spine, pelvis, and femora (particularly the proximal portion). These areas contain a high percentage of hematopoietic marrow throughout life and are most likely to show diffuse marrow abnormalities. Sagittal images are used for the spine and coronal images for the pelvis and femora. Axial images augment these screening sequences.[9] Slice thickness is generally 5 mm for sagittal and 5 mm to 1 cm for coronal screening sequences. For T1-weighted spin-echo images, a pulse sequence of 300-500/2 (repetition time ms/echo time ms) is preferable, while for T2-weighted images, 2000-2500/70 or greater is acceptable.

Spin-Echo Imaging

Fatty marrow produces bright signal on T1-weighted spin-echo images at 1.5 T due to its short T1 relaxation time.[10-12] Fat protons are predominantly made up of hydrophilic CH_2 groups within relatively large molecular complexes, leading to an efficient spin-lattice relaxation time.[4,13,14] Fatty marrow produces less signal intensity on T2-weighted spin-echo sequences relative to water protons, although brighter than muscle, due to a relatively long T2 relaxation time. The cellular make-up of hematopoietic marrow is mainly protein and water. Protein has a long T1 relaxation time due to its large molecular size. In solution, however, there is a shortening of the T1 relaxation time. The fractional contribution of protein and intracellular ("bound") water to overall signal intensity is unclear.[4,15] Interstitial/cytoplasmic water has long T1 and T2 relaxation times.

The amount of fat cells in the marrow is variable from bone to bone with aging. The relative contribution of fat to the overall marrow signal with increasing age is prominent. This is related to the decrease of red cell mass from approximately 60% in the first decade of life to less than 30% by the age of 90 due to replacement by fat.[16] Thus, the signal intensity of marrow in the first year of life is similar to muscle, becomes hyperintense to muscle by adolescence, while in the elderly even the vertebral bodies display high signal representing fatty marrow.[6,9,15,17]

Spin-echo imaging has recently been used to quantify bone marrow iron specifically. Ferric iron is stored in the bone marrow in the form of hemosiderin and ferritin. In both forms, but particularly in the former, there are superparamagnetic effects that increase local magnetic susceptibility and shorten T2 or more markedly T2*.[17-19] If sufficient concentrations of these forms of iron are present in the bone marrow, they will decrease signal intensity on T2-weighted or T2*-weighted (i.e., gradient-echo) pulse sequences.[17,18,20] Studies have been performed utilizing 16 echoes obtained simultaneously. Signal intensity was measured using operator-defined regions of interest (ROI). It has been reported that a transverse relaxation rate (1/T2) correlates strongly with iron concentrations in biologic tissues.[21-25] Using 1/T2, good correlation was found with measured histologic bone marrow iron concentration below 400 mg/mL.[21]

Fast Spin-Echo Imaging

Fast spin-echo sequences have the advantage of less sensitivity to susceptibility artifacts. In addition, relative signal intensities of fatty and hematopoietic marrow as well as iron-containing tissues may differ significantly from conventional spin-echo sequences due to factors such as effective TE and division of echo trains. These sequences have become more popular, especially with T2-weighted sequences, because of reduced acquisition times. Unfortunately, with fast T2-weighted images, fat intensity is increased, both in the marrow and subcutaneous fat, relative to conventional spin-echo T2-weighted images. Contrast between normal and abnormal marrow is diminished and marrow abnormalities with long T2 relaxation times may be difficult to detect with fast spin-echo imaging.[9] Lesion conspicuity is improved greatly if fat suppression techniques are employed with fast spin-echo sequences or fast spin-echo is replaced by STIR images of proton density fat-saturated images. The sensitivity of the latter pulse sequences for detection of free water protons, and thus marrow disease, surpasses fast spin-echo sequences.[9,26]

Fat Suppression

It is generally accepted that some type of fat suppression technique is helpful in enhancing marrow lesion conspicuity. The two forms of fat suppression employed are short tau inversion recovery (STIR) and frequency-selective fat-saturation.

On STIR images the signal from fat is nulled, while at the same time T1 and T2 signals from other tissues are additive. This greatly increases contrast sensitivity.[9,25,27] As most pathologic bone marrow conditions contain increased free water, T1 and T2 values are usually prolonged. Thus, these abnormalities display higher signal than the surrounding low signal of nulled fatty marrow. Parameters used for STIR sequences are TR 1500-2500 ms; inversion time (TI) 90-150 ms; and TE 16-60 ms. Longer values are needed at high field strength due to longer T1 relaxation times. After a 180° inversion pulse, fat will cross over the zero point before water. When a 90° pulse is applied at the crossover time of fat, net magnetization of water is tilted to the transverse plane. A subsequent 180° pulse refocuses signal from water protons only.[17] STIR images are widely used due to their high sensitivity and excellent soft-tissue contrast.[25] Disadvantages include somewhat limited anatomic definition due to loss of contrast between suppressed fatty marrow and surrounding cortical bone, as well as long imaging times (which may be circumvented with fast inversion recovery techniques).[9] In addition, specificity of bone marrow lesions is decreased because the T1 and T2 components of marrow are not separated. Thus, fibrosis, calcification, hemorrhage, and contrast-enhanced lesions have low signal intensity on STIR images. Fast spin-echo techniques can be coupled with the inversion pulse to provide fast STIR images. These are advantageous in that exam times are diminished. Another advantage of this type of sequence is the relative lack of susceptibility to field inhomogeneities which are seen with frequency-selective fat saturation techniques.

Frequency-selective fat saturation eliminates fat by presaturation of the lipid peak, allowing the remaining water portion to be imaged selectively. Fat marrow will have a low signal intensity but hematopoietic marrow and marrow lesions display high signal intensity. This is accomplished by the application of a frequency-selective radiofrequency pulse, tuned to the frequency of fat-related protons in the slice being imaged. This pulse, although having proprietary properties, generally consists of a 90° pulse to tip the proton in the X-Y plane, followed by a spoiling pulse to eliminate the transverse coherent magnetization that would normally return signal. Advantages of this technique are high lesion conspicuity as well as improved visualization of enhancing tissues post gadolinium administration. The main disadvantage is the reliance on adequate shim to ensure field inhomogeneity. Nonuniform fat suppression is often seen with large fields of view, adjacent to surface coils and in the presence of ferromagnetic elements. This leads to hyperintensity within suppressed marrow and difficulty in differentiating this hyperintensity from surrounding marrow pathology.

Chemical Shift Imaging

Chemical shift techniques utilize the different resonant frequencies of fat and water protons (approximately 3.5 parts/million).[16,28] The relative percentage of fat and water in bone marrow cannot be distinguished easily on standard spin-echo sequences because images represent the sum of in-phase signals of both fat and water. In chemical shift imaging, an image from out-of-phase water and fat magnetization is obtained. Normal cellular marrow, which contains cells with both fat and water, appears hypointense. Predominantly fatty marrow shows little change compared with in-phase images. Fractional percentages of fat and water are assessed with computer-generated measurements and T1 and T2 relaxation values are calculated.[9]

Gradient-Echo Imaging

Gradient-echo imaging offers an alternative to conventional spin-echo imaging. It is based on the use of a variable flip-angle excitation pulse (usually less than 90°)

followed by gradient reversal to refocus the echo and generate a signal.[16,29,30] Image time is reduced and motion artifact is decreased due to shortened repetition times. A critical characteristic of gradient-echo imaging is its reliance on the effective transverse relaxation time (T2*) compared with T2 dependency of conventional spin-echo sequences. The signal intensity of red marrow depends on sequence characteristics and images can be chosen at an echo time at which the phases of fat and water are either opposed (opposed-phase images) or parallel (in-phase images) due to their difference in resonance frequency.[4] With gradient-echo imaging, trabecular bone and paramagnetic substances create local field gradients where they interface with marrow, leading to artifactual signal loss. This leads to markedly hypointense marrow, regardless of underlying fatty or cellular marrow. This magnetic susceptibility effect of trabecular bone is most pronounced in the epiphysis and vertebral bodies, where trabecular density is greatest. Thus, gradient-echo imaging is most useful for evaluating the amount of trabecular bone, iron deposition, and calcification.[9] Also, this technique is useful for dynamic evaluation and quantification of contrast enhancement, especially combined with frequency-selective fat suppression.

Diffusion-Weighted Imaging

Diffusion and perfusion imaging are among the most clinically applicable of the recent imaging techniques. Although diffusion imaging has been utilized for neuroradiology, only recently has it been proposed for musculoskeletal purposes and, specifically, for imaging of bone marrow.[31,32] Diffusion-weighted (DW) sequences are sensitive to molecular motion because random motion of water molecules in gradient fields causes phase dispersion and, thus, signal attenuation. A diffusion gradient can be implemented in any MR sequence, sensitizing this sequence to the microscopic motion of water protons.[33] Sequences used for this purpose include steady-state free precession (SSFP) fat-suppressed spin-echo DW imaging, stimulated echo imaging, as well as standing DW spin-echo sequence.[31,32] The effective diffusivity of a sequence (molecular motion) is described by the b-factor. This is calculated by the equation $b = \gamma^2 G^2 \delta^2 (\Delta - \delta/3)$ (γ=gyromagnetic ratio, G=gradient strength, δ=gradient length, Δ=diffusion time). To quantify diffusion effects, the apparent diffusion coefficient (ADC) is computed from the slope of the semilog plot of the digital intensity as a function of the b-factor.

Interstitial extracellular water is more mobile than intracellular water. Extensive signal attenuation occurs with increased water diffusion (such as is seen in benign edema). Less signal attenuation is seen when there is restricted water mobility (as seen in tumor cells). Thus, benign fracture edema will appear hypointense relative to marrow infiltrated by tumor cells, which will appear hyperintense. This property has been applied to the imaging of the spine to differentiate benign osteoporotic fractures from tumor infiltration of the vertebral body.[31,34]

Contrast Enhancement

Contrast-enhanced MR imaging using gadolinium (0.1 mmol/kg) has been used for imaging of the bone marrow. Both normal fatty and hematopoietic marrow enhance mildly post contrast administration in the adult. In the infant there is marked enhancement of normal marrow after contrast administration. Gadolinium will cause shortening of T1 signal in most pathologic tissue, causing it to approach the signal intensity of surrounding fat. Thus, lesion conspicuity decreases markedly unless concomitant fat suppression is applied. Mainly for this reason, contrast enhancement has not been proven to be more sensitive than other noncontrast sequences currently being used.

There are instances when contrast enhancement is helpful in the assessment of bone marrow disease. In the assessment of osteomyelitis, gadolinium has been effective combined with fat suppression, with an overall accuracy as high as 89%.[35,36] Differentiation of benign versus pathologic fractures and transient osteoporosis/bone marrow edema versus avascular necrosis may be aided by contrast administration as well. Lesion margins may be better defined against the fatty marrow background. Schmid et al[37] performed a prospective study comparing turbo STIR and T1-weighted contrast-enhanced fat-suppressed turbo spin-echo MR in diagnostic interpretation of bone marrow abnormalities in the foot and ankle. Assessing contrast, volume, and patterns of bone marrow signal intensity in both sequences, they concluded that the addition of T1-weighted contrast-enhanced MRI does not alter diagnosis and, for most cases, they recommended performing only the STIR sequence. The indications for contrast usage in musculoskeletal MR are still controversial.

NORMAL MARROW ANATOMY

Histologic Structure and Function

Bone marrow contains three major components: myeloid tissue, adipose cells, and a support scaffolding of trabecular bone. Hematopoietic marrow contains 40% water, 40% fat, and 20% protein, while fatty marrow contains 80% fat, 15% water, and 5% protein (Fig. 108-1).[4] The hematopoietic function of the marrow includes the creation and regulation of white blood cells, red blood cells, and platelets to control the individual's need for oxygenation, cellular immunity, and coagulation.

One of the most important structural differences between red and yellow marrow is the vascular supply. In general, the vascular supply of the marrow is derived from two major arterial sources in the nutrient and periosteal arterial systems. One or more nutrient arteries per bone penetrate the cortex, enter the medullary cavity and course parallel to the long axis of the shaft of the long bone. After branching, the nutrient arteries coalesce at the capillary level with transosteal arterial branches. These then widen at the endosteal level of the diaphysis, forming an extensive sinusoidal network. The sinusoids pierce the marrow and then drain into the venous channels of the medullary foramina.[16,38,39] Red marrow contains the extensive sinusoidal network while a sparse network of capillaries, venules, and thin-walled veins is seen in fatty marrow.[9,39]

Marrow Conversion

Bone marrow is a dynamic organ which changes composition greatly during growth and development, as well as in response to physiologic stresses applied during life.[48] Conversion of red to yellow marrow is a physiologic and active process in which red marrow is progressively replaced by yellow marrow in the appendicular skeleton and in which the fraction of fat cells within the red marrow of the axial skeleton

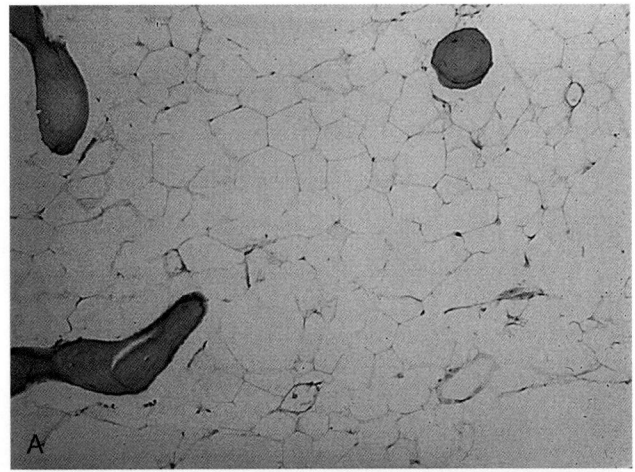

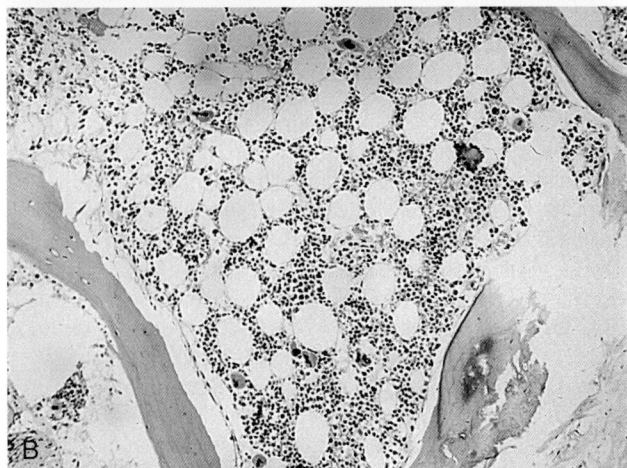

FIGURE 108-1

Normal marrow. Photomicrographs of fatty (**A**) and red (**B**) marrow show that adipocytes compose the majority of cellular elements in fatty marrow, whereas adipocytes are interspersed among precursor cells, plasma cells, and other cellular elements with higher nuclear-to-cytoplasmic ratios in red marrow. *(Reproduced with permission from Nissenbaum M: Bone marrow. In: Edelman R, Hesselink J, Zlatkin M (eds) Clinical Magnetic Resonance Imaging, 2nd edn. Philadelphia: WB Saunders, 1996.)*

progressively increases.[4,40] This process begins in the terminal phalanges shortly before birth and proceeds proximally within the appendicular skeleton in a centripetal fashion within individual bones.[41] Red marrow conversion begins in the region of the centrally located diaphyseal vessels, proceeding centrifugally with respect to central veins. A more detailed anatomic and age-related description of this process will be given later in this chapter.

Marrow Reconversion

Hematopoiesis is usually maintained adequately with available cellular marrow in the adult. However, if hemolysis, replacement or destruction of normal red marrow occurs, the demand for hematopoiesis is increased and reconversion of fatty cellular marrow may take place. In general, the process of reconversion occurs with an increase in the level of the circulating hormone erythropoietin. Reconversion extends from the central to the peripheral skeleton, with long bone changes occurring initially in the proximal femora and humeral metaphyses followed by the distal metaphyses, the diaphyses of the humeri and femora, and finally the epiphyses.[16] The process of reconversion is associated with hyperemia, capillary proliferation, and sinusoidal formation. Flat bones such as the scapula and spine reconvert more quickly as they maintain cellular marrow throughout life. Atypical, asymmetric patterns of reconversion may be seen with marrow-infiltrating disorders such as neoplasm,[42] myelofibrosis[43] or radiation changes.[44] If extreme stress is applied to red cell production, extramedullary hematopoiesis may ensue.

Age-Related Marrow Conversion—A General Overview

Knowledge of normal age-related changes in marrow distribution is critical for adequate interpretation of MR images due to similarities in appearance of normal and hematopoietic marrow on T1-weighted images.[25,12]

At birth, virtually the entire skeleton is composed of red marrow. As such, neonatal bone marrow is characteristically low signal intensity on T1-weighted images and intermediate signal intensity on T2-weighted images.[17] Soon after birth, conversion from red to yellow marrow begins in a centripetal fashion, starting first in the terminal phalanges of the hands and feet, epiphyses, and apophyses. Anatomic sections reveal conversion of marrow in the terminal phalanges by 1 year of age. Macroscopic fat is seen in the long bone midshaft by 12-14 years and the adult pattern is reached by 25 years.[8] The epiphyseal and apophyseal marrow maintains only a brief period of hematopoietic marrow, converting to yellow marrow within 3-4 months of the beginning of ossification.[8,45]

Four general MR patterns of bone marrow signal have been described in the long bones: infantile, childhood, adolescent, and adult.[8,12] Homogeneous low signal marrow in the diaphyses and metaphyses characterizes the infantile pattern, which is found during the first year of life. The childhood pattern is found from ages 1 to 10 and is characterized by higher signal in the diaphyses and metaphyses representing red to yellow marrow conversion. In patients aged 11 to 20, the adolescent pattern is seen. During this period, distal metaphyseal red marrow converts to yellow marrow, increasing the signal intensity in the distal metaphysis. Residual islands of red marrow leave a heterogeneous pattern to the metaphyseal marrow. The adult pattern (aged 25+) is characterized by predominant homogeneous high signal diaphyseal and metaphyseal marrow.[8,12] By this time, hematopoietic marrow is concentrated in the axial skeletal (skull, vertebrae, sternum, ribs, pelvis) and, to a lesser degree, the proximal appendicular skeleton (proximal humeri, femora). There is room for variability, particularly as red marrow may continue to comprise up to two-thirds of the femoral shafts.[46] After the adult pattern is reached there continues further replacement, albeit gradual, of hematopoietic marrow with fatty marrow until death. The spine and pelvis frequently appear bright on T1-weighted images in the elderly, reflecting this change.

NORMAL MARROW IMAGING

Axial Skeleton

Skull and Mandible

Within the calvarium and clivus in most infants less than 1 year of age, there is uniform low to intermediate signal intensity on T1-weighted images. Between 1 and 7 years, this hematopoietic marrow is converted to patchy low to high signal intensity marrow. By 15 years of age, most patients have homogenous high signal fatty marrow.[48] There is a gender difference with calvarial marrow, as the signal intensity of occipital, parietal, and frontal marrow in males tends to be greater than that in females during the second decade of life.[8,48]

In the mandible, prior to 10 years of age, marrow conversion is first seen in the anterior (mentalis) region of the mandibular body on MR. Red marrow remains in the ramus and condyle during this time period. From 10 to 15 years of age, marrow conversion is increasingly seen in the anterior region, followed by the premolar/molar region, angle, ramus, and condyle.[49] From 15 to 30 years of age, areas of high signal spread beyond the angle and ramus in most patients. Over 30 years of age, the majority of mandibular bone marrow show high signal on T1-weighted images. No red marrow is recognized in the body of the mandible after 30 years of age.[50]

Spine

The patterns of marrow distribution in the spine have been classified. Homogeneous red marrow is referred to as pattern 1. Linear zones of predominantly fatty marrow paralleling the endplates or triangular zones of fatty marrow excepting the vertebral body corners comprise pattern 2. Pattern 3 is characterized by multiple islands of yellow marrow, either small and indistinct (type 3a) or up to 1.5 cm in diameter (type 3b), superimposed on a background of hematopoietic marrow.

In the lumbar spine, the typical appearance of pattern 1 is seen in those under 30 years of age. The fourth decade is transitional; thus, by the age of 40, patterns 2 and 3 are seen in approximately 75% of people.

In the cervical spine pattern 1 is common in most people under 40 years of age. During the fifth decade, there is a transition through patterns 2 and 3, so that over the age of 50, most people demonstrate pattern 3.

In the thoracic spine, pattern 1 is most common under the age of 30. Transition occurs during the fourth and fifth decades, so that by age 50, most people have pattern 2 or 3.

In general, the signal intensity of marrow should be higher than adjacent vertebral disks on T1-weighted images in patients older than 10 years of age.[9]

Sternum and Clavicle

Patients younger than 1 year of age demonstrated hypointense bone marrow on T1-weighted images in all children. This remained unchanged from ages 1 to 5. Signal heterogeneity developed in the clavicle and sternum in patients 6 to 10 years of age, intermediate in intensity, and remained with this appearance into adulthood.

Pelvis

Signal intensity of marrow increases from birth to adulthood in all pelvic regions except the acetabulum.[51] The "infant pattern" is seen during the first years of life and is represented by homogeneous low to intermediate signal intensity in all ossified portions of the pelvis (the acetabulum is mostly cartilaginous at this age). From 1 to 10 years, heterogeneous intermediate to slightly hyperintense signal is seen in the acetabulum (as early as 2 years of age) and anterior ileum. The remainder of the pelvis during these years is of homogeneous intermediate signal intensity. From 11 to 20 years, intermediate signal is seen throughout the pelvis, although marked heterogeneity may be seen at this age, especially in the anterior ileum and acetabulum (Figs. 108-2 and 108-3). From 21 to 24 years, marrow with increased signal intensity is seen in the anterior ileum and acetabulum in the majority of patients. Marrow heterogeneity, which may be seen in this period, is most prominent in the acetabulum and least prominent in the posterior ileum. Anterior ileum heterogeneity is less prominent in this age than during the adolescent period.[51]

Appendicular Skeleton

In the femur, even the earliest ossified epiphyses may be of increased signal intensity, as are the greater and lesser trochanters.[12] The marrow of the proximal metaphyses, diaphysis, and distal metaphysis is all of homogeneous low T1-weighted signal, representing hematopoietic marrow. By the age of 1 year, the increased signal

intensity of yellow marrow can be seen within the ossified femoral epiphysis surrounded by a rim of low signal intensity cortical bone. Between the ages of 1 and 5, diaphyseal marrow begins to convert to yellow marrow. This may be seen as early as 1 to 2 years of age. Fatty marrow within the ossifying greater trochanter is seen by 3 years of age. Proximal and distal metaphyses remain predominantly of red marrow (Fig. 108- 4).

Between 6 and 10 years, femoral diaphyseal marrow completes its conversion to yellow marrow, as seen on MRI. Proximal and distal metaphyses remain of intermediate signal. The adolescent pattern is seen between 11 and 15 years and is most notable for transition within the distal metaphyseal marrow from red towards a more adult yellow pattern. The distal metaphysis appears inhomogeneous and slightly increased in signal relative to that seen at 6 to 10 years of age, but still lower than yellow marrow. The proximal metaphysis remains intermediate to slightly hyperintense. By 21 years of age, the adult pattern is seen with the proximal epiphysis, diaphysis, distal metaphysis, and distal epiphysis showing homogeneous yellow marrow. The proximal metaphysis is seen as either homogeneous or heterogeneous marrow of intermediate to increased signal intensity (Fig. 108-5).[12,52]

In the humerus, marrow conversion patterns are similar to femoral conversion patterns.[10] Zawin and Jaramillo[10] demonstrated that conversion from red to yellow marrow occurs earlier in the proximal epiphysis of the humerus than in the proximal epiphysis of the femur (seen in the humerus as early as 3 months of age). This most likely is related to the earlier appearance of the epiphyseal center of the humerus than in the femur. The conversion pattern in the remainder of the other anatomic regions of the humerus is similar to those reported in the femur,[52] although diaphyseal conversion may occur slightly earlier in the humerus.

Gender, Lifestyle, and Activity-Related Changes

As a response to internal and external stresses applied to the bone marrow, yellow marrow will reconvert to active hematopoietic (red) marrow. Knowledge of the "normal variant" appearances of the marrow in these individuals is important for the adequate interpretation of their MRI scans.

Poulton et al evaluated MR images of the knee and assessed for a possible relationship between marrow reconversion and age, sex, weight, and smoking. Their results showed marrow reconversion at the knee is most prevalent in heavy smokers, younger patients and, most prominently, obese women who smoke heavily. In these groups of patients, marrow reconversion can be a normal finding on MRI.[53]

Another group of patients that appear to undergo changes in their bone marrow related to physiologic stresses are elite athletes. Shellock et al found a high prevalence of hematopoietic hyperplasia in the knees of asymptomatic marathon runners within the distal femur.[54] Caldemeyer et al[55] showed that bone mineral

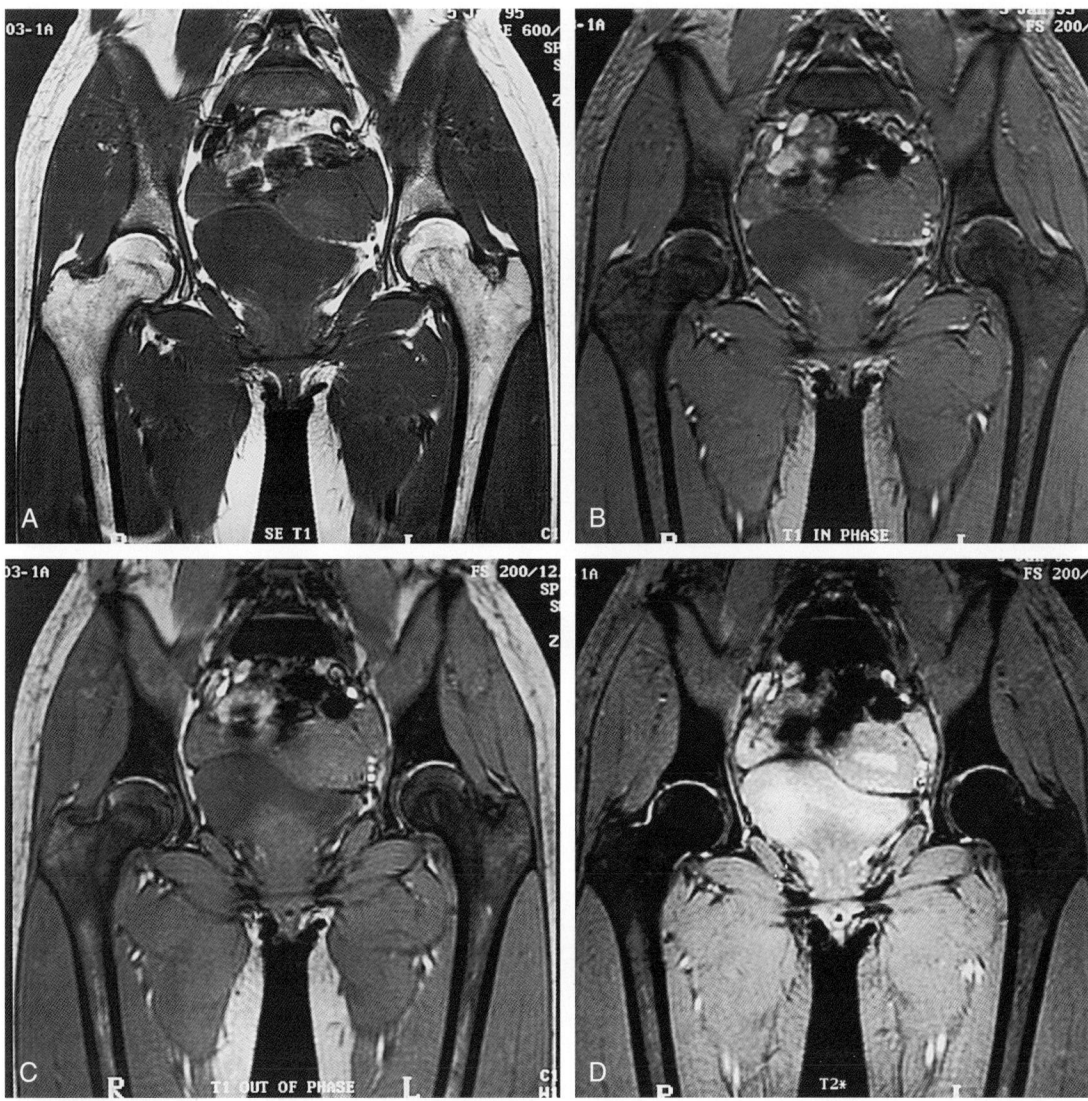

FIGURE 108-2

Normal marrow distribution. This patient was a 24-year-old woman. **A,** T1-weighted image shows islands of fatty marrow interspersed with red marrow in the femoral neck and intertrochanteric regions. **B,** T1-weighted gradient-echo image, in phase (repetition time [TR]/echo time [TE]/flip angle [FA] = 200/10.5/90°), demonstrates typical in-phase contrast relationships. Note signal intensity in the supra-acetabular and femoral diaphyseal regions. **C,** T1-weighted gradient-echo image, out of phase (200/12.5/90°), demonstrates greater loss of marrow signal intensity compared with the in-phase study. **D,** T2*-weighted gradient-echo image (200/16/20°) shows further loss of marrow signal intensity related to increased susceptibility effects. Note profoundly hypointense zones of red marrow as well as susceptibility artifact adjacent to gas-filled bowel loops. *(Reproduced with permission from Nissenbaum M: Bone marrow. In: Edelman R, Hesselink J, Zlatkin M (eds) Clinical Magnetic Resonance Imaging, 2nd edn. Philadelphia: WB Saunders, 1996.)*

density does not contribute to observed marrow changes of hematopoietic hyperplasia in the spine of endurance athletes. They hypothesized that iron store depletion or increased hematopoiesis ("sports anemia") contributed to the hematopoietic hyperplasia.

Another study looked at 20 male professional cyclists and 44 volunteers. Sagittal T1-weighted spin-echo sequence and gradient-echo with out-of-phase echo time and a turbo inversion recovery sequence was performed and the averaged bone marrow signal of three adjacent vertebrae was obtained. In addition, laboratory values such as hemoglobin, ferritin level, and VO_{2max} were obtained. They found professional male cyclists had MR findings consistent with hematopoietic hyperplasia in the lumbar spine compared with age-matched male volunteers. These cyclists had slightly less hyperplasia than did female volunteers. As there was a wide variability of imaging appearances that was largely independent of laboratory and performance data, MR signs of hematopoietic hyperplasia should be considered a normal finding in this population which is most likely multifactorial.[56]

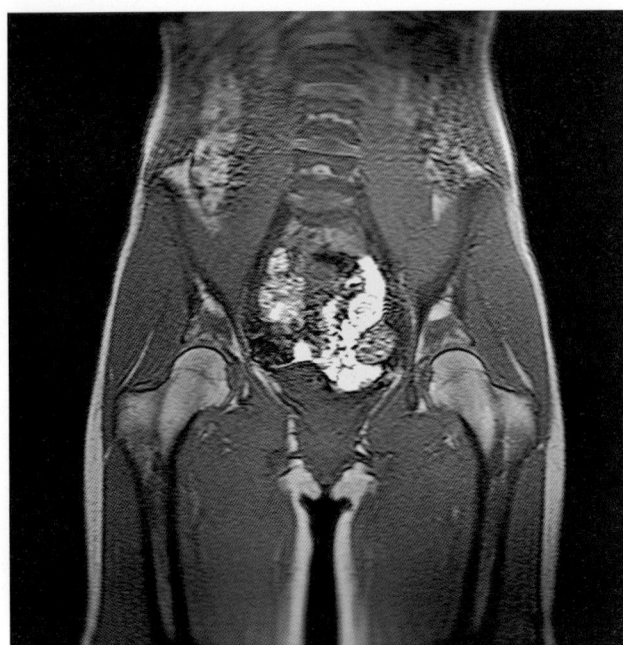

FIGURE 108-3

Distribution of normal hematopoietic marrow. Coronal gradient-echo image, pelvis. There is low signal intensity within the spine, pelvis and the proximal femurs bilaterally in a 17-year-old female.

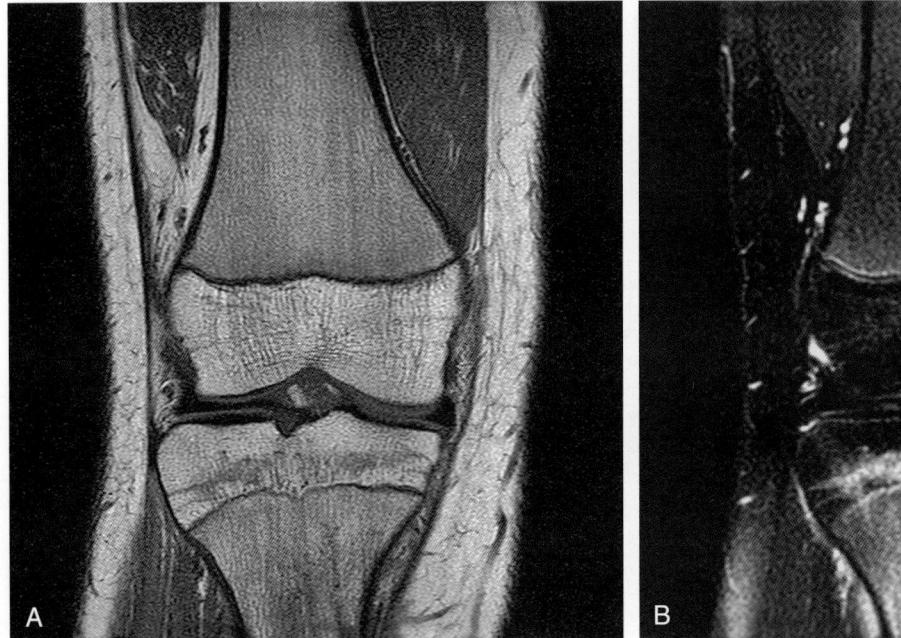
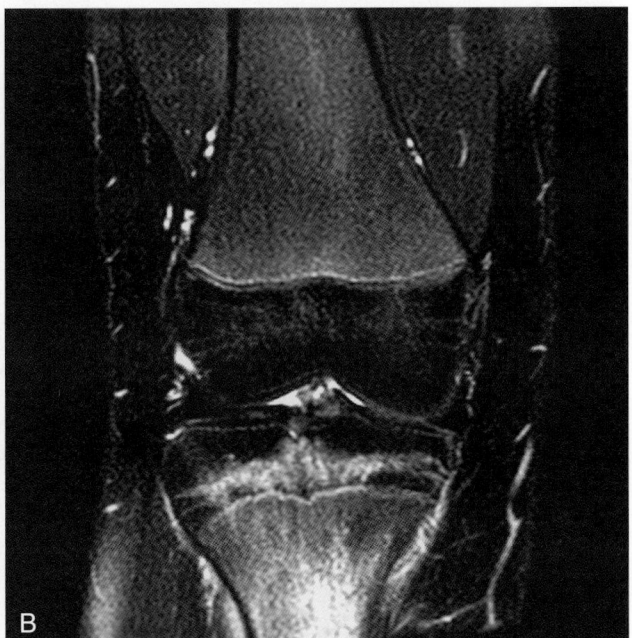

FIGURE 108-4

Normal and abnormal pattern of marrow distribution in a child. **A,** Coronal T1-weighted image, knee. The marrow is slightly hypointense within the femoral metaphysis as compared to the epiphysis. This is a normal finding in an 11-year-old male as the transition to yellow marrow is under way. **B,** Coronal T2-weighted fat-suppressed image, knee. In the same patient normal marrow is seen within the distal femoral metaphysis. The marrow in this location is slightly hyperintense as compared to the epiphysis. The proximal tibial epiphysis and metaphysis are more hyperintense than normal. This is due to a stress fracture.

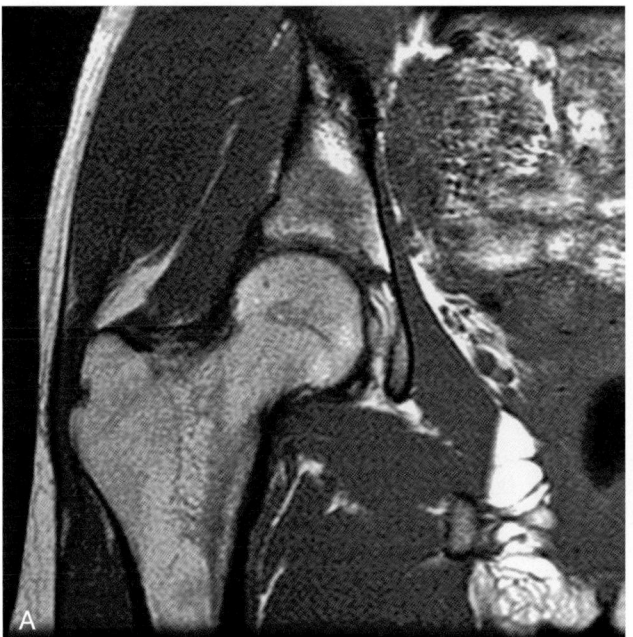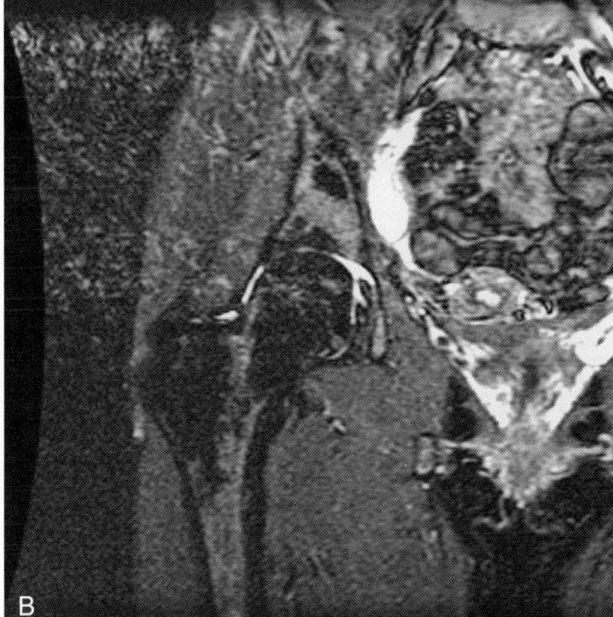

FIGURE 108-5

Normal hematopoietic marrow. **A,** Coronal T1-weighted image, hip. This is a 19-year-old female. There is marked inhomogeneity of the acetabular marrow and low signal intensity within the base of the femoral neck. **B,** Coronal STIR image, hip. The same areas are mildly increased in signal intensity, not significantly different from the intensity of the adjacent musculature. These hyperintense areas represent normal hematopoietic marrow.

Gender differences in normal bone marrow have been identified. Duda et al studied possible sex-related differences in sacral bone marrow in patients aged 17 to 42.[57] They found a higher fat content in the lateral masses of the sacrum in males than in females. In both sexes, the signal of fatty marrow is higher in the lateral masses, as is the heterogeneity, but without sex-related differences. Selective water imaging revealed a greater proportion of hematopoietic marrow in the sacrum of females compared with males in this age group.

Regarding activity levels, Le Blanc et al tried to assess whether marrow composition was altered by space flight. Four space lab crew members were imaged using a gradient inversion spectroscopy technique. T2 relaxation times were obtained for the L3 vertebral body. The T2 of the cellular and fat components and apparent cellular fraction were analyzed. Crew members were imaged before launch and after landing. The authors found no significant change in apparent cellular function of bone marrow. However, the T2 of the cellular, but not fat component increased following flight in all crew members. These increases returned to baseline in an inordinately long time period (up to 4 months after landing). During microgravity (space flight) rat studies have documented reduced osteoblastic activity.[58] Loss of red cell mass begins within the first few weeks of space flight or bedrest.[59-61] The authors surmise that the T2 changes may reflect increased osteoblastic activity following flight, reflecting an increase in bone formation.[62]

MARROW PATHOLOGY

Bone Marrow Edema

Magnetic resonance imaging allows the routine evaluation of previously unidentified bone marrow edema. This so-called edema may be seen in multiple disorders including trauma (both acute and stress related), arthritis, neuropathy, avascular necrosis and in association with benign and malignant bone lesions. Due to the presence of increased free water, edema will appear hyperintense on both inversion recovery and frequency-selective fat-suppressed images, as well as revealing increased diffusion on diffusion-weighted sequences.[63]

The primary cause of fluid accumulation in extracellular marrow space is capillary leakage. The edema will most often be seen in capillary-rich red marrow in cancellous bone, such as is seen in the vertebral body, metaphysis of long bones and within the small bones of the wrist and foot. There are different causes of capillary leakage. It may occur as a result of capillary wall changes or secondary to either increased delivery or decreased clearance of blood. Marrow edema resulting from increased blood flow is termed hyperemic, marrow edema resulting from decreased vascular drainage is termed congestive and capillary leakage resulting from tumor or direct insult is termed tumorigenic or traumatic.[64,65]

Hyperemic edema may occur as a result of local increases in blood flow due to the release of inflammatory

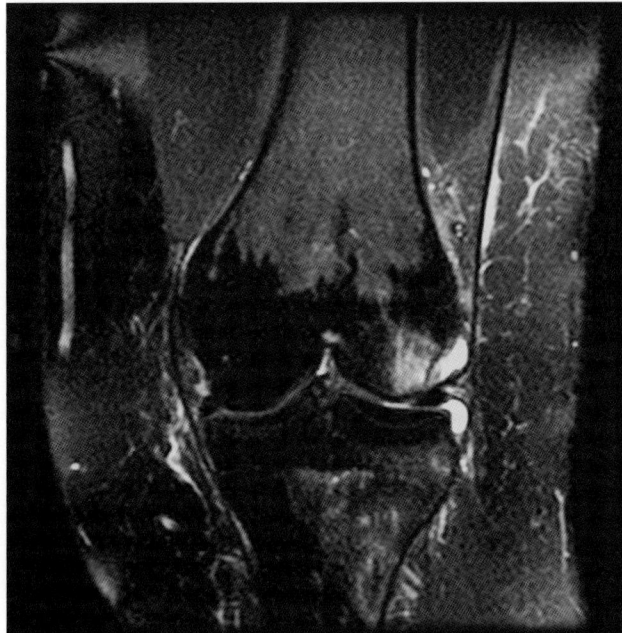

FIGURE 108-6

Bone contusion. Coronal T2-weighted fat-suppressed image, knee. The patient is a 27-year-old female. There is a focus of increased signal intensity within the lateral femoral condyle due to contusion. Note the normal hematopoietic marrow within the distal femoral metaphysis and proximal tibial metaphysis.

mediators in marrow infection or as a result of synovitis. Additionally, changes in autonomic vascular regulation in reflex sympathetic dystrophy may cause diffuse patchy marrow edema.[64,66] Steroid-induced avascular necrosis is a common cause of congestive marrow edema. Elevation of intramedullary pressure and associated venous congestion lead to rapid accumulation of interstitial fluid.[67] Tumorigenic edema is predominantly a result of local trabecular destruction, increased intramedullary pressure or release of inflammatory mediators such as occurs in osteoid osteoma.[68] As tumors contain largely water, utilization of fat-suppressed pulse sequences may cause difficulty in differentiating tumor from surrounding edema. Gadolinium administration will result in rapid tumor enhancement in distinction from the relatively low-grade enhancement of the reactive edema.[69]

Trauma is the most common cause of bone marrow edema and will be the main focus of this section. Usually the changes are confined to the subchondral bone. In the absence of radiographically apparent fracture lines, these changes are usually the result of microfractures, hyperemia, and hemorrhage.[70-72] This constellation of findings has been termed a bone contusion or bone bruise (Fig. 108-6). Evaluation of the pattern and distribution of these bone marrow changes often allows determination of the mechanism of injury on the joint or bone involved.

Patterns of Bone Marrow Edema

Bone Marrow Edema Related to Fractures

Occult fracture is a term used for a fracture not initially identifiable by radiographs. This term applies even if or when the fracture is detected by other imaging modalities or eventually on the initial radiographs retrospectively. Magnetic resonance imaging often, but not invariably, reveals a fracture line. MR reveals poorly defined or patchy areas of bone marrow edema with high signal intensity on T2-weighted, fat-suppressed or STIR images. These changes are also present on T1-weighted sequences.[73,74]

Stress fractures are categorized into fatigue and insufficiency fractures. Fatigue fractures occur in normal healthy bone subjected to repetitive trauma. If bone which possesses sufficient mineral content and elasticity is exposed to excessive muscular action or abnormal torque, fatigue fractures may occur.[75,76] Stress response may be considered a subclinical stress fracture.[73,74] A fracture line is not seen either radiographically or on MRI. However, with both a stress fracture and stress response, MR may reveal patchy decreased signal on T1-weighted sequences within the marrow fat which becomes hyperintense on STIR and frequency-selective fat suppression pulse sequences. Insufficiency fractures occur when normal physiologic load is applied to weak, deficiently mineralized bone,[76] as is seen in osteoporosis and osteomalacia (Fig. 108-7). In general, the terms fatigue fractures and stress fractures are used interchangeably and the remainder of this section will use the term stress fracture for fatigue fracture.

Stress fractures are more commonly seen in the lower extremities. They are often seen in the metatarsal and tarsal bones as well as the tibia. More recently, stress fractures of the sacrum have been described in athletes such as marathon runners. These fractures appear to be more common in women.[77] Oblique coronal MR images through the sacrum with STIR or fat-suppressed T2-weighted FSE sequences are necessary for evaluating the young athlete with buttock pain.[76] MR can play a critical role in assessing for stress fractures in certain situations. Tarsal navicular stress fractures are a diagnostic challenge due to diffuse and vague midfoot pain. Initial radiographs usually reveal no fracture. Radionuclide bone scanning may be used as a screening procedure but is nonspecific. Other entities such as stress reaction, injury to an accessory navicular (congenital variant) or posterior tibialis tendinopathy may give a similar clinical and radionuclide appearance. MRI will reveal a linear fracture line with surrounding decreased T1-weighted and increased T2-weighted fat-suppressed or STIR signal (Fig. 108-8).[78]

Vertebral Compression Fractures—Benign Versus Malignant

Atraumatic vertebral body compression fractures of the spine are a commonly encountered clinical problem seen in the elderly. The most common cause of compression

FIGURE 108-7

Sacral insufficiency fractures. Coronal T2-weighted fat-suppressed image, pelvis. There are regional areas of abnormal increased signal intensity within the sacral ala bilaterally. A vertically oriented low signal intensity line is also seen bilaterally representing the fractures.

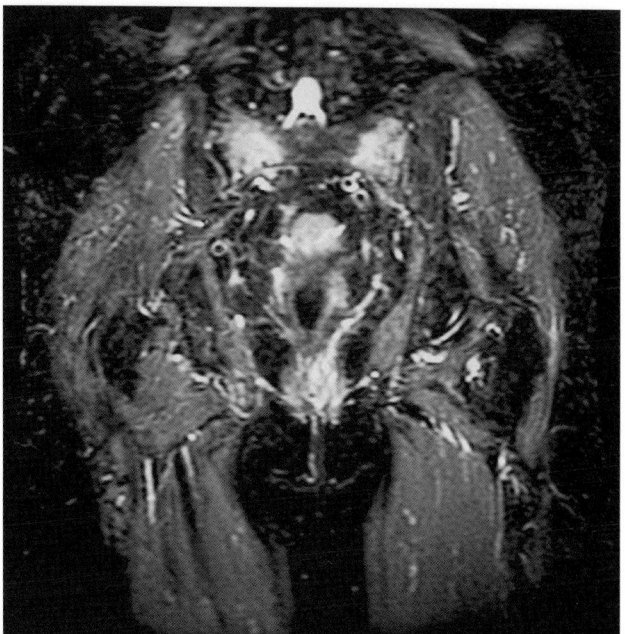

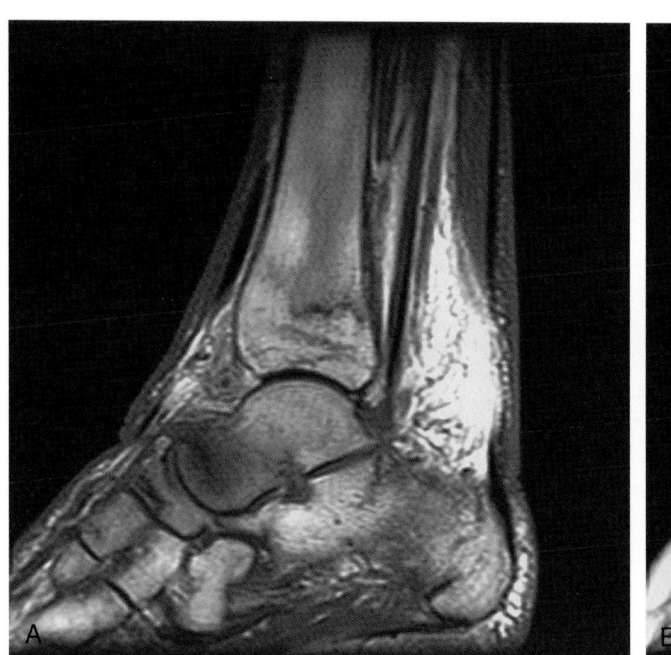

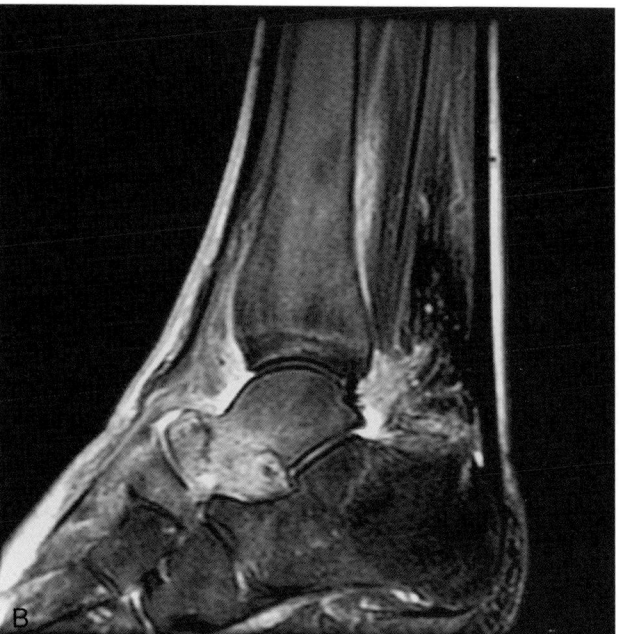

FIGURE 108-8

Stress fractures. **A,** Sagittal T1-weighted image, ankle. This is a 14-year-old male soccer player with pain and soft-tissue swelling. There is a curvilinear area of low signal intensity within the distal tibia, talar head, and the navicular compatible with stress fractures. **B,** Sagittal T-2 weighted fat-suppressed image, ankle. Low signal intensity fracture lines are re-identified. There is high signal intensity bone marrow edema within the affected bones.

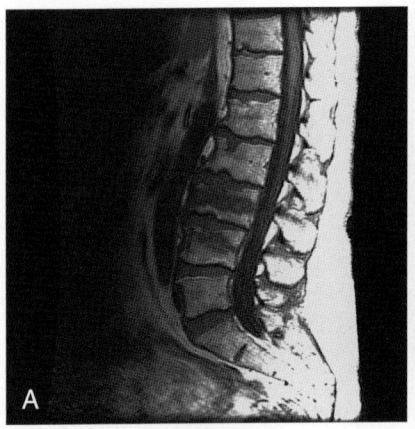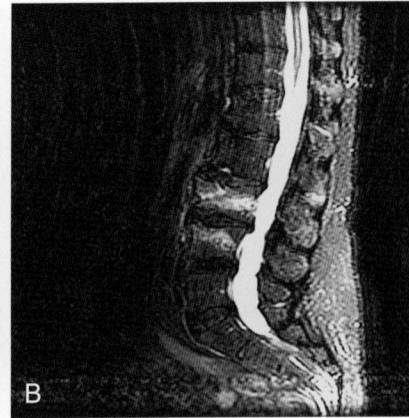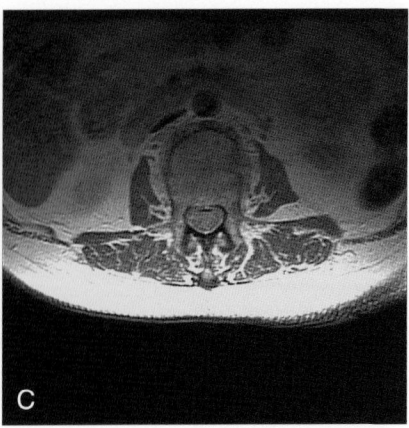

FIGURE 108-9

Benign vertebral body compression fractures. **A,** Sagittal T1-weighted image, lumbar spine. This is a 79-year-old patient with abnormal horizontally oriented decreased signal within the L3 and L4 vertebral bodies. There is mild loss of vertebral body height. **B,** Sagittal STIR image, lumbar spine. The same vertebral bodies show increased signal. No retropulsed fragments are seen extending into the spinal canal. **C,** Axial proton density image, lumbar spine. The L3 vertebral body of the same patient maintains normal signal intensity within the posterior elements. No associated soft-tissue mass is identified.

fractures in this age group is osteoporosis. Another major cause of vertebral body compression fractures is metastatic disease; 39% of all bone metastases are found in the spine.[79,80] The differentiation between acute osteoporotic and compression fracture due to metastatic lesion is critical for clinical staging, treatment planning, and prognosis.[79,81]

There are MRI findings which are helpful in distinguishing between benign versus malignant causes of acute compression fractures of the spine. Baur et al studied 87 consecutive patients with acute vertebral fractures due to osteoporotic (n = 52) or neoplastic (n = 35) infiltrations. MRI protocol included non-enhanced T2-weighted spin-echo and STIR images on a 1.5 T system. The authors evaluated the presence, location, and shape of the fluid sign in acute compression fractures. The fluid sign was defined as a focal, linear or triangular area of strong hyperintensity on STIR images on a background of diffuse hyperintensity in the vertebral body as a result of acute collapse. They found the fluid sign was adjacent to the endplates and was regarded as an additional morphologic feature leaning towards a benign osteoporotic nature of an acute fracture.[82]

Jung et al looked at the MR imaging findings in 27 patients with metastatic compression fractures and 55 patients with acute osteoporotic compression fractures. Findings suggestive of metastatic compression fractures included a convex posterior border of the vertebral body, abnormal signal intensity in the pedicle or posterior element, an epidural mass, an encasing epidural mass or other spinal metastases.[79] Findings suggestive of acute osteoporotic compression fractures included a low signal intensity band on T1-weighted and T2-weighted images, spared normal bone marrow signal intensity of the vertebral body, retropulsion of a posterior bone fragment, and multiple compression fractures (Fig. 108-9).[79] On the basis of these findings,

the sensitivity, specificity, and accuracy for metastatic compression fractures were 100%, 93% and 95% respectively.[79]

As previously described in this chapter, diffusion-weighted imaging (DWI) has been used to differentiate acute osteoporotic from malignant vertebral compression fractures and has proven to be a reliable means to distinguish between the two.[34,83-85] The predominant pulse sequence employed in these studies has been the diffusion-weighted SSFP (steady-state free precession) technique.

Bone Marrow Edema Patterns of the Knee

Post-traumatic bone marrow edema may be asymptomatic or symptomatic. It may be related to a single macrotraumatic insult or to repetitive microtraumatic insults. Major and Helms performed bilateral knee MRI on 17 collegiate asymptomatic basketball players. T2-weighted fast spin-echo images (TR/TE$_{EFF}$, 3500/65) with fat suppression in all three planes, as well as spin-echo proton density fat-suppressed images (TR/TE, 2000/20) in the sagittal plane, were obtained.[86] Forty-one percent of these asymptomatic athletes had bone marrow edema, seen in the medial femoral condyle, lateral femoral condyle, lateral tibial plateau or patella. These findings were not associated with any changes of osteoarthritis. The authors surmise that these marrow changes may be the result of forces being transmitted through the menisci, dissipated by the cartilage and eventually absorbed into the bone, resulting in microfractures or contusions.[86] Krample et al evaluated the knees of eight marathon runners 24 hours and 6 weeks after a marathon and found seven cases of localized high signal intensity on T2-weighted images within the condyles or patella. Assuming no underlying meniscal pathology, all these changes proved transitory.[87]

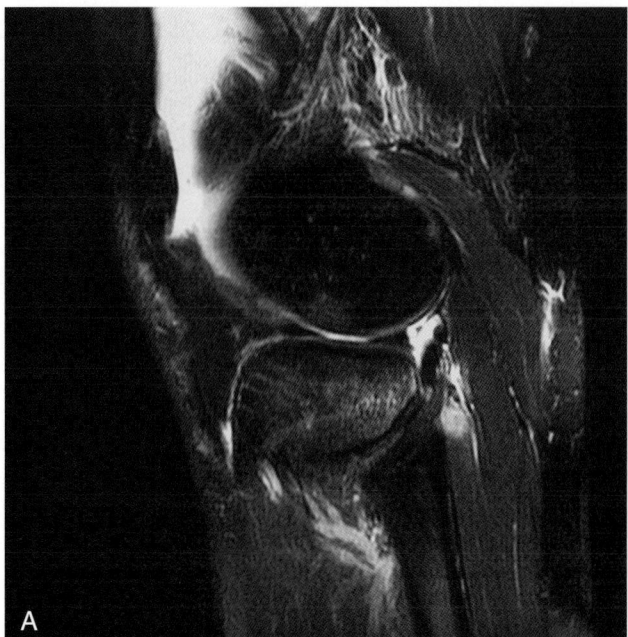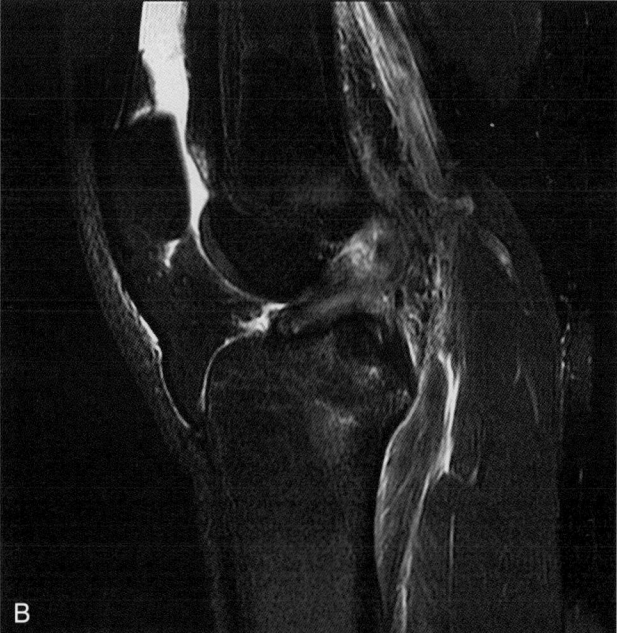

FIGURE 108-10

Bone contusion pattern of ACL rupture. **A,** Sagittal T2-weighted fat-suppressed image, knee. There is abnormal increased signal within the lateral femoral condyle and the posterolateral tibial plateau. **B,** Sagittal T2-weighted fat-suppressed image, knee. There is abnormal increased signal within the proximal anterior cruciate ligament compatible with tear.

Post-traumatic, symptomatic bone marrow edema about the knee occurs in five distinct patterns: pivot shift injury, dashboard injury, hyperextension injury, clip injury, and lateral patellar dislocation.[88] The most common of these injuries are the pivot shift and lateral patellar dislocation. The pivot shift injury is usually a non-contact injury seen often in skiers or American football players, which results from application of a valgus load to the knee while in flexion, in conjunction with external rotation of the tibia or internal rotation of the femur. This is commonly seen with a sudden deceleration and change in direction while the foot is planted. The anterior cruciate ligament is loaded and so this action may lead to its rupture. Once torn, anterior subluxation of the tibia occurs relative to the femur. This causes impaction of the lateral femoral condyle against the posterolateral tibial plateau.[89-92] The associated bone contusion pattern includes the lateral femoral condyle adjacent to the lateral femoral sulcus and posterolateral tibial plateau (Fig. 108-10). Increasing flexion of the knee at the time of injury lands the bone contusion more posteriorly in the condyle while less flexion leads to a more anterior femoral condylar contusion.[88]

Lateral patellar dislocation is seen in young athletes, usually resulting from a forced internal rotation of the femur on a fixed, externally rotated tibia while the knee is flexed.[70,88] The quadriceps mechanism pulls the patella laterally out of the trochlear groove until the medial retinaculum tears. Impaction of the patella and femur occurs, creating the classic bone contusion pattern involving the inferomedial patella and anterolateral femoral condyle (Fig. 108-11). Occasionally, edema may be seen in the adductor tubercle of the medial femoral condyle due to avulsion of the medial patellofemoral ligament.[88] The lateral femoral condyle contusion associated with ACL tears is usually more posteriorly located than that of a lateral patellar dislocation.

Post-Traumatic Bone Marrow Abnormalities of the Foot and Ankle

Ankle sprains may be associated with bone contusion.[73,93] Following a rotational or inversion injury, ankle marrow edema may be seen in the talar neck, particularly the medial portion.[73] Direct impact bone contusions are most frequently encountered in the navicular.[73]

Subtendinous bone marrow edema can occasionally be seen in association with tendinopathy on T2-weighted fat-suppressed STIR images. This may be seen at the medial malleolus associated with posterior tibialis tendinopathy, at the calcaneus, associated with peroneus brevis and longus tendon abnormalities, and the lateral cuboid, associated with peroneus longus pathology. The cause of this subtendinous marrow edema may be related to hyperemia, either in the marrow or tendon sheath, or possibly tendon friction. This edema may be associated with pain medially.[73,94]

As in the knee, bone marrow edema has been found in the foot and ankle of asymptomatic marathon runners.[95,96] Foci of T2 or STIR hyperintensity both less than and greater than 10 mm in diameter have been seen in 16% of 19 professional runners imaged.[95]

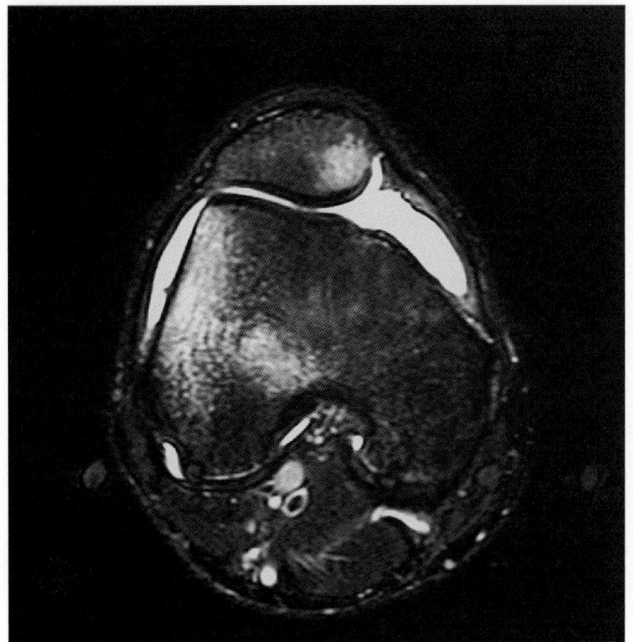

FIGURE 108-11

Transient patellar dislocation. Axial T2-weighted fat-suppressed image, knee. This is a 24-year-old male who sustained a patellar dislocation injury. Note the bone marrow edema within the medial half of the patella and the anterolateral femoral condyle characteristic of this pattern of injury.

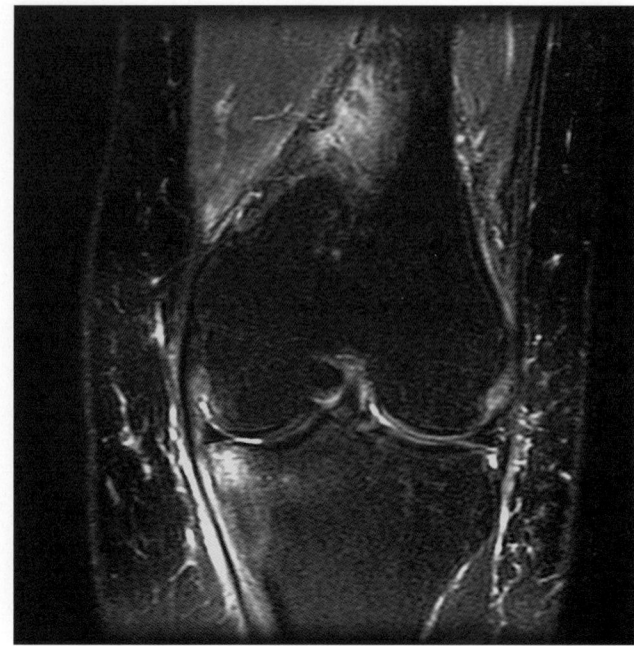

FIGURE 108-12

Osteoarthritis. Coronal T2-weighted fat-suppressed image, knee. There is mild abnormal increased signal within the medial femoral condyle and tibial plateau. Other images demonstrated joint space narrowing and thinning of the articular cartilage.

Chronic Distraction Injuries

Chronic or excessive distraction forces may be placed on trabecular bone. When placed on a focal region, this tests the elastic or plastic nature of the trabeculae and may lead to focal disruption. More diffuse distraction forces may lead to linear bruising and bone marrow edema, usually perpendicular to the longitudinal pull of the stress. If overlying cortical bone is disrupted, the term avulsion fracture is used.[64] When chronic distraction forces are applied via ligamentous insertions, painful, often linear bone edema may occur perpendicular to the pull of the ligament.[64] The term "shin splints" has been applied to overuse-related leg pain which is most likely related to traction periostitis at the soleal origin off the posteromedial tibial cortex. MRI may reveal marrow edema, cortical signal abnormalities or periosteal edema.[97-99]

Thigh splints (adductor insertion avulsion syndrome) is a similar phenomenon which occurs due to chronic traction from the large strong adductor muscle-tendon units on the proximal medial femoral shaft. Similar MRI findings are seen to those found with "shin splints".[97,100]

Osteoarthritis

It is well known that osteoarthritis of the knee is associated with multiple MRI findings. These include cartilage lesions, subchondral cysts, osteophyte formation, synovial and ligamentous abnormalities. Foci of ill-defined increased signal intensity on STIR and T2-weighted fat-suppressed images have also been commonly seen in osteoarthritic patients (Fig. 108-12). This has been referred to as bone marrow edema.

Zanetti et al looked at the bone marrow of 16 patients undergoing total knee arthroplasties. These knees were imaged 1 to 4 days prior to surgery. The tibial plateaus were assessed histologically after knee replacement to correlate the preoperative finding of bone marrow edema on MRI.[101] They found that the bone marrow edema zones consisted mainly of normal tissue (71%) with the rest composed of 11% marrow necrosis, 8% abnormal trabecular, 4% marrow fibrosis, 4% marrow edema, and 2% marrow bleeding.[101] They proposed that the term "bone marrow edema" is a misnomer, with a more accurate description of these marrow changes being "ill-defined signal intensity abnormality".

The exact cause of knee pain in patients with osteoarthritis is not known.[102-104] The characteristic feature of osteoarthritis is articular hyaline cartilage loss. However, there are no pain fibers in hyaline cartilage. There are pain fibers in other areas of the knee that are affected by osteoarthritis; these include the joint capsule, ligaments, peripheral third of the menisci, possibly the synovium as well as the periosteum and bone marrow. Creamer et al injected intra-articular anesthetic into the knees of 10 osteoarthritic patients with only 6 of 10 showing any relief.[105] This suggests that extra-articular, non-capsular causes of pain may exist. Supporting this theory is the fact that many young athletes without osteoarthritis develop very similar appearing bone marrow lesions after acute trauma (bone contusions) which are also subchondral in location and cause pain.

Several groups have looked into what relationship, if any, there is between MRI findings of bone marrow edema and osteoarthritis. Felson's group attempted to determine whether bone marrow lesions on MRI were associated with pain in knee osteoarthritis. MRI was used to identify the prevalence and size of bone marrow edema lesions in 401 patients with and without knee pain. They found that bone marrow lesions on MRI are strongly associated with the presence of pain in knee osteoarthritis, particularly large lesions.[102] A separate study by Felson et al[106] looked at patients 45 years of age and older to determine if the bone marrow edema lesions in patients with knee osteoarthritis identify knees at high risk for radiographic progression. Their results indicated that risk for medical progression of OA over a 30-month period increased six times with medial lesions. They even suggest that patients at high risk for progression of OA could be screened for bone marrow edema by MRI.[106] Pessis' group found that the absence of bone marrow edema on initial MRI exams predicted absence or worsening of chondral pathology after 1 year.[104]

There are conflicting data, however, with respect to the osteoarthritis–bone marrow edema relationship. Sowers et al found that bone marrow edema could not explain the presence or absence of knee pain only in women with full-thickness cartilage deficits accompanied by subchondral cortical defects.[103] In addition, Link's group found that MR abnormalities (including bone marrow edema) and the extent of these abnormalities correlated with radiographic abnormalities but not with clinical findings.[107] It is apparent that more work needs to be done in this important relationship.

Vascular Disorders

Vascular abnormalities (hyperemia or ischemia) of the bone marrow manifest as focal or regional areas of edema. The MR appearance is that of intermediate signal intensity on T1-weighted images and high signal intensity on T2-weighted images. Examples of vascular abnormalities include transient osteoporosis of the hip (hypcremia) and osteonecrosis (ischemia).

Transient Osteoporosis of the Hip

Initially described in 1959, transient osteoporosis of the hip is a rare disease process that has been the focus of much debate. To date, there is no consensus regarding its etiology or pathophysiology. Some believe transient osteoporosis of the hip (TOH) to be a distinct entity with a mechanism similar to reflex sympathetic dystrophy, while others claim that it represents an early reversible form of avascular necrosis.[108-112]

Originally described in pregnant women during their third trimester, TOH is now most commonly seen in young and middle-aged men. Clinically, patients experience a sudden onset of hip pain severe enough at times to significantly restrict mobility.

Plain radiographs can be normal or show osteoporosis of the femoral head and neck. MR images

reveal a nonspecific bone marrow edema pattern consisting of diffuse decreased T1- and increased T2-weighted signal within the femoral head extending into the intertrochanteric region. A joint effusion is frequently present but not necessary and the surrounding soft-tissues are normal.[113] In an attempt to differentiate irreversible from transient bone marrow edema lesions within the femoral head, Vande Berg et al[114] reviewed 72 lesions in 42 men and 25 women. The presence of a subchondral area of low T2 signal intensity at least 4 mm thick or 12.5 mm long had positive predictive values of 85% and 73%, respectively, for irreversible lesions. Lack of any subchondral change on T2-weighted images had a 100% positive predictive value for transient lesions.

Most consider TOH to be a self-limited disease with resolution of symptoms within 6 to 12 months. Therapeutic approaches to TOH range from symptomatic relief with non-steroidal anti-inflammatory drugs and protected weight bearing to core decompression. Much controversy exists over whether to treat TOH conservatively or operatively. Research has shown that core decompression, though invasive and subject to complications, can significantly reduce duration of symptoms with an almost immediate onset of effect.[112,115]

Osteonecrosis

Osteonecrosis is a dynamic process characterized by bone marrow ischemia progressing to cell death followed by attempted repair. Synonymous terms include avascular necrosis (AVN) and bone infarct. By convention, the term AVN is used with epiphyseal involvement and the term bone infarct is used with metaphyseal or diaphyseal involvement. Alcohol intake and corticosteroid use account for the majority of cases of atraumatic osteonecrosis. Other predisposing factors include trauma, sickle cell anemia, pancreatitis, and Gaucher's disease. Osteonecrosis commonly affects patients during the third, fourth, and fifth decades of life. Without early detection and therapy, these patients may suffer from secondary osteoarthritis requiring premature joint replacement.[116]

Our understanding of the pathophysiology of osteonecrosis is derived from studies focused on femoral head AVN. These studies have shown that AVN develops as a result of insufficient blood flow to the bone. In cases of trauma, it is the disruption of the normal blood supply that causes necrosis. The pathology behind atraumatic AVN is less well understood. In these cases, necrosis is likely dependent upon several factors, often working simultaneously. Occlusion of femoral head vascularity may result from altered femoral head anatomy, intravascular occlusion from thrombi or lipid emboli or extravascular compression due to intraosseous hypertension.[117] With disruption of femoral head blood flow, local PO_2 is reduced and with 2 to 3 hours of ischemia, osteocyte necrosis occurs. Following necrosis, a reparative response ensues, largely directed by the nearby viable bone. Undifferentiated mesenchymal tissue and capillaries penetrate the necrotic area for a variable distance and then differentiate into osteoblasts that coat

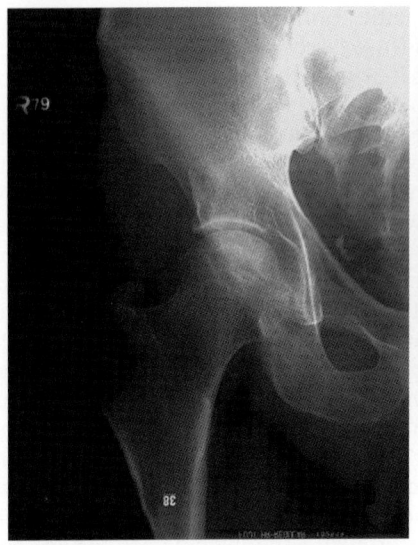 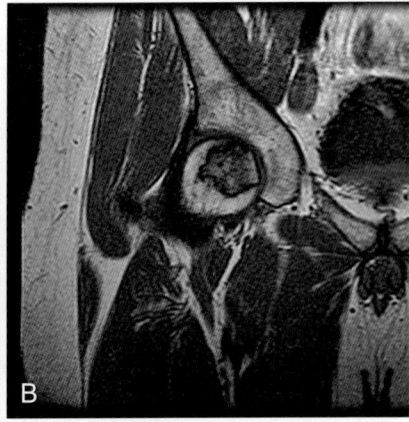 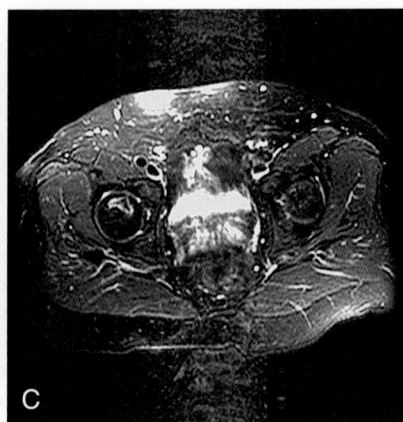

FIGURE 108-13

Femoral head avascular necrosis. **A,** Anteroposterior radiograph, hip. There is an area of mixed lysis and sclerosis within the femoral head. **B,** Coronal T1-weighted image, hip. A focal area of signal abnormality is present within the femoral head that is bound by a serpiginous low signal intensity rim. **C,** Axial T2-weighted fat-suppressed image, hip. The serpiginous rim is of high T2 signal intensity. Note the characteristic location of AVN of the femoral head within the anterosuperior aspect.

the dead trabeculae with new bone.[118] MRI can be used to examine this dynamic process of necrosis and repair. It has been determined to be the most sensitive imaging modality for the evaluation of osteonecrosis.

The MRI findings of osteonecrosis are the same regardless of the cause or location: a geographic area of variable signal intensity surrounded by a peripheral serpentine rim of T1 and T2 signal hypointensity. The peripheral hypointense rim represents sclerosis and demarcates viable from infarcted bone.[118] In up to 80% of cases, a high signal intensity band can be seen just within the hypointense rim ("double line" sign) that is virtually pathognomonic for osteonecrosis. Some investigators attribute the hyperintense inner band to hyperemic granulation tissue and others to chemical shift misregistration (Fig. 108-13).[119] On fast spin-echo T2-weighted images without fat suppression, the double line sign may be difficult to appreciate as the inner hyperintense border may be obscured by fat (Fig. 108-14).[120]

The marrow space enclosed by the hypointense serpentine band can have a variety of signal characteristics. Mitchell et al[121] proposed a classification system to describe these signal abnormalities ranging from Class A to D. Infarcted marrow with signal intensity changes similar to fat is categorized as Class A. Class B marrow abnormalities parallel the signal characteristics of blood, with high signal intensity on T1- and T2-weighted images. The signal intensity changes associated with Class C resemble fluid, with low T1- and high T2-weighted signal. Finally, Class D signal abnormalities are similar to fibrous tissue with low signal intensity on both T1- and T2-weighted images.

In reality, several classes of signal intensity changes are frequently seen in infarcted bone and, unlike radiographic staging, the MR classification system does not predict the likelihood of femoral head collapse. Instead, determining the location and percentage of

femoral head weight-bearing surface involved by AVN has proven important.[120,122] In order to predict the probability of femoral head collapse in hips affected by AVN, Shimizu et al[123] evaluated 66 hips in 50 patients by plain radiographs and MRI for an average of 44 months. Affected hips were in the early stages of AVN prior to collapse. By 32 months, 21 (74%) of the femoral heads had collapsed when AVN affected more than two-thirds of the weight-bearing surface area.

Without early recognition and treatment, the ultimate endpoint of AVN is secondary osteoarthritis eventually requiring joint replacement. Especially when involving the hip or knee joint, the diagnosis should be made before subchondral fracture or cartilage damage. Early diagnosis of AVN, however, can be difficult. Before the characteristic findings are seen, early AVN can manifest as bone marrow edema with low signal intensity on T1-weighted images and intermediate to high signal intensity on T2-weighted images. Bone marrow edema is, however, nonspecific and can be seen with other entities such as stress fracture, transient osteoporosis, infection or tumor.[114]

An entity that warrants specific mention is spontaneous osteonecrosis of the knee (SONK). This form of osteonecrosis is characterized clinically by the abrupt onset of pain in a person who lacks the typical risk factors associated with atraumatic osteonecrosis. Several features differentiate SONK from classic osteonecrosis of the knee. For example, SONK is seen in older patients, usually greater than 60 years of age. Women are affected three times more frequently than men. Spontaneous osteonecrosis is usually limited to one femoral condyle or one tibial plateau and the medial side of the joint (weight-bearing portion) is more commonly affected.[124] On MRI, a linear focus of decreased T1- and T2-weighted signal is present within the subchondral bone surrounded by extensive marrow edema.[125,126]

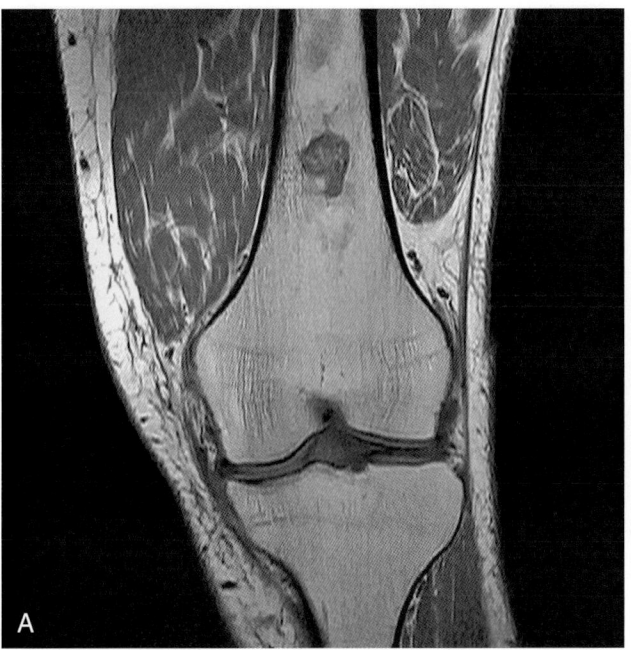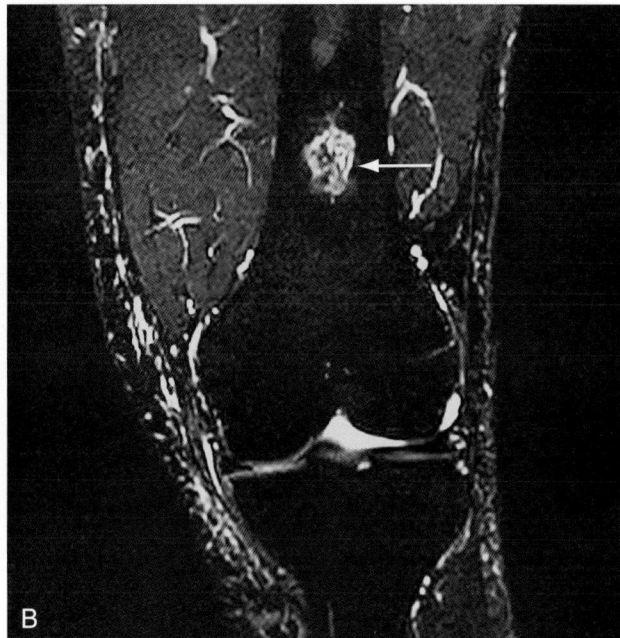

FIGURE 108-14

Bone infarct. **A,** Coronal T1-weighted image, distal femur. There is a geographic area of abnormal signal intensity within the metadiaphyseal region. A peripheral serpiginous low signal intensity rim is present. **B,** Coronal T2-weighted fat-suppressed image, distal femur. The same area is of heterogeneous signal intensity centrally. The border of the lesion is formed by two lines: an outer low signal intensity line and an inner high signal intensity line. The outer low signal intensity line is not well seen due to fat suppression (*arrow*). The inner T2-hyperintense rim is seen along the superior and lateral aspects of the lesion. This rim represents the double line sign of osteonecrosis.

The etiology of SONK remains unclear. Currently it is thought to be due to a subchondral insufficiency fracture with subsequent osteonecrosis between the fracture line and the subchondral bone. The fact that SONK occurs suddenly within the weight-bearing aspect of the joint in elderly (usually osteoporotic) individuals supports this theory.[125,126]

Marrow Proliferative Disorders

Bone marrow abnormalities may be the first indication of a focal or systemic disorder. Careful evaluation of bone marrow is necessary. MR images showing obvious marrow signal abnormalities pose little diagnostic difficulty but if signal alterations are more subtle, deciding whether or not a malignant process exists can be challenging. Hematopoietic (red) marrow, with its patchy appearance and variable signal intensity, can simulate a disease process. To differentiate normal red marrow from a pathologic process, the distribution and intensity of the signal changes should be carefully evaluated. As discussed earlier, normal hematopoietic marrow has a characteristic distribution based on age and functional status. A thorough knowledge of this pattern is essential, as any variation can represent disease. For example, if what appears to be normal red marrow is present in areas where none should exist, such as within the peripheral appendicular skeleton

or within the epiphyses/apophyses of an adult, an abnormality may be present. In processes with low tumor burden, these changes may be quite subtle and without significant alterations in signal intensity.[127] If the distribution of red marrow is normal, pathology can be identified with changes in signal intensity. Normal hematopoietic marrow is of intermediate T1- and T2-weighted signal, similar to muscle. The signal intensity of muscle can be used as an internal control; a pathologic process may exist if the red marrow signal intensity is greater than that of muscle.[113]

To complicate matters, a normal appearance of the bone marrow does not necessarily exclude pathology and diffuse signal changes do not necessarily indicate a malignant process. In 10% to 20% of patients with marrow infiltration by leukemia or myeloma, the MR appearance remains normal.[128] Diffuse signal changes can be the result of relatively benign red marrow hyperplasia. Red marrow hyperplasia can occur in response to alterations in lifestyle (athletics, smoking, and obesity), chronic anemias (sickle cell disease or thalassemia) or in patients using granulocyte colony-stimulating factor as seen with modern chemotherapy regimens.

Marrow proliferative disorders are processes that result from the proliferation of cells that normally exist within the marrow. They affect the bone marrow in a diffuse manner. Such disorders include polycythemia vera, myeloid metaplasia with myelofibrosis, mastocytosis, multiple myeloma, and leukemia.

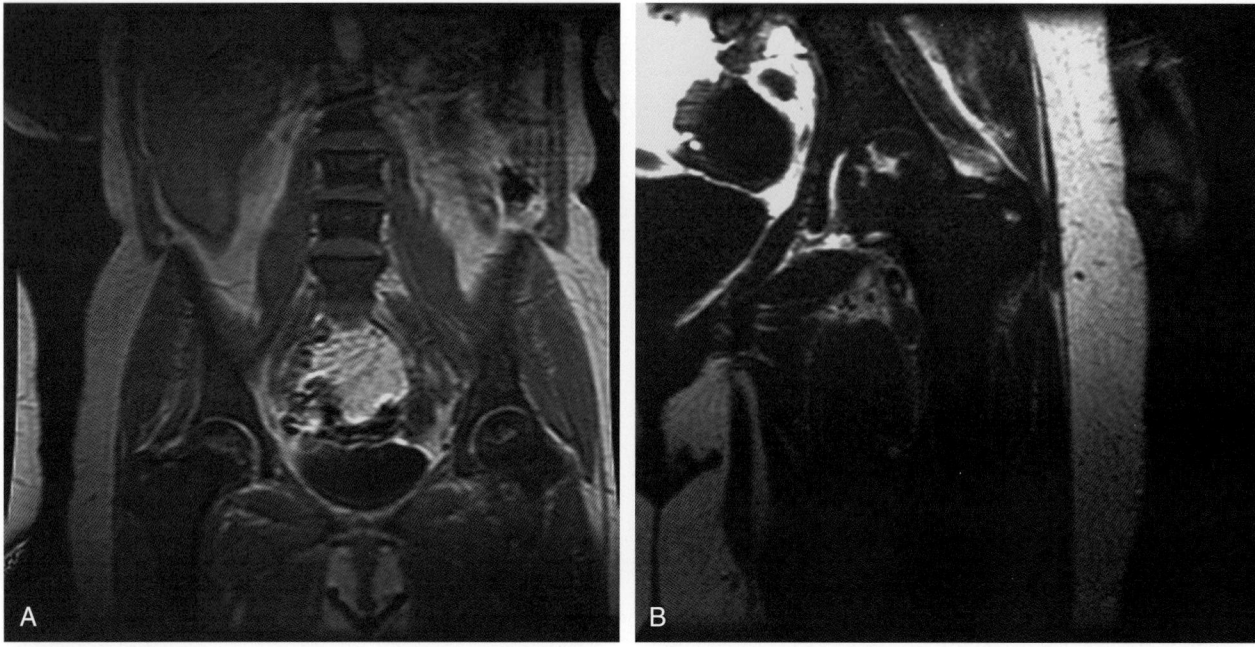

FIGURE 108-15

Myelofibrosis. **A,** Coronal T1-weighted image, pelvis. There is diffuse abnormal decreased signal intensity within the lumbar spine, pelvis, and both proximal femurs. Note that the marrow is lower in signal intensity than muscle and intervertebral disks. **B,** Coronal T1-weighted image, hip. In the same patient, there is diffuse abnormal low attenuation within the visualized femur and pelvis. There is a small remnant of normal bone marrow within the femoral head.

Polycythemia Vera and Myeloid Metaplasia with Myelofibrosis

Polycythemia vera (PV) and myeloid metaplasia with myelofibrosis (MMM) are two of the four diseases that are grouped together as the myeloproliferative disorders. Both diseases affect older patients, usually during the 6th to 8th decades of life. At the root of each disorder is the malignant transformation of a pluripotent stem cell resulting in an uncontrolled expansion of all bone marrow elements (erythroid, myeloid, and megakaryocytic lineages). In polycythemia vera the erythroid cell line is primarily affected. Patients have an elevated red cell mass with typical hematocrit values above 54%. Such a high red cell mass can potentially result in stroke, myocardial infarction or venous thromboembolism. Myeloid metaplasia is also the result of clonal myeloproliferation. As a reaction to myeloproliferation, the levels of several fibrogenic and osteogenic cytokines are altered, resulting in bone marrow fibrosis. Marrow fibrosis can be so extensive as to completely obliterate the normal marrow space. In response, extramedullary hematopoiesis within the liver and spleen develops, resulting in marked hepatosplenomegaly.[129]

Polycythemia vera and myeloid metaplasia have similar MRI findings. The involved bone marrow is of diffusely intermediate signal intensity on T1-weighted images due to cellular infiltration. Myelofibrosis can occur with both diseases. Fibrotic marrow is of low signal intensity on all MR pulse sequences (Fig. 108-15). In patients with PV and MMM, Kaplan et al[130] demon- strated a correlation between MR imaging findings and certain clinical parameters of disease severity (serum lactate dehydrogenase (LDH) and cholesterol levels). Affected patients with non-fatty hypercellular marrow within the femoral epiphyses and greater trochanters had a higher level of serum LDH and lower levels of cholesterol compared to patients with normal appearing proximal femurs.

Mastocytosis

Mast cells are located within several different organs: skin, gastrointestinal tract, spleen, liver, and bone marrow. Systemic mastocytosis (SM) is a rare disease that usually affects adults and is characterized by the abnormal proliferation of mast cells. Radiographic abnormalities are seen in 70% of patients and range from osteoporosis, mixed lysis-sclerosis, to osteosclerosis. These findings typically involve the axial skeleton and can be focal or diffuse.

Though MRI is exquisitely sensitive in detecting the cellular infiltration of bone marrow, no pattern of infiltration is specific for mastocytosis. Spin-echo T1-weighted and STIR images demonstrate a wide variety of signal abnormalities ranging from normal to focally or diffusely heterogeneous. Late in the course of the disease, diffuse osteosclerosis may develop. When this occurs, the bone marrow appears hypointense on both T1- and T2-weighted images, similar to any other diffusely sclerotic disease process.[131-133]

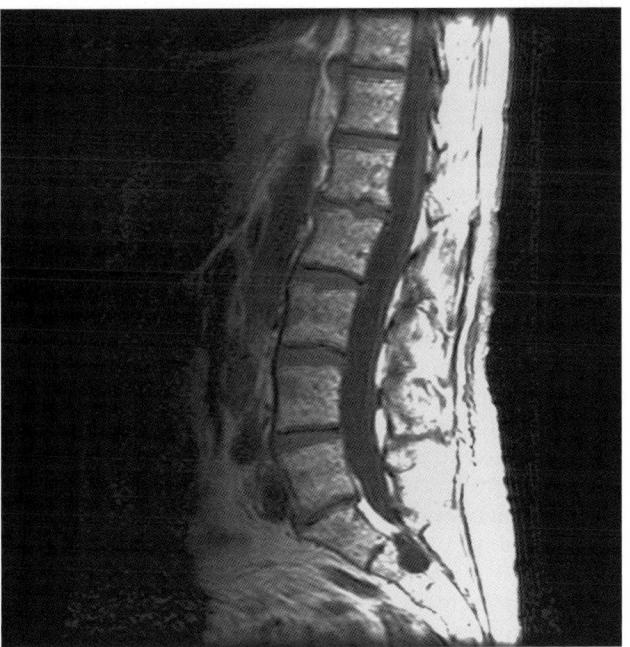

FIGURE 108-16

Variegated pattern of multiple myeloma. Sagittal T1-weighted image, lumbar spine. There are innumerable tiny foci of low signal intensity diffusely within the marrow.

Multiple Myeloma

Plasma cells, derived from B lymphocytes, are responsible for providing humoral immunity in the form of immunoglobulins. Plasma cell neoplasms are a group of diseases that result from the monoclonal proliferation of immunoglobulin-secreting cells. The spectrum of monoclonal gammopathies ranges from benign to malignant, depending on the amount of monoclonal protein detected in the blood and/or urine and the percentage of plasma cell marrow infiltration.

The relatively benign monoclonal gammopathies are further subdivided into monoclonal gammopathy of undetermined significance (MGUS) and monoclonal gammopathy of borderline significance. Affected patients are often serendipitously detected by routine blood analysis. They have no symptoms attributable to the disease and do not receive any specific form of treatment. Abnormal MR images are detected at a frequency of 19% and reveal two different patterns of marrow involvement: variegated and focal. The variegated pattern is characterized by the presence of innumerable tiny foci of low signal intensity on T1-weighted images (Fig. 108-16). The focal pattern demonstrates at least one area of well-defined low signal intensity on T1-weighted images, of high signal intensity on T2-weighted images, and of increased signal intensity on post-contrast images (Fig. 108-17). Patients with an abnormal MRI progress to more aggressive disease sooner and require treatment earlier than those with normal MRI findings.[134]

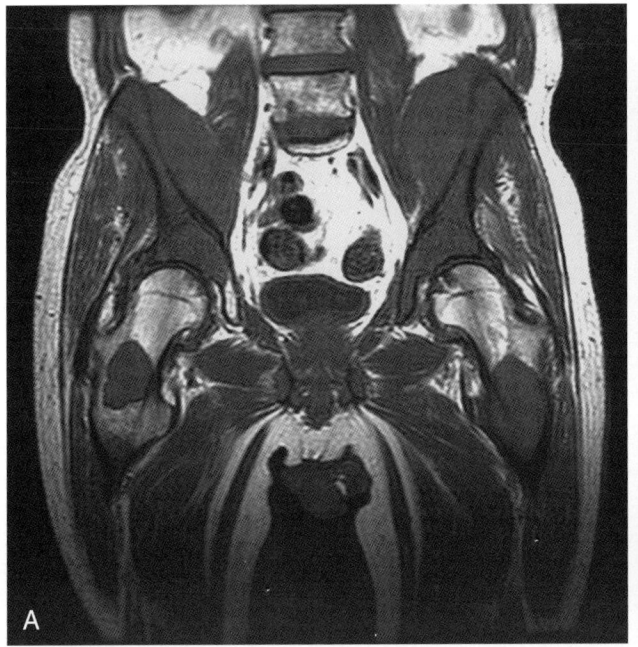
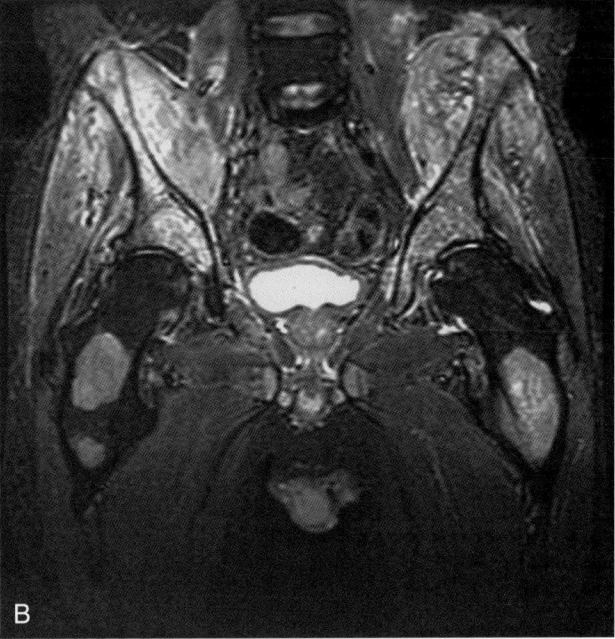

FIGURE 108-17

Multiple myeloma. **A,** Coronal T1-weighted image, pelvis. This 65-year-old patient with multiple myeloma demonstrates focal involvement of the proximal femurs bilaterally and more diffuse involvement of the pelvis. Abnormal areas are of low T1 signal intensity. **B,** Coronal T2-weighted fat-suppressed image, pelvis. The same abnormal areas are of increased T2 signal intensity. Extraosseous soft-tissue involvement surrounding the ilium bilaterally is manifested by increased signal intensity within the iliacus muscles.

Multiple myeloma (MM) represents a more aggressive form of monoclonal gammopathy. The malignant proliferation of plasma cells within the marrow space results in pain, anemia, osteoporosis, and eventually bone destruction. The classic presentation is low back pain in a patient over the age of 50. With increased screening for various diseases, multiple myeloma patients are more commonly discovered prior to the onset of symptoms.[135]

An important feature of the clinical staging system developed by Salmon and Durie is the number of lesions detected by radiographic skeletal survey (RSS). More than one documented lytic bone lesion by RSS indicates stage III disease and portends a poor prognosis with a median survival time of less than 2 years. Because MRI has been shown to be more sensitive than plain radiographs, it has been used to aid with lesion detection and staging. With early stage I multiple myeloma, the variegated and focal MRI patterns are seen, similar to patients with MGUS. Occasionally, a diffuse pattern of marrow replacement is seen with decreased T1- and variably increased T2-weighted signal intensity and post-contrast enhancement. Bone marrow changes are seen more often with stage I MM than with MGUS, with a frequency ranging from 29% to 36%.[136] Detecting marrow changes in patients with stage I MM has important prognostic significance. Patients with abnormalities detected by MRI have a significantly shorter time to disease progression than those with normal MRI exams.[137]

Stage III disease is assigned to patients with a greater tumor burden. These patients contend with lower hemoglobin values and a greater number of lytic bone lesions. At this stage, the focal and diffuse patterns of marrow involvement are more commonly seen by MRI.[138] In addition to diagnosis and staging, MRI can be used to detect complications. Vertebral compression fractures are often seen at the time of diagnosis and can be evaluated with MRI. Patients with greater than 10 focal lesions or a diffuse pattern of infiltration are six times more likely to develop vertebral compression fractures during the course of the disease.[139] In patients with neurologic symptoms, MR imaging can quickly and accurately detect spinal cord compression from an extraosseous mass arising from lytic lesions within the vertebral bodies. Permanent deficit can be avoided with prompt initiation of radiotherapy.[140]

Treatment of multiple myeloma is initiated with the onset of symptoms and involves various chemotherapy regimens. Response to treatment is usually assessed clinically by a decrease in myeloma protein levels and bone marrow plasmacytosis.[127] MR imaging provides a noninvasive means of evaluating patients post treatment. With complete response, MR images reveal one of two patterns: a total resolution of marrow abnormality, or persistent abnormality without enhancement or with peripheral rim enhancement.[141] In patients with a partial response, conversion of a diffuse to variegated or focal pattern and a decrease in the amount of marrow involvement with persistent enhancement are seen.[141] Currently, studies evaluating the response to treatment with dynamic contrast-enhanced MR imaging are being performed.

Leukemia

Leukemia is a condition that results in bone marrow infiltration by malignant clones of lymphoid or myeloid stem cells. The course of the disease may be acute or chronic but if left untreated, all cases are ultimately fatal. Diagnosis is made by laboratory analysis and bone marrow biopsy.[142]

Leukemic infiltration of bone marrow is a diffuse process, similar to other myeloproliferative disorders. In adults, chronic leukemias tend to involve areas of residual red marrow like the pelvis, proximal femurs, and spine. MR imaging of the vertebral bodies demonstrates homogeneous decreased T1-weighted signal intensity, often lower than that of the adjacent intervertebral disk. T2 signal intensity may be high, but this is not always the case. Because the cellularity and signal intensity of normal marrow are variable, differentiating normal from diseased marrow can be difficult. Without a complete understanding of the normal age-appropriate distribution of red marrow, leukemic infiltration can be overlooked. Involvement of the epiphysis or apophyses at any age is abnormal and may reflect a high tumor burden.

Initially, in response to chemotherapy, the bone marrow becomes hypocellular and edematous. With time, normal hematopoietic cells repopulate the area. Imaging at this time can be confusing as hematopoietic marrow regeneration can simulate disease relapse. The value of MRI in monitoring response to treatment remains controversial.[127]

Marrow Replacing Disorders

Marrow replacing disorders are processes in which cells of other origin come to occupy the marrow space. In contrast to marrow proliferative disorders, these abnormalities tend to affect the bone in a focal rather than diffuse manner. Examples include osteomyelitis, primary bone tumors, lymphoma, and metastatic disease.

Osteomyelitis

It is well documented that triple-phase bone scans are sensitive in the detection of uncomplicated osteomyelitis.[73,143-145] The specificity, however, is low, especially when there is superimposed neuropathic arthropathy, prior surgery or healing fractures.[73,146,147] The specificity may be greatly enhanced with the addition of either gallium 67 citrate or, more commonly, indium 111-labeled white blood cell studies to the triple-phase bone scan.[73,143] Unfortunately, the combined studies are costly as well as leading to high false-negative and -positive rates. In addition, these techniques do not give the spatial resolution necessary for presurgical planning, nor do they demonstrate soft-tissue abscess or sinus tracts.[143]

Although specific MR parameters vary with location of abnormality and age of patient, at our institution most osteomyelitis sequences include T1-weighted spin-echo short and long axis images, long axis STIR images, pre- and post-gadolinium injection images with fat suppression in short axis and either long axis or sagittal

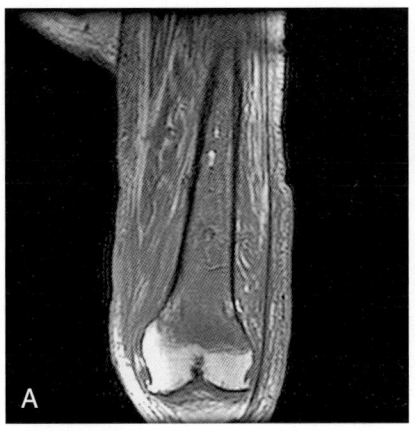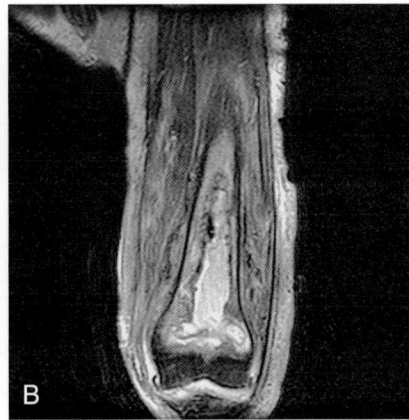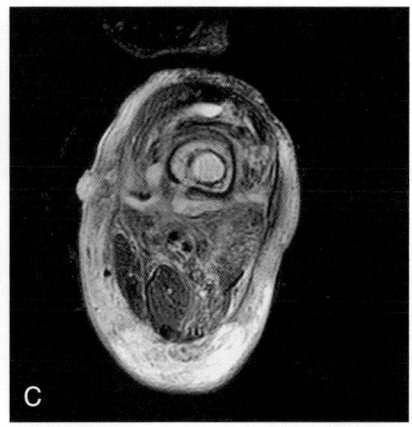

FIGURE 108-18

Osteomyelitis and abscess. **A,** Coronal T1-weighted image, distal femur. This is a 63-year-old woman with soft-tissue swelling about the thigh. There is marked decreased signal intensity within the diaphysis and metaphysis. **B,** Coronal T2-weighted fat-suppressed image, distal femur. The same area is hyperintense with fluid signal intensity within the distal diaphysis and metaphysis. The surrounding soft-tissues are edematous. **C,** Axial T2-weighted fat-suppressed image, distal femur. There is disruption of the posterior cortex due to osteomyelitis and abscess.

plane, as well as T2-weighted fat-suppressed fast spin-echo short axis images (time permitting).

The major MRI findings of osteomyelitis are due to replacement of marrow by edema, inflammatory cell infiltration, hemorrhage, fibrin, and debris. This will manifest as decreased signal on T1-weighted images with increased signal intensity on T2-weighted fat-suppressed images and STIR sequences (Fig. 108-18). The sensitivity of STIR sequences may actually lead to an overestimation of the true extent of infection within the marrow, especially if there is associated neuropathic disease or septic arthritis.[35,148,149] Overall accuracy in delineating the true extent of infection is increased by comparing these STIR sequences with post-gadolinium, fat-saturated T1-weighted pulse sequences.[35,150] Nearly all infected marrow will enhance, with the exception of a small border of sympathetic enhancement associated with osteitis. In this case the quantity of marrow enhancement, as well as the presence of abnormal T2 signal, helps to differentiate sympathetic enhancement from osteomyelitis.[35]

There are secondary signs that are helpful in increasing diagnostic accuracy and confidence when assessing for osteomyelitis.[148] These include cellulitis, cortical disruption, and periostitis. In diabetic or bedridden patients, the presence of soft-tissue ulceration or sinus tracts associated with the bone changes are critical elements in making the diagnosis. These will appear bright on T2-weighted pulse sequences.

The importance of adequate and homogeneous fat suppression cannot be overstated. This is particularly true when dealing with athletes and their post-traumatic bone marrow edema patterns, in addition to suspected cases of osteomyelitis. In the latter instance, in the best of circumstances, there is often postoperative metallic artifact present, particularly in the feet of diabetics, as well as multiple amputations and patient motion. If poor fat suppression is added to the equation, image interpretation is, to say the least, very difficult.

Benign and Malignant Primary Bone Tumors

Evaluation of benign or malignant bone tumors should begin with plain radiographs which are important to identify the presence and location of a lesion. They help to establish a lesion's aggressiveness by demonstrating cortical destruction, periosteal reaction, and soft-tissue mass development. Radiographs can aid in creating a differential diagnosis by showing calcifications and matrix mineralization. Subtle osseous findings can be better detected with CT scanning.

MRI of bone tumors is performed to supplement information provided by plain radiographs. With its multiplanar capabilities, MRI is best able to determine local extension of tumor. This information is critical for staging purposes. Tumors are assigned a higher stage if they have extended beyond the compartment of origin or have metastasized. MRI is also valuable in monitoring response to therapy.

Like other marrow replacing disorders, primary bone tumors affect the bone marrow in a focal manner (Fig. 108-19). The specific MR imaging characteristics of various bone marrow tumors are covered elsewhere.

Lymphoma

The lymphomas are a group of malignant neoplasms that arise in lymph nodes or extranodal lymphoid tissues. The two major subgroups are Hodgkin's disease and non-Hodgkin's lymphoma (NHL).[129] With widespread dissemination of disease, osseous involvement is not uncommon, occurring in 5% to 15% of patients with Hodgkin's disease and in 25% to 40% of patients with non-Hodgkin's lymphoma.[140] Clinical stage IV disease (Ann Arbor classification system) is assumed with bone marrow infiltration and is indicative of a poor prognosis.

Blind bone marrow biopsy or aspiration procedures, which are usually employed for the documentation of involvement, are subject to frequent errors due to the small sample size and the focal nature of marrow

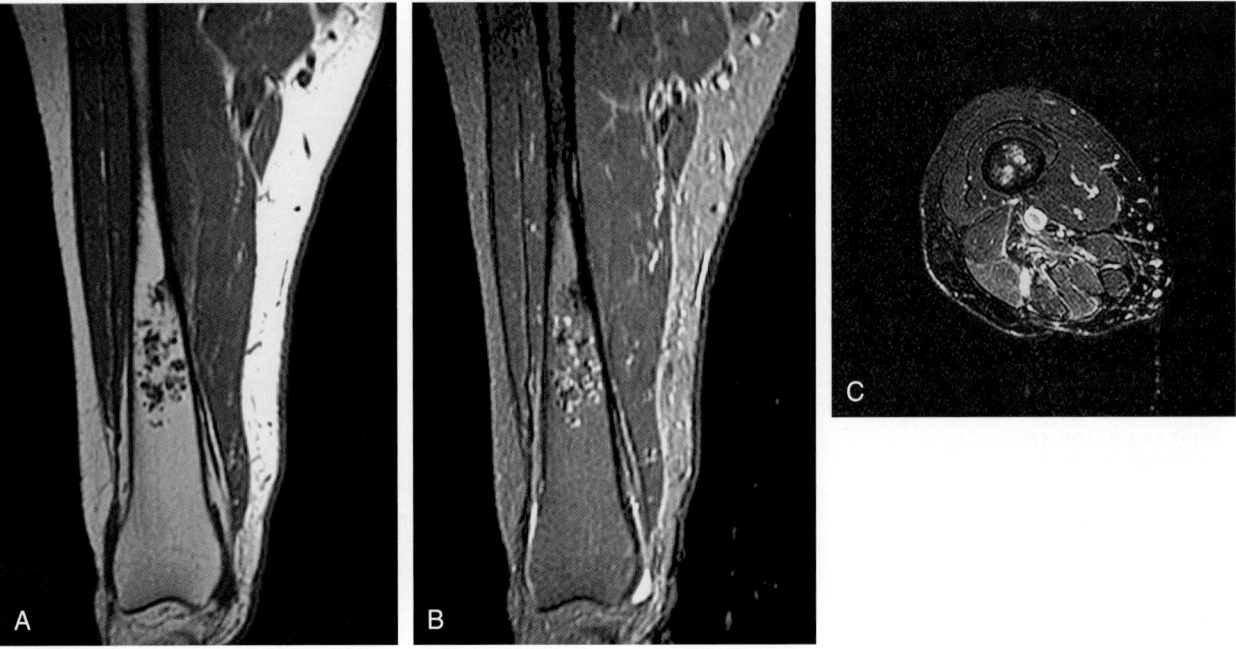

FIGURE 108-19

Enchondroma. **A,** Coronal T1-weighted image, distal femur. There is a large focal lesion within the femur that has a lobulated border. There are thin internal septations and foci of low signal intensity related to chondroid matrix. **B,** Coronal IR image, distal femur. The same lesion has foci of increased signal corresponding to cartilage. Note there is no surrounding bone marrow edema. **C,** Axial T2-weighted fat-suppressed image, femur. The area of increased signal intensity is seen within the central portion of the bone. There is no cortical destruction or associated soft-tissue mass.

involvement. Underestimation of disease could result in inadequate treatment of a potentially curable disease. To improve the yield of bone marrow biopsy, MRI can aid in selecting an appropriate biopsy site.

With its ability to assess larger volumes of marrow space, MRI is superior to bone marrow biopsy in detecting osseous infiltration by lymphoma. This has been shown to be the case with Hodgkin's disease, intermediate-grade NHL, and high-grade NHL.[151] Demonstrating infiltration by low-grade NHL with MRI can be more difficult, but femoral bone marrow imaging may improve detection. Patients with lymphoma and abnormal MRI findings within the femoral head bone marrow have an overall lower survival rate than patients with normal MRI findings.[152]

Primary lymphoma of the bone, unlike metastatic lymphoma, is a rare condition that accounts for less than 5% of all primary osseous malignancies. The majority of cases are of the non-Hodgkin's variety. MR images reveal a focal area of decreased T1-weighted signal intensity. Lesions have a variable appearance on T2-weighted images but are usually increased in signal intensity. A lesion can appear T2 hypointense if fibrosis is present. Moderate homogeneous enhancement is seen after contrast administration. While these imaging features are nonspecific, combining MRI with plain radiography can increase diagnostic accuracy. Especially in a person greater than 30 years old, the presence of a solitary, permeative metadiaphyseal lesion with a layered periosteal reaction on plain radiographs and a soft-tissue mass on MRI is highly suggestive of lymphoma.[153]

Metastatic Disease

Patients with a history of primary malignancy complaining of focal pain are initially evaluated with plain films and bone scan. Plain radiographs suffer from lack of sensitivity. Significant bony destruction must occur before a pathologic process can be identified. Radionuclide bone scans, while sensitive, lack specificity; degenerative changes or infection can mimic a metastatic deposit. MRI, with its superior sensitivity and specificity, is excellent for the evaluation of suspected metastatic disease. However, the high cost and length of the whole-body MRI screening have prevented its widespread use for this disease.

Bony metastatic disease is extremely common in adults with breast, prostate or lung cancer. Metastatic lesions are focal and usually multiple in number, but occasionally they may have a diffuse presentation. Most lesions are found within the well-vascularized red marrow space of the spine, pelvis, proximal shoulder, and hips (Figs. 108-20 and 108-21). On MRI, lesions can have a variable appearance but are generally of low T1-and high T2-weighted signal intensity. The adjacent bone marrow demonstrates some degree of edema (usually to a lesser extent than osteomyelitis or fracture) but this is not always required. Two signs have been described to assist with differentiating benign from metastatic disease. The "bull's eye" sign refers to a focus of high T1-weighted signal within the center of an osseous lesion and serves as a negative discriminator for metastasis. In contrast, the "halo" sign, a rim of high T2-weighted signal surrounding an osseous lesion, is a

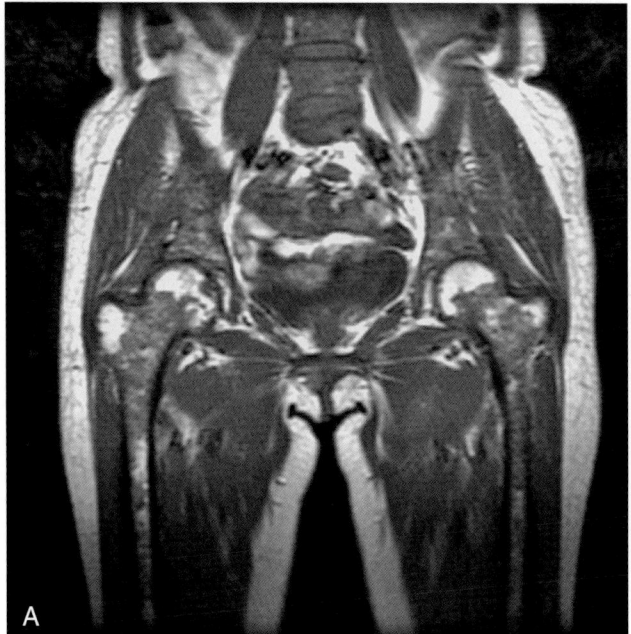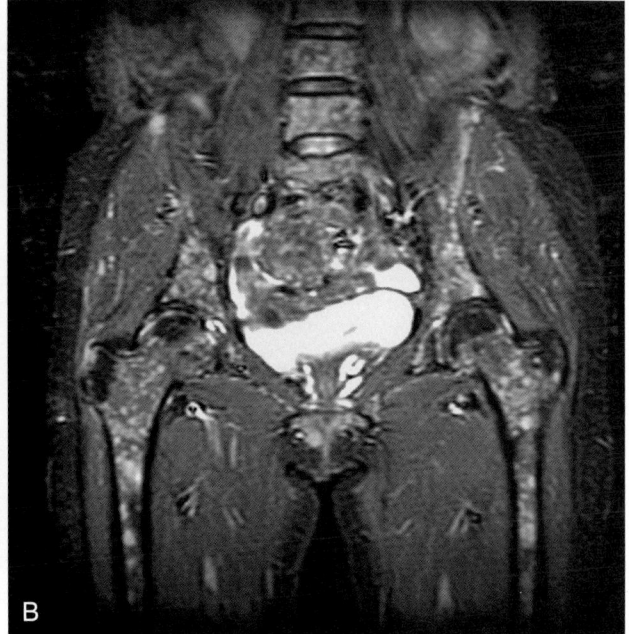

FIGURE 108-20

Diffuse osseous metastases. **A,** Coronal T1-weighted image, pelvis. Diffuse abnormal decreased signal intensity is present within the proximal femurs bilaterally, the pelvis, and within the lower lumbar spine. Portions of both femoral heads and greater trochanters have been spared. **B,** Coronal T2-weighted fat-suppressed image, pelvis. The same areas are of heterogeneous increased signal intensity.

strong indicator of metastatic disease.[154] Sclerotic metastases are commonly of decreased T1- and T2-weighted signal intensity (Fig. 108-22).

Contrast-enhanced images increase lesion conspicuity and, in cases of a solitary lesion, improve diagnostic specificity. Studies using dynamic contrast-enhanced MR imaging have shown that enhancement of metastatic lesions occurs sooner than in red marrow, a finding that can prove helpful in distinguishing the two entities.[155] Care should be taken when ascribing lesion enhancement to malignancy. Significant overlap exists between well-vascularized benign enhancing lesions and malignant lesions. In such cases, the patient's age, tumor site, and location of lesion within the bone are factors that may help with differentiation.[156] Because benign lesions such as bone islands, Paget's disease and hemangiomas can mimic metastatic disease, correlation with plain films should always be made.

Diffusion-weighted MR imaging with apparent diffusion coefficient (ADC) mapping is an additional tool helpful for differentiating benign from metastatic disease. Tissues densely packed with malignant cells demonstrate restricted diffusion capacity, resulting in increased signal intensity on DWI. Since T2 shine-through effects can be confused with true areas of restricted diffusion, apparent diffusion coefficients can be calculated to provide a more quantitative measurement of diffusion capacity. Herneth et al[157] calculated ADC in 22 patients with known or suspected vertebral metastases. The ADC for metastatic lesions measured lower than that of normal vertebral bodies (0.69×10^{-3} mm^2/s versus 1.66×10^{-3} mm^2/s). ADC mapping

consequently demonstrates low signal intensity within those vertebral bodies affected by metastatic disease as compared to normal ones. For greater accuracy, diffusion-weighted images should be evaluated in conjunction with ADC mapping.

Marrow Depleting Disorders

Aplastic Anemia

Aplastic anemia (AA), a failure of the bone marrow, can be due to an inherited defect, or an acquired insult to the stem cell line or local marrow environment. Though clinical differentiation may be difficult, an acquired etiology (infections, drugs or toxins) is the usual cause in up to 80% of cases. Congenital causes including Fanconi anemia, amegakaryocytic thrombocytopenia (thrombocytopenia-absent radius (TAR) syndrome), and Shwachman–Diamond syndrome are less common. Clinical and laboratory observatioins suggest that AA is an autoimmune process.[158]

CBC and peripheral smears demonstrate pancytopenia. Bone marrow aspirates reveal a paucity of hematopoietic elements with a varying degree of fat cell replacement. A specimen is considered hypocellular if it is either less than 30% cellular in individuals younger than 60 years old or less than 20% cellular in those greater than 60 years old. While spontaneous recovery with limited supportive therapy does occur, the disease often assumes a chronic form, requiring immunosuppressive therapy or bone marrow transplantation.[159]

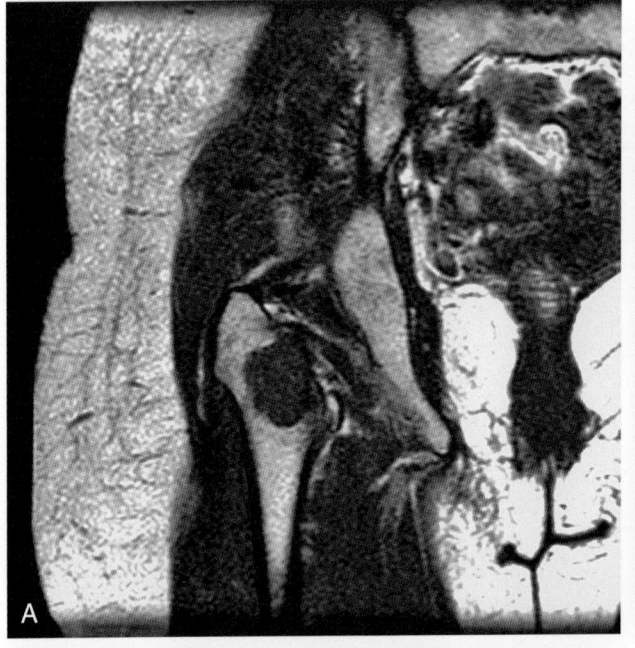

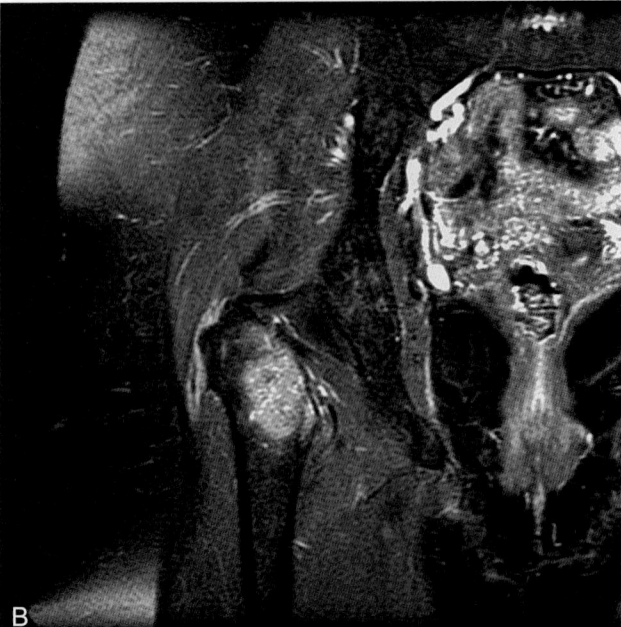

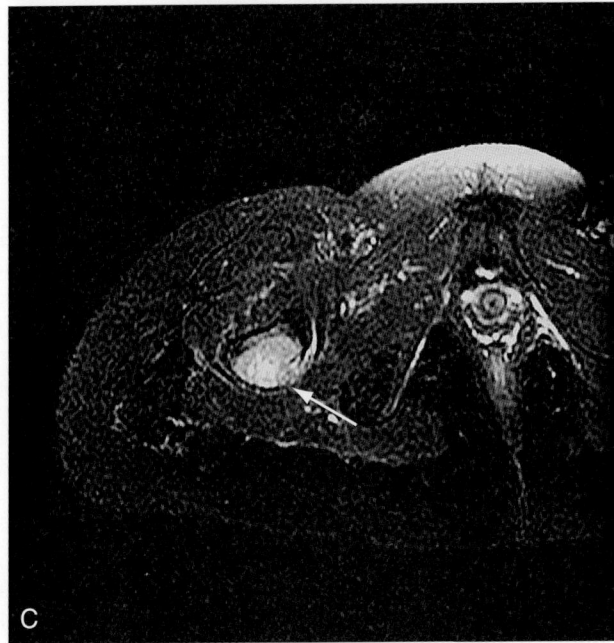

FIGURE 108-21

Focal osseous metastasis. **A,** Coronal T1-weighted image, hip. There is a focal ovoid-shaped area of decreased signal intensity within the intertrochanteric region of the femur. **B,** Coronal post-contrast T1-weighted fat-suppressed image, hip. The lesion demonstrates post-contrast enhancement. **C,** Axial T2-weighted fat-suppressed image, hip. Again, the lesion is of increased signal intensity. Medially, the low signal intensity cortex is discontinuous, indicating cortical destruction (*arrow*).

The MRI findings reflect the hypocellularity observed on bone marrow aspirates. The marrow is of diffusely increased signal on T1-weighted images, intermediate signal on T2-weighted images and dark on STIR and frequency-selective fat suppression pulse sequences. Recognizing the lack of hematopoietic marrow in areas where some should exist will help with diagnosing aplastic anemia.[159] The patient's age is also important. In an elderly person, the normally fat-predominant marrow can look similar to the diffusely abnormal pattern of aplastic anemia.[39]

The diffusely hyperintense marrow seen with aplastic anemia may be disrupted by foci of low T1-weighted signal. These foci may represent residual hematopoietic marrow or responses to therapy.[160] Alternatively they may signify the development of myelodysplastic syndrome or leukemia. Care should therefore be taken to avoid misinterpreting foci of regenerating hematopoietic marrow for clonal disease in patients with aplastic anemia who respond to treatment.[140]

Supportive therapy of patients with aplastic anemia frequently includes blood transfusions. This piece of history should be obtained prior to interpreting MR images. Excess iron deposition within the reticuloendothelial system, hemosiderosis, occurs with repeated blood transfusions. As a result, signal intensity on T1- and

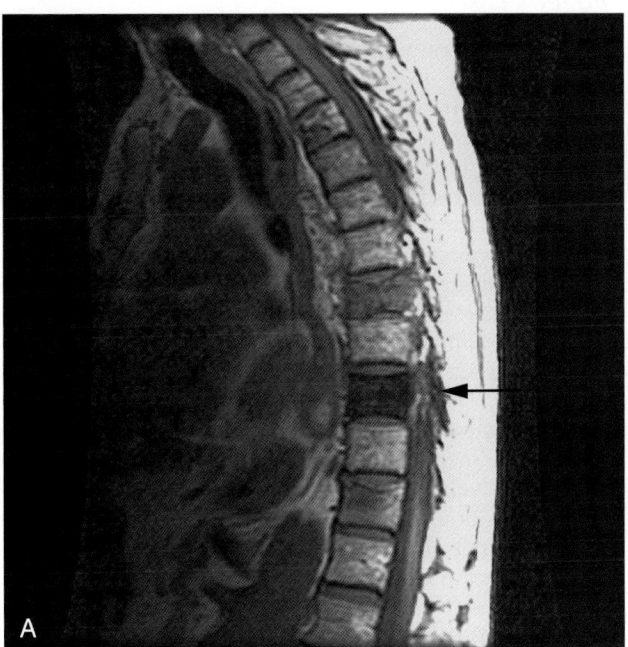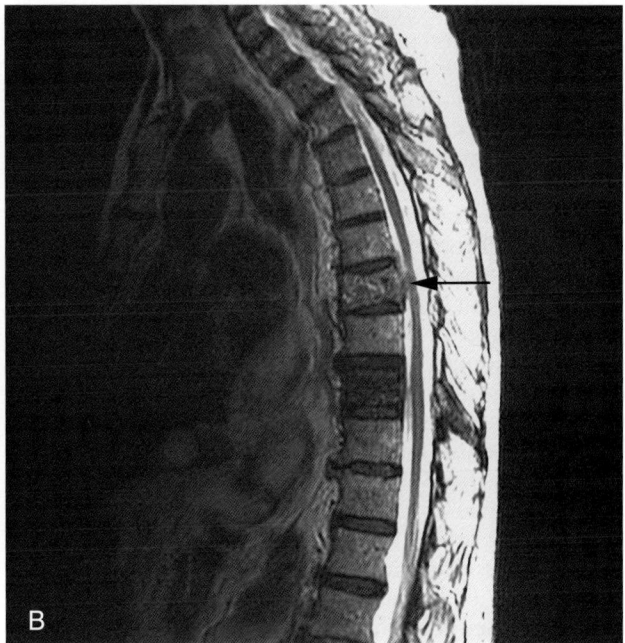

FIGURE 108-22

Vertebral metastases. **A,** Sagittal T1-weighted image, thoracic spine. Several upper and mid-thoracic vertebral bodies are of abnormal low signal intensity. One mid-thoracic vertebral body is of extremely low signal intensity (*arrow*). **B,** Sagittal T2-weighted image, thoracic spine. The same areas are of slightly increased signal intensity with the exception of the extremely low signal mid-thoracic vertebral body. This pattern of very low signal intensity on both T1- and T2-weighted images can be seen with a densely sclerotic metastasis. Note slight retropulsion of posterior aspect of the vertebral body due to tumor (*arrow*).

T2-weighted images is decreased, making the characteristic findings of untreated aplastic anemia difficult to appreciate.[140]

Chemotherapy

The histologic changes that occur within bone marrow post chemotherapy have been studied.[161] Chemotherapy works systemically, destroying both normal hematopoietic marrow and tumor cells. Within the first week of treatment, the marrow becomes hypocellular and edematous. This manifests as decreased T1- and increased T2-weighted signal intensity. After the first week, fat cells begin to arise within the marrow. The bone marrow becomes progressively hyperintense on T1-weighted images, an appearance similar to that of untreated aplastic anemia.[140,162,163] If the signal is not diffusely T1 hyperintense, consider treatment failure, relapse of disease or the use of hematopoietic growth factors, i.e., G-CSF.[164]

Radiation Therapy

The effects of radiation-induced changes of the bone marrow can be divided into acute and chronic. Acutely, radiation therapy (RT) causes edema, vascular congestion, and capillary injury.[45] Hemorrhage is also frequently seen in the acute setting. In the chronic phase, bone marrow is devoid of vascularity and hematopoietic cells and is replaced by fat.

The MR appearance of irradiated bone marrow depends upon the phase in which it was imaged. Stevens et al[45] studied signal intensity changes within lumbar bone marrow in 14 patients with various malignancies following therapy with 1500 to 5000 rads (15 to 50 Gy). Within the first 2 weeks, increased signal was seen on STIR MR images, almost certainly reflecting early edema and necrosis. Though no signal changes were appreciated on spin-echo T1-weighted images in this study, other investigators have shown slightly increased signal intensity. This early finding may be due to hemorrhage within the marrow space or very early fatty replacement.[165,166] Between weeks 3 and 6, T1-weighted images demonstrated a heterogeneous signal. Chronic changes of irradiation were seen 6 weeks to 14 months following initiation of therapy. This consisted of either the typical homogeneous pattern of increased T1 signal intensity seen with fat replacement or a band pattern of peripheral intermediate signal intensity, possibly representing hematopoietic marrow, surrounding the central marrow fat.[45] The characteristic finding of chronic RT is that of bright marrow signal that is sharply limited to the radiation portal.

Otake et al[166] studied the temporal changes in contrast enhancement of irradiated bone marrow using dynamic contrast material-enhanced imaging. Twenty-three patients who were treated with RT were prospectively evaluated with MR studies: before RT, 2 and 4 weeks after initiation of RT, and 4 weeks after completion of RT. The changes that occurred 2 weeks after the initiation of RT most likely reflected acute radiation effects. During the acute phase, a transient increase in contrast enhancement was observed within the RT field. This may be related to the dilatation of the sinusoids seen histologically during the acute phase. During the chronic phase (those images obtained at 4 and 8 weeks) there was a significant decrease in marrow contrast enhancement when compared to pre-treatment images. This decrease in contrast enhancement was thought to reflect the decreased cellularity, decreased vascularity, and increased fatty content.

Evaluation of post-radiation therapy images requires knowledge of the radiation dose to the affected bone and the time interval between treatment and imaging. For doses equal to or greater than 30 to 40 Gy, the characteristic bright appearance of irradiated bone is non-reversible. Chronic microvascular changes prevent the migration of hematopoietic cells into the radiation field. For doses less than 30 Gy, regeneration of the marrow may occur 1 year after radiation therapy. This should not be confused with tumor recurrence.[140]

Miscellaneous

Osteopetrosis

This skeletal disease represents a group of inherited disorders characterized by a defect in osteoclast function that results in increased bone density. The accumulation of sclerotic bone within the marrow space narrows cranial nerve foramina and predisposes to pathologic fractures.[167] Clinically, the types of osteopetrosis include a severe autosomal recessive form, an intermediate autosomal recessive form, and two relatively benign autosomal dominant types.[168]

The autosomal recessive type (infantile form) is usually fatal within the first few years of life. Affected patients suffer from repeated infections, cranial nerve neuropathies or bone marrow failure. MR imaging demonstrates markedly low signal intensity on T1- and T2-weighted pulse sequences corresponding to diffuse osteosclerosis. This appearance is not pathognomonic of osteopetrosis however; other processes such as hemosiderosis, diffuse metastatic disease or fibrosis may have similar findings.[169] In this form of osteopetrosis the obliteration of normal marrow spaces by sclerotic bone results in an atypical distribution of hematopoietic cells. In infants, marrow stores are shifted to the skull base and to the ends of long bones. And for patients aged 3 to 5 years, red marrow relocates to the diaphyseal segment of long bones and the calvarium. These hemato-poietically active regions of high T2 signal intensity stand out against the background of diffusely hypointense sclerotic bone.[170]

The more benign autosomal dominant form of osteo-petrosis is often incidentally diagnosed and is associated with a normal lifespan. Patients may present with pathol-ogic fractures that are readily identified by MR imaging.[168]

Paget's Disease

Exceedingly common, Paget's disease affects approx-imately 3% to 4% of the population over the age of 40 and up to 10% to 11% over the age of 80. The disease is characterized by excessive osteoclast resorption followed by ineffectual bone remodeling. Pathologically there are three distinct phases: the lytic phase, the mixed phase, and the blastic phase. The radiographic mani-festations reflect the stage of the disease.[171]

Paget's disease is most frequently imaged during the mixed phase. The MR imaging characteristics of this phase are similar to plain radiographs, demonstrating bony enlargement and thickening of the cortex and trabeculae. The normal bone marrow signal intensity is typically maintained.[172] During the lytic to early mixed phase, the marrow space signal is heterogeneous on T1- and T2-weighted images. On T1-weighted images, the marrow is of decreased signal intensity, but contains scattered foci of normal bright marrow. Observation of these foci is an important clue that excludes malig-nant transformation (Fig. 108-23).[171,173,174] Compared to normal, pagetic bone demonstrates increased gadolinium enhancement, often in a "speckled" pattern. This finding reflects the increased metabolic activity seen during the active phase of disease.[175] Finally, during the late blastic (inactive) phase, the marrow space has low signal intensity on all pulse sequences, corresponding to the bony sclerosis seen on plain radiographs.

Sarcomatous degeneration is a rare complication, occurring in approximately 1% of patients with long-standing disease. Clinically patients may experience new focal pain and swelling. MR images show masslike marrow replacement, cortical destruction, and soft-tissue masses.[171,175,176]

Iron Storage Disorders

MR imaging is useful to detect the presence and severity of iron overload states. Primary hemochromatosis is a genetic disorder characterized by increased intestinal iron absorption despite normal intake. Excess iron is deposited within parenchymal cells of the liver, heart, pancreas, and other organs. As iron deposition increases, parenchymal damage occurs, resulting in organ failure. In contrast, hemosiderosis is a condition in which excess iron is deposited within the reticuloendothelial (RE) cells of the liver, spleen, and bone marrow. The iron (hemosiderin) can be derived from chronic red blood cell hemolysis (sickle cell anemia, thalassemia) or multiple blood transfusions.[177]

Tissues overloaded by iron are of extremely low T1 and T2 signal intensity on standard spin-echo pulse sequences. This finding is accentuated on T2-weighted gradient-echo (GRE) images by a blooming effect. The GRE pulse sequence is more sensitive to the field inhomogeneities induced by paramagnetic substances, allowing for smaller amounts of parenchymal iron deposition to be detected.[178]

Evaluating the pattern of iron deposition may be helpful in distinguishing hemosiderosis from primary hemochromatosis. In hemosiderosis, iron is primarily deposited within the reticuloendothelial cells of the

171. Smith SE, Murphey MD, Motamedi K, et al: From the archives of the AFIP: radiologic spectrum of Paget disease of bone and its complications with pathologic correlation. Radiographics 22:1191-1216, 2002.

172. Roberts MC, Kressel HY, Fallon MD, et al: Paget disease: MR imaging findings. Radiology 173:341-345, 1989.

173. Tins BJ, Davies AM, Mangham DC: MR imaging of pseudosarcoma in Paget's disease of bone: a report of two cases. Skeletal Radiol 30:161-165, 2001.

174. Sundaram M, Khanna G, El-Khoury GY: T1-weighted MR imaging for distinguishing large osteolysis of Paget's disease from sarcomatous degeneration. Skeletal Radiol 30:378-383, 2001.

175. Greditzer HG, McLeod RA, Unni KK, et al: Bone sarcomas in Paget disease. Radiology 146:327-333, 1983.

176. Boutin RD, Spitz DJ, Newman JS, et al: Complications in Paget disease at MR imaging. Radiology 209:641-651, 1998.

177. Kornreich L, Horev G, Yaniv I, et al: Iron overload following bone marrow transplantation in children: MR findings. Pediatr Radiol 27:869-872, 1997.

178. Sparacia G, Iaia A, Banco A, et al: Transfusional hemochromatosis: quantitative relation of MR imaging pituitary signal intensity reduction to hypogonadotropic hypogonadism. Radiology 215:818-823, 2000.

179. Charrow J, Esplin JA, Gribble TJ, et al: Gaucher's disease: recommendations on diagnosis, evaluation, and monitoring. Arch Intern Med 158:1754-1760, 1998.

180. Maas M, Poll LW, Terk MR: Imaging and quantifying skeletal involvement in Gaucher's disease. Br J Radiol 75:A13-A24, 2002.

181. Maas M, Hollak CEM, Akkerman EM, et al: Quantification of skeletal involvement in adults with type I Gaucher's disease: fat fraction measured by Dixon quantitative chemical shift imaging as a valid parameter. Am J Roentgenol 179:961-965, 2002.

182. Negendank W, Soulen RL: Magnetic resonance imaging in patients with bone marrow disorders. Leukemia Lymphoma 10:287-298, 1993.

183. Stevens SK, Moore SG, Amylon MD: Repopulation of marrow after transplantation: MR imaging with pathologic correlation. Radiology 175:213-218, 1990.

184. Tanner SF, Clarke J, Leach MO, et al: MRI in the evaluation of late bone marrow changes following bone marrow transplantation. Br J Radiol 69:1145-1151, 1996.

185. Chim CS, Ooi C, Ma SK, et al: Bone marrow necrosis in bone marrow transplantation: the role of MR imaging. Bone Marrow Transplant 22:1125-1128, 1998.

CARTILAGE

Mark H. Awh ● Deborah Burstein ● Michael E. Stadnick

INTRODUCTION

The growth of surgical and pharmacologic treatment capabilities for cartilage disorders has significantly increased interest in the accurate diagnosis and evaluation of cartilage abnormalities. At the same time, cartilage injury due to acute trauma and cartilage degeneration associated with an aging population have led to an increased incidence of osteoarthritis. At arthroscopy, over 60% of knees are found to have cartilage injury, and as many as 4% of patients have full-thickness cartilage defects.[1] In the United States alone, total knee arthroplasty in now performed over 150,000 times a year.[2] Lost wages and productivity related to cartilage disabilities and treatment costs related to cartilage injury continue to grow. The economic impact of cartilage disease is obviously substantial. Osteoarthritis is now the second leading cause of disability in the United States,[3] trailing only cardiovascular disease. These converging trends in therapy and epidemiology have placed MR in a position of great importance in the modern medical approach to articular cartilage disorders.

Traditionally, plain radiographs have served as the initial approach in the diagnosis of cartilage disorders. Radiography, of course, only assesses cartilage indirectly, visualizing joint space narrowing, and radiographs are typically insensitive for early or mild cartilage abnormalities. Radionuclide bone scans are effective for the detection of the increased osteoblastic activity that occurs with osteoarthritis, but also rely on indirect effects for evaluation of articular cartilage. MR allows direct visualization of cartilage morphology, and with newer techniques, provides insight into the biochemistry and physiology of articular cartilage. MR's ability to non-invasively detect abnormalities and to more accurately characterize lesions has led to its status as the preferred diagnostic modality for the evaluation of articular cartilage.

STRUCTURE AND BIOCHEMISTRY OF ARTICULAR CARTILAGE

Articular cartilage is a remarkable substance, with unique biochemical and structural properties. This smooth, white, glistening material is perfectly sculpted to match the bone it covers, as well as the congruent surface of its apposing bone. Despite being very thin, a layer of articular cartilage is capable of remaining healthy and functional throughout a lifetime, absorbing extraordinary forces. The force placed upon cartilage at the knee with each step has been described as equal to the "amount of compression that would be exerted on the skin if a 300-lb person were to hang from a ledge on a fingertip."[4] Compared to other soft-tissues, articular cartilage may appear inert, particularly in light of the very low cellular volume (<10% of the tissue volume), and its lack of blood vessels, nerves, or lymphatics. Yet despite its low metabolic activity, cartilage is not a static structure, and its form and function depend upon its dynamic response to the forces placed upon it.

Articular cartilage serves several vital purposes in the function of a healthy diarthrodial joint.[5-7] The compressive forces upon weight-bearing joints are substantial, and cartilage acts to evenly distribute these forces upon underlying subchondral bone, thus decreasing peak stresses upon the joint. Perhaps more importantly, healthy articular cartilage provides a near frictionless gliding surface for the apposed motion of the joint components. Indeed, the coefficient of friction for articular

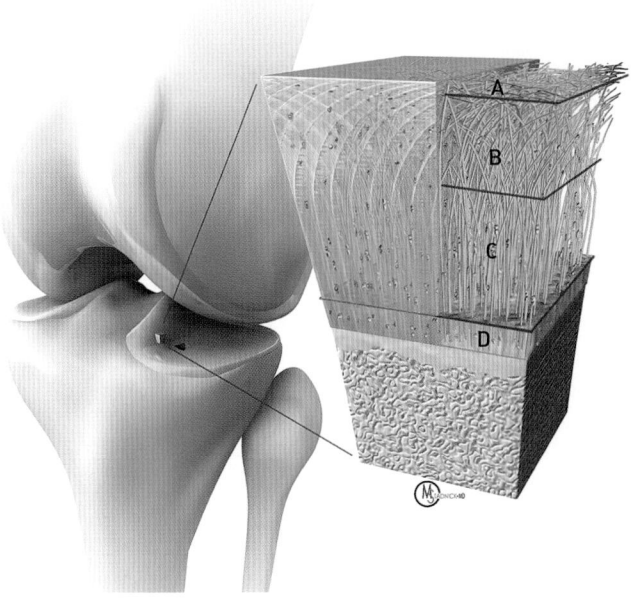

FIGURE 109-1

Three-dimensional representation of the zonal anatomy of articular cartilage at the tibial plateau. **A,** Superficial zone with collagen fibers parallel to the articular surface; **B,** transitional zone with arclike collagen fibers; **C,** radial zone containing collagen fibers that course perpendicular to the subchondral bone; and **D,** calcified zone separated from the adjacent radial zone by the tidemark.

cartilage has been calculated as less than that of ice gliding on ice.[8]

Although cartilage often appears homogeneous both grossly and on MR images, histologically and biochemically its structure is quite complex.[9,10] Articular cartilage is frequently divided into four zones (Fig. 109-1),[11] with each having a distinct composition. At the surface, a thin superficial zone contains collagen fibers that are oriented parallel to the articular surface. Below this level, the transitional zone has larger collagen fibrils that run in an arc-like configuration. The radial zone is the largest, and contains collagen fibrils that course perpendicular to the subchondral bone. These fibrils are embedded in the last layer, a calcified zone of cartilage that binds articular cartilage to subchondral bone. The calcified layer contains the tidemark, a region that straddles the boundary between calcified and noncalcified cartilage, and which serves as a preferential shear plane in the development of adult cartilage defects. In general, the collagen content of hyaline cartilage decreases slightly from the superficial zone to the tidemark.

The only cellular component of articular cartilage is the chondrocyte, which is responsible for the production and maintenance of extracellular matrix, the latter comprising approximately 90% of cartilage volume. The extracellular matrix is itself made up of water, its largest constituent, and the macromolecules collagen, proteoglycan, and glycoprotein, as well as other small macromolecules.[8] Greater than 90% of collagen within hyaline cartilage is type 2, whereas type 1 collagen predominates in fibrocartilage.[6] The major role of collagen within articular cartilage is to provide tensile strength. Mesh-

works of collagen define the shape of the articular cartilage, but collagen alone is unable to bear weight. This ability is provided by the proteoglycans. The best-known and most abundant proteoglycan in articular cartilage is aggrecan, a complex macromolecule consisting of a protein backbone attached to chondroitin sulfate and keratin sulfate. These individual aggrecan monomers in turn attach in large groups to hyaluronic acid, forming high molecular weight aggregates that become trapped in the collagen matrix (Fig. 109-2A). Because they contain multiple negatively charged carboxyl and sulfate groups, mobile ions distribute in cartilage in relation to the concentration of the proteoglycans; in turn the distribution of mobile ions impacts the distribution of water in the tissue. This interaction between proteoglycans and water accounts for much of the stiffness and resilience of articular cartilage. The last macromolecular component of the extracellular matrix, the glycoproteins and other small macromolecules, assists in the structural organization and maintenance of the matrix and the chondrocytes.

The complex and variable interplay between proteoglycans, water, and the collagen network accounts for the unique physical properties of articular cartilage.[12-14] With load bearing, articular cartilage actually compresses, causing extrusion of water from articular cartilage, with resultant compaction of the solid matrix (Figs. 109-2B and C). The solid matrix confers a resistance to water movement, resulting in resistance to further compression. In addition, the increased negative charge density of the compressed aggrecans acts as a second resistor to external force. When external loads are removed, such as at rest, cartilage swells to its fullest, bound only by the tensile strength of the collagen network. Cartilage is thus able to act as a biological shock absorber, changing its shape and resistance to deformation in response to the external forces placed upon it.

The structural design and function of articular cartilage is impressive, but is offset by a major weakness—the limited ability of articular cartilage to heal. After skeletal maturity, chondrocytes continue to synthesize and recycle aggrecans, but the collagen network is relatively static. When the collagen network is damaged (through biological or mechanical events), chondrocytes adjacent to the injury have a very limited ability to respond. With disruption of the collagen network, corresponding decreases in aggrecan and increases in water content occur.[15] These changes in the normal structural relationships hinder the ability of cartilage to respond to external stress, and a vicious cycle leading to further cartilage damage ensues. The structural and biochemical changes in articular cartilage following injury not only account for the physiologic behavior of damaged articular cartilage, but also help explain the appearance of damaged cartilage on MR images.

MR OF NORMAL ARTICULAR CARTILAGE

To optimize the ability to diagnose cartilage disorders with MR, an accurate understanding of the MR appearance of normal articular cartilage must be obtained.

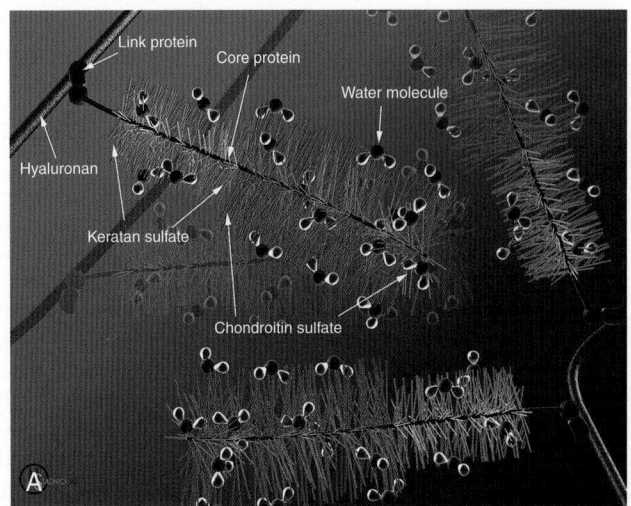

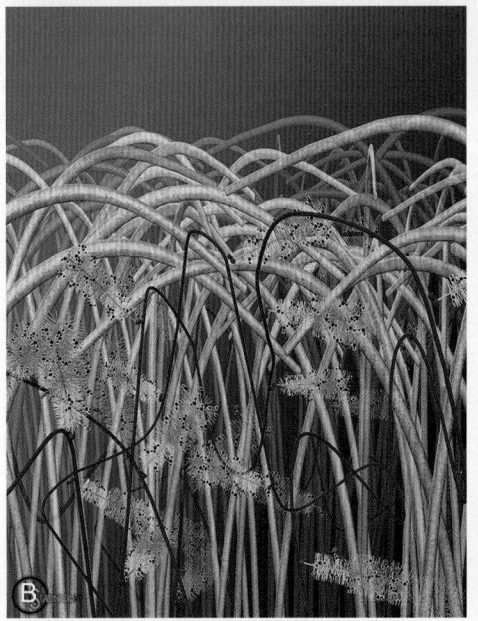

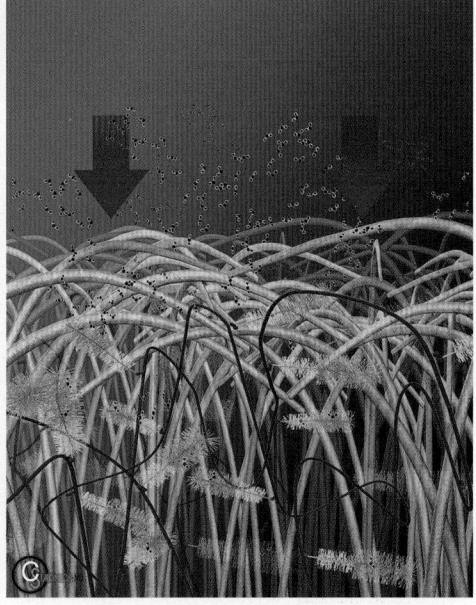

FIGURE 109-2

Structure and function of aggrecan. **A,** Each aggrecan monomer is composed of highly hydrophilic chondroitin sulfate and keratan sulfate chains attached to a protein backbone. Link proteins help bind multiple aggrecan monomers to hyaluronic acid, which in turn weaves through the collagen network. **B,** At rest, the presence of aggrecans within the collagen network results in osmotic swelling; the degree of swelling is limited by the tensile strength of the collagen network. **C,** With compression, water is "squeezed" from the cartilage matrix, resulting in compression of cartilage until osmotic pressure and the repulsion caused by the increased negative charge density of the aggrecans equals the externally applied force.

Unfortunately, the MR appearance of normal articular cartilage, and more importantly, the reasons for the MR appearance, remain controversial.

In the early days of MR, articular cartilage was somewhat poorly seen and felt to display homogeneous signal characteristics. Today, even modern systems utilizing routine pulse sequences may display uniform signal from articular cartilage. But higher performance MR systems and the use of pulse sequences optimized for the visualization of articular cartilage reveal a more complex appearance. With high-resolution T2-weighted sequences,

a three-layered appearance to articular cartilage has been described.[16-18] These layers are felt to correspond to histologic zones within articular cartilage. Along the articular surface, a low signal intensity layer signifies the tangentially oriented collagen fibers of the superficial zone. Deep to this layer, higher signal intensity is noted within the region corresponding to the transitional zone. The deepest layer, of low signal intensity, correlates with the radial zone of articular cartilage and adjacent calcified cartilage. The cause of the layered effect is thought to be primarily related to zonal differences in

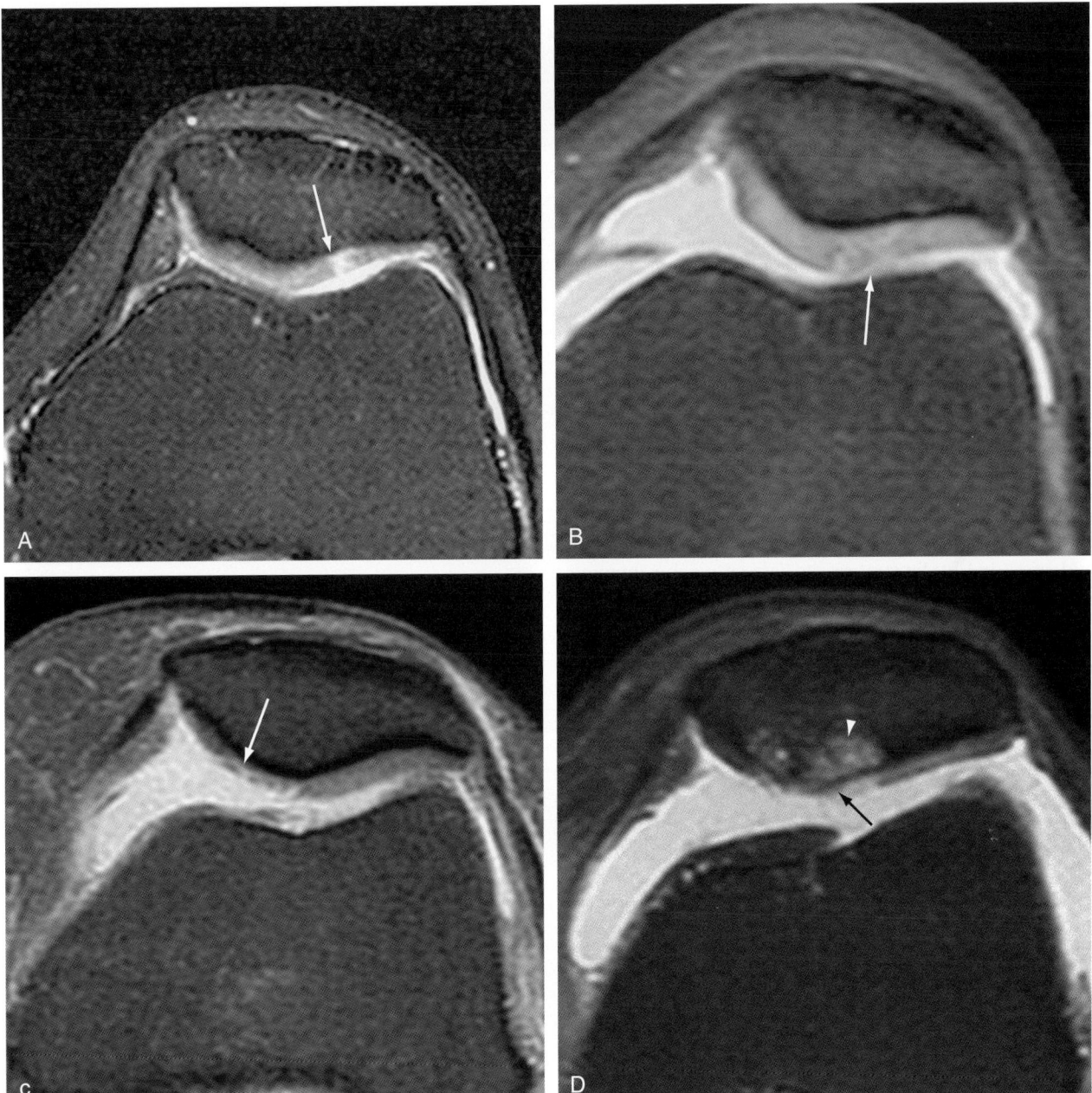

FIGURE 109-9

The Modified Outerbridge Classification of Articular Cartilage Injury, demonstrated at the patellofemoral joint. **A,** A grade 1 lesion on MR demonstrates abnormal signal intensity within articular cartilage (*arrow*), with preservation of normal cartilage morphology. **B,** Superficial fraying is apparent at the lateral facet (*arrow*) in a patient with grade 2 patellar disease. **C,** Articular cartilage is abnormally thinned and irregular (*arrow*) in a patient with a grade 3 abnormality. **D,** With grade 4 injury, full thickness loss of articular cartilage is noted (*arrow*). In such patients, subchondral degenerative changes are often present (*arrowhead*).

cartilage injury when reporting MR examinations. The location of cartilage injury must be noted, as weight-bearing injuries have a worse prognosis as compared to non–weight-bearing lesions. The size and shape of the cartilage injury should also be noted, as the choice of treatment options is heavily influenced by the morphology and size of a cartilage lesion. Associated subchondral abnormalities, when present, should be described.

The arthroscopic and MR appearance of damaged cartilage reflect the changes in matrix biochemistry and structure that occur following injury. Alterations in tissue morphology lead to progressively increasing anatomic defects, including surface fibrillation, fissures, and/or gross tissue loss. Specific compositional changes that have been detected in injured cartilage include increased water content, decreases in proteoglycan concentration,[59] and disorganization of the collagen network.[60]

These structural and biochemical changes result in an increase in T2 within injured cartilage,[61] leading to increased signal intensity within damaged cartilage on T2-weighted images. Lengthening of T1 also occurs, resulting in decreased signal intensity within lesions on T1-weighted images. Such signal changes without alteration in morphology equate to grade 1 lesions.

Reliance upon signal changes within cartilage for the detection of cartilage injury, however, is often problematic. The diagnosis of a grade 1 lesion on MR images may be subjective, and at times has been judged unreliable.[45,62] The key to the accurate diagnosis of hyaline cartilage disorders in routine clinical practice is the recognition of morphologic changes that occur within cartilage following injury. It is for this reason that most routine MR evaluations of articular cartilage at the knee utilize fat-suppressed fast spin-echo images (with its highly arthrographic appearance) or 3D-SPGR/FLASH images (with its high resolution and resultant morphologic detail). The former is more useful for detecting a broad range of knee pathology, and thus is the more commonly used technique, with the high signal intensity fluid provided by fat-suppressed fast spin-echo imaging providing high conspicuity for the detection of cartilage defects at the knee.

Articular cartilage injuries at the knee can be broadly grouped into those that are traumatic and those that are degenerative. In adults, traumatic forces tend to extend along the tidemark, the preferential shear plane between the deepest, calcified layer of cartilage and underlying subchondral bone. As a result, most traumatic cartilage injuries in adults result in full-thickness cartilage separation from subchondral bone.[63] With incomplete separation of the articular cartilage, a flaplike injury may occur (Fig. 109-10). With complete separation, a full thickness defect is noted. Such post-traumatic defects often are well defined and have sharply angled margins. With these injuries, a careful search for a displaced cartilaginous loose body should be performed, as the loose body may be an important cause of patient symptoms such as knee locking (Fig. 109-11). Subchondral marrow edema is frequently present in association with traumatic cartilage injury.[64] In particular, when the edema is focal and well defined, the probability of cartilage injury is significantly increased (Fig. 109-12). Recognition of marrow edema at articular surfaces thus serves as a useful clue in the diagnosis of cartilage lesions, serving to draw attention to areas with possible cartilage defects. However, it should be noted that marrow edema is nonspecific, frequently occurring in the absence of cartilage injury or in association with nontraumatic, degenerative cartilage lesions.[64,65]

Osteochondral Fracture

With increasing traumatic force, the injury to articular cartilage may extend into subchondral bone, resulting in an osteochondral fracture. Such injuries commonly result from twisting trauma, and often occur in conjunction with soft-tissue injuries such as anterior cruciate ligament tears. The diagnosis of an osteochondral fracture on MR images requires visualization of a fracture

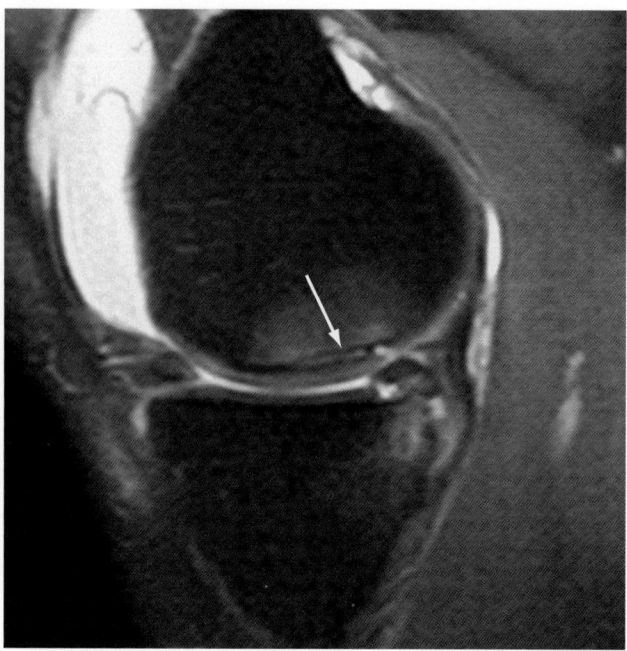

FIGURE 109-10

A fat-suppressed fast spin-echo proton-density–weighted sagittal image reveals a flaplike traumatic cartilage injury (*arrow*). As is typical, articular cartilage has separated along the tidemark.

line that extends to the articular surface. The amount of force required to generate an osteochondral fracture at the knee is substantial, and thus cartilage injuries frequently accompany osteochondral fractures (Fig. 109-13). MR is able to demonstrate features of osteochondral fractures that influence treatment decisions. Nondisplaced osteochondral fractures can often be treated conservatively. Osteochondral fractures with displaced fragments or significant depression of the articular surface may require operative intervention.

Prior to skeletal maturation, the tidemark is not defined, thus allowing traumatic forces to more easily extend into subchondral bone, and making isolated chondral lesions less likely.[63,66] An example is osteochondritis dissecans, a particular form of osteochondral fracture that occurs primarily in children and adolescents. Classic osteochondritis dissecans is limited to an epiphysis and occurs most commonly at the lateral articular surface of the medial femoral condyle, though the inferomedial or anterior aspects of the lateral femoral condyle may also be involved.[67] The exact cause of osteochondritis dissecans remains controversial, though a traumatic origin is supported by multiple studies,[68-70] and the lesion often occurs in active individuals who are subjected to repetitive microtrauma. MRI is quite useful in both the diagnosis and management of osteochondritis dissecans, as it is able to provide information on fragment size, viability of the subchondral bony fragment, and stability of the osteochondral fragment,[71] all of which influence the need for operative intervention. The most commonly used sign of fragment instability is a high signal intensity line between the

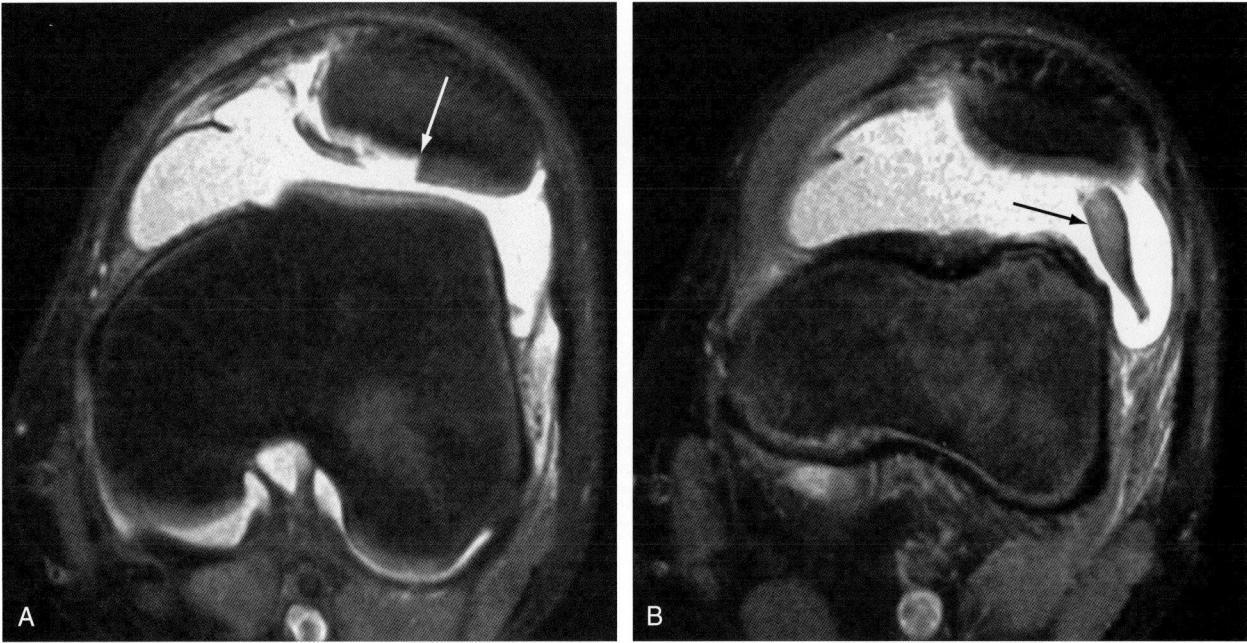

FIGURE 109-11

Acute cartilage injury following lateral patellar dislocation. **A,** A fat-suppressed fast spin-echo proton-density–weighted axial image reveals a large cartilage defect at the medial patellar facet in a patient status post lateral patellar dislocation. Note the acutely angled edge (*arrow*) at the site of the defect, typical for a post-traumatic cartilage defect. **B,** An axial image at a higher level demonstrates the avulsed cartilage loose body (*arrow*) within the lateral aspect of the suprapatellar bursa.

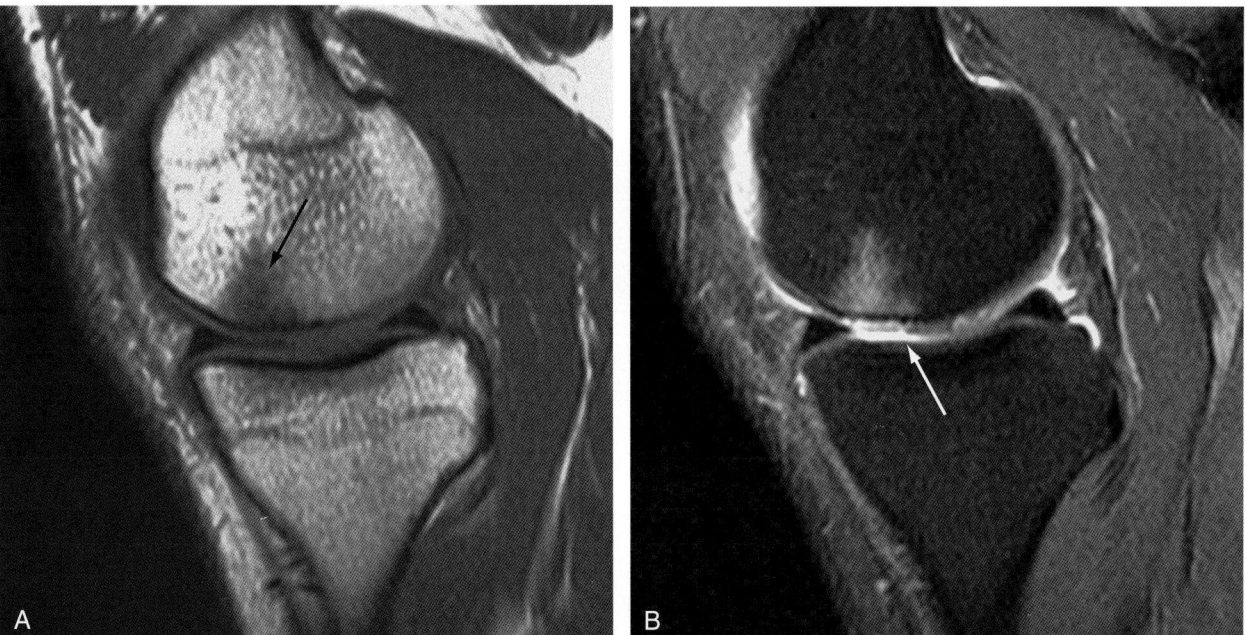

FIGURE 109-12

Subchondral marrow edema as an indicator of acute cartilage injury. **A,** Following trauma, well-defined subchondral edema (*arrow*) is identified within the medial femoral condyle on a T1-weighted sagittal image. **B,** Fat-suppressed fast spin-echo proton-density–weighted sagittal image confirms the subchondral edema, and reveals an associated full thickness cartilage defect (*arrow*).

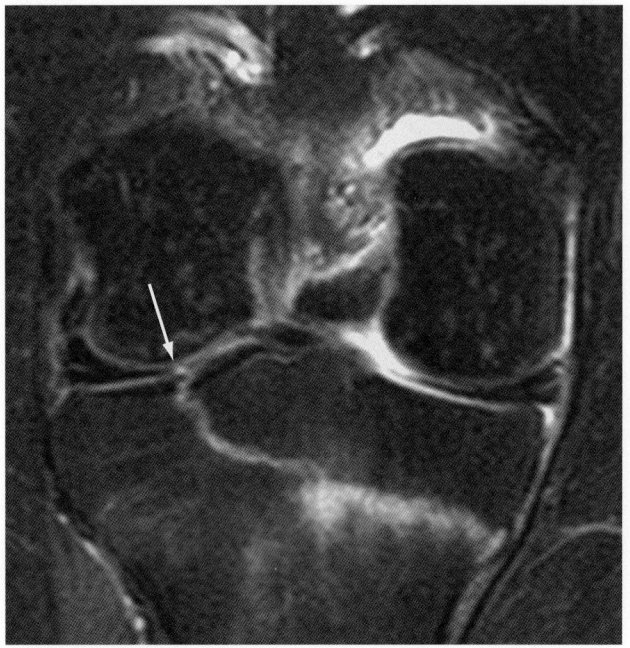

FIGURE 109-13

An osteochondral fracture extending to the articular surface of the lateral tibial plateau is identified in this 34-year–old male who sustained a sports-related injury. A subtle associated cartilage defect (*arrow*) is apparent.

fragment and underlying bone.[72] Additional signs that may indicate lesion instability include the presence of subchondral cysts and focal cartilage defects at the site of the osteochondral lesion (Fig. 109-14).[73]

Degenerative Cartilage Injury

Degenerative cartilage abnormalities are generally referred to as osteoarthritis, which is a misnomer in light of the lack of a true inflammatory component. Osteoarthritis is a multifactorial disorder, though frequently no clear cause for joint degeneration is evident. Factors known to increase the risk for the development of osteoarthritis include prior trauma, obesity, disruption of the articular surface, joint instability, and joint malalignment. In individuals with osteoarthritis, articular cartilage attempts to respond to the damage that occurs to the cartilage matrix. Chondrocytes are able to detect tissue damage and release mediators that stimulate a tissue response, often seen as clusters of chondrocytes surrounded by newly-formed matrix. Unfortunately, the matrix formed in response to cartilage injury is altered, with decreased collagen content and organization, and with lowered proteoglycan content. This altered matrix is more vulnerable to injury, in part accounting for the progressive nature of osteoarthritis.

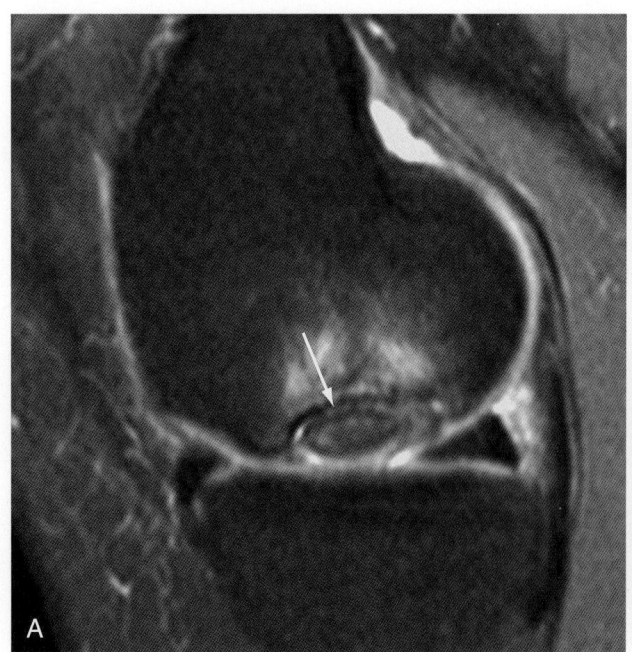
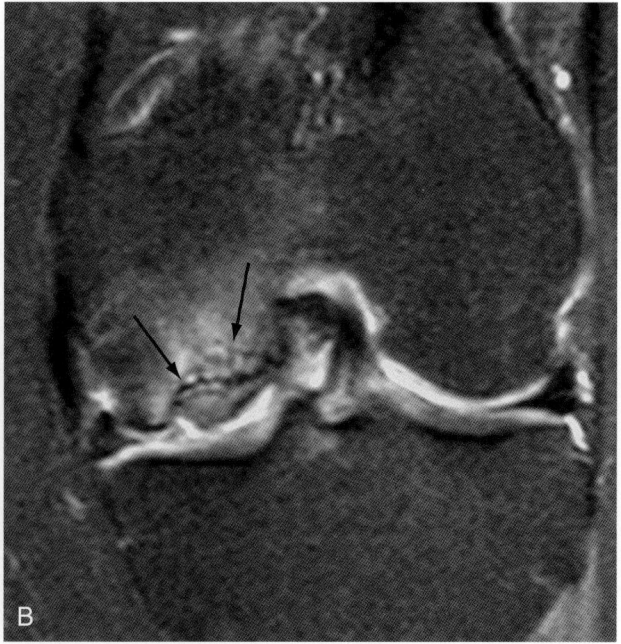

FIGURE 109-14

MR signs of lesion instability in osteochondritis dissecans. **A,** A high signal intensity interface (*arrow*) is seen between the osteochondral fragment and overlying bone on a fat-suppressed proton-density–weighted sagittal image from a patient with unstable osteochondritis dissecans. **B,** A fat-suppressed proton-density–weighted coronal image in another patient with unstable osteochondritis dissecans reveals prominent cystic changes (*arrows*) above the osteochondral fragment.

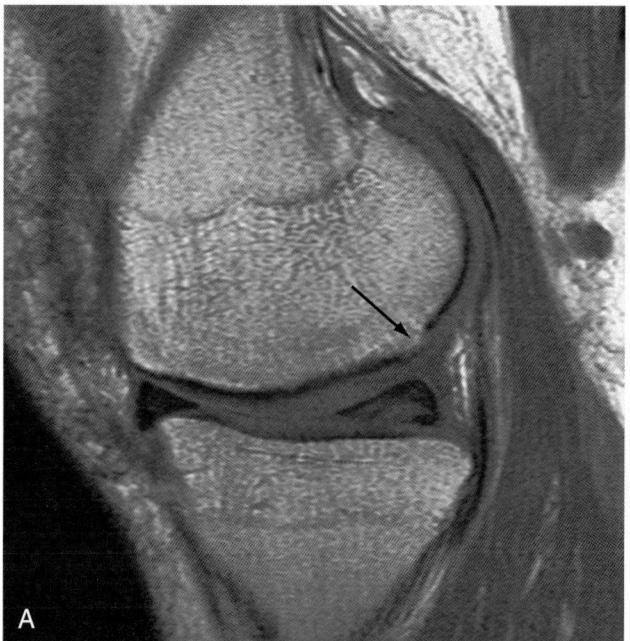
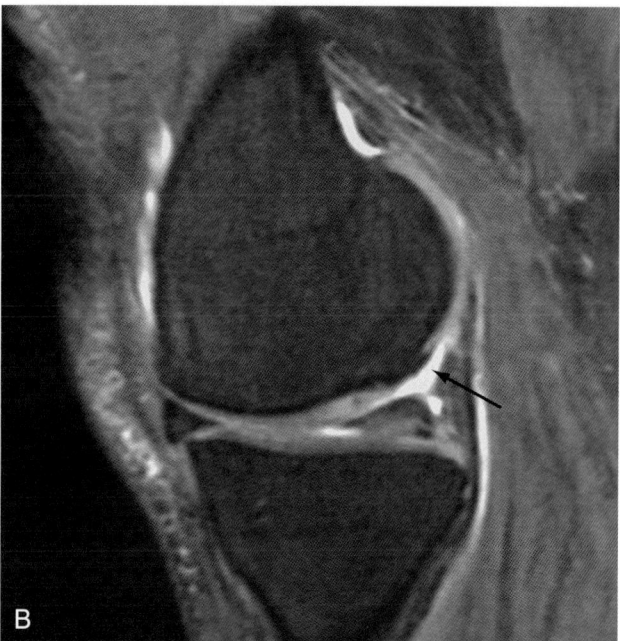

FIGURE 109-15

Central osteophytes as a sign of cartilage loss at the knee. **A,** A T1-weighted sagittal image demonstrates a central osteophyte (*arrow*) along the posterior weight-bearing surface of the medial femoral condyle. **B,** Fluid fills a full-thickness cartilage defect (*arrow*) at the site of the central osteophyte on the corresponding water excitation double-echo steady-state (WE DESS) sagittal view.

The earliest changes in arthritic cartilage are the grade 1 lesions, demonstrating intrinsic signal changes within the cartilage without alterations in surface morphology. With disease progression, morphologic alterations such as surface fibrillation, fissuring, and the development of cartilage defects occur. Accompanying changes in underlying bone, such as osteophyte formation and reactive marrow edema, may also be noted. The osteophytes that form in association with osteoarthritis may be central or marginal. The presence of central osteophytes, those that involve the articular surface, is an important marker for cartilage defects. A recent study revealed that the presence of central osteophytes correlated with a high likelihood of full-thickness or near full-thickness cartilage defects at the knee (Fig. 109-15).[74] In contrast to traumatic cartilage defects, the defects that develop secondary to osteoarthritis are often more irregular and have obtuse margins.

Cartilage defects, though they vary in character, are an important feature of both traumatic and degenerative cartilage injury. The detection of these cartilage defects plays a critical role in patient management and treatment decisions. The use of ancillary finding such as bone marrow edema and central osteophytes can increase the ability to detect cartilage defects, though accurate characterization of defects depends upon direct visualization. Most radiologists rely heavily upon the sagittal and coronal planes for the visualization of cartilage defects at the femoral-tibial articulation. We have found that fluid-sensitive axial images (such as fat-suppressed fast spin-echo proton-density–weighted

images), traditionally favored for evaluation of patellar cartilage, are quite valuable in the detection and characterization of femoral condylar or tibial plateau cartilage defects. In patients with intact articular cartilage at the femoral-tibial joint, the congruent cartilage surfaces allow only minimal amounts of fluid to collect between the surfaces. In patients with cartilage defects, fluid often fills the defect, creating a localized fluid collection that is visible en face in the axial plane. This localized fluid, referred to as the "crater sign," may be used as an indicator for the presence of a cartilage defect at the knee (Fig. 109-16). The size and shape of a cartilage defect is often more easily determined from the appearance of the crater than from direct visualization of the cartilage defect in the sagittal or coronal planes (Fig. 109-17).

MR OF POSTOPERATIVE ARTICULAR CARTILAGE

Because of articular cartilage's very limited ability to heal, nonoperative treatment of cartilage injury is largely palliative. As a result, numerous techniques have been developed for operative treatment of cartilage lesions, and the use of operative therapies has increased considerably. The surgical techniques employed generally involve transfer of cartilage or cartilage precursors into areas of cartilage loss. An exception is the treatment of unstable osteochondritis dissecans, in which fixation of an in situ osteochondral fragment is performed (Fig. 109-18). Regardless of the source of the transfer

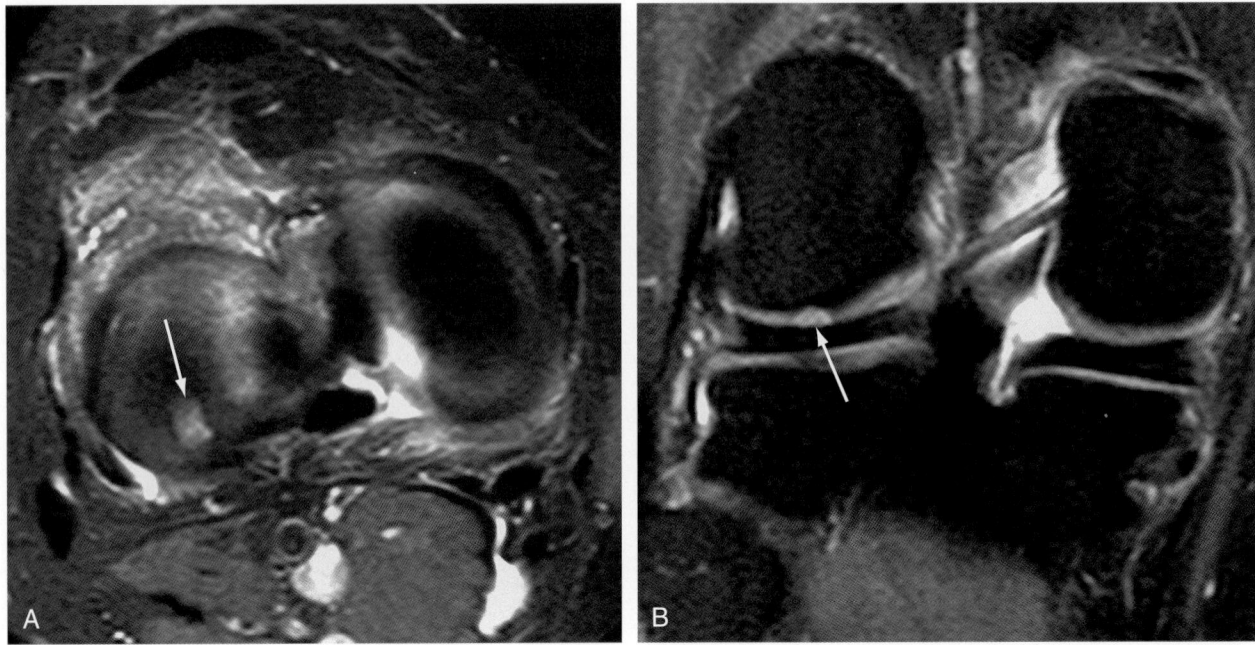

FIGURE 109-16

The "crater sign" for detection of cartilage defects at the knee. **A,** Localized fluid, compatible with the "crater sign" (*arrow*), is seen en face at the posterolateral aspect of the femoral-tibial articulation on a fat-suppressed proton-density–weighted axial image of the knee. **B,** A full thickness cartilage defect at the posterior weight-bearing surface of the lateral femoral condyle (*arrow*) is confirmed, though it is more subtle, on the fat-suppressed proton-density–weighted coronal view.

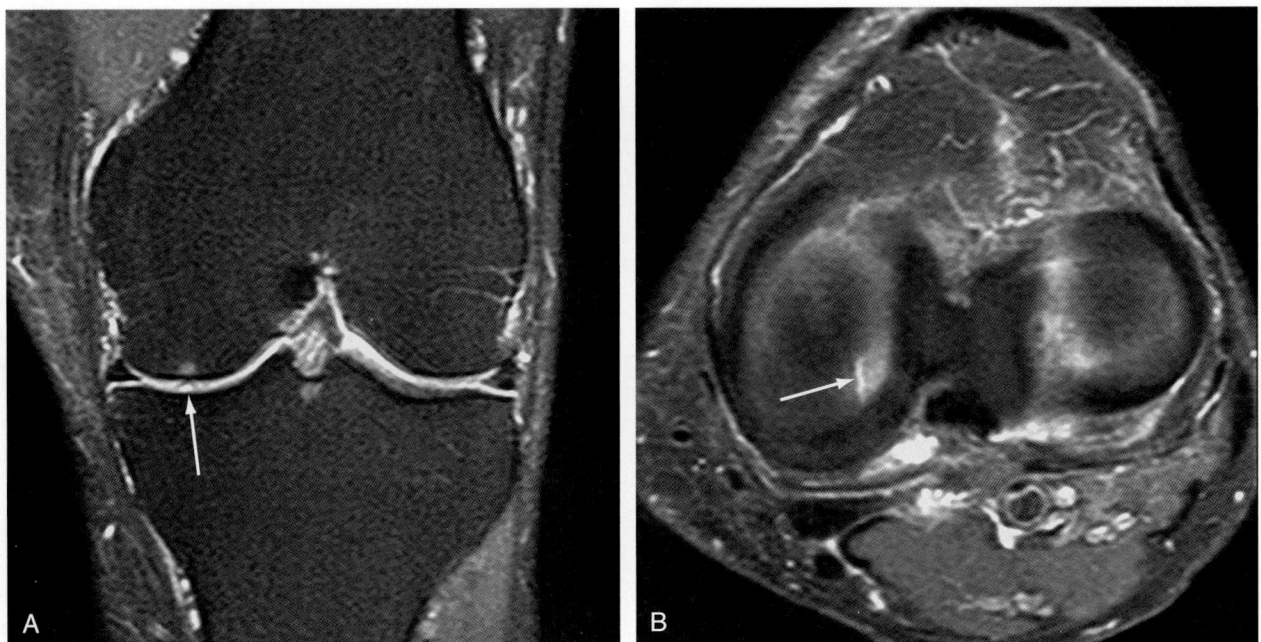

FIGURE 109-17

The "crater sign" as a means to evaluate the morphology of cartilage defects at the knee. **A,** A fat-suppressed proton-density–weighted coronal image reveals a subtle cartilage defect at the posterior weight-bearing surface of the medial femoral condyle (*arrow*). **B,** The size and linear morphology of the defect is more easily appreciated by viewing the "crater" (*arrow*) on the corresponding fat-suppressed proton-density–weighted axial image.

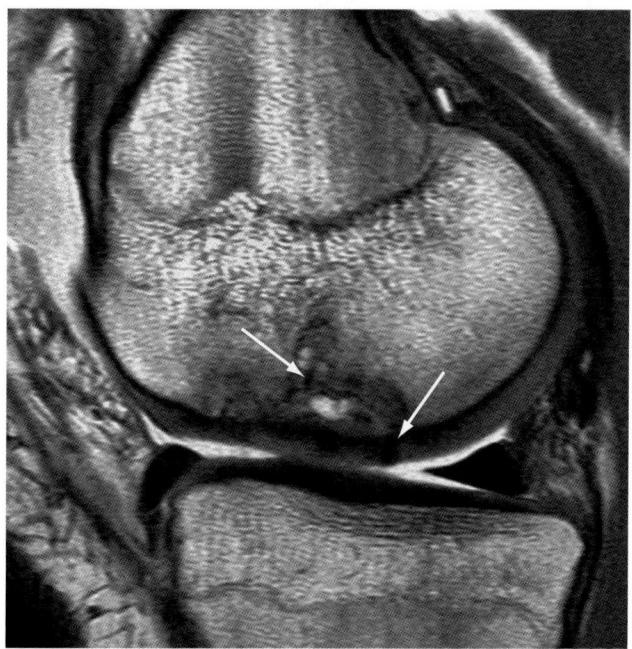

FIGURE 109-18

A fast spin-echo proton-density–weighted image without fat-suppression obtained at 3 T reveals a congruent articular surface in a patient status postoperative stabilization of osteochondritis dissecans. Only minimal metallic artifact (arrows) is present, in part because of the fast spin-echo technique utilized. (Courtesy of Lawrence N Tannenbaum, MD.)

material, the ability of MR to evaluate the chondral surface and underlying subchondral bone is invaluable in the assessment of the postoperative patient. Any of the cartilage-sensitive sequences may be utilized in the evaluation of postoperative cartilage, though routine clinical practice tends to favor fast spin-echo imaging, in part due to the reduction in metallic artifact that is obtained with this method.

One of the first and still most commonly used operative methods for the treatment of cartilage injury is the arthroscopic debridement and microfracture technique, which uses sharp surgical instruments to create holes in the subchondral bone beneath a cartilage defect. The microfractures are theorized to release stem cells from the marrow that will subsequently differentiate into fibrocartilage. When the procedure fails, MR may reveal bone marrow edema and thinned and irregular repair tissue at the site of the defect.[75] Unfortunately, even when successful, the fibrocartilage formed by this procedure is weaker than hyaline cartilage, and thus initial relief may progress to symptom recurrence as the fibrocartilage layer degrades.[76]

Given the lack of long-term success from techniques that depend upon fibrocartilage formation, orthopedists have increasingly turned to methods that are capable of generating or transplanting hyaline cartilage at the site of injury. The two most common procedures are the osteochondral autograft transplantation, also known as mosaicplasty, and autologous chondrocyte implantation. The osteochondral autograft procedure is performed by

harvesting plugs of articular cartilage and subchondral bone from non–weight-bearing areas of the knee, such as the intercondylar notch or lateral aspect of the trochlear groove, and transferring the plugs to the site of a cartilage defect. The technique can be performed with a single large plug for smaller cartilage defects (Fig. 109-19) or with multiple smaller plugs for larger lesions. Ideally, the plugs are positioned such that a smooth articular surface is created at the transfer site. MR is able to visualize the articular surface following this procedure, as well as evaluate potential complications such as donor site avascular necrosis, loose bodies, or instability at the graft site.[77,78]

Autologous chondrocyte implantation was introduced in Sweden in 1994.[79] In this treatment, chondrocytes are harvested from the patient's intercondylar notch or femoral trochlea and grown in culture for approximately 4 weeks. In a second, open procedure, the cells are reimplanted at the site of the cartilage defect with an overlying periosteal flap. Over time, these implanted cells begin to produce hyaline-like repair tissue. After 2 to 6 months, an articular surface that closely resembles normal articular cartilage is found. On follow-up MR, the congruity of the articular surface and the status of underlying subchondral bone can be assessed (Fig. 109-20). Complications of the procedure that can be demonstrated with MR include delamination, repair tissue hypertrophy, and arthrofibrosis.[75,78,80]

In patients with very large cartilage injuries (>2 cm^2), autologous chondrocyte implantation and osteochondral autograft transplantation procedures are often contraindicated. A promising technique in such patients is the use of shell osteochondral allografts obtained from cadaver bone.[81,82] With this technique, the patient's osteochondral abnormality is resected, the edges are squared off, and the subchondral bone is abraded. An osteochondral shell is then resected from an identical location on a size-matched cadaveric bone. The carefully fitted shell is pressed into the defect and thereby forms a new articular surface. MR following the procedure can assess the congruity of the articular surface and incorporation of the graft. In addition, it has been found that the presence of bone marrow edema on postoperative MR may serve as a surrogate biomarker for the patient's humoral immune response to the graft.[83] Those patients who exhibited marrow edema not only demonstrate a positive antibody response, but also are much more likely to develop graft failure (Fig. 109-21). As patients undergoing this procedure traditionally do not undergo immunosuppression, MR in such cases may affect the decision to provide immunosuppression postoperatively, or ultimately influence the routine use of immune-modulating practices in patients undergoing osteochondral shell allograft transplantation.

ADVANCED MR IMAGING TECHNIQUES

Until recently, much of the focus of clinical MR has been on acute cartilage injuries, with little known about the long-term effects of such injuries. Similarly, relatively

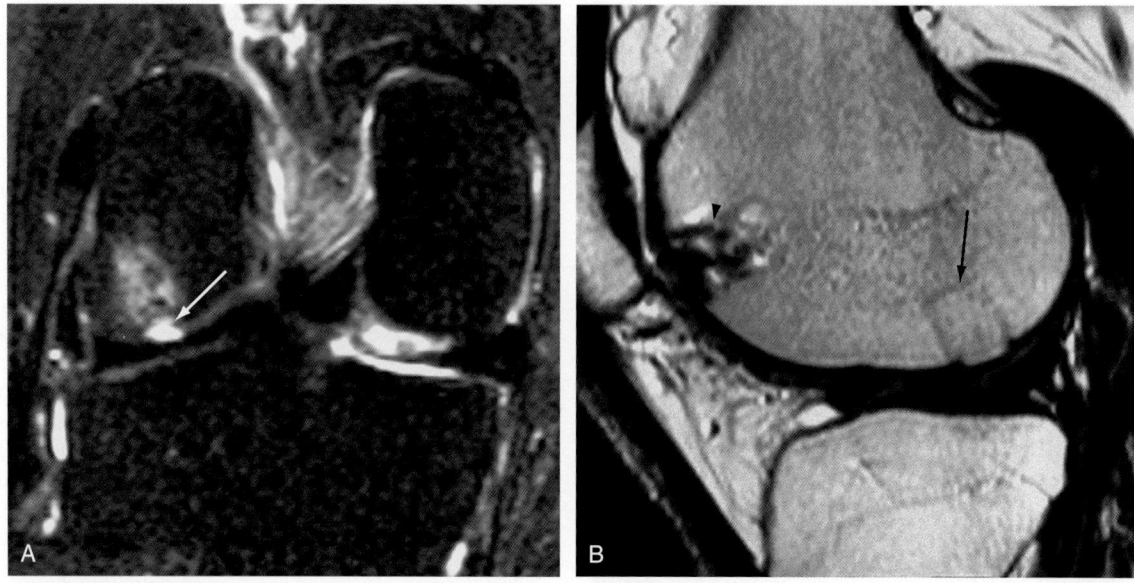

FIGURE 109-19

Osteochondral autograft transfer procedure. **A,** A cartilage defect at the lateral femoral condyle (*arrow*) is well seen on the preoperative fat-suppressed T2-weighted fast spin-echo coronal image of the knee. **B,** Postoperative fast spin-echo T2-weighted image without fat suppression reveals excellent incorporation of an osteochondral autograft (*arrow*), with a smooth articular surface noted. The donor site at the lateral trochlear groove (*arrowhead*) is also apparent.

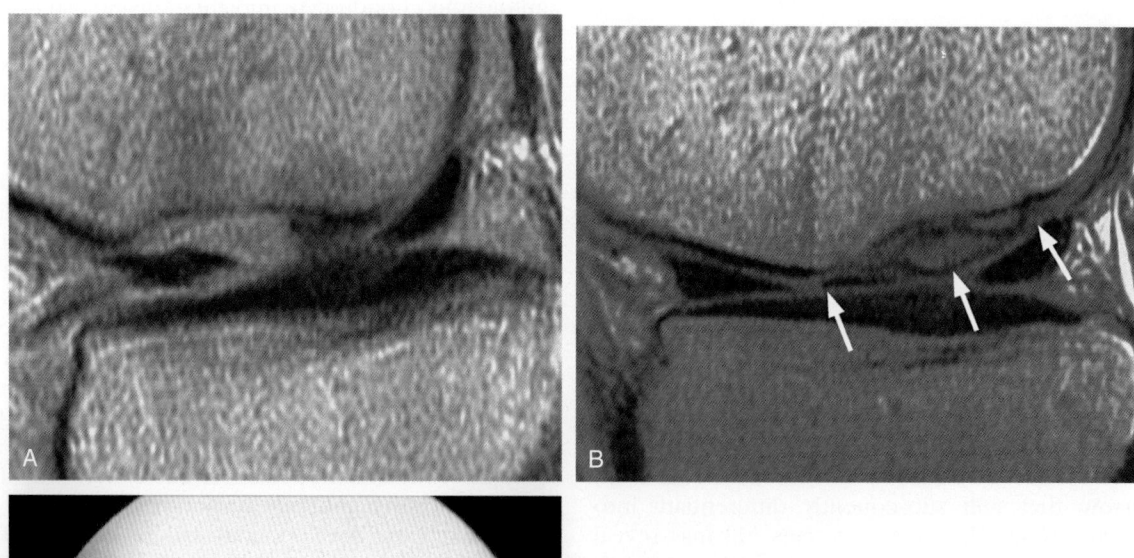

FIGURE 109-20

Autologous chondrocyte implantation. **A,** A preoperative proton-density–weighted sagittal image reveals a large, post-traumatic osteochondral defect within the lateral femoral condyle. **B,** 1.5 years after surgery, a sagittal proton-density–weighted image demonstrates fill-in of the defect with heterogeneous repair tissue (*arrows*). **C,** Second-look arthroscopy 2 years following surgery shows well-integrated tissue at the repair site. *(From Alparslan L, Minas T, Winalski CS: Magnetic resonance imaging of autologous chondrocyte implantation. Semin Ultrasound CT MRI 22:341-51, 2001, with permission.)*

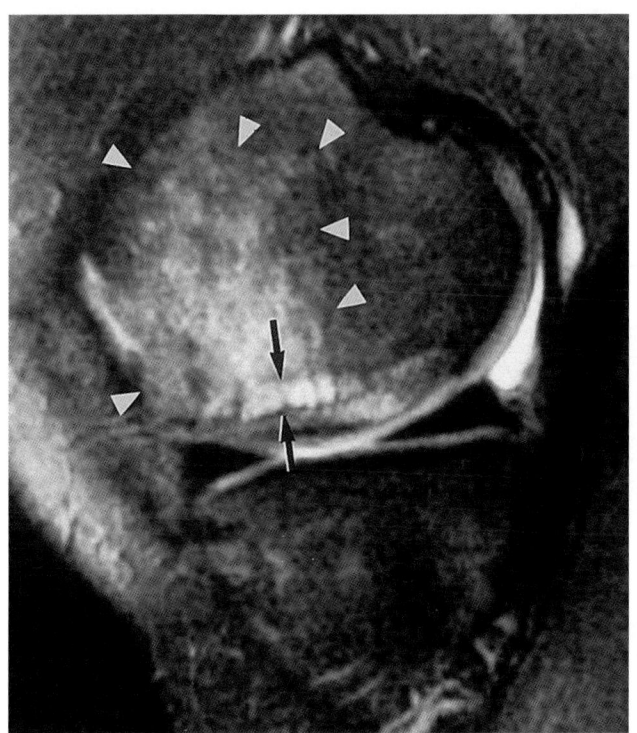

FIGURE 109-21

Following osteochondral shell allograft transplantation, a proton-density–weighted fast spin-echo fat-suppressed image reveals prominent marrow edema (*arrowheads*) within the medial femoral condyle, above the graft site. The edema is particularly intense (*arrows*) at the allograft interface. Patients with this appearance have a higher probability for the development of humoral immunity to the graft, and subsequent graft failure. (*From Sirlin CB, Brossmann J, Boutin RD: Shell osteochondral allografts of the knee; comparison of MR imaging findings and immunologic responses. Radiology 219:35-43, 2001, with permission.*)

little attention has been given to chronic degenerative disease, in part due to the inability to intervene on more than a palliative level. However, a number of pharmacologic interventions under active development focus on altering the biochemical degeneration of cartilage secondary to acute injury or chronic degeneration. Therefore, much effort is being put into developing MR techniques that provide more specific information on cartilage structure and biochemistry under clinical conditions, such that the risk factors, natural progression, and potential therapies of the disease can be better understood.

Perhaps the most straightforward method of obtaining more specific information from MR is to utilize the superb contrast between cartilage and other tissues to segment the cartilage from surrounding tissues and represent the tissue in three dimensions, from which local and global indices of cartilage thickness and volume can be obtained. Pulse sequences with better contrast and faster acquisition times are under active development (Fig. 109-22),[84] and should aid in the implementation of such studies across wider populations.

The information available from assessing local morphology and its alterations with activity or disease has recently been reviewed,[85] and the techniques validated.[86-90] Although only available over the past several years, important observations are already emerging. In one study, the rate of cartilage loss in the patella was poorly correlated to cartilage loss in the tibia, suggesting that the mechanisms for degradation of cartilage in these compartments may differ.[91] Documentation is increasing on the "baseline" rates of loss of cartilage in osteoarthritis,[92] and after injuries and interventions such as partial meniscectomy.[91] The effects of genetics on cartilage volume are also being investigated.[93]

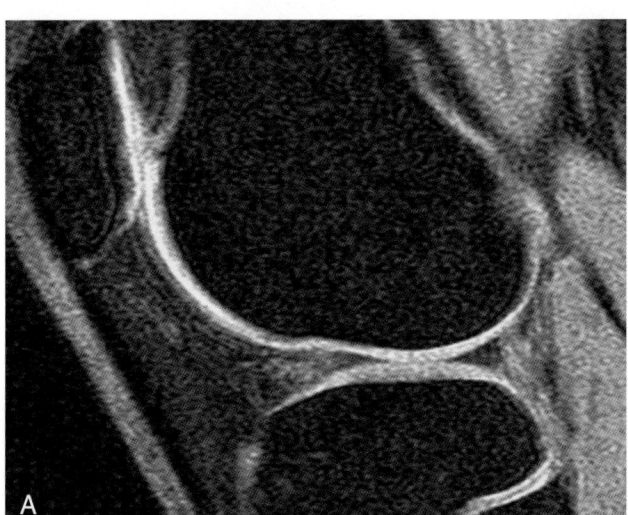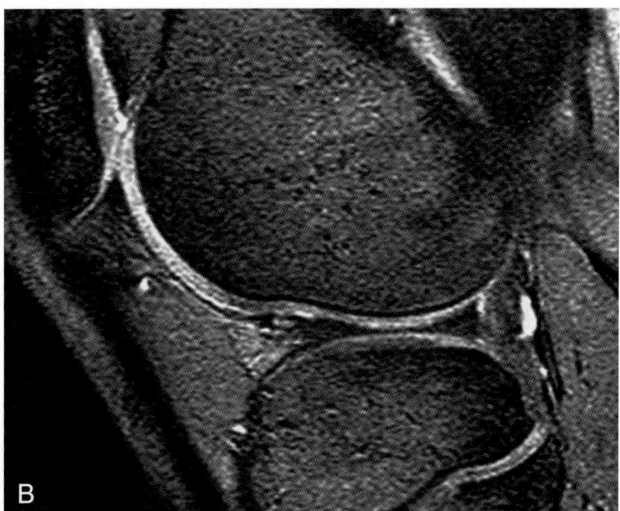

FIGURE 109-22

Fast, high-contrast cartilage imaging. Fluctuating equilibrium MR (FEMR) is a rapid fat-water imaging technique based on steady-state free precession. Images from a healthy 27-year–old volunteer. **A,** 3D spoiled gradient-recalled echo (3D-SPGR) image with fat suppression (512 × 256, 16 cm field of view, 2 mm slices, 48 sections, TR/TE 50/5 ms, 45 degree flip angle, scan time 8:56 s). **B,** FEMR water image (512 × 256, 16 cm field of view, 2 mm slices, 48 sections, TR/TE 6.6/1.2 ms, 25 degree flip angle, scan time 2:43 s). The signal-to-noise ratio in the cartilage in the FEMR image is similar to that in the SPGR image in about one third of the scan time, allowing faster cartilage volume and thickness measurements. (*From Gold GE, McCauley TR, Gray ML, Disler DG: What's new in cartilage? RadioGraphics 23:1227-1242, 2003, with permission.*)

Thus, while not providing direct biochemical information, the ability to obtain more detailed and localized metrics of cartilage morphology may enable a better understanding of the factors contributing to cartilage loss and the ability of pharmaceuticals to alter the course of disease. In addition to cartilage volume, metrics such as cartilage thickness and curvature can be analyzed (Fig. 109-23).[84] These data may aid in the understanding of how joint architecture and joint shape affect arthritis progression, as has been recently suggested.[94] These data might also help identify a population at risk for osteoarthritis, which would aid in the identification of a population for clinical trials and for therapeutic intervention.[95]

Furthermore, the ability to measure changes in cartilage morphology with activity may provide a possible

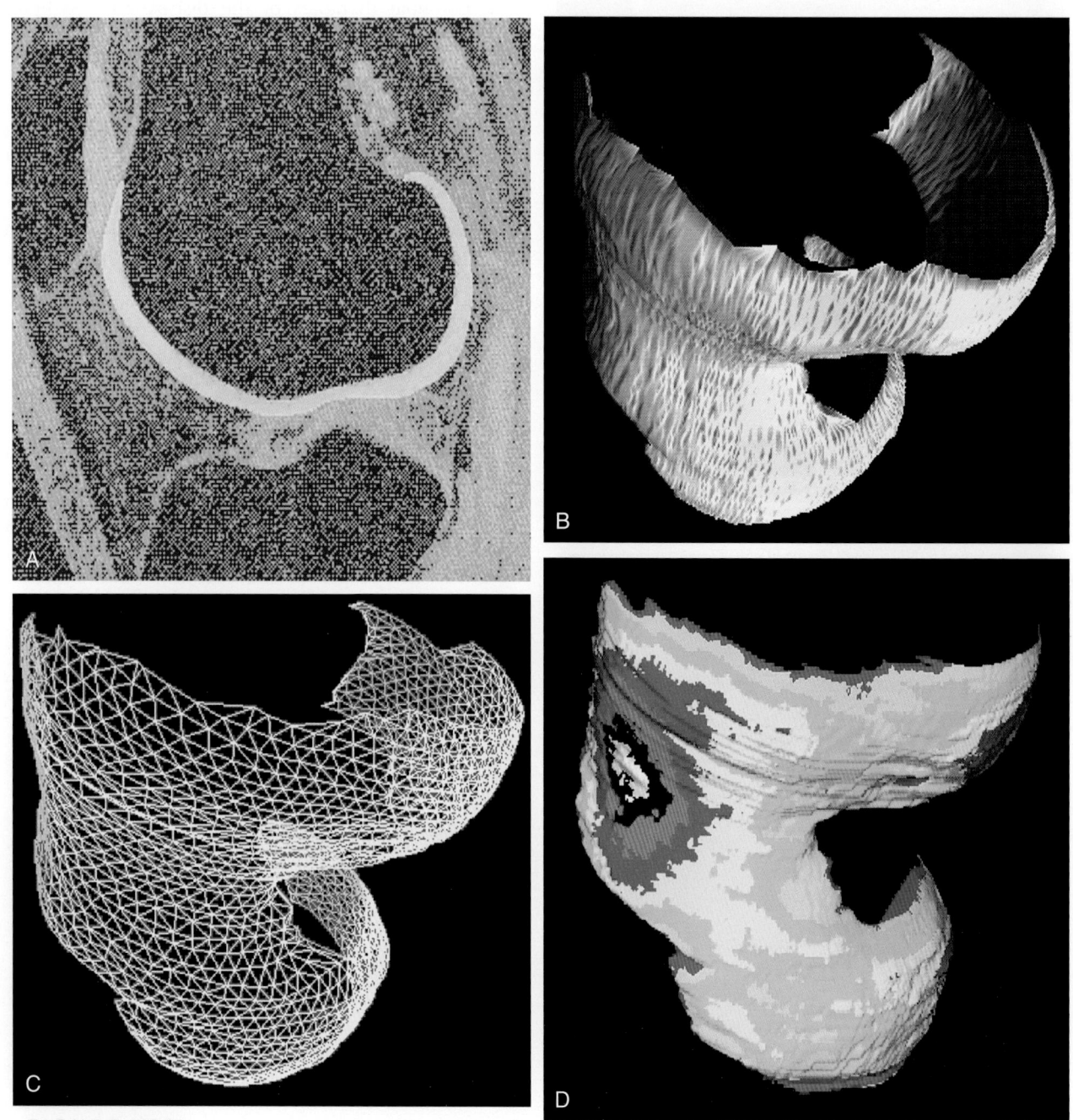

FIGURE 109-23

Morphometric analysis of cartilage from MR images. **A,** The difference in the MRI parameters among the different tissue structures allows them to be distinguished from one another and segmented for tissue-specific analysis. Here, the focus is on the cartilage; the cartilage segmentation (shown in green) allows joint parameters to be measured, such as **B,** cartilage volume; **C,** cartilage curvature; and **D,** cartilage thickness, and monitor changes in these parameters with time or following an intervention. *(From Eckstein F, Reiser M, Englmeier KH, Putz R: In vivo morphometry and functional analysis of human articular cartilage with quantitative magnetic resonance imaging—from image to data, from data to theory. Anat Embryol (Berl) 203:147-173, 2001, with permission.)*

means for relating the morphologic features to cartilage functional capacity. For example, quantification of patellar cartilage deformation with activities such as walking or squatting[96] may allow for future "cartilage stress tests," i.e., a measurement of cartilage deformation in response to joint loading, with an assessment of whether that degree of deformation was in the normal range.

In addition to morphologic detail, a number of MR parameters now have the potential to yield direct information regarding cartilage biochemical state. The most apparent is the MR T2 relaxation time, which is sensitive to a wide range of water interactions in tissue, including macromolecular concentration, macromoleculer structure, and bulk organization of the matrix. In particular, T2 has been demonstrated to be sensitive to cartilage hydration (macromolecular concentration).[97-102] While both collagen and glycosaminoglycans impact T2, since collagen is the most abundant macromolecule in cartilage and since it has a stronger effect on T2 per unit concentration,[102] it is believed that collagen is the main determinant of the baseline T2 in cartilage.

Overall tissue matrix organization can impact water mobility and hence T2. This is the basis of the "magic angle" effect in cartilage, in which the alignment of the collagen architecture relative to the main magnetic field has an impact on the T2 dipole interactions and hence the T2 relaxation time (see "MR of Normal Articular Cartilage"). The effect can be seen as vertical striations in high-resolution images obtained with T2 weighting,[22] and improved pulse sequences now allow for high-resolution images that demonstrate this architectural organization of the cartilage matrix in vivo (Fig. 109-24).[103,104] Although it is clearly not the only factor influencing T2, disruption of the collagen architecture can thus lead to alterations in T2 within cartilage (Fig. 109-25).

Molecular structure is also a determinant of T2. In several studies in which interleukin-1 (IL-1)-degraded cartilage was employed as a model system to study cartilage metabolism under osteoarthritis-like conditions, T2 was shown to decrease despite an expected increase in tissue hydration.[102,105] This decrease presumably is due to enhanced water-macromolecular interactions, with the molecular changes occurring with IL-1 degradation.

In summary, T2 is impacted by a large number of processes occurring in tissue, and a specific interpretation of baseline T2 or T2 changes is difficult. A T2 lesion (either an area of low or high T2) may be due to alteration in the hydration in that area, molecular changes, disruption of the architectural organization of the collagen fibrils, or some combination of the above (Fig. 109-26). Yet despite these uncertainties, T2 is very sensitive to tissue abnormalities, and thus may provide a sensitive indication of pathologic changes in cartilage. While a number of technical factors need to be further investigated, T2 mapping is now feasible in patellar, femoral, and tibial cartilage,[106,107] and has the potential to reveal changes in cartilage not apparent using morphologic techniques.

Another approach to obtaining specific molecular information regarding cartilage is to image the charge

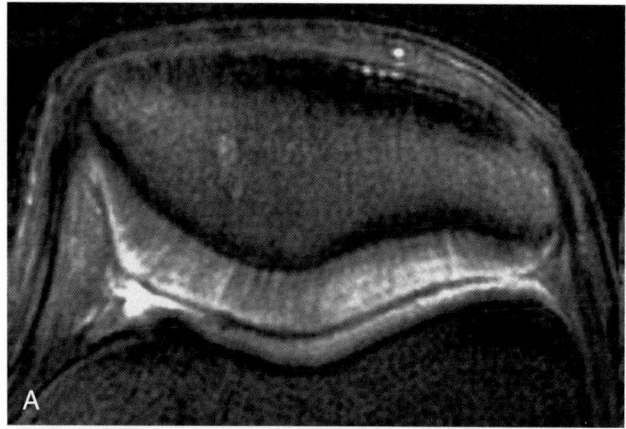
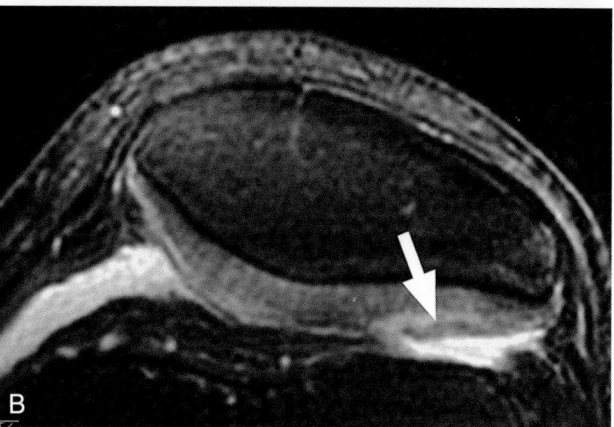

FIGURE 109-24

High-resolution in vivo imaging of cartilage architecture. Driven equilibrium Fourier transform (DEFT) imaging provides a method to get high signal from articular cartilage while maintaining good cartilage-to-fluid contrast. **A,** Healthy volunteer, demonstrating vertical collagen bundles (collections of many individual collagen fibers) in the radial zone. **B,** Patient with a horizontal fissure within patellar cartilage (*arrow*). (*Courtesy of Garry E Gold, MD.*)

associated with the glycosaminoglycan (GAG) molecules. This approach is based on the work of Maroudas et al on the theoretical description of how charged ions will distribute in cartilage in relation to the fixed charge density.[108,109] Early studies utilized MR imaging of the charged sodium ion,[110] and in vivo imaging of sodium by MRI was shown to be feasible.[111] However, due to the challenges inherent in quantitating the sodium concentration by MRI in degenerated cartilage, and the limited resolution and availability of sodium MRI, a more recent approach utilizes the charged clinical MRI contrast agent gadolinium diethylenetriamine pentetate [Gd(DTPA)$^{2-}$] (Magnevist, Berlex, NJ), which is implemented using the much more available proton MRI.

The approach is based on the premise that if Gd(DTPA)$^{2-}$ is given time to penetrate into cartilage, it will be distributed in higher concentration in areas of cartilage in which the GAG content is relatively low, and will be lower in concentration in regions rich in the negatively-charged GAG (Fig. 109-27). The MRI technique used to image GAG on the basis of the distribution

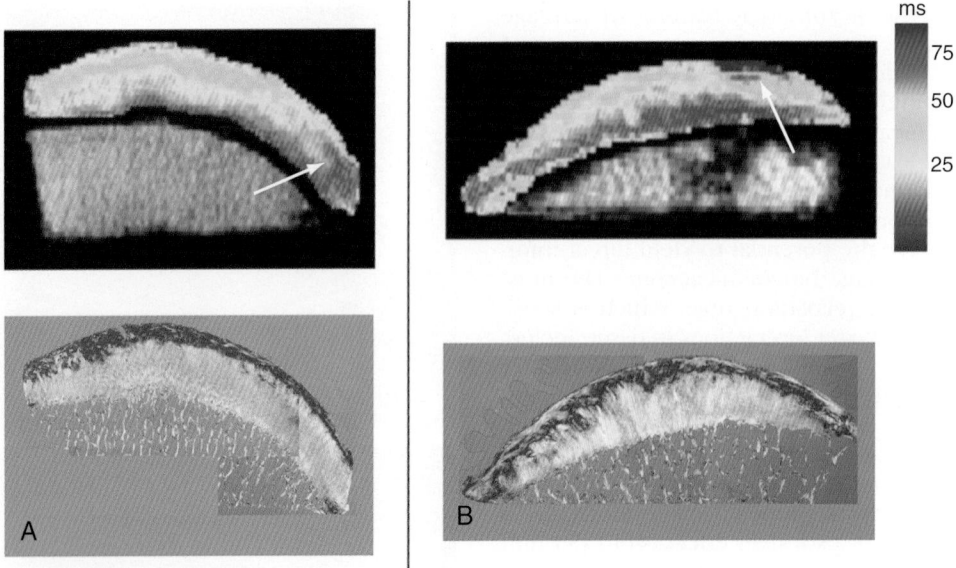

FIGURE 109-25

T2 lesions in human cartilage appear as regions of focally low or high T2. T2 (top, in ms) and polarized light microscopy (PLM, bottom), as an indicator of collagen orientation in two samples of human cartilage. **A,** Example of a relatively normal sample on PLM histology, yet there is a region of focally low T2 (*arrow*). **B,** Example of complex human disease. On the left-hand side of the sample, T2 appears mottled, corresponding to the disorganization seen on PLM. On the right-hand side of this sample, there is a region of focally high T2 (*arrow*) that corresponds to normal PLM. These examples suggest that T2 is influenced both by architectural factors and by factors not visualized on standard histologic measures of collagen orientation. *(From Menezes NM, Gray ML, Hartke JR, Burstein D: T2 and T1-rho MRI in articular cartilage systems. Magn Reson Med 51:503-509, 2004, with permission.)*

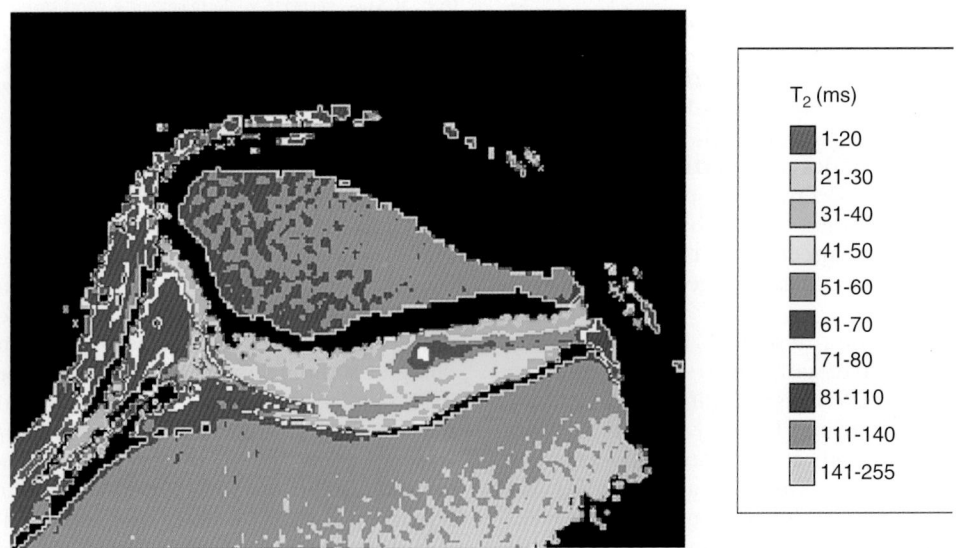

FIGURE 109-26

In vivo T2 mapping of cartilage lesions. T2 is dependent upon the concentration and structure of macromolecules, as well as overall architecture. Focal variations in T2 as seen in this figure may be due to local alterations in the collagen content and/or molecular structure, as well as some contribution from glycosaminoglycan concentration and alterations in the collagen architectural structure. *(From Burstein D, Bashir A, Gray ML: MRI techniques in early stages of cartilage disease. Invest Radiol 35:631, 2000, with permission.)*

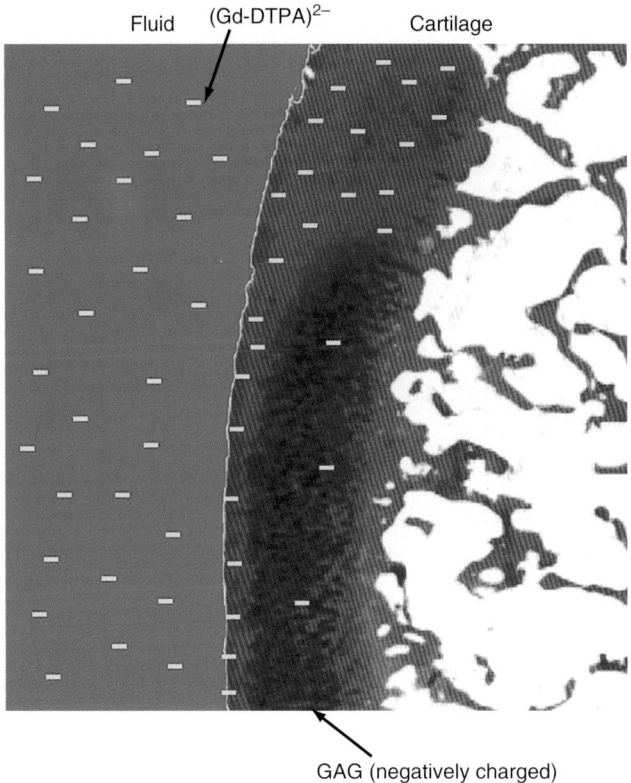

Fluid   (Gd-DTPA)$^{2-}$ Cartilage

GAG (negatively charged)

FIGURE 109-27

Molecular imaging of cartilage glycosaminoglycan (GAG). The basis of the delayed gadolinium-enhanced MRI of cartilage (dGEMRIC) technique is shown schematically here. An area is shown of cartilage that is depleted of GAG (top region of cartilage and along surface) and one high in GAG (lower region). The gadolinium diethylenetriamine pentetate [Gd(DTPA)$^{2-}$] (shown as yellow negative signs) distributes in inverse relation to the concentration of the negatively charged GAG, with higher Gd(DTPA)$^{2-}$ in the GAG-depleted area. *(From Burstein D, Gray ML: Potential of molecular imaging of cartilage. Sports Med Arth Rev 11:182-191, 2003, with permission.)*

of Gd(DTPA)$^{2-}$ is referred to as delayed gadolinium-enhanced MRI of cartilage (dGEMRIC) [the "delay" referring to the time required to allow the Gd(DTPA)$^{2-}$ to penetrate the cartilage tissue]. Since Gd(DTPA)$^{2-}$ inversely affects the MRI parameter T1, T1 measured after full penetration of contrast (T1$_{Gd}$) is used as a dGEMRIC index (T1$_{Gd}$). Lower GAG is associated with a higher Gd(DTPA)$^{2-}$ concentration and is measured as lower T1$_{Gd}$. Therefore, the dGEMRIC index varies directly with GAG concentration.

The dGEMRIC technique has been applied in both basic science and clinical studies, and the dGEMRIC measurement corresponds to "gold standard" measures for GAG of biochemistry and histology.[112-115] Clinical studies have demonstrated that dGEMRIC images show "lesions" in cartilage that are not observable in the presence of the nonionic contrast agent ProHance (Bracco Diagnostics, NJ),[116] further validating that the dGEMRIC image corresponds to the distribution of the negatively-charged GAG molecules.

This approach of imaging the concentration of one of the molecular constituents of cartilage may yield insight into the physiologic and pathologic processes occurring in vivo. For example, a recent study reported that individuals who exercise on a regular basis have higher dGEMRIC indices (denoting higher GAG) than those who are sedentary.[117] In a finding that is consistent with previous ex vivo biochemical studies, the medial compartment, in comparison with the lateral compartment, has been shown to have generally lower values for the dGEMRIC index,[118] possibly reflecting a response to the different mechanical environment for the different compartments.

Regarding pathology, relatively little is known about the temporal changes in GAG concentration during the evolution of arthritic disease in vivo. It is generally thought that GAG is lost and collagen damaged before there is frank loss of cartilage tissue. Interestingly, in several case studies of asymptomatic individuals, large "GAG lesions" can be seen in anatomically intact tissue.[119] In others, the GAG in cartilage appears relatively high or low overall (Fig. 109-28).[120] In a recent study, arthroscopically diseased compartments had lower dGEMRIC index than reference compartments.[121] Long-term studies during which such individuals are monitored over time are necessary to determine whether the existence of regions of low GAG is tantamount to being on the road to developing arthritis.

While the above studies illustrate the possibility of detecting cartilage degeneration earlier than previously possible, and of monitoring the evolution of arthritis and interventions, an exciting possibility is the use of such methods to explore and validate strategies for *repairing* cartilage. The repair process of cartilage in culture studies has been demonstrated previously by dGEMRIC.[122,123] Increases in the dGEMRIC index have also been observed clinically in cartilage implants,[124] and in the cartilage in several case studies of patients recovering from surgery and taking nutritional supplements.[120]

SUMMARY

In recent years, the clinical importance and capabilities of MR in the evaluation of articular cartilage have increased considerably. Increased clinical awareness of hyaline cartilage injury and new pharmacologic and surgical treatments mandate the sensitive evaluation of articular cartilage in routine musculoskeletal MR examinations. With proper MR technique and interpretive skills, articular cartilage injuries can now be diagnosed with high sensitivity. Though to date morphologic evaluation has dominated clinical practice, newer techniques promise to add biochemical and molecular information to the diagnostic armamentarium. Combined techniques and longer-term monitoring have the potential to provide enormous insights into the temporal and spatial evolution of cartilage degeneration and into the factors that modulate this degeneration. Indeed, we appear to be on the leading edge of a paradigm shift where, rather than focusing on the late stages of disease with palliative therapy, we can recognize early cartilage injury, and intervene with appropriate preventive and disease-reversing therapies.

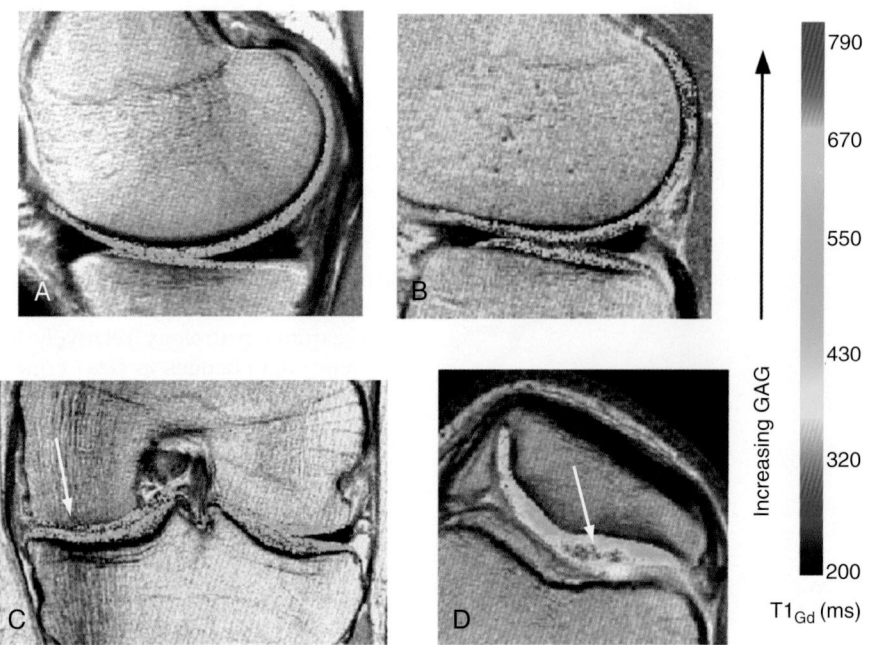

FIGURE 109-28

What is the distribution of glycosaminoglycan (GAG) in vivo? **A,** Image from an asymptomatic individual with uniformly high delayed gadolinium-enhanced MRI of cartilage (dGEMRIC) index. **B,** Individual with chronic knee problems has generally low dGEMRIC index across the cartilage, with "pockets" of very low values. **C,** Example where the medial compartment (*arrow*) has a lower dGEMRIC index than the lateral, possibly due to degeneration of cartilage secondary to a prior meniscectomy. **D,** Example of a large area of focally low dGEMRIC index (*arrow*) in anatomically intact cartilage. The areas of biochemical degeneration in intact cartilage may be amenable to pharmacologic intervention. Overall, these images illustrate the types of information that can be investigated in more depth in the study of the molecular effects in the disease process of osteoarthritis. *(From Burstein D, Gray ML: Potential of molecular imaging of cartilage. Sports Med Arth Rev 11:182-191, 2003, with permission.)*

REFERENCES

1. Peyron JG, Altman RD: The epidemiology of osteoarthritis. In Moskowitz RW, Howell DS, Goldberg VM, Mankin HJ, eds: Osteoarthritis: Diagnosis and Medical/Surgical Management, 2nd ed. Philadelphia: WB Saunders, 1992.
2. Curl WW, Krome J, Gordon ES, et al: Cartilage injuries: a review of 31,516 knee arthroscopies. Arthroscopy 13:456-460, 1997.
3. Wroble RR: Articular cartilage injury and autologous chondrocyte implantation: Which patients might benefit? Physician Sports Med 28(11):43-49, 2000.
4. Nelson FRT, Wagner J: An update on articular cartilage transplantation. J Musculoskel Med 15:56-66, 100, 1998.
5. Mankin HJ, Brandt KD: Biochemistry and metabolism of articular cartilage in osteoarthritis. In Moskowitz RW, Howell DS, Goldberg VM, Mankin HJ, eds: Osteoarthritis: Diagnosis and Medical/Surgical Management, 2nd ed. Philadelphia, WB Saunders, 1992.
6. Buckwalter JA, Mankin HJ: Articular cartilage. I. Tissue design and chondrocyte matrix interactions. J Bone Joint Surg Am 79:600-611, 1997.
7. Akeson WH, Amiel DA, Gershuni DH: Articular cartilage physiology and metabolism. In Resnick D, ed: Diagnosis of Bone and Joint Disorders, 3rd ed. Philadelphia: WB Saunders, 1995.
8. Minas T, Nehrer S: Current concepts in the treatment of articular cartilage defects. Orthopedics 20:525-538, 1997.
9. Suh JK, Scherping S, Marui T, et al: Basic science of articular cartilage injury and repair. Oper Tech Sports Med 3:78-86, 1995.
10. Newman AP: Articular cartilage repair. Am J Sports Med 26:309-324, 1998.
11. Recht MP, Resnick D: Imaging of articular cartilage: Current status and future directions. Am J Roentgenol 163:283-290, 1994.
12. Mow VC, Kuei SC, Lai WM, Armstron CJ: Biphasic creep and stress relaxation of articular cartilage in compression? Theory and experiments. J Biomech Eng 102:73-84, 1980.
13. Mow VC, Holmes MH, Lai WM: Fluid transport and mechanical properties of articular cartilage: a review. J Biomech 17:377-394, 1984.
14. Woo SLY, Simon BR, Kuei SC, Akeson WH: Quasi-linear viscoelastic properties of normal articular cartilage. J Biomech Eng 102:85-90, 1980.
15. Bollet AJ, Nance JL: Biochemical findings in normal and ostoeoarthritic articular cartilage II: chondroitin sulfate concentration and chain length, water, and ash content. J Clin Invest 45:1170-1177, 1996.
16. Modl JM, Sether LA, Haughton VM, Kneeland JB: Articular cartilage: correlation of histologic zones with signal intensity at MR imaging. Radiology 181:853-855, 1991.
17. Rubenstein J, Recht M, Disler DG, et al: Laminar structures on MR images of articular cartilage. Radiology 204:15-16, 1997.
18. Xia Y, Farquhar T, Burton-Wurster N, Lust G: Origin of cartilage laminae in MRI. J Magn Reson Imaging 210:843-850, 1997.
19. Goodwin DW, Wadgihiri YZ, Dunn JF: Micro-imaging of articular cartilage: T2, proton density and the magic angle effect. Acad Radiol 5:790-798, 1998.
20. Frank LR, Wong EC, Luh WM, et al: Articular cartilage in the knee: mapping of the physiologic parameters at MR imaging with a local gradient coil–preliminary results. Radiology 210:241-246, 1999.
21. Goodwin DW, Dunn JF: High-resolution magnetic resonance imaging of articular cartilage: correlation with histology and pathology. Top Magn Reson Imaging 9:337-347, 1998.
22. Goodwin DW, Zhu H, Dunn JF: In vitro MR imaging of hyaline cartilage: correlation with scanning electron microscopy. Am J Roentgenol 174:405-407, 2000.
23. Erickson SJ, Prost RW, Timins ME: The "magic angle" effect: background physics and clinical relevance. Radiology 188:219, 1993.
24. Wacker FK, Bolze X, Felsenberg D, Wolf KJ: Orientation-dependent changes in MR signal intensity of articular cartilage: a manifestation of the "magic angle" effect. Skeletal Radiol 27:306-310, 1998.
25. Rubenstein JD, Kim JK, Morava-Protzner I, et al: Effects of collagen orientation on MR imaging characteristics of bovine articular cartilage. Radiology 188:219-226, 1993.
26. Rubenstein JD, Kim JK, Henkelman RM: Effects of compression and recovery on bovine articular cartilage: appearance on MR images. Radiology 201:843-850, 1996.

27. Mosher TJ, Smith H, Dardzinski BJ, et al: MR imaging and T2 mapping of femoral cartilage—in vivo determination of the magic angle effect. Am J Roentgenol 177:665-669, 2001.
28. Lehner KB, Rechl HP, Gimeinwieser JK, et al: Structure, function, and degeneration of bovine hyaline cartilage: assessment with MR imaging in vitro. Radiology 170:495-499, 1989.
29. Paul PK, O'Byrne E, Blancuzzi V, et al: Magnetic resonance imaging reflects cartilage proteoglycan degradation in the rabbit knee. Skeletal Radiol 20:31-36, 1991.
30. Burstein D, Gray ML, Hartman AL, et al: Diffusion of small solutes in cartilage as measured by nuclear magnetic resoncance (NMR) spectroscopy and imaging. J Orthop Res 188:219-226, 1993.
31. Henkelman RM, Stanisz GJ, Kim JK, Bronskill MJ: Anisotropy of NMR properties of tissue. Magn Reson Med 32:592-601, 1994.
32. Conway WF, Hayes CW, Laughran T, et al: Cross sectional imaging of the patellofemoral joint and surrounding structures. RadioGraphics 11:195-217, 1991.
33. Vallotton JA, Meuli RA, Leyvraz PF, Landry M: Comparison between magnetic resonance imaging and arthroscopy in the diagnosis of patellar cartilage lesions: a prospective study. Knee Surg Sports Traumatol Arthrosc 3:157-162, 1995.
34. McCauley TR, Kier R, Lynch KJ, Joki P: Chondromalacia patellae: diagnosis with MR imaging. Am J Roentgenol 158:101-105, 1992.
35. Winalski CS, Minas T: Evaluation of chondral injuries by magnetic resonance imaging: repair assessments. Oper Tech Sports Med 8:108-119, 2000.
36. Potter HG, Linklater JM, Allen AA, et al: Magnetic resonance imaging of articular cartilage in the knee. An evaluation with use of fast spin-echo imaging. J Bone Joint Surg Am 80:1276-1284, 1998.
37. Bredella MA, Tirman PF, Peterfly CG, et al: Accuracy of T2-weighted fast spin-echo MR imaging with fat saturation in detecting cartilage defects in the knee: comparison with arthroscopy in 130 patients. Am J Roentgenol 172:1073-1080, 1999.
38. Yao L, Gentili A, Thomas J: Incidental magnetization transfer contrast in fast spin-echo imaging of cartilage. J Magn Reson Imaging 6:180-184, 1996.
39. Mohr A, Roemer FW, Genant HK, Liess C: Using fat-saturated proton density-weighted MR imaging to evaluate articular cartilage. Am J Roentgenol 181:280-282, 2003.
40. Mirowitz SA, Shu JJ: MR imaging evaluation of knee collateral ligaments and related injuries: comparison of T1-weighted, T2-weighted, and fat-saturated T2-weighted sequences—correlation with clinical findings. J Magn Reson Imaging 4:725-732, 1994.
41. Lal NR, Jamadar DA, Doi K, et al: Evaluation of bone contusions with fat-saturated fast spin-echo proton-density magnetic resonance imaging. Can Assoc Radiol J 51:182-185, 2000.
42. Escobedo EM, Hunter JC, Zinc-Brody GC, et al: Usefulness of turbo spin-echo MR imaging in the evaluation of meniscal tears: comparison with a conventional spin-echo sequence. Am J Roentgenol 167:1223-1227, 1996.
43. Eckstein F, Schnier M, Haubner M, et al: Accuracy of cartilage volume and thickness measurements with magnetic resonance imaging. Clin Orthop 352:137-148, 1998.
44. Disler DG, Peters TL, Muscoreil SJ, et al: Fat-suppressed spoiled GRASS imaging of knee hyaline cartilage: technique optimization and comparison with conventional MR imaging. Am J Roentgenol 163:887-892, 1994.
45. Disler DG, MaCauley TR, Kelman CG, et al: Fat-suppressed three-dimensional spoiled gradient-echo MR imaging of hyaline cartilage defects in the knee: comparison with standard MR imaging and arthroscopy. Am J Roentgenol 167:127-132, 1996.
46. Recht MP, Piraino DW, Paletta GA, et al: Accuracy of fat-suppressed three-dimensional spoiled gradient echo FLASH MR imaging in the detection of patellofemoral articular cartilage abnormalities. Radiology 198:209-212, 1996.
47. Recht MP, Dramer J, Marcellis S, et al: Abnormalities of articular cartilage in the knee: analysis of available MR techniques. Radiology 187:473-478, 1993.
48. Erickson SJ, Waldschmidt JG, Czervionke LF, Prost RW: Hyaline cartilage: truncation artifact as a cause of trilaminar appearance with fat-suppressed three-dimensional spoiled gradient-recalled sequences. Radiology 201:260-264, 1996.
49. Disler DG, McCauley TR, Wirth CR, Fuchs MD: Detection of knee hyaline cartilage defects using fat-suppressed three-dimensional spoiled gradient-echo MR imaging: comparison with standard MR imaging and correlation with arthroscopy. Am J Roentgenol 165:377-382, 1995.
50. Ruehm S, Zanetti M, Romero J, Hodler J: MRI of patellar articular cartilage: evaluation of an optimized gradient-echo sequence (3D-DESS). J Magn Reson Imaging 8:1246-1251, 1998.
51. Speer KP, Spritzer CE, Goldner JL, Garrett WE: Magnetic resonance imaging of traumatic knee articular cartilage injuries. Am J Sports Med 19:396-402, 1991.
52. Woertler K, Strothman M, Tombach B, Reimer P: Detection of articular cartilage lesions: experimental evaluation of low- and high-field strength MR imaging at 0.18 and 1.0T. J Magn Reson Imaging 11:678-685, 2000.
53. Bredella MA, Losasso C, Moelleken SC, et al: Three-point Dixon chemical-shift imaging for evaluating articular cartilage defects in the knee joint on a low-field-strength open magnet. Am J Roentgenol 177:1371-1375, 2001.
54. Kramer J, Recht MP, Imhof H, Engel A: Post-contrast MR arthrography in assessment of cartilage lesions. J Comput Assist Tomogr 18:218-224, 1994.
55. Rand T, Brossman, J, Pedowitz R, et al: Analysis of patellar cartilage. Comparison of conventional MR imaging and MR and CT arthrography in cadavers. Acta Radiol 41:492, 2000.
56. Gagliardi JA, Chung EM, Chandnani VP, et al: Detection and staging of chondromalacia patellae: relative efficacies of conventional MR imaging, MR arthrography, and CT arthrography. Am J Roentgenol 163:629-636, 1994.
57. Outerbridge RE: The etiology of chondromalacia patellae. J Bone Joint Surg Br 43:752-767, 1961.
58. Yulish BS, Montanez J, Goodfellow DB, et al: Chondromalacia patellae: assessment with MR imaging. Radiology 164:763-766, 1987.
59. Bollet AJ, Nance JL: Biochemical findings in normal and ostoearthritic articular cartilage, II: chondroitin sulfate concentration and chain length, water, and ash content. J Clin Invest 45:1170-1177, 1966.
60. Burstein D, Bashir A, Gray ML: MRI techniques in early stages of cartilage disease. Invest Radiol 35:622-638, 2000.
61. Mosher TJ, Dardzinski BJ, Smith MB: Human articular cartilage: influence of aging and early symptomatic degeneration on the spatial variation of T2-preliminary findings at 3T. Radiology 214:259-266, 2000.
62. Hayes CW, Sawyer RW, Conway WF: Patellar cartilage lesions: in vitro detection and staging with MR imaging and pathologic correlation. Radiology 176:479-493, 1990.
63. Terry GC, Flandry F, Van Manen JW, Norwood LA: Isolated chondral fractures of the knee. Clin Orthop 234:170-177, 1988.
64. Rubin DA, Harner CD, Costello JM: Treatable chondral injuries in the knee: frequency of associated focal subchondral edema. Am J Roentgenol 174:1099-1106, 2000.
65. Turner DA: Subchondral bone marrow edema in degenerative chondrosis. Am J Roentgenol 175:1749-1750, 2000.
66. Bradley J, Dandy DJ: Osteochondritis dissecans and other lesions of the femoral condyles. J Bone Joint Surg 71-B:518-522, 1989.
67. Obedian RS, Grelsamer RP: Osteochondritis dissecans of the distal femur and patella. Clin Sports Med 16:157-175, 1997.
68. Federico DJ, Lynch JK, Jokl P: Osteochondritis dissecans of the knee: a historical review of etiology and treatment. Arthroscopy 6:190-197, 1990.
69. Green WT, Banks HH: Osteochondritis dissecans in children. J Bone Joint Surg 255:3-12, 1990.
70. Mubarak SJ, Carroll NC: Juvenile osteochondritis dissecans of the knee: etiology. Clin Orthop 157:200-211, 1981.
71. Dipaola JD, Nelson DW, Colville MR: Characterizing osteochondral lesions by magnetic resonance imaging. Arthroscopy 7:101-104, 1991.
72. De Smet AA, Ilahi OA, Graf BK: Reassessment of the MR criteria for stability of osteochondritis dissecans in the knee and ankle. Skeletal Radiol 25:159-163, 1996.
73. Boutin RD, Januario JA, Newberg AH, et al: MR imaging features of osteochondritis dissecans of the femoral sulcus. Am J Roentgenol 180:641-645, 2003.
74. McCauley TR, Kornaat PR, Jee WH: Central osteophytes in the knee: prevalence and association with cartilage defects on MR imaging. Am J Roentgenol 176:359-364, 2001.
75. Alparsian L, Winalski C, Boutin R, Minas T: Post-operative magnetic resonance imaging of articular cartilage repair. Semin Musculoskeletal Radiol 5:345-363, 2001.
76. Gillogly SD, Voight M, Blackburn T: Treatment of articular cartilage defects of the knee with autologous chondrocyte implantation. J Orthop Sports Phys Ther 28:241-251, 1998.
77. Sanders TG, Mentzer KD, Miller MD, et al: Mosaicplasty for the treatment of articular cartilage defects: postoperative MR appearance with clinical correlation. Skeletal Radiol 30:570-578, 2001.
78. Recht MP, Kramer JF: MR imaging of the postoperative knee: a pictorial essay. RadioGraphics 22:765-774, 2002.
79. Brittberg M, Lindahl A, Nilsson A, et al: Treatment of deep cartilage defects in the knee with autologous chondrocyte transplantation. N Engl J Med 331:889-895, 1994.
80. Alparslan L, Minas T, Winalski CS: Magnetic resonance imaging of autologous chondrocyte implantation. Semin Ultrasound CT MRI 22:341-51, 2001.
81. Convery FR, Meyers MH, Akeson WH: Fresh osteochondral allografting of the femoral condyle. Clin Orthop 273:139-145, 1991.
82. Bugbee W, Convery FR: Osteochondral allograft transplantation. Clin Sports Med 18:67-75, 1999.
83. Sirlin CB, Brossmann J, Boutin RD: Shell osteochondral allografts of the knee; comparison of MR imaging findings and immunologic responses. Radiology 219:35-43, 2001.
84. Gold GE, McCauley TR, Gray ML, Disler DG: What's new in cartilage? RadioGraphics 23:1227-1242, 2003.
85. Eckstein F, Reiser M, Englmeier KH, Putz R: In vivo morphometry and functional analysis of human articular cartilage with quantitative magnetic resonance imaging—from image to data, from data to theory. Anat Embryol (Berl) 203:147-173, 2001.
86. Burgkart R, Glaser C, Hyhlik-Durr A, et al: Magnetic resonance imaging-based assessment of cartilage loss in severe osteoarthritis: Accuracy, precision, and diagnostic value. Arthritis Rheum 44:2072-2077, 2001.

87. Eckstein F, Heudorfer L, Faber SC, et al: Long-term and resegmentation precision of quantitative cartilage MR imaging (QMRI). Osteoarthritis Cartilage 10:922-928, 2002.

88. Burgkart R, Glaser C, Hinterwimmer S, et al: Feasibility of t and z scores from magnetic resonance imaging data for quantification of cartilage loss in osteoarthritis. Arthritis Rheum 48:2829-2835, 2003.

89. Glaser C, Burgkart R, Kutschera A, et al: Femoro-tibial cartilage metrics from coronal MR image data: Technique, test-retest reproducibility, and findings in osteoarthritis. Magn Reson Med 50:1229-1236, 2003.

90. Raynauld JP, Kauffmann C, Beaudoin G, et al: Reliability of a quantification imaging system using magnetic resonance images to measure cartilage thickness and volume in human normal and osteoarthritic knees. Osteoarthritis Cartilage 11:351-360, 2003.

91. Cicuttini FM, Wluka AE, Wang Y, et al: Compartment differences in knee cartilage volume in healthy adults. J Rheumatol 29:554-556, 2002.

92. Cicuttini FM, Wluka AE, Stuckey SL: Tibial and femoral cartilage changes in knee osteoarthritis. Ann Rheum Dis 60:977-980, 2001.

93. Hunter DJ, Snieder H, March L, Sambrook PN: Genetic contribution to cartilage volume in women: a classical twin study. Rheumatology (Oxford) 42:1495-1500, 2003.

94. Bullough PG: The role of joint architecture in the etiology of arthritis. Osteoarthritis Cartilage 12(Suppl A):2-9, 2004.

95. Lohmander LS, Felson D: Can we identify a "high risk" patient profile to determine who will experience rapid progression of osteoarthritis? Osteoarthritis Cartilage 12(Suppl A):49-52, 2004.

96. Eckstein F, Lemberger B, Stammberger T, et al: Patellar cartilage deformation in vivo after static versus dynamic loading. J Biomech 33:819-825, 2000.

97. Fragonas E, Mlynarik V, Jellus V, et al: Correlation between biochemical composition and magnetic resonance appearance of articular cartilage. Osteoarthritis Cartilage 6:24-32, 1998.

98. Lusse S, Claassen H, Gehrke T, et al: Evaluation of water content by spatially resolved transverse relaxation times of human articular cartilage. Magn Reson Imaging 18:423-430, 2000.

99. Nieminen MT, Toyras J, Rieppo J, et al: Quantitative MR microscopy of enzymatically degraded articular cartilage. Magn Reson Med 43:676-681, 2000.

100. Liess C, Lusse S, Karger N, et al: Detection of changes in cartilage water content using MRI T2-mapping in vivo. Osteoarthritis Cartilage 10:907-913, 2002.

101. Mlynarik V, Trattnig S, Huber M, et al: The role of relaxation times in monitoring proteoglycan depletion in articular cartilage. J Magn Reson Imaging 10:497-502, 1999.

102. Menezes NM, Gray ML, Hartke JR, Burstein D: T2 and T1-rho MRI in articular cartilage systems. Magn Reson Med 51:503-509, 2004.

103. Hargreaves BA, Gold GE, Lang PK, et al: MR imaging of articular cartilage using driven equilibrium. Magn Reson Med 42:695-703, 1999.

104. Hargreaves BA, Gold GE, Beaulieu CF, et al: Comparison of new sequences for high-resolution cartilage imaging. Magn Reson Med 49:700-709, 2003.

105. Henkelman RM, Stanisz GJ, Menezes N, Burstein D: Can MTR be used to assess cartilage in the presence of Gd-DTPA2⁻? Magn Reson Med 48:1081-1084, 2002.

106. Dardzinski BJ, Mosher TJ, Li S, et al: Spatial variation of T2 in human articular cartilage. Radiology 205:546-550, 1997.

107. Smith HE, Mosher TJ, Dardzinski BJ, et al: Spatial variation in cartilage T2 of the knee. J Magn Reson Imaging 14:50-55, 2001.

108. Maroudas A: Physicochemical properties of cartilage in the light of ion exchange theory. Biophys J 8:575-595, 1968.

109. Maroudas A, Thomas H: A simple physicochemical micromethod for determining fixed anionic groups in connective tissue. Biochim Biophys Acta 215:214-216, 1970.

110. Lesperance LM, Gray ML, Burstein D: Determination of fixed charge density in cartilage using nuclear magnetic resonance. J Orthop Res 10:1-13, 1992.

111. Shapiro EM, Borthakur A, Gougoutas A, Reddy R: 23-Na MRI accurately measures fixed charge density in articular cartilage. Magn Reson Med 47:284-291, 2002.

112. Bashir A, Gray ML, Hartke J, Burstein D: Nondestructive imaging of human cartilage glycosaminoglycan concentration by MRI. Magn Reson Med 41:857-865, 1999.

113. Bashir A, Gray ML, Burstein D: Gd-DTPA2⁻ as a measure of cartilage degradation. Magn Reson Med 36:665-673, 1996. (Published erratum appears in Magn Reson Med 36:964, 1996.)

114. Trattnig S, Mlynarik V, Breitenseher M, et al: MRI visualization of proteoglycan depletion in articular cartilage via intravenous administration of Gd-DTPA. Magn Reson Imaging 17:577-583, 1999.

115. Nieminen MT, Rieppo J, Silvennoinen J, et al: Spatial assessment of articular cartilage proteoglycans with Gd-DTPA-enhanced T1 imaging. Magn Reson Med 48:640-648, 2002.

116. Bashir A, Gray ML, Boutin RD, Burstein D: Glycosaminoglycan in articular cartilage: In vivo assessment with delayed Gd(DTPA)(2⁻)-enhanced MR imaging. Radiology 205:551-558, 1997.

117. Tiderius CJ, Svensson J, Leander P, et al: dGEMRIC (delayed gadolinium enhanced MRI of cartilage) indicates adaptive capacity of human knee cartilage. Magn Reson Med 51:286-290, 2004

118. Tiderius CJ, Olsson LE, De Verdier H, et al: Gd-DTPA2⁻-enhanced MRI of femoral knee cartilage: a dose-response study in healthy volunteers. Magn Reson Med 46:1067-1071, 2001.

119. Burstein D, Velyvis J, Scott KT, et al: Protocol issues for delayed Gd(DTPA) (2⁻)-enhanced MRI (dGEMRIC) for clinical evaluation of articular cartilage. Magn Reson Med 45:36-41, 2001.

120. Williams A, Gillis A, McKenzie C, et al: Glycosaminoglycan distribution in cartilage as determined by delayed gadolinium-enhanced MRI of cartilage (dGEMRIC): Potential clinical applications. Am J Roentgenol 182:167-172, 2004.

121. Tiderius CJ, Olsson LE, Leander P, et al: Delayed gadolinium-enhanced MRI of cartilage (dGEMRIC) in early knee osteoarthritis. Magn Reson Med 49:488-492, 2003.

122. Allen RG, Burstein D, Gray ML: Monitoring glycosaminoglycan replenishment in cartilage explants with gadolinium-enhanced magnetic resonance imaging. J Orthop Res 17:430-436, 1999.

123. Williams A, Oppenheimer RA, Gray ML, Burstein D: Differential recovery of glycosaminoglycan after IL-1-induced degradation of bovine articular cartilage depends on degree of degradation. Arthritis Res Ther 5:R97-105, 2003.

124. Gillis A, Bashir A, McKeon B, et al: Magnetic resonance imaging of relative glycosaminoglycan distribution in patients with autologous chondrocyte transplants. Invest Radiol 36:743-748, 2001.

CHAPTER 110

PEDIATRIC MUSCULOSKELETAL SYSTEM

Caroline L. Hollingsworth ● George S. Bisset III

Magnetic resonance imaging (MRI) offers exquisite soft-tissue contrast and multiplanar evaluation of musculoskeletal disorders. Cartilaginous components of the immature skeleton such as nonossified epiphyses and physes are better visualized by MRI than by plain radiographs or computed tomography (CT). Advantages of MRI in the pediatric patient include no known adverse biologic effect, no ionizing radiation, and no absolute requirement for intravenous contrast in order to obtain superb spatial resolution and soft-tissue contrast. However, pediatric MRI presents a unique set of challenges, including smaller structures of interest, developmental variants, a unique group of pathologic processes, and issues relating to sedation.

This chapter seeks to address procedural issues specific to the pediatric population, as well as outlining some of the uses of MR in the evaluation of musculoskeletal disorders. Bone tumors and bone marrow disorders are covered in Chapters 107 and 108; therefore, only nuances specific to the pediatric population are addressed in this chapter.

TECHNIQUE

Sedation

Conscious sedation is a fundamental and necessary part of successful MR imaging in young patients. Most children under the age of 6 years will require sedation while undergoing an MR examination. Occasionally older children will also require sedation. The practice of responsible conscious sedation is difficult and time consuming but because of potentially devastating deleterious effects, the establishment of safe sedation protocols and procedures is paramount.

Patient preparation is an integral component of a successful sedation protocol. Prior to conscious sedation for any procedure, the patient must undergo a screening evaluation and informed consent must be obtained. The purpose of the screening examination is to elicit potential factors that may increase the risk of complication, including presence and extent of current medical conditions such as cardiovascular, respiratory, metabolic or central nervous system disease.[1] It is also important to identify current medications, recent illnesses (e.g., upper respiratory infection), any allergies and previous history of adverse response to particular sedative agents.

Patients should be informed of fasting requirements for conscious sedation prior to the day of their procedure. Clear liquids in moderation can be allowed up to 2 hours before sedation at any age. Solid food and semisolid liquids (formula and breast milk) should be withheld for 4 hours prior to sedation in children under 6 months old, 6 hours prior to sedation in children 6 months to 3 years old and 8 hours prior in children over 3 years of age. Adhering to this protocol will help minimize risks of aspiration, while helping to avoid dehydration and hypoglycemia.

Parental consent for conscious sedation is an integral part of the preprocedural process. In fact, signed informed consent has been incorporated into the minimum standard of care for sedated patients by the

Joint Commission on Accreditation of Healthcare Organizations.[2] At a minimum, this process familiarizes the patient and parent or guardian with the procedure, the importance of conscious sedation, associated risks, and alternatives. In addition, safe and responsible sedation practices include immediate access to resuscitation equipment and drugs appropriate for children of all sizes from the preterm infant to an adult-sized teenager. Protocols for routine surveillance of equipment are necessary to ensure supplies are updated and replaced as needed.

It is important to determine which personnel will be responsible for sedation. Many institutions employ radiology nurses for this purpose. This allows the technologist and radiologist to focus on obtaining an adequate exam. The radiology nurse may be responsible for obtaining a pertinent history, performing a limited, focused physical exam, administering appropriate medications for sedation after consultation with the radiologist, post-procedural monitoring and discharge instructions. However, it should be clear that the ultimate responsibility of practicing safe and successful conscious sedation rests on the radiologist or the clinician assigned to this task.

As a general rule, conscious sedation can be utilized in children whose current medical condition and past medical history place them within the definition of the American Society of Anesthesia (ASA) class I or II (ASA Task Force). In select patients who are classified as ASA class III, conscious sedation may be provided at the radiologist's discretion. Many children in ASA classes III, IV or V will require sedation or anesthesia by an anesthesiologist.[3]

Monitoring of the patient is a critical component of a successful sedation program. One trained practitioner must be assigned to sedate, monitor, and attend to the child.[4,5] Monitoring a sedated child involves both physical observation (allowing for limitations due to the exam) and monitoring devices. Although a variety of monitoring techniques have been employed, at a minimum, continuous pulse oximetry and heart rate monitoring should be part of a standard protocol. The simplest and most direct way to accomplish this is with the pulse oximeter, which provides continuous measurement of transcutaneous oxygen saturation with minimal disturbance to the patient. Oxygen supplementation by blow-by technique should be considered during scanning.[3,5] However, occasionally this practice may arouse the child. Mobile MR-compatible equipment is important, as it allows continuous monitoring of the sedated child before, during and after the procedure. Vital signs including heart rate, respiratory rate, and oxygen saturation should be recorded at a maximum interval of every 5 minutes during the exam.[4]

Post-procedural monitoring is necessary until the patient is ready for discharge. Discharge criteria recommended by the American Academy of Pediatrics, Committee on Drugs include: satisfactory and stable cardiovascular system and airway, awake or easily arousable patient, intact protective reflexes, patient can talk and sit up (when age appropriate). For infants and handicapped children who are not capable of these

responses, the goal at discharge should be to regain normal activity and level of consciousness for that child.[4]

Although there is an extensive armamentarium of pharmacologic agents available for sedation in children, optimal sedation protocols usually employ only a few sedatives and analgesics.[3] A single agent or combination of two agents should suffice. In general, the use of multiple agents to achieve sedation increases the risk of adverse effects.[6] It is the radiologist's responsibility to be aware of both desired and adverse effects as well as antagonists (when available) for any medication given to a child for the purpose of conscious sedation. Table 110.1 summarizes the more frequently used pediatric sedative agents.[3]

Chloral hydrate is a sedative agent frequently used in both pediatrics and diagnostic imaging. This sedative has a low rate of side-effects and a long safety record. Oral chloral hydrate in doses of 75 to 100 mg/kg given 20 to 40 minutes before the examination is generally effective in patients younger than 18 months. The total dose should not exceed 2 g. This relatively high dose is necessary because of relatively long examination times and repetitive loud noises produced by alternating currents in the coils. Intravenous pentobarbital sodium may be used with a high degree of success in patients older than 18 months. This agent is given by slow injection of 2 to 3 mg/kg doses and titrated approximately every 10 minutes until sedation is achieved or until a total dose of 8 to 9 mg/kg is reached. Hyperesthesia is a well-known side-effect and the addition of intravenous fentanyl citrate as an analgesic in doses of 1 to 2 μg/kg (not to exceed a total of 4 μg/kg) may be useful.

Occasionally (approximately 2% of the time), patients fail this sedation regimen, either from an inability to maintain sedation within safe dose limits or from an adverse reaction to the medications (respiratory compromise or paradoxical hyperactivity reaction). In these instances, it may be necessary to perform the study with the use of general anesthesia (if compatible anesthesiology equipment is available) or pursue heavier sedation under the guidance of an anesthesiologist.

Immobilization and Coil Selection

One of the most important aspects of patient preparation when performing an exam on a child is patient comfort. Exam times are often long and many children experience difficulty maintaining a motionless state for the duration of the examination. Even the most sophisticated motion reduction techniques have difficulty compensating for gross motion. Immobilization should be considered when gross motion is a potential problem, especially in young children. Immobilization should help the child remain motionless, not serve as a restraining device during the exam.

Because of the range of shapes and sizes of the anatomic regions of interest in the pediatric population, it is important to have a variety of volume and surface coils available to optimize image quality. Ideally, one would like to use the smallest coil available that will

TABLE 110-1 Sedative Agents for Pediatric Imaging

Agents	Class	Effect	Dose	Route[a]	Onset	Duration[b]
Chloral hydrate[c]	NA	Sedative	50-100 mg/kg, up to 120 mg/kg reported, max single dose 2 g	PO (PR)	20-30 min (rarely up to 60 min)	30-90 min
Sodium pentobarbital	Barbiturate	Sedative	2-3 mg/kg doses titrated q 5-7 min until sedated or max cumulative amount of 8 mg/kg, not to exceed 200 mg	IV (PO, IM)	5-10 min	40-60 min
Fentanyl citrate	Narcotic	Analgesic with sedative properties	1 µg/kg slowly IV q 5-7 min, adult-size patients 25-50 µg per dose, max cumulative dose 4.0 µg/kg	IV	1-2 min	30-60 min for analgesia; sedation may be shorter
Midazolam	Benzodiazepine	Sedative, anxiolytic, amnestic	0.02-0.05 mg/kg IV, titrate using ½ original dose (2-4 min) based on effect and oxygen saturation, max bolus dose 1.0 mg	IV (PO)	1-5 min (IV)	20-30 min
Diazepam	Benzodiazepine	Sedative, anxiolytic, amnestic	0.05-0.1 mg/kg IV, max cumulative dose 5.0 mg; 0.2-0.3 mg/kg PO, max cumulative dose 10 mg	IV (PO)	5-15 min (IV)	30-120 min
Methohexital	Barbiturate	Sedative	20 mg/kg in 10% solution	PR	10-15 min	45 min
Morphine	Narcotic	Analgesic with sedative properties	0.1-0.2 mg/kg, max dose 3-4 mg	IV (IM)	3-5 min	Analgesia up to 4 hr; sedation is variable but shorter
Meperidine	Narcotic	Analgesic with sedative properties	1-2 mg/kg, max dose 100 mg	IV (IM)	5-10 min	Analgesia 1-2 hr; sedation is variable but shorter
Naloxone hydrochloride	NA	Narcotic antagonist	0.01-0.1 mg/kg (lower antagonist dose for infant); repeat 2-3 min; titrate to reversal, max dose 2 mg	IV	1-2 min	Max to 20-30 min
Flumazenil	NA	Benzodiazepine antagonist	0.01 mg/kg, max dose (adult) 0.2 mg, max cumulative dose 1 mg	IV	1-3 min; peak effect 6-10 min	Max 60 min but usually <30 min depending on benzodiazepine dose

Note: IM = intramuscular, max = maximum, NA = not applicable, PO = per oram, PR = per rectum.
[a]Preferred route listed first with alternative route(s) in parentheses.
[b]Duration of sedative effect for imaging purposes. Drowsiness, ataxia, and other effects may have variable durations depending on the agent, dose, and route of administration.
[c]Thioridazine or hydroxyzine have been reported as adjuncts in children difficult to sedate with chloral hydrate alone.
Adapted from Frush D: Pediatric sedation in radiology: the practice of safe sleep. Am J Roentgenol 167:1383, 1996.

include the entire area of interest. This allows optimization of both spatial resolution and the signal-to-noise ratio. It is also best, particularly with sedated patients, to select a single-coil set-up for the entire examination, because changing coils in the midst of an examination often necessitates additional sedation. Optimally, the extremity (or region) of interest should be positioned such that it lies within at least one of the three orthogonal planes with respect to the bore of the magnet. Positioning the patient in this way will decrease the need for double-oblique imaging. It is also important to place the area of interest as close to the center of the magnetic field as possible in order to optimize the homogeneity of the magnetic field.

Pulse Sequences

A thorough discussion of pulse sequences is beyond the scope of this chapter. However, a brief overview of the more commonly used sequences is worthwhile. Conventional spin-echo sequences are still the most commonly used pulse sequences. T1-weighted images (repetition time <800 ms, echo time <30 ms), in which fat produces a high signal intensity and most infiltrative processes produce low signal intensity, provide excellent contrast between normal and abnormal marrow and between pathologic processes and adjacent subcutaneous fat. Muscle produces relatively low signal intensity on all pulse sequences, such that contrast between muscle and infiltrative processes is well seen on proton density-weighted and T2-weighted images (on which most pathologic processes produce increased signal intensity). Fast spin-echo techniques have advantages in the pediatric population primarily because of decreased scan time. Fast spin-echo inversion recovery (FSEIR) images may be useful for maximizing contrast between pathologic processes and surrounding tissues. This pulse sequence also provides increased contrast between red and yellow marrow.[7] Gradient-recalled sequences are often useful for visualizing articular cartilage and for producing T2* contrast with a relatively short imaging time. Fast GRE sequences can help combat artifact from gross motion with very quick scan times, especially in young patients.[8] Fat suppression, usually coupled with conventional or fast spin-echo T2-weighted imaging, may be a useful adjunct for improving contrast resolution in situations in which processes of high signal intensity are in contact with fat.

Contrast Administration

The indications for using Gd-DTPA as a contrast agent in the pediatric patient differ from indications in the adult population. This is due to a variety of differences in disease processes, as well as developmental maturation of the musculoskeletal system. The intravenous administration of Gd-DTPA does not require a change in monitoring practices. In general, intravenous access should be obtained prior to sedation or alternatively just prior to post-contrast imaging in older co-operative

children. EMLA (eutectic mixture of local anesthetic) cream can be used at the injection site to reduce anxiety of both the parent and child, although successful use of EMLA cream requires preprocedural planning. Prior to contrast material administration, a T1-weighted sequence with fat saturation should be obtained through the region of interest. Routinely, hand bolus administration of gadolinium (0.1 mmol/kg) is followed by repeating the same precontrast T1-weighted sequence. Alternatively, dynamic contrast images can be obtained with faster gradient-echo pulse sequences. In this situation, consider contrast-filled injection tubing to allow consistent positioning of the child within the bore of the magnet for precontrast, dynamic, and post-contrast imaging.[8]

Although the addition of post-contrast sequences does not usually affect sensitivity or specificity during primary imaging of pediatric bone or soft-tissue tumors, it has been suggested that contrast-enhanced T1-weighted images may help select biopsy sites in bulky tumors and provide superior delineation of the relationship between the tumor and the neurovascular bundle.[9] Dynamic contrast enhancement may also prove useful in the evaluation of post-therapy tumors by distinguishing differential enhancement patterns of tumor, radiation effects, and postoperative fluid collections.[10] These findings, however, remain to be proven conclusively.

The differential diagnosis of soft-tissue masses in the pediatric population is vast. When imaging pediatric soft-tissue tumors, pre- and post-gadolinium enhanced sequences may play a critical role in defining potential cystic versus solid components of a lesion. Precontrast sequences help define the extent and signal characteristics of the mass. Post-contrast images in this setting are useful in answering one important question: Does the lesion enhance? This information will define whether the mass is cystic or solid. Postoperatively, pre- and post-contrast imaging is often necessary to help differentiate residual tumor from the post-surgical sequela of the procedure.

There is controversy regarding the administration of Gd-DTPA in the setting of inflammatory and infectious disorders in the pediatric patient. Although some authors have found that paramagnetic contrast agents are not needed for routine evaluation of extraspinal musculoskeletal infections in children, this practice is not ubiquitous.[11] In the setting of suspected osteomyelitis, gadolinium-enhanced sequences may improve definition of disease extent and increase conspicuity of complications such as abscesses and devitalized tissue.[12,13] In problematic cases of osteomyelitis, gadolinium-enhanced images can help define the true extent of the disease process and help guide percutaneous drainage as well as surgical debridement. Gadolinium administration has not proven useful in the evaluation of children with sickle cell disease and the clinical question of infection versus infarction (Fig. 110-1).[14,15] Gadolinium-enhanced images have proven helpful in the evaluation of children with juvenile rheumatoid arthritis. Due to rapid diffusion of gadolinium from the synovium into the joint space, dynamic injection technique or rapid post-contrast

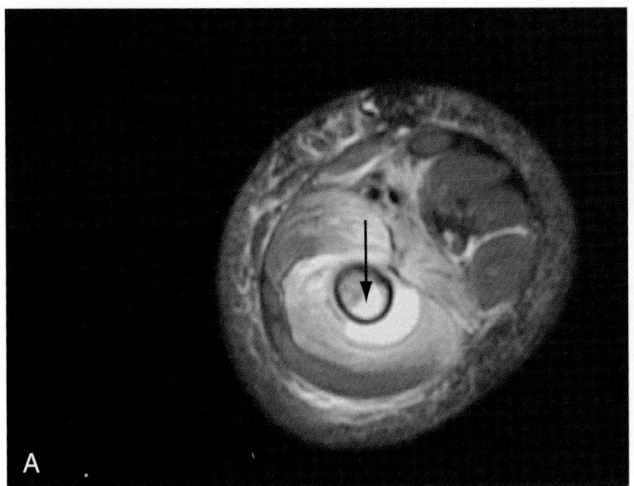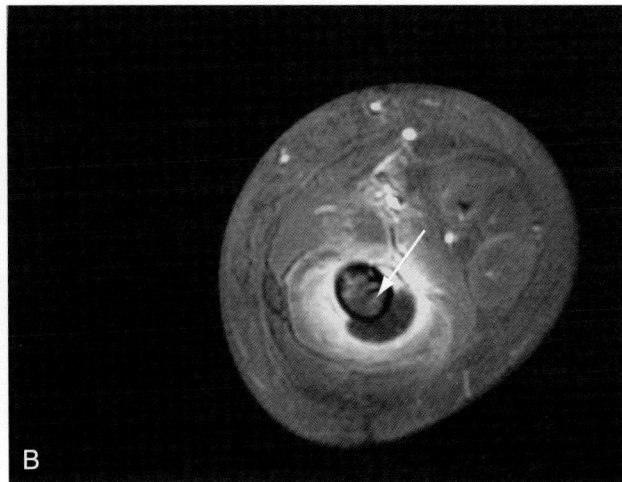

FIGURE 110-1

Sickle cell disease with sequela of acute infarction. Axial T2-weighted image (**A**) and axial T1-weighted image (**B**) demonstrate marrow edema (*arrow*), extensive soft-tissue and fascial inflammatory changes and focal fluid collection.

acquisition is crucial.[16] Post-contrast images allow better delineation of synovial hypertrophy and pannus formation. Recent research has focused on defining synovial inflammation in response to time–activity curves.[12] These investigations have shown promise with regard to assessing response to therapy.

INFECTION AND INFLAMMATION

Osteomyelitis

Osteomyelitis in children is most often the result of acute hematogenous dissemination. Direct inoculation, such as from penetrating trauma or surgery, is a less frequent cause of bone infection. *Staphylococcus aureus* is the causative agent in the majority of cases. Other organisms that have been implicated less frequently in osteomyelitis include streptococci, Haemophilus species, Salmonella (usually in patients with sickle cell disease), and Candida species. The most commonly affected anatomic area within the bones of the appendicular skeleton is the metaphysis, most likely because of its rich blood supply. Sluggish flow in the venous sinusoids probably predisposes to thrombosis and formation of an infected nidus. Subsequently, the inflammatory response produces increased intraosseous pressure, which may lead to bone necrosis with subsequent spread of infection through the Haversian system, into the cortex, and into the subperiosteal space. In the neonate, transphyseal vessels provide an avenue of spread to the epiphysis, which increases the frequency of subsequent septic arthritis as well as growth disturbance from physeal destruction.[17]

Clinical diagnosis rests on localized signs and symptoms, fever, elevated white blood cell count and erythrocyte sedimentation rate, and either bacteremia or positive bone aspirate culture. However, in younger children and neonates, signs and symptoms may be minimal or absent and leukocytosis and erythrocyte sedimentation rate elevation are not specific for osteomyelitis.

When acute osteomyelitis is suspected in a child, imaging is used to guide diagnosis and subsequent treatment. Plain radiographs are usually obtained to exclude other pathologic processes such as fracture or tumor. Early in the course of osteomyelitis, loss of normal fat planes and soft-tissue swelling may be the only findings, as bone destruction and periosteal reaction are not evident before 10 days to 2 weeks after the onset of symptoms. Radionuclide bone scintigraphy has been used extensively in the diagnosis of osteomyelitis. A multiphase ^{99}Tc methylenediphosphonate (MDP) bone scan will become positive 24 to 48 hours after the onset of symptoms.[18] Advantages include high sensitivity and the ability to image the entire skeleton. Although sensitivity has been reported as high as 95%, early in the course of disease relative ischemia from increased intraosseous pressure may cause false-negative results.[19] Tc-labeled white blood cell scanning or gallium citrate 67 scanning may be useful adjunctive tests to increase specificity. Disadvantages of radionuclide imaging include the use of ionizing radiation, low spatial resolution, relatively low specificity, and potential obscuration of metaphyseal findings by adjacent normal physeal activity. CT has limited value in the setting of acute osteomyelitis but better depicts sequelae of chronic disease such as bony sequestra and cortical destruction.

MR imaging has become a useful diagnostic tool in children with acute and chronic osteomyelitis.[20-22] Sensitivity of MR in adults and children with osteomyelitis has been reported at 88% to 100% with a specificity of 75% to 100%.[22-25] MR provides exquisite evaluation of both the marrow cavity and adjacent soft-tissues. Multiplanar capability may provide important

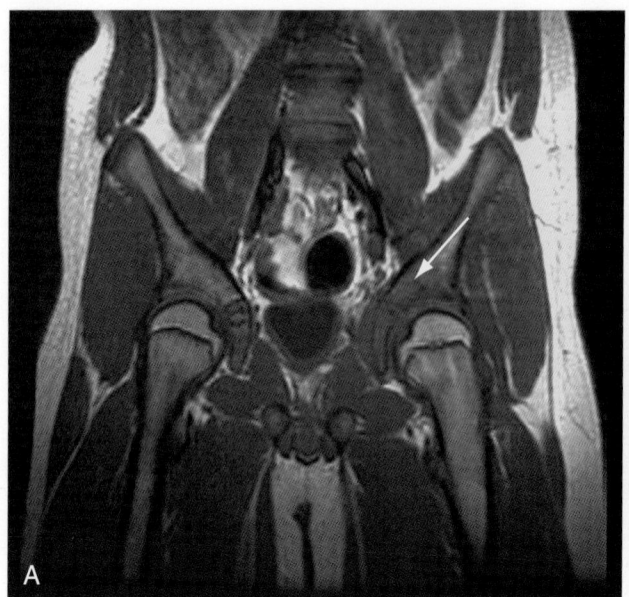 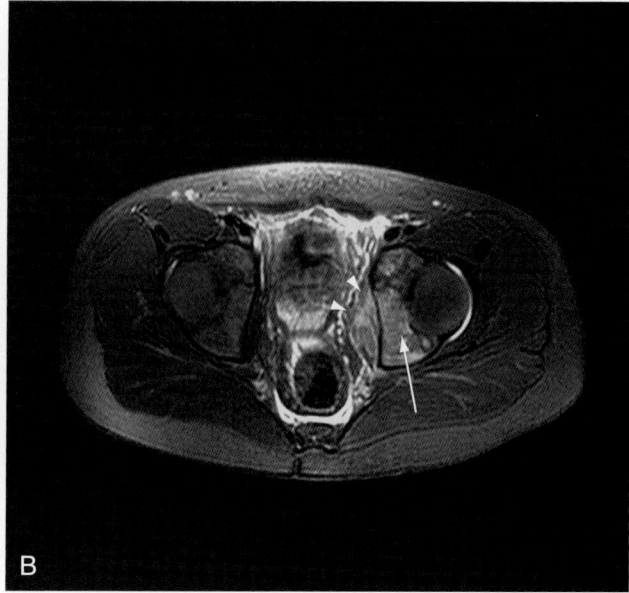

FIGURE 110-2

Acute osteomyelitis. **A,** Coronal T1-weighted image of the pelvis demonstrates decreased signal within the left acetabulum (*arrows*) as a result of acute osteomyelitis. **B,** Axial T2-weighted image at the same level demonstrates characteristic high signal from marrow edema within the left acetabulum (*arrows*) and associated soft-tissue inflammatory changes involving the left obturator internus (*arrowheads*).

anatomic information for percutaneous or open drainage and debridement.

MR imaging is capable of distinguishing acute from chronic osteomyelitis.[12] In acute osteomyelitis (Fig. 110-2), there is an ill-defined margin between normal and involved areas of bone marrow as well as between normal and involved areas of soft-tissue. There is a relative lack of cortical bone thickening but periosteal elevation may be present. In chronic osteomyelitis

(Fig. 110-3), there is a well-defined interface between normal and involved areas of marrow and soft-tissue. There is frequently evidence of cortical thickening. Brodie's abscess, a subacute form of osteomyelitis (Fig. 110-4), appears as a central area of decreased signal intensity on T1-weighted sequences and increased signal intensity on T2-weighted sequences with absent central enhancement and variable rim enhancement.[13] Sinus tracts appear as linear or curvilinear areas of increased

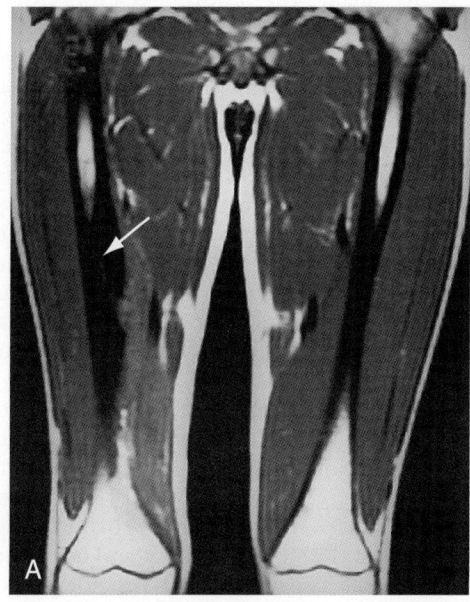 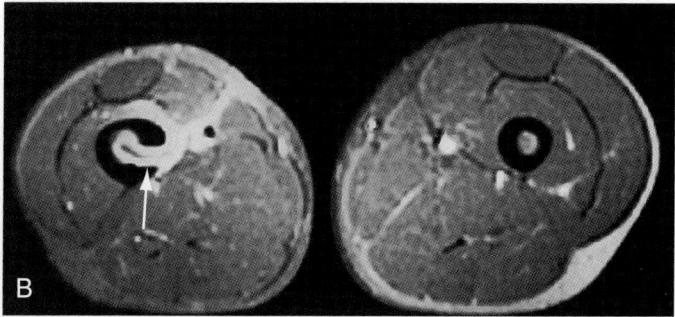

FIGURE 110-3

Chronic osteomyelitis with sinus tract formation. Coronal T1-weighted (600/20) image before contrast enhancement (**A**) and axial T1-weighted (600/12) image after contrast enhancement (**B**) demonstrate cortical thickening of the femoral diaphysis with a curvilinear sinus tract (*arrow*) extending from the marrow space to an adjacent area of soft-tissue signal abnormality. The orientation and location of the tract are well demonstrated.

signal intensity on T2-weighted sequences connecting the marrow space to the extraosseous soft-tissues. It is particularly useful to obtain longitudinal images in the plane of the sinus tract for surgical planning. T1-weighted images, usually obtained in a coronal or sagittal plane, show decreased signal intensity in areas of marrow involvement. STIR and fat-suppressed T2-weighted sequences have been reported to provide the best contrast between normal and involved marrow.[21] When obtained, contrast-enhanced images have been reported to be particularly useful in differentiating between viable areas of involvement and necrotic, devascularized zones within bone. This technique has also been used to define the margins of intraosseous and soft-tissue abscesses.[21]

Although osteomyelitis most commonly involves the metaphyses in children, epiphyseal osteomyelitis can also occur. MR imaging may help differentiate epiphyseal infection from epiphyseal neoplasms by providing information about associated soft-tissue abscess, sinus tract or sequestra. Another somewhat unusual form of osteomyelitis seen in children is chronic recurrent multifocal osteomyelitis (CRMO). This idiopathic non-pyogenic inflammatory bone disease typically has a prolonged or recurrent course.[26] Classically, multiple bones are involved, but this disease may present as a solitary lesion. CRMO commonly affects the distal tibia and femoral metaphyses but may also involve the clavicle and forearm as well as, rarely, the ribs, mandible, pelvis, and sternum.[27] MR imaging typically demonstrates decreased T1 signal adjacent to the physis and heterogeneously increased T2 signal without the soft-tissue abnormalities associated with pyogenic osteomyelitis.[12]

There is debate in the setting of suspected osteomyelitis in children regarding the utilization of conventional radiography, nuclear scintigraphy, and MR imaging. Although scintigraphy is more cost effective, more readily detects multiple foci of disease and may not require sedation, MR provides detailed evaluation of isolated or adjacent soft-tissue infection, more precisely delineates extent of periosteal and epiphyseal involvement and assesses for presence of joint effusion. Despite differing opinions regarding the initial imaging algorithm in acute osteomyelitis, most authors agree that MR provides useful information when localized disease does not respond to appropriate standard therapy or when biopsy or debridement is contemplated.[28-30] Gadolinium-enhanced imaging is recommended for complicated infections of the pelvis or extremities.[13,25,30]

Myositis

Myositis may result from bacterial or viral infection. In the absence of abscess or necrosis, muscle edema may be the only finding on MRI. Bacterial myositis often results from direct extension of osteomyelitis or subcutaneous abscess. Abscess formation in the setting of bacterial myositis is common and in this setting the inflammatory response may take on a mass-like appearance.[31] Viral myositis is not typically associated with abscess formation. MRI may be useful in defining

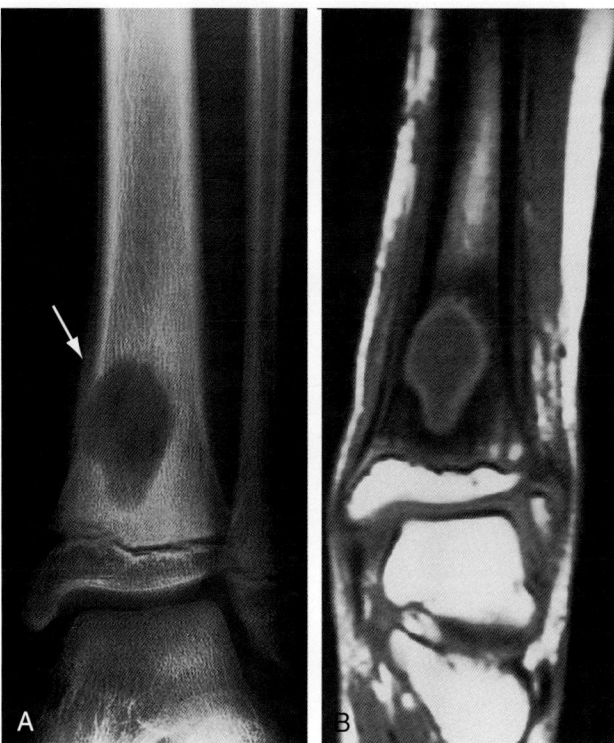

FIGURE 110-4

Brodie's abscess. **A,** Plain radiograph demonstrates localized lucent defect in the distal tibial metaphysis and adjacent periosteal reaction *(arrow)*. **B,** Coronal T1-weighted (500/12) image demonstrates abscess cavity as well as more extensive marrow signal abnormality not seen on the plain radiograph.

areas of involvement and guiding surgery or percutaneous drainage. Skeletal muscle produces relatively low signal intensities on T1- and T2-weighted sequences. Involved areas are seen as increased signal intensity on T2-weighted images (Fig. 110-5). Fat suppression may significantly enhance contrast between normal and inflamed muscle as well as excluding intramuscular fat as a source of intramuscular increased signal intensity.[32]

Dermatomyositis

Dermatomyositis is an idiopathic multisystem non-suppurative inflammatory disorder primarily affecting skeletal muscle and skin. This disease is characterized by proximal muscle weakness and a typical rash. Traditionally, confirmation of muscle involvement has been made by electromyography or muscle biopsy. MRI of the lower extremities has been shown to demonstrate signal abnormalities in affected muscle groups that correlate with disease activity.[33-35] MR imaging can be useful during initial diagnosis to define the extent of muscle abnormalities and determine the most appropriate area for biopsy. Subsequent imaging may provide information helpful in assessment of response to therapy and extent of disease.

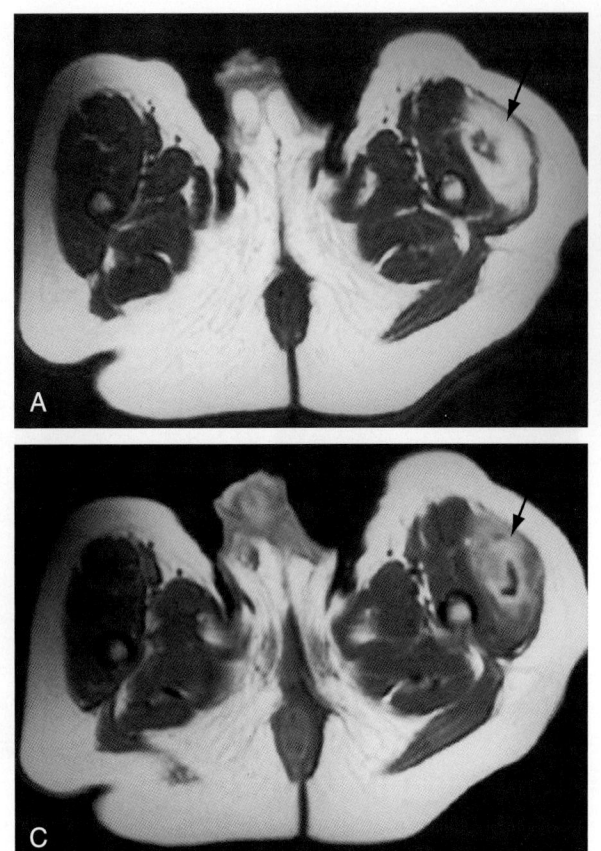

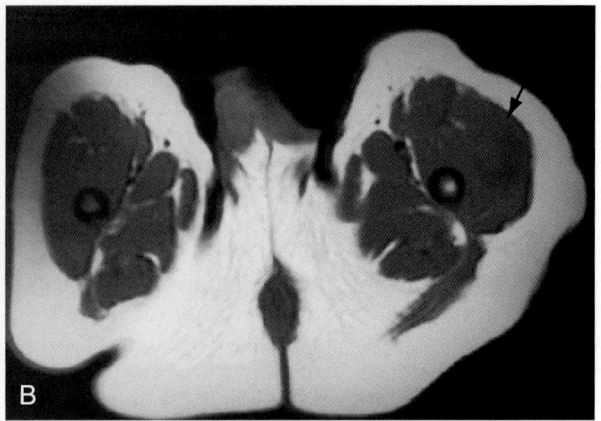

FIGURE 110-5

Myositis. **A,** Axial T2-weighted (2700/85) image of the proximal thighs demonstrates localized mixed, primarily increased muscle signal intensity and swelling *(arrow)*. T1-weighted (500/12) images before (**B**) and after (**C**) contrast enhancement demonstrate irregular ring enhancement *(arrows)*.

Muscle involvement is characterized by increased signal intensity on T2-weighted sequences (Fig. 110-6). Axial images best demonstrate relative involvement of different muscle groups. In the lower extremities, the adductors are most frequently involved, followed by the gluteus and quadriceps groups, with the hamstrings usually least involved. There may also be increased signal intensity in the subcutaneous fat on T2-weighted images thought to represent subcutaneous edema, perimuscular edema, and enhancement of chemical shift artifact at fat–muscle interfaces. All of these findings are enhanced on fat-suppressed T2-weighted images.[33,34] Patients with "inactive" disease and patients who have undergone treatment demonstrate normalization of these findings. Improvement in signal changes correlates with improvement in muscle strength assessment.[34]

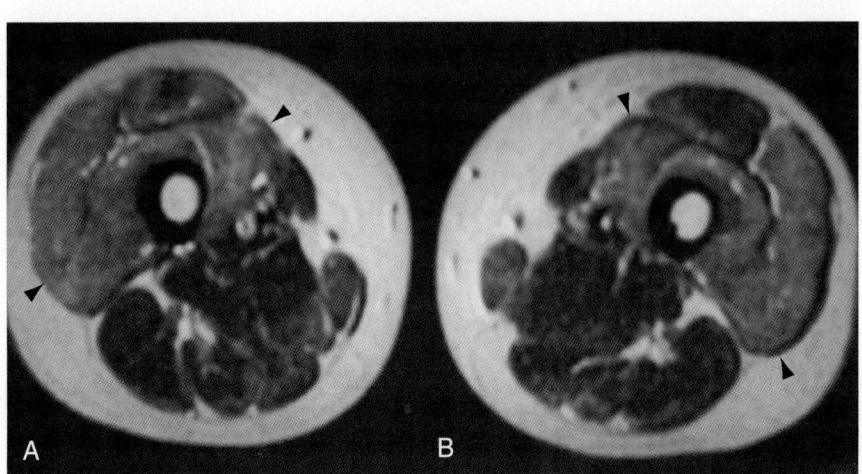

FIGURE 110-6

Dermatomyositis. Axial T2-weighted (2000/85) image of the thighs demonstrates diffuse increased signal intensity involving primarily the anterior and lateral thigh musculature *(arrowheads)*.

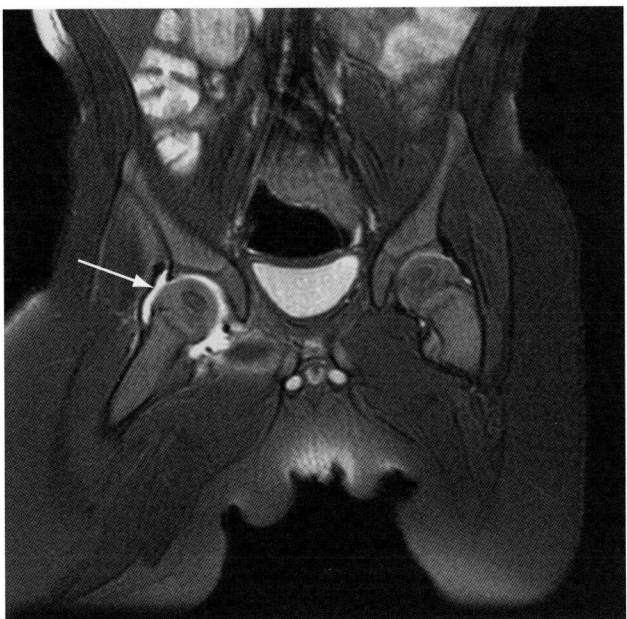

FIGURE 110-7

Septic right hip. Coronal T2-weighted image with fat saturation demonstrates a right joint effusion (*arrow*). Marrow signal is normal. The left hip is normal.

Septic Arthritis

MRI has little role in the evaluation of acute septic arthritis, although it may occasionally be used to confirm or dispute the presence of joint fluid for arthrocentesis. MR imaging can also provide detailed information about the pelvis in cases where the clinical picture is confusing.

The appearance of septic arthritis by MR imaging is nonspecific. A joint effusion (Fig. 110-7) in the presence or absence of reactive synovitis may be demonstrated by MR imaging but these findings are also seen with transient synovitis, trauma, juvenile chronic arthritis or reactive arthritis.[12] Abnormal marrow signal may be present in septic arthritis as a result of marrow edema or associated osteomyelitis.[35] Diagnosis of septic arthritis rests primarily on clinical findings and joint aspiration.

SYNOVIAL DISORDERS

MRI has become an important diagnostic tool in evaluation of synovial disorders largely because of its ability to directly visualize articular cartilage, joint effusion, menisci and ligaments, and hypertrophy of the synovium.[36,37]

Juvenile Chronic Polyarthritis

Juvenile chronic polyarthritis, or juvenile rheumatoid arthritis, is a chronic inflammatory condition of childhood that may affect many organ systems. The most prominent feature is involvement of the joints (most frequently the knee), with chronic synovitis leading to synovial hypertrophy and pannus formation. Chronic synovial inflammation results in production of joint fluid and pannus formation and eventually leads to cartilage and bony erosion. These inflammatory changes may eventually progress to bony ankylosis. Localized hyperemia causes bone overgrowth and premature physeal fusion. Meniscal atrophy in the knees has also been noted.[38-40]

The synovial hypertrophy and pannus formation appear as a thickened area of low to intermediate signal intensity on T1-weighted images with bright signal on T2-weighted images. It may be difficult to distinguish hypertrophic synovium from joint fluid on these sequences. For this reason, gadolinium-enhanced T1-weighted fat-suppressed images are needed for optimal visualization of the hypertrophic synovium, which is typically hypervascular (Fig. 110-8).[38] Prompt post-contrast imaging is crucial since there is rapid diffusion of contrast material from the synovium to the joint.[16] Synovial proliferation will manifest as enhancing linear, villous or nodular tissue within the joint spaces, readily distinguishable from the low-signal joint fluid. Cartilage loss and bone erosions may also be better demonstrated on contrast-enhanced images. It has also been suggested that joint fluid loculation is better assessed on contrast-enhanced images and this may prove useful for planning intra-articular therapy.[38]

Hemophilia

Hemophilia, an X-linked recessive chronic coagulation disorder related to deficiency of factor XIII (hemophilia A) or factor IX (hemophilia B), is associated with repeated hemarthrosis and subsequent progressive joint disease. It is thought that repeated intra-articular hemorrhage leads to absorption of red blood cell products and hemosiderin by the synovial lining, resulting in synovial inflammation and hypertrophy with subsequent pannus formation.[41] The combination of intra-articular blood products and proteolytic enzymes produced by the abnormal synovium contributes to articular cartilage destruction. In addition, subchondral cysts form, which are thought to result from intraosseous hemorrhage. These cysts may cause mechanical instability.[41] These changes are underestimated by plain film radiography owing to the inability to directly visualize synovium or articular cartilage.

MRI has been used to evaluate these changes to select patients for synovectomy or supplementary factor replacement.[42-44] Because of hemosiderin deposition, the hypertrophic synovium produces low to intermediate signal intensity on T1- and T2-weighted images and is generally readily distinguishable from intra-articular fluid without administration of contrast material. Scattered foci of increased signal intensity on T2-weighted images are thought to represent edema or acute inflammation.[42,44] Cartilage loss may be focal or diffuse. Subchondral cysts usually form along weight-bearing surfaces and have variable signal contents,

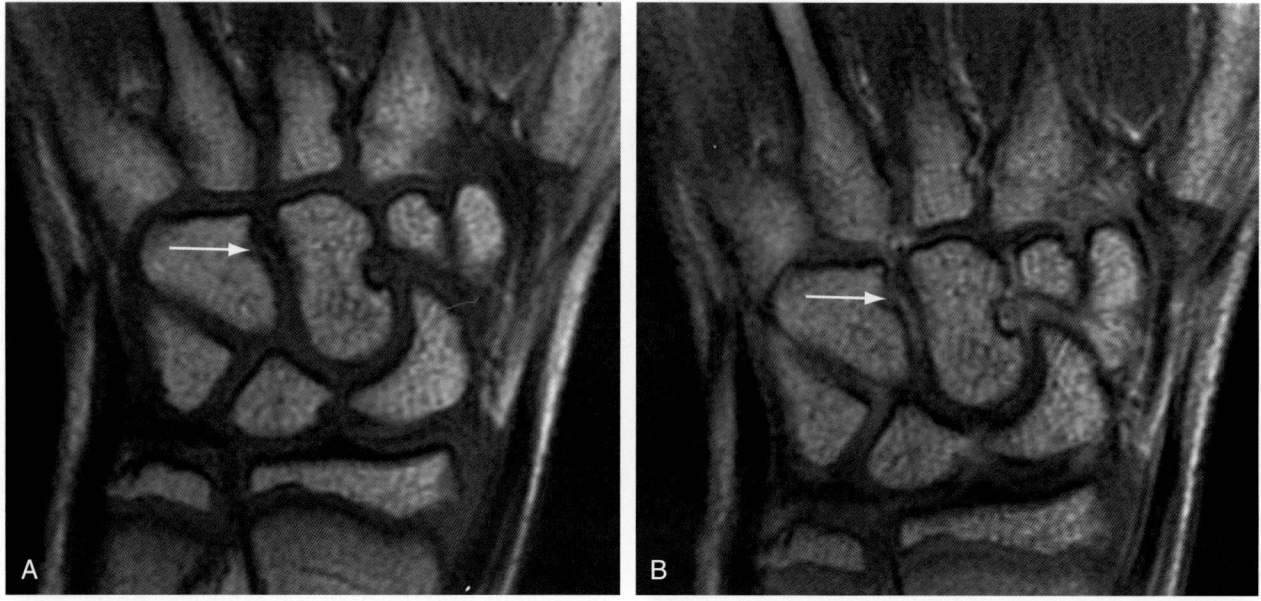

FIGURE 110-8

Juvenile rheumatoid arthritis. Coronal T1-weighted images of the left wrist pre (**A**) and post (**B**) administration of gadolinium contrast material. Precontrast image demonstrates an erosion at the medial aspect of the hamate (*arrow*). Post-contrast image demonstrates enhancement of the synovium which is typically hypervascular.

thought to represent various stages of hemorrhage resolution.[45] Joint effusions also have variable signal intensities, probably because of the presence of various blood breakdown products[45] (Fig. 110-9).

Pigmented Villonodular Synovitis

Pigmented villonodular synovitis is an idiopathic disorder generally affecting the synovial joints and synovial tendon sheaths, usually in adults. The lesion consists of nodular synovial proliferation with hemosiderin deposition. Cases occurring in the pediatric population are unusual[46] and may be suspected clinically to represent soft-tissue malignant neoplasms. MRI may be performed to evaluate the extent of the mass. Pigmented villonodular synovitis produces a characteristic mixed signal mass on T1- and T2-weighted images with areas of low signal intensity produced by hemosiderin deposition[47-49] (Fig. 110-10).

TRAUMA

MRI has had a dramatic effect on the imaging evaluation of musculoskeletal trauma, having clear advantages over plain radiography in the detection of occult osseous injury[50-53] as well as associated soft-tissue injury.[54,55]

Traumatic conditions of particular interest in the pediatric population, in which MRI may provide useful information, include physeal injury (including slipped capital femoral epiphysis and Blount's disease), stress fractures, and osteochondritis dissecans.

Physeal Injury

Salter–Harris Injuries

The physis is composed of four layers from the epiphyseal aspect to the metaphyseal aspect: resting cartilage, proliferating cartilage, hypertrophying cartilage, and endochondral ossification layer. Mechanical strength is provided primarily by collagen in a noncellular matrix. The layer of hypertrophying cartilage has relatively less collagen and a greater proportion of cellular elements and is the most frequent site of separation in injuries producing physeal separation.[56] In the immature skeleton, the physis is a point of mechanical weakness that is susceptible to injury. This structure is relatively weaker than associated tendons, ligaments, and fibrous joint capsule.[56] Injuries that tend to produce ligamentous injuries in adults (e.g., abduction injury of the knee) are more likely to produce physeal injury in children. Injuries to the growth plate have the potential to produce total or partial growth arrest, leading to progressive deformity and limb length discrepancy.[57-60] Growth disturbance may be due to disruption of physeal blood supply or intermingling of the epiphyseal and metaphyseal portions of blood supply leading to bony bridge formation.[61]

MRI is particularly well suited to the evaluation of physeal injury because of its ability to demonstrate both ossified and unossified portions of immature bones. Plain film radiography demonstrates fracture lines through ossified portions of the skeleton, but provides only indirect information about fractures of cartilaginous portions. MRI demonstrates bony and cartilaginous

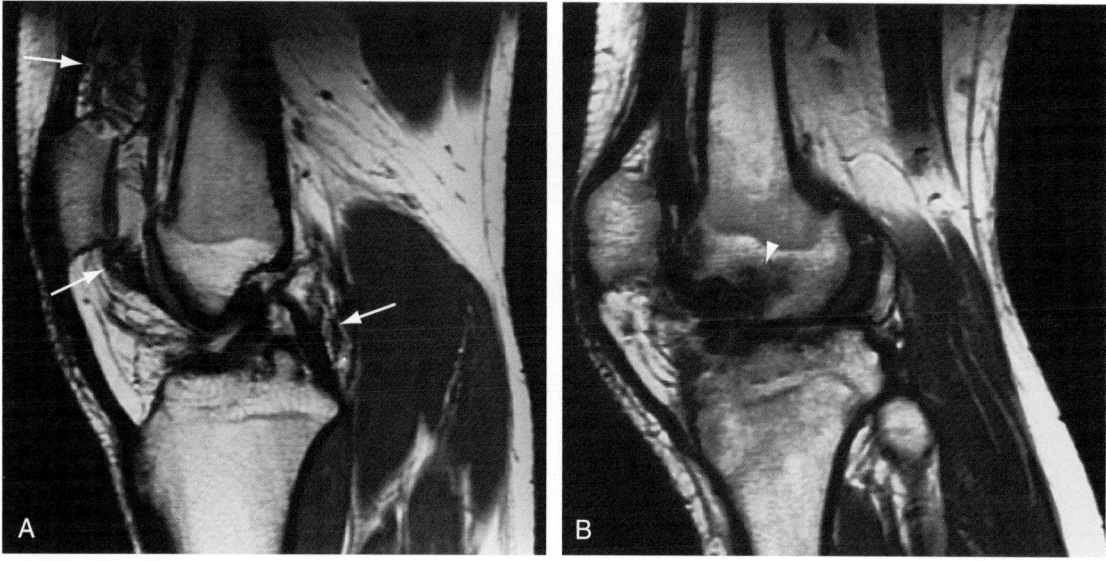

FIGURE 110-9

Hemophilic arthropathy. **A,** Sagittal proton density-weighted (2500/17) image of the knee through the intercondylar notch demonstrates a large mixed-signal joint effusion *(arrows)* resulting from intra-articular hemorrhage. **B,** Sagittal proton density-weighted (2500/17) image lateral to (**A**) demonstrates an area of decreased signal intensity in the lateral femoral condyle secondary to intraosseous hemorrhage *(arrowhead)*.

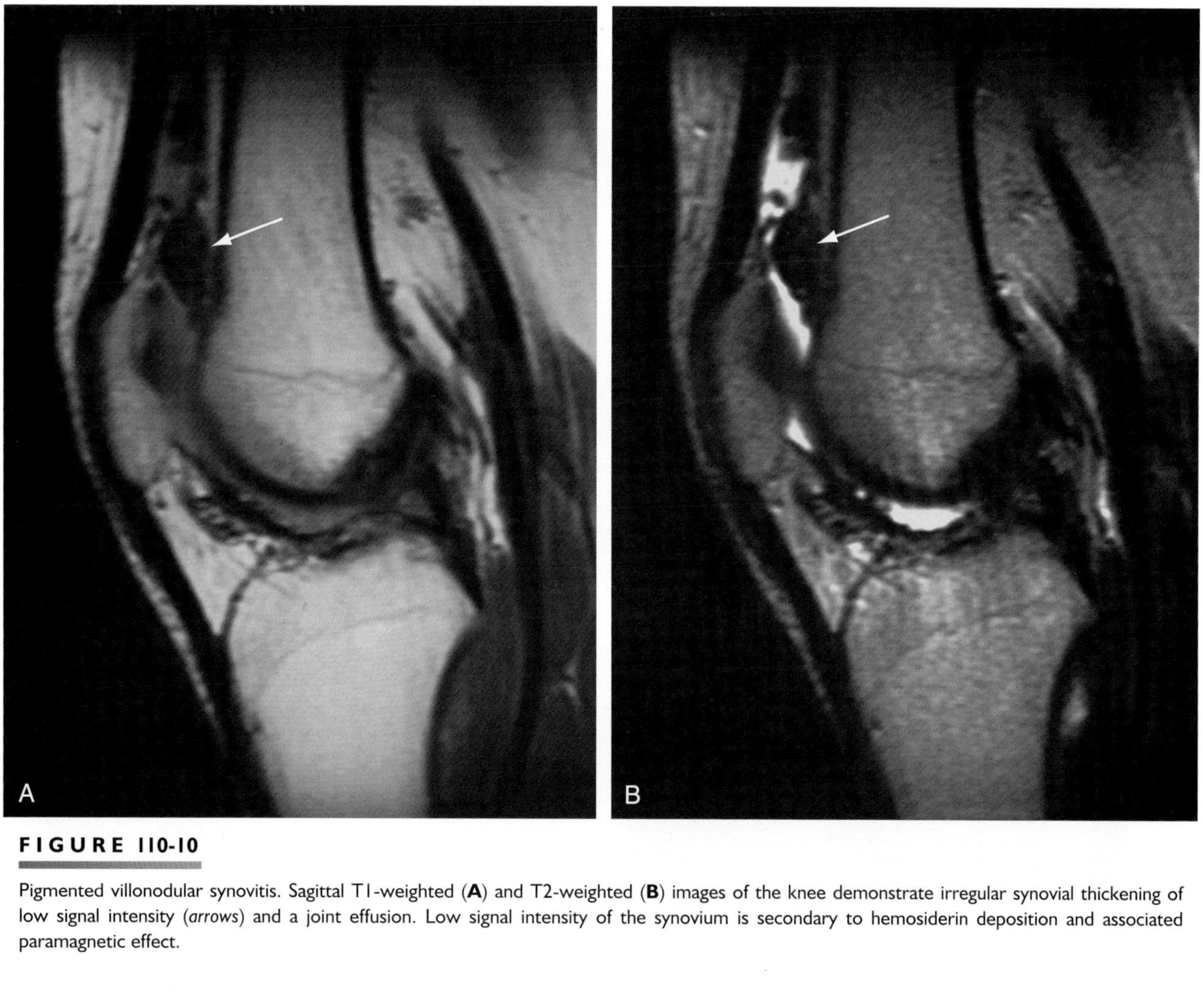

FIGURE 110-10

Pigmented villonodular synovitis. Sagittal T1-weighted (**A**) and T2-weighted (**B**) images of the knee demonstrate irregular synovial thickening of low signal intensity *(arrows)* and a joint effusion. Low signal intensity of the synovium is secondary to hemosiderin deposition and associated paramagnetic effect.

fracture planes directly (Fig. 110-11) and may alter the Salter–Harris classification of an injury previously determined by plain film radiography.[62]

In addition to better morphologic characterization of fractures, MRI may provide useful information regarding growth arrest and the development of bony bridges across the physis after injury[61] (Fig. 110-12). Contrast-enhanced examinations have demonstrated development of transphyseal enhancement corresponding to intermingling of epiphyseal and metaphyseal blood supply after experimentally produced physeal injury.[61] Bony bridge formation may ensue with one of two patterns: a narrow band of low signal intensity corresponding to dense bone or a wider band with central signal intensity matching that of surrounding marrow. The treatment of physeal bridge formation consists of surgical resection and interposition of various materials, including fat and silicone rubber, to prevent recurrence. MRI may be useful in determining the distribution and extent of bony bridge formation for surgical planning.[61]

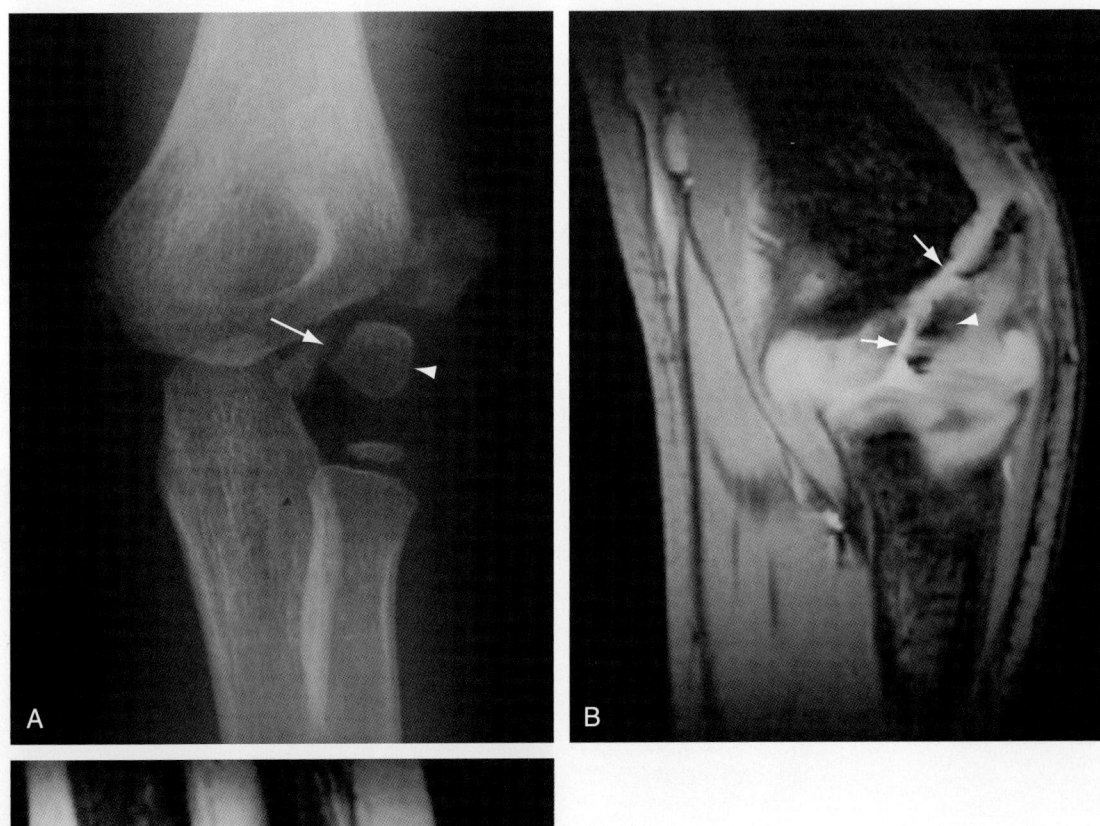

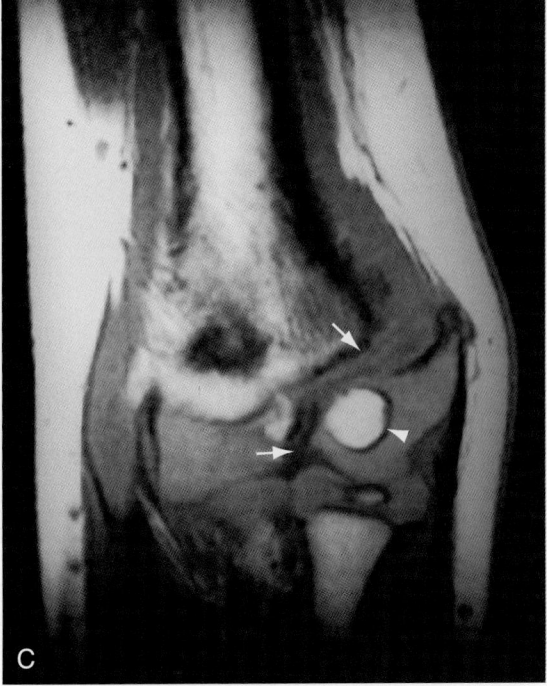

FIGURE 110-11

Salter–Harris type IV fracture of the distal humerus. **A,** Plain radiograph demonstrates fracture *(arrow)* through the capitellum *(arrowhead)*. There has also been separation of a distal humeral metaphyseal fragment laterally. Coronal oblique multiplanar gradient-recalled (500/20/30°) image **(B)** and coronal T1-weighted (500/14) image **(C)** clearly demonstrate the fracture line through the bony as well as the cartilaginous portions of the distal humerus *(arrows)*.

Slipped Capital Femoral Epiphysis (SCFE)

Slipped capital femoral epiphysis is an uncommon disorder affecting older children and adolescents, with a predilection for obese black males. The increased risk associated with obesity may be due to decreased femoral anteversion and resultant abnormal mechanical forces on the femoral head.[63] It represents a Salter–Harris type I fracture but, unlike acute physeal injuries, usually has an insidious, nonspecific clinical presentation. Complications of slipped capital femoral epiphysis include joint incongruity and associated secondary osteoarthritis, avascular necrosis of the femoral head,[64] and chondrolysis.[65,66]

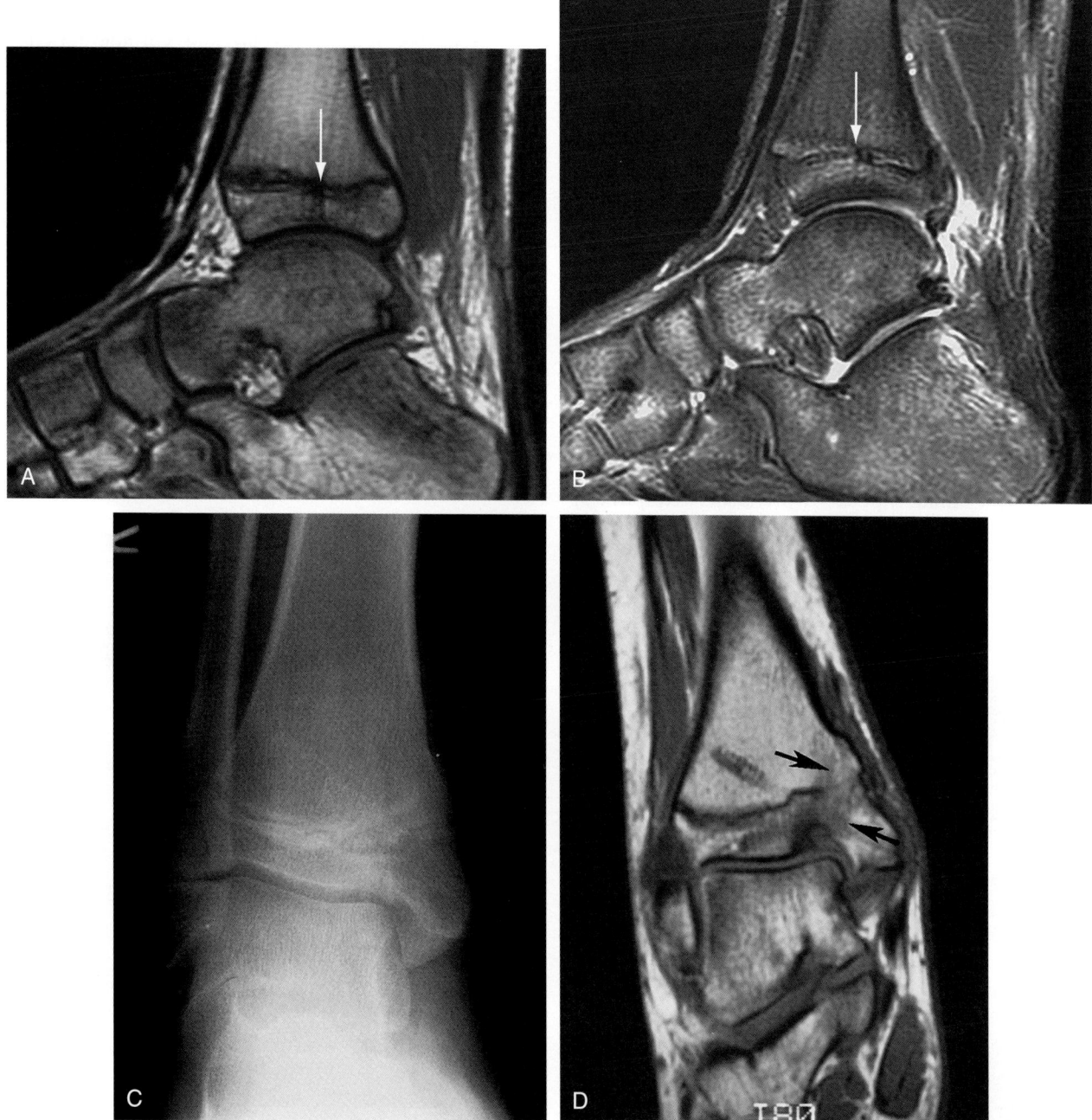

FIGURE 110-12

Physeal bridge formation after physeal injury. Sagittal T1-weighted (**A**) image and T2-weighted (**B**) image with fat saturation of the right ankle demonstrate a narrow band of low signal intensity (*arrows*) across the distal tibial physis corresponding to early bony bridge formation after physeal injury. **C,** Initial radiograph in a different patient with Salter–Harris type IV fracture of the distal tibia associated with fracture of the distal fibular metaphysis. **D,** Coronal T1-weighted (500/12) image obtained 1 year later demonstrates a broad band with signal corresponding to marrow extending obliquely across the physis (*arrows*), representing bony bridge formation. A tract from previous hardware is also present in the distal tibial metaphysis. (**C** and **D** courtesy of Diego Jaramillo MD, Children's Hospital, Boston, MA.)

Diagnosis is typically made by use of anteroposterior and frog-leg lateral radiographs of the hips, which demonstrate displacement of the femoral head along the plane of the physis. Ultrasonography has been advocated for diagnosis of slipped capital femoral epiphysis as well as for detection of associated joint effusion although this modality has not been generally embraced as an imaging tool in this entity.[67]

MRI can provide excellent three-dimensional demonstration of the direction and degree of slippage in SCFE as well as characterizing associated joint effusion. Initially, axial T1-weighted images should be obtained to select an optimal coronal plane through the proximal femurs for direct side-to-side comparison. T1- and T2-weighted images should be obtained in the coronal plane. Sagittal images may also be useful, because a component of slippage in the anteroposterior direction is common. Images demonstrate displacement of the femoral epiphysis relative to the femoral neck, with lateral and anterior displacement of the femoral neck. Hip joint effusion is best seen on T2-weighted images. In addition, MRI is an excellent imaging modality for early detection of avascular necrosis, which may complicate SCFE (Fig. 110-13). Chondrolysis has traditionally been diagnosed by detection of joint space narrowing to less than 3 mm as seen on hip radiographs.[65] Further study is required to determine whether signal changes in articular cartilage on MR images may precede joint space narrowing and allow earlier diagnosis. MRI may also be useful for screening the contralateral side, where asymptomatic, mild slippage with associated physeal widening may be seen in up to 14% of patients.[68]

Blount's Disease

Blount's disease (tibia vara, osteochondrosis deformans tibiae) is separated into an infantile form, presenting between 1 and 3 years of age,[69,70] and an adolescent form, presenting after age 8 years.[71] In both types, there is abrupt varus deformity of the proximal tibia associated with medial narrowing of the epiphysis, metaphyseal beaking, alteration and early fusion of the medial aspect of the physis, and bowing of the lower extremity. As with slipped capital femoral epiphysis, there is a reported association with obesity.[72] The disorder is probably caused by pressure necrosis of the medial aspect of the physis in the infantile group and chronic repetitive trauma or infection in the adolescent group.

The role of MRI in the evaluation of Blount's disease has yet to be defined. In the later stages of the disease, there is compromise of knee stability, and hypertrophy of the medial meniscus has been described.[70] This may predispose to meniscal injury, which is well demonstrated by MRI (Fig. 110-14). MRI may also prove useful for mapping the distribution of physeal growth disturbance for surgical planning.

Stress Fracture

Stress fractures result from repetitive injury to trabecular bone, eventually exceeding the normal reparative process. Bony stress injuries are traditionally categorized

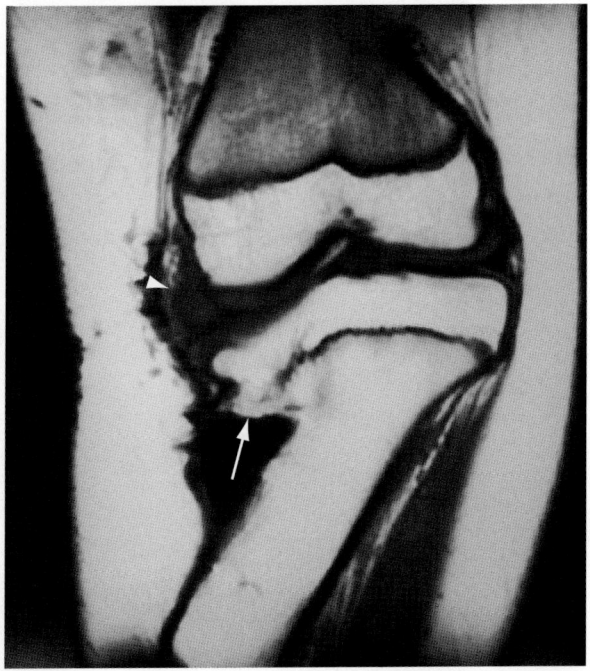

FIGURE 110-14

Blount's disease. Coronal T1-weighted (600/20) image demonstrates abrupt varus of the knee produced by localized proximal tibial bowing. There is medial physeal fusion, depression of the medial tibial plateau, and sclerosis along the medial aspect of the proximal tibial metaphysis, or "buttressing" (arrow). Also noted is a complex tear of the medial meniscus (arrowhead).

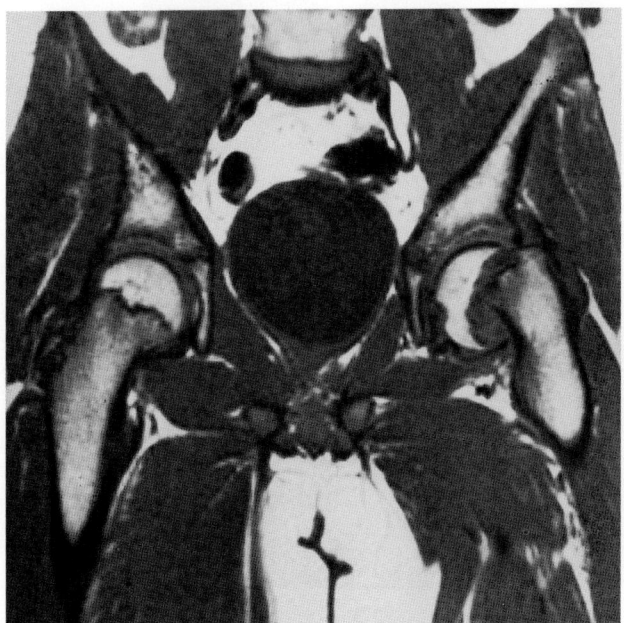

FIGURE 110-13

Slipped capital femoral epiphysis. T1-weighted (500/20) coronal image demonstrates marked displacement of the left femoral epiphysis. Marrow signal in the femoral head is normal (no evidence of avascular necrosis). The right side is normal.

as either insufficiency fractures or fatigue fractures. Insufficiency fractures occur in abnormal bones due to normal stresses and may be seen in children with osteopenia or osteoporosis, as well as after radiation therapy. Fatigue fractures occur most commonly in the lower extremities and result from new activity or abrupt increase in intensity of activity.[73] On MR imaging, stress fractures typically appear as linear low signal intensity lines on T1- and T2-weighted images. Accompanying marrow edema is often present (Fig. 110-15). When extensive marrow edema is present, the distinction between a stress fracture and a more aggressive lesion such as tumor or infection can be difficult. Soft-tissue swelling, edema, and joint effusions may be absent. Stress fractures in older children with fatty marrow are well seen on T1-weighted sequences. However, in infants and young children with predominantly hematopoietic marrow, trabecular injury is better appreciated on T2-weighted images.[7]

Osteochondritis Dissecans

Osteochondritis dissecans is a poorly understood disorder in which there is separation of an osteochondral fragment along an articular surface, usually in the femoral condyles, capitellum or talar dome. Suggested etiologic factors include trauma,[74] avascular necrosis,[75] and abnormal ossification.[76] Osteochondritis dissecans of the capitellum is of particular interest in children because it is associated with growth distur-

bance of the capitellum, trochlea, olecranon, and radial head, leading to secondary osteoarthritis.[77]

The osteochondral fragment in osteochondritis dissecans may be stable, loose in situ or free within the joint space. Children with stable osteochondral fragments respond to limited weight bearing, whereas patients with loose in situ fragments may require fragment fixation or debridement by arthroscopy or arthrotomy. Patients with loose fragments generally require arthrotomy with fragment removal.[78]

MR images demonstrate decreased signal intensity on T1-weighted images in the osteochondritis dissecans fragment and adjacent margin of parent bone, with variable increase in signal intensity on T2-weighted images (Fig. 110-16). Signs of loosening include fragment displacement, disruption of overlying articular cartilage, and a fluid interface between the fragment and adjacent parent bone. This appears as a line of intermediate signal intensity on T1-weighted images and increased signal intensity on T2-weighted images.[78] Osteochondritis dissecans is generally best demonstrated on coronal or sagittal images, depending on the location of the lesion.

DEVELOPMENTAL DYSPLASIA OF THE HIP

Developmental dysplasia of the hip (DDH) includes a spectrum of disease severity from mild acetabular dysplasia to frank hip dislocation. Normal hip development is determined by the relationship between growth

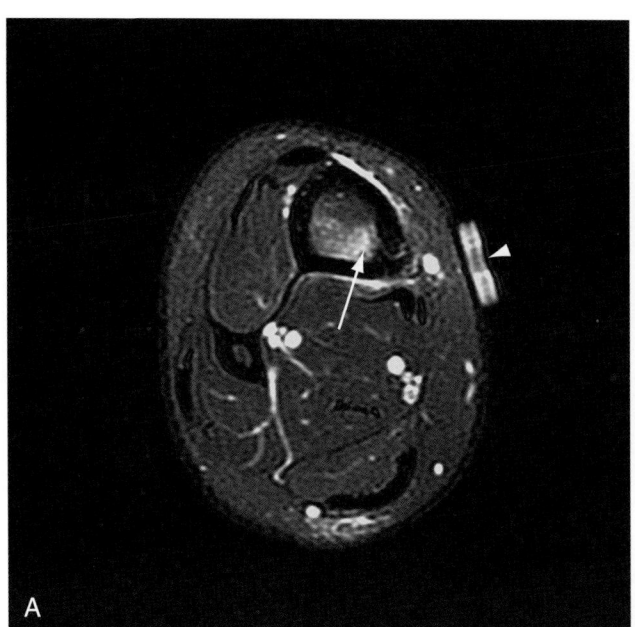

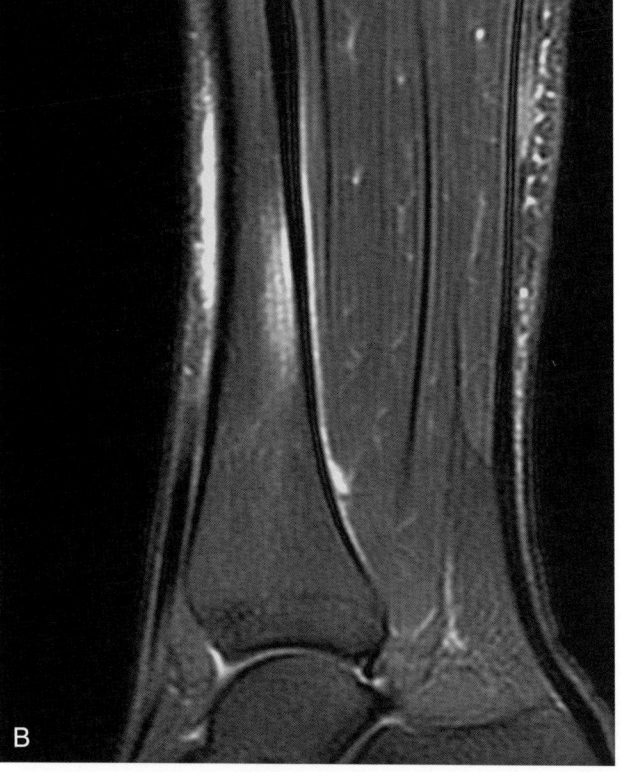

FIGURE 110-15

Stress fracture. **A,** Axial T2-weighted image of the tibia demonstrates linear high signal in the cortex (*arrow*) and marrow edema as well as adjacent soft-tissue high signal. A marker indicates site of patient's pain (*arrowhead*). **B,** Sagittal image provides better extent of marrow edema.

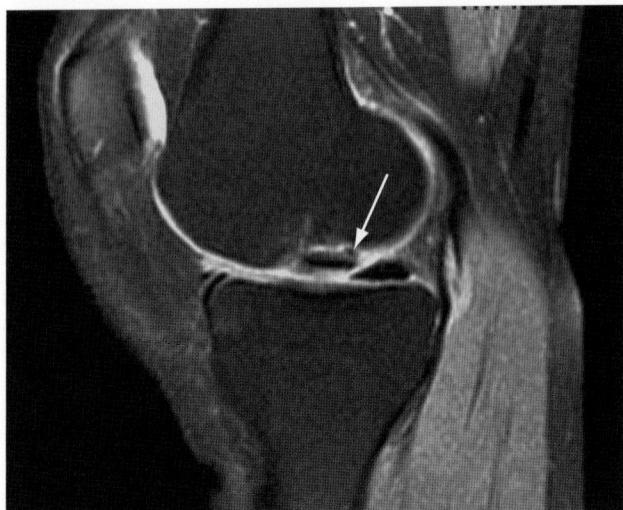

FIGURE 110-16

Osteochondritis dissecans. Sagittal fast spin-echo proton density image of the left knee demonstrates an osteochondral fragment (*arrow*) at the medial femoral condyle with surrounding high signal intensity fluid. The surrounding fluid suggests instability of the fragment.

of the acetabular triradiate cartilage and an appropriately located spherical femoral head. As many as 1 in 60 newborns may demonstrate hip instability on clinical examination.[79] The majority (88%) stabilize in a 2-month period and the remainder require treatment. The majority of these (95%) respond to abduction and flexion splinting.[79] Predisposing factors for DDH include breech intrauterine positioning, female sex, oligohydramnios, and positive family history. Children with neuromuscular disorders such as cerebral palsy have unequal muscle forces which predispose them to deformity of the proximal femur and acetabulum.

The role of imaging in the evaluation of developmental dysplasia of the hip has changed substantially with the advent of ultrasonography, CT, and MRI. Plain films provide information about the bony acetabulum, bony coverage, and femoral head position and ossification. However, there is little information provided about cartilaginous and other soft-tissue structures. In addition, because of the projective nature of plain film radiography, three-dimensional determination of hip position can be difficult. Also, hip position is best evaluated in the presence of an ossified femoral head, and femoral head ossification is often delayed in developmental dysplasia of the hip.

Arthrography provides improved soft-tissue information by demonstrating intrasynovial cartilaginous surfaces. However, arthrography is invasive and requires deep sedation or general anesthesia and still has the disadvantages of projective imaging.

Ultrasonography is widely accepted as the imaging method of choice in the evaluation of the young infant's hip. Advantages include real-time assessment of hip stability, good visualization of femoral head and some acetabular cartilage, and visualization of the fibrocarti-

laginous labrum. The utility of ultrasonography decreases with increasing ossification of the femoral head, and it is generally not useful after the age of 6 months.

CT may be particularly useful in the postoperative evaluation to confirm hip location in three dimensions and has been used to estimate femoral and acetabular anteversion.[80] CT, however, is limited in its ability to evaluate unossified portions of the hip and requires ionizing radiation.

The role of MRI in the evaluation of developmental dysplasia of the hip remains controversial. Cost, availability, and the need for sedation prohibit the routine use of MRI in the evaluation of developmental dysplasia of the hip. MRI does provide direct visualization of many soft-tissue structures of the hip, such as the articular cartilage, the labrum, the transverse acetabular ligament, the iliopsoas tendon, the ligamentum teres, and the joint capsule.[81,82] In the patient with persistent dislocation (despite conservative therapy), late diagnosis or acetabular dysplasia, MRI can provide useful information about factors preventing reduction. Additional advantages of MRI include the ability to scan through casting material, no ionizing radiation and the safety of this technique in postoperative evaluation.

Anatomic assessment is best made on axial and coronal T1-weighted images (Fig. 110-17). An axial localizer should be obtained first to select an optimal coronal plane aligned with the femoral heads and acetabula for direct side-to-side comparison. Resolution is optimized by using the smallest volume coil available in which the patient's pelvis will fit, such as the knee coil for infants or the head coil for young children. Spatial resolution on the side of interest may be further improved by the addition of a surface coil. Hip joint fluid is best imaged on T2-weighted spin-echo or T2*-weighted gradient-recalled sequences. Acetabular cartilage and femoral head cartilage produce relatively low signal intensity on T1-weighted images, with increasing signal intensity on T2-weighted images. The fibrocartilaginous labrum is seen as a triangular structure of low signal intensity along the cartilaginous margin of the acetabulum on all pulse sequences.

Other low-signal intensity structures include the joint capsule, the transverse acetabular ligament, the iliopsoas tendon, and the ligamentum teres. The joint capsule attaches superolaterally to the bony margin of the acetabulum and to the labrum, superomedially to the transverse acetabular ligament, and inferiorly to the femoral neck. Infolding of the joint capsule is a potential cause of reduction failure and is best seen in the coronal plane.[81] The transverse acetabular ligament represents a continuation of the labrum and extends across the shallow inferior portion of the normal acetabulum. It is best seen on coronal images, where it is continuous with the inferomedial portion of the joint capsule. Shortening of the transverse acetabular ligament is an infrequent cause of reduction failure.[81] The normal iliopsoas tendon may be difficult to identify because it is thin and flat and lies immediately adjacent to the anterior aspect of the labrum and femoral head, best seen on axial images. When invagination of the iliopsoas tendon into the hip joint space occurs in association with developmental

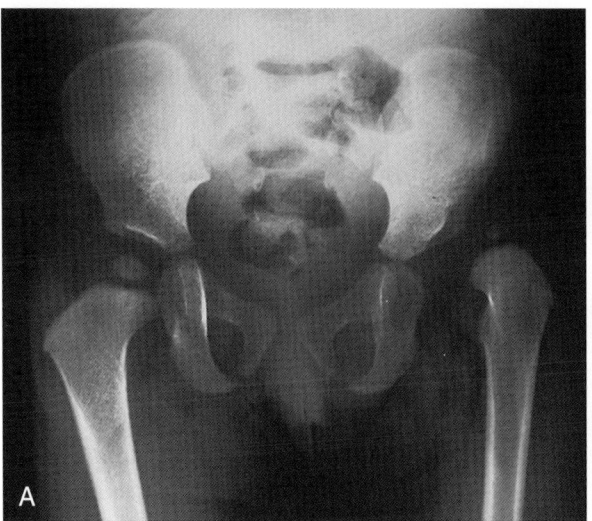

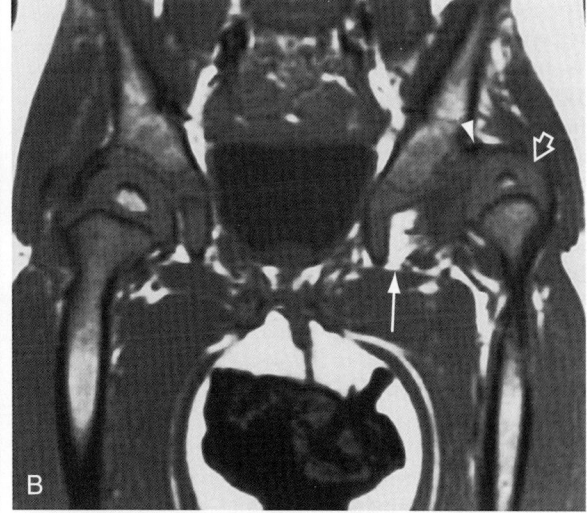

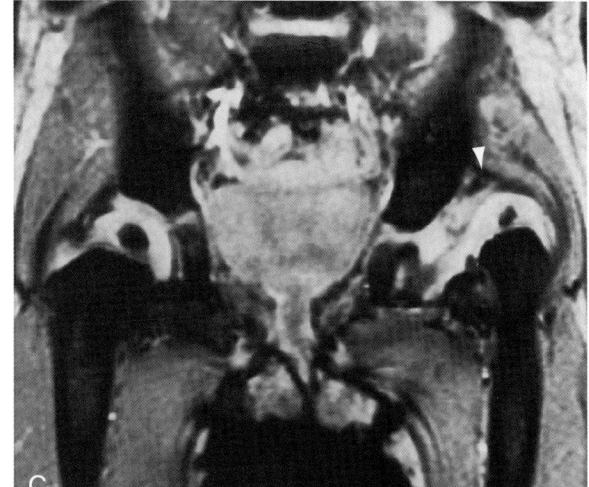

FIGURE 110-17

Developmental dysplasia of the hip. **A,** Plain radiograph demonstrates left hip dislocation, delay in femoral head ossification, and a shallow, steep bony acetabulum. Coronal T1-weighted (600/15) image (**B**) and gradient-echo (50/20/20°) image (**C**) demonstrate hypertrophy of the fatty pulvinar *(solid arrow)* and elevation without inversion of the low signal intensity fibrocartilaginous labrum *(arrowheads)*. The size and shape of the cartilaginous femoral head are well seen *(open arrow)*.

dysplasia of the hip, the tendon tends to become thickened and is more easily identified.[78] The ligamentum teres extends from the fovea of the femoral head to the transverse acetabular ligament and is best seen in the coronal plane. It is also more likely to be rounded and thickened in the presence of hip dislocation. The fibrofatty pulvinar, or acetabular fat pad, is seen on T1-weighted images as a high signal-intensity structure that expands to fill the space created by chronic hip dislocation (see Fig. 110-17).

MRI may also be useful in selecting patients for acetabular reconstruction by providing three-dimensional information about both bony and cartilaginous coverage of the femoral head. There is a subset of patients who have residual acetabular bony dysplasia at plain radiography but who have adequate cartilaginous coverage at MRI. Surgical reconstruction may be obviated in this group. This discrepancy between plain film and MRI findings is thought to be due to the delayed ossification of acetabular cartilage that may be seen in patients with developmental dysplasia of the hip.[83]

TUMORS AND TUMOR-LIKE CONDITIONS

Imaging of specific musculoskeletal tumors, including pediatric tumors, is discussed in Chapter 107. The following represents a brief overview of the role of MRI in evaluating pediatric tumors and tumor-like conditions.

Role of Magnetic Resonance Imaging in Tumor Imaging

The role of MRI in musculoskeletal tumor imaging has been the subject of many reports.[84-93] MRI has a limited role in primary evaluation of suspected bone lesions. The diagnosis is still largely based on plain film findings and confirmed by biopsy. However, evaluation of local extent of disease, detection of skip areas, and assessment of vital structure involvement, such as neurovascular bundles, adjacent muscle groups, joint capsule, and transphyseal extension, are best accomplished by MRI. MRI also provides useful information regarding tumor response to therapy, completeness of resection, and detection of local recurrence on follow-up examinations.

It is useful to obtain a combination of axial and longitudinal images to evaluate an extremity tumor. Whether coronal or sagittal images are obtained depends on the location of the mass and the geometry of the involved bone. Most bone and soft-tissue tumors produce low signal intensity on T1-weighted images and are easily differentiated from high signal intensity of marrow or subcutaneous fat on this sequence (Figs. 110-18 to 110-23). Intramedullary extent is best judged on longitudinal T1-weighted images. It is important to image the entire length of an involved bone to search for skip lesions and transphyseal extension. Invasion of adjacent musculature is best seen on axial T2-weighted images, particularly with fat suppression, on which most tumors produce high signal intensity in contrast to the low signal intensity of skeletal muscle. Involve-

ment of the neurovascular bundle is also best seen in the axial plane. Longitudinal STIR images and gradient-echo images may be useful adjuncts to standard spin-echo sequences for the demonstration of the extent of soft-tissue masses and soft-tissue components of bone tumors.

Malignant Tumors

Malignant tumors of particular interest in the pediatric population include osteosarcoma,[94-103] Ewing's sarcoma,[95,104-107] leukemia,[108-110] neuroblastoma,[111] and soft-tissue sarcomas, particularly rhabdomyosarcoma.[112]

MRI has particular utility in evaluating the local extent of malignant tumors, particularly with respect to intramedullary extension, physeal and cortical penetration, and involvement of adjacent soft-tissue structures

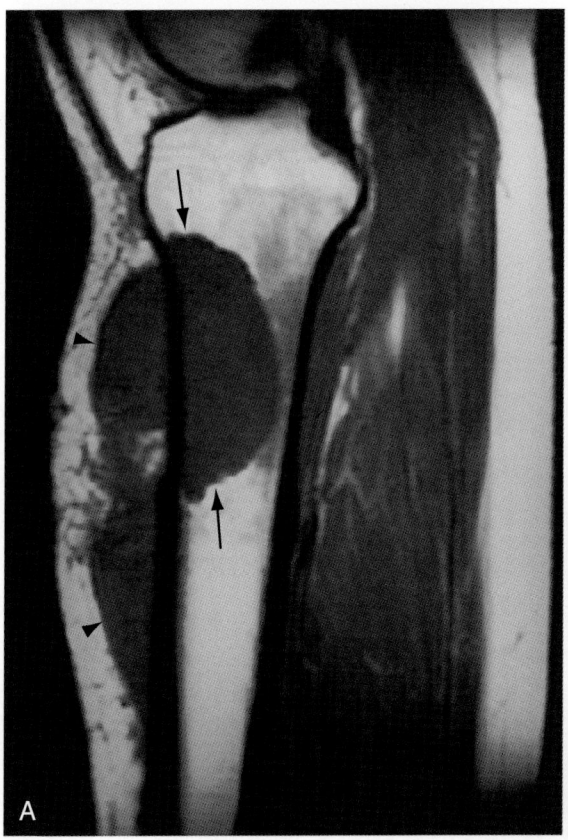
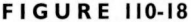
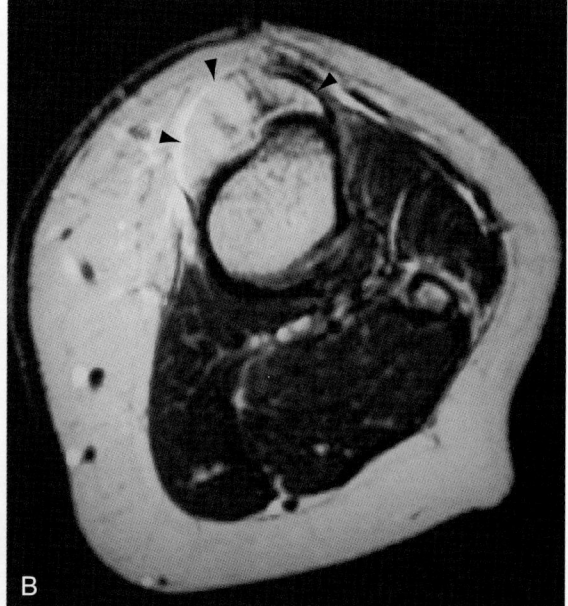
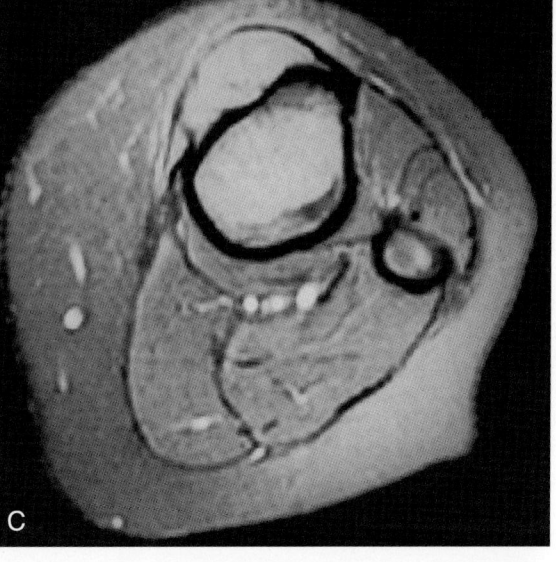

FIGURE 110-18

Osteosarcoma. Sagittal T1-weighted (600/20) image (**A**) and axial T2-weighted (2000/85) image (**B**) demonstrate intramedullary component of tumor (arrows) as well as extent of soft-tissue mass (arrowheads). **C,** Axial T1-weighted (800/30) image with fat suppression shows improved contrast between tumor and subcutaneous fat.

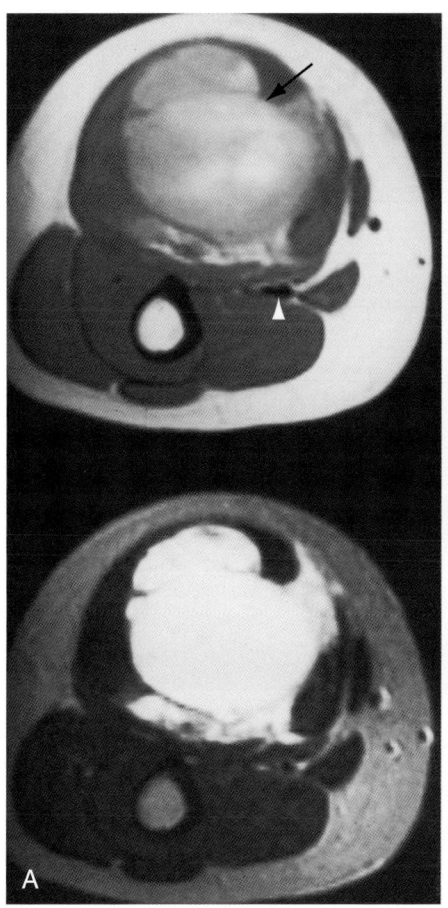

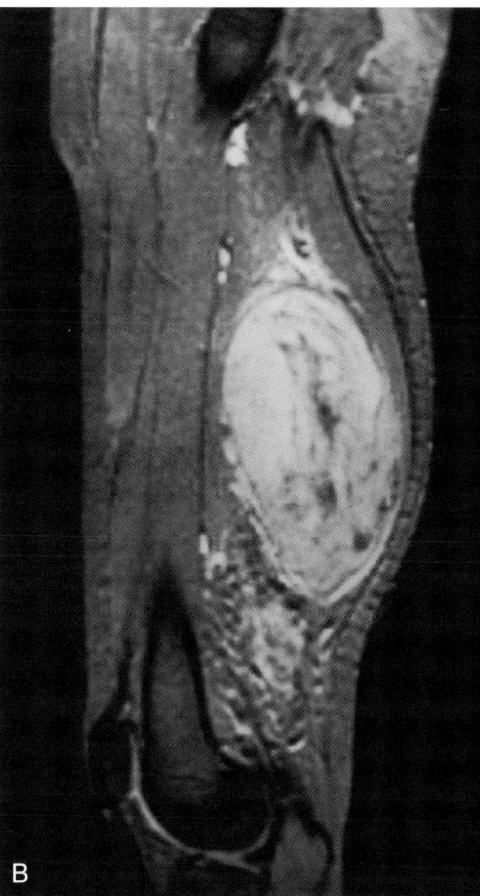

FIGURE 110-19

Soft-tissue sarcoma. **A,** Axial proton density-weighted (1900/20, *top*) and T2-weighted (1900/80, *bottom*) images of the thighs obtained with the patient prone demonstrate a large soft-tissue mass involving the posterior thigh musculature *(arrow)*. The neurovascular bundle *(arrowhead)* is clearly separate from the mass. **B,** Sagittal gradient-echo (50/12/30°) image demonstrates the superior-inferior extent of the tumor.

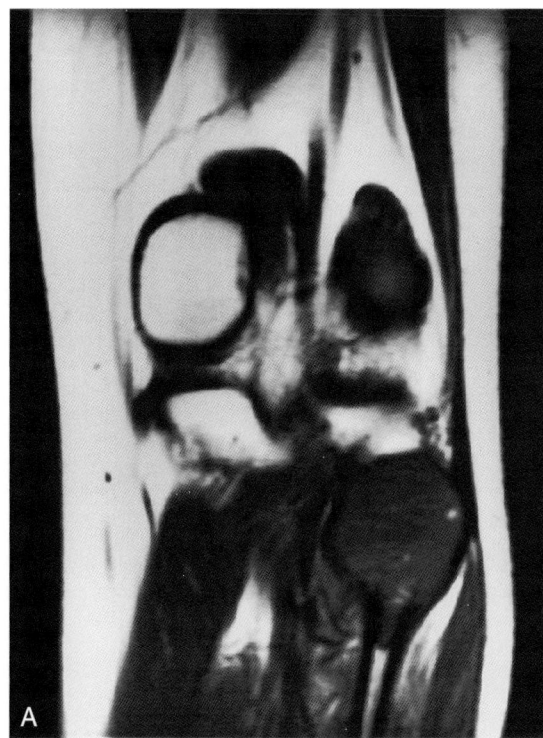

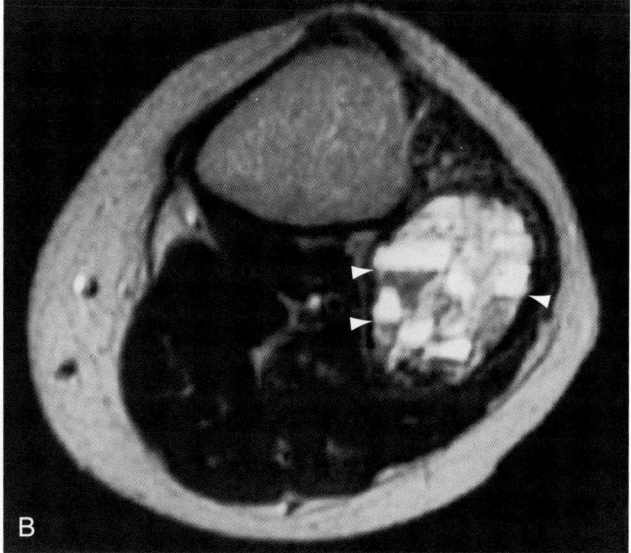

FIGURE 110-20

Aneurysmal bone cyst. **A,** Coronal T1-weighted (500/12) image of the knee demonstrates marked expansion of the fibular head with decreased signal intensity in the marrow space. **B,** Axial T2-weighted (2000/80) image demonstrates fluid–fluid levels in multiple cystic spaces within the lesion *(arrowheads)*.

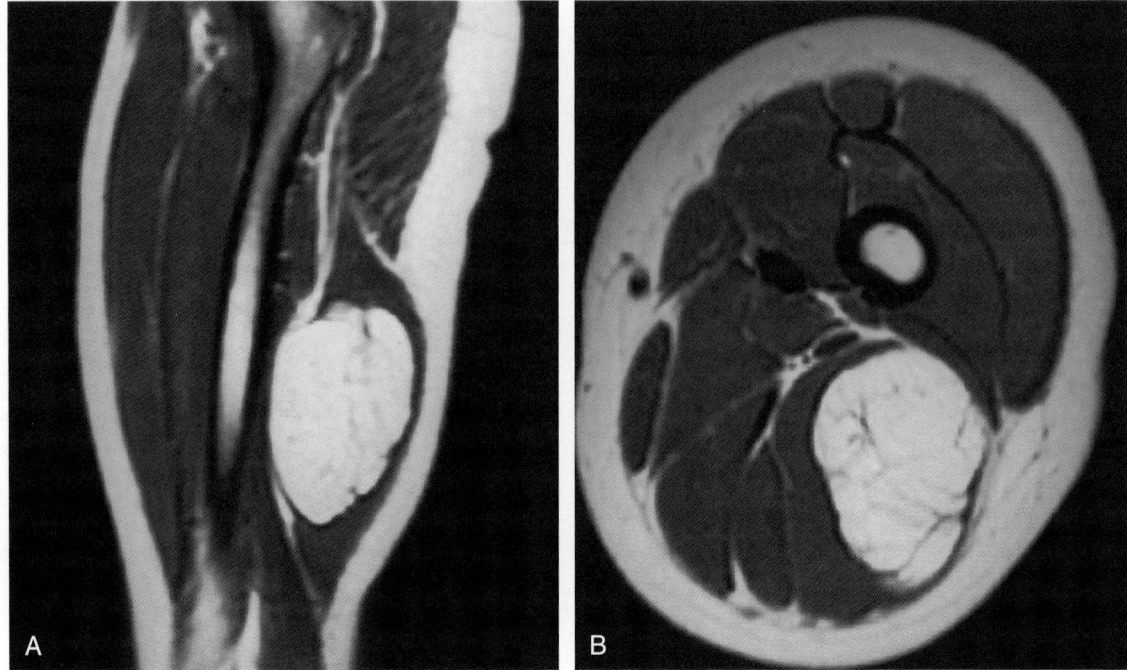

FIGURE 110-21

Intramuscular lipoma. Sagittal T1-weighted (500/30) image (**A**) and coronal proton density-weighted (2000/20) image (**B**) demonstrate a mass within the biceps femoris muscle with signal characteristics corresponding to fat. There are fine internal septa, but no significant soft-tissue component.

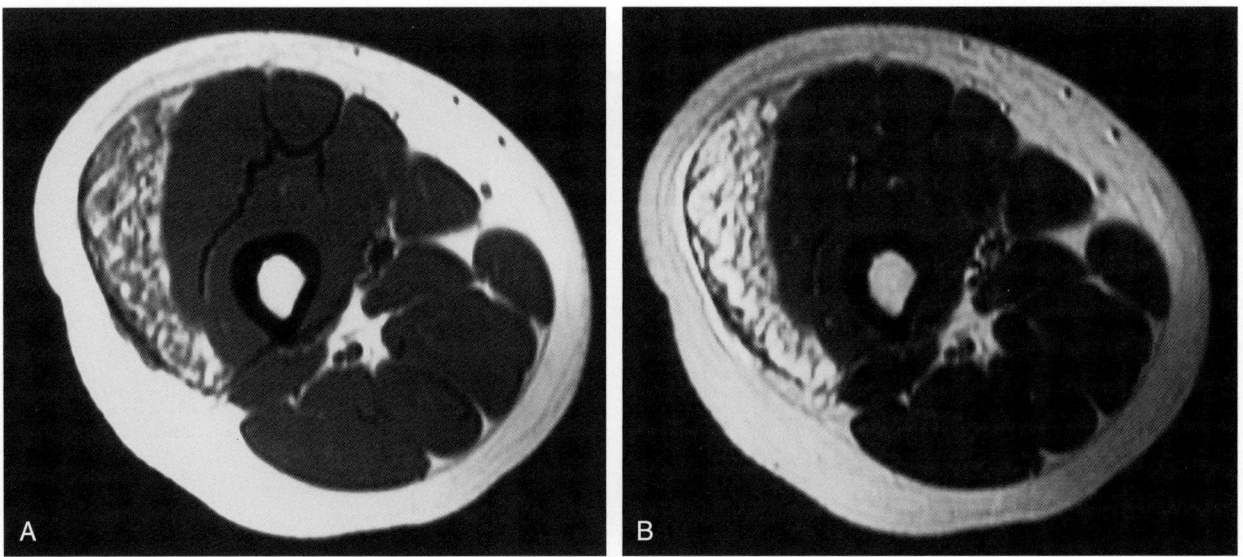

FIGURE 110-22

Venous malformation. T1-weighted (500/12) axial image (**A**) and T2-weighted (2000/80) axial image (**B**) of the thigh demonstrate a well-defined heterogeneous signal lesion that is primarily high in signal intensity on T2-weighted images. Serpiginous vascular spaces are clearly seen, particularly on the T2-weighted image.

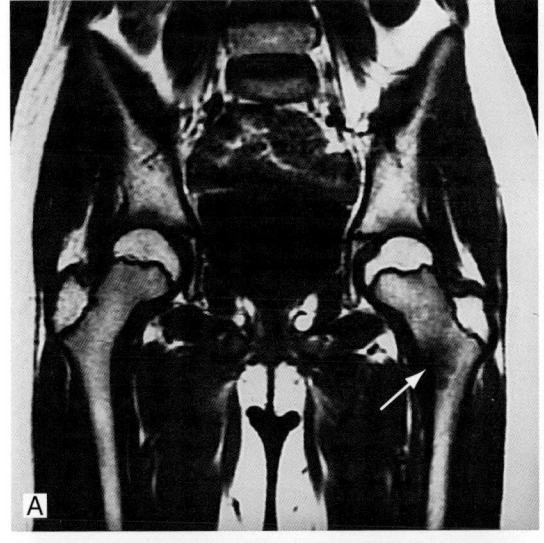

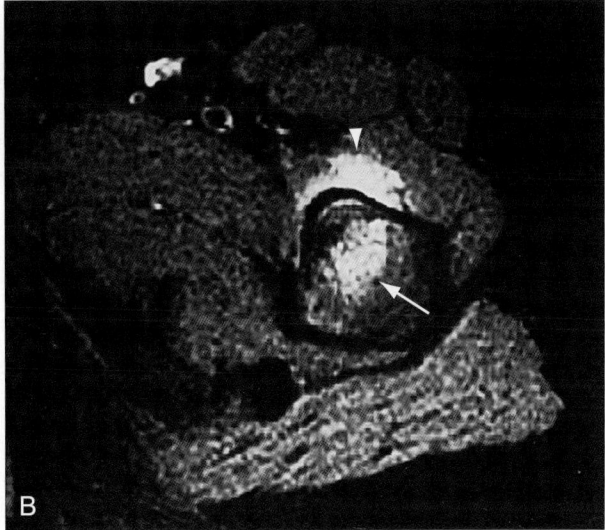

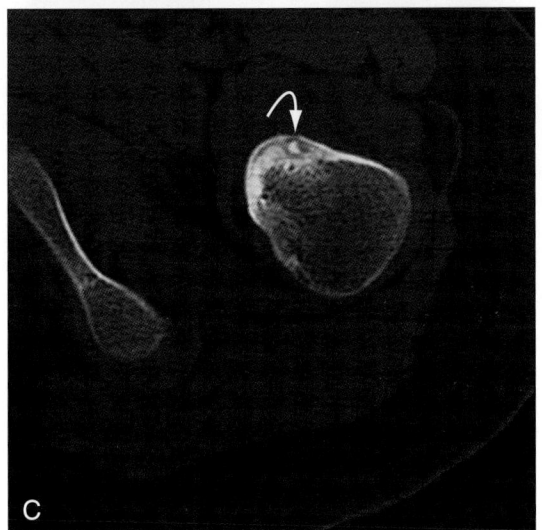

FIGURE 110-23

Osteoid osteoma. MR images obtained to evaluate chronic hip pain. **A,** Coronal T1-weighted (500/15) image demonstrates localized decrease in marrow signal in the femoral neck *(arrow)*. **B,** Axial STIR (1600/20; inversion time [TI] = 170) image demonstrates high signal intensity edema in the marrow space *(arrow)* and adjacent soft-tissue *(arrowhead)*. **C,** Axial CT image clearly demonstrates nidus in the anterior subcortical portion of the femoral neck *(arrow)*. (*A to C* from Bisset GS III: Case 26, osteoid osteoma. In: Pediatric Disease [Fourth Series] Test and Syllabus, Number 35. Reston, VA: American College of Radiology, 1993, pp T84-T87, 691-720.)

(see Figs. 110-18 and 110-19). Standard or fast spin-echo images, STIR images, and fat-suppressed T2-weighted images are generally sufficient for this purpose.

A variety of techniques have been suggested for evaluating tumor response to therapy, including evaluation of signal changes on conventional spin-echo sequences,[89,101,106,107] dynamic contrast imaging with or without subtraction techniques,[84,94,96,98,99,113] and MR spectroscopy.[102] The more elaborate techniques have not gained wide acceptance owing to factors such as the requirement for customized analysis software or pulse sequences, limitations imposed by region-of-interest selection and associated sampling errors, and a relative lack of specificity.

Benign Lesions

MRI may have a more significant role in diagnosis of some benign soft-tissue masses, in which a characteristic appearance may be diagnostic. In children, soft-tissue masses are most commonly vascular in origin. Hemangiomas usually appear in infancy as a result of pathologic angiogenesis which typically causes cellular proliferation over several years and then subsequent involution. This is in contrast to other vascular malformations which characteristically have stable endothelium in which growth of the tumor follows growth of the child and does not involute over time. Hemangiomas produce variable signal intensities on T1-weighted images (ranging from isointense with skeletal muscle to mixed, primarily high signal intensity) and bright signal on T2-weighted images. The characteristic serpiginous form of the vascular spaces and the interface of the lesion with surrounding tissues are best demonstrated on T2-weighted images.[114-120]

Although hemangiomas are the most common vascular tumor in childhood, others include infantile hemangiopericytoma, hemangioendothelioma (kaposiform and spindle cell) and tufted angioma. Although originally described in association with large infantile hemangiomas, Kasabach–Merritt syndrome has been reported

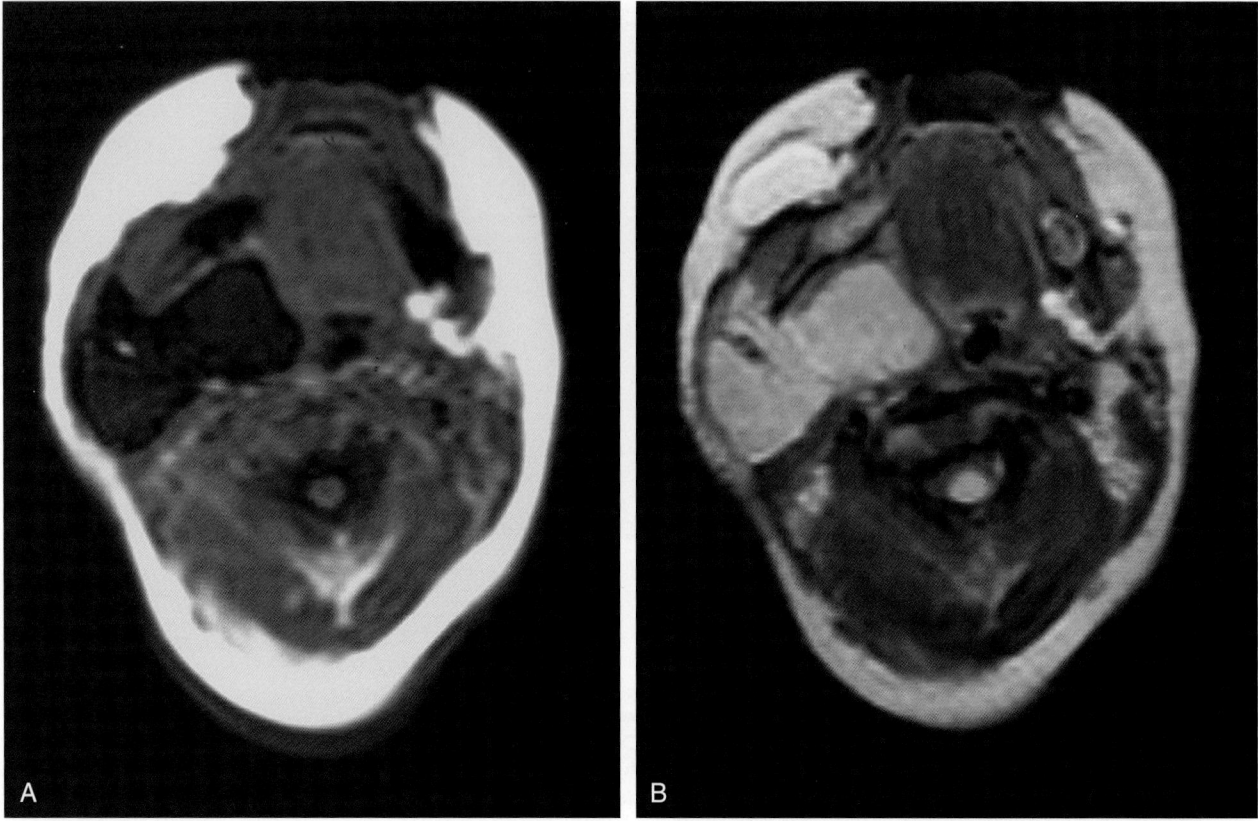

FIGURE 110-24

Lymphangioma. Axial T1-weighted (**A**) and T2-weighted (**B**) images at the level of the mandible demonstrate a lymphangioma in the right neck with low T1 and high T2 signal respectively. Several internal septations are noted.

with both kaposiform hemangioendothelioma and tufted angioma. This syndrome has a high mortality rate and is characterized by severe consumptive coagulopathy, low fibrinogen, and thrombocytopenia.[121]

Venous and lymphatic malformations result from errors of morphogenesis. This wide constellation of diseases incorporates variable combinations of abnormal arteries, veins, lymphatics, and capillaries. Vascular malformations can be categorized as lesions with low flow (venous, capillary or lymphatic) or high flow (arteriovenous malformation and fistulas). Venous malformations constitute the most common type of vascular malformation. These lesions will often have phleboliths on plain radiographs. By MRI, venous malformations are typically hypointense on T1-weighted imaging and hyperintense on T2-weighted imaging and demonstrate diffuse contrast enhancement after intravenous contrast administration (see Fig. 110-22). Lymphatic malformations will not enhance after the administration of intravenous contrast material. Very slow flow within the abnormal vascular channels of venous malformations often precludes detection of true flow voids and results in the increased signal typical of T2-weighted sequences. These lesions will often have linear bands of interspersed fat.

Lymphangioma may appear as a simple cystic structure with signal characteristics of simple fluid content (cystic hygroma) or as a complex multiloculated mass (Fig. 110-24). These lesions often present with rapid enlargement resulting from intralesional hemorrhage. Hemoglobin breakdown products may alter the signal characteristics of the lesion contents. Vascular lesions often have a mixture of both hemangiomatous and lymphangiomatous components.[118] Lipoma, which may be superficial (subcutaneous) or deep (intramuscular), produces a characteristic appearance of a mass entirely composed of tissue with signal characteristics approximating those of subcutaneous fat on all pulse sequences (see Fig. 110-21). There may be fine septa of low signal intensity in a benign lipoma, but more substantial soft-tissue components should raise the suspicion of a malignant neoplasm (liposarcoma).[90]

MRI may also be useful in delineating non-tumorous conditions that may simulate a tumor mass clinically, such as subcutaneous fat necrosis (Fig. 110-25) or arteriovenous fistula. Purely cystic structures with simple fluid contents and imperceptibly thin walls, such as synovial cysts and ganglion cysts, produce a characteristic MRI appearance and are readily distinguished from neoplastic processes. Soft-tissue hematoma

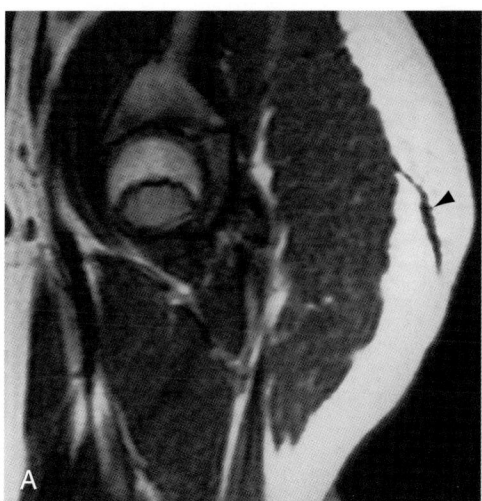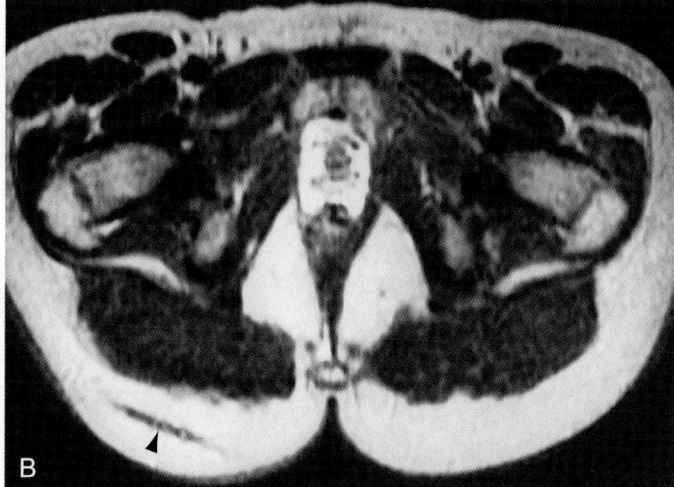

FIGURE 110-25

Subcutaneous fat necrosis. The patient presented with a palpable mass in the buttock, clinically suspected of being a soft-tissue tumor. Sagittal T1-weighted (500/20) image (**A**) and axial T2-weighted (2000/80) image (**B**) demonstrate a linear area of decreased signal intensity in the subcutaneous fat corresponding to a site of previous injury (*arrowheads*).

may be a clinically evident mass suggestive of tumor. MRI may show characteristic mixed signal intensities from various hemoglobin breakdown products, depending on the age of the hematoma.[54] Caution should be exercised, however, because tumors may present with intratumoral hemorrhage.

Benign bone lesions of interest in the pediatric population for which MRI may be useful for anatomic assessment and surgical planning include simple bone cyst,[122] aneurysmal bone cyst,[122,123] Langerhans' cell histiocytosis,[122] and fibromatosis.[124,125]

Another lesion that may be encountered in the pediatric population when MRI is performed to evaluate occult musculoskeletal pain is an osteoid osteoma (see Fig. 110-23). This lesion produces a characteristic history of pain, worse at night, that is relieved by aspirin.[126] The lesion is composed of a central, often calcified nidus surrounded by reactive bone sclerosis and variable cortical thickening. These findings are most directly visualized with CT. At MRI, the nidus may be inapparent on T1-weighted images and is usually high in signal intensity on T2-weighted sequences.[85] Reactive bone sclerosis and adjacent cortical thickening are seen as areas of low signal intensity on T1-weighted sequences. Marrow edema may produce increasing signal intensity on progressively more T2-weighted sequences.[127]

BONE MARROW DISORDERS

One of the strengths of MRI is its ability to detect the presence and distribution of disorders affecting the marrow because of the striking changes in marrow fat signal caused by most such entities. MRI of bone marrow disease has been the subject of a variety of reports.[128-131]

Normal Conversion of Hematopoietic to Fatty Marrow

To determine the significance of marrow signal changes, it is important to have an understanding of normal marrow signal changes related to conversion of red marrow to yellow marrow during development.

At birth, red marrow predominates throughout the skeleton with the exception of the phalanges of the feet and hands. In the normal adult, red marrow predominates in the proximal femurs and humeri, the pelvis, the vertebral bodies, and the skull. There is a progressive conversion from red (hematopoietic) marrow to yellow (fatty) marrow in the peripheral skeleton, which occurs in a predictable pattern. This has been documented by macroscopic inspection[132] and by MRI evaluation of the femur.[133,134] Knowledge of the expected marrow distribution at a given age is essential for the detection of primary marrow disturbances as well as other processes affecting the marrow signal, such as tumor infiltration, trauma, infection, and infarction.

On T1-weighted MR images, fatty marrow appears as a uniform high signal intensity owing to the shortened T1 relaxation time of fat. Red marrow appears as an intermediate signal intensity similar to or slightly greater than that of muscle. The conversion on MR images from red marrow signal to yellow marrow signal precedes the conversion as determined by gross inspection. This is thought to occur because as little as 10% fat content may produce a predominantly high signal intensity on T1-weighted images.[133] There is disagreement on the rate at which the progression of conversion from the low signal intensity red marrow to the high signal intensity yellow marrow takes place as assessed by MRI. A chart of red and yellow marrow distribution in various age groups is

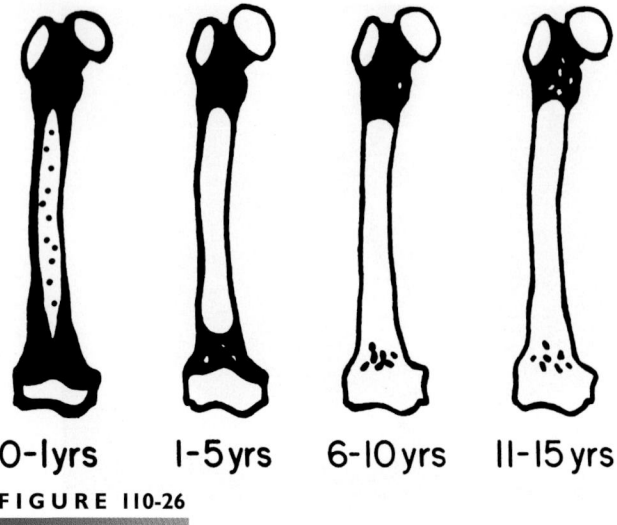

0-1yrs   1-5yrs   6-10yrs   11-15yrs

FIGURE 110-26

Normal conversion of hematopoietic marrow to fatty marrow in the developing femur as a function of age. Black areas represent hematopoietic marrow and white areas represent fatty marrow. *(From Waitches G, Zawin JK, Poznanski AK: Sequence and rate of bone marrow conversion in the femora of children as seen on MR imaging. Am J Roentgenol 162:1399-1406, 1994.)*

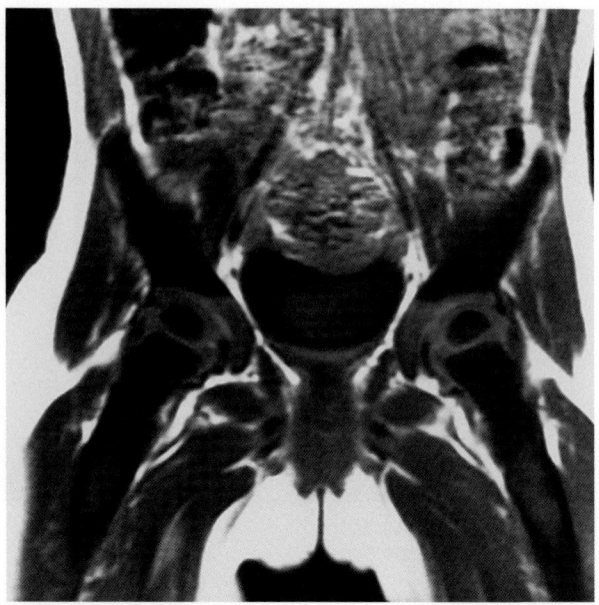

FIGURE 110-27

Sickle cell disease. Coronal T1-weighted (500/11) image demonstrates generalized low marrow signal intensity resulting from a combination of marrow hyperplasia and iron deposition from multiple transfusions.

shown in Figure 110-26. Differences in reported rates of conversion may be due to a combination of window setting variations, coil selection, and interobserver variation.[134]

Anemias

Sickle Cell Disease

Sickle cell disease includes a variety of hemoglobinopathies that have in common the production of hemoglobin S. These include homozygous hemoglobin SS disease, SC disease, and sickle cell disease combined with thalassemia (α or β). Marrow abnormalities related to sickle cell disease result primarily from red marrow expansion in response to chronic hemolytic anemia and infarction or avascular necrosis secondary to increased blood viscosity.

The marrow expansion or hyperplasia seen in sickle cell disease produces decreased marrow signal intensity on T1-weighted images with variable signal intensity noted on T2-weighted images.[135,136] In more severe cases, the combination of chronic hemolysis and multiple transfusions may lead to secondary hemosiderosis and associated marked diffuse decrease in marrow signal intensity on all pulse sequences (Fig. 110-27). Other disorders that may produce similar diffuse signal changes include Blackfan–Diamond syndrome (red blood cell aplasia) and the thalassemias. Focal areas of decreased signal intensity on T1-weighted images with increased signal intensity on T2-weighted images have been shown to correlate with pain and are thought to represent edema from acute infarction, whereas focal areas of decreased signal intensity on T1- and T2-weighted sequences are thought to represent

remote infarction.[135] However, it is important to remember that the marrow abnormalities depicted by MR with acute infarction along with associated soft-tissue changes cannot be reliably differentiated from infection. Extraosseous abnormalities seen in the setting of sickle cell disease with acute infarction include fascial, muscular, and more superficial soft-tissue inflammation, including focal fluid collections.[15]

Aplastic Anemia

Aplastic anemia, in the untreated phase, is characterized histologically by extensive fatty replacement of marrow with few hematopoietic cellular elements. MRI demonstrates bright signal on T1-weighted images corresponding to yellow marrow in a widespread distribution often including the axial skeleton.[128-130] With treatment, patchy areas of decreased signal intensity develop, often beginning in the vertebral column, corresponding to regenerating areas of red marrow.

Marrow Packing Disorders

Gaucher's Disease

Gaucher's disease represents a genetically complex group of disorders in which the common feature is relative deficiency of β-glucocerebrosidase, leading to accumulation of glucocerebroside in the reticuloendothelial system. Type 1, the most common form, is a chronic disorder with central nervous system sparing, characterized by marrow infiltration and expansion and

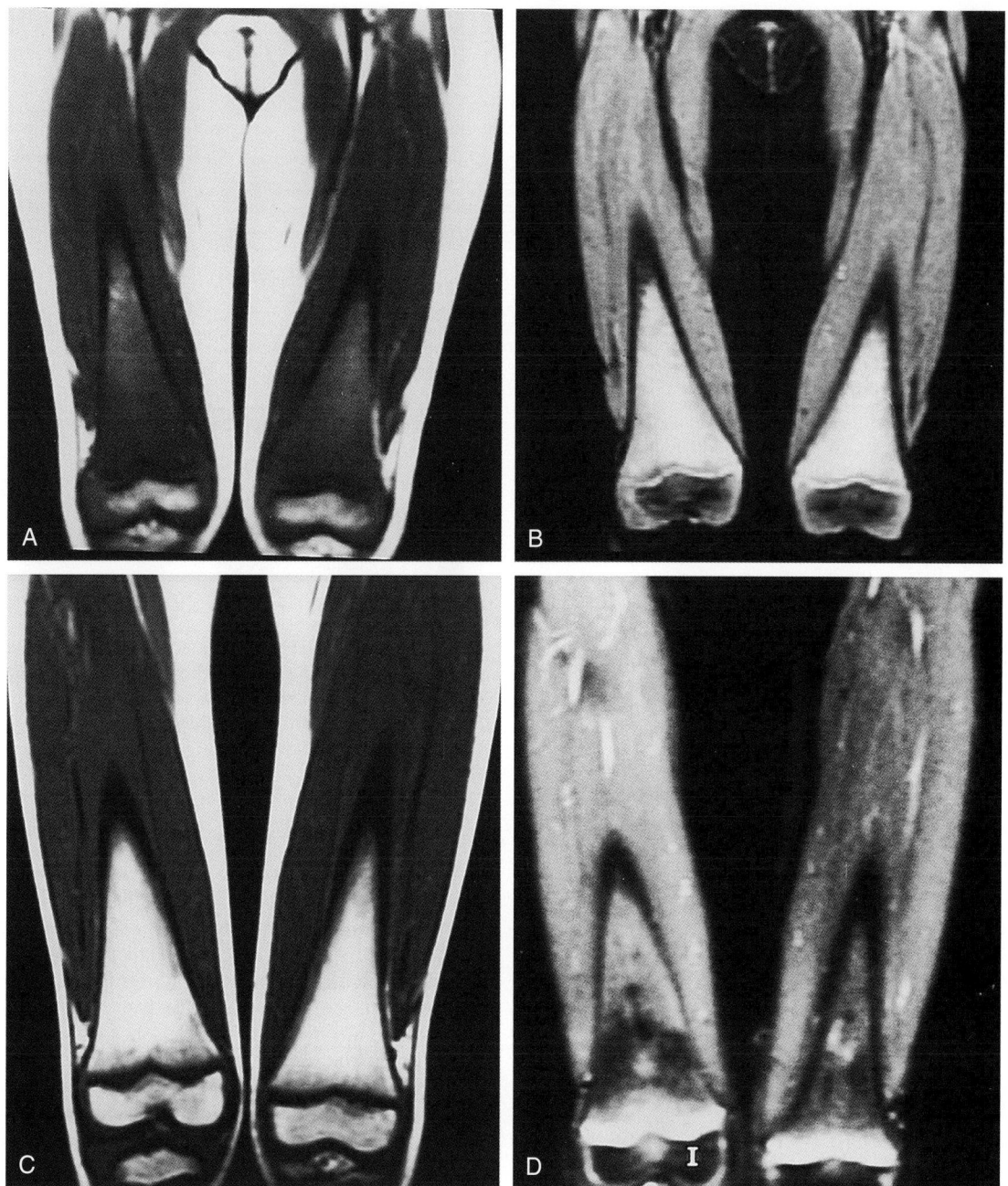

FIGURE 110-28

Gaucher's disease. Pretreatment: **A,** Coronal T1-weighted (500/12) image demonstrates widespread abnormally decreased marrow signal. **B,** Coronal STIR (1000/20, TI = 150) image demonstrates widespread abnormally increased signal. Post-treatment: Coronal T1-weighted (550/11) image (**C**) and coronal fast STIR (5000/18, TI = 155) image (**D**) demonstrate substantial improvement in marrow signal.

marked hepatosplenomegaly. Types 2 and 3 represent fatal infantile and juvenile forms, respectively, that produce progressive neurologic compromise.

Plain film findings in the extremities of patients with Gaucher's disease reflect secondary changes of marrow infiltration and include the Erlenmeyer flask deformity of the distal femurs, osteoporosis, and complications such as avascular necrosis and pathologic fracture.

Marrow infiltration produces heterogeneous decreased signal intensity on T1- and T2-weighted images (Fig. 110-28), often with sparing of the epiphyses.[137-139] Areas of increased signal intensity on T2-weighted sequences correlate with painful episodes and are thought to represent edema from recent infarction.[138,139] Patients may also suffer from episodes of bone pain crisis termed pseudo-osteomyelitis that clinically and radiographically may resemble infectious osteomyelitis. MRI demonstrates areas with decreased signal intensity on T1-weighted images and increased signal intensity on T2-weighted images with associated periosteal elevation and soft-tissue edema, the periosteal elevation and edema being indistinguishable from osteomyelitis.[137] Signal changes suggestive of subacute hemorrhage (increased signal intensity on T1- and T2-weighted images) within the medullary and subperiosteal spaces have also been reported in association with acute symptoms and may help support a diagnosis of pseudo-osteomyelitis.[140]

Avascular Necrosis

Avascular necrosis or bone infarction results from compromise of blood supply to the affected bone. The most commonly affected site in the pediatric population is the femoral head, but any location may be involved. Avascular necrosis has been associated with a wide variety of conditions. Those of particular interest in the pediatric population include sickle cell disease,[135,136,141] Gaucher's disease,[138,139] meningococcal infection with disseminated intravascular coagulation,[142] slipped capital femoral epiphysis,[64] steroid use,[143] leukemia,[144] bone marrow transplantation,[145] and trauma.[146] MRI patterns of avascular necrosis in the femoral head include preservation of a normal fat signal on all pulse sequences except for a low signal intensity reactive margin, areas of high signal intensity on both T1- and T2-weighted images, areas of low signal intensity on T1-weighted images and high signal intensity on T2-weighted images, and areas of low signal intensity on all pulse sequences.[146] Areas of involvement are often heterogeneous and may produce a ring of decreased signal intensity surrounding a central area of high signal intensity[147] (Fig. 110-29).

Legg-Calvé-Perthes Disease

Legg-Calvé-Perthes disease (LCP) is an idiopathic aseptic necrosis of the femoral head seen most commonly in children between the ages of 3 and 12 years. The disease may be bilateral in approximately 10% and affects boys more often than girls. The incidence varies widely, between 5.5 and 15.6 children per 100,000.[148]

As with adults, marrow signal changes are readily identified in the femoral head ossification center before radiographs become abnormal.[149-152] Unlike avascular necrosis in the adult, which typically progresses to joint failure necessitating hip replacement, Legg-Calvé-Perthes disease usually progresses through a predictable series of stages including condensation, fragmentation, and reparation of the capital femoral epiphysis. During reparation, there is femoral and acetabular cartilaginous hypertrophy. Femoral head cartilage thickening is least pronounced superiorly, producing a characteristic broadening of the femoral head.[153] This broadening and loss of the normal rounded contour can lead to uncovering of the femoral head and secondary degen-

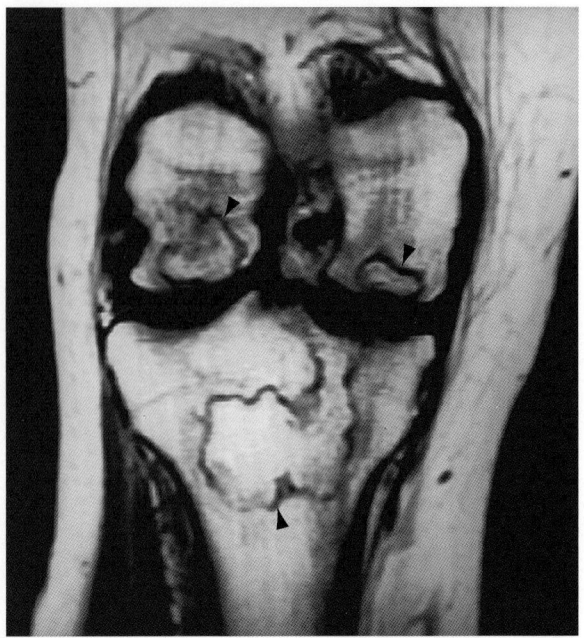

FIGURE 110-29

Bone infarcts. Coronal T1-weighted (600/20) image of the knee demonstrates sharply demarcated areas with irregular rims of low signal intensity in the femoral condyles and proximal tibia corresponding to bone infarcts *(arrowheads)*. The patient was receiving long-term steroid therapy. Plain radiographs were normal.

erative changes as well as persistent deformity. Physeal bridging at the proximal femoral physis has been found to be a significant predictor of growth arrest.[154] The bony portions of the femoral head and acetabulum are visualized with plain film radiography. However, the cartilaginous components, which are seen as relatively low signal intensity structures on T1-weighted images with increasing signal intensity on T2-weighted images, are well demonstrated by MRI.[150,151,153]

Initially, axial T1-weighted images should be obtained to select an optimal coronal plane through the proximal femurs for direct side-to-side comparison. Coronal T1-weighted images afford good anatomic assessment (Fig. 110-30). Enhanced anatomic detail may be facilitated by the addition of a surface coil on the side of interest. T2-weighted images demonstrate hip joint fluid and help characterize marrow signal changes. Visualization of cartilaginous coverage, including the low signal intensity fibrocartilaginous labrum, provides a better assessment of functional containment of the femoral head, without the discomfort and risks associated with arthrography. In cases of inadequate coverage, there may be indentation of the femoral head produced by the lateral margin of the acetabulum.[150] MRI may also be used to assess femoral head coverage in the postoperative patient in a cast. Transient changes in femoral head marrow signal have been reported in children presenting with hip pain, possibly representing transient marrow edema.[155] This may be an early, reversible precursor to Legg-Calvé-Perthes disease.

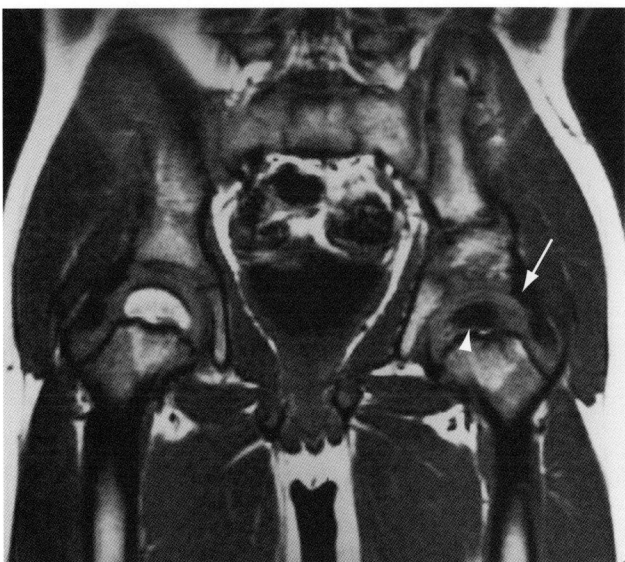

FIGURE 110-30

Legg-Calvé-Perthes disease. Coronal T1-weighted (600/20) image demonstrates decreased marrow signal intensity in the left femoral head (arrowhead). There is adequate coverage of the cartilaginous femoral head by the low signal intensity fibrocartilaginous labrum (arrow).

Other Iatrogenic Marrow Changes

Whereas MRI is sensitive for pathologic changes in the marrow space, there is a relative lack of specificity owing to similar signal changes in malignant neoplasia, inflammation, and red marrow reconversion. This may be a particular problem in patients with disseminated marrow disease related to malignant neoplasm, such as leukemia or neuroblastoma, who undergo treatment with regimens that may affect marrow signal, such as chemotherapy with or without radiation therapy,[154] bone marrow transplantation,[155,156] and administration of hematopoietic growth factors used in conjunction with chemotherapy.[157] On follow-up examinations, signal changes related to treatment may be similar to those related to recurrence.

A characteristic pattern of hematopoietic marrow reconversion in the vertebral bodies after bone marrow transplantation has been described.[158] These findings consist of peripheral bands of intermediate signal intensity on T1-weighted images (corresponding to hematopoietic marrow) surrounding a central area of bright signal (corresponding to fatty marrow). Deviations from this pattern may be suggestive of tumor recurrence. Pretransplant irradiation may limit the capacity of the affected area to reconvert to hematopoietic marrow.[159]

TARSAL COALITIONS

Tarsal coalition is a frequent cause of foot and ankle pain in children and young adults and is thought to result from faulty differentiation of primary mesenchyme leading to abnormal joint formation. Although primarily a congenital disorder, coalitions may occasionally develop secondary to trauma and rheumatoid arthritis. Tarsal coalitions may be fibrous, cartilaginous or osseous. Although some individuals remain asymptomatic, pain usually develops secondary to progressive ossification of the coalition and resultant limited mobility of the subtalar joint. Occasionally a flat foot deformity develops secondary to spasm of the peroneal and extensor tendons. Approximately 90% of tarsal coalitions are talocalcaneal or calcaneonavicular. Less common coalitions include talonavicular, calcaneocuboid, and cubonavicular. Occasionally multiple coalitions will occur in one foot.

Calcaneonavicular coalitions are more readily apparent on conventional radiographs (45° internal oblique view). When an osseous coalition is present there is a bridging bony bar across the two bones which do not normally articulate. With fibrous or cartilaginous coalition the bones have irregular surfaces with sclerosis. Due to the complex relationship of the subtalar joint, talocalcaneal coalitions may be difficult to visualize by conventional radiography. A number of secondary signs have been described, including a talar beak[160] and the "complete C" sign.[161] Both CT and MRI have proven useful for delineating tarsal coalitions.[162,163] MR imaging may have the advantage of better assessing associated or additional soft-tissue abnormalities and may provide slightly better delineation of non-osseous coalitions (Fig. 110-31).

When evaluating a painful foot by MR for possible coalition axial, coronal and sagittal T1 and FSE T2 with fat saturation images should be obtained. Calcaneonavicular coalitions are best seen on sagittal and axial planes, while the coronal plane is best for identification of talocalcaneal coalitions. Associated bone marrow edema is often present.

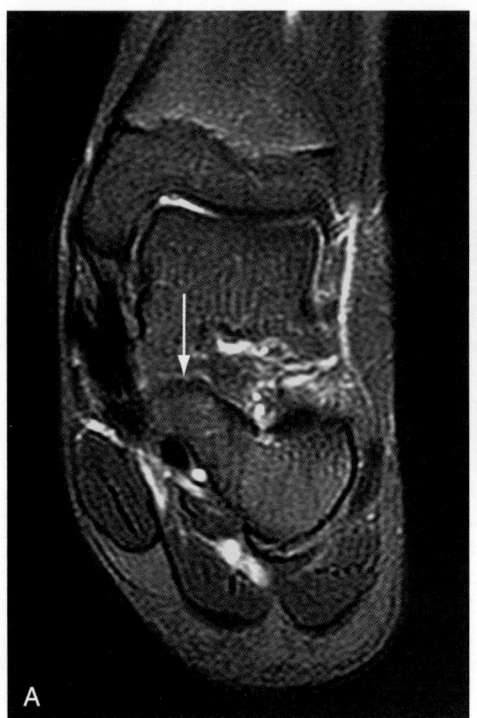

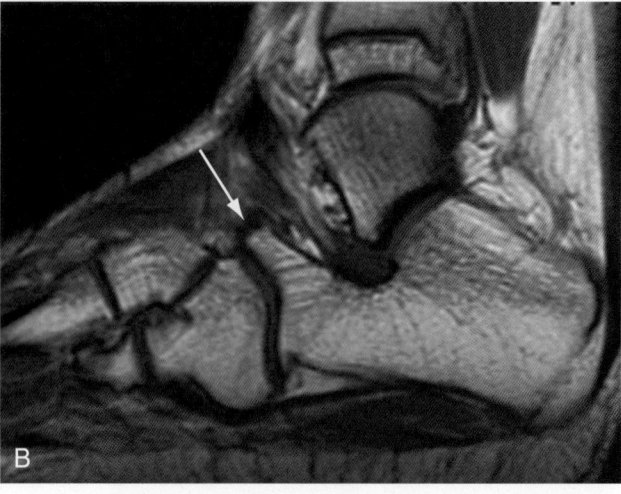

FIGURE 110-31

Tarsal coalition (calcaneonavicular). **A,** Coronal T2-weighted image with fat saturation of the ankle demonstrates irregularity of the calcaneo-navicular joint compatable with a fibrous coalition (*arrow*). **B,** Sagittal T1-weighted image of the ankle demonstrates beaking of the calcaneus (*arrow*).

REFERENCES

1. Haber D: Preanesthetic assessment of the pediatric patient. Anesthiol Clin North Am 8:759-784, 1990.
2. Joint Commission on Accreditation of Health Care Organizations: 1995 Comprehensive Accreditation Manuals for Hospitals. Oakbrook Terrace, IL: Joint Commission, 1995.
3. Frush DP, Bisset GS 3rd, Hall SC: Pediatric sedation in radiology: the practice of safe sleep. Am J Roentgenol 167:1381-1387, 1996.
4. Committee on Drugs, American Academy of Pediatrics: Guidelines for monitoring and management of pediatric patients during and after sedation for diagnostic and therapeutic procedures. Pediatrics 89:1110-1114, 1992.
5. Fisher DM: Sedation of pediatric patients: an anesthesiologist's perspective. Radiology 175:613-615, 1990.
6. Miller R, Leno T: Advances in pediatric emergency department procedures. Emerg Med Clin North Am 9:639-654, 1991.
7. Moore SG, Bisset GS, Siegel MJ, et al: Pediatric musculoskeletal MR imaging. Radiology 179:345-360, 1991.
8. Barnewolt CE, Chung T: Techniques, coils, pulse sequences, and contrast enhancement in pediatric musculoskeletal MR imaging. Magn Reson Imaging Clin North Am 6:441-453, 1998.
9. Gronemeyer SA, Kaufman WM, Rocha MS, et al: Fat-saturated contrast-enhanced T1-weighted MRI in evaluation of osteosarcoma and Ewing sarcoma. J Magn Reson Imaging 7:585-589, 1997.
10. Vanel D, Shapeero LG, De Baere T, et al: MR imaging in the follow-up of malignant and aggressive soft-tissue tumors: results of 511 examinations. Radiology 190:263-268, 1994.
11. Haddad MC, Sharif HS, Aabed SY, et al: Gadolinium DTPA: value in MR imaging of extraspinal musculoskeletal infections. Eur Radiol 3:527-535, 1993.
12. Gylys-Morin VM: MR imaging of pediatric musculoskeletal inflammatory and infectious disorders. Magn Reson Imaging Clin North Am 6:537-559, 1998.
13. Dangman BC, Hoffer FA, Rand FF: Osteomyelitis in children: gadolinium-enhanced MR imaging. Radiology 182:743-747, 1992.
14. Bonnerot V, Sebag G, de Montailembert M, et al: Gadolinium-DPTA enhanced MRI of painful osseous crises in children with sickle cell anemia. Pediatr Radiol 24: 92-95, 1994.
15. Frush DP, Heyneman LE, Ware, RE, Bisset GS: MR features of soft tissue abnormalities due to acute marrow infarction in five children with sickle cell disease. Am J Roentgenol 173: 989-993, 1999.
16. Reiser MF, Bongratz GP, Erlemann R, et al: Gadolinium DTPA in rheumatoid arthritis and related diseases: first results with dynamic magnetic resonance imaging. Skeletal Radiol 18:591-597, 1989.

17. Gold R: Diagnosis of osteomyelitis. Pediatr Rev 12:292-297, 1991.
18. Handmaker H, Leonards R: The bone scan in inflammatory osseous disease. Semin Nucl Med 6: 95-105, 1976.
19. Tuson CE, Hoffman EB, Mann MD: Isotope bone scanning for acute osteomyelitis and septic arthritis in children. J Bone Joint Surg 76:306-310, 1994.
20. Cohen, MD Cory DA, Kleiman M: Magnetic resonance differentiation of acute and chronic osteomyelitis in children. Clin Radiol 41:53-56, 1990.
21. Fletcher BD, Scoles PV, Nelson AD: Osteomyelitis in children: detection by magnetic resonance. Radiology 150:57-60, 1984.
22. Mazur JM, Ross G, Cummings J, et al: Usefulness of magnetic resonance imaging in the diagnosis of acute musculoskeletal infections in children. J Pediatr Orthop 15:144-147, 1995.
23. Stover B, Sigmund G, Langer M, et al: MRI in diagnostic evaluation of osteomyelitis in children. Eur Radiol 4:347-352, 1994.
24. Unger E, Moldofsky P, Gatenby B, et al: Diagnosis of osteomyelitis by MR imaging. Am J Roentgenol 150:605-610, 1988.
25. Hopkins KL, Li KSP, Bergman G: Gadolinium-DTPA-enhanced magnetic resonance imaging of musculoskeletal infectious processes. Skeletal Radiol 24:325-330, 1995.
26. Sundaram M, McDonald D, Engel E, et al: Chronic recurrent multifocal osteomyelitis: an evolving clinical and radiologic spectrum. Skeletal Radiol 25:333-336, 1996.
27. Brown T, Wilkinson RH: Chronic recurrent multifocal osteomyelitis. Radiology 166:493-496, 1998.
28. Jaramillo D, Treves ST, Kasser JR, et al: Osteomyelitis and septic arthritis in children: appropriate use of imaging to guide treatment. Am J Roentgenol 165:399-403, 1995.
29. Mandell GA: Imaging in the diagnosis of musculoskeletal infections in children. Curr Probl Pediatr 26:218-237, 1996.
30. Towers JD: The use of intravenous contrast in MRI of extremity infection. Semin US CT Magn Reson Imaging 18:269-275, 1997.
31. May DA, Disler DG, Jones EA, et al: Abnormal signal intensity in skeletal muscle at MR imaging: patterns, pearls and pitfalls. Radiographics special number:295-315, 2000.
32. Hernandez RJ, Keim DR, Chenevert TL, et al: Fat-suppressed MR imaging of myositis. Radiology 182:217-219, 1992.
33. Hernandez RJ, Keim DR, Sullivan DB, et al: Magnetic resonance imaging appearance of the muscles in childhood dermatomyositis. J Pediatr 117:546-550, 1990.
34. Hernandez RJ, Sullivan DB, Chenevert TL, Keim DR: MR imaging in children with dermatomyositis: musculoskeletal findings and correlation with clinical and laboratory findings. Am J Roentgenol 161:359-366, 1993.
35. Kaufman LD, Gruber BL, Gerstman DP, Kaell AT: Preliminary observation on the role of magnetic resonance imaging for polymyositis and dermatomyositis. Ann Rheum Dis 46:569-572, 1987.

36. Poznanski AK: Radiological approaches to pediatric joint disease. J Rheumatol 19(suppl 33):78-93, 1992.
37. Sebag G, Hervé-Somma C: Imaging in pediatric rheumatology. Clin Exp Rheumatol 11(suppl 9):s51-s52, 1993.
38. Hervé-Somma CM, Sebag GH, Prieur AM, et al: Juvenile rheumatoid arthritis of the knee: MR evaluation with Gd-DOTA. Radiology 182:93-98, 1992.
39. Senac MO, Deutsch D, Bernstein BH, et al: MR imaging in juvenile rheumatoid arthritis. Am J Roentgenol 150:873-878, 1988.
40. Yulish BS, Leiberman JM, Newman AJ, et al: Juvenile rheumatoid arthritis: assessment with MR imaging. Radiology 165:149-152, 1987.
41. Arnold WD, Hilgartner MW: Hemophilic arthropathy: current concepts of pathogenesis and management. J Bone Joint Surg Am 59:287-305, 1977.
42. Baunin C, Railhac JJ, Younes I, et al: MR imaging in hemophilic arthropathy. Eur J Pediatr Surg 1:358-363, 1991.
43. Nuss R, Kilcoyne RF, Geraghty S, et al: Utility of magnetic resonance imaging for management of hemophilic arthropathy in children. J Pediatr 123:388-392, 1993.
44. Yulish BS, Lieberman JM, Strandjord SE, et al: Hemophilic arthropathy: assessment with MR imaging. Radiology 164:759-762, 1987.
45. Kulkarni MV, Drolshagen LF, Kaye JJ, et al: MR imaging of hemophiliac arthropathy. J Comput Assist Tomogr 10:445-449, 1986.
46. Curtin WA, Lahoti OP, Fogarty EE, et al: Pigmented villonodular synovitis arising from the sheath of the extensor hallucis longus in an eight-month-old infant. Clin Orthop 292:282-284, 1993.
47. Jelinek JS, Kransdorf MJ, Utz JA, et al: Imaging of pigmented villonodular synovitis with emphasis on MR imaging. Am J Roentgenol 152:337-342, 1989.
48. Kottal RA, Vogler JB III, Matamoros A, et al: Pigmented villonodular synovitis: a report of MR imaging in two cases. Radiology 163:551-553, 1987.
49. Poletti SC, Gates HS, Martinez SM, Richardson WJ: The use of magnetic resonance imaging in the diagnosis of pigmented villonodular synovitis. Orthopaedics 13:185-190, 1990.
50. Berger PE, Ofstein RA, Jackson D, et al: MRI demonstration of radiographically occult fractures: what have we been missing? Radiographics 9:407-436, 1989.
51. Deutsch AL, Mink JH, Wasman AD: Occult fractures of the proximal femur: MR imaging. Radiology 170:113-116, 1989.
52. Stafford SA, Rosenthal DI, Gebhardt MC, et al: MRI in stress fracture. Am J Roentgenol 147:553-556, 1986.
53. Yao L, Lee JK: Occult intraosseous fracture: detection with MR imaging. Radiology 167:749-751, 1988.
54. Ehman RL, Berquist TH: Magnetic resonance imaging of musculoskeletal trauma. Radiol Clin North Am 24:291-319, 1986.
55. Dooms GC, Risher MR, Hricak H, Higgins CB: MR imaging of intramuscular hemorrhage. J Comput Assist Tomogr 9:908-913, 1985.
56. Salter RB, Harris WR: Injuries involving the epiphyseal plate. J Bone Joint Surg Am 45:587-622, 1963.
57. Hynes D, O'Brien T: Growth disturbance lines after injury of the distal tibial physis. J Bone Joint Surg Br 70:231-233, 1988.
58. Ogden JA: Injury to the growth mechanisms of the immature skeleton. Skeletal Radiol 6:237-253, 1981.
59. Ogden JA: The evaluation and treatment of partial physeal arrest. J Bone Joint Surg Am 69:1297-1302, 1987.
60. Riseborough EJ, Barret IR, Shapiro F: Growth disturbances following distal femoral physeal fracture-separations. J Bone Joint Surg Am 65:885-889, 1983.
61. Jaramillo D, Shapiro F, Hoffer FA, et al: Post-traumatic growth-plate abnormalities: MR imaging of bony-bridge formation in rabbits. Radiology 175:767-773, 1990.
62. Jaramillo D, Hoffer FA, Shapiro F, Rand F: MR imaging of fractures of the growth plate. Am J Roentgenol 155:1261-1265, 1990.
63. Galbraith RT, Gelberman RH, Hajek PC, et al: Obesity and decreased femoral anteversion in adolescence. J Orthop Res 5:523-528, 1987.
64. Lowe HG: Avascular necrosis after slipping of the upper femoral epiphysis. J Bone Joint Surg Br 43:688-699, 1961.
65. Ingram AJ, Clarke MS, Clark CS, Marshall WR: Chondrolysis complicating slipped capital femoral epiphysis. Clin Orthop 165:99-109, 1982.
66. Vrettos BC, Hoffman EB: Chondrolysis in slipped upper femoral epiphysis. Long-term study of the aetiology and natural history. J Bone Joint Surg Br 75:956-961, 1993.
67. Castriota-Scanderberg A, Orsi E: Slipped capital femoral epiphysis: ultrasonographic findings. Skeletal Radiol 22:191-193, 1993.
68. Carney BT, Weinstein SL, Noble J: Long-term follow-up of slipped capital femoral epiphysis. J Bone Joint Surg Am 73:667-674, 1991.
69. Johnston CE II: Infantile tibia vara. Clin Orthop 255:13-23, 1990.
70. Langenskiöld A: Tibia vara: osteochondrosis deformans tibiae. Blount's disease. Clin Orthop 158:77-82, 1981.
71. Thompson GH, Carter JR, Smith CW: Late-onset tibia vara: a comparative analysis. J Pediatr Orthop 4:185-194, 1984.
72. Dietz WH, Gross WL, Kirkpatrick JA: Blount disease (tibia vara): another skeletal disorder associated with childhood obesity. J Pediatr 101:735-737, 1982.
73. Anderson MW, Greenspan A: Stress fractures. Radiology 199:1-12, 1996.
74. Aichroth P: Osteochondral fractures and their relationship to osteochondritis dissecans of the knee: an experimental study in animals. J Bone Joint Surg Br 53:448-454, 1971.
75. Aichroth P: Osteochondritis dissecans of the knee: a clinical survey. J Bone Joint Surg Br 53:440-447, 1971.
76. Caffey J, Madell SH, Royer C, et al: Ossification of the distal femoral epiphysis. J Bone Joint Surg Am 40:647-654, 1958.
77. Jawish R, Rigault P, Padovani JP, et al: Osteochondritis dissecans of the humeral capitellum in children. Eur J Pediatr Surg 3:97-100, 1993.
78. Mesgarzadeh M, Sapega AA, Bonakdarpour A, et al: Osteochondritis dissecans: analysis of mechanical stability with radiography, scintigraphy, and MR imaging. Radiology 165:775-780, 1987.
79. Barlow TG: Early diagnosis and treatment of congenital dislocation of the hip. J Bone Joint Surg Br 44:292-301, 1962.
80. Hernandez RJ: Evaluation of congenital hip dysplasia and tibial torsion by computed tomography. J Comput Tomogr 7:101-108, 1983.
81. Johnson ND, Wood BP, Jackman KV: Complex infantile and congenital hip dislocation: assessment with MR imaging. Radiology 168:151-156, 1988.
82. Guidera KJ, Einbecker ME, Berman CG, et al: Magnetic resonance imaging evaluation of congenital dislocation of the hips. Clin Orthop 261:96-101, 1990.
83. Bos CFA, Bloem JL, Verbout AJ: Magnetic resonance imaging in acetabular residual dysplasia. Clin Orthop 265:207-217, 1991.
84. Fletcher BD, Hanna SL, Fairclough DL, Gronemeyer SA: Pediatric musculoskeletal tumors: use of dynamic, contrast-enhanced MR imaging to monitor response to chemotherapy. Radiology 184:243-248, 1992.
85. Berquist TH: Magnetic resonance imaging of primary skeletal neoplasms. Radiol Clin North Am 31:411-424, 1993.
86. Bloem JL, Taminiau AHM, Eulderink F, et al: Radiologic staging of primary bone sarcoma: MR imaging, scintigraphy, angiography, and CT correlated with pathologic examination. Radiology 169:805-810, 1988.
87. Golfieri R, Baddeley H, Pringle JS, et al: Primary bone tumors. MR morphologic appearance correlated with pathologic examinations. Acta Radiol 32:290-298, 1991.
88. Hanna SL, Fletcher BD, Parham DM, Bugg MF: Muscle edema in musculoskeletal tumors: MR imaging characteristics and clinical significance. J Magn Reson Imaging 1:441-449, 1991.
89. Holscher HC, Bloem JL, Nooy MA, et al: The value of MR imaging in monitoring the effect of chemotherapy on bone sarcomas. Am J Roentgenol 154:763-769, 1990.
90. Kransdorf MJ, Jelinek JS, Moser RP: Imaging of soft tissue tumors. Radiol Clin North Am 31:359-372, 1993.
91. Panuel M, Gentet JC, Scheiner C, et al: Physeal and epiphyseal extent of primary malignant bone tumors in childhood. Correlation of preoperative MRI and the pathologic examination. Pediatr Radiol 22:433-438, 1993.
92. Reuther G, Mutschler W: Detection of local recurrent disease in musculoskeletal tumors: magnetic resonance imaging versus computed tomography. Skeletal Radiol 19:85-90, 1990.
93. Vade A, Eisenstadt R, Schaff HB: MRI of aggressive bone lesions of childhood. Magn Reson Imaging 10:89-96, 1992.
94. Bonnerot V, Charpentier A, Frouin F, et al: Factor analysis of dynamic magnetic resonance imaging in predicting the response of osteosarcoma to chemotherapy. Invest Radiol 27:847-855, 1992.
95. Boyko OB, Cory DA, Cohen MD, et al: MR imaging of osteogenic and Ewing's sarcoma. Am J Roentgenol 148:317-322, 1987.
96. de Baere T, Vanel D, Shapeero LG, et al: Osteosarcoma after chemotherapy: evaluation with contrast material-enhanced subtraction MR imaging. Radiology 185:587-592, 1992.
97. Gillespy T III, Manfrini M, Ruggieri P, et al: Staging of intraosseous extent of osteosarcoma: correlation of preoperative CT and MR imaging with pathologic macroslides. Radiology 167:765-767, 1988.
98. Hanna SL, Parham DM, Fairclough DL, et al: Assessment of osteosarcoma response to preoperative chemotherapy using dynamic FLASH gadolinium-DTPA-enhanced magnetic resonance mapping. Invest Radiol 27:368-373, 1992.
99. Hanna SL, Reddick WE, Parham DM, et al: Automated pixel-by-pixel mapping of dynamic contrast-enhanced MR images for evaluation of osteosarcoma response to chemotherapy: preliminary results. J Magn Reson Imaging 3:849-853, 1993.
100. Lawrence JA, Babyn PS, Chan HS, et al: Extremity osteosarcoma in childhood: prognostic value of radiologic imaging. Radiology 189:43-47, 1993.
101. Pan G, Raymond AK, Carrasco CH, et al: Osteosarcoma: MR imaging after preoperative chemotherapy. Radiology 174:517-526, 1990.
102. Redmond OM, Stack JP, Dervan PA, et al: Osteosarcoma: use of MR imaging and MR spectroscopy in clinical decision making. Radiology 172:811-815, 1989.
103. Shramek JK, Kassner EG, White SS: MR appearance of osteogenic sarcoma of the calvaria. Am J Roentgenol 158:661-662, 1992.
104. Dunne Eggli K, Quiogue T, Moser RP: Ewing's sarcoma. Radiol Clin North Am 31:325-337, 1993.
105. Frouge C, Vanel D, Coffre C, et al: The role of magnetic resonance imaging in the evaluation of Ewing sarcoma. Skeletal Radiol 17:387-392, 1988.
106. Lemmi MA, Fletcher BD, Marina NM, et al: Use of MR imaging to assess results of chemotherapy for Ewing sarcoma. Am J Roentgenol 155:343-346, 1990.
107. MacVicar AD, Olliff JF, Pringle J, et al: Ewing sarcoma: MR imaging of chemotherapy-induced changes with histologic correlation. Radiology 184:859-864, 1992.

108. Benz-Bohm G, Gross-Fengels W, Bohndorf K, et al: MRI of the knee region in leukemic children. Part II. Follow up: responder, non-responder, relapse. Pediatr Radiol 20:272-276, 1990.

109. Bohndorf K, Benz-Bohm G, Gross-Fengels W, Berthold F: MRI of the knee region in leukemic children. Part I. Initial pattern in patients with untreated disease. Pediatr Radiol 20:179-183, 1990.

110. Moore SG, Gooding CA, Brasch RC, et al: Bone marrow in children with acute lymphocytic leukemia: MR relaxation times. Radiology 160:237-240, 1986.

111. Couanet D, Geoffray A, Hartmann O, et al: Bone marrow metastases in children's neuroblastoma studied by magnetic resonance imaging. Adv Neuroblastoma Res 2:547-555, 1988.

112. Shapeero LG, Couanet D, Vanel D, et al: Bone metastases as the presenting manifestation of rhabdomyosarcoma in childhood. Skeletal Radiol 22:433-438, 1993.

113. Hanna SL, Langston JW, Gronemeyer SA, Fletcher BD: Subtraction technique for contrast-enhanced MR images of musculoskeletal tumors. Magn Reson Imaging 8:213-215, 1990.

114. Buetow PC, Kransdorf MJ, Moser RP, et al: Radiologic appearance of intra-muscular hemangioma with emphasis on MR imaging. Am J Roentgenol 154:563-567, 1990.

115. Cohen EK, Kressel HY, Perosio T, et al: MR imaging of soft-tissue hemangiomas: correlation with pathologic findings. Am J Roentgenol 150:1079-1081, 1988.

116. Hawnaur JM, Whitehouse RW, Jenkins JP, Isherwood I: Musculoskeletal haemangiomas: comparison of MRI with CT. Skeletal Radiol 19:251-258, 1990.

117. Kaplan PA, Williams SM: Mucocutaneous and peripheral soft-tissue hemangiomas: MR imaging. Radiology 163:163-166, 1987.

118. Meyer JS, Hoffer FA, Barnes PD, Muliken JB: Biological classification of soft-tissue vascular anomalies: MR correlation. Am J Roentgenol 157:559-564, 1991.

119. Nelson MC, Stull MA, Teitelbaum GP, et al: Magnetic resonance imaging of peripheral soft tissue hemangiomas. Skeletal Radiol 19:477-482, 1990.

120. Yuh WTC, Kathol MH, Sein MA, et al: Hemangiomas of skeletal muscle: MR findings in five patients. Am J Roentgenol 149:765-768, 1987.

121. Laor T: MR imaging of soft tissue tumors and tumor-like lesions. Pediatr Radiol 34: 24-37, 2004.

122. Conway WF, Hayes CW: Miscellaneous lesions of bone. Radiol Clin North Am 31:339-358, 1993.

123. Munk PL, Helms CA, Holt GA, et al: MR imaging of aneurysmal bone cysts. Am J Roentgenol 153:99-101, 1989.

124. Kransdorf MJ, Jelinek JS, Moser RP, et al: Magnetic resonance appearance of fibromatosis. A report of 14 cases and review of the literature. Skeletal Radiol 19:495-499, 1990.

125. Liu P, Thorher P: MRI of fibromatosis: with pathologic correlation. Pediatr Radiol 22:587-589, 1992.

126. Jaffe HL: "Osteoid osteoma," benign osteoblastic tumor composed of osteoid and atypical bone. Arch Surg 31:709-728, 1935.

127. Glass RBJ, Poznanski AK, Fisher MR, et al: MR imaging of osteoid osteoma. J Comput Assist Tomogr 10:1065-1067, 1986.

128. Cohen MD, Klatte EC, Bachner R, et al: Magnetic resonance imaging of bone marrow disease in children. Radiology 151:715-718, 1984.

129. Kangarloo H, Dietrich RB, Taira RT, et al: MR imaging of bone marrow in children. J Comput Assist Tomogr 10:205-209, 1986.

130. Steiner RM, Mitchell DG, Rao VM, Schweitzer ME: Magnetic resonance imaging of diffuse bone marrow disease. Radiol Clin North Am 31:383-409, 1993.

131. Vogler JB, Murphy WA: Bone marrow imaging. Radiology 168:679-693, 1988.

132. Kricun ME: Red-yellow marrow conversion: its effect on the location of some solitary bone lesions. Skeletal Radiol 14:10-19, 1985.

133. Moore SG, Dawson KL: Red and yellow marrow in the femur: age-related changes in appearance at MR imaging. Radiology 175:219-223, 1990.

134. Waitches G, Zawin JK, Poznanski AK: Sequence and rate of bone marrow conversion in the femora of children as seen on MR imaging: are accepted standards accurate? Am J Roentgenol 162:1399-1406, 1994.

135. Rao VM, Fishman M, Mitchell DG, et al: Painful sickle cell crisis: bone marrow patterns observed with MR imaging. Radiology 161:211-215, 1986.

136. Sebes JI: Diagnostic imaging of bone and joint abnormalities associated with sickle cell hemoglobinopathies. Am J Roentgenol 152:1153-1159, 1989.

137. Cremin BJ, Davey H, Goldglatt J: Skeletal complications of type I Gaucher disease: the magnetic resonance features. Clin Radiol 41:244-247, 1990.

138. Lanir A, Hadar H, Cohen I, et al: Gaucher disease: assessment with MR imaging. Radiology 161:239-244, 1986.

139. Rosenthal DI, Scott JA, Barranger J, et al: Evaluation of Gaucher disease using magnetic resonance imaging. J Bone Joint Surg Am 68:802-808, 1986.

140. Horev G, Kornreich L, Hadar H, Katz K: Hemorrhage associated with "bone crisis" in Gaucher's disease identified by magnetic resonance imaging. Skeletal Radiol 20:479-482, 1991.

141. Bohrer SP: Bone changes in the extremities in sickle cell anemia. Semin Roentgenol 22:176-185, 1987.

142. Damry N, Schurmans T, Perlmutter N: MRI evaluation and follow-up of bone necrosis after meningococcal infection and disseminated intravascular coagulation. Pediatr Radiol 23:429-431, 1993.

143. Genez BM, Wilson MR, Houk RW, et al: Early osteonecrosis of the femoral head: detection in high-risk patients with MR imaging. Radiology 168:521-524, 1988.

144. Pieters R, Brenk AI, Veerman JP, et al: Bone marrow magnetic resonance studies in childhood leukemia. Evaluation of osteonecrosis. Cancer 60:2994-3000, 1987.

145. Mascarin M, Giavitto M, Zanazzo GA, et al: Avascular necrosis of bone in children undergoing allogeneic bone marrow transplantation. Cancer 68:655-659, 1991.

146. Chang CC, Grenspan A, Gershwin ME: Osteonecrosis: current perspective on pathogenesis and treatment. Semin Arthritis Rheum 23:47-69, 1993.

147. Totty WG, Murphy WA, Ganz WI, et al: Magnetic resonance imaging of the normal and ischemic femoral head. Am J Roentgenol 143:1273-1280, 1984.

148. Baker DJ, Hall AJ: The epidemiology of Perthes' disease. Clin Orthop 209: 89, 1986.

149. Bluemm RG, Falke THM, Ziedses des Plantes BG, Steiner RM: Early Legg-Perthes disease (ischemic necrosis of the femoral head) demonstrated by magnetic resonance imaging. Skeletal Radiol 14:95-98, 1985.

150. Egund N, Wingstrand H: Legg-Calvé-Perthes disease: imaging with MR. Radiology 179:89-92, 1991.

151. Henderson RC, Renner JB, Sturdivant MC, Greene WB: Evaluation of magnetic resonance imaging in Legg-Perthes disease: a prospective, blinded study. J Pediatr Orthop 10:289-297, 1990.

152. Toby EB, Koman LA, Bechtold RE: Magnetic resonance imaging of pediatric hip disease. J Pediatr Orthop 5:665-671, 1985.

153. Rush BH, Bramson RT, Ogden JA: Legg-Calvé-Perthes disease: detection of cartilaginous and synovial changes with MR imaging. Radiology 167:473-476, 1988.

154. Jaramillo D, Galen TA, Winalski CS, et al: Legg-Calvé-Perthes disease: MR imaging imaging evaluation during manual positioning of the hip—comparison with conventional arthrography. Radiology 1999; 212:519-525.

155. Pay NT, Singer WS, Bartal E: Hip pain in three children accompanied by transient abnormal findings on MR images. Radiology 171:147-149, 1989.

156. Hanna SL, Fletcher BD, Fairclough DL, Jenkins JH: Magnetic resonance imaging of disseminated bone marrow disease in patients treated for malignancy. Skeletal Radiol 20:79-84, 1991.

157. Fletcher BD, Wall JE, Hanna SL: Effect of hematopoietic growth factors on MR images of bone marrow in children undergoing chemotherapy. Radiology 189:745-751, 1993.

158. Stevens SK, Moore SG, Amylon MD: Repopulation of marrow after transplantation: MR imaging with pathologic correlation. Radiology 175:213-218, 1990.

159. Kauczor HU, Brix G, Dietl B, et al: Bone marrow after autologous blood stem cell transplantation and total body irradiation: magnetic resonance and chemical shift imaging. Magn Reson Imaging 11:965-975, 1993.

160. Conway JJ, Cowell HR: Tarsal coalition: clinical significance and roentgenographic demonstration. Radiology 92:799-811, 1969.

161. Lateur LM, Van Hoe LR, Van Ghillewe KV, et al: Subtalar coalition: diagnosis with the C sign on lateral radiographs of the ankle. Radiology 193:847-851, 1994.

162. Newman JS, Newberg AH: Congenital tarsal coalition: multimodality evaluation with emphasis on CT and MR imaging. Radiographics 20: 321-332, 2000.

163. Emery KH, Bisset GS 3rd, Johnson ND, Nunan PJ: Tarsal coalition: a blinded comparison of MRI and CT. Pediatr Radiol 28:612-616, 1998.

CHAPTER 111

SYNOVIUM

Christine B. Chung ● Neeraj J. Panchal

INTRODUCTION

Synovial membranes line the diarthrodial (movable) joints, bursae, and tendon sheaths of the body. The complex structure of this specialized, vascular tissue parallels its complex function, acting as a filter system that lubricates and nourishes the articular structures as well as serving as a shock absorber. The synovium is affected by a variety of disorders that can be localized to a specific articulation, or can be systemic in nature. These include inflammatory, infectious, degenerative, traumatic, and neoplastic categories of disease (Box 111-1).

The advent of magnetic resonance (MR) imaging, with its excellent soft-tissue contrast and multiplanar imaging capabilities, not only revolutionized the diagnostic capabilities within the musculoskeletal system in general, but provided a noninvasive means to study the anatomy and pathology in delicate structures such as the synovium. This chapter begins with a review of the general anatomy of the synovium that serves as a foundation for understanding both optimization of imaging protocols as well as pathologic processes affecting this tissue.

SYNOVIAL ANATOMY

Synovial joints are surrounded by an envelope of tissue comprised of two layers: a more superficial thick fibrous capsule and a more delicate inner layer, the synovial membrane. The fibrous capsule serves to stabilize the articulation, binding together apposing osseous structures, while the synovial membrane lines the intra-articular structures including ligaments, tendons, and intracapsular periosteal surfaces not covered by cartilage. The latter are termed the bare or unprotected

portions of the joint, due to the vulnerability of the periosteum to synovial disease processes.

Normal synovium is comprised of two layers: the synovial intima and subsynovial tissue. The synovial intima is formed by a layer of synovial cells, loosely connected, one to four cells thick. The subsynovial tissue

---

Box III-I | Synovial Disorders

General Synovial Abnormalities
Effusion
Hemarthrosis
Lipohemarthrosis
Intra-articular bodies
Synovial and ganglion cysts
Synovitis
Bursitis

Specific Synovial Abnormalities
Synovial Inflammatory Disorders
Infectious
Noninfectious
　　Rheumatologic disorders
　　Post-traumatic synovitis

Hematopoietic Disorders
Hemophilia

Tumors and Tumor-like Disorders
Pigmented villonodular synovitis
Localized nodular synovitis
Idiopathic synovial osteochondromatosis
Idiopathic lipoma arborescens
Intracapsular chondroma
Synovial chondrosarcoma
Synovial hemangioma
Amyloidosis

varies in structure depending on its location (articular, bursal, tenosynovial, etc.) and may be fibrous, areolar, fibroareolar, areolar-adipose, or adipose in character.[1] The subsynovium contains a vascular and lymphatic network, with the majority of synovial capillaries intimately associated with the synovial intima. It is through this capillary network that fluid enters an articulation as an ultrafiltrate of plasma. As this fluid passes through the leaky endothelium of the capillaries in the subsynovium, into the synovial intima en route to the articulation, synovial cells add molecules such as hyaluronic acid that, in combination with the plasma, form joint fluid as we know it. As there is no basement membrane to act as a barrier between blood vessels and joint space, joint fluid can be considered an extension of the extracellular fluid space.[1] In normal joints, there appears to be an outward flux of fluid from the vascular bed into the joint, while absorption of joint fluid occurs primarily through the lymphatic vessels.[1]

MR IMAGING CONSIDERATIONS

While it is widely accepted that MR imaging has revolutionized the ability to visualize and characterize delicate soft-tissue structures such as the synovium, debate still exists regarding the optimal imaging technique for its evaluation. Much of this debate stems from the difficulty in establishing the imaging characteristics of normal synovium, including enhancement patterns after the intravenous (IV) administration of contrast material.

The normal synovial membrane in conjunction with the fibrous joint capsule can be seen as a thin, low-signal-intensity linear structure on MR imaging. The few studies that document the imaging appearance of the synovium in an asymptomatic patient population report discrepant results with regard to the presence and degree of synovial enhancement after IV contrast administration.[1-7] In a study by Boegard et al, designed to evaluate the occurrence and extent of enhancement of synovial structures after the IV administration of a gadolinium-based contrast material in the knee joints of middle-aged, healthy, asymptomatic individuals, synovial enhancement was present in each articulation.[2] Moreover, the thickness of synovial structures within these asymptomatic articulations showed significant variability with the exception of the suprapatellar recess, in which synovial thickness was constant and minimal. This study emphasizes the difficulty in identifying a gold standard in synovial assessment and establishes that synovial enhancement can occur in the asymptomatic articulation.

In the setting of acute synovial inflammatory processes, the majority of studies contend that MR imaging in conjunction with the IV administration of gadolinium-based contrast material is beneficial in distinguishing synovial proliferation from adjacent joint fluid as both appear low in signal intensity on T1-weighted and high in signal intensity on T2-weighted, unenhanced images.[3-14] Some authors have argued against the usefulness of contrast-enhanced imaging for synovial evaluation, noting that the exact border between effusion and synovium can also be difficult to distinguish after the IV administration of contrast. This is due to the diffusion of contrast material into the joint over time, resulting in enhancement of the effusion.[1,10] It appears, however, that the signal intensity of inflamed synovial tissue on T1-weighted MR images increases markedly within the first minute after IV administration of contrast.[10,15,16] On the contrary, the rate of signal increase in effusion is slower, beginning in the periphery where contrast material diffuses into the joint space from the synovium and reaching maximum signal intensity 15 minutes after IV injection.[1] Based on the temporal relationship of synovial versus effusion enhancement, volumes of both joint fluid and synovium can be determined in a reasonably accurate fashion with a maximal analytic error of 20%.[10,11,17]

MR imaging in conjunction with the IV administration of gadolinium-based contrast material has also proven helpful in characterizing disease activity in synovial inflammation. As synovial inflammation becomes inactive, a gradual decrease in vascularization occurs with transformation to fibrous tissue.[3]

Although the use of IV contrast administration in conjunction with MR imaging portrays the synovium to best advantage, the synovium can certainly be assessed with standard MR imaging sequences. Several investigators have described areas of synovial thickening to have intermediate to high signal intensity on proton density– or T1-weighted images as compared to adjacent joint fluid.[4,8,14,18] Morphologic changes in the synovium can also be detected on T2-weighted images in inflamed synovium, appearing as frondlike densities or irregular thickening.

GENERAL SYNOVIAL ABNORMALITIES

Effusion

The imaging diagnosis of an effusion exists when a synovial articulation contains more than a physiologic amount of fluid. Although quantitative guidelines for some joints have been published, measurements are rarely used to determine the presence of effusion.[19] Fluid distribution within articulations is joint specific and requires familiarity with capsular anatomy. When an effusion represents increased production of synovial fluid, the signal characteristics will reflect those of normal joint fluid on MR imaging, intermediate signal intensity on T1-weighted images, and high signal intensity on fluid-sensitive imaging sequences. The imaging characteristics of joint fluid after the IV administration of gadolinium-based contrast material, as previously discussed, depend largely on the temporal relationship of injection and imaging.

It is unusual for an effusion to be the only abnormal finding on an MR imaging study. Most effusions are the result of traumatic, degenerative, inflammatory, and less commonly neoplastic disorders. The presence of joint effusion warrants a careful search of the MR imaging

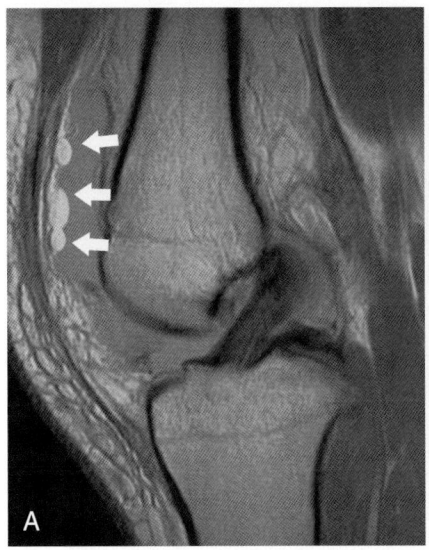 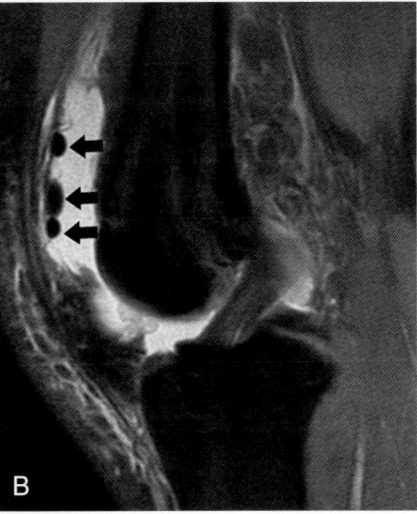

FIGURE III-I

Lipohemarthrosis. **A,** Proton density–weighted sagittal MR image of the knee in a patient presenting with a patellar dislocation shows lobular foci of high signal intensity *(arrows)* within a suprapatellar joint effusion. **B,** The corresponding T2-weighted fat-suppressed sagittal MR image shows low signal intensity within the lobules *(arrows)* consistent with complete fat suppression.

study for underlying pathology. Some studies suggest that the mere presence of joint effusion is a reflection of synovitis, and have positively correlated synovial membrane volume, effusion volume, and clinical signs of inflammation.[10,20]

Hemarthrosis

The detection of intra-articular blood requires careful clinical and radiographic examination. This is particularly important in the setting of trauma in order to exclude occult fracture or ligamentous injury. It has been suggested that trauma may lead to increased vascular permeability as well as disruption of blood vessels, both of which could contribute to a post-traumatic hemarthrosis.[21] Alternatively, hemarthrosis may accompany other disorders including hemophilia and other bleeding disorders, pigmented villonodular synovitis, intra-articular neoplasms such as synovial hemangioma, rheumatologic disorders such as gout, neuroarthropathy, and anticoagulant therapy.[22,23]

Recent hemorrhage can result in a layering effect in the effusion, with supernatant fluid floating on cellular debris.[24] Effusions that represent the subacute phase of a hemarthrosis after cell lysis will typically have higher signal intensity than water on T1-weighted images, but will usually remain isointense to fluid on fluid-sensitive sequences. Repeated bleeding into a joint causes the intra-articular deposition of hemosiderin. Hemosiderin-laden tissues will demonstrate low signal intensity on all pulse sequences, and may further demonstrate an apparent increase in size on gradient-recalled images, the so-called "blooming effect." Regardless of the stage of hemarthrosis, the effusion should not enhance in the immediate phase after IV administration of contrast. As in the case of an uncomplicated effusion, however, delayed post-contrast images will show fluid enhancement.[4,8]

Lipohemarthrosis

The presence of fat and blood within a joint cavity—lipohemarthrosis—has long been associated with intra-articular fracture. As noted in the discussion of hemarthrosis, a single fluid-fluid level can be seen with the separation of hemorrhagic fluid into its cellular and serum components. The double fluid-fluid level, however, is a more specific finding suggesting the presence of lipohemarthrosis.[24] This radiographic diagnosis can be challenging due to variations in the anatomy of the suprapatellar joint space.[25] MR imaging, however, facilitates both the identification and characterization of fluid levels, easily denoting the presence of fat signal intensity on T1-weighted images (Fig. 111-1). This issue is somewhat complicated by the evolving stages of lipohemarthrosis related to the stages of formation and lysis of blood clot. The earliest findings of lipohemarthrosis include the presence of several fluid-fluid levels with entrapment of globules of fat. The classic double fluid level can be expected several hours after injury.[26]

Intra-articular bodies

Intra-articular bodies can be detected with MR imaging, where they are optimally visualized with fluid in the joint (Fig. 111-2). In that setting they appear as filling defects within bright fluid on fluid-sensitive sequences. The signal characteristics of the bodies are a reflection of their composition. Cartilaginous bodies have low signal intensity on T1-weighted and fluid-sensitive sequences. Osseous fragments contain marrow and accordingly have high signal intensity on T1-weighted images. Signal characteristics on fluid-sensitive sequences depend on the use of spin-echo versus fast spin-echo imaging, as well as fat-suppression techniques. Mucoid and fibrinoid material is typically ill defined with heterogeneous,

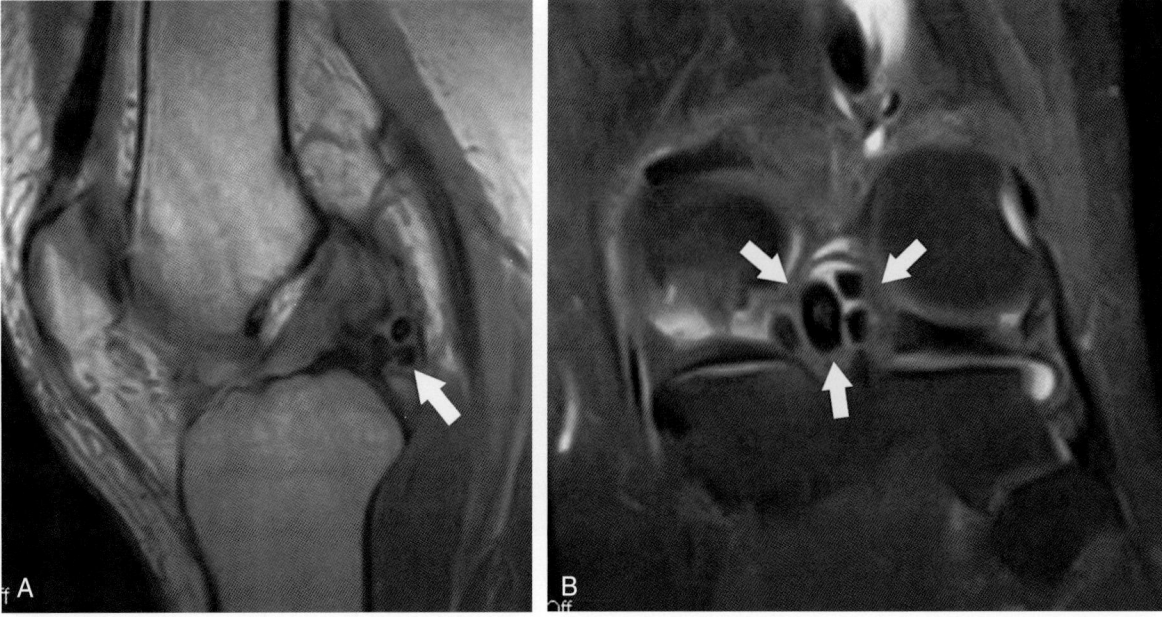

FIGURE III-2

Intraarticular bodies. **A,** Proton density–weighted sagittal MR image of the knee in a patient with a remote history of trauma shows several rounded foci of low signal intensity *(arrow)* in the posterior joint space. **B,** The corresponding proton density–weighted fat-suppressed coronal MR image through the posterior aspect of the knee shows the low-signal-intensity intra-articular bodies *(arrows)* surrounded by minimal joint fluid.

intermediate signal intensity. In the absence of native joint fluid, MR arthrography increases the sensitivity for the detection of intra-articular bodies.[27]

The composition of the intra-articular bodies provides a clue in the determination of their etiology. Severe synovial hyperplasia can lead to the formation of rice bodies, which have been associated with both synovial inflammatory processes such as rheumatoid arthritis and infectious etiologies such as tuberculosis.[28] A combination of synovial hyperplasia and cartilage metaplasia results in the intra-articular bodies associated with synovial osteochondromatosis.[29]

Synovial and Ganglion Cysts

Synovial cysts are fluid-filled masses lined with synovium that are located within or about joints (Fig. 111-3). They can be intraneural, extraneural, or develop between or within muscles.[30] The distinction between synovial cyst and ganglion cyst appears to be made primarily on the basis of the histologic nature of the lining of the cyst and the contents of the cyst, as well as the presence or absence of communication with the joint. Ganglion cysts are lined by spindle-shaped cells rather than synovium and are characterized by myxoid contents.[31] In the case of ganglia, communication with the joint or tendon sheath is considered unusual, though this is a point of debate.[31,32] In the absence of histologic confirmation of the nature of cells lining a para-articular fluid collection, the importance lies not in the nomenclature but in the

detection of any communication between cyst and articulation or tendon sheath, as failure to resect such a communication could result in recurrence of the collection.

As true synovial cysts are, by definition, lined by synovial cells, they manifest disease and are affected by the same disease processes as other synovium-lined structures. They are most commonly encountered about the knee, and occur with synovial inflammatory disorders, rheumatologic and otherwise, as a result of trauma, and in conjunction with osteoarthritis (Fig. 111-4).[33-36] They also occur with relatively high frequency in the asymptomatic, healthy population.[35,36]

Bursitis

A bursa is a synovium-lined space that arises embryologically separate from a joint, typically to provide cushioning between a bony protuberance and the overlying soft-tissues (Fig. 111-5). Some, such as the suprapatellar bursa in the knee or the subscapularis bursa in the shoulder, gain communication with the adjacent joint during development. In the case of the knee, synovial infoldings or plicae can be left behind as the vestiges of once distinct synovial spaces. Secondary bursae, or adventitial bursae, can also be encountered in and around osseous prominences (Fig. 111-6). These bursae are not part of the normal anatomy but form when abnormal friction develops between a bone and soft-tissue. They are always abnormal; the most common

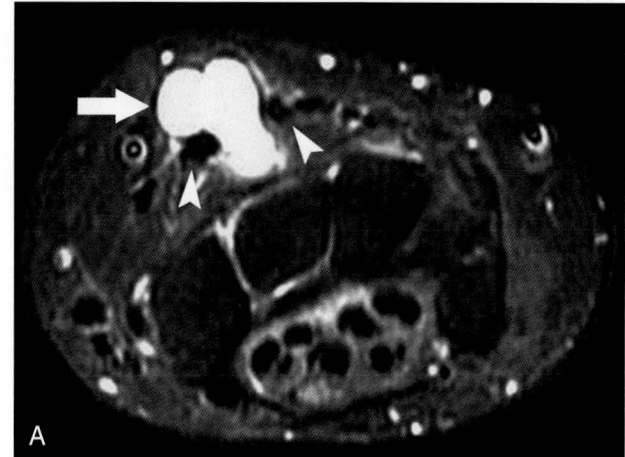

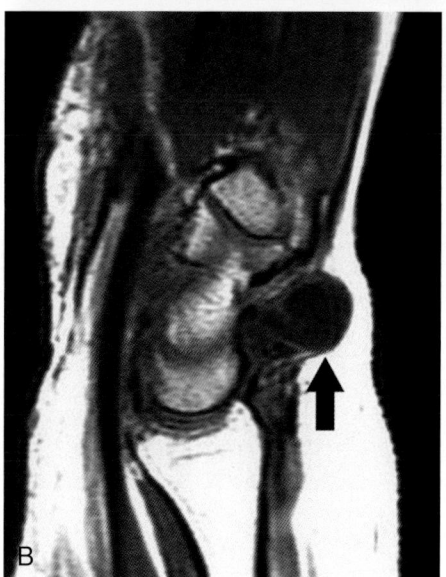

FIGURE III-3

Ganglion cyst. **A,** T2-weighted fat-suppressed axial MR image of the wrist in a patient with a wrist mass shows a polylobulated mass with high signal intensity *(arrow)* extending between the extensor tendons *(arrowheads)*. **B,** The corresponding T1-weighted fat-suppressed sagittal image acquired after IV administration of contrast shows low internal signal intensity with mild peripheral enhancement *(arrow)* consistent with a ganglion cyst.

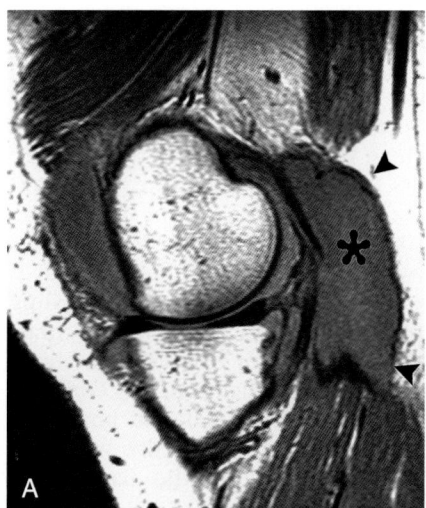
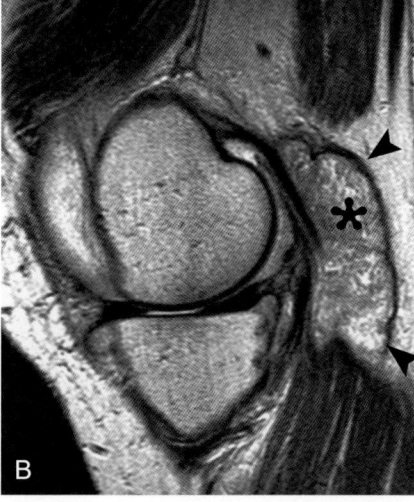

FIGURE III-4

Baker's cyst. **A,** Proton density–weighted sagittal MR image through the medial aspect of the knee shows a Baker's cyst *(arrowheads)* with homogeneous central intermediate signal intensity *(asterisk)*. **B,** The corresponding sagittal T2-weighted fast spin-echo image shows extensive low-signal-intensity debris *(asterisk)* within the inflamed cyst.

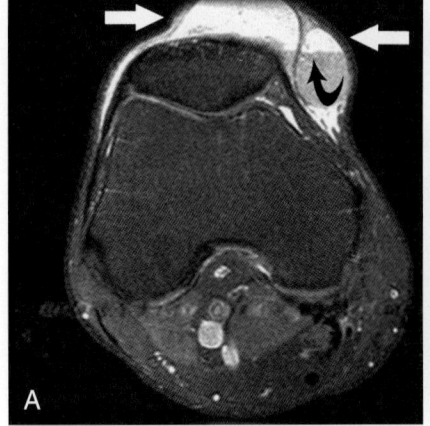
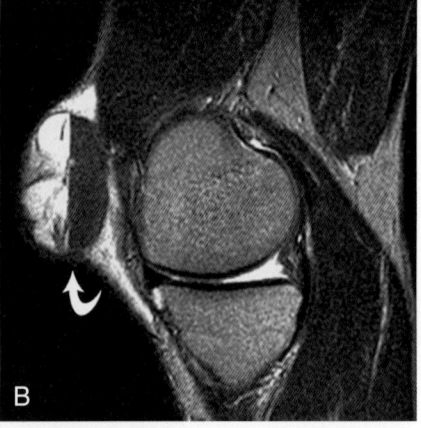

FIGURE III-5

Prepatellar bursitis. **A,** Axial T2-weighted fat-suppressed MR image of the knee in a patient with knee pain and a palpable mass shows a polylobulated mass *(arrows)* with a fluid-fluid level *(curved arrow)*. **B,** The presence of the fluid level *(curved arrow)* was confirmed on the sagittal T2-weighted fat-suppressed MR image and represented a post-traumatic hemorrhagic pre-patellar bursitis.

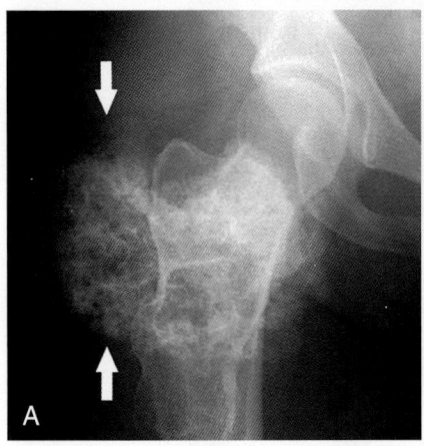
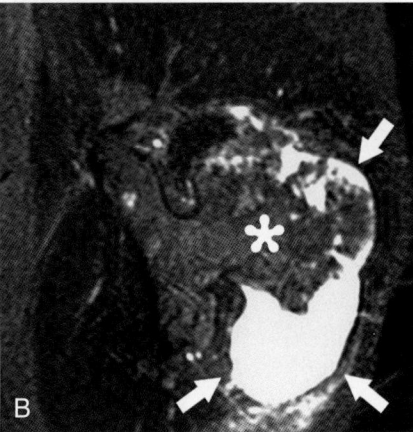

FIGURE III-6

Adventitial bursa. **A,** Oblique radiograph of the hip demonstrates a large osteochondroma projecting from the metadiaphyseal region of the femur *(arrows)*. **B,** Sagittal inversion recovery image through the osteochondroma *(asterisk)* shows the presence of a fluid collection adjacent to the osseous excrescence that represents adventitial bursa formation *(arrows)*.

example is that of the adventitial bursa that forms between the iliotibial band and the lateral femoral condyle in iliotibial band friction syndrome.[37]

As in the case of the synovial cyst, the presence of fluid within a bursa should prompt careful analysis of the surrounding soft-tissues to exclude traumatic soft-tissue abnormalities such as tendon tears.[38] Bursal inflammation has been associated with rheumatologic synovial inflammatory processes such as rheumatoid arthritis and gout, infectious synovial inflammatory processes such as tuberculosis, and trauma (acute or chronic), in which a hemorrhagic component can be seen.[39-41] Bursal distension has also been documented with relatively high frequency in asymptomatic populations.[36]

SPECIFIC SYNOVIAL ABNORMALITIES

Synovial Inflammatory Disorders

Several articular disorders are characterized by inflammation of the synovial membrane. Among these, infection, rheumatologic disorders, and post-traumatic reactive synovitis comprise the disease processes that are commonly encountered and whose accurate diagnosis is crucial to the well-being of the patient. The

aforementioned synovial inflammatory processes share a common pathologic expression that is nonspecific in nature. This includes soft-tissue swelling due to synovial proliferation, periarticular osteopenia due to increased hyperemia in the proliferative synovial tissue, joint space narrowing due to destruction of the articular surface by inflammatory, hypertrophic synovium, and marginal erosion of bone as a result of the proliferation of synovial tissue in the periphery of the joint where bone is not protected by a covering of cartilage.

When applying the strengths of MR imaging to the evaluation of synovial inflammatory disorders, it is clear that this imaging technique allows the creation of a window through which to see the internal architecture of an articulation, its osseous infrastructure as well as supporting soft-tissues. The magnitude of this development should not be underestimated for it represents the difference between detecting the sequelae of a disease process versus the detection of its inciting pathology. With respect to the former, the role of contrast administration in the diagnosis of synovitis has been previously discussed. The application of contrast-enhanced MR imaging attempts to make an important distinction in the diagnosis—that of an active versus an inactive process. This affects not only the diagnosis of disease but also its response to therapy.

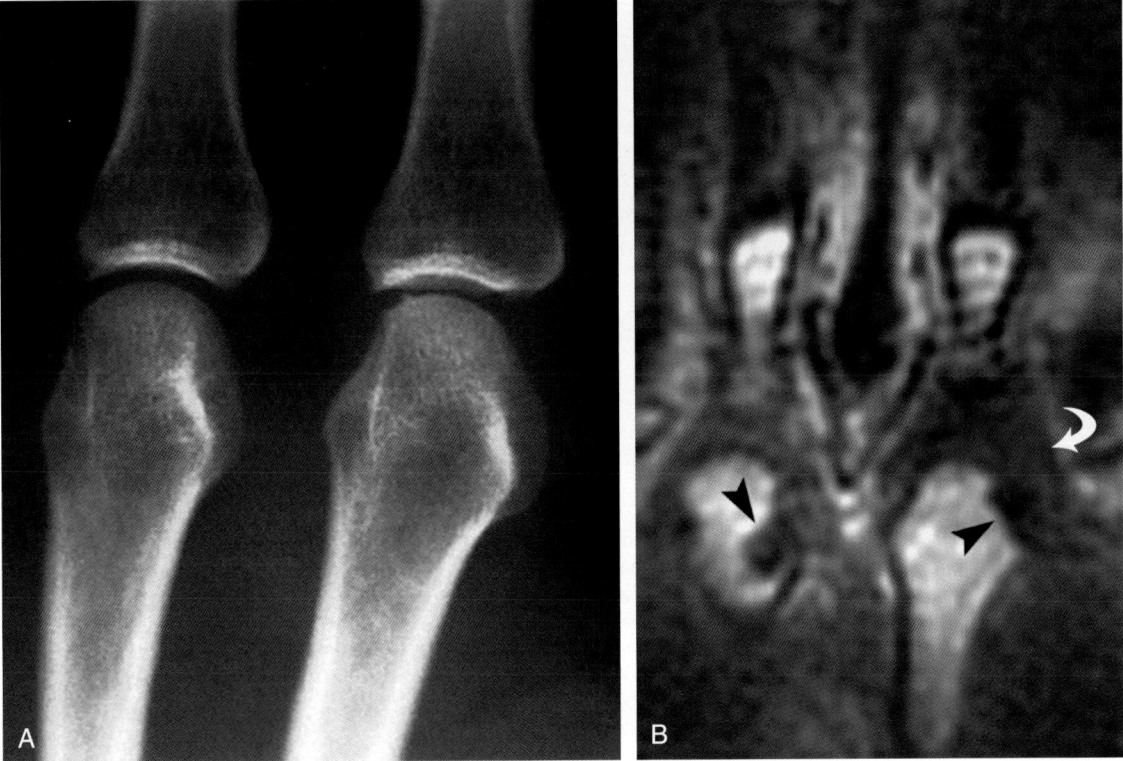

FIGURE III-7

Radiographically occult erosions. **A,** Normal frontal radiograph of the metacarpophalangeal joints in a patient who presented with joint pain. **B,** The corresponding coronal T1-weighted MR image at the time of the radiograph shows erosive change *(arrowheads)* at the margins of the joints as well as synovial proliferation *(curved arrow)*.

Not only can MR imaging aid in the diagnosis and characterization of synovitis, it can also be used to quantitatively assess synovial volume. Two primary techniques are implemented to this end. The first involves a measurement of synovial volume with comparison to a group of normal controls.[42,43] The second technique involves measuring the rate of contrast enhancement of diseased synovium in a series of consecutive and rapidly acquired images. This method results in an enhancement ratio calculated from the values of the signal intensities obtained prior to and at a fixed time after contrast administration.[44] Different rates of enhancement have proven characteristic of different tissues.[15] In addition, decreased rates of enhancement of pannus have been associated with states of remission in rheumatoid arthritis.[44]

Despite the fact that synovitis reflects the causative process in the destruction seen in many synovial inflammatory processes, the detection of bone erosions is important for the determination of disease prognosis and institution of therapy. Numerous studies have established the increased sensitivity of MR imaging compared to that of conventional radiography for the detection of bone erosions (Fig. 111-7).[44-47] MR imaging has been found to allow visualization of bone erosions that are not evident with conventional radiography. Bone erosions are defined as partial or complete loss of the low signal intensity that characterizes cortical bone in both T1-weighted and fluid-sensitive sequences (Fig. 111-8). The erosion can be further characterized as active when there is significant post-contrast enhancement of adjacent bone. Identification of bone erosion in at least two MR imaging planes increases the specificity of the abnormality.[45,48,49]

Finally, bone marrow edema may prove important in the prediction of sites of ultimate erosive change as well as in narrowing the differential diagnosis of synovial inflammatory processes. Bone marrow edema involves no disruption of cortex; rather, it occurs in the trabecular bone within the marrow cavity. Edema is characterized by low signal intensity on T1-weighted images, and high signal intensity on fluid-sensitive sequences. This finding is the result of increased water in the marrow, and may represent the internal osseous response to an external attack by inflamed synovium. Marrow edema occurring early in the course of synovial inflammatory disease has been found to be strongly associated with subsequent bone erosion at the same site and is actually believed to be the strongest individual predictor of the development of such erosions when compared to adjacent synovitis and tenosynovitis. Clearly, however, bone marrow edema and bone erosions are two singular processes that can occur either in an isolated fashion or in tandem. The relationship between the two has yet to be completely elucidated.

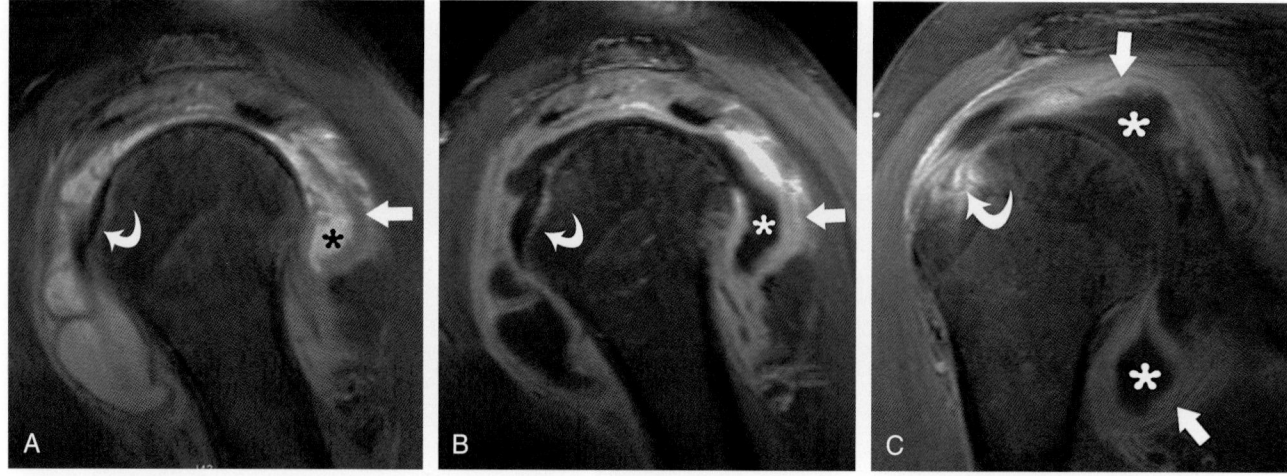

FIGURE 111-8

Septic arthritis. **A,** Sagittal T2-weighted fat-suppressed MR image of the shoulder in a patient with bacterial septic arthritis (anterior noted by the region of the lesser tuberosity, *curved arrow*) shows high signal intensity within the joint (*asterisk*) as well as capsular thickening (*arrow*). **B,** T1-weighted fat-suppressed sagittal MR image of the shoulder obtained after IV administration of gadolinium-based contrast material verifies the presence of low-signal-intensity fluid within the articulation (*asterisk*) as well as synovitis. The latter is manifested by synovial thickening and intense enhancement (*arrow*). **C,** Coronal T1-weighted fat-suppressed post-contrast MR image demonstrates the intra-articular fluid (*asterisk*), synovial thickening and enhancement (*arrows*), and osseous erosion in the greater tuberosity (*curved arrow*). The erosion is characterized by both marrow enhancement and cortical loss.

Infectious Synovitis

The routes of contamination implicated in the development of infectious synovitis include hematogenous spread, spread from a contiguous source, direct implantation, or postoperative infection. The diagnosis of septic arthritis is crucial in that any delay may increase morbidity and lead to complications such as bone and cartilage destruction, osteomyelitis, and ultimately ankylosis. The provenance of the synovitis, infectious or noninfectious, can be challenging and at times impossible to elucidate by imaging. Several small series have shown the MR imaging findings in septic arthritis to be nonspecific, with overlap of findings seen in inflammatory arthropathies.[50-53] There have been unsuccessful attempts to identify criteria that may be indicative of joint infection including changes in the signal intensity of joint effusion and bone marrow edema involving both sides of an articulation (Fig. 111-9).[54,55] A study by Graif et al analyzed the MR imaging signs related to the joint space, synovium, cartilage, bone, and peri-articular soft-tissues in patients with both infectious and noninfectious synovitis. They found the combination of bone erosions with marrow edema to be highly suggestive for septic arthritis (see Fig. 111-8). The coexistence of synovial thickening, synovial edema, and soft-tissue edema or bone marrow enhancement increased the level of confidence for the diagnosis of infectious synovitis. The study concluded, however, that no single imaging finding or combination could be either pathognomonic for, or exclude the presence of, a septic arthritis.[50]

Although the imaging findings of infectious synovitis are nonspecific in nature, variations in disease manifestation can be seen in accordance with the infecting organism. Rapid destruction of bone and cartilage is characteristic of bacterial arthritis, whereas tuberculosis and fungal diseases have a more indolent course. In addition, in tuberculosis, subchondral extension of pannus, masslike intra-articular protrusion of granulation tissue, and fibrous ankylosis predominate.[51,52,56]

The nonspecific nature of imaging findings in infectious synovitis emphasizes the need for precise clinical correlation, laboratory findings, and joint aspiration to make the accurate and timely diagnosis of a septic joint. Any destructive monoarticular process should be regarded as infection until proven otherwise.

Rheumatologic Disorders

Among the disorders that are characterized by synovial inflammation, rheumatoid arthritis and the seronegative spondyloarthropathies (psoriasis, Reiter syndrome, ankylosing spondylitis, inflammatory bowel disease) must be emphasized. In both these disease processes, the predominant target area in the synovial joint is the synovial membrane. The expression of the inflammation in this target tissue is, as previously described, largely nonspecific in nature and includes synovitis, periarticular osteopenia, diffuse loss of joint space, and marginal erosion (Fig. 111-10).

In the case of rheumatoid arthritis, increasing attention has been focused on the use of MR imaging for diagnosis, prognostication, and monitoring of disease progression and response to therapy. It has been suggested that incorporation of MR imaging signs of synovitis into the diagnostic criteria for rheumatoid arthritis would not only increase diagnostic accuracy but lead to a diagnosis earlier in the course of the disease.[13] The MR imaging signs used included periarticular enhancement in the wrist or finger joint.[57,58]

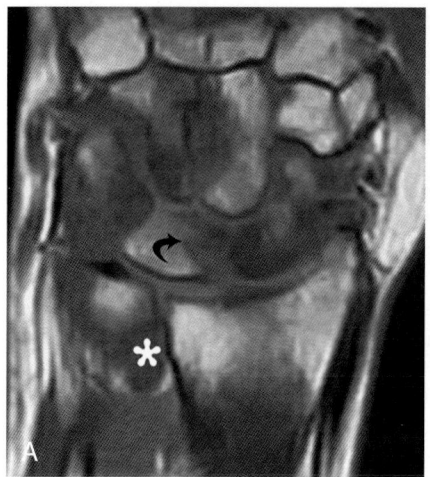
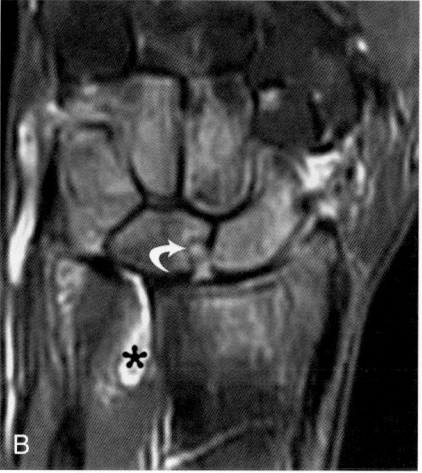
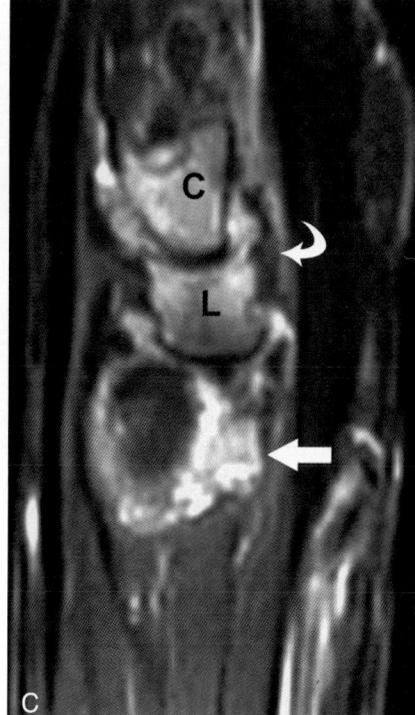

FIGURE III-9

Tuberculous arthritis. **A,** Coronal T1-weighted MR image in a patient with tuberculous arthritis shows patchy bone marrow edema (low signal intensity) throughout the carpus, erosive change on the lunate side of the scapholunate interspace *(curved arrow)*, and synovitis in the distal radioulnar joint *(asterisk)*. **B,** On the T2-weighted image, the bone marrow edema appears bright in signal intensity, as does the erosive change *(curved arrow)* and synovitis *(asterisk)*. **C,** The corresponding T1-weighted fat-suppressed sagittal image acquired after IV administration of contrast shows the low signal intensity of the joint fluid *(curved arrow)* adjacent to the capitate (C) and lunate (L) and enhancing soft-tissue of the active synovial inflammation *(arrow)*.

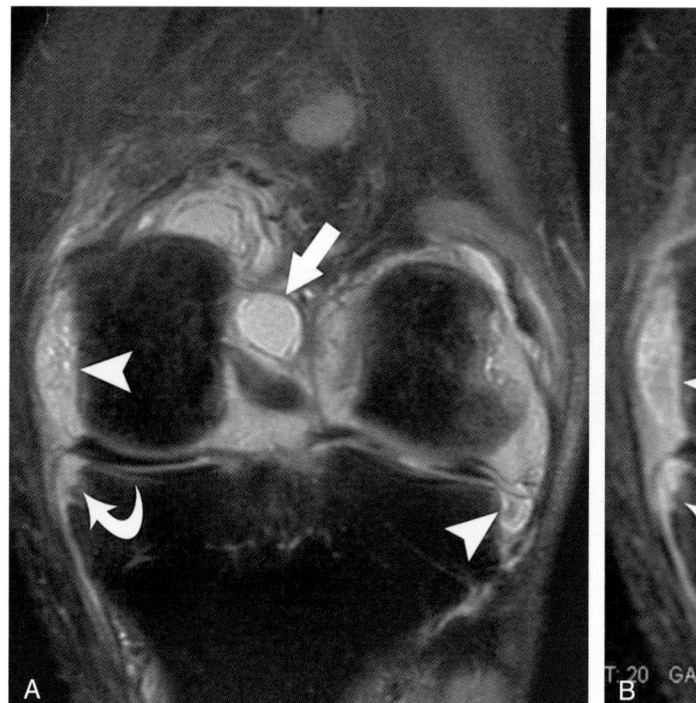
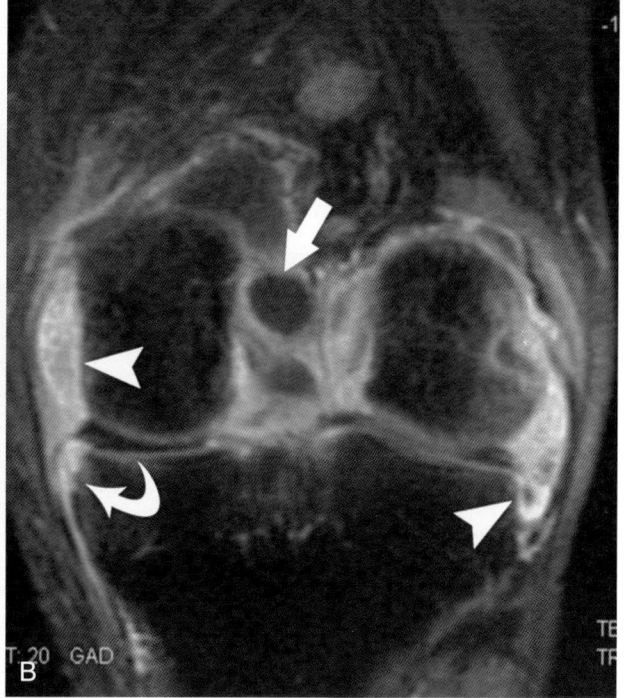

FIGURE III-10

Rheumatoid arthritis. **A,** Coronal T2-weighted fat-suppressed MR image in a patient with rheumatoid arthritis shows areas of high signal intensity, with internal stranding *(arrowheads)* surrounding the articulation. Marginal cortical irregularity is noted at the medial tibial plateau *(curved arrow)*, as well as high signal intensity in the region of the posterior cruciate ligament *(arrow)*. **B,** Coronal T1-weighted fat-suppressed MR image obtained after IV administration of contrast material shows diffuse enhancement of the material surrounding the articulation *(arrowheads)*, consistent with synovial inflammation and hypertrophy. On the post-contrast image, the uncomplicated joint fluid adjacent to the posterior cruciate ligament demonstrates low signal intensity.

As previously discussed, MR imaging has proven useful in the detection and characterization of synovial hypertrophy, the quantification of synovial hypertrophy, and the detection of both bone marrow edema and osseous erosion (Fig. 111-11). In the case of rheumatoid arthritis, MR imaging can also be used to evaluate clinical problems derived from local extra-articular involvement such as tenosynovitis, "rice-bodies" bursitis, and Baker's cyst rupture. Tendinous rupture, osteonecrosis, and stress fracture (complications of rheumatoid arthritis) can be evaluated by MR imaging.[59]

Although the seronegative spondyloarthropathies share with rheumatoid arthritis nonspecific synovitis as the hallmark of disease in the appendicular skeleton, the degree of inflammatory change is of less intensity. Therefore, periarticular osteopenia is less common, as is the extent of osseous erosion, when compared with rheumatoid arthritis. While synovitis and erosions are considered the hallmarks of inflammatory arthritis, the finding of marrow edema may prove to be the most promising imaging finding for narrowing the differential

diagnoses for synovial inflammatory processes. In contradistinction to rheumatoid arthritis, the seronegative spondyloarthropathies have a proclivity to osseous fusion of synovial joints, perhaps related to enthesopathy at capsuloligamentous attachments. The work of McGonagle et al has implied that the distribution of marrow edema may prove helpful in distinguishing between the seronegative spondyloarthropathies and rheumatoid arthritis. These investigators demonstrated a perientheseal distribution of marrow edema in a cohort of patients who presented with a recent onset of knee effusion, while this pattern was not seen in rheumatoid patients.[60]

Calcium pyrophosphate dihydrate crystal deposition disease is a rheumatologic disease initially characterized by the occurrence of intermittent episodes of synovial inflammation, the so-called "pseudo-gout" attacks. Over time, several categories of clinical expression of the disease have emerged including intermittent, episodic bouts of synovial inflammation, chronic, indolent joint degeneration with joint-specific distribution patterns, and

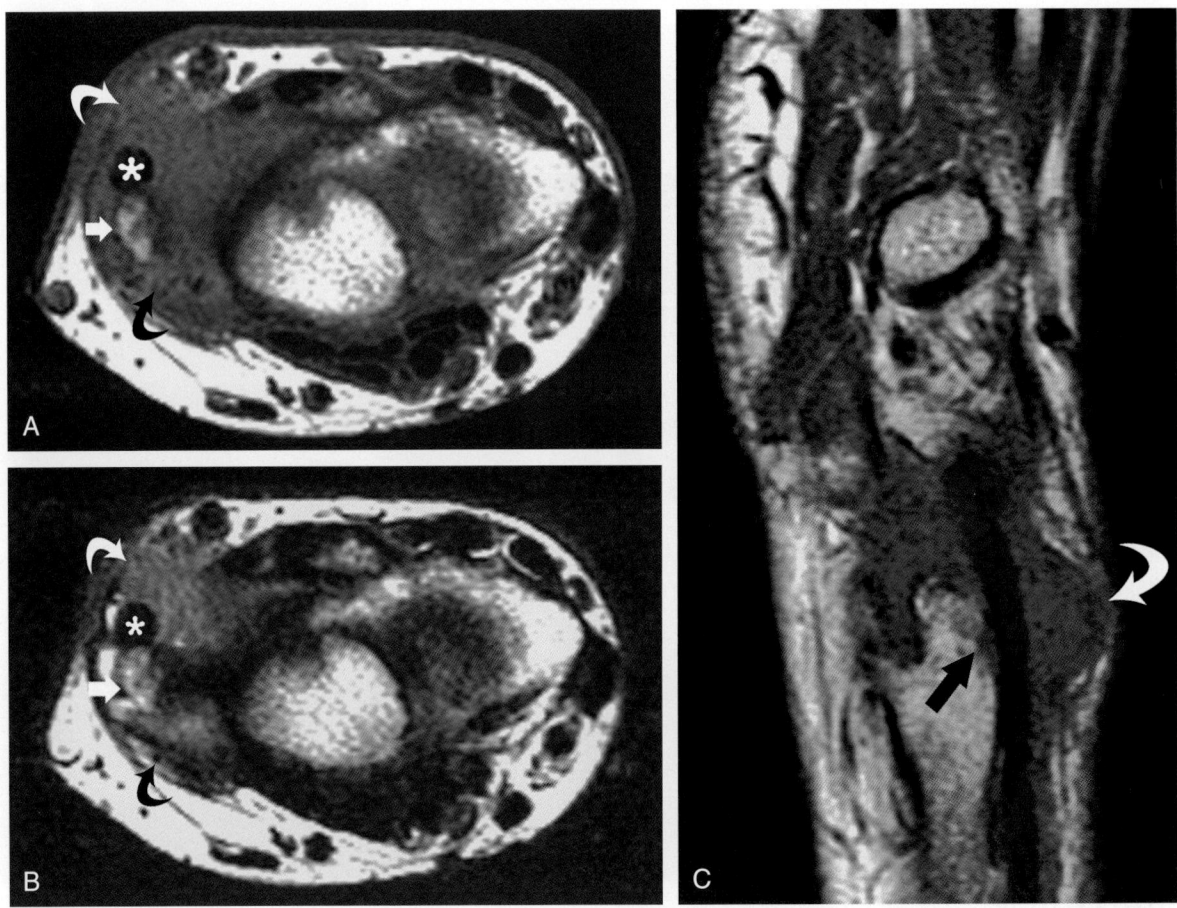

FIGURE III-II

Synovitis. **A,** Axial T1-weighted image through the wrist shows soft-tissue proliferation of intermediate signal intensity consistent with synovial inflammation (*curved arrows*) around the ulnar styloid (*arrow*) and extensor carpi ulnaris (*asterisk*) tendon. **B,** The corresponding T2-weighted fast spin-echo axial image identifies the intermediate to low signal intensity character of the synovial proliferation (*curved arrows*) around the ulnar styloid (*arrow*) and extensor carpi ulnaris tendon (*asterisk*) suggesting its quiescent nature. **C,** Sagittal T1-weighted image through the ulna shows the soft-tissue component of the synovitis (*curved arrow*) as well as an osseous erosion (*arrow*).

asymptomatic disease. The general radiographic features of calcium pyrophosphate dihydrate crystal deposition disease include calcification of articular and periarticular structures and pyrophosphate arthropathy. While a predominance of subchondral cysts can be encountered in this disease process, erosive changes are not characteristic. During acute attacks, the MR imaging findings are simply those of a nonspecific synovial inflammation. In some cases, calcium pyrophosphate dihydrate crystal accumulation can lead to masses of low signal intensity on both T1-weighted and fluid-sensitive sequences. Variable enhancement is seen after the IV administration of contrast material. When calcifications occur in intra-articular soft-tissues such as hyaline cartilage, meniscus, labrum, or ligamentous structures, they can be easily overlooked on MR imaging as they are low in signal intensity on all sequences as is the tissue in which they reside.[61] In some cases in the meniscus of the knee, however, regions of crystal deposition may produce intermediate signal intensity that can simulate meniscal pathology.[62]

Calcification within periarticular soft-tissues and tendons associated with pain is a commonly encountered entity. The calcifications are often comprised of calcium hydroxyapatite crystals.[63] The deposition of calcium hydroxyapatite appears to follow a sequence described by clinical symptoms, precise location of calcification, and the response of surrounding structures to the calcification.[63,64] Although soft-tissue calcification is often perceived to be static, it is, indeed, dynamic in nature. The consistency of the calcification may range from liquid to a dense, solid form. The size may change

with resorption or growth over time. The location may change, with migration from tendon to a periarticular, intra-articular, or intraosseous location. The calcification may be inert, or incite an intense inflammatory response in tendon sheath, bursa, or articular structures, in some cases even resulting in erosion of bone and bone marrow edema.[64,65] On MR imaging, the calcification will appear low signal intensity on all imaging sequences. The synovitis provoked by this disease process is nonspecific in nature and can involve tendon sheaths, bursae, or articular synovium (Fig. 111-12).

Gout is a rheumatologic disorder resulting from a metabolic imbalance characterized by episodic attacks of synovial inflammation with the development of characteristic erosive changes, as well as articular and periarticular soft-tissue calcifications. MR imaging is not routinely used for the evaluation of gout; however, this disease process has been referred to as "the great deceiver" in that it can mimic infection or neoplasm. Manifestations of gout occur in three clinical stages: acute, intercritical (interval phase between attacks), and chronic tophaceous gout. In an acute attack, the MR imaging findings are those of nonspecific synovitis. With repeated attacks, the development of erosive changes with the classic morphology of the overhanging edge occurs in conjunction with soft-tissue calcification (Fig. 111-13). Studies have shown that tophi show predictable low signal intensity on T1-weighted images, but heterogeneous signal intensity on fluid-sensitive sequences (Fig. 111-14).[66-68] There is variable enhancement in the tophus after the IV administration of contrast material.

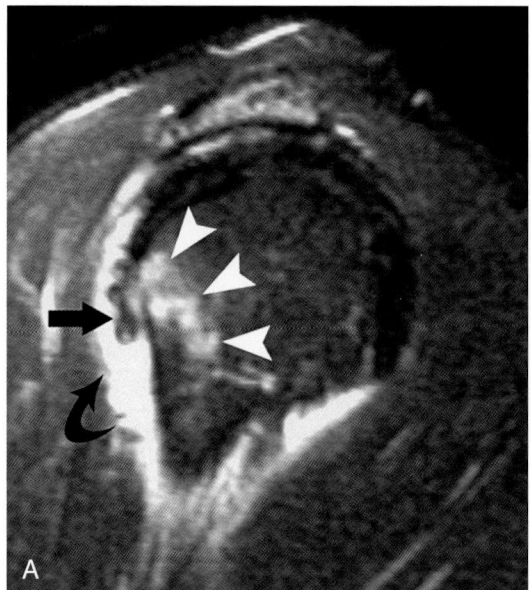
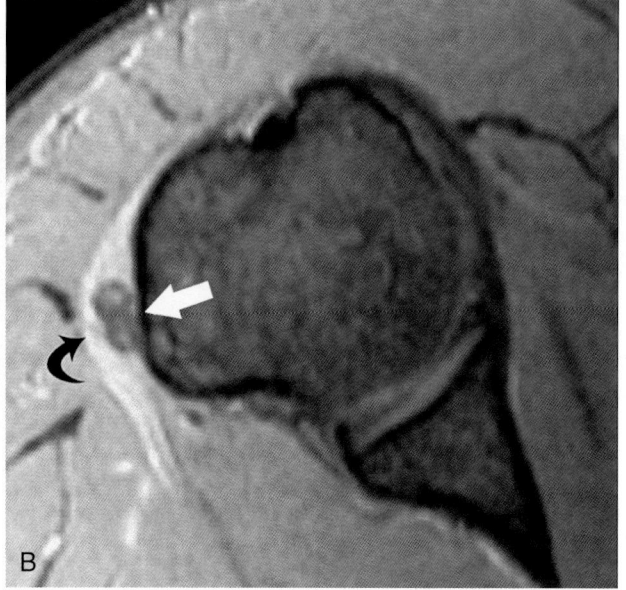

FIGURE III-12

Calcium hydroxyapatite crystal deposition. **A,** Sagittal T2-weighted fat-suppressed MR image in a patient who presented with shoulder pain shows a focus of low signal intensity *(arrow)* adjacent to the vertical facet of the greater tuberosity with adjacent bone marrow edema *(arrowheads)* and high signal intensity in the subdeltoid bursa *(curved arrow)*. **B,** The gradient-echo axial image confirms the finding of calcium hydroxyapatite crystal deposition in the attachment of the teres minor with reactive inflammation in the adjacent humerus and bursa.

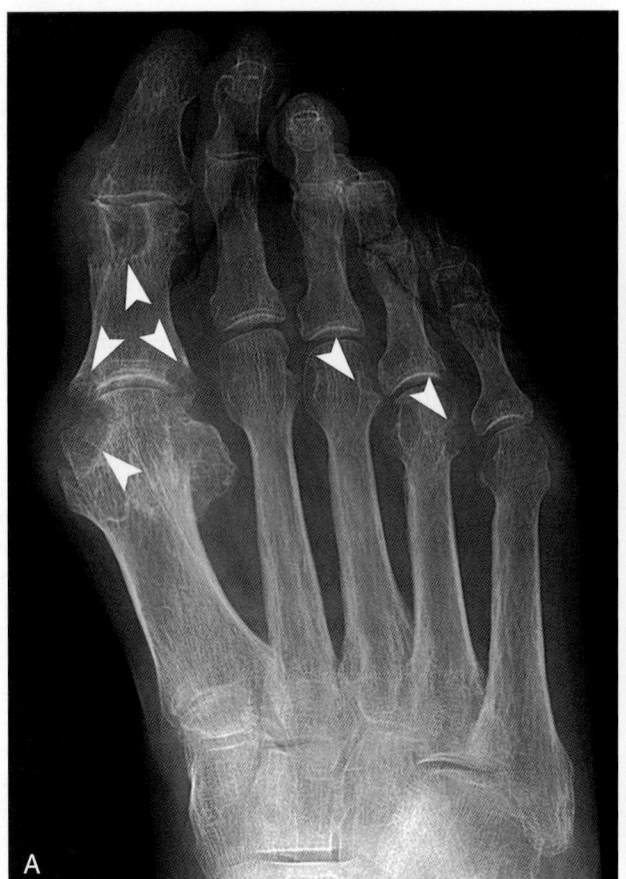
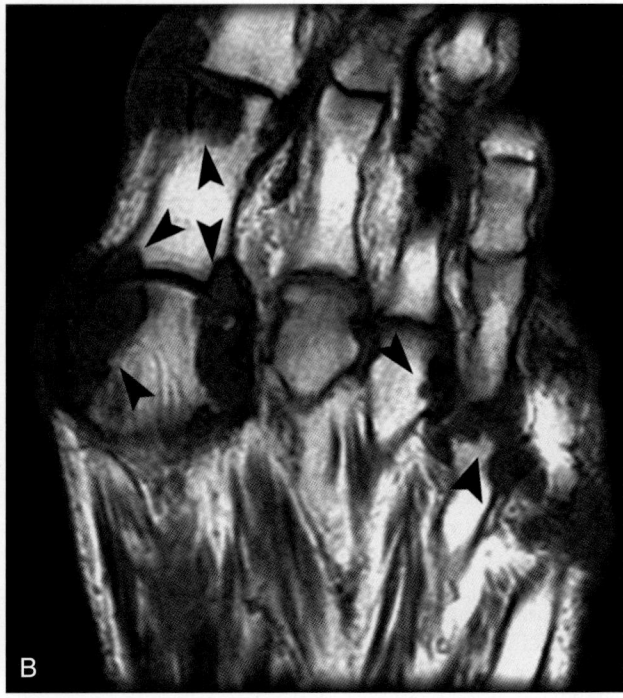

FIGURE III-13

Gout. **A,** Frontal radiograph of the forefoot shows osseous erosions *(arrowheads)* characteristic of gout. **B,** The corresponding T1-weighted axial MR image verifies the presence of erosive change *(arrowheads)*.

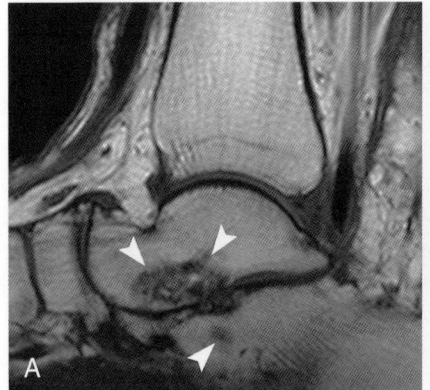
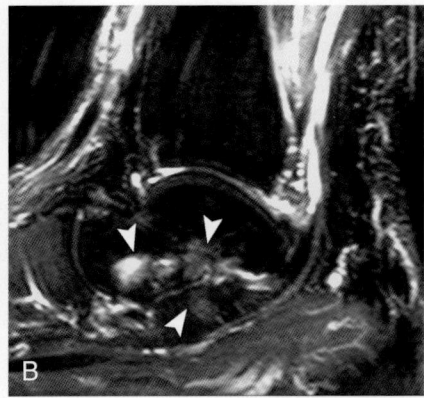
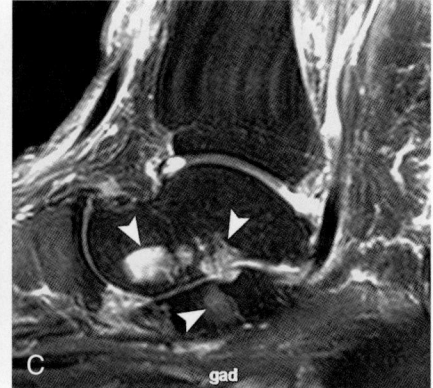

FIGURE III-14

Gout. **A,** Sagittal T1-weighted MR image in a patient with chronic renal failure and known gout shows areas of low signal intensity surrounding the sinus tarsi *(arrowheads)*. **B,** The corresponding T2-weighted fat-suppressed sagittal MR image shows the areas to be intermediate to high signal intensity *(arrowheads)*. **C,** The T1-weighted fat-suppressed post-contrast image shows variable enhancement, consistent with the diagnosis of gout. Subsequent aspiration of the sinus tarsi confirmed the diagnosis.

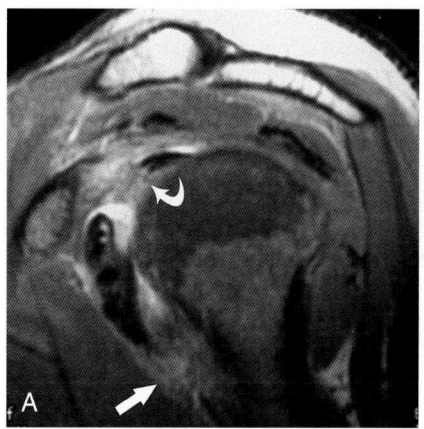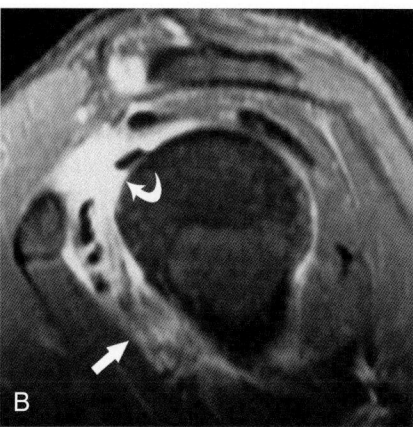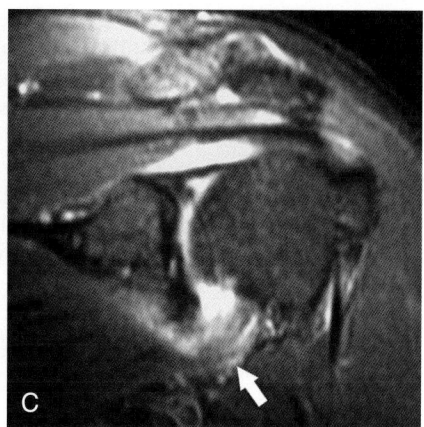

FIGURE III-15

Adhesive capsulitis. **A,** Proton density–weighted sagittal MR image of the shoulder in a patient who presented with chronic shoulder pain and decreased range of motion shows thickening of the rotator cuff interval capsule *(curved arrow)* with intermediate-signal-intensity material surrounding the biceps tendon. In addition, thickening of the capsule in the region of the axillary pouch is noted *(arrow)*. **B,** T1-weighted fat-suppressed post-contrast sagittal MR image through the shoulder in which intense, homogeneous enhancement is seen in the thickened rotator cuff interval capsule *(curved arrow)* consistent with synovitis and the clinical entity of adhesive capsulitis. **C,** Coronal T1-weighted fat-suppressed post-contrast MR image through the anterior aspect of the articulation shows the thickened enhanced axillary capsulitis pouch capsule *(arrow)*.

Osteoarthritis is the most frequent type of arthritis. It can be primary or secondary to previous inflammatory process, metabolic disorder, or traumatic injury. This is a disease associated with cartilage degeneration in the early stages, joint space narrowing, subchondral sclerosis, and osteophytosis in the later stages. Low-grade synovial inflammation, joint effusion, and popliteal cysts have been described in osteoarthritis.[9,69] Moreover, it appears that large effusions and synovial thickening are more frequent in those patients with symptomatic knee pain.

Post-traumatic Synovitis

Post-traumatic synovitis is often associated with acute injury, chronic repeated microtrauma, and overuse syndromes.[9,18] These injuries may result in inflammation, localized synovitis, and subsequent fibrosis. Although the detection of structural abnormalities is prioritized in the assessment of the post-traumatic MR imaging study, attention should also be focused on the synovium, for both the detection and quantification of synovitis. In cases of post-traumatic synovitis that prove refractory to conservative therapy, arthroscopic debridement has been shown to be helpful.

The clinical entity of "frozen shoulder" or adhesive capsulitis of the shoulder is a specific example of a post-traumatic synovitis. The clinical finding of decreased range of motion is suggestive of, but not specific for, this diagnosis. Histologically, the disease demonstrates inflammation of the joint capsule, particularly the synovial capsule of the axillary recess and the rotator cuff interval, those portions of the capsule not reinforced by rotator cuff tendon. MR imaging findings include synovial thickening in the aforementioned regions of the

capsule. In addition, the hypertrophic synovium can encase the biceps tendon as it moves from an extra-articular position within the intertubercular sulcus to an intra-articular position en route to its attachment to the supraglenoid tubercle. Finally, images after IV administration of gadolinium show intense enhancement of the hypertrophic synovial tissue, consistent with the diagnosis of synovitis (Fig. 111-15).[70] Recent studies have explored the use of MR arthrography for the evaluation of adhesive capsulitis. This imaging method showed thickening of the joint capsule and synovium with a diminished filling ratio (of contrast) of the axillary recess to posterior joint cavity.[71]

Hematopoietic Disorders

Hemophilia is a disease manifested by abnormality of the coagulation mechanism and caused by functional deficiencies of specific clotting factors.[72] It is a chromosomal X-linked recessive disorder manifested in males and carried by females. Severity of the disease correlates to the degree of factor deficiency. Patients with severe or moderately severe disease can suffer repeated hemarthroses either spontaneously or secondary to minor trauma. These repeated hemarthroses lead to a severe and disabling arthropathy that appears to be propagated through the synovium. The hemarthrosis results in absorption of hemosiderin and red cell products by the synovial membrane, which, in turn, becomes hypertrophic, hyperplastic, hypervascular, and inflamed. This pannus not only extends throughout the joint but also is a source of proteolytic enzymes that destroy the articular cartilage and result in erosions, subchondral cyst formation, and ultimately endstage degeneration.

The MR imaging findings parallel the pathologic process, and in the acute phase demonstrate hemarthrosis and synovitis. Areas of low signal intensity on T1-weighted and fluid-sensitive sequences correlate to areas of hemosiderin-laden synovium. Gradient-echo imaging has been advocated as a more sensitive means to detect blood products in the synovium in the early phases of the disease.[73] Erosions and subchondral cysts are seen and demonstrate low signal intensity on T1-weighted images and high signal intensity on fluid-sensitive sequences. In the chronic stage of the disease, the joints become disorganized, contracted, and fibrotic with exposure of subchondral bone.

Tumors and Tumor-like Disorders

Pigmented Villonodular Synovitis

Pigmented villonodular synovitis (PVNS) is a rare, benign synovial proliferative process whose distribution is usually monoarticular. The disorder is idiopathic. There are two primary forms, localized and diffuse. The diffuse form usually involves large joints and may affect the synovial lining, bursae, or tendon sheaths. Although any synovial joint may be involved, the knee is most frequently affected. Other sites of involvement in decreasing order of frequency include the hip, the ankle, the hands and feet, the shoulder, and the elbow. Patients usually present with nonspecific symptoms such as monoarticular pain and decreased range of motion. Affected individuals are typically between the ages of 20 and 40 years; there is a slight male preponderance. Histopathologically, the disease is characterized by the presence of abundant hemosiderin-laden macrophage deposition in a bulky, masslike synovium.[74-78]

MRI is the imaging method of choice for the diagnosis, surgical planning, and evaluation of recurrence. Although not pathognomonic, MR imaging features in PVNS provide the diagnosis in over 95% of cases. Clumps of hemosiderin-laden macrophage deposits demonstrate low signal intensity on T1- and T2-weighted images due to the paramagnetic effects of the iron in the ferric (3+) state (Fig. 111-16). This is the most reliable diagnostic feature. Gradient-echo imaging, as in the case of hemophilia, may further enhance imaging of these findings due to the magnetic susceptibility effects.[75,77] A large joint effusion is usually present but is nonspecific in nature.

Less characteristic MR imaging findings in PVNS include bone erosions and extra-articular spread of lesions. T2-hyperintense signal may also be seen due to subchondral cysts or reactive bone marrow edema. Additionally, focal deposits of lipid-laden macrophages can result in fat signal intensity.

In addition to facilitating the diagnosis, MR imaging is useful in characterizing the extent of disease by the detection of extra-articular spread, as well as assessing the status of the adjacent ligamentous and fibrocartilaginous structures. Common extra-articular sites of spread include the popliteus tendon sheath, posterior to the posterior cruciate ligament, the semimembranosus bursa, and previous arthroscopy portals.

The treatment of diffuse PVNS is a complete synovectomy. The high recurrence rate, reported to range from 33% to 46%, precludes localized surgical treatment. The exact reasons for such a high rate of recurrence are unclear but may be related to the difficulty in performing a complete synovectomy. A recent hypothesis also suggests a high rate of recurrence due to the failure to identify and resect extra-articular lesions. The latter hypothesis, if correct, increases the importance of carefully addressing the bursa and tendon sheaths about the joint.[76]

Localized Nodular Synovitis

Localized nodular synovitis, like its more diffuse counterpart, pigmented villonodular synovitis, is a rare synovial inflammatory disorder whose etiology is uncertain. Although this disorder shares similar histopathologic characteristics and patient population as PVNS, the MR imaging characteristics of the localized form are distinct from PVNS. Moreover, the reader should be aware that it is of paramount importance to distinguish these two entities because their surgical planning, treatment, and response to treatment differ dramatically.[75,79,80]

The MR imaging characteristics of localized nodular synovitis vary. The classic appearance is a rounded or ovoid solitary lesion that demonstrates different degrees of low signal on T1- and T2-weighted images depending upon the concentration of hemosiderin occupying the lesion. The lesion typically is more conspicuous on gradient-echo imaging due to the paramagnetic effect of iron molecules in the ferric state. There is usually heterogeneous enhancement following IV administration of contrast material which likely relates to the rich capillary network occupying the fibrous stroma.[75]

The most commonly affected regions are tendon sheaths about small articulations of the fingers and toes. When intra-articular disease is present it is almost always localized to the knee joint (Fig. 111-17). Specifically, the most common location is the infrapatellar (Hoffa's) fat pad. Other affected areas about the knee are the suprapatellar pouch and the intercondylar notch.

The importance of distinguishing localized nodular synovitis from PVNS cannot be overemphasized. MR imaging of PVNS usually shows a more exuberant pattern of hemosiderin deposition manifested as frondlike irregularities of low signal intensity residing within the joint spaces. This finding is absent in localized nodular synovitis; in fact, only a small portion of the synovium is involved. In addition, PVNS-induced masses insinuate themselves throughout the articulation resulting in marked constriction. The localized form manifests as a solitary mass that grows outward and may have an associated pedicle. In a recent study by Huang et al, it has been noted that when the lesion grows in excess of 5 cm, knee extension is more likely to be restricted. Joint effusions in this disease are usually small or absent.[80]

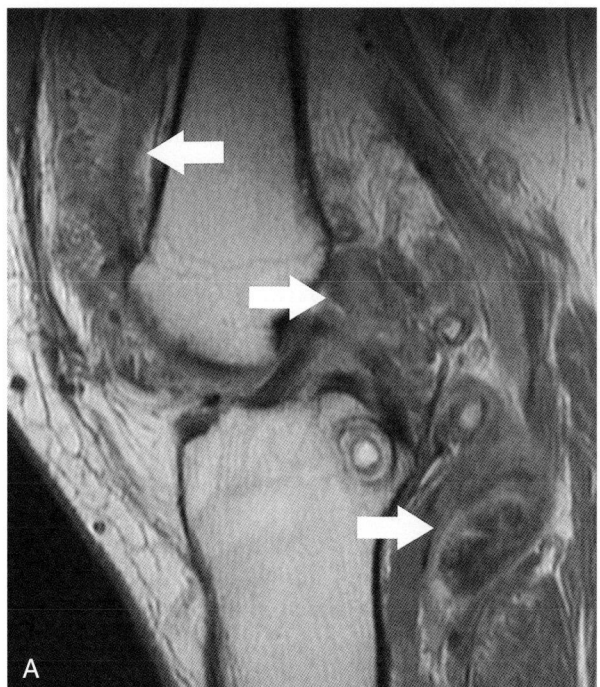

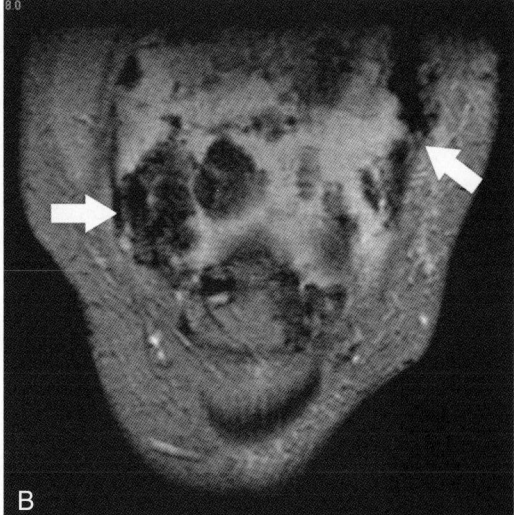

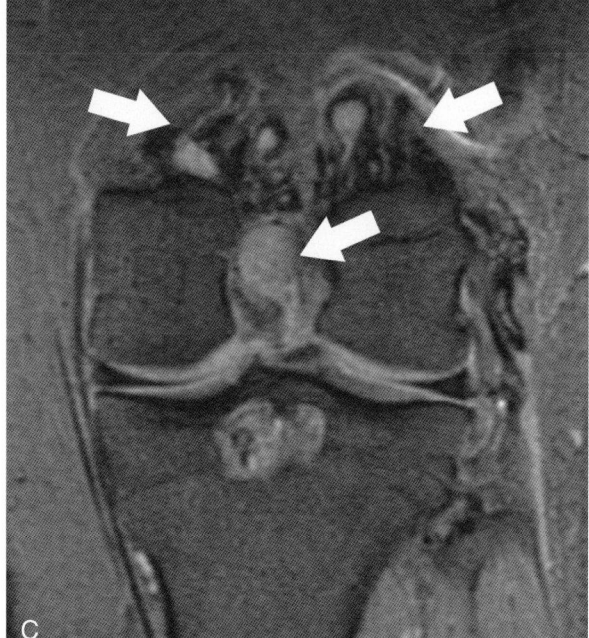

FIGURE III-16

PVNS. **A,** Proton density–weighted sagittal MR image of the knee in a patient with chronic knee pain demonstrates heterogeneous material of intermediate to low signal intensity distending the knee joint *(arrows)*. **B,** Gradient coronal MR image through the anterior aspect of the knee reveals the blooming artifact associated with the thickened, irregular capsule *(arrows)* consistent with the diagnosis of pigmented villonodular synovitis. **C,** Gradient coronal MR image through the posterior aspect of the knee shows similar findings in the posterior joint space and intercondylar notch *(arrows)*. The foci of blooming low signal intensity represent hemosiderin deposition within the capsule.

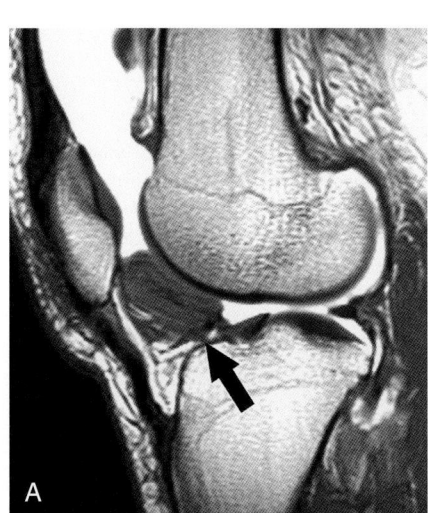

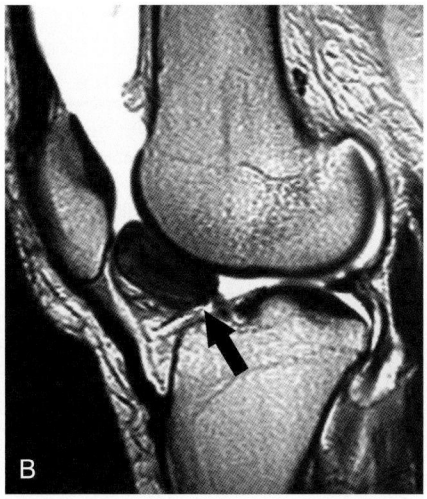

FIGURE III-17

Focal nodular synovitis. T1-weighted (**A**) and T2-weighted (**B**) sagittal fast spin-echo MR arthrogram images through the knee show a well-defined nodular density *(arrow)* at the inside margin of Hoffa's fat pad in an infrapatellar location. The signal characteristics are low on T1- and T2-weighted images. In conjunction with the location, these findings are consistent with focal nodular synovitis.

Differential considerations of localized nodular synovitis affecting Hoffa's fat pad include cartilaginous lesions, namely intracapsular chondroma, osteochondroma, and Hoffa's disease. Like localized nodular synovitis, these entities present as a solitary mass. Chondromas, however, demonstrate a flocculent cartilaginous matrix that is well appreciated on both conventional radiographs and MR imaging. On MR imaging these lesions are classically hypointense relative to muscle on T1-weighted images and show heterogeneous signal intensity on T2-weighted images. Areas of punctate low signal intensity correspond to areas of calcification or ossification, and T2-hyperintense foci represent chondroid matrix. Hoffa's disease, as the name implies, is a post-traumatic process localized to Hoffa's fat pad. It is characterized on MR imaging by an ill-defined heterogeneous mass surrounded by a zone of edema.[79]

The treatment of choice for localized nodular synovitis is local excision of the solitary mass. When compared to PVNS, localized nodular synovitis never requires a total synovectomy and the rate of recurrence is exquisitely low, usually less than 5%. Excision can usually be accomplished with arthroscopic guidance; however, an open procedure may be warranted in certain instances.

Idiopathic Synovial Osteochondromatosis

Idiopathic synovial osteochondromatosis is a nonneoplastic, proliferative, metaplastic disorder of the synovium characterized by the presence of multiple cartilaginous or osteocartilaginous bodies within an articulation or adjacent synovium-lined structure (Fig. 111-18). Two forms of the condition occur, the first of

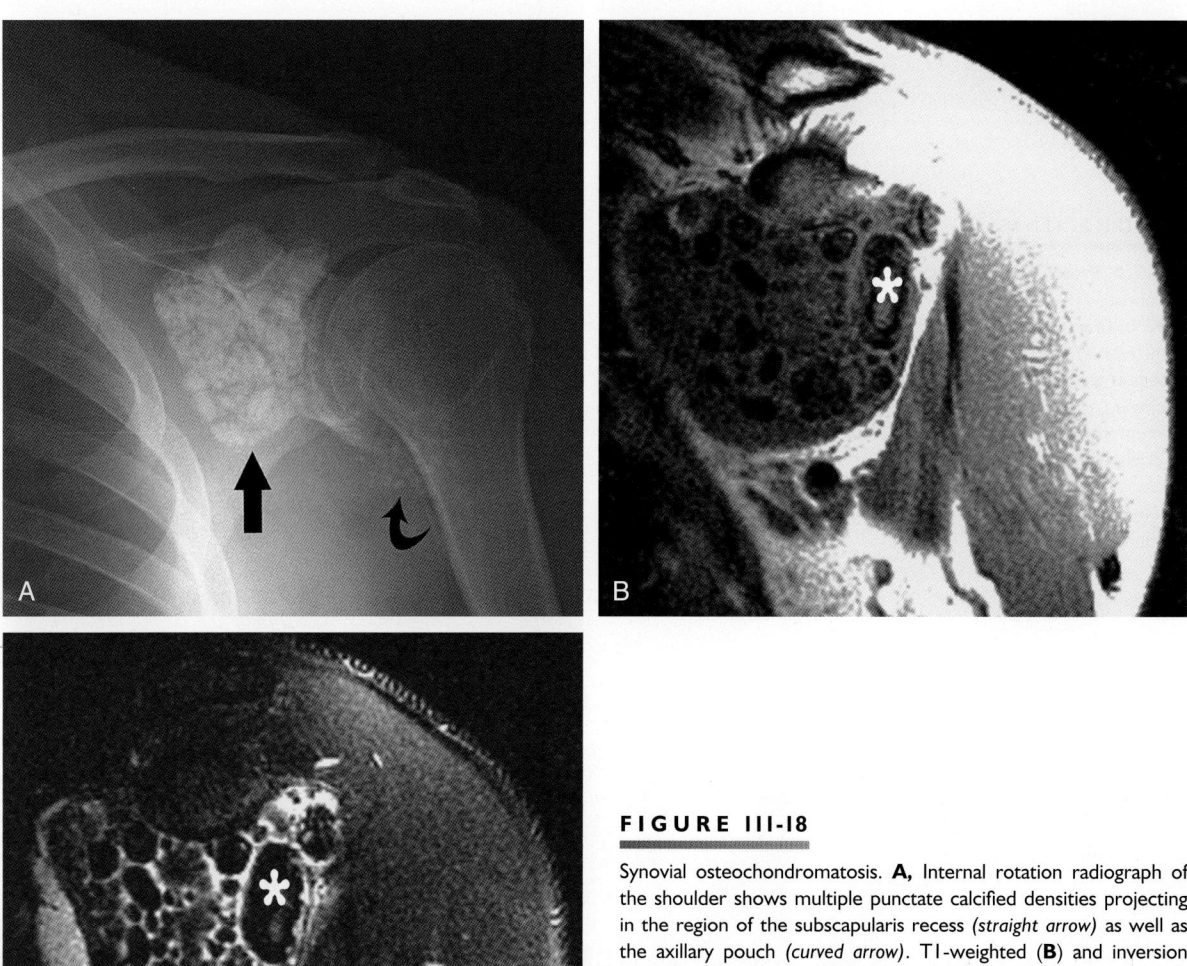

FIGURE 111-18

Synovial osteochondromatosis. **A,** Internal rotation radiograph of the shoulder shows multiple punctate calcified densities projecting in the region of the subscapularis recess *(straight arrow)* as well as the axillary pouch *(curved arrow).* T1-weighted (**B**) and inversion recovery (**C**) coronal images through the shoulder show multiple intra-articular bodies within the fluid-filled articulation *(arrow)* consistent with synovial osteochondromatosis. Some of the bodies are ossified with central matrix *(asterisk).*

which, secondary osteochondromatosis, is fairly common and typified by the presence of intra-articular osteocartilaginous bodies against a backdrop of degenerative joint disease. The second type, primary synovial osteochondromatosis, is relatively uncommon and characterized by the presence of multiple intra-articular bodies, uniform in size, distributed proportionally throughout the joint. The condition is usually progressive, leading to early osteoarthritis. Treatment includes removal of intra-articular bodies with complete synovectomy, though local recurrence is not uncommon.

The MR imaging characteristics depend on the sequence used and the presence and extent of calcification and/or ossification in the bodies (Fig. 111-19). One series reported that 85% of cases of synovial osteochondromatosis demonstrated radiographic evidence of fine cartilaginous calcification.[81] In the case of intra-articular bodies comprised primarily of cartilage, the bodies are lobulated in appearance with intermediate to low signal intensity on T1-weighted sequences with high signal intensity on fluid-sensitive sequences.[82] In the case of calcified intra-articular bodies, the signal characteristics are described as foci of low signal intensity on both T1-weighted and fluid-sensitive sequences.[83] Marrow-containing bodies will show the high signal intensity of the marrow within the bodies on T1-weighted images. Heterogeneous enhancement of cartilaginous bodies

can be seen after IV administration of contrast material, aiding in the distinction between uncalcified cartilage-containing masses and synovial fluid.[81]

Idiopathic Lipoma Arborescens

Lipoma arborescens, or villous lipomatous proliferation of the synovial membrane, is a rare intra-articular lesion that usually involves the knee but has been reported in the hips, shoulders, wrists, and elbows.[65,84] It is characterized by villous proliferation of the synovium and extensive replacement of the subsynovial tissue by mature adipose cells. It is usually a monoarticular condition, however it may occur bilaterally. The etiology of this entity is unknown, and while some cases appear to arise de novo, other cases suggest an association with nonspecific reactive processes to various inflammatory disorders, such as rheumatoid arthritis.

MR imaging shows a frondlike morphology with high signal intensity (isointense to subcutaneous fat) on T1-weighted images. No magnetic susceptibility artifact is present. Lack of enhancement after IV injection of contrast material excludes the diagnosis of other synovial inflammatory or neoplastic processes. Although there is no significant enhancement after contrast administration, enhancement in the connective tissue septa of the villous projections has been described.[84]

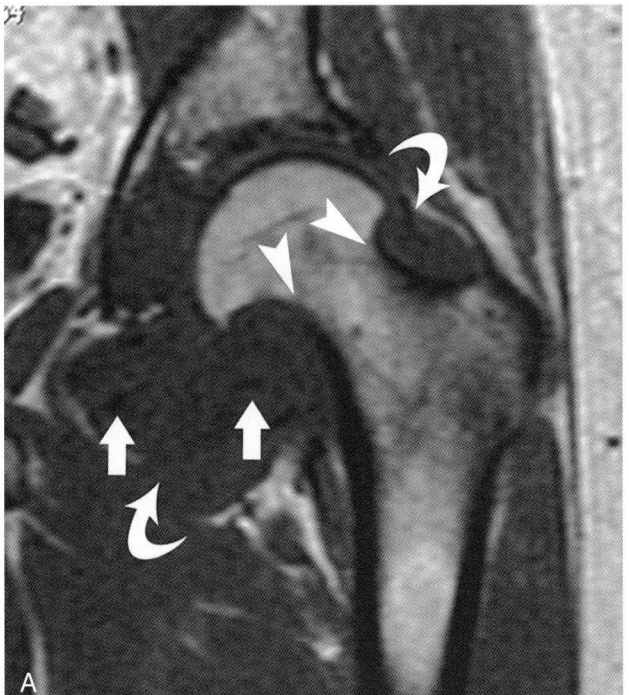 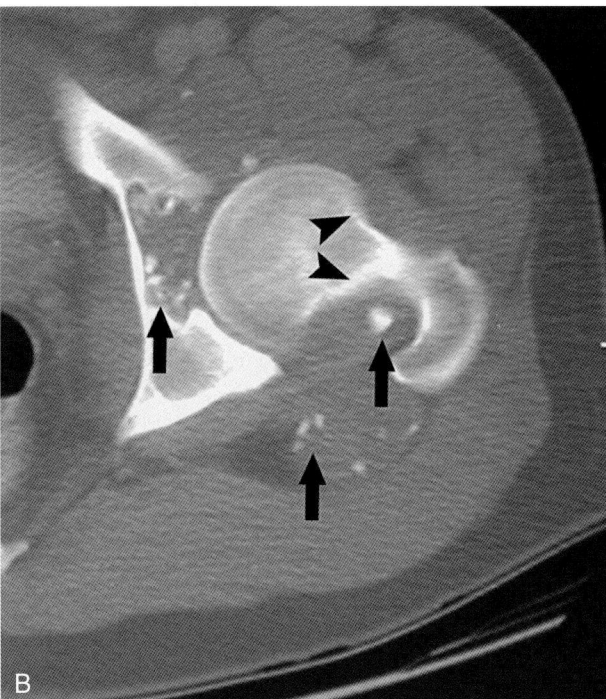

FIGURE III-19

Synovial osteochondromatosis. **A,** T1-weighted coronal MR image through the hip in a patient with chronic hip pain shows abnormal morphology of the proximal femur with constriction at the femoral head-neck junction *(arrowheads)*. There is distension of the joint capsule *(curved arrows)* with intermediate signal intensity material, and internal punctate foci of low signal intensity *(arrows)*. **B,** Axial computed tomography image verifies that the punctate foci of low signal intensity on the MR image represented the calcifications *(arrows)* of synovial osteochondromatosis. The remodeling of the proximal femur due to the chronic pressure erosion of this synovial disorder can also be appreciated *(arrowheads)*.

Lipoma arborescens should be distinguished from synovial lipoma. The former is characterized by diffuse subsynovial deposition of fat and a villous appearance, associated joint effusion, and in some cases bone erosion, whereas the latter is a solitary localized mass of adipose tissue with a round or oval contour without synovial changes.[85]

Amyloidosis

Amyloidosis is an infiltrative disorder characterized by the deposition of a pathologic proteinaceous substance (amyloid) in various tissues and organs in the body ultimately resulting in physiologic derangement. Amyloidosis is further characterized into multiple subtypes depending upon the chemical nature of the protein that makes up the amyloid fibril. Fifteen different biochemical subtypes of amyloid have been described to date. The histopathologic appearance, however, is uniformly characterized by apple green birefringence of Congo red–stained amyloid on polarized light microscopy, irrespective of the biochemical subtype. The most common biochemical subtype in amyloid arthropathy is β_2-microglobulin.[86-88]

Amyloid arthropathy has been well documented as a complication in long-term hemodialysis patients. This disorder develops due to accumulation of high concentrations of the normal serum protein β_2-microglobulin in the synovium, bone, and soft-tissues about the joint. Although amyloid deposition can be histologically documented in the joints of short-term hemodialysis patients, radiographic manifestations usually occur at least 5 years after treatment begins. Joint involvement is bilateral and fairly symmetric; although any joint may be involved, this entity has a predilection for the shoulders, wrists, hips, and knees. MR imaging characteristics of amyloid are not unlike those of other deposition diseases that involve the synovium.[86-88]

MR imaging demonstrates soft-tissue nodules of low to intermediate signal intensity on all pulse sequences with associated joint effusions. These nodules are most commonly seen around the elbow, hand, and wrist joints. In fact, amyloid deposition has been implicated as the cause of carpal tunnel syndrome in long-term dialysis patients.

Additionally, discrete periarticular intraosseous lytic foci and subchondral cystic changes are a characteristic finding on conventional radiographs. On MR imaging, these lesions are dark on T1-weighted images and dark, bright, or intermediate signal on T2-weighted images. The exact nature of these lesions is not known. Some experts speculate that these lesions may represent focal amyloid deposits. Others believe these are synovial fluid collections that develop as a result of extrinsic compression from the pericapsular soft-tissue deposits.

Involvement of fibrocartilaginous structures has also been documented on MR imaging. Specifically, thickening of the supraspinatus and infraspinatus tendons of the rotator cuff as well as the iliofemoral portion of the hip joint capsule have been reported. Tendon rupture or tears however, are not associated with this disease.[86-88]

Synovial Sarcoma

Synovial sarcoma is a malignant neoplasm of mesenchymal origin, named for its histologic similarity to synovium. In actuality, synovial sarcoma has no relationship with synovial tissue, except for the misleading similarity on light-microscopic examination. Therefore, it is not entirely surprising that an intra-articular location is exceedingly rare.[89]

This lesion presents as a large, deep-seated, rapidly growing mass. Symptoms and physical examination findings are nonspecific and mimic those of a benign lesion. It is a lesion of young adults or children and affects predominantly the extremities, more frequently the lower extremities near articulations.

The MR imaging characteristics of synovial sarcoma are nonspecific and include a relatively well-defined, large, juxta-articular mass with signal intensity that is intermediate on T1-weighted images, and intermediate to high signal intensity on T2-weighted images (Fig. 111-20). Heterogeneous signal intensity, mainly on T2-weighted images, predominates in large lesions. Synovial sarcomas show intense but heterogeneous gadolinium enhancement, which may help to differentiate these lesions from their benign counterparts. The existence of hemorrhagic components, fluid-fluid levels and areas that are hyper-, hypo- and isointense to fat (triple signal) on T2-weighted images in a mass located close to a synovium-lined structure suggest this diagnosis. Irregular calcifications are present within the lesion in 10% to 25% of cases. MR imaging demonstrates bone infiltration in 21% to 28% of cases.[89-91]

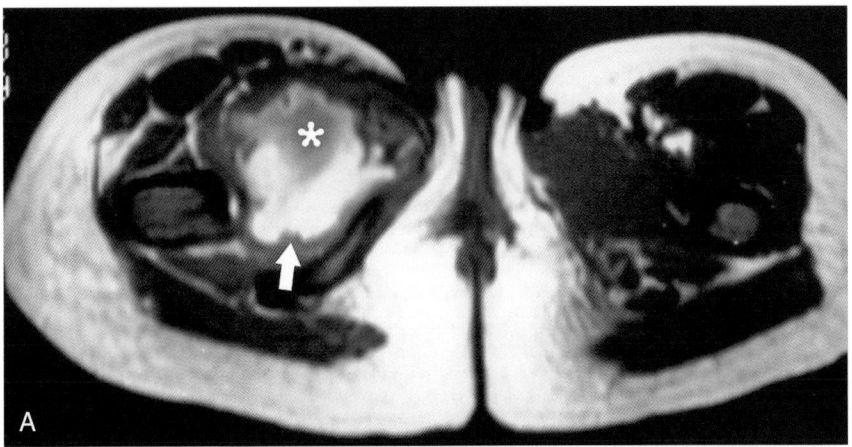

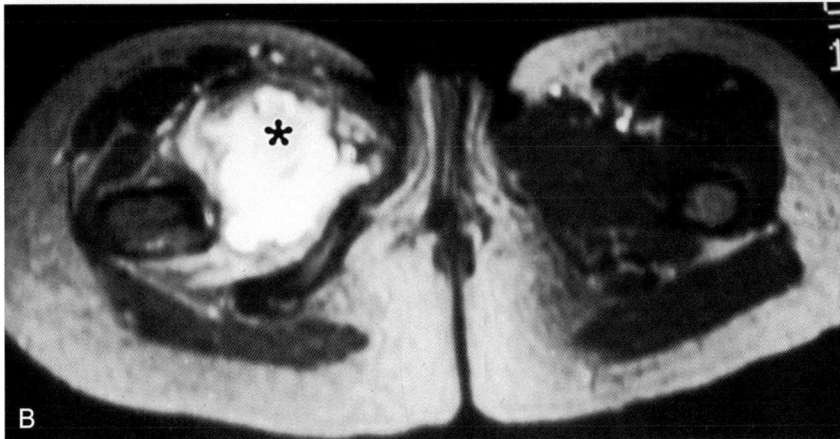

FIGURE III-20

T1-weighted (**A**) and T2-weighted (**B**) axial MR images in a patient with a synovial sarcoma showed a periarticular mass (*) with irregular margins (*arrow*) and foci of bright and dark signal on both T1- and T2-weighted images.

REFERENCES

1. Winalski CS, Aliabadi P, Wright RJ, et al: Enhancement of joint fluid with intravenously administered gadopentetate dimeglumine: technique, rationale, and implications. Radiology 187:179-185, 1993.
2. Boegard T, Johansson A, Rudling O, et al: Gadolinium-DTPA-enhanced MR imaging in asymptomatic knees. Acta Radiol 37:877-882, 1996.
3. Konig H, Sieper J, Wolf KJ: Rheumatoid arthritis: evaluation of hypervascular and fibrous pannus with dynamic MR imaging enhanced with Gd-DTPA. Radiology 176:473-477, 1990.
4. Kursunoglu-Brahme S, Riccio T, Weisman MH, et al: Rheumatoid knee: role of gadopentetate-enhanced MR imaging. Radiology 176:831-835, 1990.
5. Ostergaard M, Gideon P, Henriksen O, et al: Synovial volume—a marker of disease severity in rheumatoid arthritis? Quantification by MRI. Scand J Rheumatol 23(4):197-202, 1994.
6. Ostergaard M, Lorenzen I, Henriksen O: Dynamic gadolinium-enhanced MR imaging in active and inactive immunoinflammatory gonarthritis. Acta Radiol 35:275-281, 1994.
7. Whitten CG, Moore TE, Yuh WT, et al: The use of intravenous gadopentetate dimeglumine in magnetic resonance imaging of synovial lesions. Skeletal Radiol 21:215-218, 1992.
8. Adam G, Dammer M, Bohndorf K, et al: Rheumatoid arthritis of the knee: value of gadopentetate dimeglumine-enhanced MR imaging. Am J Roentgenol 156:125-129, 1991.
9. Bjorkengren AG, Geborek P, Rydholm U, et al: MR imaging of the knee in acute rheumatoid arthritis: synovial uptake of gadolinium-DOTA. Am J Roentgenol 155:329-332, 1990.
10. Ostergaard M, Stoltenberg M, Henriksen O, et al: The accuracy of MRI-determined synovial membrane and joint effusion volumes in arthritis. A comparison of pre- and post-aspiration volumes. Scand J Rheumatol 24:305-311, 1995.
11. Ostergaard M: Different approaches to synovial membrane volume determination by magnetic resonance imaging: manual versus automated segmentation. Br J Rheumatol 36:1166-1177, 1997.
12. Ostergaard M, Klarlund M: Importance of timing of post-contrast MRI in rheumatoid arthritis: what happens during the first 60 minutes after IV gadolinium-DTPA? Ann Rheum Dis 60:1050-1054, 2001.
13. Ostergaard M, Szkudlarek M: Magnetic resonance imaging of soft tissue changes in rheumatoid arthritis wrist joints. Semin Musculoskelet Radiol 5:257-274, 2001.
14. Beltran J, Caudill JL, Herman LA, et al: Rheumatoid arthritis: MR imaging manifestations. Radiology 165:153-157, 1987.
15. Reiser MF, Bongartz GP, Erlemann R, et al: Gadolinium-DTPA in rheumatoid arthritis and related diseases: first results with dynamic magnetic resonance imaging. Skeletal Radiol 18:591-597, 1989.
16. Tamai K, Yamato M, Yamaguchi T, et al: Dynamic magnetic resonance imaging for the evaluation of synovitis in patients with rheumatoid arthritis. Arthritis Rheum 37:1151-1157, 1994.
17. Clunie G, Hall-Craggs MA, Paley MN, et al: Measurement of synovial lining volume by magnetic resonance imaging of the knee in chronic synovitis. Ann Rheum Dis 56:526-534, 1997.
18. Bredella MA, Tirman PF, Wischer TK, et al: Reactive synovitis of the knee joint: MR imaging appearance with arthroscopic correlation. Skeletal Radiol 29:577-582, 2000.
19. Schweitzer ME, Falk A, Berthoty D, et al: Knee effusion: normal distribution of fluid. Am J Roentgenol 159:361-363, 1992.
20. Segami N, Nishimura M, Kaneyama K, et al: Does joint effusion on T2 magnetic resonance images reflect synovitis? Comparison of arthroscopic findings in internal derangements of the temporomandibular joint. Oral Surg Oral Med Oral Pathol Oral Radiol Endod 92:341-345, 2001.
21. Resnick D: Common disorders of synovium-lined joints: pathogenesis, imaging abnormalities, and complications. Am J Roentgenol 151:1079-1093, 1988.
22. Blyth T, Hunter J, Madhok R, et al: Subsynovial vascular abnormality causing recurrent hemarthrosis in an 84-year-old man. J Rheumatol 22:552-553, 1995.
23. Martin DJ, Merenda G, McDonald DJ, et al: Recurrent hemarthrosis associated with gout. Clin Orthop 277:262-265, 1992.
24. Lugo-Olivieri CH, Scott WW Jr, Zerhouni EA: Fluid-fluid levels in injured knees: do they always represent lipohemarthrosis? Radiology 198:499-502, 1996.
25. SanDretto MA, Carrera GF: The double fat fluid level: lipohemarthrosis of the knee associated with suprapatellar plica synovialis. Skeletal Radiol 10:30-33, 1983.
26. Ryu KN, Jaovisidha S, De Maeseneer M, et al: Evolving stages of lipohemarthrosis of the knee. Sequential magnetic resonance imaging findings in cadavers with clinical correlation. Invest Radiol 32:7-11, 1997.

27. Brossmann J, Preidler KW, Daenen B, et al: Imaging of osseous and cartilaginous intraarticular bodies in the knee: comparison of MR imaging and MR arthrography with CT and CT arthrography in cadavers. Radiology 200:509-517, 1996.

28. Chung C, Coley BD, Martin LC: Rice bodies in juvenile rheumatoid arthritis. Am J Roentgenol 170:698-700, 1998.

29. Boles CA, Ward WG Sr: Loose fragments and other debris: miscellaneous synovial and marrow disorders. Magn Reson Imaging Clin N Am 8:371-390, 2000.

30. Pagnoux C, Lhotellier L, Marek JJ, et al: Synovial cysts of the proximal tibiofibular joint: three case reports. Joint Bone Spine 69:331-333, 2002.

31. Ortega R, Fessell DP, Jacobson JA, et al: Sonography of ankle ganglia with pathologic correlation in 10 pediatric and adult patients. Am J Roentgenol 178:1445-1449, 2002.

32. Ehara S: Communication of the ganglion with the joint and the tendon sheath. Am J Roentgenol 180:541-542, author reply 542, 2003.

33. Niki Y, Matsumoto H, Otani T, et al: Gigantic popliteal synovial cyst caused by wear particles after total knee arthroplasty. J Arthroplasty 18:1071-1075, 2003.

34. Andonopoulos AP, Meimaris N, Yiannopoulos G, et al: Large synovial cysts originating from the sternoclavicular joints in a patient with rheumatoid arthritis. Ann Rheum Dis 62:1119-1120, 2003.

35. Hill CL, Gale DR, Chaisson CE, et al: Periarticular lesions detected on magnetic resonance imaging: prevalence in knees with and without symptoms. Arthritis Rheum 48:2836-2844, 2003.

36. Tschirch FT, Schmid MR, Pfirrmann CW, et al: Prevalence and size of meniscal cysts, ganglionic cysts, synovial cysts of the popliteal space, fluid-filled bursae, and other fluid collections in asymptomatic knees on MR imaging. Am J Roentgenol 180:1431-1436, 2003.

37. Muhle C, Ahn JM, Yeh L, et al: Iliotibial band friction syndrome: MR imaging findings in 16 patients and MR arthrographic study of six cadaveric knees. Radiology 212:103-110, 1999.

38. Bond JR, Sundaram M, Beckenbaugh RD: Radiologic case study. Partial tear of the distal biceps tendon with mass-like bicipitoradial bursitis and associated hyperostosis of the radial tuberosity. Orthopedics 26:376, 448-450, 2003.

39. Donahue F, Turkel D, Mnaymneh W, et al: Hemorrhagic prepatellar bursitis. Skeletal Radiol 25:298-301, 1996.

40. Dawn B, Williams JK, Walker SE: Prepatellar bursitis: a unique presentation of tophaceous gout in a normouricemic patient. J Rheumatol 24:976-978, 1997.

41. Kataria RK, Chaiamnuay S, Jacobson LD, et al: Subacromial bursitis with rice bodies as the presenting manifestation of rheumatoid arthritis. J Rheumatol 30:1354-1355, 2003.

42. Cimmino MA, Bountis C, Silvestri E, et al: An appraisal of magnetic resonance imaging of the wrist in rheumatoid arthritis. Semin Arthritis Rheum 30:180-195, 2000.

43. Ostergaard M, Hansen M, Stoltenberg M, et al: Quantitative assessment of the synovial membrane in the rheumatoid wrist: an easily obtained MRI score reflects the synovial volume. Br J Rheumatol 35:965-971, 1996.

44. Lee J, Lee SK, Suh JS, et al: Magnetic resonance imaging of the wrist in defining remission of rheumatoid arthritis. J Rheumatol 24:1303-1308, 1997.

45. Ostergaard M, Gideon P, Sorensen K, et al: Scoring of synovial membrane hypertrophy and bone erosions by MR imaging in clinically active and inactive rheumatoid arthritis of the wrist. Scand J Rheumatol 24:212-218, 1995.

46. Tonolli-Serabian I, Poet JL, Dufour M, et al: Magnetic resonance imaging of the wrist in rheumatoid arthritis: comparison with other inflammatory joint diseases and control subjects. Clin Rheumatol 15:137-142, 1996.

47. Foley-Nolan D, Stack JP, Ryan M, et al: Magnetic resonance imaging in the assessment of rheumatoid arthritis—a comparison with plain film radiographs. Br J Rheumatol 30:101-106, 1991.

48. McQueen FM, Stewart N, Crabbe J, et al: Magnetic resonance imaging of the wrist in early rheumatoid arthritis reveals a high prevalence of erosions at four months after symptom onset. Ann Rheum Dis 57:350-356, 1998.

49. Klarlund M, Ostergaard M, Gideon P, et al: Wrist and finger joint MR imaging in rheumatoid arthritis. Acta Radiol 40:400-409, 1999.

50. Graif M, Schweitzer ME, Deely D, et al: The septic versus nonseptic inflamed joint: MRI characteristics. Skeletal Radiol 28:616-620, 1999.

51. Imhof H, Nobauer-Huhmann IM, Gahleitner A, et al: Pathophysiology and imaging in inflammatory and blastomatous synovial diseases. Skeletal Radiol 31:313-333, 2002.

52. Lund PJ, Chan KM, Unger EC, et al: Magnetic resonance imaging in coccidioidal arthritis. Skeletal Radiol 25:661-665, 1996.

53. Strouse PJ, Londy F, DiPietro MA, et al: MRI evaluation of infectious and non-infectious synovitis: preliminary studies in a rabbit model. Pediatr Radiol 29:367-371, 1999.

54. Erdman WA, Tamburro F, Jayson HT, et al: Osteomyelitis: characteristics and pitfalls of diagnosis with MR imaging. Radiology 180:533-539, 1991.

55. Brown JJ, vanSonnenberg E, Gerber KH, et al: Magnetic resonance relaxation times of percutaneously obtained normal and abnormal body fluids. Radiology 154:727-731, 1985.

56. Sawlani V, Chandra T, Mishra RN, et al: MRI features of tuberculosis of peripheral joints. Clin Radiol 58:755-762, 2003.

57. Sugimoto H, Takeda A, Hyodoh K: Early-stage rheumatoid arthritis: prospective study of the effectiveness of MR imaging for diagnosis. Radiology 216:569-575, 2000.

58. Sugimoto H, Takeda A, Masuyama J, et al: Early-stage rheumatoid arthritis: diagnostic accuracy of MR imaging. Radiology 198:185-192, 1996.

59. Narvaez JA, Narvaez J, Roca Y, et al: MR imaging assessment of clinical problems in rheumatoid arthritis. Eur Radiol 12:1819-1828, 2002.

60. McGonagle D, Gibbon W, Emery P: Classification of inflammatory arthritis by enthesitis. Lancet 352:1137-1140, 1998.

61. Bencardino JT, Hassankhani A: Calcium pyrophosphate dihydrate crystal deposition disease. Semin Musculoskelet Radiol 7:175-185, 2003.

62. Burke BJ, Escobedo EM, Wilson AJ, et al: Chondrocalcinosis mimicking a meniscal tear on MR imaging. Am J Roentgenol 170:69-70, 1998.

63. Hayes CW, Conway WF: Calcium hydroxyapatite deposition disease. Radiographics 10:1031-1048, 1990.

64. Yang I, Hayes CW, Biermann JS: Calcific tendinitis of the gluteus medius tendon with bone marrow edema mimicking metastatic disease. Skeletal Radiol 31:359-361, 2002.

65. Soler T, Rodriguez E, Bargiela A, et al: Lipoma arborescens of the knee: MR characteristics in 13 joints. J Comput Assist Tomogr 22:605-609, 1998.

66. Yu JS, Chung C, Recht M, et al: MR imaging of tophaceous gout. Am J Roentgenol 168:523-527, 1997.

67. Ruiz ME, Erickson SJ, Carrera GF, et al: Monoarticular gout following trauma: MR appearance. J Comput Assist Tomogr 17:151-153, 1993.

68. Chung CB, Mohana-Borges A, Pathria M: Tophaceous gout in an amputation stump in a patient with chronic myelogenous leukemia. Skeletal Radiol 32:429-431, 2003.

69. Hill CL, Gale DG, Chaisson CE, et al: Knee effusions, popliteal cysts, and synovial thickening: association with knee pain in osteoarthritis. J Rheumatol 28:1330-1337, 2001.

70. Connell D, Padmanabhan R, Buchbinder R: Adhesive capsulitis: role of MR imaging in differential diagnosis. Eur Radiol 12:2100-2106, 2002.

71. Lee MH, Ahn JM, Muhle C, et al: Adhesive capsulitis of the shoulder: diagnosis using magnetic resonance arthrography with arthroscopic findings as the standard. J Comput Assist Tomogr 27:901-906, 2003.

72. Yulish BS, Lieberman JM, Strandjord SE, et al: Hemophilic arthropathy: assessment with MR imaging. Radiology 164:759-762, 1987.

73. Rand T, Trattnig S, Male C, et al: Magnetic resonance imaging in hemophilic children: value of gradient echo and contrast-enhanced imaging. Magn Reson Imaging 17:199-205, 1999.

74. Hughes TH, Sartoris DJ, Schweitzer ME, et al: Pigmented villonodular synovitis: MRI characteristics. Skeletal Radiol 24:7-12, 1995.

75. Masih S, Antebi A: Imaging of pigmented villonodular synovitis. Semin Musculoskelet Radiol 7:205-216, 2003.

76. Ohnuma M, Sugita T, Kawamata T, et al: Pigmented villonodular synovitis of the knee with lesions of the bursae. Clin Orthop 414:212-218, 2003.

77. Patkar D, Prasad S, Shah J, et al: Pigmented villonodular synovitis: magnetic resonance features of an unusual case of bilateral hip joint involvement. Australas Radiol 44:458-459, 2000.

78. Steinbach LS, Neumann CH, Stoller DW, et al: MRI of the knee in diffuse pigmented villonodular synovitis. Clin Imaging 13:305-316, 1989.

79. Stacy GS, Heck RK, Peabody TD, et al: Neoplastic and tumorlike lesions detected on MR imaging of the knee in patients with suspected internal derangement: Part 2, articular and juxtaarticular entities. Am J Roentgenol 178:595-599, 2002.

80. Huang GS, Lee CH, Chan WP, et al: Localized nodular synovitis of the knee: MR imaging appearance and clinical correlates in 21 patients. Am J Roentgenol 181:539-543, 2003.

81. Wittkop B, Davies AM, Mangham DC: Primary synovial chondromatosis and synovial chondrosarcoma: a pictorial review. Eur Radiol 12:2112-2119, 2002.

82. Kim SH, Hong SJ, Park JS, et al: Idiopathic synovial osteochondromatosis of the hip: radiographic and MR appearances in 15 patients. Korean J Radiol 3:254-259, 2002.

83. Tuckman G, Wirth CZ: Synovial osteochondromatosis of the shoulder: MR findings. J Comput Assist Tomogr 13:360-361, 1989.

84. Tiao WM, Yeh LR, Lu YC, et al: Lipoma arborescens of the knee: a case report. J Formos Med Assoc 100:412-415, 2001.

85. Ryu KN, Jaovisidha S, Schweitzer M, et al: MR imaging of lipoma arborescens of the knee joint. Am J Roentgenol 167:1229-1232, 1996.

86. Sheldon PJ, Forrester DM: Imaging of amyloid arthropathy. Semin Musculoskelet Radiol 7:195-203, 2003.

87. Escobedo EM, Hunter JC, Zink-Brody GC, et al: Magnetic resonance imaging of dialysis-related amyloidosis of the shoulder and hip. Skeletal Radiol 25:41-48, 1996.

88. Amoroso E, Vitale C, Silvestro A: Spinal-cord compression due to extradural amyloidosis of the cervico-occipital hinge, in a hemodialysed patient. A case report. J Neurosurg Sci 45:120-124, 2001.

89. Narvaez JA, Narvaez J, Aguilera C, et al: MR imaging of synovial tumors and tumor-like lesions. Eur Radiol 11:2549-2560, 2001.

90. Blacksin MF, Siegel JR, Benevenia J, et al: Synovial sarcoma: frequency of nonaggressive MR characteristics. J Comput Assist Tomogr 21:785-789, 1997.

91. Jones BC, Sundaram M, Kransdorf MJ: Synovial sarcoma: MR imaging findings in 34 patients. Am J Roentgenol 161:827-830, 1993.

EXTREMITY SCANNERS

John V. Crues III

Since its introduction into medical imaging in the early 1980s, the complexity and robustness of magnetic resonance imaging (MRI) has repeatedly surprised physicists and clinical radiologists alike. New pulse sequences, new applications, and new hardware continue to create an ever-changing landscape in musculoskeletal MRI. Whereas the excitement of new sequences and high-resolution imaging at ultra-high fields is covered in other chapters, this chapter describes imaging at low and medium field strengths using small, low-cost, easily-installed scanners for use in imaging centers and treating physician offices. The four commercially available extremity scanners that are currently approved by the Food and Drug Administration (FDA) will be described, and their financial, medical, and social implications discussed.

THE SCANNERS

Extremity scanners are designed to provide MR imaging of the arms and legs using small magnets to limit construction and installation costs. Three FDA-approved magnets image at 0.2 T, where permanent magnets are cost-effective, and the fourth operates at 1.0 T, using a superconducting magnet. Because of the sophisticated design of these imaging systems, including the surface coils used, we have found joint imaging to be equal to or better than that obtained at similar field strengths using multipurpose, whole-body scanners, with the exception that the high-field scanner is somewhat limited in spectral fat suppression due to field inhomogeneity at the periphery of the field of view (FOV). Decreased costs, low weight, and ease of installation in limited space differentiate these devices from standard whole-body scanners and allow placement in office locations where large magnets are not practical, opening up markets not addressed by standard MR offerings. Use of extremity MRI poses potential advantages and disadvantages for patients, treating physicians, radiologists, and payers.

Applause

Table 112-1 lists the four FDA-approved extremity scanners currently on the market. The Applause, manufactured by MagneVu, Carlsbad, CA, and currently distributed by General Electric Medical Systems, is the only commercial MR scanner which images in a nonuniform magnetic field and is the least expensive but most restrictive of the four devices (Fig. 112-1). Imaging in a nonuniform field requires a three-dimensional Fourier transform (3DFT) technique for spatial encoding, since a slice-selection gradient cannot be used. Phase-encoding in two dimensions substantially increases the imaging time, so to conserve time and limit the physical size of the magnet, the imaging volume is restricted to a $1.0 \times 5.0 \times 7.5$ cm slab. A local surface coil is built into the scanner, optimizing the signal-to-noise ratio (SNR)

TABLE 112-1 PDA-Approved Extremity Scanners

Model	Manufacturer	Field Strength
Applause	MagneVu (Marketed by GE Medical Systems)	0.2 T inhomogeneous
C-Scan	Esaote (Marketed in the US by GE Medical Systems)	0.2 T homogeneous
E-Scan	Esaote (Marketed in the US by GE Medical Systems)	0.2 T homogeneous
OrthoOne	ONI	1.0 T homogeneous

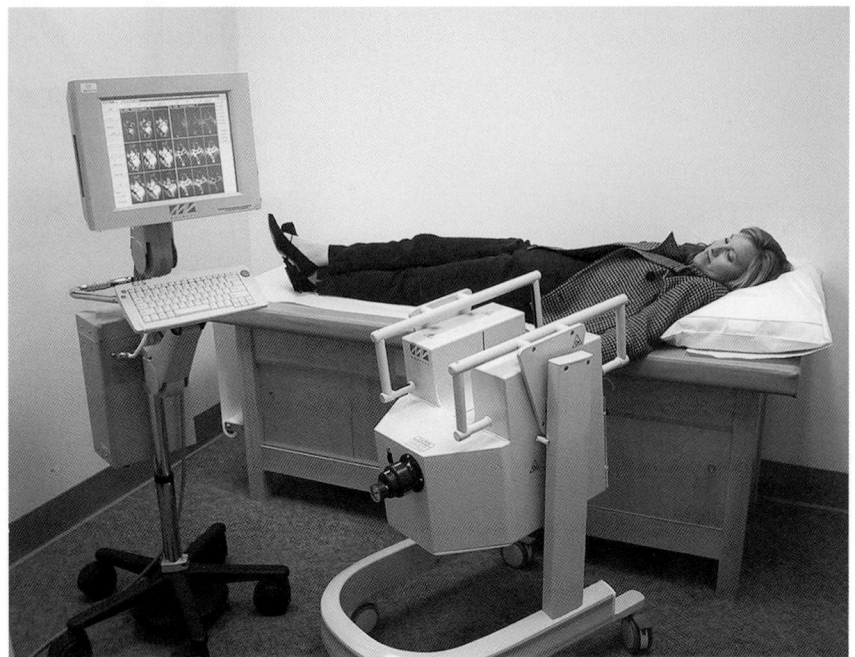

FIGURE 112-1

The open design of the MagneVu extremity scanner allows patients to be scanned in comfortable positions, recumbent or seated.

and placing the acquisition FOV in a fixed position between 1 and 2 cm from the magnet face, limiting imaging to body regions adjacent to the skin. Because of its compact design, this device does not require magnetic field or radiofrequency shielding, reducing installation costs and allowing it to be rolled from room to room. The magnet is a permanent magnet operated by a standard PC, but cryogens are needed to cool the magnet during operation.

The optimization of the signal-to-noise factor by using a small, locally applied surface coil and 3DFT imaging allows imaging at resolutions substantially higher than those normally achieved on high-field scanners. Our standard hand MR imaging protocol for evaluation of rheumatoid arthritis (RA) is comprised of four acquisitions, which are displayed for image interpretation in the coronal plane. Two are centered at the lunocapitate articulation, one with T1-weighted and the other with a short-tau inversion recovery (STIR) technique (Table 112-2). The spatial resolution is 1 mm in-plane and 0.6 mm through-plane. Two additional acquisitions are centered between the second and third metacarpophalangeal joints, as the wrist and second and third metacarpophalangeal joints are the most commonly involved regions of the hand in RA. In the foot, similar imaging is performed with centering between the fourth and fifth metatarsal joints and the second and third metatarsal joints.

Current applications for the Applause include foot, wrist, and hand imaging for the detection and characterization of bone erosions in inflammatory arthropathies.[1,2] With the success of the tumor necrosis factor inhibitors in the treatment of RA and other inflammatory arthropathies,[3-7] objective evidence of active inflammation and erosive disease is of value in staging and assessing

disease activity. Multiple studies have shown MRI to be significantly more sensitive than plain radiographs in evaluating soft-tissue and bone changes in RA[8-19]; however, the specificity of focal cortical defects seen with high-resolution MRI is still being evaluated.[1,20,21] Despite the extensive literature documenting the clinical advantages of MRI in the evaluation of RA, the use of MRI in clinical rheumatologic practice is uncommon. This may be in part due to scientific disagreements,[16] but the delay in embracing MRI by the rheumatologic community also stems from its expense and the difficulty older arthritic patients experience in lying in a traditional magnet. With the cost of the new therapeutic

TABLE 112-2 Applause Imaging Protocols*

Series	Weighting	Anatomic Centering
Hand for Rheumatoid Arthritis		
1	T1	Between 2nd and 3rd MCP
2	STIR	Between 2nd and 3rd MCP
3	T1	Medial margin of the lunate
4	STIR	Medial margin of the lunate
Foot for Rheumatoid Arthritis		
1	T1	Between 2nd and 3rd MTP
2	STIR	Between 2nd and 3rd MTP
3	T1	Between 4th and 5th MTP
4	STIR	Between 4th and 5th MTP

*All sequences are performed using a 3D Fourier transform spin-echo technique. The FOV is 7 cm in distal to proximal length, 5 cm in medial to lateral length, and 1 cm in anteroposterior dimension. Sixteen contiguous slices are obtained and displayed in the coronal plane of the hand and axial plane of the foot (parallel to long axis of metatarsals).

Box 112-1	Percentage of Treated Patients with Inflammatory Arthropathy in a Rheumatologist's Practice with Detectable Erosions[1]
Number of patients:	132
Number with erosions by MRI:	125 (95%)
Number by radiography:	78 (59%)

Box 112-2	Treated Rheumatoid Arthritis Patients with Detectable Changes in Erosions by MRI at 6-Month Intervals[21]
Number of patients:	128
Number of intervals:	176
Progression:	63 (36%)
No change:	80 (45%)
Regression:	21 (12%)
Both:	9 (5%)
Artifacts:	3 (2%)

agents being in excess of $10,000 per year, the economic and medical value of MRI in helping to determine timing and dosage of TNF-alpha inhibitors is being actively investigated.[1,2,4,13,16,19] As seen in Figure 112-1, the openness of the Applause makes it far more comfortable for arthritic patients than other currently available scanners. As will be discussed below, the economic advantages to rheumatologic practices may be a further incentive for the use of the MagneVu scanner in clinical practice.

Whereas the low mean field strength (0.2 T) of the Applause provides tissue contrast similar to other low-field scanners, the submillimeter resolution is essential for sensitive evaluation of changes in size of erosions typically measuring 2 to 5 mm in diameter. This combination, along with the small imaging volume, allows higher resolution imaging (1.0 × 1.0 × 0.6 mm) than is customary with spin-echo sequences on traditional scanners (0.8 × 0.8 × 3.0 mm). Since the detection of very early erosions or small increases in size of erosions may lead to intensive intervention, sub-millimeter resolution will probably be essential for effective use of MRI in inflammatory arthropathies. Using this technique, we have found 95% of 132 consecutive patients in the office of a single rheumatologist to have erosions, whereas 59% were positive by three-view radiographs interpreted with the knowledge of the MR findings (Box 112-1).[1] Information obtained at 6-month follow-up shows detectable changes in bone erosions in over 50% of RA patients treated with disease-modifying antirheumatic drugs (Box 112-2; Figs. 112-2 and 112-3).[20]

C-Scan

The C-scan is an updated version of the Artoscan, the only original extremity scanner still on the market. With over 1000 sold, it accounts for more machines than all other extremity scanners combined (Fig. 112-4). Manufactured by the Esaote Company in Genoa, Italy, and marketed in the United States by General Electric Medical Systems, the C-scan operates at a uniform 0.2 T. The device uses a permanent magnet, which does not need magnetic field shielding. Radiofrequency shielding is supplied by flexible material placed around the aperture of the magnet, eliminating the need for expensive shielding in the walls. This magnet is not portable. Although the C-Scan is not FDA approved for use in patients with internal ferromagnetic objects or pacemakers, data indicate that patients with aneurysm clips

and pacemakers can be safely scanned in the older Artoscan magnet, as the chest and brain cannot be placed in areas where the magnetic radiofrequency fields would adversely affect these medical devices.[22,23]

The C-scan is designed to image the extremities from the elbow to the fingers and the knee to the toes. Unlike the MagneVu scanner, the 12 cm 3D FOV of this device allows imaging of entire joints with accuracy typical of full-body scanners at similar field strength, making this scanner a good orthopedic imager.[24,26] Care must be taken in using this device not to make up for the poor SNR inherent at 0.2 T with voxel dimensions too large to provide adequate spatial resolution for evaluation of joint structures of interest. In-plane resolution should be no greater than 0.8 mm and through-plane resolution no greater than 4 mm for typical knee imaging (American College of Radiology [ACR] accreditation recommendations) (Table 112-3; Fig. 112-5). Meniscal tears (Fig. 112-6), anterior cruciate ligament (ACL) injuries (Fig. 112-7), cartilage injuries (Fig. 112-8), anterior talofibular ligament tears (Fig. 112-9), calcaneal fracture (Fig. 112-10), common extensor tendon injuries of the elbow (Fig. 112-11), cartilage injury (Fig. 112-12), and carpal tunnel syndrome from a ganglion cyst (Fig. 112-13) are some of the common musculoskeletal injuries well evaluated with the C-scan. Because of the confined imaging space, the ankle must be imaged in plantarflexion. Radiologists familiar with imaging this joint in dorsiflexion on whole-body scanners may find the anatomy confusing until experience is gained. An advantage of plantarflexion is minimization of magic-angle artifact of the tendons.

The major disadvantage with the C-scan MR scanner is that it images at 0.2 T where most radiologists believe intrinsic contrast and the SNR lead to poorer image quality than imaging at higher fields. This has led to a lack of success of this magnet in radiology practices in the United States: consequently the vast majority of C-scan machines in the US are located in orthopedic offices where they are owned by the orthopedic practice and supervised and interpreted by an associated radiology group. Outside the United States, C-scan machines can be very successful in radiology practices, especially in Italy where 40% of installed MR scanners are extremity devices.

Text continues on page 3659

TABLE 112-3 Imaging Protocols for the Esaote C-scan

Pulse Sequence	Mode	Contrast	Plane	TR (ms)	No. of Slices	Gap (mm)	Thickness (mm)	TE (ms)	TI (ms)	FOV (mm)	Matrix	Acquisitions	Time (min)	%
						Standard Knee								
SE		T1	Sag	680	20	0.4	4.0	18		160	192 × 192	3	6:34	79
SE		T2	Sag	3000	20	0.4	4.0	80		160	192 × 160	1	8:06	117
SE		T1	Cor	650	19	0.4	4.0	18		160	192 × 192	3	6:17	78
STIR			Cor	1470	15	1.0	5.0	24	75	170	192 × 160	2	7:53	96
SE		T2	Axial	3000	13	1.0	5.0	100		160	192 × 160	1	8:06	98
SE		T1	Sag	550	9	0.3	3.0	34		180	192 × 160	4	6:30	96
						Calf/Long Bone								
SE		T1	Axial	500	11	0.4	4.0	18		160	192 × 192	4	6:27	69
STIR			Axial	1340	14	0.5	4.0	24	75	170	192 × 160	2	7:11	63
SE		T1	Sag	500	14	0.4	4.0	18		180	192 × 176	4	5:55	91
SE		T2	Cor	2670	17	0.4	4.0	90		160	192 × 160	1	7:12	80
SE		T1	Cor	500	14	0.4	4.0	18		180	192 × 176	4	5:55	91
						Ankle and Heel								
SE		T1	Axial	600	17	0.4	4.0	18		140	192 × 176	3	5:20	61
SE		T2	Axial	3000	17	0.4	4.0	100		140	192 × 160	1	8:06	60
SE		T1	Sag	600	16	0.4	4.0	18		140	192 × 176	3	5:20	61
STIR			Sag	1340	14	0.5	5.0	24	75	140	192 × 160	2	7:11	64
SE		T1	Cor	600	13	0.4	4.0	24		140	192 × 192	3	5:49	68
STIR		T1	Cor	1190	11	0.4	4.0	24	75	180	192 × 160	3	9:33	103
						Foot								
SE		T1	Axial	680	20	0.5	3.5	18		150	192 × 192	3	6:34	51
SE		T2	Axial	2800	19	0.5	3.5	80		160	192 × 160	1	7:33	86
SE		T1	Cor	450	10	0.4	4.0	24		170	192 × 160	3	3:38	82
STIR			Cor	1080	10	0.4	4.0	24	85	190/140	192 × 144	3	5:45	77
SE		T1	Sag	620	18	0.5	3.5	18		160	192 × 192	3	5:59	56
						Elbow								
SE		T1	Axial	620	18	0.4	4.0	18		140	192 × 192	3	5:59	59
SE		T2	Axial	3000	13	1.0	5.0	100		140	192 × 160	1	8:06	75
SE		T1	Cor	600	13	0.4	4.0	24		140	192 × 192	3	5:49	68
STIR			Cor	900	10	0.8	4.0	16	75	140	192 × 160	2	4:51	53
SE		T1	Sag	580	15	0.4	4.0	18		140	192 × 192	4	7:28	67
						Wrist or Hand								
SE		T1	Axial	550	16	0.4	4.0	18		120	192 × 160	4	5:55	53
SE		T1	Cor	500	12	0.4	4.0	20		120	192 × 176	4	5:55	52
STIR			Cor	1150	12	0.4	4.0	24	75	140	192 × 160	2	6:10	50
GE		TE	Cor	540	12	0.4	3.5	16	Flip angle 45	130	192 × 176	4	6:23	47
SE		T1	Sag	690	18	0.4	4.0	20		120	192 × 192	3	6:40	48
SE		T2	Axial	3000	16	0.4	4.0	90		120	192 × 160	1	8:06	54

Cor, coronal; FOV, field of view; GE, gradient-echo; Sag, sagittal; SE, spin-echo; STIR, short-tau inversion recovery.

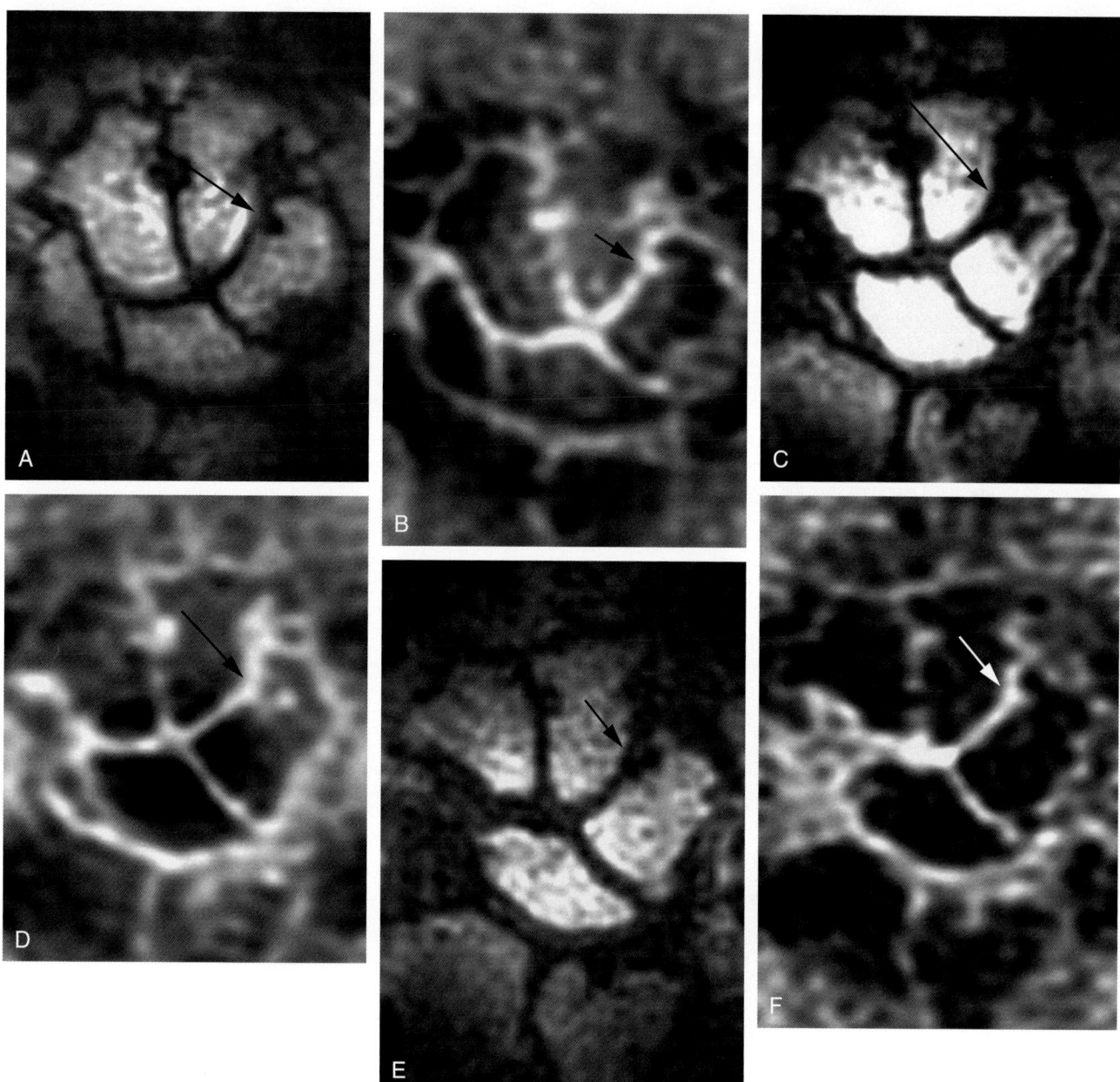

FIGURE 112-2

Change in triquetral erosion in a rheumatoid arthritis patient started on infliximab in August, 2002. **A,** T1-weighted coronal MagneVu image acquired on August 26, 2002, with 1.0 mm isotrophic resolution shows a distal triquetral erosion *(arrow).* **B,** The STIR image shows typical increased signal of an untreated erosion *(arrow).* **C,** Follow-up T1-weighted image on January 21, 2003, shows enlargement of the erosion in spite of intensive treatment *(arrow).* **D,** The follow-up STIR shows loss of signal intensity *(arrow).* **E** and **F,** T1-weighted 0.6 mm isotrophic images performed on July 7, 2003, show marked improvement after 11 months of treatment *(arrows).*

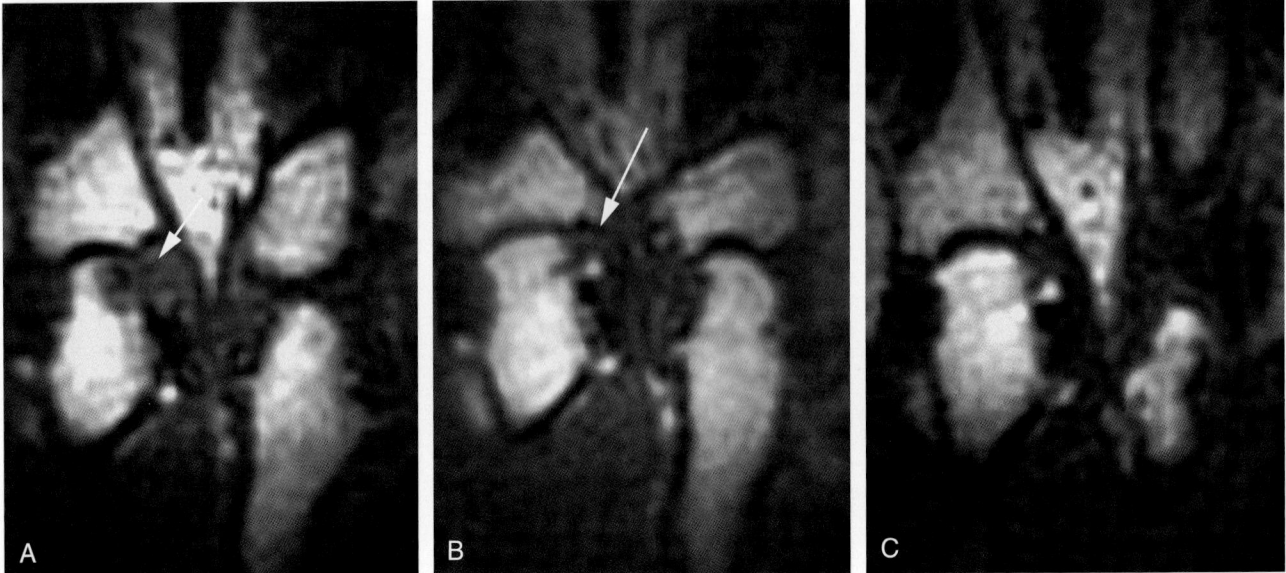

FIGURE 112-3

Progressive improvement in third metacarpal head erosion over two 6-month intervals in a rheumatoid arthritis (RA) patient on TNF-alpha inhibitors. **A,** Initial T1-weighted image shows a typical acute RA erosion *(arrow).* **B,** Marked decrease in erosion after 6 months of therapy is shown *(arrow).* **C,** Continued improvement is present over the next 6-month period on persistent therapy.

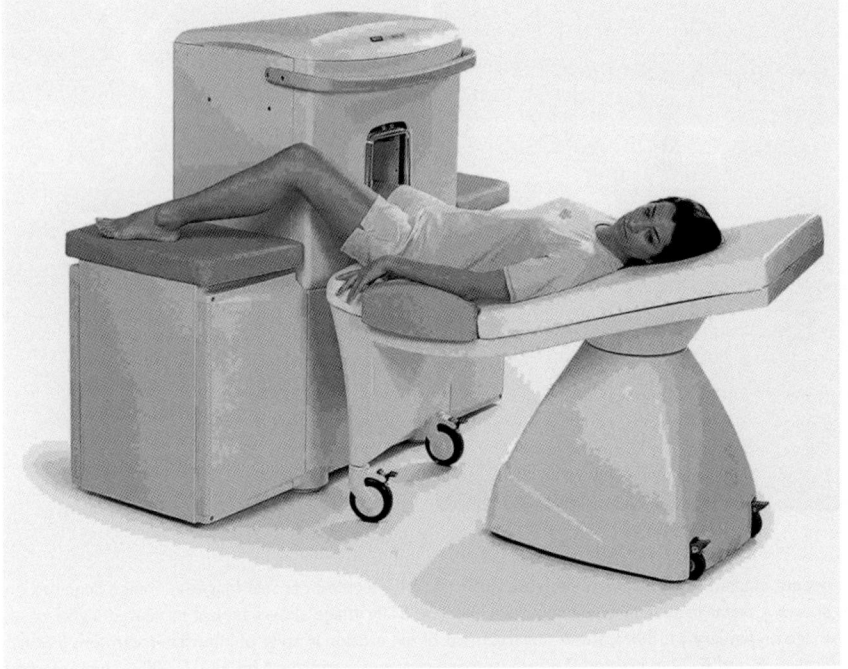

FIGURE 112-4

The Esaote C-Scan is a compact extremity MR scanner with internal shielding, requiring a dedicated room.

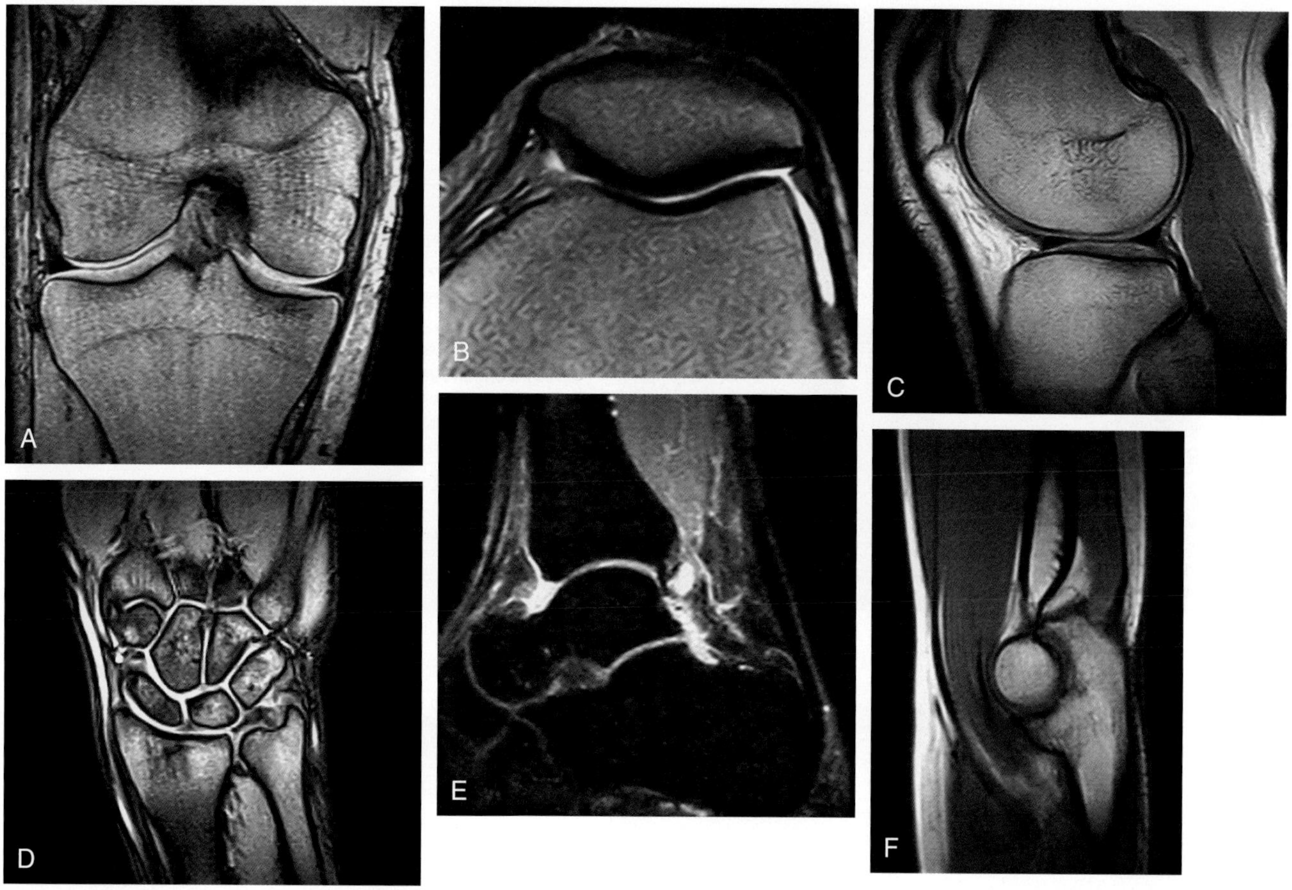

FIGURE 112-5

Images from the C-Scan extremity scanner. **A,** T1-weighted gradient-echo coronal image displays detailed knee anatomy. **B,** T2-weighted axial sequence clearly shows normal patellar and trochlear articular cartilage. **C,** The menisci are well seen with a T1-weighted sagittal technique. **D,** The triangular fibrocartilage is well seen on this coronal gradient-echo image of the wrist. **E,** A STIR sagittal sequence depicts the bone of the normal ankle without marrow edema. **F,** This sagittal T1-weighted image is typical of the image quality of the C-Scan in evaluating the elbow.

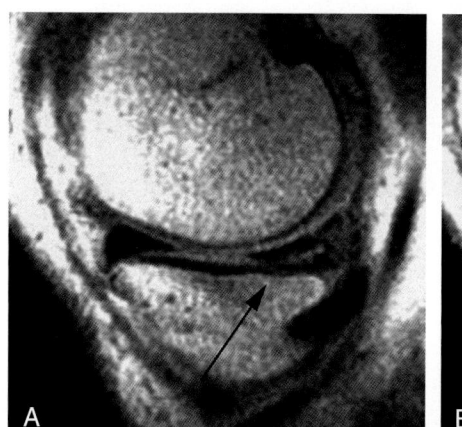
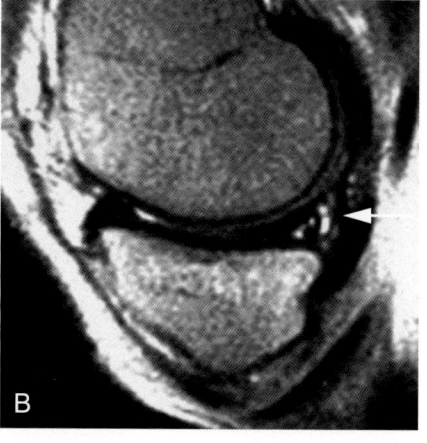

FIGURE 112-6

Image from an Esoate Artoscan of a tear of the posterior horn of the medial meniscus. **A,** T1-weighted sagittal image shows linear increased signal intensity within the posterior horn extending to the inferior articular surface *(arrow)*. **B,** T2-weighted image shows joint fluid extending through the tear into a small parameniscal cyst *(arrow)*.

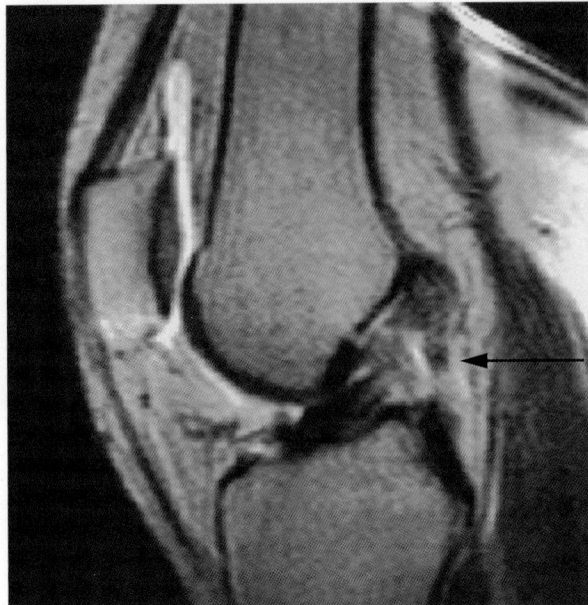

FIGURE 112-7

Anterior cruciate ligament (ACL) injury. An acute tear of the ACL is detected on this T2-weighted sagittal image *(arrow)* from an Artoscan.

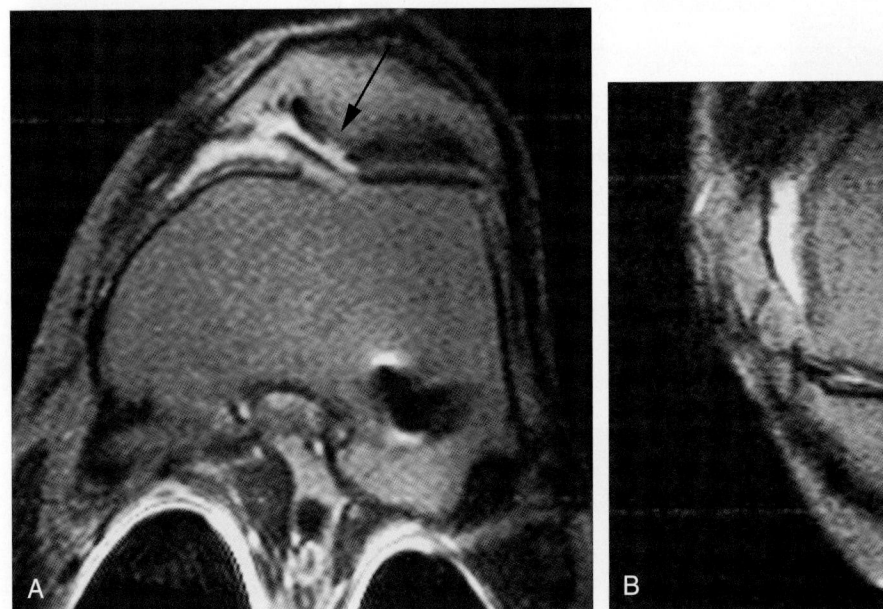

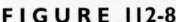

FIGURE 112-8

Articular cartilage injuries. **A,** T2-weighted axial sequence from an Artoscan evaluates an injury to the articular cartilage of the patella *(arrow)*. **B,** Diffuse articular cartilage thinning is well visualized on this sagittal T2-weighted image of the medial femoral condyle *(arrows)*.

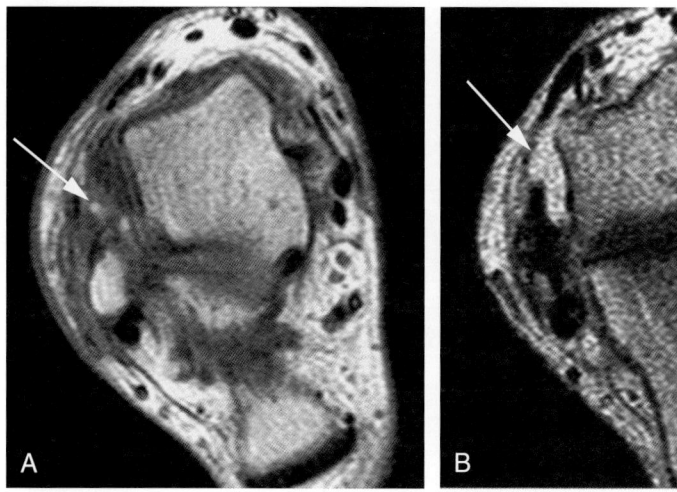

FIGURE 112-9

Anterior talofibular ligament tear. **A,** T1-weighted axial image shows disruption of the anterior talofibular ligament *(arrow)*. **B,** The acute tear is seen with improved contrast on the T2-weighted image *(arrow)*.

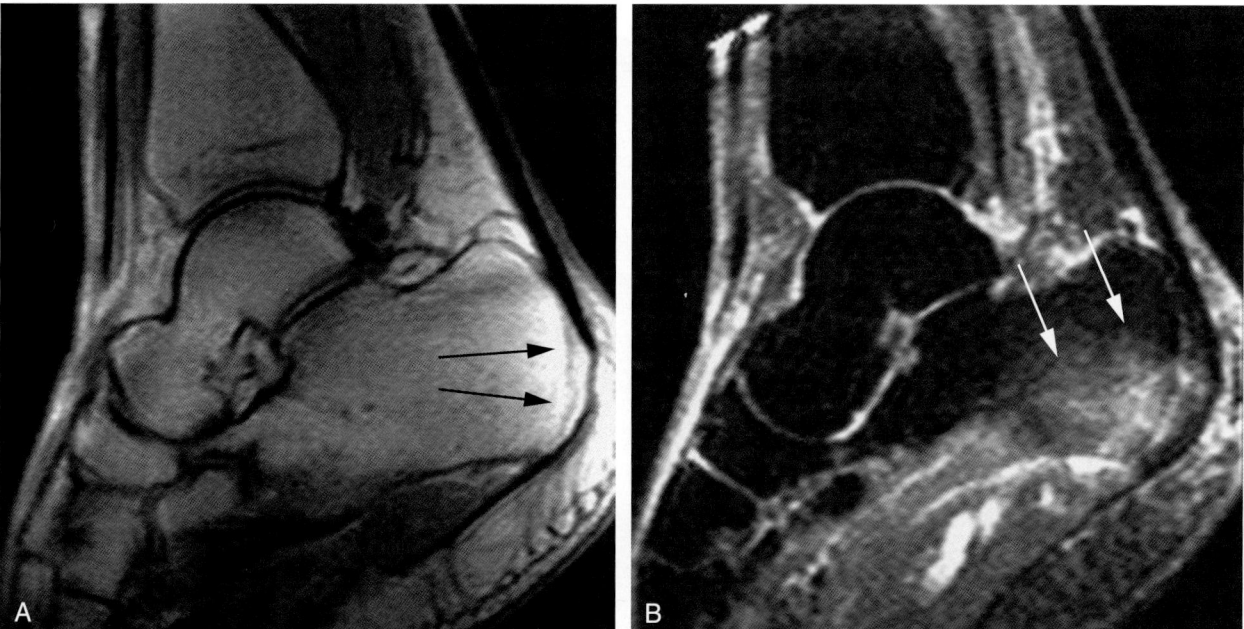

FIGURE 112-10

Calcaneal stress fracture. **A,** A subtle low-signal-intensity line may represent a nondisplaced fracture on T1-weighted sagittal images *(arrows)*. **B,** Marrow edema is much more evident within the injured calcaneus on the STIR sequence *(arrows)*.

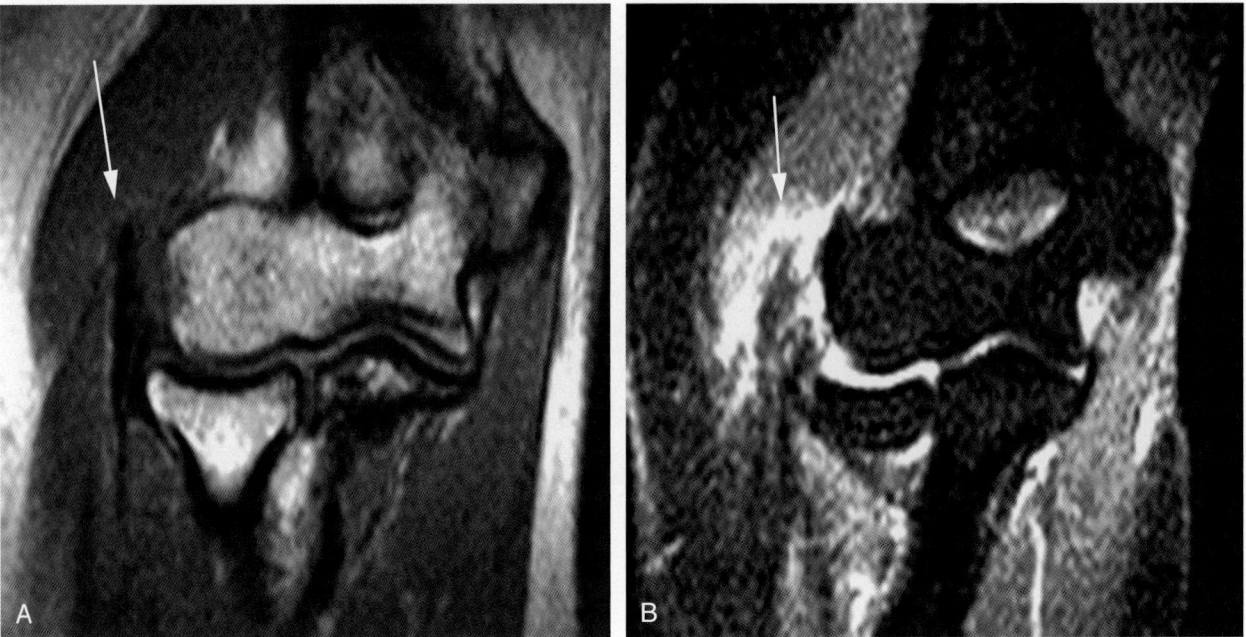

FIGURE 112-11

Common extensor tendon tear. **A,** Increased signal intensity is seen at the origin of the common extensor tendon on the T1-weighted coronal sequence *(arrow)*. **B,** STIR images display greater contrast in delineating the injury *(arrow)*.

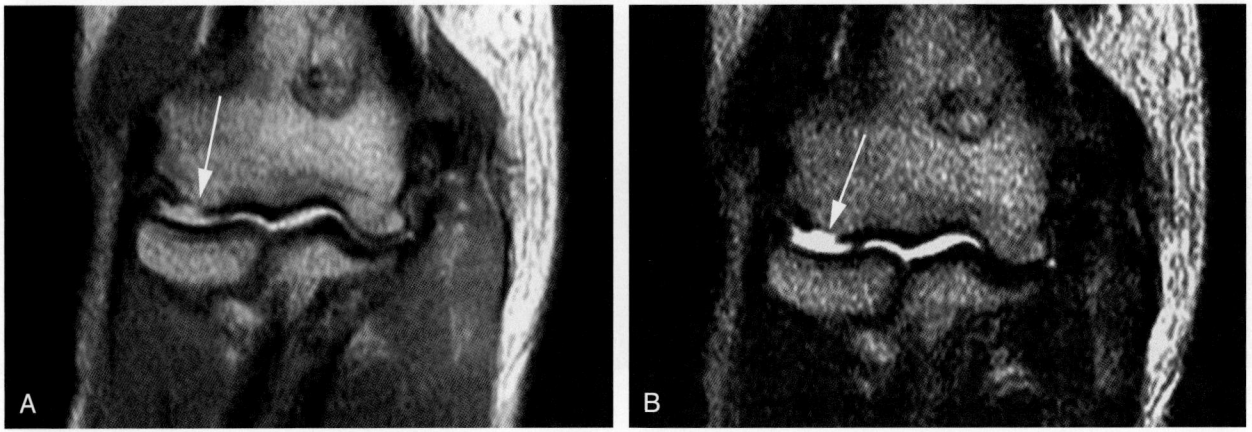

FIGURE 112-12

Capitular articular cartilage injury. **A,** A focal full-thickness defect in the articular cartilage of the capitulum is shown on this T1-weighted coronal image *(arrow)*. **B,** Fluid filling the defect is better seen on the T2-weighted image *(arrow)*.

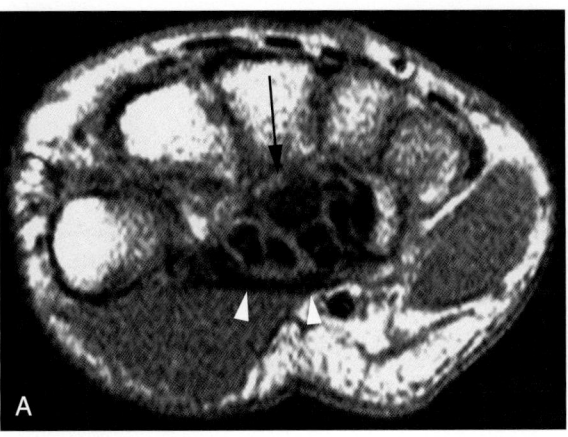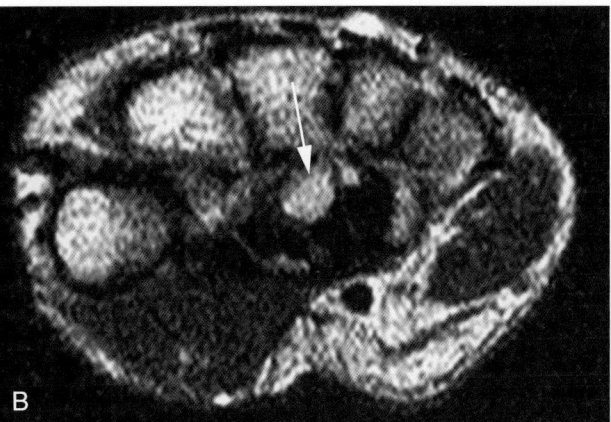

FIGURE 112-13

Carpal tunnel syndrome from mass effect of a ganglion cyst. **A,** A low-signal-intensity cyst *(arrow)* in the carpal tunnel produces mass effect and bowing of the flexor retinaculum *(arrowheads)* in a patient with symptoms of carpal tunnel syndrome. **B,** The cyst is high signal intensity on T2-weighted axial images *(arrow)*.

E-Scan

The E-scan MRI device is also manufactured by the Esaote Company in Genoa, Italy, and marketed in the United States by General Electric Medical Systems. The protocols we use with this scanner are given in Table 112-4. Specifically designed with open access to the imaging volume (Fig. 112-14), the E-scan allows examination of not only the distal extremities like the C-scan, but also the shoulder (Fig. 112-15) and the hip, with image quality and accuracy at least as good in our experience as 0.2 T whole-body scanners.[27] The permanent magnet poles are located above and below the table, making this a vertical field scanner with magic-angle artifacts similar in location to those seen on typical whole-body open MRI devices. The table rotates around the magnet poles, which helps in positioning patients, especially those who experience claustrophobia in whole-body units.

The E-scan allows for evaluation of numerous musculoskeletal pathologies, including flexor tenosynovitis of the wrist (Fig. 112-16), supra- and infraspinatus tendon tears (Fig. 112-17),[27] little league elbow injury (Fig. 112-18), and anterior cruciate ligament graft tears (Fig. 112-19). We have found T2-weighted images in patients scanned on the Artoscan and E-scan devices to correlate well with arthroscopic findings in over 70% of lesions showing grade III or IV changes at surgery (unpublished data) (Fig. 112-20).[25]

The E-scan has a larger acquisition FOV than the C-scan, and thus evaluates larger areas around the major joints with less peripheral distortion. For medium-sized orthopedic practices the additional ability to scan shoulders can have significant impact on financial performance as discussed below.

Text continues on page 3665

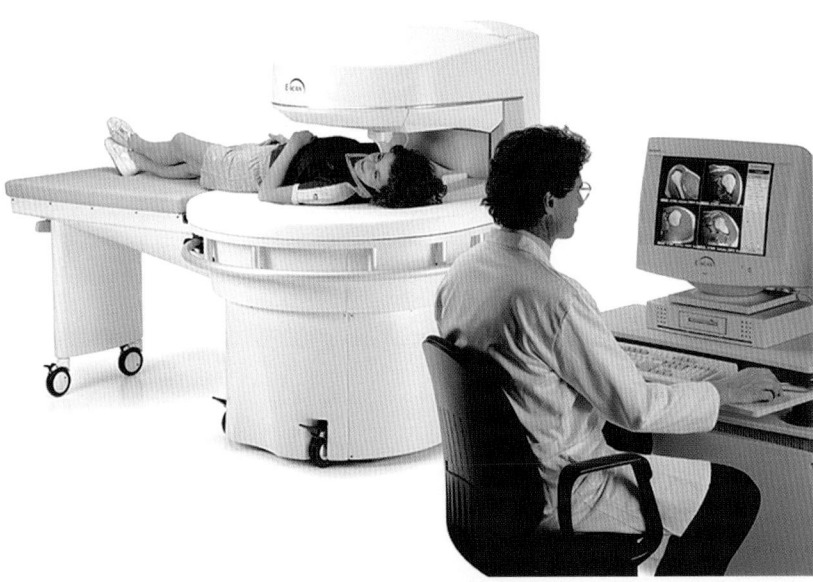

FIGURE 112-14

Esaote E-Scan. The open design of the Esaote E-Scan allows imaging of the hip and shoulder in addition to extremity joints. This design requires radiofrequency shielding of the walls of a dedicated room, and is thus more expensive to install than the MagneVu or the C-Scan.

TABLE 112-4 Imaging Protocols for the Esaote E-scan

Pulse Sequence	Mode	Contrast	Plane	TE (ms/deg)	TI/Flip (ms)	No. of Acquisitions	FOVs (mm)	Samples (ms)	Phases (ms)	Hamming Filter	Thickness	Gap	No. of Slices	TR
Shoulder														
SE HF	2D	T1	Ax Ref	18		1	160/160	192	128		5	1	11	400
SE	2D	T1	Cor	24		2	140/140	192	160		5	0.5	12	580
SE	2D	T2	Cor	80		1	140/140	192	160		5	0.5	12	2400
GE	2D	T2	Ax	74	75	2	140/140	192	160		5	0.5	14	630
SE	2D	T1	Ax	24		2	140/140	192	160		5	0.5	14	680
SE	2D	T2	Sag	80		1	140/140	192	160		5	0.5	12	2400
STIR	2D	Fat up	Cor	24	80	2	140/140	192	128		5	0.5	12	1850
Ankle/Heel														
SE HF	2D	T1	Ax Ref	18		1	140/140	192	128		4	1	11	400
SE	2D	T1	Axial	24		2	130/130	192	160		4	1	16	775
TSE	2D	T2	Axial	80		1	130/130	192	160		4	1	16	2360
SE	2D	T1	Cor	24		2	120/120	192	160		4	1	16	770
SE	2D	T1	Sag	24		2	130/130	192	160		4	1	12	580
STIR	2D	Fat Sup	Sag	24	75	2	140/140	192	160		5	1	10	1200
Knee														
SE HF	2D	T1	Ax Ref	18		1	160/160	192	128		4	1	11	400
SE	2D	T1	Sag	24		2	140/140	192	152		4	1	18	870
SE	2D	T2	Sag	80		1	140/140	192	152		4	1	18	2650
SE	2D	T1	Cor	24		2	140/140	192	152		4	1	18	870
STIR	2D	Fat Sup	Cor	30	75	1	140/140	192	128		6 or 7	1	13	1970
TSE	2D	T2	Axial	80		1	140/140	192	152		4	1	18	2650
Forefoot/Midfoot														
SE HF	2D	T1	Ax Ref	18		1	140/140	192	128		4	1	11	400
SE	2D	T1	Axial	24		2	140/140	192	160		4	1	16	
TSE	2D	T2	Axial	80		1	140/140	192	160		4	1	16	2360
SE	2D	T1	Cor	24		1	140/140	192	160		4	1	16	720
STIR	2D	T2	Cor	24	75	2	140/140	192	160		4	1	16	2560
SE	2D	T1	Sag	24		2	140/140	192	160		4	1	16	770
STIR	2D	Fat Sup	Sag	24	75	2	140/140	192	160		4	1	16	2260
Wrist/Hand														
SE HF	2D	T1	Ax Ref	18		1	120/120	192	128		4	1	11	400
SE	2D	T1	Axial	24		2	110/110	192	160		4	0.5	16	770
SE	2D	T1	Cor	24		2	130/130	192	160		3.5	0.5	11	560
STIR	2D	Fat Sup	Cor	24	75	2	130/130	192	128		3.5	0.5	11	1100
GE	3D	T1	Cor	16	40	1	110/110	192	176-24		2.5	0	52	32
SE	2D	T1	Sag	18		2	110/110	192	160		3.5	0.5	74	510
TSE	2D	PD/T2	Axial	80/90		1	110/110	192	160		4	0.5	15	

Continued

TABLE 112-4 Imaging Protocols for the Esaote E-scan—cont'd

Pulse Sequence	Mode	Contrast	Plane	TE (ms/deg)	TI/Flip (ms)	No. of Acquisitions	FOVs (mm)	Samples (ms)	Phases (ms)	Hamming Filter	Thickness	Gap	No. of Slices	TR
Finger														
SE HF	2D	T1	Ax Ref	18		1	120/120	192	128		4	1	11	400
SE	2D	T1	Axial	24		3	110/110	192	160		3	0.3	25	680
TSE	2D	T2	Axial	80		1	120/120	192	160		3	0.3	15	2360
SE	2D	T1	Sag	24		3	110/110	192	160		3	0.3	10	
STIR	2D	Fat Sup	Cor	24	75	2	110/110	192	160		3	0.3	10	1000
SE	2D	T1	Cor	18		2	130/130	192	160		3	0.3	10	680
Elbow														
GE	3D		Cor	16	40	1	130/130						52	
SE HF	2D	T1	Ax Ref	18		1	130/130	192	128		4	1	11	400
SE	2D	T1	Axial	24		2	130/130	192	152		4	1	18	870
TSE	2D	T2	Axial	80		1	130/130	192	152		4	1	18	2650
STIR	2D	Fat Sup	Cor	24	75	2	140/140	192	160		4	1	12	1410
SE	2D	T1	Cor	24		2	140/140	192	160		4	1	14	680
Hip														
SE	2D		Sag	24		2	140/140						14	
SE HF	2D	T1	Cor Ref	18		1	220/220	192	128		6	1	11	400
SE	2D	T1	Cor	26		3	220/220	192	176		6	0.6	11	560
TSE SE	2D	FT2	Sag	80		1	220/220	192	160		6	0.6	11	3000
SE	2D	T1	Sag	26		3	230/230	192	176		6	0.6	13	660
STIR	2D	Fat Sup	Cor	25	75	3	230/200	192	144		6	0.6	11	1100
Long Bone/Masses														
SE HF	2D	T1	Ax Ref	18		1	230/230	192	128		5	1	11	400
SE	2D	T1	Axial	24		3	230/230	192	160		5	1	15	680
TSE	2D	PD/T2	Axial	80		1	230/230	192	160		5	1	15	2300
STIR	2D	Fat Sup	Axial	24	75	2		192	160		5 or 6	1	10	1410
SE	2D	T1	Sag	24		3		192	160		5	1	12	540
SE	2D	T1	Cor	24		3		192	160		5	1	12	540
STIR	2D	STIR	Cor	24	75	2		192	160		5	1	12	1410

Ax Ref, axial reference image; Cor, coronal; Cor Ref, coronal reference image; Fat Sup, fat suppressed; FOV, field of view; FT2, fast spin-echo T_2; GE, gradient-echo; PD, proton density; Sag, sagittal; SE, spin-echo; SE HF, spin-echo half fourier transform; STIR, short-tau inversion recovery; TME, turbo multi-echo.

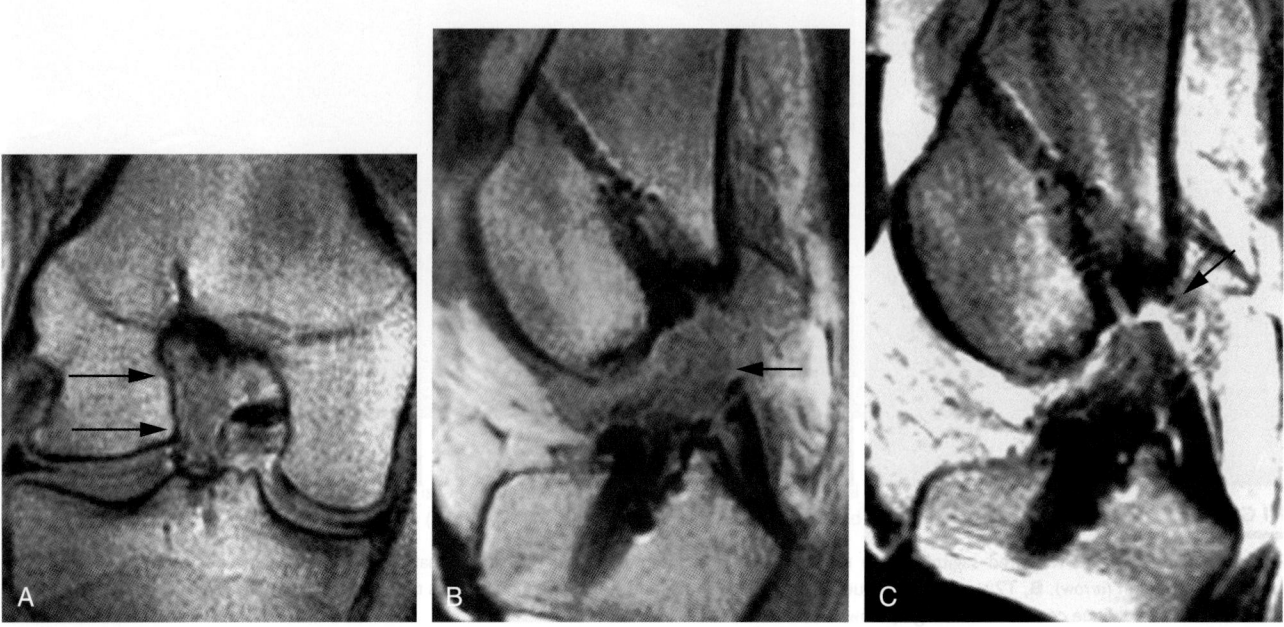

FIGURE 112-19

Anterior cruciate ligament graft tear. **A** and **B,** Diffuse high signal intensity is seen along the course of the ACL graft in the notch of the knee on T1-weighted coronal (**A**) and sagittal (**B**) images *(arrows)*. **C,** High signal intensity interrupting the graft is well displayed on the T2-weighted sagittal sequence *(arrow)*.

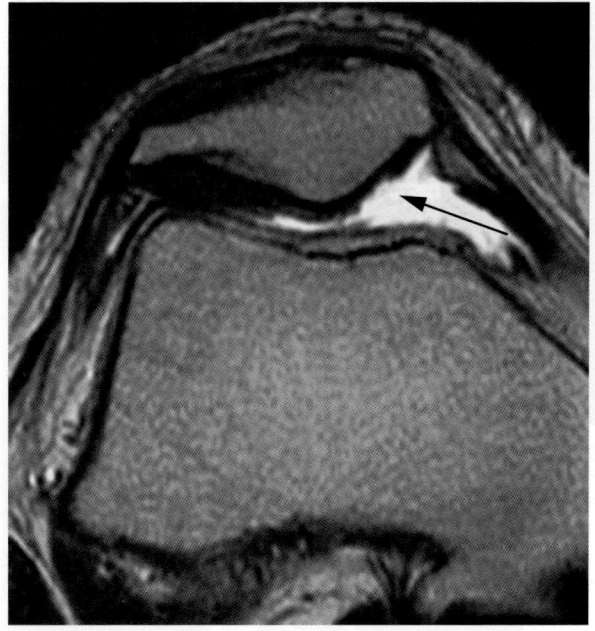

FIGURE 112-20

Patellar chondromalacia. T2-weighted axial and sagittal (not shown) images clearly delineate the surface irregularity and loss of articular cartilage in this patient with grade IV patellar chondromalacia *(arrow)*.

OrthoOne

The first three extremity scanners discussed use permanent magnets near 0.2 T. ONI's OrthoOne scanner is the only current extremity magnet known to the authors to image at a high magnetic field (1.0 T), thus benefiting from superior intrinsic contrast and SNR. Reminiscent of an over-grown beer keg with a hole through the long axis, the OrthoOne is a superconducting magnet with a restricted imaging volume, limiting its use to peripheral extremities similar to the C-scan device (Fig. 112-21). The image quality is in line with whole-body 1.0 T machines (Fig. 112-22), and our protocols are similar to those used in our whole-body scanners (Table 112-5), a few exceptions being noted below. Although to our knowledge its diagnostic accuracy has not been reported, we have found it to perform similarly to our 1.0 T whole-body magnets with two exceptions: 1. because of the restricted imaging volume the ankle must be scanned in plantar-flexion as in the C-scan (Fig. 112-23); 2. the magnet field is not sufficiently uniform across the imaging volume to allow spectral fat suppression across the entire knee or ankle, but uniform fat suppression is routinely obtained in small joints such as the wrist (Fig. 112-24). We find neither of these limitations a significant hindrance to superb imaging, as the anatomy of the ankle in plantar-flexion is easily learned and STIR imaging gives excellent fat suppression for detection of subtle soft-tissue and bone edema on the OrthoOne scanner.

The wide spectrum of extremity joint pathology displayed above and in other chapters of this textbook is also well evaluated by the OrthoOne. Figure 112-25 shows a rupture of the common extensor tendon of the elbow; however, subtle ankle injuries (Fig. 112-26) and wrist injuries (Fig. 112-27) are also well seen with the OrthoOne.

TABLE 112-5 Imaging Protocols for the ONI OrthoOne

Plane	Contrast	TR	TE	TI (ms/deg)	FOV	Freq Phase
Elbow						
Cor	IR	3800	15.3	90	15	256 × 192
Cor	T1	800	14		15	288 × 192
Axial	T1	900	15.6		12	288 × 192
Axial	T2	3000	120		12	256 × 192
Sag	T1	800	15		15	288 × 192
Wrist						
Cor	IR	4400	16.9	90	100	256 × 192
Cor	T1	950	18		100	288 × 192
Cor	T2*	50	15		100	256 × 224
Axial	T2	3800	120	30	100	256 × 192
Axial	T1	950	18.8		100	288 × 224
Sag	T1	900	17.4		100	288 × 224
Knee						
Axial	T2	3000	120		150	256 × 192
Sag	PD	2300	15.2		150	320 × 224
Sag	T2	2600	120		150	320 × 192
Cor	T1	850	14.8		150	320 × 192
Cor	IR	5000	14	90	150	256 × 192
Obl Cor (ACL)	T2	1800	120		140	256 × 192
Ankle						
Sag	T1	800	15		150	288 × 192
Sag	IR	4000	15.3	90	150	256 × 192
Obl Cor	PD	2000	19		140	288 × 224
Axial	T2	3000	120	90	140	256 × 192
Axial	T1	950	14		140	288 × 192
Foot						
Sag	IR	4200	14	90	150	256 × 192
Sag	T1	900	15.4		150	288 × 224
Cor	IR	3600	14	90	150	256 × 192
Cor	T1	700	15.9		150	320 × 192
Axial	T1	950	15.4		120	320 × 192
Axial	T2	3000	120		120	256 × 192
Hand/Finger						
Sag	T1	650	18.1		140	320 × 192
Sag	IR	2800	17.6	90	140	256 × 192
Cor	T1	650	20.2		140	320 × 192
Cor	IR	3000	17.6	90	140	
Cor	T1	50	15	30	100	256 × 192
Axial	T1	900	17.4		100	
Axial	T2	3000	120	90	100	

Cor, coronal; FOV, field of view; IR, inversion recovery; Obl Cor, oblique coronal; PD, proton density; Sag, sagittal.

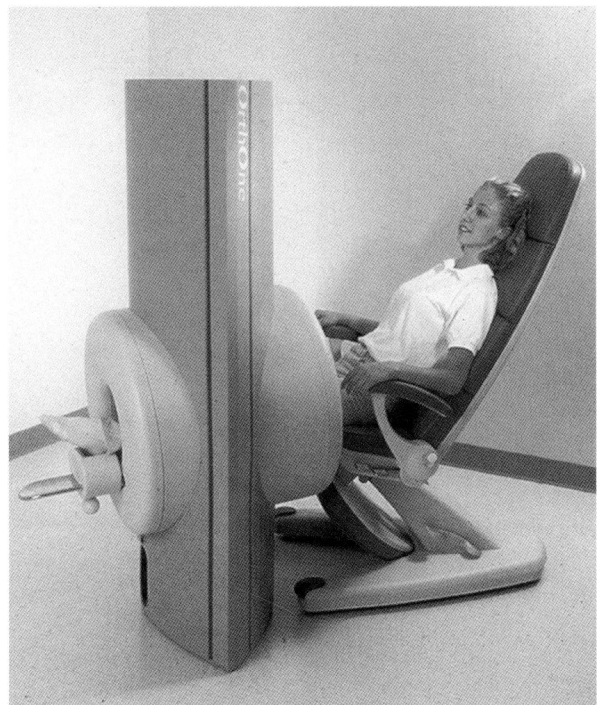

FIGURE 112-21

The OrthoOne scanner from ONI. The OrthoOne is a high-field (1.0 T) superconducting MR scanner with an open arrangement in which only the patient's extremity is placed within the device.

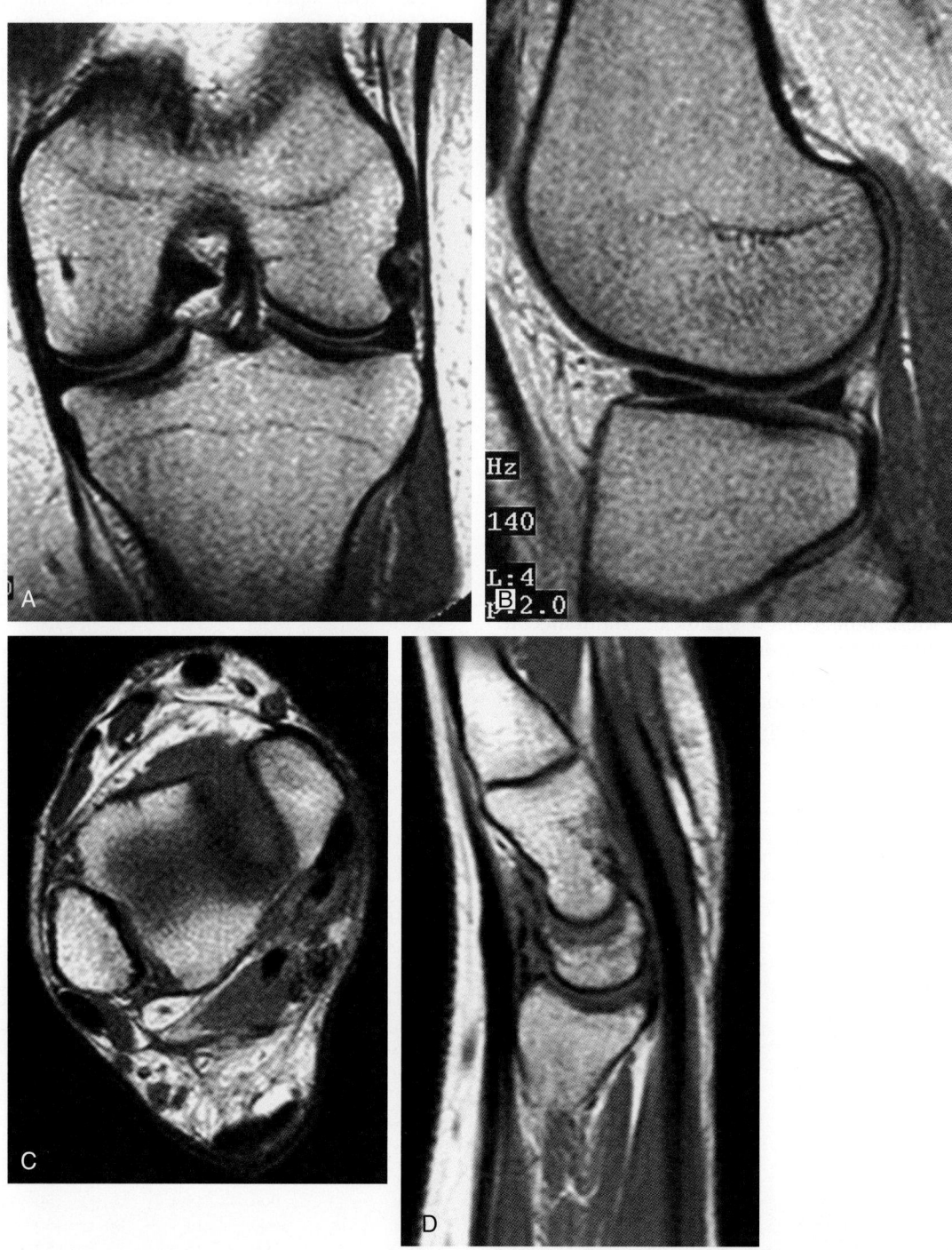

FIGURE 112-22

OrthoOne images. **A,** T1-weighted coronal images of the knee show signal-to-noise ratios and contrast similar to whole-body 1.0 T imagers. **B,** Sagittal proton density–weighted images allow excellent visualization of the menisci. **C,** Axial images through the ankle show exquisite anatomic detail. **D,** The lunate is normally oriented with respect to the capitate on this normal T1-weighted sagittal image through the wrist.

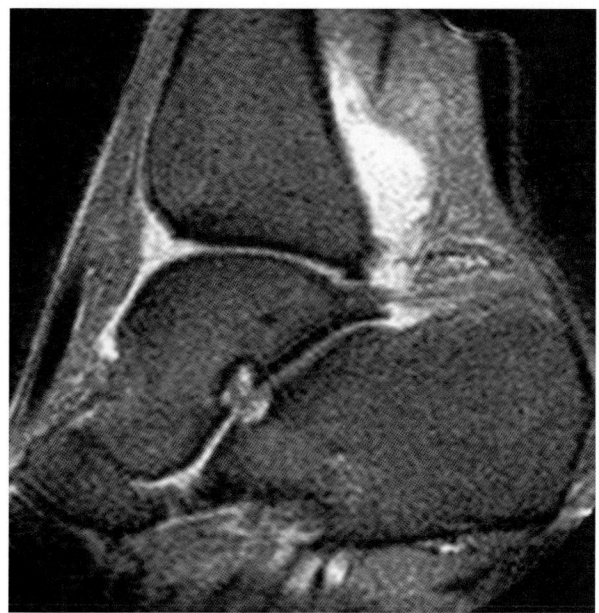

FIGURE 112-23

Mortise joint effusion. This T2-weighted OrthoOne image shows a large effusion in the mortise joint.

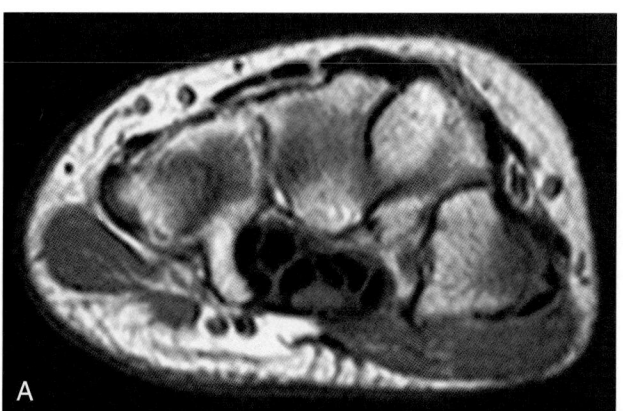

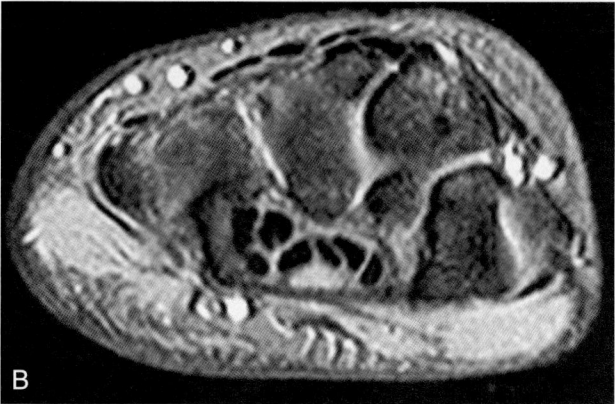

FIGURE 112-24

T1 and spectral fat-suppressed proton density–weighted image of the wrist using the ONI scanner. **A,** Non–fat-suppressed axial T1-weighted image clearly depicts the anatomy of the wrist. **B,** Uniform spectral fat suppression is seen on this proton density–weighted fat-suppressed image in the same location as in **A.**

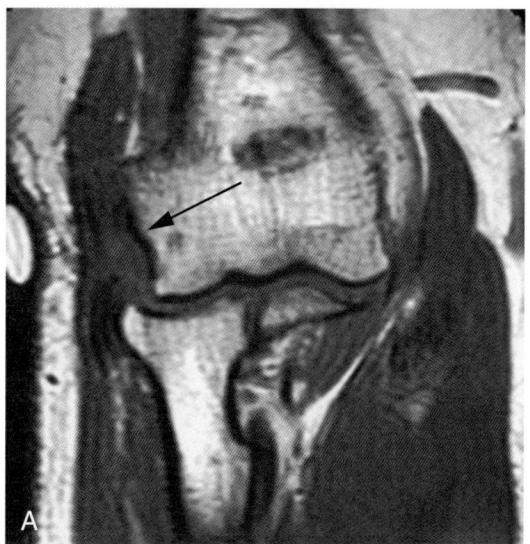

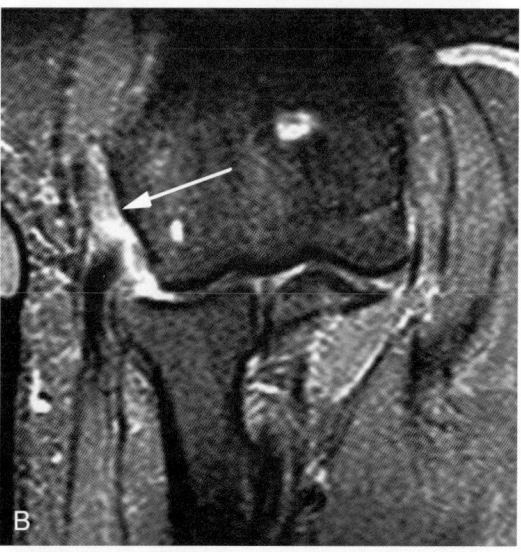

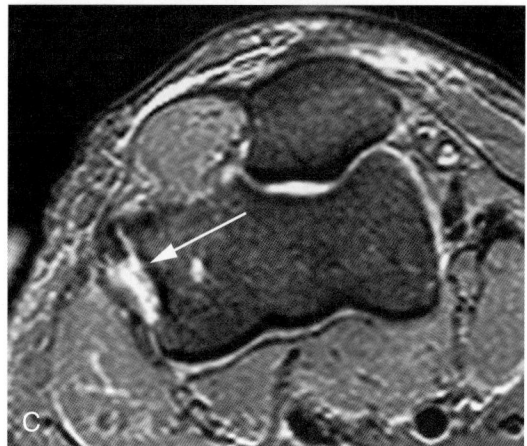

FIGURE 112-25

Common extensor tendon rupture using the ONI scanner. **A,** A marker placed on the skin on the lateral side of the elbow joint shows where the patient's pain is located, perfectly consistent with the common extensor tendon rupture seen as high signal intensity interrupting the origin of the tendon with the lateral epicondyle *(arrow)*. **B,** The edema is readily apparent on the T2-weighted images *(arrow)*. **C,** The fat-saturated T2-weighted axial image shows high signal intensity in the region of the tear *(arrow)*.

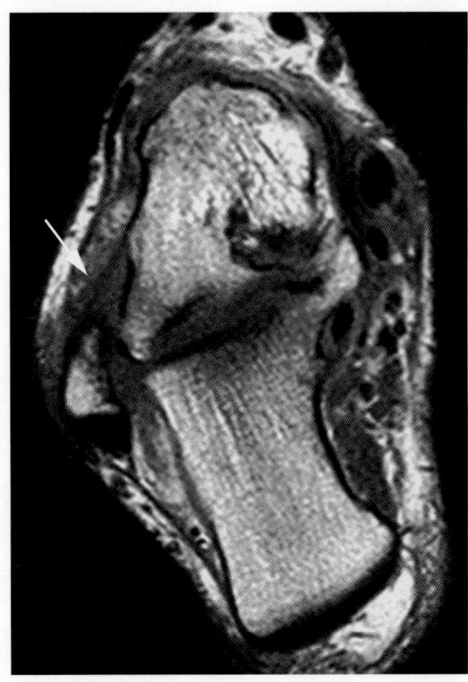

FIGURE 112-26

Anterior talofibular ligament sprain on ONI scanner. This T1-weighted axial image shows indistinctness of the margins of the anterior talofibular ligament and increased signal intensity within the ligament *(arrow)*.

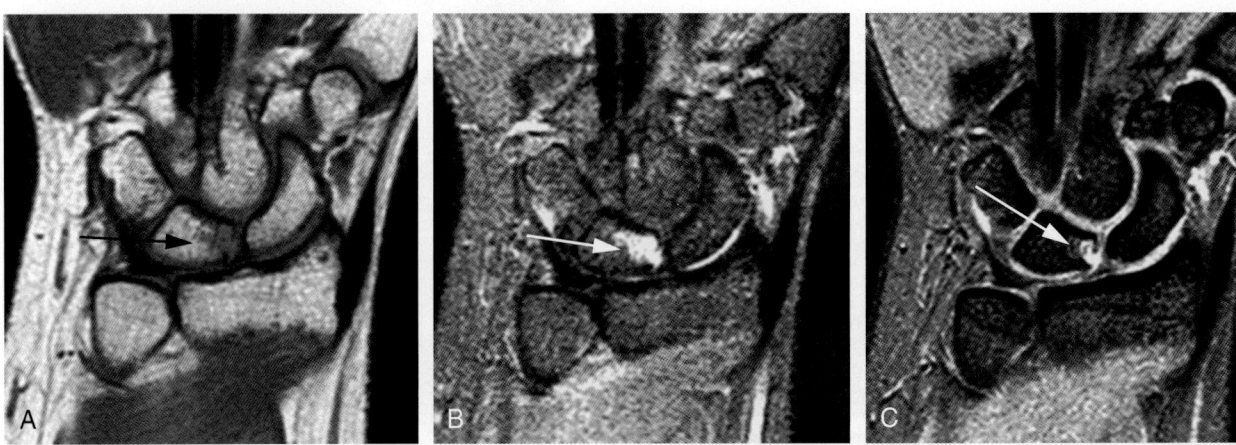

FIGURE 112-27

Lunate injury on ONI scanner. **A,** Low signal intensity consistent with edema is seen in the lunate in a patient with subacute trauma *(arrow)*. **B** and **C,** The edema is better depicted as high signal intensity on fat-suppressed T2-weighted images *(arrows)*.

IMPLEMENTATION

Why Use Extremity Scanners?

The major forces driving the use of extremity scanners are medical, patient acceptance, and financial. In numerous musculoskeletal injuries, such as X-ray–occult, subchondral bone injuries, delay in diagnosis causing a delay in treatment can be detrimental.[28-30] The presence of the MR scanner in the treating orthopedic clinic may lead to more rapid diagnosis and immediate treatment. "One-stop shopping," where the patient can get diag-

nostic and therapeutic care in one location and in one visit, is convenient for patients, can decrease time away from work, and allows the treating physician more control over the patient's entire medical encounter, providing a public relations advantage in competitive medical markets. The most compelling reason to install extremity magnets in treating physicians' offices is financial. Established offices can accurately determine the volume of MR imaging they have sent to imaging centers and hospitals, as well as the percentage of patients whose medical plans require their imaging to be performed at contracted imaging facilities. Knowing patient volume can minimize the financial risk of installing an in-office scanner, not unlike hospital decisions in implementing imaging for inpatients. Much of the uncertainty inherent in decision-making in outpatient imaging centers where the referral sources are not controlled by the investor is eliminated.

The impact on radiologists is somewhat more complicated. For groups who own MR scanners, in-office scanners are direct competitors, though many radiology groups continue to work with their referring physicians and perform the professional interpretation of the imaging of in-office scanners to maintain important relationships. For radiologists who do not own imaging equipment, in-office scanners constitute a source of expansion of the practice requiring little capital investment. In the United States and most of Western Europe, the standard of practice is for trained radiologists to interpret all MR imaging studies.

Although the lower costs associated with extremity scanners provide the potential for smaller charges to patients, insurers, and government agencies, this has not yet been realized due to several factors. First, the reimbursement has to reflect not just the fixed and variable costs of providing the service, but also the amount of revenue generated. Since the daily volume of many in-office scanners is low, per-study reimbursement remains high to cover fixed costs. Second, the reimbursement system in the United States and other Western countries has become excessively rigid with billing codes and reimbursements controlled by federal governments, essentially fixing reimbursements for approved services and making any attempts at changing pricing cumbersome, occasionally (as with mammography) requiring an Act of Congress in the United States.

Pitfalls in the Use of Extremity Scanners

In spite of the advantages of in-office MR imaging, numerous potential problems loom over any such business venture including: the potential for suboptimal image quality, loss of quality control by the radiologist, loss of referral base by radiologists, loss of income, and risk of over-utilization. As discussed above, image quality with modern scanners is primarily determined by field strength. With both high- and low-field-strength scanners on the market, image quality should be integrated into equipment selection, as will be described below. Quality control is a much more important and potentially troublesome problem in the operation of any MRI device. Lawsuits have already made their way through US courts from alleged patient losses due to poor quality control. Treating physicians and their office managers are not well schooled in MRI quality control; therefore, it is essential for the radiologist to recognize that part of his or her responsibility, as the professional component of the imaging team, is the supervision of quality control. As such, I believe that the radiologist should be responsible for establishing the imaging protocols, determine appropriate indications (with assistance from ACR guidelines), supervise the technologists, ensure the ability to obtain accurate clinical histories from the referring

physicians, design mechanisms to ensure the correct body parts are imaged, and maintain frequent, robust communications with the technologists and referring physicians. The owning physician group must institute policies and procedures to ensure that the equipment is maintained and operated according to the manufacturer's instructions.

Despite all of the political rhetoric flooding the airwaves since the Clinton administration, there has been little objective evidence documenting over-utilization of MRI in musculoskeletal medicine.[31-33] An unpublished study funded by the American Academy of Orthopedic Surgeons performed by the Battelle Medical Technology Assessment and Policy Research Center in 1993 showed that increased use of MRI of the knee would decrease the cost of treating knee injuries as long as the cost for MRI was less than $2000 per examination. This supports independent cost-efficacy analyses of MRI of the knee from Yale,[34,35] as well as others.[36] Since publication of these studies, utilization of MRI for joint evaluation has increased in the United States, and many experts have become concerned that ownership of MRI scanners by referring physicians may cause over utilization.[37-47] With over 400 extremity scanners operating in referring physician offices in the United States alone, studies evaluating utilization of in-office scanners would be valuable, but to our knowledge none has been published. Therefore, it is important that ACR guidelines for the use of MRI in musculoskeletal imaging be followed.

The Business of In-Office Extremity MRI

State and federal laws within the United States and other countries concerning ownership and financial relationships in medicine are complex and unlike regulations in other forms of commerce. It is essential therefore that local expertise in medical law be obtained before installing and operating an extremity MRI. Restrictions concerning joint ventures in diagnostic imaging equipment usually prohibit joint ventures between referring physicians and other professional organizations, so the most common business relationship for in-office MRI in the United States is for the treating physician to own the scanner and for the radiologist to contract to provide professional services to the ownership entity, similar to contractual relationships between radiology groups and hospitals. As opposed to inpatient services, the radiologist is often paid a per-scan fee by the owning corporation, allowing the patient to receive a single bill when reimbursement is from private sources. Separate billing for technical services from the treating physician and professional services from the radiologist may be prudent for all patients covered under government healthcare programs, such as Medicare and Medicaid.

Once the relationship between the physician groups has been finalized, proper selection of equipment is essential for success. Table 112-6 lists the specific joints imaged for each of the four extremity scanners. For rheumatology practices the selection is relatively straightforward, as most rheumatologists do not perform sufficient large joint MRI examinations to justify the

TABLE 112-6 Body Regions Imaged by Extremity Scanners

Scanner	Body Regions Imaged
MagneVu	Small joints of hand, wrist, and foot
C-Scan	Knee, ankle, foot, elbow, wrist, and hand
E-Scan	Knee, ankle, foot, elbow, wrist, hand, shoulder, and hip
OrthoOne	Knee, ankle, foot, elbow, wrist, and hand

TABLE 112-7 Estimates of Extremity Scanner Costs

Scanner	List Price ($)	Installation
MagneVu	150,000	Minimal
C-Scan	295,000	Minimal
E-Scan	547,680	Room shielding required
OrthoOne	495,000	Room shielding and vibration shielding required

added purchase cost and operational expenses of scanners designed for orthopedic evaluations. The MagneVu device is currently the optimal choice for most small rheumatology practices. Larger rheumatology practices, especially those interested in contrast-enhanced studies to follow changes in synovial volume, should also consider the C-Scan and OrthoOne, both of which are being actively used by rheumatology practices in the United States and Europe. Equipment selection is more involved for orthopedic practices, with three extremity and numerous whole-body magnets to consider. Table 112-7 lists the approximate costs for the four extremity scanners known to the author. For the small orthopedic practice limited primarily to treating distal extremity abnormalities, the C-scan is a highly effective and practical device when the practice can support at least two studies per day. For larger groups, especially if shoulder diseases constitute 15% or greater of the practice, the E-scan's ability to image shoulders can add significant volume. Both the purchase and installation costs of the E-scan are higher than the C-scan, so detailed financial analyses of the impact of increased volume versus increased costs are necessary to maximize profit when considering these two scanners from Esaote. For many groups the ability to provide a higher percentage of their patients' imaging needs in house favors purchase of the E-scan, even if the profit may not exceed that from a C-scan.

The in-office market for high-field scanners is driven by factors other than purely financial. The costs of the OrthoOne scanner are similar to the E-scan, but the joints imaged are the same as the C-scan. However, because of the improved image quality, the OrthoOne is a good choice for orthopedic groups predominantly treating extremity injuries where personal, medical, or competitive reasons require high-field imaging. In the United States few 0.2 T extremity scanners are successful in hospitals or outpatient imaging centers; however, half of the ONI installed base are in hospitals and imaging centers, where operators of busy high-field whole-body scanners can relieve backlogs by transferring joint imaging to an OrthoOne device at a fraction of the cost of installing an additional whole-body machine. For large orthopedic groups that have spine diseases as an extensive part of their practice, a whole-body scanner may be the appropriate in-office choice. When installing a whole-body unit, most practices in our experience have found high-field scanners to be preferable to low-field, open scanners, despite their higher costs.

As with any diagnostic imaging practice, effective communication between patients, technologists, radiologists, and treating physicians is essential. We have found the use of film as the medium for conveying image information to be problematic. Film is expensive; even simple image manipulation, such as windowing and leveling, is impossible, which in our experience limits diagnostic accuracy when interpreting low-field images. Film is not easily or rapidly transferred to other geographic locations, often severely impeding rapid interpretations when the radiologist and the scanner are in different locations, compromising one of the most important advantages for both the patient and the treating physician—the ability to diagnose and begin treatment on a single office visit. Therefore, most implementations of in-office scanners use PACS—electronic picture archiving and communications systems. Policy and procedures of in-office diagnostic imaging must also use the telephone and FAX equipment to maximize efficiency and accuracy of information transfer. Frequent communication between the entire imaging team makes possible the quality control supervision discussed above, even when the radiologist and scanner are in separate locations.

SUMMARY

A spectrum of MR scanners is now FDA approved and commercially available for in-office imaging for a wide range of rheumatologist and orthopedic practices. Successful implementation requires a well-organized team composed of the treating physician, MR technologist, radiologist, and support personnel using equipment matched to the practice's patient population. Expert legal advice, sophisticated communications systems, and well-thought-out policies and procedures are essential for proper quality control to maximize medical efficacy and financial success.

REFERENCES

1. Crues JV, Shellock FG, Dardashti S, et al: Identification of wrist and metacarpophalangeal joint erosions using a portable-MR system compared to conventional X-ray. J Rheumatol, 31(4):676-685, 2004.
2. Crues JV, Troum O, Dardashti S, et al: Identification of wrist and MCP joint erosions using a portable, low-field, extremity MR system: Results compared to conventional X-ray. In ISMRM, July 2003, Toronto.
3. Bresnihan B: Rheumatoid arthritis: Principles of early treatment. J Rheumatol 29(suppl 66):9-12, 2002.

4. Emery P: Evidence supporting the benefit of early intervention in rheumatoid arthritis. J Rheumatol 29(suppl 66):3-8, 2002.

5. Guidelines for the management of rheumatoid arthritis: 2002 update. Arthritis Rheum 46:328-346, 2002.

6. Kalden JR: Expanding role of biologic agents in rheumatoid arthritis. J Rheumatol 29(suppl 66):27-37, 2002.

7. Smolen JS, Emery P, Bamron V, et al: Treatment of early rheumatoid arthritis with infliximab plus methotrexate or methotrexate alone: Preliminary results of the ASPIRE trial. In European League Against Rheumatism 2003, Lisbon, Portugal.

8. Goldbach-Mansky RT, Murphy M, Flemming D, et al: T2-weighted MRI may define "active" carpal bone erosions in patients with early rheumatoid arthritis. In American College of Rheumatology, October 29, 2002, New Orleans.

9. Ostergaard M, Hansen M, Stoltenberg M, et al: MRI bone erosions in radiographically non-eroded rheumatoid arthritis wrist joint bones give a 4-fold increased risk of radiographic erosions five years later category: 16 RA–clinical aspects. In American College of Rheumatology, October 2002, New Orleans.

10. Benton NM, Perry D, Crabbe V, et al: Magnetic resonance scanning at first presentation predicts modified Sharp score at six years in patients with rheumatoid arthritis category: 16 RA—clinical aspects. In American College of Rheumatology, October 2002, New Orleans.

11. Lindegaard HM, Horgler-Petersen K, Vallo V, et al: Baseline MRI erosions in early rheumatoid arthritis MCP and wrist joint bones markedly increase the risk of radiographic erosions at 1 year follow-up category: 16 RA–clinical aspects. In American College of Rheumatology, October 2002, New Orleans.

12. Bird P, Lassere M, Carlton K, et al: MRI demonstrates progression of erosive damage in RA patients with disease duration greater than two years. In American College of Rheumatology, October 2002, New Orleans.

13. Conaghan PG, O'Connor P, McGonagle D, et al: Elucidation of the relationship between synovitis and bone damage: A randomized magnetic resonance imaging study of individual joints in patients with early rheumatoid arthritis. Arthritis Rheum 48:64-71, 2003.

14. Strand V, Sharp JT: Radiographic data from recent randomized controlled trials in rheumatoid arthritis: What have we learned? Arthritis Rheum 48:21-34, 2003.

15. Bird P, Lassere M, Shnier R, et al: Computerized measurement of magnetic resonance imaging erosion volumes in patients with rheumatoid arthritis. Arthritis Rheum 48:614-624, 2003.

16. Goldbach-Mansky RT, Woodburn J, Yao L, et al: Magnetic resonance imaging in the evaluation of bone damage in rheumatoid arthritis: A more precise image or just a more expensive one? Arthritis Rheum 48:585-589, 2003.

17. Boutry N, Larde A, Lapegue F, et al: Magnetic resonance imaging appearance of the hands and feet in patients with early rheumatoid arthritis. J Rheumatol 30:671-679, 2003.

18. Cimmino MA, Innocenti S, Livrone F, et al: Dynamic gadolinium-enhanced magnetic resonance imaging of the wrist in patients with rheumatoid arthritis can discriminate active from inactive disease. Arthritis Rheum 48:1207-1213, 2003.

19. McQueen FM, Benton N, Perry D, et al: Bone edema scored on magnetic resonance imaging scans of the dominant carpus at presentation predicts radiologic joint damage of the hands and feet six years later in patients with rheumatoid arthritis. Arthritis Rheum 48:1814-1827, 2003.

20. Crues JV, Troum O: Detection of change in size of erosions in inflammatory arthritis using high-resolution in-office MRI. Arth Rheum 95:S169, 2004.

21. Ejbjerg B, Narvestad E, Szkudlarek M, et al: MRI of healthy wrist and finger joints occasionally shows changes resembling RA erosions and synovitis. In American College of Rheumatology, October 29, 2002, New Orleans.

22. Shellock FG, Crues JV: Aneurysm clips: Assessment of magnetic field interaction associated with a 0.2-T extremity MR system. Radiology 208:407-409, 1998.

23. Shellock FG, O'Neil M, Ivans V, et al: Cardiac pacemakers and implantable cardioverter defibrillators are unaffected by operation of an extremity MR imaging system. Am J Roentgenol 172:165-170, 1999.

24. Franklin PD, Lemon RA, Barden HS: Accuracy of imaging the menisci on an in-office, dedicated, magnetic resonance imaging extremity system. Am J Sports Med 25:382-388, 1997.

25. Shellock FG, Stone K, Crues JV: Evaluation of the knee using an extremity MRI system: Diagnostic findings compared to arthroscopy. Med Sci Sports Med 30:S123, 1998.

26. Peterfy CG, Roberts T, Genant HK: Dedicated extremity MR imaging: An emerging technology. Radiol Clin North Am 35:1-20, 1997.

27. Shellock FG, Bert JM, Fritts HM, et al: Evaluation of the rotator cuff and glenoid labrum using a 0.2-Tesla extremity magnetic resonance (MR) system: MR results compared to surgical findings. J Magn Reson Imaging 14:763-770, 2001.

28. Blum GM, Tirman PFJ, Crues JV III: Osseous and cartilaginous trauma. In Mink JH, Reicher MA, Crues JV, et al (eds): MRI of the Knee. New York: Raven Press, 1993, pp 295-332.

29. Delzell PB, Schils JP, Recht MP: Subtle fractures about the knee: Innocuous-appearing yet indicative of significant internal derangement. Am J Roentgenol 167:699-703, 1996.

30. Vellet AD: The evolution of post-traumatic osteoarthritis: Its relationship to occult post-traumatic subcortical fractures identified on MRI. Bildgebung 59:121-122, 1992.

31. Powe NR: Economic and cost-effectiveness investigations of radiologic practices. Radiology 192:11-18, 1994.

32. Saini S, Seltzer SE, Bramson RT, et al: Technical cost of radiologic examinations: Analysis across imaging modalities. Radiology 216:269-272, 2000.

33. Tigges S, Sutherland D, Manaster BJ: Do radiologists use the American College of Radiology Musculoskeletal Appropriateness Criteria? Am J Roentgenol 175:545-547, 2000.

34. Ruwe PA, Wright J, Randall RL, et al: Can MR imaging effectively replace diagnostic arthroscopy? Radiology 183:335-339, 1992.

35. Ruwe PA, McCarthy S: Cost-effectiveness of magnetic resonance imaging. In Mink JH, Reicher MA, Crues JV, et al (eds): MRI of the Knee. New York: Raven Press, 1993, pp 463-466.

36. Bui-Mansfield LT, Youngberg RA, Warme W, et al: Potential cost savings of MR imaging obtained before arthroscopy of the knee: Evaluation of 50 consecutive patients. Am J Roentgenol 168:913-918, 1997.

37. Armsrrong JDI: Self-referral: Opportunity for ethical dialogue, appropriate prohibition, and quality assessment. Radiology 186:73-74, 1993.

38. Evens RG: What to do about self-referral? Radiology 186:75-76, 1993.

39. Hillman BJ, Bernhardt LB, Rial WY, et al: 1991 RSNA special focus session on "The New Health Care": Impact on radiologists. Radiology 184:309-314, 1992.

40. Hillman BJ: Self-referral for diagnostic imaging. Radiology 185:633-634, 1992.

41. Kouri BE, Parsons RG, Alpert HR: Physician self-referral for diagnostic imaging: Review of the empiric literature. Am J Roentgenol 179:843-850, 2002.

42. Levin DC, Spettell CM, Rao VM, et al: Impact of MR imaging on nationwide health care costs and comparison with other imaging procedures. Am J Roentgenol 170:557-560, 1998.

43. Mitchell JM, Sunshine JH: Consequences of physicians' ownership of health care facilities—Joint ventures in radiation therapy. N Engl J Med 327:1497-1501, 1992.

44. Morreim EH: Unholy alliances: Physician investment for self-referral. Radiology 186:67-72, 1993.

45. Morreim EH: What to do about self-referral prohibition: A rejection that is long overdue. Radiology 186:79-82, 1993.

46. Muroff LR: Anti-self-referral legislation: A solution that is long overdue. Radiology 186:76-78, 1993.

47. Relman AS: "Self-referral"—What's at stake? N Engl J Med 327:1522-1524, 1992.

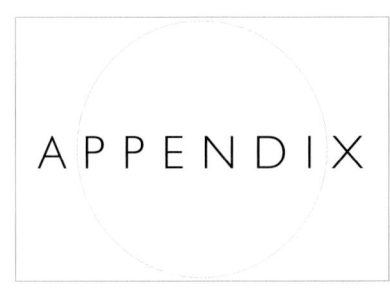

APPENDIX

MRI Scan Protocols

Robert R. Edelman, John R. Hesselink, Michael B. Zlatkin, and John V. Crues

Please note that the protocols should be read across two pages (double-page spread layout). The relevant protocol for each volume appears in the appendix for that volume only. The following protocols have been used on a General Electric Signa, 1.5-T magnet, software version 4.8, or a Siemens 1.5-T Vision, software version B2.5. Criteria used in developing these protocols include

1. Coverage of area of interest with appropriate slice thickness
2. Optimization of tissue contrast
3. Optimization of tradeoffs among signal-to-noise (S.N) ratio, spatial resolution, and scan time
4. Minimization of artifact induced by the patient
5. Maximization of safety of the patient
6. Maximization of throughput of patients

These are examples of protocols in use today and may not be optimal for a particular MRI system or clinical indication; their clinical efficacy is not guaranteed. Variations on these protocols are encouraged; sequence parameters should be selected that work best for the particular clinical setting and for the particular software and hardware configurations in use. Some sequences are not yet approved by the U.S. Food and Drug Administration for routine use and may require IRB permission.

RECOMMENDATIONS

- If fast spin-echo (FSE) sequences are not available, conventional SE sequences can be used but scan times are lengthened.
- Repetition time (TR) should be modified to accommodate adequate numbers of slices to span region of interest.
- For SE sequences, the TR and echo time (TE) can usually be varied substantially without degrading image contrast or S/N ratio.
- Depending on gradient capabilities, the TE may need to be increased to accommodate a lengthened readout (lower bandwidth) for small fields of view (FOVs).
- Number of excitations (NEX) varies depending on field strength, receiver coil, sequence bandwidth, and so on.
- Matrices are assumed to be number $\times$ 256 unless 128 $\times$ 128 or number $\times$ 512 acquisition is specified.
- Rectangular FOV should be used routinely for axial and sagittal acquisitions; reduce the number of phase-encoding steps accordingly to maintain the level of spatial resolution and decrease the scan time.
- Presaturation regions should be applied as needed to eliminate vascular signal. Minimal TR increased.
- If a multicoil array is not available for body applications, use a body coil; FOV or NEX may need to be increased to obtain adequate S/N ratio.
- Orient the phase-encoding gradient to minimize motion and wraparound artifact.
- For abdominal imaging, use respiratory motion compensation techniques (e.g., breath-hold, respiratory gating, navigator echoes, respiratory-ordered phase encoding [ROPE]).

Body MRI

Protocols from F Scott Pereles MD, John Salanitri MD, Charles Facanati BS RT, Terry Cunningham BS RT, Northwestern Memorial Hospital

Examination	Indications	Coil	Plane	Sequence	TR (ms)	TE (ms)
Chest wall		Body phased array		Scout		
			Axial (both sides chest)	T1 FS GRE	132	2.47
			Axial (both sides chest)	T2 HASTE	1000	57
			Sagittal (lesion side only)	T2 HASTE	1000	55
			Sagittal (lesion side only)[a]	T1 FS GRE	117	2.47
			Coronal (lesion side only)[b]	T1 FS GRE	100	2.47
			Axial (lesion side only)	T1 FS GRE	132	2.47
			Axial (lesion side only)[c]	T1 FS GRE	132	2.47
			Sagittal (lesion side only)[d]	T1 FS GRE	117	2.47
			Coronal (lesion side only)[e]	T1 FS GRE	100	2.47
Optional						
			Coronal[f]	T2 FS HASTE	785	100

Comments:
Mark lesion with Vitamin E capsule.
Contrast dose 20 mL (not to exceed 0.2 mmol/kg).
[a]Plane of lesion determines section plane. For anterior or posterior lesion do sagittals.
[b]Plane of lesion determines section plane. For lateral lesion do coronals.
[c]Breath-hold.
[d]Acquire 90 s after injection.
[e]Acquire 120 s after injection.
[f]Fat saturated. Use if lesion is lateral in position.

Protocols from Robert R Edelman MD, Wei Li MD, Roland Bejm RT, Eugene E Dunkle RT, Evanston Northwestern Hospital

Examination	Indications	Coil	Plane	Sequence	TR (ms)	TE (ms)
Chest wall and sternum	Mass Infection Trauma	8 Channel torso phased array	Coronal	Localizer	100	Min
			Sagittal	T1 SE	500	Min
			Axial	T1 SE	600	Min
			Axial	T2 FSE	5200	85
			Sagittal	FS T2 FSE	4225	85
			Coronal	FS T2 FSE	4000	85
			Coronal	T1 SE	550	Min
			Coronal	STIR FSE	5325	34
			Axial[a]	T1 FS 3D GRE	3.1	Min Full
			Axial[b]	T1 FS 3D GRE	3.1	Min Full

Comments:
[a]Pre-contrast.
[b]Post-contrast.

TI (ms)	FA (degrees)	FOV (cm)	SLTHK (mm)	SLSP (mm)	Matrix	NEX	Freq	BW	ET	Contrast
	70	36–40	4	1	256 × 164	1	LR	63.6		–
	150	36–40	5	0	256 × 206	1	LR	63.6	256	–
	150	28	5	0	256 × 197	1	SI	63.6	256	–
	70	28	4	1	256 × 140	2	SI	63.6		–
	70	28	4	1	256 × 164	1	SI	63.6		–
	70	28	4	1	256 × 164	1	LR	63.6		–
	70	28	4	1	256 × 164	1	LR	63.6		+
	70	28	4	1	256 × 140	2	SI	63.6		+
	70	28	4	1	256 × 164	1	SI	63.6		+
	150	36–40	5	1	256 × 154	1	SI	63.6		–

TI (ms)	FA (degrees)	FOV (cm)	SLTHK (mm)	SLSP (mm)	Matrix	NEX	Freq	BW	ET	Contrast
–	60	46	9	2	512 × 160	1	SI	62.5	–	–
–	–	30	5	1	256 × 128	3	SI	15.63	–	–
–	–	24	5	1	256 × 128	3	RL	15.63	–	–
–	–	24	5	1	256 × 160	3	RL	15.63	12	–
–	–	30	5	1	256 × 160	3	SI	15.63	12	–
–	–	26	3	1	256 × 160	4	SI	15.63	12	–
–	–	26	3	1	256 × 128	3	SI	15.63	–	–
150	–	26	3	1	256 × 160	3	SI	15.63	8	–
Auto	12	36	4	ZIP 2	256 × 160	1	RL	62.5	–	–
Auto	12	36	4	ZIP 2	256 × 160	1	RL	62.5	–	+

Protocols from F Scott Pereles MD, John Salanitri MD, Charles Facanati BS RT, Terry Cunningham BS RT, Northwestern Memorial Hospital

Examination	Indications	Coil	Plane	Sequence	TR (ms)	TE (ms)
Breast (bilateral)	Cancer	Breast phased array		Scout	3.75	1.88
			Axial	SE T1	525	17
			Axial	STIR	4870	63
			Coronal	STIR	5130	63
			Sagittal	STIR	8200	63
			Sagittal[a]	3D VIBE T1 FS GRE	4.3	1.76
			Sagittal[b]	3D VIBE T1 FS GRE	4.3	1.76

Comments:
Have a 40 s delay after the 1st measurement, then inject Gd (0.1 mmol/kg) at 2 mL/s. No delay between the remaining 4 measurements.
Subtract the 1st measurement from each of the remaining 4 measurements, make axial MPR and MIPs.
Send source data and STIR data to work station.
[a]Done to check fat saturation.
[b]Rerun the VIBE as 5 measurements.

Protocols from Robert R Edelman MD, Wei Li MD, Roland Bejm RT, Eugene E Dunkle RT, Evanston Northwestern Hospital

Examination	Indications	Coil	Plane	Sequence	TR (ms)	TE (ms)
Breast (bilateral)	Cancer	Phased array	3 planes[a]	Localizer	–	–
			Axial	ASSET calibration	–	–
			Sagittal[b]	T1 SE	600	Min
			Sagittal[c]	FS STIR FSE	4175	42
			Sagittal[d]	T1 FS 3D GRE	3.1	Min Full
			Sagittal[e]	T1 FS 3D GRE	3.1	Min Full
			Axial[f]	T1 High res SPGR	–	Min Full

Comments:
[a]Both breasts; center frequency on water.
[b]Do both breasts separately.
[c]Do both breasts separately; fat saturation.
[d]Pre-contrast FS GRE sequence of both breasts.
[e]Post-contrast FS GRE sequence of both breasts.
[f]High res. post-Gd axial.

Protocols from Robert R Edelman MD, Wei Li MD, Roland Bejm RT, Eugene E Dunkle RT, Evanston Northwestern Hospital

Examination	Indications	Coil	Plane	Sequence	TR (ms)	TE (ms)
Breast	Silicon gel implants	Breast phased array	Axial, both breasts	Scout	100	Min
			Sagittal, 1 breast[a]	T2 FSE	4475	85
			Sagittal, 1 breast[a,b]	STIR FSE Silicon sat	5150	34
			Axial, 1 breast[a,b]	STIR FSE Silicon sat	5150	34
			Axial, 1 breast[a]	T2 FSE	4475	85

Comments:
[a]Center on water frequency.
[b]Silicon saturation.

TI (ms)	FA (degrees)	FOV (cm)	SLTHK (mm)	SLSP (mm)	Matrix	NEX	Freq	BW	ET	Contrast
	60		6		128 × 102	1		63.6		−
		27	4	0.4	256 × 230	1	LR	63.6		−
160	180	27	4	0.4	256 × 205	1	LR	63.6	7	−
160	180	27	4	0.4	256 × 205	1	SI	63.6	7	−
160	180	20	4	0.4	256 × 192	1	SI	63.6	7	−
	12	20	1	288 images/slab	256 × 189	1	SI	63.6		−
	12	20	1	288 images/slab	256 × 189	1	SI	63.6		+

TI (ms)	FA (degrees)	FOV (cm)	SLTHK (mm)	SLSP (mm)	Matrix	NEX	Freq	BW	ET	Contrast
−	−	48	10	2	256 × 128	1	−	−	−	−
−	−	48	10	0	−	1	RL	−	−	−
−	−	20	4	0	256 × 192	2	AP	15.63	−	−
150	−	20	4	0	256 × 160	2	AP	20.83	8	−
−	12	18	3	ZIP 2	256 × 160	1	AP	62.5	−	−
−	12	18	3	ZIP 2	256 × 160	1	AP	62.5	−	+
−	12	30	3	0.5	384 × 224	1	AP	31.25	−	+

TI (ms)	FA (degrees)	FOV (cm)	SLTHK (mm)	SLSP (mm)	Matrix	NEX	Freq	BW	ET	Contrast
−	30	40	5	2	256 × 160	0.75	RL	15.63	−	−
−	−	16	5	1	256 × 160	2	SI	15.63	−	−
150	−	20	5	1.5	256 × 160	2	AP	20.83	−	−
150	−	18	5	1	256 × 160	2	AP	20.83	−	−
−	−	16	5	1	256 × 160	2	RL	15.63	−	−

Protocols from Fergus Coakley MD, University of California, San Francisco

Examination	Indications	Coil	Plane	Sequence	TR (ms)	TE (ms)
Abdomen	General	Torso	Axial	T1 FGRE dual	90–150	2.1, 4.2
			Axial[a]	FS T2 FRFSE	25–3000	100
			Coronal[b]	T2 SSFSE	Infinity	100
			Axial	Test bolus (FGRE)	Min	Min
			Axial[c]	T1 3D SPGR	Min	Min
Optional						
Abdomen	General	Torso	Axial[d]	SPGR	130	20
			Axial[e]	GRASS	30	6
			Axial[f]	FMPSPGR	90–150	4.2

Comments:
[a]Breath-hold.
[b]Non-fat sat T2 overview.
[c]Do pre- and post-Gd as per dynamic instructions.
[d]Breath-hold T2* if using feridex.
[e]Vasc evaluation. 2–3 slices/breath-hold, can substitute FFE/FIESTA/TrueFISP.
[f]Do before Gd if suspect AML/myelolipoma.

Dynamic contrast instructions
1. Precontrast scan. Use 3D spoiled GE sequence (Vasc TOF SPGR or FAME—GE: VIBE (fl3d_itn)—Siemens)
2. Test bolus sequence: oblique axial. Set to run for 2 min. Pt holds breath for as long as possible then quiet resp and another breath-hold for as long as possible at 1 mib. Start scan and injector simultaneously.
3. Review images to find time to peak (within 1st 30 s)
   GE/Phillips (centrically ordered k space): delay = time to peak + 2 s
   Siemens (sequential k space): delay = time to peak + (½ injection time) − (½ acquisition time).

Protocols from F Scott Pereles MD, John Salanitri MD, Charles Facanati BS RT, Terry Cunningham BS RT, Northwestern Memorial Hospital

Examination	Indications	Coil	Plane	Sequence	TR (ms)	TE (ms)
Abdomen	Liver and general	Body phased array	3 Plane	Scout	4.87	2.44
			Axial[a]	T1 GRE	224	2.4/4.76
			Coronal[b]	T2 HASTE	1000	54
			Axial	T2 HASTE	1000	54
			Coronal	FS T1 GRE	185	2.47
			Axial[c]	FS T1 GRE	250	2.47
			Coronal[d]	FS T1 GRE	185	2.47
Optional						
Abdomen	Liver and general	Body phased array	Axial[e]	TrueFISP	4.73	2.37
			Coronal	TrueFISP	4.73	2.37
			Axial[f]	GRE T2*		
			Axial[g]	FS T1 GRE	250	2.47

Comments:
Cover entire liver and pancreas.
20 mL Gd not to exceed 0.2 mmol/kg.
[a]In and opposed phases, saturation band placed above diaphragm.
[b]Non-breath-hold interleaved.
[c]Use fluoro prep for arterial phase, repeat at 60, 90, 120, and 180 s post-injection.
[d]Do at 90 s.
[e]Useful for portal vein thrombosis.
[f]Optional for hemochromatosis, hemosiderosis. Several slices through liver, spleen and pancreas.
[g]Do at 5, 10, 15 min delay if suspect cholangiocarcinoma, PSC, slow filling hemangioma.

TI (ms)	FA (degrees)	FOV (cm)	SLTHK (mm)	SLSP (mm)	Matrix	NEX	Freq	BW	ET	Contrast
40	46	10			256 × 128	1		63.6		
160	36–40	5	0		256 × 198	1	SI	63.6	256	−
160	36	5	0		256 × 198	1	LR	63.6	256	
160	36–40	3	0		256 × 198	1	SI	63.6	256	−
160	36	3	0		256 × 198	1	LR	63.6	256	
70	36	7	2		256 × 160	1	LR	63.6		−
150	36	20–40			320 × 320	1	SI	63.6	256	−
150	36	40			320 × 320	1	LR	63.6	256	−
180	36–40	1.5	40 images/slab		384 × 384	1	LR	63.6	127	−
80	36	6	1.8		256 × 128	1	LR	63.6		−
80	36–40	6	1.8		256 × 128	1	SI	63.6		−
80	36	6	1.8		256 × 128	1	LR	63.6		+
80	36–40	6	1.8		256 × 128	1	SI	63.6		+
60–90	36–40	5	0		256 × 180	1	SI	63.6		+
60–90	36–40	5	0		256 × 180	1	LR	63.6		+
80	36	6	1.8		256 × 128	1	LR	63.6		+
80	36–40	6	1.8		256 × 128	1	SI	63.6		+

TI (ms)	FA (degrees)	FOV (cm)	SLTHK (mm)	SLSP (mm)	Matrix	NEX	Freq	BW	ET	Contrast
	75	32–40	8	1	256 × 128–192	1	LR	16		
		32–40	5–6	1	256 × 160	1	LR	32	17	
		32–40	6	1	256 × 160–192	0.5	SI	62.5	100+	
		32–40	4	0	256 × 160–192	0.5		62.5	100+	
		32–40	20–40		320 × 320	0.5		62.5	100+	
		36	5	0	256 × 64	1	LR	62.5		
	15–20	32–40	6	50% overlap	320 × 160	0.5	LR	31		
	15–20	20–28	8	1	256 × 128–192	1	LR	16		
		32–40	5	1	256 × 128–192	1	LR	15		
	70	32–40	5–8	1	256 × 128–192	1	LR	16		
		32–40	4	0	256 × 160–192	0.5	SI	62.5	100+	

Protocols from F Scott Pereles MD, John Salanitri MD, Charles Facanati BS RT, Terry Cunningham BS RT, Northwestern Memorial Hospital

Examination	Indications	Coil	Plane	Sequence	TR (ms)	TE (ms)
Abdomen	Liver donor	Body phased array		Scout		
			Axial	TrueFISP	3.52	1.76
			Coronal	TrueFISP	3.52	1.76
			Axial[a]	T1 GRE	174	2.38/4.76
			Axial[b]	RARE	2800	1100
			Coronal[b]	RARE	2800	1100
			Axial[c]	FS T2 HASTE	1000	67
			Coronal[c]	FS T2 HASTE	1680	111
			Coronal[d]	3D 2D TSE	4206	673
			Sagittal[e]	Tming bolus	1000	1.16
			Coronal[f]	3D CE MRA	3.26	1.03

Comments:
18 g cannula in antecubital fossa vein; 40 mL Gd at 2 mL/s.
Post processing: Create two subtracted numbered sets from MRA—arterial and portal venous phases. AP MIP with aorta. AP MIP with aorta edited out. AP MIP of portal vein phase with aorta and IVC edited out. VR images as required.
[a]In/opposed phase.
[b]Thick slab RARE in AP, oblique orientations.
[c]Breath-hold sequence.
[d]Respiratory gated, cover biliary birfucation.
[e]2 mL Gd @ 2 mL/s.
[f]Do timing bolus, 1 pre-contrast and 2 post-contrast acquisitions. Breath-hold (insp.).

Protocols from F Scott Pereles MD, John Salanitri MD, Charles Facanati BS RT, Terry Cunningham BS RT, Northwestern Memorial Hospital

Examination	Indications	Coil	Plane	Sequence	TR (ms)	TE (ms)
Hepatic and mesenteric MRA		Body phase array		Scout		
			Axial[a]	T2 HASTE	1000	63
			Coronal[b]	T2 HASTE	1000	59
			Axial	T1 FS GRE	250	2.47
			Coronal	T1 FS GRE	187	2.47
			Sagittal	Timing bolus	1000	1.19
			Coronal[c]	3D CE MRA	3.26	1.08
			Axial	T1 FS GRE	250	2.47
			Coronal	T1 FS GRE	187	2.47

Comments:
Post processing: Two subtracted 3D sets from MRA (arterial and venous). Coronal arterial phase MIP. Sagittal MPR through mesenterics. VR as needed.
40 mL Gd not to exceed 0.3 mmol/kg.
[a]Non-breath-hold; cover liver and kidneys.
[b]Anterior spine to front of liver.
[c]One pre-contrast and two post-contrast acquisitions; center slab on anterior wall of aorta; 72–90 mm slab; 40 mL Gd @ 2 mL/s.

TI (ms)	FA (degrees)	FOV (cm)	SLTHK (mm)	SLSP (mm)	Matrix	NEX	Freq	BW	ET	Contrast
	70	36-40	5	0	256 × 179	1	RL	63.6		no
	70	36-40	5	0	256 × 179	1	SI	63.6		no
	70	36-40	7	2.1	256 × 154	1	LR	63.6		no
		30-40	10-50		256 × 256	1	LR	63.6	256	no
		30-40	40-60		256 × 256	1	SI	63.6	256	no
		36-40	4	0	256 × 179	1	LR	63.6	256	no
		36-40	4-5	0	256 × 197	1	SI	63.6	256	no
		36-40	1.5	40 slices	384 × 380	1	SI	63.6	127	no
500	8	35	15		192 × 192	1	SI	63.6		yes
	25	40	1.7	40-64 slices/slab	512 × 281	1	SI	63.6		yes

TI (ms)	FA (degrees)	FOV (cm)	SLTHK (mm)	SLSP (mm)	Matrix	NEX	Freq	BW	ET	Contrast
		36-40	5	0	256 × 197	1	LR	63.6	256	–
		40	5	0	256 × 197	1	SI	63.6	256	–
	70	36-40	6	2	256 × 128	1	LR	63.6		–
	70	40	6	2	256 × 128	1	SI	63.6		–
500	8	40	10		192 × 192	1	SI	63.6		+
	25	40	1.5	64 slices/slab	512 × 280	1	SI	63.6		+
	70	36-40	6	2	256 × 128	1	LR	63.6		+
	70	40	6	2	256 × 128	1	SI	63.6		+

Protocols from F Scott Pereles MD, John Salanitri MD, Charles Facanati BS RT, Terry Cunningham BS RT, Northwestern Memorial Hospital

Examination	Indications	Coil	Plane	Sequence	TR (ms)	TE (ms)
Portal and superior mesenteric MRV		Body phase array		Scout		
			Axial[a]	T1 GRE	174	2.38/4.76
			Axial	T2 HASTE	1000	63
			Coronal	T2 HASTE	1000	59
			Axial	TrueFISP	3.52	1.76
			Coronal	TrueFISP	3.52	1.76
			Axial	T1 FS GRE	250	2.47
			Coronal	T1 FS GRE	187	2.47
			Axial	T1 FS GRE	250	2.47
			Coronal	T1 FS GRE	187	2.47

Comments:
[a]In and opposed phase; sat band above diaphragm.
[b]Do at 25, 60 and 90 s post contrast.
[c]Do at 120 and 300 s post contrast.

Protocols from Robert R Edelman MD, Wei Li MD, Roland Bejm RT, Eugene E Dunkle RT, Evanston Northwestern Hospital

Examination	Indications	Coil	Plane	Sequence	TR (ms)	TE (ms)
Hepatic and superior mesenteric MRA	Stenosis Occlusion Pre-surgical planning	8 Channel torso phased array	3 Planes	Scout	–	–
			Axial	T2 SSFSE	Min	90
			Sagittal	T2 SSFSE	Min	90
			Coronal	T2 SSFSE	Min	90
			Axial	T1 FS 3D GRE	3.1	Min Full
			Sagittal[a]	CE 3D MRA	3.6	1.3
			Axial[b]	T1 FS 3D GRE	3.1	Min Full
Hepatic and superior mesenteric MRA			Axial	T1 2D GRE	100	Min

Comments:
[a]Do a non-contrast mask run, followed by arterial and portal venous phase runs. Use test bolus of MR fluoroscopic triggering.
[b]Post-contrast GRE sequence.

Protocols from Fergus Coakley MD, University of California, San Francisco

Examination	Indications	Coil	Plane	Sequence	TR (ms)	TE (ms)
Portal MRV		Torso	Coronal[a]	T2 SSFSE	Infinity	100
			Axial[b]	T1 FGRE dual	90–150	2.1/4.2
			Axial[c]	FS T2 FRFSE	25–3000	100
			Coronal[d]	GRASS	34	13
			Axial[e]	Test bolus	Min	Min
			Coronal[f]	3D MRA	Min	Min
			Axial[g]	3D T1 SPGR	Min	Min
Options (if available, substitute FFE, FIESA or TrueFISP for GRASS)						
			Axial[h]	GRASS	30	6

Comments:
Post processing: Image subtractions for all post contrast phases. Create rotating MIPs.
[a]Non-FS localizer.
[b]In/opposed phase; cover liver.
[c]FS T2 axial, cover liver.
[d]With and without sat band (perpendicular to PV) for portal venous direction.
[e]FGRE sequence.
[f]Set up using fast vasc loc TOF squence on GE for localizer or stack of FFE axials on Phillips. FS dynamic 3D MRA.
[g]T1 axial post-Gd.
[h]For vasc evaluation, try 2-3 slices/breath-hold. For IVC, consider coronal/sagittal.

TI (ms)	FA (degrees)	FOV (cm)	SLTHK (mm)	SLSP (mm)	Matrix	NEX	Freq	BW	ET	Contrast
70		36–40	7	2.1	256 × 154	1	LR	63.6		no
		36–40	5	0	256 × 197	1	LR	63.6	256	
		40	5	0	256 × 197	1	SI	63.6	256	
70		36–40	5	0	256 × 179	1	LR	63.6		
70		40	5	0	256 × 179	1	SI	63.6		
70		36–40	6	2	256 × 128	1	LR	63.6		no
70		40	6	2	256 × 128	1	SI	63.6		no
70		39–40	6	2	256 × 128	1	LR	63.6		yes
70		40	6	2	256 × 128	1	SI	63.6		yes

TI (ms)	FA (degrees)	FOV (cm)	SLTHK (mm)	SLSP (mm)	Matrix	NEX	Freq	BW	ET	Contrast
–	–	48	9	2	256 × 128	1	–	62.5	100+	–
–	–	36–40	7–9	1–2	256 × 160	0.5	RL	62.5	100+	–
–	–	40	6	1	256 × 160	0.5	SI	62.5	100+	–
–	–	36–40	7–9	1–2	256 × 160	0.5	SI	62.5	100+	–
Auto	12	34	4	ZIP 2	256 × 128	1	RL	62.5	–	–
–	25	34	3	ZIP 2	320 × 192	1	SI	125	–	+
Auto	12	34	4	ZIP 2	256 × 128	1	RL	62.5	–	+
–	60	36	9	2	512 × 160	1	RL	62.5	–	+

TI (ms)	FA (degrees)	FOV (cm)	SLTHK (mm)	SLSP (mm)	Matrix	NEX	Freq	BW	ET	Contrast
		32–40	6	1	256 × 160–192	0.5	SI	62.5	100+	
	75	32–40	8	1	256 × 128–192	1	LR	16		
		32–40	5–6	1	256 × 160/0.75	1	LR	32	17	
	20	36–40	10	0	256 × 128–192	1	SI	15		
	30+	36	5	0	256 × 64	1	LR	62.5		
	45	32–40	3	32 slab	512 × 192	0.5	SI	3		
	15–20	32–40	6–8	50% overlap	320 × 160/0.75	0.5	LR	31		+
	33	32–40	5	1	256 × 128–192	1	LR	15		

Protocols from Russell N Low MD, Sharp and Children's MRI Center for the GE Signa

Examination	Indications	Coil	Plane	Sequence	TR (ms)	TE (ms)
Abdomen	Bowel and peritoneum	Body	Coronal	Localizer		
		Body	Axial	SSFSE	inf	90
		Body	Axial[a]	2D T1 SGE	165	2.1
		Body	Axial[a]	3D T1 SGE	4	1.2
		Body	Axial[a]	T2 TSE	2500	77
		Body	Coronal[a]	T2 TSE	2500	77

Comments:
[a]Fat saturated.

Protocols from Russell N Low MD, Sharp and Children's MRI Center for the Phillips Integra

Examination	Indications	Coil	Plane	Sequence	TR (ms)	TE (ms)
Abdomen	Bowel and peritoneum	Body	Coronal[a]	SSTSE		
		Body	Axial[a]	SSTSE		
		Body	Axial[b]	T2 TSE	1600	70
		Body	Axial[c]	T1 THRIVE	shortest	shortest
			Coronal[d]		shortest	shortest
		Body	Axial[c]	T1 HiRes WATS	shortest	shortest

Comments:
[a]Breath-hold sequence.
[b]Respiratory triggered sequence, 24 slices, time to acquire 3 min 28 s.
[c]Breath-hold sequence, use Mobitrak with 2 stations each of 24 images.
[d]Breath-hold sequence. Use Mobitrak, 3 stations of 50 slices done as 1 breath-hold of 18 s each.

Protocols from F Scott Pereles MD, John Salanitri MD, Charles Facanati BS RT, Terry Cunningham BS RT, Northwestern Memorial Hospital

Examination	Indications	Coil	Plane	Sequence	TR (ms)	TE (ms)
Abdomen	Kidneys			Scout[a]		
			Axial[b]	T2 HASTE	1200	86
			Coronal[c]	T2 HASTE	1000	57
			Axial[d]	T1 GRE	178	2.38/4.76
			Axial[e]	T1 FS GRE	193	2.47
			Coronal[f]	T1 FS GRE	125	2.47
			Axial[g]	T1 FS GRE	193	2.47
			Sagittal[h]	T1 FS GRE	250	2.47
			Coronal[i]	T1 FS GRE	125	2.47

Comments:
[a]Breath-hold inspiration.
[b]Non-breath-hold.
[c]Spine to front of liver.
[d]In and opposed phase; breath-hold.
[e]Cover liver and kidneys.
[f]Cover kidneys only.
[g]Use fluoro prep, do corticomedullary phase, 60 s venous phase, 360 s MR IVU phase.
[h]90 s corticomedullary phase (kidney to kidney).
[i]180 s excretory phase.

TI (ms)	FA (degrees)	FOV (cm)	SLTHK (mm)	SLSP (mm)	Matrix	NEX	Freq	BW	ET	Contrast
	60	40	6		128 × 128	1		63.6		–
		25–28	5	1.5	256 × 192	2	LR	63.6		–
150		30–40	5	0	256 × 198	1	LR	63.6	256	–
180		25–28	4	0.8	384 × 269	2	SI	63.6	23	–
150		25–28	4	0.8	512 × 204	3	SI	63.6	23	–
70		30–40	6	2	256 × 128	1	LR	63.6		–
70		30–40	6	2	256 × 128	1	SI	63.6		–
70		30–40	6	2	256 × 128	1	SI	63.6		+
70		30–40	6	2	256 × 128	1	LR	63.6		+
70		30–40	6	2	256 × 141	1	SI	63.6		+
150		30–40	5	0	256 × 198	1	SI	63.6	256	–
150		30–40	4	0.8	512 × 256	3	LR	63.6	23	–

TI (ms)	FA (degrees)	FOV (cm)	SLTHK (mm)	SLSP (mm)	Matrix	NEX	Freq	BW	ET	Contrast
		32–40	6	1	256 × 160–192	0.5	SI	62.5	100+	–
		24–28	5	1	512 × 256	2	AP	16	8	–
		24–28	5	1	512 × 256	2	AP	16	8	–
		24–28	8	2	256 × 192	1	LR	16		–
15–20		32–40	8	50% overlap	320 × 160/0.75	0.5	LR	31		–
30+		36	5		256 × 64	1	LR	62.5		+
		32–40	3	32 slab	512 × 192	0.5	SI	3		+
15–20		32–40	8	50% overlap	320 × 160/0.75	0.5	LR	31		+

TI (ms)	FA (degrees)	FOV (cm)	SLTHK (mm)	SLSP (mm)	Matrix	NEX	Freq	BW	ET	Contrast
–	60	44	8	0	256 × 128	1	SI	31	–	–
–	–	42	6	1	512 × 192	2	AP	15	–	–
–	–	34	5	1	256 × 192	2	SI	15	12	–
–	–	28	6	1	256 × 192	2	AP	15	12	–
–	–	28	6	1	512 × 192	2	RL	15	–	+

Protocols from Robert R Edelman MD, Wei Li MD, Roland Bejm RT, Eugene E Dunkle RT, Evanston Northwestern Hospital

Examination	Indications	Coil	Plane	Sequence	TR (ms)	TE (ms)
Pelvis	Metastatic disease	8 Channel torso phased array	Coronal	Localizer	100	Min
			Axial	T1 SE	500	Min
			Sagittal	T2 FSE	4000	102
			Coronal	T1 SE	500	Min
			Axial	T2 FS SSFSE	Min	90
			Coronal	T2 FS SSFSE	Min	90
			Axial	T1 FS SE	500	17
			Axial	T1 FS SE	500	17
			Coronal	T1 FS SE	500	17

Protocols from Fergus Coakley MD, University of California, San Francisco

Examination	Indications	Coil	Plane	Sequence	TR (ms)	TE (ms)
Pelvis	Rectosigmoid cancer staging			Localizer		
			Coronal[a]	SSFSE	Infinity	100
			Axial	T2 FSE	4000	85
			Sagittal	T2 FSE	4000	85
			Coronal[b]	T1 SE	5–700	10–15
			Axial[c]	T1 FS SE	5–700	10–15
			Axial[d]	T1 FS SE	5–700	10–15

Comments:
[a]Breath-hold; non-FS T2; overview.
[b]For levator ani assessment.
[c]FS axial pre-Gd
[d]FS axial post-Gd.

Protocols from Fergus Coakley MD, University of California, San Francisco

Examination	Indications	Coil	Plane	Sequence	TR (ms)	TE (ms)
Pelvis	Bladder tumor			Localizer		
			Coronal[a]	T2 SSFSE	Infinity	100
			Axial[b]	T1 SE	5–700	10–15
			Axial[b]	T2 FSE	4000	85
			Sagittal[b]	T2 FSE	4000	85
			Best[c]	FS T1 FMPSPGR	90–150	4.2
			Best[d]	FS T1 FMPSPGR	90–150	4.2
			Axial[e]	T1 SE	5–700	10–15
			Axial[f]	T1 SE	5–700	10–15

Comments:
[a]Cover pelvis.
[b]No FS.
[c]Pre-Gd.
[d]Dynamic post-Gd through bladder. 20, 60, 120, 180, 300 s post-injection.
[e]Delayed post-Gd series. Same coverage as prior T1 SE sequence.
[f]Delayed post-Gd series. Incremental coverage to include renal hila.

Notes
Main components are axial T1, high resolution axial and sagittal T2, delayed post-Gd T1 in best plane. Incremental T1 axial images to renal hila for adenopathy and HN. Bladder is NOT emptied for 2 hours prior to the study.

TI (ms)	FA (degrees)	FOV (cm)	SLTHK (mm)	SLSP (mm)	Matrix	NEX	Freq	BW	ET	Contrast
–	–	40	7	1	256 × 128	1	SI	15.63	–	–
–	–	32	6	1	256 × 160	4	RL	15.63	–	–
–	–	38	6	1	256 × 160	2	SI	20.83	12	–
–	–	38	6	1	256 × 160	4	RL	15.63	–	–
–	–	38	6	1	256 × 160	0.5	RL	62.5	100+	–
–	–	40	5	1	256 × 160	0.5	SI	62.5	100+	–
–	–	40	6	1	256 × 160	1	RL	15.63	–	–
–	–	40	6	1	256 × 160	1	RL	15.63	–	+
–	–	38	5	1	256 × 160	2	SI	15.63	–	+

TI (ms)	FA (degrees)	FOV (cm)	SLTHK (mm)	SLSP (mm)	Matrix	NEX	Freq	BW	ET	Contrast
		32–40	6	1	256 × 160–192	0.5		62.5	100+	–
		32–40	5	1	512 × 256	2	AP	30	8	–
		24–28	5	1	512 × 256	2	AP	16	8	–
		32–40	5	1	256 × 192	1	SI	16		–
		32–40	5	1	256 × 192	1	LR	16		–
		32–40	5	1	256 × 192	1	LR	16		+

TI (ms)	FA (degrees)	FOV (cm)	SLTHK (mm)	SLSP (mm)	Matrix	NEX	Freq	BW	ET	Contrast
		32–40	8	2	256 × 160–192	0.5	SI	62.5		
		24–28	8	2	256 × 192	1	LR	16		–
		24–28	5	1	512 × 256	2	LR	16	8	
		24–28	5	1	512 × 256	2	SI	16	8	
	70	24	5–10	1–2	256 × 128–192	1		16		–
	70	24	5–10	1–2	256 × 128–192	1		16		+
		32–40	5	0	256 × 192	1	LR	16		+
		32–40	8	2	256 × 192	1	LR	16		+

Protocols from Fergus Coakley MD, University of California, San Francisco

Examination	Indications	Coil	Plane	Sequence	TR (ms)	TE (ms)
Pelvis	Ovarian or adnexal mass	Torso		Localizer		
			Coronal[a]	T2 SSFSE	Infinity	100
			Axial[b]	T2 FSE	4000	85
			Sagittal[b]	T2 FSE	4000	85
			Axial	T1 SE	5–700	10–15
			Axial[c]	T1 FS SE	5–700	10–15
			Axial[d]	T1 SE	5–700	10–15
			Coronal[e]	FS T1 FMPSPGR	90–150	4.2
			Sagittal[f]	FS T1 FMPSPGR	90–150	4.2
			Axial[g]	T2 SSFSE	Infinity	100
			Coronal[g]	T2 SSFSE	Infinity	100

Comments:

Similar to routine pelvis, addition of post-Gd images. As ovarian septae and nodules have delayed enhancement, do dynamic post-Gd images.

[a]Non-FS, overview.

[b]No FS.

[c]Do FS to characterize bright T1 lesions seen in prior sequence. May be optional.

[d]Match to prior sequence done pre-Gd; no FS.

[e]Abdominal localizer; center on umbilicus.

[f]Non-dynamic breath-hold FS axial T1.

[g]Breath-hold T2 through abdomen.

Protocols from F Scott Pereles MD, John Salanitri MD, Charles Facanati BS RT, Terry Cunningham BS RT, Northwestern Memorial Hospital

Examination	Indications	Coil	Plane	Sequence	TR (ms)	TE (ms)
Pelvis	Ovarian or adnexal mass	Body phase array		Scout	3.75	1.88
			Axial	SE T1	550	11
			Axial[a]	T2 HASTE	1800	64
			Sagittal	T2 HASTE	1800	64
			Uterine long axis[b]	T2 TSE	3500	83
			Uterine short axis[b]	T2 TSE	3500	83
			Axial[c]	T1 FS GRE	234	2.3
			Sagittal	T1 FS GRE	172	2.08
			Sagittal[d]	T1 FS GRE	172	2.08
			Axial[e]	T1 FS GRE	234	2.3
			Coronal[f]	T1 FS GRE	146	1.94

Comments:

[a]Non-breath-hold; interleaved; cover entire pelvis.

[b]High resolution; small FOV.

[c]Hip joint to hip joint.

[d]45 and 60 s delay.

[e]90 s delay.

[f]120 s delay.

TI (ms)	FA (degrees)	FOV (cm)	SLTHK (mm)	SLSP (mm)	Matrix	NEX	Freq	BW	ET	Contrast
		32–40	6	1	256 × 160-192	0.5		62.5	100+	−
		24–28	5	1	512 × 256	2	AP	16	8	−
		24–28	5	1	512 × 256	2	SI	16	8	−
		24–28	8	2	256 × 192	1	LR	16		−
		24–28	8	2	256 × 192	1	LR	16		−
		24–28	8	2	256 × 192	1	LR	16		+
	70	32–40	10	2	256 × 128-192	1	SI	30		−
	70	32–40	8	2	256 × 128-192	1	SI	30		+
		32–40	8	2	256 × 160-192	0.5	LR	62.5	100+	+
		32–40	8	2	256 × 160-192	0.5	SI	62.5	100+	+

TI (ms)	FA (degrees)	FOV (cm)	SLTHK (mm)	SLSP (mm)	Matrix	NEX	Freq	BW	ET	Contrast
	60	6			128 × 128	1		63.6		−
		36–40	6	2	512 × 358	2	LR	63.6		−
	150	36–40	5	0	256 × 198	1	LR	63.6	256	−
	150	25–28	5	0	256 × 198	1	SI	63.6	256	−
	150	25–28	4	0.8	512 × 256	3		63.6	23	
	150	25–28	4	0.8	512 × 256	3		63.6	23	
	80	25–30	6	1.8	320 × 160	1	LR	63.6		−
	80	25–30	6	1.8	256 × 204	1	SI	63.6		−
	80	25–30	6	1.8	256 × 204	1	SI	63.6		+
	80	25–30	6	1.8	320 × 160	1	LR	63.6		+
	80	30–35	6	1.8	320 × 192	1	SI	63.6		+

Protocols from F Scott Pereles MD, John Salanitri MD, Charles Facanati BS RT, Terry Cunningham BS RT, Northwestern Memorial Hospital

Examination	Indications	Coil	Plane	Sequence	TR (ms)	TE (ms)
Pelvis	Endometrial or cervical cancer	Body phase array		Scout	3.75	1.88
			Axial	SE T1	434	11
			Axial[a]	HASTE	1000	58
			Sagittal[b]	T2 TSE	4500	117
			Axial	T2 TSE	4630	114
			Axial[c]	T1 FS GRE	170	1.94
			Sagittal	T1 FS GRE	158	1.85
			Sagittal[d]	T1 FS GRE	158	1.85
			Axial[e]	T1 FS GRE	170	1.94
			Coronal[f]	T1 FS GRE	158	1.85

Optional if uterine anomaly

			Uterine long axis[b]	T2 TSE	4520	102
			Uterine short axis[b]	T2 TSE	4520	102

Comments:
[a]Non-breath-hold, interleaved; cover entire pelvis.
[b]High resolution; small FOV.
[c]Hip joint to hip joint.
[d]45 and 60 s delay.
[e]90 s delay.
[f]120 s delay.

Protocols from Robert R Edelman MD, Wei Li MD, Roland Bejm RT, Eugene E Dunkle RT, Evanston Northwestern Hospital

Examination	Indications	Coil	Plane	Sequence	TR (ms)	TE (ms)
Pelvis	Endometrial or cervical cancer	8 Channel torso phased array	Coronal	T1 SPGR	150	Min Full
			Axial	T1 SE	525	Min
			Sagittal	T2 FS FSE	4500	102
			Oblique axial	T2 FS FSE	4500	102
			Oblique coronal	T2 FS FSE	4500	102
			Axial	T1 FS SPGR	225	4.2
			Sagittal	T1 FS SPGR	225	4.2
			Sagittal[a]	T1 FS SPGR	225	4.2
			Axial[b]	T1 FS SPGR	225	4.2

Comments:
[a]20, 40, and 90 s post-Gd.
[b]160 s post-Gd.

Protocols from F Scott Pereles MD, John Salanitri MD, Charles Facanati BS RT, Terry Cunningham BS RT, Northwestern Memorial Hospital

Examination	Indications	Coil	Plane	Sequence	TR (ms)	TE (ms)
Pelvis	Maternal pathology in the pregnant female	Body array coil		Scout		
			Axial[a]	SE T1	434	11
			Axial[b]	T2 HASTE	1000	58
			Coronal[c]	T2 HASTE	1000	58
			Sagittal[d]	T2 TSE	4500	117
			Any plane	TrueFISP	3.52	1.76

Comments:
Do after 12 weeks gestation. Supine patient; empty bladder before exam.
[a]Entire pelvis.
[b]Non-breath-hold, interleaved; cover entire pelvis.
[c]Breath-hold.
[d]Non-breath-hold; place sat. band over anterior abdominal wall; cover pelvic side wall to side wall.

TI (ms)	FA (degrees)	FOV (cm)	SLTHK (mm)	SLSP (mm)	Matrix	NEX	Freq	BW	ET	Contrast
	60		6		128 × 128	1		63.6		−
		25–28	5	1.5	256 × 192	2	LR	63.6		−
	150	36–40	5	0	256 × 198	1	LR	63.6	256	−
	180	25–28	4	0.8	384 × 269	2	SI	63.6	23	−
	180	25–28	4	0.8	512 × 204	4	LR	63.6	23	
	80	36–40	6	1.8	320 × 224	1	LR	63.6		−
	80	36–40	6	1.8	256 × 204	1	SI	63.6		
	80	36–40	6	1.8	256 × 204	1	SI	63.6		+
	80	36–40	6	1.8	320 × 224	1	LR	63.6		+
	80	36–40	6	1.8	256 × 204	1	SI	63.6		+
	180	25–28	4	0.8	512 × 256	3		63.6	23	
	180	25–28	4	0.8	512 × 256	2		63.6	23	

TI (ms)	FA (degrees)	FOV (cm)	SLTHK (mm)	SLSP (mm)	Matrix	NEX	Freq	BW	ET	Contrast
−	70	44	8	0	256 × 128	1	SI	31	−	−
−	−	32	6	1	512 × 192	2	RL	15	−	−
−	−	34	5	1	256 × 192	2	SI	15	12	−
−	−	28	6	1	256 × 192	2	RL	15	12	−
−	−	42	6	1	256 × 192	2	AP	15	12	−
−	70	38	5	1	256 × 128	1	RL	62	−	−
−	70	30	5	1	256 × 128	1	SI	62	−	−
−	70	30	5	1	256 × 128	1	SI	62	−	+
−	70	38	5	1	256 × 128	1	RL	62	−	+

TI (ms)	FA (degrees)	FOV (cm)	SLTHK (mm)	SLSP (mm)	Matrix	NEX	Freq	BW	ET	Contrast
		25–28	5	1.5	256 × 192	2	LR	63.6		−
	150	30–40	5	0	256 × 198	1	LR	63.6	256	−
	150	30–40	5	0	256 × 198	1	SI	63.6	256	−
	180	25–28	4	0.8	384 × 269	2	SI	63.6	23	−
	70	30–40	5	0	256 × 179	1		63.6		−

Protocols from Julia R Fielding MD, University of North Carolina

Examination	Indications	Coil	Plane	Sequence	TR (ms)	TE (ms)
Pelvic floor			3 planes	Localizer	15	5
			Sagittal[a]	HASTE	4.4	90
			Axial[b]	T2 TSE	5000	132
			Coronal[c]	T2 TSE	5000	132

Comments:
60 mL ultrasound gel in rectum prior to start of study.
Repeat HASTE at maximal strain in valsalva.
[a]Center low in pelvis.
[b]Center on cervix.
[c]Center on anal canal.

Protocols from Fergus Coakley MD, University of California, San Francisco

Examination	Indications	Coil	Plane	Sequence	TR (ms)	TE (ms)
Pelvic floor			Coronal[a]	T2 SSFSE	Infinity	100
			Axial[b]	T2 FSE	4000	85
			Sagittal[b]	T2 FSE	4000	85
			Axial	T1 SE	5–700	10–15
			Sagittal midline[c]	T2 SSFSE	Infinity	100
			Axial[d]	T2 SSFSE	Infinity	100
			Sagittal midline[e]	T2 SSFSE	Infinity	100

Comments:
[a]No FS, overview.
[b]No FS.
[c]Screen for pelvic floor relaxation. Obtain one image in rest, coach patient to bear down and strain as hard as they can and repeat the image in maximal strain. Do as single acquisition.
[d]Axial at level below symphysis. Follow instructions for prior sequence.
[e]Patient relaxed for 1st 5 measurements; instruct to strain maximally over next 10 measurements and relax for last 5 measures. Do total of 20 measurements.

Protocols from F Scott Pereles MD, John Salanitri MD, Charles Facanati BS RT, Terry Cunningham BS RT, Northwestern Memorial Hospital

Examination	Indications	Coil	Plane	Sequence	TR (ms)	TE (ms)
Pelvic MRV		Body phase array		Scout		
			Axial[a]	TrueFISP	3.52	1.76
			Coronal[b]	TrueFISP	3.52	1.76
			Axial	T1 FS GRE	250	2.47
			Coronal	T1 FS GRE	185	2.47
			Axial[c]	T1 FS GRE	250	2.47
			Coronal	T1 FS GRE	185	2.47

Comments:
[a]Mid abdomen to SFV.
[b]Include IVC.
[c]Can repeat multiple times between 2-8 min post-injection.

TI (ms)	FA (degrees)	FOV (cm)	SLTHK (mm)	SLSP (mm)	Matrix	NEX	Freq	BW	ET	Contrast
	1	35-40	10	0	160 × 256					−
	180	30	10	single slice	128 × 256	1	SI			−
	180	20	3	interleaved	270 × 256	2	LR			−
	180	20	3	interleaved	270 × 256	2	SI			−

TI (ms)	FA (degrees)	FOV (cm)	SLTHK (mm)	SLSP (mm)	Matrix	NEX	Freq	BW	ET	Contrast
		32-40	6	1	256 × 160-192	0.5		62.5	100+	−
		24-28	5	1	512 × 256	2	AP	16	8	
		24-28	5	1	512 × 256	2	SI	16	8	
		24-28	8	2	256 × 192	1	LR	16		−
		24-32	10	single slice	256 × 160-192	0.5	SI	62.5	100+	
		24-32	10	single slice	256 × 160-192	0.5	LR	62.5	100+	
		24-32	10	20 acquisitions/series	256 × 160-192	0.5	SI	62.5	100+	

TI (ms)	FA (degrees)	FOV (cm)	SLTHK (mm)	SLSP (mm)	Matrix	NEX	Freq	BW	ET	Contrast
	70	36-40	5	0	256 × 179	1	LR	63.6		−
	70	36-40	5	0	256 × 179	1	SI	63.6		−
	70	36-40	6	2	256 × 128	1	LR	63.6		−
	70	36-40	6	2	256 × 128	1	SI	63.6		−
	70	36-40	6	2	256 × 128	1	LR	63.6		+
	70	36-40	6	2	256 × 128	1	SI	63.6		+

Protocols from Fergus Coakley MD, University of California, San Francisco

Examination	Indications	Coil	Plane	Sequence	TR (ms)	TE (ms)
Pelvic MRV		Torso		Localizer		
			Coronal	T2 SSFSE	Infinity	100
			Axial	T2 SSFSE	Infinity	100
			Sagittal	T2 SSFSE	Infinity	100
			Axial[a]	T1 FGRE	90–150	4.2
			Axial[b]	Test bolus	Min	Min
			Coronal[c]	3D MRA	Min	Min
Options						
			Axial[d]	2D GRE TOF		
			Axial[e]	GRASS	30	6
			Sagittal[f]	T2 FSE	4000	85

Comments:
[a]In phase only, no FS.
[b]FGRE sequence.
[c]Set up using Fast vasc loc TOF sequence on GE for localizer or stack of FFE axials on Phillips. FS dynamic 3D MRA.
[d]Superior traveling sat band for veins.
[e]For vasc evaluation try 2–3 slices/breath-hold. For IVC, coronal/sagittal.
[f]Evaluate incidental uterine findings.
Post processing: Image subtractions for all post contrast phases, create rotating MIPs.

Protocols from Fergus Coakley MD, University of California, San Francisco

Examination	Indications	Coil	Plane	Sequence	TR (ms)	TE (ms)
Fetal MRI		Torso		Localizer		
			Coronal[a]	FMPSPGR	90–150	4.2
			Coronal[b]	T2 SSFSE	Infinity	100
			As needed[c]	T2 SSFSE	Infinity	100
			As needed[d]	FMPSPGR	90–150	4.2
Options						
			As needed[e]	SPGR	130	20

Comments:
T2 SSFSE and T1 FMPSPGR images through fetal ROI in planes prescribed by radiologist.
Always use a surface coil—torso works best (consider pelvic in earlier pregnancy).
Use small FOV to increase spatial resolution, however, be aware that noise increases and may have wrap.
Prescribe slice number and thickness so that obtained in a single maternal breath-hold. Avoid split acquisitions (fetus can move).
Acquire T2-weighted images first as these have better quality than T1 images (FMPSPGR prone to poor SNR, therefore has larger slice thickness, lower phase-encode steps, and lower bandwidth).
Consider left decubitus position in late pregnancy to avoid IVC compression and syncope.
Gadolinium not to be used.
[a]Localizer; coronal to mother.
[b]Breath-hold T2, coronal to fetus.
[c]Breath-hold T2, multiple planes as needed.
[d]Breath-hold T1, multiple planes to fetus as needed.
[e]Breath-hold T2* for suspected congenital hemochromotosis.

TI (ms)	FA (degrees)	FOV (cm)	SLTHK (mm)	SLSP (mm)	Matrix	NEX	Freq	BW	ET	Contrast
		32–40	4–6	1	256 × 160–192	0.5	SI	62.5	100+	
		32–40	4–6	1	256 × 160–192	0.5	LR	62.5	100+	
		32–40	4–6	1	256 × 160–192	0.5	SI	62.5	100+	
75		32–40	8	1	256 × 128–192	1	LR	16		
30+		36	5	0	256 × 64	1	LR	62.5		
45		32–40	3	32 slab	512 × 192	0.5	SI	3		
			3–4	1 mm overlap			LR			
33		32–40	5	1	256 × 128–192	1	LR	15		
		24–28	5	1	512 × 256	2	SI	16	8	+

TI (ms)	FA (degrees)	FOV (cm)	SLTHK (mm)	SLSP (mm)	Matrix	NEX	Freq	BW	ET	Contrast
	70	32–40	8	1	256 × 128–192	1	SI	16		
		32–40	6–8	1	256 × 128–192	1	SI	31	100+	
		20–28	3–5	0–1	256 × 128–192	1		31	100+	
	70	20–28	8	1	256 × 128–192	1		16		
	15–20	20–28	6–8	1	256 × 128–192	1		16		

Protocols from Fergus Coakley MD, University of California, San Francisco

Examination	Indications	Coil	Plane	Sequence	TR (ms)	TE (ms)
Prostate MRI and MRS		Endorectal		Localizer		
			Sagittal[a]	T2 FSE	1000	90
			Axial[b]	T1 SE	766	8

If spectral data are acquired obliquely to match angle of prostate in SI dimension, the axial and coronal images must also be acquired obliquely to overlay spectra and reference images.

			Axial[c]	FSE	6000	96
			Coronal[d]	FSE	5000	98
			Axial[e]	PROSE	1000	130

Comments:
[a]Localizer; check coil position; no FS.
[b]Pelvis.
[c]Axial or axial oblique of prostate.
[d]Acquired perpendicular to axial images.
[e]Axial or axial oblique covering prostate; spectroscopy.

Protocols from Fergus Coakley MD, University of California, San Francisco

Examination	Indications	Coil	Plane	Sequence	TR (ms)	TE (ms)
Penis				Localizer		
			Axial[a]	T1 SE	5-700	10-15
			Axial[a,b]	T2 FSE	4000	85
			Sagittal[c]	T2 FSE	4000	85
			Coronal[c]	T2 FSE	4000	85

Comments:
Penis positioned prior to study by taping to anterior abdominal wall (not directly but with towels or 4 × 4s arranged about penis). Empty bladder before scan.
[a]Coverage 5 cm below to 3 cm above prostate.
[b]No FS.
[c]No FS; center on prostate.

Penis	Urethral trauma			Localizer		
			Axial[a]	T1 SE	5-700	10-15
			Axial[a,b]	T2 FSE	4000	85
			Sagittal[c]	T2 FSE	4000	85
			Coronal[c]	T2 FSE	4000	85

Comments:
Penis positioned prior to study by taping to anterior abdominal wall (not directly but with towels or 4 × 4s arranged about penis). Empty bladder before scan.
[a]Coverage 5 cm below to 3 cm above prostate.
[b]No FS.
[c]No FS; center on prostate.

Testis and scrotum				Localizer		
			Axial[a]	T1 SE	5-700	10-15
			Sagittal[b]	T2 FSE	4000	85
			Coronal[b]	T2 FSE	4000	85
			Best[c]	FS T1 FMPSPGR	90-150	4.2
			Best[d]	FS T1 FMPSPGR	90-150	4.2
			Axial[e]	T1 SE	5-700	10-15

Comments:
[a]Coverage 5 cm below to 3 cm above prostate.
[b]No FS; center on prostate.
[c]Pre-Gd.
[d]Dynamic post-Gd through testis or mass. 20, 60, 120, 180, 300 s post-injection.
[e]Same coverage as dynamic series.

TI (ms)	FA (degrees)	FOV (cm)	SLTHK (mm)	SLSP (mm)	Matrix	NEX	Freq	BW	ET	Contrast
		24	5	1.5	256 × 192	1	SI	16	8	
		24	5	1.5	256 × 192	1	AP	16		
		14	3	0	256 × 192	3	AP	20	16	
		16	3	0	256 × 192	3	RL	20	16	
		11	25-40		16 × 8	1				

TI (ms)	FA (degrees)	FOV (cm)	SLTHK (mm)	SLSP (mm)	Matrix	NEX	Freq	BW	ET	Contrast
		24-28	5	1	256 × 192	1	LR	16		−
		24-28	3-4	0	512 × 256	2	LR	16	8	
		24-28	3	0	512 × 256	2	AP	16	8	
		24-28	3	0	512 × 256	2	AP	16	8	
		24-28	5	1	256 × 192	1	LR	16		−
		24-28	4	0	512 × 256	2	LR	16	8	
		24-28	3	0	512 × 256	2	AP	16	8	
		24-28	3	0	512 × 256	2	AP	16	8	
		24-28	8	2	256 × 192	1	LR	16		−
		24-28	4	0	512 × 256	2	AP	16	8	
		24-28	4	0	512 × 256	2	SI	16	8	
	70	24	5	1	256 × 128-192	1		16		−
	70	24	5	1	256 × 128-192	1		16		+
		32-40	5	0	256 × 192	1	LR	16		+

Protocols from Javier Beltran, Maimonides Medical Center

Examination	Coil	Plane	Pulse Sequence	TR (ms)	TE (ms)	TI (ms)	FA (degrees)	FOV (cm)
Ankle	Extremity	Axial	TSE T2	3630	83		90	15
		Axial	TSE T1	437	9.8		90	15
		Coronal	TSE T1	877	12		90	17
		Sagittal	STIR	3410	25	150	90	18
		Sagittal	FLASH 2D	910	1		60	18
Foot	Extremity	Axial	TSE T2	3630	83		90	15
		Axial	TSE T1	437	9.8		90	15
		Sagittal	FI2D FS	679	11		60	18
		Sagittal	STIR	3800	25	130	90	18
		Coronal	T1	785	12		90	18
		Coronal	STIR	3780	24	150	90	18

Protocols from John Crues for the ARTOSCAN

Examination	Plane	Pulse Sequence	TR (ms)	TE (ms)	TI (ms)	FOV (cm)	# of slices	SLTHK (mm)
Standard knee	Sagittal	SE	680	18		160	20	4.0
	Sagittal	SE	3000	80		160	20	4.0
	Coronal	SE	650	18		160	19	4.0
	Coronal	STIR	1470	24	75	170	15	5.0
	Axial	SE	3000	100		160	13	5.0
Calf/long bone	Axial	SE	500	18		160	11	4.0
	Axial	STIR	1340	24	75	170	14	4.0
	Sagittal	SE	500	18		180	14	4.0
	Coronal	SE	2670	90		160	17	4.0
	Coronal	SE	500	18		180	14	4.0
Ankle and heel	Axial	SE	600	18		140	17	4.0
	Axial	SE	3000	100		140	17	4.0
	Sagittal	SE	600	18		140	16	4.0
	Sagittal	STIR	1340	24	75	140	14	5.0
	Coronal	SE	600	24		140	13	4.0
	Coronal	STIR	1190	24	75	180	11	4.0
Foot	Axial	SE	680	18		150	20	3.5
	Axial	SE	2800	80		160	19	3.5
	Coronal	SE	450	24		170	10	4.0
	Coronal	STIR	1080	24	85	190/140	10	4.0
	Sagittal	SE	620	18		160	18	3.5
Elbow	Axial	SE	620	18		140	18	4.0
	Axial	SE	3000	100		140	13	5.0
	Coronal	SE	600	24		140	13	4.0
	Coronal	STIR	900	16	75	140	10	4.0
	Sagittal	SE	580	18		140	15	4.0
Wrist coronal hand	Axial	SE	550	18		120	16	4.0
	Coronal	SE	500	20		120	12	4.0
	Coronal	STIR	1150	24	75	140	12	4.0
	Coronal	3D-GE	540	16	FA 45°	130	12	1.0
	Sagittal	SE	690	20		120	18	4.0
	Axial	SE	3000	90		120	16	4.0

SLTHK (mm)	Matrix	NEX	Freq	Distance factor (%)
5	512	2	RL	20
5	256	4	RL	20
4	512	4	RL	20
3	256	1	AP	30
3	256	1	AP	30
5	512	2	RL	20
5	256	3	RL	20
4	384	1	RP	20
4	256	1	RP	20
4	512	3	RP	20
4	256	1	RL	20

SLSP (mm)	Matrix	NEX	Time (min)	%	Contrast
0.4	192 × 192	3	6:34	79	T1
0.4	192 × 160	1	8:06	117	T2
0.4	192 × 192	3	6:17	78	T1
1.0	192 × 160	2	7:53	96	
1.0	192 × 160	1	8:06	98	T2
0.4	192 × 192	4	6:27	69	T1
0.5	192 × 160	2	7:11	63	Fat Sup
0.4	192 × 176	4	5:55	91	T1
0.4	192 × 160	1	7:12	80	T2
0.4	192 × 176	4	5:55	91	T1
0.4	192 × 176	3	5:20	61	T1
0.4	192 × 160	1	8:06	60	T2
0.4	192 × 176	3	5:20	61	T1
0.5	192 × 160	2	7:11	64	Fat Sup
0.4	192 × 192	3	5:49	68	T1
0.4	192 × 160	3	9:33	103	Fat Sup
0.5	192 × 192	3	6:34	51	T1
0.5	192 × 160	1	7:33	86	T2
0.4	192 × 160	3	3:38	82	SE
0.4	192 × 144	3	5:45	77	Fat Sup
0.5	192 × 192	3	5:59	56	T1
0.4	192 × 192	3	5:59	59	T1
1.0	192 × 160	1	8:06	75	T2
0.4	192 × 192	3	5:49	68	T1
0.8	192 × 160	2	4:51	53	Fat Sup
0.4	192 × 192	4	7:28	67	T1
0.4	192 × 160	4	5:55	53	T1
0.4	192 × 176	4	5:55	52	T1
0.4	192 × 160	2	6:10	50	Fat Sup
0.4	192 × 176	4	6:23	47	T2*
0.4	192 × 192	3	6:40	48	T1
0.4	192 × 160	1	8:06	54	T2

Protocols from John Crues for the E-SCAN

Examination	Plane	Mode	Pulse Sequence	TE (ms/deg)	TI/FA (ms)	NEX	FOV (cm)	# of slices
Shoulder	Axial reference	2D	SE HF	18		1	16/16	11
	Coronal	2D	SE	24		2	14/14	12
	Coronal	2D	TSE	80		1	14/14	12
	Axial	2D	GE	74	75	2	14/14	14
	Axial	2D	SE	24		2	14/14	14
	Sagittal	2D	SE	80		1	14/14	12
	Coronal	2D	STIR	24	80	2	14/14	12
Ankle/heel	Axial reference	2D	SE HF	18		1	14/14	11
	Axial	2D	SE	24		2	13/13	16
	Axial	2D	TSE	80		1	13/13	16
	Coronal	2D	SE	24		2	12/12	16
	Sagittal	2D	SE	24		2	13/13	12
	Sagittal	2D	STIR	24	75	2	14/14	10
Knee	Axial reference	2D	SE HF	18		1	16/16	11
	Sagittal	2D	SE	24		2	14/14	18
	Sagittal	2D	SE	80		1	14/14	18
	Coronal	2D	SE	24		2	14/14	18
	Coronal	2D	STIR	30	75	1	14/14	13
	Axial	2D	TSE	80		1	14/14	18
Forefoot/midfoot	Axial reference	2D	SE HF	18		1	14/14	11
	Axial	2D	SE	24		2	14/14	16
	Axial	2D	TSE	80		1	14/14	16
	Coronal	2D	SE	24		1	14/14	16
	Coronal	2D	STIR	24	75	2	14/14	16
	Sagittal	2D	SE	24		2	14/14	16
	Sagittal	2D	STIR	24	75	2	14/14	16
Wrist/hand	Axial reference	2D	SE HF	18		1	12/12	11
	Axial	2D	SE	24		2	11/11	16
	Coronal	2D	SE	24		2	13/13	11
	Coronal	2D	STIR	24	75	2	13/13	11
	Coronal	3D	GE	16	40	1	11/11	52
	Sagittal	2D	SE	18		2	11/11	74
	Axial	2D	TSE	80		1	11/11	15
Finger	Axial reference	2D	SE HF	18		1	12/12	11
	Axial	2D	SE	24		3	11/11	25
	Axial	2D	TSE	80		1	12/12	15
	Sagittal	2D	SE	24		3	11/11	10
	Coronal	2D	STIR	24	75	2	11/11	10
	Coronal	2D	SE	18		2	13/13	10
	Coronal	3D	GE	16	40	1	13/13	52
Elbow	Axial reference	2D	SE HF	18		1	13/13	11
	Axial	2D	SE	24		2	13/13	18
	Axial	2D	TSE	80		1	13/13	18
	Coronal	2D	STIR	24	75	2	14/14	12
	Coronal	2D	SE	24		2	14/14	14
	Sagittal	2D	SE	24		2	14/14	14
Hip	Coronal reference	2D	SE HF	18		1	22/22	11
	Coronal	2D	SE	26		3	22/22	11
	Sagittal	2D	TSE SE	80		1	22/22	11
	Sagittal	2D	SE	26		3	23/23	13
	Coronal	2D	STIR	25	75	3	23/20	11
Long bone/masses	Axial reference	2D	SE HF	18		1	23/23	11
	Axial	2D	SE	24		3	23/23	15
	Axial	2D	TSE	80		1	23/23	15
	Axial	2D	STIR	24	75	2		10
	Sagittal	2D	SE	24		3		12
	Coronal	2D	SE	24		3		12
	Coronal	2D	STIR	24	75	2		12

SLTHK (mm)	SLSP (mm)	Frequency (ms)	Phase (ms)	TR	Contrast
5	1	192	128	400	T1
5	0.5	192	160	580	T1
5	0.5	192	160	2400	T2
5	0.5	192	160	630	T2*
5	0.5	192	160	680	T1
5	0.5	192	160	2400	T2
5	0.5	192	128	1850	Fat sup
4	1	192	128	400	T1
4	1	192	160	775	T1
4	1	192	160	2360	T2
4	1	192	160	770	T1
4	1	192	160	580	T1
5	1	192	160	1200	Fat sup
4	1	192	128	400	T1
4	1	192	152	870	T1
4	1	192	152	2650	T2
4	1	192	152	870	T1
6	1	192	128	1970	Fat sup
4	1	192	152	2650	T2
4	1	192	128	400	T1
4	1	192	160	720	T1
4	1	192	160	2360	T2
4	1	192	160	720	T1
4	1	192	160	2260	Fat sup
4	1	192	160	770	T1
4	1	192	160	2260	Fat sup
4	1	192	128	400	T1
3.5	0.5	192	160	770	T1
3.5	0.5	192	160	560	T1
3.5	0.5	192	128	1100	Fat sup
0.9	0	192	176-24	32	T1
3.5	0.5	192	160	510	T1
3.5	0.5	192	160	2360	PD/T2
4	1	192	128	400	T1
3	0.3	192	160	680	T1
3	0.3	192	160	2360	T2
3	0.3	192	160	680	T1
3	0.3	192	160	1000	Fat sup
3	0.3	192	160	680	T1
1	0	192	176-24	50	T1
4	1	192	128	400	T1
4	1	192	152	870	T1
4	1	192	152	2650	T2
4	1	192	160	1410	Fat sup
4	1	192	160	680	T1
4	0.9	192	160	700	T1
6	1	192	128	400	T1
6	0.6	192	176	560	T1
6	0.6	192	160	3000	T2
6	0.6	192	176	660	T1
6	0.6	192	144	1100	Fat sup
5	1	192	128	400	T1
5	1	192	160	680	T1
5	1	192	160	2300	T2
5	1	192	160	1410	Fat sup
5	1	192	160	540	T1
5	1	192	160	540	T1
5	1	192	160	1410	STIR

Protocols from John Crues for the ONI OrthoOne

Examination	Plane	TR (ms)	TE (ms)	TI (ms/deg)	FOV (cm)	Freq Phase	Contrast
Elbow	Coronal	3800	15.3		15	256 × 192	IR
	Coronal	800	14	90	15	288 × 192	T1
	Axial	900	15.6		12	288 × 192	T1
	Axial	3000	120		12	256 × 192	T2
	Sagittal	800	15		15	288 × 192	T1
Wrist	Coronal	4400	16.9	90	10	256 × 192	IR
	Coronal	950	18		10	288 × 192	T1
	Coronal	50	15	30	10	256 × 224	T2*
	Axial	3800	120		10	256 × 192	T2
	Axial	950	18.8		10	288 × 224	T1
	Sagittal	900	17.4		10	288 × 224	T1
Knee	Axial	3000	120		15	256 × 192	T2
	Sagittal	2300	15.2		15	320 × 224	PD
	Sagittal	2600	120		15	320 × 192	T2
	Coronal	850	14.8		15	320 × 192	T1
	Coronal	5000	14	90	15	256 × 192	IR
	Oblique coronal (ACL)	1800	120		14	256 × 192	T2
Ankle	Sagittal	800	15		15	288 × 192	T1
	Sagittal	4000	15.3	90	15	256 × 192	IR
	Oblique coronal	2000	19		14	288 × 224	PD
	Axial	3000	120	90	14	256 × 192	T2
	Axial	950	14		14	288 × 192	T1
Foot	Sagittal	4200	14	90	15	256 ×192	IR
	Sagittal	900	15.4		15	288 × 224	T1
	Coronal	3600	14	90	15	256 × 192	IR
	Coronal	700	15.9		15	320 × 192	T1
	Axial	950	15.4		12	320 × 192	T1
	Axial	3000	120		12	256 × 192	T2
Hand/finger	Sagittal	650	18.1		14	320 × 192	T1
	Sagittal	2800	17.6	90	14	256 × 192	IR
	Coronal	650	20.2		14	320 × 192	T1
	Coronal	3000	17.6	90	14	256 × 192	IR
	Coronal	50	15	30	10	256 × 192	T1
	Axial	900	17.4		10	320 × 192	T1
	Axial	3000	120	90	10	256 × 192	T2

Protocols from Michael B Zlatkin NMSI, Weston, Florida

Examination	Indication	Coil	Plane	Options	TR (ms)	TE (ms)	FOV (cm)	SLTHK (mm)	SLSP (mm)	Matrix	NEX	Freq	Contrast
Temporomandibular joint (TMJ)	Derangement	TMJ PA	Sagittal	SE	650	15	14	2	0.5	256 × 192	2	SI	
			Coronal	SE	650	15	14	2	0.5	256 × 192	2	SI	
			Sagittal	FSE (ET 8)	3000	20/75	14	2	0.5	256 × 192	2	SI	
			Sagittal	GRE (FA 15)	50	15	14	7	0	256 × 128	4	SI	

Comments:

Sagittal DE—perform open and closed sides at same time. Approx 6–8 slices through R and L. Coronal done bilateral.

Sagittal GRE—each scan is approximately 10–20 seconds. Do one side at a time same series, opening mouth wider each time. Start with mouth closed.

Protocols from Paul Clifford MD, Jose Rodriguez RT MR, University of Miami, Florida

Examination	Indication	Coil	Plane	Options	TR (ms)	TE (ms)	FOV (cm)	SLTHK (mm)	SLSP (mm)	Matrix	NEX	Freq	Contrast
General mass protocol	Mass	Body or torso[a]	Sagittal or Coronal[b]	SE T1	600	15	To cover	6	1	192	1	AP/LR	No
				FSE STIR (ET 7)	3000	40	To cover	6	1	160	1	HF/LR	No
				TI 150 at 1.5 T									
	Contrast?	Surface coil covering 2 × tumor	Axial	SE T1, ST-SI	600	15	2 × tumor	5	1	224	2	AP/LR	No
			Axial[c]	FSE STIR (ET 7), ST-SI	3500	40	2 × tumor	5	1	160	2	AP/LR	No
			Axial	SE T1, Fat Sat	600	15	2 × tumor	5	1	192		AP/LR	No
			Axial	SE T1, Fat Sat	600	15	2 × tumor	5	1	192	2	AP/LR	Yes
			Sagittal or Coronal[b]	SE T1, Fat Sat	600	15	2 × tumor	5	1	192	2	AP/LR	Yes

Comments:

Place a skin marker over the area of palpable or suspected mass. Small and superficial masses may be marked with a small amount of petroleum jelly.

Sequences in each plane should be identical in terms of location of slices.

[a]Smaller masses in the distal extremities may be evaluated performing all sequences in a surface coil and utilizing smaller slice thickness.

[b]To cover from joint to joint or entire compartment in which a mass resides: sagittal for anterior and posterior masses; coronal for medial or lateral masses.

[c]FSE FS T2 or SE dual echo sequences may replace the axial STIR sequence. A sagittal STIR or T2 FSE may be added here particularly if gadolinium is not to be utilized.

Matrix: phase selectable at 128, 192, 256 and 512. The frequency direction is fixed at 256 data points.

Protocols from Michael B Zlatkin NMSI, Weston, Florida

Examination	Indications	Coil	Plane	Options	TR (ms)
Ankle ARTHROPOST	OCD	Extremity PA	C/A/S	FSE(ET2)(FS)	500
	Loose body		C/A	FSE(ET8)(FS)	4000
	Ligament injury		Sagittal	FSE(ET8)	3000
Hip ARTHROPOST	Labral tear	PA Pelvic	C/A/S	SE(FS)	500
			C/S	FSE(ET6)(FS)	4000
Knee ARTHROPOST	Recurrent men tear	PA extremity	C/A/S	SE(FS)	600
	chodromalacia		Sagittal	SE	600
			Sagittal	FSE(ET4)(FS)	3000
Shoulder ARTHROPOST (Labrum)	Labral tear	Shoulder PA	A/C	FSE(ET2)(FS)	500
	Slap lesion		Coronal	FSE(ET8)(FS)	4000
	Instability		Sagittal	FSE(ET8)	3000
			Axial	FSE(ET2) high resolution	600

Comments:
For labrum use ABER as option as indicated by MD. 600/15, 256 × 192, 3 mm, 2 nex. 14 FOV

Examination	Indications	Coil	Plane	Options	TR (ms)
Shoulder ARTHROPOST (Rotator cuff)	Rotator cuff tear	Shoulder PA	A/C	FSE(ET2)(FS)	500
			C/A	FSE(ET8)(FS)	4000
			Sagittal	FSE(ET8)	3000
			Coronal	FSE(ET2) high resolution	600
Wrist ARTHROPOST	TFCC tear	Wrist PA	C/A/S	SE(FS)	500
	Lig tear		Coronal	FSE(ET8)(FS)	4125
			Axial	FSE(ET10)(FS)	3000
			Coronal	SE high resolution	600
Elbow ARTHROPOST	UCL tear	Elbow PA	C/A/S	FSE(ET2)(FS)	500
	Loose body		C/A	FSE(ET8)(FS)	4000
			Sagittal	FSE(ET8)	3000

KEY: The following are definitions of headings and abbreviations used in the protocols above.

CONTRAST : Gd (gadolinium, 0.2ml/kg, 1/200 dilution in saline). 35 cc for Knee, 12–15 cc for shoulder, Hip. 8–10 cc for elbow, ankle. 3 cc for wrist.

ET : Echo train for fast spin echo sequence

FC : Flow compensation technique which utilizes additional gradients to refocus protons out of phase as a result of flow

FOV : Field of view for the acquisition

FREQ : Frequency encoding selection; SI, RL, AP

FS : Fat saturation, "chem sat"

FSE : Fast spin echo

GRE : Gradient recalled echo; also known as fast scan, GRASS, or FISP. /## refers to the flip angle

MATRIX : Number of data points acquired in the phase direction, program selectable at 128, 192, 256 and 512. The frequency direction is fixed at 256 data points

STIR : Short Tau inversion recovery

NEX : Number of excitations. The number of times the acquisition sequence is repeated to increase signal to noise ratio

TE (ms)	FOV (cm)	SLTHK (mm)	SLSP (mm)	Matrix	NEX	Freq	Contrast
17	12	3	0	256 × 256	2	SI	
35–45	12	3	0.5	384 × 224	2	SI	
55	14	4	1	320 × 224	2	SI	
21	22	4	0	256 × 256	2	RL	
40	8	4	0	256 × 192	2	SI	
17	12	3	0	256 × 256	1.5	SI	
20	12	3	0	256 × 256	2	AP	
40	12	3	0.5	384 × 256	2	AP	
17	12	3	0	256 × 256	2	SI	
35–45	12	3	0.5	384 × 224	2	SI	
55	14	3	0	320 × 224	2	SI	
15	12	2	0/0	512 × 256	2	SI	
17	12	3	0	256 × 256	2	SI	
35–45	12	3	0.5	384 × 224	2	SI	
55	14	4	1	320 × 224	2	SI	
15	12	2	0	512 × 256	2	SI	
21	8	3	0	256 × 256	2	RL	
35–45	8	3	0	256 × 256	2	SI	
35–45	8	3	0	256 × 256	2	SI	
Min	6	2	0	512 × 384	2	SI	
17	12	3	0	256 × 256	2	SI	
35–45	12	3	0.5	384 × 224	2	SI	
55	14	4	1	320 × 224	2	SI	

NP	:	No phase wrap; eliminates wrap around artifact, or aliasing, in the phase encoding direction
ST	:	Saturation subroutine which utilizes additional radiofrequency pulses to saturate spins outside the imaging volume immediately, prior to each slice select gradient to reduce artifacts. Pulses can be applied in one or all of 6 planes: S – superior, I – inferior, A – anterior, P – posterior, R – right, L – left, C/S or C/I – moving sat pulses for time-of-flight MR angio sequences
PLANE	:	Anatomic plane of imaging desired
SLSP	:	Interslice spacing (mm). INTERLV – interleaving results in a 100% slice gap between images with an automatic second acquisition that images the slice gaps. Results in images with no slice gaps but without crosstalk artifact
SLTHK	:	Slice thickness (mm)
TE	:	Echo time
TR	:	Pulse repetition time
PA	:	Phased array coil
A	:	Axial plane
C	:	Coronal plane
S	:	Sagittal Plane

INDEX I 17

Intracranial hemorrhage—cont'd
putaminal, 1306, *1307*, 1330
relaxation mechanisms, 177, 1288,
    1289-1290
secondary, 1287
signal intensity effects, 1289-1290
    evolution of imaging appearances,
        1290-1295, *1291, 1292, 1292t,
        1293, 1294*
    spin-echo pulse sequences, 1290-1295,
        1291, 1292t, *1293, 1294*
subacute hematoma, *1291*, 1292, 1295,
    1423
subarachnoid hemorrhage, 1423
subchronic hematoma, 1423
thalamic, *1291*, 1306-1307, *1309*, 1330
therapeutic aspects, 1330
time course of bleeding, 1303-1304
treatment, 1552
undetermined cause, 1327
vascular malformations, 1313, 1315,
    1316-1319, 1330
venous malformations (angiomas), 1442
Intracranial vascular malformations, 1936,
    1937
Intracranial vasculitis, 1525, *1526*
Intracranial venous thrombosis, 1531-1533
    magnetic resonance venography, 1532,
        1534, 1535
Intraductal papillary mucinous tumors, 2666,
    2668-2669, *2669, 2670*
Intradural disease, 2159-2189
Intraluminal contrast agents
    bowel obstruction imaging, 2740
    colorectal cancer imaging, 2734
    female pelvis imaging, 2997
    gastrointestinal tract imaging, 2684-2685,
        2686, 2687
    peritoneal imaging, 2751
Intramural hematoma, aorta, 781-782
Intramuscular hematoma, 3386, *3387*
Intranuclear ophthalmoplegia, *1140*, 1158,
    1159
Intraocular tumors, 1914
Intraoperative imaging
    applications, 525
        neurologic surgery, 523-524, *526*
        3D Slicer applications, 517, *518*
    guidance, 512, 517
        magnet design, 514
        see also Interventional imaging
    three-dimensional planning, 517
Intraspinal electrodes, 2193
Intrauterine device, pelvic actinomycosis,
    3036
Intrauterine growth restriction, 3080
Intravaginal coils, female pelvis imaging,
    2998
Intravascular contrast agents *see* Blood pool
    contrast agents
Intravascular tracers, 333
    brain perfusion imaging, 334-336, *335*
        diffusion effects, 334
        see also Blood pool contrast agents
Intravenous access, 64, 66
Intravenous drug abusers, pyogenic infectious
    spondylitis, 2338
Intraventricular hemorrhage, 1326-1327,
    1330, *1331*
    anoxic-ischemic perinatal brain injury,
        1791, 1793, *1793*
    head injury, 1338, *1356*, 1359
    intracranial aneurysm rupture, 1422
    maternal cocaine use, 1690, *1691*
Intra-view motion artifacts, 586-587, *587*

Intussusception, 2720-2721
Inverse Fourier transform, 14, 42, 43
Inversion recovery, 30, 68, 76-81, 77, 144,
    153, *153*
    blood nulling (black blood preparation),
        276
    cardiac perfusion imaging, 860-861
        delayed-enhancement imaging, 864, 865
    cerebral hemorrhage imaging, 1298
        head injury, 1350
    fat suppression, 219-220, *219*
    orbital imaging, 1913
    see also Short-tau inversion recovery (STIR)
Inversion recovery-fast spin-echo
    epilepsy, 1392
    muscle imaging, 3467
Inversion time (TI), 76
iPAT
    diffusion tensor imaging with echo-planar
        imaging, 1617
    functional magnetic resonance
        imaging/BOLD, 1399
Iris, 1953
Iron
    magnetic properties, 175
        arterial blood, 175, *175*
        desaturated hemoglobin, 175-176, *176*
        extracellular protein-bound iron, 177
        intracellular storage forms, 177, 181
        methemoglobin, 176-177
    salvage pathway in hemorrhage/cerebral
        hematoma, 174-177, *175*
    storage forms
        body iron status evaluation in
            hemochromatosis, 2592
        chronic hematoma imaging, 1295
        tissue content quantification, 178
    toxicity in free form, 175
Iron overload, 2591-2593
    bone marrow appearances, 3570-3571
    skull base, 1993
Iron oxide-based contrast agents, 370t, 372t
    blood pool imaging, 373, 382
    bone marrow imaging, 380
    cell labeling, 380
    coronary stem cell therapy evaluation, 929
    intraluminal administration
        colorectal cancer imaging, 2734
        gastrointestinal tract imaging, 2684
    liver imaging, 371
    lymph node imaging, 379
    magnetic resonance
        cholangiopancreatography, 2486
    relaxivity, 366
    renal perfusion imaging, 430, *432*
    tumor transferrin receptor imaging,
        442-443
    see also Superparamagnetic iron oxides
        (SPIO); Ultrasmall particles of iron
        oxide (USPIO)
Iron oxide-containing cosmetics, 596
    permanent/tattoos, 657-658
Iron oxide-containing hair products, 596,
    597
Iron-EHPG, 2487
Iron-HBED, 2487
Irritable bowel syndrome, 2702
    imaging features, 2704, *2704*
Irritable hip syndrome, 3390
ISAT study, 1429-1430
Ischemic cardiomyopathy, 1024
Ischemic cholangitis
    chemotherapy-related, 2511
    postliver transplatation complication,
        2510, *2510*

Ischial tuberosity stress fracture, 3377, 3384,
    3384, 3385
Ischiocavernosa muscles, 2921
Ischiofemoral ligament, 3366
ISIS (image-selected in-vivo spectroscopy),
    473, 1841
Islet cell tumors, 2675, *2677, 2678*, 2705
    classification, 2675
    liver metastases, 2569, 2572
    octreotide nuclear medicine scintigraphy,
        2675, *2678*
Isocenter of magnet, 39
Isoniazid, 1388
Isotopes, 461
    gyromagnetic ratios, 24t
    reonant frequencies, 26
    spin, 24t

J

J coupling, 193
Jacobson's nerve, 2004, 2129
JC virus, 1283, 1589
Jefferson bursting fracture, 2348, *2349*
Jejunal diverticulum, 2717
Jejunum, 2684
Jugular bulb
    dehiscence, 2007, *2009*
    diverticulum, 2007, *2010*
    variants, 2007, 2009, *2009*
Jugular foramen, 1141
    anatomy, 2003-2004, *2007*
    neuroma, 1166, *1166*
    paragangliomas, 2011-2012, *2016, 2017*
        see also Glomus jugulare
    schwannoma, 2010, 2011, *2015*
    tumors, 1973
    vascular variants, 2005-2006, 2007, 2009
    venous anatomy, 1973
Jugular megabulb deformity, 2007, *2009*
Jugular vein obstruction, 2405
Juvenile angiofibroma, 1995-1997, 2037,
    2040, 2042, 2070, 2074
    olfactory (I) nerve region involvement,
        1142
Juvenile aponeurotic fibroma, 3525
Juvenile arteriovenous malformation, spinal
    cord, 2170
Juvenile chronic polyarthritis (juvenile
    rheumatoid arthritis), 3607, *3608*
Juvenile dermatomyositis, 3478
Juvenile glaucoma (buphthalmos), 1956
Juvenile pilocytic astrocytoma, 1755, *1757*,
    1762, *1762, 1763*
    cortical, 1775, *1775*
    orbit, 1938, *1939, 1940*, 1941
Juvenile polyposis, 2716
Juxta-articular bone cyst, glenoid fossa,
    3269
Juxtaglomerular cell tumor (reninoma),
    2825, *2826*
Juxtapapillary diverticulum, 2528-2529,
    2529

K

k-space, 13-14, *14*, 42-44, *44*, 145-146,
    206, *206*
    contrast-enhanced magnetic resonance
        angiography, 743, 744, 746, 748,
        766-767, 1515
    elliptic-centric recording, 711, 748,
        767, 1515, 1516